General Thoracic Surgery

General Thoracic Surgery

Edited by

Thomas W. Shields, M.D., D.Sc. (Hon.)

Professor of Surgery
Northwestern University Medical School
Chief of Thoracic Surgery
Veterans Administration Lakeside Medical Center
Attending Surgeon
Northwestern Memorial Hospital
Chicago, Illinois

Third Edition

LEA & FEBIGER   *Philadelphia* • *London* • 1989

Lea & Febiger
600 Washington Square
Philadelphia, PA   19106-4198
U.S.A.
(215) 922-1330

Technical note: The "original magnifications," listed with each of the photographs of microscopic material, represent the ratio between the size of the photographic image on the original negative and the size of the microscopic specimen itself, and should be used only as an approximate indication, since they do not reflect subsequent magnifications and/or reductions in the final reproduction of the photographs.

Library of Congress Cataloging-in-Publication Data

General thoracic surgery.

   Includes bibliographies and index.
   1. Chest—Surgery.   I. Shields, Thomas W., 1922–
[DNLM: 1. Thoracic Surgery.   WF 980 G326]
RD536.G45   1989   617'.54   88-32578
ISBN 0-8121-1159-1

First Edition, 1972
Second Edition, 1983
Third Edition, 1989

PRINTED IN THE UNITED STATES OF AMERICA

Print No. 3   2   1

To the three Chairmen of the Department of Surgery of Northwestern University Medical School whom I have had the pleasure and good fortune to work with during my thoracic surgical career:

the late Dr. Loyal Davis
Dr. John M. Beal
Dr. David L. Nahrwold

Preface

The third edition of *General Thoracic Surgery* has been prepared to thoroughly update the material presented in the second edition and to present additional information of interest and importance to thoracic surgeons of the world community. The aim has been to achieve extensive and complete coverage of the specialty of general thoracic surgery and of all the allied areas that the general thoracic surgeon should be cognizant of to be the "compleat surgeon." Twenty-five new chapters have been incorporated into the text. These include chapters on computed tomography, magnetic resonance imaging, jet ventilation, additional and newer operative techniques, trauma, complications of cystic fibrosis, paragonimiasis of the pleura and lungs, chylothorax, and additional chapters on chemotherapy. Many of the previous chapters have been rewritten by new authors who, like the former authors, are recognized to be among the contemporary authorities in their respective fields.

The organization of the text remains the same as that of the second edition, which appears to have been well accepted as a readable and easy-to-follow unified approach to the subjects identified as important to the thoracic surgeon. Cross-references have been added to facilitate access to additional information of value on the subjects specifically covered in other chapters. The index has been expanded and hopefully will be of greater value for ready reference to the material in the text. Again, a major effort has been made to decrease the repetition so often seen in a multiauthored text, but, as in the past, complete success has not been achieved. I hope the repetition will be of educational value.

As with the previous editions, I have been fortunate to have been able to enlist the aid of outstanding thoracic surgeons, radiologists, anesthesiologists, oncologists, and physicians in the preparation of the text. I wish to thank each for their contributions, each of which is of inestimable value to the overall soundness and importance of the text.

Chicago, Illinois   Thomas W. Shields

Contributors

Joseph Aisner, M.D.
Professor of Medicine
University of Maryland School of Medicine
Baltimore, Maryland

Homeros Aletras, M.D.
Professor of Surgery
University of Thessalonica
Thessalonica, Greece

Leslie B. Arey, Ph.D.*
Professor of Anatomy, Emeritus
Northwestern University Medical School
Chicago, Illinois

Carl L. Backer, M.D.
Instructor in Clinical Surgery
Northwestern University Medical School
Chicago, Illinois

Timothy E. Baldwin, M.D.
Assistant Professor of Surgery
University of Washington School of Medicine
Seattle, Washington

Arthur E. Baue, M.D.
Professor of Surgery
St. Louis University School of Medicine
St. Louis, Missouri

Maurice Beaulieu, M.D.
Division of Thoracic Surgery
Laval University Faculty of Medicine
Sainte-Foy, Québec, Canada

Ronald Belsey, M.S.
Visiting Professor of Surgery
University of Chicago Pritzker School of Medicine
Chicago, Illinois

Charles E. Blevins, Ph.D.
Professor and Chairman, Department of Anatomy
Indiana University School of Medicine
Indianapolis, Indiana

Anita King Bowes, M.D.
Instructor in Otorhinolaryngology
Rush Medical College of Rush University
Chicago, Illinois

Ralph Braunschweig, M.D.
Clinical Assistant Professor of Anesthesiology
Columbia School of Medicine, University of Missouri
Columbia, Missouri

———————————

*Deceased.

Lewis W. Britton, III, M.D.
Assistant Professor of Surgery
Albany Medical College of Union University
Albany, New York

Edward A. Brunner, M.D., Ph.D.
Professor and Chairman, Department of Anesthesia
Northwestern University Medical School
Chicago, Illinois

Peter H. Burri, M.D.
Professor of Anatomy
Institute of Anatomy
University of Berne
Berne, Switzerland

James C. Carrico, M.D.
Professor and Chairman, Department of Surgery
University of Washington School of Medicine
Seattle, Washington

Martin H. Cohen, M.D.
Professor of Medicine
George Washington University School of Medicine
Washington, DC

Joel D. Cooper, M.D.
Professor of Surgery
Washington University School of Medicine
St. Louis, Missouri

James D. Cox, M.D.
Physician in Chief
M.D. Anderson Cancer Center
University of Texas Medical School at Houston
Houston, Texas

David W. Cugell, M.D.
Professor of Medicine
Northwestern University Medical School
Chicago, Illinois

Thomas R. DeMeester, M.D.
Professor and Chairman, Department of Surgery
Creighton University School of Medicine
Omaha, Nebraska

Jean Deslauriers, M.D.
Clinical Professor of Thoracic Surgery
Laval University Faculty of Medicine
Sainte-Foy, Québec, Canada

Ronald B. Dietrick, M.D.
Formerly Director of Medical Services
Kwangju Christian Hospital
Kwangju, South Korea

André Duranceau, M.D.
Professor of Surgery
University of Montreal Faculty of Medicine
Montreal, Québec, Canada

Forrest C. Eggleston, M.D.
Formerly Professor and Head, Department of Surgery
Christian Medical College
Ludhiana, Punjab, India

Nabil M. El-Baz, M.D.
Associate Professor of Anesthesiology
Rush Medical College of Rush University
Chicago, Illinois

F. Henry Ellis, Jr., M.D., Ph.D.
Clinical Professor of Surgery
Harvard Medical School
Boston, Massachusetts

David M. Epstein, M.D.
Associate Professor of Radiology
University of Pennsylvania School of Medicine
Philadelphia, Pennsylvania

L. Penfield Faber, M.D.
Professor of Surgery
Rush Medical College of Rush University
Chicago, Illinois

Andrew E. Filderman, M.D.
Assistant Professor of Medicine
Yale University School of Medicine
New Haven, Connecticut

James E. Fish, M.D.
Assistant Professor of Medicine
Johns Hopkins University Medical School
Baltimore, Maryland

Jack Fisher, M.D.
Assistant Clinical Professor of Surgery
Vanderbilt University School of Medicine
Associate Clinical Professor of Surgery
Meharry Medical College School of Medicine
Nashville, Tennessee

Willard A. Fry, M.D.
Associate Professor of Clinical Surgery
Northwestern University Medical School
Chicago, Illinois

Gordon Gamsu, M.D.
Professor of Radiology
University of California, San Francisco School of Medicine
San Francisco, California

Warren B. Gefter, M.D.
Professor of Radiology
University of Pennsylvania School of Medicine
Philadelphia, Pennsylvania

Gary G. Ghahremani, M.D.
Professor of Radiology
Northwestern University Medical School
Chicago, Illinois

Joan Gil, M.D.
Professor of Pathology
Mt. Sinai School of Medicine of the City University of New York
New York, New York

Robert J. Ginsberg, M.D.
Professor of Surgery
University of Toronto Faculty of Medicine
Toronto, Ontario, Canada

Jeffrey Glassroth, M.D.
Associate Professor of Medicine
Northwestern University Medical School
Chicago, Illinois

William W.L. Glenn, M.D.
Professor of Surgery, Emeritus
Yale University School of Medicine
New Haven, Connecticut

Douglas R. Gracey, M.D.
Professor of Medicine
Mayo Medical School
Rochester, Minnesota

F. Anthony Greco, M.D.
Professor of Medicine and Oncology
Vanderbilt University School of Medicine
Nashville, Tennessee

Hermes C. Grillo, M.D.
Professor of Surgery
Harvard Medical School
Boston, Massachusetts

Renee S. Hartz, M.D.
Associate Professor of Surgery
Northwestern University Medical School
Chicago, Illinois

John D. Hainsworth, M.D.
Assistant Professor of Medicine and Oncology
Vanderbilt University School of Medicine
Nashville, Tennessee

Robert D. Henderson, M.B.*
Professor of Surgery
University of Toronto Faculty of Medicine
Toronto, Ontario, Canada

Lauren D. Holinger, M.D.
Associate Professor of Otorhinolaryngology
Rush Medical College of Rush University
Chicago, Illinois

R. Maurice Hood, M.D.
Professor of Clinical Surgery
New York University School of Medicine
New York, New York

Babette J. Horn, M.D.
Assistant Professor of Clinical Anesthesiology
Northwestern University Medical School
Chicago, Illinois

*Deceased.

Guo Jun Huang, M.D.
Professor of Thoracic Surgery
Chinese Academy of Medical Sciences and China Union Medical University
Beijing, People's Republic of China

Glyn G. Jamieson, M.B.
Professor and Chairman, Department of Surgery
University of Adelaide Medical School
Adelaide, South Australia

Robert W. Jamplis, M.D.
Clinical Professor of Surgery
Stanford University School of Medicine
Stanford, California

Thomas Keane, M.D.
Associate Professor of Radiology
University of Toronto Faculty of Medicine
Toronto, Ontario, Canada

R. Keenan, M.D.
Instructor in Surgery
University of Toronto Faculty of Medicine
Toronto, Ontario, Canada

Merrill, S. Kies, M.D.
Associate Professor of Clinical Medicine
Northwestern University Medical School
Chicago, Illinois

James Kilman, M.D.
Professor of Surgery
Ohio State University College of Medicine
Columbus, Ohio

Hiroyuki Koda, M.D.
Research Fellow Cardiothoracic Surgery
Yale University School of Medicine
Mito National Hospital
Mito, Japan

Pierre Leblanc, M.D.
Department of Chest Medicine
Laval University Faculty of Medicine
Sainte-Foy, Québec, Canada

Joseph LoCicero, III, M.D.
Assistant Professor of Surgery
Northwestern University Medical School
Chicago, Illinois

Susan R. Luck, M.D.
Associate Professor of Clinical Surgery
Northwestern University Medical School
Chicago, Illinois

André McClish, M.D.
Department of Anesthesia
Laval University Faculty of Medicine
Sainte-Foy, Québec, Canada

Patricia M. McCormack, M.D.
Associate Professor of Surgery
Cornell University Medical College
New York, New York

P. Michael McFadden, M.D.
Head, Department of Cardiovascular Surgery
Palo Alto Medical Clinic
Palo Alto, California

Martin F. McKneally, M.D., Ph.D.
Professor and Chief, Cardiothoracic Surgery
Albany Medical College of Union University
Albany, New York

Nael Martini, M.D.
Professor of Surgery
Cornell University Medical College
New York, New York

Richard A. Matthay, M.D.
Professor of Medicine
Yale University School of Medicine
New Haven, Connecticut

Lawrence L. Michaelis, M.D.
Professor of Surgery
Northwestern University Medical School
Chicago, Illinois

Joseph I. Miller, Jr., M.D.
Associate Professor of Cardiothoracic Surgery
Emory University School of Medicine
Atlanta, Georgia

Wallace T. Miller, M.D.
Professor and Vice-Chairman, Department of Radiology
University of Pennsylvania School of Medicine
Philadelphia, Pennsylvania

Darroch W.O. Moores, M.D.
Assistant Professor of Surgery
Albany Medical College of Union University
Albany, New York

Gordon F. Murray, M.D.
Professor and Chairman, Department of Surgery
West Virginia University School of Medicine
Morgantown, West Virginia

Keith S. Naunheim, M.D.
Assistant Professor of Surgery
St. Louis University School of Medicine
St. Louis, Missouri

H. Christian Nohl-Oser, M.A., D.M.
Late Hunterian Professor
Royal College of Surgeons
London, England

Andranik Ovassapian, M.D.
Professor of Clinical Anesthesia
Northwestern University Medical School
Chicago, Illinois

Peter C. Pairolero, M.D.
Professor of Surgery
Mayo Medical School
Rochester, Minnesota

G. Alexander Patterson, M.D.
Assistant Professor of Surgery
University of Toronto Faculty of Medicine
Toronto, Ontario, Canada

Donald L. Paulson, M.D., Ph.D.
Clinical Professor of Thoracic and Cardiovascular Surgery
University of Texas Health Science Center at Southwestern
   Medical School
Dallas, Texas

W. Spencer Payne, M.D.
Professor of Surgery
Mayo Medical School
Rochester, Minnesota

Michail Perelman, M.D.
Professor of Surgery
Academy of Medical Science and First Moscow Medical Institute
Moscow, USSR

Carlos A. Perez, M.D.
Professor of Radiology
Washington University School of Medicine
St. Louis, Missouri

Ronald B. Ponn, M.D.
Clinical Instructor of Cardiothoracic Surgery
Yale University School of Medicine
New Haven, Connecticut

James A. Radosevich, M.D.
Assistant Professor of Medicine
Northwestern University Medical School
Chicago, Illinois

Marleta Reynolds, M.D.
Assistant Professor of Surgery
Northwestern University Medical School
Chicago, Illinois

Charles L. Rice, M.D.
Assistant Professor of Surgery
University of Washington School of Medicine
Seattle, Washington

Roy E. Ritts, M.D.
Professor of Microbiology and Oncology
Mayo Medical School
Rochester, Minnesota

Philip G. Robinson, M.D.
Assistant Professor of Clinical Pathology
Northwestern University Medical School
Chicago, Illinois

Steven T. Rosen, M.D.
Associate Professor of Medicine
Northwestern University Medical School
Chicago, Illinois

Martin Rothberg, M.D.
Department of Surgery
Creighton University School of Medicine
Omaha, Nebraska

G. Edward Rozar, Jr., M.D.
Assistant Professor of Surgery
West Virginia University School of Medicine
Morgantown, West Virginia

Steven A. Sahn, M.D.
Professor of Medicine
Medical University of South Carolina
Charleston, South Carolina

Frank L. Seleny, M.D.
Professor of Clinical Anesthesiology
Northwestern University Medical School
Chicago, Illinois

David M. Shahian, M.D.
Assistant Clinical Professor of Surgery
Harvard Medical School
Boston, Massachusetts

Robert C. Shamberger, M.D.
Assistant Clinical Professor of Surgery
Harvard Medical School
Boston, Massachusetts

H. Shennib, M.D.
Instructor in Surgery
University of Toronto Faculty of Medicine
Toronto, Ontario, Canada

Thomas W. Shields, M.D., D.Sc. (Hon.)
Professor of Surgery
Northwestern University Medical School
Chicago, Illinois

David B. Skinner, M.D.
President and Prof. of Surgery
The New York Hospital
Cornell University Medical College
New York, New York

Herbert M. Sommers, M.D.
Professor of Pathology
Northwestern University Medical School
Chicago, Illinois

William G. Spies, M.D.
Assistant Professor of Radiology
Northwestern University Medical School
Chicago, Illinois

Bryan H.R. Stack, M.B., Ch.B.
Consultant Physician
Western Infirmary
Glasgow, Scotland

Harold Stern, M.D.
Associate Clinical Professor of Cardiothoracic Surgery
Yale University School of Medicine
New Haven, Connecticut

Jeffrey Swanson, M.D.
Assistant Professor of Surgery
Oregon Health Sciences University
Portland, Oregon

Panagiotis N. Symbas, M.D.
Professor of Cardiothoracic Surgery
Emory University School of Medicine
Atlanta, Georgia

Timothy Takaro, M.D.
Clinical Professor of Surgery
Duke University School of Medicine
Durham, North Carolina

Thomas R. Todd, M.D.
Associate Professor of Surgery
University of Toronto Faculty of Medicine
Toronto, Ontario, Canada

Allan L. Toole, M.D.
Associate Clinical Professor of Cardiothoracic Surgery
Yale University School of Medicine
New Haven, Connecticut

Victor F. Trastek, M.D.
Assistant Professor of Surgery
Mayo Medical School
Rochester, Minnesota

Donald D. Trunkey, M.D.
Professor and Chairman, Department of Surgery
Oregon Health Sciences University
Portland, Oregon

Harold C. Urschel, Jr., M.D.
Clinical Professor of Thoracic and Cardiovascular Surgery
University of Texas Health Sciences Center and Baylor University
    Medical Center
Dallas, Texas

Robert Vanecko, M.D.
Associate Professor of Clinical Surgery
Northwestern University Medical School
Chicago, Illinois

Mohan Verghese, M.D.
Professor of Surgery
Christian Medical College
Ludhiana, Punjab, India

William H. Warren, M.D.
Assistant Professor of Surgery
Rush Medical College of Rush University
Chicago, Illinois

Paul F. Waters, M.D.
Assistant Professor of Surgery
University of Toronto Faculty of Medicine
Toronto, Ontario, Canada

Ewald R. Weibel, M.D.
Professor and Chairman, Department of Anatomy
University of Berne
Berne, Switzerland

Kenneth J. Welch, M.D.
Professor of Surgery
Harvard Medical School
Boston, Massachusetts

Earle R. Wilkins, Jr., M.D.
Clinical Professor of Surgery
Harvard Medical School
Boston, Massachusetts

Hak Y. Wong, M.D.
Associate in Clinical Anesthesiology
Northwestern University Medical School
Chicago, Illinois

Contents

Section 6. Anesthetic Management of the Thoracic Surgical Patient

Section 7. Postoperative Management

Section 8. Operative Procedures

Section 9. Thoracic Trauma

Section 10. The Chest Wall

Section 11. The Diaphragm

Section 12. The Pleura

Section 13. The Trachea

Section 14. The Lung

Section 15.   The Esophagus

Section 16.   The Mediastinum

Section 17.   Radiation Therapy

Section 18.   Chemotherapy

Section 19.   Immunotherapy

Anatomy

CHAPTER 1

EMBRYOLOGY OF THE LUNGS AND ESOPHAGUS

Leslie B. Arey

THE LUNGS

Evolutionary Advances

The first appearance of lungs among vertebrates was in *Dipnoi*, or lungfishes. With the exception of the *Dipnoi*, lungs occur only in tetrapods and are a basic characteristic of all such vertebrates. The proximal segment of the trachea in tailed amphibians and higher vertebrates specialized as a larynx, and the wall of the trachea became strengthened by cartilage. The actual respiratory portion of the system shows progressive complexity in the several classes of vertebrates through bushlike branching and reduplication of the mucosal lining. The interior of the lungs in some urodeles is wholly smooth; in others, the lining is only partially smooth. Anuran amphibians have internally ridged lungs, and the resulting recesses are lined with still smaller recesses, the alveoli. In some lizards, and in all turtles and crocodiles, septa extend inward and subdivide the lung into a spongy mass supplied by branching ducts. The lungs of birds are not arranged as blindly ending respiratory trees. Instead, anastomosing tubules produce complete air circuits, and smoothly lined extensions—the so-called air sacs—invade every major part of the body. Successive reduplication of the inner respiratory surfaces achieves the high degree of complexity of the mammalian lung, which is characteristically lobated except in some types, such as whales and elephants. The mechanisms by which air is made to enter and leave the lungs differ in the several groups of tetrapods, and only in mammals are there paired pleural cavities separated from a peritoneal cavity by a single, complete diaphragm.

Development of the Human Lung

Early Development

The earliest indication of the future respiratory tract occurs in human embryos 3 mm long. Such specimens possess about 20 mesodermal somites and are in the fourth week of development (Fig. 1–1). The respiratory primordium is then in the form of a groove that runs lengthwise in the floor of the pharynx, just caudal to the region where paired pharyngeal pouches are developing (Fig. 1–1*A*). Lateral furrows next cut off a short tube (Fig. 1–1*B, C*). The larynx soon organizes about the cranial end of this tube, whereas the caudal end becomes rounded, and, in 4-mm embryos, this so-called lung bud begins to bifurcate (Fig. 1–1*D*). At the 5-mm stage it is easy to recognize a cranial laryngeal region, an intermediate tracheal tube, and two primary bronchi (Fig. 1–2*A*). The latter are potentially more than bronchi, since by growth and repeated bifurcation they ultimately will produce all the branches, twigs, air sacs, and alveoli of the respiratory tree. The right primary bronchus extends more directly caudad than does the veering left bronchus, and this difference is maintained in subsequent branchings.

The smaller left branch of the two primary ones diverges more from the parent stem than does the larger right branch. This early difference has a practical sequel. The conducting airways of the future left lung come to occupy as little room as possible, and, as noted by Barnett (1957), space in the thorax is thereby made for the off-center heart. This outcome is not the result of simple, mechanical crowding because the asymmetry occurs much too early.

In an embryo 7 mm long—about 5 weeks old—the right primary bronchus gives rise to two side buds, or lateral bronchi (Fig. 1–2*B*), while the left bronchus forms but one. The blind end of each main tube is known as the stem bronchus. Even at this early stage the plan of the future gross lobation becomes apparent, since these buds presage the upper, middle, and lower lobes on the the right side and the upper and lower lobes on the left side. Subsequent branching gives rise to bushlike systems of epithelial tubes (Fig. 1–2*C, D*). The manner of progressive division is asymmetrically or irregularly dichotomous.

As early as the stage of the third order of branching from the trachea, axes are being established for the first of the intralobar, segmental bronchi—ten for the right lung and eight for the left. The longer bronchopulmonary

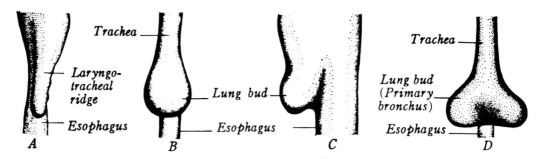

Fig. 1–1. Early stages of the human respiratory primordium (after Grosser and Heiss). ×75. A, At 2.5 mm, in ventral view; B and C, at 3 mm, in ventral and lateral views; D, at 4 mm in ventral view. (Reproduced with permission from Arey, L.B.: Developmental Anatomy, 7th ed. Philadelphia, W.B. Saunders Co., 1965, p. 265.)

segments require more time to develop than do shorter ones, so that the former continue to branch until the end of the sixteenth week. Yet, as described by Bucher and Reid (1961), about 70% of the total branching of the respiratory tree is accomplished between the tenth and fourteenth weeks of development.

Later Development

According to Loosli and Potter (1959), during the total prenatal period the lung advances through three stages in preparation for respiratory functioning (Fig. 1–3). First, until nearly the sixteenth week of fetal life, the human lung resembles an early exocrine gland in appearance because of the ordinary cuboidal epithelium of its lining. Second, during the next eight weeks, capillaries become abundant and seem to interrupt the epithelium of the more distal air passages; this period of development has been called the canalicular phase. Third, in the final fetal months, and as early as 26 weeks,

prototypes of alveolar sacs and alveoli appear; during this so-called alveolar phase the patterns within the lung come to resemble those at birth. It is in the final four to six generations of branchings that the airway volume and the expanse of the airway lining increase by the formation of the forerunners of air sacs and their component alveoli.

The establishment of a primary axis for each lung is initiated and completed with the formation of branches for the secondary bronchi. Thereafter, each bronchus develops its own pattern of branching, but variations from the common pattern are common. Such departures, as noted by Heiss (1919), usually begin in subsegmental bronchi, and these are branches of the fourth or fifth order. Wells and Boyden (1954) have pointed out that these departures result from displacements at predictable sites and bring about alterations in adjacent regions. In general, the original bronchial tree incurs some remodeling before it reaches its definitive, adult configuration.

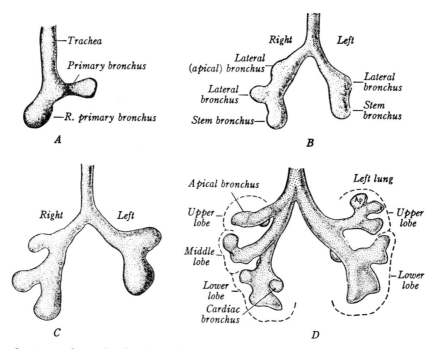

Fig. 1–2. Development of primary and secondary bronchi of the human lung, in ventral views (after Heiss and Merkel). ×50. A, At 5 mm; B, at 7 mm; C, at 8.5 mm; D, at 10 mm. (Ap, apical bronchus—homologue of left lung.) (Reproduced with permission from Arey, L.B.: Developmental Anatomy, 7th ed. Philadelphia, W.B. Saunders Co., 1965, p. 265.)

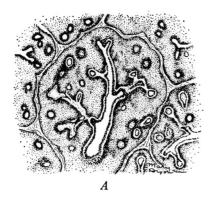 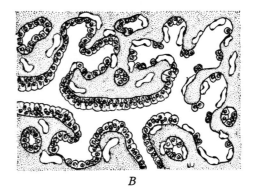

A   B

Fig. 1–3. Sections of local regions within the human lung. *A*, Developing lobules in "glandular phase," at 4 months (×75); *B*, seeming loss of lining epithelium in early "alveolar phase," at 7 months (×125). (Reproduced with permission from Arey, L.B.: Developmental Anatomy, 7th ed. Philadelphia, W.B. Saunders Co., 1965, p. 267.)

Bucher and Reid (1961) have shown that in the end the nonrespiratory airways of the lingula and middle lobe, and those of the anterior and basal segments, have 20 to 25 generations, in comparison to the approximately 15 generations of the shorter segments (Fig. 1–4). It has

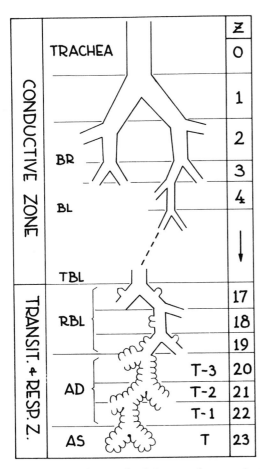

Fig. 1–4. Diagram indicating the dichotomy of airways during the prenatal period of some 23 generations of branching. BR, bronchi; BL, bronchioles; TBL, terminal bronchioles; RBL, respiratory bronchioles; AD, alveolar ducts; AS, alveolar sacs. (Reproduced with permission from Weibel, E.R.: Morphometry of the Human Lung. Heidelberg, Springer-Verlag, 1963, p. 111.)

been claimed frequently that no new tubular airways are formed after birth, but Boyden and Tompsett (1965) concluded that segments are variable and "one may not state with certainty whether the nonrespiratory generations increase or decrease after birth." According to Reid (1965), all of the airways demonstrable in the best obtainable bronchogram of an adult are already present, although in miniature, in a fetus of 16 weeks.

Surprisingly, after the sixth fetal month, the total number of nonrespiratory generations of tubules is diminished by two to four branchings. This results from the transformation of a corresponding number of ordinary bronchioles into respiratory bronchioles by the interposition of scattered alveoli in their walls. Boyden and Tompsett (1965) found that a similar conversion continues after birth when respiratory bronchioles, already present, add more alveoli to their walls and, in so doing, become alveolar ducts (Fig. 1–5).

The early, main bronchus of the right upper lobe gains the name of eparterial bronchus because it alone lies upon the corresponding pulmonary artery. Originally this bronchus is dorsal—that is, posterior—to the artery, as the name implies. Later, when the heart descends, it is located cranially with respect to this vessel; yet, with respect to the upright posture of man, the name—"upon the artery"—is again wholly appropriate. It has been stated frequently that this bronchus was anciently a secondary branch in what was then the upper lobe of a bilobed right lung. Flint (1906) theorized that, later in the course of evolutionary advance, it migrated upward onto the main bronchial stem and induced the formation of a new lobe about it. Others, such as Huntington (1920), regard the eparterial bronchus as an entirely independent outgrowth, arising at a higher level, that became the basis for a new and definitive upper lobe.

The left upper lobe contains a bronchial branch that seems to be the rudimentary equivalent of the entire bronchial tree in the upper lobe on the right side (Fig. 1–2*D*, Ap). Since, however, this branch remains small and fails to produce a separate lobe about it, the left upper lobe is said to be the equivalent of both the upper and middle lobes of the right side. Such a suppression of a homologous left upper lobe has been interpreted by

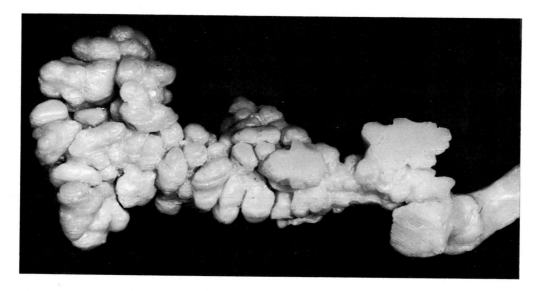

Fig. 1–5. Model of a branch peripheral to a terminal bronchiole in a 2-month old infant (×50). At left, several clusters of alveolar sacs; adjoining is a short region of suddenly differentiating alveolar ducts; next follows a relatively long stretch of respiratory bronchioles; at far right, a terminal bronchiole. (Reproduced with permission from Boyden, E.A., and Tompsett, D.H.: The changing patterns in the developing lungs of infants. Acta Anat. *61*:164, 1965.)

Flint (1906) as an adaptation to facilitate the normal, caudal recession of the aortic arch. An alternative explanation, advanced by Huntington (1920), stresses the lessened opportunity for pulmonary expansion on the left side, resulting from the rotations of the heart and esophagus in opposite directions. As a contributory factor, Heiss (1919) and Ekehorn (1921) suggested that the more caudal position of the left cardinal vein is perhaps significant. Also on the left side, an important bronchial branch is suppressed in the lower lobe, owing to the position of the heart and pulmonary vein. This suppression, however, affords opportunity for an excessive development of the corresponding right ramus, which then projects into the space between the heart and diaphragm as the so-called cardiac bronchus.

Development of Alveoli

In the fifth fetal month, the epithelial lining of the more terminal branches of the respiratory tree is still cuboidal. Early in the sixth month, as shown by Short (1950), the adjoining capillaries begin to crowd against the epithelium, which then seems to disappear locally, so that the capillaries lie exposed (Fig. 1–3B). It is more probable that the local epithelial lining merely flattens to extreme thinness and remains. At least, as first demonstrated by Low and Sampaio (1957), a complete layer of this sort, continuous with the ordinary endodermal lining of the tract, exists throughout later life; it is demonstrable convincingly only with the electron microscope.

Still other distinctive cells, known as the "great alveolar cells" or "type II cells," occupy niches in the epithelial lining. They are interpreted by Sorokin (1965) and others as specially differentiated components of the pulmonary epithelium, although some, including Bertalanffy (1964), consider them to be macrophages that wandered inward from the interalveolar septa. The osmiophilic surfactant that coats alveolar epithelium and acts to decrease surface tension is, in all likelihood, a derivative of these great alveolar cells. Buckingham and Avery (1962) found that great alveolar cells contain lipoidal inclusion bodies that become abundant when the surfactant coating first appears. Campiche and his associates (1963) recorded that type I and type II cells are recognizable by the end of the sixth fetal month.

A period of alveolar development begins at 26 weeks. As already described, the postnatally developing alveolar ducts are the earliest respiratory units to approximate the concentrated adult state of typical alveoli. In sharp contrast, the studies of Boyden and Tompsett (1965) have shown that the terminal saccules, each a cluster of alveolar prototypes, are still in a relatively undifferentiated state in an infant (Fig. 1–6). Moreover, within the saccules the recesses that represent alveoli are still small and shallow. Later, the alveoli become large and deeper, contiguous ones being separated by higher interalveolar partitions, known as interalveolar septa. There is no evidence of new sacs and component alveoli being formed postnatally.

Weibel (1962) set the number of alveoli, counted at 8 years and thereafter, at about 300 million, whereas Dunnill (1962) counted only some 20 million in the newborn. The discrepancy seems to lie in a failure to recognize that an apparent decrease in size, coupled with an apparent increase in number, results from confusing the larger air sacs with the smaller, gradually deepening component alveoli. The alveoli of young and middle-aged individuals, as determined by Weibel (1962), occupy 62% of the total lung volume, which is 2700 ml; they have an alveolar surface of 70 to 80 square meters, as does also the accompanying capillary surface (see Chapter 2). The

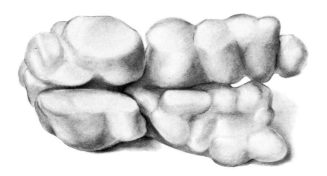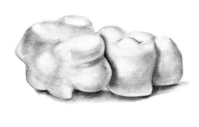

Fig. 1–6.   Models of six terminal air sacs in a 2-day old infant (×85). Well illustrated are the shallowness and variations in size of pulmonary alveoli during the perinatal period. (Reproduced with permission from Boyden, E.A., and Tompsett, D.H.: The changing patterns in the developing lungs of infants. Acta Anat. *61*:182, 187, 1965.)

weight of the lung increases from 20 g at birth to 200 g at 12 years. Its volume doubles after childhood.

Mesodermal Components

The trachea and both of the early primary bronchi lie within a median mass of mesenchyme located cranially, and more or less dorsal to the peritoneal cavity. This tissue mass resembles a broad mesentery; somewhat later it becomes the mediastinum. The primary bronchial buds grow laterocaudad into their respective pleural cavities, carrying before them—right and left—dome-shaped investments of mesenchyme surfaced with mesothelium. The subsequent branching of each bronchial tree takes place within these simultaneously growing tissue masses. The mesenchyme adapts itself to the shape of each bronchial tree and, accordingly, the external lobation of the two lungs gradually takes form, including the subdivision of each lobe into its characteristic numbers of bronchopulmonary segments. Internally, each lobe becomes subdivided by connective tissue septa into incompletely demarcated major lobules. The mesenchyme that is most intimately related to the branching respiratory tree differentiates into smooth muscle, supporting tissue, blood vessels, and lymphatics.

Each early lung comes to lie in a primordial pleural cavity, separated from the heart by a common pleuropericardial membrane. Since the lungs enlarge rapidly, they progressively require more room. Thus, each gains during the seventh week of development at the expense of the spongy tissue of the adjacent body wall. Such a burrowing advance proceeds at first laterally and then ventrally. It splits off an increasingly expansive membrane from the general thoracic wall, and progressively permits the lungs to flank the heart on each side. Each final membrane is a joint product consisting of the original pleuropericardial membrane and its supplemental addition. The two compound membranes join ventrally and, thus, produce a complete sac, the pericardium. The mesothelium and the subjacent connective tissue that covers the external surface of each lung are called the visceral pleura. The facing layer, which largely came into being when the pericardium split away, lines the thoracic wall and constitutes the parietal pleura.

The original pleuropericardial membranes incom-

pletely separate the coelomic space occupied by the heart and lungs. During the sixth week each membrane becomes a complete partition, and henceforth the heart occupies a wholly separate chamber. For a brief time, each pleural cavity still communicates with the peritoneal cavity, but shortly the pair of hitherto incomplete pleuroperitoneal membranes seals off the corresponding communicating foramen by becoming incorporated into the developing diaphragm (see Chapter 8).

Perinatal Events

Movements of the chest, simulating those of respiration, sometimes occur late in the fetal period, and these movements tend to aspirate some amniotic fluid into the lungs. Windle and his associates (1939) suggest that such activity is best interpreted not as a practice in breathing, but rather as a response to oxygen lack in the fetus. In any event, the lungs are said by Lind and Hirvensalo (1966) to have the same gross size before birth as after postnatal breathing occurs. Aeration would then be a matter of the replacement of pulmonary fluid by air.

The pulmonary tissue, previously relatively compact, slowly becomes spongy owing to a great terminal increase in the size of its alveoli and blood vessels. For weeks the alveoli remain small and shallow, but eventually they deepen and press against each other until the interlocking arrangement is both intimate and intricate.

At term, each lung contains about 40 ml of fluid. This fluid seems to be mostly a secretion of the lung itself, since, as established by Adams (1963) and Fujiwara (1964) and their associates, its composition differs from that of amniotic fluid. Various explanations have been advanced concerning the absorption and disappearance of this fluid.

One proposal involved the increase in blood circulation at birth, since the oncotic pressure of plasma exceeds that of the accumulated pulmonary fluid and should act to promote its removal by that route. Still another causative factor, suggested by Aherne and Dawkins (1964) is the neighboring rich lymphatic network, which dilates greatly after a few breaths have been taken, and also shows, as demonstrated by Boston and his associates (1965), a measured increase in lymph flow. A more appropriate explanation of the fate of the lung liquid was forwarded by Lagercrantz and Slotkin (1986). These investigators reported that the absorption of lung liquid appears to depend on a sustained increase in plasma catecholamines in the hours immediately before birth. Olver (1981), in studies in fetal sheep, noted that liquid is secreted into and moves out of the lungs at a rate of 200 to 300 ml per 24 hours. With the injection of epinephrine, the secretion of lung liquid was stopped immediately and the lung liquid was promptly absorbed. The administration of beta-2-receptor blockers by Slotkin and associates (1986), preventing the effects of epinephrine on surfactant production and lung-liquid absorption, severely compromised the ability of one-day-old rats to survive low-oxygen conditions, as compared to control animals, which did not receive the beta blockers. Irestedt and colleagues (1982, 1984, 1986) at the Karolinska Institute indirectly confirmed the effect of catecholamine on lung liquid absorption in man by measuring lung compliance and plasma catecholamine concentration shortly after birth. They found a greater increase in lung compliance associated with higher levels of catecholamines and a lesser increase in lung compliance with lower levels of catecholamines.

When initial inflation of the lungs has been completed, and pulmonary fluid has been absorbed—at 3 days after birth—the lungs, if not larger, as stated by Lind and Hirvensalo (1966), are said by others at least to have more rounded margins. The lungs increase markedly in weight after birth, owing to the greater amount of blood admitted to them. Premature babies, born before the air sacs have developed properly, apparently accomplish respiratory exchanges through the terminal system of ducts; these substitutes function well enough to sustain life. Prematurity does not affect the outcome of subsequent maturative completion.

Histogenesis

Tissue differentiation of various kinds within the respiratory tree proceeds in a proximodistal direction. Hence these specializations spread in a wave-like manner down the airways from the highest level of the larynx and trachea to the last formed terminal twigs. Some data on these matters have been provided by Bucher and Reid (1961). A gradation in the endodermal epithelium from pseudostratified to columnar, and then to cuboidal, is seen throughout the bronchial tree of embryos of 10 weeks, and, at 13 weeks, all such cells are ciliated. At 24 weeks the cells in the most peripheral twigs are flattened and nonciliated, with capillaries seemingly penetrating between these cells (p. 6). Goblet cells in the epithelium and the evaginated primordia of deeper seromucous glands can be detected at 13 weeks in the trachea and main bronchi; by the twenty-fourth week these compound glands attain typical acinar structure, but a differentiation between mucous and serous cells occurs later. A basement membrane can be recognized at 10 weeks, but it is not a continuous sheet until 2 weeks later. Campiche and his associates (1963) have supplied some information on the differentiation of the human lung as observed by electron microscopy.

Condensations of mesenchyme about the epithelial tube of the emerging trachea are recognizable at 7 weeks. At 10 weeks, large, precartilaginous cells have appeared throughout the trachea and primary bronchi and, at the twelfth week, similar differentiation reaches the level of the segmental bronchi; this is about 6 weeks after these bronchi arose. Thereafter, cartilaginous plates appear in steady succession until the twenty-fifth week, when the smallest bronchi are supplied. Bucher and Reid (1961) found that full histogenesis of cartilage, at any particular site, is achieved on the average in 2 weeks' time. Bronchioles and still smaller divisions of the respiratory tree lack cartilages and glands.

The mesenchymal investment of the epithelial tubes also gives rise to other types of tissue. Pulmonary blood vessels are arising in the fifth week of development, whereas the lymphatics of this region develop considerably later. Smooth muscle appears in the primary bronchi before the twelfth week, and this differentiation spreads progressively down the bronchioles, respiratory bronchioles, and alveolar ducts. Elastic fibers and collagenous fibers, already present at higher levels, differentiate in the peripheral airways during the canalicular period—17 to 24 weeks. At any level, collagenous fibers precede the appearance of elastic fibers. The waves of specialization in both mesenchyme and endodermal epithelium illustrate well the existence and operation of histogenetic gradients in development.

Most of the cells entering into the fabric of the airways are nonspecific. Fibroblasts, smooth muscle cells, endothelial cells, and the epithelial cells that line much of the tubular system are all similar structurally to those found in other regions of the body. By contrast, the principal cells that line the pulmonary alveoli are highly specialized for effecting diffusive interchanges, and do not have structural counterparts elsewhere. Moreover, the greater alveolar cells of the lining—type II cells, which are presumably also of epithelial origin, have distinctive qualities since, among other things, they are thought by Dannenberg (1963) and Oren (1963) and their associates to be parent to the alveolar phagocytes, which are metabolically different from other macrophages of the body. Little of a comprehensive nature is known concerning sequential changes in the ultramicroscopic structure of cell constituents. Nevertheless, the great alveolar cells do become recognizable in the terminal, prealveolar epithelium of the sixth month by the appearance in the cytoplasm of phospholipid-containing, lamellated bodies. These bodies are believed by Gautier and his associates (1962) to be identical with the later surfactant material on the epithelial lining. Perhaps it is significant that the course of differentiation in the airways proceeds in a centrifugal direction, so that cells most specific to the lung are not only far removed from the pluripotent pharynx, but also are late in the time-order of differentiation.

Histochemistry

Some attention has been directed to the chemistry of the developing lungs and to the specificity of their cellular constituents; Sorokin (1965) has reviewed these investigations briefly. In particular, studies have been pursued on elastin and on the patterns of deposition of glycogen and lipids. Enzymatic identification supports the view that visible change occurs first in epithelium and that here the direction of chemical differentiation, like that occurring in structure, proceeds peripherally along the pulmonary trees in a progressive manner. Yet, only in some instances has it been possible to ascribe a significant role to a specific enzyme.

Chemical differentiation within the general area of the initial lung bud presages the onset of visible morphologic changes. Sharing similar phenomena in other cephalic primordia are the following intracellular changes: glycogen accumulation; enzymatic activities, especially involving alkaline phosphatase in the epithelium; and an increase in cytoplasmic ribonucleoprotein. Experimental attacks have revealed some information underlying pulmonary morphogenesis. It is known that the fetus develops at low oxygen tension and that the lung can develop to an advanced stage under an anaerobic environment in organ culture. Activity of the citric-acid cycle and the rate of oxidative metabolism appear to increase from the eighth week to term.

Causal Development

Experiments designed to determine the extent of dependent and independent development of the lung buds have been reviewed by Sorokin (1965). One line of approach has focused on discovering the degree to which the lung is a self-developing entity. Using the isolation method, the pioneering experiments included the excision of a neighboring region of the embryo along with the lung buds. Later refinements limited the in vitro cultures to the lungs alone. Such cultured material from birds and mammals develops to a fair likeness of the normal lung, with all of the essential cellular elements of the adult, including a respiratory region with alveoli. Even parts of the respiratory tract, such as the syrinx and trachea of birds, develop well under these conditions.

Improved technical methods have extended the maintenance of cultures into longer periods of time, and thereby have brought success with the use of younger starting material. It is true, however, that the older the starting stage, the closer the end product is to adult conditions. Yet, the general conclusion has emerged that many, at least, of the characteristics of pulmonary structure—and especially that of the branching, epithelial, respiratory tree—are inherent in the endodermal epithelium of the so-called primary lung bud. Once started, development in vitro proceeds in a self-governing manner.

To be sure, blood vessels are less abundant in cultured specimens, and growth falls behind after a few days. Such slackening growth results from a progressively slowing mitotic rate, especially in epithelium in contrast to the developing mesenchyme. The result is that branching occurs less often, since branching of the epithelial tubes under any set of conditions is a function of its mitotic

rate. It is important to emphasize that it is growth rather than differentiation that becomes limited in cultured specimens. Actually, both the structural and the chemical differentiation of pulmonary epithelial cells are so well matched under in vivo and in vitro conditions that the relative independence of differentiation from growth becomes apparent.

It has been commonly assumed that a specific chemical induction is responsible for producing the initial appearance of the primordial "lung bud," but definite proof of such a specific influence at that time is lacking. On the other hand, various experiments performed on later, definitive lung buds indicate the dependence of orderly epithelial, tubular branching on the presence of factors residing in the enveloping mesenchyme.

Removal of the mesenchyme from a developing lung bud interrupts the branching of the epithelial bronchial tubes, but branching resumes as soon as regeneration replaces the portion of mesenchyme that was removed. Isolated epithelium, cultured in vitro, either spreads about or gathers in spherical aggregations, but it is incapable of tubular morphogenesis. When recombined, however, with the pulmonary mesenchyme, characteristic development proceeds. Moreover, such bronchial-tree mesenchyme, grafted onto a denuded tracheal tube, can even induce the formation of a supernumerary, branching lung bud at that level. That this inductive pulmonary mesenchyme has a specific influence is proved by the fact that substituted mesenchyme, taken from other regions of the body, is incompetent. In general, such "foreign" mesenchyme serves only to check the spread of bronchial development or at best, in the case of metanephrogenic mesenchyme, it permits only an inferior degree of development.

Incidentally, pulmonary epithelium has the potentiality of budding for some time after it normally ceases this activity. This continuing potential is proved by subjecting such a developed site to the influence of inciting mesenchyme. The capability of induction is strongest in mesenchyme nearest to normally budding regions of the bronchial tree.

Dissociated, cultured cells of a lung primordium reaggregate, with the epithelial cells gathered at the center of a mesenchymal mass, and then they resume the branching type of development. The effectiveness of this response, however, decreases with the increasing age of the donor embryo. Separated mesenchyme, placed at some distance from the denuded epithelial tree, migrates toward the latter and reinvests it; following this restoration, branching resumes. Trials show that the best results depend on the right amount of reinvesting mesenchyme used at a certain stage in its maturation.

From the preceding review it follows that diverse experiments on the developing lung bud indicate, first, the operation, at an appropriate time, of a true inductive influence; second, the ability of dissociated cells of epithelium and mesenchyme to "recognize" others of the same kind and to reassociate separately into homogeneous tissue masses; third, the existence of a chemotactic influence, quite different from induction, that leads spatially separated mesenchyme into a mass movement toward epithelium; and fourth, the ability of such recombined components then to resume the branching type of tubular, bronchial development.

Anomalies

A greatly reduced lung, or even its total absence, is a rare occurrence. Equally remarkable is the presence of an accessory lung. Variations occur in the size and number of the major pulmonary lobes. Rarely there is a third—that is, true—upper lobe and a corresponding eparterial bronchus on the left side. The right upper bronchus at times arises directly from the lower trachea, as it does normally in the sheep, hog, and ox. On the other hand, the right upper bronchus may imitate the reduced condition normal for the left side. The presence of a definite cardiac lobe of the lung, although infrequent, is of special interest since such a lobe occurs regularly in some mammals, including certain primates. Variations occur in the bronchopulmonary segments and in their component bronchi. Congenital cysts arise as derivatives of the bronchioles.

The lungs may be transposed in position, as in a mirror image. This reversal, known as situs inversus, may affect the thoracic viscera alone, or it may be a part of a large transposition that involves the abdominal viscera as well. Positive information on the cause of such reversals is lacking, but this abnormal condition is merely a part of the larger problems of how bilateral symmetry and how asymmetries are established in the body normally.

A serious anomaly results when the esophagus becomes atretic or discontinuous at some point along its course, thereby producing a blind sac at its upper end. Another type of anomaly occurs when the esophagus makes a fistulous connection with the trachea; this occurrence is said to represent an incomplete separation of the early laryngotracheal groove from the foregut.

Development of the Pulmonary Vessels

Pulmonary Arteries

The origin and relations of the pulmonary arteries have been studied extensively by Congdon (1922). Before the primitive aortic sac—or truncus arteriosus region—of the early heart has subdivided into an ascending aorta and pulmonary trunk, it sends forth two well-developed vascular plexuses. These extend caudad along the right and left sides of the short tracheopulmonary bud, which still is not separate along its cranial extent, from the esophagus. This stage occurs in human embryos 4 mm long, and nearly 5 weeks old (Fig. 1–7A). Promptly thereafter, a vascular sprout from each dorsal aortic root grows ventrad toward the corresponding primitive pulmonary artery, and by the 6-mm stage, at least, it joins the artery not far from its point of origin (Fig. 1–7A, B). When this joining occurs, the distal portion of each pulmonary vessel, so tapped, then appears as a mere offshoot set at a right angle to an aortic arch—which is, however, composite in origin (Fig. 1–7C).

This most caudal and tardiest pair of aortic arches in the total series of arches to appear is often numbered as the sixth (Fig. 1–8). Some observers, however, number them five since the pair just cranial is so inconstant, incomplete, and transitory that these vascular pathways may not really qualify as true arches. Still others avoid the controversy by designating the most caudal pair as pulmonary arches, instead of assigning them a number.

By the time the definitive pair of pulmonary aortic arches comes into existence, the truncus arteriosus is subdividing by means of two merging internal ridges. These ridges take a spiraling course and produce a separate ascending aorta and pulmonary trunk. As a consequence, the newly derived main pulmonary trunk supplies this most caudal pair of aortic arches, and, necessarily, also supplies the pulmonary artery that extends lungward from each arch.

In a human embryo 11 mm long, and nearly 6 weeks old, the pair of pulmonary arches and the arterial extensions stemming from them are well established. On the left side this condition persists until birth; the dorsal portion of the arch beyond the point of origin of its pulmonary artery is known as the ductus arteriosus (Fig. 1–8B). Most of the fetal blood leaving the heart through the pulmonary trunk bypasses the pulmonary circulation because the lungs are not yet respiratory in function. Hence, the blood shunts through the ductus arteriosus and is delivered directly into the aorta (Fig. 1–9). After birth, with the onset of breathing and the establishment of a vigorous pulmonary circulation, the ductus collapses. During the succeeding 2 or 3 postnatal months it gradually obliterates, leaving as a vestige the fibrous ligamentum arteriosum.

On the right side the dorsal portion of the pulmonary arch that corresponds to the ductus arteriosus undergoes early degeneration and disappears (Figs. 1–8B, 1–9).

The distribution of the main arterial branches within the lung follows a quite regular pattern. In fact, anomalies in the entire arterial supply seem to be relatively rare and minor in nature.

Pulmonary Veins

Since lungs are new acquisitions in vertebrate phylogeny, it is not surprising that the paired pulmonary veins arise independently rather than by the conversion of vascular channels originally present for other temporary purposes. Neil (1956) has provided a careful account of the early development of the human pulmonary veins.

A single vascular sprout begins to bud from the cranial wall of the left atrium in human embryos of 4 to 5 mm—about 4 weeks old. Slightly later this main stem connects with a still incomplete vascular plexus forming in the region of the so-called primary lung buds (Fig. 1–7C). In 7- to 8-mm embryos—about 5 weeks old—there is an indication of the later branching of the stem vein into individual channels that will thereafter drain each pulmonary plexus (Fig. 1–10A). At this time the common venous stem enters the left atrium caudal to the entrance of the sinus venosus into the right atrium.

A subsequent bifurcation of the original venous branch

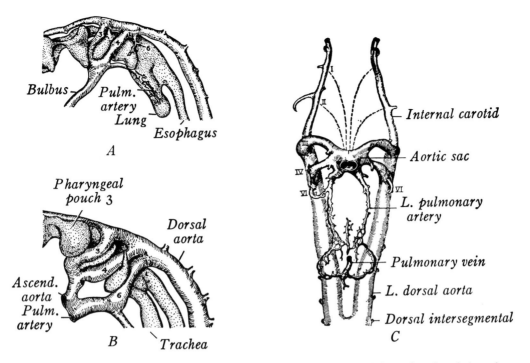

Fig. 1–7. Reconstructions of the aortic arches, with special reference to the development of the sixth arch and the pulmonary artery (after Congdon). *A,* Lateral view, at 5 mm, ×23; *B,* ventral view, at 5 mm, ×23, showing also the relation of the arteries to the early pulmonary vein; *C,* lateral view, at 11 mm, ×17. (Reproduced with permission from Arey, L.B.: Developmental Anatomy, 7th ed. Philadelphia, W.B. Saunders Co., 1965, p. 351.)

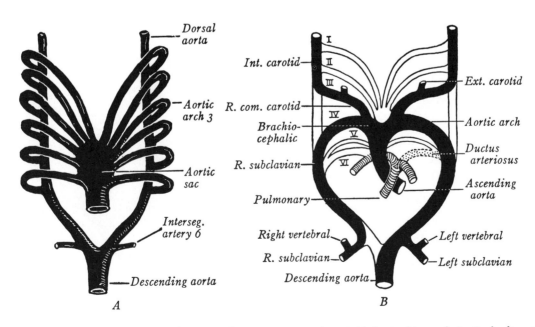

Fig. 1–8. Diagram showing the transformation of the aortic arches. Persisting vessels are in black; atrophic vessels, in stipple; discontinued vessels, in white. (Reproduced with permission from Arey, L.B.: Developmental Anatomy, 7th ed. Philadelphia, W.B. Saunders Co., 1965, p. 352.)

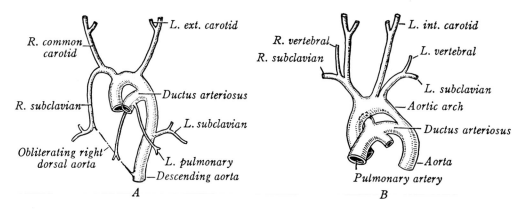

Fig. 1–9. Changing relations of the aortic arch derivatives, shown in ventral views. *A,* At 17 mm, ×20; *B,* at birth, ×½. (Reproduced with permission from Arey, L.B.: Developmental Anatomy, 7th ed. Philadelphia, W.B. Saunders Co., 1965, p. 353.)

to each lung produces a total of four drainage vessels from the pair of lungs. As the atrium continues its growth, the stem vessel and its four main branches are progressively taken up into the atrial wall. As a result, first the stem vein, then two, and finally four tributary pulmonary veins open separately into the left atrium and at some distance from each other (Fig. 1–10*B*). The extent of the absorbed tissue of these vessels is recognizable permanently as a smooth area in the lining of the atrial wall.

Not uncommonly, less than the usual degree of absorption results in fewer than four pulmonary veins entering the left atrium. Abnormal openings into the right atrium are presumably related to the presence of an atrial septum that arose too far to the left. More bizarre endings of the pulmonary drainage relate to a retention of some primitive connections with venous plexuses in the im-

mediate neighborhood. Communication with the right common cardinal system can result in drainage into the derived superior vena cava or azygos vein. Similarly, persistent relations with the left common cardinal system can produce drainage into derivatives such as a left superior vena cava, a left innominate vein, or into the coronary sinus. Primitive connections with the vitello-umbilical system can lead to drainage into the portal vein or ductus venosus. Apparently there are few instances of complete anomalous pulmonary return that do not fit into the categories already discussed—and the basic explanations as set forth. When such rare aberrations do occur, they tend to be associated with other gross cardiac malformations.

THE ESOPHAGUS

The esophagus, as a part of the primitive tubular gut, originates through the folding of the entodermal layer in

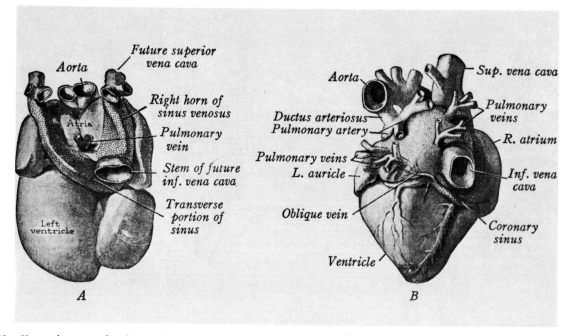

Fig. 1–10. Human hearts, in dorsal view, showing the absorption of the pulmonary veins into the left atrium. *A,* At 7 mm, ×28 (Braus); *B,* in newborn, ×⅔. (Arey, L.B.: Developmental Anatomy, 7th ed., revised. Philadelphia, W.B. Saunders Co., 1974, p. 385.)

early somite stages of the human embryo. The literature covering all phases of esophageal development was reviewed and evaluated by Lewis (1912). Smith (1957) added data relative to the separation of the lung from the foregut.*

Development of the Esophagus

The Epithelium

At first a simple, single layer (Fig. 1–11A), it shows two rows of nuclei by the fourth week of development, and this condition remains through the ninth week (Fig. 1–11B). By the eleventh week stratification into three layers has occurred, and the superficial layer of cells is ciliated (Fig. 1–11C). These cells are eventually desquamated, although some may persist even to the time of birth when there are about 10 layers of cells (compare Fig. 1–13). Eventually the stratification reaches some 25 layers.

In human embryos of 6 to 7 weeks, large vacuoles appear in the epithelium, so that in transverse sections the lumen may appear to be double or triple (Fig. 1–12A, B). Some superficial vacuoles communicate with the main lumen (Fig. 1–12C). Three weeks later such local cavitations have been lost as the process seemingly con-

---

*Editor's footnote: Early in embryonic development, the primitive gut acquires a double-layered wall. This consists of the entodermal layer and the closely associated splanchnic mesoderm, which together constitute the spanchnopleura. At the same time, the embryo begins to be bounded by definite folds. Cephalad, the central gutter of the splanchnopleura becomes the tubular foregut. The cephalic portion, which is to become the pharynx, appears compressed dorsoventrally and has a wide lateral extent. A series of pouchlike diverticula appears on either side—the developing pharyngeal pouches. Caudal to the level of the pouches, the foregut becomes abruptly narrowed in its lateral extent. Just cephalic to this point, at the level of the fourth pouches, the foregut gives rise to the lung bud. From this point to the dilation that marks the beginning of the stomach, the foregut remains of relatively small and uniform diameter and becomes the esophagus. Keith (1933) suggested that the esophagus is derived from two different segments of the foregut. The upper or retrotracheal portion originates from the pharyngeal segment and the lower or infratracheal part arises from the pregastric segment of the foregut.

The stages of development involving the separation of the trachea and esophagus in the upper portion were described well by Smith (1957). He stated that in the 21- to 23-day embryo, the first primordium of the respiratory system is seen in the midline of the ventral wall of the foregut between the thyroid primordium cranially and the anterior intestinal portal caudally. With further cellular proliferation, a ridge develops on the external surface of the foregut and a corresponding groove, the laryngotracheal sulcus, develops on the internal surface. The ridge widens as it extends caudally. During the next 12 days, the foregut and the laryngotracheal groove lengthen. A definite thickening of the ventral wall of the foregut occurs cephalad to the liver primordium. Near the end of this period—25 to 27 days—a knob-like lung bud appears adjacent to the sinus venosus. Ridges of entodermal cells develop from the lateral walls at the caudal end of the lung bud region of the foregut. The union of these proliferating ridges within the lumen of the foregut divides it into a ventral respiratory and a dorsal digestive portion. Next is the development of lateral esophageal grooves. These run caudally from just dorsal to the tracheoesophageal ridges to the dorsal wall of the esophagus. In the 27- to 29-day embryo, the diameter of the esophagus just caudal to the tracheoesophageal separation diminishes markedly. The elongation of the esophagus apparently causes this reduction in the lumen. Independent development of the trachea and esophagus continues, and in the 34- to 36-day embryo, separation of the respiratory tree from the esophagus is essentially complete.

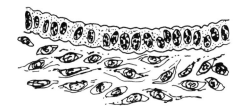

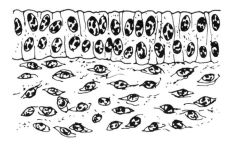

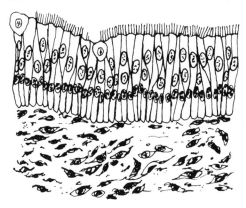

Fig. 1–11. Histogenesis of the epithelial lining of the esophagus, ×550. *A*, At 3 weeks; *B*, at 4 weeks; *C*, at 11 weeks. (Redrawn after Patten, B.M.: Human Embryology. New York, Blakiston, 1953.)

tributes to the enlargement of the esophageal lumen. The vacuoles do not result from cellular degeneration, but are probably caused by the active moving apart of local epithelial cells. Vacuolation produces bulges and ridges into the main lumen, but at no time is there a solid epithelial cord, as occurs temporarily in the duodenum of various vertebrates and regularly in the developing human duodenum.

At about 3 months of development pale groups of mucus-containing cells begin to appear at laryngeal and cardiac levels. A month later they bud into the adjacent mesenchyme as the characteristic superficial glands of the lamina propria. The lower group comprises the so-called cardiac glands, continuous with similar glands in the cardiac portion of the stomach. The deep glands of the tunica submucosa are indicated at 5 months (Fig.

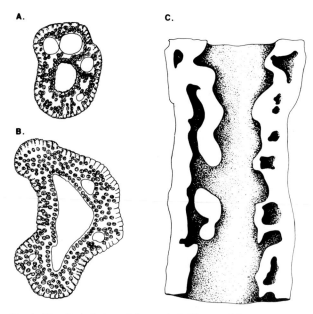

Fig. 1–12. Vacuolation of the epithelial lining of the esophagus. *A, B,* Transverse sections at 6.5 weeks and 7 weeks, ×160; *C,* Longitudinal hemisection of a model at 7 weeks, ×130. (Redrawn after Keibel, F., and Mall, F.P.: Manual of Human Embryology. Philadelphia, J.B. Lippincott Co., 1912.)

1–13) as short ingrowths, but even at birth they are laggard in their final stages of development.

The Accessory Layers

The early epithelial tube lies within a bed of undifferentiated mesenchyme. In embryos of 7 weeks the tunica muscularis is differentiating, thereby separating a tunica submucosa from a tunica adventitia (Fig. 1–14*A*). The muscular coat, subdivided into a circular and a longitudinal layer (Fig. 1–14*B, C*), differs lengthwise in its composition. The upper third is composed of striated muscle; the lower third is smooth muscle; the middle third is mixed—both striated and smooth. The development of the striated muscle has not been studied sufficiently, since smooth muscle originally extends to the

larynx and possibly transforms. There is no evidence that the striated fibers of the pharynx downgrow onto the esophagus. There is no developmental or anatomic basis for the presence of a pharyngo-esophageal or a gastro-esophageal sphincter; the basis of activity is wholly physiologic.

Folds of the tunica mucosa, also involving the tunica submucosa, produce the star-shaped lumen as seen in transverse sections. The original circular contour of the lumen has become quadripartite at 8 weeks of development.

By the third month the longitudinally coursing fibers of the lamina muscularis mucosae are appearing, and this feature establishes the deep boundary of the tunica mucosa and hence the presence of a definite lamina propria (Fig. 1–14*C*). In embryos of 2 months the mesenchyme of this layer is beginning to differentiate slowly into typical areolar connective tissue. Sometime after birth the superficial portion of the lamina propria begins to indent the stratified epithelium locally, and in a child of 12 months it has produced characteristic, tall connective-tissue papillae.

Anomalies

Stenosis or local atresia may occur. The latter abnormality usually involves the trachea also and exhibits diverse variations. Commonly there is a fistulous communication between the esophagus and trachea: the upper esophagus usually is atretic and ends as a blind sac; the trachea opens into the separate lower segment of the esophagus. The cause seems to relate to an incomplete separation of the early laryngotracheal groove from the foregut in an embryo of the fourth week. The investigations of Smith (1957) have helped to clarify the stage of development involving the separation of the trachea and esophagus. These studies suggest that a possible mechanism of development is an overgrowth of the ridges forming the tracheoesophageal septum, but the specific embryologic cause remains unknown. Traction diverticula and pulsion diverticula do not have a convincing developmental basis.

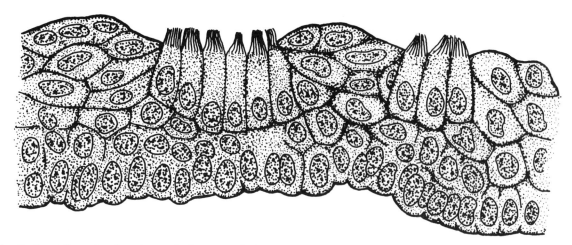

Fig. 1–13. Section at 5 months, through a patch of mucous cells that will become a cardiac gland within the mucous membrane of the esophagus, ×1200. (Redrawn after Keibel, F., and Mall, F.P.: Manual of Human Embryology. Philadelphia, J.B. Lippincott Co., 1912.)

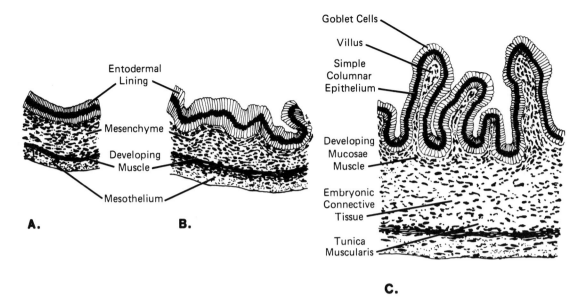

Fig. 1–14. Histogenesis of the accessory layers of the digestive tube, ×140. *A*, At 7 weeks; *B*, at 10 weeks; *C*, at 11 weeks. (Redrawn after Patten, B.M.: Human Embryology. New York, Blakiston, 1953.)

REFERENCES

Adams, F.H., et al.: The nature and origin of the fluid in the fetal lamb lung. J. Pediatr. *63*:881, 1963.

Aherne, W., and Dawkins, M.J.R.: The removal of fluid from pulmonary airways after birth. Biol. Neonate *7*:214, 1964.

Barnett, C.H.: A note on the dimensions of the bronchial tree. Thorax *12*:175, 1957.

Bertalanffy, F.D.: Respiratory tissue. Int. Rev. Cytol. *17*:213, 1964.

Boston, R.W., et al.: Lymph flow and clearance of liquid from the lungs. Lancet *2*:473, 1965.

Boyden, E.A., and Tompsett, D.H.: The changing patterns in the developing lungs of infants. Acta Anat. *61*:164, 1965.

Bucher, U., and Reid, L.: Development of the intrasegmental bronchial tree. Thorax *16*:207, 219, 1961.

Buckingham, S., and Avery, M.E.: Time of appearance of lung surfactant in the foetal mouse. Nature (London) *193*:688, 1962.

Campiche, A., et al.: An electron microscope study of the development of the human lung. Pediatrics *32*:976, 1963.

Congdon, E.D.: Transformation of the aortic-arch system of the human embryo. Contrib. Embryol. *14*:47, 1922.

Dannenberg, A.M., Jr., et al.: A histochemical study of enzymatic functions of exudate cells and alveolar macrophages. J. Cell Biol. *17*:465, 1963.

Dunnill, M.S.: Postnatal growth of the lung. Thorax *17*:329, 1962.

Ekehorn, G.: Über die Entwicklung der Lungen beim Menschen. Z. Anat. Entwicklungsgesch. *62*:271, 1921.

Flint, J.M.: The development of the lungs. Am. J. Anat. *6*:1, 1906.

Fujiwara, T., et al.: Fetal lamb amniotic fluid: Relationship of lipid composition to surface tension. J. Pediatr. *65*:824, 1964.

Gautier, A., et al.: Pulmonary epithelium in the human fetus and newborn. Proc. 5th Int. Congr. Electron Micro., Vol. 2. New York, Academic Press, 1962.

Heiss, R.: Zur Entwicklung und Anatomie der menschliche Lunge. Arch. Anat. Physiol. (Anat. Abt.) Jahrgang 1, 1919.

Huntington, G.S.: A critique of the theories of pulmonary evolution in mammals. Am. J. Anat. *27*:99, 1920.

Irestedt, L., Lagercrantz, H., and Belfrange, P.: Causes and consequences of maternal and fetal symphoadrenal activation during parturition. Acta Obstet. Gynecol. Scand. (Suppl.) *118*:111, 1984.

Irestedt, L., et al.: Fetal and maternal plasma catecholamine levels at elective cesarian section under general or epidural anesthesia versus vaginal delivery. Am. J. Obstet. Gynecol., *142*:1004, 1982.

Irestedt, L., et al.: Quoted by Lagercrantz, H., and Slotkin, T.A.: The "stress" of being born. Scientific American *254*(4):100, 1986.

Keith, A.: Human Embryology and Morphology, 5th ed. London, Edward Arnold, 1933, pp. 303–305.

Lagercrantz, H., and Slotkin, T.A.: The "stress" of being born. Scientific American *254*(4):100, 1986.

Lewis, F.T.: The development of the esophagus. *In* Manual of Human Embryology, Vol. 2. Edited by F. Keibel and F.P. Mall. Philadelphia, J.B. Lippincott Co., 1912, p. 355.

Lind, J., and Hirvensalo, M.: Roentgenologic studies of the size of the lungs of the newborn baby before and after aeration. Ann. Paediatr. Fenn. *12*:20, 25, 1966.

Loosli, C.G., and Potter, E.L.: Pre- and postnatal development of the human lung. Am. Rev. Respir. Dis. *80* (Part 2):5, 1959.

Low, F.N., and Sampaio, M.M.: The pulmonary alveolar epithelium as an entodermal derivative. Anat. Rec. *127*:51, 1957.

Neil, C.A.: Development of the pulmonary veins. Pediatrics *18*:880, 1956.

Olver, R.E.: Of labour and the lungs. Arch. Dis. Child. *56*:659, 1981.

Oren, R., et al.: Metabolic patterns in three types of phagocytizing cells. J. Cell Biol. *17*:487, 1963.

Reid, L.: The embryology of the lung. *In* Ciba Foundation Symposium Development of the Lung. Boston, Little, Brown and Co., 1965, p. 109.

Short, R.H.D.: Alveolar epithelium in relation to growth of the lung. Philos. Trans. R. Soc. London (Ser. B) *235*:35, 1950.

Slotkin, T.A., et al.: Quoted by Lagercrantz, H., and Slotkin, T.A.: The "stress" of being born. Scientific American *254*(4):100, 1986.

Smith, E.I.: The early development of the trachea and esophagus in relation to atresia of the esophagus and tracheoesophageal fistula. Contrib. Embryol. *36*:43, 1957.

Sorokin, S.: Recent work on developing lungs, Chapter 18. *In* Organogenesis. Edited by R.L. DeHaan and H. Ursprung. New York, Holt, Rinehart and Winston, 1965.

Weibel, E.R.: Morphometrische Analyse der menschlichen Lunge. Z. Zellforsch. *57*:648, 1962.

Wells, L.J., and Boyden, E.A.: The development of the bronchopulmonary segments in human embryos. Am. J. Anat. *95*:163, 1954.

Windle, W., et al.: Aspiration of amniotic fluid by the fetus. Surg. Gynecol. Obstet. *69*:705, 1939.

CHAPTER 2

ULTRASTRUCTURE AND MORPHOMETRY OF THE HUMAN LUNG

Peter H. Burri, Joan Gil, and Ewald R. Weibel

ORGANIZATION OF THE LUNG

The application of electron microscopy and of quantitative methods in morphology—morphometry—has markedly widened the general understanding of lung structure and has set the course for a more functional approach to the study of pulmonary architecture.

It cannot be the aim of this chapter, however, to cover all aspects of lung microanatomy; in this respect, the reader is referred to the specialized literature. We would rather present the morphologic and quantitative background needed to understand the functioning of the gas exchange apparatus.

The lung is composed of three phases: air, tissue, and blood. The tissue forms a complete barrier between air and blood; it is a stable structural framework, whereas air and blood are continuously exchanged. In describing the ultrastructure of the lung, we will emphasize the specializations of the tissue in forming boundary spaces for air and blood. Morphometry will deal with the quantitative relations among these three phases.

From the functional point of view the organization of the lung may be defined in relation to the hierarchy of airways and blood vessels, from the trachea down to alveoli, or from the main stem of the pulmonary artery through the capillary network to the pulmonary veins entering the left atrium.

All of this is jointly considered in the scheme of Figure 2–1. Besides showing the three phases, the diagram introduces the three major functional zones of the lung; first, the *conductive zone* consisting of air channels and blood vessels whose function is to guide and distribute air or blood into the peripheral lung units; second, the *respiratory zone* comprised of alveoli and capillaries; and third, the *intermediate* or *transitory zone* containing elements of both.

FINE STRUCTURE OF THE LUNG

Fine Structure of Conducting Airways

The conducting airways are a system of hollow, flexible tubes, which multiply toward the periphery according

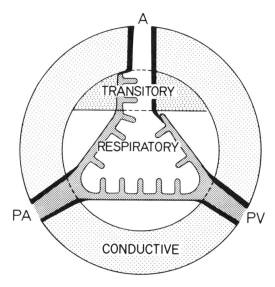

Fig. 2–1. Schematic representation of lung zones. A = airways, PA = pulmonary artery, PV = pulmonary vein.

to the principle of irregular dichotomy. From the trachea to bronchi to bronchioles, the structure of the airway wall gradually changes. What is common to all is the general scheme of a three-layered wall made of a *mucosa*, a *muscle layer*, and a *connective tissue sheath* (Fig. 2–2), and the presence of a typical ciliated epithelium, which is described first.

The Lining Epithelium of Conductive Airways

The inspired air must be humidified and warmed before it reaches the delicate gas-exchange area; furthermore, air pollutants and dust, as well as airborne microorganisms, must be removed. Though the upper respiratory tract—especially the nasal portion—is especially designed for these functions, the respiratory epithelium (Fig. 2–3) of all conducting airways shows spe-

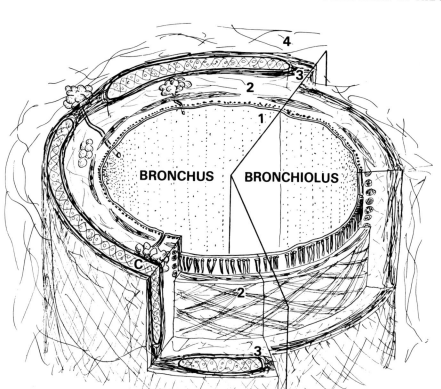

Fig. 2–2. Structure of bronchi and bronchioles. 1, Mucosa with epithelium and elastic fibers; 2, smooth muscle layer; 3, fibrous layer contains cartilage (C) in the bronchi; 4, peribronchial sheath of loose connective tissue.

cial features for the handling of airborne particles: It is a ciliated pseudostratified columnar epithelium with numerous scattered goblet cells. Ciliated cells occur from the trachea down to the last respiratory bronchiole, but their height decreases with the reduction of the airway diameter; ciliated cells of the trachea are columnar (Fig. 2–4), whereas those of the respiratory bronchioles are cuboidal (Fig. 2–5). The frequency of goblet cells also decreases toward the periphery; in bronchioles they are replaced by Clara cells (Fig. 2–5), whose secretory role is not yet clear. Cytologic, kinetic, and histochemical studies by Breeze and Wheeldon (1977), Jeffery and Reid (1977), Jeffery (1983), and Spicer (1983) and St. George (1985) and their co-workers, have provided insights into the cell types of the airway epithelium of various species, including man. Great emphasis is also being put on the investigation of the endocrine cells interspersed in the epithelium, often called Feyrter, Kulchitsky, APUD—*a*mine *p*recursor *u*ptake and *d*ecarboxylation—or small granule cells. These endocrine cells are present in the respiratory tract of all vertebrate species investigated so far. Lauweryns and Cokelaere (1973) found them thinly scattered along the airways, either isolated or clustered in neuroepithelial bodies. Suspected to be involved in the secretion of vasoactive substances in the lung, they most likely represent, according to Sorokin and co-workers (1983), a heterogeneous population of cells.

The frequently found basal cells represent a prolifer-

ative pool of undifferentiated cells, which are thought to replace the overlying cells upon differentiation and maturation. Less common are the brush cells and migratory cells. Finally, one should mention the occurrence of naked nerve endings between individual cells, more frequently in the trachea and large bronchi. They are thought to be irritant receptors.

Figure 2–3 shows a schematic representation of a portion of the respiratory epithelium of a bronchus. The function of this epithelium is to capture airborne particles in a sticky mucous layer and to remove them efficiently from the lung. For this purpose, cilia show a synchronized rhythmic beat within a thin layer of fluid of low viscosity. On top of this a blanket of mucus is moved in the direction of the pharynx, carrying along intercepted particles. This cleaning mechanism can be compared with a conveyor belt and is often called the "mucociliary escalator." The mucous layer is secreted onto the epithelial surface by goblet cells and by seromucous glands located in the walls of trachea and bronchi (Fig. 2–2). The small bronchioles are most likely devoid of mucus, as their wall contains neither goblet cells nor glands; but we (J.G. and E.R.W.) (1971) found that their surface is formed by a fluid layer of low viscosity that is sometimes topped by a thin osmiophilic film. Finally, the presence in the bronchial secretion of several humoral agents, which would protect the airways against infections, has been reported.

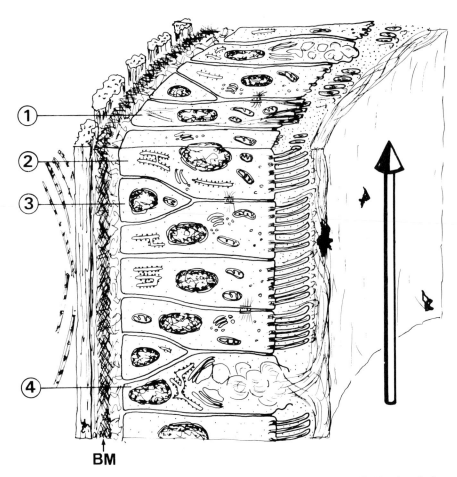

Fig. 2–3. Pseudostratified epithelium of bronchus with brush (1), ciliated (2), basal (3), and goblet cells (4). The cilia beat in a serous fluid which is topped by a mucous layer secreted partly by goblet cells. A strong basement membrane (BM) and a layer of longitudinal elastic fibers form the basis of the epithelium.

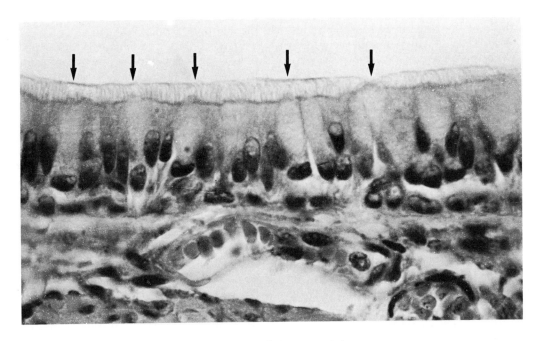

Fig. 2–4. Pseudostratified epithelium from bronchus. Note goblet cells (arrows). ×600.

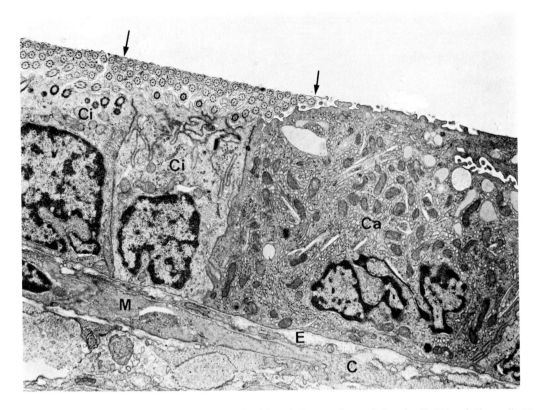

Fig. 2–5. Electron micrograph of bronchiolar wall with simple cuboidal epithelium made up of ciliated cells (Ci) and Clara cells (Ca). In place of the mucous layer there is a fine osmiophilic film (arrows) at the air-liquid interface. A smooth muscle cell (M) and collagenous (C) and elastic (E) fibers are seen in the subepithelial tissue. Rat lung fixed by vascular perfusion. ×9200.

Trachea and Bronchi

Trachea and bronchi are characterized by the presence of cartilage within the fibrous sheath of their walls (Fig. 2–2). In the trachea and stem bronchi the cartilage is in the form of incomplete rings; in the trachea these cover the ventral and lateral aspects, whereas the dorsal wall contains a strong layer of transverse smooth muscle. After about the second or third generation, these rings are gradually replaced by irregular cartilage plates and a layer of smooth muscle appears between mucosa and cartilage.

All conducting airways are surrounded by an external, loose connective tissue sheath (Fig. 2–2), which is continuous with the other connective elements of the lung. It is a structure of considerable physiologic significance, as it contains bronchial vessels, to supply the bronchial wall with blood from the systemic circulation, as well as nerves and lymphatic vessels. Only a small part of the arterial bronchial flow, in some species as little as 25%, is drained by the bronchial veins. Most of it goes into the peribronchial venous plexus and from there into the pulmonary veins forming a small right-to-left shunt. The bronchus is usually accompanied by a branch of the *pulmonary artery*, which is enveloped by connective tissue continuous with the peribronchial sheath.

Lymphatic vessels contained in these peribronchial and perivascular sheaths, as well as in the subpleural and septal connective tissue, constitute the main drainage path for the interstitial fluid.

Bronchioles

A bronchiole is an airway devoid of cartilage and seromucous glands; goblet cells are rare. Because airway structure does not change abruptly, either seromucous glands or goblet cells may still be present in transitional zones. Bronchioles are rather small conducting airways, measuring about 1 mm or less in diameter. However, their added cross-sectional area is such that they are not supposed to contribute substantially to the flow resistance of the airways in the normally breathing healthy individual. Their walls are generally thin and molded into the surrounding parenchyma. They are supplied with blood from the lesser circulation, rather than from bronchial arteries. The bronchiolar mucosa is lined by a simple cuboidal epithelium (Fig. 2–5) composed of ciliated cells and of Clara cells, which have the characteristic features of secreting cells: their cytoplasm contains many mitochondria, rough and smooth endoplasmic reticulum, and typical membrane-bounded granules of low electron density that are considered storage vacuoles for a secretory product of still unknown composition. These cells seem to take the place of goblet cells of larger airways.

In bronchioles the *smooth muscle cells* form a well-developed, relatively thick layer arranged in a geodesic network, capable of narrowing the airway.

Fine Structure of Transitory Airways

Respiratory Bronchioles

The last generation of exclusively conducting bronchioles is the *terminal bronchioles*. These branch to form about three generations of *respiratory bronchioles* (see Fig. 2–22), which have essentially the same structure as other bronchioles except that here and there and increasingly toward the periphery the continuity of their wall is interrupted by areas of typical gas-exchanging tissue. Contrary to common textbook descriptions, the cuboidal epithelial cells of respiratory bronchioles are in most cases ciliated; short cilia can even be demonstrated in close proximity to alveoli.

Alveolar Ducts and Sacs

The mammalian airways form a blind-ending system. Dichotomy as a branching pattern can be demonstrated up to the last ranks of the airway system, the *alveolar ducts* and *alveolar sacs* (see Fig. 2–22). These structures differ from the bronchioles described previously in that they lack a proper wall; instead, their wall is formed by the openings of alveoli (Fig. 2–6A and B); their epithelial lining is nothing more than extensions of squamous alveolar epithelial cells. It is generally admitted that usually three generations of alveolar ducts immediately follow the last respiratory bronchioles. Finally, the last ducts give rise to two alveolar sacs. An alveolar sac represents the blind end of the airway branching system (see Fig. 2–22).

Fine Structure of the Gas-Exchange Region

In the respiratory zone of the lung, the blood is spread in capillaries in the walls of the alveoli. The air-blood contact becomes intimate and gas exchange can take place.

The Alveoli

Alveoli are small pouches placed in groups around respiratory bronchioles, alveolar ducts, and alveolar sacs. They are polyhedral structures lacking one side—the mouth, which opens into the airways—and they have been compared with the cells of a honeycomb (Fig. 2–6 A and B) or with the air bubbles in a foam. A polygonal shape in general is economical, for it allows a close packing of the alveoli. Haefili-Bleuer's and one of our (E.R.W.) (1987) studies on human pulmonary acini have revealed that the shape of alveoli is not simple and that often an "alveolus" appears like a cluster of several connected pouches, as in Figure 2–6B. Furthermore, alveolar shape also depends on the degree of lung inflation, according to one of us (J.G.) and co-workers (1979). Only in fully inflated lungs has the alveolar configuration some similarity with the cells of a honeycomb. At lower inflation degrees alveoli are often cup-like.

The alveolar wall is always common to two adjacent alveoli and is called the *alveolar septum* (Fig. 2–6B). The most conspicuous feature of the septum is a single but dense network of capillaries, which is shown in Figure 2–7 in face view. Sometimes the septa are interrupted by *pores of Kohn*, which provide a path of communication between adjoining alveoli. The septa also contain a skeleton of connective tissue fibers that is specially well developed around the mouth of alveoli, where it forms a polygonal ring (Fig. 2–6) and may contain smooth muscle fibers. The collagenous and elastic fibrous elements form a three-dimensional continuum that extends from the pleura to the hilus. This assures transmission of chest and diaphragmatic movements into the deeper regions of the lung; but it contributes only a smaller part to the retractive force of the lung, the major part being due to surface forces. We (E.R.W. and J.G.) (1977) and I (E.R.W.) (1984) discussed the arrangement of the connective tissue in detail.

The Alveolocapillary Tissue Barrier

Figure 2–8 shows a section of a small portion of an interalveolar septum with a capillary. The septum is lined on both sides by alveolar epithelial cells which, in this instance, are thin. The capillary is also lined by a single squamous cell layer, the endothelium. Together with the intercalated connective tissue, these two cell layers constitute the alveolocapillary tissue barrier, which is the structure separating air and blood in the pulmonary gas-exchange region. It is supplemented by an extremely thin extracellular lining layer that contains macrophages (Figs. 2–9 and 2–10). The morphometric characteristics of the cell population that constitutes this tissue barrier in the human lung are shown in Table 2–2.

Epithelium. The epithelium of the alveoli is continuous, although its thickness in places only reaches 0.1 to 0.3 μm, which is at the limit of resolution of the light microscope. The study by Low (1952) brought the first conclusive evidence for an uninterrupted epithelial lining of alveoli. It consists of the following cell types (Table 2–1).

Alveolar epithelial cells type I (Fig. 2–11), also called *squamous cells*, send out broad, thin cytoplasmic extensions. Though they are some 30 to 40% less numerous than the type II cells, they cover between 92 and 95% of the total alveolar surface. The nuclei lie in depressions between two capillaries. These cells are poor in organelles—such as mitochondria or endoplasmic reticulum—which are confined to the perinuclear cytoplasm, whereas the cytoplasmic extensions essentially contain only pinocytotic vesicles. Crapo and associates (1982) found that in man a single type I cell covers some 5000 μm² of the alveolar surface, on the average.

Alveolar cells type II are cuboidal cells (Fig. 2–12). These cells have also been called *granular pneumocytes, septal cells, alveolar cells,* and *great alveolar cells* although they are much smaller than type I cells. They have no cytoplasmic extensions and typically are in niches between capillaries of the alveolar septum. Their free surface is covered by somewhat irregular microvilli. The cells occupy from 5 to 8% of the alveolar surface and form junctional complexes with neighboring alveolar

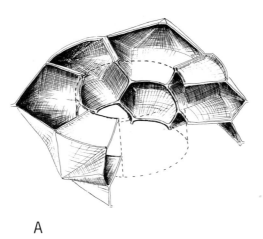

A

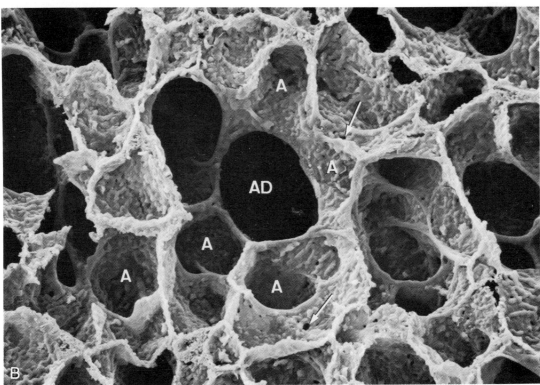

Fig. 2–6. *A*, Schematic representation of arrangement of alveoli around alveolar duct. (Reproduced with permission from Weibel, E.R.: Morphometry of the Human Lung. Heidelberg. Springer-Verlag, 1963, p. 57.) *B*, Scanning electron micrograph of human lung, ×150. AD = alveolar duct; A = alveoli; arrows point to pores of Kohn.

cells type I. Compared with alveolar cells type I, the granular pneumocyte is rich in mitochondria, endoplasmic reticulum, Golgi apparatus, and multivesicular bodies. Their most distinctive morphologic feature, however, is the presence of lamellar osmiophilic inclusions— "lamellated bodies"—which I (J.G.) and Reiss (1973) supposed are the sites of storage of the surface-active phospholipids. At the light microscopic level, alveolar cells type II may be easily confounded with macrophages.

A *third pneumocyte, the brush cell*, has been described by Meyrick and Reid (1968). In the rat this cell can easily be found in terminal bronchioles; it is, however, rare in the gas exchange zone. The brush cell is

characterized by a spray of rather thick and regular cylindrical microvilli at the surface and by thick bundles of microfibrils in the cytoplasm. Brush cells are large, but only a small part of their membrane reaches the epithelial surface. Similar cells occur in larger airway epithelia and in other organs also; their significance is still obscure.

Alveolar macrophages—dust cells—are the cells of the alveolar lining layer (Fig. 2–11). They are large cells exhibiting many vacuolar inclusions and lysosomes. Most of their phagosomes are filled with dark, lipid-rich inclusions. In their functional location they are closely apposed to the alveolar epithelial surface and are sub-

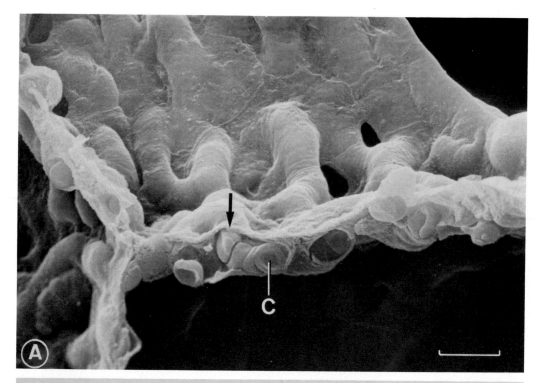

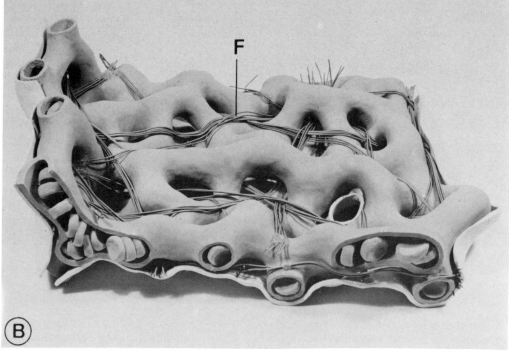

Fig. 2–7. Capillaries in the alveolar wall of human lung are shown in a scanning electron micrograph (A) and in a model (B). Note thin tissue barrier separating air and blood (arrow) and fibers (F) interwoven with capillary network (C). Scale marker 10 μm. (Reproduced with permission from Weibel, E.R.: The Pathway for Oxygen. Cambridge MA, Harvard University Press, 1984.)

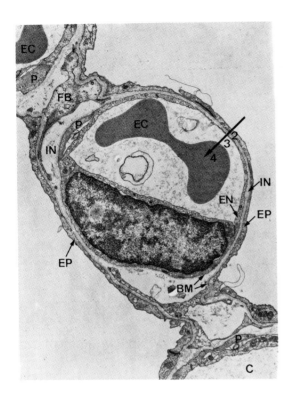

Fig. 2–8. Electron micrograph of alveolar capillary (C) from monkey lung with erythrocyte (EC). Note endothelial cell lining of capillary (EN), processes of pericytes (P) and the thin extensions of squamous alveolar epithelial cells (EP) covering the alveolar surface. The interstitial space (IN) is bounded by two basement membranes (BM) and contains some fibroblast processes (FB) as well as a few connective tissue fibrils. This lung was fixed by instillation of fixative into airways resulting in a loss of the surface lining layer; hence only parts 2 (tissue barrier), 3 (blood plasma), and 4 (erythrocyte) of the gas exchange pathway are preserved. × 8600. (Reproduced with permission from Weibel, E.R.: Morphometric estimation of pulmonary diffusion capacity. I. Model and method. Respir. Physiol. *11*:54, 1970/71.)

mersed under the surfactant film of the lining layer (Fig. 2–10); their bodies are in depressions of the alveolar wall and they send out large extensions. In conventional histologic preparations, they have been removed from their original position on the alveolar wall; they appear to float in the alveolar space and their surface is generally rounded-off so that they acquire the appearance of large, spherical cells. Contrary to previous views that alveolar macrophages are derivatives of the epithelium it has been convincingly shown that they derive from blood monocytes.

Interstitium. The interstitium is the space between the basal laminae of alveolar epithelium and capillary endothelium (Fig. 2–8). It contains connective tissue and interstitial fluid. The connective tissue comprises cells, fibers, and amorphous substance containing proteoglycans allegedly in a gel matrix. Its distribution can vary considerably. In places where the air-blood barrier is very thin, connective tissue may be reduced to a few isolated, fine fibrils or may even be absent, in which instance the adjoining basement membranes fuse. These latter regions are particularly important for gas exchange.

In lung edema they usually are not widened by interstitial fluid and can therefore be called "restricted" as opposed to those "unrestricted" thicker portions of interstitium between capillaries, where interstitial fluid can accumulate under pathologic conditions. The interstitial fibroblasts have been clearly demonstrated to contain contractile filaments (Fig. 2–11), so Kapanci and coworkers (1974, 1976) suggested that they can regulate blood flow through the alveolar septum. In view of the interstitial structure described, I (E.R.W.) and Bachofen (1979) proposed an alternative function for these cells: they could control the compliance of the unrestricted interstitial regions by regulating the width of the septum. In the postnatal rat lung it has been established that the interstitial cells form two distinct populations of cells: a lipid-containing—LIC, and a non-lipid-containing type—NLIC. The lipid droplets of LIC disappear, however, before weaning; the fate of the LIC remains unclear, according to Maksvytis and co-workers (1984). Lymphatic vessels are never found in alveolar septa; nevertheless a continuous path of the interstitial fluid toward the lymphatics of the subpleural space and of the peribronchial and perivascular connective sheaths has been postulated; the fluid probably follows connective fibers.

Endothelium. The endothelial cells form a capillary wall that is similar in structure to the endothelium in some other organs (Figs. 2–8, 2–9, 2–13). The cells form thin cytoplasmic extensions and hence resemble the alveolar epithelial cells of type I. A single cell covers between 1000 and 1500 μm² of the capillary lumen. Lung capillaries have no fenestrations. Further details will be discussed subsequently.

Extracellular Lining Layer and Pulmonary Surfactant

On the basis of theoretic considerations, as early as 1929 von Neergaard predicted that the alveolar surface must be lined by a layer of surface-active fluid, now commonly called *pulmonary surfactant*. It is an essential element assuring the stability of the air-filled lung. Its basic characteristics are twofold: first, it lowers the surface tension at the air-liquid interface of the alveoli; and second, its surface tension is variable with the degree of inflation of alveoli.

Morphologic demonstration of pulmonary surfactant is only possible with the electron microscope. In routine preparations, usually no traces of this material are found (Fig. 2–8). In lungs fixed by vascular perfusion, an extracellular duplex lining layer on the alveolar surface can be preserved (Fig. 2–9), which we (J.G. and E.R.W.) (1969/70) supposed to contain the alveolar surfactant system fixed in situ. Much of this material forms pools in pits and irregularities of the alveolar wall, which it smooths out. These pools are polymorphous: sometimes they are of moderate electron density with dark specks, or they may contain lipid micelles or tubular myelin, a liquid crystal made up of surface active lipoproteins.

The synthesis and secretion of pulmonary surfactant is the function of the type II pneumocytes. Figure 2–12*B*

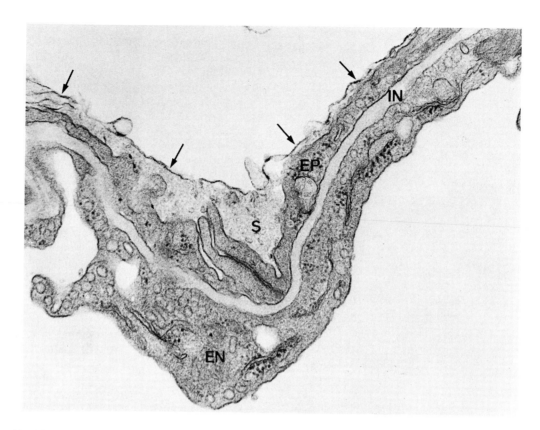

Fig. 2–9. Air-blood barrier of rat lung fixed by vascular perfusion to preserve surface lining layer (S) made up of base layer and osmiophilic surface film (arrows). IN = interstitial space; EP = squamous alveolar epithelial cells; EN = endothelial cell lining of capillary. ×38,700. (Reproduced with permission from Weibel, E.R.: Morphometric estimation of pulmonary diffusion capacity. I. Model and method. Respir. Physiol. *11*:54, 1970/71.)

shows how the organelles of this cell are involved in synthesizing, storing and secreting the two main components: the phospholipid dipalmitoyl-phosphatidyl-choline—DPPC—and the specific apoprotein to which DPPC is bound to form the lipoprotein, constituting the actual surfactant film. It appears that tubular myelin figures (Fig. 2–10) are an extracellular reserve form of surfurcant, which can spread on the surfce when alveoli enlarge. For further details and references, see Weibel (1985).

Fine Structure of Pulmonary Blood Vessels

Alveolar Capillaries

The dense capillary network (Fig. 2–7) that is intercalated between adjoining alveoli and forms part of the interalveolar septa is lined by an uninterrupted endothelial cell layer (Fig. 2–8). Characteristically, these endothelial cells are formed of two parts: (1) a region of cytoplasm surrounding the nucleus and containing the vast majority of cellular organelles, such as mitochondria, endoplasmic reticulum, Golgi complex, and various granules; and (2) thin cytoplasmic extensions, which are 0.1 μm thick and virtually free of organelles. In the thinnest regions—<0.1 μm—they are composed of two cell membranes and some intercalated cytoplasm (Fig. 2–8); the portions of average thickness contain numerous pinocytotic vesicles that are, in part, attached to either of the cell membranes (Figs. 2–8, 2–13). These vesicles are involved in the transport of materials, mainly of proteins, across the endothelial cell. In connection with pas-

Table 2–1. Morphometric Characteristics of Cell Population in the Human Alveolar Septal Tissue

	Cell Number		Average Cell	
	Absolute n × 10⁹	Relative %	Volume μm³	Apical Surface μm²
Pneumocytes I	19	8.3	1,763	5,098
Pneumocytes II	37	15.9	889	183
Endothelial cells	68	30.2	632	1,353
Interstitial cells	84	36.1	637	—
Macrophages	23	9.4	2,491	—

After Crapo, J.D., et al.: Cell numbers and cell characteristics of the normal human lung. Am. Rev. Respir. Dis. *126*:332, 1982.

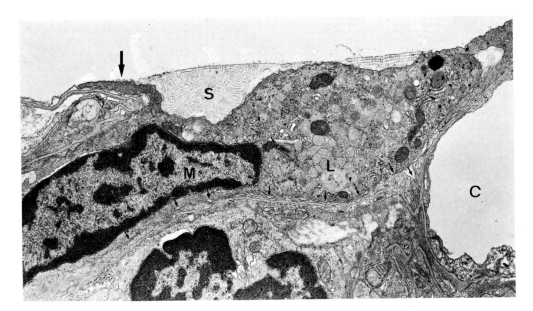

Fig. 2–10. Alveolar macrophage (M) with pseudopods and groups of lysosomal vesicles (L) in cytoplasm submerged beneath surface lining layer (S) and closely stuck to the alveolar epithelium (arrows). The base-layer of the surface lining layer contains so-called tubular myelin figures. The capillary (C) is empty because of fixation by vascular perfusion. ×10,500. (Reproduced with permission from Gil, J.: Ultrastructure of lung fixed under physiologically defined conditions. Arch. Intern. Med. *127*:896, 1971.)

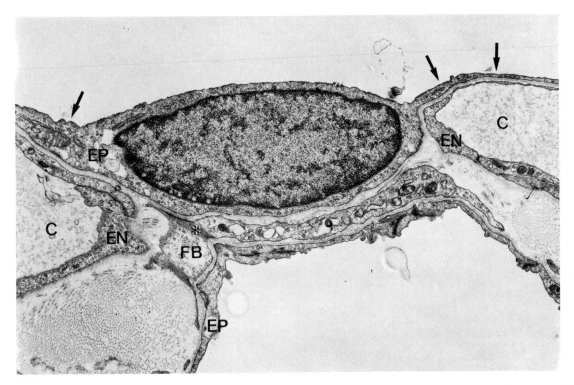

Fig. 2–11. Type I alveolar cell with thin cytoplasmic extensions (arrows). C = alveolar capillary; EP = squamous alveolar epithelial cells; EN = endothelial cell lining of capillary; FB = fibroblast process with an intracytoplasmic bundle of contractile filaments (*). ×8600.

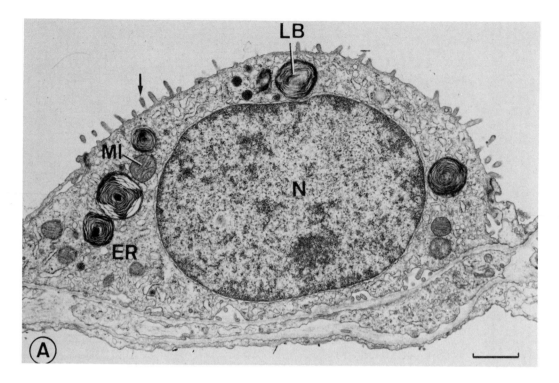

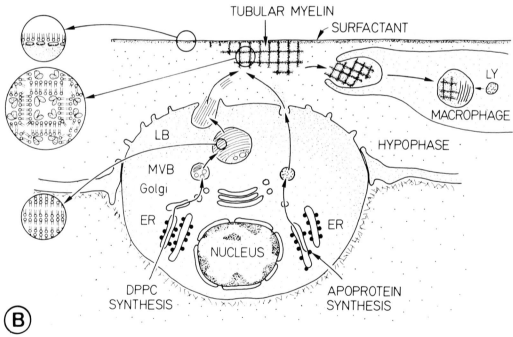

Fig. 2–12. *A,* In a type II epithelial cell the abundant cytoplasm surrounding the nucleus (N) contains the characteristic osmiophilic lamellar bodies (LB), which store surfactant, and a rich complement of organelles such as endoplasmic reticulum (ER) and mitochondria (MI). The surface membrane carries microvilli (arrow), and junctions (J) with neighbouring type I cells as seen. (Reproduced with permission from Weibel, E.R.: Design and structure of the human lung. *In* Pulmonary Diseases and Disorders. Edited by A.P. Fishman. New York, McGraw-Hill, 1971.) *B,* Schematic diagram of pathways for synthesis and secretion of surfactant DPPC and apoproteins by a type II cell, and for their removal by macrophages. Note the arrangement of phospholipids in the lamellar bodies, in tubular myelin, and in the surface film. (Reproduced with permission from Weibel, E.R.: The Pathway for Oxygen. Cambridge MA, Harvard University Press, 1984.)

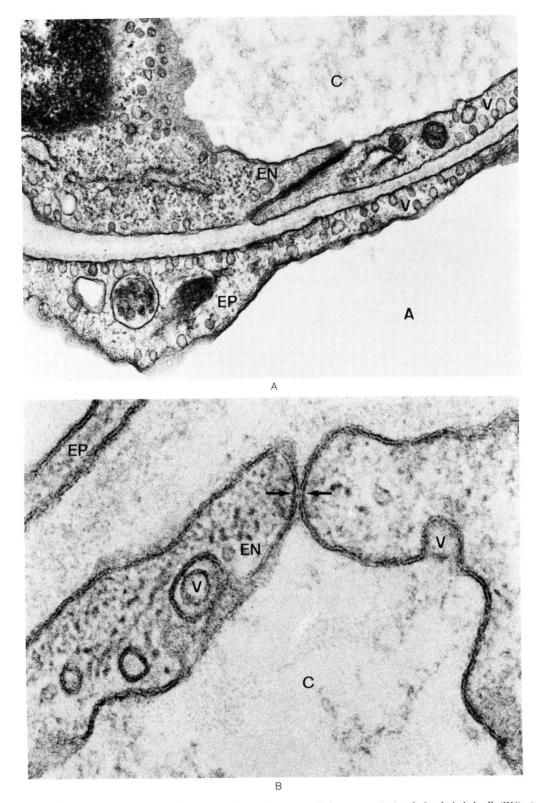

Fig. 2–13. *A*, Air-blood barrier showing thin cytoplasmic extensions of alveolar epithelium type I (EP) and of endothelial cells (EN) with intercellular junction. Note abundance of pinocytotic vesicles (V). ×37,000. *B*, High-power view of junction between two capillary endothelial cells. The triple-layered structure of the cell membranes is apparent. In the junction the membranes are closely apposed over a very short stretch (arrows). Note pinocytotic vesicles (V). A = alveolus; C = capillary, ×184,800.

sage of macromolecules the main problem, however, is the different permeability between endothelium and epithelium. There is general agreement that the epithelium represents the chief permeability barrier of the lung. Endothelium can be permeated under a variety of circumstances. The explanation for this difference was provided by comparative freeze-fracture studies of endothelial versus epithelial junctions. The epithelial tight junctions consist of a continuous network of three to five interconnected ridges and grooves, while the endothelial junctions have only one to three rows of particles with few interconnections and even some discontinuities, as discussed by Schneeberger (1979). Since it is believed that there is an inverse correlation between the number of strands constituting a tight junction and its permeability, it follows that epithelial junctions are "tight" while endothelial junctions are relatively "leaky."

Alveolar capillaries are associated with pericytes. Pericytes seem to be less frequent in the alveolar capillaries than in the systemic capillaries and less densely branched. Their function is still debated: they are supposed to be contractile cells, phagocytic elements, or both.

Ultrastructure of Larger Pulmonary Vessels

The endothelial lining of pulmonary arteries and veins differs from that of alveolar capillaries in that the cytoplasmic extensions are thicker (Fig. 2–14). They are likewise rich in pinocytotic vesicles and may contain numerous cellular organelles. These endothelial cells also contain a characteristic rod-shaped granule (Fig. 2–15) known to occur in all vascular endothelia of all vertebrate species thus far investigated by me (E.R.W.) and Palade (1964). In the mammalian vascular system these organelles are particularly numerous in medium-sized and larger branches of pulmonary arteries and veins, whereas they occur less frequently in systemic vessels of the same size. Based on indirect evidence, we (P.H.B. and E.R.W.) (1968) had proposed that these organelles contain a procoagulative substance. This assumption proved to be correct. Wagner and associates (1982) and Warhol and Sweet (1984), using immunocytochemical techniques, demonstrated that the endothelial specific organelles contained Factor VIII-related antigen, also called von Willebrand factor.

The electron microscopic study of intima and media of pulmonary vessels does not reveal many features that are not manifest by light microscopy. The circular smooth muscle cells of peripheral vessels of the muscular type are long, slender, and rather densely arranged (Fig. 2–14). In elastic vessels—larger pulmonary arteries—the connective tissue elements prevail (Fig. 2–16); the space between the prominent elastic laminae contains much collagenous tissue and relatively short smooth muscle cells, which extend from one elastic lamina to the next in an oblique course and appear to insert on the elastic laminae with ramified ends (Fig. 2–16). In Figure 2–15 a portion of a longitudinal section of a medium-sized

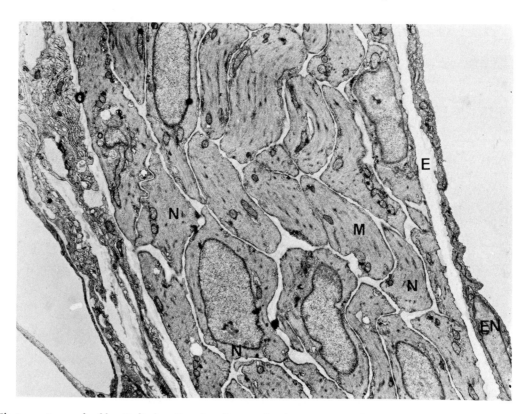

Fig. 2–14. Electron micrograph of longitudinal section of medium-sized pulmonary artery of muscle type. The endothelium (EN) lies over a strong elastic membrane (E). The smooth muscle fibers (M) are obliquely sectioned; their cytoplasm shows a very fine filamentous structure. Some muscle cells (labeled N) show intercellular contacts (nexus), serving spread of excitation among the cells. × 5850.

pulmonary vein is shown; its thin wall is made up of an endothelium, a few irregularly arranged smooth muscle fibers, and collagenous as well as elastic fibers.

One interesting feature is that smooth muscle cells of these vessel walls not only form close intercellular contacts in form of patches or nexus (Figs. 2–14, 2–16), but also have close cell-to-cell contact with endothelial cells by means of short extensions across the internal elastic membrane (Fig. 2–15). It is assumed that cell-to-cell contacts between endothelial or epithelial cells and smooth muscle or interstitial cells are important in inducing and regulating various cell functions.

Bronchial Vessels. The arteries of the bronchial wall are of the "muscle type." Figure 2–15 shows a small bronchial arteriole with one layer of circular smooth muscle and typically thick endothelial layer. Note the many contacts between muscle and endothelial cells. Bronchial arteries are often characterized by intimal longitudinal smooth muscle bundles that I (E.R.W.) (1959) found to be related to the stretch strain to which these vessels are frequently exposed rather than to a special regulatory function.

MORPHOMETRY OF THE LUNG

The application of morphometric methods in analyzing lung tissue has yielded new insights into lung structure and its dimensions and has opened the possibility of a morphologic approach to the study of lung function.

Compartmental Distribution of Lung Volume

Any morphologic analysis of the functional capacity of the gas exchange apparatus involves exact knowledge of the total lung volume and of its compartmental distribution.

To illustrate the distribution of the lung volume among the various zones and constituents we shall consider the lung of a medium-sized adult inflated to about three-fourths total lung capacity; the total lung volume would then amount to about 5.7 L. Table 2–2 gives the approximate distribution of this volume among the lung compartments as derived from morphometric analysis of fixed lungs. The greatest compartment is the air space, of which about two-thirds is in alveoli, and only a small fraction in conductive airways—representing the anatomic dead space.

Number and Size of Alveoli and Capillaries

Alveoli

In spite of its ability to supply the organism with enough oxygen, the lung of the newborn is structurally still immature. Besides primitive air sacs, which have often been misinterpreted as alveoli, only a fraction of the final number of alveoli is present at birth. We (P.H.B., E.R.W.) with a co-worker (1974), and Kauffman and associates (1974), had studied the postnatal development of alveoli previously, using the rat lung as a model. It could be shown that alveoli were formed by outgrowth of new, so-called secondary septa from the sides of the primary ones present at birth. This occurrence transformed the smooth-walled channels and saccules of the newborn lung into alveolar ducts and alveolar sacs. This process was followed by an important remodeling of the septal structure. Indeed, in contrast to the

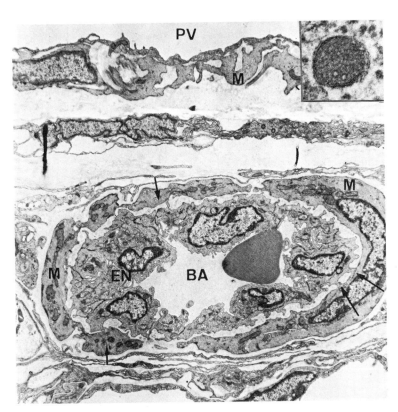

Fig. 2–15. Bronchial arteriole (BA) in semi-contracted state with thick endothelium (EN), and simple layer of smooth muscle cells (M). Note numerous contacts between endothelial and muscle cells (arrows). At top, section of wall of small pulmonary vein (PV) with loose smooth muscle layer (M) and endothelium. ×4850. Inset shows sample of specific endothelial organelles (also called Weibel-Palade bodies) at higher power. Note membrane and internal tubules. ×83,200.

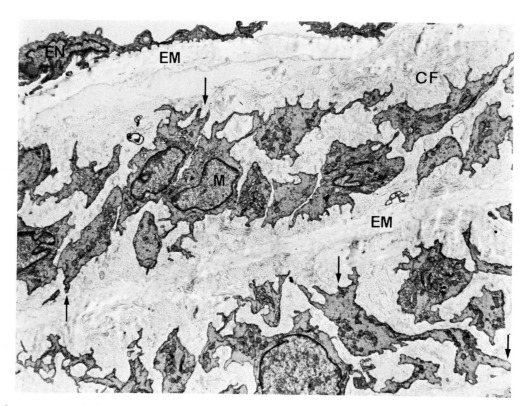

Fig. 2–16. Electron micrograph of pulmonary artery of elastic type. Note three strong elastic membranes (EM) paralleling the endothelium (EN), and ramified smooth muscle cells (M), which take an oblique course reaching from one elastic membrane to the next (arrows). Direction of muscle fibers alternates from one layer to the next. Collagen fibrils (CF) are abundant and mixed with elastic fibers. ×4850.

mature septum containing a single capillary network interlaced with a fibrous skeleton, the primary and secondary septa presented a three-layered structure: a capillary network was found on both sides of a thick central sheet of connective tissue. The restructuring now consisted in a massive reduction of the interstitial tissue, probably accompanied by fusions of capillary segments. Zeltner and co-workers and Zeltner and I (P.H.B.) (1987) obtained similar findings in studies on human lung growth. At about 1 month of age, a human lung compared well structurally with a 1-week-old rat lung. Although alveolar formation in man starts during late fetal life,

according to Langston and co-workers (1984), more than 80% of all alveoli are formed postnatally. Following alveolization, the septal structure is altered much in the same way as in the rat lung: a remodeling of the parenchymal microvasculature reduced the double capillary network to a single one. Figure 2–17 summarizes the findings of these studies and proposes a new staging and timing of lung development and growth. It appears that alveolization proceeds at a faster pace than assumed so far: bulk alveolar formation seems to be terminated at about 1½ years of age. It is further accompanied and followed, respectively, by a stage of microvascular mat-

Table 2–2. Approximate Distribution of Total Lung Volume in Milliliters for Adult Human Lung at Three-Fourths Total Lung Capacity*

Zones	Compartments			
	Air Channels	Tissue	Blood	
Conducting	Bronchi 170	Walls Septa	Arteries 150	Veins 150
Transition	Respiratory bronchioles Alv. ducts 1500	Fibers Lymph 200	Arterioles 60	Venules 60
Respiratory	Alveoli 3150	Barrier 150	Capillaries 140	

*Total lung volume = 5.7 liters.

Reproduced with permission from Weibel, E.R.: Normal Values for Respiratory Function in Man. Edited by P. Arcangeli et al. Milano, Panminerva Medica, 1970, p. 242.

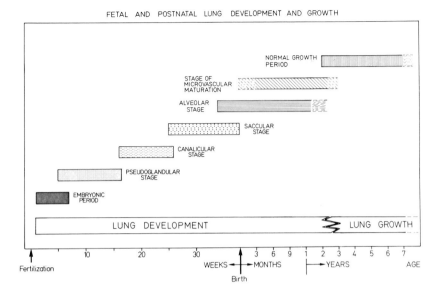

FETAL AND POSTNATAL LUNG DEVELOPMENT AND GROWTH

Fig. 2–17. Stages and timing of human lung development. Open-ended bars indicate that exact start and end of the stages are still unknown. (Reproduced with permission from Zeltner, T.B. and Burri, P.H.: The postnatal development and growth of the human lung. II. Morphology. Respir. Physiol., 67:269, 1987.)

uration lasting from a few months after birth to the age of 2 or 3 years. I (E.R.W.) (1963) found that in the adult the number of alveoli averages 300 million. According to Angus and Thurlbeck (1972), the number is related to body length and varies largely between 200 and 600 million.

For a lung of an adult inflated to three fourths of its maximal volume, I (E.R.W.) (1963) found that the average alveolar diameter lies between 250 and 290 μm. However, Glazier and his associates (1967) demonstrated, on dog lungs, that alveolar size is not identical in all parts of the lung, but that in an erect lung the upper parts contain larger alveoli than the dependent parts, owing to the weight of the lung tissue.

Capillaries

As shown previously, capillaries form a dense network spreading over the surface of alveoli (Fig. 2–7). On the average, this network is made up of hexagonal meshes, which means that usually three capillary segments are connected to each other at a junction point. The capillary network seems to be continuous over many interalveolar facets, perhaps even over a whole lobule or more. The number of small capillary segments in the adult human lung is of the order of 300×10^9. I (E.R.W.) (1963) noted that this figure implies that each alveolus is surrounded by a network composed of 1800 to 2000 capillary segments. In an electron microscopic morphometric analysis of eight normal human lungs by Gehr and co-workers (1978a), the total capillary volume was found to vary between 125 and 387 ml—mean 213 ml—and the capillary surface area from 74 to 189 m²—mean 126 m². During lung growth, capillary volume showed the steepest increase among all the parameters relevant for gas exchange. During the first 6 months, capillaries held only 22% of the volume of the interalveolar septa, while this

value reached 42% in adult lungs according to Zeltner and co-workers (1987).

The Gas Exchange Surface and the Air-Blood Barrier

The alveolocapillary air-blood barrier is composed of a surface-lining layer, epithelium, interstitium, and endothelium that have to be crossed by the oxygen molecules on their way from air to blood. As it will be developed, the following dimensions of this barrier are of greatest importance for gas exchange: first, the surface area of air-tissue interface; second, the surface area of tissue-blood interface; and third, the thickness of the barrier and of its components.

The alveolar surface area of the adult human lung has been found to vary between 97 and 194 m²—mean 143 m².

This range is in contrast to previously published results, where, by light microscopic morphometry, values between 70 and 80 m² had been obtained. This discrepancy is due to the higher resolution of the electron microscope, which allows one to measure the complex free surface of the epithelial cells. With the light microscope one could analyze only a smoothed surface of the alveolar wall.

In most species investigated, the total capillary surface area did not differ from the alveolar surface area by more than 10 to 12%: In the rat lung the capillary-to-alveolar surface ratio is 1.05 to 1.1, which means that the capillary surface area of the rat lung is 5 to 10% higher than the alveolar surface. In the human and in the dog lung, where the capillaries are less dense, the quotient is about 0.88.

Thickness and Composition of the Alveolocapillary Barrier

From Figure 2–8 it is evident that the width of the alveolocapillary barrier can vary from about 0.3 to several microns. The thickness of this tissue barrier is important because it determines, together with other parameters, the diffusion resistance of the barrier that oxygen molecules moving from the alveolus to the capillary must overcome. This resistance is very low in thin and higher in thick parts, so that the flux of gas at each point is inversely proportional to local barrier thickness. Hence, the thin parts of the barrier contribute most to gas exchange. In estimating an overall average thickness, this factor is best taken into account by determining the harmonic mean thickness of the air-blood barrier, that is, the average of the reciprocal value of thickness, rather than the arithmetic mean, which estimates the tissue mass building the barrier. The arithmetic and harmonic mean thickness vary relatively little in various mammalian species. It appears that on the average the harmonic mean thickness is about one-third of the arithmetic mean thickness. Estimates on human lungs give values of about 0.6 μm for the harmonic mean barrier thickness, whereas the arithmetic mean thickness lies around 2 μm.

Morphometric Estimation of Diffusing Capacity

The term "diffusing capacity of the lung"—D_L—has been introduced by physiologists, as noted by Forster (1964), to estimate the conductance of the pulmonary gas exchange apparatus for gaseous diffusions between alveolar air and capillary blood. The physiologic definition uses Ohm's law and states that, for oxygen,

$$D_{L_{O_2}} = \dot{V}_{O_2}/\Delta P_{O_2}$$

where $\dot{V}_{O_2}$ is the O_2 uptake and ΔP_{O_2} the mean gradient of O_2 partial pressure between alveoli and capillaries.

It is implicit in the definition that a major part of D_L is determined by structural properties of the lung, mainly by the available gas exchange surfaces, by the thickness of the air-blood barrier, and by the capillary blood volume. I (E.R.W.) (1970/71) noted that refinements in morphometric methods have made it possible to estimate D_L from measurements of lung structure performed on electron micrographs. To this end, the air-hemoglobin barrier must be subdivided into three partial resistances—or conductances, that is, the reciprocal of the resistances—which are arranged in series, as shown in Figure 2–18. We then find D_L from the sum of the partial resistances

$$\frac{1}{D_L} = \frac{1}{D_t} + \frac{1}{D_p} + \frac{1}{D_e}$$

whereby D_t, D_p, and D_e are the diffusion conductances in tissue, plasma, and erythrocytes, respectively. D_L can be calculated if we measure the alveolar and capillary

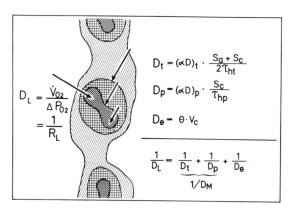

Fig. 2–18. Model for estimating pulmonary diffusing capacity from physiologic (left) and morphometric information (right).

surface areas, S_a and S_c, the capillary volume V_c, and the harmonic mean thicknesses τ_h of tissue—t—and plasma—p. In addition, we need to know appropriate values for the physical coefficients of permeability—αD—and of the rate of O_2 binding by the blood—θ.

Table 2–3 presents the results obtained by Gehr and associates (1978a) in a morphometric study of adult human lungs. Using "most reasonable" estimates of the physical coefficients I (E.R.W.) (1984) found $D_{L_{O_2}}$ to amount to about 205 ml O_2/min/mm Hg.

For comparison, the currently available or accepted physiologic values of D_L at rest amount to about 30 ml O_2/min/mm Hg. This value is hence far below the morphometric estimates. Here it should be noted that two different things are measured: morphometry estimates the size of the gas exchange apparatus that is maximally available for gas exchange. Its values refer to a fully expanded lung. This can lead to an overestimation of D_L by as much as 25 to 50% because I (J.G.) and associates (1979) showed that in lungs inflated with air and fixed by vascular perfusion, parts of the diffusion barrier are folded away from the surface even at highest inflation and thus do not contribute to gas exchange. Furthermore we suppose that a gradient from air to blood exists at every point along the alveolar capillary. Under resting conditions, this is most certainly not the case; in fact, it is probable that the capillary blood is saturated before it leaves the capillary, as Karas and associates (1987) showed for the lungs of animals performing heavy exercise. We would therefore expect that the physiologic estimates of D_L at rest should amount to only 20 to 40%

Table 2–3. Basic Morphometric Parameters and Diffusing Capacity in Human Lung

Weight	74	kg
Alveolar surface	143	m²
Capillary surface	126	m²
Capillary volume	213	ml
Tissue barrier	0.62	μm
Plasma barrier	0.15	μm
$D_{L_{O_2}}$	205	ml O_2 / min/mm Hg

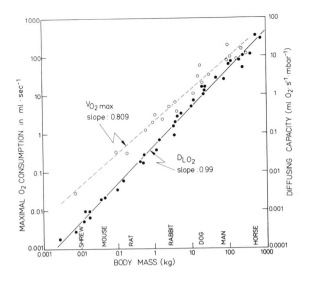

Fig. 2–19. The pulmonary diffusing capacity (full dots) and maximal O_2 consumption (open circles) scale with body mass at a different slope on a double-logarithmic plot. (Reproduced with permission from Weibel, E.R.: The Pathway for Oxygen. Cambridge MA, Harvard University Press, 1984.)

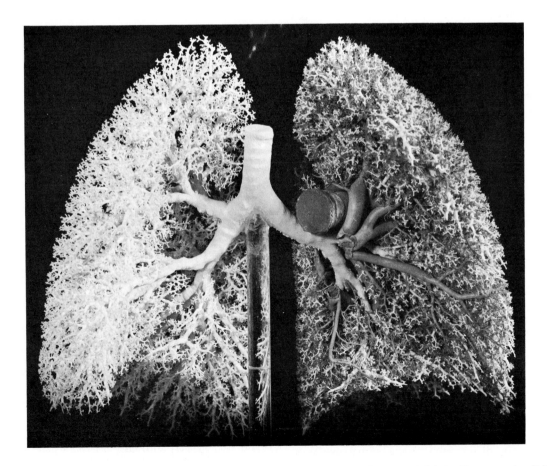

Fig. 2–20. Cast of human lung, showing airways in right lung and pulmonary arteries and veins in left lung. Note irregular dichotomy of all branches.

of the maximal or "true" diffusing capacity. That this reasoning is probably correct is shown by the findings of Bitterli and co-workers (1971) in man that, in exercise, physiologic estimates may yield values of DL between 70 and 100 ml O_2/min/mm Hg. The morphometric estimate of pulmonary diffusing capacity in man is therefore about two times larger than the physiologic estimate. I (E.R.W.) and my colleagues (1983) confirmed this difference by direct measurement of the physiologic and morphometric values of DL in animals. We concluded from this that the lung provides a gas exchange apparatus that is large enough to allow O_2 to diffuse to the blood in sufficient quantity when O_2 consumption is elevated owing to work. Destruction of lung tissue, as occurs in emphysema, would tend to reduce the "true" diffusing capacity by reduction of the gas exchange surfaces and, possibly, by thickening of the barrier.

Figure 2–19 shows the results of a comparative study of DL in mammalian species ranging from the smallest mammal, the Etruscan shrew, weighing only 2 g, to the horse. It is apparent that DL is directly related to body mass; in contrast, maximal O_2 consumption—$\dot{V}O_2$ mass— varies with the 0.8 power of body mass. Consequently, the lung's capacity for O_2 uptake is not matched to the body's need for O_2 when one compares animals of different body size.

On the other hand, the lung can respond to increased O_2 demands, or to reduced environmental O_2 at high altitude, by enlarging the pulmonary diffusing capacity, as we (P.H.B. and E.R.W.) (1971) and Hugonnaud (1977) and Gehr (1978b) and their associates showed. I (E.R.W.) (1987) and my colleagues found that athletic animals, such as dogs or horses, have a larger diffusing capacity than animals of the same size but lower O_2 needs. The question of how the lung's morphometric properties are related to the body's O_2 needs is still a matter of scientific debate, as I (E.R.W.) (1984) and Taylor and co-workers (1987) noted.

Morphometry of Conducting and Transitory Airways and Blood Vessels

Figure 2–20 shows a plastic cast of a human lung; in the right lung only the airways have been modeled, whereas, in the left lung, pulmonary arteries and veins have also been demonstrated. It is apparent, that the airways branch toward the periphery by systematically dividing in two, that is, by dichotomy. This dichotomy is, however, not regular; the two branches arising from a parent branch may differ considerably in both length and diameter. This is called irregular dichotomy. Figure 2–21 shows a similar cast of an acinus from a human lung in which the casting material, silicon rubber, has filled the airways out to the most peripheral alveoli. On such preparations Haefeli-Bleuer and I (E.R.W.) (1987) showed that the most peripheral airways, the respiratory bronchioles and alveolar ducts, also branch by irregular dichotomy.

The pattern of dichotomous branching provides a scheme with respect to which the systematic progression of the increase in the number of branches and of the

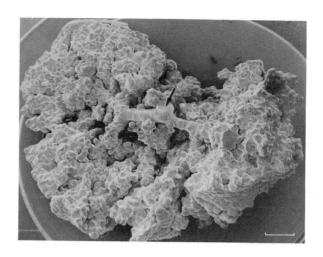

Fig. 2–21. Silicon rubber cast of a human pulmonary acinus shown in a scanning electron micrograph. Part of the alveolar ducts have been trimmed off to show the transitional bronchiole (arrow) and the first few orders of respiratory bronchioles. Note that alveolar ducts and sacs are densely covered by alveoli. Scale marker 1 mm.

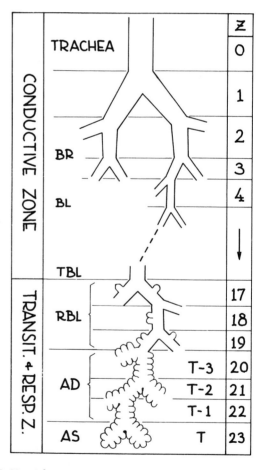

Fig. 2–22. Schematic representation of sequence of airway branches as function of generation z. Bronchi (BR), bronchioles (BL), terminal (TBL) and respiratory (RBL) bronchioles are followed by alveolar ducts (AD) and sacs (AS) in the terminal generation T = 23. (Reproduced with permission from Weibel, E.R.: Morphometry of the Human Lung. Heidelberg, Springer-Verlag, 1963, p. 111.)

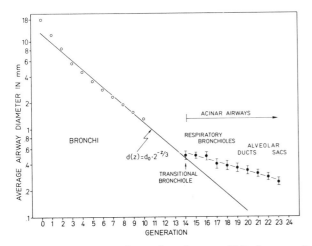

Fig. 2–23. Progressive reduction by cube root of 1/2 of average diameter of conducting airways in regularized dichotomy model contrasts with slow decrease of diameter of acinar airways with progressive generations of branching. Compare text. (Reproduced with permission from Haefeli-Bleuer, B., and Weibel, E.R.: Morphometry of the human pulmonary acinus. Anat. Rec., *220*:401, 1988.

reduction in dimensions can be described. If we first disregard the irregularities, we can estimate the average number of generations necessary to provide a sufficient number of terminal airway channels to carry alveoli for gas exchange, namely, alveolar ducts and sacs. I (E.R.W.) (1963) and Haefeli-Bleuer and I (E.R.W.) (1987) estimated this average number of generations at 23. Figure 2–22 shows in schematic form that the first 16 generations are purely conducting airways, leading from the trachea to the terminal bronchioles. From generation 17 on, alveoli are progressively incorporated into the airway wall until, in the twentieth generation, the entire wall is occupied by them. On the basis of more recent information the transition from terminal to alveolated bronchioles may occur at generation 14, so that a total of nine generations carry alveoli. It must be stressed that these are average values and that, because of the irregularity, airways will terminate in alveolar sacs anywhere from about generations 15 to 30.

This irregularity becomes apparent if length and diameter of the bronchial branches are measured on casts. Nevertheless, average dimensions can be calculated from these size distributions. If the average diameters—d—are plotted semilogarithmically against generations—z (Fig. 2–23), we find them to follow an exponential function, namely,

$$d(z) = d_o \cdot 2^{-z/3}$$

This means that with each generation the average airway diameter is reduced by $\sqrt[3]{1/2}$—which, as pointed out by Thompson (1942), is known in hydrodynamics to be a function of optimal size relationship between parent and daughter branches. But Figure 2–23 also reveals that the diameters of peripheral or transitory airways that are provided with alveoli do not fit on this function; they are considerably larger than one would expect from their position in the bronchial tree. This difference can be

explained by their different roles in conveying oxygen from ambient air to alveoli. In conducting airways, air is transported en masse; that is, a solution of O_2 in nitrogen is flowing through the tubes, and hydrodynamic principles prevail. Toward the periphery, however, O_2 molecules will have to advance toward the alveolar surface by diffusion in the gas phase—and this, as emphasized by Gomez (1965), requires a greater cross-sectional area of the peripheral airways.

From this detailed information, we can construct a first model of the lung that may be useful for some general considerations on structure-function relationship in the airway system. The model assumes regular dichotomy over 23 generations. Its most pertinent dimensional properties are given in Table 2–4. It may be noted that the anatomic dead space of 150 ml, as estimated by physiologic methods, is reached at about generation 16, which corresponds to terminal bronchioles.

Irregular dichotomous models can also be constructed. Figure 2–24 reveals the numbers of generations necessary to arrive at airways of 2-mm diameter, as well as the distribution of distances from these branches to the trachea; these branches were located between generations 4 and 13 and at 18 to 31 cm from the root of the trachea. Each of these about 400 branches of 2-mm diameter leads through an average of 14 subsequent branchings until alveolar sacs are reached. The units of lung tissue that they supply have a volume of some 12 ml and contain approximately 740,000 alveoli each. This consideration of irregularity can be carried further, but one should refer to the original publications by me (E.R.W.) (1963) and Haefeli-Bleuer and me (E.R.W.) (1987) for additional information.

The blood vessels undergo, in principle, the same sequence of branching as the airways, with some differences in detail. Pulmonary arteries are topographically very closely associated with the airways (Fig. 2–20); down to the respiratory bronchioles their branching would therefore seem to parallel that of the airways, but this is only partially true. It is well known that relatively large pulmonary arteries may send smaller branches to the capillary network of adjacent groups of alveoli. These "accessory" branches are called supernumerary arteries and cause, on the one hand, a more rapid progression of arterial branching and, on the other, a greater irregularity in the arterial dimensions per generation.

At present, no extensive data on the morphometry of the pulmonary vascular tree are available. A preliminary model can be derived by comparing pulmonary arteries with airways and by determining the average generation number of dichotomous branching. The larger branches of the pulmonary artery, perhaps down to 2-mm diameter and reaching to the eighth generation on the average, have dimensions closely approximating those of the accompanying bronchi. In a first approximation, we may therefore use the measurements obtained on the bronchial tree to describe the major pulmonary arterial tree. We would therefore claim that these branches reduce their dimension with each generation to obey the

Table 2–4.   Dimensions of Human Airway Model (Average Adult Lung with Volume 4800 ml at about Three-fourths Maximal Inflation)

Generation z	Number per Generation $n(z)$	Diameter $d(z)$ cm	Length $l(z)$ cm	Total Cross Section $A(z)$ cm²	Total Volume $V(z)$ cm³	Accumul. Volume $\sum_{i=0}^{z} V(i)$ cm³
0	1	1.8	12.0	2.54	30.50	30.5
1	2	1.22	4.76	2.33	11.25	41.8
2	4	0.83	1.90	2.13	3.97	45.8
3	8	0.56	0.76	2.00	1.52	47.2
4	16	0.45	1.27	2.48	3.46	50.7
5	32	0.35	1.07	3.11	3.30	54.0
6	64	0.28	0.90	3.96	3.53	57.5
7	128	0.23	0.76	5.10	3.85	61.4
8	256	0.186	0.64	6.95	4.45	65.8
9	512	0.154	0.54	9.56	5.17	71.0
10	1024	0.130	0.46	13.4	6.21	77.2
11	2048	0.109	0.39	19.6	7.56	84.8
12	4096	0.095	0.33	28.8	9.82	94.6
13	8192	0.082	0.27	44.5	12.45	106.0
14	16384	0.074	0.23	69.4	16.40	123.4
15	32768	0.066	0.20	113.0	21.70	145.1
16	65536	0.060	0.165	180.0	29.70	174.8
17	131072	0.054	0.141	300.0	41.80	216.6
18	262144	0.050	0.117	534.0	61.10	277.7
19	524288	0.047	0.099	944.0	93.20	370.9
20	1048576	0.045	0.083	1600.0	139.50	510.4
21	2097152	0.043	0.070	3220.0	224.30	734.7
22	4194304	0.041	0.059	5880.0	350.00	1084.7
23*	8388608	0.041	0.050*	11800.0	591.00	1675.0

*Adjusted for complete generation.

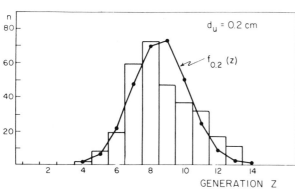

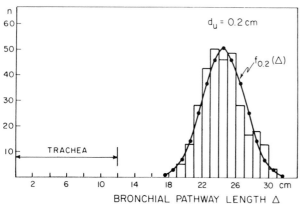

Fig. 2–24.   Distribution of airways of 2-mm diameter with respect to generation z and distance from larynx Δ. (Modified with permission from Weibel, E.R.: Morphometry of the Human Lung. Heidelberg, Springer-Verlag, 1963, p. 126.)

hydrodynamic law of optimal size reduction described previously (Fig. 2–23). Next we may determine the total number of precapillaries, that is, of the terminal arterial branches that lead into the capillary network, and calculate from that the average generation number of dichotomous branching needed to reach this number; I (E.R.W.) and Gomez (1962) found this to be of the order of 28 generations, hence about five generations more than the airways. The diameter of these precapillaries is between 20 and 30 μm; if this range is plotted on Figure 2–23, it is noted that it falls on the function for dimensional reduction by $\sqrt[3]{\frac{1}{2}}$ fitted to the major branches. This suggests that the pulmonary arterial tree reduces the dimension of its branches progressively following a hydrodynamic law for optimal reduction of diameters in a dichotomous branching system all the way out to the terminal branches. This seems logical, as there is mass flow of blood throughout, the diffusion of gases in the blood phase playing a negligible role for transport along the vessel axis. All this is highly conjectural as long as it is not substantiated by more extensive actual measurement.

REFERENCES

Angus, G.E., and Thurlbeck, W.M.: Number of alveoli in the human lung. J. Appl. Physiol. 32:483, 1972.

Bitterli, J., et al.: Repeated measurements of pulmonary O_2 diffusing capacity in man during graded exercise. In Pulmonary Diffusing Capacity on Exercise. Edited by M. Scherrer. Stuttgart, H. Huber, 1971, p. 139.

Breeze, R.G., and Wheeldon, E.G.: The cells of the pulmonary airways. Am. Rev. Respir. Dis. 116:705, 1977.

Burri, P.H.: The postnatal growth of the rat lung. III. Morphology. Anat. Rec. 180:77, 1974.

Burri, P.H., and Weibel, E.R.: Beeinflussung einer spezifischen cytoplasmatischen Organelle von Endothelzellen durch Adrenalin. Z. Zellforsch, 88:426, 1968.

Burri, P.H., and Weibel, E.R.: Morphometric estimation of pulmonary diffusion capacity. II. Effect of P_{O_2} on the growing lung. Respir. Physiol. 11:247, 1971.

Burri, P.H., Dbaly, J., and Weibel, E.R.: The postnatal growth of the rat lung. I. Morphometry. Anat. Rec. 178:711, 1974.

Crapo, J.D., et al.: Cell numbers and cell characteristics of the normal human lung. Am. Rev. Respir. Dis. 125:332, 1982.

Forster, R.E.: Diffusion of gases. In Handbook of Physiology, Section 3, Respiration, Vol. I. Edited by W.O. Fenn and H. Rahn. Washington, D.C. American Physiological Society, 1964, p. 839.

Gehr, P., Bachofen, H., and Weibel, E.R.: The normal human lung: ultrastructure and morphometric estimation of diffusion capacity. Respir. Physiol. 32:121, 1978a.

Gehr, P., et al.: Adaptation of the growing lung to increase $\dot{V}_{O_2}$: III. The effect of exposure to cold environment in rats. Respir. Physiol. 32:345, 1978b.

Gil, J., and Reiss, O.K.: Isolation and characterization of lamellar bodies and tubular myelin from rat lung homogenates. J. Cell Biol. 58:152, 1973.

Gil, J., and Weibel, E.R.: Improvements in demonstration of lining layer of lung alveoli by electron microscopy. Respir. Physiol. 8:13, 1969/70.

Gil, J., and Weibel, E.R.: Extracellular lining of bronchioles after perfusion-fixation of rat lungs for electron microscopy. Anat. Rec. 169:185, 1971.

Gil, J., et al.: The alveolar volume to surface area relationship in air and saline filled lungs fixed by vascular perfusion. J. Appl. Physiol. 47:990, 1979.

Glazier, J.B., et al.: Vertical gradient of alveolar size in lungs of dogs frozen intact. J. Appl. Physiol. 23:694, 1967.

Gomez, D.M.: A physico-mathematical study of lung function in normal subjects and in patients with obstructive pulmonary diseases. Med. Thorac. 22:275, 1965.

Haefeli-Bleuer, B., and Weibel, E.R.: Morphometry of the human pulmonary acinus. Anat. Rec. 220:401, 1988.

Hugonnaud, C., et al.: Adaptation of the growing lung to increased oxygen consumption. II. Morphometric analysis. Respir. Physiol. 29:1, 1977.

Jeffery, P.K.: Morphologic features of airway surface epithelial cells and glands. Am. Rev. Respir. Dis. 128:14S, 1983.

Jeffery, P.K., and Reid, L.M.: The respiratory mucous membrane. In Respiratory Defense Mechanisms, Part I. Edited by J.D. Brain, D.F. Proctor, and L.M. Reid. New York, Marcel Dekker, 1977.

Kapanci, Y.: Location and function of contractile interstitial cells of the lungs. In Lung Cells in Disease. Edited by A. Bonhuys. New York, Elsevier North-Holland, 1976, p. 69.

Kapanci, Y., et al.: "Contractile interstitial cells" in pulmonary alveolar septa. J. Cell Biol. 60:375, 1974.

Karas, R.H., et al.: Adaptive variation in the mammalian respiratory system in relation to energetic demand. VII. Flow of oxygen across the pulmonary gas exchanger. Respir. Physiol. 69:101, 1987.

Kauffman, S.L., Burri, P.H., and Weibel, E.R.: The postnatal growth of the rat lung. II. Autoradiography. Anat. Rec. 180:63, 1974.

Langston, C., et al.: Human lung growth in late gestation and in the neonate. Am. Rev. Respir. Dis. 129:607, 1984.

Lauweryns, J.M., and Cokelaere, M.: Hypoxia sensitive neuroepithelial bodies. Intrapulmonary secretory neuroreceptors modulated by the CNS. Z. Zellforsch. 145:521, 1973.

Low, F.N.: Electron microscopy of the rat lung. Anat. Rec. 113:437, 1952.

Maksvytis, H.J., et al.: In vitro characteristics of the lipid-filled interstitial cell associated with postnatal lung growth: evidence for fibroblast heterogeneity. J. Cell. Physiol. 118:113, 1984.

Meyrick, B., and Reid, L.: The alveolar brush cell in rat lung: a third pneumocyte. J. Ultrastruct. Res. 23:71, 1968.

St. George, J.A., et al.: An immunohistochemical characterization of Rhesus monkey respiratory secretions using monoclonal antibodies. Am. Rev. Respir. Dis. 132:556, 1985.

Schneeberger, E.E.: Barrier function of intercellular junctions in adult and fetal lungs. In Pulmonary Edema. Edited by A.P. Fishman and E.M. Renkin. Bethesda, American Physiological Society, 1979.

Sorkin, S.P., et al.: Comparative biology of small granule cells and neuroepithelial bodies in the respiratory system: short review. Am. Rev. Respir. Dis. 128:26S, 1983.

Spicer, S.S., et al.: Histochemical properties of the respiratory tract epithelium in different species. Am. Rev. Respir. Dis. 128:20S, 1983.

Taylor, C.R., et al.: Adaptive variation in the mammalian respiratory system in relation to energetic demand. VIII. Structural and functional limits to oxidative metabolism. Respir. Physiol. 69:117, 1987.

Thompson, D'Arcy W.: Growth and Form. New York, Cambridge University Press, 1942, p. 448.

Von Neergaard, K.: Neue Auffassungen über einen Grundbegriff der Atemmechanik. Die Retraktionskraft der Lunge, abhängig von der Oberflächenspannung in den Alveolen. Z. Gesamte Exp. Med. 66:373, 1929.

Wagner, D.D., Olmsted, J.B., and Marder, V.J.: Immunolocalization of von Willebrand protein in Weibel-Palade bodies of human endothelial cells. J. Cell Biol. 95:355, 1982.

Warhol, M.J., and Sweet, J.M.: The ultrastructural localization of von Willebrand factor in endothelial cells. Am. J. Pathol. 117:310, 1984.

Weibel, E.R.: Die Blutgefässanastomosen in der menschlichen Lunge. Z. Zellforsch. 50:653, 1959.

Weibel, E.R.: Morphometry of the Human Lung. Heidelberg, Springer-Verlag, 1963.

Weibel, E.R.: Morphometric estimation of pulmonary diffusion capacity. I. Model and method. Respir. Physiol. 11:54, 1970/71.

Weibel, E.R.: The Pathway for Oxygen: Structure and Function in the Mammalian Respiratory System. Cambridge MA, Harvard University Press, 1984, pp. 1–425.

Weibel, E.R.: Lung cell biology. In Handbook of Physiology. Section

3, The Respiratory System, Vol. I. Edited by A.P. Fishman and A.B. Fisher. Bethesda, American Physiological Society, 1985, p. 47.

Weibel, E.R., and Bachofen, H.: Structural design of the alveolar septum and fluid exchange. *In* Pulmonary Edema. Edited by A.P. Fishman and E.M. Renkin. Bethesda, American Physiological Society, 1979.

Weibel, E.R., and Gil, J.: Structure function relationship at the alveolar level. *In* Bioengineering Aspects of the Lung. Edited by J.G. West. New York, Marcel Dekker, 1977.

Weibel, E.R., and Gomez, D.M.: Architecture of the human lung. Science 137:577, 1962.

Weibel, E.R., and Palade, G.E.: New cytoplasmic components in arterial endothelia. J. Cell Biol. 23:101, 1964.

Weibel, E.R., et al.: Maximal oxygen consumption and pulmonary diffusing capacity: a direct comparison of physiologic morphometric measurements in canids. Respir. Physiol. 54:173, 1983.

Weibel, E.R., et al.: Adaptive variation in the mammalian respiratory system in relation to energetic demand. VI. The pulmonary gas exchanger. Respir. Physiol. 69:81, 1987.

Zeltner, T.B., and Burri, P.H.: The postnatal development and growth of the human lung. II. Morphology. Respir. Physiol. 67:269, 1987.

Zeltner, T.B., et al.: The postnatal development and growth of the human lung. I. Morphometry. Respir. Physiol. 67:247, 1987.

READING REFERENCES

Ballard, P.L.: Hormones and Lung Maturation. Berlin, Springer-Verlag, 1986.

Burri, P.H.: Development and growth of the human lung. *In* Handbook of Physiology, Section 3, The Respiratory System, Vol. I. Edited by A.P. Fishman and A.B. Fisher. Bethesda, American Physiological Society, 1985, p. 1.

Murray, J.F.: The Normal Lung, 2nd Ed. Philadelphia, W.B. Saunders Co., 1986.

Scarpelli, E.M., and Mantone, A.J.: The pulmonary surfactant system. *In* Pulmonary Surfactant. Edited by B. Robertson, L.M.G. van Golde and J.J. Batenburg. Amsterdam, Elsevier Science Publishers, 1984; p. 119.

Von Hayek, H.: Die menschliche Lunge. 2. Auflage. Heidelberg, Springer-Verlag, 1970.

Weibel, E.R.: The Pathway for Oxygen: Structure and Function in the Mammalian Respiratory System. Cambridge MA, Harvard University Press, 1984, pp. 1–425.

Weibel, E.R.: Lung cell biology. *In* Handbook of Physiology, Section 3, The Respiratory System, Vol. I. Edited by A.P. Fishman and A.B. Fisher. Bethesda, American Physiological Society, 1985, p. 47.

Weibel, E.R.: Functional morphology of lung parenchyma. *In* Handbook of Physiology, Section 3, The Respiratory System, Vol. III. Part 1. Edited by P.T. Macklem and J. Mead. Bethesda, American Physiological Society, Bethesda, 1986; p. 89.

CHAPTER 3

ANATOMY OF THE THORAX AND PLEURA

Charles E. Blevins

The thorax is a flexible, airtight cage whose framework comprises the most continuously active combination of skeletal, muscular, and articulating tissues in the body. Its primary function is to produce movements responsible for ventilation of the lungs. It also affords protection for thoracic viscera and support for the upper extremities, but such responsibilities are secondary to the vital function of producing the alternating changes in pressure required for inflation and deflation of the lungs. Such pressure changes must be orderly, well-coordinated, and accompanied by close compliance of the lungs with changes in thoracic dimensions. The volume and rate of air movement must be compatible with vital needs for oxygen under a variety of conditions. To meet such requirements a uniquely functional anatomic apparatus is required.

RESPIRATORY MOVEMENTS

Movements of the thorax are the result of both active and passive events. During inspiration the thorax is actively enlarged by coordinated muscle contractions. As a direct result of increased thoracic dimensions, intrathoracic, intrapleural, and intrapulmonic pressures are sequentially reduced so that atmospheric air is forced into the lungs. Expiration is a passive event, largely owing to the relaxation of forces generated during inspiration. It is marked by the return of thoracic dimensions to resting levels, and by increased pressure within the chest, pleural cavities, and lungs. Muscle activity may facilitate the expiratory phase of breathing, but it is not essential.

Inspiratory movements enlarge the thorax in all dimensions. They are a blend of efforts directed in the anteroposterior, bilateral, and supero-inferior axes. Increase in anteroposterior dimensions is marked by forward and upward movement of the lower part of the sternum, which is called the "pump-handle" movement. The sternum is more firmly anchored at its upper extent by relatively short ribs and costal cartilages than at its lower limits where both ribs and cartilages are longer.

Since the points of pivot of the ribs are located at their vertebral articulations, elevation of the ribs lifts the body of the sternum outward and forward. The greatest excursion occurs at the level of the longest ribs, that is, ribs five to seven. The axis for such movement is on a line drawn through the head, neck, and tubercle of each rib (Fig. 3–1).

During normal quiet respiration the ribs are elevated by contraction of the intercostal muscles. Taylor (1960) and Campbell (1955) reported that the scalene muscles also aid in elevation in some individuals. Jones and associates (1953) reported that the effect of muscles within

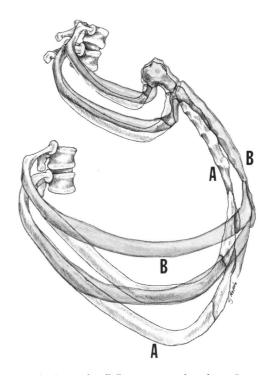

Fig. 3–1. The "pump-handle" movement in breathing. Compare position of sternum and ribs at the beginning (A) and the end (B) of inspiration. Note the increase in anteroposterior dimensions.

39

individual intercostal spaces is apparently small, but synchronous contraction of all intercostal muscles is sufficient to elevate the rib cage as a unit. The resultant increase in anteroposterior dimension is greatest at the level of ribs five to seven (Fig. 3–1).

Increase in bilateral dimensions is marked by upward and lateral excursion in the vicinity of the midaxillary line. The greatest degree of movement is noted in ribs seven to ten, whose costal cartilages descend and then ascend before articulation with the sternum. Since the middle of each rib-cartilage unit is lower than either costovertebral or costosternal articulations, elevation swings each unit upward and laterally much like the action of lifting a bucket handle upward toward the middle of its arc of swing (Fig. 3–2). This action is accomplished by contraction of intercostal muscles also, but Cherniack and Cherniack (1961) suggested that it is facilitated by muscle fibers of the diaphragm that are perpendicular to the costal margin.

The greatest increase in thoracic dimensions during inspiration is in the supero-inferior dimensions. It is accomplished by contraction of the diaphragm, which is generally described as "dome-shaped." The dome, however, is uneven; its anterolateral attachments are at higher levels than its posterolateral attachments. Fur-

thermore it is indented by the heart and may present two domes, one related to the liver and one related to the stomach and spleen. Contraction of the majority of its muscle fibers flattens the diaphragm against the abdominal viscera thereby increasing vertical intrathoracic dimensions. Contraction of its peripheral or costal muscle fibers may also produce an outward flaring of the lowest costal margin. During quiet respiration the diaphragm undergoes an excursion of about 1 to 2 cm, but it may move as much as 6 to 7 cm during deep breathing. The lower ribs are believed to be helpful in resisting upward and medial pull of the diaphragm as a result of stabilization by the serratus posterior inferior muscles. The quadratus lumborum may stabilize the twelfth rib, but its effect on respiration is probably insignificant.

The diaphragm and intercostal muscles are therefore the primary muscles of inspiration. Movements of the diaphragm account for 75 to 80% of pulmonary ventilation during quiet respiration compared to 20 to 25% contributed by the intercostal muscles—mainly the external intercostals and the anterior portions of the internal intercostals. During severe or labored breathing, however, other skeletal muscles may be utilized. The sternocleidomastoid, serratus posterior superior, and levatores costarum may be active in elevation of the ribs. Muscles of the extremities may also be helpful in moments of severe need. With the torso in fixed position, movement of the arms and shoulders away from the thorax may be sufficient to enlarge thoracic dimensions to a small but sometimes necessary degree. Deltoid, trapezius, pectoral, and latissimus dorsi muscles are involved in such activity.

Expiration can occur only when intrapulmonic pressure exceeds that of the atmosphere. At the end of inspiration, the lungs are inflated and stretched. Inspiratory muscles have reached optimal efficiency in expanding the rib cage against atmospheric pressure. At this point, elastic resistance of lung tissue is at first equal to and then greater than muscular forces that would retain the expanded state of the thorax. The lungs recoil elastically and the consequent rise in intrapulmonic pressure is sufficient to force air out of the lungs. Both soft and hard tissues of the thoracic wall comply passively with the reduction of lung volume, aided by atmospheric pressure directed against them. Expiration stops when intrapulmonic pressure is once again equal to atmospheric pressure. In quiet breathing, expiration is accomplished almost exclusively by elastic recoil of the lungs and the rib cage. However, during vigorous or carefully controlled expiration, such as while singing, shouting, abdominal straining, or playing a wind instrument, muscles of the abdominal wall may aid in the reduction of thoracic dimensions by compression of abdominal viscera against the diaphragm.

Although the change from inspiratory to expiratory efforts thus represents a shift from active to passive events, the change in airflow is not a chaotic event. Rather, it is well regulated by the diaphragm, which continues to contract with decreasing efficiency, but does not reach the zero point until the middle of expiration.

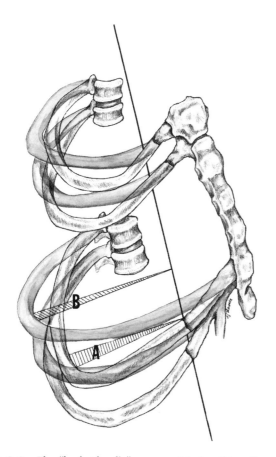

Fig. 3–2. The "bucket-handle" movement in breathing. Compare distance of the ribs from central axis of the thorax at the beginning (A) and the end (B) of inspiration. Note increase in lateral dimensions.

In this respect, it is not entirely unlike the action of limb musculature, in which gradual relaxation of flexor muscles prevents uncoordinated movement of an extremity in the opposite direction by antagonistic extensors. As described by Agostini and Torri (1962), during maximal breathing efforts the diaphragm also contracts toward the end of vigorous expiration, limiting the extent to which the lungs can collapse.

SURFACE LANDMARKS AND STRUCTURES SUPERFICIAL TO THE THORAX

The thoracic surgeon is primarily concerned with the thoracic wall and the thoracic contents. However, a few overall considerations of structures related to surface features will be helpful in orientation to deeper structures of the thorax itself (Fig. 3–3). In all but the most obese subjects, the outline of the sternum can be visualized in the thoracic midline. Extending laterally and slightly upward from the jugular notch of the sternum, the clavicles curve forward and then backward toward the shoulders. From the lowermost margin of the body of the sternum, the lower margin of the rib cage diverges bilaterally to reach its lowest level at the midaxillary line.

The outline of the sternocleidomastoid muscles may be seen extending diagonally upward from the upper part of the anterior surface of the manubrium of the sternum and the medial third of the clavicle toward the base of the skull. Immediately below the clavicle, the outline of the pectoralis major muscle is evident. These muscles extend bilaterally from broad clavicular, sternal, and costal origins, converge toward the axilla, and form a bilaminar, U-shaped tendon that attaches to the lateral lip of the intertubercular sulcus of the humerus. The lower margin of each pectoralis major muscle forms the anterior fold of the axilla. The pectoralis major muscles are supplied by medial and lateral pectoral nerves from the brachial plexus and are versatile in function. They adduct and rotate the arm medially and in addition may elevate it—clavicular portion—or depress it—sternocostal portion. If the shoulder girdle is held in fixed position, these muscles may also elevate the upper ribs in forced inspiration. During artificial respiration, pulling the flexed upper extremity toward the head may also force the pectoralis major muscles to elevate the upper ribs.

Deep to the pectoralis major muscles lie the pectoralis minor muscles. They originate by slips from the second to fifth ribs and converge upward to a tendon that inserts on the coracoid process of the scapula. Supplied also by the medial and lateral pectoral nerves, these muscles are active in depressing and rotating the shoulders downward.

In thin, muscular subjects the serratus anterior muscles can be visualized along the anterolateral aspects of the thoracic wall. They originate by slips from the upper

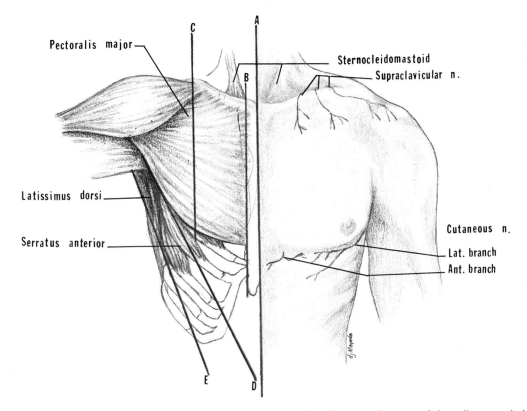

Fig. 3–3. Surface features and details of structures superficial to the thoracic wall in the pectoral region and the axilla. Musculoskeletal features are shown on the left. Surface features and cutaneous innervation are shown on the right. Cutaneous branches of the fifth intercostal space are illustrated as typical of other intercostal spaces not shown. Common lines of reference are shown. A = midsternal line; B = lateral sternal line; C = midclavicular line; D = anterior axillary fold; E = posterior axillary fold.

eight ribs. They are closely applied to the thoracic wall as they pass upward and laterally to attach to the anterior surface and medial border of the scapula on either side. They hold the scapulae toward the thoracic wall and are important in adduction and elevation of the arms above the horizontal position during scapulohumeral movement. On each side, the serratus anterior is supplied by the long thoracic nerve, which passes downward in the midaxillary line on the external surface of the muscle.

In men, the nipple lies near the lower border of the pectoralis major muscles, just lateral to the midclavicular line, over the fourth intercostal space or fourth or fifth ribs. Nipple position is inconsistent in women owing to the variable size of the mammary gland, which lies generally over the second to sixth ribs. The "axillary tail" extends upward into the axilla along the lower border of the pectoralis major muscle.

Cutaneous innervation of the anterolateral thoracic wall is supplied by supraclavicular nerves and terminal filaments of thoracic spinal nerves. Skin above, overlying, and slightly below the clavicle is supplied by supraclavicular nerves, which arise as terminal filaments of spinal nerves C3 and C4. The remainder of the thoracic wall is supplied by anterior cutaneous and lateral cutaneous branches of thoracic spinal nerves.

The posterior aspect of the thorax is almost completely covered by superficial muscles of the back, but a few bony landmarks are either visible or palpable (Fig. 3–4).

In the midline, the spinous process of the seventh cervical vertebra—vertebra prominens—stands out clearly. Below this, the spine of the first thoracic vertebra may be equally visible. Spines of the remaining 11 thoracic vertebrae extend downward so that the tip of each overlies the body of the vertebra below. In the midthoracic levels the vertebral spines may be sufficiently long to overlie the intervertebral disc below the subjacent vertebra. The medial border of each scapula lies lateral to the midline at the level of the second to seventh ribs. The spine of the scapula extends diagonally upward from the medial border at about the third thoracic vertebra to end in the acromion at the shoulder.

Surface contours of the back of the thorax are formed by muscles of the shoulder and scapular region; these muscles support and help move the upper extremity. Posterolateral margins of the neck and uppermost limits of the shoulder are marked by the trapezius muscles. Each of these arises from broad origins, including the superior nuchal line of the occipital bone, the ligamentum nuchae of the neck, the spine of the seventh cervical vertebra, and spines and supraspinous ligaments of all thoracic vertebrae. Fibers sweep downward, laterally, and upward toward the shoulder, where they insert on the spine and acromion of the scapula and on the lateral third of the clavicle. In lower cervical and upper thoracic levels, their aponeurotic origin is sufficiently devoid of muscle fibers to allow spines of thoracic vertebrae to be

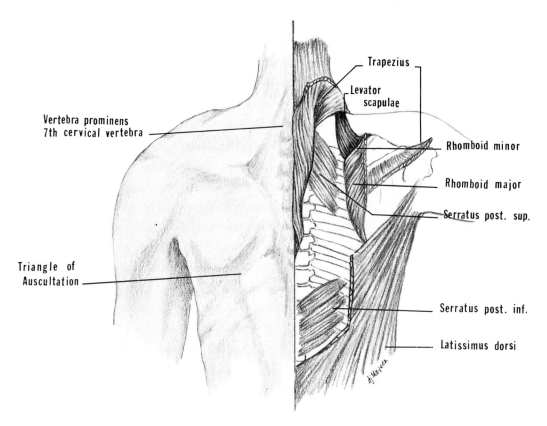

Fig. 3–4. Surface features and details of structures superficial to the posterior aspect of the thorax. The scapula has been displaced upward and laterally on the right side to permit a better view of muscles superficial to the thorax.

easily palpable. The trapezius muscles are supplied by spinal accessory nerves and by filaments from cervical spinal levels C3 and C4. They are powerful stabilizers of the scapulae and shoulders and can elevate, depress, or adduct the scapulae, thereby aiding in the entire spectrum of scapulohumeral movements.

Lower and lateral parts of the back of the thorax are covered by the latissimus dorsi muscles. These muscles arise by broad aponeurotic origins, from spines of lower thoracic vertebrae, the lumbodorsal fascia, and the iliac crests. Additional slips of muscle also arise from outer surfaces of the lower three or four ribs and blend with overlying components. Muscle fibers converge upward to insert by tendons into the intertubercular groove of the humerus on each side. In their upper thirds, these muscles converge with the teres major muscles to form the posterior folds of the axillae. The latissimus dorsi muscles are adductors, extensors, and medial rotators of the arm. Each is supplied by a thoracodorsal nerve from the posterior cord of the brachial plexus. Because of attachment to the ribs, the latissimus dorsi muscles can also be considered accessory muscles of respiration.

The lower border of the trapezius muscle overlies the upper border of the latissimus dorsi. Near the point of overlap a triangle is formed by the lateral border of the trapezius, the upper border of the latissimus dorsi, and the medial border of the scapula. Save for lower fibers of the rhomboid muscles, this area is free of an intervening mass of muscle tissue. Since a stethoscope placed over this triangle can detect respiratory sounds relatively free of distortion, it is called the *triangle of auscultation*.

Deep to the trapezius and latissimus dorsi muscles lies a layer of muscles involved in scapular movements and, to a lesser degree, movements of the ribs. Those related to the scapula are the levator scapulae, rhomboid major, and rhomboid minor muscles. The thin levator scapulae extends from the transverse processes of the first three or four cervical vertebrae diagonally downward to attach at the superior angle of the scapula on each side. The rhomboid minor may be fused with the rhomboid major. It extends from spines of the seventh cervical vertebra and first thoracic vertebra to the medial border of the scapula near the base of its spine. The rhomboid major arises from the spines of the second to the fifth thoracic vertebrae and the supraspinous ligament between these vertebrae and is attached to the medial border of the scapula, usually below the spine of the scapula. The levator scapulae, rhomboid major, and rhomboid minor elevate, adduct, and retract the scapula. All are supplied by the dorsal scapular nerve, but the levator scapulae is supplied also by branches from C4 and C5.

The serratus posterior muscles are said to be inspiratory muscles and thus merit brief attention. The serratus posterior superior muscles arise by aponeuroses from the ligamentum nuchae and spinous processes of the seventh cervical vertebra and the first to third thoracic vertebrae, and are attached to the upper borders of the first three to the first five ribs. They are supplied by ventral rami of segmental spinal nerves—intercostal nerves—and are said to be active in elevation of the upper ribs. The serratus posterior inferior muscles take aponeurotic origins from spinous processes of the lower two thoracic and upper two lumbar vertebrae; they insert by muscular slips on the lower three or four ribs. They are also supplied by ventral rami of segmental spinal nerves and are presumably able to prevent upward displacement of their ribs during inspiration.

Innervation of skin over the back is provided by medial cutaneous branches of dorsal rami of C4, C5, C8, T1, and T2 and by medial and lateral cutaneous branches of T3 to T10. Considerable overlap and asymmetry of these nerves have been described by Johnston (1908).

ANATOMIC FEATURES OF THE THORAX

Firm structural support for the thorax is provided by the sternum, ten pairs of costae—ribs and costal cartilages, two pairs of ribs without cartilage, and twelve thoracic vertebrae and their intervertebral discs. Collectively these components surround a cavity that is reniform in cross section, related to the neck above by a narrow thoracic inlet, and to the abdominal cavity below by a larger thoracic outlet. The inlet is surrounded by the manubrium of the sternum, the first ribs, and the first thoracic vertebra. Its anterior boundaries lie about 1 inch below the posterior limits. The inlet is roofed by bilateral thickened endothoracic fascia—Sibson's fascia or suprapleural membrane—and and subjacent parietal pleura which project upward into the base of the neck. Additional details of soft tissue relations of the thoracic inlet are considered at the end of this chapter in the section on *Pleura and Lungs in Relation to the Thoracic Wall.* The outlet is formed by the xiphoid process, fused costal cartilages of ribs seven to ten, the anterior portions of the eleventh ribs, the shafts of the twelfth ribs, and the body of the twelfth thoracic vertebra. The anterior margin of the outlet is at the level of the tenth thoracic, the lateral limits at the second lumbar, and the posterior margin at the twelfth thoracic vertebra. The outlet is therefore higher at its anterior margin than at its posterior limit and reaches its lowest level in the lateral aspect near the midaxillary line. It is sealed off from the abdominal cavity by the diaphragm.

The Sternum and Its Joints

The sternum is an elongated, flat bone that lies in the anterior midline. It is 15 to 20 cm long and is formed from cartilaginous precursors that ossify separately to form three components: the manubrium, the body, and the xiphoid process (Fig. 3–5).

The manubrium is about 5 cm wide in its upper half and 2.5 to 3 cm wide in its lower half. Its upper border is thickened and marked on either side by a notch for articulation with the clavicle. Centrally, an indentation is present, which together with the sternal ends of each clavicle forms the jugular—suprasternal—notch. The widest portion of the manubrium is marked by bilateral indentations—costal incisura—to accommodate articulation of the first costal cartilage. At the lower limits, each lateral margin of the bone is indented by a demifacet

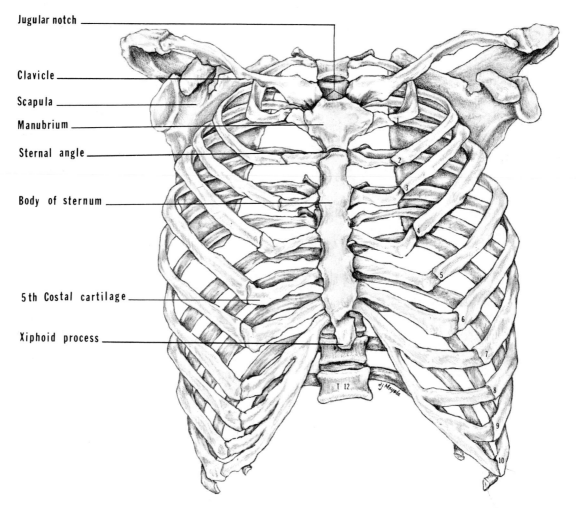

Jugular notch

Clavicle

Scapula

Manubrium

Sternal angle

Body of sternum

5th Costal cartilage

Xiphoid process

Fig. 3–5. Anterior view of the skeleton of the thorax and bones of the pectoral girdle. Bilateral asymmetry is evident in the body and xiphoid process of the sternum. The left subcostal arch is slightly higher than the right one.

for articulation of the upper half of the second costal cartilage. The lower margin of the manubrium articulates with the body of the sternum.

The body or longest portion of the sternum is slightly more than twice the length of the manubrium. It is slanted at a steeper angle than the manubrium; hence its articulation with that bone forms an angle, called the sternal angle. The outer border of this angle is readily palpable and lies at the level of the fourth to fifth thoracic vertebrae or their intervening intervertebral disc. The joint is a synchondrosis: articular surfaces of each bone are covered with hyaline cartilage and are united by fibrocartilage. It is sufficiently flexible to allow movement of the body on the more stable manubrium during respiratory movements. Ossification of the joint may form a synostosis during adult years, thus limiting flexibility, but, as noted by Trotter (1934), correlation is not observed between age and its incidence.

Lateral margins of the body exhibit segmental incisurae for articulation of costal cartilages two to seven. The incisura for the second costal cartilage is incomplete, for it represents only the lower half of the articulation

surface that is completed by the demifacet on the lower margin of the manubrium. The body ends at about the level of the tenth to eleventh thoracic vertebrae, where it forms a cartilaginous joint with the xiphoid process.

The xiphoid is a cartilaginous process that is usually ossified by middle age. It is the shortest and thinnest part of the sternum and may occasionally be bifid or perforated. It extends downward for a variable distance to end in the sheath of the rectus abdominis muscle. Its posterior surface is even with that of the sternal body; its anterior surface is somewhat recessed. The xiphoid is flexible at the xiphisternal joint, but it moves with the sternum during respiratory movements. Supportive costoxiphoid ligaments, extending from its anterior surface to the front of the seventh costal cartilage, prevent its backward displacement by contractions of the diaphragm.

The midline of the sternum is almost completely subcutaneous and is therefore easily accessible for sternal puncture, sternal transfusion, or incision during thoracic surgery. Its lateral margins are covered by origins of the sternal components of the pectoralis major muscles.

Ribs and Their Joints

The size and shape of the thorax are largely determined by the ribs and costal cartilages. A rib and its associated cartilage are properly termed a costa. The costae form continuous arches that extend backward for a short distance in relation to the vertebrae, turn forward at the angle, and extend toward the sternum, with which all but two pairs of them articulate directly or indirectly. Developmentally, the costae arise as arched, cartilaginous struts extending serially and horizontally from their respective vertebral bodies to the sternum. As development proceeds, the vertebral ends of each costal pair migrate cephalad. This shift in position is more pronounced in costal pairs two to nine and, as a result, the head of each of these ribs becomes pressed against the body of the vertebra immediately above. At the end of the growth period, ribs two to nine articulate with both their own and the immediately suprajacent vertebrae. The tenth rib may migrate sufficiently to articulate with the ninth and tenth thoracic vertebrae or it may remain low enough to articulate only with the body of the tenth thoracic vertebra. The eleventh and twelfth ribs migrate only slightly and thus form joints only with their own vertebrae. The angle of costal elements of the thoracic wall relative to the vertebrae and the sternum is therefore the result of cephalic migration of vertebral extremities and relative retention of sternal extremities at their original levels.

Ossification is initiated at the bend or angle of the costae. It spreads posteriorly toward the vertebrae and anteriorly toward the sternum. By the time bone deposition stops, the short vertebral portion is completely ossified. Since that part of the costa from the angle forward is longer, its ossification is not complete by the time bone formation ceases. The ossified portion of each costa becomes the rib proper and the unossified part remains as costal cartilage.

Relations of ribs and their costal cartilages to the sternum and to each other vary at different levels (Figs. 3–5, 3–6). The upper seven pairs of ribs articulate directly with the sternum by way of costal cartilages and are therefore called "true" or vertebrosternal ribs. In contrast, the lower five pairs are called "false" ribs since they do not articulate with the sternum at all. Of the false ribs, three pairs—the eighth, ninth, and tenth—

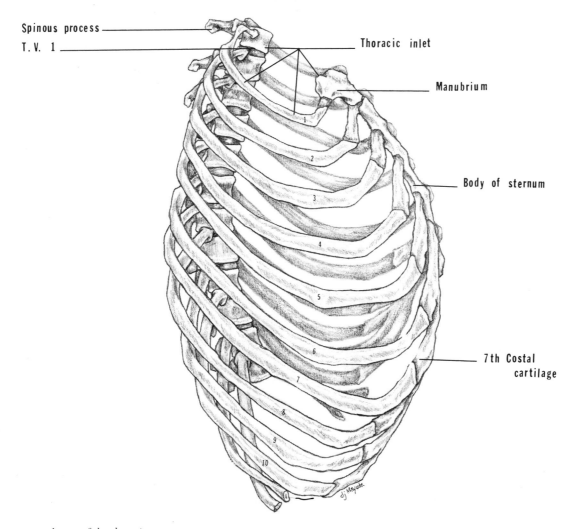

Fig. 3–6. Lateral view of the thoracic cage.

are called vertebrocostal since their associated cartilages articulate with immediately suprajacent cartilages. The remaining pairs—eleven and twelve—terminate in cartilaginous tips, ending in muscles of the abdominal wall. Since their only articulation is with the vertebrae, they are called vertebral ribs.

The costal cartilages change sequentially in length and direction. The first and second costal cartilages are short and follow a slightly downward course. The third and fourth gradually increase in length and are horizontal, or nearly so. The fifth to seventh cartilages extend downward from the tip of their ribs and then turn upward to meet the sternum. Since both ribs and cartilages of these costae are the longest and most flexible, they are maximally involved in the "bucket-handle" rib movement. The fused cartilages of ribs seven to ten course diagonally upward to the lower end of the sternum to form the infrasternal angle.

Ribs exhibit many similar features, but their form is variable at different levels. They increase in length from the first to the seventh and then gradually shorten to the twelfth. The most common features are characteristic of ribs three to nine which are frequently called "typical ribs." From their vertebral to sternal ends, each of these ribs is formed by a head, a neck, and a shaft (Fig. 3–7). The head is enlarged and marked by two facets, separated by an interarticular crest. The upper facet articulates with a facet on the body of the suprajacent vertebra. A slightly larger inferior facet articulates with a facet on the body of the adjacent vertebra whose number corresponds with that of the rib. The joint formed between costal facets, suprajacent, and adjacent vertebral bodies is termed a costovertebral joint.

The neck of each rib extends dorsolaterally for about 2.5 cm, and is marked by a crest on its upper border. The end of the neck and beginning of the shaft are marked by a tubercle. The tubercle bears a roughened elevation and a smooth articular surface. The elevation serves as an attachment for costotransverse ligaments. The articular surface meets a facet on the transverse process of the corresponding vertebra to form the costotransverse joint.

The shaft of the rib extends dorsolaterally for an additional 5 to 7.5 cm and then turns gradually forward and downward. The accentuated portion of this forward curvature is called the angle of the rib. The angle marks the lateral extent of the erector spinae muscles of the back. Throughout its course the shaft is twisted slightly so that its superolateral border is rounded and convex. The lower margin of the inferomedial surface is scored by a costal groove for the intercostal vessels and nerves. This groove is most clearly defined on the inner aspect of the posterior half of each rib. The shaft terminates in a small indentation which forms a hyaline-cartilaginous joint with its costal cartilage.

The less typical ribs differ in the following respects. The first rib is shorter than the rest and, beyond its neck, is wider and more curved. The head is small and bears only one facet for articulation with the body of the first thoracic vertebra. The upper and lower surfaces of the shaft are flat and its edges are sharp. Near the middle of the shaft a rounded tubercle is present that serves as an attachment for the anterior scalene muscle. Behind the tubercle is a depression where the first rib is crossed by the subclavian artery. A smaller depression for the subclavian vein may sometimes be noted in front of the tubercle (see Fig. 25–4).

The second rib is nearly twice the length of the first and articulates with the bodies of the first and second thoracic vertebrae. Its shaft is curved but not twisted and is marked by a roughened tubercle for upper digitations of the serratus anterior muscle.

The eleventh and twelfth ribs are sequentially shorter than suprajacent ones and bear only one articular surface for their corresponding vertebrae. They exhibit poorly defined or completely absent necks, angles, and costal grooves. The length of the twelfth rib is of consequence in renal surgery. While it is often shorter in a woman than in a man, Hughes (1949) has shown that longer ones, 11 to 14 cm, are more common than shorter ones, 1.5 to 6 cm. The posterior margin of parietal pleura normally crosses the twelfth rib at the lateral margin of the erector spinae muscles. If the twelfth rib is short, the surgeon may inadvertently palpate the lower border of the eleventh rib to determine the level for the initial incision. Such an incision risks entering the thoracic cavity instead of extraperitoneal tissue or renal fascia behind the kidneys.

Variations in rib structure may be of clinical significance. The first rib may be fused with the second at the scalene tubercle. This is usually associated with other variations in the second rib, sternum, or associated thoracic vertebrae. The seventh cervical vertebra may bear a cartilaginous or ossified rib called a cervical rib. Such a rib may be very short or it may be attached to the first costal cartilage or to the manubrium. Variations in the thoracic inlet or the presence of a cervical rib can produce compression of the subclavian artery and the brachial plexus resulting in compromise of neurovascular supply to the upper extremity. Occasionally the sternal extremity of the third or fourth rib may be bifid, and the eighth rib may reach the sternum on one or both sides. A lumbar rib may be associated with the first lumbar vertebra.

The structure of the heads of ribs two through nine and the associated vertebrae shows that the costovertebral joints consist of two joint cavities, each composed of costal and vertebral facets. The cavities are separated by a ligament extending from the interarticular crest of the rib to the intervertebral disc. Articular surfaces are covered with fibrous cartilage; joint cavities are surrounded by a synovial articular capsule. The capsule is thickened by radiate ligaments that fan out from the head of the rib to adjacent vertebral bodies.

Costotransverse joints, between the articular tubercle and the transverse process of the rib, are also synovial. Articular surfaces are covered with hyaline cartilage and the joint is enclosed by a fibrous capsule. The capsule is reinforced by costotransverse ligaments, which connect the neck and tubercle of the rib to the transverse process of its own vertebra and to that immediately

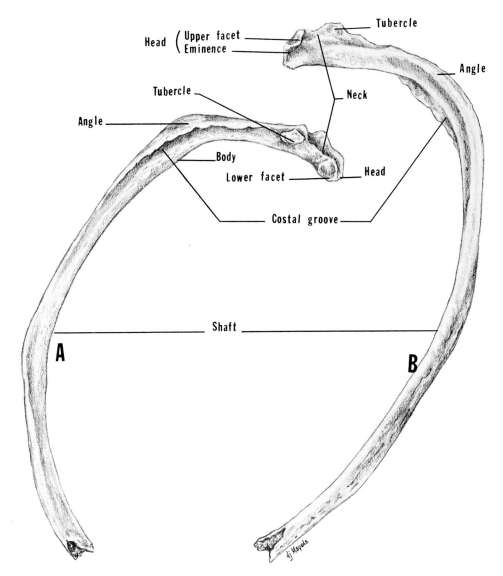

Fig. 3–7. A "typical rib." *A,* Inferior view; *B,* superior view.

above. Motions involved in both the "bucket-handle" and "pump-handle" movements of breathing are permitted by the flexibility of both the costovertebral and costotransverse joints. Fixation of these joints adversely affects pulmonary function.

Intercostal Spaces

The frequency with which the spaces between ribs are used in surgical approaches to the thorax prescribes an understanding of their muscular, fascial, and neurovascular features (Figs. 3–8 to 3–11). Lying deep to the skin, superficial fascia—tela subcutanea—and muscles related to the thoracic girdle and upper extremity, each intercostal space is traversed by three layers of muscle and their related deep fascia. Both muscles and fascia are attached to periosteum at the upper and lower borders of the ribs. During thoracoplasty an incision over the body of the rib and subsequent retraction of its per-

iosteum during removal of the rib will not violate the contents of the intercostal spaces.

From the surgical approach, the first layer of tissue to be encountered within the intercostal space is composed of the external intercostal muscles. Their fibers extend diagonally downward and forward from the lower margin of each rib to the upper margin of the subjacent rib. Musculature of this layer is continuous from a posterior position at the tubercle of the rib and posterior fibers of the costotransverse ligament (Figs. 3–9, 3–11, 3–12) to an anterior position at or near the costal cartilages. At this point, the investing fascia of the muscle continues further anteriorly to the sternum as the external—anterior—intercostal membrane (Figs. 3–12, 3–13). Intercostal muscles of the lower seven intercostal spaces interdigitate with the external oblique muscle of the abdominal wall. The next layer encountered consists of the internal intercostal muscles and their fascia. Muscle

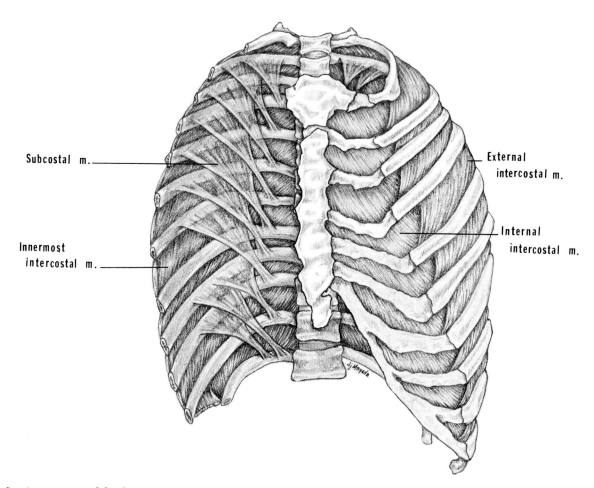

Subcostal m.

Innermost intercostal m.

External intercostal m.

Internal intercostal m.

Fig. 3–8. Anterior view of the thoracic wall and muscles of the intercostal spaces. The left side of the thorax is intact. The anterior half of the right side has been removed to demonstrate the inner aspect of the posterolateral thoracic wall.

fibers extend downward and backward between costal cartilages in the anterior-medial part of the intercostal space and between the ribs proper further laterally and posteriorly in the intercostal space. The reverse direction of these muscle fibers from those of the external intercostal muscle lends a cross-diagonal supportive force. Musculature of this layer extends from the sternum (Figs. 3–12, 3–13) as far posteriad as the angle of the ribs (Figs. 3–11, 3–12). At this point their investing fasciae form the internal-posterior-intercostal membrane, which attaches to the tubercle of each rib and the adjacent vertebra (Fig. 3–11).

Neurovascular components of the intercostal spaces are encountered immediately deep to these two layers. From above downward. The intercostal vein, artery, and nerve enter the posterior part of the intercostal space (Figs. 3–11, 3–12). In this region they lie within the endothoracic fascia deep to the internal intercostal membrane and just superficial to parietal pleura (Fig. 3–12). They remain in this position for a distance of 4 to 6 cm whereupon they gain the space between the internal and innermost intercostal muscles along the costal groove near the angle of the ribs (Figs. 3–7, 3–10 to 3–12). The neurovascular component, therefore, lies in the upper

limits of the intercostal space, in contrast to the collateral branches, which lie in the lower limits. The origin and distribution of these neurovascular elements are considered in detail later. Their position with respect to the ribs is important during incision of the intercostal space. Since major intercostal vessels and nerves lie in close relation to the lower border of each rib, incisions near this level are to be avoided. A preferable site is along the upper margin of each rib. Although accessory nerves and vessels may be sectioned at this level, there is negligible loss of function or sensitivity. It is equally important, however, to understand that the overlap of adjacent nerves is so great that paralysis and complete anesthesia are seldom produced within one intercostal space unless its nerve, the one above, and the one below are all severed.

The next layer of tissue encountered is less well defined. It consists of the innermost intercostal, subcostal, and transversus thoracis muscles and their fasciae. The innermost intercostals are best developed in the middle portion of the intercostal space (Figs. 3–9 to 3–12) and may be absent completely in the upper regions of the thoracic wall. They extend between adjacent ribs in the same direction as the internal intercostal muscles. Davies

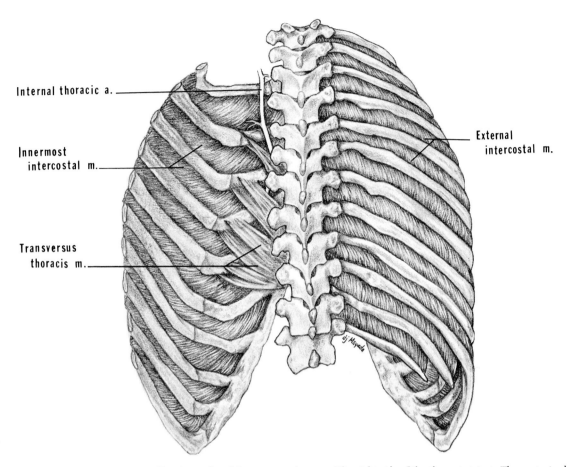

Internal thoracic a.

Innermost
intercostal m.

Transversus
thoracis m.

External
intercostal m.

Fig. 3–9. Posterior view of the thoracic wall and muscles of the intercostal spaces. The right side of the thorax is intact. The posterior half of the left side has been removed to show the inner aspect of the anterior thoracic wall.

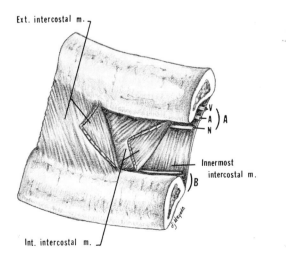

Ext. intercostal m.

V
A) A
N

Innermost
intercostal m.

B

Int. intercostal m.

Fig. 3–10. Relations of structures within an intercostal space. Intercostal vessels and nerves are shown at A. Collateral vessels are shown at B. V = vein, A = artery, N = nerve.

and associates (1932) considered them to be inner laminae of the internal intercostal muscles. The subcostal muscles extend as a variable number of slips from the lower margin of the angle of the ribs, diagonally across more than one intercostal space to the upper margin of the second or third rib below. The transversus thoracis is a thin layer of muscle on the inner aspect of the anterior thoracic wall. Aponeurotic slips of this muscle extend diagonally upward from the body and xiphoid process of the sternum to costal cartilages. The lowermost fibers of the transversus thoracis are almost horizontal and are continuous with the transversus abdominis muscle of the abdominal wall.

Deep to the third layer of muscles is the endothoracic fascia. It consists of variable amounts of areolar connective tissue, affording a natural cleavage plane for separation of the subjacent pleura from the thoracic wall.

The arterial supply of the intercostal spaces consists of posterior and anterior intercostal arteries. The posterior intercostal arteries of the first and second intercostal spaces arise from the highest intercostal arteries, which are branches of the subclavian artery; those of the remaining nine intercostal spaces are branches of the thoracic aorta. These arteries supply most of their respective intercostal spaces except the anteriormost limits. Each gives rise to a posterior branch supplying the spinal cord and deep muscles and skin of the back, an anterior branch running between the vein and nerve in the costal groove, and a collateral branch arising near the angle of the rib and descending to the upper border of the rib below. In the midaxillary line each anterior branch gives rise to a lateral cutaneous branch, which perforates the intercostal space to supply overlying skin. The posterior intercostal artery coursing below the twelfth rib is called the subcostal artery. It follows a course similar to those above but has no collateral branches.

The anterior intercostal arteries arise as segmental branches of the internal thoracic arteries in the first five or six intercostal spaces and as branches of the musculophrenic arteries in the lower intercostal spaces. Two such arteries are given off in each intercostal space, one passing toward the upper rib and one toward the lower. They continue laterally to anastomose with terminal branches of anterior and collateral branches of the posterior intercostal arteries.

The intercostal spaces are drained by eleven pairs of posterior intercostal veins and one pair of subcostal veins.

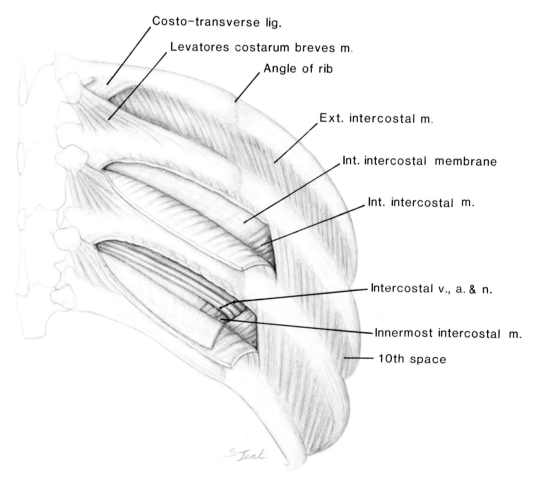

Costo-transverse lig.

Levatores costarum breves m.

Angle of rib

Ext. intercostal m.

Int. intercostal membrane

Int. intercostal m.

Intercostal v., a. & n.

Innermost intercostal m.

10th space

Fig. 3–11. Exposure of the posterior part of intercostal spaces 8, 9, and 10. Note that the intercostal vein, artery and nerve lie between the internal intercostal muscle and the innermost intercostal muscle layers. From the intervertebral foramen to the angle of the rib, the intercostal vessels and nerves are covered by the internal intercostal membrane.

These vessels follow the course of the posterior intercostal arteries and for the most part are tributary to the azygos or hemiazygos venous system. They lie above the nerve and artery throughout their course. Major blood flow is directed posteriorly by valves, but terminal vessels may also be tributary to the internal thoracic veins by way of small anterior intercostal veins. Posterior intercostal veins of the first intercostal space may be tributary to the brachiocephalic, vertebral, or superior intercostal veins. The second, third, and fourth posterior intercostal veins drain into the superior intercostal vein on each side; these in turn drain into the brachiocephalic vein on the left and into the azygos vein on the right. Right and left subcostal veins join the ascending lumbar veins on their respective sides of the thorax and ascend as the azygos and hemiazygos veins respectively.

Lymphatic drainage of the anterior limits of the upper four or five intercostal spaces enters the sternal—internal thoracic—nodes, which lie along the internal thoracic arteries. Their efferent vessels are tributary to a single vessel that joins the bronchomediastinal trunk. These nodes may commonly be invaded by metastases from breast carcinoma. Posterolateral portions of the intercostal spaces are drained by lymphatics that are tributary to one or two nodes near the vertebral ends of each intercostal space. Such nodes also receive lymphatic tributaries from the pleura. Nodes of upper intercostal spaces drain into the thoracic duct; those of the lower spaces are tributary to the cisterna chyli.

The thoracic wall is innervated segmentally by twelve pairs of thoracic spinal nerves. Upper thoracic spinal nerves also supply innervation to the axilla and upper extremity. Lower thoracic spinal nerves also supply portions of the abdominal wall and are called thoracoabdominal nerves. The midthoracic spinal nerves—T4 to T6—exhibit the most common pattern and are considered as typical nerves to the thoracic wall. Each spinal nerve is formed from a dorsal and a ventral root. The dorsal root contains sensory neurons which are distributed to posterior gray columns of the spinal cord. The ventral root contains somatic motor neurons originating in anterior gray columns of the spinal cord. Near the intervertebral foramen the dorsal and ventral roots unite to form a mixed spinal nerve. Each spinal nerve gives rise to a small meningeal nerve and then passes out of

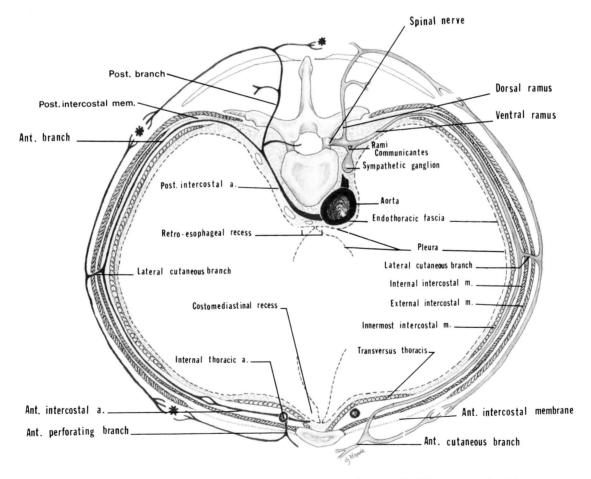

Fig. 3–12.   Summary scheme of structures within an intercostal space. Arteries are shown on the left, nerves on the right.

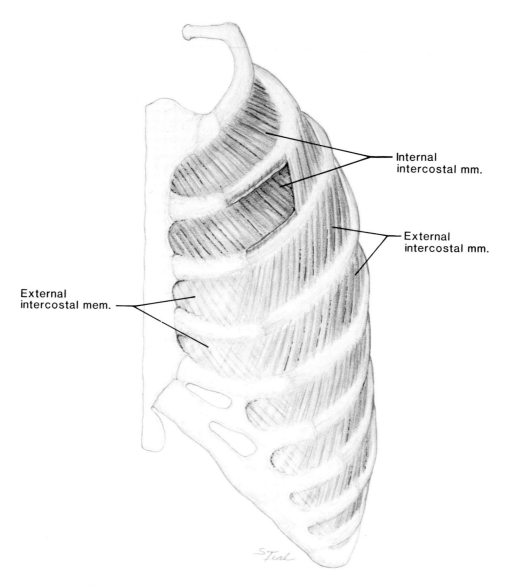

Internal
intercostal mm.

External
intercostal mm.

External
intercostal mem.

Fig. 3–13. Anterior view of the left half of the thorax. Note the opposing diagonal course of the external intercostal muscle fibers vs. those of the internal intercostal muscle fibers. The external–anterior–intercostal membrane extends from the costochondral junction to the sternum in the intercostal spaces.

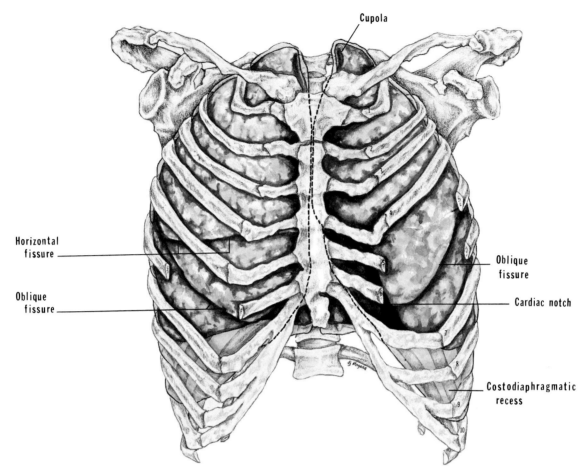

Fig. 3–14. Anterior view of thorax showing surface relations of pleura and lungs. Pleural borders subjacent to bone are shown by interrupted lines.

the intervertebral foramen, to branch into a dorsal and ventral ramus (Fig. 3–12).

The dorsal ramus of the thoracic spinal nerve passes backward to supply paravertebral back muscles and skin of the back. It forms medial and lateral cutaneous branches. Medial branches supply periosteum, ligaments, and joints of the vertebra, as well as deep muscles of the back before terminating in cutaneous filaments. Lateral branches supply the small levator costae muscles and deep back muscles, and follow a long descending course before becoming cutaneous. Extensive terminal overlap and anastomoses occur among medial and lateral cutaneous branches of dorsal rami from different spinal levels. Consequently, cutaneous pain is difficult to localize in this region.

Just lateral to the intervertebral foramen, the ventral ramus of the thoracic nerve establishes communications with the sympathetic chain by two branches or rami communicantes (Fig. 3–12). The white ramus contains preganglionic sympathetic fibers, and the gray ramus contains postganglionic sympathetic fibers. Beyond this point the ramus continues as the intercostal nerve and

is responsible for segmental distribution to skin, muscle, and serous membranes of the thoracic wall. Each intercostal nerve passes backward below the rib in the vicinity of costotransverse ligaments and then gains the costal groove. It continues its course in the plane between the innermost intercostal and internal intercostal muscles. Near the angle of the rib a collateral branch is given off. This branch passes laterally and then forward in the lower part of the intercostal space, terminating as a lower anterior cutaneous nerve.

Near the midaxillary line a lateral cutaneous branch is given off. It pierces the intercostal muscles, passes through the serratus anterior muscles, and then forms anterior and posterior cutaneous branches.

Just lateral to the sternal margin, the intercostal nerve lies between transversus thoracis and internal intercostal muscles. At this point it pierces overlying internal and external intercostal muscles, becomes subcutaneous, and forms anterior and median cutaneous branches.

Each segment of the thoracic wall is thus supplied circumferentially from behind forward by branches of the dorsal ramus and collateral, lateral, and anterior

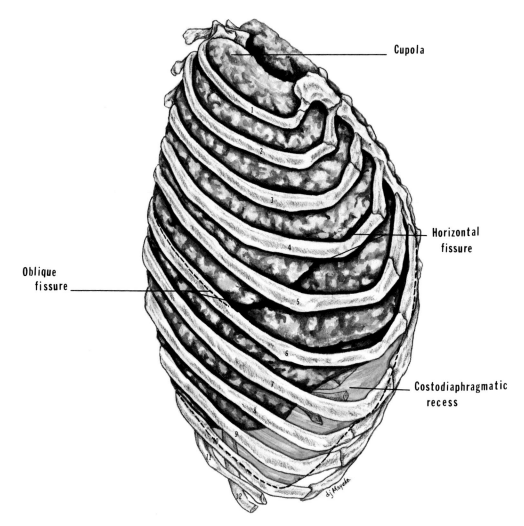

Fig. 3–15. Lateral view of thorax showing surface relations of pleura and lungs.

branches of the ventral ramus. The ventral rami—intercostal nerves—supply the intercostal, subcostal, serratus posterior superior, and tranversus thoracis muscles and the skin overlying the intercostal spaces. While the pattern of innervation for each intercostal space is basically similar, considerable intersegmental overlap is characteristic. For that reason, complete paralysis or anesthesia in only one intercostal space does not occur unless the nerve of that space, as well as those of the intercostal spaces above and below, is sectioned.

PLEURA AND LUNGS IN RELATION TO THE THORACIC WALL

Developmentally the lungs arise as bilateral diverticula of the foregut. The diverticula progressively enlarge and grow into the thoracic cavity, invaginating the pleural sac with them. That part of the pleural sac applied to the thoracic wall forms the parietal pleura; that applied to the invaginated lung primordia becomes the visceral pleura. Parietal pleura and visceral pleura are continuous at the root of the lung and the pulmonary ligament.

Lying deep to and adhering to the endothoracic fascia, the parietal pleura is a continuous, serous membrane divided into three regions, named in relation to surrounding structures. Costal pleura is related to the inner surface of the sternum, ribs, and bodies of thoracic vertebrae, thus forming anterior, lateral, and posterior walls of the pleural cavities; mediastinal pleura is related to the pericardial sac and other mediastinal structures, forming the medial wall of the pleural sac; diaphragmatic pleura is related to the diaphragm and thus forms the floor of the pleural sac.

Borders of the pleura are formed by continuity of the outer surfaces of costal, mediastinal, and diaphragmatic pleurae. For example, a sharp anterior border of the pleura is defined along the line at which costal and mediastinal pleurae meet, subjacent to the sternum. The inferior border of the pleura is formed by the line of union between costal and diaphragmatic pleurae. The posterior border is outlined by the meeting of costal pleura with the posterior margin of mediastinal pleura near the thoracic vertebrae. The anterior reflection of

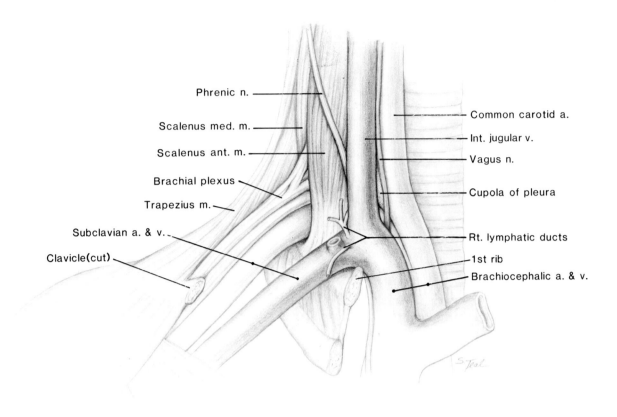

Fig. 3–16. Relations of the pleural cupola on the right side. Note the position of the cupola near the inferior and medial border of the scalenus anterior muscle, where it is crossed by the phrenic nerve and the vagus nerve. The subclavian artery passes anterior to the insertion of the scalenus anterior muscle on the first rib. The subclavian artery and the brachial plexus lie posterior and lateral to the muscle.

mediastinal and costal pleurae forms a thin, sharp costomediastinal recess within the pleural sac. A similar recess, the costodiaphragmatic recess, is formed at the base of the pleural sac by reflections of costal and diaphragmatic pleurae (Figs. 3–12, 3–14, 3–15).

The anterior, inferior, and posterior borders of the pleura may be related to overlying structures of the thoracic cage. Their topographic localization varies slightly, but it will be helpful for the thoracic surgeon to bear the following generalization in mind. The anterior pleural borders of the pulmonary cupolae are separated by visceral structures at the base of the neck. As they descend medially behind the sternum, they come to appose one another at the sternal angle. The right anterior border continues downward close to the midline. At the lower limits of the body of the sternum it diverges laterally along the sixth or seventh costal cartilage to become the inferior pleural border. The left anterior pleural border may follow a similar course, but more commonly it diverges laterally at the fourth costal cartilage, lies at the lateral sternal margin at the fifth, still further laterally at

the sixth cartilage, and then diverges laterally with increasing severity at the seventh costal cartilage. The lateral displacement of the left anterior pleural border between the fourth and sixth costal cartilages forms the cardiac notch. If the cardiac notch is well defined far enough laterally, it is possible to withdraw fluid from the pericardial sac without entering the pleural sac.

The inferior borders of both pleural sacs diverge laterally along the seventh costal cartilage and then cross ribs eight, nine, and ten. Their lowest level is reached about the middle of the eleventh rib in the midaxillary line. From this point they follow an almost horizontal course, cutting across the twelfth rib to meet the posterior pleural border at the twelfth thoracic vertebra. If the twelfth rib is short, the posterior pleural border may lie below it. In such instances, an incision along the twelfth rib will enter the pleural sac. In some individuals, as noted by Melnikoff (1923), the inferior border may be sufficiently high so that it does not cross the twelfth rib at all, but, instead, meets the posterior borders of the pleura at the eleventh thoracic vertebra.

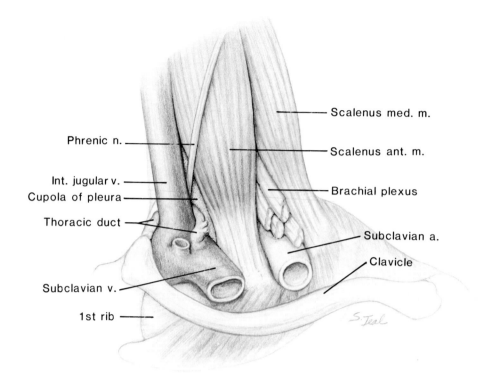

Phrenic n.

Int. jugular v.
Cupola of pleura

Thoracic duct

Subclavian v.

1st rib

Scalenus med. m.

Scalenus ant. m.

Brachial plexus

Subclavian a.

Clavicle

Fig. 3–17. Relations of the pleural cupola on the left side. Note the position of the cupola near the inferior and medial border of the scalenus anterior muscle. The cupola is crossed by the phrenic nerve and vagus nerve. The vagus nerve lies bewteen the internal jugular vein and the common carotid artery but is not visible in this dissection.

The posterior pleural borders ascend alongside or in front of the bodies of thoracic vertebrae until they diverge superiorly near the pulmonary cupolae. They are rounded, in contrast to either anterior or inferior borders. Right and left posterior borders may be in close apposition in front of the vertebral bodies. Where this occurs, thin retroesophageal recesses are formed behind the esophagus and in front of the aorta, hemiazygos, and azygos veins.

Knowledge of the surface relations of lobes and fissures of the lungs is important in percussion, auscultation, and roentgen evaluation of the pulmonary field. Although the lungs are in constant motion during respiration, the surface relations observed by Brock (1954) are essentially as described in Chapter 4. Knowledge of the topography of the various fissures of the lung is helpful in localizing abnormal pulmonary sounds as well as in localizing abnormal densities in roentgenograms of the chest (Figs. 3–14, 3–15).

For surgical purposes the lungs and pleura may be considered to be coextensive, with their respective costal, mediastinal, and diaphragmatic surfaces separated only by a film of serous fluid. In quiet respiration those portions of the lung within the costomediastinal and costodiaphragmatic recesses are insufficiently inflated to be identified by percussion. Percussible limits of the lower border of the lung normally lie at slightly higher levels than the lower limits of the pleura. The frequency with

which indwelling lines or catheters are surgically inserted into the subclavian veins and the consequence of damaging nearby pleura or neurovascular structures require special knowledge of soft tissue relations at the thoracic inlet (Figs. 3–16, 3–17). On both sides of the thorax, the subclavian vein lies deep to the clavicle and crosses the first rib anterior to the attachment of the serratus anterior muscle on the scalene tubercle of the first rib. The second part of the subclavian artery passes posterior to the scalenus anterior muscle and its third part lies lateral to the attachment of muscle on the first rib. Likewise, components of the brachial plexus pass behind and then lateral to the scalenus anterior muscle. More importantly, in relation to pulmonary function, the cupola of the pleura is consistently related to the inferior and medial border of the scalenus anterior muscle. In this position, the cupola reaches its most superficial position and therefore is susceptible to damage during invasive surgical procedures. This portion of the cupola is also crossed superficially by the phrenic nerve and the vagus nerve. On the right side the vagus nerve descends within the carotid fascia between the internal jugular vein and the common carotid artery and subsequently crosses the first part of the subclavian artery to enter the thorax between the common carotid and subclavian arteries. On the left side, the vagus nerve lies on the cupola of the pleura between the internal jugular vein and the common carotid artery to enter the thorax between the common carotid and subclavian arteries.

REFERENCES

Agostini, E., and Torri, G.: Diaphragm contraction as a limiting factor to maximum expiration. J. Appl. Physiol. *17*:427, 1962.

Brock, R.C.: The Anatomy of the Bronchial Tree: With Special Reference to the Surgery of Lung Abscess, 2nd ed. London, Oxford University Press, 1954.

Campbell, E.T.M.: The role of the scalene and sternomastoid muscles in breathing in normal subjects. an electromyographic study. J. Anat. *89*:378, 1955.

Cherniack, R.M., and Cherniack, L.: Respiration in Health and Disease. Philadelphia, W.B. Saunders Co., 1961, p. 7.

Davies, F., Gladstone, R.J., and Stibbe, E.P.: Anatomy of intercostal nerves. J. Anat. *66*:323, 1932.

Hughes, F.A.: Resection of twelfth rib in surgical approach to renal fossa. J. Urol. *61*:159, 1949.

Johnston, H.M.: The cutaneous branches of the posterior primary divisions of the spinal nerves and their distribution in the skin. J. Anat. Physiol. *43*:80, 1908.

Jones, D.S., Beargie, R.T., and Pauly, T.E.: Electromyographic study of some muscles of costal respiration in man. Anat. Rec. *117*:17, 1953.

Melnikoff, A.: Die chirurgische Anatomie des Sinus costodiaphragmaticus. Arch. Klin. Chir., Berl. *123*:133, 1923.

Taylor, A.: The contribution of the intercostal muscles to the effort of respiration in man. J. Physiol. (Lond.) *151*:390, 1960.

Trotter, M.: Synostosis between manubrium and body of sternum in Whites and Negroes. Am. J. Phys. Anthropol. *18*:439, 1934.

READING REFERENCES

Gardner, E., et al.: Anatomy, 3rd ed. Philadelphia, W.B. Saunders Co., 1969.

Basmajian, J.V.: Grant's Method of Anatomy, 10th ed. Baltimore, Williams & Wilkins, 1980.

Healy, J.E., and Seybold, W.D.: A Synopsis of Clinical Anatomy. Philadelphia, W.B. Saunders Co., 1969.

Hollinshead, W.H. and Rosse, C.: Textbook of Anatomy, 4th ed. Philadelphia, J.B. Lippincott Co., 1985.

Lachman, E.: Comparison of posterior boundaries of lungs and pleura as demonstrated on cadaver and on roentgenogram of the living. Anat. Rec. *83*:521, 1942.

Mainland, D., and Gordon, E.T.: Position of organs determined from thoracic radiographs of young adult males, with study of cardiac apex beat. Am. J. Anat. *68*:457, 1941.

Woodbourne, R.T.: Essentials of Human Anatomy, 7th ed. New York, Oxford University Press, 1983.

CHAPTER 4

SURGICAL ANATOMY OF THE LUNGS

Thomas W. Shields

Until recent decades the anatomy of the lungs was a little understood and seemingly unimportant subject. With the development of roentgenographic and endoscopic techniques and the advancement of pulmonary surgery, detailed anatomic knowledge of the lungs became a necessity.

The essential anatomic unit of the lung, the bronchopulmonary segment, was established as that portion of the lung substance that represents the total branching of a major—segmental—subdivision of a lobar bronchus. These units are named for their topographic position in the lung.

THE LOBES AND FISSURES

The right lung is composed of three lobes—the upper, middle, and lower—and is the larger of the two lungs. The left is made up of only two lobes—the upper and lower. Two fissures are usually present on the right. The oblique—major—fissure separates the lower lobe from the upper and middle lobes, and the horizontal—minor—fissure separates the other two (Fig. 4–1). In life the oblique fissure on the right begins posteriorly at the level of the fifth rib or intercostal space, runs downward and forward approximating the course of the sixth rib, and ends at the diaphragm in the vicinity of the sixth costochondral junction. The horizontal fissure begins in the oblique fissure in the region of the midaxillary line at the level of the sixth rib and runs anteriorly to the costochondral junction of the fourth rib. On the left, the oblique—major—fissure is found (Fig. 4–2). This begins at a somewhat higher level posteriorly, between the third and fifth ribs, and runs downward and forward to end in the region of the sixth or seventh costochondral junction.

Variations in the fissures do occur, and often there is a failure of development of part or all of a fissure. This is commonly seen as a more or less complete fusion of the middle lobe and the anterior portion of the upper lobe in over 50% of lungs examined. Accessory fissures occur also, and certain portions of the lung may be demarcated into so-called accessory lobes. On occasion,

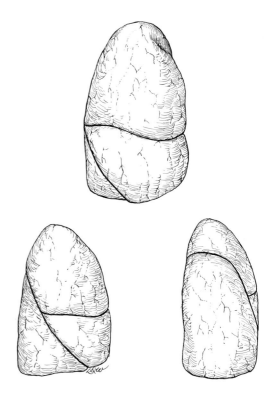

Fig. 4–1. Anterior, lateral, and posterior aspects of right lung. (Redrawn and modified by permission from Anson, B.J.: Atlas of Human Anatomy. Philadelphia, W.B. Saunders Co., 1950, p. 199.)

such fissures are visible as linear shadows on the roentgenogram, and the accessory lobe may appear less radiolucent than the surrounding portions of the lung. The usual accessory lobes are the posterior accessory, the inferior accessory, the middle lobe of the left lung, and the azygos lobe (Fig. 4–3). In contrast to the first three named, which are true accessory lobes made up of specific bronchopulmonary segments, the azygos lobe is not a true accessory lobe because it is formed of varying portions of one or two segments—apical and posterior— of the right upper lobe. The fissure is formed by an

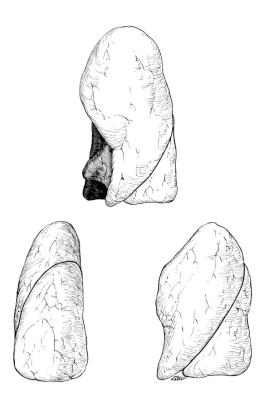

Fig. 4–2. Anterior, lateral, and posterior aspects of left lung. (Redrawn by permission from Anson, B.J.: Atlas of Human Anatomy. Philadelphia, W.B. Saunders Co., 1950, p. 199.)

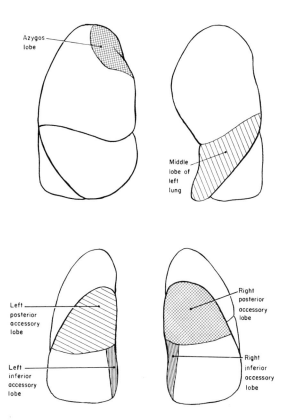

Fig. 4–3. Accessory lobes of the lungs.

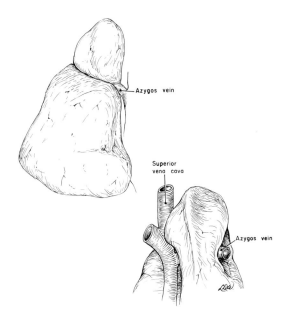

Fig. 4–4. Anterior and posterior views of the azygos lobe formed by an aberrant loop of the azygos vein. (Redrawn and modified by permission from Anson, B.J.: Atlas of Human Anatomy. Philadelphia, W.B. Saunders Co., 1950, pp. 203–204.)

aberrant loop of the azygos vein and its mesentery of two layers of the parietal pleura and two of the visceral pleura (Fig. 4–4). On the roentgenogram, this fissure may appear as an inverted comma to the right of the mediastinum (Fig. 4–5). This anomaly is seen in 0.5 to 1.0% of the anatomic dissections and routine roentgenograms of the chest.

BRONCHOPULMONARY SEGMENTS

Each lobe of the right and left lungs is subdivided into several individual anatomic units, the bronchopulmonary segments. The general pattern is that of 18 segments, 10 in the right lung and 8 in the left. The terminology proposed by Jackson and Huber (1943) is accepted by

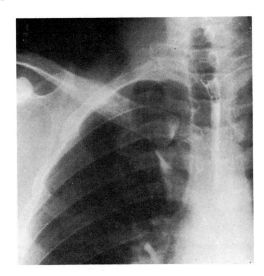

Fig. 4–5. Roentgenogram of the chest showing an azygos lobe.

Table 4–1. Bronchopulmonary Segments

Right Lung		Left Lung	
		Upper Lobe	
Apical	1	Superior Division	
Anterior	2	Apical Posterior	1 + 3
Posterior	3	Anterior	2
		Inferior Division—Lingula	
		Superior Lingular	4
		Inferior Lingular	5
		Middle Lobe	
Lateral	4		
Medial	5		
		Lower Lobe	
Superior	6	Superior	6
Medial Basal	7	Anteromedial Basal	7 + 8
Anterior Basal	8	Lateral Basal	9
Lateral Basal	9	Posterior Basal	10
Posterior Basal	10		

most and is listed in Table 4–1. The topographic positions of the segments are shown in Figures 4–6A and B. Knowledge of the detailed anatomic features of the bronchial distribution and the vascular supply of each segment is essential for the surgeon. Although there is a general pattern to the anatomic features in each segment, variation is the rule. The usual pattern and the most common deviations from it are best portrayed by separate descriptions of the bronchial, arterial, and venous systems.

BRONCHIAL TREE*

The trachea bifurcates at about the level of the seventh thoracic vertebra into the right and left main-stem bronchi. Compared with the left bronchus, which arises at a sharper angle, the right one arises in a more direct line with the trachea—an important factor in the localization of aspirated material.

The Right Bronchial Tree

The length of the right main bronchus from the trachea to the point where the right upper lobe bronchus branches from its lateral wall is about 1.2 cm. The upper lobe bronchus, approximately 1 cm in length, in turn gives off three segmental bronchi, one to the apical, one to the posterior, and one to the anterior segment. The branching may be a simple trifurcation or with varying combinations of the three major branches. The segmental bronchi further subdivide to supply the various portions of the segments.

Proceeding distally from the takeoff of the upper lobe bronchus, the primary bronchus is known as the bronchus intermedius, over which the main stem pulmonary artery crosses, thus giving rise to the term "eparterial bronchus" to designate the right upper lobe bronchus.

*The described anatomic patterns and variations of the bronchi and pulmonary arteries and veins have been selected by the author primarily from the studies of Birnbaum (1954), Bloomer, Liebow, and Hales (1960), and Boyden (1955).

After a distance of approximately 1.7 to 2 cm, the middle lobe bronchus arises from the anterior surface of the bronchus intermedius. It varies in length between 1.2 and 2.2 cm before it bifurcates into lateral and medial branches. The superior segmental bronchus of the lower lobe arises from the posterior wall of the bronchus intermedius, slightly distal to the middle lobe bronchus. The superior segment is called the posterior accessory lobe when a fissure is present. This bronchus most often arises as a single branch and divides into three rami, usually by bifurcation or rarely by trifurcation. Distal to the superior bronchus, the basal stem bronchus sends off segmental bronchi to the medial—the inferior accessory lobe when a fissure is present—anterior, lateral, and posterior basal segments. The medial basal bronchus arises anteromedially and is distributed to the anterior and paravertebral surfaces of the lower lobe. The anterior basal branch arises on the anterolateral aspect of the basal trunk approximately 2 cm distal to the superior segmental bronchus and divides into two major rami. The lateral basal bronchus and the posterior basal bronchus most often arise as a common stem. Each of these bronchi, in turn, divides typically into two major subdivisions (Fig. 4–7A and 4–7B).

Numerous variations occur, but the basic pattern encountered is as described. Infrequently, the upper lobe bronchus on the right undergoes two separate bifurcations to form the three bronchopulmonary segments. Of more interest is the rare occurrence of a tracheal bronchus that arises above, or at the level of, the main stem carina and supplies the apical bronchopulmonary segment of the right upper lobe (Fig. 4–8). The variations in the middle lobe bronchus and its branchings, other than an occasional supero-inferior spatial relationship of the segments rather than lateral and medial arrangements, are of little interest. In the division of the lower lobe bronchus, the presence of a subsuperior or an accessory subsuperior bronchus is not an uncommon finding. One to three such bronchi may be identified.

The Left Bronchial Tree

The left main bronchus is longer than the right and its first branch arises anterolaterally as the left upper lobe bronchus approximately 4 to 6 cm distal to the main stem carina. This bronchus is approximately 1 to 1.5 cm long and divides into a superior and an inferior—lingular—branch. The superior division ascends and the inferior descends. The superior branch most often bifurcates into an apical posterior segmental bronchus and an anterior segmental bronchus. Occasionally, the anterior segment migrates inferiorly to create a trifurcate pattern. The inferior or lingular bronchus—the analog of the middle lobe—is variable in length—1 to 2 cm—and subsequently divides into superior and inferior divisions, the former of which in turn subdivides into posterior and inferior rami.

Approximately 0.5 cm distal to the left upper lobe orifice, the lower lobe stem bronchus gives off its first branch, the superior segmental bronchus. This bronchus arises posteriorly and bifurcates in most instances, but

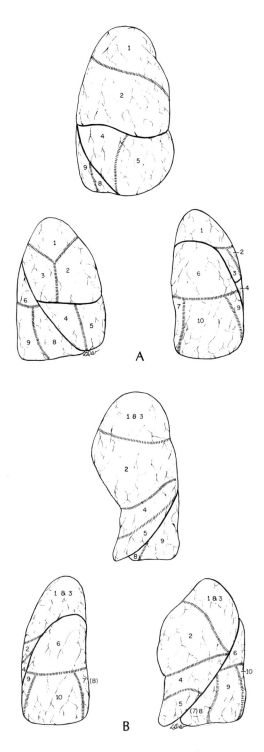

Fig. 4–6. *A,* Schematic representation of the topographic positions of the bronchopulmonary segments of the right lung seen in anterior, lateral, and posterior views. *B,* Schematic representation of the topographic positions of the bronchopulmonary segments of the left lung seen in anterior, lateral, and posterior views.

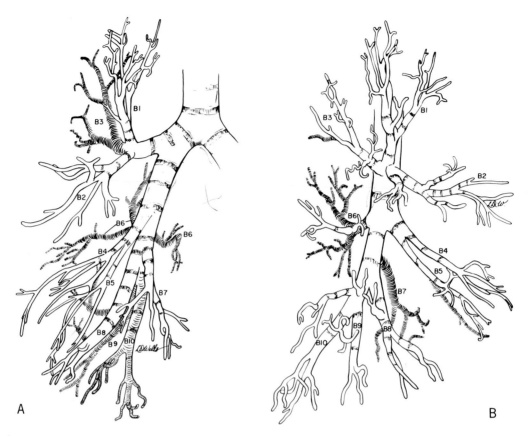

Fig. 4–7. *A* and *B*, Right bronchial tree, anterior and lateral views. Boyden's modification of numerical nomenclature used. (Redrawn and modified from Brock, R.C.: The Anatomy of the Bronchial Tree, 2nd ed. London, Oxford University Press, 1954, pp. 190–191.)

trifurcation does occur. After giving off the superior branch the basal trunk continues for an average distance of 1.5 cm as a single trunk. The bronchus then usually bifurcates into an anteromedial basal segmental bronchus and a common stem bronchus for the lateral basal and posterior basal bronchi. These branches further subdivide into numerous rami for their respective segments (Figs. 4–9A and 4–9B).

On the left side, the common variations are in the distribution of the segmental bronchi from the superior and inferior divisions of the left upper lobe bronchus and the presence of a subsuperior or accessory subsuperior bronchus arising from the lower lobe bronchus. Many of these deviations from normal have little clinical importance, but are significant at the time of surgical resection of the various portions of the lungs.

THE PULMONARY ARTERIAL SYSTEM

The main pulmonary artery arises to the left of the aorta and passes superiorly and to the left. It occupies a position anterior to the left main bronchus and divides into the right and left main pulmonary arteries. These two vessels lie in an oblique line that is parallel, and slightly superior, to the pulmonary veins. The right main pulmonary artery is longer than the left, but its extra-pericardial length up to its first branch is less than that

of the left. The branching pattern of the pulmonary arteries is more variable than that of the bronchi, although the arteries tend to lie closely adjacent to the segmental bronchus and to follow their branching. No one pattern for either the right or the left pulmonary artery may be described as the standard one. However, a relatively typical distribution of the segmental arteries is often encountered, and, from this, the multitude of variations may be readily understood (Figs. 4–10, 4–11).

The Right Pulmonary Artery

As it leaves the pericardial sac, the right pulmonary artery is anterior and inferior to the right main bronchus and posterior and superior to the superior pulmonary vein. The first branch is the truncus anterior; this is the major vessel carrying blood to the right upper lobe. It arises superolaterally and shortly divides into two branches. The more superior branch of the truncus anterior again divides to form an apical branch that loops posteriorly over the upper lobe bronchus to supply a variable portion of the posterior segment. This latter vessel is known as the posterior recurrent artery. The more inferior branch of the truncus anterior goes to the anterior segment, but also may give off a branch to the apical segment. The truncus anterior carries the entire blood supply to the right upper lobe in one out of ten individuals. In the majority of persons, one or more as-

The major variations in the right arterial system occur with almost each of the aforementioned branchings. In as many as 20% of the population, two arteries arise from the anterior trunk. These vessels are designated as the truncus anterior superior and the truncus anterior inferior. When they are present, the recurrent posterior branch is almost always a branch of the truncus anterior superior. Infrequently more than one ascending branch to the upper lobe arises from the interlobar portion of the artery; the more proximal branch supplies a portion of the anterior segment. On occasion, the posterior ascending artery may be found to arise from the superior segmental artery or, even more rarely, from the middle lobe artery. The middle lobe artery, as well as the superior segmental artery, although usually a single vessel, may be represented by two or, at times, even three vessels. Last, in addition to the variable branchings of the common basal trunk, a subsuperior or accessory subsuperior artery may arise from either the common stem or the posterior basal branch.

The Left Pulmonary Artery

The left pulmonary artery ascends to a higher level, passes more posteriorly, and has a greater length before giving off its first segmental branch to the lung than does the right pulmonary artery. The branches to the left upper lobe arise from the anterior, the posterosuperior, and the interlobar portions of the vessel. The number of branches may vary from two to seven, but four branches to the lobe form the most common pattern. Generally, the first branch arises from the anterior portion of the artery to supply the anterior segment, a part of the apical segment, and occasionally, the lingular division of the lobe. The first branch of this anterior segmental artery supplies the anterior segment and also may give off a lingular branch. Usually it also branches to provide a vessel carrying blood to the apical segment. The second and, infrequently, a third branch from this first anterior trunk give rise to a vessel, or vessels, going to the anterior segment, to the apical segment, and uncommonly, to the posterior segment. This anterior trunk is generally quite short, and often the branches may appear as separate vessels arising from a common opening from the main artery. A second branch from the main artery as it passes distally and posterosuperiorly over the left upper lobe bronchus and into the interlobar fissure is present in almost 80% of instances. This second arterial branch, and occasionally a third, is given off anterosuperiorly to the apical posterior segment. Posteriorly, as the artery passes into the interlobar fissure, it branches to form a vessel going to the superior segment of the lower lobe. This vessel usually is a single one that bifurcates or, infrequently, trifurcates at a variable distance from its takeoff from the main stem arterial trunk. Most often, the lingular artery originates from the interlobar portion of the pulmonary artery distal to the superior segmental artery and constitutes the lingular arterial supply in toto in 80% of persons. At a variable distance from the origin of the lingular vessel, the pulmonary stem artery, now the common basal trunk, most commonly divides into two major

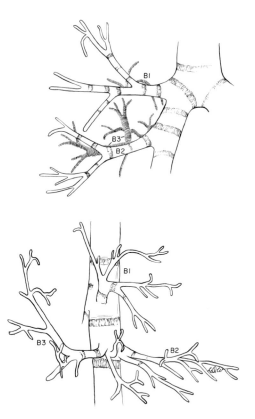

Fig. 4–8. Tracheal bronchus supplying the apical segment of the right upper lobe. (Redrawn and modified with permission from Bloomer, W.E., Liebow, A.A., and Hales, M.R.: Surgical Anatomy of the Bronchovascular Segments. Springfield, IL, Charles C Thomas, 1960, p. 25.)

cending vessels from the interlobar portion of the pulmonary artery are also present. The interlobar portion crosses over the bronchus intermedius. Generally, only one ascending vessel to the upper lobe is present. This branch, frequently quite small in caliber, supplies almost exclusively the posterior segment and is referred to as the posterior ascending artery. At the same level, or even either slightly proximal or distal to the posterior ascending artery, the middle lobe artery arises anteromedially from the interlobar portion of the pulmonary artery. The site of origin is usually at the level of the junction of the horizontal and oblique fissures. The artery is usually single and bifurcation of the vessel is the rule, but the subdivisions are quite variable. The arterial branch to the superior segment of the lower lobe arises posteriorly and opposite to the middle lobe artery at the same level or slightly distal to it. The superior segmental artery is usually a single trunk that bifurcates. Distal to the aforementioned branchings of the interlobar portion of the artery, the vessel is considered the common basal trunk. The medial basal segmental artery may arise independently or may arise in common with the anterior basal branch. The remainder of the basal trunk then terminates with its division into the lateral and posterior segmental branches, the mode of actual branching being quite variable.

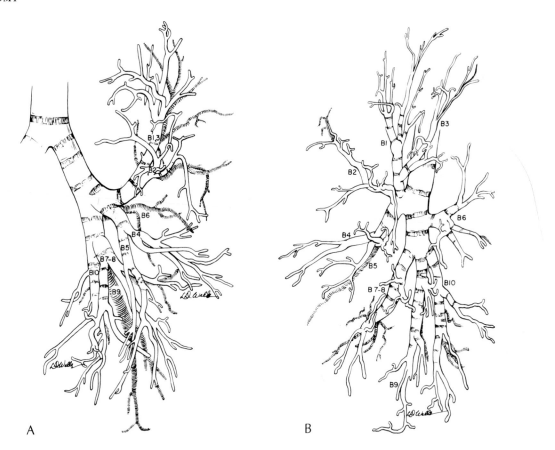

Fig. 4–9. *A* and *B*, Left bronchial tree, anterior and lateral views. Boyden's modification of numerical nomenclature used. (Redrawn and modified from Brock, R.C.: The Anatomy of the Bronchial Tree, 2nd ed. London, Oxford University Press, 1954, pp. 191–192.)

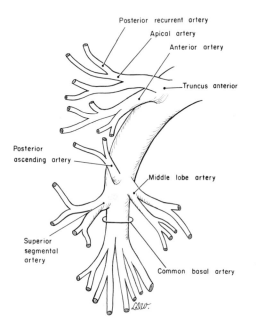

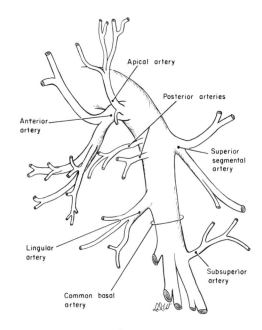

Fig. 4–10. Common pattern of branching of the right pulmonary artery.

Fig. 4–11. Common pattern of branching of the left pulmonary artery.

branches. The more anterior branch supplies the anteromedial basal segment, and the posterior one supplies the lateral basal and posterior basal segments. The patterns of branching of the common basal trunk and its major divisions are quite variable.

Likewise, major variations may occur in all the segmental branches of the left pulmonary artery. As mentioned, the first anterior branch may supply the lingular division as well as other portions of the upper lobe, and, although in less than one in ten individuals, this branch may carry all the blood supplying the lingular division. Another variation is that the first anterior branch may carry only the blood supplying the apical segment; the anterior segment in this situation receives its arterial supply from the interlobar portion of the artery. As noted, the superior segmental artery usually arises proximal to the branch, or branches, going to the lingula, but in as many as one in three persons, the superior segmental branch may be distal to the lingular artery takeoff. Both these vessels may be multiple. Again, in one in three persons, a branch of one of the lingular vessels or even a direct branch from the interlobar portion of the artery may supply some blood to the anterior segment of the left upper lobe. Rarely, this vascular branch carries the entire arterial supply to this segment. As on the right, branches to the subsuperior segmental region are often found arising as single or multiple vessels from the common basal stem or, more frequently, from the posterior basal branch. Last, a vessel may arise from the common basal stem or one of its branches to contribute to the lingular blood supply.

PULMONARY VENOUS SYSTEM

The venous drainage pattern of the lung reveals a greater number of variations than does the arterial pattern. There are usually two major venous trunks from both lungs: the superior and inferior pulmonary veins. The tributaries of these veins are intersegmental and form various combinations to create the major trunks (Figs. 4–12, 4–13).

Right Pulmonary Veins

The superior pulmonary vein lies anterior and somewhat inferior to the pulmonary artery. It usually is made up of four major branches, which drain the upper and middle lobes. The first three branches from above downward drain the upper lobe and are identified as the apical anterior, anterior–inferior, and posterior branches. The posterior branch is composed of central and interlobar divisions. The fourth and most inferior trunk drains the middle lobe and generally is made up of two branches. Although the middle lobe vein most often joins the superior pulmonary vein, on occasion it may enter the pericardium and drain into the atrium as a separate vessel. Rarely, it becomes a tributary of the inferior pulmonary vein.

The inferior pulmonary vein is inferior and posterior to the superior vein. It drains the lower lobe and as a rule is made up of two major trunks. The first is the

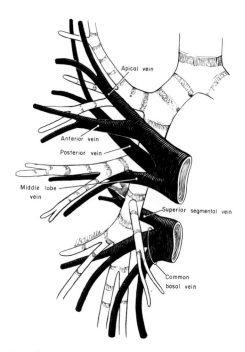

Fig. 4–12. Schematic representation of the tributaries of the right superior and inferior pulmonary veins. (Adapted with permission from Kubick, S.: Klinische Anatomie, Ein Farbfoto-Atlas der Topographie 2. Aufl (Band III-Thorax). Stuttgart, Georg Thieme Verlag, 1971, p. 97.)

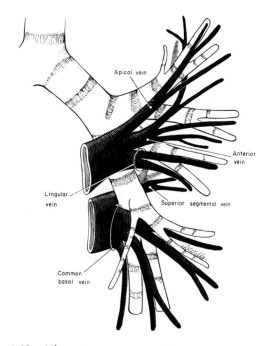

Fig. 4–13. Schematic representation of the tributaries of the left superior and inferior pulmonary veins. (Adapted with permission from Kubick, S.: Klinische Anatomie, Ein Farbfoto-Atlas der Topographie 2. Aufl (Band III-Thorax). Stuttgart, Georg Thieme Verlag, 1971, p. 97.)

superior segmental vein, which drains the superior segment. The other branch, known as the common basal vein, is made up of superior basal and inferior basal tributaries, and these vessels drain the various basal segments of the lower lobe.

Left Pulmonary Veins

On the left, the superior pulmonary vein is closely applied to the anteroinferior aspect of the pulmonary artery, and, as a result, obscures the anterior branches of the artery. This vein is made up of three to four tributaries that drain the entire upper lobe. The first division, the apical posterior vein, is made up of an apical ramus and a posterior ramus. The second division represents the anterior vein, which may have three rami: a superior, inferior, and posterior rami. The third and fourth divisions represent the superior and inferior lingular veins. A single trunk may represent these veins in about 50% of persons. This trunk, as seen with the middle lobe vein on the right, may drain into the inferior pulmonary vein; this variant occurs more commonly on the left than on the right.

The inferior pulmonary vein, as on the right, is located inferior and posterior to the superior vein and has two similar tributaries: the superior segmental and the common basal veins. The latter is made up of superior and inferior basal divisions, which drain the basal segments of the lobe.

INTRAPERICARDIAL ANATOMY

The right pulmonary artery passes from the left to the right behind the ascending aorta and constitutes the superior border of the transverse sinus. It then lies behind the superior vena cava and forms the superior border of the postcaval recess of Allison (Fig. 4–14); the medial and inferior borders of this recess are the superior vena cava and right superior pulmonary vein. Although the right pulmonary artery is longer than the left pulmonary artery, it is not as accessible as the left. The left pulmonary artery passes inferior to the aortic arch and forms the superior border of the left pulmonary recess. The medial border of this recess is formed by the fold of Marshall (Fig. 4–15).

The superior and inferior pulmonary veins bulge into the pericardium and are invested to a greater, or lesser, extent by the pericardium's serous layer. On the right, these two vessels most often enter into the left atrium separately, although rarely they form one vessel. In contrast, on the left the two veins form a common trunk in one out of four persons.

The serous—parietal—pericardial investments of the vessels are important because these fibrous tissue layers must be divided to obtain free access to the entire circumference of the individual vessel. On the right, the serous layer leaves the lateral and posterior surfaces of the superior vena cava and comes to lie upon the artery in the postcaval recess. At this point, only about one fifth of the circumference of the vessel is free. In contrast, three fourths of the circumference is free in the trans-

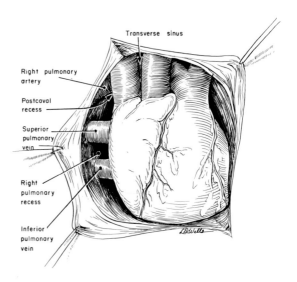

Fig. 4–14. Intrapericardial anatomy on the right. (Redrawn with permission from Healey, J.E., Jr., and Gibbon, J.H., Jr.: Intrapericardial anatomy in relation to pneumonectomy for pulmonary carcinoma. J. Thorac. Surg. *19*:864, 1950.)

verse sinus medial to the superior vena cava. From the artery, the serous layer passes inferiorly and reflects upon the superior, anterior, and inferior surfaces of the superior vein; approximately one third of this vessel is not free posteriorly. The layer then descends to cover most of the inferior pulmonary vein and then passes down to envelop the inferior vena cava. On the left, the reflection of the serous pericardium passes over the anterior and inferior surfaces of the left pulmonary artery, and approximately one half of the vessel is free in the pericardial sac. The layer then descends inferiorly to the superior vein, so that only the posterior surface is not free in the sac. It then passes downward to envelop the inferior vein, which is subsequently almost totally free within the sac, except for a small surface located posteriorly.

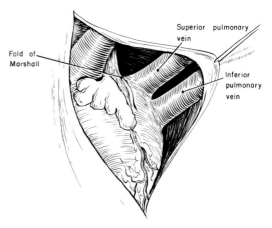

Fig. 4–15. Intrapericardial anatomy on the left. (Redrawn with permission from Healey, J.E., Jr., and Gibbon, J.H., Jr.: Intrapericardial anatomy in relation to pneumonectomy for pulmonary carcinoma. J. Thorac. Surg. *19*:864, 1950.)

BRONCHIAL ARTERIES AND VEINS

The bronchial arterial system arises from the systemic circulation and accounts for approximately 1% of the cardiac output. It empties mainly into the pulmonary veins and a lesser bronchial vein system that enters the azygos venous system on the right and the hemiazygos on the left. The origins of the arteries are variable from the aorta, intercostal arteries, and, occasionally, from the subclavian or innominate arteries. According to Olson and Athanasoulis (1982) in 40% of persons the pattern is one bronchial artery on the right side with two on the left. In 21% there is one bronchial artery on each side and in 20% there are two on each side. The remaining 10% have two arteries on the right and only one on the left. On the right, according to Nathan and his associates (1970), the major source is from the first or, at times, the second right aortic intercostal artery. Distally on the right, as well as on the left, the other bronchial arteries take their origin directly from the aorta, the level of origin varying between the third and the eighth thoracic vertebrae, but most commonly the origins are between the levels of the fifth and sixth thoracic vertebrae.

The arteries to either side enter the hilus of the lung and form a communicating arc around the main bronchus. From here, the main arterial divisions radiate along the major bronchi. These vessels are closely applied to the bronchial wall. There are generally two divisions, an anterior and posterior branch, along each bronchus. The vessels follow the course of the bronchus and divide as do the bronchi. Networks of intercommunicating vessels are often present on the bronchial walls. It has been assumed that two thirds of this blood supply empties into the pulmonary veins, and that the rest empties into the bronchial veins. The bronchial veins are present in the mucosa and also external to the bronchial cartilage. The direction of flow is to the venous plexus of the perihilar regions and then subsequently into either the azygos or hemiazygos systems.

REFERENCES

Birnbaum, G.L.: Anatomy of the Bronchovascular System. Its Application to Surgery. Chicago, Year Book Medical Publishers, 1954.

Bloomer, W.E., Liebow, A.A., and Hales, M.R.: Surgical Anatomy of the Bronchovascular Segments. Springfield, IL, Charles C Thomas, 1960.

Boyden, E.A.: Segmental Anatomy of the Lungs. New York, McGraw-Hill Book Co., 1955.

Jackson, C.L., and Huber, J.F.: Correlated applied anatomy of bronchial tree and lungs with system nomenclature. Dis. Chest 9:319, 1943.

Nathan, H., Orda, R., and Barkay, M.: The right bronchial artery, anatomical considerations and surgical approach. Thorax 25:328, 1970.

Olson, P.R., and Athanasoulis, C.A.: Hemoptysis: treatment with transcatheter embolizations of the bronchial arteries. *In* Interventional Radiology. Edited by C.A. Athanasoulis, et al.: Philadelphia, W.B. Saunders Co., 1982, p. 196.

READING REFERENCES

Allison, P.R.: Intrapericardial approach to the lung root in the treatment of bronchial carcinoma by dissection pneumonectomy. J. Thorac. Surg. *15*:99, 1946.

Barrett, R.J., Day, J.C., and Tuttle, W.M.: The arterial distribution to the left upper pulmonary lobe. J. Thorac. Surg. *32*:190, 1956.

Barrett, R.J., O'Rourke, P.V., and Tuttle, W.M.: The arterial distribution to the right upper pulmonary lobe. J. Thorac. Surg. 36:117, 1958.

Brock, R.C.: The Anatomy of the Bronchial Tree, 2nd ed. London, Oxford University Press, 1954.

Caudwell, E.W., et al.: The bronchial arteries. An anatomic study of 150 human cadavers. Surg. Gynecol. Obstet. 86:395, 1948.

Cory, R.A.S., and Valentine, E.J.: Varying patterns of the lobar branches of the pulmonary artery. Thorax 14:267, 1959.

Cudkowicz, L.: The Human Bronchial Circulation in Health and Disease. Baltimore, Williams & Wilkins, 1968.

Healey, J.E., Jr., and Gibbon, J.H., Jr.: Intrapericardial anatomy in relation to pneumonectomy for pulmonary carcinoma. J. Thorac. Surg. *19*:864, 1950.

Kent, E.M., and Blades, B.: The surgical anatomy of the pulmonary lobes. J. Thorac. Surg. *12*:18, 1942.

Kubik, S., and Healey, J.E.: Surgical Anatomy of the Thorax. Philadelphia, W.B. Saunders Co., 1970.

Milloy, F.J., Wragg, L.E., and Anson, B.J.: The pulmonary arterial supply to the right upper lobe of the lung based upon a study of 300 laboratory and surgical specimens. Surg. Gynecol. Obstet. *116*:35, 1963.

Milloy, F.J., Wragg, L.E., and Anson, B.J.: The pulmonary arterial supply to the upper lobe of the left lung. Surg. Gynecol. Obstet. *126*:811, 1968.

CHAPTER 5

LYMPHATICS OF THE LUNG

H. Christian Nohl-Oser

A thorough knowledge of the lymphatic drainage of the lungs is important when treating patients with lung cancer. Many other conditions also involve the intrathoracic lymph nodes, such as tuberculosis, sarcoidosis, silicosis, Hodgkin's disease, and other forms of lymphoma—a fact upon which diagnostic procedures such as scalene node biopsy and mediastinoscopy are based. Moreover, the adoption of the TNM—tumor-nodal involvement-metastases—system of staging of lung cancer makes the exact location of lymph node metastases essential. For this purpose various diagnostic methods are available in the clinical—prethoracotomy—staging, such as computed tomography—CT—scanning, magnetic resonance imaging—MRI, lymphatic scintigraphy and mediastinoscopy. Employment of one or all of the techniques makes it possible to relate the involved regional nodal stations to the larger anatomic structures in the chest.

The lung has a rich network of lymphatic vessels, which permeates its loose interstitial connective tissue. For some time it has been uncertain whether true alveolar lymphatics exist at the level of the "air-blood barrier." Lauweryns (1971), among others, has confirmed by electron microscopy that lymphatic capillaries are not present in the interalveolar septa. He found them, however, in the interlobular, pleural, peribronchial, and perivascular connective tissue sheaths, abutting the adult's alveolar wall. He therefore terms these microscopic vessels "juxta-alveolar lymphatic capillaries." They have monocuspid, conically shaped valves and their structure is entirely compatible with great permeability and active transport.

Without doubt, absorption of fluid, whether intra-alveolar fluid, transudate, or exudate, takes place through these "juxta-alveolar lymphatics." Meyer and associates (1969) had previously shown that ^{131}I tagged human albumin instilled into the alveoli is chiefly absorbed into the bloodstream at the level of the "air-blood barrier," but some is also taken up by the lymphatics. The efficiency of lymphatic absorption was actually found to be 37 times that of the blood.

Some knowledge of these microscopic channels has a bearing on certain clinical problems. That lymphatic obstruction alone can result in pleural effusions is shown by the rare but nonmalignant yellow nail syndrome. In the early stages, however, pulmonary extra-alveolar interstitial edema occurs; is recognizable in the chest roentgenograms as Kerley's B lines, as Steiner (1973) noted. These fine radiopaque lines are best seen in the costophrenic angles and are due to the increased opacity of the interlobular septa. They are caused either by lymphatic obstruction or by increased pulmonary capillary pressure and are, therefore, sometimes seen in association with malignant disease or with any cardiovascular condition leading to chronic pulmonary venous hypertension.

Malignant infiltration of the peribronchial or bronchial submucosal lymphatics is important to the surgeon, because spread along these vessels may be more advanced than is perceived by the naked eye. Cotton (1959), in an extensive study of the bronchial spread of lung cancer, showed that peribronchial spread is more common than submucosal extension, whereas Lange-Cordes (1956/57) found submucosal malignant infiltration at the point of section in over one fourth of 100 resected specimens. The practical implication from these studies is that section of the bronchus during lung resection for malignant disease should ideally be more than 2 cm proximal to the edge of the macroscopic growth.

Ultimately all these lymphatic channels drain into the various lymph node stations.

For anatomic description, the lymph nodes draining the lungs may be conveniently divided into two main groups: the pulmonary lymph nodes, which are confined within the visceral pleural reflections and are, therefore, invariably removed by a simple pneumonectomy—an extrapericardial resection without the removal of the mediastinal nodes; and the mediastinal lymph nodes. A published statement by Tisi and colleagues (1983), however, acting as members of a committee set up by the American Thoracic Society—ATS, proposes significant modifications in the conventional anatomic definitions of lymph node stations with special reference to clinical staging of lung cancer. By incorporating knowledge gained by the widespread use of mediastinoscopy and computed tomography, the reclassification aims at relating the location of certain lymph node stations to those major anatomic landmarks that can be identified by these diagnostic means. For instance, it is suggested that the traditional terms of "hilar" or "mediastinal" nodes be "avoided, because they lack clinical-anatomic specificity." A careful study of this lengthy and detailed document is recommended.

Of course, the ultimate object of any complex tumor staging is not merely the pursuit of accuracy for its own sake, but for the bearing that it may have on case selection for different forms of treatments. It may be that the ATS reclassification may succeed in its aims, but this will only become apparent with time. Meanwhile it seems reasonable to adhere to the established anatomic description until time proves that it does need modification.

PULMONARY LYMPH NODES

The pulmonary lymph nodes are divided into intrapulmonary and bronchopulmonary nodes, the latter being subdivided into hilar and interlobar nodes.

The intrapulmonary lymph nodes may be related to division of segmental or small bronchi, or may lie in the bifurcation of the branches of the pulmonary artery. Occasionally they are found under the pleura. The bronchopulmonary lymph nodes are situated either alongside the lower portions of the main bronchi, that is, within the pleural reflections—hilar lymph nodes—or in the angles formed by the bifurcation into lobar bronchi—interlobar nodes. The latter are, therefore, found in the depths of the interlobar fissures. These interlobar nodes make up the "lymphatic sump," first described by Borrie (1952). Because all lobes of the corresponding lung drain into this region, the nodes belonging to it warrant further description.

Anatomic Disposition of the Lymphatic Sumps

Right Sump

The lymph nodes pertaining to this region lie in relation to the bronchus intermedius. This area lies between the right upper lobe above and the right middle lobe and right superior segmental bronchus below. It is indicated in Figure 5–1 by a circle.

During lobar resection, a constant lymph node at the upper and posterior end of the great fissure forms an important landmark. It is invariably found in the angle between the right upper lobe bronchus and the bronchus intermedius. A bronchial artery coursing over the posterior aspect of the right main bronchus leads to it (Fig. 5–2). By careful dissection this node will be found on the interlobar portion of the pulmonary artery, where the artery gives off the posterior ascending segmental branch to the upper lobe and the superior—apical—branch to the lower lobe. This lymph node is contiguous—below—with a constant node lying above the su-

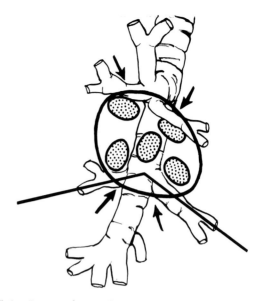

Fig. 5–1. Diagram showing the collection of lymph nodes comprising the right lymphatic sump (see text). The line drawn through the axis of the superior–apical–segmental bronchus of the lower lobe and the middle lobe bronchus represents the level below which nodes are not involved by malignant disease in the upper lobe. Arrows indicate tendency of lymphatic drainage.

perior—apical—segmental bronchus of the lower lobe (Fig. 5–3).

Other lymph nodes of the sump are found in the main fissure lying closely alongside the interlobar portion of the pulmonary artery or in the bifurcation of its branches, thus providing a useful guide to the artery during dissection of the fissure. These nodes have frequent connections with others lying more anteriorly among the upper lobe branches of the superior pulmonary vein (Fig. 5–4), and are related to the anterior segmental bronchus of the upper lobe. They are known to cause bronchiectasis of this segment by compression. Above they have

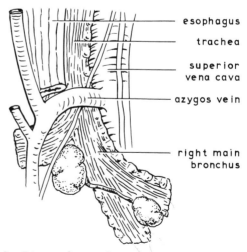

esophagus

trachea

superior vena cava

azygos vein

right main bronchus

Fig. 5–2. Diagram showing the posterior aspect of the right main bronchus, as seen when the lung is pulled forward during dissection. The subcarinal lymph node and the node below the right upper lobe bronchus are seen. A constant bronchial artery leading to the latter node is shown.

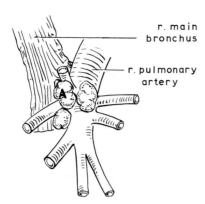

Fig. 5–3. Diagram showing the lymph nodes exposed when the main fissure of the right lung has been opened up. The node (A), which lies posteriorly in the angle between the upper lobe bronchus and the intermediate stem bronchus, is seen to cover the branches of the pulmonary artery to the posterior segement of the upper lobe and the superior segment of the lower lobe.

connections with the large node lying under the vena azygos (Fig. 5–5). Similarly, the middle lobe bronchus is surrounded by lymph nodes, which may compress it and cause atelectasis of the middle lobe, the so-called middle lobe syndrome, first described by Brock and co-workers (1937).

All three lobes of the right lung drain into this sump region. The drainage from the upper lobe involves the nodes lying on the lateral aspect of the bronchus inter-medius, whereas the lower lobe drains not only to these nodes, but also to those lying on its medial surface. These nodes are contiguous with the inferior tracheobronchial or subcarinal nodes.

Significantly, malignant tumors in the upper lobe do not metastasize to any nodes lying below a line drawn through the axis of the middle and superior segmental bronchus of the lower lobe (Fig. 5–1). This fact makes an upper lobectomy for early growths a sound procedure anatomically and pathologically. The nodes in the sump, however, have to be dissected from the pulmonary artery and its branches during an upper lobectomy. In the pres-

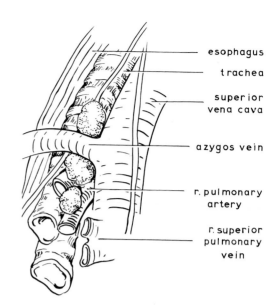

Fig. 5–5. Diagram illustrating the connections between the lymph nodes anterior to the right upper lobe bronchus and the right superior tracheobronchial node, which is situated medial to the azygos vein.

ence of obviously malignant nodes, a pneumonectomy achieves a better clearance.

For right lower lobe growths, a right lower and middle lobectomy provides complete ablation of all nodes in the sump; a simple lower lobectomy would not achieve this result.

Left Sump

The collection of lymph nodes that forms the left sump lies between the upper and lower lobes in the main fissure. This region is indicated by an oval circle in Figure 5–6. The following nodes are invariably present. A large constant node lies in the bifurcation between the upper and lower lobe bronchi and is, therefore, close to the origin of the bronchus of the lingula segment (Fig. 5–7). A bronchial artery, passing across the soft posterior part of the main bronchus, always leads to it. Other nodes are found lying on the pulmonary artery in the main fissure and in the angles formed by its branches. Another large constant node is found above and posterior to the main pulmonary artery, lying on the left main bronchus; on lifting it from these two structures a large bronchial artery is seen to course along the superolateral edge of the bronchus. This lymph node has connections below with a node lying in the angle between the superior— apical—segmental bronchus of the lower lobe and the stem bronchus. When dissecting the hilum of the left lung from behind, one frequently sees a large node lying between the inferior pulmonary vein and the main bron-chus. This node is contiguous above with the inferior tracheobronchial or subcarinal nodes.

The sump on the left side is confined to the main fissure, and since there is no bronchus intermedius as on the right, it is difficult to clear the nodes by lobectomy. As on the right side, however, few upper lobe growths metastasize below the level of the sump (Fig. 5–6).

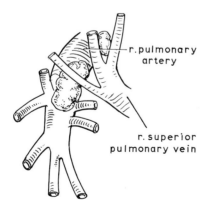

Fig. 5–4. Diagram showing the contiguity of lymph nodes lying on the right pulmonary artery in the main fissure with nodes lying higher up among the branches of the superior pulmonary vein.

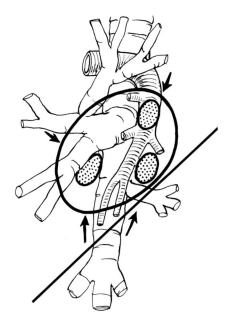

Fig. 5–6. Diagram illustrating the left lymphatic sump (see text), found by opening the main fissure. The straight line, drawn through the superior—apical—segmental bronchus of the left lower lobe, represents the level below which lymphatic drainage from the upper lobe does not occur. Arrows indicate tendency of lymphatic drainage.

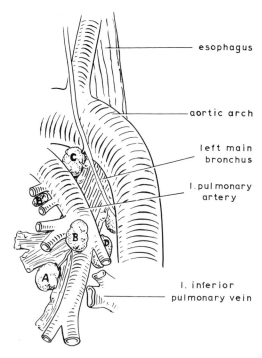

esophagus

aortic arch

left main bronchus

l. pulmonary artery

l. inferior pulmonary vein

Fig. 5–7. Diagram showing the lymph nodes most frequently seen on opening the main fissure of the left lung. A constant node (A) lies in the angle between the upper and lower lobe bronchi, with a bronchial artery leading to it. Other lymph nodes (B and B′) are found on the main pulmonary artery and in the angles of the branches. The constant node (C) behind and above the pulmonary artery, before it enters the fissure, is shown. Another node (D) above the inferior pulmonary vein is seen with its connections to the inferior tracheobronchial nodes higher up.

MEDIASTINAL LYMPH NODES

The mediastinal lymph nodes can be divided into the following groups: anterior mediastinal group, posterior mediastinal group, tracheobronchial nodes, and paratracheal nodes.

Anterior Mediastinal Nodes

These lymph nodes overlie the upper portions of the pericardium. On the right side they lie parallel and anterior to the phrenic nerve, whereas on the left they are in close proximity to the origin of the pulmonary artery and the ligamentum arteriosum. They extend upward near the phrenic nerve to nodes lying along the inferior border of the left innominate vein in the region where the left superior intercostal vein joins the left innominate vein (Fig. 5–8). The anterior mediastinal nodes lie, therefore, anterior to the great vessels in the superior mediastinum and are not accessible during conventional mediastinoscopy.

Posterior Mediastinal Nodes

These nodes are largely paraesophageal. They are less evident in the superior than in the inferior mediastinum. In the latter region they are found in the pulmonary ligament. These pulmonary ligament nodes, two to three in number, lie below the inferior pulmonary vein. The largest is in close proximity to this vein. They are far more frequently found on the left than on the right side and have connections with the para-aortic nodes in the abdomen. On the right side a paraesophageal node is occasionally found to lie retrotracheally in the region of the vena azygos arch.

Tracheobronchial Nodes

These nodes constitute the most important group of mediastinal nodes, especially since they are accessible

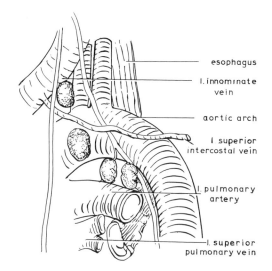

esophagus

l. innominate vein

aortic arch

l superior intercostal vein

l. pulmonary artery

l. superior pulmonary vein

Fig. 5–8. Diagram showing the mediastinal nodes on the left side. The superior tracheobronchial nodes, in relation to the recurrent laryngeal nerve, have connections with the anterior mediastinal group, which ascends upward to the left innominate vein.

for biopsy during mediastinoscopy. They lie in three groups about the bifurcation of the trachea.

The inferior tracheobronchial nodes are in the angle of the bifurcation of the trachea. They are, therefore, also known as bifurcation or subcarinal nodes (Fig. 5–9). They lie within the pretracheal fascial envelope but cannot be reached during mediastinoscopy without breaching the dense fibrous bronchopericardial membrane, which lies in front of them. This group may consist of several nodes, some of which lie on the posterior aspect of the carina and are, therefore, inaccessible to mediastinoscopic biopsy, as pointed out by Pearson (1968). The subcarinal nodes are contiguous with the hilar nodes on either side.

The superior tracheobronchial nodes, right and left, are located in the obtuse angle between the trachea and corresponding main bronchus. They lie, in contrast to the subcarinal nodes, outside the pretracheal fascia and can, therefore, only be reached by breaking through this fascia. On the right side the superior tracheobronchial nodes are medial to the arch of the vena azygos and above the right pulmonary artery. Brock and Whytehead (1955) describe in addition an anterior tracheal group, which lies in front of the lowest part of the trachea. This group constitutes the bridge of lymphatic tissue between the inferior tracheobronchial and the right superior tracheobronchial nodes. The left superior tracheobronchial nodes lie in the concavity of the aortic arch and are in a less compact group. Some are closely related to the left recurrent laryngeal nerve. Others are situated slightly more anteriorly and form a continuous link with the anterior mediastinal nodes in the region of the ligamentum arteriosum and the root of the left pulmonary artery.

Paratracheal Nodes

These nodes appear higher in the superior mediastinum. Those on the right lie anterolaterally to the trachea, inferior and to the right of the innominate artery, and are overlapped laterally by the superior vena cava. They are larger and more numerous than those on the left, which tend to be scanty. The right paratracheal nodes form the link between the superior tracheobronchial nodes below and the inferior deep cervical lymph nodes above. The latter lie outside the chest, and it is the medial group of the inferior deep cervical nodes that is frequently the site of metastases from bronchial carcinoma. These lymph nodes are on the scalenus anterior muscle, below the omohyoid, and are therefore also known as the scalene nodes.

LYMPHATIC DRAINAGE OF THE LUNGS TO THE MEDIASTINUM

The introduction of mediastinoscopy by Carlens (1959) has made it possible to study the lymphatic spread of lung cancer, from which some inferences on the lymphatic drainage of the lungs can be made. In 1972 I undertook and reported an analysis of 749 persons with bronchial carcinoma, in whom a mediastinoscopy or scalene node biopsy was performed. Figures 5–10 and 5–11 show the lymphatic spread of lung cancer to the nodes in the mediastinum from the right and left lung respectively, as found in this investigation. The figures given within each lymph node relate to the number of patients to have this particular group of nodes involved, each patient being represented only once in the diagram. If

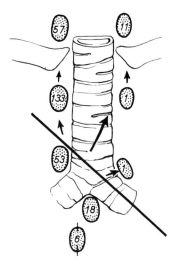

SUPERIOR MEDIASTINAL SPREAD

Ipsilateral —— 190 cases —— 45 %

Contralateral — 13 cases — 3 %

Fig. 5–10. Diagram showing the number and situation of nodes involved by cancer of the right lung in 423 patients, found either at scalene node biopsy or at mediastinoscopy. Superior mediastinal spread was considered to be present if any of the nodes above the straight line were involved. (Nohl-Oser, H.C.: An investigation of the anatomy of the lymphatic drainage of the lungs. Ann. R. Coll. Surg. Engl. 51:157, 1972.)

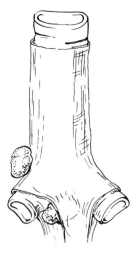

Fig. 5–9. Diagram illustrating the location of the inferior tracheobronchial nodes within the pretracheal fascial envelope and the superior tracheobronchial nodes outside this fascial layer. (Redrawn with permission from Sarrazin, R., and Voog, R.: La Mediastinoscopie. Paris, Masson et Cie, 1968, p. 8.)

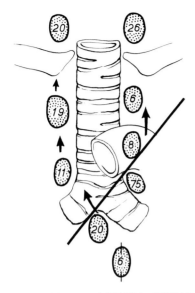

SUPERIOR MEDIASTINAL SPREAD

Ipsilateral —— 40 cases — 12·2 %

Contralateral — 50 cases — 15·3 %

Fig. 5–11. Diagram showing the number and situation of nodes involved by cancer of the left lung in 326 patients. For further explanation see legend of Fig. 5–10. (Nohl-Oser, H.C.: An investigation of the anatomy of the lymphatic drainage of the lungs. Ann. R. Coll. Surg. Engl. 51:157, 1972.)

in one patient more than one node was involved, only the farthest node from the primary growth was charted.

Maassen (1967) and Greschuchna and Maassen (1973) examined this problem in a similar way, so that a comparison between my series and those of Greschuchna and Maassen is possible. The findings of the two series are represented in Figures 5–12 and 5–13, where malignant spread to the mediastinum from each individual lobe is shown. The incidence of mediastinal spread in this instance is expressed in terms of the percentage of the total number of patients with mediastinal node involvement. Significant agreement on the general trend of mediastinal spread is apparent. This combined series comprises a total of 1356 patients.

Several conclusions can be drawn from these two series. Malignant disease in the right lung spreads mainly to the ipsilateral nodes of the mediastinum (Figs. 5–10 and 5–12). The superior tracheobronchial nodes, being the regional lymph node station, are readily involved. From there the lymphatic pathways lead up to the paratracheal nodes and finally to the right scalene or inferior deep cervical nodes. Growths in the lower and middle lobes often give rise to metastases in the inferior tracheobronchial—subcarinal—nodes. These are intermediate lymph node stations from which contralateral spread can also occur. According to the previously mentioned statement by the American Thoracic Society: "carinal involvement can be viewed, for all intents and purposes, as bilateral node involvement." Greschuchna and Maas-

sen (1973) noted spread to the opposite mediastinum in a quarter of the cases when the middle lobe was involved. The limited number of patients—12—in my series precludes any deductions. Tumors in the lower and middle lobes may also involve the nodes in the pulmonary ligament, which in turn have a direct connection with the para-aortic nodes in the abdomen. Sarrazin and associates (1974) confirmed this subdiaphragmatic spread by routine abdominal exploration, while Bethune and colleagues (1978) demonstrated the existence of lymphatic pathways to the para-aortic nodes by endobronchial lymphoscintigraphy.

In contrast, when malignant disease involves the left lung, contralateral lymphatic spread occurs as frequently as spread on the same side (Figs. 5–11 and 5–13). The regional left superior tracheobronchial nodes are often involved. The mode of spread differs also in other respects from that of the right side. Upper lobe tumors metastasize often to the inferior tracheobronchial—subcarinal—nodes and also to the anterior mediastinal group. The spread of left upper lobe tumors to the anterior mediastinal nodes has also been commented upon by both Pearson and associates (1972) and Sarrazin and associates (1974). It can also be verified preoperatively by anterior mediastinotomy, as these nodes are inaccessible by cervical mediastinoscopy. For that reason some authors, among them Bowen and colleagues (1978) and Pagé and collaborators (1980) advise an anterior mediastinotomy in addition to a mediastinoscopy in the preoperative assessment of patients with left upper lobe tumors. Upward spread to the left scalene nodes probably takes place through the anterior mediastinal nodes, because the left paratracheal nodes are rarely involved (Fig. 5–14).

Malignant lesions in the left lower lobe have an even greater tendency to contralateral spread. They may also involve the posterior mediastinal nodes in the pulmonary ligament, which are, as already mentioned, much more prominent on the left than on the right side. From here descending spread to the para-aortic nodes was found by Sarrazin and associates (1974) in 15% of patients with right lower and middle lobe tumors and in 20% in the presence of a left lower lobe growth.

Finally, a more recent study by Hata and collaborators (1981) tackled this problem in an entirely different way. They investigated the lymphatic drainage of the bronchial system by in-vivo experiments in humans, using the method of endobronchial lymphoscintigraphy as elaborated by Bethune and colleagues (1978). In 142 normal individuals, with no hilar or mediastinal node enlargement on the chest radiogram, a depot of ^{99m}Tc antimony sulfide in colloidal form was injected into the chosen segmental bronchus through a flexible fiber-optic bronchoscope. Hourly scanning of the chest over a period of 6 hours completed the examination. In all 160 scintigrams were carried out, approximately eight investigations for each segment. The data of this study largely support the evidence gained from the above clinical findings.

In conclusion, both investigations must be considered

GRESCHUCHNA and MAASSEN (1973)   NOHL-OSER (1972)

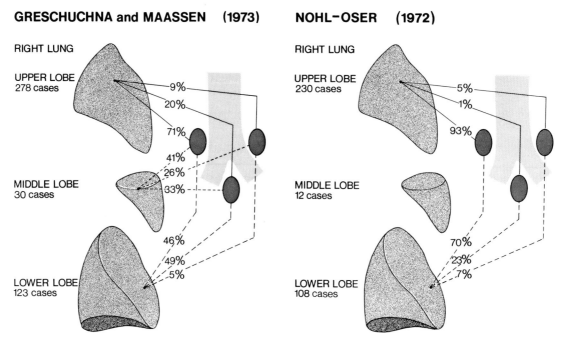

Fig. 5–12. Comparison between two large series showing the mediastinal spread of bronchial carcinoma, as determined by mediastinoscopy or scalene node biopsy, when involving the right lung. The incidence of spread from each lobe to the various mediastinal nodes is here expressed as the percentage of the total number of patients with mediastinal node involvement.

GRESCHUCHNA and MAASSEN (1973)   NOHL-OSER (1972)

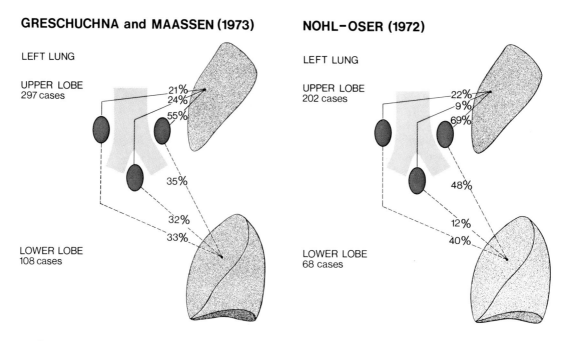

Fig. 5–13. Mediastinal spread of bronchial carcinoma involving the left lung. For further explanation see legend for Fig. 5–12.

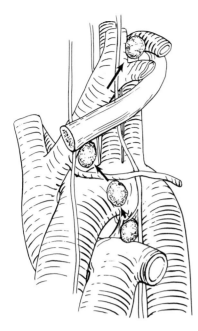

Fig. 5–14. Diagram showing the ascending lymphatic pathways toward the left scalene node region via the anterior mediastinal nodes.

to have considerable practical implications in the surgical assessment of patients with lung cancer.

REFERENCES

Bethune, D.C.G., Mulder, D.S., and Chiu, R.C.J.: Endobronchial lymphoscintigraphy (LEBS): new diagnostic modality. J. Thorac. Cardiovasc. Surg. 76:446, 1978.

Borrie, J.: Primary carcinoma of the bronchus: prognoses following surgical resection. Ann. R. Coll. Surg. Engl. 10:165, 1952.

Bowen, T.E., et al.: Value of anterior mediastinotomy in bronchogenic carcinoma of the left upper lobe. J. Thorac. Cardiovasc. Surg. 76:269, 1978.

Brock, R.C., Cann, R.J., and Dickinson, J.R.: Tuberculous mediastinal lymphadenitis in childhood, secondary effects on the lung. Guy's Hosp. Rep. 87:295, 1937.

Brock, R.C., and Whytehead, L.L.: Radical pneumonectomy for bronchial carcinoma. Br. J. Surg. 43:8, 1955.

Carlens, E.: Mediastinoscopy: a method of inspection and tissue biopsy in the superior mediastinum. Dis. Chest 36:343, 1959.

Cotton, R.E.: The bronchial spread of lung cancer. Br. J. Dis. Chest 53:142, 1959.

Greschuchna, D., and Maassen, W.: Die lymphogenen Absiedlungswege des Bronchialkarzinoms. Stuttgart, Georg Thieme Verlag, 1973.

Hata, E., Troidl, H., and Hasegawa, T.: In vivo Untersuchungen der Lymphdrainage des Bronchialsystems beim Menschen mit der LymphoSzintigraphie: eine neue diagnostische Technik. In Behandlung des Bronchialkarzinoms. Resignation oder neue Ansätze. Symposium Kiel. Stuttgart, G. Thieme Verlag, 1981.

Lange-Cordes, E.: Über die intramuköse Ausbreitung der Bronchialcarcinome. Thoraxchirurgie 4:327, 1956/57.

Lauweryns, J.M.: The blood and lymphatic microcirculation of the lung. Pathol. Annu. 6:365, 1971.

Maassen, W.: Die Tuberkulose und ihre Grenzgebiete in Einzeldarstellungen, Band 19. Ergebnisse und Bedeutung der Mediastinoskopie und anderer thoraxbioptischer Verfahren. Berlin, Springer-Verlag, 1967.

Meyer, E.C., Dominguez, E.A.M., and Bensch, K.G.: Pulmonary lymphatic and blood absorption of albumin from alveoli, a quantitative comparison. Lab. Invest. 20:1, 1969.

Nohl-Oser, H.C.: An investigation of the anatomy of the lymphatic drainage of the lungs. Ann. R. Coll. Surg. Engl. 51:157, 1972.

Pagé, A., et al.: Parasternal mediastinoscopy in bronchial carcinoma of the left upper lobe. Canad. J. Surg. 23:171, 1980.

Pearson, F.G.: An evaluation of mediastinoscopy in the management of presumably operable bronchial carcinoma. J. Thorac. Cardiovasc. Surg. 55:617, 1968.

Pearson, F.G., et al.: The role of mediastinoscopy in the selection of treatment for bronchial carcinoma. J. Thorac. Cardiovasc. Surg. 64:382, 1972.

Sarrazin, R., Voog, R., and Dyon, J.F.: Contribution à l'étude des lymphatique du poumon. Poumon. Coeur 30:289, 1974.

Steiner, R.E.: The radiology of the pulmonary circulation. In A Textbook of X-ray Diagnosis, 4th ed., Vol. 2. Edited by S.C. Shanks and P. Kerley. London, H.K. Lewis & Co., Ltd., 1973, p. 121.

Tisi, G.M., et al.: Clinical staging of primary lung cancer. Am. Rev. Resp. Dis. 127:659, 1983.

CHAPTER 6

SURGICAL ANATOMY OF THE ESOPHAGUS

Martin Rothberg and Thomas R. DeMeester

RADIOGRAPHIC AND ENDOSCOPIC ANATOMY OF THE ESOPHAGUS

The esophagus starts as the continuation of the pharynx and ends at the cardia of the stomach. When the head is in normal anatomic position, the transition from pharynx to esophagus occurs at the lower border of the sixth cervical vertebra. Topographically this corresponds to the cricoid cartilage anteriorly and the carotid tubercle, the palpable transverse process of the sixth cervical vertebra, laterally (Fig. 6–1A,B). Flexion and extension of the neck will shift this point craniad or caudad by the length of one cervical vertebral body. After traversing the thorax and passing through the diaphragm, the esophagus terminates in the stomach at the level of the eleventh thoracic vertebra. The esophagus is firmly attached only at its upper and lower ends; during swallowing, these points of fixation move craniad the distance of one cervical vertebral body.

The configuration of the resting esophagus is determined by the contiguous structures it passes and the environmental pressure of the cavities it traverses. On a barium esophagogram, the cervical portion of the esophagus is flattened, owing to compression by adjacent structures; the thoracic portion is more rounded, owing to the negative intrathoracic pressure; and the abdominal portion is flattened, owing to the positive intra-abdominal pressure.

On the anteroposterior roentgenogram, the esophagus lies in the midline with a deviation to the left in the lower portion of the neck and upper portion of the thorax, and returns to the midline in the midportion of the thorax near the bifurcation of the trachea (Fig. 6–2A). In the lower portion of the thorax, the esophagus again deviates to the left to pass through the diaphragmatic hiatus.

On the lateral roentgenogram, the esophagus follows the curve of the vertebral column, except in the lower thoracic area where it curves anteriorly to pass through the diaphragmatic hiatus (Fig. 6–2B). This posterior curve and its terminal left anterior deviation is of importance in the performance of rigid esophagoscopy. The patient should be positioned to allow extension of the cervical and thoracic spine so that the rigid scope can be manipulated through this terminal arc. This region is the second most common site for traumatic esophageal perforation during rigid endoscopy, the first being the narrow entrance of the esophagus at the level of the cricopharyngeus.

Three normal areas of esophageal narrowing appear on the barium esophagogram and at esophagoscopy. The uppermost narrowing is located at the entrance into the esophagus and is caused by the cricopharyngeal muscle. Its luminal diameter is 1.5 cm and it is the narrowest point of the esophagus. The middle narrowing is due to an indentation of the anterior and left lateral esophageal wall caused by the crossing of the left main stem bronchus and aortic arch. The luminal diameter at this point is 1.6 cm. The lowermost narrowing of the esophagus is at the hiatus of the diaphragm and is caused by the gastroesophageal sphincter mechanism. The luminal diameter at this point varies somewhat depending on the distention of the esophagus by the passage of food, but has been measured at 1.6 to 1.9 cm. These normal constrictions tend to hold up swallowed foreign objects, and the overlying mucosa is subjected to injury by swallowed corrosive liquids because of their slow passage through these areas.

Measurements obtained during endoscopic examination (Fig. 6–3) show the average distance from the incisor teeth to the cardia of the stomach is 38 to 40 cm in men and generally 2 cm shorter in women. These distances are proportionately shorter in children, being 18 cm at birth, 22 cm at age 3 years, and 27 cm at 10 years. In men, the length of the esophagus from the cricopharyngeus muscle to the cardia ranges from 23 to 30 cm with an average of 25 cm. In women the range is 20 to 26 cm with an average of 23 cm. The distance from the incisor teeth to the cricopharyngeus is 15 cm in men and 1 cm shorter in women. The bifurcation of the trachea and the indentation of the aortic arch ranges between 24 and 26 cm from the incisor teeth. It is helpful to locate an intraluminal lesion in reference to this landmark in

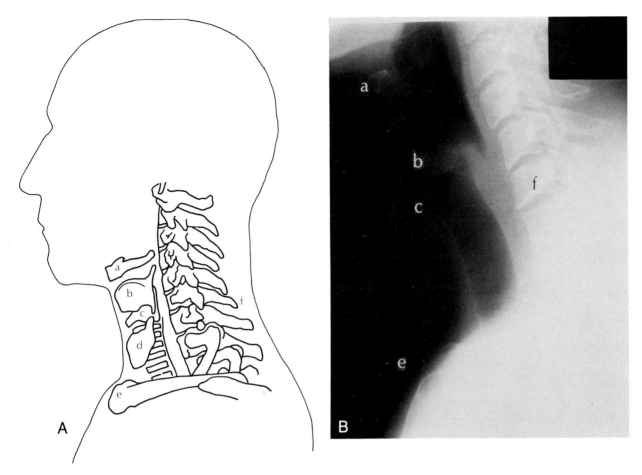

Fig. 6–1. *A*, Topographic relationships of the cervical esophagus: (a) hyoid bone, (b) thyroid cartilage, (c) cricoid cartilage, (d) thyroid gland, (e) sternomanubrial joint, (f) C6. *B*, Lateral radiographic appearance.

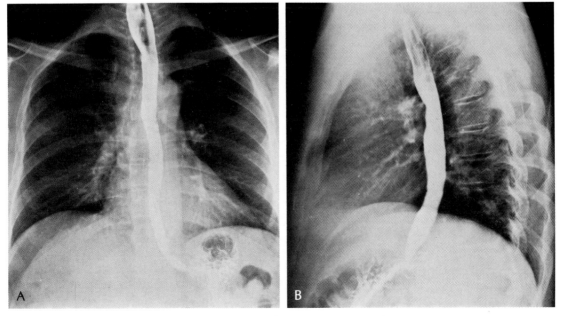

Fig. 6–2. Barium esophagogram. *A*, Anteroposterior view. *B*, Lateral view.

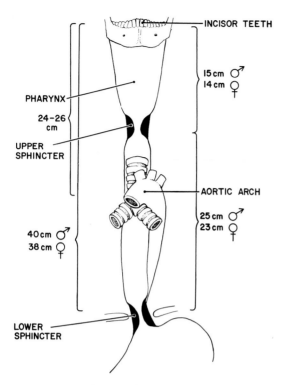

Fig. 6–3. Important clinical endoscopic measurements of the esophagus in adults.

order to decide on a left or right thoracotomy approach and avoid interference from the aortic arch.

RELATIONSHIP OF THE ESOPHAGUS TO THE HYPOPHARYNX

The esophagus serves as a conduit between the pharynx and the stomach. As such, the esophagus represents an extension of the hypopharynx beginning at the lower border of the larynx at the level of the sixth cervical vertebra. The pharyngeal musculature consists of three overlapping, broad, flat, fan-shaped constrictors (Fig. 6–4). They are the superior constrictor arising mainly from the medial pterygoid plate, the middle constrictor arising from the hyoid bone, and the inferior constrictor arising from the thyroid and cricoid cartilages. These muscles insert with their corresponding muscle from the opposite side into a median posterior raphe.

The opening of the esophagus is collared by the cricopharyngeal muscle, which arises from both sides of the cricoid cartilage of the larynx and forms a continuous transverse muscle band without an interruption by a median raphe. The fibers of this muscle blend inseparably with those of the inferior pharyngeal constrictor above and the inner circular muscle fibers of the esophagus below. Thus, some investigators believe that the cricopharyngeus is part of the inferior constrictor; that is, the inferior constrictor has two parts, an upper or retrothyroid portion having diagonal fibers, and a lower or retrocricoid portion having transverse fibers. Keith (1910) has shown that these two parts of the same muscle

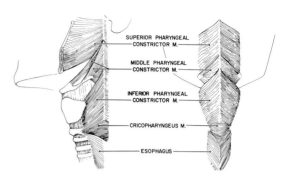

Fig. 6–4. External muscles of the pharynx.

serve totally different functions. The retrocricoid portion serves as the upper sphincter of the esophagus and relaxes when the retrothyroid portion contracts to force the swallowed bolus from the pharynx into the esophagus.

RELATIONSHIP OF THE CERVICAL ESOPHAGUS TO STRUCTURES AND FASCIAL PLANES OF THE NECK

The cervical portion of the esophagus is approximately 5 cm long and descends between the trachea and the vertebral column from the level of the sixth cervical vertebra to the level of the interspace between the first and second thoracic vertebrae posteriorly, or the suprasternal notch anteriorly. It is separated from the posterior wall of the trachea by loose fibrous tissue, and from the prevertebral fascia by loose alar fascia. The recurrent laryngeal nerves lie in the right and left grooves between the trachea and the esophagus. The left recurrent nerve lies somewhat closer to the esophagus than the right owing to the slight deviation of the esophagus to the left and the more lateral course of the right recurrent nerve around the right subclavian artery. Laterally, on the left and right side of the esophagus are the carotid sheaths and the lobes of the thyroid gland.

Anteriorly, the cervical esophagus and trachea are bounded by the pretracheal fascia, which splits to envelop the thyroid gland, then continues down to the aortic arch. Posteriorly, both are bound by the prevertebral fascia, and laterally by the fascia forming the carotid sheath (Fig. 6–5A, B). The buccopharyngeal fascia, which lies over the posterior pharyngeal muscles, extends inferiorly, directly on the posterior wall of the esophagus and laterally to the carotid sheaths, and separates the esophagus from the prevertebral fascia. These fascial planes form two spaces: a paraesophageal space containing the thyroid gland, larynx, trachea, and part of the pharynx, and a retroesophageal space. This latter space is continuous with the retropharyngeal space at the base of the skull above and the superior mediastinum below. These spaces allow an access for extension of infection into the mediastinum.

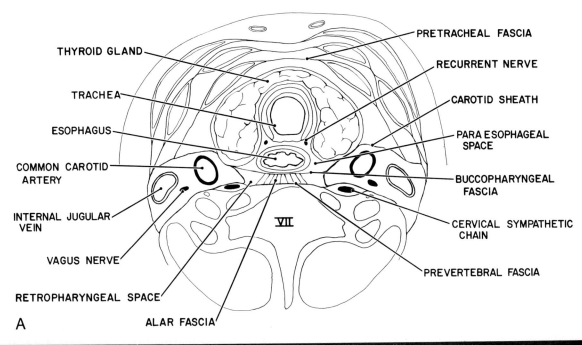

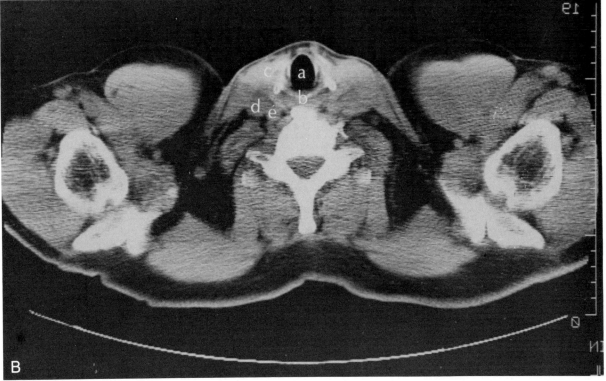

Fig. 6–5. *A*, Cross section of the neck at the level of the thyroid isthmus. *B*, CT appearance viewed from above: (a) trachea, (b) esophagus, (c) left thyroid lobe, (d) internal jugular vein, (e) common carotid artery.

RELATIONSHIP OF THE THORACIC ESOPHAGUS TO MEDIASTINAL STRUCTURES

From the thoracic inlet to the tracheal bifurcation the thoracic esophagus remains in intimate relationship with the posterior wall of the trachea and the prevertebral fascia. Just above the tracheal bifurcation, the esophagus passes to the right of the aorta. This anatomic positioning can cause a notch indentation in its left lateral wall on a barium swallow roentgenogram. Immediately below this notch the esophagus crosses both the bifurcation of the trachea and the left main stem bronchus, owing to the slight deviation of the terminal portion of the trachea to the right by the aorta (Fig. 6–6A,B). From there down the esophagus passes over the posterior surface of the subcarinal lymph nodes, and then descends over the pericardium of the left atrium to reach the diaphragmatic hiatus (Fig. 6–7A,B).

The right lateral surface of the thoracic esophagus is completely covered by the parietal pleura except at the level of the fourth thoracic vertebra where the azygos vein turns anteriorly over the esophagus to join the superior vena cava. The left lateral surface of the upper portion of the thoracic esophagus is covered anterolaterally by the left subclavian artery and posterolaterally by the parietal pleura. The distal portion of the esophagus, from the aortic arch down, lies to the right of the descending thoracic aorta. At the level of the eighth thoracic vertebra, the aorta disappears behind the esophagus, and its left lateral wall is covered only with the parietal pleura of the mediastinum and is the common site of perforation in Boerhaave's syndrome. From the bifurcation of the trachea downward, both the vagal nerves and the esophageal nerve plexus lie on the muscular wall of the esophagus.

Posteriorly, the thoracic esophagus follows the curvature of the spine and remains in close contact with the vertebral bodies (Figs. 6–6 and 6–7). From the eighth thoracic vertebra downward the esophagus moves ventrally away from the spine and passes through the esophageal hiatus of the diaphragm in front of the aorta (Fig. 6–8). The inferior vena cava, while not in apposition to the esophagus, lies anterior and to its right. Dorsally, the esophagus is crossed by the first five intercostal arteries and the hemiazygos vein. The thoracic duct passes through the hiatus of the diaphragm on the anterior surface of the vertebral column behind the aorta and under the right crus. In the thorax it lies dorsal to the esophagus between the azygos vein on the right and the descending thoracic aorta on the left. From the level of the fifth thoracic vertebra upward, the thoracic duct gradually moves to the left and settles between the esophagus and the left parietal pleura, dorsal to the aortic arch and the intrathoracic part of the subclavian artery. In the neck it turns away from the esophagus and joins the venous system at the junction of the subclavian and internal jugular veins.

RELATIONSHIP OF THE TERMINAL ESOPHAGUS TO THE DIAPHRAGMATIC HIATUS AND STOMACH

The muscular fibers forming the crura of the diaphragm arise by tendinous bands from the anterolateral surface of the first three or four lumbar vertebrae and their intervening fibrocartilages (Fig. 6–8). The right crus is longer and thicker than the left and the inferior extension of its fibers gives rise to the ligament of Treitz. The upper abdominal aorta lies at the base of the diaphragmatic hiatus just anterior to the vertebral bodies. The celiac and superior mesenteric arteries, as they arise from the upper abdominal aorta, separate the muscle bundles of the right and left crura. In many situations, a well-marked median arcuate ligament or tendinous rim of the diaphragm unites the two crura anterior to the aorta just above the celiac artery. The cadaver dissections described by Lindner and Kemprud (1971) show that in most situations the median arcuate ligament was a firm, well-defined ligamentous structure, but in several cadavers it was difficult to identify any definite connective tissue structure.

As the right crus ascends, it divides into a superficial and deep muscle layer. The superficial layer, by a gradual anterior curve, forms the muscular rim of the right edge of the esophageal hiatus. The deep layer inclines obliquely to the left over the anterior surface of the abdominal aorta and then ascends to form the left margin of the esophageal hiatus. The left crus ascends vertically against the fibers to the left margin of the hiatus. This anatomy is found in only about 46% of individuals, and marked variability exists. The most common anatomic variant is a shift to the left of various degrees depending on the extent to which the margins of the hiatus are formed by muscle fibers from the left crus.

As the esophagus passes through the diaphragmatic hiatus, it is surrounded by the phrenoesophageal membrane, a fibroelastic ligament arising from the subdiaphragmatic fascia as a continuation of the transversalis fascia lining the abdomen (Fig. 6–9). The phrenoesophageal membrane divides at the lower margin of the esophageal hiatus into a stout elongated ascending leaf that surrounds the terminal segment of the esophagus in a tent-like fashion, and into a shorter, thin, descending leaf, which merges as the visceral peritoneal covering of the stomach. The upper leaf of the membrane attaches itself in a circumferential fashion around the esophagus, about 1 to 2 cm above the level of the hiatus. Between the upper leaf of the membrane and the cardia is a ring of fatty tissue interspersed with fibers from the lower leaf of the membrane. These fibers blend in with the elastic-containing adventitia of the distal 2 cm of the esophagus and the cardia of the stomach. This makes up the abdominal portion of the esophagus and is subjected to the positive pressure environment of the abdomen.

At the gastroesophageal junction the outer longitudinal muscle fibers of the esophagus are continuous with the outer longitudinal muscle fibers of the stomach, and the inner circular fibers of the esophagus interlace with and

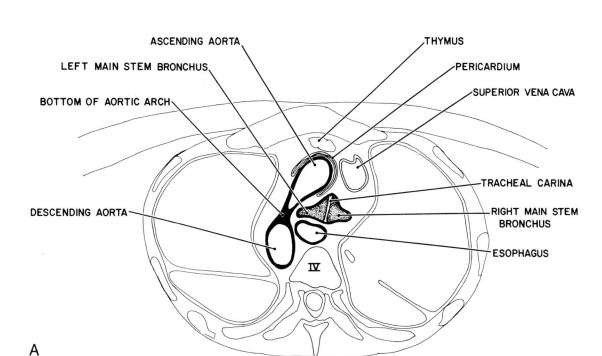

ASCENDING AORTA
THYMUS
LEFT MAIN STEM BRONCHUS
PERICARDIUM
BOTTOM OF AORTIC ARCH
SUPERIOR VENA CAVA
TRACHEAL CARINA
DESCENDING AORTA
RIGHT MAIN STEM BRONCHUS
ESOPHAGUS

A

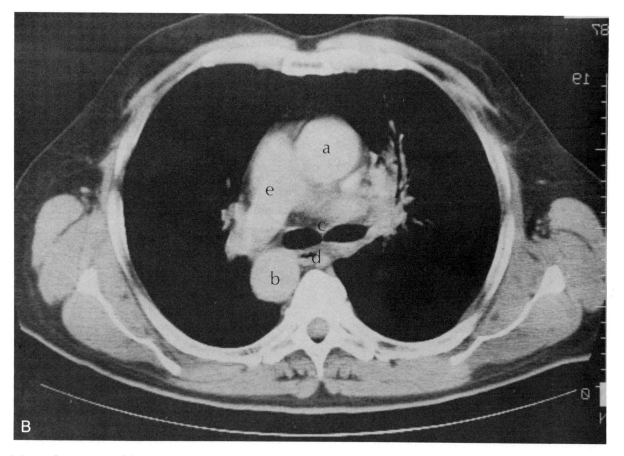

B

Fig. 6–6. *A*, Cross section of the thorax at the level of the tracheal bifurcation. *B*, CT appearance viewed from above: (a) ascending aorta, (b) descending aorta, (c) tracheal carina, (d) esophagus, (e) pulmonary artery.

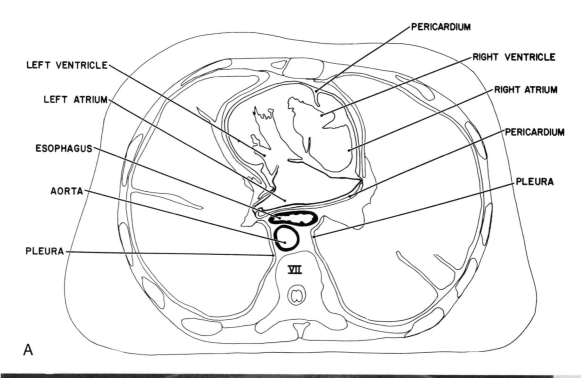

LEFT VENTRICLE

LEFT ATRIUM

ESOPHAGUS

AORTA

PLEURA

PERICARDIUM

RIGHT VENTRICLE

RIGHT ATRIUM

PERICARDIUM

PLEURA

VII

A

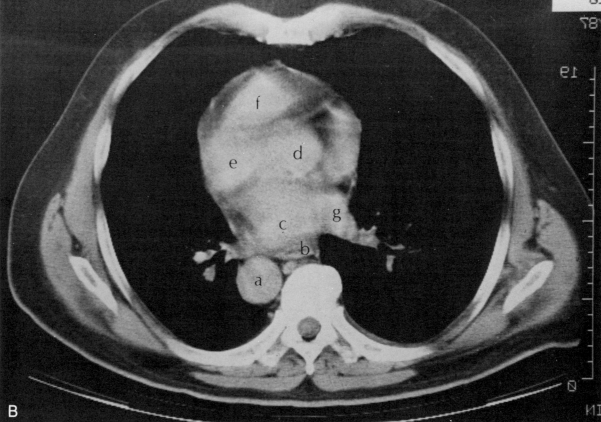

B

Fig. 6–7. *A*, Cross section of the thorax at mid-left arterial level. *B*, CT appearance viewed from above: (a) aorta, (b) esophagus, (c) left atrium, (d) right atrium, (e) left ventricle, (f) right ventricle, (g) pulmonary vein.

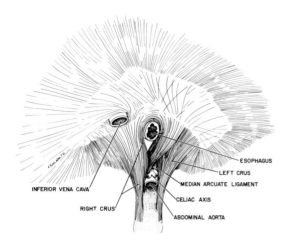

Fig. 6–8. The diaphragm and esophageal hiatus seen from below.

are eventually replaced by the inner oblique gastric fibers that arise in the direction of the gastric fundus (Fig. 6–10). For a distance of 1.5 cm caudad from the insertion of the upper phrenoesophageal membrane the muscular wall of the cardia gradually becomes thicker because of increased density of the esophageal circular musculature on the lesser curvature side and the gastric oblique musculature on the greater curvature side. The line of maximal muscular thickness has an oblique orientation so that on the greater curvature side it is more cephalad than on the lesser curvature side. It is also asymmetrical in that the muscle mass on the side of the greater curvature is larger (Fig. 6–10). The function of this asymmetrical oblique muscle thickening is difficult to determine but Liebermann-Meffert and her associates (1979) have pointed out some relationships of interest. The manometrically defined distal esophageal high pressure zone is located in this area, and the length of the high pressure zone is similar to that of the thickening. The highest pressure in the high pressure zone is found in the area of the greatest thickening, that is, on the side of the greater curvature of the stomach. Therefore, this muscle thickening might, at least in part, coincide with the lower esophageal sphincter. Some authors ascribe to this muscular arrangement a role in the anti-reflux mechanism. Other factors contributing to the closing mechanism of the cardia are: the intra-abdominal portion of

the esophagus, the rosette-like configuration of the gastric mucosa around the orifice of the cardia, the sharp angle between the lower esophagus and the gastric fundus, and the phrenoesophageal membrane and its configuration with the esophageal hiatus at the diaphragm. None of these latter structures, however, can be considered a definite anatomic sphincter.

MUSCULATURE OF THE ESOPHAGUS

The musculature of the esophagus can be divided into an outer longitudinal and an inner circular layer. The upper 2 to 6 cm of the esophagus contains only striated muscle fibers. From there on smooth muscle fibers gradually become more abundant and at a distance of 4 to 8 cm from the superior end, or at the junction of the upper and lower two-thirds, the smooth musculature constitutes 50% of the esophageal muscle. The transition of striated to smooth muscle in the inner circular layer is at a higher level than in the outer longitudinal layer. Most of the clinically significant esophageal motility disorders involve only the smooth muscle in the lower two thirds of the esophagus. When a surgical esophageal myotomy is indicated, the incision usually needs only to extend this distance.

The longitudinal muscle fibers originate from a cricoesophageal tendon arising from the dorsal upper edge of the anteriorly located cricoid cartilage. The two bundles of muscles diverge and meet in the midline on the posterior wall of the esophagus about 3 cm below the cricoid (Fig. 6–4). From this point on, the entire circumference of the esophagus is covered by a layer of longitudinal muscle fibers. This configuration of the longitudinal muscle fibers around the most proximal part of the esophagus leaves a V-shaped area in the posterior wall covered only with circular muscle fibers. In the upper third of the esophagus the longitudinal muscle layer is thicker on the lateral surface than on the ventral or dorsal surfaces. In the lower two-thirds the longitudinal layer becomes more uniform and its overall thickness decreases distally. The course of the longitudinal muscle fibers is that of an elongated spiral, turning to the left around one quarter of the esophageal circumference—90 degrees—as they descend.

The circular muscle layer of the esophagus is thicker than the outer longitudinal layer. These fibers run horizontally only in the isolated and retracted esophagus. In situ, their course is elliptical and spiral with an inclination that varies according to the level of the esophagus: in the cervical portion the highest point of the ellipse is dorsal, in the upper thoracic portion the highest point is right lateral, behind the heart ventral, and in the abdomen the fibers are horizontal. The arrangement of both the longitudinal and circular muscle fibers makes the peristalsis of the esophagus assume a worm-like drive as opposed to segmental and sequential squeezing. As a consequence, severe motor abnormalities of the esophagus assume a corkscrew-like pattern on the barium swallow roentgenogram.

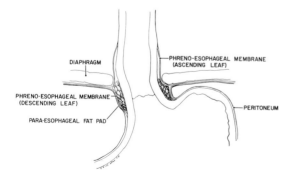

Fig. 6–9. Attachments and structure of the phrenoesophageal membrane.

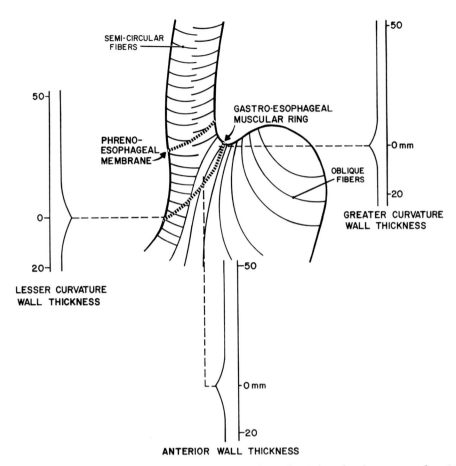

Fig. 6–10. The inner muscular fiber arrangement, and muscular thickness at the cardia. (Adapted with permission from Lieberman-Meffert, D., et al.: Muscular equivalent of the lower esophageal sphincter. Gastroenterology 76:31, 1979.)

ARTERIAL BLOOD SUPPLY OF THE ESOPHAGUS

The cervical portion of the esophagus receives its main blood supply from the inferior thyroid artery with smaller accessory branches from the common carotid, subclavian and superficial cervical arteries. The thoracic portion receives its blood supply from the bronchial arteries with 75% of individuals having one right-sided and one or two left-sided branches. Two esophageal branches arise directly from the aorta. The upper branch is usually the shorter and originates at the level between the sixth and seventh thoracic vertebrae; the lower is longer and originates at the level between the eighth and ninth thoracic vertebrae. The abdominal portion of the esophagus receives its blood supply mainly from esophageal branches of the left gastric and inferior phrenic arteries (Fig. 6–11). On entering the wall of the esophagus the arteries assume a T-shaped division to form longitudinal anastomoses giving rise to an intramural vascular network in the muscular and submucosal layers. As a consequence the esophagus can be mobilized from the stomach to the level of the aortic arch without fear of devascularization and ischemic necrosis. Caution should be exercised as to the extent of esophageal mobilization in patients who have had a previous thyroidectomy and ligation of the

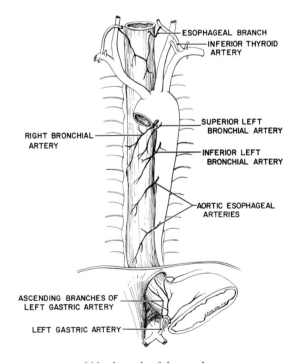

Fig. 6–11. Arterial blood supply of the esophagus.

inferior thyroid arteries proximal to the origin of the esophageal branches.

VENOUS DRAINAGE OF THE ESOPHAGUS

Blood from the capillaries of the esophagus flows into a submucosal venous plexus and then into a periesophageal venous plexus from which the esophageal veins originate. In the cervical region, the esophageal veins empty into the inferior thyroid vein; in the thoracic region into the bronchial, azygos, or hemiazygos veins; and in the abdominal region into the coronary vein (Fig. 6–12). The submucosal venous networks of the esophagus and stomach are in continuity with each other, and in patients with portal venous obstruction, this communication functions as a collateral pathway for portal blood to enter the superior vena cava via the azygos vein.

NERVE SUPPLY OF THE ESOPHAGUS

The constrictor muscles of the pharynx receive branches from the pharyngeal plexus, which is on the posterior lateral surface of the middle constrictor muscle and is formed by pharyngeal branches of the vagus nerves with a small contribution from the ninth and eleventh cranial nerves (Fig. 6–13).

The complete parasympathetic innervation of the esophagus is provided by the vagus nerves. The cricopharyngeal sphincter and the cervical portion of the esophagus receive branches from both recurrent laryngeal nerves, which originate from the vagus nerves; the right recurrent nerve at the lower margin of the subclavian artery, the left at the lower margin of the aortic arch. They are slung dorsally around these vessels and ascend in the groove between the esophagus and trachea giving branches to each. Damage to these nerves not only interferes with the function of the vocal cords but

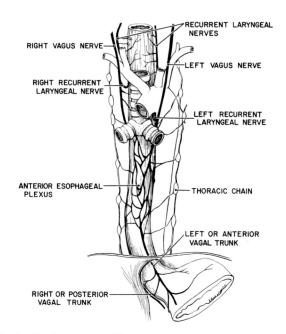

Fig. 6–13. Innervation of the esophagus.

also interferes with the function of the cricopharyngeal sphincter and the motility of the cervical esophagus, causing a predisposition to pulmonary aspiration on swallowing.

The upper thoracic esophagus receives branches from the left recurrent laryngeal nerve and directly from both vagus nerves as they descend through the superior mediastinum. The lower thoracic esophagus is innervated by the esophageal plexus located directly on both the anterior and posterior esophageal wall and formed by both vagal nerves after they pass behind the hilum of the lung and turn medially to reach the esophagus. The esophageal plexus also receives fibers from the thoracic sympathetic chain. The left vagus nerve splits before the esophageal plexus to form two branches: the first branch runs through the ventral esophageal plexus and constitutes the main element of the anterior or left abdominal vagal trunk; the second branch runs around the left esophageal wall, to join the dorsal esophageal plexus, and contributes to the formation of the posterior or right abdominal vagal trunk. As a result of the intertwining of fibers from both the left and right vagus in the esophageal plexus, both the left or anterior and right or posterior abdominal vagal trunks contain fibers of the original left and right vagus. The average distance above the diaphragm at which the left or anterior vagal trunk becomes a single nerve is 5.13 cm, and the right or posterior vagal trunk is 3.7 cm.

The preganglionic sympathetic fibers supplying the esophagus take origin from the fourth to the sixth spinal cord segments and terminate in the cervical and thoracic sympathetic ganglions. The pharyngeal plexus receives sympathetic fibers that arrive directly from the superior cervical ganglion via vagal nerves. The postganglionic fibers reach the esophagus via nerve branches that veer off from the cervical and thoracic sympathetic chain:

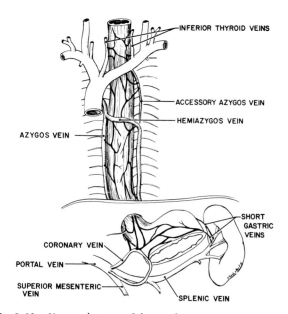

Fig. 6–12. Venous drainage of the esophagus.

some reach the esophageal wall directly; others join the vagal trunks. Thus the vagal nerves caudad from their entrance into the neck always contain a number of post-ganglionic sympathetic fibers. The distal esophageal segments also receive direct sympathetic fibers coming from the celiac ganglion. These fibers reach the esophagus via the periarterial plexus around the left gastric and phrenic arteries.

Afferent visceral sensory pain fibers from the esophagus end without synapse in the first four segments of the thoracic spinal cord by using a combination of sympathetic and vagal pathways. These pathways are also occupied by afferent visceral sensory fibers from the heart; hence, both organs have similar symptomatology.

LYMPHATIC DRAINAGE OF THE ESOPHAGUS

The detailed lymphatic anatomy of the esophagus and its lymphatic drainage is discussed in Chapter 7.

REFERENCES

Keith, A.: A demonstration on diverticula of the alimentary tract of congenital or of obscure origin. Br. Med. J. *1*:376, 1910.

Liebermann-Meffert, D., et al.: Muscular equivalent of the lower esophageal sphincter. Gastroenterology *76*:31, 1979.

Lindner, H.H., and Kemprud, E.: A clinicoanatomical study of the arcuate ligament of the diaphragm. Arch. Surg. *103*:600, 1971.

READING REFERENCES

Abel, W.: The arrangement of the longitudinal and circular musculature at the upper end of the oesophagus. J. Anat. Physiol. *47*:381, 1913.

Arey, L.B., and Tremaine, M.J.: The muscle content of the lower esophagus of man. Anat. Rec. *56*:315, 1933.

Bowden, R.E.M., and El-Ramli, H.A.: The anatomy of the oesophageal hiatus. Br. J. Surg. *54*:983, 1967.

Butler, H.: The veins of the oesophagus. Thorax *6*:276, 1951.

Demel, R.: The blood supply of the esophagus: a study of surgery of the esophagus (Die Gefassversorgung der Speiserohre. Ein Beitrag zur Oesophaguschirurgie). Arch. Klin. Chir. *128*:453, 1924.

Eliska, O.: Phreno-oesophageal membrane and its role in the development of hiatal hernia. Acta Anat. (Basel) *86*:137, 1973.

Liebermann-Meffert, D., et al.: Muscular equivalent of the lower esophageal sphincter. Gastroenterology *76*:31, 1979.

Shapiro, A.L., and Robillard, G.L.: Gastroesophageal vagal and sympathetic innervation: in relation to an anatomic approach to combined gastric vagal sympathectomy. J. Int. Coll. Surg. *13*:318, 1950a.

Shapiro, A.L., and Robillard, G.L.: The esophageal arteries: their configurational anatomy and variations in relation to surgery. Ann. Surg. *131*:171, 1950b.

Swigart, L.L., et al.: The esophageal arteries: an anatomic study of 150 specimens. Surg. Gynecol. Obstet. *90*:234, 1950.

CHAPTER 7

LYMPHATIC DRAINAGE OF THE ESOPHAGUS

Thomas W. Shields

ANATOMY

Anatomically the esophagus is divided readily into three portions: a cervical segment, a thoracic segment, and an abdominal segment. The cervical esophagus extends from the level of the cricopharyngeus to the thoracic inlet—the level of the first thoracic vertebra and the clavicle—approximately 18 cm from the upper incisor teeth. The thoracic segment extends from the thoracic inlet to the esophageal hiatus, approximately 38 cm from the upper incisor teeth. The abdominal segment extends from the esophageal hiatus to the gastroesophageal junction, approximately 40 cm from the upper incisor teeth.

Unfortunately there is no general agreement about the appropriate divisions of the thoracic esophagus. Some authors divide it into three and others into two sections. In some systems the boundaries of these divisions vary with the relationship of the esophagus to other intrathoracic structures—aortic arch, tracheal bifurcation, inferior pulmonary veins—and in other systems the boundaries are placed at varying distances from the cardioesophageal junctions as visualized during endoscopic examination. The suggestion of Sarrazin and associates (1984), however, based on their anatomic findings and the lymphographic findings of Laslo and Szabo quoted by them, is that for the purposes of initial lymphatic drainage, the thoracic portion of the esophagus be divided into a superior—retrotracheal—segment and an inferior segment. The former segment extends from the thoracic inlet to the tracheal bifurcation—readily identifiable on roentgenograms of the chest—and the latter from this site to the esophageal hiatus.

No matter how the segments are defined, such divisions are arbitrary at best since the lymphatics of the esophagus are composed of two large, interconnecting networks that mainly course in a longitudinal manner. This was initially investigated by Sakata (1903) and subsequently confirmed by others. The first is a mucosal network that extends into the second, the submucosal network, which along with the first, is continuous cephalad with lymphatics of the pharynx and caudad with those of the stomach. Thus lymphatic drainage from any site may occur in any direction and the direction of flow is longitudinal rather that segmental. In contrast studies, the longitudinal flow is at least six times that of the transverse or segmental flow.

The mucosal and submucosal lymphatic networks pierce the muscular layers of the esophagus at various sites and are connected to a smaller muscular lymphatic network in the esophageal wall or closely applied to its surface. The initial lymph node groups are minute superficial nodes contained in the connective adventitial sheath (Fig. 7–1). Such nodes are termed epiesophageal nodes by Sarrazin and associates (1984) and paraesophageal nodes by Mannell (1982). These include the nodes juxtaposed to the esophagus. They may be considered nodal station number 1. From these nodes efferent channels traverse the adventitia to the areas of the vagus nerves and the associated vessels to empty into the periesophageal nodes within the mediastinum.

These periesophageal groups are the mediastinal nodes described in Chapter 5 and consist of the paratracheal, superior tracheobronchial, inferior tracheobronchial—subcarinal—and posterior mediastinal node groups. The drainage pattern continues either upwards to the deep cervical nodes or inferiorly to the nodes beneath the diaphragm. The more proximal nodal groups below the diaphragm, the diaphragmatic, celiac, and left gastric nodes and those on the lesser curvature of the stomach are considered a continuation of the periesophageal nodes by Mannell (1982). The data of the Japanese Committee for Registration of Esophageal Cancer (1985) support this contention. Both the periesophageal and these proximal subdiaphragmatic abdominal nodes may be considered nodal station number 2 and along with the nodes of station number 1—the paraesophageal nodes—may be considered regional nodes of the thoracic esophagus. Drainage may also progress upward to the cervical area, laterally to the hilar nodes in the chest or inferiorly to more distant nodes in the abdomen—in the suprapyloric area, on the common hepatic artery, and along the greater curvature or splenic hilum. These may be considered station number 3 nodes

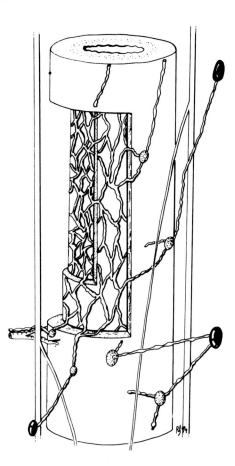

Fig. 7–1. Schematic illustration of mucosal and submucosal lymphatic esophageal networks with connections to the epiesophageal lymph nodes stapled in the adventitial layer and then to the periesophageal lymph nodes (solid) of the mediastinum. (Reproduced with the permission of Sarrazin, R., et al.: *In* Giuli, R., ed.: Cancer of the Esophagus 1984: One Hundred and Thirty-Five Questions. New York, Scientific Medical Publications of France, Inc., 1984.)

or distant or lateral nodes of the thoracic esophagus (Table 7–1) (Fig. 7–2).

CLASSIC LYMPHATIC DRAINAGE PATTERN OF THE ESOPHAGUS

A rational approach to the lymphatic drainage of the esophagus based on the aforementioned observations and the evaluation of Sarrazin and associates (1984), as well as those of Ide (1974), Sannohe (1981) and Tanabe (1986) and their associates, may be described as follows. Drainage from the cervical portion of the esophagus is into the internal jugular nodes and the supraclavicular node groups. Inferior drainage into the superior paratracheal nodes—nodes on the innominate artery—may occur, but is infrequent unless the aforementioned nodal groups are grossly involved (Fig. 7–3A). Drainage from the superior or retrotracheal portion of the thoracic esophagus is into the paraesophageal and periesophageal nodes—the superior and inferior tracheobronchial and the paratracheal node groups—and inferiorly to the regional nodes beneath the diaphragm. This area also drains superiorly

Table 7–1. Lymph Nodes of the Thoracic Esophagus

Regional Nodes	Station No. 1	Paraesophageal Nodes
		    Epiesophageal nodes
		    Paracardial nodes

	Station No. 2	Periesophageal Nodes
		    Paratracheal nodes
		    Tracheobronchial nodes
		    Posterior mediastinal
		        nodes
		    Diaphragmatic nodes
		    Left gastric nodes
		    Lesser curvature nodes
		    Celiac nodes

Distant Nodes	Station No. 3	Lateral Esophageal Nodes
		    Cervical nodes
		    Pulmonary hilar nodes
		    Suprapyloric nodes
		    Common hepatic nodes
		    Greater curvature nodes
		    Splenic hilar nodes

into the supraclavicular nodes (Fig. 7–3B). The inferior thoracic esophagus drains into the paraesophageal and periesophageal nodes. The subcarinal nodes may become involved; more consistently, however, the drainage is into the inferior periesophageal nodes and into the nodes of the region of the cardia below the diaphragm. From there the drainage is into the nodes of the celiac region: the nodes along the left gastric artery, celiac axis and lesser curvature of the stomach (Fig. 7–3C). More distant drainage is then into the nodes in the suprapyloric area—common hepatic artery—and infrequently into those along the splenic artery on the superior aspect of the pancreas into the splenic hilum. The abdominal portion of the esophagus drains primarily into the aforementioned nodes of the cardia and celiac region. On occasion, this area also may drain into the subcarinal nodes via the lymphatic pathways in the pulmonary ligament (Fig. 7–3D). Akiyama (1984) noted that nodal involvement at the hepatoduodenal ligament or at the hilum of the spleen is rare in squamous cell carcinoma but may occur more readily with adenocarcinoma. Incidentally, Sarrazin and associates (1984) have never observed a dye injection into the esophagus enter the thoracic duct or the described posterior mediastinal paravertebral lymphatic chain.

LYMPHATIC SPREAD IN ESOPHAGEAL CARCINOMA

Akiyama and his colleagues (1981) reported the results of extensive lymph node dissection in 205 patients with squamous cell carcinoma of the esophagus at the time of esophagectomy. A total of 6,258 nodes were examined; 398 were found to contain tumor and were present in 121 of the 205 dissections carried out. The positive rate was therefore 59% of all patients. The exact number of lymph nodes identified in each patient was not recorded, but Siewert (1984), who carried out similar extensive nodal dissections, reported the removal of 12 to 18 nodes

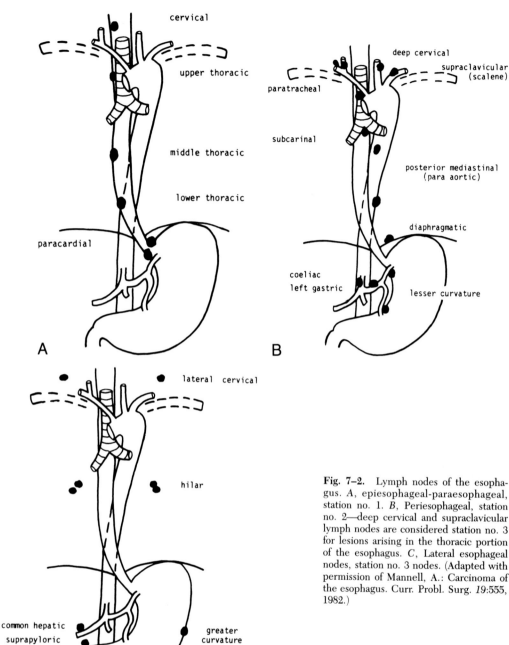

Fig. 7–2. Lymph nodes of the esophagus. *A*, epiesophageal-paraesophageal, station no. 1. *B*, Periesophageal, station no. 2—deep cervical and supraclavicular lymph nodes are considered station no. 3 for lesions arising in the thoracic portion of the esophagus. *C*, Lateral esophageal nodes, station no. 3 nodes. (Adapted with permission of Mannell, A.: Carcinoma of the esophagus. Curr. Probl. Surg. *19*:555, 1982.)

in the tracheobronchial area, 12 to 18 in the paraesophageal tissues, and 15 to 22 in the splenic hilar area. Unfortunately, the number along the lesser and greater curvatures of the stomach was not given.

Akiyama and associates (1981) divided the lymph node groups and drainage areas slightly differently than Sarrazin and his associates (1984). The definition of the upper esophagus—superior or retrotracheal segment—is the same, but the inferior segment is divided equally into a middle and a lower portion—the dividing line being approximately at the level of the inferior pulmonary vein. The lower thoracic portion is considered to include the abdominal portion of the esophagus. The

main lymph nodal areas that were involved are seen in Figure 7–4. The rate of lymph node involvement is seen in Table 7–2. The incidence of involvement of the various lymph nodal groups from tumors located in the three areas is shown in Table 7–3 and in Figure 7–5.

Unfortunately, the incidence of spread to the supraclavicular area was unrecorded because such disease was considered to indicate nonresectability, as it is by most. Postlethwaite (1986), however, reported that in a compilation of a number of autopsy series, cervical or supraclavicular metastases were identified in 199 of 2,850 autopsies, an incidence of 6.9%. In a small surgical series of 36 patients reported by Sannohe and associates (1981),

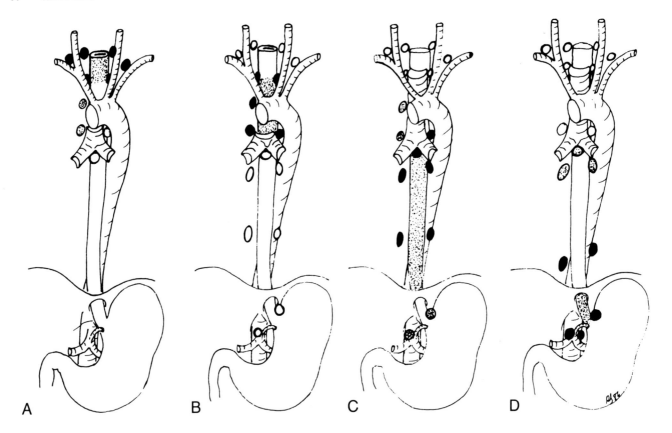

Fig. 7–3. Major lymph node groups draining the various segments of the esophagus. Solid color indicates nodes most often involved, stippled pattern indicates nodes less frequently invaded, white indicates nodes infrequently involved. *A*, cervical esophagus. *B*, superior portion of thoracic esophagus. *C*, inferior portion of thoracic esophagus. *D*, abdominal portion of esophagus. (Adapted with permission from Sarrazin, R., et al.: *In* Giuli, R., ed.: Cancer of the Esophagus in 1984: One Hundred and Thirty-Five Questions. New York, Scientific Medical Publications of France, Inc., 1984.)

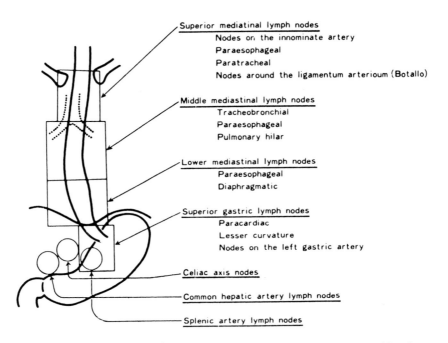

Fig. 7–4. Mapping of possibly involved nodes in patients with carcinoma of the thoracic esophagus suggested by Akiyama, H., et al. (Reproduced with permission from Akiyama, H. et al.: Principles of surgical treatment for carcinoma of the esophagus: analysis of lymph node involvement. Ann. Surg. *194*:438, 1981.)

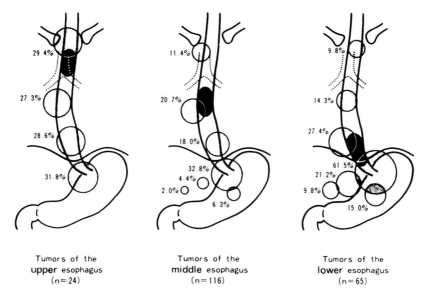

Tumors of the
upper esophagus
(n=24)

Tumors of the
middle esophagus
(n=116)

Tumors of the
lower esophagus
(n=65)

Fig. 7–5. Ratio of positive lymph nodes per number of resected cases. (Reproduced with permission of Akiyama, H., et al.: Principles of surgical treatment for carcinoma of the esophagus: analysis of lymph node involvement. Ann. Surg. *194*:438, 1981.)

Table 7–2. Rate of Positive Lymph Nodes in Squamous Cell Carcinoma of the Thoracic Esophagus

Location of Tumor	Number of Patients	Number Positive	Percentage
Superior Segment	24	16	66.7
Inferior Segment*	181	105	58.0
Middle	116	59	50.9
Lower*	65	46	70.8
Total	205	121	59.0

*Includes abdominal portion

Adapted with permission from Akiyama, H., et al.: Principles of surgical treatment for carcinoma of the esophagus: analysis of lymph node involvement. Ann. Surg. *194*:438, 1981.

Table 7–3. Lymph Node Groups Involved in Squamous Cell Carcinoma of the Thoracic Esophagus

Lymph Node Groups	Location of Tumor Superior Portion	Location of Tumor Inferior Portion*
Thoracic		
Superior mediastinal	29.4%	10.7%
Middle mediastinal	27.3%	18.3%
Lower mediastinal	28.6%	21.3%
Abdominal		
Superior gastric	31.8%	43.0%
Coeliac axis	0.0%	10.3%
Common hepatic artery	0.0%	4.7%
Splenic artery	0.0%	9.3%

*Includes middle and lower thoracic portions and abdominal portion of the esophagus

Adapted with permission from Akiyama, H., et al.: Principles of surgical treatment for carcinoma of the esophagus: analysis of lymph node involvement. Ann. Surg., *194*:438, 1981.

however, metastatic disease was present in the supraclavicular nodes in 7 of 22 patients with squamous cell carcinoma of the thoracic esophagus in whom supraclavicular node dissection was done either unilaterally or bilaterally as a part of the resectional procedure—an incidence of 31.8%. When the other 14 patients in their series are included, however, the incidence falls to 19.4% for the entire group of patients. These data are similar to those reported by Ide and his associates (1974). These authors found that supraclavicular involvement was present in 20% of patients with lesions in the superior portion of the thoracic esophagus. However, such involvement was present in only 4% of patients with lesions in the upper half of the inferior portion—mid esophagus—and in none of the patients in whom the lesions were in the lower half of the inferior portion–the lower third of the esophagus. In contrast, spread to the nodes below the diaphragm was noted in 30% of patients with lesions in the upper third, 38% with lesions in the middle third and 48% with lesions in the lower third of the esophagus.

Comment

This information, along with the aforementioned data of Akiyama and his colleagues (1981) and the recent reports of Tanabe and associates (1986) of lymphoscintigraphic studies of the esophagus, confirms the longitudinal spread of lymphatic metastases. Also it may be generalized that although there is a greater tendency for the lesions in the superior portion of the thoracic esophagus than those in the inferior portion to spread cephalad, the highest incidence of spread from either area is caudal. Thus, regardless of the site of the esophageal tumor, lymphatic metastasis other than to the nodes in the mediastinum has a greater propensity to involve the nodes below the diaphragm than those in the supraclavicular region.

REFERENCES

Akiyama, H.: Which groups of lymph nodes draining the esophagus could be usually excised during operation. *In* Cancer of the Esophagus 1984: One Hundred & Thirty-Five Questions. Edited by R. Giuli. New York, Scientific Medical Publications of France, Inc., 1984.

Akiyama, H., et al.: Principles of surgical treatment for carcinoma of the esophagus: analysis of lymph node involvement. Ann. Surg. *194*:438, 1981.

Ide, H., et al.: Lymph node metastases of thoracic esophageal cancer. *Shujutsu, 18*:1355, 1974.

Mannell, A.: Carcinoma of the esophagus. Curr. Probl. Surg. *19*:555, 1982.

Postlethwait, R.W.: Surgery of the Esophagus, 2nd ed., Norwalk, CT, Appleton-Century-Crofts, 1986, p. 385.

Sakata, K.: Über die Lymphgefässe des Oesophagus und über seine regionaren Lymphdrüsen mit Berucksichtigung der Verbreitung des Karzinoms. Mitt. Grenzgeb. Med. Chir. *11*:634, 1903.

Sannohe, Y., Hiratsuka, R., and Doki, K.: Lymph node metastases in cancer of the thoracic esophagus. Am. J. Surg. *141*:216, 1981.

Sarrazin, R., et al.: Lymph node anatomy and physiology still leave a lot of unknowns. *In* Cancer of the Esophagus 1984: One Hundred & Thirty-Five Questions. Edited by R. Giuli. New York, Scientific Medical Publications of France, Inc., 1984.

Siewert, J.R.: Quality of resection, lymph nodes, neighboring organs. *In* Cancer of the Esophagus 1984: One Hundred & Thirty-Five Questions. Edited by R. Giuli. New York, Scientific Medical Publications of France, Inc., 1984.

Tanabe, G., et al.: Clinical evaluation of esophageal lymph flow system based on I uptake of dissected regional lymph nodes following lymphoscintigraphy (in Japanese). Nippon Kyobu Geka Gakkai Zasshi, *87*:315, 1986.

CHAPTER 8

EMBRYOLOGY AND ANATOMY OF THE DIAPHRAGM

Thomas W. Shields

The diaphragm serves as the anatomic division between the thoracic and the abdominal cavities and, as such, is a muscular structure that is dealt with by both abdominal and thoracic surgeons. The surgical correction of acquired and congenital abnormalities of the diaphragm may be made from either abdominal or thoracic approaches, depending on the nature of the lesion, the location of the lesion, other abnormalities of the chest or abdomen, and the particular training and experience of the involved surgeon. The diaphragm exists as an anatomic barrier but is not a surgical barrier, since the competent surgeon should be able to handle any surgical problem involving the diaphragm and, therefore, should be versatile enough to approach diaphragmatic lesions from either above or below.

EMBRYOLOGY

The diaphragm originates from an unpaired ventral portion—the septum transversum; from paired dorsal lateral portions—the pleuroperitoneal folds; and from an irregular medial dorsal portion—the dorsal mesentery (Fig. 8–1). The septum transversum, formed during the third week of gestation, separates the pericardial region from the rest of the body cavity. This part of the diaphragm grows dorsad from the ventral body wall and moves caudad with the other contributors to the diaphragm to reach the normal position of the diaphragm at about 8 weeks. The pleuroperitoneal folds arise on the lateral body walls, at the level where the cardinal veins swing around to enter the sinus venosus of the heart. These folds extend medially and somewhat caudally to join with the septum transversum and the dorsal mesentery to complete the development of the diaphragm at about the seventh week; the right pleuroperitoneal canal closes somewhat earlier than the left. Muscle fibers migrate from the third, fourth, and fifth cervical myotomes, carrying along their innervation, and grow between the two membranes to complete the structures of

the diaphragm. During the tenth week, the intestines return from the yolk sac to the abdominal cavity and, at about 12 weeks, rotation and fixation of the intestines occur.

A delay or variation in the described timetable may result in a variety of congenital hernias with or without a hernial sac, or may even result in a congenital "eventration" of a hemidiaphragm. Early return of the intestines to the abdomen prior to closure of the pleuroperitoneal membrane results in a hernia through this opening—a so-called foramen of Bochdalek hernia. A sac usually is not present, but if it is, the return of the intestines may have occurred after the closure of the pleuroperitoneal membrane but prior to the migration of the cervical myotomes between the membranes. Foramen of Morgagni hernias occur anteriorly, almost always have a sac, and therefore are probably due to the lack of ingrowth of the cervical myotomes. A congenital short esophagus is related to late closure of the diaphragm and early return of the intestine to the abdomen. Congenital "eventration" may be a total error of ingrowth of cervical myotomes in one or both hemidiaphragms, and therefore, is really a large congenital diaphragmatic hernia and not an eventration. An absent diaphragm probably represents an error of growth of the septum transversum and other embryologic elements. Duplication of a hemidiaphragm can occur. The fusion and formation timetable variations also may involve defects in the diaphragm in association with certain vascular anomalies of the lungs and heart.

ANATOMY

Gross Features

The diaphragm is a dome-shaped structure of muscular fibers radiating out from either side of an irregularly shaped central tendon; it consists of the right and the left hemidiaphragms. In structure and function the di-

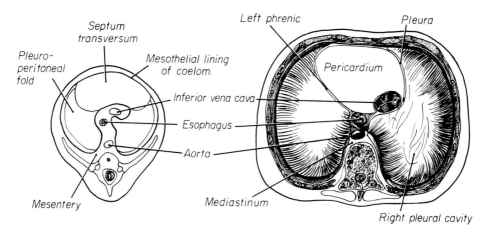

Fig. 8–1. Schematic illustration of embryologic components of the diaphragm. (Redrawn from Shields, T.W.: The diaphragm. *In* Nora, P.: Operative Surgery: Principles and Techniques. Philadelphia, Lea & Febiger, 1972.)

aphragm differs from any other muscle in the body. It is a muscular septum between the abdominal and thoracic cavities, serving as the major muscle of respiration. Its dome-like shape allows important abdominal structures, such as the liver and the spleen, to have the protection of the lower ribs and the chest wall. Voluntary muscular fibers originate from the xiphisternum, from the lateral lower six ribs on each side, and from the external and internal arcuate ligaments that arise from the upper three lumbar vertebrae. Bilaterally, the muscle fibers insert into the central tendon of the diaphragm.

The central tendon is a thin aponeurosis of closely interwoven fascial fibers in the form of a three-leaf clover. The two lateral leaves form the dome of the diaphragm and the third—anterior—leaf is fused with the diaphragmatic surface of the pericardium.

Major interest in the muscular portion of the diaphragm centers about the two crura, which play varying roles in the formation of the esophageal hiatus. The right crus arises from the bodies of the first and second lumbar vertebrae, and the fibers divide as they pass to the left, normally overlapping in front and behind to form the entire esophageal hiatus. Collis and associates (1954), however, found this arrangement in only a little more

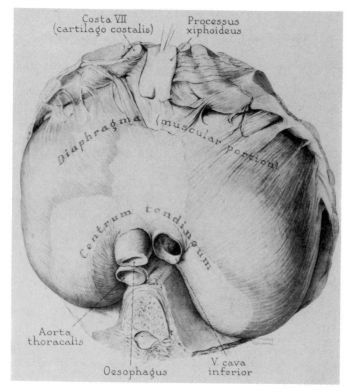

Fig. 8–2. The diaphragm as seen from above. Normal apertures and topographic landmarks shown. (Reproduced with permission from Anson, B.J.: Atlas of Human Anatomy. Philadelphia, W.B. Saunders Co., 1950, p. 210.)

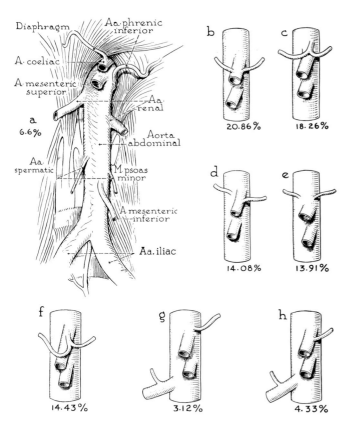

Fig. 8–3. The arterial supply of the diaphragm from the abdominal aorta with variations in the origin of the inferior phrenic arteries. (Redrawn with permission from Anson, B.J. and McVay, C.: Surgical Anatomy, 5th Edition, W.B. Saunders Co., 1971.)

than half of their subjects. In the others, the left crus contributed to a varying degree to the makeup of the hiatus, and in approximately 2%, the left crus made up the major portion of the esophageal hiatus.

The hiatal opening is situated at the level of the tenth thoracic vertebra just to the left of the midline and just ventral to where the aorta passes into the abdomen. The inferior vena cava passes through the tendinous portion of the right side of the diaphragm between the anterior leaf and the right lateral leaf at the level of the eighth thoracic vertebra. The other normal openings are the parasternal foramina—the foramina of Morgagni— through which the internal mammary arteries pass into the abdomen to become the superior epigastric arteries (Fig. 8–2).

The thoracic side of the diaphragm is covered with the parietal pleura, and the abdominal surface with peritoneum, except at the naturally occurring openings.

Blood Supply

The principal blood supply of the diaphragm is derived directly from the aorta or from its most superior abdominal branches (Fig. 8–3), and its venous drainage empties into the inferior vena cava. Both the arterial supply and the venous drainage—the right and left inferior phrenic veins—are found on the undersurface of the diaphragm (Fig. 8–4). The inferior phrenic artery usually bifurcates

posteriorly near the dome of the diaphragm and the branches course along the margins of the central tendon. The smaller posterior division courses laterally above the dorsal and lumbocostal origin of the diaphragm, where it has collateral anastomes with the lower five intercostal arteries. The larger anterior division runs anterosuperiorly to the edge of the central tendon, where it anastomoses freely with the pericardiacophrenic artery. The venous pattern is similar except that the veins generally course along the posterior aspect of the central tendon to join the inferior vena cava. Veins on the inferior surface of the diaphragm communicate with the hepatic veins through the left triangular and coronary ligaments of the liver.

Nerve Distribution

The right and left phrenic nerves arise from their respective third, fourth, and fifth cervical nerve roots and constitute the total nerve supply for the ipsilateral hemidiaphragm. The distribution of each nerve is important in reference to incisions into the diaphragm. The course of each has been described by Merendino and his coworkers (1956). The right phrenic nerve reaches the diaphragm just lateral to the inferior vena cava, and the left just lateral to the left border of the heart. Generally, the nerves divide, either just above or at the level of the diaphragm, into several terminal branches. Some are distributed to the pleural and peritoneal surfaces, but the great bulk of each nerve passes into, or through, the diaphragm and most often divides into four major rami to supply the various muscular portions. Usually, two of the rami share a common trunk for a varying distance so that three muscular branches arise from each phrenic nerve: one anteromedially, one laterally, and the remaining one posteriorly (Fig. 8–5). Injury to any of these branches causes paralysis of the supplied portion of the hemidiaphragm.

Surgical Incisions

Incisions into the diaphragm must be made so as to avoid injury to the major branches of the phrenic nerves. Incision through the central tendon rarely causes diaphragmatic paralysis (Fig. 8–6a,b), but this approach provides only minimal exposure of the adjacent compartment. A more satisfactory access is provided by a circumferential incision at the periphery of the diaphragm, which permits excellent exposure of the upper abdominal contents from the thorax and vice versa with little or no possibility of injury to any major branch of the ipsilateral phrenic nerve (Fig. 8–6c). On the left, the incision may be started at the esophageal hiatus and carried from behind forward circumferentially 2.5 to 3 cm away from the attachment of the diaphragm to the chest wall. The crural or posterior branch of the phrenic nerve is divided but this division is of little consequence. The main branch of the left inferior phrenic artery is usually encountered with this incision and requires division and ligation. Alternatively the incision may be started anteriorly just lateral to the pericardium and extended circumferentially as far posteriorly as necessary.

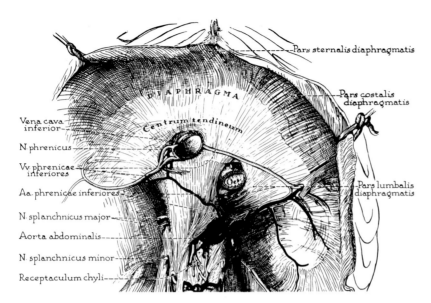

Fig. 8–4. The arterial and venous distribution on the undersurface of the diaphragm. (Redrawn with permission from Anson, B.J. and McVay, C.: Surgical Anatomy, 5th Edition, W.B. Saunders Co., 1971.)

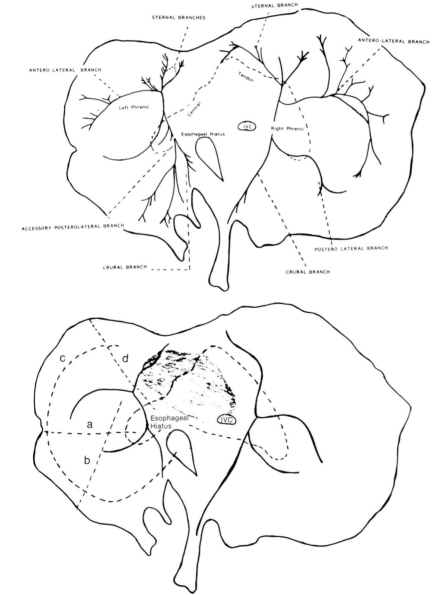

Fig. 8–5. Distribution of the phrenic nerves as seen from above. (Redrawn with permission from Merendino, K.A., et al.: The intradiaphragmatic distribution of the phrenic nerve with particular reference to the placement of diaphragmatic incisions and controlled segmental paralysis. Surgery 39:189, 1956.)

Fig. 8–6. Safe areas for incision into the diaphragm. (Redrawn with permission of Merendino, K.A., et al.: The intradiaphragmatic distribution of the phrenic nerve with particular reference to the placement of diaphragmatic incisions and controlled segmental paralysis. Surgery 39:189, 1956.)

The ipsilateral hemidiaphragm may then be raised as a trap-door and retracted medially for exposure. Closure of the incision is accomplished readily by approximating the cut edges of the hemidiaphragm with multiple interrupted simple or mattress sutures of 0 or 2-0 nonabsorbable material of the surgeon's choice. A similar incision may also be carried out on the right.

When a combined abdominothoracic approach is used, the incision in the diaphragm may be extended medially between the pericardial attachment to the diaphragm and the entrance of the phrenic nerve into the diaphragm, with severence of only the small sternal division of the nerve (Fig. 8–6d). The incision is then carried to the apex of the eosphageal hiatus. To ensure adequate exposure, the phrenic nerve and pericardiacophrenic vessels must be freed from the pericardium proximally and retracted laterally. Care must be exercised to prevent injury to these structures while this retraction is being carried out. This incision is closed the same as a circumferential incision. Incisions in the diaphragm other than a circumferential or a very medial one must be avoided because the anterolateral and posterolateral branches of the nerve are likely to be divided.

REFERENCES

Collis, J.L., Kelly, T.D., and Wiley, A.M.: Anatomy of the crura of the diaphragm and the surgery of hiatus hernia. Thorax 9:175, 1954.

Meredino, K.A., et al.: The intradiaphragmatic distribution of the phrenic nerve with particular reference to the placement of diaphragmatic incisions and controlled segmental paralysis. Surgery 39:189, 1956.

READING REFERENCES

Patten, B.: Human Embryology, 3rd ed. New York, McGraw-Hill Book Co., 1968, p. 406.

Physiology of the Lungs

CHAPTER 9

PULMONARY GAS EXCHANGE

Jeffrey Glassroth, Douglas R. Gracey, and David W. Cugell

LOCUS OF BLOOD-GAS INTERFACE

The alveolocapillary membrane is where inspired air and pulmonary blood meet and gas transfer occurs. This membrane is made up of the attenuated cytoplasm of an alveolar lining cell—alveolar type I cell—and its basement membrane plus the attenuated cytoplasm of the capillary endothelial cell and its basement membrane. Divertie and Brown (1964) have described a space of variable width between the two basement membranes, the interstitial space. The majority of disease processes that alter the alveolocapillary membrane interfere with gas transport across this membrane and probably produce their deleterious effects by interfering with pulmonary ventilation, pulmonary blood flow, or the homogeneous distribution of blood and air, or by some combination of these distribution defects.

PHYSICS AND PHYSIOLOGY OF GASES

Pressure and temperature changes alter the volume of all gases in a predictable manner. Because of marked variation in solubility and chemical reaction rates in body fluids, the behavior of different gases in a liquid phase in vivo varies widely.

Laws Pertaining to Gases in the Gas Phase

At constant pressure the volume of a gas is directly proportional to the temperature—Charles' law. At constant temperature the volume is inversely proportional to the pressure—Boyle's law.

The combination of Charles' and Boyle's laws gives the relationship:

$$PV = nRT$$

n = the number of moles of gas
R = a constant having the same value for all perfect gases
T = the absolute temperature in degrees Kelvin (K).
    $T = t° C + 273$.

At 0°C and 760 mm Hg pressure 1 mole of any perfect gas will have a volume of 22.41 liters.

The partial pressure of one gas in a mixture of gases of volume V is equal to the pressure that the gas would exert if it occupied the same volume V in the absence of other gases—Dalton's law. The partial pressure of each gas in a mixture is proportional to the fraction of the mixture made up by that gas; for example, the fraction of oxygen in room air is 0.21, and the sum of the partial pressures of all the gases in a mixture equals the total pressure of the gas mixture.

The partial pressure of any gas in a mixture is the product of the total or barometric pressure—P_B—times the fraction of the gas in the mixture—F.

$$P = P_B \times F$$

If there is water vapor in the mixture, the partial pressure of water vapor must be subtracted from the barometric pressure. Water vapor pressure is assumed to equal 47 mm Hg when a gas is fully saturated at 37°C.

$$P = (P_B - 47) \times F$$

For example:
Barometric pressure = 760 mm Hg
Oxygen concentration = 20.93%
$P_{O_2} = (760 - 47) \times 0.2093 = 149$ mm Hg

Environmental Conditions and Measurement of Gases

Body Temperature and Pressure, Saturated With Water Vapor—BTPS

Under this condition the temperature of the gas is 37°C and the partial pressure of water vapor is 47 mm Hg.

Ambient Temperature and Pressure, Saturated—ATPS

Under most circumstances, the ambient temperature is lower than body temperature. A gas at ambient conditions usually contains less water vapor than under BTPS conditions, depending upon ambient temperature and relative humidity.

Standard Temperature and Pressure, Dry—STPD

Oxygen, carbon dioxide, and carbon monoxide volumes are expressed at Standard Temperature and Pressure, Dry—STPD conditions. This manner of expression is customary for any gas undergoing metabolic exchange. Lung volumes and ventilation are expressed at BTPS conditions. A minute ventilation of 10 L/min STPD is equivalent to 12 or 13 L/min BTPS.

Conversion from ATPS Volumes to BTPS Volumes

As air temperature increases from ambient—ATPS—to BTPS conditions, gas volumes increase because of thermal expansion. If a fluid reservoir such as that within the lung is present, there will be an increase in the water vapor pressure to 47 mm Hg. The expansion due to heat and the increase in volume due to the addition of water vapor are expressed in the formula:

$$V_{BTPS} = V_{ATPS} \times \frac{273 + 37}{273 + t_A} \times \frac{P_B - P_{H_2O}}{P_B - 47}$$

273 = melting point of ice in °K
37 = body temperature in °C (degrees centigrade)
t_A = ambient temperature °C
P_B = barometric pressure, in mm Hg
P_{H_2O} = water vapor pressure at t_A
47 = water vapor pressure at 37°C (saturated)

Laws Pertaining to Gases in Liquids

Partial Pressure of Gases in Liquids

A gas in contact with a liquid will exchange molecules with the liquid. When equilibrium is reached, the number of gas molecules entering the liquid phase equals the number leaving to enter the gas phase, and the partial pressures of the gas in both the liquid and the gas phase are equal.

Volume of Gas in Liquids

The volume of a gas contained in a liquid is expressed in volumes percent—ml per 100 ml of liquid. These volumes are usually expressed under STPD conditions. The gas may be merely physically dissolved, in chemical combination, or both. For example, the oxygen content of the arterial blood of a healthy subject with a hemoglobin concentration of 14 g percent while he breathes room air will be about 19 volumes percent—19 ml oxygen STPD per 100 ml of whole blood. All but 0.3 volumes percent of the oxygen is in chemical combination with hemoglobin.

UNIQUE PROPERTIES OF SPECIFIC GASES

Different gases have special biologic properties. Some gases—oxygen and carbon dioxide—undergo metabolic exchange, other gases are insoluble in the pulmonary membrane and remain in the gas phase, and other gases have specific effects on the body that make them valuable as anesthetic agents.

Gases That Undergo Metabolic Exchange

Oxygen

This essential component of cellular respiration is carried in the blood in two forms: in physical solution in the plasma and in chemical combination with hemoglobin. The quantity of oxygen that can be carried in physical solution is minimal—about 1.5% of the total—compared with the large amount of oxygen that exists in chemical combination with hemoglobin. The quantity of oxygen combined with hemoglobin depends on the partial pressure of oxygen in the blood. This relationship (Fig. 9–1), the oxyhemoglobin dissociation curve, has a sigmoid shape with a steep slope between 10 and 60 mm Hg P_{O_2}. The curve is comparatively flat between 70 and 100 mm Hg (Fig. 9–1). The characteristics of this curve must be considered when treating hypoxemia.

Marked changes in P_{O_2} at the upper portion of the curve have little effect upon the arterial oxygen saturation. At the lower end of the curve where the oxygen pressures are equivalent to the P_{O_2} in the capillaries, large quantities of oxygen are available for tissue metabolism. Both acidosis and temperature elevation shift the oxyhemoglobin saturation curve to the right (Fig. 9–1). This rightward shift makes oxygen more readily available in the more acid environment of the tissues. The quantity of dissolved oxygen is directly proportional to the partial pressure of oxygen in blood and equals 0.003 ml of oxygen per 100 ml of blood per mm Hg P_{O_2}. With an arterial P_{O_2} of 90 mm Hg, the amount of dissolved oxygen in the blood is equal to 0.27 ml per 100 ml; but if the subject breathes 100% oxygen and achieves an arterial P_{O_2} of 600 mm Hg, the amount of dissolved oxygen would be 1.8 ml per 100 ml of blood.

Even during 100% oxygen breathing the dissolved oxygen contributes little to the total blood oxygen content if hemoglobin values are near normal. One gram of hemoglobin combines chemically with 1.34 ml of oxygen. If the blood hemoglobin is 15 g/100 ml, then 20.1 ml of oxygen/100 ml of blood can be carried in association with hemoglobin at saturation. The actual quantity of oxygen in combination with hemoglobin depends on the partial

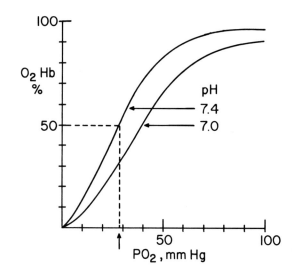

Fig. 9–1. Oxyhemoglobin (O_2 Hb) dissociation curve. The sigmoid relationship between P_{O_2} and percent saturation of hemoglobin with oxygen is shown together with the rightward shift of the curve that occurs with acidosis. The arrow denotes the p50 (see text).

pressure of oxygen and the amount of available hemoglobin (Fig. 9–2). The blood hemoglobin that is combined with oxygen—oxyhemoglobin—divided by the oxygen capacity of the blood sample—hemoglobin concentration × 1.34—gives the percent saturation of the hemoglobin with oxygen. Oxygen partial pressures in excess of 60 mm Hg add comparatively little to the oxygen content of the blood (Fig. 9–1).

The oxygen combining characteristics of hemoglobin may be expressed in terms of the p50 (see Fig. 9–1). The p50 is the partial pressure of oxygen at which hemoglobin is 50% saturated. When measured under the following conditions: temperature 37°C, pH 7.40, and P_{CO_2} 40 mm Hg, the p50 is normally 27 mm Hg. Certain diseases or conditions may change the p50. For example, as noted previously, an increase in either hydrogen ion concentration, temperature, or both, will shift the oxygen-hemoglobin dissociation curve to the right and increase the p50. An increase in carbon dioxide tension or in the enzyme 2,3 diphosphoglycerate—2, 3 DPG— will also shift the curve to the right. The opposite change in temperature, hydrogen ion concentration, carbon dioxide tension or 2,3 DPG shifts the curve to the left and lowers the p50 below 27 mm Hg. An increase in 2,3 DPG occurs in the presence of chronic hypoxemia, for example, at high altitudes and in chronic severe anemia, and shifts the curve to the right. This action facilitates the release of oxygen in the tissues since rightward movement of the oxygen-hemoglobin dissociation curve results in a lower saturation of hemoglobin at higher partial pressures of oxygen. In addition to an increase in 2,3 DPG, other compensations for chronic hypoxemia improve the delivery of oxygen to the tissues, such as an increase in cardiac output and secondary polycythemia. Substantial carboxyhemoglobinemia, as in acute carbon monoxide poisoning, has a physicochemical effect on the oxygen-hemoglobin curve and shifts it to the left and up. This action lowers the p50, increases the affinity of hemoglobin for oxygen, and compounds the problem of tissue hypoxemia initially caused by the combination of a significant amount of hemoglobin with carbon monoxide. The shift in the oxygen-hemoglobin dissociation curve contributes to the acute lactic acidosis that often follows tissue hypoxia irrespective of the cause.

Carbon Dioxide

Contrary to its limited capacity for oxygen, blood can accommodate enormous quantities of carbon dioxide (Fig. 9–3). Carbon dioxide is carried in the blood as a dissolved gas, as bicarbonate ions, carbonic acid, and carbaminohemoglobin, and as other carbamino compounds. Reduced—unoxygenated—hemoglobin has a greater affinity for carbon dioxide than does oxyhemoglobin. This upward shift in the carbon dioxide dissociation curve at low P_{O_2} is called the Haldane effect and facilitates transfer of carbon dioxide from tissue to capillary blood, where the P_{O_2} is low, and transfer of carbon dioxide from the capillary into the pulmonary alveolus where the P_{O_2} is higher (Fig. 9–3).

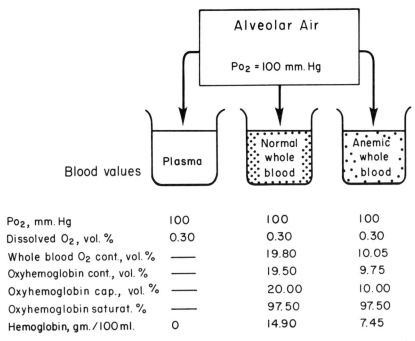

Blood values	Plasma	Normal whole blood	Anemic whole blood
P_{O_2}, mm. Hg	100	100	100
Dissolved O_2, vol. %	0.30	0.30	0.30
Whole blood O_2 cont., vol. %	——	19.80	10.05
Oxyhemoglobin cont., vol. %	——	19.50	9.75
Oxyhemoglobin cap., vol. %	——	20.00	10.00
Oxyhemoglobin saturat. %	——	97.50	97.50
Hemoglobin, gm./100 ml.	0	14.90	7.45

Fig. 9–2. Oxygen solubility and hemoglobin binding. Plasma in contact with oxygen contains only that amount of gas that can dissolve (0.00003 ml oxygen/ml plasma/mm Hg P_{O_2}). Each gram/100 ml blood of hemoglobin combines with 1.34 ml oxygen. With 14.90 g percent hemoglobin, the oxygen capacity is 20.00 volumes percent. At a P_{O_2} of 100 mm Hg and with this hemoglobin, blood will contain 19.50 volumes percent oxygen. When the oxygen dissolved in the plasma is added to the oxygen bound to hemoglobin, the total oxygen content becomes 19.80 volumes percent. Were this patient anemic with only 7.45 g percent of hemoglobin, the saturation at the same P_{O_2} would be identical. The whole blood oxygen content exceeds the oxyhemoglobin capacity in the anemic patient because of the relatively greater contribution of dissolved oxygen to the whole blood oxygen content. (From Preston, F.W., and Beal, J.M., eds.: Basic Surgical Physiology. Chicago, Year Book Medical Publishers, 1969.)

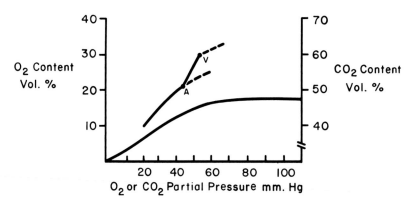

Fig. 9–3. Oxygen and carbon dioxide dissociation curves for whole blood. Oxyhemoglobin saturation of this blood at any P_{O_2} can be determined by dividing the corresponding oxygen content into the oxygen capacity (18.0 volumes percent in this case). The carbon dioxide dissociation curve is relatively linear over the range of partial pressures usually encountered in clinical practice. The difference in the carbon dioxide curve for the arterial (A) and venous (V) blood is due to a greater carbon dioxide carrying capacity of unoxygenated hemoglobin—Haldane effect. (From Preston, F.W., and Beal, J.M., eds.: Basic Surgical Physiology. Chicago, Year Book Medical Publishers, 1969.)

Gases That Are Soluble but Metabolically Inactive

Carbon Monoxide

Coburn (1970) has noted that carbon monoxide is produced by the body in small quantities and is therefore involved in metabolic exchange, but we will consider it a foreign and inactive gas. Carbon monoxide is moderately soluble in the pulmonary membrane and has an affinity for hemoglobin 210 times greater than does oxygen. Because of these properties carbon monoxide in low concentrations and for brief exposure periods is highly useful in the measurement of the diffusion capacity. Even brief exposure to high concentrations or prolonged exposure to relatively low levels of carbon monoxide can be highly toxic, because large amounts of carboxyhemoglobin, which is a stable compound, are produced and prevent hemoglobin from participating in oxygen transport.

Nitrogen

Nitrogen diffuses across the pulmonary membrane and is present in body tissues at the same partial pressure as in alveolar air. Inhalation of 100% oxygen rapidly eliminates nitrogen from the alveolar air, but a small amount of nitrogen continues to diffuse into the alveolar air from the large body tissue stores. Prolonged breathing of 100% oxygen eventually eliminates nitrogen stores from the body.

Gases That Are Insoluble in the Pulmonary Membrane

Helium and Neon

At low concentrations, helium and neon are essentially insoluble in tissue and within brief time intervals do not diffuse across the pulmonary membrane. Because they can be confined to the pulmonary gas compartment, concentration changes of these gases can be used to calculate the size of lung volume compartments.

Anesthetic Gases

All gases used for inhalation anesthesia are highly soluble in both blood and tissue and therefore diffuse rapidly through the pulmonary membrane. Nitrous oxide and ethyl ether are two commonly employed examples.

Nitrous Oxide

This is the most widely used inorganic gas in anesthesia. The blood concentration required to produce surgical anesthesia in man varies but is approximately 23 volumes percent. To achieve this concentration the inspired nitrous oxide percentage must be high, so an increased inspired oxygen concentration must be given along with it to avoid hypoxemia. Nitrous oxide is carried in solution in the blood, not in combination with hemoglobin, and is almost completely eliminated from blood and tissue promptly upon termination of nitrous oxide inhalation. A minute quantity diffuses through the skin of anesthesized subjects.

Ethyl Ether

Over 90% of the inhaled concentration of ether is eliminated by the lung. Although the concentration of ether in the urine parallels the plasma concentration, the amount eliminated by the kidney is small. The inspired concentration of ether required for surgical anesthesia is around 3.5 to 4.5 volumes percent. This relatively low concentration permits the use of room air as the source of oxygen in inhaled mixtures since the presence of ether decreases the partial pressure of oxygen in the inhaled mixture to a minimal degree.

Multiple Inert Gases

A variety of other inert gases of varying solubilities—e.g., ethane, sulfur hexafluoride—have been used in the study of ventilation and perfusion relationships within the lung. Tests using this so-called multiple inert gas technique popularized by Wagner (1974) are generally available only in research laboratories, but in that setting have proved to be useful in increasing our understanding of gas exchange in the lung.

MEASUREMENTS OF GAS EXCHANGE

Total pulmonary gas exchange may be measured by collecting expired air and calculating the amount of oxygen consumed and carbon dioxide produced per unit of time. The normal resting adult male consumes approximately 275 ml of oxygen and produces 230 ml of carbon dioxide per minute. Such measurements give little information about the actual efficiency of gas exchange.

Pulmonary Diffusing Capacity

Whether in the gas phase, dissolved in the plasma, or in chemical association, gases move from regions of higher to lower pressures. The diffusing capacity is a measure of the capacity of the pulmonary membrane to transfer gas between alveolar air and pulmonary capillary blood. Carbon dioxide diffuses from the pulmonary capillary blood into the alveolar air because the capillary P_{CO_2} is higher than the alveolar P_{CO_2}. Carbon dioxide is highly soluble in the pulmonary membrane, and its diffusion is rarely impaired despite extensive lung disease. Retention of carbon dioxide occurs whenever alveolar ventilation is ineffective, resulting in an alveolar P_{CO_2} increase and a reduction of the gradient for carbon dioxide across the pulmonary membrane. Limitations of oxygen diffusion do result in clinically significant disease. Although oxygen diffusion can be determined, carbon monoxide is a more convenient agent for diffusion measurements.

Carbon monoxide has three basic diffusion methods: single breath, rebreathing, and steady state or continuous breathing. The term "diffusion capacity" may well be a misnomer. Many processes are involved in the transfer of carbon monoxide from inspired air to pulmonary capillary blood. Diffusion is only one part of this system, and diffusion may not be measurable apart from other factors that influence gas transfer.

Results of measurements of the carbon monoxide diffusing capacity are influenced by the method employed, the volume of blood in the pulmonary capillary bed, the blood hemoglobin level, and the breathing pattern. Said (1960) and Finley and their colleagues (1962) have noted that abnormal carbon monoxide diffusion values may result from ventilation/perfusion imbalance. As an example of this concept—exaggerated to absurdity—consider a patient with completely normal lungs, one of which is perfused but not ventilated and the other ventilated with air containing trace amounts of carbon monoxide but not perfused. There will be no carbon monoxide uptake even though the pulmonary membrane is normal. As pointed out by one of us (D.R.G.) and co-workers (1968), a reduction in the blood gas interface secondary to a loss of capillary surface area, as occurs when there is a reduction in pulmonary capillary volume, is one basis for the impaired diffusion in some lung diseases. Because the diffusing capacity measures more than just gas diffusion, the term "transfer factor" has been adopted to describe the overall process. Irrespective of the gas used, the diffusion capacity or transfer factor calculation requires a determination of gas uptake per unit of time and a measurement of the pressure difference between the alveolus and the pulmonary capillary. The result is expressed in ml/min/mm Hg.

The diffusion defects noted in diffuse lung diseases are due to a combination of factors including a reduction in the pulmonary capillary bed volume, a decrease in the surface area of the blood gas interface, and imbalances in the ventilation and perfusion of the pulmonary parenchyma secondary to nonuniform distribution of the pathologic changes within the lung parenchyma (see Chapter 73). The classic concept of the "alveolar capillary block"—a uniform increase in the thickness of the pulmonary membrane that retards the movement of gas—is probably inaccurate, particularly in the resting state.

Arterial Blood Gases

An indirect but useful method of estimating the adequacy of pulmonary gas exchange is the measurement of arterial blood gas tensions and pH. In the normal resting state, with the subject breathing room air, blood gas and pH values are maintained within narrow limits. The arterial P_{O_2} is greater than 75 to 80 mm Hg; depending upon the subject's age, the arterial P_{CO_2} is between 38 and 42 mm Hg, the pH is 7.38 to 7.42, and the plasma bicarbonate ion is 20 to 28 mEq/L. The position of the normal subject at the time the blood sample is taken has little effect upon the results, but in persons with considerable abdominal obesity or diaphragmatic paralysis, significant changes in arterial blood gas composition may occur when the individuals move from the erect to the supine position. Hyperventilation reduces alveolar P_{CO_2}, increases alveolar P_{O_2}, and has similar effects on arterial blood gas composition. In the normal subject, mild exercise has no significant effect on the arterial P_{O_2}; a mild rise in the P_{O_2} occurs if the exercise is vigorous. However, in diseases associated with ventilation/perfusion imbalance there may be an acute fall in the arterial P_{O_2} with exercise. The arterial blood gas and pH in various states are illustrated in Table 9–1.

When interpreting arterial P_{O_2}—Pa_{O_2}—measurements, the alveolar oxygen tension—PA_{O_2}—should be estimated. This can be accomplished as follows:

$$PA_{O_2} = FI_{O_2} \times (P_B - 47) - \frac{(PA_{CO_2})}{R}$$

where: FI_{O_2} is the inspired fraction or percentage of oxygen, P_B is barometric pressure—assume 760 mm Hg at sea level, 47 is water vapor pressure at 37°C, PA_{CO_2} is the alveolar CO_2, which is assumed to equal the measured arterial CO_2—Pa_{CO_2}, and R is the respiratory quotient, assumed to be 0.8.

The equation may be simplified to:

$$PA_{O_2} = PI_{O_2} - (Pa_{CO_2} \times 1.25)$$

Table 9–1. Blood Gases and Acid-Base Status in Various Conditions

Condition (Clinical Example)	Breathing Pattern	Status	P_{O_2} (mm Hg)	P_{CO_2} (mm Hg)	pH	HCO_3^- (mEq/L)
Normal	—	—	75–90	38–42	7.38–7.42	20–28
Resp. alkalosis (anxiety)	Hypervent.	Acute	High	Low	High	Normal
Resp. acidosis (narcotic overdose)	Hypovent.	Acute	Low	High	Low	Normal
Resp. alkalosis (pulm. fibrosis)	Hypervent.	Chronic	Low or normal	Low	High norm	Low
Resp. acidosis (obstructive dis.)	Hypovent.*	Chronic	Low	High	Low norm	High
Metab. acidosis (diabetic acid.)	Hypervent.	Acute	High	Low	Low	Low
Metab. alkalosis (prolonged vomiting)	Hypovent.*	Chronic	Low	High	High	High

*May not be clinically apparent.

The alveolar-arterial oxygen difference—$P_{A_{O_2}} - P_{a_{O_2}}$—of a person breathing room air averages about 8 mm Hg in young persons and increases with age to values over 20 mm Hg in the eighth decade. Calculation of this difference will correct for changes in level of ventilation—i.e., $P_{a_{CO_2}}$. A $P_{A_{O_2}} - P_{a_{O_2}}$ value should never be negative or near zero. Such a calculation suggests a laboratory error.

Acid-Base Balance

An acute change in arterial P_{CO_2} is accompanied by an acute change in arterial pH in the opposite direction. The pH shift approximates 0.01 units per mm Hg change in P_{CO_2}. Under acute conditions the serum bicarbonate exerts little influence upon the relationship of pH and P_{CO_2}. It takes from hours to days for the renal compensatory mechanisms to alter the bicarbonate and thus correct the pH following an abrupt and persistent change in P_{CO_2}. Such compensation does not occur with brief changes in ventilation, but is present whenever hyperventilation or alveolar hypoventilation is chronic. Renal buffering mechanisms respond to chronic increases in arterial P_{CO_2} and concomitant decreases in pH by retaining bicarbonate. Chronic hyperventilation leading to sustained hypocapnia and an elevated pH stimulates compensatory renal bicarbonate excretion. Some examples of acid-base derangements are shown in Table 9–1. Acid-base balance and its relationship to pulmonary gas exchange will be described further. It may be misleading to attempt an interpretation of arterial blood gas and pH changes without some knowledge of the status of the patient and prior treatment. Combined respiratory and metabolic acid-base problems may become quite complex and the acid-base status can be unraveled only with full knowledge of the clinical condition of the patient.

FACTORS AFFECTING PULMONARY GAS EXCHANGE

Partition of Ventilation

Each inspiration has a useful component that bathes the alveoli with fresh air and a component that "goes along for the ride" and ventilates only the conducting tubes—alveolar and dead-space fractions of the tidal volume. That portion of the ventilation distributed to alveoli where gas exchange occurs is the alveolar ventilation. Ventilation of lung regions with anatomically intact but nonfunctioning alveoli is equivalent to ventilation of the conducting airways—dead-space ventilation. In the normal subject, breathing quietly at rest, there is approximately 1 ml of dead-space volume per pound of body weight. The total minute ventilation measured at the mouth reveals little regarding effective alveolar ventilation. But, if one also knows the respiratory rate, it is possible to estimate alveolar ventilation, assuming that most alveoli are functioning. For example, two patients breathe a total of 5 L/min. However, one patient breathes 25 times per minute with a tidal volume of 200 ml whereas the other patient breathes 10 times a minute with a tidal volume of 500 ml. The patient with a 200-ml tidal volume mainly ventilates his dead space. The actual dead-space volume—V_D—and the ratio between dead space and tidal volumes—V_D/V_T—can be measured if the alveolar and expired concentrations of a gas undergoing metabolic exchange and the tidal volume are known. Carbon dioxide is customarily used, and it is assumed that the arterial and alveolar P_{CO_2} are equivalent. The formula for these measurements, as shown, merely states that the ratio of dead-space volume to tidal volume is the same as the ratio of alveolar—arterial—CO_2 to expired CO_2.

$$V_D/V_T = \frac{P_{CO_2} \text{ (arterial)} - P_{CO_2} \text{ (expired)}}{P_{CO_2} \text{ (arterial)}}$$

Distribution of Ventilation

Several methods are available to evaluate the uniformity or nonuniformity of the distribution of inspired air. One method requires that the patient inhale 100% oxygen for 7 minutes, thereby washing out the nitrogen in his lungs. With a nitrogen meter and continuous sampling of the expired air stream a continuous plot of the breath-by-breath exhaled nitrogen concentration is obtained. In the normal subject, a rapid decrease of nitrogen occurs within the first minute or two of oxygen breathing. Patients with gross alveolar hypoventilation or marked maldistribution of ventilation will have a slow washout curve. When ventilation abnormalities are marked, the washout curve has an erratic pattern with much variation in the breath-to-breath concentration of exhaled nitrogen. In the presence of localized areas of marked hypoventilation, as in bullous disease, the nitrogen concentration in the forced expiratory air sample delivered at the end of the 7-minute washout period will be markedly elevated. Another method for evaluating ventilation uniformity uses a single-breath nitrogen washout. The patient inspires 100% oxygen to total lung capacity and exhales completely while the nitrogen concentration and volume of the single expirate are monitored. The alveolar portion of the expiration should have a nearly constant nitrogen concentration if inspired oxygen is uniformly distributed within the lung.

A single-breath nitrogen washout curve is shown in Figure 9–4. The initial portion of the expirate contains no nitrogen as it consists solely of the terminal portion of the previous inhaled oxygen—phase 1. As expiration continues, the nitrogen concentration rises rapidly as the dead space is rinsed with alveolar gas—phase 2. A nitrogen plateau then appears, which rises slowly, at a rate of 1.0 to 1.5% nitrogen per liter expired, in normal subjects—phase 3. A steep—concentration increase of greater than 1.5% N_2/L— or irregular phase 3 occurs whenever ventilation is nonuniform. In obstructive lung disease values of 10% N_2/L or greater are not unusual. Most adults have a fourth phase. The onset of phase 4 is apparent from an abrupt increase in nitrogen concentration. This sudden rise occurs when the lung volumes are small and airways to the dependent portions of the lung close. The lung volume corresponding with the onset of phase 4 is known as the closing volume. Because there is a gradation of intrapleural pressure from apex to base in the upright subject, small airways in the de-

pendent lung zones are subjected to higher transpulmonary pressures than those at the apex. The basal airways close at small lung volumes, producing the characteristic phase 3–4 junction that defines the closing volume. The rise in nitrogen concentration during phase 4 is due to the lesser dilution of upper zone nitrogen during the previous oxygen inhalation. Also, basal lung zones, with a lower N_2 concentration, cease contributing to expiration after the onset of phase 4. The closing volume enlarges and the phase 4 onset moves up in the vital capacity, toward total lung capacity with age and in the presence of small airway pathology. As the closing volume point rises progressively in the patient's lung volume, it eventually exceeds the resting end-expiratory lung volume, which is the functional residual capacity—FRC. Thus some dependent airways will close at the end of every breath. During normal resting tidal ventilation, ventilation of dependent lung zones is reduced, creating a ventilation/perfusion imbalance. This imbalance increases with age and is one of the factors responsible for a decline in the arterial oxygen tension of the elderly.

Distribution of Blood Flow

Pulmonary blood flow can be considered uniform in anatomic terms if every alveolus receives equivalent blood flow. In functional terms, physiologic uniformity exists when blood flow is distributed to each alveolus in proportion to its ventilation. Blood flow nonuniformity occurs to some degree in normal individuals. In the erect man, breathing normally at rest, the lung bases are perfused whereas the apices are minimally perfused owing to gravity and the low hydrostatic pressures in the pulmonary circuit. The apical areas of the lung receive considerable ventilation but are poorly perfused. This mismatch is not sufficiently great to be physiologically significant in the normal individual.

The distribution of blood flow to various portions of the lung can be evaluated by several methods. The roentgenogram of the chest may demonstrate relative hyperlucency of one parenchymal region, suggesting a local reduction in pulmonary blood flow as may occur with a pulmonary embolus. Perfusion scans using radioactive tagged macroaggregated albumin that lodges in the pulmonary capillaries provides good evidence of the gross distribution of blood flow within the pulmonary vascular bed (see Chapter 15). More precise visualization of pulmonary blood flow requires catheterization and contrast visualization of the vascular bed. Arterial blood gas determinations are not particularly useful for estimating abnormalities in the distribution of pulmonary blood flow. In most instances in which nonuniformity of blood flow is the sole functional abnormality, arterial blood gas values are within normal limits.

Relationship of Ventilation and Perfusion

Effective gas exchange within the lung requires a close approximation of the distribution of ventilation and pulmonary capillary blood flow. Major nonuniformity or mismatching between ventilation—V—and perfusion—Q—will be reflected in arterial blood gas abnormalities. In

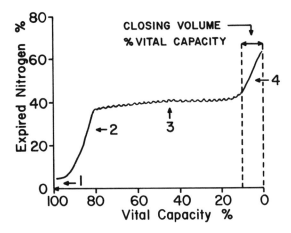

Fig. 9–4. Tracing of expired nitrogen concentration and expired volume from total lung capacity to residual volume. The four phases of the curve (see text) are shown. Oscillations of the nitrogen tracing during phase 3 are synchronous with the heart beat and are caused by cardiac churning of gases in the airways.

normal individuals the distribution of blood flow and ventilation to various areas of the lung is neither completely homogeneous nor equally matched. Some regions of lung, for example, tend to receive relatively more ventilation than blood flow. Normally, no adverse consequences follow from this relationship. Major physiologic disturbances occur primarily when blood flow to regions that are relatively underventilated, i.e., low V/Q, is substantial. In such situations, of which atelectasis and pneumonitis are examples, severe hypoxemia may occur. Elimination of carbon dioxide tends to be unaffected because other, more normal, lung regions are usually overventilated in compensation. This allows maintenance of a normal or low arterial carbon dioxide tension. Compensation for a fall in oxygen tension, on the other hand, is limited by the shape of the oxyhemoglobin dissociation curve (Fig. 9–1).

Shunts and Venous Admixture

A "right-to-left shunt" exists whenever blood passing through the pulmonary capillaries is not exposed to ventilated alveoli and is not oxygenated. Thus, as noted by Robin and associates (1977), a shunt can be considered an area of lung where V/Q is zero. Shunts occur in such conditions as lobar pneumonia and with acute atelectasis of a lobe or entire lung. The fraction of total pulmonary blood flow that is shunted can be approximated by measurement of arterial Po_2. With minor degrees of shunting the Po_2 with the subject at rest and breathing room air may be normal. Up to 6% right-to-left shunt occurs in healthy subjects, and this "physiologic" shunt results from venous blood normally entering the pulmonary veins, left atrium, or left ventricle. Whenever there is a greater than normal degree of shunting, hypoxemia will be present and inhalation of 100% oxygen for 10 to 20 minutes will fail to increase the Po_2 above 550 mm Hg, which would be expected in normal individuals. The ratio of shunted to total pulmonary blood flow can be estimated as follows if the arterial Po_2 is greater than 150 mm Hg during oxygen breathing:

$$\frac{\text{Shunt Flow}}{\text{Total Flow}} = \frac{[Po_2 \text{ (alv.)} - Po_2 \text{ (art. blood)}] \times 0.003}{(\text{art.} - \text{mixed ven. } O_2 \text{ cont.}) + [Po_2 \text{ (alv.)} - Po_2 \text{ (art.)}] \times .003}$$

Po_2 (alv.) = the alveolar Po_2 while breathing 100% oxygen.

It is estimated from the barometric pressure minus water vapor pressure (47 mm Hg) and alveolar Pco_2 (approximately 40 mm Hg).

Thus, Po_2 (alv.) = (760 − 47) − 40 = 673 mm Hg.

0.003 = the solubility factor for converting Po_2 into oxygen content in volume percent (see Fig. 9–2).

Art.-mixed ven. O_2 cont. = the difference in oxygen content between mixed venous and arterial blood. It is usually from 4 to 6 volumes percent and can be assumed for the purpose of estimating shunt flow.

The assumed value for the difference between mixed venous and arterial oxygen content has a definite effect upon the calculated shunt. The larger the difference be-

tween alveolar and arterial Po_2, the greater the effect of the assumed value of arterial-mixed venous difference upon the calculated shunt flow.

Venous admixture is a variant of right-to-left shunt in which there is a relative but not total lack of ventilation to the involved area, i.e., V/Q is low but greater than zero. Ventilation of a lung region may be normal, but, if blood flow is markedly increased, ventilation may be relatively inadequate; or ventilation may be markedly decreased in the presence of normal blood flow. Venous admixture results from relative ventilation/perfusion imbalances. Unlike a true shunt, the arterial Po_2 deficit of venous admixture can be corrected by 100% oxygen breathing. Studies with the multiple inert gas technique of Wagner and co-workers (1974) have shown that, contrary to past assumptions, extremely low ventilation/perfusion ratios can produce hypoxemia that is not corrected with 100% oxygen breathing. Furthermore, the use of high oxygen concentrations to measure shunt may cause absorptive atelectasis in those regions with a low V/Q and, thereby, increase the shunt. Nevertheless, measurement of the "shunt fraction" has practical application; for example, for monitoring the progress of acutely ill patients with the adult respiratory distress syndrome. This is especially true when samples of mixed venous blood are available from a central—i.e., Swan-Ganz—catheter line allowing accurate determination of the mixed venous and arterial oxygen content difference.

MANAGEMENT OF PATIENTS WITH IMPAIRED GAS EXCHANGE

The diagnosis and proper management of impaired gas exchange requires accurate measurement of arterial blood gases and pH. Minimal or subclinical defects in gas transport or distribution may require measurements of diffusion, and alveolar and arterial Po_2 at rest and with exercise. It has been estimated that a 50% reduction in the exercise carbon monoxide diffusing capacity is needed before a significant reduction in the exercise arterial Po_2 will be noted. Nevertheless, the majority of clinically significant problems can be evaluated by a careful history and physical examination supplemented by arterial blood measurements.

Proper interpretation of arterial blood gas and pH values requires a thorough knowledge of the patient's previous history of lung disease, or other medical and surgical problems that might alter pulmonary gas transport. Diuretics, steroids, and sedative drugs are frequent causes of abnormal arterial blood gas composition. Knowledge of prior use of sedatives and analgesics is most important in evaluating blood gas data, particularly in patients with pulmonary disease, because they may be unduly sensitive to respiratory depression from small doses that are usually well tolerated. Calculation of the $Pa_{O_2} - Pa_{O_2}$ difference assists the clinician in identifying aberrations in arterial blood gas values that are due to primary disturbances of ventilation without accompanying changes in the lung parenchyma. Patients with abnormal breathing patterns who are thought to have abnormal gas transport may have acid-base disturbances instead. For example, hypoventilation with an attendant rise in arterial P_{CO_2} and fall in P_{O_2} may occur because of severe metabolic alkalosis.

There are many therapeutic options for the management of patients with alterations in pulmonary gas exchange. Selection of the appropriate program should be based on a careful evaluation of the patients and their metabolic status, particularly their arterial blood gases. Important goals include optimization of tissue oxygenation and maintenance of relatively normal acid-base balance. To achieve adequate oxygenation, oxygen-carrying capacity—i.e., hemoglobin concentration, cardiac output, and regional blood flow must be maintained. Arterial P_{O_2} should, ideally, be at least 65 to 75 mm Hg to completely saturate hemoglobin. This may be achievable with relatively low concentrations of F_{IO_2}. When gas exchange is seriously deranged, concentrations exceeding an F_{IO_2} of 0.50 may be needed, raising the possibility of pulmonary oxygen toxicity. As pointed out by Weisman and co-workers (1982), positive airway pressure, either as continuous positive airway pressure—CPAP—or positive end-expiratory pressure—PEEP, may allow significant reductions in the amount of supplemental oxygen needed to maintain acceptable arterial P_{O_2} levels. However, excessive levels of positive pressure, particularly in patients with volume depletion, may cause a reduction

in cardiac output. Thus, careful monitoring of these patients is essential. In patients who appear unlikely to maintain adequate levels of ventilation, as indicated by a rising arterial P_{CO_2} or unusual degree of ventilatory effort, mechanical ventilation is advisable. Modes such as control, assist-control, and intermittent mandatory ventilation—IMV—are available to facilitate optimal mechanical support.

REFERENCES

Coburn, R.F.: Current concepts: endogenous carbon monoxide production. N. Engl. J. Med. *282*:207, 1970.

Divertie, M.B., and Brown, A.L., Jr.: The fine structure of the normal human alveolar-capillary membrane. J.A.M.A. *187*:938, 1964.

Finley, T.N., Swenson, E.W., and Comroe, J.H., Jr.: The cause of arterial hypoxemia at rest in patients with "alveolar-capillary block syndrome." J. Clin. Invest. *41*:618, 1962.

Gracey, D.R., Divertie, M.B., and Brown, A.L., Jr.: Alveolar-capillary membrane in idiopathic interstitial pulmonary fibrosis: electron microscopic study of 14 cases. Am. Rev. Respir. Dis. *98*:16, 1968.

Robin, E.D., Laman, P.D., Goris, M.L. and Theodore, J.: A shunt is (not) a shunt is (not) a shunt. Am. Rev. Respir. Dis. *115*:553, 1977.

Said, S.I., et al.: Shunting effect of extreme impairment of pulmonary diffusion. Bull. Johns Hopkins Hosp. *107*:255, 1960.

Wagner, P.D., Saltzman, H.A., and West, T.B.: Measurement of continuous distributions of ventilation-perfusion ratios: Theory. J. Appl. Physiol. *36*:588, 1974.

Weisman, I.M., Rinaldo, J.E., and Rogers, R.M.: Current concepts: positive end-expiratory pressure in adult respiratory failure. N. Engl. J. Med. *307*:1381, 1982.

CHAPTER 10

MECHANICS OF BREATHING

David W. Cugell, James E. Fish, and Jeffrey Glassroth

The term "mechanics of breathing" refers to the elastic properties of the lung and chest wall and to airflow resistance. These properties will be described and related to lung volume and airflow measurements—the standard tests of ventilatory function. For more detailed mathematical descriptions of these properties and for the methodology of testing, see the general references. The subdivisions of the lung volume referred to are shown in Figure 10–1.

GAS VOLUMES COMMONLY REPORTED:
Vital capacity (VC) is the maximum volume that can be expired following a maximal inspiration.
Total lung capacity (TLC) is the volume in the lungs after a maximal inspiration.
Residual volume (RV) is the volume remaining in the lungs after a maximal expiration. In normal individuals RV is approximately 25 to 30% of TLC.
Functional residual capacity (FRC) is the volume in the lungs at the end of a normal expiration.
Tidal volume (TV) is the volume of a spontaneous breath.
OTHER VOLUMES:
Inspiratory capacity (IC) is the maximal volume that can be inspired from the resting end-*ex*piratory position to TLC.
Expiratory reserve volume (ERV) is the volume that can be expired from a spontaneous end-expiratory position—i.e., from FRC to RV.
Inspiratory reserve volume (IRV) is the volume that can still be inspired from a spontaneous end-*in*spiratory position.

ELASTIC PROPERTIES OF THE LUNG

The inflated lung is an elastic structure that tends to deflate itself. The deflation force exerted by an expanded lung is the *elastic recoil pressure*. This recoil pressure increases with increasing lung volume, and the pressure required to maintain inflation equals the elastic recoil pressure. Irrespective of the manner in which it is measured, the recoil pressure of the lung is always considered positive because it is always directed toward deflation. The elastic recoil pressure is expressed as the pressure difference between the alveolar lumen and the pleural space. Alveolar pressure is equivalent to atmospheric

pressure when the glottis and mouth are open and there is no airflow. Therefore, under these conditions, the intrapleural pressure is equal but opposite in sign to the elastic recoil pressure.

Pleural pressure changes can be conveniently and reliably measured in the upright subject by placing a small tube with an attached balloon in the esophagus. Under static conditions, that is, when there is no airflow, a given degree of lung inflation is maintained either by inspiratory muscle contraction, by the elasticity of the chest wall resisting inward collapse, or both. The "resting" lung volume or FRC is the result of the balance between equal but opposite forces generated by the inward elastic recoil of the lungs and the outward recoil of the chest cage.

A *pressure-volume* plot made under static conditions (Fig. 10–2) defines the elastic properties of the lung. Multiple measurements of the elastic recoil pressure or the intrapleural pressure and corresponding intrathoracic gas volume over the entire range of lung volumes are necessary to describe the entire pressure-volume curve of the lung. Elastic recoil pressures are frequently reported as the static recoil pressure at total lung capacity—*maximum retractive force*—or at some fraction of total lung capacity—*static recoil pressure, 90% of total lung capacity.* The pressure-volume relationship of the lung is often described in terms of *lung compliance*. If measured over the tidal volume portion of the curve, it is almost linear, and is expressed as the change in volume per unit change in pressure—ml/cm H_2O.

The pressure-volume relationship is basic to an understanding of the fundamental relation between the work of breathing and lung mechanics. The "stiffer" lung will display a more horizontal curve (Fig. 10–2C), meaning that it takes a greater pressure to achieve the same inflation volume compared with a normal lung (Fig. 10–2A). These lungs are called less compliant. At lung volumes approaching total lung capacity, considerably more pressure per liter of inspired volume is required than at smaller lung volumes. In both health and disease, the tidal volume occurs on the steepest part of the pres-

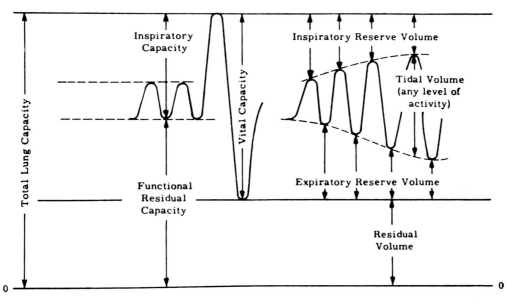

Fig. 10–1. Lung volumes. (Standardization of definitions and symbols in respiratory physiology. Fed. Proc. 9:602, 1950.)

sure-volume curve where the largest volume change is accomplished with a minimal pressure change. For any given ventilatory requirement, every person has an optimal pattern of tidal volume and breathing frequency at which his work of breathing is minimal. When the lungs are stiff, a pattern of rapid, shallow breathing is adopted and this pattern minimizes the work of breathing. Even so, more effort than normal is required to ventilate stiff lungs (Fig. 10–2C). Although it would appear that the patient with emphysema is at an advantage because he requires less effort to deform his lungs (Fig. 10–2B), his work of breathing is increased because of obstruction to airflow and because hyperinflation requires that tidal breathing be shifted to a less advantageous position on the pressure-volume curve.

mechanical disadvantage

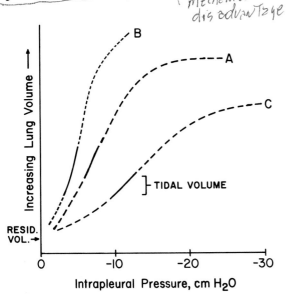

Fig. 10–2. Pressure-volume curves: A, normal; B, emphysema; C, pulmonary fibrosis. The solid line represents the tidal volume in these three conditions.

The elastic properties of the lung reside mainly in the alveolar walls and their liquid lining. The walls contain a network of collagen, elastic, and reticular fibers in addition to their capillary network and epithelial lining. The thin liquid film on the luminal surface of the alveolar epithelium creates a *surface tension* that accounts in part for lung elasticity. Surface tension forces tend to reduce the surface to the smallest possible area. In the bubble-like alveolus, surface tension increases as the size of the bubble decreases, and, if unopposed, would lead to alveolar collapse. A lipid substance in the alveolar lining fluid reduces surface tension at the gas-liquid interface, thereby protecting the lungs against alveolar collapse. This substance, *surfactant*, can be extracted from normal lung tissue and is absent or reduced in persons with pulmonary atelectasis, hyaline membrane disease, or infarction. Surfactant maintains surface-tension forces relatively constant despite varying degrees of lung inflation and alveolar size.

Although pressure changes in the lung are similar everywhere during inflation, ventilation is not evenly distributed throughout the normal organ. At successive horizontal levels of the lung, from apex to base, the volume change produced by a given pressure change becomes progressively greater. The most dependent portions of the lung receive more ventilation per unit of lung tissue than the uppermost levels. The reason for this discrepancy is the effect of gravity. While pressure changes producing inflation are essentially the same over the normal lung surface, the absolute pressure is not. In the erect position the weight of the lung makes the intrapleural pressure at the lung base less negative than it is at the apex. With a less negative intrapleural pressure at the bases the elastic recoil pressure and the volume of each alveolus at the base are less than in higher regions at the onset of inspiration (Fig. 10–3). With inflation the pressure change transmitted to all lung tissue is the same, but different regions will inflate to different volumes

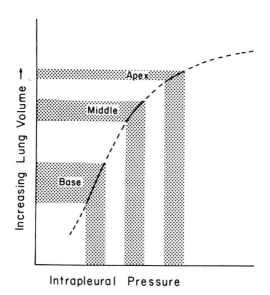

Fig. 10-3. Effect of gravity in the upright position. As one approaches the base of the lung, there is a greater volume change per unit of lung tissue for the same pressure change.

depending upon where, on the pressure-volume curve, inflation commences. A dependent portion has a lesser recoil pressure to begin with; therefore, a normal breath will inflate a basal region more than other areas because its behavior is confined to a steeper portion of the pressure-volume curve. Fortunately, perfusion of the normal lung is similarly affected by gravity so that a fairly good match between ventilation and perfusion is maintained throughout the lung.

In diseases of the lungs in which the elastic properties are not uniformly the same, regional ventilation becomes nonuniform. Adjacent lung regions, even neighboring alveoli, have different pressure-volume characteristics. Thus, the same pressure change, even when beginning at the same absolute level of intrapleural pressure, produces different volume changes in neighboring areas. The pressure-volume characteristics as measured with an esophageal balloon are those of the whole lung and are averages that may obscure regional differences. Diffuse infiltrative disease, such as diffuse pulmonary fibrosis, produces not only inequalities in inspired gas distribution but also inequalities in the distribution of blood flow, resulting in abnormal gas exchange. The overall adverse effects of these diseases can best be assessed by measurements of gas exchange and arterial blood gas content (Chapter 9).

ELASTIC AND MECHANICAL PROPERTIES OF THE CHEST WALL

Lung inflation and deflation are accomplished by changes in the dimensions of the chest wall. These dimensional changes are determined by the elastic properties of the bony and soft tissue structures of the thorax and by the muscle forces that impart motion to the respiratory system. Like the lung, the chest wall exerts a recoil pressure proportional to its volume of expansion.

This recoil pressure is measured as the difference between pleural pressure and body surface pressure under static conditions when the muscles of respiration are completely relaxed. By plotting this pressure against the thoracic gas volume, one obtains the pressure-volume relationship of the chest wall. The *compliance* of the chest wall, as described by the slope of this relationship, is normally high enough so that the rib cage and soft tissue structures do not restrict respiratory movement.

Certain factors, however, may restrict movement of the chest wall and reduce its compliance. For instance, an increase in the longitudinal dimension of the thorax is primarily determined by movement of the diaphragm. Diaphragmatic movement may be restricted by conditions that increase intra-abdominal pressure, such as pregnancy, obesity, ascites, and intra-abdominal tumors. Changing from the erect to the supine position may also restrict the diaphragm by shifting the weight of the abdominal contents toward the diaphragm. These conditions generally reduce vital capacity, total lung capacity, and functional residual capacity.

Changes in the anteroposterior and transverse dimensions of the chest wall are primarily effected by the intercostal muscles and accessory muscles of respiration, and are dependent on the mobility of the rib cage. Thus, conditions that result in deformation or fixation of the thorax, such as kyphoscoliosis or ankylosing spondylitis, may also restrict expansion. Obesity may also reduce chest wall compliance by increasing the soft tissue mass of the thorax. Moreover, because respiratory movement is ultimately dependent on the action of the respiratory muscles, conditions that result in paralysis or weakness of the respiratory muscles severely limit ventilation and often cause respiratory failure. Because of the difficulties of measuring chest wall compliance, muscle strength, and leverage, as well as intra-abdominal pressure and gravitational forces, it is customary to rely upon measurements of their consequences, such as changes in lung volumes, gas exchange, ventilation, and perfusion. The results of these tests plus knowledge of the clinical status of the patient are usually adequate to determine whether the chest wall or underlying lung disease is at fault.

LUNG VOLUME MEASUREMENTS

An isolated decrease in a lung volume does not affect health as long as adequate volume remains to permit normal ventilation of the alveoli. Although the tidal volume normally increases with exercise, the ventilation necessary for a given level of exercise can be achieved by increasing either tidal volume or breathing frequency. Thus, compensation for a limited lung volume can be attained by increasing the breathing frequency. In the presence of lung diseases characterized by airway obstruction, however, ventilation is maintained by a relatively greater increase in tidal volume than in frequency. This interrelation between tidal volume and frequency is further considered subsequently in the section: *Work of Breathing.*

The reduction of lung volumes occurring with diseases

of the chest wall, lungs, or pleura provides a crude guide to the severity of the disease. Thus, volume measurements may be useful for deciding when therapeutic intervention is appropriate or in judging the response or lack of response to therapy. Lung volume measurements are easily made, and their reproducibility renders them useful for longitudinal studies in a given patient. For example, a loss of 500 ml upon serial testing of a patient with an initial vital capacity of 4 or 5 L would be significant. Unfortunately, a single measurement is not a sensitive indicator of early disease because there is approximately a 20% variation in lung volumes among persons of the same age, height, and sex.

Although no specific diagnosis is suggested by a lung volume decrease, simple volume measurements, particularly the vital capacity, are just as sensitive an index of disease as the direct measurement of mechanical factors that determine static lung volumes, such as the lung compliance.

Vital Capacity

The vital capacity can be determined either by adding separate measurements of the maximal expired volume and maximal inspired volume starting from the resting lung volume, or by using a single expiratory effort starting from total lung capacity (Fig. 10–1). The maneuver may be performed in a leisurely or "slow" manner as distinct from the "forced" vital capacity. In the forced maneuver the patient empties his lungs as rapidly as possible starting from total lung capacity. In patients with obstructive lung disease, this forced maneuver may increase expiratory obstruction and produce a spuriously low measurement of vital capacity (see section *Airway Resistance During Expiration*).

Functional Residual Capacity

This is the volume of gas remaining in the lungs at the end of expiration. Two methods are commonly used for measurements of functional residual capacity: inert gas dilution or washout and body plethysmography. Nitrogen, argon, and helium are the inert gases customarily employed. For an accurate determination, the gas must be evenly distributed or washed out from all air-containing units of the lung. This may not occur, or may occur only slowly, in the presence of bullous disease, airway obstruction, or other conditions in which portions of the lung are poorly ventilated.

For the plethysmographic method of measuring functional residual capacity, the subject sits in an airtight cabinet, the body plethysmograph. Measurements of changes in alveolar pressure and lung volume are made simultaneously while the patient is panting against an obstruction to airflow that is interposed briefly at the mouth. Alveolar pressure is equivalent to the pressure at the mouth under these circumstances. With this method all of the gas within the chest, even in the presence of airway obstruction or bullous disease, is measured. The test is simple to perform but relatively elaborate and costly equipment is required. However, the same apparatus can be used for the direct measurement of airway resistance. Discrepancies between plethysmographic and inert gas volume determinations may reflect the volume of poorly ventilated lung that is present.

Residual Volume

The residual volume, air remaining in the lungs following a complete expiration, is calculated by subtracting the expiratory reserve volume (Fig. 10–1) from the functional residual capacity determined by any of the preceding methods and is therefore no more accurate than the functional residual capacity.

Total Lung Capacity

The total lung capacity is usually computed by merely adding the separately determined vital capacity and residual volume. It is less reproducible than the vital capacity because the variability in the separately measured volume components may be additive. The *total lung capacity* can also be calculated from roentgenograms of the chest and includes all the gas within the lungs, similar to the plethysmographic measurements.

AIRFLOW RESISTANCES

To generate airflow, the bellows action of the chest wall must overcome the elastic properties of the lungs and chest wall plus frictional resistances to motion. These frictional resistances consist of pressure losses due to air flowing through the airways and to friction within the tissues of the lung and chest wall during breathing movements. Unlike measurements of elastic recoil pressures made under static conditions, resistances are a dynamic property and must be measured while there is airflow. The components of total airflow resistance within the lungs and thorax are: *airway resistance, lung tissue resistance, and chest wall resistance.* The sum of the last two resistances is about equal to the airway resistance. The resistances of lung tissue and chest wall tend to be minimally affected by disease and are overshadowed by the magnitude of the changes in airway resistance. The majority of airway resistance occurs in large airways— i.e., those 2 mm or larger in diameter.

Increases in airflow resistance are due primarily to increases in airway resistance; thus indirect measurements of airflow resistance, such as the maximum midexpiratory flow rate, volume expelled in the first second of the forced vital capacity maneuver, and maximum voluntary ventilation, may be used as an index of airway resistance. Inertia is still another mechanical property of the respiratory system, but it is a negligible quantity and can be ignored.

Measurements of airflow resistance provide an "average" value for the entire system of airways. In any generalized obstructive lung disease, some airways have a higher resistance to airflow than others, and there will be greater flow into alveoli whose conducting airways have the lowest resistance. The result is a nonuniform distribution of inspired air creating a mismatch between ventilation and perfusion and impairment of gas exchange.

Airway Resistance During Inspiration

Airway diameter varies depending upon the gradient between intra- and extra-lumenal airway pressures. These gradients function in an opposite manner for intrathoracic and extrathoracic airways. The extrathoracic airway diameter increases during *ex*piration whereas the intrathoracic airway increases in diameter on *in*spiration. An exception is a fixed orifice type of obstruction such as occurs in association with a tumor completely encircling an airway. Airway dilatation on inspiration is produced by radial traction provided by elastic forces of the lung tissue surrounding the airway (Fig. 10–4). A loss of elastic recoil, such as that occurring in emphysema, results in a decrease of airway caliber. Conversely, an increase in elastic forces increases traction on the airway, enlarging airway dimensions.

Inspiratory airflow increases in direct proportion to the force or effort applied. Patients with chronic obstructive pulmonary disease, in whom impaired expiratory airflow is invariably present, may have decreased inspiratory flow as well. Inspiratory flow is reduced in patients with chronic bronchitis and in those with asthma because the bronchial lumen is narrowed by secretions and edema or bronchospasm or both. Inspiratory flow is also reduced when airways become stiff and less expansile because of inflamed bronchial walls or become narrow owing to decreased radial traction (Fig. 10–4). Inspiratory flow measurements, usually made from an inspiratory flow-volume loop (Fig. 10–7), are primarily useful in unusual, but often remedial, localized obstructions of major airways because limitation of inspiratory flow may equal or exceed expiratory flow limitation. In patients with the usual types of obstructive lung diseases, inspiratory flow limitation is not clinically important, whereas expiratory flow limitation is invariably severe.

Airway Resistance During Expiration

Unlike inspiratory flow, which depends to a major extent on the muscular effort generated, expiratory flow depends primarily on the mechanical properties of the lungs and is related to effort only up to a certain point. Beyond this point further increases in effort do not increase expiratory flow and in some instances may decrease it. This concept is illustrated in the isovolume pressure-flow curves in Fig. 10–5. These curves are ob-

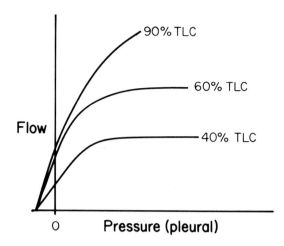

Fig. 10–5. Isovolume pressure flow plot at three different lung volumes.

tained by performing a series of active expirations with increasing effort at a particular lung volume and by plotting flow rates against corresponding pleural pressure. In this instance pleural pressure represents the driving pressure or force related to muscular effort. In Figure 10–5 curves obtained at three different lung volumes are represented. Between total lung capacity—TLC—and 75% of TLC, flow increases with effort and is dependent not only on effort but on the patency of airways and high elastic recoil of the lung at high volumes. At volumes below approximately 75% of TLC, expiratory flow increases with effort up to a point, at which further increases in effort do not lead to a higher flow rate. Flow reaches a maximal level at this point because further increases in pleural pressure due to effort tend to compress airways and limit flow to the same extent that they tend to drive flow. This dynamic compression occurs because intrathoracic airways are exposed to pleural pressures. This concept is illustrated by the model in Figure 10–6. In this model the "lung" or "alveolus" and airway are suspended in a box representing the thorax. The lung is separated from the chest wall for descriptive purposes only, and the space between the lung and chest wall should be considered the airless pleural space. The numbers represent pressure in centimeters of water. In Figure 10–6A the pleural pressure is equal to the pressure surrounding the airways. At this level of lung inflation the pleural pressure is equal and opposite in sign to the elastic recoil pressure of the lung— +10; there is no pressure gradient to produce airflow, and net alveolar pressure is atmospheric, or zero. During active expiration (Fig. 10–6B) pleural pressure becomes less negative. Since alveolar pressure is equal to the sum of pleural pressure and lung recoil pressure, it will increase by an amount equal to the increase in pleural pressure. At this point the difference between alveolar pressure— +20— and airway opening pressure—0—represents the total pressure producing expiratory flow. It follows that there must be some point between the alveolus and the airway opening at which airway intraluminal pressure is equal

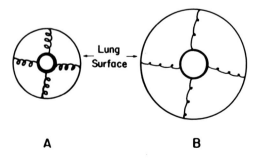

Fig. 10–4. Effect of inspiration on an intrapulmonary airway: *A*, end-expiration; *B*, end-inspiration. The inner circle could also represent an alveolus.

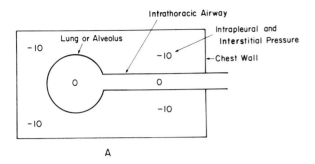

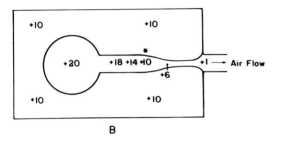

Fig. 10–6. See text for discussion. Static recoil pressure is + 10 cm H₂O. *A,* Static conditions; *B,* dynamic conditions. Airway is compressed downstream from point marked by asterisk.

to pleural pressure, and intraluminal pressures downstream from this point will be less than pleural pressure. This downstream segment will tend to collapse and limit flow. If there is a further increase in effort, the downstream segment tends to collapse even further. In this case any additional increase in driving pressure resulting from greater effort is merely dissipated in keeping the collapsed segment open.

Maximal flow over most of the vital capacity is thus effort-independent, but it is dependent on the lung recoil pressure and the resistance of peripheral airways upstream from the collapsible segment. Therefore, diseases such as emphysema that reduce the elasticity of airways and lung tissue tend to produce flow limitation by reducing the driving pressure and by making airways more collapsible. Diseases such as chronic bronchitis and asthma produce flow limitation by increasing the resistance of upstream or peripheral airways. Because maximal expiratory flow over the effort-independent range of the vital capacity—below 75% of TLC—depends on the resistance of peripheral airways, tests of forced expiration have become a useful means of detecting airway disease in its early stages.

Because of the pressure, volume, and flow relationships of the lung, the presence of airway obstruction can be determined by measuring maximal expiratory flow. Because maximal flow is relatively independent of effort, and primarily dependent on the recoil pressure of the lung, and because the recoil pressure of the lung is dependent on lung volume, one need only relate the measured flow to the lung volume at which it is measured;

this relationship is called a flow-volume curve (Fig. 10–7).

The initial acceleration phase of the expiratory half of the loop represents the inertia of the system. Thereafter, maximal flow decreases as lung volume decreases. The initial portion of the curve between TLC and approximately 75% of TLC is the effort-dependent portion. Beyond this point, maximal flow is relatively independent of effort and dependent on lung recoil and the resistance of airways upstream from the collapsible segment. By measuring flow at a particular volume, such as 50% or 25% of the vital capacity, and comparing it to established normal standards, one can detect the presence of airflow limitation. Measurements made from the maximal expiratory flow-volume curve can identify patients with early expiratory airflow limitation before abnormalities occur in their timed vital capacity measurements. Although such measurements are more sensitive, they are neither as reproducible nor specific as spirometric tests of forced expiration that relate expired volume to the time of expiration, such as the *timed vital capacity.*

Timed Vital Capacity

This measurement is obtained from the conventional spirogram, a graph of expired volume and time. The patient makes a forced expiration from total lung capacity (Fig. 10–8). Because the effort must be maximal, the patient must be cooperative and the technician capable of coaxing the patient to do his best. The slope of a tangent to the volume-time curve at any point represents airflow at that point. Because airflow is maximal as long as a certain minimal effort is exceeded, portions of the forced vital capacity curve are very reproducible provided the patient exerts his best effort. Both reproducibility and appearance of the tracing can be used to judge the dependability of the results obtained.

Other analyses from the timed vital capacity include the volume expired in the first second of the forced vital capacity maneuver, the FEV_1. It includes the earliest part of expiration, which is effort-dependent, and a later portion, which is less so. If airflow is diminished because of disease, flow tends to decrease throughout expiration. Measurement of airflow in the first 2 and first 3 seconds of the expiratory effort helps verify the 1-second value. If the 1-second volume is low but the 2- and 3-second volumes are normal, one suspects poor performance. Some laboratories report the volume expired at 0.75 or even 0.5 second. These volumes have the same significance as does the 1-second volume. Reduced 1-second volumes are particularly meaningful when the patient's total vital capacity is normal since airflow obstruction is then very likely. If the total vital capacity is reduced, then the forced 1-second volume may also be reduced, whether or not airflow obstruction is present. Therefore, it is useful to report the 1-second volume, or other timed fractional volumes, as a percentage of the total forced vital capacity, the so-called FEV_1/FVC ratio.

Another derived index of airflow is the forced expiratory flow between 25 and 75% of vital capacity, $FEF_{25-75\%}$, also called the maximum mid-expiratory flow

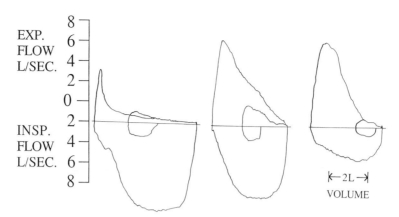

Fig. 10–7. Flow-volume loops from three subjects. The small, inner loop represents flow and volume changes during a normal, resting tidal breath. For each tracing the residual volume is to the right, and total lung capacity to the left. The patient shown on the left has a large vital capacity, severe expiratory airflow limitation throughout the entire vital capacity, but no problem with inspiratory airflow. Note that dynamic airway compression occurs during a forced expiratory maneuver—airflow in the mid vital capacity is greater during a relaxed, tidal breath than it is during the forced vital capacity. A normal, healthy subject is shown in the middle panel. The patient on the right has inspiratory airflow limitation, but very good expiratory airflow. This pattern is observed when there is an extrathoracic airway defect which can occur with tracheal tumors, vocal chord lesions, or tracheomalacia.

rate—MMF. This rate is calculated by measuring the time required to expire the middle 50% of the vital capacity. Because it is an estimate of the average rate of airflow over the middle half of the vital capacity, it is expressed in units of flow. Hence, the middle 50% of the vital capacity in liters is divided by the time taken to expire it (Fig. 10–8). Because this measurement is derived from the effort-independent portion of the forced vital capacity, it primarily reflects the flow characteristics in peripheral airways upstream from or proximal to the collapsible segment. For this reason the $FEF_{25-75\%}$ is considered a useful test of small airway function.

Peak Flow

Peak flow can be measured either from the flow-volume loop (Fig. 10–7) or with a simple hand-held ane-

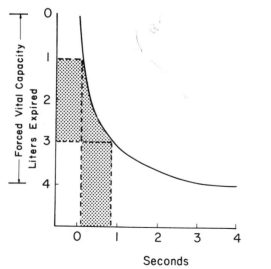

Fig. 10–8. The forced vital capacity curve. Both the mid-half of the forced vital capacity and the time required to deliver this mid-half volume are shaded.

mometer type of device such as the Wright Peak Flow Meter. These two methods do not give comparable results and both depend on patient effort. Despite these limitations, determination of peak flow is one test that young children are often able to perform well and may be the only way of measuring their airflow.

Maximum Voluntary Ventilation

Maximum voluntary ventilation—MVV—is determined by having the patient breathe as fast and as deep as possible for a fraction of a minute. The expired volume is measured and the ventilation expressed in liters per minute. The determination depends on both adequate inspiratory and expiratory airflow plus considerable endurance and patient cooperation. When properly performed, it provides an excellent index of overall ventilatory ability. It also serves as an alternate test of airflow and as a check on the results of other expiratory flow measurements. Since the maximum mid-expiratory flow rate and timed fractions of the forced vital capacity are calculated from the same volume-time curve (Fig. 10–8), both will be spuriously low if the performance is poor.

Relation of the Functional Residual Capacity and Residual Volume to Airflow Obstruction

Functional residual capacity and residual volume may increase in obstructive lung disease by two mechanisms. First, there may be a loss of lung tissue and therefore lung elasticity. The chest wall forces that counterbalance lung elastic recoil are less opposed and expand the thorax to a larger volume. Second, if airway resistance is increased to such a degree that the patient cannot exhale his inspired volume before inspiring his next breath, he will increase his intrathoracic gas volume until expiratory resistance has decreased sufficiently to enable him to exhale satisfactorily (Fig. 10–9).

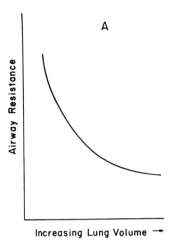 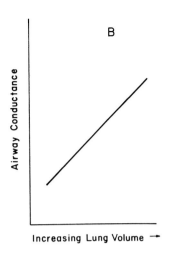

Fig. 10–9. *A*, The airway resistance is dependent on the lung volume at which it is measured and is non-linear. *B*, The reciprocal of airway resistance, airway conductance, is linearly related to lung volume. The slope of this line is the specific conductance.

Measurements of Airway Resistance and Airflow

The pressure drop from the alveoli to the mouth and the airflow at the mouth can be measured and provide a direct measure of *airway resistance*—resistance = pressure/flow. The airway resistance—R_{aw} depends on the lung volume at which it is measured, as would be expected since airways narrow at decreasing lung volumes (Fig. 10–4) independent of the dynamic narrowing previously described. Proper interpretation of an airway resistance value requires knowledge of the lung volume at which it was measured, particularly when there is airflow obstruction, because lung volumes are often increased. Lung volumes range so widely among normal subjects that both airway resistance and the corresponding lung volume must be measured. With the body plethysmograph method both volume and resistance are determined simultaneously. The relationship between airway resistance and lung volume (Fig. 10–9A) is curvilinear, whereas the relationship between the reciprocal of airway resistance, *airway conductance*, and lung volume is nearly linear (Fig. 10–9B). The slope of this conductance-lung volume plot is the *specific conductance*. The specific conductance is relatively insensitive to changes of resistance in the peripheral airways until it has increased severalfold because changes in small airway resistance are masked by the relatively higher resistance of the upper airways. Direct resistance or conductance measurements are seldom more sensitive for defining airway obstruction than is a well-performed forced vital capacity determination.

WORK OF BREATHING

Breathing requires that the respiratory muscles or a mechanical ventilator generate a pressure—force—sufficient to move the volumes of air required for ventilation. Force is required to stretch tissue, to counteract gravity, and to overcome frictional resistances of tissues and airways. There is an optimal combination of breathing frequency and tidal volume at which the work of breathing is minimal. This combination varies between subjects and for specific metabolic requirements. If tidal volume is increased, the pressures required become disproportionately large (see pressure-volume curve in Fig. 10–2). If breathing frequency increases, the airway resistance increases owing to additional flow turbulence and to increased expiratory airway narrowing because of dynamic airway compression. Attempts to drive the respiratory system faster than it will respond, using pressures greater than those required for maximum expiratory airflow, represent wasted effort. In both health and disease each person spontaneously selects whatever combination of tidal volume and breathing frequency achieves the required ventilation at a minimal work of breathing. In normal man the work of breathing requires little energy, approximately 1 ml of oxygen per liter of ventilation. In disease the oxygen cost of breathing increases greatly and may represent a large portion of the metabolic needs of the patient, thereby limiting the proportion of total oxygen uptake available for muscles not involved in ventilation. Thus, exercise capacity is limited when lung disease causes a substantial increase in the work of breathing.

READING REFERENCES

General

Chusid, E.L.: The Selective and Comprehensive Testing of Adult Pulmonary Function. Mt. Kisco, NY, Futura Publishing, 1983.

Murray, J.F.: The Normal Lung. Philadelphia, W.B. Saunders Co., 1986.

West, J.B.: Respiratory Physiology: The Essentials, 2nd ed., Baltimore, Williams & Wilkins, 1979.

Chest Wall and Lung Elasticity

Gibson, G.J., and Pride, N.B.: Lung distensibility. Br. J. Dis. Chest 70:143, 1976.

Rahn, H., et al.: The pressure-volume diagram of the thorax and lung. Am. J. Physiol. *146*:161, 1946.

Turner, J.M., Mead, J., and Wohl, M.E.: Elasticity of human lungs in relation to age. J. Appl. Physiol. *25*:664, 1968.

Airflow Resistance

Fry, D.Q., and Hyatt, R.E.: Pulmonary mechanics: a unified analysis of the relationship between pressure, volume and gasflow in the lungs of normal and diseased human subjects. Am. J. Med. 29:672, 1960.

Hogg, J.C., Macklem, P.T., and Thurlbeck, W.M.: Site and nature of airway obstruction in chronic obstructive lung disease. N. Engl. J. Med. 278:1355, 1968.

Hyatt, R.E., Rodarte, J.R., Wilson, T.A., and Lambert, R.K.: Expiratory flow limitation. J. Appl. Physiol. 55:169, 1983.

Mead, J., et al.: Significance of the relationship between lung recoil and maximum expiratory flow. J. Appl. Physiol. 22:95, 1967.

Pride, N.B., et al.: Determinants of maximum expiratory flow from the lungs. J. Appl. Physiol. 23:646, 1967.

Radiologic and Imaging Studies of the Chest

CHAPTER 11

ROENTGENOGRAPHIC EVALUATION OF THE CHEST

Wallace T. Miller

For the physician interested in diseases of the chest, the roentgenogram of the chest is of paramount importance in identifying the presence of such disease and in providing clues about its nature.

THE ROUTINE EXAMINATION

Adequate roentgenographic examination of the chest necessitates at least two projections to provide a three-dimensional view of the thorax. The number of projections considered adequate varies with the individual physician. The views commonly employed are straight posteroanterior—PA—and lateral projections.

The PA roentgenogram can be made at 60 to 80 kilovolts—kV—at a tube film distance of 72 inches without a grid. However, a high kilovoltage technique has been employed by an increasing number of radiologists. This technique employs x rays above the 125-kV range with a fine line grid, creating a roentgenogram that has more information by providing less contrast but more penetration. An added advantage of this high kV technique is the decreased time required for exposure, reducing patient motion.

The lateral roentgenogram is of considerable importance in the routine examination of the chest, since many lesions in the chest are apparent only in the lateral view. Examples include small mediastinal lesions, some masses in the anterior portions of the lung adjacent to the mediastinum (Fig. 11–1), lesions in the vertebral column, lesions behind the heart and diaphragm on the PA view, and small pleural effusions (Fig. 11–2). Thus, adequate examination of the chest in other than routine screening procedures requires a lateral film.

SUPPLEMENTARY ROENTGENOGRAMS

The routine examination of the chest will allow discovery of most chest lesions. However, additional projections or different types of roentgenograms may be necessary to make an accurate assessment of the character of a particular lesion.

Oblique views are quite helpful in localizing a suspected lesion and then projecting it free from overlying structures. The oblique roentgenogram is particularly helpful in determining whether a lesion is in the lung or in the chest wall. It is also quite helpful in investigating mediastinal lesions, particularly with barium in the esophagus (Fig. 11–3). The oblique roentgenogram is designated right or left anterior or right or left posterior on the basis of the patient's relationship to the film cassette. In a right anterior oblique position, the right side of the patient is closer to the film and the patient is facing the film cassette.

The oblique view can be confusing to interpret. It is helpful to remember that the heart is an anterior structure and thus will move to the left in a right anterior oblique or to the right in the left anterior oblique view. The aortic arch appears "closed" in the right anterior oblique and "open" in the left anterior oblique view.

It is helpful when examining oblique roentgenograms to remember that posteriorly placed lesions in the lung will maintain a constant relationship with the spine and anteriorly placed lesions in the lung will maintain a constant relationship with the heart.

Figures 11–4C and 11–4D demonstrate some of the normal anatomic structures seen on the oblique roentgenogram.

Lateral decubitus roentgenograms are extremely important in the investigation of suspected pleural effusion or in demonstration of air fluid levels in pulmonary cavities. The decubitus roentgenogram is made with the beam projected in a horizontal plane, with the patient lying on his side. In a right lateral decubitus roentgenogram, the patient lies on his right side and free pleural fluid will layer along the right lateral chest wall (Fig. 11–2C). Amounts of fluid as small as 50 to 100 ml can be identified in the lateral decubitus position. If pneumothorax is present and examination is being made to

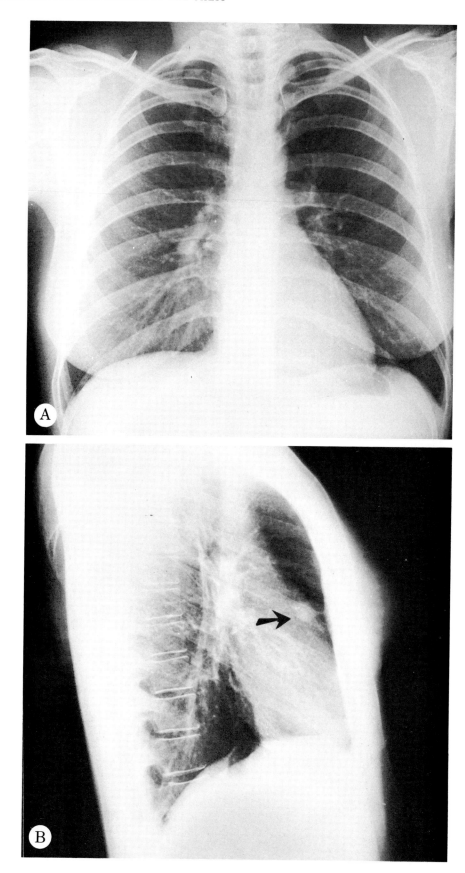

Fig. 11–1. Carcinoma of the lung. The posteroanterior (PA) roentgenogram (*A*) apparently shows no abnormality, but the lateral roentgenogram (*B*) demonstrates an unsuspected mass adjacent to the anterior mediastinum (arrow). This mass was subsequently seen to lie in the right upper lobe and was a primary carcinoma of the lung. This finding demonstrates the value of the lateral roentgenogram in the survey examination.

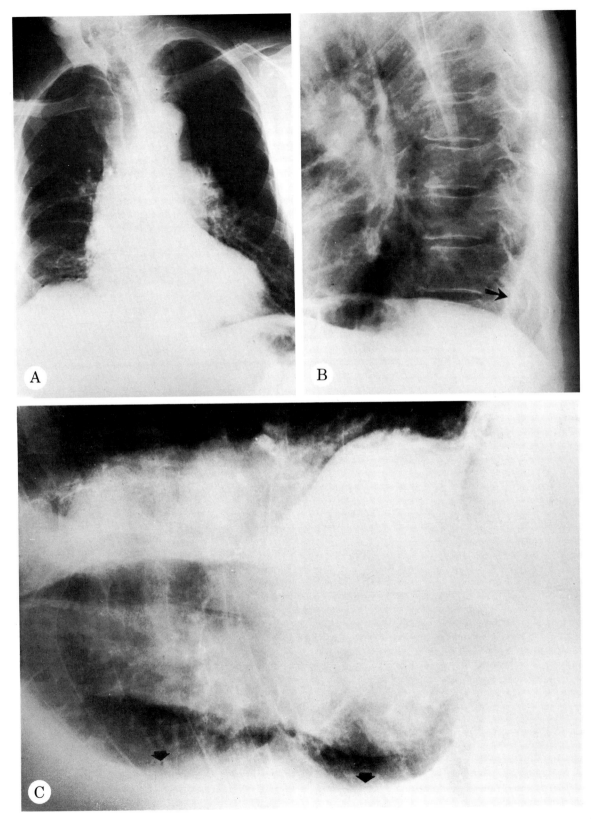

Fig. 11–2. Pleural effusion. No apparent abnormality is noted on the PA roentgenogram (A). The lateral roentgenogram (B) demonstrates blunting of the posterior costophrenic sulcus (arrow), suggesting a pleural effusion. The right lateral decubitus view (C) demonstrates a large effusion on the right (arrows).

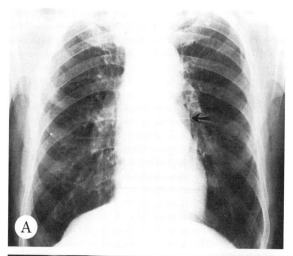

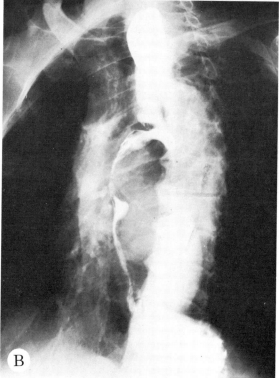

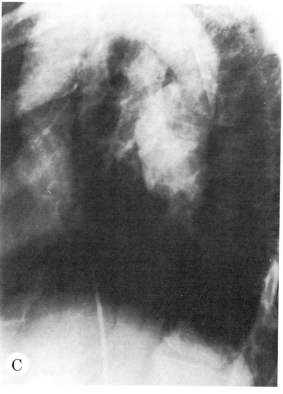

Fig. 11–3. Aortic aneurysm. The PA roentgenogram *(A)* demonstrates a mass in the area of the left hilus. The oblique roentgenogram *(B)* shows the marked displacement of the esophagus by the mass and also shows intimate relationship of the mass to the descending aorta. An aortogram *(C)* made in the lateral projection confirms the diagnosis of an aortic aneurysm.

investigate the air-outlined pleura, the x-ray beam should be centered on the elevated rather than the recumbent side.

The *lordotic* view is a useful projection in investigating the apical portions of the lungs that may be obscured by overlying shadows of the anterior first rib and the clavicle in the routine PA projection. It is employed for confirmation of a suspected lesion identified in the apex (Fig. 11–5). In this view, lesions located anteriorly appear to move upward and those located posteriorly appear to move downward. A lordotic roentgenogram may also be useful in demonstrating disease in the right middle lobe, particularly if the right middle lobe is collapsed.

Stereoscopic views of the chest may be useful in studying lesions adjacent to the mediastinum or partially ob-

scured by overlying bony structures. Stereoscopy can be particularly useful in investigating apical lesions and in recognizing cavities. The physician experienced in stereoscopy may prefer stereoscopic roentgenograms for localization of lesions of the chest rather than oblique or lordotic projections.

Expiratory roentgenograms may be helpful in assessing pulmonary air trapping, either local or diffuse. They can be helpful in the investigation of endobronchial neoplasms or particularly useful in the localization of endobronchial foreign bodies in children. A foreign body will usually be manifest as an emphysematous lobe or lung so that, on the expiratory roentgenogram, the mediastinum will shift to the side opposite the lesion. The expiratory roentgenogram is also useful in investigating

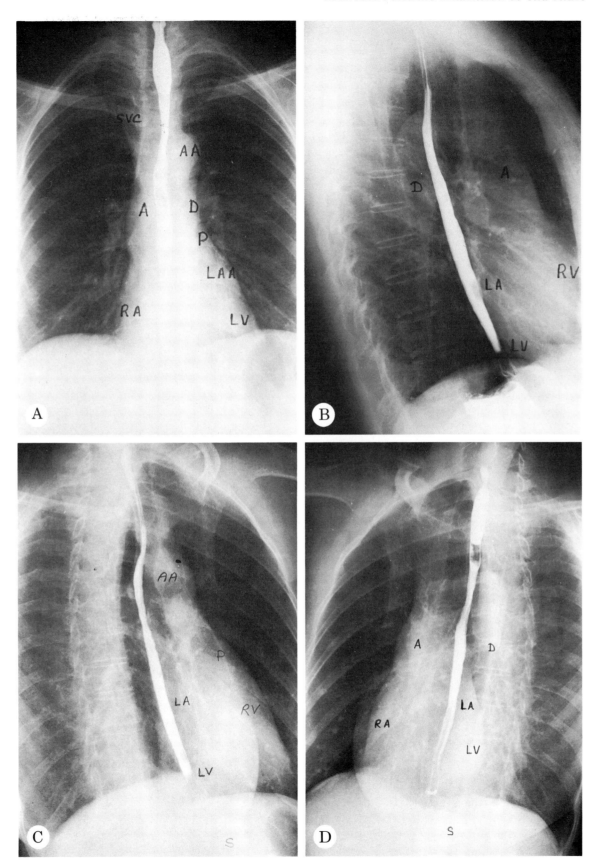

Fig. 11–4. Normal PA *(A)*, lateral *(B)*, right anterior oblique *(C)*, and left anterior oblique *(D)* roentgenograms. A = ascending aorta, D = descending aorta, AA = aortic arch, RA = right atrium, RV = right ventricle, LA = left atrium, LV = left ventricle, LAA = left atrial appendage, P = main pulmonary artery, SVC = superior vena cava, S = stomach.

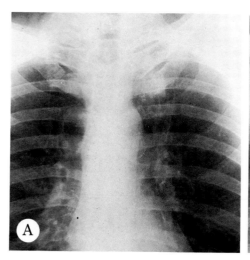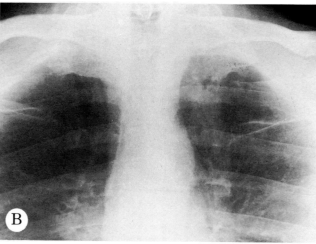

Fig. 11–5. Carcinoma of the lung. The presence of the mass in the left apex can only be suspected on viewing the PA roentgenogram *(A)*. There is an increased density under the first anterior rib on the left. An apical lordotic view *(B)* demonstrates a definite mass in the left apex, which subsequently proved to be a carcinoma of the lung.

a suspected pneumothorax that is poorly recorded with routine inspiration.

Penetrated grid roentgenograms are exposed at higher kV or ma, or both, and utilize a fixed or moving—Bucky—grid between the patient and the film to remove scattered radiation. This practice allows better penetration and improved radiographic contrast, aiding in investigation of mediastinal or bony lesions. This roentgenogram is useful in identifying a suspected lesion behind the heart or diaphragm and poorly seen on the routine roentgenogram because of inadequate penetration (Fig. 11–6).

The *supine* roentgenogram is made when the patient is unable to sit or stand and is the routine projection in infants, owing to the difficulty of obtaining satisfactory erect films in the very young. Interpretation of this roentgenogram should take into consideration the magnification of mediastinal structures that occurs with the subject in the recumbent position and also the increase in pulmonary perfusion in the upper lobes, which may give the appearance of pulmonary vascular engorgement. The supine roentgenogram can be helpful in investigating pleural effusion, although decubitus films are much more reliable.

Magnification roentgenograms can be made by using a very small focal spot— 0.3 mm— and increasing the patient-film distance, thus magnifying pulmonary structures without undue sacrifice of detail. Magnification techniques can occasionally be helpful in evaluating diffuse lung disease.

LAMINOGRAPHY

Laminography—tomography, body section radiography, planigraphy—utilizes reciprocal movement of the x-ray tube and film about a fixed fulcrum to create a roentgenogram in which a plane of several millimeters' thickness is in focus and the remainder of the details of the anatomy of the patient are blurred. This study es-

sentially allows roentgenographic investigations of a thin slice of the body of the patient and it is extremely useful in the study of chest lesions, both pulmonary and mediastinal. Laminographs are useful: (1) to obtain better visualization of a poorly understood shadow seen on the chest roentgenogram; (2) to demonstrate the presence or absence of calcification within a pulmonary nodule; and (3) to demonstrate the presence or absence of cavitation within a pulmonary lesion. Laminography is extremely important in the study of pulmonary tuberculosis (Fig. 11–7). Favis (1955) showed that laminography revealed cavitation in 10.7% of patients in whom no suggestion of a cavitation was seen on the conventional roentgenogram. The primary role of laminography is in better demonstration of a lesion poorly shown or poorly understood on the routine roentgenogram. It is of little value in a blind search for a clinically suspected lesion not shown on the routine roentgenograms.

Laminograms are usually made in the AP or lateral position, but the oblique position can sometimes be useful, particularly when evaluating the hilum. Oblique hilar tomography may clearly demonstrate or exclude adenopathy in a hilum that is suspiciously large on routine films.

Laminography was widely used in the study of pulmonary and mediastinal lesions. It has largely been supplanted by computed tomography. It may still be used to demonstrate cavitation or calcification within a lesion. It may also be used to demonstrate additional nodules where a solitary pulmonary nodule is identified. Computed tomography is more useful in this regard.

COMPUTED TOMOGRAPHY

Computed tomography—CT—is a recently introduced roentgenologic technique for imaging cross-sectional anatomy of the body. In this technique, a pencil-thin beam of x-rays passes through the body, and the transmitted radiation is measured by a sodium iodide

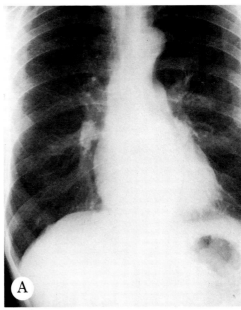

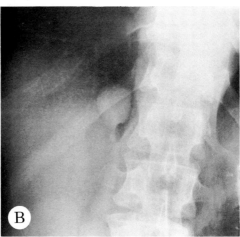

Fig. 11–6. Pulmonary granuloma. The routine PA roentgenogram (A) appears normal. An overpenetrated grid roentgenogram (B) demonstrates a pulmonary nodule seen through the left diaphragm.

crystal. A series of measurements is made as the beam rotates around the body. These measurements are then fed into a computer, which reconstructs the x-ray absorption characteristics of each small area in the plane of the scan. The resultant image is an accurate measurement of the x-ray transmission of each part of the imaged body plane. Density differences of 1 to 2% can be recognized by this technique, whereas density differences of 4 to 5% are necessary for recognition on the usual roentgenogram.

In the chest, CT scanning is particularly useful in the mediastinum, where absorption characteristics of various masses may yield useful information. It is more useful in identifying mediastinal nodes when the routine roentgenogram of the chest is equivocal or even normal.

CT scanning is sensitive in detecting pulmonary nodules, identifying 48% more nodules than whole lung tomography in a study by Schaner and associates (1978).

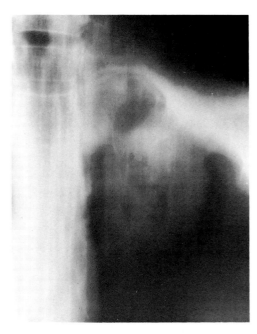

Fig. 11–7. Tuberculosis. Laminogram demonstrates cavitation in pulmonary tuberculosis. This cavity is very thick-walled and is much more characteristic of carcinoma than tuberculosis. Resection proved this mass to be a large tuberculoma.

However, 60% of the newly detected nodules were granulomata or subpleural lymph nodes, and the CT scan is unable to differentiate these from metastases.

CT scanning is helpful in assessing the degree of mediastinal but not chest wall involvement of a peripheral carcinoma of the lung (Fig. 11–8). Computed tomography will be discussed in greater detail in Chapter 13.

MAGNETIC RESONANCE

Magnetic resonance uses radio waves modified by a magnetic field to produce images that contain somewhat different information than is obtained in the standard roentgenogram or CT scan. By varying the excitation time of the radio signal and the repetition time between the signals, information can be obtained about the material that is being imaged that may be useful in assessing the character of the tissue being evaluated—it may allow one to distinguish between tumor, cyst, blood, and various normal tissues. It also allows one to assess blood flow in various vessels, because the flowing blood contains no signal and usually shows as a void (Fig. 11–9A and C).

Magnetic resonance imaging in the chest is particularly useful in studying mediastinal structures, for which it competes with CT in degree of usefulness. It has major applications and potential in imaging the heart, the cardiac chambers, and great vessels.

Magnetic resonance will be discussed in greater detail in Chapter 14.

FLUOROSCOPY

Historically, fluoroscopy of the chest has been used as a screening procedure in the determination of disorders

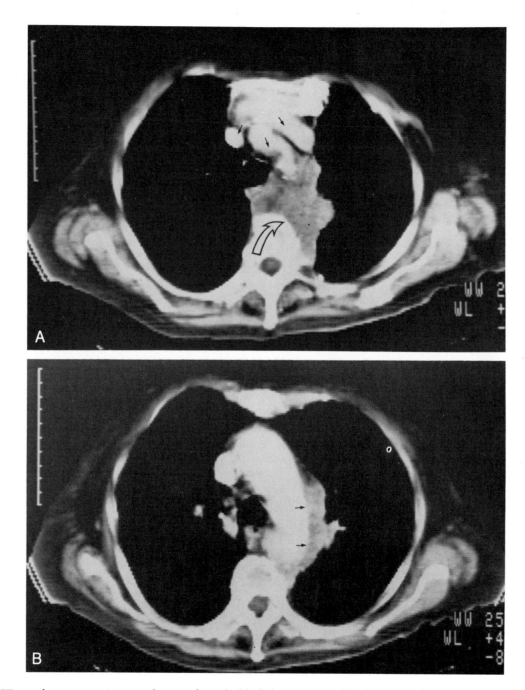

Fig. 11–8. CT scan demonstrating invasion of aorta and vertebral body by carcinoma of the lung. *(A)*, a large mass invading the T3 vertebral body (open arrow). This mass was not apparent on the routine chest film. The great vessels are opacified by contrast material (small arrows). *(B)*, A section made lower in the patient showing opacification of the aortic arch with tumor adherent to the aortic arch (arrows).

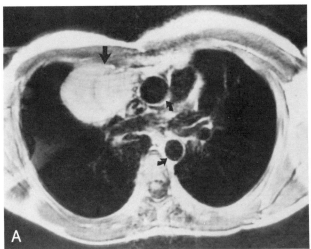

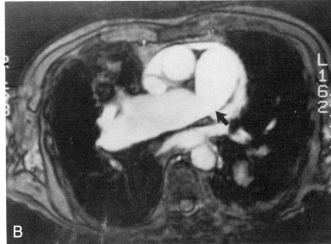

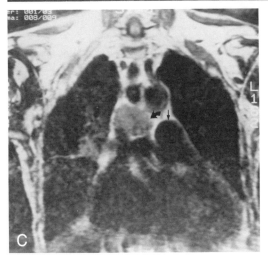

Fig. 11–9. MRI scan in patient with carcinoma of the lung and atrial septal defect. *A* shows a large mass (large arrow) invading the mediastinum. The ascending and descending aorta (curved arrows) show no signal and are seen as a dark image or void. The pulmonary artery and its branches are also visible as dark structures between the ascending and descending aorta. These are surrounded by mediastinal fat, which appears white. *B* uses a different technique, which allows the blood vessels to show as white structures rather than black. No contrast material is used. A massively dilated pulmonary artery (arrow) is noted, secondary to this patient's atrial septal defect. *C* is a coronal section that shows metastatic adenopathy (curved arrow) adjacent to the dilated main pulmonary artery (small arrow) and above the right main pulmonary artery. The distinction between adenopathy and the normal vascular structures had been difficult to see on a CT scan but is easy to see on this MR image.

and diseases of the chest. It is no longer acceptable for screening. Small lesions are easily missed and no permanent record of the fluoroscopic procedure is usually made. The amount of visual information available on a roentgenogram is infinitely greater than that available even with an image-intensified fluoroscope. In addition, the patient radiation exposure is many times greater with fluoroscopy.

Fluoroscopy is still useful in evaluating a lesion that has been identified by roentgenography; and it is especially useful in studying pulmonary or cardiac dynamics. Fluoroscopic observation of the patient during breathing and rotation can localize a lesion to the lung or to the chest wall and can also identify the position of the lesion.

Air-trapping is readily identified fluoroscopically, and limitation of diaphragmatic motion or paralysis of a hemidiaphragm can be appreciated. These observations are helpful in investigation of an elevated hemidiaphragm seen on the routine roentgenogram of the chest or in investigating a suspected subphrenic abscess.

Evaluation of diaphragmatic motion fluoroscopically must be done with the subject in both the PA and lateral positions. Partial eventration of the diaphragm is a common finding and it is frequently misinterpreted as diaphragmatic paralysis if the patient is fluoroscoped only in the PA position. The dome of the diaphragm may move paradoxically with the patient in this position, but in the lateral position, a portion of the diaphragm—usually the posterior—will be seen to move normally. This indicates a localized diaphragmatic weakness—eventration—rather than true paralysis.

True paralysis of the diaphragm may be overlooked if fluoroscopy is done with the patient breathing quietly. Asking the patient to take a quick "sniff" may demonstrate a previously overlooked paralysis.

Fluoroscopy may also be useful in recognizing pulmonary emphysema and in evaluating the extent of this disease. Intracardiac calcification can be readily identified fluoroscopically, and occasionally a pericardial effusion can be seen fluoroscopically or in a cinefluorographic film strip.

The character of a mediastinal lesion may be much better understood following fluoroscopy, particularly when the esophagus is outlined with barium sulfate. The esophagus is a mobile structure and is frequently displaced by mediastinal masses. The character and the location of the displacement can aid in the differential diagnosis of a mediastinal mass and in determining the surgical approach to such a mass.

It is useful to observe a mediastinal mass for pulsation since many middle mediastinal masses are vascular. Unfortunately, it is frequently impossible to differentiate between the true expansile pulsation of a vascular mass and the transmitted pulsation of a mass adjacent to the aorta. The Valsalva and Müller maneuvers can sometimes be useful in distinguishing between an avascular and a vascular mass. A nonvascular mass will not change with the Valsalva or Müller maneuver, while the vascular mass may become smaller with the Valsalva and larger with the Müller maneuver.

THE LUNG

The anatomic positions of the lung and the normal fissures are described in Chapter 4. The interlobar septa are frequently visible on the chest roentgenogram (Fig. 11–10) and are of great help in assessing loss of volume in any of the lobes. Anomalous septa are not uncommon. Any pulmonary segment may have an anomalous fissure between that segment and the remainder of the lobe, resulting in an accessory lobe. The most common anomalous fissures are the superior and inferior accessory fissures. The superior accessory fissure occurs in 5% of anatomic specimens and separates the superior segment of the lower lobe from the basilar segments. The inferior accessory fissure occurs in approximately 30% of anatomic specimens and separates the medial basal segment of the right lower lobe from the remainder of the right lower lobe. Another commonly seen anatomic fissure is the azygos fissure, which extends supralaterally from the azygos vein to the apex of the right lung. This fissure is seen in 1% of specimens and does not create a true accessory lobe, as do most other anomalous fissures.

Each lobe of the lung is divided into several pulmonary segments, each of which is supplied by a segmental bronchus. Various names have been applied to the pulmonary subsegments. The widely used classification of Jackson and Huber (1943) and the numeric classification of Boyden (1955) are presented in Table 4–1 (p. 60) and are

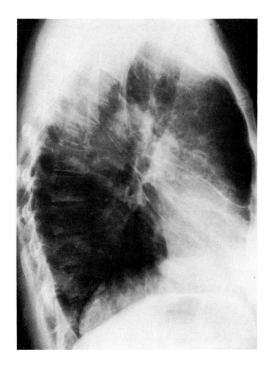

Fig. 11–10. Interlobar septa. The major fissures bilaterally and the minor fissure on the right are seen in this roentgenogram of the patient with interstitial edema and fluid in the fissures.

illustrated in Figure 4–6 (p. 61). The pulmonary segments may undergo consolidation or atelectasis. The characteristic configuration of pulmonary consolidation of the various segments is schematically presented in Figures 11–11 through 11–15. Occasionally, consolidation of an anomalous pulmonary segment can be recognized on the routine roentgenogram. More commonly, segmental variations are demonstrated by bronchography.

The pulmonary arteries accompany the bronchial tree and exhibit a segmental distribution similar to that of the bronchial tree. The pulmonary veins are slightly larger than the arteries and lie lateral to them in the upper lobes and somewhat more horizontal in the lower lobes. It is frequently possible to distinguish between the arteries and veins on the routine roentgenogram of the chest. Laminography makes this identification simple.

THE MEDIASTINUM

The heart occupies the major portion of the lower half of the mediastinum anterior to the spine. On the PA roentgenogram, the transverse diameter of the heart is normally one-half of the transverse diameter of the chest or less. Detailed discussion of the anatomy and pathology of the heart is beyond the scope of this text. Figure 11–4 demonstrates the normal position of the cardiac chambers and the great vessels in the PA and lateral projections.

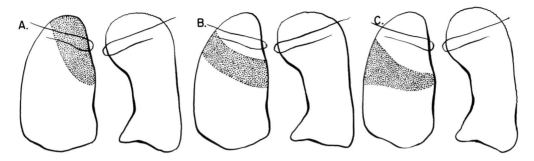

Fig. 11–11. Consolidation of right upper lobe. *A*, Apical segment; *B*, posterior segment; *C*, anterior segment.

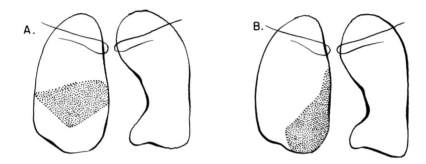

Fig. 11–12. Consolidation of right middle lobe. *A*, Lateral segment; *B*, medial segment.

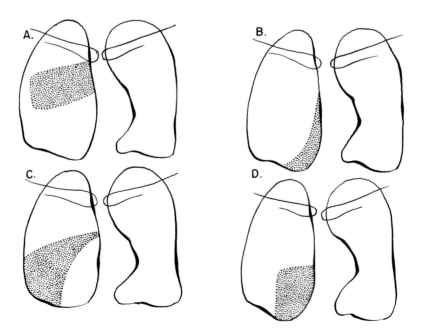

Fig. 11–13. Consolidation of right lower lobe. *A*, Superior segment; *B*, medial basal segment; *C*, lateral basal segment; *D*, posterior basal segment.

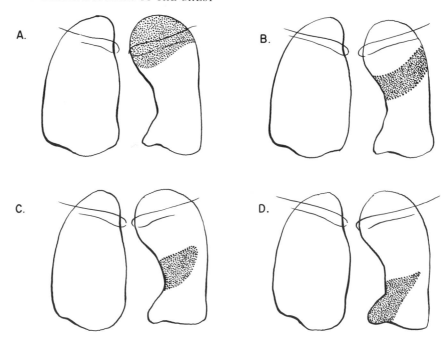

Fig. 11–14. Consolidation of the left upper lobe. *A,* Apical posterior segment; *B,* anterior segment; *C,* lingular segment, superior division; *D,* lingular segment, inferior division.

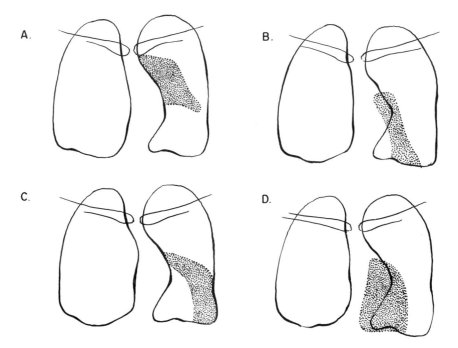

Fig. 11–15. Consolidation of left lower lobe. *A,* Superior segment; *B,* lateral basal segment; *C,* anteromedial basal segment; *D,* posterior basal segment.

The mediastinum is divided by anatomists into the superior and inferior mediastinum and into the anterior, middle, and posterior compartments. For the surgeon, designation of superior and inferior compartments is of little importance. What is important, however, is the division of the mediastinum into three compartments: the anterior, middle—visceral—and paravertebral compartments, as seen on the lateral roentgenogram.

In the anatomic division of the mediastinum, the anterior compartment is bounded anteriorly by the sternum and posteriorly by the heart, aorta, and brachiocephalic vessels. The middle mediastinum contains the heart, ascending aorta, great vessels, trachea and main bronchi, and the esophagus. The "posterior mediastinum" in reality is nonexistent and should be considered to be the two paravertebral sulci.

The roentgenographic classification of mediastinal lesions becomes a simple one when one includes the descending aorta and the esophagus in the middle—visceral—compartment and those structures that lie posterior to the anterior spinal ligament in the paravertebral areas or posterior compartment. Thus, arbitrary divisions can be made on the lateral roentgenogram (Fig. 11–16) to divide the mediastinum into these three compartments.

Various lines or stripes occur about the mediastinum on the PA roentgenogram. Displacement of these stripes is often indicative of mediastinal pathology.

The paraspinal line, as Brailsford (1943) described, is a longitudinal density lying to the left of the thoracic spine (Fig. 11–17). It is related to the left-sided position of the descending aorta and will be seen on the right side if the descending aorta is present on the right. Ordinarily, no paraspinal line is seen on the right, but in patients with large hypertrophic spurs, the spurs may push the paraspinal line out, making it visible. Tumors or inflammatory processes involving the paravertebral bodies will characteristically displace the paraspinal line

(Fig. 11–18). The line is ordinarily less than 1 cm from the left border of the vertebral column, but in some people it may lie normally as far as 3 cm to the left of the vertebral column (Fig. 11–17).

The anterior mediastinal stripe is an oblique linear density presenting from right to left downward over the trachea for a distance of several centimeters (Fig. 11–19). This stripe is produced by the contiguous pleura of the right and left upper lobes as they touch anterior to the great vessels.

The inferior esophageal pleural stripe lies posterior to the heart and represents the right side of the distal esophagus (Fig. 11–19). The superior esophageal pleural stripe is slightly higher than the anterior mediastinal stripe and is slightly to the left. It represents the apposition of the two lungs against the esophagus in the retrotracheal area of the upper mediastinum. All of these mediastinal stripes can be displaced by lesions in the adjacent mediastinum.

THE DIAPHRAGM AND CHEST WALL

The diaphragm is a musculotendinous structure that separates the thorax from the abdomen. It is divided into right and left hemidiaphragms. The hemidiaphragm is usually lower on the side where the heart is anatomically placed in the absence of displacement due to some pathologic process. Thus, the right hemidiaphragm is usually higher than the left. Felson (1973) found, in a series of 500 normal chests, that the left hemidiaphragm was at a level even with or higher than the right in 9% of the subjects.

Variations of diaphragmatic contour are frequent. Most commonly, there is elevation of a segment of the diaphragm due to lack of muscle in the segment—localized eventration. Fluoroscopically, paradoxical motion will often be observed in such a localized segment and, in all instances, that portion of the diaphragm will move less well than the normal diaphragm.

The chest wall is composed of the bones and muscles

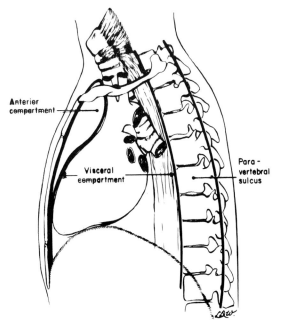

Anterior
compartment

Visceral
compartment

Paravertebral
sulcus

Fig. 11–16. The mediastinal compartments. Imaginary lines drawn along the anterior border of the trachea extended to the xiphoid and the anterior border of the spine will divide the mediastinum into three compartments: anterior, visceral (middle), and paravertebral (posterior).

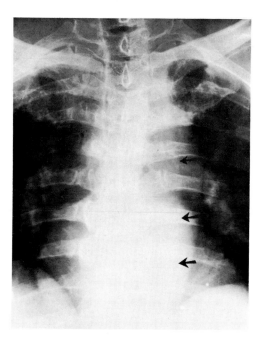

Fig. 11–17. Paraspinal line is seen only on the left in most patients and in this patient is unusually wide but normal.

of the thoracic cage. The bones are readily identifiable on the roentgenogram owing to the differences in density, but the muscular shadows are not readily identifiable unless a large mass of muscle is absent, either owing to a surgical procedure or to congenital anomaly. Thus bony abnormalities can be easily identified on the roentgenogram of the chest, but soft-tissue abnormalities are seldom seen. The soft tissues of the chest wall can be studied by CT scanning.

THE ABNORMAL CHEST

Abnormalities of the Lung

Roentgenographic images are made possible by the different coefficients of absorption of the various body tissues. Thus air, fat, bone, and soft tissues can be distinguished one from another. The chest is admirably suited for detection of pathology for one major reason. The lung contains air in the bronchi and alveoli, making excellent contrast between the lung and the adjacent structures. In addition, the lung is a common site of pathology—manifest on the roentgenogram as areas of increased or decreased density—and frequently gives clues to the nature of systemic diseases as well as localized pulmonary conditions. It is important for the radiologist and the surgeon to recognize certain primary pat-

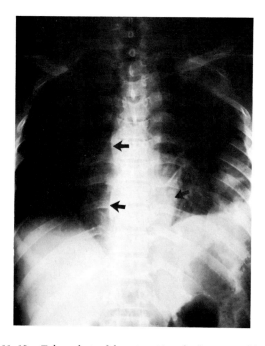

Fig. 11–18. Tuberculosis of the spine. Note displacement of the paraspinal line on the left and also on the right by tuberculous abscess.

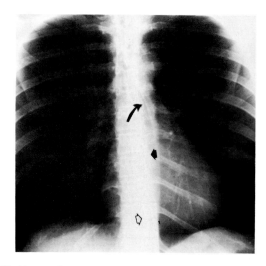

Fig. 11–19. Mediastinal stripes. Anterior mediastinal stripe (curved arrow). Paraspinal stripe (short closed arrow). Inferior esophageal stripe (short open arrow).

terns occurring in the lungs as these patterns often indicate the nature of the patient's illness.

Atelectasis

Atelectasis is loss of volume of the lung, lobe, or segment from any cause. Fraser and Paré (1978) list five mechanisms of atelectasis. Resorption atelectasis occurs secondary to obstruction of a major bronchus or multiple small bronchi. For the surgeon, this type of atelectasis is the most important because it is often secondary to obstruction of a major bronchus by tumor, foreign body, or bronchial plug. Passive atelectasis occurs secondary to a space-occupying process in the thorax, particularly pneumothorax or hydrothorax. Compression atelectasis is a localized parenchymal collapse contiguous to a space-occupying pulmonary mass or bulla. Adhesive atelectasis or mitral atelectasis denotes collapse occurring in the presence of patent bronchi, presumably secondary to abnormalities of surfactant. This form of atelectasis occurs in association with pneumonia. Cicatrization atelectasis results from pulmonary fibrosis, either localized or general.

Several roentgenographic signs suggest atelectasis. The most reliable sign of collapse is displacement of interlobar fissures. Localized increase in density of the collapsed lobe is another reliable sign of atelectasis. Indirect signs of atelectasis include: elevation of the hemidiaphragm of the ipsilateral side; deviation of the trachea and other mediastinal structures toward the involved side; compensatory hyperaeration of the rest of the ipsilateral lung, and sometimes of the contralateral lung, with herniation of the contralateral upper lobe across the mediastinum; displacement of the hilum toward the collapsed lobe or segment; and decrease in size of the bony hemithorax of the involved side. These indirect signs are ordinarily seen only with atelectasis of major segments of the lung. They are less reliable than the direct signs and can occasionally be simulated by normal anatomic variations.

Certain fundamental observations can be made about lobar collapse. The proximal portion of the lobe is tethered to the hilus and consequently the radiographic shadow of the collapsed lobe will always point toward the hilus. Lobar collapse always occurs toward the mediastinum on the PA film. On the lateral film, the upper lobe collapses anteriorly, the lower lobe collapses posteriorly, and the middle lobe symmetrically decreases in volume.

Robbins and Hale (1945), as well as Lubert and Krause (1951), have described clearly the roentgenographic patterns of lobar collapse. The patterns of lower lobe collapse are similar on the right and left sides, whereas the patterns of upper lobe collapse are slightly different. Figures 11–20 through 11–24 show schematic representations of lobar collapse, as described by Lubert and Krause (1951).

Recognition of the presence of a collapsed lobe is frequently difficult, particularly if the collapse is almost complete (Figs. 11–25 through 11–28). Of great help in identifying the presence of atelectasis is the silhouette

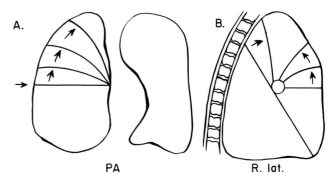

Fig. 11–20. Schematic representation of lobar collapse of the right upper lobe. (After Lubert, M., and Krause, G.R.: Patterns of lobar collapse as observed radiographically. Radiology, 56:165, 1951.)

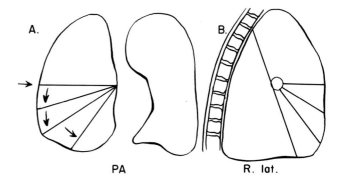

Fig. 11–21. Schematic representation of lobar collapse of the right middle lobe. (After Lubert, M., and Krause, G.R.: Patterns of lobar collapse as observed radiographically. Radiology 56:165, 1951.)

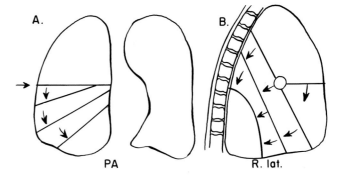

Fig. 11–22. Schematic representation of lobar collapse of right lower lobe. (After Lubert, M., and Krause, G.R.: Patterns of lobar collapse as observed radiographically. Radiology 56:165, 1951.)

sign, popularized by Felson (1973). The sign is based on the premise that consolidation of a segment or lobe of a lung contiguous with the border of the heart, aorta, diaphragm, or mediastinum will obliterate that portion of the border of the roentgenogram. Frequently, this obliteration of a heart border or a fuzziness of the diaphragm is the first clue leading one to suspect the presence of atelectasis.

Diffuse Pulmonary Disease

Pulmonary pathology can be manifest as density occurring in the pulmonary alveoli or in the interstitial

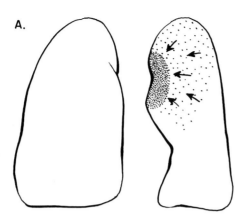
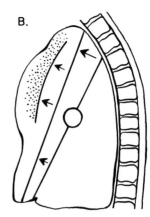

Fig. 11–23. Schematic representation of lobar collapse of left upper lobe. (After Lubert, M., and Krause, G.R.: Patterns of lobar collapse as observed radiographically. Radiology 56:165, 1951.)

space or both. It is frequently helpful to distinguish alveolar form interstitial disease, although in some instances, this distinction cannot be made or can be made only with great difficulty. In pure alveolar or interstitial disease, certain roentgenographic appearances aid in the distinction.

The roentgenographic findings that can be helpful in recognizing alveolar disease are, first and frequently, a confluence of alveolar consolidation creating large homogeneous densities (Fig. 11–29). Second, an air bronchogram is frequently present (Fig. 11–30). The air bronchogram was originally described by Fleischner (1948) and has been popularized by Felson (1973). Parenchymal consolidation results in visualization of the bronchi when the air in the bronchi is not displaced by endobronchial fluid, such as in pneumonia. The air in the bronchi—usually not visible because of surrounding alveolar air—is now quite obvious because the alveoli are filled with fluid. Third, a small fluffy, rosette-shaped shadow may be seen diffusely through the lungs. This is the "acinar

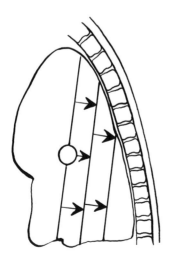

Fig. 11–24. Schematic representation of lobar collapse of left lower lobe (PA) view same as Figure 10–22. (After Lubert, M., and Krause, G.R.: Patterns of lobar collapse as observed radiographically. Radiology 56:165, 1951.)

shadow" Aschoff (1924) described and is probably representative of consolidation of a single pulmonary acinus. Fourth, certain patterns of distribution may be seen in alveolar disease, for example, lobar or segmental consolidation and the "butterfly" pattern of perihilar increase in density (Fig. 11–29). Fifth, rapidity of change of pulmonary lesions favors alveolar disease over interstitial disease, which tends to change more slowly.

Common causes of a diffuse alveolar pattern are pneumonia, pulmonary edema, bleeding into the alveoli, or aspiration of blood or gastric contents into the alveoli. Less common causes of diffuse alveolar consolidation include parenchymal sarcoidosis, pulmonary alveolar proteinosis, metastatic carcinoma—breast—and occasionally bronchioloalveolar cell carcinoma.

Interstitial disease has several roentgenographic characteristics. Kerley lines are frequently present, creating a series of fine linear densities throughout the lungs (Fig. 11–31). Shanks and Kerley (1951) described A, B, and C lines, which they attributed to lymphatic dilatation. The A lines are thin, straight lines several centimeters in length radiating from the hili. The B lines are transverse lines 1 to 2 cm long, seen at the lung bases and extending to the pleura. The C lines form a fine, interlacing network throughout the lungs, producing a reticular pattern. These lines may indicate dilatation of lymphatics, but may also represent interstitial fibrosis or edema.

Discrete nodules of varying sizes are also indicative of interstitial disease. These nodules may vary from minute to large and usually show a lack of confluence and have sharply defined margins (Fig. 11–32). A reticulonodular pattern may also be present in interstitial disease. A slow rate of change of a diffuse process favors interstitial over alveolar disease.

Common diseases causing a diffuse interstitial pattern include interstitial pulmonary edema, pneumoconiosis, sarcoidosis, metastatic tumor—both nodular and lymphangitic form, diffuse interstitial pneumonia, collagen disease—scleroderma and rheumatoid lung, eosinophilic granuloma of the lung, and idiopathic pulmonary fibrosis.

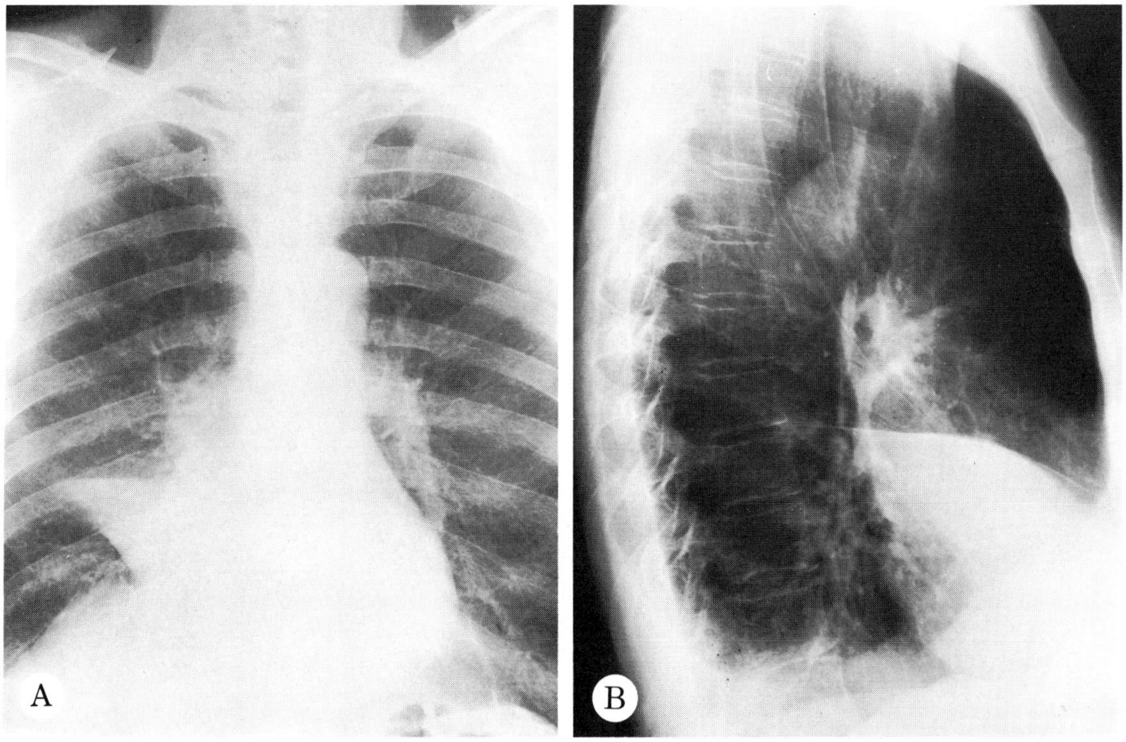

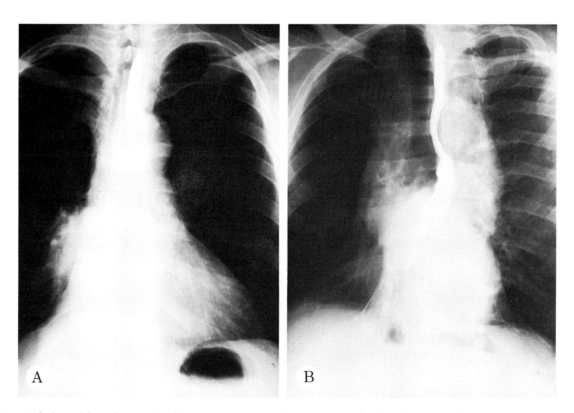

Fig. 11–25. Carcinoma with right middle lobe collapse. The PA roentgenogram (*A*) shows obliteration of the right cardiac border by the collapsed right middle lobe (silhouette sign) with an associated mass in the right hilus. The approximation of major and minor fissures can be noted on the lateral roentgenogram (*B*).

Fig. 11–26. Right lower lobe atelectasis. On the PA roentgenogram (*A*), a mass is noted in the right hilus and there is increased density behind the right side of the heart indicating right lower lobe collapse. (Note preservation of the silhouette of the border of the right side of the heart). Right lower lobe collapse is confirmed on the oblique roentgenogram (*B*).

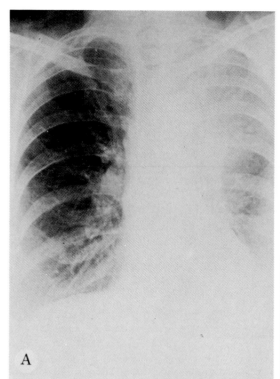

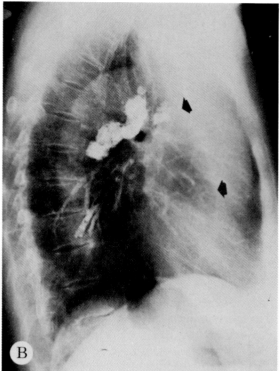

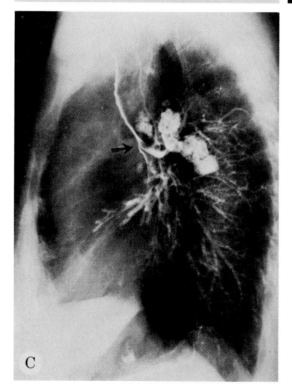

Fig. 11–27. Left upper lobe atelectasis. The hazy increased density of the collapsed left upper lobe is seen over the left apex on the PA roentgenogram *(A)*. The curvilinear line of the displaced major fissure (arrows) can be seen behind the increased density of the collapsed left upper lobe on the lateral roentgenogram *(B)*. A bronchogram (lateral projection) *(C)* shows filling of only the left lower lobe bronchi with cutoff of the upper lobe bronchus (arrow). The left upper lobe collapse was due to chronic inflammatory disease.

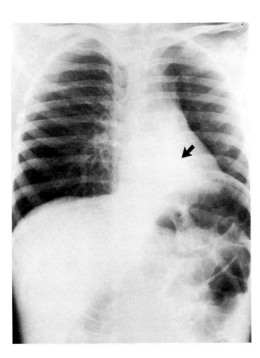

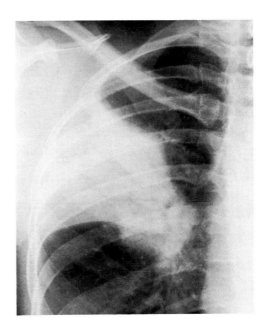

Fig. 11–30. Pneumonia. Notice the confluence of this alveolar pattern with the prominent air bronchogram. Lobar distribution is also in favor of an alveolar process.

Fig. 11–28. Postoperative left lower lobe atelectasis. The wedge-shaped density of the collapsed left lower lobe is seen behind the heart (arrow). There is also shift of the mediastinum and elevation of the left hemidiaphragm. The silhouette of the medial border of the left hemidiaphragm behind the heart is lost.

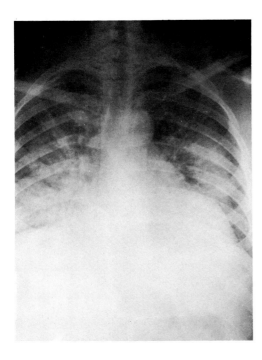

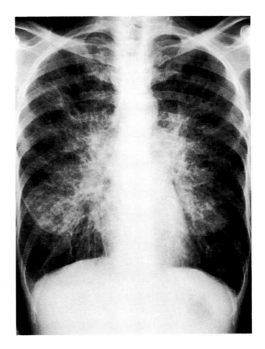

Fig. 11–29. Pulmonary edema. Note the patchy confluence of this diffuse alveolar pattern.

Fig. 11–31. Interstitial spread of metastatic pancreatic carcinoma. Note the reticular and linear pattern of this diffuse interstitial disease. Prominent Kerley lines are present.

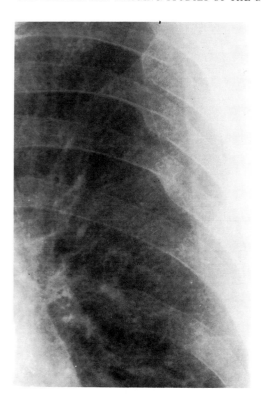

Fig. 11–32. Silicosis. Notice the fine nodular pattern of this interstitial process.

Localized Pulmonary Densities

These densities may have poorly circumscribed or discrete margins. If the margins are poorly circumscribed, a solitary density most likely denotes pneumonia or pulmonary infarction. Primary lung tumor may present in this fashion so that it is important to follow a poorly circumscribed density to complete clearing to be certain that it does not represent a tumor. Pulmonary tuberculosis and other chronic inflammatory diseases also present as poorly localized pulmonary density. A chronic infiltrate in the apical or posterior segment of the upper lobe or in the superior segment of the lower lobe should make one suspect tuberculosis. Cavitation is also suggestive of tuberculosis.

The sharply circumscribed pulmonary density most likely is due to a tumor or a granuloma. Primary or metastatic carcinoma commonly presents in this fashion. Tuberculous granuloma, histoplasmosis and other fungal diseases, benign pulmonary tumors, and occasionally pneumoconiosis may present as a sharply circumscribed pulmonary density. Also to be considered are pulmonary infarct, pneumonia, arteriovenous malformation (Fig. 11–33), bronchial cyst, and bronchial adenoma. It is sometimes possible to ascertain the nature of a solitary pulmonary nodule by appropriate clinical tests, but a transthoracic lung biopsy or thoracotomy is usually necessary to make a definitive diagnosis (see Chapter 19).

Multiple sharply circumscribed densities almost invariably indicate metastatic malignant disease. Occasionally, however, rheumatoid nodules, fungal disease,

Wegener's granulomatosis, or alveolar sarcoidosis may produce a similar pattern. Septic emboli may present as multiple pulmonary nodules, but these are usually cavitary (Fig. 11–34).

Cavitation of a solitary pulmonary density usually indicates a lung abscess, primary bronchial carcinoma, tuberculosis (Fig. 11–35), or fungal disease. Tumors and lung abscesses ordinarily have thick, shaggy walls, whereas lung tissue with fungal disease and tuberculosis have thin, smooth walls. If a lung abscess is chronic, the wall that initially was thick and shaggy generally becomes thin and smooth. Multiple cavitary lesions in the chest suggest septic emboli, metastatic tumor, tuberculosis, fungal disease, or Wegener's granulomatosis.

Calcification within a solitary pulmonary nodule can help to point to its etiologic basis. Certain types of calcification are strong evidence of benign disease. Central calcification or concentric ringlike calcification suggests granuloma. Multiple punctate calcifications throughout the lesion suggest granuloma or hamartoma. Eccentric calcification is most commonly seen in granuloma, but can also be seen in primary lung carcinoma. Thus, an eccentric calcification cannot be taken as an indication of benign disease. Multiple pulmonary calcifications usually indicate healed pulmonary infections such as histoplasmosis, tuberculosis, and varicella pneumonia.

In the study of localized pulmonary densities, laminography is helpful in identifying suspected or unsuspected cavitation or calcification within the density (Fig. 11–36).

Determination of the rate of change of a pulmonary density is also important. If early roentgenograms can be obtained for comparison, they may reveal that the lesion is changing rapidly or slowly or not at all. If prior roentgenograms cannot be obtained, follow-up examination in one or several weeks may reveal the growth rate of the pulmonary process.

Abnormalities of the Pleura

Pleural Effusion

A collection of fluid within the pleural space is the most common pleural abnormality. Fluid in the pleural cavity appears roentgenographically as a homogeneous opacity that is ordinarily in a dependent position in the pleural cavity. The fluid may be exudate, transudate, blood, pus, or chyle. Small amounts of free pleural fluid may be difficult to detect roentgenographically. Careful observation of the posterior costophrenic sulcus on the lateral roentgenogram often shows minor blunting of the sulcus with as little as 50 to 100 ml of fluid. A lateral decubitus roentgenogram confirms the presence of free pleural fluid (see Fig. 11–2).

With larger pleural effusions, the lateral costophrenic sulcus is also blunted. On occasion, the fluid may remain infrapulmonary and displace the lung upward so that the lateral costophrenic angle remains sharp (Fig. 11–37). This infrapulmonary location of fluid can be suspected if the apparent hemidiaphragm is elevated, if the costophrenic sulcus is blunted posteriorly, or if the gas bubble

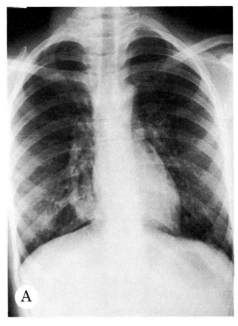

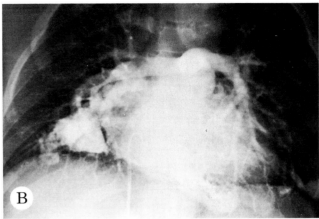

Fig. 11–33. Pulmonary AV malformation. Several nodular densities are seen in the lung fields, the largest of which is along the right cardiac border (A). A pulmonary angiogram (B) demonstrates multiple arteriovenous malformations.

in the gastric fundus lies some distance below the dome of the apparent hemidiaphragm. Decubitus films demonstrate that fluid is free and not loculated.

As the amount of pleural effusion increases, passive atelectasis occurs in the underlying lung and eventually the mediastinum may be displaced to the contralateral side.

Fluid may become loculated in the pleural space, in which instance it may be difficult to differentiate from localized pleural thickening. Loculated pleural fluid generally has a convex border toward the hilus. Pleural thickening is more likely to have a concave border toward the hilus. Loculated pleural effusion may appear in the interlobar fissure, where it assumes a cigar-shaped configuration. Localized pleural tumor may masquerade as localized pleural thickening or pleural fluid. On occasion, loculated fluid may assume a lobar shape (Fig. 11–38) or simulate a mass (Fig. 11–39).

Common causes of pleural effusion are tuberculosis, pneumonia, viral pleural infection, metastatic tumor, primary lung or primary pleural tumor, lymphoma and leukemia, pulmonary infarction, chest trauma, collagen vascular disease, congestive heart failure, and intra-abdominal problems such as subphrenic abscess or pancreatitis.

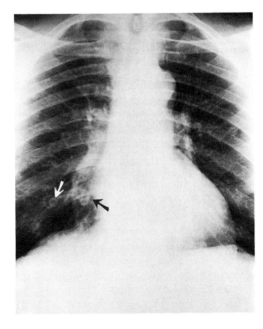

Fig. 11–34. Septic emboli. Several pulmonary nodules are present in both lungs with cavitation of two right lower lobe nodules (arrows).

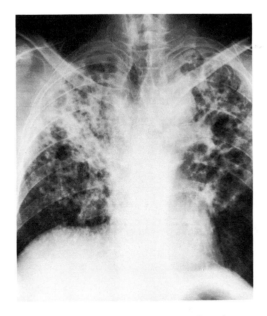

Fig. 11–35. Widespread cavitary pulmonary tuberculosis.

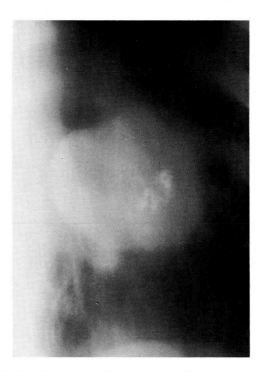

Fig. 11–36. Hamartoma. A laminogram shows "popcorn" calcification in this large hamartoma.

Pleural Thickening

Pleural thickening represents a localized fibrosis of the pleura that may be secondary to several causes. It is commonly seen at both apices, at the costophrenic angles, and occasionally along the lateral chest wall. It can be distinguished from free pleural fluid in a roentgenogram made with the subject in the decubitus position. Distinguishing pleural thickening from loculated pleural fluid may be more difficult. The lack of change over a long period of time suggests pleural thickening rather than loculated fluid.

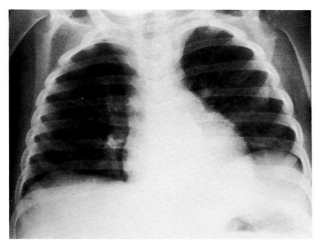

Fig. 11–37. Left pleural effusion. The separation of the stomach bubble from the lung is due to a large left pleural effusion in this child who has nephrosis. Note that the costophrenic sulcus is not blunted laterally by this free "infrapulmonary" effusion.

Causes of localized pleural thickening are usually old infection, particularly tuberculosis, or remote pulmonary infarction. Generalized pleural thickening occurs following the healing of hemothorax or pyothorax and is commonly associated with tuberculosis. Asbestosis or talc pneumoconiosis may also cause diffuse pleural thickening. Diffuse pleural mesothelioma may be difficult to distinguish from pleural thickening although pleural effusion and pleural nodulation are often present with mesothelioma. Diagnostic pneumothorax (Fig. 11–40) may help make the differentiation.

Apical pleural thickening may be difficult to distinguish from superior sulcus tumor. This distinction can be made radiographically only if rib destruction can be demonstrated or if the pleural density shows significant change over a short period of time.

Calcification of the pleura is usually secondary to old hemothorax, pyothorax, or tuberculosis. It is seen in asbestos exposure in the diaphragmatic pleura, pericardium, and chest walls. It may occur in one or multiple areas.

Pneumothorax

The presence of air within the pleural cavity is easily detected roentgenographically by identifying a thin line of visceral pleura surrounding the partially collapsed lung. This feature is best seen at the apex of the lung. It may be necessary to obtain a roentgenogram following expiration to be absolutely certain that a small pneumothorax is present. The expiratory roentgenogram accentuates the pneumothorax because the pleural cavity is decreased in volume in expiration. Fluid in the pleura in association with pneumothorax will demonstrate the straight line of an air-fluid level rather than the curved line—meniscus—seen when no pneumothorax is present. A straight air-fluid level may on occasion be the finding that makes the radiologist aware that a pneumothorax is present.

Abnormalities of the Mediastinum

The roentgenographic features of mediastinal tumors are discussed in detail in Chapter 90 and are not dealt with here. Several aspects of mediastinal disease might be emphasized, however. In all mediastinal lesions, it is important to determine the location of the mass because the differential diagnosis varies considerably for each of the three mediastinal compartments. The one mass that commonly occurs in all three compartments is lymph node enlargement. It is often possible to determine the probable etiologic basis for the enlargement of lymph nodes by using certain helpful roentgenographic criteria.

Sarcoidosis has a characteristic pattern when it causes enlarged nodes. This pattern has been called the 1–2–3 sign because three prominent areas of enlarged nodes are identified—in both hili and in the right paratracheal area. In sarcoidosis, the hilar nodes also tend to be more peripherally situated or peribronchial with discrete nodes identifiable rather than one large amorphous mass tight against the mediastinum as is more commonly seen in association with metastatic tumor or lymphoma.

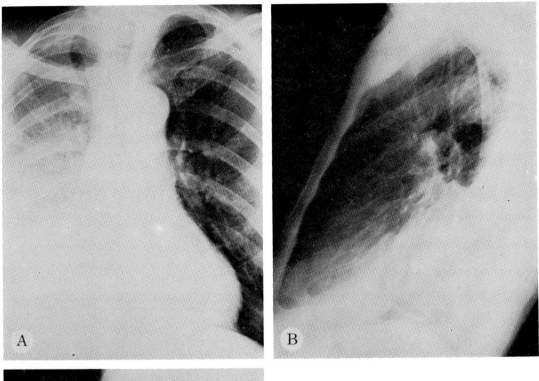

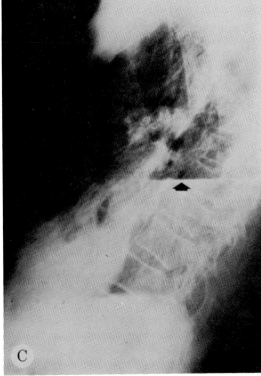

Fig. 11–38. Tuberculosis with loculated pleural effusion. The loculated effusion seen on the PA (*A*) and the lateral roentgenogram (*B*) simulated collapse of the right lower lobe. A right lateral decubitus roentgenogram showed no evidence of free effusion. However, following thoracentesis, a large collection of loculated fluid with an air fluid level (arrow) was apparent (*C*).

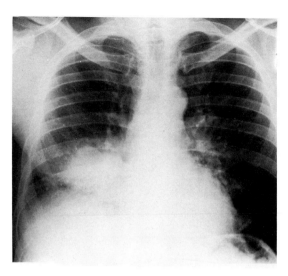

Fig. 11–39. Loculated empyema. This loculated collection of fluid near the border of the right side of the heart simulates a lung mass.

Lymphoma usually presents in only one node-bearing area rather than in several, and this area is commonly the anterior mediastinum. Lymph node enlargement in one nodal area alone or in one hilus and the mediastinum in a younger individual should make the clinician suspect lymphoma. In an older person, this same pattern should make one suspect an anaplastic carcinoma of the lung.

Middle mediastinal node enlargement may be identifiable only on films exposed during barium swallow. Enlargement of nodes in the middle mediastinum is usually indicative of metastatic tumor, most commonly from the lung. It is useful to examine the patient with primary carcinoma of the lung by barium swallow technique to be certain that middle mediastinal nodal metastases are not present. CT scanning is more reliable in revealing occult mediastinal lymph node enlargement.

Primary tuberculosis commonly presents as node enlargement in one hilus or in the mediastinum, but it usually occurs in children and commonly in association

with a parenchymal pulmonary lesion. It may occur on occasion in the adult, in which instance the pattern is similar to that seen with lymphoma.

Early lymph node enlargement may be difficult to detect. The importance of previous roentgenograms for comparison must be emphasized once again. A slightly widened mediastinum that has not changed for several years is not significant, whereas a minor alteration of mediastinal outline can be important if not present on roentgenograms made at an earlier date.

Masses occurring in the anterior cardiophrenic angle are almost invariably benign and so probably do not merit further investigation. These masses include pericardial cysts, foramen of Morgagni hernia, prominent pericardial fat pad, and pericardial fat necrosis.

Abnormalities of the Diaphragm and Chest Wall

The roentgenographic features of abnormalities of the diaphragm are covered in Chapters 52 to 55 and are not discussed here.

The most common chest wall abnormalities identifiable roentgenographically involve the ribs. Abnormalities of the chest wall that protrude into the thorax create a characteristic roentgenographic appearance that has been labeled the extrapleural sign by Felson (1973). These extrapleural lesions are smooth, seen well in only one projection—in which they are tangential to the roentgenographic beam—and usually have an acute angle at their borders, where the parietal pleura is being stripped from the thoracic cage (Fig. 11–41). Metastatic malignant disease of the rib is the most common cause of the extraplerual sign. Myeloma, primary rib tumor, fracture, or osteomyelitis may be responsible for this finding. Primary tumor of the chest wall or extrapleural hematoma may also present in this fashion.

Abnormalities of the soft tissues of the chest may also

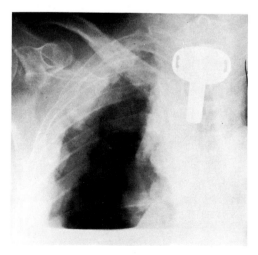

Fig. 11–40. Pleural mesothelioma. Diagnostic pneumothorax demonstrates diffuse pleural involvement by mesothelioma.

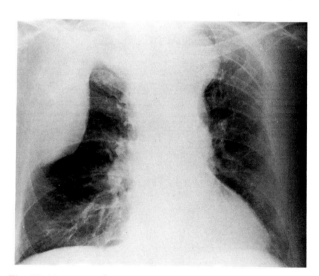

Fig. 11–41. Aortic dissection with extrapleural collection of blood. The widened contour of the aortic arch is strong presumptive evidence of a dissecting aneurysm in this patient with back pain. The mass in the right side of the chest has the characteristic configuration of an extrapleural lesion and in this instance represents a large extrapleural hematoma. A left-side hematoma would be much more characteristic.

occasionally be discernible on the roentgenogram of the chest but are much better visualized by CT scanning. The nipple of the breast frequently creates a shadow simulating a pulmonary nodule and must be considered when the nodule overlies the breast area.

CONTRAST EXAMINATIONS

Air in the bronchi and in the pulmonary alveoli provides an excellent contrast medium and makes the plain film examination of the chest fruitful. Nonetheless, in many instances artificial contrast material introduced into a thoracic structure yields information that cannot be obtained from the routine roentgenogram of the chest. Positive contrast material can be readily introduced into the esophagus, trachea and bronchi, pulmonary vasculature, aorta and mediastinal arteries, superior vena cava, and mediastinal veins—and, with some degree of difficulty, into the mediastinal lymphatics. Negative contrast material—air or other gases—can be introduced into the pleural cavity, the peritoneal cavity, the mediastinum, or the heart.

Barium Swallow

Contrast examination of the esophagus is made by means of a simple technique that is best carried out under fluoroscopic guidance. A thick mixture of barium outlining the esophageal contour readily demonstrates any displacement of the esophagus by adjacent mediastinal structures on routine films. Abnormalities of the esophagus itself, such as achalasia or esophageal tumor, can be readily demonstrated. Considerable information about the location and nature of a mediastinal mass, particularly one in the visceral compartment, can be obtained by studying the displacement of the esophagus by such a mass. Barium swallow is useful in evaluating patients with primary bronchial carcinoma in that it may identify previously unsuspected mediastinal lymph node metastases. Barium in the esophagus is also helpful in evaluating enlargement of the cardiac chambers.

Bronchography

Instillation of positive contrast material into the trachea for visualization of the bronchial tree may be accomplished by one of several methods. The contrast material can be dripped over the patient's extended tongue into the trachea; it can be introduced by a catheter inserted through the patient's nose or mouth into the trachea; or it can be introduced by an indwelling catheter inserted into the trachea through a puncture made in the cricothyroid membrane. The contrast medium generally used is aqueous or oily propyliodone—Dionosil.

Since the advent of fiberoptic bronchoscopy, bronchography is used almost exclusively to identify bronchiectasis or to assess the extent of known bronchiectasis. Bronchoscopy is ordinarily employed as the primary investigative procedure for suspected bronchial abnormalities.

Angiography

Opacification of the vasculature of the chest is often helpful in investigation of a pulmonary or mediastinal abnormality.

Pulmonary Angiography

Pulmonary angiography can be accomplished by introducing a catheter into the main pulmonary artery or one of its branches or by introducing a catheter into the great veins or heart proximal to the pulmonary artery. It can also be carried out by direct injection into the veins of one or both arms.

Pulmonary angiography is most commonly used to investigate thromboembolic disease of the lungs. Large thrombi are seen as negative filling defects within the opacified pulmonary arterial tree and poor perfusion of the vessels distal to these thrombi is usually evident (Fig. 11–42).

Congenital abnormalities of the pulmonary vascular tree, such as hypoplasia or agenesis of the pulmonary artery, arteriovenous malformation (see Fig. 11–33), pulmonary varix, or anomalous pulmonary venous return, also are identified by angiography. These abnormalities ordinarily can be suspected on the routine roentgenographic examination of the chest, but angiography may be necessary for confirmation. Pulmonary angiography may be useful in determining resectability of primary carcinoma of the lung by demonstrating invasion of important mediastinal structures (Fig. 11–43).

Opacification of the chambers of the heart—angiocardiography—is used to study intracardiac malformations and pericardial effusions. Discussion of angiographic findings of intracardiac abnormalities is beyond the scope of this text.

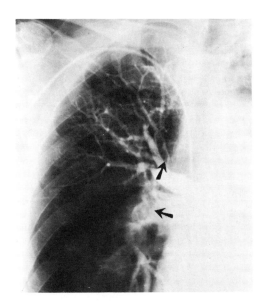

Fig. 11–42. Pulmonary embolus. Multiple large emboli (arrows) in the right pulmonary artery are demonstrated by pulmonary arteriogram. Lack of perfusion of the right middle and lower lobes is apparent.

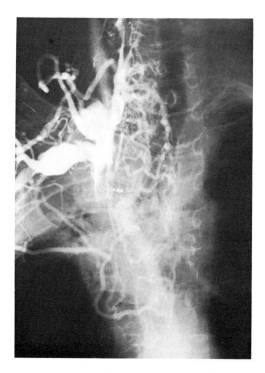

Fig. 11–43. Carcinoma of the lung. Superior vena cavagram demonstrates complete obstruction of the superior vena cava with extensive collateral circulation in this patient with a nonresectable bronchial carcinoma.

Aortography

Positive contrast material can be used to opacify the aorta by either selective catheterization of the aorta itself or by injection of the venous system, either directly or by catheter, and study of opacification of the aorta after contrast material passes through the heart. Since the aorta is an important structure in the visceral mediastinal compartment, opacification of the aorta can be useful in evaluating masses in this area.

Aneurysms of the thoracic aorta are usually readily identifiable by routine chest roentgenography. Most aortic aneurysms are fusiform and conform to the shape of the aorta. Dissecting aneurysm of the aorta and saccular aneurysms of the aorta, however, may present difficult diagnostic problems. Dissecting aortic aneurysms can usually be suspected on clinical grounds. The routine roentgenogram is helpful if it shows a change in the aortic contour from earlier roentgenograms or widening of the aortic shadow even without earlier roentgenograms. Aortography is necessary to be certain that a dissection is present, however. The false channel of the dissection can ordinarily be shown as a negative defect that subsequently opacifies (Fig. 11–44).

Most aneurysms of the aorta are fusiform but they may on occasion take a saccular form, in which case they can pose a diagnostic problem. An aortic aneurysm can be suspected by proximity of a mass to the aorta and by ringlike calcification in the wall of the mass. Aortography is usually necessary to make certain that this mass is an aneurysm. It is important to recognize that an aneurysm

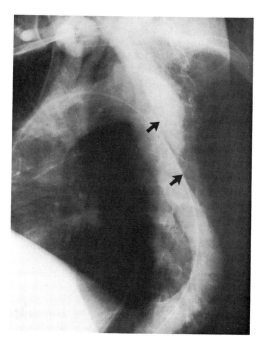

Fig. 11–44. Dissecting aneurysm of the aorta. Aortography clearly demonstrates the presence of the false channel of the aortic dissection (arrows).

may be filled with clot and may not opacify during aortic injection. Irregularities of the contour of the aortic wall in the area of the aneurysm usually indicate its presence.

Aortography may also be useful in identifying aneurysms of the great vessels or anomalies of the great vessels. Tortuous great vessels may simulate superior mediastinal masses (Fig. 11–45).

Selective Catheterization of the Aortic Branches

Catheterization of the bronchial arteries was initially thought to be helpful in the diagnosis of primary carcinoma of the lung. However, subsequent investigation revealed changes in patients with inflammatory lesions of the lung that are difficult to distinguish from those due to tumor. Bronchial arteriography may be helpful in documenting bronchial collateral circulation in patients with pulmonary artery stenosis. Bronchial artery embolization has been performed to control massive bleeding in patients with tumor or pulmonary aspergilloma.

Venography

The *superior vena cava* can easily be opacified by injecting the veins of one or both upper extremities. This opacification may yield information about masses in the superior mediastinum. Invasion of the superior vena cava by bronchial carcinoma or displacement of vena cava by enlarged mediastinal lymph nodes ordinarily indicates inoperability. Superior vena cavagraphy may also be useful in investigation of the superior vena cava syndrome.

The *azygos vein* is another thoracic vein that can be opacified readily. This opacification is accomplished by injecting contrast material into a rib or a vertebral spinous process or by refluxing contrast material into the

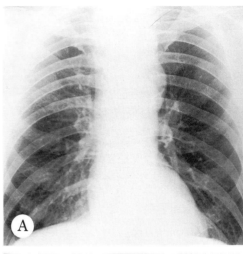

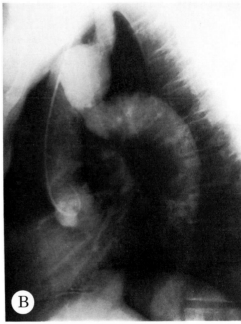

Fig. 11–45. Pseudocoarctation of the aorta. Aortography (B) demonstrates that a suspected mediastinal mass (A) is a tortuous and kinked aorta.

azygos vein following direct catheterization of this vein from the superior or inferior vena cava. Azygography can be useful in evaluating the operability of primary carcinoma of the lung and may also be helpful in investigating other mediastinal masses or in the investigation of liver disease.

Selective catheterization of the thymic vein was described by Kreel (1967) and has been used in the investigation of thymic masses.

Air Contrast Studies

Air contrast studies can be made by injecting air or some other gas into various compartments of the chest. These procedures are not as popular as the angiographic techniques, but often can yield equally important information.

Diagnostic Pneumothorax

This procedure is useful in investigating pleural lesions (Fig. 11–40). It is simple to introduce some air into the pleural space following diagnostic thoracentesis. Roentgenograms made with the patient in various positions may yield helpful clues about the nature of the disease involving the pleura.

Diagnostic Pneumoperitoneum

This study may be used to investigate anomalies of the diaphragm. It is most useful in investigating diaphragmatic hernias or subphrenic abscess.

Diagnostic Pneumomediastinum

Although infrequently used, diagnostic pneumomediastinum has been employed to investigate anterior mediastinal masses, particularly those in the thymus. In patients with myasthenia gravis, in whom a thymic tumor is strongly suspected, pneumomediastinography may reveal a tumor where none could be seen on the routine roentgenogram. CT, however, is the procedure of choice in searching for occult thymomas.

REFERENCES

Aschoff, L.: Lectures on Pathology. New York, Paul B. Hoeber, 1924.
Boyden, E.A.: Segmental Anatomy of the Lungs. A Study of the Patterns of the Segmental Bronchi and Related Pulmonary Vessels. New York, McGraw-Hill Book Co., 1955.
Brailsford, J.F.: The radiographic posteromedial border of the lung or the linear thoracic paraspinal shadow. Radiology, 41:34, 1943.
Favis, E.A.: Planigraphy (body section radiography) in detecting tuberculous pulmonary cavitation. Dis. Chest 27:688, 1955.
Felson, B.: Chest Roentgenology. Philadelphia, W.B. Saunders Co., 1973.
Fleischner, F.G.: The visible bronchial tree: a roentgen sign in pneumonic and other pulmonary consolidations. Radiology 50:184, 1948.
Fraser, R.G., and Paré, J.A.P.: Diagnosis of Diseases of the Chest. Philadelphia, W.B. Saunders Co., 1978.
Jackson, C.L., and Huber, J.F.: Correlated applied anatomy of the bronchial tree and lungs with a system of nomenclature. Dis. Chest 9:319, 1943.
Kreel, L.: Selective thymic venography. New method for visualization of the thymus. Br. Med. J. 1:406, 1967.
Lubert, M., and Krause, G.R.: Patterns of lobar collapse as observed radiographically. Radiology 56:165, 1951.
Robbins, L.L., and Hale, C.H.: The roentgen appearance of lobar and segmental collapse of the lung. Radiology 44:107; 45:120, 260, 347, 1945.
Schaner, E.G., et al.: Comparison of computed and conventional whole lung tomography in detecting pulmonary nodules. Am. J. Roentgenol. 131:51, 1978.
Shanks, S.C., and Kerley, P.: A Textbook of X-ray Diagnosis, Vol. II. Philadelphia, W.B. Saunders Co., 1951.

READING REFERENCES

Bauman, R., Lodwick, G., and Tavaras, J.: The digital computer in medical imaging: a critical review. Radiology 153:73, 1984.
Brock, R.C.: The Anatomy of the Bronchial Tree. London, Oxford University Press, 1954.
Cimmino, C.V.: Further notes on the esophageal-pleural stripes. Radiology 77:974, 1961.
Felson, B.: The roentgen diagnosis of disseminated pulmonary alveolar disease. Semin. Roentgenol. 2:3, 1967.

Foster-Carter, A.F., and Hoyle, C.: The segments of the lungs: a commentary on their investigation and morbid radiology. Dis. Chest *11*:511, 1945.

Fraser, R.G., Breatnach, E., and Barnes, C.T.: Digital radiography of the chest: clinical experience with a prototype unit. Radiology *148*:1, 1983.

Gefter, W.B., et al.: Semi-invasive aspergillosis: a new look at the spectrum of *Aspergillus* infection of the lung. Radiology *140*:313, 1981.

Genereaux, G.P.: Radiologic assessment of diffuse lung disease. *In* Radiology: Diagnosis, Imaging, Intervention. Edited by J.M. Tavaras and J.T. Ferrucci. Philadelphia, J.B.Lippincott Co., 1986.

Genereaux, G.P.: The posterior pleural reflections. AJR *141*:141, 1983.

Godwin, J.D.: The solitary pulmonary nodule. Radiol. Clin. North Am. *21*:709, 1983.

Heitzman, E.R.: The Lung: Radiologic-Pathologic Correlations. St. Louis, C.V. Mosby, 1984.

Heitzman, E.R.: The Mediastinum: Radiologic Correlations with Anatomy and Pathology. St. Louis, C.V. Mosby, 1977.

Kreel, L., Blendis, L.M., and Piercy, J.E.: Pneumomediastinography by the trans-sternal method. Clin. Radiol. *15*:219, 1964.

Liebow, A.A., et al.: The genesis and functional implications of collateral circulation of the lungs. Yale J. Biol. Med. *22*:637, 1950.

Lynch, P.A.: A different approach to chest roentgenography: triad technique (high kilovoltage, grid, wedge filter). AJR *93*:965, 1965.

Miller, W.T., and MacGregor, R.R.: Tuberculosis: The frequency of unusual radiographic findings. AJR *130*:867, 1978.

Naidich, D.P., Zerhouni, E.A., and Siegelman, S.S.: Computed Tomography of the Thorax. New York, Raven Press, 1984.

Ormond, R.S., Jaconette, J.R., and Templeton, A.W.: The pleural esophageal reflection: an aid in the evaluation of esophageal disease. Radiology *80*:738, 1963.

Osborne, D.R., et al.: Comparisons of plain radiography, conventional tomography, and computed tomography in detecting intrathoracic lymph node metastases from lung carcinoma. Radiology *142*:157, 1982.

Parkes, W.R.: Occupational Lung Disorders. London, Butterworths, 1982.

Ravin, C.E.: Pulmonary vascularity: radiographic considerations. Journal of Thoracic Imaging *3*:1, 1988.

Reid, L.: The lung: its growth and remodeling in health and disease. AJR *129*:777, 1977.

Rosai, J., and Levine, G.D.: Tumors of the thymus. Fascile 13, Atlas of Tumor Pathology, AFIP (Armed Forces Institute of Pathology), 1975.

Schatz, M., Patterson, R., and Fink, J.: Immunologic lung disease. N. Engl. J. Med. *300*:1310, 1979.

Storch, C.B.: Fundamentals of Clinical Fluoroscopy. New York, Grune & Stratton, 1951.

Tuddenham, W.J., et al.: Supervoltage and multiple simultaneous roentgenography: new techniques in roentgen examination of the chest. Radiography *63*:184, 1954.

Viamonte, M., Jr.: Angiography evaluation of lung neoplasm. Radiol. Clin. North Am. *3*:529, 1965.

Wittenborg, M.H., and Aviad, I.: Organ influence on a normal posture of the diaphragm: a radiological study of inversions and heterotaxis. Br. J. Radiol. *136*:280, 1963.

CHAPTER 12

ROENTGENOGRAPHIC EVALUATION OF THE ESOPHAGUS

Gary G. Ghahremani

Fluoroscopic examination of the esophagus during ingestion of radiopaque contrast media serves as the primary diagnostic method for evaluating both esophageal motility and structural abnormalities. According to statistical data reported by Mettler (1987), a total of 7.6 million barium studies of the esophagus and upper gastrointestinal tract are performed in the United States each year. Although the conventional barium esophagograph remains a simple, cost-effective screening technique, a wide spectrum of other imaging methods are currently available for better demonstration and more accurate diagnosis of esophageal lesions. This chapter provides an overview of the value and limitations of such roentgenologic procedures.

The majority of functional and organic disorders affecting the pharynx or esophagus manifest with dysphagia. Their optimal assessment and differential diagnosis by the various modalities requires a tailored approach. Selection of the appropriate test often depends on pertinent clinical information about the character and duration of the patient's symptoms, and their potential relationships to any coexistent systemic diseases, administered medications, and previous surgical, diagnostic or therapeutic procedures.

ROENTGENOGRAPHIC METHODS OF EXAMINATION

Plain Chest Roentgenograms

The esophageal body contained within the posterior mediastinum has a 3 to 5-mm thick muscular wall, but it is normally invisible on plain films of the chest. This is partly due to the fact that the esophagus collapses during its resting phase while the upper and lower esophageal sphincters maintain their tonic contraction to prevent aspiration of air and retrograde flow of gastric contents into the esophagus. Nevertheless, the standard PA and lateral chest radiographs may provide significant clues to the diagnosis of an underlying pathology when the esophageal lumen contains an abnormal collection of air, fluid, or food particles, or harbors an ingested radiopaque object. Furthermore, chest films may show a retrocardiac soft tissue density with an air-fluid level, and thereby suggest an otherwise unsuspected hiatal hernia.

The term "air esophagogram" denotes the plain film visualization of an atonic, noncollapsing esophagus by virtue of retained air in its lumen. This finding was initially observed in patients with esophageal involvement by scleroderma. Proto and Lane (1977), however, noted that the same phenomenon occurs with mediastinal fibrosis secondary to inflammation or irradiation, following thoracic surgery, or when esophageal motility and intraluminal pressure are disturbed by extensive pulmonary infiltrates, causing diminished compliance of the lungs and poor respiratory excursion.

On chest roentgenograms a diffuse mediastinal widening in the absence of normal gas collection in the gastric fundus might be a manifestation of a dilated esophagus, usually containing a foamy mixture of air, food, or secretions. These features are highly suggestive of achalasia, but may also be seen with a peptic stricture or infiltrating tumor of the gastroesophageal junction. Carcinoma of the esophagus may also be visible on chest films as a soft tissue mass thickening the esophagopleural stripe, indenting the trachea, or causing mediastinal adenopathy and pulmonary metastasis. Furthermore, plain roentgenograms of the chest and neck continue to play an important role in the evaluation of suspected esophageal perforation and pneumomediastinum as recently emphasized by Han and associates (1985).

Single-Contrast Esophagography

The standard contrast material for opacification of the esophageal lumen is a colloidal suspension of a micropulverized barium sulfate in water (Fig. 12–1). Commercial products of various densities and viscosities are

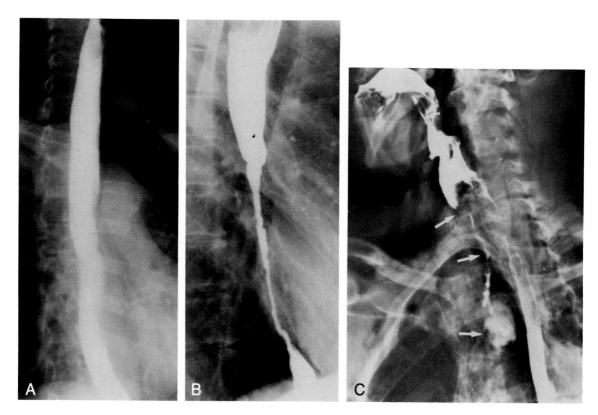

Fig. 12–1. Conventional single-contrast esophagography. *A,* Normal appearance of the barium-filled esophagus with its uniformly tubular shape and smooth margins. *B,* Long esophageal stricture complicating chronic reflux esophagitis in a patient with Zollinger-Ellison syndrome. *C,* Perforation of the right pyriform sinus during esophagoscopy. The orally administered barium has clearly outlined the origin and course of a narrow extraluminal passage into the mediastinum (arrows).

available; they usually contain flavoring agents as well as chemical additives such as aluminum hydroxide, sorbitol, and methyl cellulose. Iodinated water-soluble preparations—such as Gastrografin or Hypaque—may be used in instances of suspected esophageal perforation and anastomotic leakage. These aqueous contrast media are readily absorbed after extravasation into the mediastinal soft tissues and pleural or peritoneal spaces, whereas extraluminal barium sulfate carries the potential risk of inducing foreign body reaction and fibrotic changes. As documented by Foley and associates (1982), however, the mucosal tears and transmural perforations of the upper gastrointestinal tract are better diagnosed with barium than with iodinated contrast media. These authors have pointed out that 25 to 50% of esophageal perforations are unrecognizable or inadequately shown during initial evaluation with water-soluble agents because their low density and rapid transit time impairs an optimal mucosal coating and visualization of minimal leakage. Furthermore, the aspiration of such iodinated hypertonic solutions into the lungs can lead to chemical pneumonia and pulmonary edema, particularly among patients with esophageal dysmotility or obstruction.

Roentgenologic examination of the esophagus is performed under fluoroscopic observation. In conventional single-contrast esophagography, the patient is first examined in upright and then in recumbent positions while taking sequential swallows of relatively diluted barium—

40 to 80% weight/volume of barium sulfate in water. Spot films of the well-distended esophagus are obtained, including views of the gastroesophageal segment during suspended respiration, which accentuates any existing hiatal hernia or Schatzki's ring. In infants a nursing bottle is used for oral administration of contrast material, but controlled instillation through a soft feeding tube is recommended if esophageal atresia or tracheoesophageal fistula is suspected.

The uniform tubular shape of opacified esophageal lumen and the repetitive nature of its peristaltic activity permit an accurate fluoroscopic analysis of both motility and structural changes. In addition, permanent record of the observed normal or pathologic findings is almost routinely obtained. This is usually done with serial spot films or 100-mm photocamera views of the esophagus in various projections. Large roentgenograms covering the entire length of the esophagus can also be obtained while the patient is continually drinking barium (Fig. 12–1), but such blindly exposed overhead films should not be substituted for fluoroscopically guided roentgenograms.

A continuous dynamic recording is the preferred technique for the evaluation of the pharyngeal and esophageal motility. For this purpose, cineradiography using 8-mm or 16-mm films at the speed of 15 to 30 frames per second was previously used in most institutions. The availability of high-resolution videotape attachment to television monitors of fluoroscopic units has simplified the recording of esophageal motility. This method offers the advantage of reduced radiation exposure to the patient while permitting immediate replay and detailed analysis of the recorded findings.

Roentgenographic study of esophageal peristalsis and motility disorders is conducted with the patient in prone-oblique position. The horizontal placement eliminates the interference of gravity with the passage of contrast material, and permits better visibility of the esophagus by projecting it away from the thoracic spine. The patient is instructed to swallow one mouthful of barium at a time. The initiated primary peristaltic wave appears as a lumen-obliterating contraction that propagates distally at 2 to 4 cm per second. In normal adults the bolus transit through the 20 to 24 cm long esophagus is completed in 6 to 8 seconds. Patients with esophageal dysmotility, however, usually show considerable retention and delayed clearing of barium. The associated fluoroscopic findings are decreased incidence and amplitude of peristaltic waves following deglutition, failure of once-initiated contraction to progress distally, and repetitive nonpropulsive waves commonly referred to as tertiary contractions. In contrast to the dilated atonic esophageal body in achalasia, the entity of "nutcracker esophagus" described by Benjamin (1979) and Ott (1986) and their colleagues is characterized by recurrent high-amplitude contractions of the distal esophagus, which cause dysphagia and cramping retrosternal pain.

Double-Contrast Esophagography

This technique permits an accurate demonstration of mucosal abnormalities that are usually the hallmark of inflammatory or neoplastic processes. As described by Balfe (1981), Koehler (1980), and others, the examination requires especially formulated high-density barium for coating the esophageal mucosa while the lumen is fully distended by gas. For this purpose, carbon dioxide released by ingested effervescent agents such as citrocarbonate granules is used together with swallowed air. This serves as a radiolucent intraluminal gas collection to expand the lumen and provide a detailed view of the esophageal inner surface. Any areas of narrowing or rigidity are also better recognizable when the otherwise pliable esophageal wall is maximally stretched.

Double-contrast roentgenograms of the normal esophagus typically show a smooth, featureless mucosa and the well-demarcated walls of this tubular structure (Fig. 12–2A). In older individuals, however, a finely nodular surface pattern may be seen, owing to glycogenic acanthosis of the esophagus. As described by Ghahremani and Rushovich (1984), this benign degenerative condition is characterized by glycogen deposits within multifocal plaques of hyperplastic squamous epithelium.

Multiple longitudinal folds are commonly visible in a partially collapsed esophagus, but they become totally effaced and obliterated with progressive luminal distention. Hence the detection of prominent thickened folds on air-contrast views indicates their loss of pliability caused by submucosal edema and diffuse inflammatory changes. Superficial ulcerations and extensive mucosal irregularities are found in severe esophagitis caused by reflux, caustic injury, and infections such as moniliasis (Fig. 12–2B). Itai (1978), Levine (1986), and their co-workers have demonstrated that carcinoma of the esophagus can be recognized in its early nonobstructive stage on double-contrast swallows. It appears as a localized area of mucosal nodularity of superficially ulcerated plaque-like lesion, with distinct borders separating it from the normally flat mucosa (Fig. 12–2C).

Modified Esophagography Methods

Most radiologists currently use a biphasic technique that includes upright double-contrast views as well as fluoroscopy and spot filming of the barium-filled esophagus in prone-oblique positions. In selected cases, however, special tests and maneuvers might be employed to resolve a particular diagnostic problem.

Water Siphonage Test. This simple test improves the fluoroscopic detection of gastroesophageal reflux. Following oral administration of barium the patient is placed in a supine position and asked to drink approximately 30 ml of water. The test is positive when the opening of the gastroesophageal junction leads to fluoroscopically visible regurgitation from the barium-filled stomach. The limiting factors are a 5% false-negative rate and occasional transient reflux in normal persons.

Acid-Barium Test. This test is based on the use of a barium sulfate and hydrochloric acid mixture at a pH of 1.7. The appearance of abnormal esophageal contractions and reflux indicates a positive test for peptic esophagitis.

Solid Bolus Test. Subtle areas of narrowing and symptomatic lower esophageal rings can be evaluated by the use of barium tablets or capsules of predetermined diameter. They permit more accurate measurement of the narrowed lumen and its functional significance.

Pharmacoradiologic Tests. Various drugs affecting the esophageal motor function can enhance the diagnostic value of barium studies. The author and associates (1972a) used anticholinergic drugs such as atropine or propantheline bromide—Pro-Banthine—for hypotonic esophagography. The resultant spasmolysis and transient abolishment of peristalsis permitted a clear distinction between the functional and organic narrowing of the lumen. Furthermore, the drug-induced aperistalsis caused engorgement and better visibility of esophageal varices.

Ennis and Lewicki (1973) used Mecholyl-aided esophagography. These authors noted that the subcutaneous injection of methacholine at a dose of 2.5 mg induces severe esophageal contractions of the barium-filled esophagus in patients with achalasia. The positive test serves to distinguish the latter entity from other causes of esophageal dilatation, including scleroderma, peptic stricture, or cancer of the gastroesophageal junction.

COMPUTED TOMOGRAPHY

This imaging technique is primarily used for preoperative staging of esophageal carcinoma, radiation treatment planning of unresectable tumors, and evaluation of

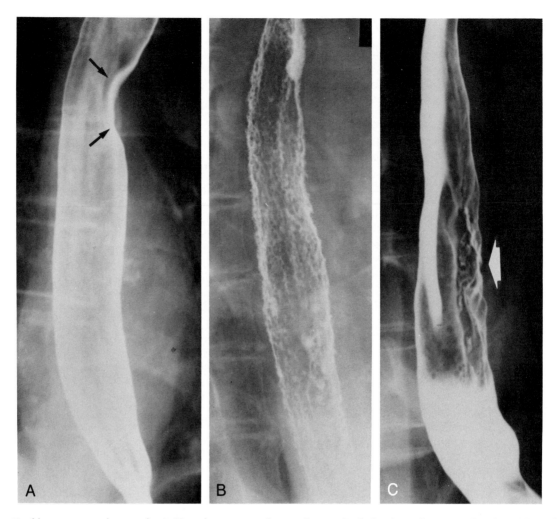

Fig. 12–2. Double-contrast esophagography. *A,* Normal examination showing the completely flat, featureless mucosal surface of the well-distended and almost transparent esophagus. The tubular lumen is slightly indented by the aortic arch and left mainstem bronchus (arrows). *B,* Monilial esophagitis causing a diffusely granular and ulcerated mucosa of the entire esophagus. *C,* Early esophageal carcinoma mainfested as a localized area of mucosal nodularity and superficial ulcerations (arrow).

pathologic processes involving the esophagus and its adjacent mediastinal organs.

For pretherapy CT scanning of patients with carcinoma of the esophagus, serial transverse sections of the chest and upper abdomen are obtained immediately following intravenous administration of iodinated contrast material to opacify the vascular structures. With modern, high-resolution scanners the normal esophageal wall is clearly identified and measures 3 to 5 mm in thickness (Fig. 12–3A). Tumors extending beyond the muscular layers cause distortion and increased density of periesophageal fat. The examination permits assessment of the tumor size, its extraluminal extent, mediastinal invasion, regional lymphadenopathy, and distant metastases to the lungs, liver, and skeleton (Fig. 12–3B, C). Many radiologists use the CT scanning system advocated by Moss and associates (1981). Stage I denotes a localized esophageal carcinoma projecting into the lumen without visible wall thickening, whereas Stage II tumors cause infiltration and thickening of the esophageal wall. These lesions are potentially resectable for cure. CT scans of Stage III carcinomas, however, show direct extension into the adjacent organs, and Stage IV tumors are characterized by distant metastases.

The overall accuracy of CT in staging esophageal carcinoma is about 80 to 90%, according to the data reviewed by Picus (1983), Halvorsen (1986), and their associates. Local extraesophageal extension is detected in 76 to 86% of cases at the time of initial presentation, and approximately one third of the patients show liver or subdiaphragmatic metastases. Considerable difficulty, however, exists in accurate staging of mediastinal or celiac lymph nodes because their enlargement alone is not a reliable indication for metastatic involvement. Furthermore, tumors of the gastroesophageal junction pose a diagnostic challenge since a coexistent hiatal hernia or pseudomass often distorts the anatomic landmarks.

Magnetic Resonance Imaging

This new modality has already established its value in assessing abnormalities of the thorax and mediastinum.

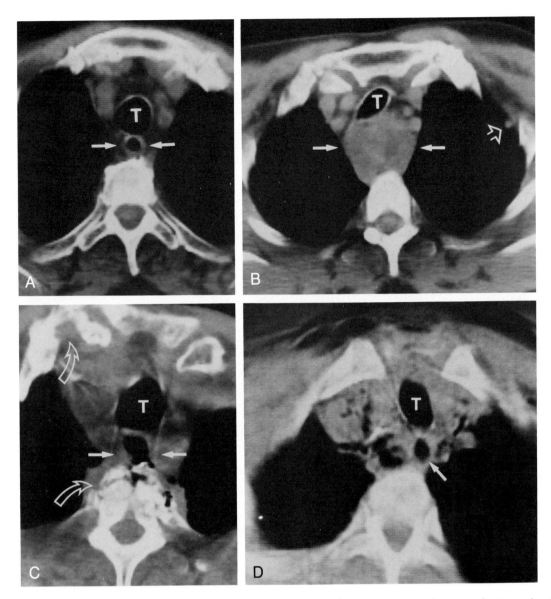

Fig. 12–3. Computed tomography of the esophagus in 4 different patients. *A*, Normal transverse section of upper mediastinum showing the thin-walled esophagus (arrows), located directly behind the circular outline of the trachea (T) and anterior to the vertebral body of T4. *B*, Leiomyosarcoma of the esophagus presenting as a bulky tumor (arrows) which has obliterated the esophageal lumen and mediastinal fat planes. It has also caused deformity and anterior displacement of the trachea (T) and pulmonary metastasis (open arrow). *C*, Ulcerated carcinoma of the proximal esophagus with multiple fistulous tracts extending into the posterior mediastinum (arrows). Note the metastatic lesions destroying the adjacent vertebral body as well as the left sternoclavicular joint (curved arrows). *D*, Computed tomographic appearance of massive pneumomediastinum following endoscopic perforation of the cervical esophagus. There are numerous air collections around the esophagus (arrow) and the trachea (T), causing a widened mediastinum with irregular margins.

Quint and colleagues (1985) have shown that benign and malignant tumors arising from the esophageal wall can be visualized and differentiated from other mediastinal lesions. This technique offers the advantage of direct cross-sectional and sagittal imaging (Fig. 12–14). Such multiplanar three-dimensional views permit better visualization of the tumor's length, bulk, and internal characteristics as well as its extraluminal extension and vascular invasion. Motion artifacts produced by esophageal peristalsis, respiration, and the pulsations of the heart and aorta can degrade the magnetic resonance images. Additional clinical experience is needed to determine

diagnostic applications and relative value of MRI compared to the more established method of computed tomography.

RADIONUCLIDE SCINTIGRAPHY

Gastroesophageal reflux can be detected and quantitatively analyzed in symptomatic patients by chest scanning after oral administration of technetium—^{99m}Tc—sulfur colloid solution. This technique is also useful for the evaluation of esophageal transit time in patients with gastrointestinal motility disorders as reported by Malmud and Fisher (1982).

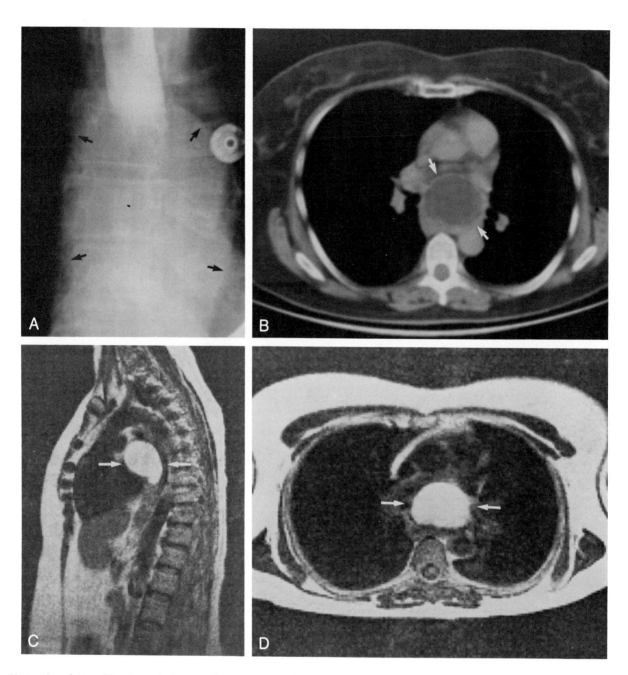

Fig. 12–4. Correlation of imaging techniques used in preoperative diagnosis of an esophageal duplication cyst in a 61-year-old woman. *A,* Close-up view of barium esophagogram reveals extrinsic compression of midesophagus by a soft tissue mass (arrows). *B,* CT scan of the same level illustrates obliteration of the esophagus by a thin-walled cystic lesion (arrows). *C,* Magnetic resonance image of the chest in sagittal section demonstrates a pear-shaped duplication cyst with high intensity due to its fluid content (arrows). *D,* Cross-sectional MR image clearly shows the lesion (arrows), but the anatomic details of the thorax and mediastinum are better visible on CT. (Courtesy of Anthony R. Lupetin, M.D., Allegheny General Hospital, Pittsburgh, Pennsylvania.)

ANGIOGRAPHY

The multiplicity of sources for arterial and venous circulation of the esophagus has limited the application of angiographic methods to this organ. Selective catheterization of the left gastric or splenic arteries can demonstrate the site of hemorrhage from esophageal varices or Mallory-Weiss tears. Such hemorrhages may also be treated by transcatheter infusion of vasoconstrictive agents and controlled embolization. Percutaneous transhepatic catheterization of the portal vein and its branches has been widely used for diagnosis and treatment of esophageal varices by Lunderquist (1974), Keller (1983), and their associates. Azygography and selective mediastinal venography were previously advocated by Yune and Klatte (1972) for the evaluation of tumors involving midesophageal and other mediastinal structures. MRI and contrast-enhanced CT, however, are more accurate, noninvasive methods for diagnosing such lesions.

REFERENCES

Balfe, D.M., et al.: Routine air-contrast esophagography during upper gastrointestinal examinations. Radiology *139*:739, 1981.

Benjamin, S.B., Gerhardt, D.C., and Castell, D.O.: High amplitude, peristaltic esophageal contractions associated with chest pain and/or dysphagia. Gastroenterology 77:478, 1979.

Ennis, J.T., and Lewicki, A.M.: Mecholyl esophagography. Am. J. Roentgenol. *119*:241, 1973.

Foley, M.J., Ghahremani, G.G., and Rogers, L.F.: Reappraisal of contrast media used to detect upper gastrointestinal perforations. Comparison of ionic water-soluble media with barium sulfate. Radiology *144*:231, 1982.

Ghahremani, G.G., et al.: Esophageal varices: enhanced radiologic visualization by anticholinergic drugs. Am. J. Dig. Dis. *17*:703, 1972a.

Ghahremani, G.G., Heck, L.L., and Williams, J.R.: A pharmacologic aid in the radiologic diagnosis of obstructive esophageal lesions. Radiology *103*:289, 1972b.

Ghahremani, G.G., and Rushovich, A.M.: Glycogenic acanthosis of the esophagus: radiographic and pathologic features. Gastrointest. Radiol. 9:93, 1984.

Halvorsen, R.A., Jr., et al.: Esophageal cancer staging by CT: long-term follow-up study. Radiology *161*:147, 1986.

Han, S.Y., et al.: Perforation of the esophagus: correlation of site and cause with plain film findings. Am. J. Roentgenol. *145*:537, 1985.

Itai, Y., et al.: Superficial esophageal carcinoma: radiological findings in double-contrast studies. Radiology *126*:597, 1978.

Keller, F.S., Rosch, J., and Dotter, C.T.: Transhepatic obliteration of gastroesophageal varices with absolute ethanol. Radiology *146*:615, 1983.

Koehler, R.E., Weyman, P.G., and Oakley, H.F.: Single- and double-contrast techniques in esophagitis. Am. J. Roentgenol. *135*:15, 1980.

Levine, M.S., et al.: Early esophageal cancer. Am. J. Roentgenol. *146*:507, 1986.

Lunderquist, A., and Vang, J.: Transhepatic catheterization and obliteration of the coronary vein in patients with portal hypertension and esophageal varices. N. Engl. J. Med. *291*:646, 1974.

Malmud, L.S., and Fisher, R.S.: Radionuclide studies of esophageal transit and gastroesophageal reflux. Semin. Nucl. Med. *12*:104, 1982.

Mettler, F.A., Jr: Diagnostic radiology: usage and trends in the United States, 1964–1980. Radiology *162*:263, 1987.

Moss, A.A., et al.: Esophageal carcinoma: pretherapy staging by computed tomography. Am. J. Roentgenol. *136*:1051, 1981.

Ott, D.J., et al.: Radiologic and manometric correlation in "nutcracker" esophagus. Am. J. Roentgenol. *147*:692, 1986.

Picus, D., et al.: Computed tomography in the staging of esophageal carcinoma. Radiology *146*:433, 1983.

Proto, A.V., and Lane, E.J.: Air in the esophagus: a frequent radiographic finding. Am. J. Roentgenol. *129*:433, 1977.

Quint, L.E., Glazer, G.M., and Orringer, M.B.: Esophageal imaging by MR and CT: study of normal anatomy and neoplasms. Radiology *156*:727, 1985.

Yune, H.Y., and Klatte, E.C.: Mediastinal venography: selective transfemoral catheterization technique. Radiology *105*:285, 1972.

READING REFERENCES

Halpert, R.D., et al.: Radiological assessment of dysphagia with endoscopic correlation. Radiology *157*:599, 1985.

Heiken, J.P., Balfe, D.M., and Roper, C.L.: CT evaluation after esophagogastrectomy. Am. J. Roentgenol. *143*:555, 1984.

Laufer, I.: Double-Contrast Gastrointestinal Radiology with Endoscopic Correlation. Philadelphia, W.B. Saunders Co., 1979.

Taylor, C.R.: Carcinoma of the esophagus—current imaging options. Am. J. Gastroenterol. *81*:1013, 1986.

CHAPTER 13

COMPUTED TOMOGRAPHY OF THE CHEST

David M. Epstein and Warren B. Gefter

Computed tomography—CT—is now firmly established as an indispensable radiologic modality for the evaluation of the chest. CT can provide cross-sectional images with exceptional anatomic detail and far greater tissue contrast than can be obtained by conventional roentgenography. Although the major contribution of CT in the thorax is in the evaluation of the mediastinum, CT has also found applications in the evaluation of the lung, pleura, and chest wall.

TECHNIQUE

CT passes multiple, highly collimated x-ray beams at various angles through the anatomic plane of interest to expose an array of electronic detectors rather than a radiographic film. The density of the tissue that each beam traverses determines the beam's degree of attenuation and consequently the ouput from the detectors. These projections of tissue density obtained from the detectors are then mathematically reconstructed by a computer into an image that is essentially a map of tissue densities. Density differences of only 1 to 2% can be recognized by this technique, whereas differences of 4 to 5% are required for recognition on standard roentgenograms.

Thoracic CT is not a screening procedure. Each CT examination should be tailored to address a particular clinical problem. Several operator-dependent variables need to be addressed on each examination to create optimally informative images. These variables include selection of the appropriate slice thickness, slice spacing, and field of view. The judicious and appropriately timed administration of intravenous iodinated contrast agents is particularly important in evaluating the pulmonary hila and mediastinum. Intravenous contrast enhancement is also critical to proper evaluation of the aorta and great vessels, particularly in patients with suspected dissection of those vessels.

Differences in tissue density are expressed in terms of CT numbers. Typical CT numbers range from approximately −1000—air—to +1000—dense cortical bone. Structures of the same density as water have a CT number of approximately zero; in contrast, fat is approximately −100. Because many technical variables can affect a CT number, a relative comparison of CT numbers between structures is usually far more informative than any absolute value. The full scale of CT numbers generated by the CT reconstruction process cannot be displayed in a single image because current electronic display systems use only a limited number of shades of gray. The operator has to select, through manipulation of the electronic windows at the CT console, the portion of the CT number range he wishes to display. All CT images of the chest should be viewed with at least two, and optimally three window settings: one for the lungs, one for the mediastinum and chest wall, and one for the bony structures.

CLINICAL APPLICATIONS

Mediastinum

Mediastinal Masses

The evaluation of mediastinal masses seen on conventional roentgenography is enhanced by CT by more subtle density discrimination as well as clarification of relationships to other vital structures and visualization of tissue planes. Solid lesions can be separated from those that are cystic or fatty and areas of necrosis or calcification are more easily detected with CT than with plain films.

The thymus gland normally appears as a bilobed arrowhead-shaped structure, often best visualized at the level of the aortic arch but frequently seen extending from the left brachiocephalic vein to the root of the aorta and pulmonary artery. Moore and colleagues (1983) reported that normal thymic measurements vary with age. Because of fatty infiltration, patients older than 30 years tend to have atrophic glands; however, the thymic contours are usually preserved. In patients over 40, the presence of a spherical or ovoid mass in the expected location of the thymic gland or deformity of the adjacent pleura suggests a thymoma (Fig. 13–1). Diffuse enlargement of the thymic gland with preservation of its normal

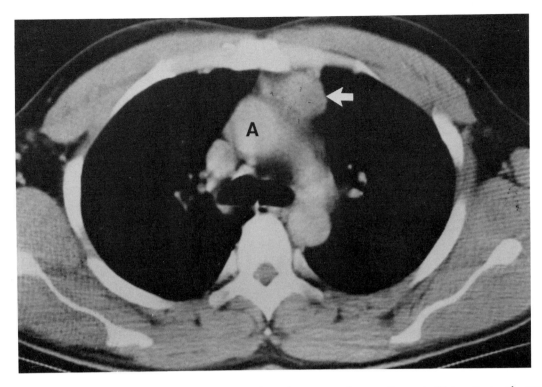

Fig. 13–1. Thymoma. A well-circumscribed ovoid soft tissue mass (arrow) anterior to the ascending aorta (A) in patient with myasthenia gravis is consistent with thymoma.

shape is more suggestive of hyperplasia. Well-circumscribed thymic tumors are almost always benign, whereas tumors showing infiltration into adjacent fat are usually malignant. However, CT cannot consistently differentiate benign from malignant thymoma unless there is evidence of metastatic disease to the mediastinum, pleura, or lungs (Fig. 13–2). Thymoma is seen in 10 to 15% of patients with myasthenia gravis. It is also associated with red cell aplasia.

Brown and associates (1982) reported CT to be helpful in localizing thymic carcinoid tumors in patients suspected of having ectopic production of ACTH. CT may also be used to identify mediastinal parathyroid adenomas in patients with unexplained hypercalcemia.

Teratomas are difficult to distinguish from thymic lesions by CT criteria alone. Both are usually solid masses and may contain calcifications. Teratomas, however, more frequently than thymomas, show areas of low density within the mass because of either cystic or fatty components. A predominently low-density mediastinal mass suggests a cystic teratoma or mediastinal germ cell tumor (Fig. 13–3).

The iodine content of a substernal thyroid on CT scans that are not contrast-enhanced is diagnostically helpful because of its higher density than other solid mediastinal masses. CT can also confirm the presence of a substernal thyroid by showing direct extension of the mass from the neck into the mediastinum or contiguous sections. Occasionally, a substernal thyroid may appear to have low density because of a relative lack of iodine in areas of cystic degeneration. CT cannot exclude malignancy of the thyroid gland.

Perhaps the greatest utility of CT in evaluation of the mediastinum has been in the detection of lymphadenopathy. The extent and distribution of lymphadenopathy is accurately assessed with CT. Lymph nodes appear as discrete or confluent regions of soft tissue density separable from other mediastinal structures, particularly when intravenous contrast has been administered. Lymphadenopathy may contain regions of lower density because of necrosis of high-density calcification from granulomatous disease or radiation therapy. The identification of lymph nodes does not indicate their histologic characteristics or even the presence of disease. Anatomic and pathologic studies reported by Genereux and Howie (1984) of patients with no known chest disease frequently identified lymphadenopathy in all regions of the mediastinum. Lymph node size tended to vary with location; however, 95% of normal lymph nodes were less than 11 mm in diameter. Enlarged lymph nodes may have a variety of causes, including metastatic tumor, lymphoma, sarcoidosis, and other granulomatous or inflammatory causes.

The CT assessment of mediastinal lymphadenopathy is important in the preoperative staging of bronchial carcinoma, particularly in comparison to surgical staging. One inherent difficulty posed for CT in this regard is that even though lymph nodes containing tumor are apt to be larger than normal, there is no absolute size criterion above which a lymph node must contain tumor, and conversely microscopic metastases occur in lymph nodes that are normal in size. Another inherent problem in CT imaging of lymphadenopathy is that some lymph nodes are vertically disposed and the technique does not

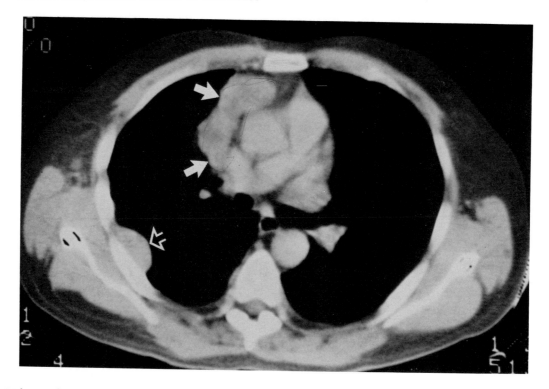

Fig. 13–2. Malignant thymoma. Inhomogeneous, slightly irregular anterior mediastinal mass (closed arrows) with a pleural metastasis on the right (open arrow) indicates a malignant thymoma.

provide reliable estimates of their longitudinal dimension. The sensitivity and specificity of CT in detecting enlarged lymph nodes caused by metastatic disease have been variably reported in the literature, as noted by Libschitz and colleagues (1984) and is influenced by patient selection, prevalence of disease, lymph node size construed as abnormal, and method of surgical sampling.

Most surgeons now recognize that enlarged lymph nodes need not harbor metastases, and that normal-sized lymph nodes may contain metastases, as confirmed by us (D.M.E.) and our co-workers (1986). The advantage of CT over the chest roentgenogram is its ability to identify the precise mediastinal location of enlarged lymph nodes that should be surgically evaluated for the presence of metastasis prior to resection (Fig. 13–4). A normal mediastinum on CT frequently eliminates the need for surgical staging, mediastinoscopy, or mediastinotomy. In 10% of these patients, however, histologic evidence of metastatic tumor in nodes may be anticipated at thoracotomy. To summarize, enlarged lymph nodes identified by CT require histologic confirmation. CT should serve as a guide for selecting the appropriate surgical staging procedure to sample enlarged lymph nodes. No patient should be denied surgery on the basis of nodal size alone.

Most benign cystic lesions of the mediastinum are homogeneous and water-equivalent in density (Fig. 13–5). They are not enhanced following intravenous contrast administration. Bronchogenic cysts are typically round or ovoid low-density structures—water-equivalent—in the subcarinal or right paratracheal regions. Pericardial cysts occur in both the right and left cardiophrenic angle.

Either mass may occasionally be higher in density owing to hemorrhage or proteinaceous contents.

Homer and associates (1978) reported that localized benign mediastinal fat collections can be diagnosed with absolute certainty using CT. Their low density permits easy distinction from lymphadenopathy. Epicardial fat pads, and paravertebral and retrocrural lipomatosis are easily identified by their low CT numbers in the fat range.

Neurogenic tumor, the most common posterior mediastinal mass, is well evaluated by CT. CT allows precise localization, detection of vertebral body destruction, and recognition of intraspinal tumor extension.

Mediastinal Widening

The evaluation of a widened mediastinal contour on the plain film is ideally suited for CT as reported by Baron and colleagues (1981a). CT can distinguish normal variants—abundant fat or tortuous vessel—from aneurysms, aortic dissections, or soft tissue masses. Abundant fat in the mediastinum is readily diagnosed because of its characteristic low CT density. It is common in patients taking corticosteroids or with Cushing's syndrome. With the administration of intravenous iodinated contrast material, Baron and associates (1981b) noted that tortuous great vessels and congenital vascular anomalies of the aortic arch were readily demonstrated (Fig. 13–6).

Gross and co-workers (1980) found CT to be useful in detecting aortic dissection in individuals who are hemodynamically stable. Medial displacement of intimal calcification may be identified on the precontrast CT scan. Following the administration of intravenous con-

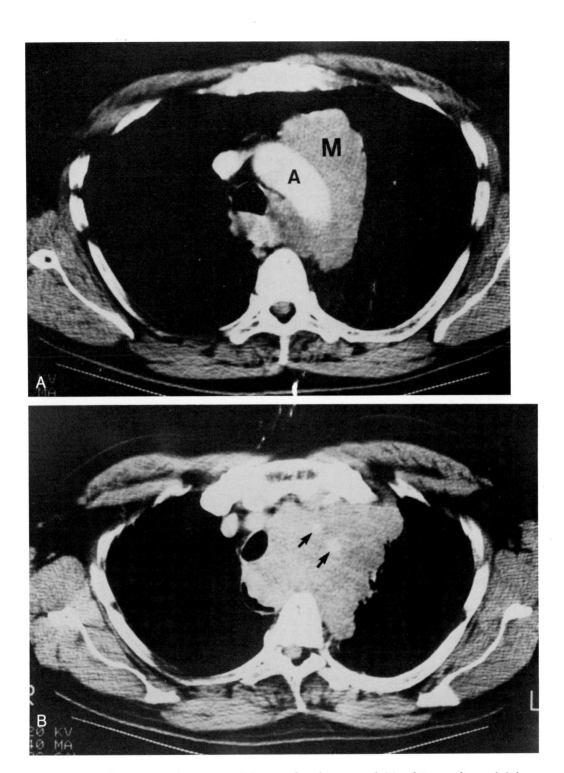

Fig. 13–3. Mediastinal germ cell tumor. *A,* Soft tissue mass (M) surrounding the aortic arch (A) and *B,* extending cephalad to encase the great vessels (arrows) and displace the trachea to the right. This mass cannot be distinguished from extensive lymphadenopathy due to lymphoma or metastatic tumor.

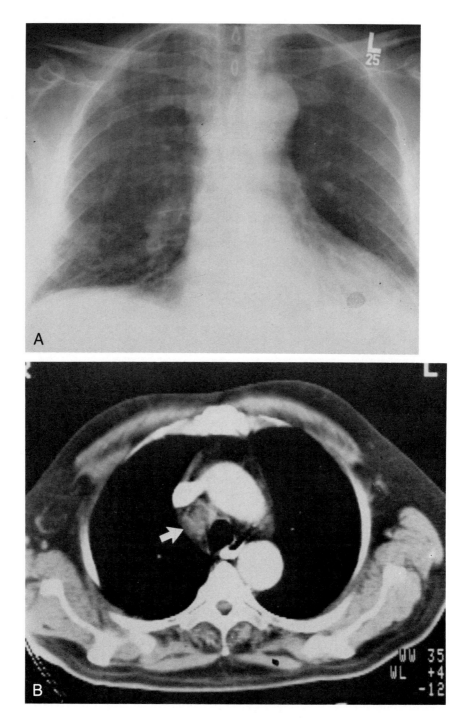

Fig. 13–4. Carcinoma of the lung. *A,* PA chest radiograph reveals no evidence of mediastinal adenopathy. *B,* CT scan reveals a 2 cm right paratracheal lymph node (arrow) behind the superior vena cava. At mediastinoscopy, this lymph node contained metastatic tumor.

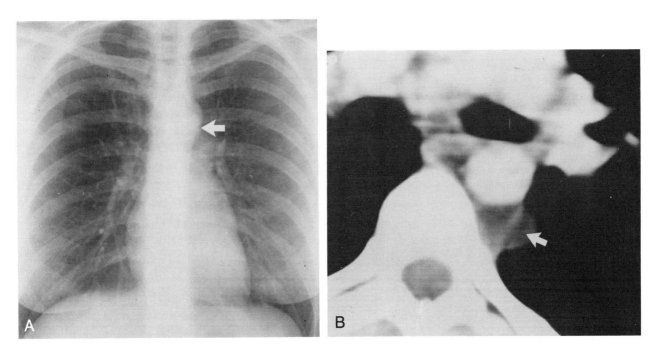

Fig. 13–5. Foregut cyst of the mediastinum. *A,* PA chest radiograph reveals a subtle contour deformity (arrow) in the region of the aortic arch. *B,* CT scan shows a well-circumscribed fluid-containing density (arrow) posterior to the descending aorta. Its fluid density is typical of a benign mediastinal cyst.

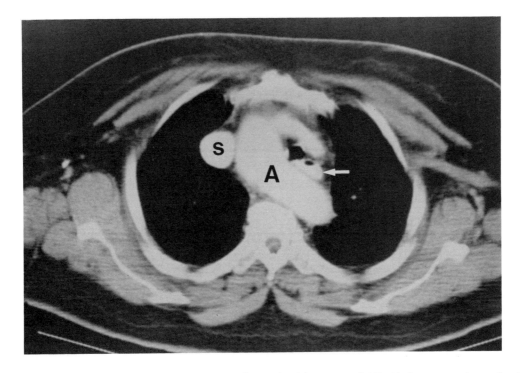

Fig. 13–6. Circumflex right aortic arch. CT scan shows a congenital anomaly of the aortic arch (A) with the aorta passing to the right and behind the trachea and esophagus (arrow). The superior vena cava (S) is identified laterally on the right.

trast, one may identify a thickened aortic wall, a septum between two opacifying lumens, or a differential time density between opacification of the two lumens suggesting an aortic dissection. The origin of the dissection, as well as any associated hemothorax or hemopericardium, can be visualized (Fig. 13–7). If the patient is hemodynamically unstable, it is advisable to resort directly to aortography rather than CT.

Diffuse mediastinal infection or fibrosing mediastinitis is difficult to distinguish from infiltrating metastatic tumor or lymphoma in the mediastinum. The confirmation of infiltrating soft tissue abnormality, however, should lead to appropriate tissue diagnosis by biopsy.

Mediastinal contours may be distorted by esophageal neoplasms. Thompson and associates (1983) have advocated CT as a useful preoperative staging procedure for esophageal carcinoma (Fig. 13–8). Although CT may provide the best preoperative nonsurgical estimate of the extent of esophageal carcinoma, its accuracy in the identification of periesophageal lymph nodes and extraesophageal tumor extension has been disputed by Quint and colleagues (1985).

Following esophagectomy with gastric interposition, the mediastinal contour is widened in most patients, owing to the intrathoracic stomach. CT has been helpful in detecting postoperative complications including mediastinal abscess or hematoma in these patients and in distinguishing these lesions from the normal postoperative intrathoracic stomach. Becker and associates (1987) found CT to be the most effective imaging modality for the detection of tumor recurrence in such patients (Fig. 13–9).

Lungs

Pulmonary Nodule

Advances in CT technology have concentrated on various disorders of the pulmonary parenchyma. Using conventional radiology, the distinction between a benign and malignant solitary pulmonary nodule depends on its growth pattern and the presence of calcification. A nodule that fails to grow over a two-year interval, or a nodule that has "popcorn" or concentric rings of calcification, is presumed to be benign. CT has been advocated as a method for distinguishing between benign and malignant lung nodules on the basis of density.

Initially, Siegelman and co-workers (1980) developed a technique using thin-section—2 to 5-mm—CT with a computerized data printout to distinguish benign from malignant lung nodules on the basis of density numbers. Although this technique has been substantiated by Proto and Thomas (1985), technical problems have precluded its widespread use.

An alternative approach relies on a commercially available phantom that mimics the environment of any given lung nodule. In a multi-institutional study of 384 nodules not considered calcified by conventional methods, Zerhouni and associates (1986) reported that the phantom technique permitted the identification of occult calcification in 37 nodules, thereby suggesting a benign cause.

CT was most effective in establishing the benign character of nodules 3 cm or less in diameter and those with discrete or smooth margins (Fig. 13–10). CT rarely yielded a confident diagnosis of benign disease in larger nodules and in those with an irregular or spiculated border.

In those patients in whom calcification is not demonstrated, thoracotomy or biopsy is usually required to exclude malignancy. Occasionally, a carcinoma may contain an area of calcification. Therefore interpretation of thin-section CT must be both qualitative and quantitative.

Pulmonary Metastases

In patients known to have an extrapulmonary malignancy, CT provides a sensitive means of identifying small pulmonary metastases (Fig. 13–11). Many pulmonary metastases are located subpleurally so that detection by conventional tomography is impractical because of the obscuring density of the overlying chest wall. The capability of visualizing the lung apex, the retrocardiac and retrosternal regions, and the posterior inferior lung recesses near the diaphragm make CT the most sensitive imaging modality in the detection of pulmonary nodules less than 6 mm in diameter. Schaner and colleagues (1978) noted that the major problem in using CT imaging for the detection of occult metastasis is its lack of specificity. Granulomas or subpleural lymph nodes may constitute up to 25% of lung nodules in geographic areas endemic for histoplasmosis. These nodules, unless calcified, are generally indistinguishable from pulmonary metastases.

Cystic and Cavitary Disease

Computed tomography may be helpful in localizing and characterizing cystic and cavitary parenchymal lung disease. In a study by Müller and co-workers (1984), correlation was made between the CT and bronchographic findings in 13 lungs. In only six bronchograms did CT give an accurate assessment of the presence and extent of disease. More recently, however, Grenier and collaborators (1986), using thin—1.5 mm sections—in 36 patients, reported excellent correlation of bronchiectasis with CT scans and bronchography. Moreover, in two cases the lung findings were better appreciated on the CT scans than on bronchography. This series had only one false-negative CT examination and concluded that CT was a reliable, noninvasive method for the assessment of bronchiectasis (Fig. 13–12). These authors suggest that the demonstration of diffuse bronchiectasis by CT may exclude surgery, while focal bronchiectasis requires further confirmation with bronchography.

CT has also been helpful in defining the extent of bullae in patients with both emphysema and congenital bullous disease. It is particularly useful in those patients for whom surgical bullectomy is being contemplated. Occasionally patients present with hemoptysis and cystic or bullous disease in the lung. Such patients are often suspected of having a mycetoma caused by secondary noninvasive aspergillosis. In these patients, CT some-

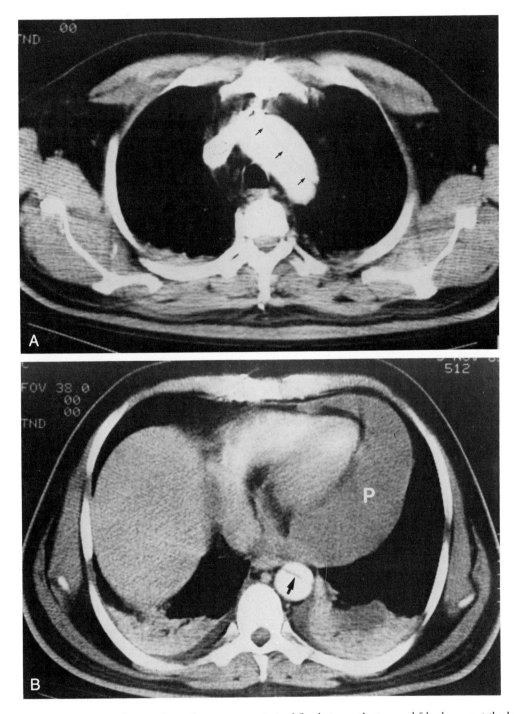

Fig. 13–7. Aortic dissection. *A*, Linear lucency (arrows) represents an intimal flap between the true and false lumens at the level of the aortic arch. *B*, The intimal flap (arrow) is again identified in the descending aorta. A large pericardial effusion (P) is also identified. Posteriorly, there are small bilateral pleural effusions and passive atelectasis in the lung bases.

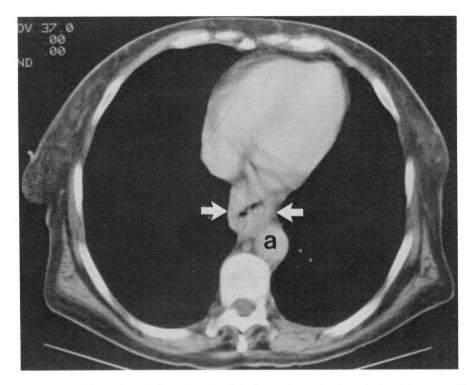

Fig. 13–8. Esophageal carcinoma. CT reveals marked esophageal wall thickening (arrows) and contiguity of the mass with the descending aorta (a). These findings suggest extraesophageal tumor extension.

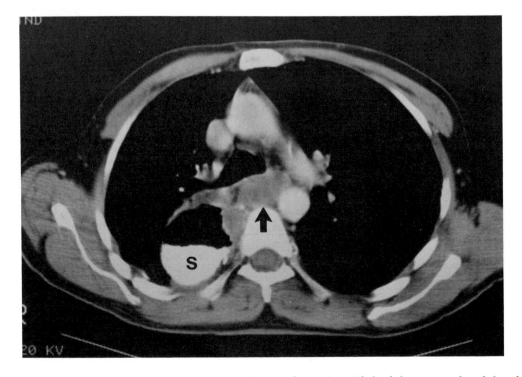

Fig. 13–9. Recurrent tumor post esophagectomy. CT scan shows soft tissue density (arrow) behind the carina and medial to the intrathoracic stomach (S) post esophagectomy. These findings are characteristic of recurrent tumor.

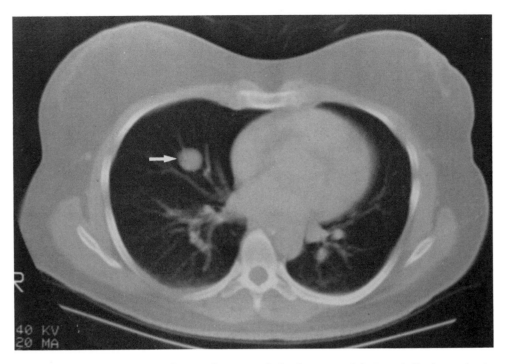

Fig. 13–10. Pulmonary nodule. CT scan shows a solitary well-circumscribed pulmonary nodule (arrow). Further evaluation with thin section computed tomography or the commercially available phantom would be helpful to search for occult calcification suggestive of benignancy.

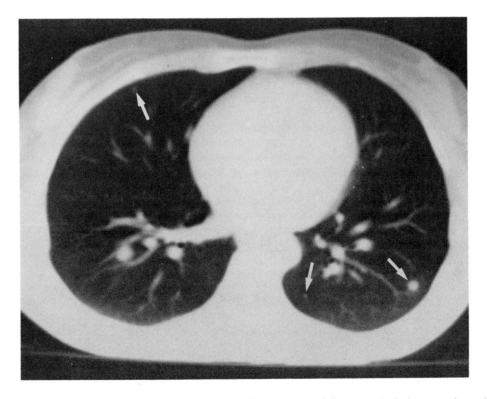

Fig. 13–11. Multiple pulmonary nodules. CT scan reveals multiple small pulmonary nodules (arrows) which were radiographically occult with conventional radiography. In a patient with a known extrathoracic malignancy, these are highly suggestive, though not definitive, for metastatic disease.

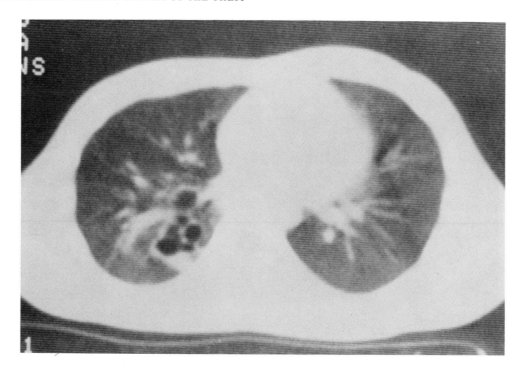

Fig. 13–12. Bronchiectasis. CT scan reveals focal cystic bronchiectasis in the right lower lobe.

times makes it possible to identify an intracavitary mycetoma that is occult by conventional roentgenography.

Interstitial Disease

The application of CT, particularly high-resolution CT, to the study of interstitial and air-space disease in the lung is still in a developmental stage. Although conventional roentgenography remains unequivocally the best method for routine screening, evaluation, and follow-up of parenchymal lung disease, CT with its greatly enhanced contrast resolution and unobstructed cross-sectional visualization of lung anatomy has the potential to add significantly to the display of parenchymal lung processes.

Recognizing that most pathologic processes involve both air-space and interstitial components and that the roentgenographic appearances of these can overlap, Zerhouni and associates (1985) defined four CT categories of observable abnormalities in interstitial lung disease in a study of 89 patients: (1) thickened and irregular interfaces caused by both bronchial wall thickening and irregular interfaces between the bronchi, vessels, and aerated parenchyma were the most common sign of interstitial disease, seen in 89% of cases; (2) normally invisible linear and reticular structures were observed in 78% of cases; (3) ground-glass appearance caused by an overall increase in density was seen in 35% of cases; and (4) nodules of approximately 1 mm or more in diameter were often identified in association with an underlying reticular pattern.

In a study of 23 patients, Bergin and Müller (1985) found the CT pattern helpful in the characterization of interstitial lung disease. Nodular patterns were identified in patients with sarcoidosis, silicosis, and lymphangitic spread of malignancy. In Zerhouni and associates' (1985) experience, nodularity with a large reticular meshwork suggests lymphangitic carcinomatosis; they also identified nodularity in patients with miliary tuberculosis. Non-nodular reticular patterns were seen in patients with fibrosing alveolitis, rheumatoid lung, and hypersensitivity pneumonitis.

The distribution of interstitial densities may also be helpful in clarifying the nature of interstitial lung disease. A peripheral reticular CT pattern is seen in patients with fibrosing alveolitis or collagen vascular disease, whereas a more central pattern is seen in patients with hypersensitivity pneumonitis.

Air-space Disease

Naidich and associates (1985) described the CT appearance of air-space disease. The findings include: (1) air-space nodules that are poorly marginated opacities ranging up to 1 cm in size, caused by sublobular accumulations of fluid, hemorrhage, or cells; (2) coalescent densities that are usually the result of confluence of air-space nodules; (3) air bronchograms and air alveolargrams; and (4) ground-glass opacity that is defined as a zone of increased lung density presumably caused by focal hypoaeration. Several disease processes can produce air-space patterns identified with CT. Pneumonia or aspiration, hemorrhage, pulmonary edema, alveolar proteinosis, and alveolar cell carcinoma may all have an identical CT appearance (Fig. 13–13). CT adds little to the characterization of these diverse disease processes. CT may, however, better define the extent of disease than plain films. This is particularly important for demonstrating the spread of lobar alveolar cell carcinoma to the contralateral lung as reported by Epstein and asso-

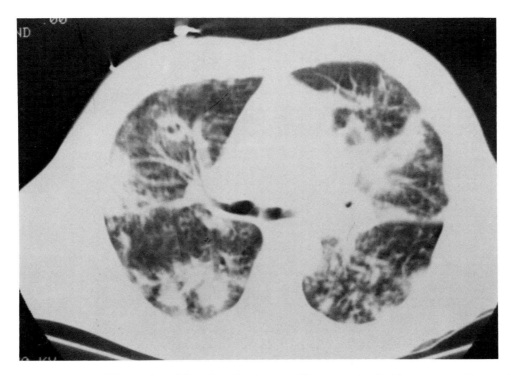

Fig. 13–13. Aspiration pneumonia. CT scan shows bilateral patchy airspace infiltrates consistent with pneumonia. Airspace infiltrates from a variety of etiologies are indistinguishable with CT.

ciates (1982). Several disease entities that pathologically involve the interstitium may resemble air-space disease, including sarcoidosis, desquamative interstitial pneumonitis, and *Pneumocystis carinii* pneumonia. This often makes it impossible to distinguish air-space nodules from interstitial nodules by CT, hampering further narrowing of the differential diagnosis.

Airways

The trachea is usually well visualized with CT. Tracheal diameter can be assessed and tumors both intrinsic and extrinsic to the trachea, as well as tracheal strictures, are easily identified. Extratracheal extension of tumor is best assessed with the cross-sectional images of CT (Fig. 13–14).

The ability to visualize a given bronchus by CT depends on the size and orientation of that bronchus. The origin and proximal portion of every major bronchus that courses horizontally often can be identified by CT provided careful scanning technique is employed. Bronchi having a vertical course are seen only in cross-section, and appear as circular lucencies. The most difficult bronchi to visualize are those that run obliquely. This is especially true of the lingular bronchus as well as the basilar segmental bronchi. Only the proximal portions of the bronchial tree, specifically the proximal portions of the segmental bronchi, can be visualized on CT. Subsegmental bronchi are not identified.

Although fiber-optic bronchoscopy remains the principal modality for evaluation of the airways, CT may be a useful adjunct in patients with suspected occult endobronchial neoplasms. Specifically, in some patients with cryptic hemoptysis or cytologically positive sputa, meticulous CT scanning of the airways may help guide the bronchoscopist to subtle endobronchial abnormalities.

Miscellaenous

Bronchial adenomas are low-grade malignancies that are often endobronchial and frequently extend beyond the bronchus into the surrounding lung or mediastinum. Characteristically they are extremely vascular tumors and most endoscopists will not biopsy such a lesion because of the danger of extensive bleeding. Since most bronchial adenomas arise in the central airways, CT can identify these lesions and define extrabronchial extension. Moreover, because of their vascular nature, contrast enhancement has been reported by Aronchick and collaborators (1986) in three bronchial carcinoids. This enhancement pattern should alert the endoscopist to the possibility of a bronchial adenoma.

CT is a sensitive, noninvasive method for establishing the diagnosis of a pulmonary varix—usually in patients with mitral stenosis—obviating the need for angiography. Pulmonary arteriovenous malformations—AVMs—are occasionally identified by CT when the draining vein can be traced through sequential scans to the hilum. Contrast-enhancement has also been used to confirm the vascular origin of these lesions. Nonetheless, we have found plain film tomography to be adequate for diagnosis of most cases of suspected AVM. Angiography is indicated for those AVMs requiring therapeutic embolization.

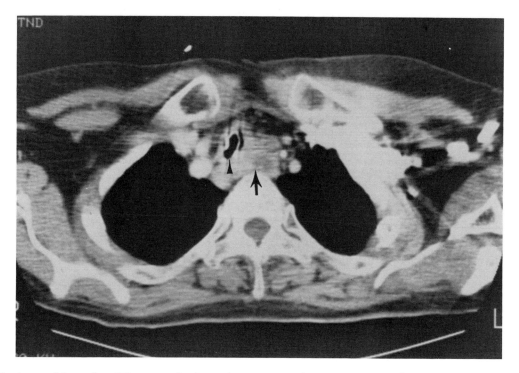

Fig. 13–14. Carcinoma of the trachea. CT scan reveals a large inhomogeneous soft tissue mass (arrow) distorting the tracheal lumen (arrowhead) and separable from the contrast-enhanced vessels in the region. This mass proved to be tumor extension from carcinoma of the trachea.

Pleura

Abscess versus Empyema

CT may provide valuable information in evaluating disease processes of the pleura and in distinguishing pleural from parenchymal lung disease. Familiarity with the CT appearance of the pleural fissures is helpful in localizing lung infiltrates and nodules and in distinguishing loculated pleural fluid from parenchymal consolidation. This application is particularly helpful in differentiating lung abscesses from empyema with bronchopleural fistula. Empyemas are enclosed within the pleural cavity and conform to the shape of the chest wall. Most empyemas have thin, smooth walls, especially along their inner margins. Abscesses, however, because they originate within the pulmonary parenchyma, retain a spherical shape (Fig. 13–15). Most abscesses tend to have thickened, irregular walls and margins. Ancillary findings of empyema include compressed lung adjacent to the inner margin of an empyema, as well as displacement of vessels and bronchi by large pleural fluid collections. The accurate identification of loculated empyemas by CT also provides useful guidance for tube thoracostomy.

Effusion versus Ascites

The differentiation of pleural effusion from ascites is sometimes difficult. Halvorsen and colleagues (1986) reported four CT signs that were useful. The following criteria suggest ascites: (1) fluid is inside—below— the diaphragm; (2) fluid does not elevate the crus of the diaphragm; (3) the interface between fluid and the liver is distinct; and (4) fluid is only posterior or lateral to the liver at the level of the bare area. Pleural effusion, on the other hand, is suggested by the following criteria: (1) fluid is outside—above—the diaphragm; (2) fluid elevates the crus of the diaphragm; (3) the interface between fluid and the liver is indistinct; and (4) fluid is posterior or medial to the liver at the level of the bare area. Used individually, each of these signs may be indeterminate or misleading. If all four criteria are fulfilled, accurate distinction of pleural fluid from ascites can be made (Fig. 13–16).

Mesothelioma

Malignant mesothelioma appears on CT as a thick, pleurally based rind of soft tissue encasing the lung (Fig. 13–17). A variable quantity of fluid, usually loculated, is generally present. The density of this fluid is usually less than that of the rind of soft tissue. Malignant mesothelioma may spread directly to involve the mediastinum, pericardium, contralateral lung, or chest wall. It may also spread through the diaphragm to involve the abdominal and retroperitoneal viscera. CT is the most effective imaging modality available to identify the extent of involvement with malignant mesothelioma.

Miscellaneous

Some benign processes involving the pleura can be well evaluated with CT. CT is useful in confirming subtle pleural plaques suspected from the chest film in patients who have a history of exposure to asbestos. The pleural plaque caused by asbestos disease can also be confidently

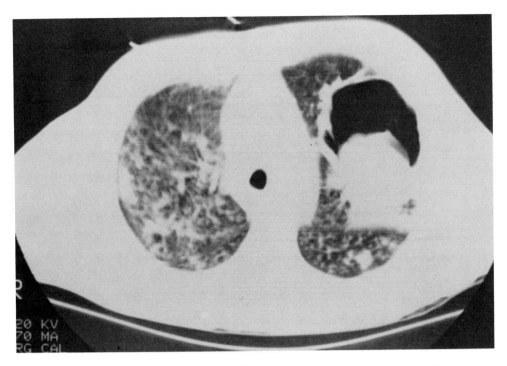

Fig. 13–15. Lung abscess. A large necrotic left lung abscess with debris has a thickened and irregular wall while retaining its spherical shape. An empyema would conform to the shape of the chest wall.

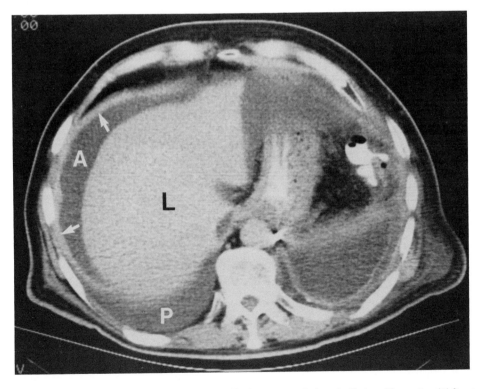

Fig. 13–16. Ascites and pleural effusion. CT scan shows evidence of both ascites and pleural effusion. The ascites (A) lies inside the diaphragm (arrows) and has a distinct interface with the liver (L). Pleural fluid (P) is identified posteriorly behind the diaphragm and has an indistinct interface with the liver.

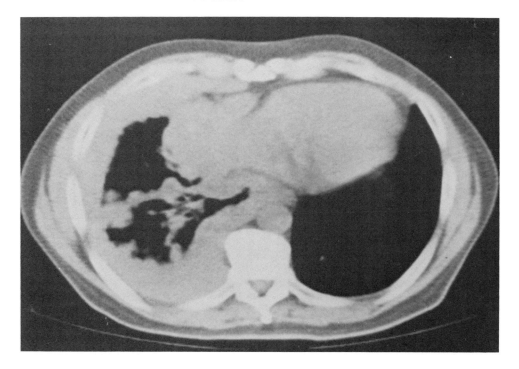

Fig. 13–17. Mesothelioma. A thick rind of pleural based soft tissue encases the entire right hemithorax and is consistent with a malignant mesothelioma.

distinguished from pulmonary nodules. CT may be useful in distinguishing rounded atelectasis from carcinoma in patients with evidence of asbestos-related pleural disease, as described by Mintzer and associates (1981). Our experience indicates that this is a difficult distinction, most often requiring biopsy confirmation. Well-circumscribed, localized pleural tumors such as fibrous mesothelioma can be identified with CT. However, only in the case of a lipoma can a specific diagnosis be made (Fig. 13–18). CT is useful in identifying a lipoma because of its characteristic lower density.

Chest Wall

Lung Cancer

CT has been used to detect chest wall invasion in patients with bronchial carcinoma. The importance of detecting chest wall invasion in lung cancer is unclear. In the absence of mediastinal metastases, a 35% 5-year survival may be anticipated with en bloc resection of peripheral lung carcinoma and the adjacent chest wall as reported by Paone and co-workers (1982). Thus, chest wall invasion from a peripheral tumor in and of itself may not be a contraindication to surgery and its preoperative detection may be of minor clinical significance. Chest wall invasion is suggested on CT by pleural thickening adjacent to the tumor, increased density in the extrapleural fat, rib destruction, and the presence of soft tissue mass in the chest wall (Fig. 13–19). With regard to these criteria, a normal CT scan has a greater predictive value than a positive study. The most sensitive finding—pleural thickening—is least specific for chest wall invasion, while the more specific finding of rib destruction is detected

far less often, as reported by Pennes and associates (1985). Depending on which criteria are accepted as suggestive for chest wall invasion, the sensitivity of CT ranges from 12 to 100% with a specificity of 44 to 96%. The presence of chest pain seems to correlate better than any of the CT findings in predicting chest wall invasion. One concludes that CT has limited predictive value in separating those patients who have parietal pleura and chest wall involvement from those who do not.

Metastatic Tumor

As with primary lung cancer, mesothelioma and metastatic tumor from extrathoracic primary tumors may cause rib destruction. The oblique orientation of the ribs on axial images, however, hampers the accurate evaluation of rib destruction.

CT does provide precise anatomic definition of many chest wall lesions. In patients with chest wall neoplasia, previously unsuspected areas of involvement may be visualized. Gouliamos and colleagues (1980) have shown CT to be especially valuable in the assessment of patients with breast cancer (Fig. 13–20).

It may difficult to distinguish between chest wall tumor and infection, since these may have similar CT appearances. Biopsy is often required in such cases.

Postoperative Evaluation

CT has been used to evaluate complications of median sternotomy. Goodman and associates (1983) reported CT was able to distinguish six patients without significant postoperative infection from six with major infections (Fig. 13–21). In the latter group, CT was of great value in determining whether the infection was limited to the presternal tissues or anterior mediastinum or present in

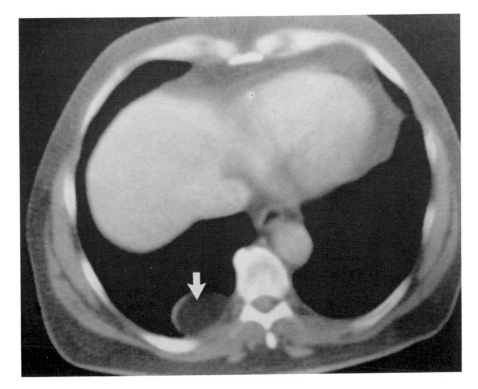

Fig. 13-18. Pleural lipoma. The characteristic low fatty density of this posterior pleural-based mass (arrow) is typical of a pleural lipoma.

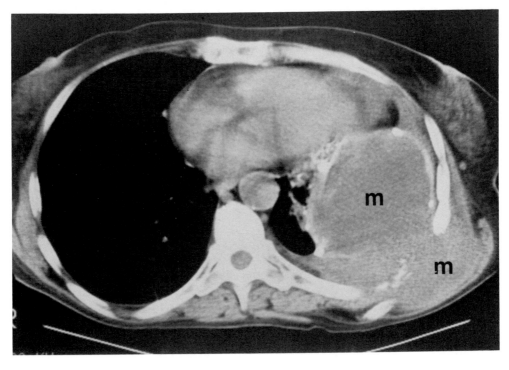

Fig. 13-19. Carcinoma of the lung. CT scan shows extension of a large mass (m) originating in the left lung through the chest wall with rib destruction. The presence of soft tissue mass within the chest wall and rib destruction are the most specific CT findings for chest wall invasion.

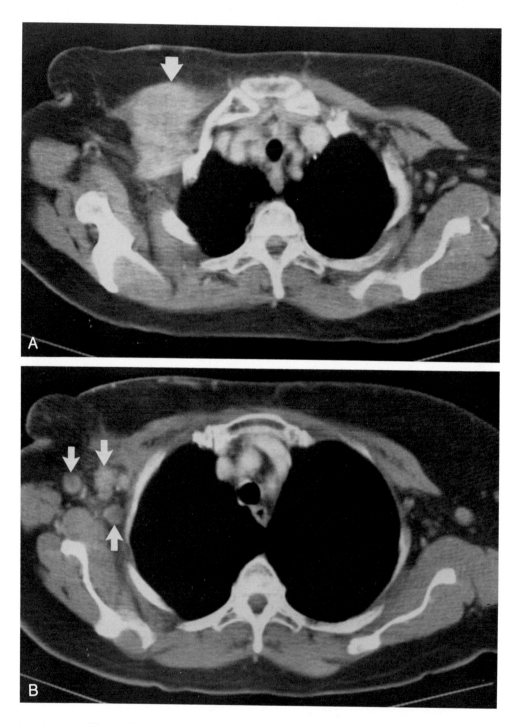

Fig. 13–20. Breast carcinoma. *A*, Chest wall recurrence (arrow) in a patient with breast carcinoma. *B*, CT scan also shows axillary lymphadenopathy (arrows) in the same patient.

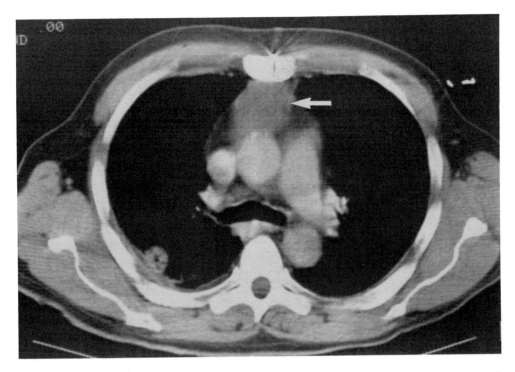

Fig. 13–21. Postoperative infection. Soft-tissue density in the mediastinum (arrow) two weeks post-median sternotomy. This proved to be a localized mediastinal abscess.

both. CT has also been useful in the detection of tumor recurrence following pneumonectomy for lung cancer, as reported by Glazer and colleagues (1984).

Miscellaneous

Evaluation of the posterior paraspinal region is facilitated by CT. Distinction can usually be made between enlarged lymph nodes, vessels, and anatomic variants such as lipomatosis. Paraspinal hematomas and involvement of vertebral bodies by extension of paraspinal masses caused by infection or metastatic tumor can also be identified with CT.

It is often difficult, however, to distinguish paraspinal infection from tumor and CT-guided biopsy may provide a definitive diagnosis in this instance.

REFERENCES

Aronchick, J., et al.: Computed tomography of bronchial carcinoid. J. Comput. Assist. Tomogr. 10:71, 1986.

Baron, R.L., et al.: Computed tomography in the evaluation of mediastinal widening. Radiology 138:107, 1981a.

Baron, R.L., et al.: CT of anomalies of the mediastinal vessels. AJR 137:571, 1981b.

Becker, C.D., et al.: Patterns of recurrence of esophageal carcinoma after transhiatal esophagectomy and gastric interposition. AJR 148:273, 1987.

Bergin, C.J., and Müller, N.L.: CT in the diagnosis of interstitial lung disease. AJR 145:505, 1985.

Brown, L.R., et al.: Roentgenologic diagnosis of primary corticotropin-producing carcinoid tumors of the mediastinum. Radiology 142:143, 1982.

Epstein, D.M., Gefter, W.B., and Miller, W.T.: Lobar bronchioloalveolar cell carcinoma. AJR 139:463, 1982.

Epstein, D.M., et al.: Value of CT in the preoperative assessment of lung cancer: a survey of thoracic surgeons. Radiology 161:423, 1986.

Genereux, G.P., and Howie, J.L.: Normal mediastinal lymph node size and number: CT and anatomic study. AJR 142:1095, 1984.

Glazer, H.S., et al.: Utility of CT in detecting postpneumonectomy carcinoma recurrence. AJR 142:487, 1984.

Goodman, L.R., et al.: Complications of median sternotomy: computed tomographic evaluation. AJR 141:225, 1983.

Gouliamos, A.D., Carter, B.L., and Emami, B.: Computed tomography of the chest wall. Radiology 134:433, 1980.

Grenier, P., et al.: Bronchiectasis: assessment by thin-section CT. Radiology 161:95, 1986.

Gross, S.C., et al.: Computed tomography in dissection of the thoracic aorta. Radiology 136:135, 1980.

Halvorsen, R.A., et al.: Ascites or pleural effusion? CT differentiation: four useful criteria. RadioGraphics 6:135, 1986.

Homer, M.J., Wechsler, R.J., and Carter, B.L.: Mediastinal lipomatosis. Radiology, 128:657, 1978.

Libshitz, H.I., et al.: Mediastinal evaluation in lung cancer. Radiology 151:295, 1984.

Mintzer, R.A., et al.: Rounded atelectasis and its association with asbestos-induced pleural disease. Radiology 139:567, 1981.

Moore, A.V., et al.: Age-related changes in the thymus gland: CT-pathologic correlation. AJR 141:241, 1983.

Müller, N.L., et al.: Role of computed tomography in the recognition of bronchiectasis. AJR 143:971, 1984.

Naidich, D.P., et al.: Computed tomography of the pulmonary parenchyma. Part 1. Distal air-space disease. J. Thorac. Imag. 1:39, 1985.

Paone, J.F., et al.: An appraisal of en bloc resection of peripheral bronchogenic carcinoma involving the thoracic wall. Chest 81:203, 1982.

Pennes, D.R., et al.: Chest wall invasion by lung cancer: limitations of CT evaluation. AJR 144:507, 1985.

Proto, A.V., and Thomas, S.R.: Pulmonary nodules studied by computed tomography. Radiology 153:149, 1985.

Quint, L.E., et al.: Esophageal carcinoma: CT findings. Radiology 155:171, 1985.

Schaner, E.G., et al.: Comparison of computed and conventional whole lung tomography in detecting pulmonary nodules: a prospective radiologic-pathologic study. AJR *131*:51, 1978.

Siegelman, S.S., et al.: CT of the solitary pulmonary nodule. AJR *135*:1, 1980.

Thompson, W.M., et al.: Computed tomography for staging esophageal and gastroesophageal cancer: re-evaluation. AJR *141*:951, 1983.

Zerhouni, E.A., et al.: Computed tomography of the pulmonary parenchyma. Part 2. Interstitial disease. J. Thorac. Imag. *1*:54, 1985.

Zerhouni, E.A., et al.: CT of the pulmonary nodule: a cooperative study. Radiology *160*:319, 1986.

READING REFERENCES

Naidich, D.P., Zerhouni, E.A., and Siegelman, S.S.: Computed tomography of the thorax. New York, Raven Press, 1984.

CHAPTER 14

MAGNETIC RESONANCE IMAGING OF THE THORAX

Gordon Gamsu

Magnetic resonance imaging—MRI—has since the late 1970s generated considerable interest as a safe technique for human imaging. As Pykett (1982) and Crooks and colleagues (1982a) showed, the sensitivity of MRI for demonstrating human disease is impressive. MRI uses physical properties of matter that are markedly different from those that result in x-ray-based roentgenographic images, and thus can provide unique diagnostic information. MRI has outstanding tissue contrast resolution and excellent separation of blood vessels from soft tissues. Thoracic imaging has been inhibited by cardiorespiratory motion, which tends to degrade image quality. Sufficient information is now available to detail MRI's advantages over the other diagnostic modalities and its relative strengths and weaknesses.

TECHNIQUES

General Principles

Atomic nuclei with an odd number of nucleons—protons and neutrons—act as magnetic dipoles. They align within a strong magnetic field, producing a net magnetic vector parallel to the magnetic field. To date, most MR imaging uses hydrogen protons. Perturbation of the aligned protons by a radio frequency—RF—pulse of a specific frequency displaces the magnetic vector by a predictable amount, dependent on the strength and duration of the RF pulse. As the protons return to their original orientation they emit a detectable RF signal. If the magnetic field contains a gradient, the emitted RF signal varies with the proton's position within the magnetic field. By suitable signal detection, the proton's precise position within the magnetic field can be plotted. In biologic tissues, various MR imaging techniques are used to define the position of protons in three dimensions within the imaged body part.

Several nuclei valuable in biological systems can be imaged with MR including hydrogen, phosphorus-31,

sodium-23, carbon-13, and fluorine. Hydrogen is by far the most commonly used because of its abundance and suitability for MR imaging. The MR image represents the intensity of the MR signal with the imaged volume, and depends on a variable combination of four parameters. These parameters are hydrogen density, two relaxation times called T1 and T2, and motion of the hydrogen protons within the imaged volume.

As the hydrogen density increases, increasing numbers of hydrogen nuclei align within the magnetic field, producing a more intense MR signal. The T1 or "spin-lattice" relaxation time depends on the interaction of the hydrogen nucleus with its molecular environment. The T1 relaxation time characterizes a time within which the proton aligns itself in a given magnetic field. The T2 or "spin-spin" relaxation time reflects magnetic interactions between protons. During realignment of the perturbed proton, the MR signal decays as the resonance of the protons becomes unsynchronized. The time of decay of the MR signal is the T2 relaxation time. The last parameter affecting the intensity of the image signal is bulk motion of the protons within the imaging volume. For instance, in thoracic imaging, rapidly flowing blood or the beating heart are not imaged with the usual imaging sequences. The time required for MR in the human is between 10 and 60 msec for the shortest component of an imaging sequence. Moving protons are subjected to different events than stationary protons are. Their emitted signal thus differs, depending on the MR sequence used to obtain the image. Motion of protons within the imaging volume increases or decreases the intensity of the MR signal.

Imaging Techniques

Roentgenographic images reveal little intrinsic contrast between normal and abnormal soft tissues. Changing roentgenographic imaging parameters produces only small changes in tissue contrast. MRI, on the other hand, uses tissue properties that can be extensively manipulated. Crooks and colleagues (1982b) demonstrated that hydrogen density varies only by about 20% for most soft tissues. The T1 and T2 relaxation times of different tissues, however, can vary by over 1000%. MRI uses techniques that allow these differences in tissue properties to be translated into major differences in tissue contrast. Techniques such as free induction decay, spin-echo, inversion recovery, and partial saturation can change the extent to which the T1 and T2 relaxation properties of different tissues affect the relative contrast between these tissues. The most commonly used technique for MRI is the spin-echo technique, which is both T1- and T2-dependent over a wide range of tissue relaxation times. Spin-echo imaging is also sensitive to flow and hydrogen density.

Contrast between tissues is relative when a spin-echo technique is employed. The degree to which T1 and T2 affect tissue intensity can be altered by two excitation properties called the repetition time—TR—and echo time—TE. The TR is the time between excitations. The specific time used for the TR allows differences in T1 relaxation of the tissues to be expressed. The TR can be set on MR units at times between 25 and 3000 msec. If two tissues have different T1 relaxation times, the appropriate TR setting allows images that demonstrate contrast differences between the two tissues. The tissue with the longer T1 does not have sufficient time to completely realign itself within the magnetic field before the next pulse sequence is initiated and it will have less signal strength than a tissue with a shorter T1 relaxation time. For instance, as I and co-workers (1983) showed, most malignant neoplasms have a longer T1—800 to 1200 msec—than mediastinal fat—<400 msec—when imaged at field strengths of 0.3 to 1.5 tesla. With a TR of 500 msec, mediastinal fat is more intense than a mediastinal neoplasm and the latter is readily identified. Images performed with a short TR are thus called T1-dependent. On spin-echo images performed with a long TR—>2000 msec, tissues with both short and long T1 relaxation times have equal signal intensity and may not be distinguishable.

The TE or echo time can also be controlled and is set in milliseconds. On most MRI units it can be varied between 10 and 200 msec. Provided the TR is sufficiently long, the decay differences—T2 relaxation times—between tissues control their contrast. This is demonstrated by varying the TE, and the subsequent images are called "T2-dependent" or "T2-weighted." Thus, with a long TE—>60 msec, the signal from a tissue with a short T2 time diminishes more than the signal from a tissue with a long T2 relaxation time. The tissue with a long T2 shows greater signal intensity on the T2-weighted image.

With most MRI units, spin-echo images are obtained at multiple levels during any single scanning sequence. The levels that can be obtained and the time taken for image acquisition depend on the TR and TE being used. Typically, 5 to 15 slices or levels are obtained, each slice being 1.5 to 10 mm thick. The usual time for the multiple image acquisition is about 5 to 15 min. For most body imaging purposes, the MR scan is composed of a 256^2

matrix with each pixel element about 1.5 mm². During MR scanning, information is being derived from multiple sites at any one time.

Cardiac and Respiratory Gating

Because of the time required for MR imaging, pulsation and respiratory motion perturb the cardiomediastinal structures and degrade the MR image. Unlike the artifacts seen with CT, motion during MRI decreases spatial resolution and diminishes signal intensity, similar to the diminution seen with flowing blood. These motions can also cause "ghosting" artifacts that also degrade the MR image. Both cardiac and respiratory synchronization are possible, but both forms of "gating" prolong image acquisition. At present, respiratory gating has not gained widespread acceptance. Lanzer and colleagues (1983) showed that cardiac gating with image acquisition timed to the cardiac cycle using an electrocardiogram—ECG—does improve resolution of cardiac, mediastinal, and hilar structures. Masses within the lower mediastinum and around the heart are also better imaged. Although cardiac gating prolongs imaging time, it is widely accepted and I advocate its routine use in thoracic MRI. A problem with ECG-cardiac gating is that the heart rate determines the TR time for the image. In most circumstances this results in a TR of around 0.7 sec, with a relatively T1-weighted image. A prolonged TR can be produced by gating the image to every other cardiac beat. The TR of about 1.5 sec, if used in combination with longer TE, produces a T2-weighted image.

Respiratory gating that acquires information only during periods of apnea between breaths is feasible but does not improve MR image quality as significantly as would be expected. It also markedly prolongs imaging time. Software improvement in MRI scanners has improved image quality by suppressing some of the artifacts produced by respiratory motion without prolonging scan time. Experimental imaging sequences allow imaging of single slices within 15 sec, permitting breath holding during the acquisition period. Respiratory degradation of the MR image should not be an important factor in the near future with the newer imaging sequences.

Sagittal and Coronal Imaging

An advantage of MRI over CT is its ability to acquire images in the sagittal and coronal planes, without reformatting of multiple transaxial images (Fig. 14–1). With most images, the matrix size is less for coronal and sagittal images than for the more commonly used transaxial images. The imaging sequences as well as cardiac gating are similar to those described for the transaxial plane. Usually 10 slices 7 mm thick with 2 to 4 mm interscan gap cover the mediastinum from front to back in the coronal plane. In the sagittal plane, 10 scans display the mediastinum and both hila, and 15 scans extend coverage to the paramediastinal lung and entire heart. In Webb and colleagues' (1984a) experience, both sagittal and coronal images occasionally display abnormalities that are not evident on transaxial scans and help to confirm suspected abnormalities. Sagittal images have been less

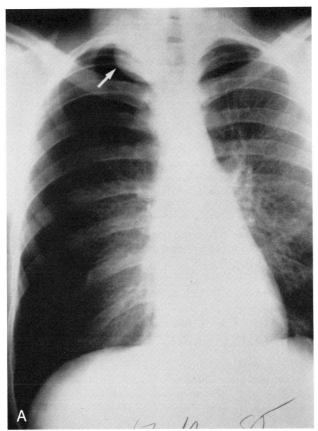

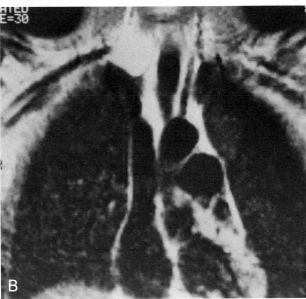

Fig. 14–1.   Coronal image of an extrapleural schwannoma. *A*, A chest roentgenogram after a spontaneous pneumothorax shows a mass at the right apex (arrow). *B*, An ECG-gated coronal MRI (T1-weighted) shows the mass, which has high intensity, suggesting that it is lipid-containing and neurogenic.

helpful than coronal images and are not widely used except at the thoracic inlet. Coronal images can show lesions around the lower trachea and in the subcarinal, paracardiac, and paradiaphragmatic regions—areas that are not well imaged in the transaxial plane. Both coronal and sagittal scanning planes are an adjunct and should be used in addition to the usual transaxial images.

Cine Magnetic Resonance Images

Cine magnetic resonance imaging is a fast MRI process that uses rapid imaging sequences. Haase and co-workers (1986) described how long flip angles and gradient refocused echoes are employed. Several versions are used, and all refer acquired image data to the ECG. Information from about 20-msec segments of the cardiac cycle are used to create a cine-formatted image with a framing rate of 20 to 40 frames per min. In the GRASS—gradient-recalled acquisition in steady state—version, the TR is set at 21 msec and the TE at 12 msec. The major thoracic application of cine-MRI has been to evaluate cardiac and great vessels morphology, function, and blood flow. For a complete series of 8 to 10 10-mm thick slices, imaging time is about 20 min. The resultant images, when displayed in a cine mode on a TV monitor, have the spatial resolution of cine-angiocardiograms, but less than that of conventional MRI, CT, or roentgenograms. A major difference between conventional MRI and cine-MRI is the visibility of rapidly flowing blood with the latter technique. A signal void from the intravascular compartment at the appropriate site is an indirect measure of vascular turbulence seen with stenosis or regurgitation.

Sechtem and colleagues (1987) showed that the cardiac functions that can be evaluated with cine-MRI are ventricular volumes and their derivations, including stroke volume; regional ventricular function, including segmental wall motion and wall thickening; valvular regurgitation through incompetent cardiac valves; and valvular stenoses. Imaging of coronary artery bypass grafts and of sites of acute myocardial infarction remains controversial. Evaluation of congenital heart disease is beyond the scope of this chapter, but at present is better with conventional spin-echo imaging than with cine-MRI. The resolution of cine-MRI precludes imaging of abnormalities in caliber of the coronary circulation.

Because of the short TR and TE used in cine-MRI, tissue contrast is low. Combined with the poor spatial resolution, the images are not useful for imaging thoracic structures apart from the cardiovascular system. Improvements in temporal resolution with this system do not compensate for the loss of the other imaging parameters.

NORMAL MRI FINDINGS

Tissue Contrast and Characterization

The relative MRI intensity of thoracic tissues is completely different from their relative x-ray density as depicted on the CT scans. For instance, fat is the most intense normal tissue found on MRI, whereas on CT its density is lower than that of normal solid tissues. Alterations in the MRI parameters used to obtain the image can also change the relative intensity of tissues, and thus the contrast between them. On T1-weighted images, mediastinal, subcutaneous, and auxiliary fat have slightly different image signal intensities, but for practical purposes their intensities can be considered to be equal. The normal involuted thymus gland in the adult has a slightly lower MRI intensity than fat, and can be readily distinguished from mediastinal fat within the prevascular space. Normal mediastinal lymph nodes, the esophagus, and many neoplasms have an intermediate signal intensity like cardiac or skeletal muscle. The normal lung and the large airways contain air and have essentially no MR signal. Cortical bone similarly has few protons susceptible to MR, and essentially no measurable MR signal. The mucosa of the trachea and esophagus can demonstrate high signal intensity on T2-weighted images. The tracheal cartilages and the laryngeal cartilages have variable signal intensity.

The mediastinum and hila have a limited variety of normal tissue and thus tissue intensities. Generally, T2-weighted images employing long TR and TE imaging sequences eliminate most contrast between normal thoracic tissues, and between normal and abnormal tissues. The tissue intensities and the T1 and T2 relaxation times of abnormal thoracic tissues have been studied intensively. Abnormal tissues within the mediastinum and hila, whether inflammatory or neoplastic, generally have longer T1 relaxation times than mediastinal fat and the thymus have, and they can be recognized on images with the appropriate imaging sequence, usually those with T1-weighting. At present, detection of a mass or lymphadenopathy within the mediastinum depends on morphologic distortions. Fatty masses such as lipomas or thymolipomas have specific MRI characteristics. Fibrous masses, such as a focal mediastinitis, have low intensity on T1- and T2-weighted images. Discrimination of other benign inflammatory masses or nodes from neoplastic ones based on their MRI signal intensity or relaxation times remains controversial. Provisional studies indicate that neoplastic tissue may have slightly longer T1 and T2 relaxation times than benign tissue.

Table 14–1.   Factors Influencing Intravascular MR Signal

Technical
Pulse sequence
Sectional position in multisection sequence
Spin-echo type
Imaging gradient
Cardiac synchronization
Biologic
Direction of flow
Velocity of flow
Acceleration/deceleration
Velocity profile

Blood Flow Effects

As von Schulthess and co-workers (1985) showed, the intravascular compartment most commonly has no evident signal on spin-echo image sequences, if blood is flowing through the vessel. MR signal can, however, be seen in vessels, depending on several factors (Table 14–1). Moving nuclei observe a disrupted imaging sequence and produce little or no signal. For instance, if the imaging plane is 8 mm thick and the imaging sequence takes 80 msec, blood with a velocity of 10 cm/sec will flow across the plane during one sequence. The velocity at which signal disappears will thus be close to 10 cm/sec. Most blood flow in large vessels exceeds 10 cm/sec, and thus on ungated images will not be visible. Blood flowing at lower velocities, especially less than 3 cm/sec, will be imaged and may demonstrate what is called "paradoxical enhancement," demonstrating MR signal intensity that is greater than stationary blood. Paradoxical enhancement is more apparent when TR is short and TE is long. This enhancement occurs when slowly flowing blood enters the imaging field only partially unperturbed by the RF pulses and thus more fully magnetized. The enhancement on longer echo—TE—images is caused by the longer echoes being even-numbered, not because of the time involved. An artifact on MR imaging, unrelated to slow flow and producing an intravascular signal, is known as an even-echo rephasing artifact and must be differentiated from slowly flowing blood. Thus, MR can image flowing blood, and both noninvasive angiography and measurement of regional blood flow and perfusion are being actively developed.

Normal MRI Anatomy

In normal subjects, mediastinal and hilar structures usually seen on CT scans are readily identified on spin-echo images. The best anatomic detail is obtained from images with a short TE and a long TR, because the signal-to-noise ratio is optimal. Cardiac gating of the images by reducing motion distortions, however, provides better anatomic appearances, even though the signal-to-noise ratio may not be optimal.

The great arteries arising from the aortic branch always appear, as well as the ascending aorta, aortic arch, and descending aorta (Fig. 14–2). The walls of the aorta and great vessels, but not the contents of these vessels, are visible. The systemic venous system of the thorax, including the subclavian veins, brachiocephalic veins, and venae cavae are also demonstrated. The ascending segment and arch of the azygos vein are evident in most normal subjects. The portions of the airway demonstrated on spin-echo images are the trachea, main bronchi, intermediate bronchus, and lobar bronchi. The spatial resolution of MRI permits visualization of only an occasional segmental bronchus. Airway caliber may be distorted by respiratory motion on the usual MR images obtained during breathing.

The vessels, trachea, and central bronchi are easily distinguished from high intensity fat within the mediastinum. The esophagus is evident behind the trachea.

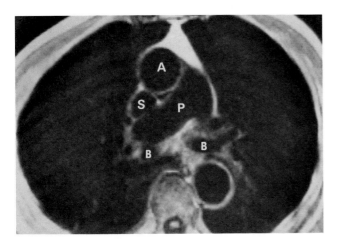

Fig. 14–2. Normal MRI through the midthorax. The aortic (A), pulmonary arteries (P), superior vena cava (S), and bronchi (B), are all seen. The vessels appear empty because flowing blood is not seen at this portion of the cardiac cycle.

On T2-weighted images, the mucosa of the esophagus and occasionally of the trachea demonstrates high intensity. On T1-weighted images, normal lymph nodes less than 10 mm in diameter are readily identified in the prevascular, pretracheal, and subcarinal regions.

The thymus, within the prevascular space, is more easily recognized by MRI than by CT. The shape, size, and signal intensity of the normal thymus is age-dependent. In the infant and child, the thymus has intermediate intensity similar to muscle or lymph nodes. In the adult, the MRI intensity of the thymus increases with fatty replacement, although it is variable among individuals. It is considerably more intense than lymph nodes or most tumors. The thymus is more distinctive and appears larger in MRI than in CT.

The pericardium is distinctly displayed in gated MRI through the heart, especially anteriorly and to the right of the great vessels (Fig. 14–3). It appears as a thin, low intensity line less than 4 mm thick. The superior peri-

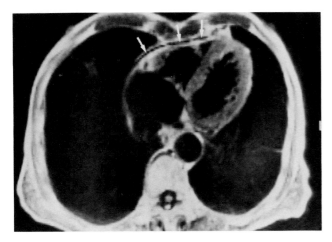

Fig. 14–3. Normal ECG-gated MRI through the heart. The cardiac chambers, myocardium, and pericardiac space (arrows) are well depicted.

cardial recesses are distinctive by MRI through the base of the heart.

The aorta and ventricles, together with their valves, are well displayed by MRI. Segments of the coronary arteries are frequently imaged. The present resolution of MRI does not permit evaluation of the caliber of vessels the size of the coronary arteries.

Within the hila, the blood vessels and bronchi usually produce no MR signal, and are distinguished by their known anatomic locations. Collections of fat are visible at three locations in the hila: lateral to the right pulmonary artery where it bifurcates in the midhilum; at the origin of the right middle lobe bronchus in the lower right hilum; and where the left pulmonary artery descends and gives origin to its left upper lobe branches in the left midlung hilum.

The right pulmonary artery is sectioned longitudinally on transaxial images. Anterior to the pulmonary artery are the upper lobe pulmonary veins and superior vena cava, whereas the right main stem bronchus and intermediate bronchus are behind the right pulmonary artery. On the left side, the pulmonary artery is 1 to 2 cm higher than on the right, with the superior pulmonary veins anterior, and the left main stem bronchus posterior. The top of the left atrium and the left atrial appendage are in front of the left superior pulmonary vein. At a slightly superior level, the left pulmonary artery originates from the main pulmonary artery to course posteriorly above the left main bronchus. Medial to the left pulmonary artery is the tracheal carina.

Structures that are particularly well displayed in the sagittal and coronal projections are the venae cavae and their connections to the right atrium, the azygos veins, the central pulmonary arteries, and the descending aorta. The ascending aorta, the aortic arch, and the descending aorta can be demonstrated in continuity on oblique lateral images if the patient is correctly positioned.

The central bronchi and their positions within the hila are particularly well imaged in coronal images through the midthorax.

The pulmonary circulation resembles the systemic circulation on spin-echo images. Only the walls of the central pulmonary vessels are demonstrated. No signal is usually seen within the pulmonary arteries or veins unless it is caused by technical factors, gating, or slice position. Pulmonary arteries beyond the hila are not visible in normal subjects. Of the pulmonary veins, only those close to the mediastinum and left atrium are routinely demonstrated.

The pulse sequences used in most thoracic images preclude obtaining a signal from the lungs. T1 and T2 relaxation measurements from the lungs are not different from background values in ungated images. With cardiac gating, MRI signal intensity increases during portions of the cardiac cycle. This signal represents intravascular blood imaged during vascular diastole because of pulsatile flow in the pulmonary circulation. With the new intravascular contrast agents for MRI, such as gadolinium-DTPA, intravascular signal can be detected with the currently available imaging systems.

ABNORMAL FINDINGS

Mediastinum and Hila

Lymphadenopathy

Within the mediastinum, detection of normal and abnormal lymph nodes depends critically on their size and their contrast with surrounding structures. MRI can detect many normal-sized lymph nodes and most abnormal nodes. On T1-weighted images, normal nodes can be found throughout the mediastinum. Those in the lower pretracheal and subcarinal spaces tend to be slightly larger than at other sites. The contrast between high intensity mediastinal fat and intermediate intensity lymph nodes allows for their identification. In early studies without cardiac gating, cardiac pulsation during the 10 to 15 min image acquisition time resulted in occasional summation of several small lymph nodes into a mass-like appearance that was misinterpreted as a single large lymph node or a mediastinal mass. In general, nodes less than 1 cm in transverse diameter are considered normal in size. Nodes larger than 1 cm in diameter are abnormal. The appearance of abnormally large lymph nodes and their changes in intensity with changes in imaging sequences cannot reliably distinguish between benign and malignant lymphadenopathy. Dooms and colleagues (1984) and von Schulthess and co-workers (1986) demonstrated some provisional data indicating that the actual measured T1 and T2 relaxation times of tissues may allow discrimination between neoplastic and inflammatory tissue. How this will be translated into a practical test in clinical MRI will be studied intensively. An additional advantage of MRI is the ready distinction between blood vessels and lymph nodes, and between the superior pericardial recess and the azygos lymph nodes. In various studies, although retrospective and unblinded, CT and MRI showed comparable accuracies for detecting mediastinal lymphadenopathy (Fig. 14–4). MRI can detect hilar lymph nodes not shown with CT, especially when ECG-gated images are used. Evaluation of the aorto-pulmonic window and lower left paratracheal lymph nodes is easier in coronal MRI than with transaxial CT scans.

Mediastinal Masses

The relationship between a mediastinal mass and adjacent vessels is better demonstrated with MRI than with contrast-enhanced CT; largely because of the excellent contrast between vessels and mass and the absence of streak artifacts on MRI. On contrast-enhanced CT scans, streaking artifacts can obscure small mediastinal vessels. Similarly, vascular compression or invasion by a mediastinal mass is excellently demonstrated by MRI. Flow signal from a compressed vessel must, however, be differentiated from vascular invasion by the compressing mass.

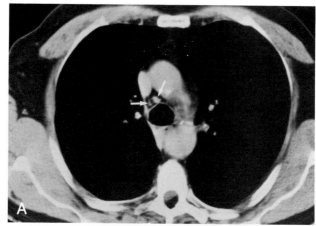
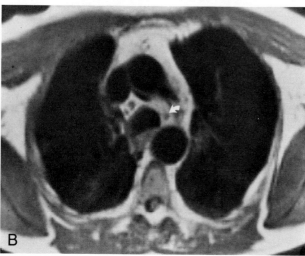

Fig. 14–4. Normal mediastinal lymph nodes comparably seen on CT and ECG-gated MRI. A, The CT scan demonstrates two small pretracheal lymph nodes (arrows). B, The MRI demonstrates the same two lymph nodes and a third lymph node (curved arrow) in the aortopulmonic window.

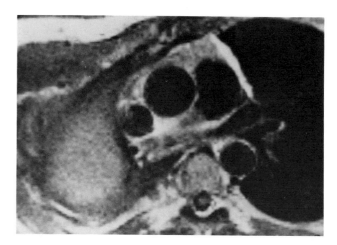

Fig. 14–5. Mediastinal metastatic tumor on MRI. A T1-weighted MR image demonstrates replacement of high intensity mediastinal fat by low intensity metastatic carcinoid from the right lung. The patient has had a right pneumonectomy.

Tumor is usually distinguished from normal mediastinal fat by using T1-weighted images (Fig. 14–5). For example, in a group of benign and malignant mediastinal masses, T1 values of the masses were about 1500 msec, whereas the T1 values of surrounding mediastinal fat averaged between 300 and 400 msec. The T2 relaxation values of inflammatory mediastinal lymph nodes differ significantly from those of neoplastic masses. This difference, however, does not produce a characteristic difference in appearance on either T1- or T2-weighted images. In fact, MRI with a T2-weighted technique of a mediastinal mass shows that both the tumor and mediastinal fat have similar signal intensities, and the mass may be impossible to distinguish from normal mediastinal fat.

Webb and Moore (1985) showed that volume averaging of high intensity mediastinal fat and low intensity blood flow can occasionally cause an area of intermediate signal intensity that mimics a mediastinal mass. This occurs, for instance, in the aortopulmonic window with volume averaging of the left pulmonary artery. Imaging with two different TR times allows volume averaging and allows mass to be distinguished. Although the intensity of volume averaging and mass can appear the same on T1-weighted images, a mass increases in intensity relative to fat on a T2-weighted image, whereas volume averaging does not change in relative intensity.

The detection and evaluation of a mediastinal mass and its edge depends both on the contrast between the mass and surrounding tissues, and also on the spatial resolution of the image. The spatial resolution of MRI is less than that of CT, and small masses, or the edges of larger masses, can be more difficult to evaluate by MRI. In comparison with CT, however, MRI, because of its high contrast resolution, allows the detection of most if not all mediastinal masses larger than 1 cm in diameter. In some instances, mediastinal masses that are not seen on CT are visible on MRI. This occurs most commonly because streak artifacts degrade the CT image or a small mass is mistaken for a vessel on CT.

Benign neoplasms of the mediastinum apparently do not differ significantly from malignant neoplasms either in intensity or in relaxation values. Fluid-filled or necrotic masses may be diagnosed as such by MRI based on their longer T1 and T2 relaxation times. MRI performed with T2-weighted images results in a significant increase in signal from the fluid or necrotic components of the mass, and can demonstrate heterogeneous areas not visible on T1-weighted images, as I and my co-workers (1984) showed.

Calcification within a mediastinal mass has diagnostic significance in many circumstances. On MRI, calcifications appear as low intensity areas, and are indistinguishable from other causes of low intensity. The clinical significance of this observation requires further clarification.

Using both T1- and T2-weighted MRI, recurrent tumor has been distinguished from post-treatment radiation damage or fibrosis. Glazer and colleagues (1985) demonstrated that post-treatment fibrosis tends to have a lower signal intensity on both T1- and T2-weighted images, whereas recurrent tumor tends to have a higher signal intensity, especially on T2-weighted images. Differentiation between the two is limited by overlap in the measurements and by the known imprecision of MRI data.

Hilar Masses

Webb and colleagues (1984b), in their studies, showed that the normal pulmonary hilum consists of pulmonary arteries, pulmonary veins, small amounts of fat at specific sites, and a few inconsistent small lymph nodes. The diagnosis of hilar mass requires the distinction between normal vessels and abnormal soft tissues. Secondary features include distortion and displacement of the bronchial tree. At some sites within the hilum, this differentiation can be made on anatomic grounds, but at other sites, masses and vessels are difficult to distinguish. Rapidly flowing blood results in little MRI signal and thus only the walls of the pulmonary arteries and veins are visible on MRI. Hilar masses are readily detected against the background of the walls of the bronchi and vessels (Fig. 14–6). The small amount of fat and small lymph nodes are not a significant problem in detecting hilar

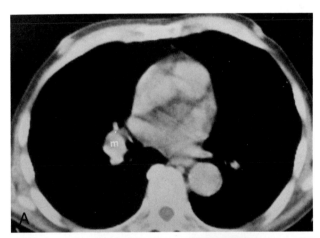

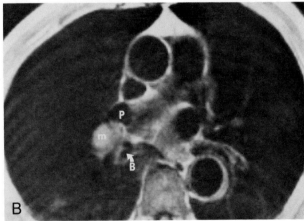

Fig. 14–6. Right hilar bronchial carcinoma. A, On the CT scan at the level of the origin of the middle lobe bronchi, the right hilar mass (m) cannot be distinguished from the adjacent interlobar pulmonary artery. B, On the MR image at the same level, the mass (m) is readily separated from artery (P) and bronchus (B).

masses. Normal hilar lymph nodes are only 3 to 5 mm in diameter and are evident within the hilar fat. The most common causes for a hilar mass are bronchial carcinoma, lymphoma, metastatic lymphadenopathy, or inflammatory lymphadenopathy. MRI allows a confident diagnosis of hilar mass, and clearly shows the relationship of the mass to normal vessels and central bronchi. Hilar masses are considerably more conspicuous and the relationship of the mass to vessels is demonstrated better at multiple levels in MRI than in CT. In several instances, hilar lymph nodes larger than 1 cm in diameter that were not clearly imaged with CT have been detected by MRI.

In many circumstances, a roentgenographic evaluation of the pulmonary hilum also requires evaluation of the bronchial tree within the hilum. Bronchial narrowing is an important indication of disease and important in guiding endoscopic evaluation of the central airways. The present resolution of MRI does not permit detailed evaluation of the bronchial tree, which is better performed with CT. MRI performed within the time of a single breath holding may improve the spatial resolution and allow evaluation of the central bronchi, although these techniques are not yet perfected.

Thymus and Thymoma

De Geer and co-workers (1986), in their description of the normal thymus, showed that it is readily demonstrated by MRI because it contrasts with anterior mediastinal fat on T1-weighted images because of its longer T1 relaxation time. The average thymus-to-fat hydrogen density ratio is 0.60. Although the T1 relaxation time of the thymus is much longer then that of fat in patients under 30 years of age, the difference decreases in the older age group. The T2 relaxation time of the thymus is similar to that of fat, and does not change with age. The normal thymus measures about 2.8 × 1.9 cm and is 5 to 7 cm in a craniocaudad direction. The thymus appears thicker in MRI than on CT scans in patients older than 20. MRI may be better than CT in distinguishing between thymus involuted with fat and mediastinal fat.

The MR imaging characteristics of thymomas are not well described, but gated MRI should be an excellent method for defining the extent of thymic tumors. The malignant potential of thymomas is closely related to their capsular invasion and mediastinal extension. Detection of mediastinal extension and transpleural spread of the tumor is important for prognosis and therapy. MRI for evaluation of possible thymic tumors should embrace the entire thorax to include the posterior costophrenic extent of the pleural space. Ten to fifteen percent of patients with myasthenia gravis have thymomas. These tumors are usually resected because up to half of them are malignant. MRI, like CT, can be used to screen for thymic masses in myasthenia gravis. MRI can theoretically also be useful for following the patient after treatment with radiation therapy for nonresectable thymic tumors. MRI may be able to differentiate between radiation changes and recurrent or residual tumor. On T2-weighted images, thymic tumor should be high in intensity, whereas radiation fibrosis remains low in intensity.

Fibrosing Mediastinitis

Fibrosing mediastinitis most commonly is caused by radiation therapy or histoplasmosis. The fibrosing process may be diffuse, or focal and mass-like. The focal form is more likely to cause compression or obstruction of mediastinal veins, arteries, or bronchi. Rholl and co-workers (1985), in their work on the MRI appearance of fibrosing mediastinitis, described a focal mass that is low in intensity both on T1- and T2-weighted images. On CT, most cases of fibrosing mediastinitis demonstrate calcification within the mass. Unfortunately, these calcifications cannot be appreciated on the usual spin-echo MRI. The collateral channels that develop with obstruction to the normal mediastinal venous pathways are evident on MRI as abnormal tubular structures without intraluminal signal. Slow flow within stenotic vessels may be appreciated by a paradoxical enhancement of the MRI signal. Obstruction of a central pulmonary artery can be appreciated from narrowing and distortion of the vessel's lumen. Bronchial obstruction is more difficult to appreciate on MRI. The rare complication of fibrosing mediastinitis with pulmonary vein obstruction and focal pulmonary edema has been demonstrated by MRI.

Esophagus

The normal esophagus is inconsistently imaged in the mediastinum by MRI as Quint and colleagues (1985) described. It can usually be seen near the thoracic inlet and the diaphragm. It can be distinguished from mediastinal fat surrounding it on T1-weighted images. The lumen of the esophagus may contain low intensity air and the mucosal lining can be recognized by its high intensity. Bulky esophageal carcinomas can be detected by MRI, and their relationship to mediastinal structures demonstrated. Extraesophageal extension of the tumor may be detected by encasement of mediastinal vessels, distortion or compression of the trachea, or contact of the esophageal mass with more than one quarter of the aortic wall. Minor degrees of extracapsular extension of esophageal tumors cannot be recognized with certainty by MRI. Subtle obliteration of fat planes is not a reliable finding, especially in the middle third of the esophagus where it is flattened against the left atrium. MRI does not have advantages over CT in staging esophageal carcinoma.

Pulmonary Parenchyma

Focal Lesions

Neoplastic lung masses appear as regions of substantially higher intensity than normal lung parenchyma on both T1- and T2-weighted images. Exceptions are heavily calcified or fibrotic masses or arterial venous malformations. These can be as low in intensity as the surrounding lung. For most lung lesions, T2-weighted images improve demonstration of the mass, as lung tissue remains dark and the lesion usually becomes brighter because of its longer T2 relaxation time. Primary and metastatic malignant masses tend to have long T2 relaxation times.

Distinction between a central bronchial carcinoma and peripheral obstructive pneumonitis may be possible with MRI using T2-weighted images. The distal fluid-filled lung, because of its high water content, can display a higher signal intensity than the proximal tumor. The detection of tumor extension to the pleura or mediastinum within a collapsed lobe has not been adequately studied. Theoretically, MRI could detect tumor within a collapsed lobe, which is potentially clinically important. Necrosis within a tumor mass has low intensity on T1-weighted images and an increase on T2-weighted images, although this may not have clinical importance except in a few specific circumstances.

Pulmonary Nodules

The greater spatial resolution of CT enables better detection of nodules close to the diaphragm, the pleura, or to each other, whereas the better contrast resolution of MRI enables the detection of nodules close to blood vessels, according to Müller and co-workers (1985). With MRI, nodules are best seen on T2-weighted images with a long TR and TE. Most pulmonary nodules are seen using both CT and MRI. CT generally enables the detection of more small nodules than does MRI. Respiratory motion further degrades resolution of MRI. Motion of the lung can also cause movement of nodules within the imaging plane, and can decrease their signal intensity by a partial-volume effect. Because blood vessels containing flowing blood result in little MRI signal, differentiation of solid nodules from normal vessels or arteriovenous malformations can be made more easily with MRI than with CT. Normal pulmonary bronchi, vessels, and fissures, however, are not visible in MRI, and the lobar or segmental origin of abnormalities are more difficult to localize. Frequently, localization of a lesion's relationship to the bronchial tree can be important in guiding a transbronchial biopsy or surgery. For this reason, MRI does not compare with CT for detection or localization of pulmonary nodules.

Diffuse Lung Disease

The normal lung shows no MRI signal above background in most adults. Signal can, however, be detected in the posterior dependent portion of the normal lung in some individuals. This may reflect atelectasis, condensed lung parenchyma, or increased dependent blood flow to the lung bases in the supine position.

Pulmonary consolidation can be recognized using MRI, but differences in signal intensity or MRI signal characteristics among atelectasis, pneumonia, and pulmonary edema have not been found. The MRI characteristics overlap substantially in the different causes of lung consolidation, although alveolar proteinosis is notable for its low T1 value. McFadden and colleagues (1987) studied a group of patients with interstitial lung disease. The most severely affected patients had the greatest signal intensity on MRI. Improvement, as indicated by a decrease in signal intensity, was seen following treatment in these patients. In this study, qualitative MRI was useful in predicting clinical course. Relaxation times, however, were not sufficiently precise to differentiate between active and inactive interstitial lung disease. In experimental studies in rats, Vinitski and co-workers (1986) found that MRI signal intensities were significantly elevated in both bleomycin-induced alveolitis and fibrosis. Both T1 and T2 values in alveolitis were the same as in controls, but were significantly decreased in fibrotic lung disease. Changes in T1 and T2 values correlated with changes in water content of the diseased lung. In practical terms, MRI for diagnosis and evaluation of diffuse lung disease is an exciting area for future investigation but cannot be considered of present clinical value.

Bronchial Carcinoma

The MRI signal intensity from bronchial carcinomas varies. Most bronchial carcinomas will yield low intensities on T1-weighted images, and higher intensities on T2-weighted images. Some tumors, however, show low intensities on both T1- and T2-weighted images, whereas others show high intensities on T1-weighting. The best contrast between lung carcinomas and surrounding mediastinum or hilar tissues has been with T1-weighted images. The adjacent tissues are usually fat or blood vessels, and T1-weighted imaging distinguishes between the bronchial mass or metastatic lymph nodes and fat.

The radiologic staging of bronchial carcinoma requires the evaluation of several intrathoracic structures. Most important in determining the resectability of the tumor is the presence and distribution of mediastinal lymph node metastases. In spin-echo MRI, normal or abnormal mediastinal lymph nodes can be distinguished from surrounding mediastinal tissues because of differences in their T1 values. With MRI using a T1-sensitive technique, the lymph nodes appear less intense than surrounding fat (Fig. 14–7). With a longer TR value, the intensities of the nodes increase relative to fat, contrast decreases, and nodes may not be detected.

In comparison with CT, MRI more often provides comparable information regarding the presence and size of mediastinal lymph nodes. Webb and colleagues (1985) showed that CT and MRI usually classify nodes identically: as normal—<1.0 cm, suspicious—1.0 to 1.5 cm, or abnormal—>1.5 cm. When MRI and CT interpretations differ, MRI may more readily discriminate between tumor and vessels.

The relative changes in the intensity of mediastinal lymph nodes with different imaging sequences—their T1 and T2 characteristics—apparently do not help distinguish lymph nodes that are involved or uninvolved by tumor. Reports have shown controversial differences or no clear differences in the T1 values of benign and malignant lesions. In the diagnosis of hilar mass or lymph node enlargement, MRI is superior to intravenous contrast material-enhanced CT, largely because hilar vessels and soft tissue can easily be distinguished by MRI. Care

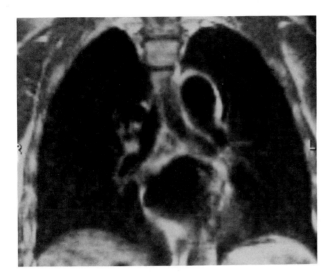

Fig. 14–7. Subcarinal metastatic lymph nodes from bronchial carcinoma. Coronal MRI demonstrates several slightly enlarged subcarinal lymph nodes not seen with CT or transaxial MRI, and suspicious for metastasis.

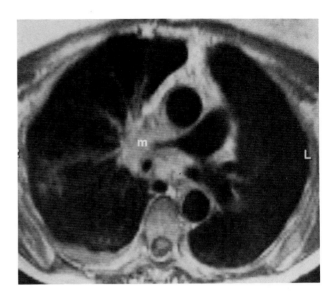

Fig. 14–8. Right hilar bronchial carcinoma invading the mediastinum. The MRI demonstrates the lower intensity mass (m) narrowing the right pulmonary artery and surrounding the intermediate bronchus.

must, however, be taken not to diagnose normal hilar tissue as abnormal.

Bronchial abnormalities are better seen on CT than on MRI, primarily because of its better spatial resolution. MRI may show only a suspicious lesion while CT shows definitely abnormal central bronchi. Because not all lobar or segmental bronchi are visible on MRI in healthy subjects, a small bronchus that is not clearly seen on MRI is difficult to interpret with certainty.

With direct invasion of the mediastinum by a lung mass, CT and MRI may both suggest invasion. Heelan and colleagues (1985) showed that direct invasion of the mediastinum adjacent to a hilar mass is usually better demonstrated on MRI because of the ease with which tumor and mediastinal vessels and fat can be distinguished (Fig. 14–8).

In patients with a superior sulcus tumor invading and destroying the upper ribs, rib destruction is often visible on plain roentgenographs and CT scans. MRI and CT usually provide similar information about the presence of pleural fluid or involvement by tumor. MRI in the sagittal plane can more clearly show tumor extension into the axilla, brachial plexus, and spinal canal, all key elements in the evaluation of patients with superior sulcus tumors.

MRI can also show invasion of the chest wall. Invasion of thoracic muscle causes an increase in signal intensity that is best demonstrated on T2-weighted images. Determination of chest wall invasion, however, remains difficult. The criteria considered in the interpretation of CT may also be applicable to MRI. These findings include an obtuse angle of the lung mass with the chest wall; more than 3 cm of contact between the mass and the pleural surface; and thickening of the pleura adjacent to the mass. None of these signs, however, are sensitive or specific. Rib destruction by a mass involving the chest wall is specific but has little sensitivity, and rib destruc-

tion is more easily discerned on conventional roentgenograms or CT images.

New surgical techniques that allow resection of focal chest wall involvement by tumor may obviate the need for detection of subtle invasion. Proximity to the chest wall and the need for probable chest wall resection may be sufficient information prior to resection.

Invasion or encroachment on mediastinal cardiovascular and aerodigestive structures is important with the new TNM staging system—stage IIIb—as Mountain (1986) described. MRI and CT have similar difficulties in distinguishing between tumor contiguity with mediastinal structures and subtle invasion into the wall of these structures. Encasement or distortion of mediastinal organs is generally better imaged by MRI. Further studies of the sensitivities and specificity of MRI in demonstrating direct invasion of the mediastinum are necessary.

Bronchial carcinoma commonly metastasizes to upper abdominal organs, notably the adrenal glands and liver. Many authors recommend scanning the upper abdomen when staging the tumor with CT. This is not generally possible with MRI because of time constraints. With more rapid imaging sequences, however, this may not be a problem.

In one study, the adrenal glands were the most frequent site of metastases at autopsy performed within a month of a "curative" resection and were present in 38% of subjects. In a study by Falke and co-workers (1987), an adrenal mass was seen at CT in 21% of patients with non-small cell bronchial carcinoma. Because up to two thirds of adrenal masses in patients with lung cancer are adrenal adenomas, however, biopsy of an enlarged gland is necessary before denying the patient surgery. MRI with T2-weighted images can distinguish adrenal metastases and other significant neoplasms—carcinomas, pheochromocytomas—from adrenal adenomas in many patients, according to Glazer and colleagues (1986). In general, although there is some overlap between groups, nonfunctioning adrenal adenomas are low in intensity, similar to the liver, on T2-weighted sequences. Functioning adenomas, carcinomas, pheochromocytomas, and metastases, as well as some inflammatory lesions, are more intense than the liver.

Pulmonary Vasculature

Pulmonary Hypertension

The appropriate MRI technique for detecting and quantifying intravascular signal in suspected pulmonary vascular abnormalities is with gated MRI. With cardiac gating, the MRI scans are obtained during specific preselected short portions of the cardiac cycle. MR images can be obtained at up to ten levels simultaneously. Imaging at multiple levels during multiple phases of the cardiac cycle is the best manner of displaying pathologic blood flow patterns in the pulmonary circulation.

The severity of the anatomic and functional abnormalities demonstrated by MRI in patients with pulmonary hypertension is proportional to the severity of the hypertension. The central pulmonary arteries in the mediastinum and hila can be measured precisely on CT scans. O'Callaghan and co-workers (1982) found that the diameter of the right pulmonary artery was 16.6 to 26.6 mm in a small group of patients with pulmonary hypertension. Accurate CT measurements of the interlobar and proximal lung arteries can also be obtained. I found that the caliber of the main pulmonary artery, measured from CT scans, accurately predicts pulmonary artery pressure. Kuriyama and co-workers (1984) showed that pulmonary artery diameter correlates with pulmonary artery pressure with a coefficient of 0.89. The upper limit of normal for the main pulmonary artery is 28.6 mm. A diameter above 28.6 mm readily predicts pulmonary hypertension. Gated MRI is as precise as or more precise than CT in determining caliber of the central pulmonary vessels.

Right ventricular hypertrophy, frequently with flattening or convexity of the intraventricular septum toward the left ventricular chamber, is invariably present with severe pulmonary hypertension. Gated MRI readily demonstrates right ventricular enlargement and displacement of the intraventricular septum.

MRI can also evidence decreased velocity of pulmonary blood flow in pulmonary hypertension. Von Schulthess and colleagues (1985) demonstrated intraluminal signal during a major portion of the cardiac cycle as the MRI manifestation of decreased blood velocity. In most patients with a pulmonary systolic pressure above 90 mm Hg, intraluminal signal is visible in gated MRI during systole. In those with a pressure below 90 mm Hg, this finding is evident in only 30%. In normotensive subjects, MR signal is evident during late diastole when blood flow is slow. During systole and early diastole, blood flow is normally too rapid to be imaged (Fig. 14–9). In MRI of normal persons the flow patterns are similar in the

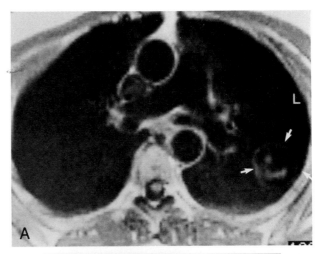

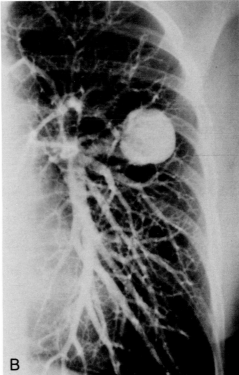

Fig. 14–9. Pulmonary arteriovenous malformation. *A*, MRI through the lungs demonstrates a mass (arrows) in the left lung containing a signal void. *B*, The pulmonary angiogram demonstrates that the lesion is an arteriovenous malformation.

aorta and central pulmonary arteries. Patients with pulmonary arterial hypertension also show a linear correlation between the intensity of the MR signal from the central pulmonary arteries and pulmonary vascular resistance.

Pulmonary Embolism

Blood flowing at normal velocity shows a signal void in the pulmonary arteries on ECG-gated images in systole. Emboli within the pulmonary arteries therefore can be detected on systolic images. The intensity of pulmonary emboli varies, depending upon the age of the clot. Chronic emboli produce low to medium intensity, and acute emboli cause high intensity (Fig. 14–10). Intraluminal signal may also be caused by slow flow in the pulmonary arteries, as in pulmonary arterial hypertension. Differentiation of emboli from flow signal is from the absence of change in signal on even—second—compared with odd—first—spin-echo images, and also the small change in appearance of clots on systolic compared with diastolic images. Slow blood flow shows the opposite findings.

Phase images show a difference in gray scale between stationary protons and protons in motion. Emboli show a gray scale level equal to that of stationary structures, whereas flowing blood has an increased intensity. A diagnosis of embolism is made based upon the findings of a focal intraluminal area of medium signal intensity within the main, hilar, or segmental pulmonary arteries. Little or no change of intensity from first to second echo images and a constant appearance on images obtained at different phases of the cardiac cycle are important.

White and colleagues (1987) made the diagnosis of pulmonary embolism in several cases with MRI, based on an intraluminal area of high signal intensity that was "fixed" during the cardiac cycle. Signal evident on both first-echo and second-spin-echo images is most consistent with thrombus. Absence of these findings in the central or segmental pulmonary arteries has also excluded pulmonary emboli by MRI. Nevertheless, MRI is not considered adequate for exclusion of emboli in more distal vessels, and the role of MRI for clinical evaluation of pulmonary thromboembolic disease remains controversial.

Pulmonary Edema

The lung parenchyma demonstrates no signal above background noise on ungated spin-echo sequences with the usual imaging parameters. On images gated to pulmonary vascular diastole, signal is evident from intravascular blood within small vessels. Pulmonary edema

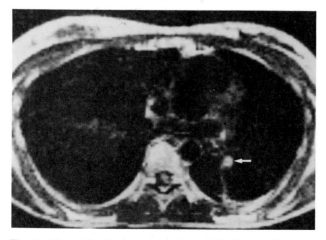

Fig. 14–10. MRI of pulmonary embolus. MRI (nongated) demonstrates an intraluminal high signal-intensity lesion (arrow) in the left descending pulmonary artery, caused by a pulmonary embolus. The embolus was confirmed by an angiogram.

is associated with an increase in lung water, both in the interstitium and intra-alveolar space. Wexler and colleagues (1985) in dogs and Schmidt and co-workers (1986) in rats, showed an increase in MRI signal intensity emanating from the lungs in pulmonary edema. The distribution of fluid may be diffuse, central or asymmetric, depending on the cause of the pulmonary edema and the presence of concomitant lung disease in humans.

The intensity of the MRI signal in experimental pulmonary edema correlates with total lung water content. Both permeability and hydrostatic pulmonary edema appear to have similar T1 relaxation times, and it appears that MRI cannot distinguish between the two. Similarly, the MRI intensity from inflammatory lesions in the lungs resembles that of pulmonary edema. The difficulty and expense, at present, of obtaining satisfactory MR relaxation measurements and their overlap for most diseases precludes MRI use for distinguishing between different types of diffuse lung diseases.

The Aorta

Aortic Aneurysm and Aortic Rupture

White and colleagues (1986) described that both CT and MRI have advantages over aortography in detecting thoracic aortic aneurysms. Both can assess the thickness of the aortic wall, accurately measure the size of the aorta, and characterize the extent of the abnormality. The excellent delineation of calcifications available from CT is advantageous in assessing the aortic wall. Aortic rupture can be seen on CT scans as a mediastinal soft tissue density or wall thickening, or a pleural effusion. The appearance of blood in MRI is usually more specific than with CT, particularly at higher magnetic field strength, and with gradient-echo techniques. The MRI characteristics of blood clot, however, vary with age, organization, and MRI technique, and can in some instances be similar to those of fat. A major advantage of MRI over CT is the ability of cine-MRI to detect and estimate the degree of aortic valve insufficiency. Thus MRI is particularly useful in assessing aneurysms of the sinuses of Valsalva, for which CT is ill suited. Although duplex ultrasonography can also provide this capability, MRI can evaluate the thorax more completely.

Aortic rupture secondary to trauma is still best evaluated with aortography. False-negative diagnosis with CT appears to be unacceptably high, although good results have been reported. There is little experience with MRI in this setting; it will probalby suffer from similar diagnostic limitations. In addition, the problems of patient monitoring and life support systems in a magnetic environment would seem to preclude MRI in most such patients. Chronic pseudoaneurysms in survivors of aortic injury can be evaluated by MRI.

Aortic Dissection

The principal diagnostic tasks in imaging patients suspected of having aortic dissection are to document the presence of dissection and to establish the extent of involvement if dissection is present. Both sensitivity and specificity of the primary diagnosis must be high, as false-positive and false-negative errors are unacceptable. Assignment of the type of dissection must also be accurate, because patients with type A dissections are immediate surgical candidates, whereas those with type B dissections are usually managed medically in the acute phase.

Current imaging methods in aortic dissection include angiography, CT, ultrasound, and MRI. Although ultrasound is accurate in assessing the ascending aorta, its limited field of view precludes its use as a general diagnostic test. Angiography is still the reference standard method for patients who have dissection, although it has limitations. It is invasive, carrying the risk of further traumatizing the vessel by the necessary catheter manipulations and compromising the patient by the need for injection of large volumes of contrast material, with potential hemodynamic and renal toxicity. Angiography also is attended with a small incidence of both false-positive and false-negative diagnoses, and its field of view is limited to the opacified vascular lumina. CT is an accurate and increasingly used imaging procedure for evaluating aortic dissection; the intimal flap and the true and false lumina can be identified in many cases. The pericardium can be assessed and renal function can be roughly estimated by contrast enhancement of the kidneys. CT requires a large volume of contrast material, cannot evaluate the aortic valve or reliably identify branch vessel involvement; and is limited in its ability to distinguish thrombus from slow flow in the false lumen. The most significant technical problem with CT is the necessity of rapid-sequence scans at the correct anatomic levels during the peak vascular opacification by a compact bolus of contrast material. If any of the technical factors are suboptimal, or if artifacts are present, diagnostic accuracy will be compromised.

Direct multiplanar MRI is advantageous in providing a cross-sectional view of the intimal flap (Fig. 14–11). Because of the orientation and frequent tortuosity of the aorta and the tendency of flaps to spiral, detecting the

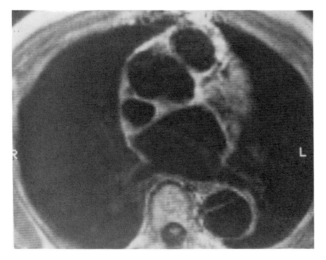

Fig. 14–11. Aortic dissection, type B. MRI through the descending aorta demonstrates a flap across the vessel lumen with rapid flow (signal void) in both the true and false lumens.

entire extent of a dissection using only the transaxial plane is occasionally difficult. Clot and slow flow in the false lumen can usually be differentiated by their differing behavior on second-echo and gradient-echo images. The presence of pericardial effusion or hemopericardium can also be identified. Using a cine-gradient-echo technique such as cine-GRASS, the presence and degree of aortic insufficiency can be identified. The relationship of arch and abdominal branch vessels to the dissection often can be delineated. Mediastinal hematoma from complicating aortic rupture can be detected.

MRI of patients with suspected dissection must include at a minimum cardiac-gated spin-echo images in the transaxial plane. One typical routine is to gate to each R wave, and acquire two echoes—20 to 28 msec and 56 to 60 msec, using 1-cm section thickness with 5-mm intersection gaps. Coronal, sagittal, or oblique planes can be acquired if necessary, in individual cases. Images obtained in this manner through the entire course of the thoracic and upper abdominal aorta can demonstrate the intimal flap as a linear or curvilinear structure of medium signal intensity within the aortic lumen. This will either be outlined on both sides by low intensity flowing blood, or on the true luminal side by low intensity and on the false luminal side by higher signal caused by slow flow or thrombus. The pericardium and mediastinum can be adequately evaluated with such images as well. In many cases, cine-GRASS or similar methods can be advantageous in detecting the site of intimal perforation and can help in distinguishing the flap from phase-encoding artifacts—particularly important in high magnetic field strength devices, in distinguishing thrombus from slowly flowing blood, and in assessing the functional competence of the aortic valve and left ventricle.

MRI has high sensitivity and specificity for detecting and typing aortic dissections. A study of MRI in aortic dissection by Kersting-Summerhof and co-workers (1988) demonstrated for an experienced reader a sensitivity of 100% and a specificity of 90%, whereas an inexperienced reader had an 83% sensitivity and a 90% specificity. About 20% of the images in this study were rated as suboptimal to inadequate. It was considered that experience is required to recognize flow artifacts and differentiate slow blood flow from thrombus. This study, however, included only standard spin-echo images; and it is likely that the addition of cine-GRASS images in potentially confusing cases would have permitted a more confident diagnosis in cases with prominent flow artifacts.

A limitation of MRI in assessing dissections is its yet unquantified and possibly limited accuracy in determining small branch vessel involvement, such as the coronary arteries. Some surgeons, however, feel that this information is not critical in preoperative assessment.

MRI may also be useful in the follow-up of patients with chronic dissection to determine the development of complications and monitor the results of surgical treatment.

Pleura

Pleural effusion generally has long T1 and T2 values. The intensity of pleural effusions is therefore low to very low on T1-weighted images. Small pleural effusions may thus go undetected on T1-weighted images when the adjacent lung is normal and thus also very low in signal intensity. Many pleural effusions, however, become markedly increased in intensity on T2-weighted images, and thus their recognition is easier on these images. Fluid within the lung has an intensity similar to that of fluid within the pleural space, and the recognition of pleural fluid is then based on the position and shape of the area of high signal intensity. Tscholakoff and colleagues (1988) showed that MRI has limited capability for determining the nature and type of fluid within the pleural space. In general, effusions with little protein have low intensity. With increasing concentrations of protein, T1 decreases. Protein-containing exudates tend to become more intense on T2-weighted images. Thus far, MRI has not been able to reliably distinguish between exudates and transudates, both because of the difficulty of obtaining reliable T1 and T2 relaxation times at the lung bases, and because of the degradation of the relaxation information from respiratory and fluid movement.

Hemorrhagic pleural effusions can, however, be distinguished from other pleural fluid collections. Hemothorax present for longer than a few days shows high signal intensities on both T1- and T2-weighted images because of a short T1 value. These findings have to be related to the magnetic field strength of the MR imager. Pleural hematoma can present as a multicompartmented image on T1-weighted studies, with nonhomogeneous, low intensity areas interspersed with high intensity regions.

Brachial Plexus

Developments in imaging coils and narrow-slice techniques have improved the MRI demonstration of small superficial structures such as the organs within the neck and the brachial plexus. Castagno and Shuman (1987) studied 47 patients with suspected brachial plexus involvement by tumor. Using various imaging planes and techniques, they were able to demonstrate tumor involvement of the brachial plexus in many cases, and to exclude involvement in those without disease. The contrast between soft tissues and the brachial vessels and nerves allows detailed evaluation of anatomy and pathology in this region. On T2-weighted images, tumors tend to have higher intensity than the scalene muscles of the neck. The display of displacement and encasement of the subclavian artery by tumor is especially important. Improvement in imaging techniques will further facilitate imaging in this area.

MR Spectroscopy

MR spectroscopy is an exciting new method for the noninvasive measurement of biochemical processes. By taking advantage of the different radiofrequency signals from nuclei within different molecules, the relative abundance of these molecules can be determined. At present, phosphorus—^{31}P—is the most widely used element; and cellular energy metabolism can be studied. Spectra of the relative quantities of high energy metabolites and metabolic pathways can be generated, and the chemical environment in living tissues can be measured. For instance, intracellular pH is readily measured. Dynamic measurement of the concentrates of the metabolites adenosine triphosphate, phosphocreatinine, and inorganic phosphate, among others, is feasible. In vivo MR spectroscopy of the thorax is experimental. Cardiac ischemia and related functions have been studied. MR spectroscopy requires magnets with high field strength, of 1.5 tesla or above, and its availability is still limited. Theoretically, MR spectroscopy could assist in evaluating therapy of focal lung lesions or diffuse lung disease, or allow differentiation between benign and malignant tissues. Its final role in medical evaluation has yet to be established.

Future Directions

MRI is undergoing rapid development and transition. Statements about its future prospects must be tentative. It is probably comparable to CT for evaluating the mediastinum and hila in most situations. Occasionally, one or the other shows better images of thoracic pathology and is more diagnostic. For cardiac abnormalities and for the central vascular structures of the thorax, MRI is frequently better than CT and does not necessitate the injection of potentially allergenic contrast materials. Direct sagittal and coronal imaging has limited application, except under special circumstances. At present, applications in the lungs are limited to research activities, although technical improvements may overcome the present drawbacks. The noninvasive measurement of blood flow and regional perfusion; imaging following the uptake of tissue-specific contrast agents; and measurement of intracellular processes are all likely future applications. Ultrafast scanning sequences, and compensated sequences that eliminate motion artifacts and image degradation, will greatly advance the application of MRI for thoracic conditions.

REFERENCES

Castagno, A.A., and Shuman, W.P.: MR imaging in clinically suspected brachial plexus tumor. AJR *149*:1219, 1987.

Crooks, C., et al.: NMR whole body imager operating at 3.5 KGauss—0.35T. Radiology *143*:169, 1982a.

Crooks, L.E., et al.: Visualization of cerebral and vascular abnormalities by NMR imaging: the effects of imaging parameters on contrast. Radiology *144*:843, 1982b.

de Geer, G., Webb, W.R., and Gamsu, G.: Normal thymus: assessment with MR and CT. Radiology *158*:313, 1986.

Dooms, G., et al.: Magnetic resonance imaging of lymph nodes: comparison with CT. Radiology *153*:719, 1984.

Falke, T.H.M., et al.: Magnetic resonance imaging of the adrenal glands. Radiographics *7*:343, 1987.

Gamsu, G., et al.: Nuclear magnetic resonance imaging of the thorax. Radiology *147*:473, 1983.

Gamsu, G., et al.: Magnetic resonance imaging of benign mediastinal masses. Radiology *151*:709, 1984.

Glazer, H.S., et al.: Radiation fibrosis: differentiation from recurrent tumor by MR imaging. Radiology *156*:721, 1985.

Glazer, G.M., et al.: Adrenal tissue characterization using MR imaging. Radiology *158*:78, 1986.

Haase, A., et al.: Flash imaging. Rapid NMR imaging using low flip angle pulses. J. Magnetic Resonance *67*:258, 1986.

Heelan, R.T., et al.: Carcinomatous involvement of the hilum and mediastinum: computed tomographic and magnetic resonance evaluation. Radiology *156*:111, 1985.

Kersting-Summerhof, B.A., et al.: Aortic dissection: sensitivity and specificty of MR imaging. Radiology *166*:651, 1988.

Kuriyama, K., et al.: CT-determined pulmonary artery diameters in predicting pulmonary hypertension. Invest. Radiol. *19*:16, 1984,

Lanzer, P., et al.: Cardiac imaging using gated magnetic resonance. Radiology *150*:121, 1983.

McFadden, R.G., et al.: Proton magnetic resonance imaging to stage activity of interstitial lung disease. Chest *92*:31, 1987.

Mountain, C.F.: A new international staging system for lung cancer. Chest *89*:225S, 1986.

Müller, N.L., Gamsu, G., and Webb, W.R.: Pulmonary nodules: detection using magnetic resonance and computed tomography. Radiology *155*:687, 1985.

O'Callaghan, J.P., et al.: CT evaluation of pulmonary artery size. J. Comp. Assist. Tomogr. *6*:101, 1982.

Pykett, I.L.: NMR imaging in medicine. Sci. Am. *246*:78, 1982.

Quint, L.E., Glazer, G., and Orringer, M.B.: Esophageal imaging by MR and CT: study of normal anatomy and neoplasms. Radiology *156*:127, 1985.

Rholl, K.S., Levitt, R.G., and Glazer, H.S.: Magnetic resonance imaging of fibrosing mediastinitis. AJR *145*:255, 1985.

Schmidt, H.C., Tsay, D.G., and Higgins, C.B.: Pulmonary edema: a MR study of hydrostatic and permeability types. Radiology *158*:297, 1986.

Sechtem, U., et al.: Cine-MRI: potential for the evaluation of cardiovascular function. AJR *148*:239, 1987.

Tscholakoff, D., et al.: Evaluation of pleural and pericardial effusion by magnetic resonance imaging. Eur. J. Radiol. (in press).

Vinitski, S., et al.: Differentiation of parenchymal lung disorders with *in vitro* proton nuclear magnetic resonance. Magnetic Resonance Med. *3*:120, 1986.

von Schulthess, G.K., Fisher, M.R., and Higgins, C.B.: Pathologic blood flow in pulmonary vascular disease as shown by gated magnetic resonance imaging. Ann. Intern. Med. *103*:317, 1985.

von Schulthess, G.K., et al.: Mediastinal masses: MR imaging. Radiology *158*:289, 1986.

Webb, W.R., Gamsu, G., and Crooks, L.E.: Multisection sagittal and coronal magnetic resonance imaging of the mediastinum and hila. Radiology *150*:475, 1984a.

Webb, W.R., et al.: Magnetic resonance imaging of the pulmonary hila: normal and abnormal. Radiology *152*:89, 1984b.

Webb, W.R., and Moore, E.H.: Differentiation of volume averaging and mass on magnetic resonance imaging of the mediastinum. Radiology *155*:413, 1985.

Webb, W.R., et al.: Bronchogenic carcinoma: staging with MR compared with staging with CT and surgery. Radiology *156*:117, 1985.

Wexler, H.R., et al.: Quantitation of lung water by nuclear magnetic resonance imaging: a preliminary study. Invest. Radiol. *20*:583, 1985.

White, R.D., Doooms, G.C., and Higgins, C.B.: Advances in imaging thoracic aortic disease. Invest. Radiol. *21*:761, 1986.

White, R.D., Winkler, M.L., and Higgins, C.B.: MR imaging of pulmonary arterial hypertension and pulmonary emboli. AJR *149*:15, 1987.

CHAPTER 15

RADIONUCLIDE STUDIES OF THE LUNG

William G. Spies

Ventilation/perfusion—V/Q—imaging of the lungs remains the most commonly performed radionuclide procedure of the chest in most nuclear medicine laboratories; it is most often performed for the detection of pulmonary thromboembolism. Since the introduction of these techniques in the early 1960s, considerable refinements of the method have been developed, in terms of new radiopharmaceuticals, newer instrumentation and techniques, and more sophisticated methods of interpretation.

V/Q imaging has also been used for a variety of other clinical indications, such as the detection and quantification of obstructive airways disease, quantitation of right-to-left cardiac shunts, assessment of pulmonary trauma and inhalation injury, and monitoring of therapy in childhood asthma. The technique has also been used for the preoperative assessment of resectability of pulmonary neoplasms and prediction of postoperative pulmonary function. It may also be used in other clinical situations in which lung resection is contemplated in patients with compromised pulmonary function.

Gallium imaging of the chest is a sensitive but somewhat nonspecific method for the detection of neoplastic or inflammatory disorders. In the detection and staging of neoplasms such as bronchial carcinoma and lymphomas, it is used in conjunction with other techniques, including roentgenography, CT scanning, and lymphangiography. Gallium imaging has assumed an important role in the assessment of acute opportunistic infections, such as *Pneumocystis carinii* pneumonia, in patients with acquired immune deficiency syndrome—AIDS, and other entities associated with decreased immunocompetence. It can also be used for the quantification of pulmonary involvement with sarcoidosis, tuberculosis, and pneumoconioses.

Iodine-131 imaging is used to assess the presence of functioning metastases in patients with well-differentiated thyroid carcinomas and also therapeutically to ablate pulmonary metastases.

Radionuclide angiography is a useful noninvasive technique for evaluating vascular disorders of the chest, such

as the superior vena cava syndrome, and for assessment of the vascularity of intrathoracic masses.

Newer methods of pulmonary radionuclide imaging are focusing on assessment of function and metabolism, such as alveolar-capillary permeability, amine receptor function, and pulmonary fluid balance. Radiolabeled monoclonal antibodies are being developed for the detection and treatment of a variety of intrathoracic neoplasms.

VENTILATION/PERFUSION IMAGING

Perfusion Imaging

Pulmonary perfusion imaging is performed by intravenously injecting radioactive particles that are large enough to be trapped in the pulmonary vasculature, specifically in the pulmonary arterioles and capillaries. The distribution of these particles is proportional to regional pulmonary blood flow. Technetium-99m—^{99m}Tc—is the radionuclide of choice for these studies, because of its favorable gamma energy for imaging with a nuclear medicine gamma scintillation camera—140 keV—low radiation dose to the patient, and short half-life of 6 hours.

The most commonly used radiopharmaceutical for pulmonary perfusion imaging is macroaggregated albumin—MAA—labeled with ^{99m}Tc. This agent is available commercially in kit form and provides particles in the range of approximately 10 to 60 μm in diameter. Human albumin microspheres—HAM—can also be labeled with ^{99m}Tc, resulting in a more uniform particle size, but also associated with a longer biological half-life and greater cost. The usual dose given to an adult patient is 2 to 4 mCi of activity, which corresponds to approximately 200,000 to 500,000 particles injected. At this dose range, Harding and colleagues (1973) have shown that less than 0.1% of the pulmonary arterioles are temporarily occluded, and therefore no physiologic effects are anticipated. In patients known to have severe pre-existing pulmonary arterial hypertension or having undergone prior pneumonectomy, the dose may be lowered to 1 to

1.5 mCi. Doses of more than 1 million particles are avoided, as are doses less than 100,000 particles, at which point the images may show areas of inhomogeneity on the basis of poor count statistics, in the absence of actual perfusion abnormalities. The particles are broken down and leave the pulmonary vasculature with a biological half-life of 6 to 8 hours and are phagocytized by the reticuloendothelial system.

Adverse reactions such as allergic responses to the radiopharmaceutical have been reported, but are extremely rare. In addition to severe pulmonary arterial hypertension, other relative contraindications to pulmonary perfusion imaging with particulate radiopharmaceuticals include right-to-left intracardiac shunts and pregnancy. None of these is an absolute contraindication, and in fact these agents are even used clinically to quantitate known right-to-left shunts, as discussed subsequently. Rhodes and co-workers (1971) reported several occurrences of transient ischemic episodes following injection of radiolabeled MAA, but not with HAM. In pregnancy, a lower dose is used to minimize the radiation dose to the fetus.

^{99m}Tc-MAA is injected intravenously with the patient in the supine position to minimize gravitational effects on the distribution of the particles in the pulmonary vasculature. After injection, the patient may be moved without affecting particle distribution. Imaging may be performed in either the upright or supine position. At least six views are routinely obtained: anterior, posterior, right and left posterior oblique, and right and left lateral. Some laboratories also obtain anterior oblique views. Both Caride and colleagues (1976) and Nielsen and associates (1977) have shown that the posterior oblique views are particularly important in detecting and localizing lower lobe perfusion defects, the commonest site of involvement in pulmonary embolism.

Imaging is performed with a gamma scintillation camera, most often using a large-field-of-view camera with a low-energy parallel-hole collimator, or a standard-field-of-view camera with a low-energy diverging collimator in the case of portable examinations. Each image is generally obtained for 300,000 to 1,000,000 counts. A normal perfusion lung scan is illustrated in Figure 15–1.

Ventilation Imaging

Ventilation imaging is performed by having the patient inhale either a radioactive gas or a fine, uniform radiolabeled aerosol. The most widely used agent is xenon-133 gas—^{133}Xe. Standard spirometric apparatus may be used for the study, but a system for venting or trapping, or both, of the exhaled gas must be used because of the relatively long half-life of the radionuclide—5.3 days.

The ^{133}Xe ventilation study is usually performed in three phases. The patient first inhales deeply as 10 to 20 mCi of ^{133}Xe is injected into the intake port of the spirometer. The patient holds his breath as long as possible while a posterior image of the lungs is obtained for 25,000 to 250,000 counts. This single breath image reflects regional ventilatory rates. Areas of lung that are well ventilated accumulate activity, and areas that are poorly ventilated appear as photopenic—cold—defects. This image may not be obtainable in patients who are extremely dyspneic.

The patient then breathes a mixture of ^{133}Xe and oxygen in a closed system with a carbon dioxide absorber for 3 to 5 minutes, in order to achieve an equilibrium in the distribution of the radioactive gas in the lungs. A 300,000 to 600,000 count equilibrium wash-in image is obtained at the conclusion of this phase. This image reflects the total ventilated lung volume, and all areas of lung that are ventilated show activity on the image. In some laboratories, serial images are also obtained during the wash-in phase.

The final and most important phase is the washout, during which the patient breathes room air and the exhaled ^{133}Xe is trapped in a charcoal system or vented away by an exhaust system. Serial washout images are obtained, typically at intervals of 1 minute, for at least 5 minutes. On these images, the activity normally disappears from the lungs within 3 to 4 minutes, in a symmetrical fashion. Areas of obstructive airways disease appear as focal or diffuse zones of xenon-133 retention or asymmetrical washout. Many nuclear medicine physicians include posterior oblique images in the washout study to better localize ventilatory abnormalities in the anteroposterior dimension. Ventilation studies are shown in Figure 15–2. Alderson and associates (1974, 1976) and Alderson and Line (1980) have shown that the ventilation study is nearly twice as sensitive as the routine roentgenograms and at least as sensitive as spirometric pulmonary function tests for the detection of obstructive airways disease. The washout portion of the study is the most sensitive part of the exam, and the duration of ^{133}Xe retention is qualitatively related to the severity of obstructive airways disease, as measured by pulmonary function studies.

^{133}Xe imaging has certain disadvantages. Ventilation studies with ^{133}Xe are normally performed prior to perfusion scans, because the energy of the photopeak of ^{133}Xe is lower—81 keV—than the ^{99m}Tc photopeak—140 keV. If the perfusion study were performed first, then degradation of the ventilation images would result from downscatter of ^{99m}Tc photons into the ^{133}Xe window. This effect is most detrimental to the relatively count-poor washout portion of the study, which is the most important phase of the ventilation scan, as previously discussed. The low energy of the ^{133}Xe photopeak is also not optimally suited to imaging with the gamma camera, resulting in relatively low resolution images. In addition, the long half-life requires the use of special disposal techniques, as mentioned, and usually precludes the performance of portable ventilation studies. Finally, because of the dynamic nature of the study, multiple projections are not routinely obtainable, with the exception of the aforementioned oblique washout views.

Other ventilatory agents have been used in an attempt to overcome these shortcomings. ^{127}Xe is another isotope of xenon gas having the advantage of higher gamma energies—172 keV, 203 keV, and 375 keV—enabling ventilation imaging to be performed after perfusion imaging.

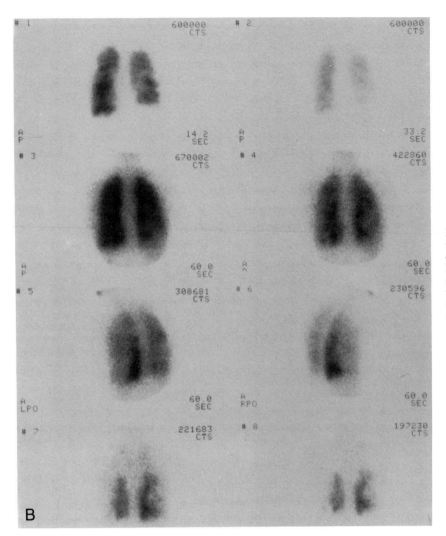

Fig. 15–2 Continued. *B*, Abnormal ¹³³Xe ventilation study in a 52-year-old woman with chronic obstructive pulmonary disease. Diffusely irregular ventilation on the single-breath image with diffuse, severe ¹³³Xe retention during 0–6 minute washout views (same views as Figure 15–2A). Retention persisted on images obtained up to 14 minutes after the onset of the washout study.

abnormalities such as subsegmental atelectasis, elevation of a hemidiaphragm, or small pleural effusions. Often the chest roentgenogram is normal. The chest roentgenogram is nevertheless important, as it may reveal other causes for the patient's symptoms, and as discussed subsequently, plays an important role in the interpretation of V/Q scans. The roentgenogram is normally obtained immediately prior to the V/Q scan and should never be more than 24 hours removed from the time of the scan.

Pulmonary angiography is considered the "definitive" test for PE, but is an invasive, expensive procedure that may be associated with significant morbidity and mortality, especially when performed by inexperienced personnel or in critically ill patients. Furthermore, the accuracy of pulmonary angiography varies with the techniques used and method of interpretation. It is most often reserved for patients having equivocal V/Q scans or those for whom measures such as pulmonary embolectomy or thrombinolytic therapy are contemplated. When necessary, pulmonary angiography should be performed no later than 72 hours and preferably within 24 hours after the lung scan to avoid a false negative angiogram secondary to clot lysis. In experienced hands, using the V/Q scan as a guide, pulmonary angiography

is a safe and accurate procedure for the confirmation or exclusion of significant PE in selected patients.

Digital subtraction angiography is a less invasive alternative to standard pulmonary angiography, as reported by Goodman and Brant-Zawadzki (1982). While promising in some instances, this technique at present lacks adequate spatial resolution to detect small emboli, and encounters significant problems related to artifacts from patient motion and cardiac and respiratory motion.

V/Q imaging is the screening procedure of choice for the evaluation of suspected PE. The system of interpretation devised by Biello and co-workers (1979b) and refined by Alderson and colleagues (1981) has become the de facto standard for evaluating these studies. The principles upon which this system is based include the overwhelming incidence of multiple emboli in patients with PE—in greater than 85% of cases—and the observation that PE usually produces perfusion defects in areas of normal ventilation, i.e., V/Q mismatch. While transient ventilatory abnormalities are demonstrated in experimental PE, such findings are fleeting, and Alderson and associates (1978) have shown that they are rarely observed. Clinically, such findings are rare, except in the case of PE with infarction. Pulmonary infarction occurs

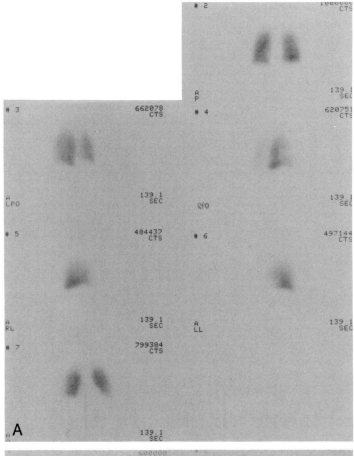

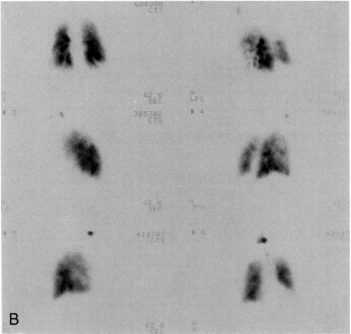

Fig. 15–3. *A,* Normal ^{99m}Tc-DTPA aerosol ventilation study. Clockwise from upper right: posterior, right posterior oblique, left lateral, anterior, right lateral, left posterior oblique. The activity inferior to the left lung represents swallowed aerosol in the stomach. *B,* Abnormal aerosol study in a 67-year-old female with chronic congestive heart failure and obstructive airways disease. Clockwise from upper left: posterior, left posterior oblique, right posterior oblique, anterior, right lateral, left lateral. Note the central deposition of aerosol in the central airways and diffusely irregular ventilation, especially in the upper lobes. The activity superior to the lungs is aerosol adherent to the mask and tubing system.

in less than 10% of cases, and is usually associated with roentgenographic abnormalities.

Perfusion defects are categorized by number, size, and location. Large defects involve 75% of a bronchopulmonary segment or more; moderate subsegmental defects, 25 to 75% of a segment; and small defects less than 25% of a segment. V/Q scan findings are usually reported as high probability—greater than 90%; low probability—less than 5%; or intermediate probability of PE.

Low probability studies demonstrate either normal findings, limited areas of ventilation/perfusion mismatch, or areas of mismatched perfusion abnormality that are in areas of roentgenographic abnormality, but are significantly less extensive. Small subsegmental perfusion defects are also not associated with angiographically demonstrable PE, even if unmatched. Less than 5% of patients with low probability scans have PE on angiography (Fig. 15–4).

High probability scans reveal two or more unmatched defects that are moderate or large in size, or unmatched defects that correspond to roentgenographic abnormalities but are substantially larger. Approximately 90% of these scans are associated with PE on angiography (Fig. 15–5). The significance of a single segmental mismatch is controversial. Although orginally considered high probability, many experts have suggested that such studies be read as intermediate probability. Other entities producing perfusion abnormality out of proportion to ventilatory abnormality may occasionally mimic PE, such as vasculitides, radiation therapy, pulmonary artery stenoses, and some infectious processes. The most common mimic is bronchial carcinoma, which may produce either V/Q match or mismatch, secondary to vascular compression or invasion, with or without bronchial obstruction. This possibility should be given strong consideration in the case of a whole-lung V/Q mismatch. An example of whole-lung mismatch secondary to pulmonary vasculitis associated with Takayasu's arteritis is illustrated in Figure 15–6. These conditions can often be suspected on clinical grounds.

Intermediate probability is assigned to cases in which extensive obstructive airways disease involves greater than 50% of the lung fields, perfusion defects correspond to roentgenographic abnormalities of comparable size, or only a single moderate or large unmatched defect is present (Fig. 15–7). In such cases, the V/Q scan has failed to produce definitive evidence for or against the presence of PE, and the decision regarding further workup or therapy must be based upon the level of pretest clinical suspicion and the clinical status of the patient. In patients with high pretest suspicion for PE, treatment with anticoagulants may proceed, with a repeat V/Q scan often obtained in 10–14 days to assess resolution. In patients with low pretest suspicion, the V/Q results should be considered in conjunction with other clinical data, and other diagnostic possibilities explored. Patients with moderate clinical suspicion or relative contraindications to anticoagulation should undergo pulmonary angiography to confirm or exclude the presence of PE.

In most centers, most pulmonary angiograms are performed in patients having intermediate probability scans. Patients with high or low probability scans do not require angiographic confirmation, unless there is overwhelming clinical suspicion to the contrary with a low probability scan, or a contraindication to anticoagulation in the case of a high probability scan. Angiographic proof is also usually obtained when measures such as pulmonary embolectomy or thrombinolytic therapy are contemplated. I and my associates (1986a) found that less than 15% of patients referred for lung scans over nearly a 6-year period ultimately required angiography.

Robin (1977) severely criticized lung scanning, claiming that it grossly overdiagnosed PE, especially in young, previously healthy patients, leading to unnecessary and potentially dangerous overuse of anticoagulants. These remarks came at a time when lung scans were usually performed without ventilation studies, and frequently comprised only 2 to 4 views. No distinctions were made regarding the size or number of perfusion defects, nor consideration given to findings on the roentgenogram. The nonspecificity of perfusion-only lung scanning is well known, since virtually all cardiopulmonary diseases may produce perfusion defects, including pneumonia, pleural effusion, congestive heart failure. The limited accuracy of the diagnosis of PE with perfusion-only imaging was demonstrated by McNeil (1976) and by me and my associates (1986a).

The criticisms of lung scanning voiced by Robin (1977) and others have largely become irrelevant with the advent of modern techniques for lung imaging, including the routine use of ventilation imaging, comparison with chest roentgenograms, and use of the Biello criteria for interpretation. Comparisons between the Biello criteria and other interpretive schemes by the groups of Carter (1982) and Sullivan (1983) have shown it to be overall the most accurate system.

Additional refinements have been introduced in the past several years by several investigators to further improve the accuracy of lung scanning in PE. Examples of such refinements include the "stripe sign" of Sostman and Gottschalk (1982), use of follow-up chest roentgenograms, as suggested by Vix (1983), assessing the age of roentgenographic abnormalities corresponding with perfusion defects, as evaluated by me and my co-workers (1986a), and comparison of V/Q scans with prior scans, as described by Alderson (1983) and by me and my co-workers (1986a). Use of these refinements has resulted in a further slight improvement in diagnostic accuracy and decrease in the number of equivocal or intermediate probability scans.

Another new technique being evaluated is the use of single photon emission computed tomography—SPECT—in conjunction with lung scanning. This technique involves acquiring data using a rotating gamma camera that circles the patient. Tomographic images are then reconstructed in multiple planes, as in conventional transmission x-ray CT. This approach has met with great success in other areas of nuclear medicine, such as cardiac and cerebral perfusion imaging, and may lead to

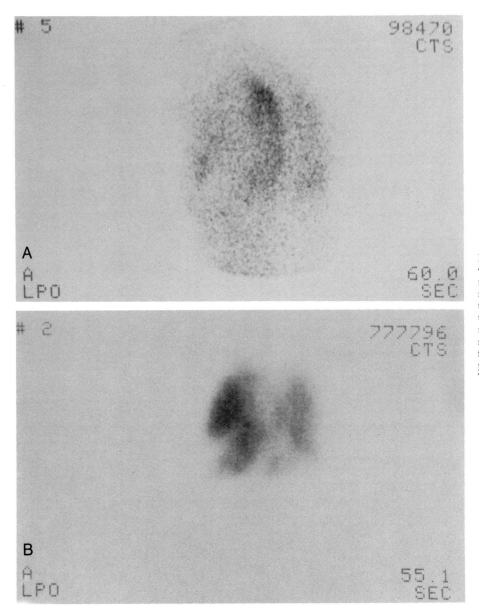

Fig. 15–4. Low probability V/Q scan with matched V/Q abnormalities. *A*, 2–3 minute left posterior oblique ^{133}Xe washout image demonstrating focal areas of retention in the lingula, posterior segment of the left upper lobe and posterior basal segment of the left lower lobe. *B*, Corresponding left posterior oblique ^{99m}Tc perfusion image demonstrates matching perfusion defects in the same segments. The chest roentgenogram was normal.

more accurate detection and localization of V/Q abnormalities, as suggested by Touya and co-workers (1986b).

Remaining criticisms of V/Q imaging have centered around the fact that the data used to validate the Biello criteria are all derived from retrospective studies. Hull and associates (1983) have conducted prospective clinical trials in suspected deep venous thrombosis and PE, and have obtained somewhat poorer results with V/Q imaging, although patient selection biases may have been present, and the techniques and interpretation used were not standard. A large multicenter prospective trial for the diagnosis of PE is ongoing, and the data from this study should shed further light on this issue. Nevertheless, it is clear that at present, V/Q imaging remains the screening procedure of choice in suspected PE, since it is the safest and most accurate noninvasive currently available.

Other Applications of V/Q Imaging

Although V/Q scans are frequently abnormal in patients with bronchial carcinoma, the scan is now rarely used for purposes of diagnosis or staging. Secker-Walker and Provan (1969) demonstrated perfusion defects associated with bronchial carcinoma, quantitated them using digital computers, and found that if the perfusion defect resulted in the abnormal lung's providing less than 33% of total pulmonary perfusion, the lesion was always unresectable. Subsequent exceptions to this rule have been reported. Ventilation can also be quantitated for various lung zones, allowing calculation of regional ventilation/perfusion ratios. Abnormalities in regional ventilation/perfusion ratio are also associated with nonresectability in most cases. Note that these are indirect approaches to the assessment of tumor extent. Furthermore, these techniques are not sensitive for the detection

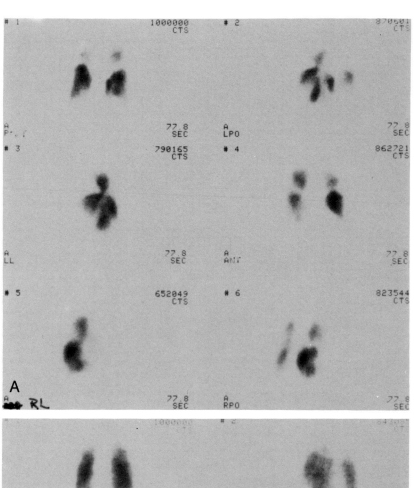

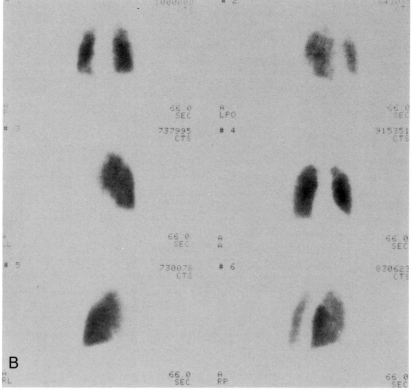

Fig. 15–5. High probability V/Q scan in a 79-year-old female with acute onset of tachycardia, tachypnea and hypoxia. *A*, ^{99m}Tc perfusion study demonstrating multiple segmental perfusion defects bilaterally. The ventilation study (not shown) was normal. *B*, Follow-up study performed after 16 days of anticoagulation therapy, showing significant resolution of the pulmonary emboli. Reprinted with permission from Spies, W.G., et al.: Radionuclide imaging in diseases of the chest. Part 1. Chest 83:122, 1983.

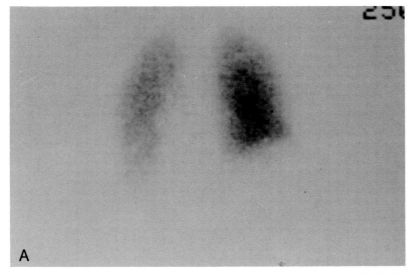

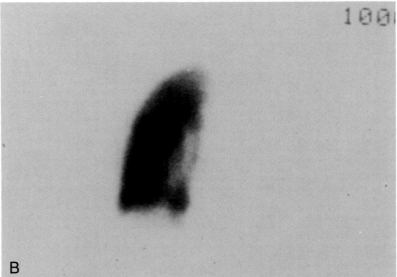

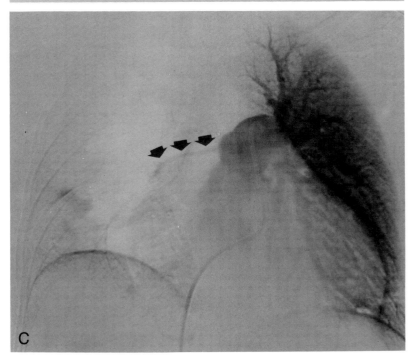

Fig. 15–6. Whole-lung V/Q mismatch in a 28-year-old female with known Takayasu's arteritis and acute chest pain and dyspnea. *A*, Posterior single-breath ^{133}Xe ventilation image demonstrating ventilation to both lungs, right greater than left. *B*, Posterior ^{99m}Tc perfusion image demonstrating normal perfusion to the left lung with a prominent hilar defect and complete absence of perfusion to the right lung. *C*, Subtraction angiographic image from a main pulmonary artery injection demonstrating severe stenosis of the main right pulmonary artery (arrows) secondary to severe arteritis. Other views showed multiple areas of aneurysmal dilatation of the proximal left pulmonary artery branches. No pulmonary emboli were identified. Reprinted with permission from Spies, W.G., et al.: Ventilation-perfusion scintigraphy in suspected pulmonary embolism: correlation with pulmonary angiography and refinement of criteria for interpretation. Radiology *159*:383, 1986.

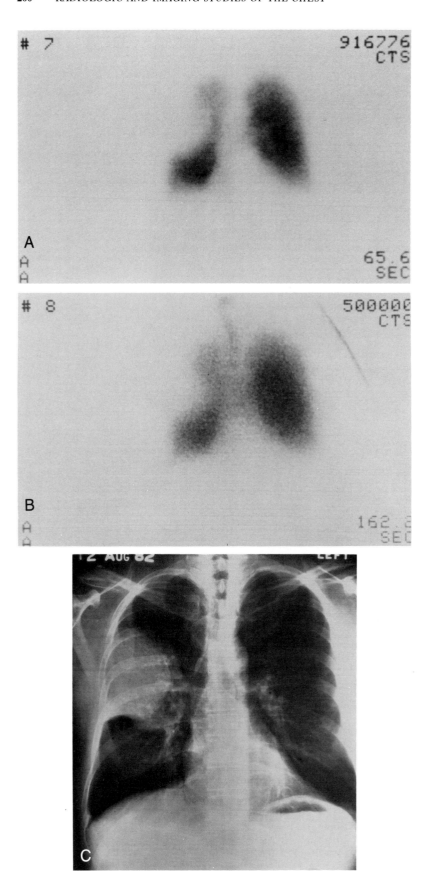

Fig. 15–7. Intermediate probability V/Q scan with a perfusion defect corresponding to a radiographic abnormality. The patient is a 42-year-old male with acute dyspnea and fever. The V/Q scan was performed using [81m]Kr as the ventilatory agent. *A,* Anterior perfusion image demonstrates a large perfusion defect in the right mid lung field. *B,* The anterior [81m]Kr image demonstrates a matching ventilation defect in the right mid lung field. *C,* The PA chest roentgenogram shows a corresponding area of consolidation in the right upper lobe that was not present one month prior. Although the ventilation and perfusion defects are matched, the findings are indicative of intermediate probability of pulmonary embolism, because of the corresponding radiographic infiltrate. While pulmonary embolism is not highly likely, particularly with only one area of involvement, an embolus with associated infarction in the right upper lobe cannot totally be excluded. Further workup established the diagnosis of Legionnaire's disease. There was no further clinical evidence suggestive of pulmonary embolism.

of small or peripheral lesions. Fiber-optic bronchoscopy and computed tomography of the chest, in conjunction with standard roentgenograms and tomograms, are now the procedures of choice for staging bronchial carcinoma. In some institutions, gallium imaging is also used for staging, as subsequently discussed.

V/Q imaging, in conjunction with quantitation using digital computers, can be used to predict postoperative pulmonary function. This determination may be critically important, because many patients with bronchial carcinoma have underlying chronic lung disease and may not be able to tolerate extensive pulmonary resection. Both Kristersson (1974) and Olsen and co-workers (1974) demonstrated a good correlation between relative pulmonary perfusion, assessed by prepneumonectomy perfusion lung scans, and postoperative pulmonary function, as measured by forced vital capacity and other pulmonary function indices. Kristersson (1974) and Boysen and co-workers (1977) have recommended pneumonectomy in patients with bronchial carcinoma and compromised lung function when the predicted postoperative FEV_1 is 800 ml or more. Such quantitation may also be used prior to resection of benign pulmonary lesions, such as bullae. The most recent application of quantitative radionuclide lung imaging has been in the preoperative and postoperative evaluation of patients undergoing unilateral pulmonary transplants, as described by the Toronto Lung Transplant Group (1986). Changes in perfusion or ventilation of the transplanted lung may be useful in monitoring pulmonary rejection.

In primary airway obstruction caused by foreign bodies, mucous plugging, or endobronchial masses, V/Q scans show striking ventilatory abnormalities. Often there are also corresponding but less severe reductions in perfusion, secondary to reflex vasoconstriction. These findings usually revert to normal when the airway obstruction is relieved, provided that irreversible lung damage has not resulted.

V/Q imaging may also be useful in the evaluation of lung injury, as reviewed by Lull and associates (1983). Perfusion defects may be identified in patients who have undergone blunt or penetrating trauma, in some cases before the changes are identifiable on a roentgenogram. Both perfusion and ventilation defects may be observed in patients with pneumothorax or hemothorax, although such entities are usually diagnosed on the chest roentgenogram.

[133]Xe ventilation studies are useful in the evaluation of inhalation injuries. Inhalation injuries often occur in conjunction with burns, and may result in a two- to fivefold increase in mortality, depending on the extent of the burn. In the early hours after the injury, the patient may be asymptomatic and have normal roentgenographic findings. Within several days, edema and inflammation of the airways may result in progressive airway obstruction, leading to atelectasis, infection, or adult respiratory distress syndrome—ARDS. Intravenous administration of ^{133}Xe in saline solution during the early stages of inhalation injury demonstrate areas of abnormal washout corresponding to sites of early obstructive airways in-

volvement. In this regard, ^{133}Xe is superior to fiber-optic bronchoscopy for evaluating the distal airways, while bronchoscopy is better for the trachea and proximal bronchi. Agee and associates (1976) reported that there is both proximal and distal involvement in most cases; thus either test alone is diagnostic in about 90% of cases, and both tests together detect virtually all cases. The results of these studies are used in conjunction with clinical probability factors to help guide patient management.

A new application for ventilation imaging with radiolabeled aerosols involves the evaluation of lung disorders associated with alterations in alveolar-capillary membrane permeability. Examples of such disorders include various interstitial lung diseases, hyaline membrane disease in neonates, and ARDS. Damage to the pulmonary capillary membrane or a change in the Starling forces may result in increased alveolar-capillary permeability. Radioaerosols are normally cleared from the alveoli into the circulation and excreted by the kidneys with a pulmonary clearance half-time of approximately 90 minutes. In the presence of ARDS or other interstitial lung disease, this half-time may be substantially shortened. By measuring ^{99m}Tc-DTPA aerosol washout using digitally acquired images, time-activity washout curves can readily be generated. Coates and O'Brodovich (1986) reviewed this technique. Smokers have faster aerosol clearance rates than nonsmokers. Clearance rates are normal in patients with asthma, pneumonia, and pulmonary edema secondary to left heart failure. This technique is simple and noninvasive, and has a potential role in the evaluation of patients at risk for developing ARDS or hyaline membrane disease, and in the detection and monitoring of patients with other forms of interstitial lung disease or alveolitis.

Whole body imaging with pulmonary perfusion agents is also used to detect and quantitate right-to-left cardiac shunts. In the presence of a shunt, some particles bypass the pulmonary vascular bed via the shunt and enter the systemic circulation, where they are trapped in end-organs in proportion to blood flow. ^{99m}Tc-human albumin microspheres—HAM—are frequently used for this application, since they are more stable in vivo than MAA, resulting in less potentially confusing activity in the kidneys and bladder secondary to the presence of free pertechnetate. In patients with significant shunts, the images demonstrate deposition of particles in the brain, kidneys, and extremities (Fig. 15–8). The data are quantitated by computer and the shunt is expressed as a percent. Normal subjects have approximately a 4% physiologic right-to-left shunt. Gates and associates (1974) obtained a good correlation with results obtained using the Fick oxygen technique at cardiac catheterization.

GALLIUM IMAGING

Gallium-67 citrate is a radiopharmaceutical used for the evaluation of inflammatory and certain neoplastic diseases. It is a cyclotron-produced radionuclide with a half-life of 78 hours and several gamma photopeaks, of which the ones commonly used for imaging include 93,

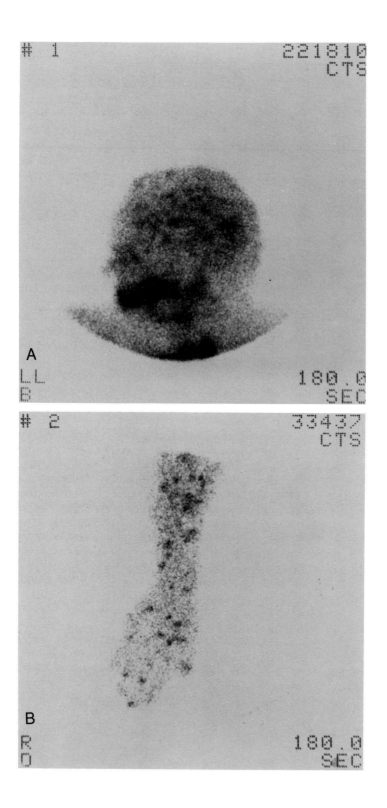

Fig. 15–8. Large right-to-left shunt. ⁹⁹ᵐTc HAM study. *A*, Left lateral skull image demonstrating marked particle deposition in the brain. Some free ⁹⁹ᵐTc pertechnetate is present in the saliva in the mouth, salivary glands and thyroid. *B*, Image of the right forearm and hand showing diffuse particle deposition. Quantitative analysis revealed a 49% right-to-left shunt.

184, and 296 keV. An iron analogue, it is largely bound to serum transferrin after intravenous injection. Gallium imaging is a sensitive but nonspecific procedure, with increased activity noted in many inflammatory and neoplastic processes. Normal sites of uptake include the liver, skeleton, salivary glands, kidneys, spleen, breasts, and large bowel. Simon and associates (1980) demonstrated that faint diffuse lung uptake may be present in about 50% of normal individuals at 24 hours, which should not be confused with a diffuse pulmonary inflammatory process. For this reason, gallium imaging of the chest is usually performed 48 to 72 hours after injection, although earlier imaging may be performed in cases of suspected acute thoracic infection to facilitate earlier diagnosis and treatment. In children, prominent uptake may be seen in the normal thymus gland, limiting the usefulness of gallium scanning for the evaluation of mediastinal masses in the pediatric age group. During the first 24 hours after injection, 20 to 30% of the dose is excreted, primarily by the kidneys. Subsequent excretion occurs primarily by way of the colon.

Hoffer (1980a) has reviewed the mechanisms of gallium uptake in disease processes. Gallium accumulation in infectious processes is related to several factors, including uptake in white blood cells—primarily bound to lactoferrin in lysosomes and other cytoplasmic organelles; increased blood flow and capillary permeability at sites of inflammation, with binding to tissue lactoferrin; and direct bacterial uptake within iron-binding organelles called siderophores. Uptake in neoplastic processes is less well understood, but may involve hyperpermeability of tumor vessels, increased extracellular fluid spaces in tumors, and uptake by iron-binding proteins, tumor cell surface receptors, or possibly other as yet unknown mechanisms.

Tumors having a high affinity for gallium include bronchial carcinoma, malignant mesothelioma, hepatocellular carcinoma, Hodgkin's disease, histiocytic and Burkitt's lymphoma, melanoma, and certain testicular neoplasms. Gallium scanning in the staging of Hodgkin's disease is highly sensitive in the detection of mediastinal involvement, with a sensitivity of 90% or greater, particularly in the nodular-sclerosing type. Evaluation of the abdomen and pelvis is less accurate, because of interfering normal colonic activity, which may obscure sites of lymphadenopathy or simulate abnormalities. CT is usually used for evaluation of abdominal or pelvic lymphadenopathy. Lymphangiography also plays a role, because it can detect involvement in lymph nodes that are not enlarged on CT. Detection of histiocytic and Burkitt's lymphoma by gallium imaging is at least as good as that of Hodgkin's disease, with virtually all metastatic foci of Burkitt's lymphoma demonstrating increased gallium uptake, as noted by Hoffer (1980b).

The overall sensitivity of gallium imaging in the staging of bronchial carcinoma is approximately 90%, without significant differences in different cell types, except for a possibly slightly lower sensitivity for adenocarcinoma. In general, primary lesions as small as 2 cm in diameter can be detected. The utility of gallium imaging in the assessment of mediastinal spread of tumor is controversial. Although it appears that gallium imaging is superior to standard roentgenograms and plain tomography in this regard, the results of clinical trials have been variable. Alazraki and colleagues (1978) suggested that the absence of gallium uptake in the mediastinum in patients whose primary lesion concentrated gallium may obviate the need for preoperative mediastinoscopy. Other investigators, such as DeMeester and associates (1976), have had less impressive results. Savage and co-workers (1976), have pointed out that since gallium uptake is nonspecific, false positives related to inflammatory disorders in the mediastinum may occur. The sensitivity of gallium imaging may be improved by using tomographic techniques, such as SPECT imaging. Nevertheless, as previously discussed, CT of the chest has become the primary imaging modality for the staging of bronchial carcinoma in most centers. The search for metastases outside the chest is best approached using other radionuclides, such as bone and liver-spleen scanning agents, and other techniques, such as CT of the abdomen. Examples of tumor uptake on gallium scans are shown in Figure 15–9.

Gallium imaging of the chest has also assumed an important role in the evaluation of infectious and other inflammatory disorders of the chest. Although the standard chest roentgenogram remains the primary imaging modality for the detection of primary inflammatory disease, gallium scanning plays a complementary role. It is more sensitive for the detection of early infectious processes, better delineates mediastinal involvement, and allows better follow-up of the response to therapy.

Diffusely increased pulmonary uptake is seen in opportunistic infections such as *Pneumocystis carinii* pneumonia—PCP—or cytomegalovirus pneumonia in immunocompromised hosts prior to the appearance of radiographic changes. Although previously a problem encountered mainly in patients with leukemia or lymphoma, this problem became important in the 1980s with the proliferation of the acquired immune deficiency syndrome—AIDS. Barron and associates (1985) confirmed the utility of gallium imaging in AIDS patients with suspected PCP, particularly in those with normal or equivocal chest roentgenograms. Kramer and associates (1986) described their experience with gallium imaging in a large series of AIDS patients presenting with acute fever or respiratory symptoms. In addition to confirming the utility of gallium imaging in the diagnosis of *Pneumocystis* and other opportunistic pneumonias, they pointed out patterns of focal lymph node uptake, seen primarily in cases of atypical tuberculosis, e.g., *Mycobacterium avium intracellulare*, and lymphoma, and focal pulmonary uptake, often seen with acute bacterial pneumonias. Negative findings were associated with Kaposi's sarcoma or the absence of identifiable infection. Examples of normal and abnormal gallium images of the chest are shown in Figure 15–10. Hattner and co-workers (1986) have emphasized the favorable economic impact of gallium scanning in this clinical setting, in which they realized a potential cost savings of 38%, as a result of obviating

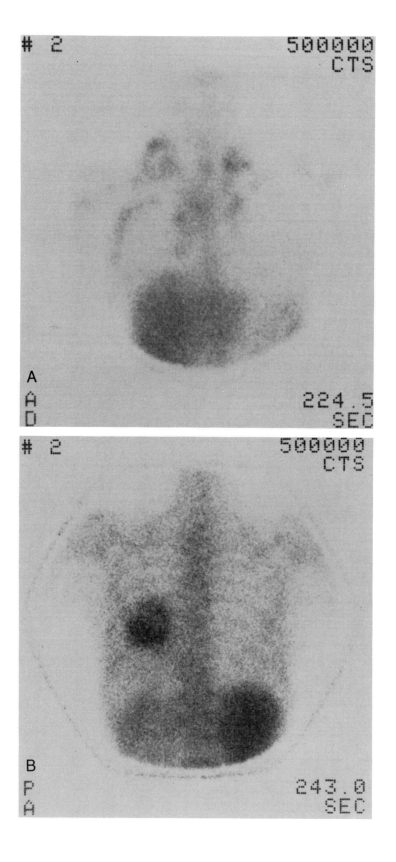

Fig. 15–9. Gallium uptake in thoracic neoplasms. *A*, 72-hour anterior chest image demonstrating gallium uptake in bilateral supraclavicular, right hilar, superior mediastinal and right axillary lymphadenopathy in a 39-year-old female with Hodgkin's disease. The activity at the inferior aspect of the image is due to normal hepatic and splenic gallium uptake. *B*, 72-hour posterior chest image demonstrating increased gallium activity in a left lower lobe adenocarcinoma in a 50-year-old female. This case is reprinted with permission from Spies, W.G., et al.: Radionuclide imaging in diseases of the chest. Part 2. Chest 83:250, 1983.

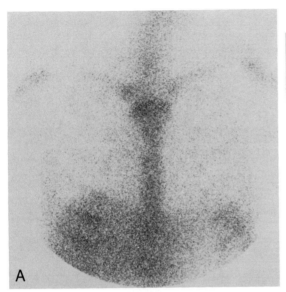

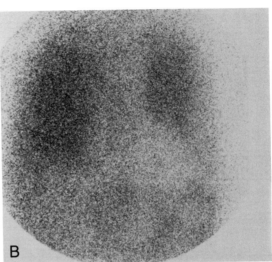

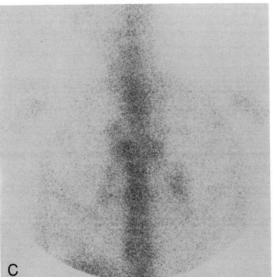

Fig. 15–10. Gallium imaging in immunocompromised patients. *A,* Normal 48-hour anterior gallium image of the chest. *B,* 72-hour anterior chest image demonstrating diffuse bilateral increased pulmonary uptake in a 61-year-old male patient with AIDS and fever. Note the negative cardiac silhouette. The abnormality was also evident on 24-hour images. Initial chest roentgenograms were negative, but later films showed perihilar infiltrates. Bronchial aspirates were positive for *Pneumocystis carinii* pneumonia. *C,* 72-hour anterior chest image showing bilateral hilar and right paratracheal lymphadenopathy in a 36-year-old male patient with AIDS who presented with nonproductive cough and fever. The patient proved to have *Mycobacterium avium intracellulare* infection, which also involved the liver and bone marrow.

the need for bronchoscopy in cases of negative gallium scans. Although diffuse pulmonary uptake is highly suspicious for the presence of acute opportunistic infection in this clinical setting, the finding is nonetheless nonspecific. The differential diagnosis of diffuse pulmonary uptake of gallium includes other diffuse bacterial and viral pneunomias, tuberculosis, sarcoidosis, pulmonary toxicity from chemotherapeutic agents or other drugs, idiopathic pulmonary fibrosis, lymphangitic metastases, pneumoconiosis, and chemical pneumonitis following lymphangiography. Bronchoscopy and biopsy are therefore generally obtained in positive cases to establish the specific diagnosis.

Although not of major importance in surgical practice, gallium imaging has also been used in the diagnosis and follow-up of granulomatous processes, such as tuberculosis and sarcoidosis, and pulmonary fibrotic disorders. Increased activity correlates with the presence of biologically active disease. Pulmonary uptake can be quantitated using a computer, resulting in excellent correlation with more invasive techniques, such as bronchoalveolar lavage in sarcoidosis, which Fajman and co-workers (1984) described. Correlation with clinical symptoms and assessment of therapy, however, is weaker.

^{131}I IMAGING

^{131}I whole-body imaging is a standard procedure for the postoperative evaluation of patients with well-differentiated thyroid carcinoma. The whole-body scan detects the presence of residual normal thyroid tissue and functioning metastases in regional lymph nodes, the lungs, or the skeleton. Uptake of ^{131}I in pulmonary metastases may be demonstrated even in the absence of identifiable lesions in the chest roentgenogram (Fig. 15–11). The scan findings are used to determine whether a therapeutic dose of ^{131}I should be administered for the ablation of residual thyroid tissue, as well as to determine the dose required. Beierwaltes (1978) suggested that the scan be performed approximately 6 weeks following total thyroidectomy without thyroid hormone replacement, to induce maximal endogenous TSH stimulation of ^{131}I uptake by metastases. The usual scan dose is 5 to 10 mCi. Administration of exogenous TSH to stimulate tumor uptake is not recommended, since it generally results in less effective and shorter-lasting stimulation, and may be associated with severe allergic reactions, including anaphylaxis. Typical therapy doses for functioning pulmonary metastases range from about 175 to 200 mCi, with follow-up whole-body scanning performed one year later. Patients given doses in this range must be hospi-

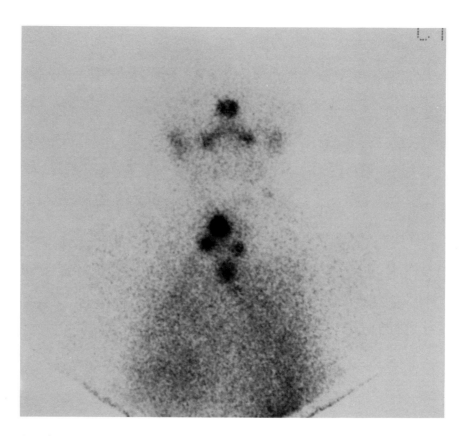

Fig. 15–11. Metastatic thyroid carcinoma. The patient is a 14-year-old white female, status: post total thyroidectomy for well-differentiated mixed papillary-follicular thyroid carcinoma. An anterior ^{131}I image of the head and chest demonstrates 4 foci of metastatic disease in the thyroid bed and diffuse bilateral pulmonary uptake, consistent with lung metastases. A subtle focus of activity in the left neck may represent a cervical lymph node metastasis. The activity in the nasal region and mouth represents normal uptake by the nasal mucosa and salivary glands.

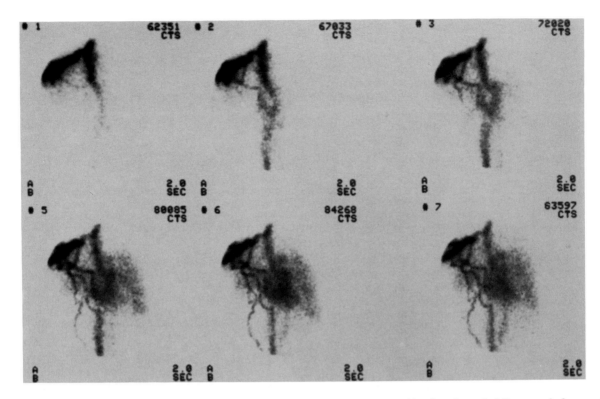

Fig. 15–12. Radionuclide angiography in superior vena cava syndrome. The patient is a 65-year-old male with poorly differentiated adenocarcinoma of the lung, brain and liver metastases, and clinical signs suggestive of superior vena cava obstruction. Selected anterior images of the chest from a radionuclide angiogram performed after injection of ⁹⁹ᵐTc DTPA in a right antecubital vein demonstrate high-grade partial obstruction of the superior vena cava, with marked flow into dilated collateral veins in the right axilla and anterior chest wall. Mild reflux into the right internal jugular vein and early visualization of the inferior vena cava via collateral flow are also noted. A small amount of activity is directly entering the superior vena cava and right heart.

talized until the retained dose drops below 30 mCi. Post-therapy repeat whole-body images are obtained prior to hospital discharge in many institutions, and may provide additional diagnostic information in up to 50% of cases, as reported by me and my associates (1986b). If necessary, repeat therapy may be given at yearly intervals. With this dose schedule, the incidence of toxicity related to radiation-induced pulmonary fibrosis or significant bone marrow suppression is very low. Follow-up scans may be obtained at longer intervals in patients with no evidence of recurrent disease.

RADIONUCLIDE ANGIOGRAPHY

Radionuclide angiography—RA—is a simple, safe, noninvasive method for evaluating blood flow to various organs. It can be used to delineate vascular anatomy and patency and to evaluate the vascularity of masses, as reviewed by Muroff (1976). RA is performed by obtaining a rapid sequence of images—0.5 to 3 sec/image—over an area of interest, immediately following the intravenous injection of a radiopharmaceutical. It is a routine part of many nuclear medicine procedures, such as renal scans, brain scans, and bone scans performed for suspected osteomyelitis. In the case of the chest, such studies may be obtained alone or in conjunction with other standard nuclear medicine examinations. Almost any ra-

diopharmaceutical may be used except MAA or HAM, which would, or course, be trapped in the pulmonary vasculature. The examination is most often performed for evaluation of suspected vascular obstruction, as in superior vena cava syndrome (Fig. 15–12). The data may be quantitated using a digital computer. RA may obviate the need for more invasive procedures, such as contrast venography or arteriography. Other potential diagnostic uses include the noninvasive demonstration of aortic aneurysms and vascular masses, such as hemangiomas and arteriovenous malformations. The major limitation of RA relates to its relatively poor spatial resolution compared to other standard techniques, such as contrast angiography and digital subtraction angiography. Technically inadequate studies occur in a small percentage of cases, because of poor bolus geometry or poor patient positioning.

FUTURE DEVELOPMENTS IN PULMONARY NUCLEAR MEDICINE

Developments in nuclear medicine have been directed toward more sophisticated evaluation of physiologic processes. Major advances usually result from the development of new radiopharmaceuticals, with the introduction of newer instrumentation following. Advances in pulmonary nuclear medicine have been no exception.

Several approaches to improvement of the scintigraphic diagnosis of PE were previously discussed. Another improvement is the use of ^{111}In-labeled autologous platelets. This technique is useful in the detection of deep vein thrombosis in the lower extremities, the precursor of PE. Investigations led by Davis (1980) and Moser and associates (1980) have suggested that imaging of PE in humans by this technique may be limited to emboli less than 12 hours old, and only in patients not on heparin.

"Hot spot" imaging of PE may be accomplished using radioactive gases labeled with positron-emitting radionuclides of carbon or oxygen, as reported by Nichols and associates (1978). In this case, inhaled radioactive gases diffuse across the alveolar-capillary membrane and are cleared from the lungs via pulmonary blood flow. As a result of decreased blood flow, the gas is retained in areas of PE, resulting in easily identified "hot spots." Although apparently sensitive, this technique is not practical for widespread use at present, because it requires an expensive, specialized positron scanner—PET scanner—and an on-site cyclotron for production of these extremely short-lived radiopharmaceuticals.

Ongoing investigations are using new radiopharmaceuticals for evaluation of pulmonary metabolic functions, which Touya (1986a) and Budinger (1982) and their colleagues reported. In addition to its respiratory function, the lung is involved in the regulation of several circulating vasoactive substances, including the activation, deactivation, release, or removal of such substances as amines, hormones, drugs, and polypeptides. Examples of such substances would include bradykinin, serotonin, prostaglandins, angiotensin I, histamine, and many others. One such line of research involves measuring the pulmonary uptake, extraction, and washout of ^{123}I-IMP, an iodoamphetamine derivative. Such studies may lead to better understanding of pulmonary metabolic functions and the ability to quantitate pulmonary endothelial amine receptors. Potential clinical applications would include the diagnosis and follow-up of treatment of such disorders as hypertension, adult and neonatal respiratory distress syndrome, cystic fibrosis, asthma, and even certain psychiatric disorders. Slutsky and Higgins (1984) have evaluated the use of thallium-201, the agent used for myocardial perfusion imaging, in the evaluation of pulmonary extracellular fluid balance, as related to the development of pulmonary edema.

A final area of research not limited to pulmonary nuclear medicine is the evaluation of radiolabeled monoclonal antibodies for the detection and treatment of various neoplasms, reported by Keenan and associates (1985). This technique has been applied by Zimmer and colleagues (1985) to the detection of small-cell lung carcinoma, using an ^{131}I-labeled antibody developed in mice. Future developments in this field will involve the development of more specific antibodies and the use of human rather than mouse monoclonal antibodies.

REFERENCES

Agee, R.N., et al.: Use of Xenon-133 in early diagnosis of inhalation injury. J. Trauma *16*:218, 1976.

Alazraki, N.P., et al.: Reliability of gallium scan chest radiography compared to mediastinoscopy for evaluating mediastinal spread in lung cancer. Am. Rev. Respir. Dis. *117*:415, 1978.

Alderson, P.O., and Line, B.R.: Scintigraphic evaluation of regional pulmonary ventilation. Semin. Nucl. Med. *10*:218, 1980.

Alderson, P.O., Secker-Walker, R.H., and Forrest, J.V.: Detection of obstructive pulmonary disease. Radiology *111*:643, 1974.

Alderson, P.O., et al.: The role of ^{133}Xe ventilation studies in the scintigraphic detection of pulmonary embolism. Radiology *120*:633, 1976.

Alderson, P.O., et al.: Ventilation-perfusion lung imaging and selective pulmonary angiography in dogs with experimental pulmonary embolism. J. Nucl. Med. *19*:164, 1978.

Alderson, P.O., et al.: Comparison of ^{133}Xe single-breath and washout imaging in the scintigraphic diagnosis of pulmonary embolism. Radiology *137*:481, 1980.

Alderson, P.O., et al.: Scintigraphic detection of pulmonary embolism in patients with obstructive pulmonary disease. Radiology *138*:661, 1981.

Alderson, P.O., et al.: Serial lung scintigraphy: Utility in diagnosis of pulmonary embolism. Radiology *149*:797, 1983.

Alderson, P.O, et al.: ^{99m}Tc-DTPA aerosol and radioactive gases compared as adjuncts to perfusion scintigraphy in patients with suspected pulmonary embolism. Radiology *153*:515, 1984.

Barron, T.F., et al.: *Pneumocystis carinii* pneumonia studied by gallium-67 scanning. Radiology *154*:791, 1985.

Beirwaltes, W.H.: The treatment of thyroid carcinoma with radioactive iodine. Semin. Nucl. Med. *8*:79, 1978.

Biello, D.R., et al.: Ventilation-perfusion studies in suspected pulmonary embolism. Am. J. Rad. *133*:1033, 1979a.

Biello, D.R., et al.: Interpretation of indeterminate lung scintigrams. Radiology *133*:189, 1979b.

Boysen, P.G., et al.: Prospective evaluation for pneumonectomy using the technetium-99m quantitative perfusion lung scan. Chest *72*:422, 1977.

Budinger, T.F., McNeil, B.J., and Alderson, P.O.: Perspectives in nuclear medicine: pulmonary studies. J. Nucl. Med. *23*:60, 1982.

Caride, V.J., et al.: The usefulness of the posterior oblique views in perfusion lung imaging. Radiology *121*:669, 1976.

Carter, W.D., et al.: Relative accuracy of two diagnostic schemes for detection of pulmonary embolism by ventilation-perfusion scintigraphy. Radiology *145*:447, 1982.

Coates, G., and O'Brodovich, H.: Measurement of pulmonary epithelial permeability with ^{99m}Tc-DTPA aerosol. Semin. Nucl. Med. *16*:275, 1986.

Cooper, J.D., et al.: Unilateral lung transplantation for pulmonary fibrosis. N. Engl. J. Med. *314*:1140, 1986.

Dalen, J.E., and Alpert, J.S.: Natural history of pulmonary embolism. Prog. Cardiovasc. Dis. *17*:259, 1975.

Davis, H.H., et al.: Scintigraphy with ^{111}In-labeled autologous platelets in venous thromboembolism. Radiology *136*:203, 1980.

DeMeester, T.R., et al.: Gallium-67 scanning for carcinoma of the lung. J. Thorac. Cardiovasc. Surg. *72*:699, 1976.

Fajman, W.A., et al.: Assessing the activity of sarcoidosis: quantitative ^{67}Ga-citrate imaging. Am. J. Rad. *142*:683, 1984.

Gates, G.F., Orme, H.W., and Dore, E.K.: Cardiac shunt assessment in children with macroaggregated albumin technetium-99m. Radiology *112*:649, 1974.

Goodman, P.C., Brant-Zawadzki, M.: Digital subtraction pulmonary angiography. Am. J. Rad. *139*:305, 1982.

Goris, M.L., et al.: Applications of ventilation lung imaging with [81m]krypton. Radiology *122*:399, 1977.

Harding, L.K., et al.: The proportion of lung vessels blocked by albumin microspheres. J. Nucl. Med. *14*:579, 1973.

Hattner, R.S., Golden, J.A., and Fugate, K.: Cost/benefit of real versus "ideal" management strategies of AIDS patients suspected of *P. carinii* pneumonia: effect of Ga-67 pulmonary imaging. J. Nucl. Med. *27*:914, 1986.

Hoffer, P.: Galluim: mechanisms. J. Nucl. Med. *21*:282, 1980a.

Hoffer, P.: Status of gallium-67 in tumor detection. J. Nucl. Med. *21*:394, 1980b.

Hull, R.D., et al.: Pulmonary angiography, ventilation lung scanning, and venography for clinically suspected pulmonary embolism with abnormal perfusion lung scan. Ann. Intern. Med. 98:891, 1983.

Keenan, A.M., Harbert, J.C., and Larson, S.M.: Monoclonal antibodies in nuclear medicine. J. Nucl. Med. 26:531, 1985.

Kramer, E.L., et al.: Chest gallium scans in patients with KS and/or AIDS. J. Nucl. Med. 27::914, 1986.

Kristersson, S.: Prediction of lung function after lung surgery. A 133Xe-radiospirometric study of regional lung function in bronchial cancer. Scand. J. Thorac. Cardiovasc. Surg. 18(Suppl.):5, 1974.

Lull, R.J., et al.: Radionuclide evaluation lung trauma. Semin. Nucl. Med. 13:223, 1983.

McNeil, B.J.: A diagnostic strategy using ventilation-perfusion studies in patients suspect for pulmonary embolism. J. Nucl. Med. 17:613, 1976.

Moser, K.M., et al.: Study of factors that may condition scintigraphic detection of venous thrombi and pulmonary emboli with indium-111-labeled platelets. J. Nucl. Med. 21:1051, 1980.

Muroff, L.R., and Freedman, G.S.: Radionuclide angiography. Semin. Nucl. Med. 6:217, 1976.

Nichols, A.B., et al.: Scintigraphic detection of pulmonary emboli by serial positron imaging of inhaled 15O-labeled carbon dioxide. N. Engl. J. Med. 299:279, 1978.

Nielsen, P.E., Kirchner, P.T., and Gerber, F.H.: Oblique views in lung perfusion scanning: Clinical utility and limitations. J. Nucl. Med. 18:967, 1977.

Olsen, G.N., Block, A.J., and Tobias, J.A.: Prediction of postpneumonectomy pulmonary function using quantitative macroaggregate lung scanning. Chest 66:13, 1974.

Rhodes, B.A., et al.: Lung scanning with 99mTc-microspheres. Radiology, 99:613, 1971.

Robin, E.D.: Overdiagnosis and overtreatment of pulmonary embolism: the emperor may have no clothes. Ann. Intern. Med. 87:775, 1977.

Rosen, J.M, et al.: 81mKr ventilation imaging: clinical utility in suspected pulmonary embolism. Radiology 154::787, 1985.

Rosenow, E.C., III, Osmundson, P.J., and Brown, M.L.: Pulmonary embolism. Mayo Clin. Proc. 56:161, 1981.

Savage, P., Carmody, R., and Highman, J.: Evaluation of gallium-67 in the diagnosis of bronchial carcinoma. Clin. Radiol. 27:197, 1976.

Schor, R.A., et al.: Regional ventilation studies with 81mKr and 133Xe: a comparative analysis. J. Nucl. Med. 19:348, 1978.

Secker-Walker, R.H., and Provan, J.L.: Scintillation scanning of lungs in preoperative assessment of carcinoma of bronchus. Brit. Med. J. 3:327, 1969.

Simon, T.R., Li, J., and Hoffer, P.B.: The nonspecificity of diffuse pulmonary uptake of 67Ga on 24-hour imaging. Radiology 135:445, 1980.

Slutsky, R.A., and Higgins, C.B.: Thallium scintigraphy in experimental toxic pulmonary edema: Relationship to extravascular pulmonary fluid. J. Nucl. Med. 25:581, 1984.

Sostman, H.D., and Gottschalk, A.: The stripe sign: a new sign for diagnosis of nonembolic defects on pulmonary perfusion scintigraphy. Radiology 142:737, 1982.

Spies, W.G., et al.: Ventilation-perfusion scintigraphy in suspected pulmonary embolism: correlation with pulmonary angiography and refinement of criteria for interpretation. Radiology 159:383, 1986a.

Spies, W.G., and Wojtowicz, C.H., and Spies, S.M.: Value of post-therapy whole-body scans in the evaluation of patients with thyroid carcinoma having undergone high-dose 131I therapy. Radiology 161(P):224, 1986b.

Sullivan, D.C., et al.: Lung scan interpretation: effect of different observers and different criteria. Radiology 149:803, 1983.

Susskind, H., et al.: Efficacy of 81mKr and 127Xe in evaluating nonembolic pulmonary disease (abstr.) J. Nucl. Med. 21:11, 1980.

Taplin, G.V., and Poe, N.D.: A dual lung-scanning technic for evaluation of pulmonary function. Radiology 85:365, 1965.

Toronto Lung Transplant Group: Unilateral lung transplantation for pulmonary fibrosis. N. Engl. J. Med. 314:1140, 1986.

Touya, J.J., et al.: The lung as a metabolic organ. Semin. Nucl. Med. 16:296, 1986a.

Touya, J.J., et al.: Single photon emission computed tomography in the diagnosis of pulmonary thromboembolism. Semin. Nucl. Med. 16:306, 1986b.

Vix, V.A.: The usefulness of chest radiographs obtained after a demonstrated perfusion scan defect in the diagnosis of pulmonary emboli. Clin. Nucl. Med. 8:497, 1983.

Zimmer, A.M., et al.: Radioimmunoimaging of human small cell lung carcinoma with 131I tumor specific monoclonal antibody. Hybridoma 4:1, 1985.

READING REFERENCES

Mettler, F.A., Jr., and Guiberteau, M.J.: Respiratory system. In Essentials of Medicine Imaging, 2nd ed. Orlando, FL, Grune & Stratton, Inc., 1986.

Mettler, F.A., Jr., and Guiberteau, M.J.: Tumor and abscess imaging. In Essentials of Nuclear Medicine Imaging, 2nd ed. Orlando FL, Grune & Stratton, Inc., 1986.

Spies, W.G., Spies, S.M., and Mintzer, R.A.: Radionuclide imaging in diseases of the chest. Part 1. Chest 83:122, 1983.

Spies, W.G., Spies, S.M., and Mintzer, R.A.: Radionuclide imaging in diseases of the chest. Part 2. Chest 83:250, 1983.

Wellman, H.N.: Pulmonary thromboembolism: Current status report on the role of nuclear medicine. Semin. Nucl. Med. 16:236, 1986.

Diagnostic Procedures

CHAPTER 16

LABORATORY PROCEDURES IN THE DIAGNOSIS OF THORACIC DISEASES

Herbert M. Sommers

Pathology has been described as "the study of the harm that disease causes," in terms of both structure and function. The purpose of this chapter is to acquaint the surgeon with different ways of collecting this evidence, with comment on the limitations of each.

TISSUE SPECIMENS FROM BIOPSY AND SURGICAL OPERATIONS

When selecting a site for biopsy or excision of tissue, one should consider several general principles. Benign tumors grow as an expanding mass, compressing and displacing adjacent structures. Expansion of the tumor tends to create either a real or an apparent capsule that may facilitate recognition and delineate the margin of the tumor. In contrast to benign tumors, malignant tumors invade adjacent tissue by irregular infiltration, tending to become fixed to normal structures and making the margins of the tumor irregular and difficult to define. In performing a biopsy of a tumor, one should include a portion of the tumor as well as adjacent tissue that may have been grossly distorted and displaced by the expanding mass. Inclusion of the tumor and adjacent tissue in the same biopsy specimen is helpful in determining whether the tumor is benign or malignant. Occasionally, primary disease processess, such as small tumors of the bronchus, can cause extensive pneumonia in lobes or in the entire lung that is far more impressive than the endobronchial tumor. All biopsy specimens should include a portion of the primary disease as well as secondary changes resulting from obstruction or other complications.

Biopsies at the time of endoscopy can present special problems. If the tumor extends into the lumen of the bronchus, the surface of the tumor may be partially necrotic. For this reason, several "bites" should be taken with the biopsy forceps to obtain enough tissue for good histologic detail. Ulcerating tumors of the bronchus may present another problem as they may excavate and

spread by submucosal lymphatics. When a biopsy forceps cannot be used effectively, a direct smear taken from the ulcer may provide the diagnosis when studied by cytologic methods. Occasionally, a tumor will extend under the adjacent normal mucosa, making it difficult if not impossible to localize. Carcinoma extending along submucosal bronchial lymphatics will usually produce a slight narrowing of the bronchus despite a normal-appearing mucosal surface. In such instances, random biopsy specimens from bronchi in these regions may show small collections of tumor in lymphatics (Fig. 16–1). In general, the larger the portion of tissue taken for a biopsy, the more likely a correct diagnosis can be made. If biopsies do not reveal anticipated findings, the possibility of inadequate sampling should be considered and additional tissue obtained.

In the selection of lymph nodes for biopsy, size and firmness are usually sufficient to differentiate nodes secondarily involved with tumor from those enlarged from infection or other causes. Metastatic carcinoma in a lymph node is typically associated with varying amounts of connective tissue, resulting in an increased firmness to palpation. Occasionally enlarged lymph nodes containing secondary tumor may be soft and appear hyperplastic owing to necrosis of the tumor due to rapid growth. A normal-appearing lymph node included with an abnormal node can act as a "control" for changes found in the abnormal node. The changes found in lymph nodes at different stages of a disease may be helpful in predicting the prognosis. Examination of several lymph nodes can help in differentiating generalized from focal disease.

Frozen Sections

The development of improved cryostats has made the preparation of frozen sections a more reliable procedure than it was in the past. Requests for a "frozen section" should be restricted to two situations: when it is necessary to ensure that biopsy examination has been ade-

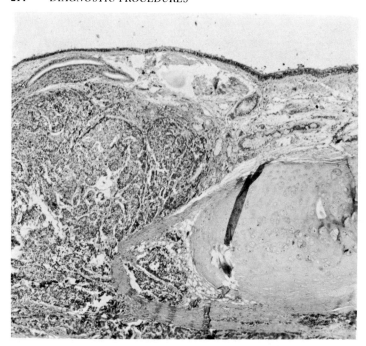

Fig. 16–1. Metastatic tumor beneath normal bronchial mucosa. Biopsy of this region would show tumor despite the intact mucosa. × 250.

quate to establish a diagnosis, and when the type of operation depends on the diagnosis made on the basis of the biopsy specimen. In most instances, tissues from epithelial tumors can be diagnosed rapidly with a high degree of reliability. By contrast, tumors of the reticuloendothelial system pose a more difficult problem, as differentiation from atypical inflammatory or hyperplastic processes may depend on subtle changes in cellular composition or structural components, such as reticulum. Asking for a frozen section as a matter of interest when the result will not influence the operation is not warranted, as freezing the tissue induces artifacts that can make the subsequent interpretation of paraffin sections more difficult.

When taking a biopsy specimen for frozen section, include as much tissue as is prudent under the circumstances. In order to cut a frozen section, one destroys a certain amount of the biopsy specimen, and, in rare instances, tumor that may have been seen in the frozen section of a small specimen may not be found in the paraffin sections. This occurrence is usually a consequence of removal of an inadequate portion of tissue for examination. If a frozen section is needed, the biopsy specimen should not be placed in a fixative solution to send to the laboratory because coagulation by formalin and other tissue fixatives changes the water content of the tissue and lowers its freezing temperature. Most mechanically refrigerated cryostats cannot achieve temperatures low enough to freeze fixed tissue.

Consultation Between Pathologist and Surgeon

The pathologist prefers to examine the tissue and microscopic sections without being prejudiced by the clinical history and physical findings. Since this is not always practical, specimens should be accompanied by a short history along with pertinent physical findings. Even more desirable is a conference between the surgeon and the pathologist at the time the frozen section is examined.

The surgeon can describe the operative findings and answer any questions the pathologist may have.

Consultation prior to biopsy may also be helpful for selected patients to arrange for special studies, such as immunofluorescence or electron microscopy. Collection and handling of specimens for such studies require specific reagents or prompt freezing. Advance notice of an unusual problem alerts the laboratory to be ready for the specimen and facilitates processing the tissue for any special procedures indicated. With good communication, an excellent understanding develops between the pathologist and the surgeon, with a direct reflection on the quality of patient care.

Cultures

When biopsy or excision has been completed, the specimen should be sent immediately to the laboratory in a *sterile container.* Unless the clinician has no question about the etiologic basis of the disease, the specimen should be cultured as well as examined histologically. Both studies can be done by giving portions of the specimen to both the microbiology and pathology laboratories, or by sending the specimen to one laboratory with explicit instructions to forward it to the other. In many instances, the recovery of infectious organisms depends on inoculation of the specimen to specific culture media. Any information concerning the clinical diagnosis or history of recent travel by the patient can be helpful in selecting media and incubation conditions for recovery of an infectious organism.

Smears

In addition to obtaining material for culture, one should place three to four smears of exudate or fluid on glass slides at the time of the operation. One should be prepared with Gram's stain and the others retained, should stains for detection of tuberculosis, fungi, or parasites be necessary. It is easy to discard unneeded slides.

Frequently the diagnosis of a specific infection can be made from a stained smear long before tissue sections are ready or the organism is identified in culture: examples include nocardiosis, actinomycosis, pneumocystis, and legionnaires' disease.

Care of Tissues Removed During the Operation

After cultures have been obtained and frozen sections made, tissues removed at operation should be placed in fixative as soon as possible. Optimal fixation requires a 10:1 ratio of formalin to tissue. When large specimens are placed in small containers, autolytic changes take place, making cellular detail much less discrete and reliable. Portions of lung may float on the surface of a fixative if residual air is trapped in the specimen. To avoid floating and achieve optimal fixation, such specimens should be partially sectioned and kept submerged below the surface of the fixative. In selected pulmonary specimens, injection of formalin into the proximal bronchus can achieve prompt fixation. If a lobe or complete lung is injected with formalin, care should be taken to weigh and measure the specimen first and not to distort it by injecting fluid under pressure.

CYTOLOGIC STUDIES OF BRONCHIAL SECRETIONS AND PLEURAL FLUID

Morning Sputum Specimens

Cytologic examination of sputum specimens is helpful and may provide the diagnosis of malignant pulmonary tumors. Specimens obtained immediately after arising in the morning are preferred, although they can be collected at any time. The patient should be instructed concerning the difference between sputum and saliva and given a small container of 50% alcohol so that all cells will be fixed promptly and autolytic changes stopped. Fixatives containing ether, acetone, or alcohol in concentrations greater than 50% should not be used. Precipitation of protein in such fluids produces hardening of the sediment and makes preparation of smears almost impossible. Rapid fixation of expectorated cells is important because cells in the sputum have been completely or partially separated from their blood supply for varying periods of time and usually have undergone some autolysis in vivo. The practice of collecting sputum in fixative solutions at the bedside also decreases autolytic changes that may develop with delayed transportation of the specimen to the laboratory. Any interval between the time of collection of the specimen and the fixation of the cells decreases the quality of cellular detail and the validity of the report (Fig. 16–2).

In patients who cannot produce sputum spontaneously, the use of a heated aerosol or ultrasonic nebulizer can frequently stimulate sufficient sputum to yield satisfactory specimens. For this purpose, 10% hypertonic saline solution or 15% propylene glycol is used in the aerosol. Three specimens on three successive days should be collected to ensure maximum accuracy. Koss (1968) has summarized the methods for obtaining cytologic specimens from the respiratory tract and given recommendations for the use of heated aerosol for sputum induction. If the specimen will be used for culture as well as for cytologic studies, propylene glycol should not be used in the aerosol. Singh and Garrison (1964) found that propylene glycol inhibited or killed certain types of microorganisms. A negative culture from a specimen collected using propylene glycol as a cytologic fixative may give a false sense of security.

Pleural Fluid

Malignant tumors extending to the pleural surfaces may exfoliate varying numbers of cells (Fig. 16–3). Individual tumors vary in this respect and occasionally the tumor incites a marked inflammatory reaction without shedding a significant number of malignant cells. The interpretation of cellular changes in pleural fluids can present a difficult problem to the cytologist, as the rapid proliferation of mesothelial and inflammatory cells often shows many of the changes characteristic of tumor cells, such as mitoses, large, prominent nuclei, and increased nuclear-cytoplasmic ratio. The accumulation of high protein-containing fluid within the pleural space serves as an excellent tissue culture system for free cells and consequently mitotic figures may be common. The period of time that an exfoliated cell is present within a fluid before removal by thoracentesis has a direct effect on its appearance, with older cells showing swelling and degenerative changes. Because of the accumulation of degenerating cells, the first fluid withdrawn by thoracentesis in a patient with suspected tumor in the pleural space is less satisfactory for cytologic studies than a fluid sample removed several days later. This fluid should be sent to the cytology laboratory to look for obvious malignant cells. The second thoracentesis should contain a younger and metabolically more active cellular population, providing a more representative sample of the different cellular elements.

Although it is preferable to centrifuge the pleural fluid immediately to prepare smears and cell block specimens, this may not be possible. The addition of ethyl alcohol to result in a 30 to 50% final concentration stops autolytic changes. Making a cell block as well as smears from centrifuged sediment can be helpful in identifying cellular arrangements not apparent on smears. Cell blocks are also useful for histochemical studies, such as the demonstration of intracellular mucin or the accumulation of glycogen.

Fine Needle Aspiration

Fine needle aspiration—FNA—as noted by Frable (1983), is an easy, safe, and inexpensive diagnostic technique well tolerated by patients in the office or other outpatient setting. A thin—No. 21 to 23 gauge—needle is used to aspirate suspicious masses anywhere in the body and the specimen obtained is processed for cytologic or histologic diagnosis. Although surgical biopsy offers greater likelihood of arriving at a more certain diagnosis, FNA offers less risk, less cost, and more convenience. FNA should be strongly considered when: (1)

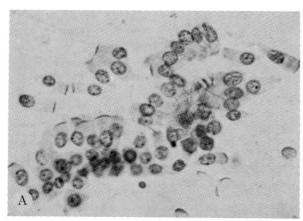

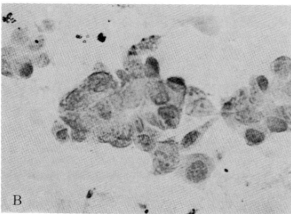

Fig. 16–2. *A*, Smear of normal cells obtained at bronchoscopy and fixed promptly in ether alcohol. Note discrete cell margins, nuclear detail, and cilia on bronchial cells. *B*, Cells from bronchoscopy allowed to dry prior to fixation in ether alcohol. Cell margins are indistinct and nuclear detail is blurred. Occasional nuclei are hyperchromatic and suggest atypical changes. Delay of fixation of bronchial smears seriously decreases the value of the specimen. ×650. (Courtesy of Pacita Manalo-Estrella, M.D.)

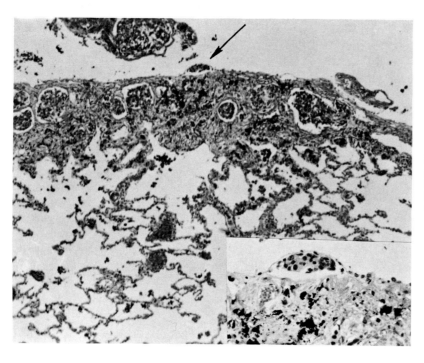

Fig. 16–3. Secondary carcinoma in subpleural lymphatics (see arrow). Groups of tumor cells shed from this surface can be identified from centrifuged pleural fluid. *Inset:* Clump of tumor cells immediately beneath pleural mesothelial membrane.

patients cannot tolerate major surgery; (2) the tumors are clearly unresectable; (3) new masses appear in a patient with multiple previous primary tumors; (4) metastases must be proven or unresectability of tumor must be documented; or (5) deep infections must be diagnosed. Aspiration is performed using fluoroscopy, ultrasound, and CT scan imaging equipment for locating deep lesions. The major limitation of FNA is the risk of a negative report caused by sampling error. Multiple samples obtained by movement of the needle during aspiration produce a more uniform sample and may offer an advantage over the core needle biopsy. Linsk (1986) stressed that improved localization technique increases the yield by assuring aspiration of the intended site.

COLLECTION OF SPECIMENS FOR CULTURE

Specimens for culture may be collected in several ways. Unless due care is taken to minimize contamination from sites other than the one under study, overgrowth by organisms not associated with the infection may occur and result in inappropriate therapy.

The easiest specimen to obtain for culture is sputum. A significant disadvantage of sputum lies in contamination by oral and pharyngeal organisms. Many sputum specimens contain only salivary and oropharyngeal secretions and frequently represent an honest but ineffective effort by the patient to raise secretions from the lower respiratory tract. In one study, collection of sputum by expectoration and culture for pneumococci by standard procedures resulted in isolation of *Streptococcus pneumoniae* in only 55% of patients with both clinical pneumonia and pneumococcal bacteremia. Although all the reasons for the poor recovery of *S. pneumoniae* by culture are not known, evidence suggests that interaction with other organisms or products from organisms found in the oropharynx, such as the alpha-hemolytic streptococci, may suppress growth of the pneumococcus. Dilworth and associates (1975) have reported that partial suppression of the endogenous flora in culture using gentamicin-containing blood agar has resulted in marked improvement in recovery of *S. pneumoniae* from sputum in patients with pneumonia.

Similary, Sanders and Sanders (1982) reported isolating from *Streptococcus salivarius* a compound they call enocin that may contribute to the protection from infection from group A *Streptococcus*. *Streptococcus salivarius* is part of the normal flora of the oropharynx.

Another method for collection of material for culture from the lower respiratory tract is the induction of sputum by ultrasonic or heated saline nebulization. Aerosolization increases the moisture content of the air going to the lower respiratory tract and improves the ability of the tracheobronchial cilia to bring up otherwise thick, viscid, or partially dehydrated secretions. Nebulization is particularly well suited for the recovery of *Mycobacterium tuberculosis* but can also be used for inducing sputum in patients with other types of pulmonary infection.

To determine whether a sputum specimen represents true secretions from an acutely inflamed portion of the bronchopulmonary tree rather than saliva or oropharyngeal secretions, it has been recommended that Gram's stain be used to evaluate the quality of the specimen before it is cultured. If the majority of cells present are neutrophils or other types of inflammatory cells, the specimen should be inoculated to culture media, but if most of the cells appear to be from squamous epithelium, presumably from the oropharynx, the laboratory should request an additional specimen. Finding large numbers of segmented neutrophils indicates a cellular response to an acute injury, most often associated with an acute bacterial infection. Van Scoy (1977) suggested that the different types and relative numbers of bacteria should be noted also, as well as whether there is evidence of bacterial phagocytosis.

The value of the Gram stain is to determine the number and type of bacteria in the area adjacent to segmented neutrophils. If a true infection is present, most bacteria are the same type rather than mixed. Assuming the patient has a bacterial pneumonia, the bacterial morphotype seen on the Gram stain should correlate with the causative agent of the pneumonia and aid the technologist in selecting the optimal isolation media. In an immunosuppressed, neutropenic patient, a Gram stain showing large numbers of the same type of bacteria may be the only guide available in the early diagnosis of the infectious agent causing pneumonia.

Tracheal cannulation, bronchoscopy, and bronchial brushing guided by fluoroscopy are additional methods for the collection of cytologic and culture specimens from the lower respiratory tract. All of these procedures are subject to some degree of oropharyngeal microbial contamination. An additional limitation to using material collected at bronchoscopy for culture has been shown by Conte and Laforet (1962) as well as by Kleinfield and Elliss (1967), who found that local anesthetic agents used in bronchoscopy may inhibit the growth of non-acid fast and anaerobic bacteria as well as fungi.

One of the best ways to collect a specimen for culture from the lower respiratory tract is translaryngeal aspiration. In this procedure, a large-bore needle is passed percutaneously between the cricothyroid and thyroid cartilages of the larynx, and a small plastic catheter is introduced into the trachea. Saline is administered through the catheter and then quickly aspirated along with tracheobronchial secretions. The saline used for injection must not contain bacteriostatic agents such as benzyl alcohol or methyl- or propylparaben. These agents are incorporated into saline used for injection of medication to prevent growth of contaminants and, as noted by Rein and Mandell (1973), may quickly kill the bacteria that cause acute pneumonia. The tracheobronchial tree below the larynx normally is sterile, and organisms found usually reflect bacterial or fungal agents associated with infection in the lower respiratory tract. Translaryngeal aspiration can cause considerable discomfort to the patient, who may be seized with intense coughing spasms following injection of saline into the trachea. The procedure should be done only after careful consideration of the potential advantages and disadvantages.

BACTERIAL INFECTIONS OF THE LUNG

Aerobic Infections

Streptococcus pneumoniae

The discovery of penicillin has removed pneumococcal pneumonia as one of the leading causes of death. Despite the availability of penicillin, the pneumococcus is still a significant cause of pneumonia and can be difficult to isolate. The diagnosis of pneumococcal pneumonia is made on the basis of sputum smears showing lancet-shaped, gram-positive diplococci and recovery of the organism from cultures. Rathbun and Govani (1967) have shown that recovery of pneumococci from sputum can be increased 47% by using intraperitoneal mouse inoculation. Presumably this improvement results for a combination of the susceptibility of the mouse to virulent pneumococci and the ability of the animal to reject the contaminating "normal" bacterial flora that otherwise overgrow the fastidious pneumococcus. Barrett-Connet (1971) noted that blood cultures from patients seriously ill with acute pneumonia were positive for pneumococci in 45% of patients when the organism could not be recovered from a sputum culture. Such a study serves to illustrate the problem of obtaining a true sputum specimen and the effect of contaminating oropharyngeal bacteria on the isolation of agents causing bacterial pneumonia.

Staphylococcus aureus

Primary staphylococcal pneumonia is not common in adults. When present, staphylococcal pneumonia is usually a complication of aspiration or sequela of virus diseases such as influenza or measles. It is a potentially very dangerous infection, owing to the high incidence of abscess formation, and the not infrequent resistance of the organism to penicillin and other antibiotics. In infants, staphylococcal lung infections may be associated with hemorrhagic pneumonia rather than abscess formation.

Klebsiella pneumonia

Of all the Enterobacteriaceae, the organism most often causing pneumonia is *Klebsiella pneumoniae*. Like the staphylococcus, it concerns the thoracic surgeon because of the high incidence of associated abscess and cavity formation. It is important to distinguish *Klebsiella pneumoniae* from the similar-appearing *Enterobacter* species, as the enterobacter organisms are rarely associated with pulmonary infections.

Anaerobic Infections

Although infection in the lung with anaerobic bacteria may seem to be a paradox, it represents one of the more serious types of infections encountered by the thoracic surgeon. Anaerobic bacteria are normally present in the upper and lower respiratory tract, usually outnumbering aerobic bacteria. Since proliferating anaerobic bacteria can rapidly reduce the oxygen content of their surrounding micro-environment, growth may occur at any point within the lung where inflammation or necrosis is present. Usually some initiating factor precedes growth of anaerobic bacteria, such as aspiration of oral or gastric contents or an obstructing foreign body.

Bartlett and Finegold (1974) analyzed 143 patients with anaerobic bacterial infections of the lung and suggested a classification of four clinical types of infection: lung abscess—arbitrarily defined as a solitary or dominant cavity measuring at least 2 cm in diameter; necrotizing pneumonia—multiple small areas of cavitation within one or more pulmonary segments or lobes; pneumonitis—pulmonary infiltrate with no evidence of cavitation; and empyema—infected pleural exudate. The last category, empyema, usually overlaps one of the other types of infection and is best treated by surgical drainage. In a further review, Bartlett (1979) compared anaerobic bacterial pneumonitis to pneumococcal pneumonia and noted that patients with the former condition were more likely to develop an abscess, even when being treated with appropriate antibiotics. Patients with pneumonia from anaerobic bacteria were also more likely to have an occult bronchial carcinoma than patients with pneumococcal pneumonia.

Many anaerobic bacteria metabolize proteins in the tissues of the host to form aromatic, volatile amines and produce strong and offensive odors. Most abscesses caused by anaerobic bacteria contain several types of organism, contributing to the difficulty of therapy. Recovery and identification of the invading bacteria in the laboratory are difficult and slow, requiring special procedures, prereduced culture media, and prolonged incubation times. For optimal recovery of anaerobic bacteria, sputum or tracheal aspirates from patients with pulmonary abscesses should be taken to the laboratory in special oxygen-free containers immediately after collection. Exposure of the culture specimen to air for even short periods may rapidly inactivate fastidious anaerobes and result in a false impression of the cause of the infection. Gram's stain on the abscess fluid should be made and correlated with the morphotypes of the bacteria isolated from the culture.

Legionnaires' Disease

In July, 1976, a strange and virulent form of pneumonia struck 182 members of the Pennsylvania branch of the American Legion during their annual meeting in Philadelphia; 18 legionnaires died. During the next 6 months an intensive investigation resulted in the isolation of a new, completely different bacterial organism, now known as *Legionella pneumophila*. This organism differs from other medically significant bacteria in that it does not stain by Gram's method and is unique in having an absolute growth requirement for cysteine. An adequate amount of this compound to grow *Legionella* is not present in blood agar, chocolate agar, or other types of primary culture media. The organism also requires an increased concentration of CO_2 for growth and may take 7 to 12 days to appear on artificial culture media.

The diagnosis of *Legionella pneumophila* pneumonia is best established by recovering the organism in culture and then following procedures for identification. More commonly the diagnosis is made by immunologic procedures, including direct fluorescent antibody staining of the organism in lung biopsies or pleural fluid as reported by Cherry and associates (1978). The most commonly used method to establish the diagnosis of legionnaires' disease has been to demonstrate a fourfold or greater rise in titer or specific antibody to the organism.

Clinically, the disease may occur in epidemics, such as was seen in Philadelphia, or as sporadic cases acquired in the community. As noted by Balows and Fraser (1979), it has been recognized as a major cause of serious or fatal pneumonia in immune-suppressed or immune-defective patients, many of whom develop the disease while in the hospital.

As an increased awareness of *Legionella pneumophila* has stimulated efforts to recover the organism, similar although distinctly non-*Legionella pneumophila* organisms have been isolated from patients with severe respiratory infections. Most of these related organisms, like *Legionella pneumophila*, were first found by passage of blood or sputum through guinea pigs or embryonated hens' eggs, or both. Since these procedures are used to isolate rickettsia, many of these organisms have been called "rickettsia-like." Feeley and his co-workers (1979) reported that with more experience and knowledge it has become possible to grow many of these organisms on a charcoal yeast-extract culture medium, allowing a much more detailed study for classification. Examples of these rickettsia-like organisms that are similar to, yet distinct from *Legionella pneumophila* included *Legionella micdadei*—the Pittsburgh Pneumonia Agent—reported by Meyerowitz and his colleagues (1979) and WIGA reported by Thomason and his associates (1979).

With continued efforts to look for and identify *Legionella pneumophila* and the *Legionella*-like organisms, additional species have been isolated from humans and environmental sources. These are summarized in Table 16–1. Although not all species have been isolated from humans at this time, Cherry and co-workers (1982) have shown that detection of antibodies in human patients to species isolated only from the environment suggest that they are the cause of disease in humans as well. Stout and co-workers (1982) showed that the isolation of *Legionella pneumophila* and related species initially from the water in air-conditioning cooling towers and subsequently from the faucets, shower heads, and hot water storage tanks in hospitals has emphasized the ubiquitousness of this group of organisms. Since the organisms are widespread, it is clear that mere exposure to contaminated water is an insufficient condition for the occurrence of legionnaire's disease. Host susceptibility is undoubtedly a critical factor for the development of infection. Patients undergoing immunosuppression for organ transplantation or other therapeutic reasons are at high risk and should be followed carefully for the sudden

Table 16–1.   Legionella species described as of January 1985

Species	Source	Species	Source
L. pneumophila	Lung	L. maceachernii	Water
L. bozemanii	Lung	L. maceachernii	Water
L. micdadei	Blood	L. jamestowniensis	Soil
L. dumoffi	Lung/E	L. rubrilucens	Water
L. gormanii	Soil	L. erythra	Water
L. longbeachae	Lung	L. hackeliae	Lung
L. jordanis	Lung	L. parisiensis	Water
L. oakridgensis	Water	L. cherri ORW^T	Water
L. wadsworthii	Lung	L. steigerwaltii	Water
L. feeleii	Lung	L. santicrucis	Water
L. sainthelensi	Water		
L. anisa	Hot water		

Adapted from Brenner, D.J., et al.: Ten new species of Legionella. Int. J. Syst. Bacteriol. 35:50, 1985.

onset of severe and rapidly developing pneumonia. Diagnosis can be made most effectively by open lung biopsy and direct fluorescent antibody studies. Although culture on enriched and selected media has been helpful, growth may require from 11 to 14 days, and contaminants can be troublesome. Serologic tests to identify bacterial products are under development and may become a valuable, rapid, and specific method for making the diagnosis. Reagents are available to make the diagnosis of legionellosis using recombinant DNA probes. Although expensive, these probes offer an alternative to standard serologic cultural methods not available in many laboratories.

Mycobacteria

Before the discovery of streptomycin and subsequently other chemotherapeutic agents, the diagnosis of tuberculosis was made on the basis of the clinical picture, a roentgenogram of the chest compatible with that of tuberculosis, and the demonstration of acid-fast bacilli in the sputum. Isolation of the organism by culture was done in few hospitals but not routinely because the culture medium was expensive, bacterial contaminants were troublesome, and little was to be gained in treating the patient by recovery of the organism. With the development of antituberculous drugs, however, it became necessary to isolate the organism so that drug susceptibility studies could be made and resistance detected. As more cultures were made, variant strains from the typical type of organism—*Mycobacterium tuberculosis*—responsible for tuberculosis in human beings were found. In 1954, Timpe and Runyon described 100 such strains, proposing a grouping for "atypical" organisms. Although the variant strains have been called by several names, including atypical, anonymous, and unclassified, all of these terms should now be dropped.

In 1959, Runyon published a more complete description of the variant mycobacteria, and for convenience classified them into four groups, I to IV. Members of group I were called *photochromogens*, because of the yellow pigment made by young colonies after exposure to light. *Mycobacterium kansasii* was the most important member of this group, which includes *M. simiae* and *M. marinum*—an organism causing "swimmers' granuloma." Group II organisms were called *scotochromogens* because of the production of pigment by colonies when grown in either the dark or the light. In some strains, exposure to light was noted to intensify pigment from yellow to orange. *M. scrofulaceum*, isolated from cervical adenitis in children, and *M. gordonae*, the so-called tap-water bacilli, were classified in this group. Group III were called *nonphotochromogens*, and ordinarily were nonpigmented although some strains may be a pale yellow. The most important group of organisms in the group III nonphotochromogenic mycobacteria are derived from *Mycobacterium avium*, an organism that causes infection in swine and birds, and the closely related *Mycobacterium intracellulare*, a similar organism that causes infection in humans, also known as the Battey bacillus. The similarity between these two groups of organisms has been known for many years and is reflected in part by the increasing tendency to refer to them as the *M. avium-intracellulare*—MAI—complex or, more simply, as the organisms in the *M. avium* complex. Group IV organisms were characterized by growth within several days and were therefore called *rapid growers*. Mycobacteria classified in group IV included *M. smegmatis*, *M. phlei*, *M. fortuitum* and *M. chelonei*. Only *M. fortuitum* and *M. chelonei* have been known to cause infection in man. Levy and associates (1977) reported several outbreaks of infections with these two organisms that occurred following cardiac surgery and mammoplasty.

For many years the Runyon groups I to IV served as a helpful outline for use in classifying newly isolated, variant strains of mycobacteria on the basis of pigment production, colonial appearance, and rate of growth. With time, exceptions to the original criteria became more numerous, and biochemical and metabolic tests enabling a more reliable identification were developed. Even the terms photochromogen and scotochromogen have less significance since it was found that *M. szulgai* is photochromogenic when grown at 24°C and scotochromogenic at 37°C. Similarly, *M. xenopi*, long placed in the group III nonphotochromogens, is usually considered a scotochromogen on initial isolation because of its intense yellow pigmentation. It is now recommended that all mycobacteria isolated from man be completely identified and that individual organisms be referred to by specific names rather than as members of groups I to IV. Recommended names with synonyms and relative pathogenicity are listed in Table 16–2. The clinical significance of the nontuberculous mycobacteria has been well summarized by Wolinsky (1979).

Specimen Collection in Pulmonary Tuberculosis

Sputum is the most easily collected specimen for use in making the diagnosis of pulmonary tuberculosis. A series of three to five early-morning specimens is recommended because experience shows that the number of bacilli shed varies from day to day in patients excreting low numbers of organisms. This variation is probably related to intermittent focal ulceration of the bronchial mucosa, releasing different numbers of tubercle bacilli in the bronchi over irregular periods. Krasnow and Wayne (1969) showed that specimens collected by heated aerosol or nebulization after the patient arises in the morning produce positive cultures after shorter incubation and with fewer contaminants than do specimens collected over 24-hour intervals. The 24-hour specimens yielded more positive cultures although they required longer incubation times and were more likely to be contaminated. Both types of specimens are of value. Collection at bronchoscopy of secretions for culture is best done by using bronchial washings or bronchial lavage, but these specimens should be processed immediately if local anesthetics have been used to facilitate passage of the bronchoscope. The use of small sponges for recovery of tubercle bacilli at bronchoscopy is not satisfactory, owing to the difficulty in removing mycobacteria from the matrix of the sponge. Bronchial brushes, used in collecting specimens for cytology, provide good specimens for culture. Note that following bronchoscopy, recovery of myocbacteria increases in sputum specimens collected over the succeeding 24 to 48 hours. Early-morning gastric aspiration for organisms swallowed during the night is recommended only for infants or children or for those patients whose sputum cannot be obtained naturally or by heated aerosol. The recovery of saprophytic, nonpathogenic species of mycobacteria from gastric aspirates can mislead the clinician until such time as identification of the organism is complete. In early stages of disseminated miliary tuberculosis, sputum specimens may not show the organism prior to invasion and ulceration of the bronchial tree. Demonstration or isolation of the organism in miliary tuberculosis may best be accomplished by liver biopsy, by bone marrow aspiration, or possibly by cerebrospinal fluid examination. Lung biopsy is helpful frequently.

Concentration Procedures

Isolation of *M. tuberculosis* and other mycobacteria from sputum and other types of contaminated clinical specimens is facilitated by a digestion procedure to release mycobacteria from mucin, kill contaminating bacteria, and concentrate the number of mycobacteria to a smaller volume.

Inoculation of the concentrated specimen should be made to a minimum of two and preferably three different types of culture media, with an egg base—Lowenstein-Jensen—and an agar base—Middlebrook 7H11 agar—currently the most popular. A third culture medium containing one or more antibiotics is strongly recommended to suppress nonmycobacterial organisms. Incubation of all media in 5 to 10% carbon dioxide results in an increased yield and rate of growth.

Stained smears of the concentrate should be made to search for the orgnisms as well as to observe the numbers shed—an indication of the activity of the infection. Sputum smears are positive for mycobacteria in approximately 60 to 70% of specimens yielding positive cultures. Smears may be stained by one of the classic acid-fast

Table 16–2. Nomenclature of mycobacteria

Legitimate Name	Relative Pathogenicity for Man	Equivalent Runyon Group	Acceptable Common Name	Names Without Legitimate Standing and Comments
M. africanum	+ + +			Intermediate form between *M. bovis* and *M. tuberculosis*. Found in North and Central Africa
M. asiaticum	+ +	Group I photochromogen		Similar to *M. simiae* but differs antigenically
M. bovis	+ + +		Bovine tubercle bacillus	Causes bovine and human tuberculosis; avirulent strains are used for BCG vaccines
M. chelonei	+	Group IV rapid grower		May cause occasional skin disease. Includes two subspecies, ss. *chelonei* and ss. *abscessus*
M. flavescens	0	Group II scotochromogen, sometimes placed with group IV rapid growers		Grows rapidly. It should be differentiated from *M. scrofulaceum*
M. fortuitum	+	Group IV rapid grower		*M. ranae; M. minetti*—wound, skin, and lung infections. It may cause disease in immunosuppressed host
M. gastri	0	Group III nonphoto-chromogen		Not known to be pathogenic for man. It may be found in gastric aspirates
M. gordonae	0	Group II scotochromogen	Tap-water scotochromogens	*M. aquae*—rarely, if ever, pathogenic for man
M. haemophilum	+ + +	None		Requires hemin for growth. Causes skin disease. Grows at 32°C
M. avium-intracellulare complex	+ + +	Group III nonphoto-chromogen	Battey bacillus	*M. batteyi, M. battey*—frequently drug-resistant
M. kansasii	+ + +	Group I photochromogen		Rare, nonpigmented, scotochromogenic, and niacin-positive strains
M. malmoense	+ + + +	Group III nonphoto-chromogens		Causes pulmonary disease similar to *M. tuberculosis*
M. marinum	+ + +	Group I photochromogen		*M. balnei, M. platypeocilus*—associated with skin infections
M. scrofulaceum	+ +	Group II scotochromogens		*M. marianum*—may cause cervical lymphadenitis
M. simiae	+ +	Group I photochromogen		*M. habana*—facultatively pathogenic; photoreactivity may be unstable; it is niacin-positive
M. szulgai	+ + +	Group I photochromogen at 25°C; Group II scotochromogen at 37°C		Associated with chronic pulmonary and extrapulmonary disease; distinctive lipid composition of cell walls
M. terrae	Rare	Group III nonphoto-chromogen	"Radish bacillus"	May be closely related to *M. triviale*
M. triviale	0	Group III nonphoto-chromogen	"V" bacillus	Has been called "atypical-atypical" mycobacterium for rough colonies
M. tuberculosis	+ + +	Human tuberculosis	Human tubercle bacillus	Causes human tuberculosis—highly contagious
M. ulcerans	+ + +			Associated with skin infections in tropics—*M. buruli*
M. xenopei	+ +	Group III nonphoto-chromogens (scoto-chromogen)		*M. littorale, M. xenopei*—grows slowly; best at 42°C; may contaminate hot-water system

techniques—Ziehl-Neelsen—or by a fluorochrome—auramine or a combination of auramine and rhodamine. The advantage of the fluorochrome stain is that it enables the microscopist to scan a larger field in a shorter period of time without loss of specificity. Although experienced microscopists may be able to tell different species of mycobacteria by their shape on a stained smear, identifying characteristics are subtle and usually not dependable unless the observer sees many smears from patients with different species of mycobacteria.

Identification of Mycobacteria

In the identification of all mycobacteria it is essential that the organisms demonstrate the characteristic size, shape, and staining reaction of the genus *Mycobacterium*. The rate of growth, both at room temperature and 37°C, should be determined with inocula sufficiently dilute to show individual colonies. Photoreactivity and pigment production can be easily determined by wrapping cultures in aluminum foil and incubating at both 24° and 37°C.

M. tuberculosis is characterized by slow growth—3 weeks at 37°C. Inoculation of large numbers of organisms may produce visible growth in shorter periods. Slow growth may occur at slightly lower or higher temperatures, but variations in growth rate are unusual and can be determined by repeating the cultures with a diluted inoculum and controlled incubation temperature. Colonies of *M. tuberculosis* grown on Lowenstein-Jensen medium are buff in color, irregular, rough, and raised above the surface of the medium. Growth in a small, tightly packed colony is considered due in part to the high lipid content of the bacterial cell wall, producing a hydrophobic reaction. In contrast to the small, "breadcrumb"-like colonies on egg-base media, early growth of *M. tuberculosis* on 7H11 agar is thin, filmy, and spreading. Certain strains of *M. bovis* are similar in appearance to *M. tuberculosis* on both types of media but, for comparable growth, usually require longer incubation periods than does *M. tuberculosis*.

The definitive identification of *M. tuberculosis* depends on several easily performed biochemical tests. The most important characteristic of *M. tuberculosis* is production of niacin in culture media. In addition to the niacin test, tests for nitrate reductase and catalase are helpful in the identification of *M. tuberculosis*. The semiquantitative catalase test is helpful in ruling out other members of the mycobacteria, because *M. tuberculosis* gives only a weakly positive reaction. Of more importance, strains of *M. tuberculosis* resistant to isoniazid—INH—are catalase negative.

The complete identification of all mycobacterial isolates is almost mandatory, as the distinction between organisms known to cause disease and those not associated with disease is important in selecting proper therapy. The use of a Runyon group designation is not adequate for this purpose. Species identification can usually be accompanied by determining relatively few characteristics. Although the incidence of tuberculosis has continued to decline, the incidence of disease from myco-

bacteria other than *M. tuberculosis* is becoming more common.

The proper determination of antimycobacterial drug susceptibility is a highly technical and expensive procedure. Primary drug resistance of *M. tuberculosis*, defined as resistance by an organism to one or more drugs in a previously untreated patient, was thought to be less than 5%. Kopanoff and his associates (1978), however, have noted that a more widely selected group of patients has shown primary drug resistance of *M. tuberculosis* in 8 to 20% of isolates, depending upon geographic location and ethnic group sampled. This previously unrecognized primary drug resistance of *M. tuberculosis* has suggested the need for more frequent routine determination of susceptibility studies than was considered necessary in the past.

Radiometric Procedures for the Mycobacteriology Laboratory

Middlebrook and associates (1977) described a broth culture medium—7H12—containing 1-^{14}C palmitic acid that could be used for the detection of the growth of *M. tuberculosis*. The method relies upon the measurement of ^{14}C-labeled carbon dioxide released during the metabolism of palmitic acid by mycobacteria in an ion chamber system (Bactec, Johnston Laboratories, Towson, MD). Initial studies with this system indicated that an inoculum of 200 viable units of *M. tuberculosis* could be detected in 12 to 14 days. The results led to further studies for the application of the technique to routine laboratory procedures to include detection, identification, and susceptibility testing with primary antituberculosis drugs by Siddiqui and associates (1981) (Fig. 16–4). A multicenter, collaborative study reported by Snider and associates (1981) found that although the results of drug susceptibility tests of *M. tuberculosis* with the radiometric and standard methods were similar, there was better agreement with the Bactec and the agar dilution procedure when comparing drug-susceptible

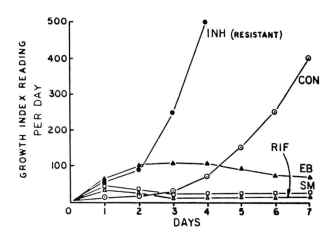

Fig. 16–4. Radiometric drug susceptiblity test pattern of an INH-resistant strain of *M. tuberculosis*. (CON: Control) (Reproduced with permission from Laszlo, A., and Siddiqi, S.H.: Evaluation of a rapid radiometric method for drug susceptibility testing of *Mycobacterium tuberculosis*. J. Clin. Microbiol., *13*:908, 1981.)

strains than with drug-resistant strains. Overall, Siddiqui and associates (1981) found results with the new procedure were better when determined in a specialty laboratory for mycobacteria than in a routine clinical laboratory. Agreement for drug susceptiblity testing between radiometric and standard agar dilution methods for *M. tuberculosis* was 95%. In addition, test results were reportable on 98% of the tests in 5 days. Although several problems were encountered with the determinations of *M. tuberculosis* susceptibility to ethambutol, these were believed to be due to test vials containing an inappropriate concentration of the drug.

Using the Bactec, *M. tuberculosis* can usually be detected rapidly in decontaminated clinical specimens by inoculation to a selective Middlebrook 7H12—medium containing polymyxin B, amphotericin B, carbenicillin, and trimethoprim—PACT. Damato and associates (1983) showed that 70% of smear-positive specimens are culture positive in the radiometric procedure within 14 days, with or without the addition of PACT to the medium, compared with 21 days by the standard procedure. Similarly, Morgan and associates (1983) found that detection times for recovery of *M. tuberculosis* from smear-negative specimens with radiometric and conventional culture systems were 13.7 and 26.3 days, respectively. Radiometric and conventional culture procedures were approximately equivalent for the recovery of *M. tuberculosis* from, 5,375 clinical specimens, but Takahashi and Foster (1983) found the recovery of *M. avium* complex was better using the radiometric procedure. In another collaborative study reported by Roberts and associates (1983) involving five laboratories, recovery and drug susceptibility tests of *M. tuberculosis* were completed in 18 days using the radiometric procedure, as opposed to 38.5 days for the conventional method.

Throughout these early developmental periods, the *Mycobacterium* species isolated by Bactec were unknown until routine identification procedures were completed. Therefore, the initial time saved in detection of mycobacteria might have been of little benefit, since 4 to 8 weeks were still needed for species identification. Another problem was the recognition by several laboratories that an absolute increase occurred in the isolation by the radiometric procedure of nonpathogenic mycobacteria—e.g., *M. gordonae*. Initially, it was recommended that all isolates recovered from the radiometric procedure should be subcultured and streaked for isolation before individual colonies could be obtained for identification by standard methods.

Fortunately, a procedure using the radiometric method provides rapid identification of *M. tuberculosis*. *M. tuberculosis* can be identified in 4 to 5 days by this method, in contrast to nontuberculous mycobacteria. This procedure was described by Morgan and associates (1985) by measuring the susceptibility of the isolate to p-nitro-d-acetylamino-β-hydroxypropiophenone—NAP. Both the rate of $^{14}CO_2$ evolution and susceptibility to NAP are used as identification criteria. The rate of CO_2 evolution is helpful because it is directly proportional to the number of cells in culture. This makes it possible to presumptively identify isolates of the *M. tuberculosis* complex—more apt to be pathogenic—and to promptly distinguish the *M. tuberculosis* strains from the increased numbers of nontuberculous mycobacteria that are NAP-test-negative.

Mycobacterium Avium Complex and AIDS

With the recognition of the acquired immune deficiency syndrome—AIDS—Greene and associates (1982) found that one of the most common opportunistic infections in this group of patients is from organisms of the *Mycobacterium avium* complex—MAC. Presenting symptoms may include chronic diarrhea, associated with extensive invasion of the mucosal villi of the small and large intestine by the bacilli. Hawkins (1986) reported that there may also be diffuse dissemination of MAC organisms to the reticuloendothelial system, including the liver, bone marrow, and spleen, as well as, but not always, to the lungs. Diagnosis of MAC infection can often be made by positive acid-fast stained smears and cultures from the stool or biopsies of the intestinal mucosa, liver, or bone-marrow, or cultures of the sputum or blood. Often positive blood cultures can establish the diagnosis of MAC infection before any changes are noted in the chest roentgenogram. Blood cultures should be drawn from the high risk patient on the basis of fever and malaise.

Blood Cultures for Mycobacteria

Recently, through the use of the lysis centrifugation—Isolator—and radiometric—Bactec—blood culture procedures, it has been possible to recover mycobacteria from blood specimens in 6 to 12 days. Recovery of mycobacteria by the Isolator blood culture system is based on the principle of lysis of both the red and white blood cells in a 10 ml sample of blood followed by centrifugation and sedimentation of mycobacteria in the blood collection tube.

The centrifuged pellet containing any organisms is then inoculated directly to egg-base or 7H11 mycobacterial culture media as well as 7H12A, a broth medium containing 1-^{14}C-palmitic acid for use with the radiometric growth detection ion chamber, Bactec.

Macker and associates (1982) and Gill and Stock (1987) reported that combined use of the lysis centrifugation and radiometric systems provides the most rapid recovery of mycobacteria from blood. Although the radiometric detection system does not distinguish between all the different mycobacterial species, members of the *Mycobacterium tuberculosis* complex can be identified by the NAP test. When the same blood sample is processed, first by the lysis-centrifugation and then by the radiometric procedure, positive results can be found in 6 to 12 days. If the mycobacterial blood culture isolate is not a member of the *M. tuberculosis* complex, identification is accomplished by subculture and isolation to egg-base or agar medium using standard procedures.

Nucleic Acid Hybridization of Mycobacteria

In addition to the radiometric instrument to help isolate and identify *M. tuberculosis*, the use of nucleic acid and hybridization has been applied to the identification and differentiation between *M. tuberculosis* and *M. avium* complex. This procedure has been found by Kiehn and Edwards (1987) to be rapid, and quite specific. To date most studies have been made on pure isolates of mycobacteria but tests are currently being conducted using genetic probes for the direct detection of pathogenic mycobacteria in clinical specimens of sputum and urine.

FUNGAL INFECTION OF THE LUNG

Fungal infection of the lung is best established by recovery of the infecting organism by culture. Morphologic changes in tissue biopsy specimens may be adequate to establish a diagnosis without culture. Histochemical staining, with periodic acid—PAS, methenamine silver, mucicarmine, or Gram's stain, of histologic sections is helpful and may afford specific identification of different fungi, but all too often it is not possible to find pathognomonic organisms in the stained specimens and only a presumptive diagnosis can be made. Perhaps the two best stains for demonstration of fungi in tissue are PAS and methenamine silver, but there is no one stain that will demonstrate all organisms. Figure 16–5 illustrates a gram-stained section of material taken from a pulmonary abscess due to *Nocardia asteroides*. Since *Nocardia asteroides* is not stained by hematoxylin or eosin, or the periodic acid-Schiff stain, it cannot be recognized unless Gram's stain or a methenamine silver stain is used. Although some strains of Nocardia may show an ability to retain an acid-fast or auramine stain, smears or sections have to be decolorized by a much milder solution of acid—1% sulfuric versus 3% hydrochloric. The ability to identify Nocardia in acid-fast and auramine-stained specimens will vary considerably between different strains.

Cultures of fungi can be made from tissues, sputum, pleural fluid, bronchial aspirates, or other clinical specimens. For optimal recovery, all specimens should be inoculated on several different types of culture media. Sabouraud's dextrose agar is an excellent general-purpose culture medium. It is able to inhibit many strains of contaminating bacteria because its high dextrose content—4%—reduces the pH to 5.6. Specimens should also be inoculated to a second medium containing antibiotics and cycloheximide to suppress less fastidious bacteria and the contaminating molds. Since the cycloheximide and antibiotics in the second medium will also inhibit certain pathogenic fungi, such as *Cryptococcus neoformans*, *Nocardia asteroides*, and *Aspergillus fumigatis*, use of Sabouraud's or a similar noninhibitory agar should not be omitted. Sabouraud's medium should be incubated at both 25° and 37°C, because different fungi may have varying rates of growth and different morphologic forms when grown at different temperatures. Fungi with more than one form are called "dimorphic," showing a yeast-like morphology at 37°C and a mycelial growth when incubated at room temperature—25°C. Examples of "dimorphic" fungi are *Histo-

plasma capsulatum*, *Blastomyces dermatitidis*, and *Sporothrix schenckii*. Growth of pathogenic fungi may take from 2 to 14 days, depending on the number of organisms present in the specimens and characteristics of the individual organism. For some fungi, unique growth requirements have led to special media. Any clinical information that may indicate the most likely organism will help in selecting the medium most likely to produce growth in the minimal time.

Members of the Candida and Cryptococcus species are easily identified by means of fermentation and carbohydrate assimilation tests. The use of several other biochemical tests in the speciation of fungi is helpful, but most pathogenic fungi are identified by morphologic characteristics noted on culture, such as septate or nonseptate mycelia, unique macro-or microconidia, and the gross and microscopic appearance of the growth nurtured on different types of media at 37°C and at room temperatures. Identification is usually made by examining portions of the culture under the microscope and by preparing small "growing mounts," where the developing pattern of growth is followed by microscopic examination over a period of several days. Unfortunately, some fungi lose certain of their specific features in culture, with the result that identification may take a prolonged period of time. Disseminated disease has been diagnosed by Musial and associates (1987). They used the lysis-centrifugation procedure, confirming that the mode of spread in the acute case is similar to tuberculosis.

Skin tests to detect hypersensitivity to fungi should be restricted to persons suspected of having histoplasmosis or coccidioidomycosis. Cross reactions and lack of specificity of antigens have made skin tests for blastomycosis, candidiasis, and cryptococcosis unreliable. A positive reaction to histoplasmin or coccidioidin indicates only that the patient has had contact with the antigen at some time in the past. It may be of little value in determining whether a current illness is caused by a specific fungus unless it is known that the patient's reaction to that antigen was negative at some time in the recent past. If the reaction to the skin test becomes negative in a patient with known, active histoplasmosis or coccidioidomycosis, this change may indicate a state of anergy and a dim prognosis.

Many patients have had subclinical infections with different fungi, so a positive reaction to a serologic test for a fungal antigen in a random specimen may have little significance. To differentiate between an old and a current fungal infection on the basis of serologic tests, antibody titers are determined on serum obtained early in the course of illness—acute phase—and at least 2 to 3 weeks later—convalescent phase. Laboratory precision in most serologic tests is seldom better than 1 dilution—twofold change—so that the results of most serologic tests should not be considered significant unless there is an increase or decrease of at least two dilutions—fourfold change—such as any from 1:4 to 1:16. In some patients, fungal infections may develop during immunosuppressive therapy for tumors or organ transplants. In these patients, both humoral and cell-bound immune re-

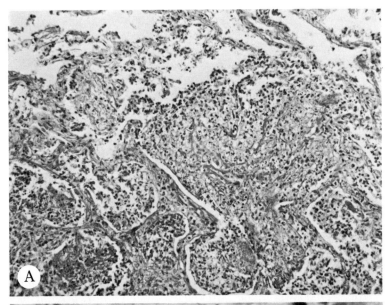

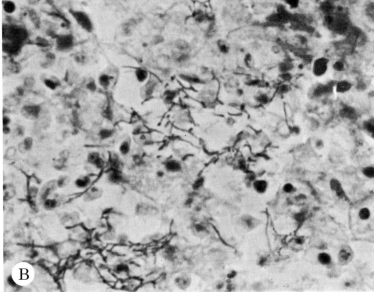

Fig. 16–5. Pulmonary abscess due to *Nocardia asteroides.* The nocardial infections cause suppuration with abscess formation. *A*, Section stained with hematoxylin and eosin or PAS does not demonstrate the organism. *B*, Gram-stained section shows thin, branching rods. × 650.

sponses may be modified by drugs so that these responses to serologic tests may not be valid. Because of the infrequent need for such tests in most hospitals, requests for fungal serology are usually forwarded to municipal or state public health laboratories, resulting in some delay in obtaining the report. Direct communication with the reference laboratory usually hastens receipt of the report.

Of serologic tests for all the so-called deep fungal infections, those for blastomycosis are the least satisfactory. Cross reactions with other antigens are most prone to occur. The immunodiffusion—ID—test for blastomycosis is specific, and a positive reaction can result in immediate treatment of the patient. The test has a sensitivity of approximately 80% and detects more blastomycosis cases than the complement-fixation test. Negative tests do not exclude a diagnosis. In contrast to blastomycosis, the serologic diagnosis of histoplasmosis can be made by either of two types of serologic tests, depending on the stage of the illness. In the early phase of the disease, reaction to a latex agglutination test may be positive, probably because an IgM antibody is present. As the infection progresses, the reaction to the agglutination test fades and becomes negative. Somewhat later in the infection, complement-fixing antibodies develop; these correlate well with the activity of the disease. Titers of 1:8 to 1:16 may be considered presumptive evidence of histoplasmosis, whereas titers of 1:32 are highly suggestive of this infection. Cross reactions with antigens from other fungi can occur in the complement-fixation test and be misleading. In some patients, the antigenic stimulation from a skin test with histoplasmin may be sufficient to stimulate an increase in complement-fixing antibody titer, but usually not before 15 days. For this reason, the initial or acute, serum for complement-fixation studies should be obtained before skin tests are performed. Kaufman and his associates (1985) found that if reaction to a skin test is positive in 72 hours, serum drawn for complement fixation will not reflect any change in titer at this time, although the possibility of a rise in the convalescent serum should be considered. Under these conditions, there must be at least a fourfold or greater change in titer to establish the diagnosis of active infection.

A micro-immunodiffusion procedure is also recommended for detecting infection by *Histoplasma capsulatum*. The results are qualitative. Two precipitin bands have diagnostic value. One, designated "h," is not influenced by skin testing and is consistently found in the serum of patients with active histoplasmosis. The second, designated "m," is found in both acute and chronic histoplasmosis and also appears after normal, sensitized individuals have been skin tested with histoplasmin. The "m" band has been considered presumptive evidence of infection with *H. capsulatum*. Finding only "m" antibodies in sera may be attributed to active or inactive disease or to skin testing. Therefore, if the patient has not had a recent histoplasmin skin test, detection of an "m" band may serve as an indicator of early disease, since this band appears before the "h" band and disappears more slowly. Kaufman and associates (1985) stated that the demonstration of both the "m" and "h" bands is highly suggestive of active histoplasmosis, regardless of other serologic results.

In coccidioidomycosis, reaction to a precipitin test may be positive in early stages of the infection. As in histoplasmosis, the complement-fixation antibody titer tends to rise as the disease becomes more advanced and falls with control of the infection. Should the infection disseminate, a state of anergy may develop with a loss of all serologic evidence of the disease. In contrast to histoplasmin, skin testing with coccidioidin does not appear to stimulate humoral antibody formation.

Cryptococcosis is one of the most common fungal infections of the lung, although in most of its subjects it may be present in a subclinical form. The disease usually becomes apparent in patients who have some defect in their host defense mechanism, particularly those who are under therapy for malignant lymphomas and those who have experienced immune suppression. The causative organism may proliferate in large numbers in the lung or brain. In many instances, the cellular reaction is minimal (Fig. 16–6), and the detection of circulating polysaccharide antigen is possible prior to the formation of circulating antibodies. When the infection appears to be controlled, either spontaneously or as a result of therapy, the polysaccharide antigen disappears, and circulating antibodies may be demonstrated by the indirect immunofluorescent antibody test or a cryptococcal yeast-cell agglutination procedure. There seems to be an inverse relationship in the time between the appearance of antigen in the serum, or spinal fluid in the early or acute stage of the disease, and the appearance of antibodies in the serum as the infection is brought under control. Using indirect fluorescent antibody, tube agglutination for antibody, and latex agglutination for antigen

tests, Kaufman and Blumer (1968) were able to show serologic evidence of cryptococcosis in 92% of 66 patients.

For additional serologic tests used in the diagnosis of fungal diseases, see Kaufman and colleagues, 1985.

PARASITIC INFECTIONS OF THE LUNG

Parasitic infections of the lungs are uncommon in the United States. When found, they are usually present in patients who have previously spent time in some part of the world in which echinococcosis, schistosomiasis, or amebiasis is endemic. Unfortunately, the identification of the parasite in sputum, pleural fluid, or other clinical specimens is difficult, and recovery by culture is difficult or impossible, depending on the organism. Biopsy or excision of suspected lesions may be the most rapid and definitive procedure.

Intestinal nematodes, such as *Ascaris lumbricoides*, hookworm, and *Stronglyloides stercoralis*, may incite a severe inflammatory reaction in the lung during passage from the pulmonary circulation into the bronchi. Sputum specimens may reveal filarial forms of the worms. Clinically, such patients show a marked eosinophilia, and a mottled infiltration of the lung is demonstrated in a roentgenogram of the chest. In occasional patients, nematodes become trapped in the lungs, incite an inflammatory reaction, and form hyalinized granulomas, which may persist as "coin lesions."

The development of serologic procedures to detect antibodies to different types of parasites that can be found in the lung has been of great help in both establishing and confirming the presence of active infection with different parasites. Since many of these tests have only recently been developed and standardized, most are available only through public health laboratories. Walls (1985) summarized many of the tests available and methods for their performance. Several of the serologic tests are described briefly in the following paragraphs.

The indirect hemagglutination test for pleuropulmonary amebiasis is both sensitive and specific and is particularly valuable in the detection of tissue invasion by amebae. In contrast to its sensitivity in patients with hepatic and pulmonary involvement, Healy (1968) found the test less sensitive in those with acute amebic dysentery and relatively insensitive for asymptomatic intestinal carriers.

In hydatid disease, patients with echinococcal cysts in the liver have much better serologic correlation than do those with cysts in the lung. Kagan and his associates (1966) found that serologic tests for echinococcal cysts do not correlate well with pulmonary involvement. The reason for this discrepancy in the reliability of serologic tests between infection in the lungs and in the liver is not known, but may be because pulmonary cysts are not as closely associated with an active blood supply as are hepatic cysts.

Pulmonary schistosomiasis may develop as a further manifestation of intestinal and hepatic infection and is usually associated with pulmonary hypertension (Fig.

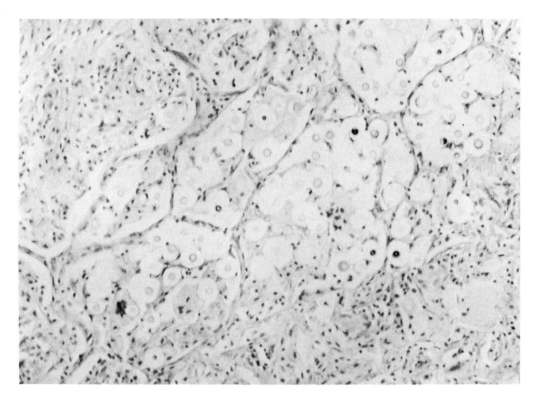

Fig. 16–6. Pneumonia from *Cryptococcus neoformans*. Note the large number of encapsulated cells filling the alveoli. The prominent capsule is well shown. In the early phase of the disease, circulating capsular polysaccharide may be demonstrated in the serum, urine, or cerebrospinal fluid before the appearance of antibodies. Periodic acid-Schiff—PAS—stain. ×450.

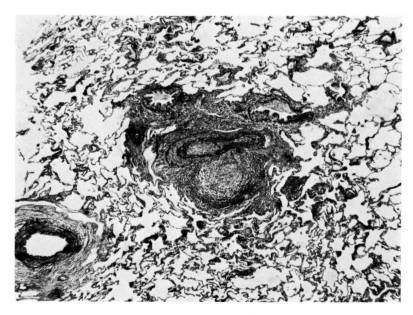

Fig. 16–7. Perivascular granuloma from *Schistosoma mansoni*. Note thickening of pulmonary vessels reflecting pulmonary hypertension. Lung biopsy is a useful means of establishing the diagnosis of schistosomal lung disease and assessing the degree of pulmonary vessel change. ×260.

16–7). Although lung biopsy is a useful means of establishing the diagnosis and assessing the pulmonary vascular disease, various serologic tests are available to help establish the diagnosis. Kagan and colleagues (1962) found the cholesterol-lecithin cercarial slide flocculation test—CL—sensitive in 77% of patients with confirmed disease, but unfortunately the test cannot be performed on contaminated or chylous sera. A bentonite flocculation test was developed to overcome this difficulty, but Kagan (1968) found this to be sensitive in only 70% of patients and gave false-positive reactions in 15% of sera from patients without schistosomiasis.

Occasional instances of infection with the oriental lung fluke, *Paragonimus westermani*, are found in persons from the Far East. This infection may be mistaken for other types of chronic disease in the lung. Although complement-fixation and other serologic tests have been described for detection of this parasite, they are generally not available in the United States owing to the infrequent need for such procedures. For a more detailed discussion on the different serologic procedures that have been described for parasitic agents, see Walls (1985).

PNEUMONITIS DUE TO PNEUMOCYSTIS CARINII

This small unicellular organism produces a rapid, consolidating pneumonitis in debilitated patients, usually after prolonged periods of therapy with antimetabolites, steroids, and antibiotics (Fig. 16–8), and is a frequent complication in patients with acquired immune deficiency syndrome—AIDS. Attempts to isolate and culture the organism have been unsuccessful. Although the disease was first recognized in malnourished infants and children in orphanages in Europe and Korea following World War II, infection with *Pneumocystis carinii* occurs in this country in patients with AIDS, with inborn immune deficiencies, or with complications caused by prolonged drug therapy for malignant tumors.

The disease is more common than in the past. Well over 50% of patients with AIDS present with this infection. The percentage varies depending on whether the patients are IV drug abusers or homosexual men; the status of the patients' T cell populations also plays a role in its incidence. Perera and his associates (1970) found 40 previously unrecognized instances on review of 301 consecutive autopsies performed in a children's hospital for leukemia or other types of cancer.

Hughes and his colleagues (1977) showed that a combination of trimethoprim and sulfamethoxazole is effective in preventing the occurrence of pneumonia from *Pneumocystis carinii* when used for prophylaxis as well as for therapy. This combination is the drug of choice for the treatment of acute infection in all patients with the disease.

Because the disease may develop and progress rapidly, causing death within 4 to 6 days, the diagnosis should be made promptly so that specific therapy can be started. Although the organism has been found in sputum smears and tracheal aspirates, dependence on this finding to establish the diagnosis is unreliable because few organisms are shed and many similar-appearing objects may be present on the smear. Jacobs and his associates (1969), as well as Johnson and Johnson (1970), showed that needle biopsy of the lung provides a rapid, effective means of determining the diagnosis. The best method is still an open lung biopsy, in which enough tissue can be obtained to culture and stain for organisms of other types as well.

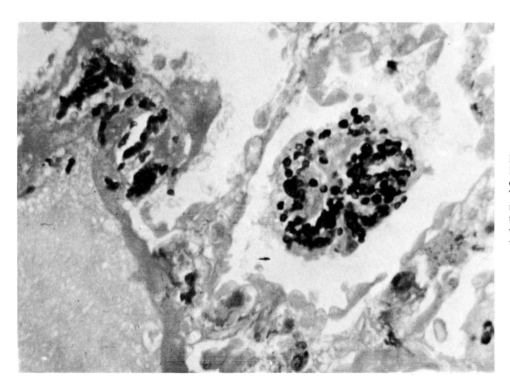

Fig. 16–8. *Pneumocystis carinii.* Large numbers of organisms are embedded in fibrin within alveoli. Tissue sections stained with hematoxylin and eosin do not show the organisms, best demonstrated with the Gomori methenamine silver stain. × 650.

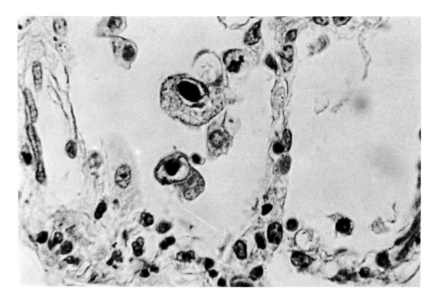

Fig. 16–9. Cytomegalovirus intranuclear inclusion body in alveolar macrophage. Not all viral diseases produce inclusion bodies, but those of the Herpes-Cytomegalovirus groups show well-formed intranuclear inclusions. ×650.

The organism is not visible on sections stained by hematoxylin and eosin; it is best demonstrated with methenamine silver stain. Since the methenamine stain requires special reagents, the laboratory should be alerted to the possibility of a *Pneumocystis* infection prior to biopsy so that sections can be stained without delay. Good results within a period of 5 to 10 minutes have been obtained with a rapid staining procedure using toluidine O, as reported by Chalvardjian (1963). Attempts to develop an immunologic test have been hampered by the inability to grow the organism in the laboratory.

VIRAL INFECTIONS OF THE LUNG

In general, the diagnosis of viral infection of the lungs is made either by isolating and identifying the organism in tissue culture or by demonstrating a fourfold or greater antibody titer rise to the antigen of a specific virus. Collection and handling of specimens for isolation of different viruses will vary, depending on the virus suspected. Isolation is carried out by inoculation into a variety of tissue cultures, including human embryonic kidney and animal cells, and, in influenza, the yolk sac of eggs.

Because of the large number of viral agents and their widely varying requirements for recovery in culture, the virus laboratory should be consulted regarding the type of specimen to be selected and the method of handling the specimen for optimal recovery of the suspected agent. Although biopsy may reveal intracellular inclusion bodies in some instances, their morphologic characteristics in tissues and cells are not specific for viral disease; their reaction with fluorescein-tagged specific antisera must be tested (Fig. 16–9). In some instances, open pulmonary biopsy should be strongly considered when the cause of a rapid progression of an infection cannot be determined. Although satisfactory drugs are not yet available for viral infections, other types of organisms, such as Nocardia, can produce infection mimicking viral pneumonitis and are susceptible to available drugs. Biopsy in these instances literally can be a lifesaving procedure.

REFERENCES

Balows, A., and Fraser, D.W.E.: International Symposium on Legionnaires' Disease. Ann. Intern. Med. *90*:489, 1979.

Barrett-Connet, E.: The nonvalue of sputum cultures in the diagnosis of pneumococcal pneumonia. Am. Rev. Respir. Dis. *103*:345, 1971.

Bartlett, S.G.: Anaerobic bacterial pneumonitis. Am. Rev. Respir. Dis. *119*:19, 1979.

Bartlett, S.G., and Finegold, S.M.: Anaerobic infections of the lung and pleural space. Am. Rev. Respir. Dis. *110*:56, 1974.

Brenner, D.J., et al.: Ten new species of Legionella. Int. J. Syst. Bacteriol. *35*:50, 1985.

Chalvardjian, A.M., and Grawe, L.A.: A new procedure for the identification of *Pneumocystis carinii* cysts in tissue sections and smears. J. Clin. Pathol. *16*:383, 1963.

Cherry, W.B., et al.: Detection of Legionnaires' disease bacteria by direct immunofluorescent staining. J. Clin. Microbiol. *8*:329, 1978.

Cherry, W.B., et al.: *Legionella jordanis:* a new species of *Legionella* isolated from water and sewage. J. Clin. Microbiol. *15*:290, 1982.

Conte, B.A., and Laforet, E.G.: The role of the topical anaesthetic agent in modifying bacteriologic data obtained by bronchoscopy. N. Engl. J. Med. *267*:957, 1962.

Damato, J.J., et al.: Detection of mycobacteria by radiometric and standard plate procedures. J. Clin. Microbiol. *17*:1066, 1983.

Damsker, B., and Bottone, E.J.: *Mycobacterium avium-Mycobacterium intracellulare* from the intestinal tract of patients with the acquired immunodeficiency syndrome. Concepts regarding acquisition and pathogenesis. J. Infect. Dis. *151*:179, 1985.

Dilworth, J.A., et al.: Methods to improve detection of pneumococci in respiratory secretions. J. Clin. Microbiol. *2*:453, 1975.

Feeley, J.C., et al.: Charcoal-yeast extract agar: primary isolation medium for *Legionella pneumophila* J. Clin. Microbiol. *10*:437, 1979.

Frable, W.J.: Thin Needle Aspiration Biopsy. Philadelphia, W.B., Saunders Co., 1983.

Gill, V.J., et al.: Use of lysis-centrifugation (Isolator) and radiometric (Bactec) blood culture systems for the detection of mycobacteremia. J. Clin. Microbiol. *22*:543, 1985.

Gill, V.J., and Stock, F.: Detection of *Mycobacterium avium-Mycobacteria intracellulare* in blood cultures using concentrated and unconcentrated blood in conjunction with a radiometric detection system. Diagn. Microbiol. Infect. Dis. *6*:119, 1987.

Good, R.C., and Snyder, D.E.: Isolation of nontuberculous mycobacteria in the United States (1980). J. Infect. Dis. *146*:829, 1982.

Greene, J.B., et al.: *Mycobacterium avium intracellulare:* a cause of disseminated life-threatening infection in homosexuals and drug abusers. Ann. Intern. Med. 97:539, 1982.

Hawkins, C.C., et al.: *Mycobacterium avium* complex infections in patients with the acquired immunodeficiency syndrome. Ann. Intern. Med. 105:184, 1986.

Healy, G.R.: The use of and limitations to the indirect hemagglutination test in the diagnosis of intestinal amebiasis. Health Lab. Sci. 5:174, 1968.

Hoeprich, P.D.: Etiologic diagnosis of lower respiratory tract infections. Calif. Med. 112:1, 1970.

Hughes, W.T., et al.: Successful chemoprophylaxis for *Pneumocystis carinii* pneumonitis. N. Engl. J. Med. 297:1419, 1977.

Jacobs, J.B., et al.: Needle biopsy in *Pneumocystis carinii* pneumonia. Radiology 93:525, 1969.

Johnson, H.D., and Johnson, W.W.: *Pneumocystis carinii* pneumonia in children with cancer. Diagnosis and treatment. J.A.M.A. 214:1067, 1970.

Kagan, I.G.: Serologic diagnosis of schistosomiasis. Bull. N.Y. Acad. Med. 44:262, 1968.

Kagan, I.G., et al.: Evaluation of intradermal and serologic tests for the diagnosis of hydatid disease. Am. J. Trop. Med. 15:172, 1966.

Kagan, I.G, et al.: A clinical, parasitologic, and immunologic study of schistosomiasis in 103 Puerto Rican males residing in the United States. Ann. Intern. Med. 56:457, 1962.

Kaufman, L., and Reiss, E.: Serodiagnosis of Fungal Disease, Chapter 96. *In* Manual of Clinical Microbiology, 4th ed. Edited by E.H. Lennette, A. Balows, W.J. Hausler, and H.F. Shadomy. Washington D.C., American Society of Microbiology, 1985.

Kaufman, L., and Blumer, S.: Value and interpretation of serological tests for the diagnosis of cryptococcosis. Appl. Microbiol. 16:1907, 1968.

Kiehn, T.E., and Edwards, F.F.: Rapid identification using a specific DNA probe of *Mycobacterium avium* complex from patients with acquired immunodeficiency syndrome. J. Clin. Microbiol. 25:1551, 1987.

Kleinfield, J., and Elliss, P.P.: Inhibition of microorganisms by topical anaesthetics. Appl. Microbiol. 15:1296, 1967.

Kopanoff, D.E., et al.: A continuing survey of tuberculosis primary drug resistance in the United States: March 1975 to November 1977. Am. Rev. Respir. Dis. 118:835, 1978.

Koss, L.G.: Diagnostic Cytology and Its Histopathologic Bases, 2nd ed. Philadelphia, J.B. Lippincott Co., 1968, p. 380.

Krasnow, I., and Wayne, L.G.: Comparison of methods for tuberculosis bacteriology. Appl. Microbiol. 18:915, 1969.

Levy, C., et al.: *Mycobacterium chelonei* infection of porcine heart valves. N. Engl. J. Med. 297:567, 1977.

Linsk, J.A: Fine Needle Aspiration for the Clinician. Phildelphia, J.B. Lippincott Co., 1986.

Macher, A.M., et al.: Bacteremia due to *Mycobacterium avium-intracellulare* in the acquired immunodeficiency syndrome. Ann. Intern. Med. 99:782, 1983.

Meyerowitz, R.L., et al.: Opportunistic lung infection due to "Pittsburgh Pneumonia Agent." N. Engl. J. Med. 301:953, 1979.

Middlebrook, G., Reggiardo, Z., and Tigert, W.D.: Automatable radiometric detection of growth of *Mycobacterium tuberculosis* in selective media. Am. Rev. Respir. Dis. 115:1066, 1977.

Morgan, M.A., et al.: Comparison of a radiometric method (Bactec) and conventional culture media for recovery of mycobacteria from smear-negative specimens. J. Clin. Microbiol. 18:384, 1983.

Morgan, M.A., et al.: Evaluation of the p-nitro-α-acetylamine-β-hydroxypropiophenone differential test for identification of *Mycobacterium tuberculosis* complex. J. Clin. Microbiol. 21:634, 1985.

Musial, C.E., et al.: Recovery of *Blastomyces dermatitidis* from blood of a patient with disseminated blastomycosis. J. Clin Microbiol. 25:1421, 1987.

Perera, D.R., et al.: *Pneumocystis carinii* pneumonia in a hospital for children: epidemiologic aspects. J.A.M.A. 214:1074, 1970.

Rathbun, H.K., and Govani, I.: Mouse inoculation as a means of identifying pneumococci in the sputum. Johns Hopkins Med. J. 120:46, 1967.

Rein, M.F., and Mandell, G.L.: Bacterial killing by bacteriostatic saline solutions—potential for diagnostic error. N. Engl. J. Med. 289:794, 1973.

Roberts, G.D., et al.: Evaluation of the Bactec radiometric method for recovery of mycobacteria and drug susceptibility testing of *Mycobacterium tuberculosis* from acid-fast smear-positive specimens. J. Clin. Microbiol. 18:689, 1983.

Runyon, E.H.: Anonymous mycobacteria in pulmonary disease. Med. Clin. North Am. 43:273, 1959.

Sanders, C.C., and Sanders, W.E.: Enocin, an antibiotic produced by *Streptococcus salivarius* that may contribute to protection against infections due to Group A streptococci. J. Infect. Dis. 146:683, 1982.

Siddiqi, S.H., Libonati, J.P., and Middlebrook, G.: Evaluation of a rapid radiometric method for drug susceptibility testing of *Mycobacterium tuberculosis*. J. Clin. Microbiol. 13:908, 1981.

Singh, M.D., and Garrison, R.G.: Propylene glycol aerosolization and the diagnosis of pulmonary histoplasmosis. Dis. Chest 46:82, 1964.

Snider, D.E., Jr., et al.: Rapid drug susceptibility testing of *Mycobacterium tuberculosis*. Am. Rev. Respir. Dis. 123:402, 1981.

Stout, J., et al.: Ubiquitousness of *Legionella pneumophila* in the water supply of a hospital with endemic Legionnaires' disease. N. Engl. J. Med. 306:466, 1982.

Takahashi, H., and Foster, V.: Detection and recovery of mycobacteria by a radiometric procedure. J. Clin. Microbiol. 17:380, 1983.

Thomason, B.M., et al.: A legionella-like bacterium related to WIGA in a fatal case of pneumonia. Ann. Intern. Med. 91:673, 1979.

Timpe, A., and Runyon, E.H.: The relationship of "atypical" acid-fast bacteria to human disease. J. Lab. Clin. Med. 44:202, 1954.

Van Scoy, R.E.: Bacterial sputum cultures. A clinician's viewpoint. Mayo Clin. Proc. 52:39, 1977.

Walls, K.W.: Serodiagnostic tests for parasitic diseases, Chapter 97. *In* Manual of Clinical Microbiology, 4th ed. Edited by E.H. Lennette, A. Balows, W.J. Hausler, H.F. Shadomy. Washington D.C., American Society of Microbiology, 1985.

Wolinsky, E.: Non-tuberculous mycobacteria and associated disease. Am. Rev. Respir. Dis. 119:107, 1979.

READING REFERENCES

Kalinske, R.W., et al.: Diagnostic usefulness and safety of transtracheal aspiration. N. Engl. J. Med. 276:604, 1967.

Sommers, H.M., and Good, R.C.: *Mycobacterium. In* Manual of Clinical Microbiology, 4th ed. Edited by E.H. Lennette, A. Balows, W.J. Hausler, and H.F. Shadomy. Washington D.C., American Society of Microbiology, 1985.

Wayne, L.G.: On the identity of *Mycobacterium gordonae* Bojalil and the so-called tap water scotochromogens. Int. J. Systematic Bacteriology 20:149, 1970.

Wayne, L.G., and Lessel, E.F.: On the synonymy of *Mycobacterium marianum* Penso 1952 and *Mycobacterium scrofulaceum* Prissick and Masson 1956 and the resolution of a nomenclatural problem. Int. J. Systematic Bacteriology 19:257, 1969.

Wayne, L.G., Runyon, E.H., and Kubica, G.P.: Mycobacteria: a guide to nomenclatural usage. Am. Rev. Respir. Dis. 100:732, 1969.

CHAPTER 17

THE PHYSIOLOGY AND PHYSIOLOGIC STUDIES OF THE ESOPHAGUS

André Duranceau and Glyn G. Jamieson

NORMAL ESOPHAGEAL FUNCTION

Pharynx

The function of the pharynx has received less attention than that of the esophagus, partly because water-infused systems do not accurately measure pressure events in the pharynx. Dodds and associates (1975), however, measured pharyngeal contractions in human subjects using intraluminal strain gauges and found average contraction pressures of 200 mm Hg with pressures recorded up to 600 mm Hg. The pharyngeal contraction lasts about 0.2 to 0.5 seconds. The rapidity of the pharyngeal contraction wave—9 to 25 cm/sec—requires it to be recorded in this fashion. Frequently, before the single pharyngeal peak an initial increase in pressure occurs. This is usually thought to be caused by the tongue thrust, the "trapped" air column, or the advancing bolus (Fig. 17–1).

Upper Esophageal Sphincter

The upper esophageal sphincter—UES—is a high pressure zone that separates the pharynx from the esophagus (Fig. 17–2). Its most important role may be to prevent esophagopharyngeal regurgitation; gastroesophageal reflux occurs in normal individuals and the sphincter may prevent the regurgitation of gastric contents into the pharynx. The sphincter may also have a role in preventing the entry of air into the esophagus, although this probably is not an important function.

The cricopharyngeus is a muscle sling attached posteriorly to both laminae of the cricoid cartilage. The configuration and location of this muscle give it a role similar to that of a bowstring, with tension exerted mostly in the anteroposterior direction. Winans (1972) documented this asymmetry within the sphincter. Using an 8-lumen catheter with all recording ports arranged circumferentially at the same level he observed 100 mm Hg pressures in the anteroposterior position and 30 mm Hg in the lateral orientation.

Although there is general agreement that the crico-

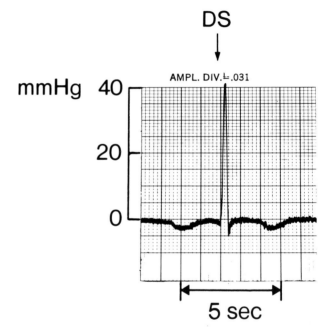

Fig. 17–1. The pharyngeal contraction lasts about 0.2 to 0.5 seconds. Pressures are recorded accurately when using intraluminal strain gauges.

pharyngeus is the major component of the UES, this muscle is only about 1 cm wide and thus cannot account totally for the 2 to 3 cm width of the high pressure zone of the UES recorded by Winans (1972) and Welch and colleagues (1979).

As suggested by Airdar (1943), passive elastic forces may play a role in the maintenance of closure of the UES in man. Certainly this appears to be true in the opossum, as reported by Asoh and Goyal (1978), in which a residual closing pressure remains in the anteroposterior direction after removing the nervous supply to the sphincter muscle. Nevertheless, UES pressure is probably predominantly due to tonic muscle contraction; sustained elec-

231

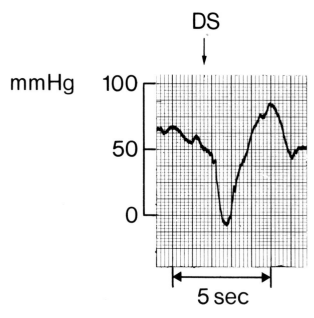

Fig. 17–2. The upper esophageal sphincter (UES) high pressure zone that separates the pharynx from the esophagus.

tromyographic activity has been recorded from the cricopharyngeus muscle in man by Shipp and co-workers (1970).

Sokol and associates (1966) have reported that during swallowing the UES moves vertically about 2 cm, and this has led to methodological problems in the study of UES function using a perfused side-hole catheter. Sampling by rapid pull-through techniques by Gerhardt (1978) and Welch and colleagues (1979) in normal controls has recorded anteroposterior basal tone in the range of 100 to 130 mm Hg.

Adaptation by Dent (1976) of the sleeve manometric technique for the study of the UES has provided further insights into UES function. Basal UES pressure was found by Kahrilas and associates (1987b) to fall during sleep to a level of 6 to 13 mm Hg, whereas in awake subjects it was of the order of 60 mm Hg.

Relaxation of the UES that allows the passage of material through it appears to occur with the onset of swallowing (Fig. 17–3) and, as noted by Kahrilas and associates (1986), it also occurs independently of swallowing to allow belching. Several stimuli that increase UES tone have been studied: balloon distention in the esophagus, reported by Creamer and Schlegal (1957), Gerhardt (1978), and Kahrilas and colleagues (1987a); acidification of the esophageal lumen, recorded by Gerhart (1978); and slow, intraesophageal gas insufflation—as opposed to rapid distention, which produces relaxation—as noted by Kahrilas and associates (1986).

Esophageal Body

The musculature of the esophageal body is not tonically contracted. The role of the longitudinal muscle in esophageal function is difficult to study. Sugarbaker and colleagues (1984) have suggested that it may improve the mechanical properties of the esophagus for bolus trans-

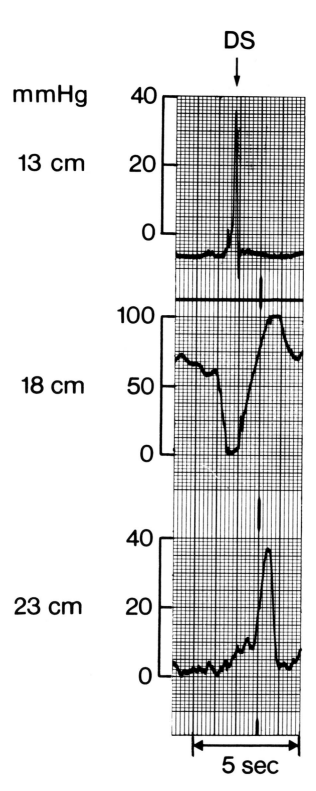

Fig. 17–3. The pharyngoesophageal junction in action. The pharynx (13 cm) contracts rapidly while the UES (18 cm) shows a complete relaxation. The pressure wave that closes the UES is seen to continue into the cervical esophagus (23 cm).

port. The circular muscle, however, is much easier to study, because of its lumen-occluding contraction, which passes down the esophageal body, pushing contents ahead of it.

Primary peristalsis is triggered voluntarily by swallowing but thereafter is not under voluntary control (Fig. 17–4). Not all peristaltic waves are complete in normal subjects. In response to dry swallows, complete waves occur only on about two thirds of occasions, with such patterns as peristaltic "fade out" at the aortic arch level, tertiary contractions in the distal esophagus, and even no detectable wave at all occurring as reported by Dodds and co-workers (1973) and Hollis and Castell (1975). As we and our associates (1983) noted, however, water swallows produce more complete peristaltic sequences. Other factors that may influence primary peristaltic activity are posture—diminution with the supine position—and age—diminution in amplitude in men over the age of 80—which have been reported by Kaye and Wexler (1981) and Hollis and Castell (1974), respectively.

The esophageal wave travels down the esophageal body at a speed of 2 to 5 cm/sec (Fig. 17–5). The wave of contraction that occurs in response to deglutition progresses slowly in the proximal striated muscle area, slows even further at the striated-smooth muscle junction, and then becomes faster in the lower half of the esophagus, except just above the lower sphincter, where it is seen to slow again. In a similar fashion, peak contraction pressures are weak in the striated esophagus and stronger in the distal esophagus. The values obtained in recording esophageal body motility vary from author to author and the influence of differing recording techniques is well documented.

Peristaltic sequences can also be modified by the rate of swallowing. Swallows at 5-second intervals or less tend to completely inhibit peristalsis; only when swallows are taken at greater than 20-second intervals do completely normal sequences occur, as reported by Ask and Tibbling (1980) and Meyer and colleagues (1981).

The control of primary peristalsis is complex. The stri-

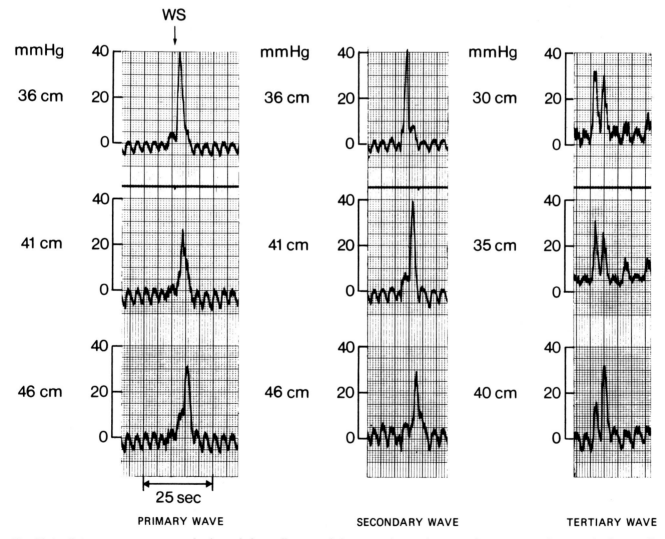

PRIMARY WAVE   **SECONDARY WAVE**   **TERTIARY WAVE**

Fig. 17–4. Primary waves are triggered voluntarily by swallowing and show normal peristalsis. Secondary waves are also peristaltic but usually result from distention or irritation. Tertiary waves are abnormal contractions and show no propulsion.

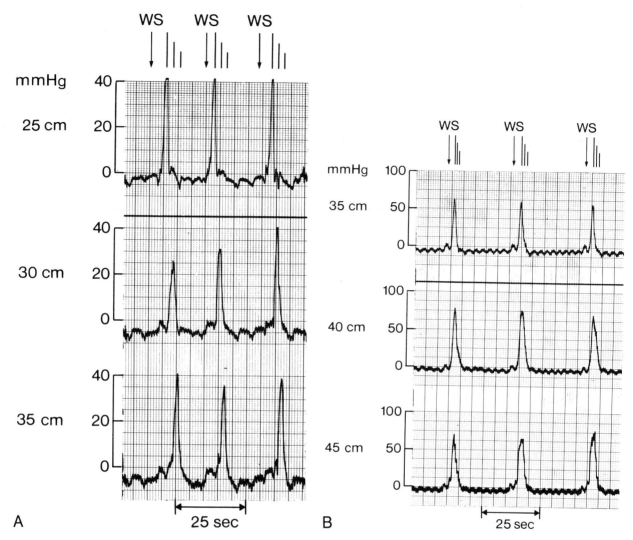

Fig. 17–5. *A*, Primary peristalsis in the proximal half of the esophagus shows weaker and slower waves. *B*, Propulsive waves in the distal esophagus are stronger and travel faster.

ated muscle is probably directly controlled by the nucleus ambiguus through the vagus, whereas the smooth muscle portion is probably controlled by a combination of extrinsic—vagal—and local neural control. Both cholinergic—excitatory—and nonadrenergic noncholinergic—inhibitory—mechanisms were suggested by Christensen (1970) and Sarna (1977) and Crist (1984) and their co-workers to be involved in normal peristalsis.

Secondary peristalsis refers to peristaltic waves that are not controlled by swallowing, but usually by esophageal distention or irritation (Fig. 17–4). These have been much less studied than primary peristaltic waves but they probably have a "housekeeper" role in clearing refluxed material from the esophagus (Fig. 17–5).

Tertiary contractions (Fig. 17–4) can be abnormal contractions in response to swallowing or can appear spontaneously between swallows (Fig. 17–6). Rubin and associates (1962) suggested a relationship between esophageal motor disorders and the emotional states of the patients during recordings. Nonpropulsive contrac-

tions and repetitive spontaneous contractions were observed when motor function of the esophageal body was recorded during "effectively charged conversation." Spontaneous tertiary contractions (Fig. 17–4) occur in healthy individuals, but are observed more often in patients with a strongly anxious personality (Fig. 17–4).

Lower Esophageal Sphincter

It is now accepted that there is both a physiologic, as emphasized by Dodds and associates (1981), and an anatomic, as documented by Liebermann-Meffert and colleagues (1979), lower esophageal sphincter and that the maintenance of basal tone is the major mechanism preventing gastroesophageal reflux.

Winans (1977) has pointed out that the pressure profile of the LES (Fig. 17–7) shows considerable radial asymmetry, with the highest pressures being recorded in the left posterior orientation. The reasons for this are not clear. As with the UES, the LES relaxes to allow passage of luminal contents in either direction, relaxation occur-

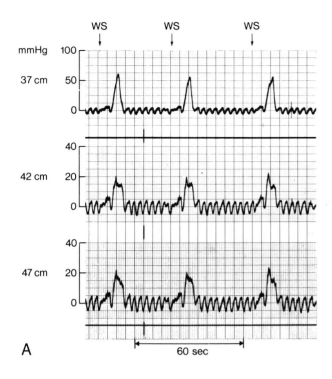

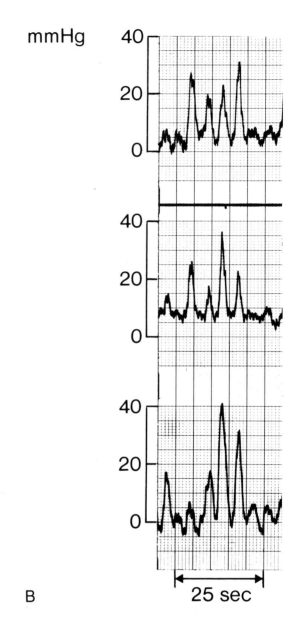

Fig. 17–6. *A,* Tertiary contractions in response to swallowing. *B,* Spontaneous tertiary contractions appearing between swallows.

ring with peristaltic activity in the esophageal body or gaseous distention in the fundus of the stomach.

The mechanisms underlying the control of basal tone in the LES are not well understood. Fisher (1977) and Dodds (1981) and co-workers wrote that cholinergic vagal drive seems a likely candidate at least in part. Circulating hormones, such as gastrin, are considered much less likely to contribute to basal tone. Basal tone varies greatly in normal individuals, and in the fasting state the migrating motor cycle may influence LES pressure, which tends to increase during the cycle, as recorded by Dent and associates (1983), and can reach high levels during phase III gastric contractions. Basal tone rises during increases in intra-abdominal pressure; it remains controversial whether this is a reflex rise in pressure or an increased diaphragmatic compression of the LES, as suggested by Boyle and Cohen (1984). Perhaps the evidence

as reported by Landers and Jamieson (1987) is beginning to favor the concept that there is a reflex involved.

LES relaxation occurs with swallowing, with esophageal body distention, and with gastric fundus distention. Transient lower esophageal sphincter relaxation— TLESR—is a phenomenon of relaxations lasting 5 to 30 seconds that was described by Dent and colleagues (1980). These probably arise as a result of gastric distention leading to nonadrenergic, noncholinergic inhibition of the LES tone. As suggested by Dent (1980) and Dodds (1980) and associates such LESRs may be the most important factor in both physiologic and pathologic reflux.

Other factors that should be mentioned, as noted by Bonavina and colleagues (1986), as contributing to pressure in the lower esophageal sphincter region are extrinsic compression by diaphragmatic muscle—which is probably most important during straining—and the intra-

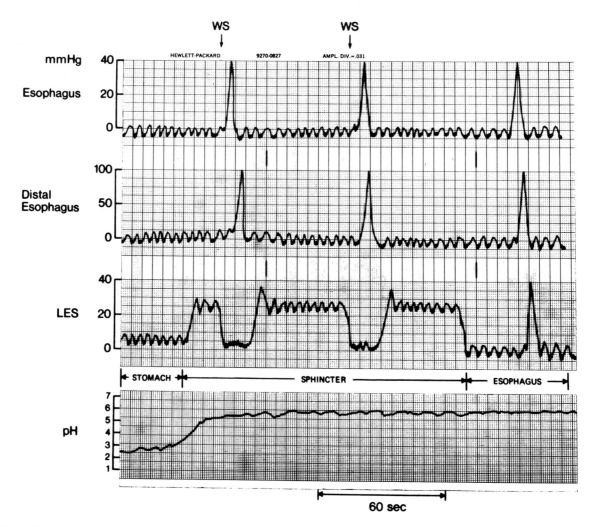

Fig. 17–7. Illustration of the lower esophageal sphincter (LES) high pressure zone between stomach and esophagus. The LES relaxes to allow the passage of the esophageal content, pushed by esophageal peristalsis.

abdominal position of the LES, which allows intra-abdominal pressure changes to buttress the LES.

EVALUATION OF ESOPHAGEAL FUNCTION

The Roles of Symptoms, Roentgenography and Endoscopy

Symptoms usually form the basis for consultation in an esophageal clinic. Dysphagia and pain on swallowing—odynophagia—are unique to the esophagus. The pain is substernal with cervical and midscapular radiation. Heartburn frequently accompanies the reflux of fluid from the gastric cavity to the esophagus. Despite the belief that careful description of symptoms can confirm the diagnosis of reflux disease, over 20% of patients with typical heartburn have in fact abnormalities of the stomach or duodenum. An esophageal disorder does not necessarily mean reflux disease. Thus symptoms can be used as a guide to esophageal investigation but cannot be used as a guide to therapy.

Symptoms should lead to roentgenologic investigation. Cine or videoroentgenologic recording of esophageal function is essential to show the normal anatomy and its variations. Curtis and associates (1984) stressed that a proper assessment of the pharyngoesophageal junction is not possible without these techniques. Such studies classify hiatus hernia types and suggest the possibility of motor disorders. Barium studies are poorly sensitive in demonstrating reflux disease. When acid barium is used, the test becomes more sensitive but shows poor specificity.

Endoscopy assesses macroscopic changes in the esophageal mucosa, whereas esophageal biopsies allow histologic assessment of these changes. In severe mucosal changes there is unanimity among various observers. In minor mucosal changes, however, there is poor correlation among endoscopists' observations. In reflux disease, histologic findings show a poor correlation with the esophagitis identified at endoscopy. Multiple biopsies at known levels are the only objective proof of the metaplastic changes in the columnar-lined esophagus. In malignant disease, biopsies and brush cytologies should succeed in clarifying the diagnosis in over 80% of patients.

Assessment of Esophageal Motility

Accurate recording of the physiologic events that occur with swallowing leads to an understanding of the pathophysiologic mechanisms of esophageal disorders. Although initial motility studies were mostly research-oriented, motility studies are now considered essential in the assessment of esophageal disease.

Esophageal motility studies record pressures simultaneously at several levels within the esophagus, allowing evaluation of the esophageal body and of the sphincters that close the upper and lower ends of the esophagus.

Intraluminal manometry is the method best suited for the study of motility in humans. Technical refinements in the last two decades, which have been discussed by Dodds (1976) and by us and our colleagues (1983), have led to greatly improved capability for accurate measurement with current techniques.

Meticulous attention to the recording technique and to the numerous factors that may affect it is necessary. For this reason it is important to have a control population evaluated with the local recording technique. This ensures more accuracy and gives a better perspective of what can be interpreted as normal in a patient population. The recording system used is usually water-perfused, and the patient is studied in a horizontal position.

Constantly perfused catheters ensure reliability in the pressures recorded. Without perfusion, marked variability is observed from patient to patient. If mechanical perfusion is used, Pope (1970) reported that the infusion rate shows a direct influence on pressure values. To overcome the inconvenience of infusing high volumes of fluid during a study and to allow more accurate changes in pressure over time—dP/dT—a constant-pressure infusion system, as described by Arndorfer (1977), that pushes small volumes of water through a noncompliant system is frequently used. Intraesophageal microtransducers are easy to use and very accurate. Their initial cost and their maintenance and repair expenses, however, have proved a major disadvantage to their routine use.

The size of the motility tube influences the recorded pressures, with an increase in size leading to an increase in the pressure recorded. The length of the recording tube may impose a "dragging" effect on the system and result in lower recorded pressures.

Both esophageal sphincters have an irregular configuration and exhibit vertical movement during deglutition. Special attention to these areas is required if reliable recordings are to be obtained. A 5-cm long perfused sleeve was devised by Dent (1976) and provides reliable lower esophageal sphincter pressure measurements despite esophageal movement. A similar sleeve catheter was developed by Kahrilas and colleagues (1987a) for the study of the upper esophageal sphincter. This catheter follows the sleeve principle and permits reliable recording despite movement of the catheter in the sphincter; this gives optimal pressure readings within the sphincter.

It is best to leave an interval of at least 30 seconds between swallows, as this ensures better organization of contractions. Dry swallows may fail to initiate contractions or result in weaker contractions, whereas liquid boluses provide longer and stronger contractions. Solid food may result in even more prolonged and vigorous waves. A cold bolus has been shown by Winship (1970) and Funch-Jensen (1981) and their colleagues to abolish contraction. Artifacts that frequently modify esophageal motility recordings are coughing, gagging, yawning, eructations, deep inspirations, and Valsalva maneuvers.

We and our associates (1983) stressed that the manometric recording technique and method of scoring motor events should be carefully standardized. Three firm indications exist for the use of esophageal manometry: (1) documentation of esophageal function in patients with suspected motor disorders, especially those with dysphagia and negative roentgenologic and endoscopic evaluation; (2) the evaluation of patients with chest pain of undetermined origin and in whom coronary artery disease has been ruled out; and (3) the documentation of physiologic abnormalities in patients with gastroesophageal reflux (Fig. 17–8).

Assessment of Esophageal Transit and Emptying

The movement of both solid and liquid boluses through the esophagus and their rate of emptying can be evaluated by roentgenologic or radioisotopic scanning techniques as pointed out by Tolin (1979), Russell (1981), and Maddern (1984) and their associates as well as by Maddern and Jamieson (1986). Bolus movement depends on several factors, such as esophageal motility, bolus consistency and size, and gravity. Roentgenographic techniques are superior to radionuclide techniques in terms of the anatomical demonstration of the esophagus and any disorder of movement, but radionuclides can measure fractional transit and emptying, and thus allow results to be quantitated. The indications for their use were reviewed by Taillefer and colleagues (1986) (Fig. 17–9).

Assessment of Intraluminal Esophageal pH

The technique of positioning one or more pH probes in the lower esophagus to record pH events has the advantage that it is easily applicable in humans and studies can be undertaken for a prolonged period of time. The technique was introduced originally to study reflux disease, but has proven useful in studying physiologic parameters such as physiologic reflux, acid clearance and lower esophageal sphincter relationships with reflux events.

Short-Term pH Studies

Tuttle and Grossman (1958), and Tuttle and colleagues (1960) measured simultaneously pressure and pH in the esophagus, at least 4 cm above the diaphragm. They observed that the pain of heartburn occurred when intraesophageal pH fell below 4.0. Piccone and associates (1965) used a pH probe in a standard fashion to document episodes of reflux in patients with hiatal hernias, in symptomatic patients without hernias, and in patients following operations to correct reflux (Fig. 17–10).

Skinner and Booth (1970) devised the standard acid

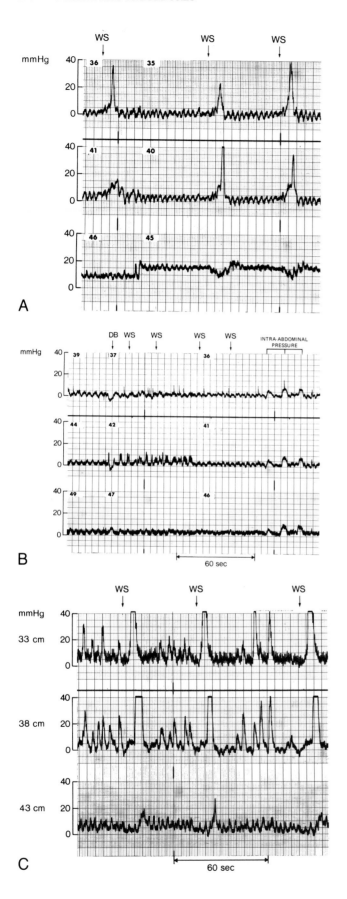

Fig. 17–8. *A*, Poor LES tone seen in reflux esophagitis in a patient with well-preserved esophageal motor activity. *B*, Absent LES and absent esophageal contractions in a patient with scleroderma. *C*, Hypotensive LES with retained primary peristalsis on swallowing (WS) but abundant spontaneous tertiary activity between deglutitions.

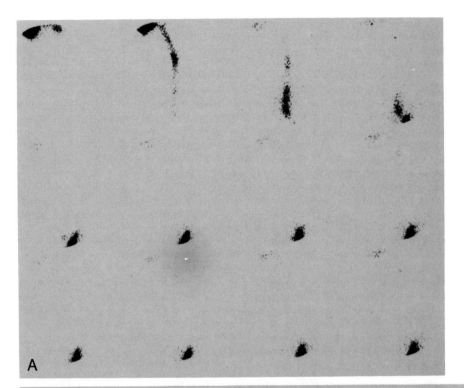

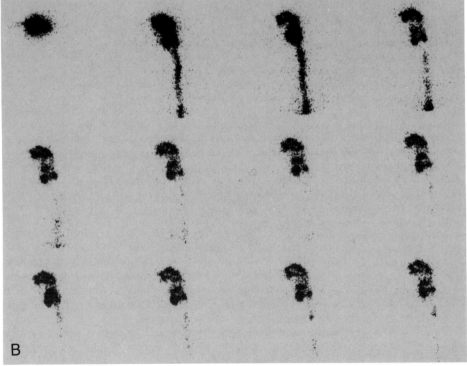

Fig. 17–9. Radionuclide assessment of esophageal transit. *A*, The normal esophagus empties its content in less than 8 seconds. *B*, Abnormal pharyngeal and hypopharyngeal retention in a patient with UES dysfunction.

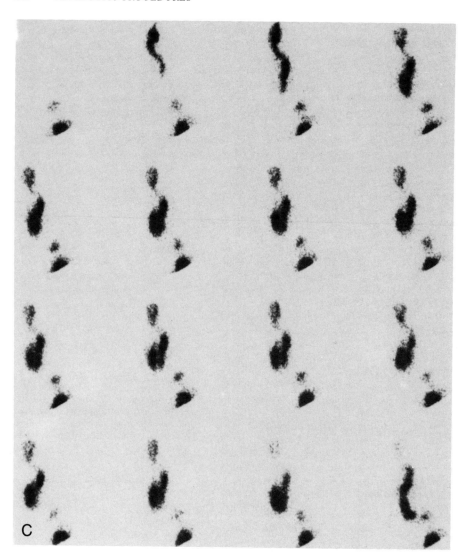

Fig. 17–9 *Continued.* C, Abnormal esophageal retention in achalasia.

reflux test: with the patient in a supine position, a pH electrode and catheter is advanced into the stomach and 300 ml of 0.1 N HCl is introduced. The pH electrode is then positioned 5 cm from the lower sphincter. The patient then performs four reflux-inducing maneuvers—deep breath, Valsalva, coughing, and Müller—while in four different positions—supine, right and left side, and Trendelenburg. A fall in pH to less than 4 is evidence of reflux. They graded reflux according to the number of reflux episodes and found the test to be semiquantitative at best, with occasional difficulties in classifying patients. Fifty-four percent of 135 patients with symptoms of reflux showed a positive test for reflux episodes. This test is still seen as a useful screening procedure when time or cost precludes the longer pH studies.

Long-Term pH Recording

Twenty-four-hour pH monitoring measures the amount and frequency of esophageal acid exposure by placing a pH electrode 5 to 6 cm above the manometric lower esophageal sphincter (Fig. 17–11). Multiple pH electrodes can measure the same events at various levels in the esophagus. Although shorter recording periods

diagnose reflux adequately, the 24-hour study permits the evaluation of a patient during a full day's normal activities, even during ambulation and during the night. Standardization and clinical application for the test were reported by Johnson and DeMeester in 1974. Its main advantages are in identifying the presence of abnormal gastroesophageal reflux and in establishing if the patient's symptoms are related to these episodes. Long-term pH monitoring combines characteristics of the initial pH studies and the sensitivity testing studies: (1) it quantitates the amount and frequency of esophageal exposure to acid; (2) it is an emptying test, as it measures the time necessary for the esophagus to clear the refluxing acid; and (3) it is a perfusion test, as it relates reflux episodes to symptoms.

Standard parameters are evaluated by the 24-hour esophageal pH recording: (1) the amount of time esophageal pH is below 4, with the total number of reflux episodes and the number of refluxes that last longer than 5 minutes; and (2) the position of the patient during these episodes of reflux—upright or supine.

When 24-hour pH recording was used by Spencer

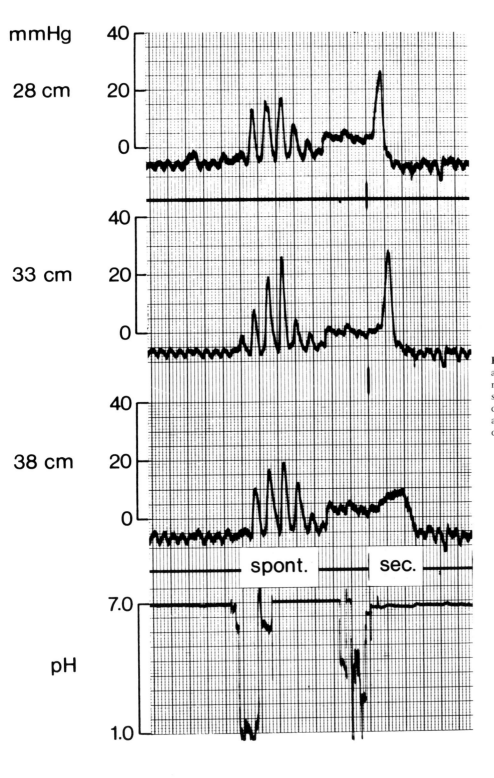

Fig. 17–10. Simultaneous short-term pH and pressure recordings in a patient with reflux. The initial reflux episode causes spontaneous repetitive and nonpropulsive contractions. This is followed by a secondary wave that clears the esophagus of its content.

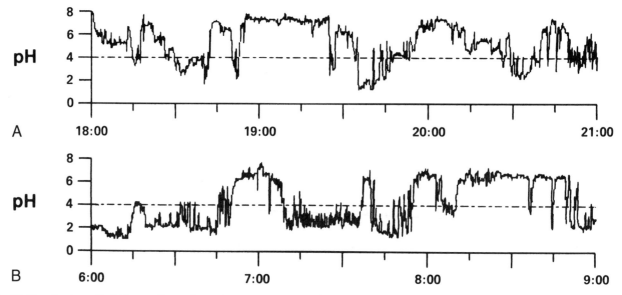

Fig. 17–11. Portions of a 24-hour pH recording. Evening: numerous reflux episodes in standing patient. *B*, In the same patient, in the supine position at the end of the night, long episodes of reflux are recorded. Endoscopy and biopsies revealed extensive columnar-lined mucosa in the esophagus.

(1969) in controls and in patients with reflux, the 15 patients with reflux showed a 5-hour mean exposure time to acid, with a majority of reflux episodes occurring during the night. The control population showed an esophageal exposure to a pH less than 4 of approximately 1 hour. Johnston (1974) and DeMeester (1976) and their associates reported that in their extensive experience in the use of 24-hour pH monitoring the total time of acid exposure in the esophagus was always less than 4.2% in a normal population. Holscher and Weiser (1984) suggested that 7% of total acid reflux exposure should be the dividing line between physiologic reflux and pathologic reflux.

The 24-hour pH studies are the most sensitive—over 90%—and the most specific—100%—evaluation to document reflux. Patients who present with suspected esophageal symptoms and who show physiologic quantities of reflux without mucosal damage and with normal esophageal function should be investigated for conditions other than reflux. This test is essential to establish unequivocal evidence of reflux as well as the results of both medical and surgical management.

Scintiscanning Reflux Studies

Fisher and colleagues (1976) were the first to use scintigraphic methods to assess gastroesophageal reflux. After they instilled or after the patient drank 300 cc of saline tagged with ^{99m}Tc sulfur colloid, they recorded radioactive counts over the esophagus and over the stomach during abdominal increases in pressure transmitted by a binder. They demonstrated increased reflux in heartburn patients mainly when increased abdominal pressure was applied. This test is only semiquantitative and loses its value whenever esophageal retention occurs. It does not demonstrate reflux consistently and has not been

shown to be superior to 24-hour pH monitoring to diagnose pathologic reflux.

Assessment of Esophageal Sensitivity

Acid Perfusion—Bernstein—Test

In 1958 Bernstein and Baker used acid perfusion to induce esophageal pain in patients with reflux disease. The test is based on reproducing symptoms by the instillation of 0.1 N HCl in the esophagus. The test is performed with the patient sitting and with a nasogastric tube passed 30 cm from the nares. With this tube in place and the patient unaware of the solutions used, infusions are started using normal saline for 15 minutes and then 0.1 N HCl at a rate of 6 cc/min until symptoms are produced. The test is positive if in two successive infusion periods acid induces pain and saline induces relief. Lazar and associates (1959) proposed that the pain was caused by simultaneous esophageal contractions during the duration of the heartburn from the perfusion. Siegel and Hendrix (1963) came to identical conclusions, documenting increased contraction and strength duration as well as an increased incidence of tertiary contractions (Fig. 17–12).

The specificity of the Bernstein test is 89%. This means that in 100 normal patients with no reflux disease, 11 will experience pain during acid infusion, thereby resulting in 11% of false positive tests. Sladen and colleagues (1975) have noted that the sensitivity of the acid perfusion test is low because the pain produced by acid infusion is not correlated with the severity of the esophagitis present.

Acid Emptying Test

This test, employed by Booth and associates (1968), measures the esophageal emptying capacity when ex-

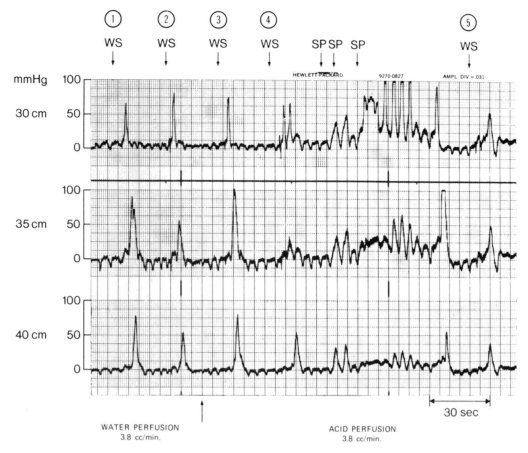

Fig. 17–12. Esophageal sensitivity as assessed by acid perfusion: increased incidence and strength of tertiary contractions are observed when acid replaces the water perfusate. The esophagus is cleared by a secondary contraction. The response to swallowing under acid perfusion (WS-5) shows a nonpropulsive contraction.

posed to an acid bolus and gives an indication of how adequate the esophageal defense mechanisms are. A bolus of 15 cc of 0.1 N HCl is introduced into the esophagus 10 cm above the pH probe. The patient performs repeated dry swallows at 30-second intervals. In the normal individual the distal esophagus is cleared of acid within 10 swallows. A prolonged clearance test indicates an impaired capacity of the esophagus to clear the irritant material from its lumen. Though the early pH studies brought attention to disordered clearance of acid by the esophagus in patients with reflux, this test lacks sensitivity.

Potential Difference Measurements

The transition zone of columnar to squamous epithelium may be accurately defined by measuring potential difference during manometric studies of the area. This is permitted by recording a higher potential difference for the esophageal mucosa when compared to the negative potential of the gastric mucosa.

Khamis and co-workers (1978) suggested that potential difference measurement may be useful to demonstrate mucosal damage in the absence of endoscopic esophagitis: a reduction in potential difference is present when injury to the esophageal mucosa has been produced. The

detection of areas of esophageal columnar epithelium in patients with chronic reflux may represent another advantage.

Orlando (1982) and Herlihy (1984) and their associates reported that the specificity for potential difference measurement is 92 to 96% but that the sensitivity is only 50 to 70%. When Eckardt and associates (1983) studied histologic findings in esophageal mucosal metaplasia, they found an underestimation of the extent of the pathologic epithelium if it was detected by potential difference measurement.

REFERENCES

Airdar, O.: Dados sebre a aque tetonica muscular da porcao inicial do esofago humano. Arquiv. Cirurg. Clin. Exp. 7:548, 1943.

Arndorfer, R.C., et al.: Improved infusion system for intraluminal esophageal manometry. Gastroenterology 73:23, 1977.

Ask, P., and Tibbling, L.: Effect of time interval between swallows on esophageal peristalsis. Am. J. Physiol. 238:G485, 1980.

Asoh, R., and Goyal, R.K.: Manometry and electromyography of the upper esophageal sphincter in the opossum. Gastroenterology 74:514, 1978.

Bernstein, L.M., and Baker, L.A.: A clinical test for esophagitis. Gastroenterology 34:760, 1958.

Bonavina, L., et al.: Length of the distal esophageal sphincter and competency of the cardia. Am. J. Surg. 151:25, 1986.

Booth, D.J., Kemmerer, W.T., and Skinner, D.B.: Acid clearing from the distal esophagus. Arch. Surg. 96:731, 1968.

Boyle, J.T., and Cohen, S.: Does intrinsic LES tone increase as an adaptive response to increased intra-abdominal pressure? Dig. Dis. Sci. 29:760, 1984.

Christensen, J.: Patterns of esophageal responses to stretch and electrical stimulation. Gastroenterology 59:909, 1970.

Creamer, B., and Schlegel, J.: Motor responses of the esophagus to distention. J. Appl. Physiol. 10:498, 1957.

Crist, J., Gidda, J., and Goyal, R.K.: Intramural mechanisms of esophageal peristalsis: roles of cholinergic and noncholinergic nerves. Proc. Natl. Acad. Sci. (USA). 81:3595, 1984.

Curtis, D.J., Cruess, D.F., and Berg, T.: The cricopharyngeal muscle: a video recording review. Am. J. Radiol. 142:497, 1984.

DeMeester, T.R., et al.: Patterns of gastroesophageal reflux in health and disease. Ann. Surg. 184:459, 1976.

Dent, J.: A new technique for continuous sphincter pressure measurement. Gastroenterology 71:263, 1976.

Dent, J., et al.: Mechanisms of gastroesophageal reflux in recumbent asymptomatic human subjects. J. Clin. Invest. 65:256, 1980.

Dent, J., et al.: Interdigestive phasic contractions of the human lower esophageal sphincter. Gastroenterology 84:453, 1983.

Dodds, W.J.: Quantitation of pharyngeal motor function in normal human subjects. J. Appl. Physiol. 39:692, 1975.

Dodds, W.J.: Instrumentation and methods for intraluminal esophageal manometry. Arch. Intern. Med. 136:515, 1976.

Dodds, W.J., et al.: A comparison between primary esophageal peristalsis following wet and dry swallows. J. Appl. Physiol. 35:851, 1973.

Dodds, W.J., et al.: Effect of atropine on esophageal motor function in humans. Am. J. Physiol. 240:G290, 1981.

Dodds, W.J., et al.: Mechanisms of gastroesophageal reflux in patients with reflux esophagitis. N. Engl. J. Med. 307:1547, 1982.

Duranceau, A.C., et al.: Esophageal motility in asymptomatic volunteers. Surg. Clin. North. Am. 63:777, 1983.

Eckardt, J.F., Janisch, H.D., and Bettendorf, U.: Barrett's syndrome: correlation of esophageal morphology with potential difference measurements. Z. Gastroenterol. 21:199, 1983.

Fischer, R.S., et al.: Gastroesophageal scintiscanning to detect and quantitate GE reflux. Gastroenterology 70:301, 1976.

Fisher, R.S., and Malmud, L.S.: The lower esophageal sphincter as a barrier to gastroesophageal reflux. Gastroenterology 72:19, 1977.

Funch-Jensen, P., and Jacobsen, E.: Esophageal peristalsis before, during and after food intake in healthy people. Scand. J. Gastroenterology 16:209, 1981.

Gerhardt, D.C.: Human upper esophageal sphincter: response to volume, osmotic and acid stimuli. Gastroenterology 75:268, 1978.

Herlihy, K.J., et al.: Barrett's esophagus: clinical endoscopic, histologic, manometric, and electrical potential difference characteristics. Gastroenterology 86:436, 1984.

Hollis, J.B., and Castell, D.O.: Esophageal function in elderly men: a new look at "presby-esophagus." Ann. Intern. Med. 80:371, 1974.

Holscher, A.H., and Weiser, H.F.: Reflux characteristics in health and disease. In Gastrointestinal Motility. Edited by C. Roman. Lancaster, England, MTP Press, 1984.

Johnston, L.E., and DeMeester, T.R.: Twenty-four hour pH monitoring of the distal esophagus. Am. J. Gastroenterol. 62:325, 1974.

Kahrilas, P.J., et al.: Upper esophageal sphincter function during belching. Gastroenterology 91:133, 1986.

Kahrilas, P.J., et al.: A method for continuous monitoring of upper esophageal pressure. Dig. Dis. Sci. 32:121, 1987a.

Kahrilas, P.J., et al.: The effect of sleep, spontaneous gastroesophageal reflux and a meal on UES pressure in normal human volunteers. Gastroenterology 92:466, 1987b.

Khamis, B., et al.: Transmucosal potential difference, diagnostic value in gastroesophageal reflux. Gut 19:396, 1978.

Kaye, M.D., and Wexler, R.M: Alteration of esophageal peristalsis by body position. Dig. Dis. Sci. 26:897, 1981.

Lazar, H.P., et al.: Nonperistaltic esophageal motility accompanying experimentally produced heartburn. J. Lab. Clin. Med. 54:917, 1959.

Landers, B.R., and Jamieson, G.G.: Response of the porcine lower esophageal sphincter to increasing intra-abdominal pressure. Dig. Dis. Sci. 32:272, 1987.

Liebermann-Meffert, D., et al.: Muscular equivalent of the lower esophageal sphincter. Gastroenterology 70:31, 1979.

Maddern, G.J., et al.: Abnormalities of esophageal and gastric emptying in progressive systemic sclerosis. Gastroenterology 87:922, 1984.

Maddern, G.J., and Jamieson, G.G.: Oesophageal emptying in patients with gastro-oesophageal reflux. Br. J. Surg. 73:615, 1986.

Meyer, G.W., Gerhardt, D.C., and Castell, D.O.: Human esophageal response to rapid swallowing: muscle refractory period or neural inhibition? Am. J. Physiol. 241:G129, 1981.

Orlando, R.C., et al.: Esophageal potential difference measurements in esophageal disease. Gastroenterology 83:1026, 1982.

Piccone, V.A., Gutelius, J.R., and McCorriston, J.R.: A multiphase esophageal pH for gastroesophageal reflux. Surgery 57:635, 1965.

Pope, C.E: Effect of infusion on force of closure measurements in the esophagus. Gastroenterology 58:616, 1970.

Rubin, J., et al.: Measuring the effect of emotions on esophageal motility. Psychosomatic Medicine 24:170, 1962.

Russell, C.O.H., et al.: Radionuclide transit: a sensitive screening test for esophageal dysfunction. Gastroenterology 80:887, 1981.

Sarna, S.K., Daniel, E.E., and Waterfall, W.E.: Myogenic and neural control systems for esophageal motility. Gastroenterology 73:1345, 1977.

Shipp, T., Deatsch, W.W., and Robertson, K.: Pharyngo-esophageal muscle activity during swallowing in man. Laryngoscope 80:1, 1970.

Siegel, C.I., and Hendrix, T.R.: Esophageal motor abnormalities induced by acid perfusion in patients with heartburn. J. Clin. Investig. 42:686, 1963.

Skinner, D.B., and Booth, D.J.: Assessment of distal esophageal function in patients with hiatus hernia and/or gastroesophageal reflux. Ann. Surg. 172:627, 1970.

Sladen, G.E., Riddell, R.H., and Willoughby, J.M.T.: Oesophagoscopy, biopsy and acid perfusion test in diagnosis of reflux esophagitis. Br. Med. J. 1:71, 1975.

Sokol, E.M., Heitmann, P., and Wolf, B.S.: Simultaneous cineradiographic and manometric study of the pharynx, hypopharynx and cervical esophagus. Gastroenterology 51:960, 1966.

Spencer, J.: Prolonged pH recording in the study of gastroesophageal reflux. Br. J. Surg. 54:912, 1969.

Sugarbaker, D.J., Rattan, S., and Goyal, R.K.: Mechanical and electrical activity of esophageal smooth muscle during peristalsis. Am. J. Physiol. 246:G145, 1984.

Taillefer, R., et al.: Nuclear medicine and esophageal surgery. Clin. Nucl. Medicine 311:4450, 1986.

Tolin, R.D., et al.: Esophageal scintigraphy to quantitate esophageal transit (quantitation of esophageal transit). Gastroenterology 76:1402, 1979.

Tuttle, S.G., and Grossman, M.I.: Detection of gstroesophageal reflux by simultaneous measurement of intraluminal pressure and pH. Proc. Soc. Exp. Biol. N.Y. 98:225, 1958.

Tuttle, S.G., Bettarello, A., and Grossman, M.I.: Esophageal acid perfusion test and a gastroesophageal reflux test in patients with esophagitis. Gastroenterology 38:861, 1960.

Welch, R.W., et al.: Manometry of the normal upper esophageal sphincter and its alterations in laryngectomy. J. Clin. Invest. 63:1036, 1979.

Winans, C.S.: The pharyngoesophageal closure mechanisms: a manometric study. Gastroenterology 63:768, 1972.

Winans, C.S.: Manometric asymmetry of the lower esophageal high pressure zone. Am. J. Dig. Dis. 22:348, 1977.

Winship, D.H., Viegas de Andrade, S.R., Zboralske, F.F.: Influence of bolus temperature on human esophageal motor function. J. Clin. Invest. 49:243, 1970.

CHAPTER 18

ENDOSCOPIC EXAMINATIONS

L. Penfield Faber and William H. Warren

The diagnostic and therapeutic capabilities of endoscopes continue to expand, and specialists who treat diseases of the esophagus and lungs must be familiar with all aspects of modern endoscopy. Flexible instrumentation, providing ease of examination, and improved anesthetic techniques have made these procedures simple, and they are accomplished with little patient discomfort and morbidity. Technical advances in instrumentation continue to provide the opportunity for new diagnostic and therapeutic procedures. The flexible instruments are now the instruments of choice for both diagnostic bronchoscopy and esophagoscopy, and they provide precise and clear visualization of both the tracheobronchial tree and esophagus. Despite their decreasing use, the open-tube bronchoscopes and esophagoscopes should remain available to the well rounded endoscopist. In specific clinical situations, they can be the instrument of choice, and familiarity with their advantages is important.

BRONCHOSCOPY

Facilities for Bronchoscopy

Ideally an area of the hospital or outpatient facility should be dedicated to endoscopic procedures. Bronchoscopy and esophagoscopy are routinely done on an outpatient basis and the logistics of the examination and postprocedure recovery for both the outpatient and inpatient must be clearly defined. The room must be large enough to store all supplies. Personnel and equipment should not be crowded during the examination, and necessary items to manage any complication must be available. It is also ideal to be able to administer general anesthesia in the endoscopic unit.

Bronchoscopy is associated with cardiac irregularities and hypoxia, and standard monitoring includes pulse oximetry and electrocardiogram. A continuous supply of oxygen is mandatory, as all patients undergoing bronchoscopy should receive supplemental oxygen. A storage area adjacent to the endoscopic room minimizes breakage, and special holding racks that allow the endoscopes to hang free and not be damaged by continued storage in a case can be devised. Different types of endoscopes are frequently used during one examination, and they must be readily accessible. Other basic equipment includes a resuscitation cart and a fluoroscopic table. The latter is used with a portable C-arm fluoroscope to assist in the obtaining of specimens from the periphery of the lung. The fluoroscope can also be used in the dilatation of esophageal strictures and to assure the proper placement of instrumentation for dilation of muscular disorders of the esophagus. A sink and storage area for cleaning solutions adjacent to the endoscopic room permits the cleaning of bronchoscopes and esophagoscopes while additional procedures are carried out.

A special cart with a flexible bronchoscope and all the necessary equipment to carry out bedside aspiration is practical. It can be returned to the storage area for cleaning and be reused several times a day.

Many endoscopic procedures are accomplished with intravenous sedation, and a recovery area is needed for the monitoring and observation of these patients following the procedure. Trained assistants are necessary to assist at the procedure, and they also clean and maintain the integrity of the equipment.

Although flexible instrumentation permits bronchoscopy to be accomplished easily, it is not recommended as an office procedure. Specific types of equipment that might not be available in an office setting may be required for a difficult procedure. It is not appropriate to have an inadequate examination because of lack of instruments, and complications are more easily managed in a dedicated facility.

Open-Tube Bronchscope

Open-tube, rigid bronchoscopes commonly used for adult bronchoscopy have an internal diameter of 6, 7, or 8 mm and a length of 40 cm (Fig. 18–1). They provide only a tunnel view, but with experience, the endoscopist becomes accustomed to this view of the bronchi. Illumination is supplied from a cold halogen light source through fiber-optic bundles inserted down a small chan-

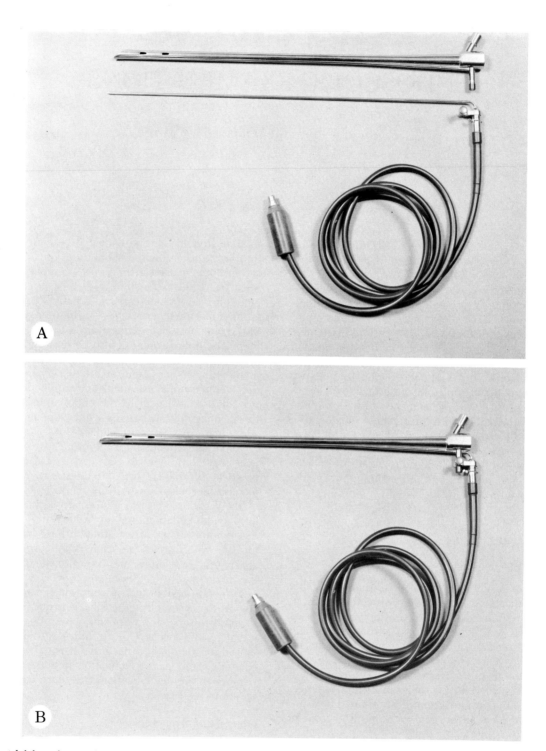

Fig. 18–1. Adult bronchscopes (A.C.M.I.), 7-mm diameter, with fiber-optic lighting. *A,* Components: bronchoscope with side channel for anesthesia equipment (above) and fiber-optic light source with attached lighting cable (below). *B,* Assembled.

nel in the wall of the bronchoscope. A side-arm channel on the open-tube bronchoscope permits assisted ventilation, and a closed system is provided by placing a lens cap over the proximal end of the bronchoscope. Visualization is significantly enhanced with forward—0°, forward oblique—30%, and right angle—90°—telescopes. The flexible fiber-optic bronchoscope can be passed through an appropriately sized open-tube bronchoscope to view fourth and fifth order bronchi. This technique replaces the need for viewing telescopes.

The Storz open-tube bronchoscope with the various Hopkin's telescopes is the optimal system for visualizing the tracheobronchial tree. A large but precise biopsy specimen can be obtained with this system because an optical biopsy forceps permits visual control of the area. With the standard open-tube bronchoscope, the view of the biopsy site is partially obscured because the forceps occludes the lumen of the bronchoscope.

Table 18–1 lists the advantages of the open-tube bronchoscope. It is the instrument of choice for the removal of foreign bodies in children and infants, the evaluation and attempted control of massive hemoptysis, and the dilatation of tracheal and bronchial strictures. Most endoscopists favor specially designed open-tube bronchoscopes for laser therapy. Although foreign bodies in adult patients can be removed with various types of snares passed through the channel of a flexible fiber-optic bronchoscope, foreign bodies can be easily and quickly removed with the open-tube endoscope. Some endoscopists use the flexible bronchoscope for foreign body retrieval in adults because they lack familiarity with the open-tube bronchoscope. The open-tube bronchoscope should always be used to remove aspirated foreign bodies from infants and children. Better control of the airway is achieved with the open-tube bronchoscope, and the various types of foreign body forceps permit firm grasp of the foreign body (Chapter 44).

Massive hemoptysis, 500 ml per 24 hours, must be assessed with the open-tube bronchoscope. Airway control with rapid and repeated suctioning is readily accomplished, and a major bronchus can be packed with gauze. Massive hemoptysis can also be evaluated using flexible fiber-optic bronchoscope through a cuffed endotracheal tube, but clots cannot be removed rapidly and the bleeding site is not clearly visible.

An open-tube bronchoscope should always be available when tracheal lesions are examined. Bleeding from biopsy or manipulation can obstruct a narrowed trachea, and in this instance, the obstruction must be forcibly bypassed with an open-tube bronchoscope. A major ad-

vantage of the specially designed open-tube bronchoscope for laser therapy is that the obstructing tumor can be rapidly debrided.

A major disadvantage of open-tube bronchoscopy is patient discomfort with topical anesthesia. General anesthesia, however, is easily accomplished for open-tube endoscopy, but does carry the disadvantage of any general anesthetic procedure.

Despite the clear view provided by angled telescopes, biopsy and brushing cannot be accomplished at the segmental level through the open-tube bronchoscope. This major disadvantage can be overcome by inserting the flexible fiber-optic bronchoscope through the open-tube bronchoscope.

Flexible Fiber-Optic Bronchoscope

This is the most commonly used instrument for diagnostic bronchoscopy. Subsegmental anatomy is easily visualized and diagnostic biopsy and brushing of lesions in the main stem bronchus as well as in the periphery of the lung are done readily. Continuing improvement in bronchoscopic design has made available smaller fiber-optic bronchoscopes for pediatric endoscopy and the flexible bronchoscope with larger channels for aspiration and larger biopsies. Table 18–2 lists general flexible fiber-optic bronchoscope specifications. Bronchoscopy through a bronchoscope can be achieved with the 1.8 mm diameter instrument.

The standard adult fiber-optic bronchoscope has an external diameter of 5.9 mm, with separate fiber-optic bundles for illumination and viewing magnification, and provides clear visualization of the tracheobronchial tree at the subsegmental level (Figs. 18–2, 18–3). A field of vision of 120° is provided. The angle of deflection is 160° in the upper direction. A channel of 2.2 mm is provided for suctioning and the passage of brush and biopsy instruments. A smaller instrument with an external diameter of 4.9 allows examination at the subsegmental level and passes through a major bronchus narrowed by stricture or tumor. Its 180° upward deflection permits visualization of a difficult-to-reach apical subsegment. The largest instrument, with an external diameter of 6.0 mm, has a 2.6 mm channel for removing thick secretions and blood clots and for the ease of bronchoalveolar lavage. The active endoscopist should have all three of these flexible fiber-optic bronchoscopes available for diagnostic and therapeutic versatility.

Flexible bronchoscopy can be accomplished in the pediatric patient with the 3.6 mm external diameter instrument that Wood and Gauderer (1984) described. It can be passed through a small endotracheal tube or alongside a small catheter delivering jet ventilation. One fiber-optic bronchoscope has a 1.8-mm outer diameter and is 100 cm long. It can be passed through a 2.6 mm fiber-optic channel into a peripheral airway. The small size limits this instrument to visualization only as it does not have a channel or control devices. This small bronchoscope may be more useful when laser photodynamic techniques become more available.

Table 18–3 lists the many advantages of the flexible

Table 18–1. Open Tube Bronchoscope

Advantages	Disadvantages
Foreign body removal	General anesthesia
Massive hemoptysis	Visualize segment
Infant endoscopy	Biopsy segment
Dilate strictures	Peripheral biopsy
Tracheal obstruction	upper lobe
Laser bronchoscopy	

Table 18–2. Fiber-Optic Bronchoscope Specifications

External Diameter (mm)	Channel (mm)	Angle of View	Upward Deflection
1.8	None	80°	None
3.6	1.2	75°–90°	160°–180°
4.9	2.2	80°–90°	180°
5.8	2.2	100°–120°	160°
6.0	2.8	80°–90°	160°
5.9	1.5	90°	100°
6.0 (double channel)	2.0	90°	160°

bronchoscope. With the flexible fiber-optic bronchoscope fourth and fifth order bronchi can be visualized and biopsy specimens can be obtained from them. Peripheral lesions can be brushed or biopsied under fluoroscopic control, and transbronchial biopsies of lung parenchyma can also be obtained. The examination is carried out in comfort under topical anesthesia, and the side effects and complications of general anesthesia do not occur.

A significant advantage is the ability to aspirate retained secretions at the bedside and in critical care units. Patients on ventilators are examined and aspirated through side-arm adaptors (Fig. 18–4) while controlled ventilation is maintained. The ability to bypass distortion of main stem bronchi and obtain a diagnosis of a distal obstructing lesion is obviously beneficial. Photography is easily accomplished through the flexible fiber-optic bronchoscope for documentation of lesions and for use at teaching conferences. Smaller television cameras have now made video bronchoscopy an excellent teaching aid. Unger (1983) described the use of the flexible broncho-

scope to debulk obstructing bronchial tumors by laser therapy. The neodymium:yttrium aluminum garnet—YAG—laser is sent through a flexible quartz fiber, which is easily passed down the channel of a flexible bronchoscope. Brachytherapy can be a valuable adjunct following the debulking of obstructing endobronchial neoplasms, according to Seagren and associates (1985). This can be accomplished either through the placement of interstitial seeds or through the use of low dose iridium-192 inserted in an intrabronchial afterloading catheter. These catheters are inserted through the flexible bronchoscope, and the calculated dose is usually achieved within 24 hours. Specialized radiation sources can also deliver brachytherapy in as little as 30 minutes. Transbronchial needle aspiration biopsy can be performed through the channel of the flexible bronchoscope, as Wang (1985) described. Cytologic sampling of paratracheal and subcarinal lymph nodes can be performed. This technique can be beneficial in the clinical staging of bronchial carcinoma, according to Shure and Fedullo (1984). Needle biopsy of thickened bronchial spurs, a widened carina, and pe-

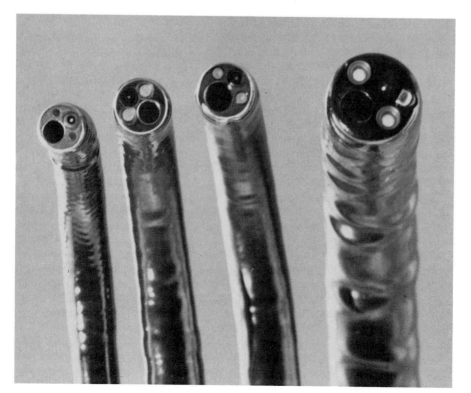

Fig. 18–2. Flexible bronchoscopes and esophagoscopes viewed on end. From left to right: 4.9-mm bronchoscope with 2-mm channel, 5.3-mm bronchoscope with 2-mm channel, 5.9-mm bronchoscope with 2.6-mm channel, 9.0-mm esophagoscope with 2.8-mm channel.

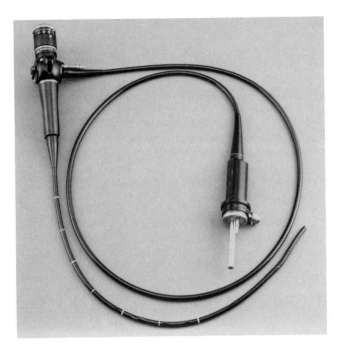

Fig. 18–3. Standard flexible bronchoscope of the Olympus type BF-10.

Table 18–3. Flexible Fiber-Optic Bronchoscope

Advantages	Disadvantages
Patient comfort	Small channel
Segmental visualization	Breakdown
Segmental biopsy	Sterilization
Peripheral biopsy	
Transbronchial needle aspiration	
Bedside aspiration	
Bronchoscopy on ventilator	
Bypass distortion	
Photography	
Increased cancer diagnosis	
Brachytherapy	
Laser bronchoscopy	

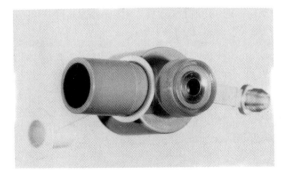

Fig. 18–4. Two-way adaptor for simultaneous flexible fiber-optic bronchoscopy and ventilation.

ripheral nodules can also be performed for cytologic examination.

Breakage is a problem if the endoscopist and nursing personnel are not careful in the use and cleaning of the instrument. In-service sessions should be required for all physicians and nurses who handle the flexible fiber-optic bronchoscope. The small channel limits biopsy size, but experience in the obtaining of multiple biopsies solves this problem. Brushing for cytologic studies supplements biopsy and can provide a diagnosis of carcinoma when the biopsy is negative. The 2.6-mm or 2.8-mm channel removes thick secretions and blood clots with repeated lavage of saline.

The flexible instrument should not be passed through a trachea narrowed by tumor or stricture, because the airway immediately becomes obstructed by the bronchoscope. In this situation, bleeding or secretions can also obstruct the narrowed lumen, and airway control with the flexible bronchoscope in place is not possible. Whenever a tracheal lesion is encountered, the endoscopist must be cautious and ask for assistance or be prepared to maintain the airway with an open-tube bronchoscope.

Gas sterilization is the only way to sterilize the flexible bronchoscope, but recommended cleaning techniques with povidone-iodine or alcohol appear adequate; Suratt and associates (1977) reported no bronchoscopy-related pneumonia in 249 procedures. Flexible bronchoscopes are now designed to permit total immersion in disinfectant solutions.

Indications

Table 18–4 lists the diagnostic and therapeutic indications for bronchoscopy. A new and persistent cough or a significant change in the cough habits of a smoker warrants a bronchoscopy. Bronchoscopic examination can rule out neoplasm as the cause of the changing cough pattern, and visualization of the severity of bronchitis and mucosal inflammation provides appropriate therapeutic guidelines. A persistent cough requires deter-

Table 18–4. Indications for Bronchoscopy

Diagnostic	Therapeutic
Severe cough	Atelectasis
Change in cough	Lung abscess
Abnormal chest roentgenogram	Foreign Body
Hemoptysis	Stricture
Wheeze	Laser
Unresolved pneumonia	Other
Abnormal sputum cytology	Following bronchoplasty
Diffuse lung disease	Prolonged intubation
Opportunistic infection	Difficult intubation
Bacteriologic sampling	Bronchography
Metastatic malignancy	Gastric aspiration
Smoke inhalation	Lobar gas sampling
Pediatric airway obstruction	Management of massive
Bronchoalveolar lavage	hemoptysis
Upper esophageal cancer	
Upper esophageal cancer	

mination of cause and treatment for the comfort and general well-being of the patient.

An abnormal roentgenogram of the chest suggesting cancer warrants evaluation of the tracheobronchial tree. Clinical judgment is always required in deciding when to use bronchoscopy for the patient with an abnormal chest roentgenogram, but the physician should err on the side of endoscopic evaluation to rule out a neoplasm. An obstructing bronchial carcinoma may be the cause of an unresolved pneumonia.

Although the most common cause of hemoptysis is bronchitis, bronchial carcinoma is common in patients with an abnormal chest roentgenogram. If the chest roentgenogram is normal and hemoptysis is present, Jackson (1985) and Poe (1988) and their associates described risk factors that indicate the need for bronchoscopy: age over 40 years, significant smoking history, repeated episodes of hemoptysis, and bleeding greater than 30 ml daily. Hemoptysis associated with wheezing may indicate the presence of a bronchial adenoma or an inflammatory bronchial stenosis. The site of massive hemoptysis must be localized to adequately prepare for possible surgical excision, bronchial tamponade, or bronchial artery embolization.

With the increasing use of sputum cytology as a screening method for high risk patients, patients with a normal chest roentgenogram and an abnormal sputum cytology are being identified. The mouth, pharynx, larynx, and tracheobronchial tree must be examined to identify the site of the early cancer. Transbronchial lung biopsies of peripheral pulmonary tissue can be performed for diagnostic information in the patient with diffuse lung disease or nodules thought to be malignant. Sarcoidosis is frequently diagnosed by transbronchial lung biopsy, alleviating the need for more invasive diagnostic procedures. This technique can also help in diagnosing mycobacterial, fungal, and viral infections.

Bronchial lavage and brushing provide the most bacteriologic information with the least morbidity in patients who are immunosuppressed or have the acquired immune deficiency syndrome—AIDS—as Springmeyer and associates (1986) reported. Special handling of all wet and dry slides and lavage fluid is required by both the pathology and bacteriology laboratories. The sheathed brush has not been significantly beneficial in obtaining bacteriologic specimens and is not recommended for routine use.

Patients with metastatic pulmonary malignancy are frequently candidates for pulmonary resection. Preoperative endoscopic assessment of bronchial extension of the tumor and diagnostic verification are indications for bronchoscopy.

Bronchoscopy is a safe and rapid method of assessing tracheal damage following smoke or caustic-fume inhalation, and provides the physician with appropriate guidelines for continued and future therapeutic direction. Necrotic mucosa and thick secretions frequently need to be debrided by bronchoscopy in these compromised patients.

The evaluation and management of the obstructed airway in infants often requires bronchoscopy. Cysts, neoplasms, tracheal malacia, webs, subglottic stenosis, and vascular rings are just some of the many types of pathologic conditions that require airway visualization.

Bronchoalveolar lavage is primarily a research tool, but can provide diagnostic information in patients with hemosiderosis, alveolar proteinosis, or eosinophilic granuloma, to evaluate the pathology of immune diseases of the lung, and to assess progression of a disease process such as sarcoidosis, according to Hunnighake and associates (1981). Bronchoalveolar lavage should not be a routine diagnostic procedure and should be used only in those centers that are prepared to appropriately handle and analyze the specimens.

Transbronchial needle aspiration cytology can be used to sample subcarinal or paratracheal lymph nodes, cytologically examine thickened spurs or a widened carina, and perform a biopsy of peripheral lung lesions. The findings must be correlated with computed tomogram so that the precise location of the enlarged lymph node is identified. In a study of 31 patients, Shure and Fedullo (1985) concluded that transbronchial needle aspiration—TBNA–increased the yield in the detection of submucosal or peribronchial bronchial carcinoma.

The flexible fiber-optic bronchoscope continues to permit an increase in the therapeutic application for bronchoscopy. Retained tracheobronchial secretions are easily removed at the bedside with minimal patient discomfort, and selective aspiration for the treatment of postoperative atelectasis is rapidly accomplished. Bronchoscopy is indicated in the early diagnosis and management of lung abscess. The passage of brushes or forceps into the abscessed cavity can promote bronchial drainage, and a neoplasm or foreign body is often identified as the cause of bronchial obstruction. The therapeutic value of bronchoscopy in gastric aspiration remains in question, but rapid and efficient bronchoscopy confirms the suspected diagnosis and may provide therapeutic benefit.

Patients requiring continuous mechanical ventilation can undergo both therapeutic and diagnostic bronchoscopic examination with the use of the two-way endotracheal tube adaptors. Pneumothorax and bleeding can be complications of this procedure, but Papin and associates (1986) described transbronchial biopsy performed during controlled ventilation. Placement of biopsy forceps and brushes must be controlled by fluoroscopic examination during the procedure to minimize visceral pleural damage. Hypoxia and hypercapnia are counteracted by increasing the F_{IO_2} to 100% and increasing the minute ventilation. Barotrauma and tension pneumothorax can be complications of biopsy during mechanical ventilation and rapid insertion of a chest tube may be necessary.

The suspicion of a foreign body in the airway is an indication for bronchoscopy and attempted removal. Weissberg and Schwartz (1987) described these techniques. With grasping and basket forceps flexible fiberoptic bronchoscopy can be used for foreign-body removal from the airway. The endoscopist must, however, be absolutely certain that he does not create a more complicated problem by either losing sight of the foreign body or impacting it distally in the tracheobronchial tree. Although Hiller and associates (1977) and Wood and Gauderer (1984) reported the successful use of the flexible bronchoscope in removing foreign bodies from both adults and children, the open-tube bronchoscope remains the instrument of choice, particularly in infants, in whom the open-tube bronchoscope permits both improved exposure and airway control.

Periodic dilatation of tracheobronchial strictures following surgery provides obvious therapeutic benefit. Endoscopic lobar and segmental lavage has proved to have therapeutic benefit in patients with cystic fibrosis and in postoperative patients with persistently thick and tenacious secretions.

Laser can effectively palliate and treat various causes of airway obstruction, as Brutinel and associates (1987) and Wolfe and Sabiston (1986) reported and are also effective in the treatment of occult but bronchoscopically visible bronchial carcinoma. Airway disease that can be effectively treated by various lasers includes tracheal stenosis, obstructing cancers, and excessive granulation tissue. The carbon dioxide laser is a cutting and vaporizing instrument and must be used with an open-tube laryngoscope or bronchoscope, because the laser beam cannot be transmitted through conventional fibers. McElvein (1981) reported good results using the carbon dioxide laser through the open-tube bronchoscope in the palliation of obstructing airway carcinomas. The carbon dioxide laser is particularly effective in the precise removal of laryngeal and vocal cord lesions. The YAG laser produces diffuse coagulation to a depth of 6 mm and vaporizes tissue and is therefore an excellent coagulating and fulgurating instrument. Personne and associates (1986) believe it is the laser of choice for the debulking of obstructive airway cancers. It also can be effective in controlling hemorrhage from necrotic airway cancers. The YAG laser beam is transmitted through a flexible quartz fiber that can be passed through the channel of the flexible fiber-optic bronchoscope, as Parr and associates (1984) described, but special rigid instruments are the bronchoscope of choice for laser therapy. The advantages of these open-tube bronchoscopes are that the tip of the instrument can be used to debulk tissue after laser coagulation, and bleeding is more effectively controlled, because simultaneous use of the laser and suction tubes is easily accomplished. Dumon (1985) and Toty (1981) and their associates and Unger (1983) all reported success in treating patients with similar airway problems using the YAG laser. Gelb and associates (1987) reported significant clinical improvement following YAG laser surgery for recurrent tracheal stenosis. Contact sapphire tips have expanded the versatility of the YAG laser. Various sizes and shapes of tips have been developed, and they permit the concentration of the laser energy into a small point. This technique results in a more precise cutting and vaporization of tissue without the deeper coagulation effects. Kato and associates (1986) and Cortese and Kinsey (1982) reported success in the treatment of small endobronchial carcinomas using a chemical photosensitizer—hematoporphyrin derivative—that is

activated by an argon dye laser transmitted through a quartz fiber. This therapy, however, is best reserved for the patient who cannot tolerate a surgical resection, because extension of tumor outside the bronchial wall and regional lymph nodes are not effectively treated by this technique. Laser instrumentation is expensive and the techniques of this type of therapy are complicated. Extensive experience is required before the endoscopist becomes competent in the use of endoscopic lasers, and continued use is required to provide complete familiarity with all of the advantages and disadvantages. The avoidance of laser complications requires particular expertise; if they occur, they can be fatal.

Palliation of obstructive endobronchial carcinomas can also be achieved by the use of brachytherapy. Radioactive seeds—[198]Au—can be implanted through the channel of the flexible fiber-optic bronchoscope, as Rabie and associates (1986) described, and afterloading catheters can also be properly positioned for the insertion of localized high energy radiation sources. This treatment is particularly effective when maximal tissue tolerance has been achieved with prior external beam radiation therapy, as Schray (1988) and Seagren (1985) and their associates described.

Bronchoscopy during a pulmonary surgical resection is significantly helpful to the thoracic surgeon. The anastomosis is easily visualized following a bronchoplastic procedure, and adequacy of the bronchial lumen is assured. Secretions or blood can be aspirated from the tracheobronchial tree during and immediately following a surgical procedure, and contamination of the dependent lung can be quickly treated under direct vision.

Complications from prolonged endotracheal intubation are well known. The flexible fiber-optic bronchoscope permits clear visualization of mucosal ulceration and developing strictures, and bronchoscopy also identifies the need for repositioning of the endotracheal tube. An endotracheal tube can be selectively placed into the opposite bronchus with the aid of the flexible bronchoscope following the development of a major bronchial fistula.

Patients with cervical arthritis or congenital maxillofacial abnormalities no longer pose the problem of difficult intubation for a general anesthetic. Endotracheal tubes are easily inserted over the properly positioned flexible fiber-optic bronchoscope. Cardiac complications should not occur in association with difficult intubations.

Contraindications

Bronchoscopy by a skilled examiner is safe. There are no absolute contraindications to the procedure, but potential complications must always be considered in evaluating the risks and benefits of performing bronchoscopy in each patient. Potential complications include cardiac arrhythmia, hypoxemia, bronchospasm, pneumothorax, bleeding, and pulmonary or systemic infection. Severely ill and debilitated patients can safely undergo bronchoscopy if it is done in an appropriate facility and by a physician who is experienced with the procedure.

Preventive measures against complications of bronchoscopy are careful evaluation and preparation of the patient and adequate facilities to carry out the procedures. Careful monitoring of each patient is also required to minimize complications. Monitoring techniques include pulse oximetry, continuous electrocardiogram, and intermittent cuff measurement of blood pressure. Hypoxemia is minimized by continuous administration of supplemental oxygen.

If the patient's history reveals allergy to any of the drugs used for topical anesthesia, general anesthesia can be used. Coagulation defects can be corrected by anticoagulant reversal or by the infusion of platelets just before and during the procedure. A brushing or bronchial biopsy should not be done unless the prothombin time is over 40% and the platelet count is greater than 50,000. Topical epinephrine in a solution of 1 to 10,000 can be instilled in the area to be brushed to minimize bleeding.

Patients with tracheal obstruction must be examined cautiously, and biopsy or manipulation of the tracheal lesion should be avoided if airway compromise is severe. Bronchoscopy must be done cautiously in a patient with bilateral vocal cord paralysis. The passage of the bronchoscope through the vocal cords can cause edema, which may produce life-threatening airway obstruction and necessitate emergency intubation or tracheostomy. Patients with hepatitis can undergo bronchoscopy if special care is taken by all personnel in the handling of biopsy specimens and all instruments used are appropriately sterilized. Similar precautions are taken when patients with AIDS are examined.

Patients with uremia bleed easily following biopsy and brushing; these procedures should be avoided in the patient with renal failure. Bronchospasm is a potential complication in patients with known asthma and can also occur in patients with obstructive lung disease. Asthmatics should be premedicated with cortical steroids and brochodilators. Sepsis following bronchoscopy is uncommon, but fever following the procedure is common. Patients with underlying valvular heart disease should receive prophylatic antibiotics before bronchoscopy because this minimizes the complication of bacterial endocarditis.

Technique

Anesthesia

Topical anesthesia is preferred for the performance of routine flexible fiber-optic bronchoscopy, but the prolonged examination in a patient with carcinoma in situ does require general anesthesia. Improved anesthetic agents and techniques have made general anesthesia the method of choice for open-tube bronchoscopy. The ability to carry out open-tube bronchoscopy under local anesthesia and achieve patient comfort is becoming a lost art.

Commonly used agents for topical anesthesia are lidocaine 2% and 4%; cocaine 3%, 5%, and 10%; and tetracaine 0.5%, 1%, and 2%. Complications from topical anesthesia result from administration of an excessive quantity of the drug. If carefully measured amounts are given and the endoscopist is always aware of the total milligram dosage instilled into the tracheobronchial tree, reactions are minimized. Lidocaine is a safe topical anesthetic agent; reactions with its use are minimal. The recommended adult dose is approximately 400 mg, but larger amounts have been given without serious side effects. Lidocaine does not provide the depth of anesthesia required for open-tube bronchoscopy.

Cocaine provides excellent topical anesthesia and is the agent of choice for open-tube bronchoscopy. The margin of safety with cocaine is not as great as with lidocaine, and a minimal amount of excessive dosage causes significant central nervous system excitation. Only a safe, measured amount should be used, to prevent other side effects of nausea, vomiting, and respiratory depression. The recommended adult dose of 300 mg of cocaine should not be exceeded.

Tetracaine is an effective local anesthetic, but side effects commonly occur when a dose in excess of 80 mg is given and it must be used with caution.

Several methods are satisfactory for the application of topical anesthesia. If the flexible bronchoscope is to be passed through the nares, the nasopharynx is initially sprayed with an atomized topical agent, and the flexible bronchoscope is then introduced to a level above the false vocal cords. With the larynx in clear view, more anesthetic agent is placed onto the vocal cords and into the trachea. The bronchoscope is then passed through the larynx into the trachea, and more of the anesthetic solution is instilled into both main stem bronchi.

A second method of topical anesthesia consists of the initial spraying of the hypopharynx with 2% or 4% lidocaine using a special atomizer (Fig. 18–5). Following this, transtracheal injection of 5 ml of 4% lidocaine is given through the cricoid membrane. It is recommended that a 21-gauge vein infusion set be used for the transtracheal injection, because the short needle prevents laceration of the posterior wall of the trachea. Bleeding from the injection site often occurs with this technique, and it should not be used when a patient is examined for hemoptysis. Anesthesia of the larynx is achieved as the patient coughs out the anesthetic agent, which has

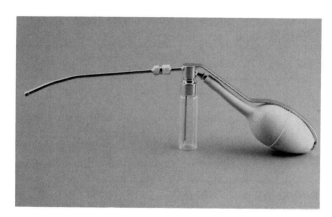

Fig. 18–5. Atomizer for topical anesthesia.

been injected into the trachea. Supplemental 2% lidocaine is then instilled into both main stem bronchi following insertion of the bronchoscope.

Successful topical anesthesia can also be obtained by forced air or oxygen nebulization of the anesthetic agent administered through the nares or mouth. The patient breathes deeply, and 0.5% tetracaine or 1% lidocaine is nebulized into the hypopharynx and tracheobronchial tree. This technique requires 15 ml to be effective, and a decreased concentration of the anesthetic agent is required. Following nebulization, the bronchoscope is positioned just above the true vocal cords and an additional aliquot of 2% or 4% lidocaine is instilled into the trachea. The bronchoscope is then inserted through the vocal cords for completion of the examination. Topical anesthetic agents inhibit bacterial growth. Care should be taken to minimize the amount aspirated into collection traps for bacteriologic analysis.

General anesthesia is easily accomplished for flexible fiber-optic bronchoscopy. In the adult patient, an endotracheal tube is inserted as for any general anesthetic. The two-way adaptor is attached to the end of the endotracheal tube, and ventilation is maintained through the side arm of the adaptor. The bronchoscope is passed through a tight-fitting plastic diaphragm attached to the second arm of the adaptor.

As large an endotracheal tube as possible should be used, because Lindholm and associates (1978) showed that airflow resistance is significantly increased when a 5.8-mm bronchoscope is inserted through an endotracheal tube smaller than 8.0 mm in diameter. The increased resistance with a smaller endotracheal tube impedes ventilation, and hypercapnia results. The 5.8-mm external diameter flexible bronchoscope can be inserted through a 7.0-mm endotracheal tube in children. The bronchoscope, however, must be withdrawn frequently to provide adequate ventilation, and if a long procedure is contemplated, blood gas monitoring is mandatory. When the endotracheal tube acts only as a sheath to provide easy access for insertion and removal of the flexible bronchoscope, the cuff of the endotracheal tube can be removed. This technique permits the patient to breathe around the endotracheal tube as well as through it and smaller endotracheal tubes can be used.

El-Baz and associates (1982) described jet ventilation anesthesia techniques through small catheters through or alongside small endotracheal tubes that can be used for flexible bronchoscopy in young children, as well as in adults with a compromised tracheal lumen. Jet ventilation techniques are not simple, and the anesthesiologist must be well experienced in their use.

General anesthesia for open-tube bronchoscopy is carried out with the use of the side arm ventilating bronchoscope (Fig. 18–6). A tight-fitting lens cap is placed over the end of the bronchoscope to enable the endoscopist to view the anatomy while ventilation is maintained through the side arm of the bronchoscope. The lens cap is removed for biopsy and aspiration. Tidal volume is lost around the bronchoscope through the larynx: this can be minimized by packing the hypopharynx with

gauze or by compression of the supraglottic area by the fingers of an assistant. The anesthesiologist must continually monitor the adequacy of ventilation. An increased minute ventilation and tidal volume are required. This method is safe for procedures lasting 15 to 20 minutes, but if a prolonged examination is necessary, other techniques of general anesthesia should be considered.

The jet technique of general anesthesia through the open-tube bronchoscope, described by Sanders (1967), is a satifactory method for general anesthesia. Carden's (1978) modification uses a jet system mounted on the bronchoscope with a commercially available adaptor. A nitrous oxide gas and oxygen mixture can be delivered with an increased pressure that provides adequate arterial oxygenation and a decreased arterial CO_2. Familiarity with the system is required before it can be routinely used.

Examination

The first phase of a diagnostic bronchoscopy is clear visualization of the larynx and vocal cords. Unsuspected leukoplakia, carcinoma in situ, and invasive carcinoma may be found, and vocal cord mobility must be assessed because invasion of the recurrent laryngeal nerve by lung cancer usually makes a patient inoperable. Examination of the larynx should be carried out before the open-tube bronchoscope is inserted; this can be done by indirect mirror examination or through the bronchoscope itself. The flexible bronchoscope can be used to inspect the larynx and vocal cords directly.

The flexible fiber-optic bronchoscope can be inserted through either the nose or mouth into the hypopharynx and then through the larynx into the trachea. Passage of the instrument through the nares does not permit easy withdrawal and reinsertion for cleaning of the lens and clearing the channel of thick mucus. Biopsy and brushing specimens must be withdrawn through the channel, and some of the specimen may be lost, decreasing diagnostic accuracy. The oral insertion of the flexible fiber-optic bronchoscope permits easy insertion of an uncuffed 8.0-mm endotracheal tube, which has previously been threaded back over the bronchoscope before its insertion (Fig. 18–7). The patient breathes around and through the endotracheal tube with the bronchoscope in place, airway control is provided, and the endotracheal tube acts as a sheath to permit rapid insertion and withdrawal of the bronchoscope. Brushing and biopsy specimens are obtained by removing the bronchoscope with the brush or forceps remaining distal to the tip of the bronchoscope and none of the specimen is lost in the channel. Placement of the endotracheal tube provides the opportunity for assisted ventilation and large catheter suctioning if bleeding is a complication. The flexible bronchoscope can also be passed through tracheostomy tubes or stomas and through side-arm adaptors on endotracheal tubes during controlled ventilation.

Open-tube bronchoscopy is done with the patient supine. An assistant positions the head with the neck slightly flexed and the chin extended. The endoscopist elevates the epiglottis with the bronchoscope and passes

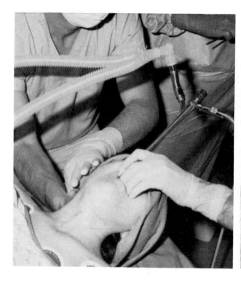
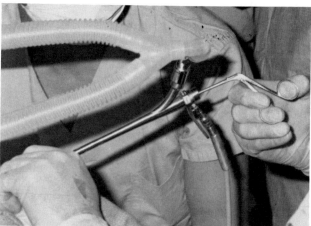

Fig. 18–6. Bronchoscopy and biopsy being carried out under general anesthesia using an open-tube ventilating bronchoscope.

the lubricated instrument through the vocal cords into the trachea. The telescope system provides a magnified field of vision at 0°, 30°, and 90°. If angle-viewing telescopes are not available, the flexible bronchoscope should be passed through the open-tube bronchoscope to view the segmental level of bronchi.

Examination of the trachea is accomplished after the bronchoscope is passed through the larynx, and the carina is next assessed for sharpness and mobility during ventilatory efforts. Widening and fixation suggest the involvement of subcarinal lymph nodes by tumor or by an inflammatory process. Biopsy of the carina is obtained if it is widened or if submucosal extension of malignancy is suspected. It is appropriate to initially examine the side of the tracheobronchial tree that is not involved by suspected disease. The uninvolved bronchus must be examined, because a second lesion not visible on the roentgenogram of the chest is often identified. All lobar

and segmental orifices must be clearly and systematically examined.

The bronchus containing the known area of disease is then examined. The character of secretions and location of lobar and segmental bronchial narrowing assist in identifying the type of pathologic process present. The extent of the anatomic change must be examined to plan the extent of a possible surgical resection. The endoscopist must be aware of the subtle manifestations of endobronchial pathology. Oho and Amemiya (1984) classified bronchoscopic findings associated with cancer, including increased submucosal vascularity, irregular bronchial folds or corrugation, mucosal thickening, stenosis, indistinct cartilage rings, and loss of circular folds.

If a lesion is identified in a main stem bronchus, a biopsy is always performed. Brushing will often cause bleeding, and it may be difficult to clearly visualize the lesion after the brushing procedure. Biopsy through the flexible bronchoscope requires persistence and practice. Although small pieces of tissue are obtained with a 1.5-mm forceps, multiple biopsies usually provide the correct diagnosis. Biopsy of segmental lesions are easily obtained with flexible instrumentation. Following each biopsy, the forceps is agitated in a solution of sterile saline in a glass test tube, and Zenker's fixative solution is added after all biopsy material has been obtained.

Kvale and associates (1976) demonstrated that the accuracy of diagnosis in lung cancer increases with the number and types of specimens obtained. Any bronchial brushing should always be done after completion of the biopsy; the routine use of a 7-mm brush is recommended because more cellular material is obtained (Fig. 18–8). The bronchial brush can be inserted into narrowed segmental bronchi to provide a positive cytologic diagnosis. Many lesions are necrotic at their peripheral aspect, and the biopsy may therefore fail to obtain viable tumor tissue.

The brush is vigorously passed over the surface of the lesion and is then quickly smeared onto the surface of a

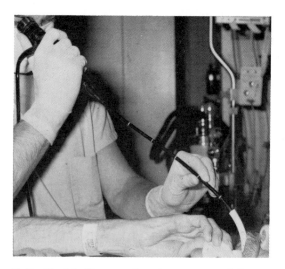

Fig. 18–7. Flexible fiber-optic bronchoscope inserted through previously passed oral endotracheal tube.

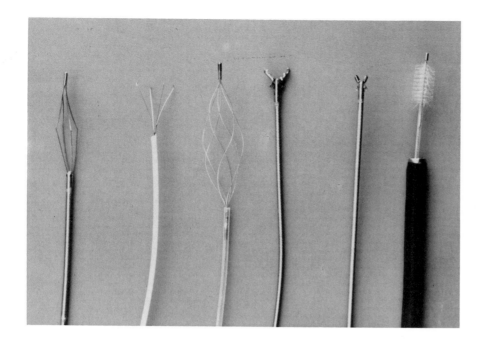

Fig. 18–8. Flexible bronchoscopy accessories. From left to right: standard basket retrieval for foreign bodies, grasping retrieval forceps, spiral basket forceps, alligator biopsy forceps, standard fenestrated biopsy forceps, and 7-mm nylon brush.

glass slide, which is immediately placed in a solution of ether/alcohol to prevent drying and cellular distortion (Fig. 18–9). Improved results are achieved if four separate brush specimens are placed on four slides. A second method of obtaining brush specimens is to agitate the brush in an isotonic solution, which is then sent to the pathology laboratory, where the suspension is passed through a millipore filter. The filter is then chemically dissolved and placed onto a glass slide, and following appropriate staining, it is examined in standard fashion. In patients with proved carcinoma, Zavala (1975) achieved a positive diagnostic accuracy of 85%, using both the brush and biopsy. Saccomanno's (1963) technique for the handling of cytologic brush specimens is also effective. Individual laboratory experience and results dictate the best method of specimen examination.

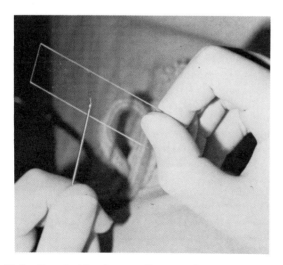

Fig. 18–9. Bronchial brush is rapidly smeared on a slide, which is immediately placed into an ether/alcohol solution for cytologic examination.

Results obtained should be systematically reviewed to achieve the best possible diagnostic accuracy and to provide laboratory efficiency and economy. Bronchial washings do not provide a high yield in malignant tumors and are not recommended for routine use.

Specimens of peripheral lesions are obtained through brushing or biopsy with the aid of C-arm fluoroscopy and image intensification. The fluoroscope permits proper placement of the brush or biopsy forceps using both the frontal and lateral projections. This technique is also used for transbronchial lung biopsy to be certain that the forceps is properly placed in the periphery of the lung.

Transbronchial biopsy is an established technique to obtain small specimens from peripheral lung lesions and from lesions of diffuse interstitial disease. This technique can be effective in establishing a diagnosis in patients with peripheral lung carcinomas, alveolar cell carcinoma, and also lymphangiectatic spread from metastatic carcinoma. The procedure is useful for diagnosis of sarcoidosis, alveolar proteinosis, tuberculosis, and pulmonary infections associated with fungal, viral, and *Pneumocystis carinii* organisms. Small biopsy size makes the procedure ineffective for the establishment of a diagnosis in patients with chronic interstitial fibrosis; in this situation, open lung biopsy is the procedure of choice. This procedure should be done under fluoroscopic control to ensure that the biopsy forceps is in the subsegment of lung tissue that contains the pathologic process and also proper peripheral placement of the biopsy forceps is ensured.

The flexible bronchoscope is initially wedged in the segmental bronchus leading to the diseased lung. The biopsy forceps is gently forced to the periphery of the lung and then withdrawn 3 to 4 mm. The jaws of the biopsy forceps are opened, advanced slightly and drawn through the bronchoscope with a quick motion. The flexible bronchoscope is left wedged in the segmental bronchus to minimize bleeding as a clot will form in the obstructed area. Five to seven transbronchial specimens provide the optimal diagnostic yield, and biopsy sites should be localized to one lung to minimize the complication of bilateral pneumothorax. Preoperative coagulation studies and platelet counts are necessary to minimize the complications of bleeding. Visual placement of the biopsy forceps under fluoroscopic control minimizes the complication of pneumothorax.

Transbronchial needle aspiration—TBNA—can be used to obtain cytologic samples from subcarinal and paratracheal lymph nodes thought to be involved by metastatic cancer, submucosal and parabronchial bronchial carcinoma, and peripheral lung nodules, as Wang (1985) and associates (1984) described. This technique can assist in the clinical staging of bronchial carcinoma and, on occasion, eliminate the need for the more invasive procedure of mediastinoscopy. Prebronchoscopic CT scan is always necessary to precisely define the location of the enlarged mediastinal lymph nodes. Needle biopsy of a peripheral lesion is always done under fluoroscopic control to ensure proper placement of the needle. An 18-gauge needle—to obtain tissue—or a 20-or 22-gauge needle—to obtain cells—attached to a flexible catheter is passed through the channel of the flexible bronchoscope and then introduced through the wall of the trachea or bronchus into any area of extrinsic compression that is visualized endoscopically or noted on the CT scan (Fig. 18–10). The needle can be reinserted several times into the area of suspicion, and saline is withdrawn through the needle and catheter to obtain an appropriate specimen for cytologic examination. The endoscopist must be familiar with the anatomy of the mediastinum and hilum to avoid damage to pulmonary arteries and major blood vessels. Wang (1986) reported a 50% diagnostic accuracy in obtaining cancer cells from mediastinal lymph nodes in patients thought to be candidates for surgical resection. Shure and Fedullo (1984) described increased diagnostic accuracy when TBNA is used with bronchoscopic evidence of submucosal or parabronchial tumor. TBNA should always be the initial biopsy procedure to

minimize the complication of a false-positive aspirate from a previously biopsied or brushed endobronchial tumor. Complications of pneumothorax, bleeding, and mediastinal infection are rare. All diagnostic endoscopists should be familiar with the techniques of TBNA.

Bronchoalveolar lavage—BAL—can be a useful diagnostic technique. It is performed by wedging the tip of a flexible bronchoscope into one of the segments of the involved lung. Aliquots of 20 cc of sterile saline are instilled into the bronchus followed by intermittent aspiration. It may be necessary to remove the tip of the bronchoscope from its wedged position to avoid collapse of the distal airway and thus obtain more of the lavage solution. Usually, approximately 100 ml of saline solution must be instilled to obtain a return of 50 ml. Complications of this technique are rare, but special care should be taken in the asthmatic patient and the administration of supplemental oxygen is always required.

BAL is the diagnostic procedure of choice in the immunocompromised patient. *Pneumocystis carinii*, cytomegalovirus, and bacterial infections all readily diagnosed used special staining techniques in the pathology laboratory. BAL has replaced transbronchial biopsy in suspected pulmonary opportunistic infection, because of greater diagnostic yield and fewer associated complications.

BAL can also be useful in the diagnosis of alveolar proteinosis, histiocytosis X, hemosiderosis, and bronchoalveolar carcinoma. It remains a research tool in defining activity of disease and prognostic information of interstitial lung disease. A central processing laboratory is required for the careful centrifuging and analysis of the obtained specimens.

Pediatric Bronchoscopy

Bronchoscopy of infants and small children requires expertise and familiarity with all available instrumentation. Smaller Storz instruments and viewing telescopes have permitted general anesthesia to become the technique of choice for infants (Fig. 18–11). A 3.0- or 3.5-mm sheath permits the passage of the 2.7-mm optical telescope, and a well illuminated view of the infant's bronchi is achieved. A small suction catheter can be passed through a channel. Secretions are readily removed for therapeutic purposes or bacteriologic study. Small biopsy and foreign-body forceps can be manipulated through this small channel with the viewing telescope in place.

The development of a flexible fiber-optic bronchoscope with an external diameter of 3.6 mm and a channel of 1.2 mm has made its use practical for pediatric endoscopy. Wood (1984) reported satisfactory results with the flexible bronchoscope in both diagnostic and therapeutic situations and has also reported success in the removal of foreign bodies. Examination of infants with the flexible fiber-optic bronchoscope is carried out using sedation and topical anesthesia. Procedures are brief but can have obvious diagnostic and therapeutic applications. Airway stenosis or obstruction would be a contraindication to the flexible fiber-optic technique because the

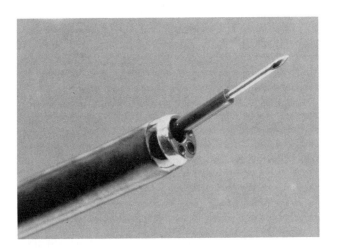

Fig. 18–10. Transbronchial needle for aspiration of mediastinal lymph nodes and thickened bronchial bifurcations.

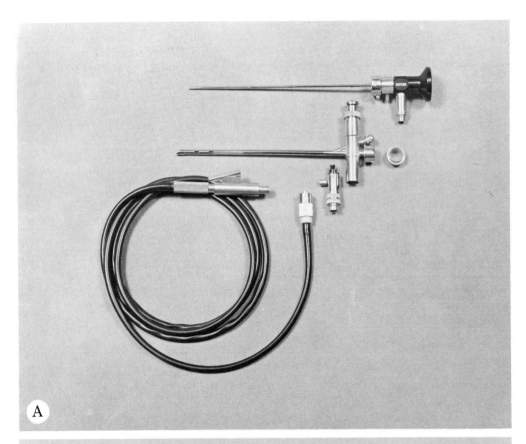

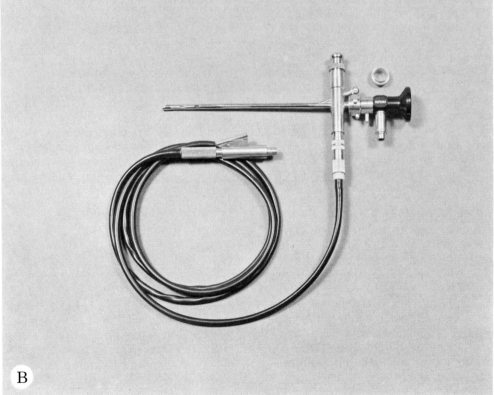

Fig. 18–11. Infant bronchoscope (Storz), 3.5-mm diameter, with fiber-optic lighting. *A*, Components (top to bottom): (1) forward-viewing endoscopic telescope (Hopkins); (2) bronchoscope with detachable windowed plus and side channels for connection to anesthesia equipment, suctioning, and insertion of proximal light; (3) proximal prismatic light carrier; and (4) fiber-optic lighting cable. *B*, assembled.

child or infant must breathe around the instrument, and a narrowed airway would not permit this. Only an experienced endoscopist should attempt pediatric flexible bronchoscopy.

Rigid infant endoscopy should be carried out in an operating room or similar well equipped facility. The infant is placed on the operating table with the neck flexed and the head hyperextended. A laryngoscope at the base of the tongue elevates the larynx, and under direct visualization, the bronchoscope sheath is carefully inserted through the glottis. The design of pediatric instrumentation allows adequate ventilation through a closed system, and general anesthesia permits a careful, unhurried examination.

Complications following pediatric endoscopy can be life-threatening. Subglottic edema from manipulation and instrumentation may obstruct the airway. Stridor after the procedure is an indication for humidification and the administration of steroids. A small bronchus may be perforated, with resultant pneumothorax or pneumomediastinum. Ventilation during the procedure must be adequate.

Complications

A careful history and examination avoids many of the complications that occur with bronchoscopy. Previous drug reactions, blood dyscrasias, and asthma are identified and appropriately prepared for. Experience with the flexible bronchoscope continues to decrease the incidence of complications since Credle and associates' (1974) report which defined a complication rate of 0.8% and a mortality of 0.1% in over 24,000 flexible examinations. Premedication and topical anesthesia were related to 11 of the 22 major complications.

Supplemental oxygen should be given to every patient undergoing bronchoscopy, as hypoxia does occur with examination. Standard monitoring includes intermittent blood pressure measurement by cuff, pulse oximetry, and electrocardiogram. Any changes in vital signs can be quickly identified and treated.

One of the most common complications associated with topical anesthesia is excessive administration of the anesthetic agent. Intravenous diazepam counteracts the systemic manifestations of excessive topical anesthesia and should be readily available. Patients who are heavy smokers and those with excessive secretions or chronic bronchitis often require supplemental anesthesia. These patients should be adequately premedicated with atropine and sedation. More dilute solutions of the topical anesthetic provide a wider margin of safety.

Laryngospasm can be avoided if the topical anesthetic is placed precisely onto the vocal cords and into the tracheobronchial tree. Complications of laryngospasm are a direct result of inadequate topical anesthesia.

Bleeding is an infrequent complication of flexible bronchoscopy and can occur when transbronchial biopsy of the pulmonary parenchyma is done. The injection of a solution of 1:10,000 epinephrine into the segmental bronchus usually decreases bleeding. Zavala (1978) recommended tamponading the bronchoscope into the seg-

mental bronchus to occlude the lumen with a blood clot. Immunosuppressed patients with suspected opportunistic pulmonary infections should routinely have clotting parameters and platelet counts done before bronchoscopic procedure. Supplemental platelet transfusion is given if the total platelet count is under 50,000. Cardiac arrhythmia is usually a result of hypoxia associated with a bronchoscopic procedure; the routine use of oxygen mimizes this problem.

Elderly and debilitated patients should receive minimal premedication, and topical anesthesia must be given in carefully measured amounts. Respiratory depression can easily occur in this group of patients; they must be carefully monitored.

Because pneumothorax is a complication of transbronchial biopsy, these procedures should be done under fluoroscopic control, with visual placement of the biopsy forceps to avoid disruption of the visceral pleura.

ESOPHAGOSCOPY

Esophagoscopy differs from bronchoscopy in two major respects. The esophagus is a more friable structure with most of its wall strength in the mucosa. It is more prone to such endoscopic injury as full-thickness mucosal tears and perforation. Secondly, a much broader spectrum of pathology affects the esophagus than affects the tracheobronchial tree, and many esophageal conditions can be managed endoscopically, which is not the case with the tracheobronchial tree.

Table 18–5 compares the advantages and disadvantages of fiber-optic and open-tube esophagoscopy. Fiber-optic esophagoscopy provides greater patient comfort, the ability to examine the entire upper gastrointestinal tract, and less danger of perforation. The major disadvantages of fiber-optic instrumentation are initial cost, mechanical failure, small biopsies, and limited instrumentation for foreign body removal. The open-tube or rigid esophagoscope has the advantages of larger biopsies, greater aspiration capacity, versatility in removing foreign bodies, and the capability of dilating a stricture directly or by passing a bougie under direct vision. Ease of sterilization and durability are also added advantages.

Open-Tube Esophagoscope

The standard open-tube esophagoscope is 9 mm in diameter and 54 cm long. Narrow and shorter instruments are available for examining children and for passing the instrument through a tight stricture. Light is transmitted through a fiber-optic light carrier inserted into the side of the channel. The Storz esophagoscope provides a magnified field of view with an optical telescope and lens system. This system is advantageous in pediatric esophagoscopy, in which the small lumen of the open-tube esophagoscope compromises visual acuity.

The open-tube esophagoscope is the instrument of choice for removing esophageal foreign bodies because the large lumen permits the passage of various types of grasping and foreign-body forceps. The foreign body frequently can be pulled into the barrel of the instrument,

Table 18–5. Fiber-Optic Versus Open-Tube Esophagoscopy

Fiber-optic esophagoscope	Patient comfort	Expensive
	Examine entire upper gastrointestinal tract	Mechanical failure
	General anesthesia not required	Dilation not possible
	Safety	Small biopsies
Open-tube esophagoscope	Deep biopsy	Patient comfort
	Aspiration capacity	Safety
	Dilate stricture	General anesthesia
	Foreign bodies	
	Ease of sterilization	

which is advantageous when sharp objects such as pins or nails have been ingested. Foreign bodies that become firmly wedged in an edematous esophageal wall can be manipulated and freed with the rigid instrument (see Chapter 44).

The open-tube esophagoscope is valuable in the initial assessment of a tight stricture of the esophagus. Biopsy samples obtained through a flexible esophagoscope are small, and if a malignancy is present, the shelf of the tumor prevents biopsy of the more distal exophytic mass. In this instance, a larger and deeper biopsy can be obtained with rigid instruments (Fig. 18–12). Esophageal mobility can also be assessed by palpating the narrowing to assess mobility. A firm stricture can be safely dilated under vision with the open-tube esophagoscope. A 12-mm gum-tipped bougie can be passed through the stricture under direct vision. The esophagoscope is then passed over the bougie, maintaining full view of the lumen as the instrument is passed through the stricture. Once the stricture has been proved to be benign and dilatable, further dilations can be performed with standard bougies. The rigid esophagoscope is also useful in the assessment of upper esophageal lesions, especially those immediately distal to the cricopharyngeus.

Foreign bodies of the esophagus in children should be removed with the open-tube esophagoscope. The quality of the image through smaller flexible instruments is not comparable, and maneuverability and types of grasping instruments are limited. On occasion, it is necessary to determine whether massive esophageal bleeding is coming from varices. In this situation, a clear field of vision cannot be obtained with the flexible instrument and the large-channel metal suction tube passed through the open tube clears the esophagus of blood and clots.

The disadvantages of open-tube esophagoscopy are the usual requirement for general anesthesia, increased incidence of perforation with its use, and the inability to examine the cardia and distal antrum of the stomach.

Flexible Esophagoscope

The standard adult flexible esophagoscope has an external diameter of 9.8 mm with a working channel of 2.8 mm (Fig. 18–13). Pediatric esophagoscopes with an external diameter of 7.9 mm and a 2.0-mm channel are also available. The active endoscopist must be familiar with the advantages and disadvantages of each model. The standard flexible instrument is a panendoscope because its length and size permit examination of the stomach and duodenum as well as the esophagus. This advantage becomes important when a patient's complaints

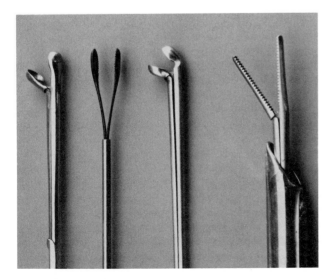

Fig. 18–12. Rigid esophagoscopy accessories. From left to right: forward biting cup biopsy forceps, foreign body forceps, angled biopsy forceps, and alligator forceps in a Jackson rigid esophagoscope.

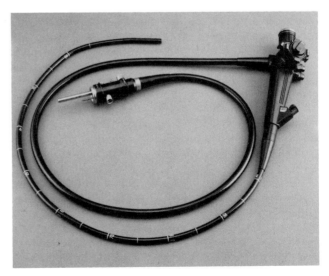

Fig. 18–13. Flexible esophagoscope. Olympus GIF type XQ-10.

are nonspecific and may be related to such conditions as gastric and duodenal peptic ulcer disease, gastritis, or carcinoma of the stomach. To provide versatility, both a large-diameter and small-diameter flexible esophagoscope should be available. The smaller instrument is ideal for pediatric patients and those difficult to intubate; it also permits examination of narrowed strictures if the instrument can be passed. When the stricture is at the esophogastric junction, it is necessary to examine the stomach and duodenum distal to the stricture. Larger diameter instruments permit larger biopsy forceps and have a wider channel for the passage of a greater variety of accessories—snares or grasping forceps—and a greater capability to irrigate and clear the lumen of retained food. Flexible fiber-optic esophagoscopy is usually performed on the awake, mildly sedated patient, and is frequently an outpatient procedure. For anatomic reasons, as in patients with a deformity of the jaw, cervical disc disease, and thoracic spinal deformity, the flexible esophagoscope is the instrument of choice.

Disadvantages include difficulty in visualizing the upper esophagus immediately below the cricopharyngeus, limits in the size of biopsy forceps, and the inability to control many foreign bodies. Flexible esophagoscopes can only be gas-sterilized, but sterilization is only required following the examination of patients with hepatitis, AIDS, and active tuberculosis. Standard cleaning of the flexible esophagoscope is carried out with an aqueous solution of 20% povidone-iodine followed by rinsing with 90% ethanol. All forceps and brushes require gas sterilization.

Indications for Esophagoscopy

The most common diagnostic indication for esophagoscopy is the investigation of persistent or recurrent upper gastrointestinal symptoms such as the substernal pain of reflux, nocturnal pulmonary aspiration, dysphagia, or undiagnosed epigastric pain. An esophagoscopic assessment is always preceded by a roentgenographic contrast study which may or may not identify esophageal or gastric disorder.

All strictures of the esophagus, when first diagnosed, should be examined esophagoscopically. Biopsies and cytologic brushing must be obtained to ascertain the benign or malignant nature of the stricture. In some instances, biopsies and cytologic brushings are negative and the endoscopist must repeat the examination because of the malignant appearance on the barium swallow. Intraluminal filling defects deserve examination as do mucosal abnormalities, which suggest the presence of esophagitis or infection of esophageal mucosa—e.g., candidal esophagitis.

Upper gastrointestinal bleeding may come from the esophagus in the form of varices, neoplasm, or esophagitis, and careful examination of the esophagus is mandatory in the examination of these patients. Particular attention should be paid to the possibility of a Mallory-Weiss mucosal tear in instances where vomiting has preceded or accompanied the appearance or gastrointestinal bleeding.

Patients who have difficulty in swallowing with normal roentgenographic studies of the esophagus require endoscopic examination. Small superficial ulcers and even a neoplasm may be missed on routine barium examination. Patients who experience pain on swallowing in the presence of a normal barium swallow have a high yield of positive endoscopic findings.

Esophagoscopy plays a pivotal role in the evaluation of patients with esophageal reflux. Those patients with endoscopic evidence of esophagitis or a stricture secondary to reflux and have not responded to medical management are candidates for antireflux surgical procedures. The success of medical or surgical therapy can be evaluated by repeat endoscopic examinations and sampling of the mucosa for histologic changes indicative of healing. Repeat examination of a Barrett's esophagus at specific intervals may detect an early malignancy.

Following the accidental ingestion of a corrosive substance, esophagoscopy should be performed within 24 hours to confirm the diagnosis and to determine the distribution and degree of injury to the esophagus and stomach. The esophagoscope is never advanced beyond the area of the first-degree burn, which is characterized by mucosal hyperemia, edema, and superficial ulceration, because of the possibility of perforation.

Esophagoscopy is always indicated when the diagnosis of achalasia is made, to rule out an associated carcinoma or the presence of reflux esophagitis. The latter finding may be an indication for an antireflux procedure in association with a surgical myotomy.

Esophagoscopy is also performed as part of a therapeutic procedure. Ingested foreign bodies can usually be removed or pushed into the stomach. The initial evaluation and dilatation of a stricture is best performed under endoscopic control. Bougies and balloon dilators passed over endoscopically inserted guide wires (Fig. 18–14) can successfully dilate many strictures, as Graham and Smith (1985) and Mangla and Kothari (1980) noted.

An esophageal lumen can be maintained by passing a rigid stent through the mouth with the aid of an esophagoscope. Complications of perforations and dislodgement of the stent do occur, as Skerik and his associates (1981) described, but successful palliation can be achieved in the inoperable patient with carcinoma of the esophagus or in the patient with an esophageal-bronchial fistula (see Chapter 87).

The technique of injecting sclerosing solution into esophageal varices has recently become more standardized. Neodymium-YAG laser therapy has been demonstrated to be a safe and effective method of palliating obstructing and unresectable carcinoma of the esophagus. Brachytherapy radiation catheters can be inserted endoscopically to deliver high dose, low penetration irradiation to the locally advanced tumor following the establishment of a lumen by laser resection.

Contraindications

There are few absolute contraindications to esophagoscopy. Rigid esophagoscopy should be avoided in the presence of a large thoracic aortic aneurysm, a Zenker's

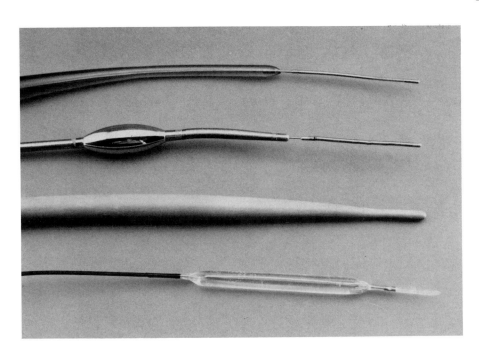

Fig. 18–14. Instruments for esophageal dilatation. From top to bottom: Savary-Guillard dilator with guide wire in place, Eder-Puestod dilator with guide wire in place, Maloney mercury dilator and balloon dilator.

diverticulum, advanced cervical hypertropic spur formation, or in the presence of bony jaw abnormalities. Other contraindications are relative and include major cardiac or pulmonary disorders.

Examination Technique

The examination is performed on a patient who has fasted overnight. In patients with achalasia, a simple overnight fast is not sufficient to clear the esophagus of retained food or liquid. Aspiration of the esophagus before the examination or 24 hours of a clear liquid diet may be necessary. Premedication varies with the situation and the patient. General anesthesia is not required. We premedicate most adult patients with 50 to 75 mg of meperidine. Atropine sulfate 0.6 mg given intramuscularly before the examination reduces secretions, prevents a vasovagal-type response to gastric distention or intubation, and reduces the incidence of ventricular arrhythmias.

Oropharyngeal anesthesia for fiber-optic esophagoscopy may be achieved in various ways. Benzocaine spray, benzonatate, viscous lidocaine, and tetracaine spray have been used successfully. The patient is positioned in the left lateral decubitus position. An assistant is required to observe the patient for any respiratory or cardiac difficulty during the examination. The assistant also aspirates any secretions accumulating in the upper airway and supports the instrument during the initial intubation. The assistant must be trained in operating the biopsy forceps and in preparing cytologic specimens.

The examiner grasps the instrument with his right hand and controls its passage by holding the instrument between the index and middle finger of his left hand. The right hand gradually advances the instrument during intubation. With the patient's head in a normal relaxed degree of flexion, the mouth wide open, and the jaw relaxed, the instrument is guided to the posterior phar-ynx and gently curved with the index finger and middle finger to approach the cricopharyngeal sphincter. The examiner seeks to glide the instrument along the posterior wall of the pharynx and control the midline orientation by placing the instrument slightly above the index and middle finger. At the same time, the index and middle fingers gently depress the tongue to facilitate establishing a gentle curve of the instrument into the cricopharyngeal sphincter. The assistant must take care not to obstruct the free movement of the control knobs of the instrument and not to allow the instrument to bend as he assists in the passage of the instrument through the cricopharyngeal sphincter. Bending the body of the instrument causes tip deflection from the midline, which makes passage through the cricopharynx more difficult. When the resistance of the cricopharyngeal sphincter is encountered, the patient is asked to swallow, and at this point the examiner's right hand gently feeds the instrument forward. A sensation of "give" tells the examiner that the instrument is past the cricopharyngeal sphincter. The instrument should not be forced, and experience must teach the examiner the limits of pressure that can be applied. In learning the technique, it is better to fail in the passage of the instrument from not applying sufficient pressure than from being too forceful.

The flexible endoscope, particularly the thinner instruments, may turn 180° in the oropharynx rather than entering the esophagus. It is also possible to enter the trachea with the pediatric-sized instruments. As soon as the criopharyngeus is passed, the endoscopist should ascertain that the instrument is not in the trachea. An immediate danger of perforating the piriform sinus exists if the tip is deflected from the midline. A plastic bite block is placed over the instrument and between the teeth to protect the instrument in patients who have teeth.

General endotracheal anesthesia is used for open-tube

esophagoscopy. The patient is supine on the operating table, and the head and shoulders are supported by an assistant. The neck is flexed and the head is extended to provide a fairly straight passage into the esophagus with the rigid instrument. A mouth guard or gauze padding is used to protect the upper teeth as the scope is inserted into the oropharynx to the right of the midline. Under direct vision, the scope is introduced to the level of the right piriform fossa. The esophageal opening has a small dimple created by the muscular ring of the cricopharyngeus. Gentle, but firm and continuous, pressure is applied under direct visual control. Care must be taken to position the esophagoscope well anterior to prevent perforation of the posterior cricopharyngeus or hypopharynx. If the lumen of the esophagus at the cricopharygeus cannot be entered or is not well visualized, a No. 12 gum-tipped bougie is passed through the scope and into the esophagus to delineate the true passage.

Visual examination begins immediately upon entering the esophagus, 16 to 18 cm from the incisor teeth. Air is insufflated to distend the esophagus while the mucosa is observed. Pulsation of the aorta may be observed at a level of 22 to 25 cm. The mucosa of the esophagus is pink like the oral cavity. Submucosal branching vessels are normally visible. The gastroesophageal junction is readily identified by the sharp change to a salmon color as the gastric mucosa is visualized. The lower 10 to 15 cm of the esophagus forms linear folds, and the lumen passes anterior and to the left. The gastroesophageal junction at 40 to 45 cm from the incisor teeth may have a linear or serrated appearance. Consequently it has been called the Z-line. There is a visual sense of increased muscular tone narrowing at the junction, and a puckering or folding of the gastric mucosa may be seen. The narrowing at the gastroesophageal junction may readily be overcome by air insufflation. Rinaldo and colleagues (1976) emphasized the role of the endoscopist in recognizing the nonrelaxing sphincter—which yields to firm pressure—as a clue to the diagnosis of achalasia.

Examination of the esophagus includes entering the stomach and retroflexing the instrument so that the fundus and entrance of the instrument itself through the gastroesophageal junction may be visualized. During the course of the examination, esophageal motility and the reflux of gastric contents, such as bile into the esophagus, may be observed. Abnormal findings should be identified descriptively and also noting the distance from the incisors. Larger instruments that can accommodate the biopsy forceps are more successful in obtaining good mucosal biopsies from the lumen of the esophagus.

Complications

The most serious complication of esophagoscopy is perforation. The incidence is reported to be 0.8% in rigid and 0.03% in flexible esophagoscopy according to Silvis and associates (1976). Although perforation can occur at any level, the most common site is just above the cricopharygeus secondary to problems of esophageal intubation. Perforation can also occur at the site of a stricture by too vigorous dilatation or full-thickness biopsy. Man-

ifestations of perforation of the upper cervical esophagus include pain, fever, and subcutaneous emphysema. Lateral roentgenograms of the neck frequently reveal air in the soft tissues as well as retrolaryngeal soft tissue edema. Intrathoracic perforations present with sepsis and shock as the initial manifestations. A small pleural effusion must be viewed with concern, especially if it is a new finding. Defects limited to the mucosa and submucosa have been reported, but with much less frequency, and this type of lesion is thought to be caused by the patient's retching during the examination (see Chapter 45).

Pulmonary aspiration may occur because of retained food in the esophagus resulting from obstruction by chronic stricture, carcinoma, or achalasia. Patients may also vomit gastric contents during introduction of the scope, but this complication can be minimized by having the patient fast for at least 8 hours before the examination. The cardiopulmonary risk of esophagogastroduodenoscopy has also been related to the endoscope diameter and the degree of systemic sedation according to Liebermann and colleagues (1985).

LASER ESOPHAGOSCOPY

Neodymium-YAG laser ablation is an increasingly practical treatment for unresectable carcinoma of the esophagus. The tumor is debulked by fulguration and coagulation. The establishment of a lumen can provide successful palliation. The flexible esophagoscope is used for this procedure.

There are two basic techniques for the laser esophagoscopy. In the first, proposed by Fleischer and Kessler (1983), the lumen is identified by barium swallow and also by a small probe passed through the lesion into the stomach. Repeated sessions are used to core out 1 to 2 cm of tumor until a satisfactory lumen is established. Tissue edema and char formation are practical limitations to the length of esophagus treated per session. Following total debridement, a 1-cm diameter lumen is established over the entire length of the cancer.

In the second method discussed by Pietrafitta and Dwyer (1986), the esophagoscope is passed through the stricture, usually following a small dilator, and the tumor is photocoagulated in a retrograde fashion. The advantage of this technique is that the lumen is re-established in a single session. This factor must be weighed against the hazards of dilating a malignant stricture, overinflation of the stomach, and the need for vigorous debridement. The incidence of perforation with this technique can be as high as 14% and a Gastrografin swallow should always be obtained before oral intake is resumed. Repeat photocoagulation sessions are usually required every 4 to 6 weeks. This technique may also be combined with endoesophageal brachytherapy or the placement of an endoesophageal prosthesis to maintain lumen potency.

ENDOSCOPIC ESOPHAGEAL SCLEROTHERAPY

Endoscopic sclerosis is an increasingly attractive therapeutic option in the management of bleeding varices, as Huizinga (1985) and Hedberg (1982) and their associates pointed out. Endoscopic sclerotherapy has decreased transfusion requirements, but has not affected long-term survival of the cirrhotic patient. Usually, sclerotherapy must be repeated at varying intervals. Twin-channel fiberscopes that provide for the simultaneous suctioning of blood and injection of the sclerosing solution have been developed. Ethanolamine oleate is injected directly into the varix using a long, flexible injector with a 25-gauge needle. Each varix is injected, proceeding circumferentially around the gastroesophageal junction. The process is repeated at 2-cm intervals until all visible varices are injected. If the patient is hemorrhaging, control may be achieved by initially injecting into the paravariceal area to reduce blood flow. Other specialized instrumentation and techniques are available for these injections. Complications include esophageal ulceration, perforation, and aspiration pneumonia.

REFERENCES

Albertini, R., Harrel, J.H., and Moser, K.M.: Hypoxemia during fiberoptic bronchoscopy. Chest 65:1, 1974.

Brutinel, W.M., et al.: A two-year experience with the neodymium-YAG laser in endobronchial obstruction. Chest 91:159, 1987.

Carden, E.: Recent improvements in techniques for general anesthesia for bronchoscopy. Chest (Suppl.) 5:697, 1978.

Cortese, D.A., and Kinsey, J.H.: Hematoporphyrin derivative phototherapy for local treatment of cancer of the tracheobronchial tree. Ann. Otol. Rhinol. Laryngol. 91:652, 1982.

Credle, W., Smiddy, J., and Elliott, R.: Complications of fiberoptic bronchoscopy. Am. Rev. Respir. Dis. 109:67, 1974.

Dumon, J.F., et al.: Endoscopic resection in bronchology using the YAG laser: evaluation of a 5-year experience. Schweitz. Med. Wochenschr. 115:1336, 1985.

El-Baz, N., et al.: High frequency positive pressure ventilation for tracheal reconstruction supported by tracheal T-tube. Anesth. Analg. 61:796, 1982.

Fleischer, D., and Kessler, F.: Endoscopic Nd:YAG laser therapy for carcinoma of the esophagus: a new form of palliative treatment. Gastroenterology 85:600, 1983.

Gelb, A.F., et al.: Nd-YAG laser surgery for severe tracheal stenosis physiologically and clinically masked by severe diffuse obstructive pulmonary disease. Chest 91:166, 1987.

Graham, D.Y., and Smith, J.L.: Balloon dilatation of benign and malignant esophageal strictures: blind retrograde balloon dilatation. Gastrointest. Endosc. 31:171, 1985.

Hedberg, S., Fowler, D., and Ryan, R.: Injection sclerotherapy of oesophageal varices using ethanolamine oleate. Am. J. Surg. 143:426, 1982.

Hiller, C., et al.: Foreign body removal with the flexible fiberoptic bronchoscope. Endoscopy 9:216, 1977.

Huizinga, W.K.J., Angorn, I.B., and Baker, L.W.: Esophageal transection versus injection sclerotherapy in the management of bleeding esophageal varices in patients at high risk. Surg. Gynecol. Obstet. 160:539, 1985.

Hunnighake, G.W., et al.: Characterization of inflammatory and immune effector cells in the lung parenchyma of patients with interstitial lung disease. Am. Rev. Respir. Dis. 123:407, 1981.

Jackson, C.V., Savage, P.J., and Quinn, D.L.: Role of fiberoptic bronchoscopy in patients with hemoptysis and a normal chest roentgenogram. Chest 87:142, 1985.

Kato, H., et al.: Five-year disease-free survival of a lung cancer patient treated only by photodynamic therapy. Chest 90:766, 1986.

Kvale, P.A., Bode, F.R., and Kini, S.: Diagnostic accuracy in lung cancer: comparison of techniques used in association with flexible fiberoptic bronchoscopy. Chest 69:752, 1976.

Lieberman, D.A., Wuerker, C.K., and Katon, R.M.: Cardiopulmonary risk of esophagogastroduodenoscopy: role of endoscope diameter and systemic sedation. Gastroenterology 88:468, 1985.

Lindholm, C.E., et al.: Cardiorespiratory effects of flexible fiberoptic bronchoscopy in critically ill patients. Chest 74:362, 1978.

Mangla, J.C., and Kothari, T.: Esophageal dilation with metal olives under fiberoptic endoscopic control: a new technic. Am. J. Gastroenterol. 73:260, 1980.

McElvein, R.B.: Laser endoscopy. Ann. Thorac. Surg. 32:463, 1981.

Oho, K., and Amemiya, R.: Practical Fiberoptic Bronchoscopy, 2nd Ed. New York, Igaku-Shoin, 1984.

Papin, T.A., Grum, C.M., and Weg, J.G.: Transbronchial biopsy during mechanical ventilation. Chest 89:168, 1986.

Parr, G.V.S., et al.: One hundred neodymium-YAG laser ablations of obstructing tracheal neoplasms. Ann. Thorac. Surg. 38:374, 1984.

Personne, C., et al.: Indications and technique for endoscopic laser resections in bronchology: a critical analysis based upon 2284 resections. J. Thorac. Cardiovasc. Surg. 91:710, 1986.

Pietrafitta, J.J., and Dwyer, R.M.: Endoscopic laser therapy of malignant esophageal obstruction. Arch. Surg. 121:395, 1986.

Poe, R.H., et al.: Utility of fiberoptic bronchoscopy in patients with hemoptysis and a nonlocalizing chest roentgenogram. Chest 92:70, 1988.

Rabie, T., et al.: Palliation of bronchogenic carcinoma with [198]Au implantation using the fiberoptic bronchoscope. Chest 90:641, 1986.

Rinaldo, J.A., Jr., Biederman, M.A., and Gelzayd, E.: The relative application of endoscopy and other diagnostic methods in achalasia. Gastrointest. Endosc. 22:145, 1976.

Saccomano, G., et al.: Concentration of carcinoma or atypical cells in sputum. Acta Cytol. 7:305, 1963.

Sanders, R.D.: Two ventilating attachments for bronchoscopy. Del. Med. J. 39:170, 1967.

Schray, M.F., et al.: Management of malignant airway compromise with laser and low dose rate brachytherapy: the Mayo Clinic experience. Chest 93:264, 1988.

Seagren, S.L., Harrell, J.H., and Horn, R.A.: High dose rate intraluminal irradiation in recurrent endobronchial carcinoma. Chest 88:810, 1985.

Shure, D., and Fedullo, P.F.: The role of transcarinal needle aspiration in the staging of bronchogenic carcinoma. Chest 86:693, 1984.

Shure, D., and Fedullo, P.F.: Transbronchial needle aspiration in the diagnosis of submucosal and peribronchial bronchogenic carcinoma. Chest 88:49, 1985.

Skerik, P., Nosek, S., and Janatova, D.: Esophageal prosthesis and its most common complications. Endoscopy 13:118, 1981.

Silvis, S.E., et al.: Endoscopic complications: results of the 1974 American Society for Gastrointestinal Endoscopy Survey. JAMA 235:928, 1976.

Springmeyer, S.C., et al.: Use of bronchoalveolar lavage to diagnose acute diffuse pneumonia in the immunocompromised host. J. Infect. Dis. 154:604, 1986.

Suratt, P.M., et al.: Absence of clinical pneumonia following bronchoscopy with contaminated and clean bronchofiberscopes. Chest 71:52, 1977.

Toty, L., et al.: Bronchoscopic management of tracheal lesions using neodymium YAG laser. Thorax 36:175, 1981.

Unger, M.: Neodymium YAG laser application in pulmonary and endobronchial lesions. In Neodymium:YAG Laser in Medicine and Surgery. Edited by S.N. Joffe. New York, Elsevier, 1983, p. 74.

Wang, K.P.: Flexible transbronchial needle aspiration biopsy for histologic specimens. Chest 88:860, 1985.

Wang, K.P.: Needle biopsy for the diagnosis of intrathoracic lesions: transbronchial needle biopsy. In Current Controversies in Thoracic Surgery. Edited by C.F. Kittle. Philadelphia, W.B. Saunders Co., 1986.

Wang, K.P., et al.: Transbronchial needle aspiration of peripheral pulmonary nodules. Chest 86:819, 1984.

Weissberg, D., and Schwartz, I.: Foreign bodies in the tracheobronchial tree. Chest 91:730, 1987.

Wolfe, W.G., and Sabiston, D.C., Jr.: Management of benign and malignant lesions of the trachea and bronchi with the neodymium-ytrium-aluminum-garnet laser. J. Thorac. Cardiovasc. Surg. 91:40, 1986.

Wood, R.E., and Gauderer, M.W.L.: Flexible fiberoptic bronchoscopy in the management of tracheobronchial foreign bodies in children: the value of a combined approach with open-tube bronchoscopy. J. Pediatr. Surg. *19*:693, 1984.

Zavala, D.C.: Diagnostic fiberoptic bronchoscopy: technique and results of biopsy in 600 patients. Chest *68*:12, 1975.

Zavala, D.C.: Flexible fiberoptic bronchoscopy: a training handbook. Iowa City, IA, The University of Iowa Publications Department, 1978.

Berci, G. (Ed.): Endoscopy. East Norwalk, CT, Appleton-Century-Crofts, 1976.

Ikeda, S., (Ed.): Atlas of Flexible Bronchofiberoscopy. Baltimore University Park Press, 1974.

Oho, K., and Amemiya, R.: Practical Fiberoptic Bronchoscopy, 2nd ed. New York, Igaku-Shoin, 1984.

Stradling, P.: Diagnostic Bronchoscopy, 4th ed. New York, Churchill Livingstone, 1981.

READING REFERENCES

Bedogni, G., et al.: Operative Endoscopy of the Digestive Tract. Padova, Italy, Piccini Medical Books, 1984.

CHAPTER 19

SURGICAL DIAGNOSTIC PROCEDURES

Joseph LoCicero, III, and Thomas W. Shields

In patients with intrathoracic pathology, the history, physical examination, and noninvasive diagnostic procedures such as chest roentgenography, computed tomography, magnetic resonance imaging and ultrasound examination frequently indicate which surgical diagnostic procedures may be important and the appropriate sequence in which to perform them. Often, as suggested by Falor (1967), several procedures may be performed sequentially during the same operative period to reduce hospital time and expense. When this is done, the pathologic material—if sufficient—is examined by frozen section or cytologic technique to ensure that a diagnosis is obtained and to determine whether other diagnostic procedures are indicated. The sequence is continued until a diagnosis is established or a definitive operation is accomplished.

PULMONARY BIOPSY

Percutaneous Needle Biopsy

Some controversy accompanies any discussion of indications for needle biopsy of the lung. Most agree that a pulmonary neoplasm with clinical or roentgenographic evidence of invasion of the chest wall represents a good indication for needle biopsy. Percutaneous biopsy of diffuse pulmonary nodular disease or solitary lesions without pleural involvement, however, has its proponents as well as its opponents. Advocates such as Khouri and associates (1985) claim that the procedure is simple to perform, has a low morbidity rate, and yields a definitive diagnosis for 95% of malignant and 88% of benign lesions. They further claim that it will reduce the unnecessary thoracotomy rate in benign nodules to 8%. Calhoun and colleagues (1986), however, followed 397 patients after transthoracic needle biopsy to determine the final diagnosis. Of 33 patients with biopsies insufficient for diagnosis, 13—40%—had cancer; of 16 patients with benign diagnoses, one—6%—had cancer; and of 83 patients with nonspecific benign biopsies, 24—29%—had cancer. They further argued that this high false negative rate was

unacceptable and that the procedure should be used only selectively. Nonetheless, this procedure has gained wide acceptance and, unfortunately, has almost become routine in the evaluation of solitary peripheral lesions.

Contraindications to needle biopsy of the lung are pulmonary hypertension, suspected arteriovenous fistula, pulmonary cysts or bullae, hemorrhagic diathesis, or an uncooperative patient.

Technique varies with the type of needle used. When the lesion is fixed to the chest wall, a true-cut needle can be used to obtain the specimen; intraparenchymal hemorrhage with hemoptysis may occur, but is not serious as a general rule in the awake patient. For diffuse lesions or for a solitary peripheral mass, a cutting type of biopsy needle is contraindicated. Most prefer a fine-needle apsiration of such lesions under fluoroscopic or computed tomographic guidance. As the sophistication of the equipment increases, more and more transthoracic needle biopsies are being performed by invasive radiologists.

A small pneumothorax occurs in 10 to 20% of patients after use of the fine-needle technique. Tube drainage of the pleural space is required in approximately one third to one half of the instances of pneumothorax—5% of all patients. Hemoptysis of varying severity—usually mild—occurs in about 6% of patients. Hemothorax rarely occurs. As reported by Berquist and associates (1980), the rate of these complications increases in central biopsies. They also noted the high incidence of hemorrhagic complications for needle biopsy of cavitary lesions—17%—and infiltrative lesions—24%. Berger and associates (1972) reported dissemination of cancer cells to the pleural space. Moloo and colleagues (1985) reported possible spread of tumor to the chest wall. Considering the number of procedures done, however, this complication must be extremely rare.

The diagnostic results of the procedure vary. Lauby and associates (1965), who routinely used this technique for the diagnosis of solitary peripheral lesions, obtained positive biopsy specimens in 45% of their 234 patients. Meyer (1977) and Sagel (1978) and their associates recorded an excellent diagnostic yield following biopsy of solitary peripheral lesions. The former authors reported an accuracy of nearly 100% in the lesions proved to be malignant, and the latter, in a much larger series of patients—896—with malignant intrathoracic neoplasms, demonstrated malignant cells in the aspirate of 96%.

With refined techniques using tomographic or ultrasound guidance, Khouri and colleagues (1985) reviewed 650 aspirations and found only 52 instances in which the sample was unsatisfactory for evaluation. Berquist and associates (1980), in evaluating 400 lesions, reported that the best yield was in cavitary lesions—100%. They had a positive diagnostic yield of 89% in infiltrates and 81% in solid nodules.

In the diagnosis of pneumoconiosis, Mann and Sinha (1966) obtained positive results by needle biopsy in approximately 50% of their patients. In other diffuse diseases and infections, the reported results have been variable. Sagel and colleagues (1978), however, demonstrated that in three fourths of 31 immunosuppressed patients, the causative agent of a focal infectious disease process was diagnosed by this method.

This technique may be applicable to the pediatric patient. Fitzpatrick and colleagues (1985) reported a definitive diagnosis in 6 of 12 biopsies performed in children and adolescents. The diagnoses included sarcoidosis, lymphoma, and eosinophilic granuloma. Sampling size in some children limited the usefulness of this technique, but the diagnostic yield should improve with experience.

Transbronchoscopic Needle Biopsy

With the development of flexible fiber-optic bronchoscopy, transbronchoscopic needle biopsy of various diffuse lesions of the lung has been carried out with or without fluoroscopic guidance. The major risks, as with percutaneous needle biopsy, have been the occurrence of pneumothorax or intraparenchymal hemorrhage with or without hemoptysis.

Transbronchoscopic needle biopsy is now commonly used to confirm a diagnosis of sarcoidosis. Pauli and associates (1984) described the procedure and reported a success rate for diagnosis of 66%. When they added transbronchoscopic forceps biopsy, their diagnostic yield rose to 78%. Transbronchoscopic needle biopsy is also used as a diagnostic adjunct in the bronchoscopic evaluation of acute pulmonary infiltrates, especially in immunosuppressed patients. This technique obviates the need for open lung biopsy in many such patients, especially when it is combined with bronchial brushing and bronchoalveolar lavage. Williams and colleagues (1985) studied 50 immunosuppressed patients by this method. They were able to obtain an accurate diagnosis confirmed by open lung biopsy, in 77% of patients. In patients in whom an infectious etiology was suspected, they showed that the sensitivity for a positive recovery of organisms was 94%. For negative results, bronchoscopy was 90% accurate in demonstrating a reasonable level of confidence that no infection was present. Using this approach as a first-line diagnostic tool has considerably reduced the need for open lung biopsy at our institution.

Open Lung Biopsy

In cases of undiagnosed pulmonary disease, a minor thoracotomy with direct biopsy of the lung may be indicated. This technique of biopsy was initially suggested by Klassen and associates (1949) as a valuable diagnostic method for such patients. It provides a more adequate representative specimen of tissue than other methods. When the cause is obscure, considerable tissue may be required for performance of the desired laboratory analyses, including electron microscopy and special bacteriologic, viral, and fungal cultures, as well as routine studies. Moreover, palpation of the lung and pleura, even through a small incision, frequently may be informative.

Incision may be made anywhere in the thorax as determined preoperatively by the roentgenographic distribution of the disease process. In most patients with diffuse lung disease, an anterior incision provides excellent exposure with minimal postoperative discomfort. The patient is anesthetized in the supine position. Next a roll is placed under the shoulder and hips to rotate the patient to a 30° angle while the arm is left comfortably by the side (Fig. 19–1). A short submammary incision is made. Because the incision is below the pectoralis major muscle, only the serratus anterior muscle fibers must be split. The chest is entered through the fifth intercostal space. This gives excellent exposure to the lateral aspects of the upper and lower lobes. A representative lapet of lung tissue is then drawn into the wound. In general, the lingula should be avoided for biopsy because of the presence of confounding pathology in this segment. Newman and co-workers (1985) removed segments of lingula, right upper lobes, and left lower lobes at 50 autopsies and discovered a high percentage of pulmonary fibrosis and vasculopathy in the lingula not found in other specimens. Although acute and chronic inflammatory changes were the same in all specimens, lingular sections were difficult to interpret. The desired piece is excised by standard wedge resection technique, usually employing a stapling device. The incision may be closed around the suction catheter, which is withdrawn at the completion of the closure. If the patient may require mechanical ventilation, however, a chest tube is always placed. Closure is accomplished by approximation of the serratus muscle, subcutaneous tissues, and skin. No sutures are needed about the ribs or in the intercostal muscles.

Depending upon the possible cause of lung disease, a histologic frozen section is usually performed. This allows the pathologist to determine what other pathologic examinations might be important and allows for submission of fresh tissue for such studies. If he determines that more tissue is required, he can immediately request additional specimens from the surgeon during the same procedure. When an infectious agent is suspected, we routinely divide a portion of the specimen to send tissue for bacterial, fungal, viral, and mycobacterial cultures.

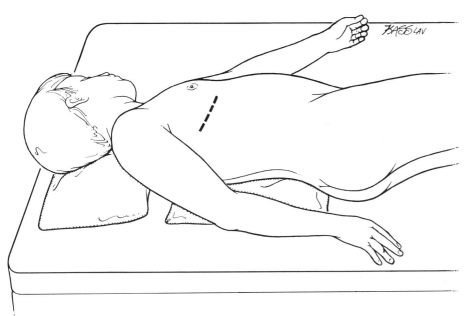

Fig. 19–1. Patient positioning for open lung biopsy. Following introduction of anesthesia, a roll is placed under the shoulder and hip on the side of the biopsy. The arm is placed comfortably at the side. This allows easy exposure for an anterolateral thoracotomy.

We also send tissues for special stains to evaluate for the presence of bacteria, fungus, *Mycobacterium*, and *Pneumocystis*.

Open lung biopsy is well tolerated even by the patient with a limited respiratory reserve, and either a local or general anesthetic may be used, depending upon the preference of the surgeon. Emergency open lung biopsy in the critically ill immunosuppressed patient may be indicated to provide necessary material to direct specific changes in medical therapy. Even though the attendant risk of morbidity is greater in such extremely ill patients than normally experienced, it may be considered an essential lifesaving procedure in the appropriate case.

Rossiter and colleagues (1979) discussed the need for proper selection of patients. Preoperatively, it must be determined that there will be benefit to the patient by making a definitive diagnosis, as well as finding the underlying primary disease state. This benefit is best measured by evaluating the change in therapy that is based upon the findings at biopsy. Cheson and co-workers (1985), in reviewing 87 cases of immunosuppressed patients in whom open lung biopsies were performed, showed that a definitive diagnosis was made in 54%. Therapy was changed in 38% of the cases and 24% of these patients eventually improved. Open lung biopsy in children, in contrast, does not appear to to be as successful. Doolin and associates (1986) reviewed the cases of 56 immunosuppressed children and found a postoperative morbidity of 52% and an operative mortality of 34%. Only 13% of children had their therapy changed and survived.

A new category of critically ill patients arose in the 1980s: those with acquired immunodeficiency syndrome—AIDS. Patients with AIDS present problems similar to those of patients with immunosuppression. Common diagnoses reported by Hopewell and Luce (1985) in 441 AIDS patients include *Pneumocystis carinii*—85%, *Mycobacterium avium* complex—17%, cytomegalovirus—17%, *Mycobacterium tuberculosis*—4%,

Legionella—4%, and other miscellaneous infections—7%. Kaposi's sarcoma was the most common noninfectious disorder—8%. Rubenstein and co-workers (1986) found *Pneumocystis* was the most common infectious diagnosis in children with AIDS as well. Nearly two thirds of the children with AIDS and AIDS related complex, however, had only lymphoid hyperplasia of the lung at the time of biopsy.

Before these patients are considered for open lung biopsy at our institution, they undergo diagnostic bronchoscopy, including bronchoalveolar lavage in segments of suspicious infiltrates, combined with transbroncial forceps biopsy. Wollschlager and Khan (1985) showed this combination had a diagnostic yield of 87%. Most patients receive empiric treatment with trimethoprim sulfisoxazole for *Pneumocystis*, the most common pathogen, before any diagnostic procedure is performed. This empiric treatment has reduced the need for open lung biopsy in AIDS patients to almost nil.

Supraclavicular Thoracotomy

Dart and colleagues (1979) advocated a supraclavicular approach for the diagnosis of indeterminate apical parenchymal or superior mediastinal lesions. The technique is similar to that described by McGoon (1964) for the biopsy of superior sulcus tumors, although a similar approach has been used by others for removal of the dorsal sympathetic chain. Even though this diagnostic procedure offers an alternative approach, its use is limited because several of the aforementioned diagnostic procedures may be accomplished more readily in almost all patients.

Thoracotomy

Solitary pulmonary lesions or a mediastinal mass not diagnosed by any of the previously described methods may necessitate a standard thoracotomy to establish diagnosis and, if feasible, to carry out definitive excision of the lesion. The incision may be limited to only the lateral portion of the thoracotomy until it can be determined whether a complete incision is required. This will decrease the procedure's morbidity. Becker and Munro (1976) have used a transaxillary thoracotomy to achieve this purpose, saving both the pectoralis major and latissimus dorsi muscles.

Complete excisional biopsy is preferable if possible. Peripheral pulmonary lesions may be excised by a wedge resection, whereas deeper lesions may require segmental resection or lobectomy to accomplish an adequate and safe excision. Needle aspiration under direct vision, as described by McCarthy and associates (1980), may permit biopsy of deep-seated lesions without the need to cut across uninvolved parenchyma or to perform a major resection to obtain tissue for examination. Pathologic examination of the specimen determines the extent of any further resection.

LYMPH NODE BIOPSY

Palpable lymph nodes or subcutaneous nodules, wherever found, should be examined by biopsy. Frequently a seemingly innocent nodule in the scalp, abdominal wall, or elsewhere proves to be a metastatic lesion.

Scalene Lymph Node Biopsy

Lymphatic drainage from the lungs and mediastinum travels superiorly by means of paratracheal lymphatics to the base of the neck. Thus, lymph nodes in the anterior scalene fat pad, even though not detectable by external palpation, may be involved by a pathologic process. According to Rouviere (1938), lymphatic drainage from the right lung travels by means of the right paratracheal system. Drainage from the upper third of the left lung proceeds by means of the left paratracheal system. The lower third's drainage, however, and to a lesser extent the middle third's drainage, may cross over to the right from the subcarinal nodes. Although these patterns are far from absolute (see Chapter 5), it is accepted policy to perform a biopsy of the right scalene nodes for disease of the right lung and the left scalene nodes for disease of the upper third of the left lung. Lesions in the lower and middle thirds of the left lung call for biopsy of both the right and left scalene areas. There are no indications for nonpalpable scalene node biopsy in patients with lung cancer. Bernstein and associates (1986) found only a 3.5% positivity rate in 57 such patients. In sarcoidosis, however, the yield is high even if the nodes are not palpable. Truedson and co-workers (1985) found an 84% yield in 167 patients with confirmed sarcoidosis.

The technique of scalene node biopsy is essentially as described by Daniels (1949), with minor modifications. An incision 4 to 6 cm long is made about 2 cm above and parallel with the clavicle, centered over the lateral edge of the sternocleidomastoid muscle. This muscle is retracted medially or partially divided, and the underlying omohyoid muscle is retracted to expose the scalene fat pad. The fat pad is excised in total, including all lymph nodes incorporated in it. The anterior scalene muscle is thus exposed, and a careful search is made for nodes

medial to this muscle and deep to the internal jugular vein. Take care to avoid injury to the thoracic duct on the left or its counterpart on the right. A portion of at least one of the nodes excised should be minced and submitted for microbiologic studies. The remainder should be processed for microscopic examination. Drainage of the wound is not done routinely, but if there should be suspicion of chylous accumulation, temporary drainage is indicated. Complications are infrequent but may result from injury to large vessels in the area or to the thoracic duct. Air embolism has been reported in rare instances, as have nerve injuries.

Any palpable supraclavicular node in patients with carcinoma of the lung should undergo biopsy. Phillips and Barker (1985) reported success in nodal aspiration for cytologic examination. In 44 patients with confirmed carcinoma of the lung, aspiration biopsy for cytologic examination of palpable supraclavicular nodes was successful 84% of the time.

Mediastinoscopy

Endoscopic visualization and biopsy of mediastinal nodes were first proposed by Harken and associates (1954) as a direct extension of scalene node dissection. Carlens (1959) demonstrated that these nodes could be exposed easily by means of an incision above the suprasternal notch and either a portion or all of a node in the paratracheal, superior tracheobronchial and subcarinal regions could be obtained by using a specially designed mediastinoscope.

The major indication for mediastinoscopy is to evaluate the mediastinal lymph nodes in patients with carcinoma of the lung. In such patients, the presence or absence of metastatic disease in the mediastinal nodes has considerable prognostic significance and such information is most helpful in planning the appropriate therapeutic approach. A full description of lung cancer staging and its prognostic significance may be found in Chapter 76. Contralateral (N3) positive nodes are an absolute contraindication for thoracotomy, whereas if only ipsilateral—N2—nodes are involved, opinion is divided as to whether pulmonary resection with radical node dissection should be recommended. Pearson (1986) reported a 25% five-year survival in a selected group of patients with involved N2 nodes identified by mediastinoscopy who then subsequently underwent resection of their tumor. In the majority of instances, however, resection is not indicated when mediastinal nodes are found to contain metastatic tumor prior to thoracotomy.

Pearson and colleagues (1968, 1982, 1986), as well as Sarin and Nohl-Oser (1969), recommended routine mediastinoscopy in the preoperative evaluation of all patients with carcinoma of the lung who have potentially resectable tumors. Numerous reports, such as that by Fishman and Bronstein (1975), supported this view. Reports by Stanford (1975) and Baker (1979) and their associates, however, questioned its routine use in patients with small peripheral lesions and a roentgenographically normal-appearing mediastinum. Fleming (1977) stressed that the procedure should be applied selectively rather than routinely in patients with carcinoma of the lung. Backer and colleagues (1987) have developed a method of applying selectivity of mediastinal exploration based on the roentgenogram and computed tomographic images of the chest. Patients with peripheral lesions and normal hilar and mediastinal shadows on the roentgenogram of the chest need no further evaluation of the mediastinum prior to thoracotomy. Those patients with an indeterminate or unevaluable mediastinum should have a CT scan of the chest. When the CT scan is negative—nodes < 1 cm in size—prethoracotomy surgical exploration of the mediastinum is unnecessary; when positive, it is always indicated. Patients with a grossly abnormal mediastinal shadow do not need a CT scan; surgical exploration of the mediastinum is the staging procedure of choice.

A small transverse incision is made 2 to 3 cm above the sternal notch, and the trachea is exposed by midline splitting of the strap muscles. The pretracheal fascia is incised and a tunnel created by gentle finger dissection along the anterior and lateral walls of the trachea into the mediastinum. The level of the aortic arch may be reached easily by the finger and any nodes at or above this level palpated. The mediastinoscope (Fig. 19–2) is then introduced and advanced farther by means of blunt instrument dissection to extend the mediastinal tunnel. Lymph nodes along the trachea and either main bronchus can be dissected bluntly and removed in total, or a biopsy specimen can be obtained with a forceps. Not all mediastinal lymph node groups are accessible for biopsy by this procedure. The inaccessible ones have been listed by Pearson (1968) as the anterior mediastinal, the subaortic, and the posterior subcarinal—posterior inferior tracheobronchial—groups (Fig. 19–3). Ginsberg and associates (1987) have described passing the mediastinoscope between the innominate and left carotid arteries

to reach the para-aortic and aortopulmonary window lymph nodes.

Take care to avoid vascular injury. In any instance of doubt, needle aspiration should be performed before biopsy specimens are taken. Minor bleeding may be controlled by insertion of silver clips or temporary application of pressure with a sponge forceps or small pack. Minor injury to the pulmonary artery may also respond to temporary packing. Should a major arterial vessel be torn, however, a thoracotomy must be performed immediately to control the bleeding and repair the tear. Injury to the left recurrent laryngeal nerve is an occasional complication of this procedure. Pleural perforation with resulting pneumothorax is also a rare complication and may require needle or tube decompression. The esophagus may also be at risk of injury. *Overzealous attempts to obtain material for biopsy, especially by one inexperienced in the operation, may end in disaster.*

The results of mediastinoscopy vary with the underlying disease process and, more importantly in patients with bronchial carcinoma, with the cell type. Sarin and Nohl-Oser (1969) reported positive mediastinal biopsy findings in approximately 50% of 296 patients with carcinoma of the lung; there was a 76% positive yield in patients with oat cell tumors, 40 to 50% yield in those with other anaplastic tumors or adenocarcinomas, and only 35% positive yield in those with squamous cell carcinoma. The diagnostic yield in patients with carcinoma of the lung also varies with patient selection, that is, with the stage of the disease and the roentgenographic features of the mediastinum in those selected for examination. Therefore it is difficult, if not impossible, to compare one series with another. Diagnostic yield in patients with diffuse lung disease, tuberculosis, or malignant disease other than bronchial carcinoma is variable with patient selection.

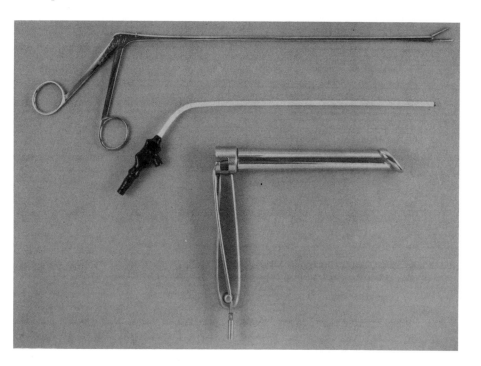

Fig. 19–2. Mediastinoscope and accessories. The scope with light source (bottom) is 20 cm long and has a rounded, blunt tip to facilitate advancement into the mediastinum. The aligator forceps (top) is used to dissect as well as grasp the lymph nodes. The guarded suction (middle) provides electrocautery capability.

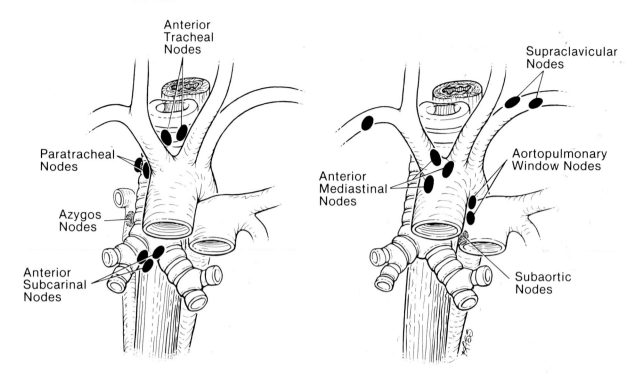

Fig. 19–3. Nodes accessible during surgical mediastinal exploration. Nodes that can be reached by the mediastinoscope are depicted on the left. Nodal groups seen on the right require separate biopsy incisions. In general, the posterior subcarinal nodes are accessible only at thoracotomy.

Mediastinotomy

In cases of mediastinal lymphadenopathy demonstrated roentgenographically, some surgeons prefer anterior mediastinotomy as described by McNeill and Chamberlain (1966) as a procedure providing a more direct approach than that afforded by mediastinoscopy. Such an approach may permit evaluation of the anterior hilar mass and its resectability. It is the procedure of choice to evaluate the mediastinal nodes on the left side when a presumably resectable carcinoma is present in the left upper lobe. This allows better access to the aortic window area.

A short transverse or hockey stick incision is made over the second costal cartilage and adjacent rib on the side chosen for biopsy. The second cartilage is dissected and blunt dissection to free the parietal pleura medially and to allow access to the mediastinum is performed. The third costal cartilage also may be removed for additional exposure. Ligation and division of the internal mammary vessels may be carried out as needed. On the right side, nodes at the hilus or along the superior vena cava and trachea may be obtained. On the left, the hilar, anterior, paratracheal, and subaortic nodes are available for biopsy (Fig. 19–2). Paraesophageal—posterior subcarinal or posterior inferior tracheobronchial—nodes occasionally can be reached for biopsy, although we have found such a biopsy to be difficult. Use of a headlight or lighted retractors enhances visibility in the depths of the operative field. Tissue from any pulmonary lesion immediately adjacent may be obtained by needle biopsy or by an open technique if desired. If even greater exposure

is necessary, the incision can be extended laterally to permit a more major anterior thoracotomy.

Complications are minimal. Bleeding may be controlled if necessary by extension of the incision. Avoid injuring the phrenic nerve. Pneumothorax may be created accidentally or deliberately and is easily managed by brief tube decompression.

Mediastinotomy has been used most often for evaluation of patients with suspected or confirmed carcinoma of the lung. Jolly (1973) and Tisi (1983) and their coworkers reported the efficacy of this procedure, especially on the left, in evaluating patients with bronchial carcinoma. On occasion, when other diagnostic measures have failed, this procedure will permit the surgeon to obtain a positive biopsy of the tumor or its lymph node metastases without resorting to a major thoracotomy if the lesion in question is clinically unresectable. It also affords access for biopsy of clinically malignant nonresectable tumors of the anterior mediastinum.

PLEURAL BIOPSY

Thoracentesis

The presence of unexplained pleural fluid is the prime indication for thoracentesis. In most instances, as much of the fluid as possible is aspirated. If, however, increasing negative pressure in the pleural space gives the patient a sensation of excessive "tightness" or oppression, aspiration should be terminated.

A local anesthetic is used for a thoracentesis. The site of aspiration is selected by roentgenographic localization and by corroborating physical findings. Ultrasound or CT scans are helpful in localizing and directing aspiration of loculated effusions. To avoid injuring the intercostal nerve and vessels, introduce the needle close to the superior border of the rib. The tip of the aspirating needle or catheter should be just inside the parietal wall of the space and secured in this position by a hemostat or other locking device. A large-bore needle is essential because the fluid may be too viscous to pass through a small needle—the tap is all too often reported as a dry one when a small needle is used. Use of a tight-fitting, 3-way stopcock facilitates aspiration and prevents ingress of air into the chest. Suction with vacuum bottles or other sources may be used, but don't evacuate the fluid too rapidly, especially in older patients. Also, the tactile sensation gained with the hands on the syringe will yield information about the degree of negative pressure obtained.

Appropriate laboratory analyses depend on the nature of the fluid and suspected clinical diagnosis. Specific gravity below 1.015 ordinarily indicates a transudate. A pH below 7 is a strong indicator of an active bacterial infection. White cell and differential counts may be helpful. Predominance of polymorphonuclear cells suggests a pyogenic infectious process, whereas a high percentage of lymphocytes is more likely to indicate granulomatous or neoplastic disease. Protein levels over 3 g/dl tend to indicate an exudate, whereas levels below 3 g indicate a probable transudate. A low sugar level suggests the possibility of tuberculosis, but certainly is not a positive indication of the presence of that disease. An elevated fat content is a strong indication of chylous infusion. Lactic acid dehydrogenase activity may be increased in neoplastic disease. Cytologic examinations may provide the diagnosis, as will positive bacteriologic findings.

Needle Biopsy of the Pleura

Percutaneous needle biopsy of the pleura frequently is indicated in the patient with undiagnosed pleural disease whether free fluid is present or not. If fluid is present, a backward-biting biopsy needle is preferable—Cope's or Abrams'. The needle is introduced in a manner and location similar to those for a thoracentesis. The hook of the biopsy unit is withdrawn by using firm lateral pressure until it impinges on the pleura. The cutting unit is advnced or rotated over the hook, and the entire unit is withdrawn with the entrapped bite of pleura within. Care must be taken to avoid taking the biopsy specimen in the superior direction, endangering the intercostal vessels.

When biopsies are performed in patients with an effusion, Cowie and co-workers (1983) showed that adequate tissue can be obtained in 90% of the specimens. When no effusion is present, the yield falls to 79%. If pleural thickening without fluid is present, a forward-biting type of biospy needle is preferred—Vim-Silverman, or others. The depth must be determined carefully by first striking a rib with the needle and then advancing the needle over this rib for another centimeter. The biopsy unit then is thrust into the thickened underlying tissue, the outer cutting sheath advanced over it, and the entire assembly withdrawn with the excised core of tissue within. Several cores should be obtained to ensure adequate material for microscopic diagnosis. Complications are infrequent, but hemorrhage, pneumothorax, and failure of lung re-expansion occur occasionally.

In 202 attempted pleural needle biopsies, Levine and Cugell (1962) were able to establish the diagnosis in 150 patients. A positive diagnosis is made by pleural biopsy in over three fourths of 28 patients with malignant effusion and four fifths of 38 patients with tuberculous effusions. In the tuberculous effusions, this diagnostic technique is the most rewarding.

The number of satisfactory results depends, as noted, not only on patient selection, but also on the number of times the procedure is used. If tuberculosis or carcinoma is suspected as the underlying cause, at least three needle biopsies should be performed before this approach is considered to have given negative results. Poe and his associates (1984) found that with repeat biospy they could increase their yield to obtain a 99% positive predictive value. When the test was negative, the predictive value fell to 77%. Thus, a negative biopsy still cannot be accepted as a final result.

Should inadequate or nondiagnostic tissue be obtained with the aforementioned methods for needle biopsy, an open pleural technique, making a small incision at the desired intercostal space with the patient under a local or general anesthetic, may be used to obtain a biopsy specimen.

Thoracoscopy

In the era of artificial pneumothorax therapy for patients with pulmonary tuberculosis, thoracoscopic inspection and lysis of pleural adhesions were commonly performed. During the late 1970s and the 1980s, there was a resurgence of interest in thoracoscopic examination of the pleural space in patients with unexplained pleural effusions, as suggested by Lloyd in 1953. Other indications include examination of the chest and evacuation of hemothorax in trauma and directed pleural biopsy when random percutaneous biopsy is inadequate or nondiagnostic. A rigid thoracoscope, a fiber-optic bronchoscope, or even a mediastinoscope may be used for the examination. We have recently used a laparoscope successfully (Fig. 19–4). The procedure is performed with local or general anesthesia. The patient is placed in the lateral decubitus position with the affected side up to facilitate the examination. Biopsy of the parietal or visceral pleura or even of the lung may be carried out under direct vision. Numerous reports on the use of thoracoscopy have been published, such as those by DeCamp (1973), Senno (1974), and Lewis (1976) and their associates. Lewis and associates (1976) described its excellent capability in confirming or excluding a diagnosis of mesothelioma. Miller and Hatcher (1978) reported a positive diagnosis of pleural-based lesions in 10 of 11 cases in which all other diagnostic procedures were negative. Boutin and colleagues (1985) described its use in over 800 cases, with a diagnostic study accuracy of 96% for

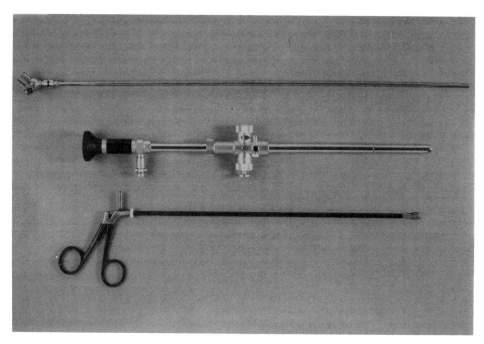

Fig. 19–4. Instrument for thoracoscopy. This Wolf laparoscope (middle), ideal for thoracoscopy, can be inserted through a trocar with a seal to prevent ingress or egress of air. The suction (top) can be used as a probe through a separate incision. The guarded biopsy forceps (bottom) gives electrocautery capability.

malignant lesions and 94% for tuberculosis. They found it unhelpful for the evaluation of bronchopleural fistulas, however. Morbidity and mortality have been reported to be remarkably low except for the occasional occurrence of bleeding, persistent air leak, and infection.

PERICARDIAL BIOPSY

Occasionally, the surgeon is called upon to assist in the diagnosis and management of pericardial effusions. With the advent of two-dimensional echocardiography, localization of the effusion is fast and accurate, facilitating drainage. Most can be managed by catheter decompression as described by Jansen and associates (1986); 87% could be managed successfully by this method. There are, however, instances in which surgical drainage and intraoperative biopsy may be important, particularly in tuberculous or malignant pericardial effusions. When necessary, a transthoracic approach is best. With the patient slightly rotated, as described earlier in this chapter for open lung biopsy and illustrated in Figure 19–1, an anterolateral left thoracotomy is made through the sixth interspace. The percardium is entered several centimeters anterior to the phrenic nerve. At least a 5 × 5 cm section of pericardium is removed for pathologic examination. As with a pleural effusion, the fluid is analyzed to enhance the diagnostic accuracy of the test. This resection creates a window for drainage into the pleura, where the fluid may be absorbed. If a pericardiectomy is required, particularly in the case of tuberculosis, it is easily accomplished through this incision. All of the pericardium anterior to the phrenic nerve is removed. Occasionally, for loculated posterior effusions, a window posterior to the phrenic nerve may be made. Using this method, Gregory and associates (1985) successfully managed 49 patients with malignant effusions. Piehler and co-workers (1985) found a much higher rate of recurrence

with subxiphoid decompression and also recommended the transthoracic approach. For tuberculous pericarditis, Quale and colleagues (1987) recommended a minimum of a pericardial window for management.

REFERENCES

Backer, C.L., et al.: Selective preoperative evaluation for possible N2 disease in carcinoma of the lung. J. Thorac. Cardiovasc. Surg. 93:337, 1987.

Baker, R.R., Lillemoe, K.D., and Tockman, M.S.: The indications for transcervical mediastinoscopy in patients with small peripheral bronchial carcinoma. Surg. Gynecol. Obstet. 148:860, 1979.

Becker, A.M., and Munro, D.D.: Transaxillary mini-thoracotomy. The optimal approach for certain pulmonary and mediastinal lesions. Ann. Thorac. Surg. 22:254, 1976.

Berger, R.L., Dargan, E.L., and Huang, B.L.: Dissemination of cancer cells by needle biopsy of the lung. J. Thorac. Cardiovasc. Surg. 63:430, 1972.

Bernstein, M.P., Ferrara, J.J., and Brown, L.: Effectiveness of scalene node biopsy for staging of lung cancer in the absence of palpable adenopathy. J. Surg. Oncol. 29:46, 1986.

Berquist, T.H., et al.: Transthoracic needle biopsy: accuracy and complications in relation to location and type of lesion. Mayo. Clin. Proc. 55:475, 1980.

Boutin, C., et al.:Thoracoscopy in lung biology in health and disease. The Pleura in Health and Disease. Edited by J. Chretien, J. Bignon, A. Hirsch, *In* Marcel Dekker, New York, 1985.

Calhoun, P., et al.: The clinical outcome of needle aspirations of the lung when cancer is not diagnosed. Ann. Thorac. Surg. 41:592, 1986.

Carlens, E.: Mediastinoscopy. Dis. Chest 36:343, 1959.

Cheson, B.D., et al.: Value of open-lung biopsy in 87 immunocompromised patients wih pulmonary infiltrates. Cancer 55:453, 1985.

Cowie, R.L., et al.: Pleural biopsy: a report of 750 biopsies using Abram's pleural biopsy punch. S. Afr. Med. J. 64:92, 1983.

Daniels, A.C.: Method of biopsy useful in diagnosing certain intrathoracic diseases. Dis. Chest 16:360, 1949.

Dart, C.H., Braitman, H.E., and Larlarb, S.: Supraclavicular thoracotomy for diagnosis of apical lung and superior mediastinal lesions. Ann. Thorac. Surg. 28:90, 1979.

DeCamp, T.P., et al.: Diagnostic thoracoscopy. Ann. Thorac. Surg. 16:79, 1973.

Doolin, E.J., et al.: Emergency lung biopsy: friend or foe of the immunosuppressed child? J. Pediatr. Surg. 21:485, 1986.

Falon, W.H.: One-staged combined diagnosis and therapy of intrathoracic tumors. Am. Rev. Respir. Dis. 95:59, 1967.

Fishman, N.H., and Bronstein, M.H.: Is mediastinoscopy necessary in the evaluation of lung cancer? Ann. Thorac. Surg. 20:678, 1975.

Fitzpatrick, S.B., et al.: Transbronchial lung biopsy in pediatric and adolescent patients. Am. J. Dis. Child. 139:46, 1985.

Fleming, W.H.: Mediastinal biopsy: selective or routine? Am. Surg. 43:74, 1977.

Ginsberg, R.J., et al.: Extended cervical mediastinoscopy: a single staging procedure for bronchogenic carcinoma of the left upper lobe. Thorac. Cardiovasc. Surg. 94:673, 1987.

Gregory, J.R., McMurtrey, M.J., and Mountain, C.F.: A surgical approach to the treatment of pericardial effusion in cancer patients. Am. J. Clin. Oncol. 8:319, 1985.

Harken, D.E., et al.: Simple cervicomediastinal exploration for tissue diagnosis of intrathoracic disease. N. Engl. J. Med. 251:1041, 1954.

Hopewell, P.C., and Luce, J.M.: Pulmonary involvement in acquired immune deficiency syndrome. Chest 87:104, 1985.

Jansen, E.W., et al.: Treatment of pericardial effusion. J. Thorac. Cardiovasc. Surg. 91:975, 1986.

Jolly, P.C., et al.: Parasternal mediastinotomy and mediastinoscopy: adjuncts in the diagnosis of chest disease. J. Thorac. Cardiovasc. Surg. 66:549, 1973.

Khouri, N.F., et al.: Transbronchoscopic needle aspiration of benign and malignant lung lesions. AJR 144:281, 1985.

Klassen, K.P., Anlyan, A.J., and Curtis, G.M.: Biopsy of diffuse pulmonary lesions. Arch. Surg. 59:695, 1949.

Lauby, W.W., et al.: Value and risk of biopsy of pulmonary lesions by needle aspiration. J. Thorac. Cardiovasc. Surg. 49:159, 1965.

Levine, J., and Cugell, D.W.: Blunt-end needle biopsy of pleura and rib. Arch. Intern. Med. 109:516, 1962.

Lewis, R.J., et al.: Direct diagnosis thoracoscopy. Ann. Thorac. Surg. 21:536, 1976.

Lloyd, M.S.: Thoracoscopy and biopsy in the diagnosis of pleurisy with effusion. Q. Bull. SEA VIEW Hosp. 14:128, 1953.

Mann, B., and Sinha, C.N.: Jack needle lung biopsy in pneumoconiosis. Dis. Chest 50:504, 1966.

McCarthy, W.J., Christ, M.L., and Fry, W.A.: Intraoperative fine needle aspiration biopsy of thoracic lesions. Ann. Thorac. Surg. 30:24, 1980.

McGoon, D.C.: Transcervical technique for removal of specimen from superior sulcus tumor for pathologic study. Ann. Surg. 159:407, 1964.

McNeill, T.M., and Chamberlain, J.M.: Diagnostic anterior mediastinotomy. Ann. Thorac. Surg. 2:532, 1966.

Meyer, J.E., et al.: Percutaneous aspiration biopsy of nodular lung lesions. J. Thorac. Cardiovasc. Surg. 73:787, 1977.

Miller, J.I., and Hatcher, C.R., Jr.: Thoracoscopy: a useful tool in the diagnosis of thoracic disease. Ann. Thorac. Surg. 26:68, 1978.

Moloo, Z., et al.: Possible spread of bronchogenic carcinoma to the chest wall after a transthoracic fine needle aspiration biopsy. Acta Cytol. (Baltimore) 29:167, 1985.

Newman, S.L., Michel, R.P., and Wang, N.S.: Lingular lung biopsy: is it representative? Am. Rev. Resp. Dis. 132:1084, 1985.

Pauli, G., et al.: Transbronchial needle aspiration in the diagnosis of sarcoidosis. Chest 85:482, 1984.

Pearson, F.G.: An evaluation of mediastinoscopy in the management of presumably operable bronchial carcinoma. J. Thorac. Cardiovasc. Surg. 55:617, 1968.

Pearson, F.G.: Lung cancer: the past 25 years. Chest 89:200S, 1986.

Pearson, F.G., et al.: Significance of positive superior mediastinal nodes identified at mediastinoscopy in patients with resectable cancer of the lung. J. Thorac. Cardiovasc. Surg. 83:1, 1982.

Phillips, M.S., and Barker, V.: Extrathoracic lymph node aspiration in bronchial carcinoma. Thorax 40:398, 1985.

Piehler, J.M., et al.: Surgical management of effusive pericardial disease: influence of extent of pericardial resection on clinical course. J. Thorac. Cardiovasc. Surg. 90:506, 1985.

Poe, R.H: Sensitivity, specificity and predictive values of closed pleural biopsy. Arch. Intern. Med. 144:325, 1984.

Quale, J.M., Lipschik, G.Y., and Heurich, A.E.: Management of tuberculous pericarditis. Ann. Thorac. Surg. 43:653, 1987.

Rossiter, S.J., et al.: Open lung biopsy in the immunosuppressed patient: is it really beneficial? J. Thorac. Cardiovas. Surg. 77:338, 1979.

Rouviere, H.: Anatomy of the Human Lymphatic System. Ann. Arbor, MI, Edwards, 1938.

Rubenstein, A., et al.: Pulmonary disease in children with acquired immune deficiency syndrome and AIDS-related complex. J. Pediatr. 108:498, 1986.

Sagel, S.S., et al.: Percutaneous transthoracic aspiration needle biopsy. Ann. Thorac. Surg. 26:399, 1978.

Sarin, C.L., and Nohl-Oser, H.C.: Mediastinoscopy. Thorax 24:585, 1969.

Senno, A., et al.: Thoracoscopy with the fiber-optic bronchoscope. J. Thorac. Cardiovasc. Surg. 67:606, 1974.

Stanford, W., et al.: Mediastinoscopy. Ann. Thorac. Surg. 19:121, 1975.

Tisi, G.M., Friedman, P.J., and Peters, R.M.: Clinical staging of primary lung cancer. Am. Rev. Respir. Dis. 127:659, 1983.

Truedson, H., Stjernberg, N., and Thunell, M.: Scalene lymph node biopsy: a diagnostic method in sarcoidosis. Acta Chir. Scand. 151:121, 1985.

Williams, O., et al.: The role of bronchoscopy in the evaluation of immunocompromised hosts with diffuse pulmonary infiltrates. Am. Rev. Respir. Dis. 131:880, 1985.

Wollschlager, C., and Khan, F.:Diagnostic value of fiber-optic bronchoscopy in acquired immune deficiency syndrome. Cleve. Clin. J. Med. 52:489, 1985.

READING REFERENCES

Bowen, T.E., et al.: Value of anterior mediastinoscopy in bronchogenic carcinoma of left upper lobe. J. Thorac. Cardiovasc. Surg. 76:269, 1978.

Oakes, D.D., Sherck, J.P., and Mark, J.B.D.: Thoracoscopy: its use for diagnosis and therapy. In Current Controversies in Thoracic Surgery. Edited by C.F. Kittle. Philadelphia, W.B. Saunders Co., 1986.

Jones, J.W., et al.: Emergency thoracoscopy: a logical approach to chest trauma management. J. Trauma 21:280, 1981.

Lincoln, C.P., Grover, F.L., and Trinkle, J.K.: Open versus needle biopsy of the lung. J. Thorac. Cardiovas. Surg. 69:507, 1975.

Assessment of the Thoracic Surgical Patient

CHAPTER 20

PREOPERATIVE PULMONARY EVALUATION

Andrew E. Filderman and Richard A. Matthay

The preoperative pulmonary evaluation of a patient is an important aspect of the overall care of the surgical candidate. Several studies have shown that respiratory difficulties constitute a large percentage of postoperative complications. This is particularly true in patients who are current smokers, or who have smoking-related diseases.

In general, the pulmonary evaluation will vary, depending on the type of surgical procedure performed. Patients undergoing thoracic surgery with pulmonary parenchymal resection will require assessment of their likely respiratory reserve following surgery. This type of evaluation may range from simple spirometric testing of air-flow rates to sophisticated pulmonary artery hemodynamic studies in an effort to predict whether the patient will tolerate pulmonary resection. In contrast, patients undergoing nonrespiratory surgical procedures require a less sophisticated evaluation to identify them as high or low risk candidates. As a rule, patients should not be rejected for required nonrespiratory surgical procedures because of high risk status. Rather, these patients need to be identified as more likely to develop problems after surgery, and given specific respiratory attention preoperatively and postoperatively. Problems that occur can be addressed more effectively if they are anticipated.

EFFECTS OF SURGERY ON THE RESPIRATORY SYSTEM

The first step in understanding the risk of a surgical procedure is to evaluate what effect, if any, this procedure will have on pulmonary function. In a review of 19 surgical series from 1922 to 1969, Latimer and co-workers (1971) showed that postoperative pulmonary complications ranged from 0.1 to 70%, with the highest incidence in thoracic or upper abdominal procedures and the lowest in nonabdominal, nonthoracic procedures. Therefore, the risk of pulmonary complications from non-abdominal, nonthoracic surgery is minimal, even in patients with abnormal pulmonary function. Abdominal

procedures, however, have been shown to result in a number of predictable changes in the lung postoperatively. These changes may include abnormalities in lung volumes, diaphragmatic function, ventilatory pattern, gas exchange, and local pulmonary defense mechanisms.

In general, upper abdominal incisions appear to result in far greater decreases in lung volumes than lower abdominal or nonabdominal procedures. Latimer and co-workers (1971) (Fig. 20–1) found that forced expiratory volume in one second—FEV_1—and the forced vital capacity—FVC—dropped over 60% on the day of operation in patients undergoing upper abdominal incisions,

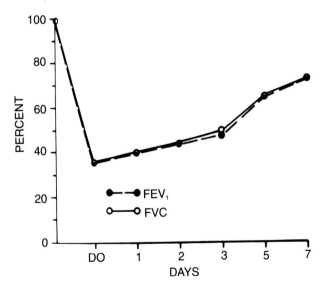

Fig. 20–1. This figure shows the mean postoperative forced expiratory volume in one second (FEV_1) and forced vital capacity (FVC) in 46 patients after upper abdominal incision. The FEV_1 and FVC are expressed as percent of the preoperative value. Both the FEV_1 and FVC fall over 60% on the day of surgery, and gradually increase towards control values over the next seven days. (DO: day of operation). (Reproduced with permission from Latimer, R.G., et al.: Ventilatory patterns and pulmonary complications after upper abdominal surgery determined by preoperative and postoperative computerized spirometry and blood gas analysis. Am. J. Surg. *122*:622, 1971.)

with a gradual increase toward preoperative levels by postoperative day seven. Factors that appear to predispose to respiratory complications include preoperatively abnormal lung function, smoking, obesity, and an anesthesia time of over 3.5 hours. Tahir (1973) and Ford (1983) and their associates noted similar decreases in lung volumes following upper abdominal procedures. In these studies, abnormalities in diaphragmatic function were documented (Fig. 20–2), with decreases in diaphragmatic excursion and a switch to predominantly rib-cage breathing. These alterations result in basilar atelectasis and decreases in tidal volume and lung volumes.

The pathogenesis of diaphragmatic dysfunction is unproven, but may include local irritation to the diaphragm, upper abdominal incisional pain with chest splinting, or abnormalities in neural control of diaphragmatic function. Adding to the change in lung volumes is a change in respiratory pattern; namely, a decrease in tidal volume with a concomitant increase in respiratory rate, as well as a decrease in sighs postoperatively. This combination of rapid, shallow breathing with diminished periodic sighing also can lead to atelectasis and arterial hypoxemia.

Gas exchange may be adversely affected in the postoperative period. Arterial hypoxemia is a frequent complication following surgery. George and colleagues (1966)

found that the mean preoperative arterial oxygen tension—PaO_2—of 88 mm Hg dropped to 63 mm Hg following laparotomy. This change appeared to be due to the development of abnormal ventilation/perfusion—V/Q—relationships secondary to micro- or macroatelectasis, particularly at lung bases. Reasons for the development of atelectasis include prolonged bed rest, poor cough mechanisms with retained secretions, inspiratory splinting, and a change in respiratory pattern with abnormal diaphragmatic function.

Finally, host defenses may be diminished postoperatively. The removal of upper respiratory tract particles may be impaired because of an ineffective cough. Coughing is decreased because of pain or respiratory muscle dysfunction. Furthermore, Harris and associates (1975) showed that in mice, hypoxia diminishes bacterial clearance from the lung. As noted, arterial hypoxemia is a frequent postoperative complication. Whether additional abnormalities occur postoperatively in mucociliary clearance, pulmonary alveolar macrophage or polymorphonuclear leukocyte—PMN—function or both, or lymphatic clearance has not been established.

Many of these same changes may also develop following thoracic surgery. For example, Braun and co-workers (1978) reported a significant decrease in lung volumes and arterial oxygenation two weeks after coronary artery bypass grafting. These changes gradually improved over the ensuing 16 weeks, but never returned to baseline preoperative values. Cain and colleagues (1979) also demonstrated a decrease in airflow rates in a group of patients requiring prolonged intensive care unit stays following open heart surgery, but were unable to predict pulmonary complications from preoperative lung function data. Asada and Yamaguchi (1971) examined lung morphology after cardiopulmonary bypass and found severe changes in lung epithelial and endothelial cell structure when perfusion time exceeded 150 minutes. Shorter pump times result in milder abnormalities. Moreover, several of the patients with significant epithelial and endothelial cell structure changes had marked decreases in arterial oxygenation. Also contributing to the development of arterial hypoxemia is the occurrence of atelectasis, which Gale and co-workers (1979) reported in 32 of 50—64%—patients undergoing cardiopulmonary bypass.

INITIAL PATIENT EVALUATION

The evaluation of the patient begins with a complete history and physical examination. Important information to be gathered includes the presence of underlying pulmonary disease such as chronic obstructive lung disease and restrictive lung disease, smoking history, and the presence and severity of such respiratory symptoms as cough, sputum production, wheezing, and dyspnea. In addition to the respiratory history, attention should also be paid to such nonpulmonary risk factors as age, obesity, disease involving the cardiovascular system, liver, and kidney, and metabolic status.

Physical examination of the chest should focus on res-

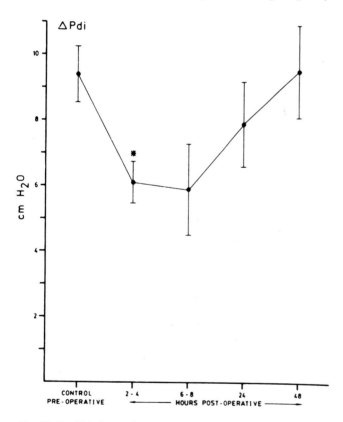

Fig. 20–2. This figure illustrates changes in the transdiaphragmatic pressure (ΔPdi) at various time periods following surgery. There is a significant decrease in Pdi at 2 to 4 hours postoperatively. (Reproduced with permission from Ford, G.T., et al.: Diaphragm function after upper abdominal surgery in humans. Am. Rev. Respir. Dis. *127*:43, 1983.)

piratory rate, quality of chest expansion, and character of airflow, with evaluation for adventitious chest sounds, rhonchi, and wheezes. As a complement to examination, the roentgenogram of the chest may be helpful in evaluating such suspected abnormalities of the respiratory system as emphysema, interstitial fibrosis, pneumonitis or pleural effusions.

PULMONARY FUNCTION EVALUATION

The degree to which a patient's respiratory status is evaluated depends upon the suspicion of underlying abnormalities and the procedure to be performed. For example, routine spirometry in a patient without a history of lung disease or cigarette smoking may be adequate for nonthoracic surgery patients. At the opposite extreme is the performance of sophisticated tests designed to measure lung reserve in patients undergoing pulmonary parenchymal resection.

As a screening test, simple spirometry measuring flow rates—FEV_1 and mid-flow rates—and FVC is a valuable tool in detecting underlying lung disease. Diament and associates (1967) have shown that simple spirometry is an excellent screening test for the presence of chronic airflow obstruction in patients with and without symptoms of chronic bronchitis. Stein and co-workers (1962) studied preoperative flow rates in 63 patients and reported that the maximum mid-expiratory flow rate was the most sensitive preoperative measure of lung function, whereas abnormalities in diffusing capacity for carbon monoxide or an elevated carbon dioxide tension—PCO_2—predicted more severe postoperative respiratory complications. In Stein's study, 21 of 30 patients with abnormal pulmonary function—decreased mid-flow rates or increased PCO_2—had postoperative respiratory complications whereas only 1 of 33 with normal lung function had problems. Similarly, Gracey and colleagues (1979) reported that preoperative abnormalities in pulmonary function predicted the development of respiratory complications. In their study, a maximal voluntary ventilation—MVV—and forced mid-expiratory flow rate—FEF_{25-75}—of less than 50% of the predicted normal, and an FVC of less than 75% of the predicted normal were the best predictors of impaired pulmonary status and postoperative complications, particularly if no improvement in function occurred after 48 hours of respiratory therapy. Milledge and Nunn (1975) have shown that patients with a low FEV_1 and an elevated PCO_2 usually have either limited lung reserve or abnormal ventilatory control, and are at high risk for development of postoperative complications. Both Mittman (1961) and Boysen and associates (1981) reported that a less-than-normal MVV may also be valuable in identifying the high risk patient. A normal MVV indicates adequate overall pulmonary function with good airflow and respiratory muscle function.

These and other studies established that the use of simple spirometry, with or without the MVV, and arterial blood gas analysis identifies the high risk patient in terms of pulmonary status. Abnormal results on these tests, however, do not absolutely preclude the performance of surgery. Rather, patients who are labeled "high risk" and who undergo surgery will need to have optimization of respiratory status preoperatively, including the cessation of smoking, treatment with bronchodilator if needed, and use of strategies to minimize sputum production. Following surgery, aggressive respiratory therapy and careful pulmonary monitoring are necessary to adequately treat any complications that arise.

PULMONARY EVALUATION FOR GENERAL THORACIC SURGERY

The majority of noncardiac thoracic procedures involve the resection of functional, as well as malignant, lung tissue, so that evaluation of pulmonary reserve in these patients is crucial in predicting the postoperative respiratory outcome. The link between cigarette smoking and lung cancer means that the presence of chronic airflow obstruction will be common in these patients. Many of these patients will have abnormal spirometry values—e.g. reduced FEV_1—and will require more sophisticated tests of pulmonary reserve prior to surgery.

As an initial screening tool, routine pulmonary function is important in identifying the low and high risk patients. The goal in evaluating the patient is to assess the amount of lung tissue that can be removed, allowing for adequate pulmonary function postoperatively. Unfortunately, there is no perfect correlation between the FEV_1 and ventilatory capacity. Segall and Butterworth (1966) studied patients with chronic obstructive bronchitis and were unable to correlate increased PCO_2 with a decrease in such parameters as FEV_1, FVC and peak flow rates. However, a majority of patients with an FEV_1 below 800 cc had elevated PCO_2. Other investigators, including Olsen and co-workers (1975) and Lockwood (1973), also stated that a predicted postoperative FEV_1 in the range of 0.8 to 1.2 L is necessary for acceptable pulmonary function without significant CO_2 retention. An FEV_1 of greater than 2 L on preoperative spirometry indicates that postoperative pulmonary function should be adequate even if a pneumonectomy is required. A preoperative FEV_1 less than 2 L suggests that more extensive pulmonary function testing to evaluate adequacy of respiratory reserve will be necessary. In general, while calculations are based on the possibility of a pneumonectomy, such procedures as lobectomy, segmentectomy, or wedge resection are being used with greater frequency in order to spare lung tissue and qualify more patients for potential curative procedures. Ali and associates (1980), however, have shown that even lesser procedures such as lobectomy will still result in an early loss of pulmonary function equivalent to that of a pneumonectomy, with gradual improvement in function over time.

Following routine spirometry, tests that have been used for further characterization of lung reserves include: (1) split-function studies measuring individual lung function using the lateral position test—LPT; (2) radioisotopic measurement of ventilation and perfusion; (3) pulmonary hemodynamic measurements assessing pulmonary vascular resistance with or without balloon occlusion of the pulmonary artery; and (4) exercise testing with measurement of maximal oxygen consumption—$\dot{V}O_2MAX$—or pulmonary vascular resistance.

Lateral Position Test—LPT

The LPT is a spirometric test used to determine unilateral lung function by comparing pulmonary function in the supine and lateral positions. This test is believed to estimate unilateral lung ventilation and thus may indicate the amount of lung function remaining after pneumonectomy. Both Marion (1976) and Walkup (1980) and co-workers showed that the LPT correlates well with isotopic measurements and provides valid preoperative measurements. A study by Jay and associates (1980), however, reported a wide variability in measurements of the same normal subject and Schoonover and co-workers (1984) found an even greater variability in LPT measurements in patients with severe COPD undergoing preoperative evaluation. Therefore, the LPT is not frequently used for routine preoperative staging.

Radioisotopic Scanning

The use of radioisotopes to measure pulmonary ventilation and perfusion has allowed for accurate evaluation of regional lung function. The technique involves inhalation of xenon-133 with scanning to measure regional lung ventilation, or injection of technetium-99m macroaggregated albumin to estimate regional lung perfusion. Postoperative lung function is then estimated by multiplying the preoperative FEV_1 by the percentage of ventilation or perfusion of the contralateral—nonsurgical—lung. When the predicted postoperative FEV_1 in the remaining lung is greater than 0.8 to 1 L it is assumed that postoperative pulmonary function will be adequate. Kristersson and associates (1972) used xenon-133 spirometry and demonstrated a correlation coefficient of 0.73 for the observed postoperative FEV_1—1 to 12 months postoperatively—compared to the predicted FEV_1. Ali and co-workers (1980) also found an excellent correlation between predicted and observed postoperative lung function using xenon-133 spirometry. Olsen and colleagues (1974) found a similar correlation using radioisotopic perfusion scans. Wernly and associates (1980) compared the efficacy of ventilation versus perfusion scanning in preoperative staging, and found a similar result with either procedure. The correlation coefficient for predicted and actual postoperative FEV_1 was approximately 0.8 for both techniques, and because of the technical ease of the technetium-99m perfusion scan, these authors recommended this procedure as the best method for assessing preoperative regional lung function.

Pulmonary Hemodynamics

The measurement of unilateral pulmonary artery pressures and pulmonary vascular resistance at rest and during exercise using balloon occlusion of the ipsilateral pulmonary artery is a useful adjunct in the preoperative pulmonary evaluation of patients requiring pneumonec-

tomy. This technique assumes that when the pulmonary artery to be resected is occluded, pressure and resistance measurements will reflect those occurring in the remaining pulmonary arterial vasculature postpneumonectomy. As with the analysis of FEV_1, the finding of pulmonary artery hypertension or arterial hypoxemia with exercise implies that a less-than-adequate pulmonary vascular reserve remains and would result in life-threatening pulmonary insufficiency. Olsen and colleagues (1975) studied 56 high risk patients prior to thoracotomy and determined that a mean pulmonary artery pressure greater than 35 mm Hg or an arterial PO_2 less than 45 mm Hg on unilateral pulmonary artery balloon occlusion implied that the patients had inadequate pulmonary reserve and were deemed physiologically inoperable. Because of the technical difficulties in performing balloon pulmonary artery occlusion, Fee and associates (1978) studied preoperative spirometry, arterial blood gases, and pulmonary vascular resistance without balloon occlusion at varying levels of exercise in 45 men scheduled for thoracotomy. The finding of a pulmonary vascular resistance greater than 190 dynes-sec-cm^{-5} during exercise identified patients at high risk for postoperative respiratory failure and death. Several of these patients had normal preoperative pulmonary function tests and arterial blood gases. All patients who had an initially elevated pulmonary vascular resistance that fell below 190 dynes-sec-cm^{-5} during exercise tolerated lung resection without difficulty. Therefore this test, which measures pulmonary vascular compliance and pulmonary capillary bed reserves, appeared to be an accurate predictor of post-thoracotomy outcome. The small number of patients evaluated with this procedure, however, led Gass and Olsen (1986) to conclude that pulmonary vascular resistance measurements may be of value in preoperatively evaluating patients, but more studies with greater numbers of patients are required prior to its routine use as a preoperative technique for assessing pulmonary reserve.

Exercise Testing

Several investigators have examined whether exercise testing with measurement of maximal oxygen consumption—$\dot{V}O_2MAX$—provides an accurate method of preoperatively predicting high risk patients. This approach may be helpful because $\dot{V}O_2MAX$ reflects an integration of pulmonary and cardiac function. Colman and associates (1982), however, preoperatively performed standard spirometry and $\dot{V}O_2MAX$, and found that the $\dot{V}O_2MAX$ was less able to predict the risk of postoperative complications than a reduced FEV_1 and FVC.

Smith and co-workers (1984) (Fig. 20–3) studied spirometry, radioisotopic lung scanning, and $\dot{V}O_2MAX$ in 22 patients prior to thoracotomy. In contrast to Colman's findings, these investigators noted a strong association between preoperative exercise capacity—$\dot{V}O_2MAX$—and the incidence of postoperative complications. Neither routine spirometry nor radioisotope perfusion scans were predictive of the postoperative course in these patients. In their study, only 1 of 10 with a $\dot{V}O_2MAX$ greater than

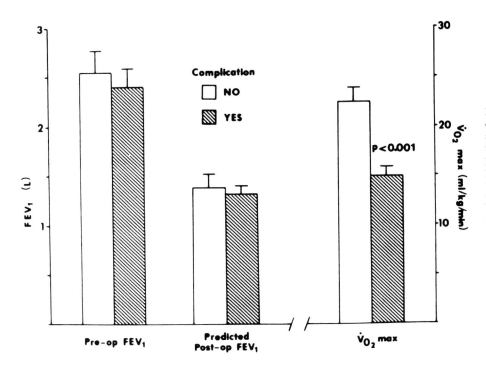

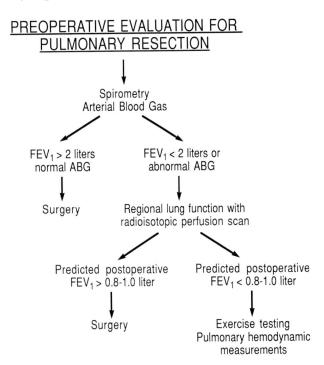

Fig. 20–3. This figure shows the preoperative forced expiratory volume in one second (FEV$_1$), the predicted postoperative FEV$_1$ (as measured by radioisotopic perfusion lung scan), and the maximal oxygen uptake ($\dot{V}O_2$MAX) on exercise in patients with (hatched bars) and without (open bars) postoperative complications. The $\dot{V}O_2$MAX was the best predictive test for postoperative complications. (Reproduced with permission from Smith, T.P., et al.: Exercise capacity as a predictor of postthoracotomy morbidity. Am. Rev. Respir. Dis. *129*:730, 1984.)

20 ml/kg/min had a complication, while all 6 patients with a $\dot{V}O_2$MAX less than 15 ml/kg/min developed postoperative problems. Similarly, Eugene and colleagues (1982) found that the $\dot{V}O_2$MAX was a sensitive predictor of post-thoracotomy mortality, with no mortality in 15 patients with a $\dot{V}O_2$MAX greater than 1 L/min, and 3 of 4 deaths in the group with a $\dot{V}O_2$MAX less than 1 L/min. The preoperative FEV$_1$ and FEV$_1$/FVC ratio did not correlate with either $\dot{V}O_2$MAX or postoperative outcome.

SUMMARY

The preoperative pulmonary evaluation of a patient involves many variables. The type of operation to be performed is an important factor. Patients undergoing nonthoracic, nonabdominal procedures are at low risk for postoperative pulmonary complications. Abdominal surgery, particularly upper abdominal incisions, may cause postoperative pulmonary dysfunction, including abnormal diaphragmatic function; a decrease in lung volumes with rapid, shallow breathing; atelectasis; arterial hypoxemia; and abnormal host defences. Even in the patient with compromised pulmonary function, however, surgery should still be carried out if absolutely necessary.

The evaluation of patients for thoracic pulmonary resection requires a more precise understanding of a patient's pulmonary function. No single preoperative test predicts with absolute certainty the postoperative respiratory outcome of an individual patient. Furthermore, it is important to withhold the final decision regarding surgery until intensive preoperative respiratory therapy is accomplished. Most investigators, however, believe that a postoperative FEV$_1$ of less than 0.8 to 1.0 L may result in postoperative pulmonary insufficiency. This must be balanced with the knowledge that surgery may

be the only curative modality for non-small cell bronchial carcinoma.

The following guidelines are useful for the preoperative determination of a patient's cardiopulmonary function and predicted postoperative pulmonary reserve. Figure 20–4 outlines this approach to the candidate for thoracic surgery.

1. The initial screening procedure of choice is spirometry. A preoperative FEV$_1$ of greater than 2 L represents

PREOPERATIVE EVALUATION FOR PULMONARY RESECTION

Spirometry
Arterial Blood Gas

FEV$_1$ > 2 liters
normal ABG

FEV$_1$ < 2 liters or
abnormal ABG

Surgery

Regional lung function with
radioisotopic perfusion scan

Predicted postoperative
FEV$_1$ > 0.8-1.0 liter

Predicted postoperative
FEV$_1$ < 0.8-1.0 liter

Surgery

Exercise testing
Pulmonary hemodynamic
measurements

Fig. 20–4. Flow diagram for the preoperative pulmonary evaluation of patients undergoing lung resection.

pulmonary function adequate to tolerate pneumonectomy. An FEV_1 of less than 2 L requires further evaluation of pulmonary reserve if pneumonectomy is planned.

2. The procedure of choice for measuring regional lung function is radioisotopic perfusion scanning coupled with preoperative spirometry. A predicted postoperative FEV_1 of greater than 0.8 to 1.0 L is usually adequate for postoperative lung function. A predicted postoperative FEV_1 of less than 800 cc may lead to postoperative respiratory insufficiency. The patient's pulmonary reserve should then be evaluated by exercise testing—$\dot{V}O_2MAX$—or measurement of pulmonary vascular hemodynamics.

3. Chronic hypercapnia—PCO_2 greater than 45 mm Hg—or arterial hypoxemia—PO_2 less than 55 mm Hg—may also be indicative of poor lung function and requires further pulmonary evaluation.

4. A mean pulmonary artery pressure greater than 35 mm Hg on unilateral pulmonary artery balloon occlusion, pulmonary vascular resistance greater than 190 dynes-sec-cm^{-5} that does not decrease with exercise, or a $\dot{V}O_2MAX$ of less than 15 ml/kg/min represents inadequate cardiopulmonary reserve with a high likelihood of postoperative complications and chronic respiratory insufficiency following pneumonectomy. Because these sophisticated tests of cardiopulmonary function have been studied in only small numbers of patients, however, their use should be limited to experimental protocols or to patients with borderline function.

REFERENCES

Ali, M.K., et al.: Predicting loss of pulmonary function after pulmonary resection of bronchogenic carcinoma. Chest 77:377, 1980.

Asada, S., and Yamaguchi, M.: Fine structural change in the lung following cardiopulmonary bypass. Chest 59:478, 1971.

Boysen, P.G., Block, A.J., and Moulder, P.V.: Relationship between preoperative pulmonary function tests and complications after thoracotomy. Surg. Gynecol. Obstet. 152:813, 1981.

Braun, S.R., Birnbaum, M.L., and Chopra, P.S.: Pre- and postoperative pulmonary function abnormalities in coronary artery revascularization surgery. Chest 72:316, 1978.

Cain, H.D., Stevens, P.M., and Adaniya, R.: Preoperative pulmonary function and complications after cardiovascular surgery. Chest 76:130, 1979.

Colman, N.C., et al.: Exercise testing in evaluation of patients for lung resection. Am. Rev. Respir. Surg. 125:604, 1982.

Diament, M.L., and Palmer, K.N.V.: Spirometry for preoperative assessment of airways resistance. Lancet 1:1251, 1967.

Eugene, J., et al.: Maximum oxygen consumption: a physiologic guide to pulmonary resection. Surg. Forum 33:260, 1982.

Fee, H.J., et al.: Role of pulmonary vascular resistance measurements in preoperative evaluation of candidates for pulmonary resection. J. Thorac. Cardiovasc. Surg. 75:519, 1978.

Ford, G.T., et al.: Diaphragm function after upper abdominal surgery in humans. Am. Rev. Respir. Dis. 127:43, 1983.

Gale, G.D., et al.: Pulmonary atelectasis and other respiratory complications after cardiopulmonary bypass and investigation of aetiological factors. Canad. Anaesth. Soc. J. 26:15, 1979.

Gass, G.D., and Olsen, G.N.: Preoperative pulmonary function testing to predict postoperative morbidity and mortality. Chest 89:127, 1986.

George, J., Hornum, I., and Mellemgard, K.: The mechanism of hypoxemia after laparotomy. Thorax 22:382, 1966.

Gracey, D.R., Divertie, M.B., and Didier, E.P.: Preoperative pulmonary preparation of patients with chronic obstructive pulmonary disease. Chest 76:123, 1979.

Harris, G.E., Johnson, W.G., and Pierce, A.K.: Bacterial lung clearance in hypoxic mice. Am. Rev. Respir. Dis. 111:910, 1975.

Jay, S.J., et al.: Variability of the lateral position test in normal subjects. Am. Rev. Respir. Dis. 121:165, 1980.

Kristersson, S., Lindell, S.E., and Svanberg, L.: Prediction of pulmonary function loss due to pneumonectomy using ^{133}xenon radiospirometry. Chest 62:694, 1972.

Latimer, R.G., et al.: Ventilatory patterns and pulmonary complications after upper abdominal surgery determined by preoperative and postoperative computerized spirometry and blood gas analysis. Am. J. Surg. 122:622, 1971.

Lockwood, P.: Lung function test results and the risk of postthoracotomy complications. Respir. 30:529, 1973.

Marion, J.M., et al.: Unilateral lung function. Comparison of the lateral position test with radionuclide ventilation-perfusion studies. Chest 69:5, 1976.

Milledge, J.S., and Nunn, J.F.: Criteria for fitness for anaesthesia in patients with chronic obstructive lung disease. Br. Med. J. 3:670, 1975.

Mittman, C.: Assessment of operative risk in thoracic surgery. Am. Rev. Respir. Dis. 84:197, 1961.

Olsen, G.N., Block, A.J., and Tobias, J.A.: Prediction of postpneumonectomy pulmonary function using quantitative macroaggregate lung scanning. Chest 66:13, 1974.

Olsen, G.N., et al.: Pulmonary function evaluation of the lung resection candidate: a prospective study. Am. Rev. Respir. Dis. 111:379, 1975.

Schoonover, G.A, et al.: Lateral position test and quantitative lung scan in the preoperative evaluation for lung resection. Chest 86:854, 1984.

Segall, J.J., and Butterworth, B.A.: Ventilatory capacity in chronic bronchitis in relation to carbon dioxide retention. Scand. J. Respir. Dis. 47:215, 1966.

Smith, T.P., et al.: Exercise capacity as a predictor of postthoracotomy morbidity. Am. Rev. Respir. Dis. 129:730, 1984.

Stein, M., et al.: Pulmonary evaluation of surgical patients. JAMA 181:765, 1962

Tahir, A.H., et al.: Effects of abdominal surgery upon diaphragmatic function and regional ventilation. Int. Surg. 58:337, 1973.

Walkup, R.H., et al.: Prediction of postoperative pulmonary function with the lateral position test. Chest 77:24, 1980.

Wernly, J.A., et al.: Clinical value of quantitative ventilation-perfusion lung scans in the surgical management of bronchogenic carcinoma. J. Thorac. Cardiovasc. Surg. 80:535, 1980.

READING REFERENCES

Boushy, S.F., et al.: Clinical course related to preoperative and postoperative pulmonary function in patients with bronchogenic carcinoma. Chest 59:383, 1971.

Gaensler, E.A., et al.: The role of pulmonary insufficiency in mortality and invalidism following surgery for pulmonary tuberculosis. J. Thorac. Cardiovasc. Surg. 29:163, 1955.

Javaheri, S., Blum, J., and Kazemi, H.: Pattern of breathing and carbon dioxide retention in chronic obstructive lung disease. Am. J. Med. 71:228, 1981.

Miller, J.I., Grossman, G.D., and Hatcher, C.R.: Pulmonary function test criteria for operability and pulmonary resection. Surg. Gynecol. Obstet. 153:893, 1981.

Rehder, K., Sessler, A.D., and Marsh, H.M.: General anaesthesia and the lung. Am. Rev. Respir. Dis. 112:541, 1975.

Reichel, J.: Assessment of operative risk of pneumonectomy. Chest 62:570, 1972.

Teculescu, D.B., Racoveanu, C., and Manicatide, M.A.: Relationships of carbon dioxide retention to ventilatory impairment and hypoxemia in chronic obstructive lung disease. Respir. 38:81, 1979.

Tisi, G.M.: Preoperative evaluation of pulmonary function. Am. Rev. Respir. Dis. 119:293, 1979.

Williams, C.D., and Brenowitz, J.B.: "Prohibitive" lung function and major surgical procedures. Am. J. Surg. 132:763, 1976.

Anesthetic Management of the Thoracic Surgical Patient

CHAPTER 21

PREANESTHETIC EVALUATION AND PREPARATION

Hak Y. Wong and Edward A. Brunner

Historically, the development of modern surgery, and of thoracic surgery in particular, was closely linked to the development of anesthesia and artificial ventilation. Until not too long ago, the possibility of an operation was often limited by the patient's ability to survive the anesthetic. With advances in our knowledge and techniques, this is now seldom the case. On the other hand, surgical procedures and demands are becoming increasingly more complex, and patients who present for thoracic surgery are increasing in age and in the complexity of their medical problems. The anesthesiologist's responsibility now consists not only of providing a complicated anesthetic to a patient, but also of becoming an integral part of the continuum of medical care that the patient has hitherto received and will require. To be able to discharge this function, the anesthesiologist must be thoroughly familiar with aspects of the patient's medical problems and the proposed operation. The preanesthetic evaluation also affords a good opportunity for the anesthesiologist to establish a rapport with the patient, which is essential to good medical practice. Current standard of care, in addition, calls for explanation of procedures and risks to the patient and obtaining informed consent.

Although a thorough history and physical examination by the patient's primary physician will provide much of the information sought by the anesthesiologist, it cannot substitute for a preanesthetic evaluation, which entails focusing on specific areas of the patient's condition in the context of the proposed operation. The thoracic surgical patient by and large has more than a single medical problem. Thoracic operations often physically interfere with the function of vital structures, and each operation has unique features. Thus, it is important that the person performing the evaluation knows the nature of the operation, the degree and manner by which it and the anesthetic will stress the patient intraoperatively, and the residual physiologic defects that will exist in the postoperative period. In addition, based on these concerns and data uncovered during the medical assessment of the patient, the anesthesiologist may need to communicate and interact with other medical specialists in order to achieve an optimal condition for the patient's course. Preanesthetic evaluation, therefore, cannot be relegated to the uninitiated.

The timing of preanesthetic evaluation depends on the condition of the patient and the nature of the operation. For the most simple surgery on healthy patients, the day before the surgery might be appropriate. Because many thoracic operations are relatively complex and performed on relatively ill patients, however, the evaluation should be initiated as far in advance of surgery as possible. This allows time for additional tests and evaluations, if unsuspected abnormalities are uncovered; consultation between specialists; and initiation of corrective therapy, if needed. In addition, the patient is allowed time to absorb and adjust to the newly acquired information and to explore any question that arises. An anesthetic outpatient clinic may serve very well in this regard for patients not requiring preoperative hospitalization.

Even in an emergency, some assessment is always possible and necessary before anesthesia is started.

SCOPE OF PREANESTHETIC EVALUATION

The fact-finding aspect of preanesthetic evaluation is centered around three objectives: (1) to detect problems and factors in the patient's physical condition that can compromise the patient's ability to cope with perioperative stress or that can be aggravated by the stress; (2) to recognize the impact of the specific pathology necessitating the surgery; and (3) to address several concerns peculiar to the practice of anesthesia.

General Medical Condition

It is beyond the scope of this text to describe general history-taking, physical diagnosis, or laboratory investigation. Because of the frequency with which they are associated with thoracic surgical patients, and the impact they have on surgical/anesthetic outcome, several conditions deserve meticulous search and emphasis. These include coronary heart disease, which may present as previous myocardial infarction, angina, arrhythmia, or congestive heart failure; cor pulmonale; obstructive airway disease; symptomatic cerebrovascular disease; electrolyte imbalance, in particular hypokalemia; diabetes mellitus; thyroid disorder; and polycythemia. Because many patients have fixed and permanent abnormalities, the evaluation should center on determining if the conditions have been optimally treated and establishing the baselines for that particular patient.

Impact of Specific Pathology

Each surgical condition necessitating an operation poses unique stress on the body and presents a different set of problems to the anesthesia team. This is particularly true in thoracic surgery because the pathologies often involve or impinge on the vital life-sustaining organs. From the standpoint of pathophysiology and preanesthetic implication, the pathologies in general thoracic surgery can be broadly categorized into three groups: esophageal diseases, surgical diseases of the lungs, and diseases of the mediastinum and pleura. Esophageal diseases include obstructive disorders predisposing patients to preoperative dehydration and malnourishment; and refluxing disorders and obstructive disorders predisposing patients to aspiration, either chronically or perioperatively, leading to pneumonitis. Surgical diseases of the lungs include abnormal source of fluid, such as abscess and hemoptysis, leading to contamination of normal lung tissues; abnormal solid tissues, such as tumor and consolidation, resulting in right-to-left venous shunting; and obstructive lesions, preventing air flow. Diseases of mediastinum and pleura include obstruction of the airway or the large veins, such as the superior vena cava syndrome; abnormal paths of communication, such as bronchopleural fistula; and abnormal collections of fluid, such as an empyema.

Anesthetic Concerns

Aside from the assessment of medical condition just discussed, the preanesthetic evaluation addresses a set of issues best described as of unique concern to the practice of anesthesia.

Anesthetic History. The patient's experience with previous anesthetics and, if possible, the old anesthetic records are reviewed. Taking note of previous difficulties, such as difficult endotracheal intubation, prolonged apnea, or postoperative jaundice, can avert potential disasters. Careful and pertinent family history may alert one to the possibility of malignant hyperpyrexia or pseudocholinesterase deficiency.

Drug History. Polypharmacy is an integral part of modern medicine, including modern anesthesia. It is particularly important in the older group of patients presenting for thoracic surgery, who may take up to five or six daily medications. To avoid adverse drug interaction, a careful drug history is mandatory (Table 21–1). This provides the opportunity to advise the patient on the continuation

or discontinuation of medications prior to surgery, and to assess special precautions dictated by the intercurrent drug therapy.

Status of the Upper Airway. This includes the evaluation of the temporomandibular joints, the cervical spine, and the vertebrobasilar arteries. Because many thoracic surgical patients are at higher risk for aspiration—full stomach—and many have coexisting heart and lung disease—limited oxygen reserve, unexpected difficulty in maintaining airway patency or endotracheal intubation is best avoided. Many thoracic surgical procedures call for special airway instrumentation, such as endobronchial tubes, making attention to the state of the upper airway even more important. Special studies, such as tomograms or CT scans of the airway, may occasionally be necessary to achieve a complete evaluation.

Intravascular Access. The ease of intravenous access should be assessed in relation to the extent and site of the proposed operation. Patients with inadequate peripheral access should be prepared for central venous cannulation. Potential arterial cannulation sites are examined and tested for adequacy of collaterals.

Postoperative Ventilation. The need for mechanical ventilation after the operation is often predictable based on the nature of the operation, the anticipated impairment of the patient's respiratory reserves, the condition of the cardiovascular system, and the anesthetic technique used. Besides advising the patient of this possibility, one may consider altering the choice of endotracheal tube—use of low pressure-high volume cuffs, the route of intubation, and the dose of respiratory depressant drugs.

Postoperative Pain-Relief. All patients should be apprised of the extent of anticipated discomfort and types of pain-relief that will be available. Two comparatively new modes of pain-relief, patient-controlled analgesia—PCA—and epidural narcotics—EN, make assessment during the preanesthetic evaluation particularly important. PCA can be most effective when the patient is motivated and can be taught how to operate the device, is expected to awake soon after surgery, and will not be too physically encumbered. EN does not require active participation from the patient, but because it is an invasive procedure, careful evaluation of contraindications and obtaining an informed consent from the patient are extremely important.

By careful review of the medical record, patient interview, and examination, and taking into consideration the nature and demand of the proposed operation, the patient can usually be assigned to one of the following three categories: (1) the patient is in optimal condition and not at excessive risk, and anesthesia and surgery can proceed; (2) the patient's condition is questionable in some areas, and specialist consultation and investigation are needed; and (3) the patient is obviously undertreated, and futher preoperative treatment and follow-up evaluation are needed.

INTERDISCIPLINARY CONSULTATION

Because the anesthesiologist approaches the patient-operation complex from a perspective slightly different

Table 21–1. Drugs Associated with Significant Interaction During Anesthesia

Drug Class and Examples	Interact With	Interaction	Comment
Theophylline Aminophylline Oxtriphylline	Cimetidine	Increased serum theophylline level	Substitute cimetidine with ranitidine
	Ketamine	Jointly reduce seizure threshold	
	Halothane and/or pancuronium	Predispose to cardiac arrhythmias when theophylline level is high	Check serum theophylline level before anesthesia
Alpha-adrenergic Blockers Prazosin (Minipress) Phenoxybenzamine (Dibenzyline) Phentolamine (Regitine)	Alpha-agonists	Decreased alpha-adrenergic effects	Chronic use of alpha-blockers up-regulates number of alpha-receptors. Exaggerated alpha response if alpha-blockers are acutely withdrawn.
Beta-adrenergic Blockers Propranolol (Inderal) Timolol (Blocadren)	Beta-agonists	Decreased beta-adrenergic effect	May need 20 × usual doses of beta-agonists
Metoprolol (Lopressor) Nadolol (Corgard) Atenolol (Tenormin)	Ketamine	Decreased sympathetic stabilization of circulation	Chronic use up-regulates number of beta-receptors
Esmolol (Brevibloc)	Enflurane/methoxyflurane	Increased cardiac depression and reduced response to hypovolemia	Do not abruptly withdraw beta-blockade perioperatively High dose beta-blockade may be reduced to equivalent of 360 mg daily of propranolol preoperatively
Calcium Channel Blockers Verapamil (Isoptin, Calan) Diltiazem (Cardizem)	Beta-blockers	Additive cardiac depression	Abrupt withdrawal may lead to coronary vasospasm
Nifedipine (Procardia)	Digitalis Volatile anesthetics High-dose Fentanyl	Increased blood digitalis level Additive cardiac depression Exaggerated vasodilation	
Antihypertensive Drugs Reserpine Guanabenz	Volatile anesthetics	Decreased anesthetic requirement MAC (except guanethedine)	Antihypertensives should be maintained throughout perioperative period
Methyldopa Clonidine Guanethedine	Direct-acting sympathomimetics	Increased sympathomimetic response	
	Indirect-acting sympathomimetics	Decreased sympathomimetic response	Clonidine withdrawal may precipitate hypertensive crisis
	Beta-blockers	May cause hypertension (due to β_2 receptor blockade)	
Monoamine Oxidase Inhibitors (MAOI) Pargyline (Eutonyl) Phenelzine (Nardil) Isocarboxazid (Marplan)	Meperidine (Demerol)	Excitement, agitation, hypertension tachycardia, rigidity, convulsions, coma	May be related to increased serotonin level
Tranylcypromine (Parnate)	Barbiturates Indirect-acting sympathomimetics	Increased sleeping time Hypertensive crisis	MAOI should be withdrawn for two weeks prior to elective surgery
	Tricyclic antidepressants	Hypertensive crisis	
	Volatile anesthetics	Hyperthermia and rigidity (reported)	
Tricyclic Antidepressants Amitriptyline (Elavil) Desipramine (Pertofrane) Imipramine (Tofranil)	Narcotic drugs	Increased analgesic and sedative response	

Table 21–1. **Drugs Associated with Significant Interaction During Anesthesia** *Continued*

Drug Class and Examples	Interact With	Interaction	Comment
Doxepin (Sinequan) Nortriptyline (Aventyl)	Barbiturates	Increased sleeping time	
Protriptyline (Vivactil)	Anticholinergics (atropine)	Increased central and peripheral cholinergic effect	
	Direct-acting sympathomimetics	Increased adrenergic response	
Phenothiazine and Butyrophenones Chlorpromazine (Thorazine) Fluphenazine (Permitil)	Volatile anesthetics	Increased hypertensive effect	Promethazine appears to have antianalgesic effect
Prochlorperazine (Compazine) Promethazine (Phenergan)	Narcotics	Increased sedation and respiratory depression	
Promazine (Sparine) Haloperidol (Haldol)	Barbiturates	Increased sleeping time	Chronic phenothiazine therapy may cause myocardial toxicity
	Anticholinergics	Increased anticholinergic effects	
	Dopamine	May have decreased response	
	Sympathomimetics	Decreased adrenergic response	
Lithium	Barbiturates	Increased sleeping time	
	Muscle relaxants (pancuronium and suxamethonium)	Increased duration of relaxation	
	Diuretics	Increased lithium level	
Digitalis	Succinylcholine	May induce ventricular dysrhythmias	
	Volatile anesthetics	May decrease digitalis-induced dysrhythmias	
	Cardioversion	Potential for ventricular fibrillation	
	Maneuvers causing hypokalemia (diuresis, hyperventilation	Potentiate digitalis toxicity	
Diuretics Furosemide (Lasix)	Digitalis	Relative toxicity due to hypokalemia	
Chlorothiazide (Diuril) Acetazolamide (Diamox)	Muscle relaxant		
	Aminoglycosides	Additive ototoxicity	
	Volatile anesthetics	Exaggerated hypotension related to fluid deficit	
Organophosphates Echothiophate Isofluorophate	Succinylcholine	Prolonged apnea	Plasma cholinesterase is inhibited by absorption of these drugs
Antiarrhythmics Quinidine Procainamide	Volatile anesthetics	Increased cardiac depression	
Bretylium Mexiletine	Muscle relaxants	Potentiates neuromuscular blockade	
Tocainide	Vasodilators	Increased hypotension	May be related to alpha-blocking action
	Volatile anesthetics	Increased cardiac depression	
	Vasodilators	Increased hypotension	May be related to ganglion-blocking action
	Direct-acting sympathomimetics	Increased beta-adrenergic response	
	Muscle relaxants	Potentiates neuromuscular blockade	

from that of other physicians, he or she frequently uncovers problems that may have been overlooked or ignored. It is most important that the anesthesia and surgical teams maintain open and equitable communication so that such problems can be satisfactorily resolved before surgery.

When there is diagnostic or therapeutic uncertainty outside the defined expertise of both the surgeon and the anesthesiologist, specific specialist consultation is indicated. Examples are evaluation of chest pain and borderline electrocardiogram, diagnosis of complex arrhythmias, testing of pacemakers, and control of severe bronchospasm. Occasionally, a consultation may be needed in anticipation of a likely postoperative problem that will require specialist management, such as renal failure or total parenteral nutrition. A consultation is most rewarding when all who are involved maintain open communication and address specific questions. The traditional carte blanche "medical clearance" type of consultation is patronizing, misleading, and seldom helpful to the anesthesia and surgical teams in their patient management. Moreover, the anesthesiologist alone has to shoulder the responsibility for the stress of anesthesia and surgery on the patient, and therefore will have to make the final judgment, together with the surgeon, on the patient's suitability for the procedure and the anesthetic technique of choice. Del Guercio and Cohn (1980) presented data that indirectly support this position. Of 148 elderly patients who had been medically "cleared" for surgery, subsequent invasive hemodynamic data showed 23.5% to have markedly increased risks. All who were in this group and had surgery died. Of special interest, these patients were readily identified by experienced anesthesiologists using physical status classification (Table 21–2).

ASSESSMENT OF RISK

Risk is defined as the chance of bad outcomes, which include death and serious morbidity. Aside from the fortunately infrequent pure anesthetic or surgical mishaps, adverse outcome after surgical procedure is largely multifactorial. Assignment of the risk to anesthesia or surgery per se is nearly impossible. Thus, as summarized by Goldstein and Keats (1970), epidemiologic studies of anesthetic risk have widely varying results and severe limitations. One of us (E.A.B.) (1975) found that at least four factors contribute to anesthetic risk: physical status of the patient; drugs used for anesthesia; site and requirement of the operation; and the surgical environment and the skill of the personnel.

More pragmatically, from the standpoint of preanesthetic evaluation and intervention to minimize risks, adverse outcomes after thoracic surgery can be broadly divided into two groups. The first group of adverse events are mostly unrelated to the preoperative state of the patient and depend only on the nature of the surgery and the skill of the personnel. In thoracic surgery, four common intraoperative threats are (1) hemorrhage; (2) cardiac arrhythmia; (3) mechanical interference with the

Table 21–2. American Society of Anesthesiologists Classification of Anesthetic Risk in Terms of Physical Status

Status	Physical Attributes
I	Patients with no organic, physiologic, biochemical, or psychologic disturbance. The pathologic process for which the operation is to be performed is localized and not related to a systemic disturbance. Examples are the physically fit for elective inguinal herniorrhaphy or hysterectomy.
II	Patients with mild systemic disturbance caused by the condition to be treated surgically or by other pathophysiologic processes. Examples are patients with mild diabetes or mild hypertension.
III	Patients with moderate systemic disturbance from whatever cause even though it may not be possible to define the degree of disability with finality. Examples are patients with recent myocardial infarction or persistent cardiac arrhythmias.
IV	Patients with severe systemic disorder already life-threatening and not always correctable by the operative procedure. Examples are patients with cardiac insufficiency or advanced pulmonary disease.
V	Moribund patients who have little chance for survival and are subject to operation in desperation. Examples are moribund patients with a ruptured aortic aneurysm or a mesenteric thrombosis.

mediastinum; and (4) ventilation/oxygenation problems. Risks not unique to thoracic surgery are anaphylaxis, adverse drug interaction, and rare occurrences such as malignant hyperpyrexia.

The second group of adverse events are reasonably predictable from the preoperative state of the patient and the nature of the operation. Interventions that change the patient's preoperative state may therefore affect the occurrence of these events. They include pulmonary complications such as atelectasis, infection, and respiratory failure and cardiac conditions including cor pulmonale, myocardial ischemic event, and heart failure. There is an extensive literature concerning attempts at predicting these events and the associated mortality and the effect of preoperative intervention.

One of the simplest systems relating outcome to preoperative status is that used by anesthesiologists, the American Society of Anesthesiologists—ASA—Physical Status Classification (Table 21–2). Although it was conceived as a simple classification of the patient's physical status at the time of preanesthetic evaluation, Dripps and co-workers (1961), Vacanti and associates (1970), and Marx and colleagues (1973) have shown it to be a fairly good indicator of general outcome after surgery (Table 21–3). Note that this classification is not a predictor of operation risks unrelated to the patient's preoperative state, such as hemorrhage and cardiac arrhythmias.

Pulmonary Complications

Pulmonary complications are common after thoracic and abdominal surgery. Anderson and associates (1963) have shown the well-known relationship between the site of operation and incidence of complication. Thoracic sur-

Table 21–3. Relation Between Physical Status and Anesthesia Mortality

Physical Status	Anesthesia Mortality Rate*
I	0
II	1:1000
III	1:150
IV	1:20
V	1:10

*Includes deaths in which anesthesia was either a primary or contributing cause.

Dripps, R.D., et al.: The role of anesthesia in surgical mortality. J.A.M.A. *178*:261, 1961. Copyright 1961, American Medical Association.

gery is at the highest risk. One particular complication, namely respiratory insufficiency secondary to loss of lung tissue by surgical resection, is fairly predictable based on preoperative pulmonary function and extent of surgery. This is dealt with in detail in Chapter 20 of this book.

Pulmonary complication not caused by lung resection is related to the effect of surgery and anesthesia on the respiratory system: mucociliary transport, mechanics of breathing, and decrease in the functional residual capacity—FRC—and forced vital capacity—FVC. Atelectasis is said to affect 10 to 80% of all surgical patients. This wide range of incidence reflects the difficulty in predicting the risk. Estimation of risk based on early epidemiological studies is less than helpful: patients and case-mix were often undefined, varying endpoints were used in morbidity measurement, the bias of preoperative treatment was ignored, and the effects of retrospective and prospective design were often not delineated in such reports. The thoracic surgical literature itself has largely focused on tuberculosis and cancer, and the risk of other types of thoracic surgery therefore has to be extrapolated from data collected from these conditions.

From the existing literature, it is clear that an abnormal expiratory spirogram is a strong predictor of postoperative complication, but there is no agreement about the cutoff point for prohibitive risks. Grossly abnormal FVC, maximum voluntary ventilation—MVV—of less than 50% of the predicted value and forced expiratory volume in 1 second—FEV_1—of less than 1 L have been shown to be a sensitive predictor of death. Gracy and colleagues (1979) found that response to bronchodilator is another index, with good response indicating a favorable outcome. Based on the expiratory spirogram and findings in the cardiovascular system, central nervous system, arterial blood gases measurement, and expected postoperative course, Shapiro and associates (1985) proposed a scoring system for predicting the risks of postoperative pulmonary complications. This is a step toward quantifying the risks and providing a basis for measurement of effects of the preoperative intervention. To date, however, there are no data verifying the score.

Cardiac Complications

Because of the age of the thoracic surgical patient population, prevalence of cardiovascular disease, predispos-

ing risk factors common to both lung and heart disease, and nature of thoracic surgery—especially lung resection, cardiovascular events are leading causes of morbidity and death, led only by pulmonary complications.

Much of the current literature is concerned with the impact of coronary artery disease, as reflected by past myocardial infarction, on perioperative cardiovascular event. Data from Topkins and Artusio (1964), Tarhan and associates (1972), Steen and associates (1976) and others show that the risk of sustaining a perioperative myocardial infarction after a previous infarction is about 6%. If the previous infarction is less than six months old, the risk increases fivefold to sixfold. The mortality of perioperative reinfarction has been uniformly higher than 50%. Rao and associates (1983) demonstrated substantial decreases in reinfarction rate and mortality and attributed these to aggressive monitoring and early correction of identified physiologic abnormalities. This attractive contribution needs independent verification. Note that the occurrence of perioperative myocardial infarction is most frequent during the second and third days after surgery, a time when many patients have already been discharged from the intensive care unit. A longer period of intensive postoperative observation may be indicated for high risk patients.

Another approach to estimation of cardiovascular risk is that of Goldman and associates (1977), wherein multivariate discriminate analysis of a thousand patients resulted in a Cardiac Risk Index (Tables 21–4 and 21–5). Aside from recent myocardial infarction, signs of congestive heart failure and ventricular arrhythmia are sig-

Table 21–4. Factors Correlated with Cardiac Risk in Surgical Patients

Criteria	Weighted Points
History	
Age over 70 years	5
Myocardial infarction in previous 6 mos.	10
Physical Examination	
S_3 gallop or jugular venous distention	11
Important valvular aortic stenosis	3
Electrocardiogram	
Rhythm other than sinus or PACs on last preoperative ECG	7
>5 PVCs/min at any time	7
General Status	3
Po_2 <60 or Pco_2 >50 mm Hg	
K <3.0 or HCO_3 <20 mEq/L	
BUN >50 or Cr >3.0 mg/dl	
Abnormal SGOT, signs of liver disease, or bedridden patient	
Operation	
Intraperitoneal, intrathoracic, or aortic	3
Emergency	4
Total Possible Points	53

Goldman, L., et al.: Multifactorial index of cardiac risk in noncardiac surgical procedures. Reprinted by permission of the New England Journal of Medicine, *297*:845, 1977.

Table 21–5.   Correlation of Cardiac Risk with Point Total

Point Total	% Cardiac Death	% Life-threatening Complication*	% No or Minor Complication
0–5 (Class I)	0.2 (1)†	0.7 (4)	99 (532)
6–12 (Class II)	2.0 (5)	5.0 (16)	93 (295)
13–25 (Class III)	2.0 (3)	11.0 (15)	86 (112)
>26 (Class IV)	56.0 (10)	22.0 (4)	22 (4)

*Intraoperative or postoperative myocardial infarction, pulmonary edema, or ventricular tachycardia without progression to cardiac deaths.

†Figures in parentheses denote number of patients.

Goldman, L., et al.: Multifactorial index of cardiac risk in non-cardiac surgical procedures. Reprinted by permission of the New England Journal of Medicine, 297:845, 1977.

nificant risk factors. Other, less weighted, factors include aortic stenosis, age above 70, emergency surgery, and poor general medical condition. The statistical analysis and conclusions of this study have been open to some questions. Nevertheless, it still stands to highlight risk factors that are potentially amenable to preoperative treatment and may therefore reduce morbidity and mortality.

Both Goldman (1977) and Steen (1978) and their associates found that intrathoracic surgery itself is a risk factor for significant cardiovascular complications.

PREANESTHETIC TREATMENT

Preanesthetic treatment of coexisting diseases uncovered during preanesthetic evaluation must be considered in the time-frame of urgency of the proposed surgery. In the best of circumstances, the objectives would be to treat acute reversible disorders, return the patient with a chronic disorder to an optimal baseline, and act to minimize the postoperative functional derangement. Although the primary responsibility for implementing treatment rests with the primary physician or surgeon, the anesthesiologist has a vested interest, because the result of such treatment may have a significant impact on the patient's intraoperative course.

The benefit of preoperative treatment of chronic obstructive lung disease in reducing postoperative pulmonary complications has been shown by Gracey (1979) Tarhan (1973), and Stein (1962) and their associates. Conditions amenable to such treatment include infection, acute exacerbation of bronchospasm, bronchorrhea, and cigarette smoking. Congestive heart failure as a result of cor pulmonale or ischemic heart disease is another situation in which adequate preoperative treatment may have a significant impact on postoperative mortality. Shields and Ujiki (1968), and Deutsch and Dalen (1969) have discussed preoperative digitalization for thoracic surgery patients. Our current practice is not to use digitalization to prevent cardiac arrhythmias caused by thoracic surgery.

Occasionally, preanesthetic treatment may call for invasive monitoring of the patient and involvement of other medical specialists. For example, a patient with unstable angina needs extensive evaluation, and treatment options such as coronary artery bypass surgery and intra-aortic balloon counterpulsation may have to be explored by a team including the cardiologist, the thoracic surgeon, and the anesthesiologist before the thoracic surgery is undertaken.

PSYCHOLOGIC PREPARATION OF THE PATIENT

Evaluation of the patient's preoperative psychological state is an important part of the preanesthetic evaluation. For the patient, the impending operation is an anxiety-generating event. The anesthesiologist, because of his ability to modify that anxiety and to offer psychological support, can establish close rapport in a very short period. Such support and rapport have a calming effect on an otherwise anxious patient. Egbert and his colleagues (1964) noted that an informative and reassuring approach from the anesthesiologist engenders patient confidence and reduces apprehension and anxiety. The patient should be encouraged to discuss his fears and to explore events that will occur on the day of operation. Frank discussion of postoperative pain and assurance of the availability of adequate doses of analgesic drugs have been found helpful. This can be augmented by appropriate drug therapy so that the patient arrives in the operating room calm, confident, and cooperative. The induction of anesthesia is safer, more controllable, and more pleasant for the calm patient than for one who is excited.

Egbert and his associates (1963, 1964) have emphasized that the need for strong postoperative narcotic analgesics, the incidence of postoperative complications, and the duration of hospital stay may be reduced significantly by an informative preoperative visit by the anesthesiologist.

INFORMED CONSENT

Before seeking a patient's consent to a particular course of anesthesia, the anesthesiologist has an obligation to adequately inform the patient of the potential benefits and risks of such a course, and other available options. The difficulty lies in striking a balance between providing enough information and unduly alarming the patient, given the inherent risks of any anesthetic and surgery. Furthermore, the specific risks of thoracic surgery previously discussed, and possible preventive and corrective measures, must be honestly disclosed where applicable. This task may be partly eased by highlighting problems and risks that are amenable to preoperative correction, advising the patient in general terms that any anesthetic poses risks, and then inquiring if the patient wishes to know the specifics of all the possible risks. Many patients would then guide the anesthesiologist as far as their coping would allow. The essence of such discussion should be documented and forms part of the proof of informed consent. On occasion, a patient may decline any discussion of risks, or the physician may find the patient in a state unsuitable to bear such an ordeal. These also should be documented.

PREANESTHETIC MEDICATION

The aim of preanesthetic medication is to decrease anxiety without producing excessive drowsiness, facilitate a smooth, rapid induction without prolonged emergence, provide amnesia for the perioperative period while maintaining cooperation prior to loss of consciousness, and relieve preoperative pain. The classes of drugs commonly used for this purpose include: (1) sedatives, hypnotics, and tranquilizers; (2) opioids; (3) anticholinergics; and (4) antihistamines and antacids. The appropriate drugs and doses can be chosen only after the psychologic and physiologic conditions of the patient have been evaluated. The type and extent of the operation, the expected postoperative course, and the anesthetic technique to be used also need to be taken into consideration. In addition, Egbert and associates (1963) found that a good preanesthetic visit may be as effective as administration of sedatives in decreasing the level of anxiety.

Several categories of patients should rarely be given preanesthetic medication before arriving in the operating room. These are patients with marginal cerebral function, patients with uncorrected hypovolemia, or patients with severe heart or lung disease, or both, whose respiratory and sympathetic drives are crucial, and those patients without informed consent.

CONCLUSION

Preanesthetic evaluation and preparation is an integral part of good anesthetic practice. It is essential for establishing physician-patient rapport and ensuring that the patient is in an optimal state for the proposed surgery. By being thoroughly familiar with the patient and the operation, the anesthesiologist can take steps to minimize intraoperative risks and postoperative problems and to facilitate the performance of surgery. The selection of techniques of monitoring and of anesthesia will follow rationally and will provide optimal safety for the patient.

REFERENCES

Anderson, W.H., Dossett, B.E., and Hamilton, G.E.: Prevention of postoperative pulmonary complications. JAMA *186*:763, 1963.

Brunner, E.A.: Factors related to anesthesia risk. Surg. Gynecol. Obstet. *141*:761, 1975.

Del Guercio, L.R.M., and Cohn, J.D.: Monitoring operative risk in the elderly. JAMA *243*:1350, 1980.

Deutsch, S., and Dalen, J.E.: Indications for prophylactic digitalization. Anesthesiology *30*:648, 1969.

Dripps, R.D., Lamont, A., and Eckenhoff, J.E.: The role of anesthesia in surgical mortality. JAMA *178*:261, 1961.

Egbert, L.D., et al.: The value of the preoperative visit by an anesthetist. JAMA *185*:553, 1963.

Egbert, L.D., et al.: Reduction of postoperative pain by encouragement and instruction of patients. N. Engl. J. Med. *270*:825, 1964.

Goldman, L., et al.: Multifactorial index of cardiac risks in noncardiac surgical procedures. N. Engl. J. Med. *297*:845, 1977.

Goldstein, A., and Keats, A.S.: The risk of anesthesia. Anesthesiology *33*:130, 1970.

Gracey, D.R., Divertie, M.B., and Dider, E.P.: Preoperative pulmonary preparation of patients with chronic obstructive pulmonary disease. Chest *76*:123, 1979.

Marx, G.F., Mateo, C.V., and Orkin, L.R.: Computer analysis of postanesthetic deaths. Anesthesiology *39*:54, 1973.

Rao, T.L.K., Jacobs, K.H., and El-Etr, A.A.: Re-infarction following anesthesia in patients with myocardial infarction. Anesthesiology *59*:499, 1983.

Shapiro, B.A., et al.: Clinical Application of Respiratory Care. Chicago, Year Book Medical Publishers, 1985, pp. 523–525.

Shields, T.W., and Ujiki, G.T.: Digitalization for prevention of arrhythmias following pulmonary surgery. Surg. Gynecol. Obstet. *126*:743, 1968.

Steen, P.A., et al.: Myocardial re-infarction after anesthesia and surgery. JAMA *239*:2566, 1976.

Stein, M., et al.: Pulmonary evaluation of surgical patients. JAMA *181*:765, 1962.

Tarhan, S., et al.: Risk of anesthesia and surgery in patients with chronic bronchitis and chronic obstructive disease. Surgery *74*:720, 1973.

Tarhan, S., et al.: Myocardial infarction after general anesthesia. JAMA *199*:318, 1972.

Topkins, M.J., and Artusio, J.F.: Myocardial infarction and surgery: A five year study. Anesth. Analg. *43*:715, 1964.

Vacanti, C.J., Van Houten, R.T., and Hill, R.C.: A statistical analysis of the relationship of physical status to postoperative mortality in 68,388 cases. Anesth. Analg. *49*:564, 1970.

READING REFERENCES

Bendixen, H.H., et al.: Respiratory Care. St. Louis, C.V. Mosby Co., 1965.

Cullen, B.F., and Muller, M.G.: Drug interaction and anesthesia: a review. Anesth. Analg. *58*:413, 1979.

Editorial views: the ASA classification of physical status—a recapitalization. Anesthesiology *49*:233, 1978.

Forrest, W.H., Brown, C.R., and Brown, B.W.: Subjective responses to six common preoperative medications. Anesthesiology *47*:241, 1977.

Peters, R.M.: The role of limited resection in carcinoma of the lung. Am. J. Surg. *143*:706, 1982.

CHAPTER 22

CONDUCT OF ANESTHESIA

Andranik Ovassapian

The needs of the surgeon for acceptable operating conditions, and those of the patient for safe anesthesia without cardiovascular depression, should be the basis for the selection and conduct of thoracic anesthesia. The anesthesiologist's responsibility begins with a careful preoperative assessment of the patient's condition. Anesthesia for thoracic surgery is complicated by several factors: opening of the chest produces a pneumothorax; manipulation of the lung, heart, and major vessels by the surgeon may interfere with ventilatory exchange and cardiovascular stability; and positioning the patient in the lateral decubitus position exposes the lower lung to contamination by secretions from the operative lung and may change the distribution of blood flow and ventilation. Thus, for safe anesthesia during thoracic surgery, the anesthesiologist should be knowledgeable about the physiology of one-lung ventilation and be skillful in techniques for isolation of the lungs.

The introduction of double-lumen endobronchial tubes for one-lung anesthesia by Bjork and Carlens in 1950 represented a major advance in thoracic anesthesia. Jenkins and Clark in 1958 advocated the routine use of double-lumen tubes for all intrathoracic operations. Yet, the difficulty in blindly positioning these tubes and the resulting possibility of life-threatening complications discouraged their use by many anesthesiologists.

Several advances have made one-lung anesthesia safer and the double-lumen tube more popular. These include the availability of disposable, and in many ways superior, double-lumen tubes; introduction of a flexible fiber-optic bronchoscope—fiberscope—by Shinnick and Freedman (1982) and the author and associates (1983) for precise positioning of endobronchial tubes; and use of different treatment modalities for management of hypoxemia during one-lung anesthesia and application of arterial blood gas or pulse oximeter for monitoring of blood oxygenation.

CHOICE OF ANESTHESIA

After thorough preoperative assessment and preparation of the patient, the anesthesiologist should choose and plan a technique that is both safe for the patient and suitable for the needs of the surgeon. An appropriate preoperative medication should be prescribed to make the patient relaxed and free of apprehension. Narcotics will minimize patient discomfort during placement of arterial cannulae and large intravenous lines. The respiratory depression caused by narcotics in patients with advanced pulmonary disease, however, should be kept in mind. Judicious use of intravenous narcotics such as fentanyl while the patient is in the operating room and prior to any procedures will provide the necessary analgesia.

Anticholinergic agents such as atropine or glycopyrrolate are prescribed with the premedication to decrease secretions during airway instrumentation, and to facilitate visualization of the airways when a fiberscope is used. Thornburn and associates (1986) have shown that anticholinergic agents also improve the pulmonary mechanics prior to general anesthesia. Because of the lower incidence of undesirable side effects, glycopyrrolate is the anticholinergic agent of choice. General endotracheal and endobronchial anesthesia with controlled ventilation is an ideal anesthetic technique for the majority of intrathoracic surgical procedures. More recently, a variety of high frequency ventilation—HFV—techniques have been developed and recommended for operations performed on the airway and for intrathoracic procedures. During HFV, ventilatory excursions of the lungs are of low amplitude. This may facilitate surgical exposure and resection during intrathoracic operations. HFV has been successfully used in situations in which access to the airway is impaired. The success or failure of HFV and its advantages and disadvantages compared to conventional mechanical ventilation depend on the following: the type of HFV used, whether one-lung or two-lung ventilation is applied, and the type of surgical procedure. There are three basic forms of HFV: high-frequency positive pressure ventilations—HFPPV, high frequency jet ventilation—HFJV, and high frequency oscillation—HFO. El-Baz and associates (1981, 1982) have successfully used one-lung HFPPV for sleeve pneumonectomy and surgical procedures on large airways. Smith and his associates (1981) reported successful use of HFPPV for pulmonary lobectomy. Hildebrand and associates (1984) applied HFJV for intrathoracic surgery, providing satisfactory operating conditions and ventilatory exchange. They indicated, however, that one-lung ventilation using a double-lumen tube provides the optimal condition if the difficulties associated with placement of double-lumen tubes and related complications can be avoided. Glenski and associates (1986) demonstrated that HFO resulted in adequate pulmonary gas exchange and excellent surgical conditions for peripheral lung procedures. However, surgical conditions for procedures on the major airway or mediastinal structures were unsatisfactory during HFO. They believe that the disadvantages of HFO outweighs the advantages during intrathoracic surgery.

A unique feature of thoracic anesthesia is the use of one-lung ventilation. The selection of an anesthetic technique and agent will be influenced by whether one-lung ventilation will be used and whether a high concentration of inspired oxygen can be delivered to the patient. The volatile halogenated anesthetic agents such as isoflurane, enflurane, and halothane permit the administration of a high inspired concentration of oxygen. In addition, halogenated agents depress the airway reflexes, cause bronchodilatation, and can rapidly be eliminated through the lungs. However, the high concentration of inhalation anesthetic agents may interfere with hypoxic vasoconstriction; this may divert blood flow from the ventilated to the nonventilated lung and worsen any hypoxemia. Another disadvantage of inhalation agents is the ease with which they may depress cardiac output when given during positive pressure ventilation. When narcotic analgesics are added to the anesthetic regimen, the concentration of inhalation agent is lowered. This helps alleviate the aforementioned problems associated with halogenated agents.

Introduction of anesthesia is achieved by the intravenous administration of 5 μg/kg fentanyl and 3 to 5 mg/kg of sodium thiopental. Anesthesia is maintained with 50% nitrous oxide and 0.5 to 1% of enflurane or isoflurane. An additional 10 to 15% μg/kg of fentanyl is given prior to and during one-lung ventilation when N_2O is discontinued and anesthesia is maintained with a low concentration inhalation agent and oxygen. At the conclusion of one-lung ventilation, nitrous oxide is started again. No additional narcotic is given from this point on. If necessary, higher concentrations of an inhalation agent are used to maintain adequate depths of anesthesia. Muscle relaxants are used for intubation of the trachea and for providing muscle relaxation and preventing diaphragmatic movement during surgery.

Weinrich and associates (1980) recommended a combination of ketamine, nitrous oxide, and muscle relaxant as an anesthetic for thoracic surgery. Ketamine has sympathomimetic properties. Thus, it supports the cardiovascular system and causes bronchodilation. It is a useful drug for the induction of general anesthesia in hypovolemic patients with an unstable cardiovascular system.

The use of epidural anesthesia to supplement a "light" general anesthetic is another approach that warrants consideration. It offers the advantage of decreasing the need to use neuromuscular blocking drugs or narcotic analgesics intraoperatively. This technique may receive more attention as epidural narcotics are increasingly used for the management of postsurgical pain. Training and experience in this technique, especially when a high or midthoracic approach is used, is needed. The technique should be used regularly to help sustain the expertise needed for its safe conduct.

During thoracic operations, it may be necessary to give various additional drugs for the control of cardiac dysrhythmias, systemic blood pressure, cardiac output, or acid-base balance. Their dosage is similar to that used in other types of anesthesia. However, caution should be exercised in the use of vasodilators and vasopressors during one-lung ventilation. Vasodilators such as sodium nitroprusside and nitroglycerin interfere with hypoxic pulmonary vasoconstriction. The vasopressors exert more vasoconstriction in oxygenated vessels than in hypoxic vessels. Consequently, both groups of drugs may divert blood flow from the ventilated to the nonventilated, hypoxic lung. This may then increase shunt and hypoxemia.

MONITORING

Various devices have been introduced to improve patient monitoring during anesthesia. As emphasized by Homi (1983), however, monitors should not affect or replace the anesthesiologist's constant touching and observation of the patient. Monitoring requirements differ among individual patients because of their general physical conditions, the presence or absence of cardiopulmonary disease, and the nature of their operative procedures. Monitoring of patients who are healthy and undergoing minor intrathoracic operations may be limited to routine monitors used in all patients undergoing general anesthesia. For most intrathoracic operations and during one-lung ventilation, monitoring of beat-to-beat arterial blood pressure and the arterial blood oxygenation is essential. Direct arterial monitoring of blood pressure not only provides beat-to-beat measurement of pressure, but also permits analysis of arterial blood gases and acid-base status during the operation and the postoperative period. The pulse oximeter provides a noninvasive, continuous monitor of the hemoglobin saturation and the heart rate. Pulse oximetry is less satisfactory in the immediate postoperative period because movement by the patient interferes with the proper functioning of this monitor.

The measurement of central venous pressure—CVP—is indicated in hypovolemic patients, when large volume shifts are anticipated, in patients with trauma and multiple injuries, and in patients with right ventricular dysfunction. Serial measurements are useful in the management of fluid and blood replacement when venous tone and myocardial function remain stable. The response of the CVP to a rapid volume infusion is a useful test of right ventricular function. CVP is subject to mechanical interference, especially during thoracic surgery.

The internal jugular and subclavian veins are common sites for central venous cannulation. It is wise to use the vein ipsilateral to the thoracotomy, because pneumothorax is a known complication of deep vein cannulation. In patients with left ventricular dysfunction, the CVP may not provide accurate information about left ventricular filling pressure. Under these circumstances, a pulmonary capillary wedge pressure should be measured by using a flow-direct pulmonary artery catheter. In most patients, the pulmonary capillary wedge pressure corresponds well with the left atrial pressure. The pulmonary artery catheter allows measurements of pulmonary artery systolic, diastolic, and mean pressures, along with the pulmonary capillary wedge pressure, CVP, and cardiac output. In addition, it provides the ability to sample mixed venous blood and to calculate the shunt. Peripheral and pulmonary vascular resistance can be calculated. Serial measurements of cardiac output can help to assess the status of the circulation and guide any necessary supportive therapy. Information derived from centrally placed catheters indicates how the myocardium manages the fluid load. However, the CVP and pulmonary wedge pressure will reflect changes in blood volume when depth of anesthesia and myocardial performance are unchanged. The combination of a fall in CVP or pulmonary wedge pressure and systemic arterial pressure suggests hypovolemia, whereas a high CVP and pulmonary wedge pressure with a low arterial pressure may indicate poor myocardial performance.

New anesthesia machines are equipped with a number of monitors and alarm systems; these include: an inspired oxygen monitor, a low and high pressure alarm system, a spirometer to measure expired tidal volume, a pressure manometer in the anesthesia circuit to monitor airway pressure, and an apnea alarm system. The use of muscle relaxants is monitored by a peripheral nerve stimulator and the body temperature is measured by a rectal or an esophageal probe. The availability of mass spectrometry and end-tidal CO_2 analysis provides additional monitoring of the patient's ventilation and confirms the proper placement of an endotracheal tube.

ONE-LUNG ANESTHESIA

One-lung anesthesia is a well-established technique with many surgical advantages. Because of its complexity, however, it adds to anesthetic difficulties. The most common indication for one-lung anesthesia is to provide the surgeon with a quiet operating field. A bronchopleural fistula, communicating empyema, bronchial hemorrhage, lung abscess, and giant air cyst represent the absolute indications for isolating the individual lungs. This prevents the spread of secretions to the healthy lung and helps ensure adequate ventilation.

Three categories of bronchial catheters are used to achieve separation of the lungs. Single-lumen endobronchial tubes with one or two inflatable cuffs were the first tubes used for one-lung anesthesia. They are intro-

duced into the bronchus of the healthy—contralateral—lung. Their major disadvantage is that the operative lung cannot be inflated or suctioned without losing the separation of the lungs. These tubes are rarely used today.

Bronchial blockers are introduced into the bronchus of the diseased lung while the healthy—contralateral—lung is ventilated through a tracheal or contralateral bronchial tube. Fogarty arterial embolectomy catheters have been employed in children by Vale (1969) and Hogg and Lorhan (1970), and well as by Cay and associates (1975). They may be positioned blindly, or more usually through a conventional bronchoscope, or with the help of a fiber-optic bronchoscope under topical or general anesthesia. Ginsburg (1981) advocated the use of Fogarty catheters in adults, while Dalens and associates (1982) used Swan-Ganz pulmonary artery catheters for this purpose in children. Aspiration of secretions or temporary ventilation of the diseased—ipsilateral—lung is not possible without losing the separation of the lungs. Dislodgement of blockers is common with coughing, change from supine to lateral position, or during surgical manipulation.

Double-lumen endobronchial tubes with two cuffs, consisting of two completely separate lumens, have their proximal ends separated into two connector limbs. A tracheal cuff is located proximal to the opening of the tracheal lumen and a bronchial cuff is located at the tip of the bronchial tube. Tubes designed for intubation of the right main stem bronchus have an opening in the bronchial cuff to permit ventilation of the right upper lobe. When a double-lumen tube is properly positioned and the bronchial and tracheal cuffs are inflated, a separate airway is formed for each lung. The main advantage of double-lumen bronchial tubes is that although isolation of the lungs is preserved one or both lungs can be ventilated. The Carlens double-lumen tube described in 1949, which has a carinal hook, and the Robertshaw double-lumen tube described in 1962, which has no carinal hook, are the most commonly used tubes. Edwards and Hatch (1965) reviewed their clinical experience with them. Burton and associates (1983) demonstrated the advantages of the Bronchocath disposable double-lumen tube. The advantages of these tubes include: a softer and more flexible structure, thin-walled tracheal and bronchial cuffs, a more gentle distal curve, and a greater inside-to-outside diameter ratio. These clear plastic disposable tubes also allow observation of the humidity of exhaled air during the respiratory cycle.

After the patient is anesthetized and paralyzed, the double-lumen tube is inserted into the trachea using a rigid laryngoscope. The tube is held such that the tip of the bronchial lumen faces anteriorly. After the tip is advanced beyond the vocal cords, the right-side Robertshaw tube is rotated 90° clockwise, whereas the left-sided Robertshaw tube is rotated 90° counterclockwise, to situate the tube in its normal position in the trachea, i.e. the bronchial lumen facing toward the intended bronchus. With the Carlens—left-sided—and White—right-sided—tubes, as the tip of the bronchial lumen passes the vocal cords, the tube is rotated 180° to bring the carinal hook anteriorly to negotiate the vocal cords.

After the carinal hook passes beyond the vocal cords, the Carlens tube is rotated 90° degrees to the right, whereas the White tube is rotated 90° to the left, in order to have the bronchial lumen face the intended bronchus. Once the double-lumen tube is placed in the trachea, the tracheal cuff is inflated. Mechanical ventilation is then begun with tidal volume of 10 ml/kg and a rate of 8 breaths/min. The bronchofiberscope is then used to evaluate the bronchial tree and position the double-lumen tube.

Fiber-optic Positioning of Double-Lumen Endobronchial Tubes

Left-sided Endobronchial Tube

A swivel adapter with a bronchoscopy port is placed in each lumen. While mechanical ventilation continues, the fiberscope is introduced first through the bronchial lumen and the patency, length, and anatomy of the left mainstem bronchus is evaluated. The tip of the fiberscope is then positioned 10 mm above the orifice of the left upper lobe bronchus. The tracheal cuff is deflated and the tube is advanced over the fiberscope into the left mainstem bronchus until it comes into view beyond the tip of the fiberscope. If the fiberscope is kept stationary during this maneuver, the tip of the endobronchial tube should lie just above the orifice of the left upper lobe. To confirm this, the fiberscope is advanced beyond the bronchial lumen to visualize both the upper and lower lobe bronchi. The fiberscope is then withdrawn from the bronchial lumen and inserted into the tracheal lumen to check the position of the bronchial cuff and the opening of the right main stem bronchus. If the bronchial cuff is seen outside the left mainstem bronchus, the tracheal cuff is deflated and the tube is advanced further until the proximal edge of the bronchial cuff lies 3 to 5 mm inside the left mainstem bronchus. This ensures separation of the lungs and stability of the tube and prevents herniation of the inflated cuff into the trachea. The bronchial and tracheal cuffs are then inflated using the minimal leak technique (Fig. 22–1).

Right-sided Endobronchial Tube

Proper positioning of right-sided double-lumen tubes is technically more difficult, because of the short and variable length of the right main stem bronchus. Rigg (1980) reported a high incidence of failure when these tubes were positioned blindly. The author and Schrader (1987) applied the following technique successfully. The fiberscope is passed through the bronchial lumen into the right mainstem bronchus. The patency, length, and anatomy of the right mainstem bronchus are evaluated. The fiberscope is rotated 90° clockwise and its tip is flexed superiorly—90° to 120°—to visualize the orifice of the right upper lobe bronchus. While the fiberscope is held stationary, its tip is returned to the neutral position. The tracheal cuff is deflated and the double-lumen tube is advanced over the fiberscope into the right main stem bronchus until it comes into view beyond the tip of the fiberscope. The fiberscope is then withdrawn inside the bronchial lumen and its tip is flexed superiorly to visualize the orifice of the right upper lobe bronchus through the slot in the bronchial cuff. Often minor adjustments of the tube are necessary to have a clear view of the right upper lobe orifice. The fiberscope is then passed through the tracheal lumen to check the position of the bronchial cuff and the opening of the left main stem bronchus (Fig. 22–2). The asymmetric design of the bronchial cuff in Bronchocath tubes makes inadequate seal of the main stem bronchus more likely with a right-sided than with a left-sided double-lumen tube. This problem is more likely to occur when the patient is placed in the lateral position during one-lung ventilation with increased airway pressure.

Another approach for positioning right-sided endobronchial tubes is to position the tip of the fiberscope at the upper level of the slot in the bronchial cuff. The tube and the fiberscope are then slowly advanced together inside the right main stem bronchus until the orifice of the right upper lobe bronchus comes into view through the slot in the broncial cuff. The tip of the fiberscope is then advanced to the middle of the slot in the bronchial cuff, and its tip flexed superiorly to visualize the right upper lobe bronchus through the slot in the bronchial cuff (Fig. 22–3).

Verifying Double-lumen Tube Placement

The following procedures will help determine whether tube placement is correct and separation of the lungs has been achieved. With a mechanical ventilator set at a tidal volume of 10 ml/kg and a rate of 8 breaths/min, the exhaled tidal volume and the peak and plateau airway pressures are measured, and the expiratory flow rate on the respirometer and the humidification of both lumens by exhaled air are observed. After the tracheal connector tube is clamped, the breath sounds should only be present on the bronchial side, and the respirometer should show a decrease of 10 to 15% in the exhaled tidal volume, whereas the expiratory flow rate should remain the same. The peak airway pressure should increase by no more than 50% when compared to two-lung ventilation. The clamp is then moved to the bronchial connector tube. Breath sounds should be present on the tracheal side. Tidal volume, expiratory flow rate and peak airway pressure should change little from one lung to another. The clamp is then removed and the tube secured. After the patient is turned into the lateral position, the breath sounds are checked once again and the measurements of tidal volume and airway pressures are repeated with each lumen occluded.

Placement is considered unsatisfactory if separation of the lungs is incomplete; if when changing from two-lung ventilation to one-lung ventilation the tidal volume decreases by more than 15%; if the expiratory flow rate of either lung slows markedly; or if the peak airway pressure increases by more than 50%.

If the tube placement is unsatisfactory, the fiberscope is used to check the position of the bronchial cuff and

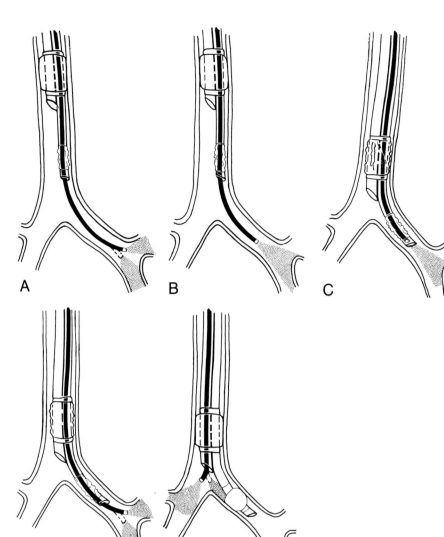

Fig. 22–1. Fiber-optic placement and positioning of left-sided double-lumen endobronchial tube. *A,* The fiberscope is passed through the bronchial lumen into the left main stem bronchus. The patency, length, and anatomy of the left main stem bronchus and the position of the orifice of the left upper lobe bronchus are evaluated. *B,* The fiberscope is withdrawn, and its tip is positioned 10 mm above the origin of the left upper lobe bronchus. *C,* The tracheal cuff is deflated, and the tube is advanced over the fiberscope into the left main stem bronchus until it comes into view beyond the tip of the fiberscope. *D,* The fiberscope is advanced beyond the bronchial lumen to visualize the left upper lobe bronchus. *E,* The fiberscope is passed through the tracheal lumen to check the position of the bronchial cuff and the opening of the right main stem bronchus.

ensure that the tip of the bronchial tube is neither pressed against the bronchial wall nor blocking the orifice to the upper lobe bronchus. For right-sided tubes, the position of the slot in the bronchial cuff with respect to the orifice of the right upper lobe must be rechecked. In the presence of advanced lung disease, loss of lung tissue, or atelectasis, more exaggerated changes in the above variables are expected when switching from two-lung ventilation to ventilation of the diseased lung. Bronchospasm may occur after bronchial intubation in lightly anesthetized patients or in patients with a reactive airway. In the presence of bronchospasm, more exaggerated changes in the variables are expected. These can be lessened by deepening the anesthesia. The peak airway pressure and tidal volume measurement during one-lung ventilation are presented in Table 22–1.

FIBER-OPTIC-AIDED PLACEMENT OF BALLOON-TIPPED CATHETERS AS BRONCHIAL BLOCKERS

The fiberscope can be used to place a Fogarty or similar balloon-tipped catheter into the desired bronchus.

As suggested by Ginsberg (1981), the distal end of the Fogarty catheter is angled to 30° to faciliate advancement into either main stem bronchus. After the patient is anesthetized and paralyzed, rigid laryngoscopy is performed and first a Fogarty catheter and then a tracheal tube are passed through the larynx into the trachea. A swivel adapter with endoscopy port is placed on the tracheal tube connector and mechanical ventilation is begun. The fiberscope is passed through the swivel adapter into the trachea to expose the catheter and the carina. The tip of the catheter is then advanced under direct vision into the desired main stem bronchus.

For left-lung blockade, the tip of the Fogarty catheter is advanced into the lower lobe bronchus so that the balloon of the catheter is positioned at the level of the orifice of the left upper lobe bronchus. For blockade of the right lung, the tip of the catheter is placed either just beyond the right upper lobe orifice in the bronchus intermedius or inside the right upper lobe bronchus.

Once the catheter is correctly positioned, the balloon is inflated with 1 to 2 ml of air. This will totally occlude

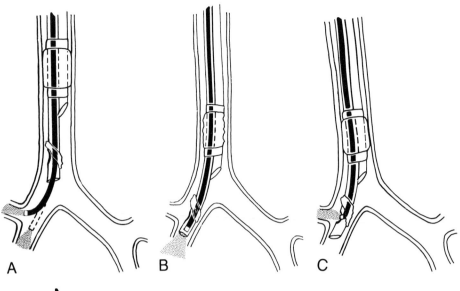

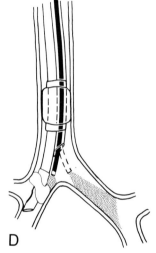

Fig. 22–2. Fiber-optic placement and positioning of right-sided double-lumen endobronchial tube. *A*, The fiberscope is passed through the bronchial lumen into the right main stem bronchus. The patency, length, and anatomy of the right main stem bronchus is evaluated. The fiberscope is then rotated 90° to the right and the tip of the fiberscope is flexed anteriorly to visualize the right upper lobe bronchus. While the fiberscope is held stationary, its tip is returned to the neutral position. *B*, The tracheal cuff is deflated, and the tube is advanced over the fiberscope into the right main stem bronchus until it comes into view beyond the tip of the fiberscope. *C*, The fiberscope is withdrawn inside the bronchial lumen to visualize the orifice of the right upper lobe bronchus through the slot of the bronchial cuff. *D*, The fiberscope is passed through the tracheal lumen to check the position of the bronchial cuff and the opening of the left main stem bronchus.

the main stem bronchus. Rao and associates (1981) placed a Fogarty catheter in the diseased lung and trachea tube in the main stem bronchus of the healthy lung in children to achieve the same objective a double-lumen tube achieves in adults. If the Fogarty catheter fails to block the diseased bronchus, the dependent lung may still be protected by the presence of the bronchial tube. Baraka and associates (1982) reported high incidence of right upper lobe collapse with blind intubation of the right main stem bronchus. This complication can be avoided by accurately positioning the tracheal tube with a fiberscope.

ONE-LUNG VENTILATION

To avoid atelectasis of the dependent lung, tidal volumes of 10 ml/kg are used. Kerr and associates (1973) have shown that if minute ventilation is not decreased during one-lung ventilation, the arterial carbon dioxide tension will be maintained at a similar level to that of two-lung ventilation. Because the compliance of the de-

pendent lung is decreased as its share of the tidal volume increases, however, peak airway pressure is increased by approximately 50%. When airway pressure increases, Cotè and colleagues (1983) showed that a larger proportion of the delivered tidal volume may be wasted because of the compression effect or distention, or both, of the breathing circuit. This may result in a slight decrease in alveolar ventilation and increase the Pa_{CO_2}.

The factors contributing to hypoxemia during one-lung ventilation are: shunting in the nonventilated lung, demonstrated by Kerr (1974) and Torda (1974) and their associates; ventilation/perfusion abnormalities in the ventilated lung; and reduction in the cardiac output. To counteract hypoxemia the ventilated—contralateral—lung should be ventilated with 100% oxygen. In a small percentage of patients, however, the Pa_{O_2} may still remain suboptimal. Various techniques have been applied to improve the Pa_{O_2} under these circumstances. One such technique is insufflation of oxygen into the ipsilateral—nonventilated—lung. Results are inconclusive, because Rees and Wansbrough (1982) showed improve-

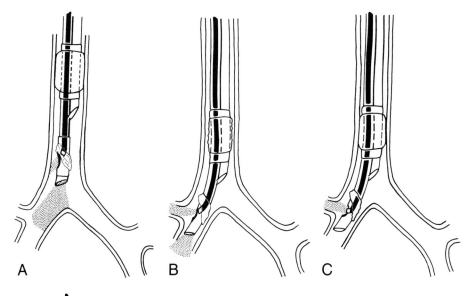

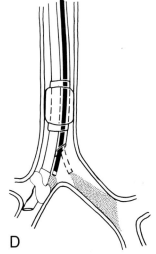

Fig. 22–3. Alternate approach to fiber-optic placement and positioning of right-sided double-lumen endobronchial tube. *A,* After evaluating the right main stem bronchus, the fiberscope is withdrawn inside the bronchial lumen until its tip is placed at the upper level of the slot of the bronchial cuff. *B,* The tube and the fiberscope are then advanced together inside the right main stem bronchus until the orifice of the right upper lobe comes just into view through the slot of the bronchial cuff. *C,* The fiberscope is advanced 2 to 3 mm inside the bronchial lumen. Its tip is flexed anteriorly to visualize the center of the right upper lobe bronchus through the slot in the bronchial cuff. *D,* The fiberscope is passed through the tracheal lumen to check the position of the bronchial cuff and the opening of the left main stem bronchus.

Table 22–1.   Tidal Volumes and Peak Airway Pressures During One-Lung Ventilation

	Supine		Lateral	
	TV	PAP	TV	PAP
Left-sided tube (N = 25)				
Two-lung ventilation	813 ± 71	22 ± 3	817 ± 76	23 ± 4
Left-lung ventilation	740 ± 81	34 ± 5	746 ± 62	35 ± 5
Right-lung ventilation	763 ± 71	32 ± 4	761 ± 65	33 ± 5
Right-sided tube (N = 8)				
Two-lung ventilation	818 ± 81	23 ± 4	821 ± 90	23 ± 4
Left-lung ventilation	750 ± 76	36 ± 5	759 ± 69	35 ± 3
Right-lung ventilation	722 ± 69	35 ± 7	758 ± 58	34 ± 4

Abbreviations: TV, Tidal volume of 10 to 12 ml/kg; PAP, peak airway pressure (cm H_2O).

ment, whereas Capan (1980) and Alfery (1981) and their associates showed that it is ineffective without application of CPAP. CPAP of the nonventilated lung improves arterial oxygenation, but it leads to overdistention of the operative lung and suboptimal surgical conditions. Applying HFJV with low driving pressure to the operative lung, Wilks and associates (1985) demonstrated improved oxygenation during one-lung ventilation while maintaining good surgical field. Gentle independent ventilation of the operative—ipsilateral—lung with small tidal volumes coordinated with surgeon's movements is a simple, inexpensive approach to improving Pa_{O_2}.

In the dependent—contralateral—lung, compression by the mediastinum and cephalad movement of the paralyzed diaphragm result in a decrease in functional residual capacity—FRC. These result in underventilation of well-perfused alveoli and an increase in airway closure. Trapped gas comes into equilibrium with mixed venous blood, contributing to arterial desaturation. Application of positive end-expiratory pressure—PEEP—to the dependent, ventilated lung may improve the situation. However, Khanam and Branthwaite (1973) observed that application of PEEP to the ventilated lung not only increases functional residual capacity, but also increases the intra-alveolar pressure, shifting higher proportion of pulmonary blood flow to the nonventilated lung, and contributes to a reduction in cardiac output. Depending on the degree of increased intra-alveolar pressure during application of PEEP and its effect on the pulmonary circulation and cardiac output, the Pa_{O_2} may increase, decrease, or remain the same, according to Katz and associates (1982). In addition to the raised intra-alveolar pressure, hypovolemia, dysrhythmias, myocardial depression, and surgical manipulation can all decrease the cardiac output and contribute to arterial desaturation. Ligation of the branches of the pulmonary artery to the collapsed section of lung will reduce the shunt and improve the arterial blood oxygenation.

Kerr (1974), Torda (1974), and Flacke (1976) and their associates have shown that the shunt through the nonventilated lung is about 20 to 25% of the cardiac output. This degree of shunt is much less than one would expect from complete collapse of an entire lung. Several factors are responsible for this. First, the effect of gravity and hydrostatic pressure in the lateral decubitus position increases the blood flow to the dependent lung. Second, the operative lung may have decreased pulmonary blood flow, because of underlying pathology. Third, Marshall and Marshall (1980) and Benumof (1978) showed that hypoxic pulmonary vasoconstriction—HPV—increases pulmonary vascular resistance in the operative—ipsilateral—lung. This diverts blood flow away from the operative lung and toward the nonoperative, dependent—contralateral—lung.

Anesthetic concentrations of inhalation agents may abolish hypoxic pulmonary vasoconstriction, thereby increasing the blood flow to the nonventilated lung, and consequently decreasing the Pa_{O_2}. Rogers and Benumof (1983) and Augustine and Benumof (1984) showed that halothane and isoflurane cause an insignificant change in the amount of shunted blood, when used in a concentration of one minimum alveolar concentration—MAC—or less. To avoid the possible inhibition of hypoxic pulmonary vasoconstriction from higher concentrations of inhalation anesthetics and to minimize the respiratory depressant effect of high doses of narcotics, a combination of a narcotic and inhalation anesthetics may be particularly useful for intrathoracic operation. It is critical that arterial oxygenation during one-lung ventilation be monitored by either frequent blood gas analyses or continuous measurement of hemoglobin saturation by an oximeter.

Complications

There are two main types of complications related to one-lung ventilation: technical and physiological (Table 22–2). Because of the shape and large size of double-lumen tubes, the incidence of difficult tracheal intubation is higher than with the use of single-lumen tubes. The practical difficulties encountered with Robertshaw tubes have been reviewed by Black and Harrison (1975). Complications included laceration of the tracheobronchial tree and malposition of the tube. The site of laceration is usually the posterior membranous wall of the trachea or a main stem bronchus. The diagnosis may be difficult to make, but can be confirmed by fiber-optic bronchoscopy. Improper positioning of double-lumen endobronchial tubes reported by Read (1977) and Oakes (1982) and their associates includes failure to advance the tube far enough down the intended bronchus. Difficulties resulting from improperly positioned endobronchial tubes include: incomplete isolation of the lungs; failure to collapse the operative lung; difficulty in ventilating one or both lungs; air entry into the wrong lung; and air trapping and unsatisfactory deflation of the lung. If not recognized, air trapping can eventually cause rupture of the lung and tension pneumothorax. If any of these circumstances arise, two-lung ventilation should be resumed, and the cause of the problem identified and corrected before one-lung ventilation is attempted once

Table 22–2. Complications of Bronchial Intubation and One-Lung Ventilation

Technical
    Unsuccessful or difficult intubation
    Trauma of the airway
        Minor trauma
        Rupture of tracheobronchial tree
    Improper position of the bronchial tube
        Tube not inserted far enough
        Intubation of wrong bronchus
        Tube inserted too far into the bronchus
    Tube dislodgement
Physiologic
    Hypoxemia
        Increased venous admixture
        Alteration of hypoxic pulmonary vasoconstriction
        Increased intra-alveolar pressure
        Decreased cardiac output
        Atelectasis of dependent lung

again. The physiological complication of one-lung ventilation is hypoxemia.

BLOOD AND FLUID REPLACEMENT

Blood and fluid replacement during thoracic surgery is a delicate task and an extremely important part of the anesthetic management. Great care must be taken not to overload the circulation, especially in patients undergoing lobectomy or pneumonectomy, because the pulmonary venous capacitance is greatly reduced. Blood loss during most intrathoracic operations does not necessitate a transfusion, but major bleeding can occur at any time. A large intravenous cannula that allows blood and fluid to be administered rapidly is essential, as is the ready availability of blood. All fluids, especially blood, should be warmed during administration.

The perioperative fluid regimen recommended by Gisecke (1986) is to replace NPO insensible loss with maintenance type solution—5% dextrose in water, 5% dextrose in 0.45 percent saline—at a rate of 2 ml/kg/hr. During surgery, in addition to 2 ml/kg/hr of insensible loss, an additional 6 ml/kg/hr of replacement-type solution—lactated Ringer's, 5% dextrose in lactated Ringer's, saline, normosal—is recommended for intrathoracic surgery.

This regimen should be followed only for the first hour or two of surgery to avoid over-hydration. Hutchin and associates (1969) discussed the danger of overhydration of patients during pneumonectomy. Infusion of large volumes of fluids may improve the urine output and circulatory dynamics, but at the risk of developing pulmonary edema and impaired lung mechanics. Twigley and Hillman (1985) stated that crystalloid solutions given during surgery go to the interstitial space. Dawidson and Ericksson (1982), and Brinkmeyer (1981) and Baek (1975) and their associates noted that excessive amounts of crystalloid solutions increase interstitial fluid, which causes peripheral and pulmonary edema without correcting the plasma volume deficit. To maintain an adequate blood volume and urine output and to avoid overhydration and congestion of the tissues, including the lungs, Twigley and Hillman (1985) suggested using colloid solutions perioperatively. This suggestion is based on the fact that most intraoperative cardiovascular changes are secondary to an absolute or relative change in intravascular circulating volume, caused by bleeding and vasodilatory effects of anesthetic drugs. These changes are ideally corrected with a colloid. Colloid solutions are useful to expand plasma volume and should be considered for replacing blood and fluid loss when the patient's blood pressure and pulse rate reflect signs of hypovolemia. The controversy of crystalloid or colloid use for blood and fluid replacement continues to be unresolved. In addition to monitoring of blood pressure, pulse rate, and urine output, monitoring of central venous pressure—CVP—and pulmonary artery wedge pressure is helpful in guiding appropriate fluid therapy. This is especially true in patients with poor general health and during operations with major blood and fluid losses.

Continuous measurement of CVP and pulmonary artery wedge pressures are helpful in patients with myocardial disease or advanced pulmonary disease. In a patient with a healthy heart, however, a serious overload of crystalloid solutions is possible without significant elevation of the CVP or pulmonary artery wedge pressure. This is particularly true if infusion of fluid is constant over a number of hours. Soft tissue edema and increased urine output are the best signs of overload with intravenous fluids. Edema is most easily seen in the scleral conjunctiva. It should be noted that congestion and edema of tissues caused by overhydration is also position-dependent. In the lateral decubitus position, the nonoperative, healthy lung is dependent, and accumulates more fluids. A moderate fluid overload can result in decreased Pa_{O_2} intraoperatively and moderate to severe hypoxemia in the immediate postoperative period.

The shortage of blood, together with transfusion hazards, has stimulated a search for alternatives to the use of homologous blood since the 1970s. Transmission of AIDS through blood transfusion has further increased the public's fear of accepting blood transfusion. Autologous transfusion by aspiration from the surgical field was reported by Bergman and co-workers (1974). Brewster and associates (1979) and Mattox (1978) showed that intraoperative autotransfusion significantly reduces the use of homologous blood transfusion. Preoperative donation of blood by the patient and the value and importance of an autologous blood program was emphasized by Haugen and Hill (1987). Normovolemic hemodilution on the day of operation may be employed if the physical condition of the patient permits.

SPECIFIC PROCEDURES AND SUGGESTED MANAGEMENT

Bronchoscopy

During bronchoscopy the airway is shared by the surgeon and anesthesiologist, and the patient's ventilation must be monitored carefully. Both rigid and fiber-optic bronchoscopy, under topical anesthesia and sedation, are performed by the surgeon. Patients with severe systemic or pulmonary disease or a severely compromised airway, however, and patients who are anxious, either at the beginning of or after sedation, however, may benefit from the expertise of an anesthesiologist. Administration of atropine 0.6 to 0.8 mg IM or glycopyrrolate 0.3 to 0.4 mg IM half an hour prior to bronchoscopy is essential, as the airway must be dry for the topical anesthesia to be effective. After conscious sedation, topical anesthesia is applied as follows: lidocaine 4% is first sprayed on the base of the tongue and tonsillar fossae; after 45 seconds, lidocaine jelly is spread on the base of the tongue with a tongue blade. Lidocaine jelly is applied to an Ovassapian intubating airway described by me (1987) (Fig. 22–4), which is then placed in patient's mouth, and the oropharynx is suctioned. The intubating airway keeps tongue anteriorly, facilitates exposure of larynx, and protects the bronchofiberscope from being bitten by the

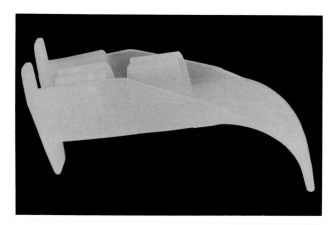

Fig. 22–4. The Ovassapian Fiberoptic Intubating Airway.

patient. The bronchofiberscope is advanced through the intubating airway to expose the larynx. The local anesthetic is now sprayed over the laryngeal vestibule, vocal cords, arytenoids, and pyriform sinuses. After 45 seconds the tip of the fiberscope is passed beyond the vocal cords and lidocaine is sprayed inside the trachea and carina.

General anesthesia for bronchoscopy must provide unconsciousness, sufficient relaxation for safe instrumentation of the airway, maintenance of adequate gas exchange, and a rapid recovery at the end of the procedure. Ventilation during rigid bronchoscopy in the paralyzed patient can be carried out by intermittent positive pressure ventilation—IPPV—using a ventilating bronchoscope; by manual jet ventilation using a venturi injector device described by Sanders (1967); by HFJV, as introduced by Ericksson and Sjostrand (1977); or by HFPPV. Manual jet ventilation can be achieved through a rigid bronchoscope or a fiber-optic bronchoscope, as described by Satyanarayana (1980). Vourc'h and co-workers (1983) compared manual jet ventilation with HFJV during bronchoscopy in patients with tracheobronchial stenosis. Arterial blood gas tensions were identical during both manual jet ventilation and HFJV at a rate of 150 per minute.

From the endoscopist's point of view, HFJV is preferable to manual jet ventilation because the tracheobronchial wall remains immobile. During HFPPV there is no air entrainment, so that anesthetic gases can be delivered at known concentration. When general anesthesia is required for fiber-optic bronchoscopy, the instrument is passed through an endotracheal tube mounted with a swivel adapter with a bronchoscopic port. This allows continuation of anesthesia and IPPV. The ratio of the external diameter of the bronchofiberscope to that of the internal diameter of the endotracheal tube is critical because the instrument reduces the effective ventilatory area of the endotracheal tube lumen.

Mediastinoscopy

Mediastinoscopy can be performed under local anesthesia, but endotracheal general anesthesia is more pleasant for the patient, provides more flexibility for the surgeon, and facilitates management of major complications that may occur during this procedure. Com-

pression of the innominate artery by the mediastinoscope can diminish or block blood flow to the right carotid and subclavian arteries. Lee and Salvatore (1976) reported a sudden loss of pulse and blood pressure in the right arm during mediastinoscopy, which was misdiagnosed as a cardiac arrest. The right radial artery pulse should therefore be monitored by palpation or finger plethysmography to detect compression of the innominate artery.

Sudden hypotension, bradycardia, or dysrhythmia may occur as a result of mechanical stimulation or compression of the trachea, vagus nerve, or great vessels. Repositioning of the mediastinoscope and intravenous administration of atropine or ephedrine may be necessary to restore the pulse rate and blood pressure. Massive bleeding caused by accidental injury to a major vessel is a distinct, but rare, possibility. The management of such bleeding necessitates thoracotomy and major surgical intervention. The anesthesiologist should be ready for massive replacement of fluids and blood. An intraoperative tension pneumothorax manifested by increased peak airway pressure, hypotension, and cyanosis is uncommon but will require immediate diagnosis and treatment, as stated by Furgang and Saidman (1972). Other reported complications associated with mediastinoscopy, reported by Ashbaugh (1970), include injury to the recurrent laryngeal nerve, phrenic nerve, or esophagus, transient hemiparesis, and air embolism.

Cysts of the Lung

IPPV or vigorous coughing might result in a dangerous rise in pressure and rupture of a cyst. Ting and associates (1963) reported that the size of a cyst will increase if it is in communication with the bronchus and has a valve-type action so that air may enter but not leave the cyst during IPPV. In a closed cyst, administration of nitrous oxide should be avoided, as was suggested by Isonhower and Cucchiara (1976), as it could rapidly increase the volume of and pressure within the cyst. As the size of the cyst increases, it may cause compression atelectasis and mediastinal shift and interfere with adequate gas exchange. Ventilation may also become inadequate if a significant portion of the tidal volume enters and leaves the communicating cyst without participating in gas exchange. Overinflation and rupture of the cyst may cause tension pneumothorax and cardiopulmonary insufficiency.

If the disease is confined to one lung, Isonhower and Cucchiara (1976) suggested that isolation of the lungs with a double-lumen endobronchial tube will avoid IPPV to the diseased side. Bilateral air cysts represent a difficult problem because of the possible increase in their size and their interference with gas exchange in the dependent lung while the upper lung is being operated upon. Bilateral thoracotomy may be necessary. Normandale and Feneck (1985) and McCarthy and associates (1987) have successfully applied HFJV for the anesthetic management of patients with bullous cystic lung disease.

Bronchopleural Fistula

The complications associated with a large bronchopleural fistula are loss of ventilation, contamination of the contralateral lung, and development of pneumothorax when IPPV is applied. These complications are best avoided by the passage of an endobronchial tube prior to induction of general anesthesia. Securing the airway with a double-lumen endobronchial tube in a conscious patient is a safe, but not always easy, approach. Placing patients in a head-up, lateral decubitus position with the affected side down will minimize the chance of secretions moving into the tracheobronchial tree while the trachea is being intubated. Dennison and Lester (1961), Francis and Smith (1962), and Parkhouse (1957) have indicated that the double-lumen endobronchial tube permits IPPV of the healthy lung, without the loss of minute ventilation through the fistula, and prevents soiling of the healthy lung. If tracheal intubation is difficult or not desirable in the conscious patient, general anesthesia with spontaneous ventilation can be used until the airway is secured with a double-lumen endobronchial tube. If a double-lumen tube cannot be applied and a single lumen tube is placed, Baker and co-workers (1971) suggested that spontaneous ventilation be maintained until the chest is opened. During surgery, the air leak can be minimized by manually packing the lung.

Carlon and co-workers (1980) successfully applied high frequency positive-pressure ventilation to provide adequate oxygenation and carbon dioxide removal in a patient with a large bronchopleural fistula. Hildebrand and associates (1984) indicated that HFJV at 100 cycles per minute was unsuitable during lobectomy with an open bronchus and resulted in a rapid deterioration in Pa_{O_2} and rise in Pa_{CO_2}. Their results conflict with those of Moulaert and Rolly (1983), who claimed that ventilation with an open bronchus was possible with HFJV at a rate of 250 cycles per minute.

Pneumothorax and Hemothorax

An important feature in the anesthetic management of these conditions is to drain them under local anesthesia prior to inducing anesthesia or administering IPPV.

Tracheal Resection

A thorough preoperative evaluation and understanding of the airway problem is essential. Good rapport must be established with the patient and heavy premedication avoided. Close communication between the surgeon and anesthesiologist must be established during tracheal reconstruction, and each one should be fully aware of the other's plan, approach, and readiness prior to the induction of anesthesia.

Various methods of maintaining adequate ventilation have been applied during operations on the trachea or bronchi. Use of a single-lumen endotracheal tube placed above the tracheal lesion before surgery is begun and advanced inside the trachea or bronchi below the tracheal lesion during surgery has been described by Belsey (1950) and Geffin and associates (1969). It is safer to secure the airway while the patient is awake.

If an awake intubation is not possible, a slow, inhalation induction with a halogenated anesthetic agent with oxygen should be performed, with spontaneous ventilation maintained until tracheal intubation is achieved. The bronchofiberscope can be used to apply topical anesthesia to the larynx and trachea, to evaluate the site and degree of tracheal stenosis, and to intubate the trachea. The instrument enables the anesthesiologist to place the tip of the tube just above the stenotic area and avoid any trauma. After exposure of the trachea, as the surgeon starts resecting the lesion, the orotracheal tube is advanced beyond the lesion into the lower section of the trachea. The surgeon completes the resection and anastomosis in the presence of the endotracheal tube. To avoid the presence of an endotracheal tube in the surgical field, Akdikmen and Landmesser (1965) and Geffin (1969) described the use of two separate endotracheal tubes. The first endotracheal tube is placed orally above the tracheal lesion. The second sterile, armored endotracheal tube is inserted by the surgeon into the distal trachea or one of the main stem bronchi after he has cut the trachea distal to the lesion. This second endotracheal tube is then connected to the anesthesia machine using sterile corrugated tubing and Y-piece, and anesthesia is continued. After resection of the lesion and placement of sutures on the posterior tracheal wall, the surgeon removes the endotracheal tube placed in the distal trachea. The original orotracheal tube is now advanced beyond the suture line into the lower trachea, or one of the main stem bronchi, until the surgeon completes the repair of the trachea.

A third approach is use of HFJV through a small-sized catheter, as described by Ericksson (1975) and Rogers (1985) and their co-workers; manual jet ventilation, as reported by Lee and English (1974); and HFPPV as applied by El-Baz (1982). Scamman and Choi (1986) have used a sterile nasogastric—NG—tube for application of low frequency jet ventilation and measurement of end tidal CO_2 during tracheal resection. The distal end of the NG tube was cut off above the highest side hole and was placed 2 cm into the distal stump of the trachea. The larger lumen was connected to a Sander's jet apparatus and the smaller to a CO_2 analyzer. Normal arterial and end tidal gas tensions were maintained while the surgeon completed the posterior and lateral wall anastomosis. Neuman and associates (1984) have described successful use of HFJV for tracheal resection in a seven-year-old child.

To avoid contamination of the operating room from inhalation agents, intravenous anesthetics are used during HFPPV or jet ventilation. Early extubation is highly desirable to minimize the compromise of blood flow to the trachea.

Woods (1961) and Coles (1976) and their associates applied extracorporeal circulation for management of tracheobronchial resection.

Laser Surgery

Laser surgery of the airway presents several potential anesthetic problems. These include ventilation and oxygenation through a compromised and shared airway and hazards introduced by the laser beam. The major hazards from laser surgery are fires and destruction of normal tissues. Fire can occur when the laser strikes a rubber or plastic endotracheal tube in an oxygen-rich anesthetic mixture. Nitrous oxide, like oxygen, supports combustion, whereas halogenated anesthetic agents are not flammable and do not support combustion.

To minimize the danger of fire, Brutinel and associates (1983) recommended using 50% oxygen or less in nitrogen, whereas Eisenman and Ossoff (1986) favor a mixture of oxygen and helium during general anesthesia. The use of metallic or noncombustible disposable endotracheal tubes and protection of standard rubber or plastic endotracheal tubes by wrapping them with aluminum or copper tape have been thoroughly reviewed by Hermens (1983) and co-workers. Endotracheal tubes wrapped with metallic tape may cause pharyngeal and laryngeal injury, caused by the presence of rough edges, and pieces of tape can loosen, break off, and be aspirated. All oil-based ointments and lubricants should be avoided because they are combustible and can be ignited.

In case of fire, the surgery should be stopped and the endotracheal tube should be removed immediately. The lungs as well as the trachea may be injured either by smoke inhalation or a direct thermal burn.

The surgical field should be immobile to minimize the chance of laser damage of normal tissue. Choice of anesthesia for bronchoscope laser surgery depends on the surgical technique and the age and condition of the patient. Rontal and associates (1986) favor topical anesthesia with sedation whenever possible, but particularly in patients with higher grade airway obstruction.

General anesthesia is the method of choice for most children and for adult patients who cannot tolerate local anesthesia. Dumon and associates (1984) favored spontaneous ventilation, whereas Brutinel (1983) and Vourc'h (1983) and their co-workers recommended controlled ventilation. If jet ventilation is chosen, scavenging of inhalation anesthetic agents is difficult, and total intravenous anesthesia must be provided. Prolonged respiratory depression, and the need for postoperative ventilatory support, is a potential complication of total intravenous anesthesia. Whatever anesthetic technique is chosen, the basic principle of anesthetic management of patients with a compromised airway should be followed. Communication between the anesthesiologist and the surgical team is essential, and a plan for management of total airway obstruction must be agreed upon prior to the induction of anesthesia. All routine safety precautions during laser surgery, both for the patient and the operating room personnel, should be observed. A sign noting that a laser is in use should be placed on the outside of the door. Finally, postoperative care is extremely important, as respiratory depression, laryngospasm, bronchospasm, airway obstruction, and hemorrhage can all occur and require immediate treatment.

REFERENCES

Akdikmen, S., and Landmesser, C.M.: Anesthesia for surgery of the intrathoracic portion of the trachea. Anesthesiology 26:117, 1965.

Alfery, D.D., et al.: Improving oxygenation during one-lung ventilation: the effects of PEEP and blood flow restriction to the nonventilated lung. Anesthesiology 55:381, 1981.

Ashbaugh, D.G.: Mediastinoscopy. Arch. Surg. 100:586, 1970.

Augustine, S.D., and Benumof, J.L.: Halothane and isoflurane do not impair arterial oxygenation during one-lung ventilation in patients undergoing thoracotomy. Anesthesiology 61:A484, 1984.

Baek, S.M., et al.: Plasma expansion in surgical patients with high central venous pressure: the relationship of blood volume to hematocrit, CVP, pulmonary wedge pressure and cardiorespiratory changes. Surgery 78:304, 1975.

Baker, W.L., et al.: Management of bronchopleural fistulas. J. Thorac. Cardiovasc. Surg. 62:393, 1971.

Baraka, A., et al.: One-lung ventilation of children during surgical excision of hydatid cysts. Br. J. Anaesth. 54:523, 1982.

Belsey, R.: Resection and reconstruction of the intrathoracic trachea. Br. J. Surg. 38:200, 1950.

Benumof, J.L.: Mechanism of decreased blood flow to atelectatic lung. J. Appl. Physiol. 46:1047, 1978.

Bergman, D., et al.: Intraoperative autotransfusion during emergency thoracic and elective open heart surgery. Ann. Thorac. Surg. 18:590, 1974.

Bjork, V.O., and Carlens, E.: The prevention of spread during pulmonary resection by the use of a double-lumen catheter. J. Thorac. Cardiovasc. Surg. 20:151, 1950.

Black, A.M.S., and Harrison, G.A.: Difficulties with positioning Robertshaw double-lumen tubes. Anaesth. Intensive Care 3:299, 1975.

Brewster, D.C., et al.: Intraoperative autotransfusion in major vascular surgery. Am. J. Surg. 137:507, 1979.

Brinkmeyer, S., et al.: Superiority of colloid over electrolyte solution for fluid resuscitation. Crit. Care Med. 9:396, 1981.

Brutinel, W.M., et al.: Bronchoscopic therapy with neodymium-yttrium-aluminum garnet laser during intravenous anesthesia. Chest 84:518, 1983.

Burton, N.A., et al.: Advantages of a new polyvinyl chloride double-lumen tube in thoracic surgery. Ann. Thorac. Surg. 36:78, 1983.

Capan, L.M., et al.: Optimization of arterial oxygenation during one-lung anesthesia. Anesth. Analg. 59:847, 1980.

Carlens, E.: A new flexible double-lumen catheter for bronchospirometry. J. Thorac. Surg. 18:742, 1949.

Carlon, G.C., et al.: High-frequency positive pressure ventilation in management of a patient with bronchopleural fistula. Anesthesiology 52:160, 1980.

Cay, D.L., et al.: Selective bronchial blocking in children. Anaesth. Intensive Care 3:127, 1975.

Coles, J.C., et al.: A method of anesthesia for imminent tracheal obstruction. Surgery 80:379, 1976.

Cotè, C.J., et al.: Wasted ventilation measured in vitro with eight anesthetic circuits with and without inlet humidification. Anesthesiology 59:442, 1983.

Dalens, B., et al.: Selective endobronchial blocking vs. selective intubation. Anesthesiology 57:555, 1982.

Dawidson, I., and Eriksson, B.: Statistical evaluation of plasma substitutes based on 10 variables. Crit. Care Med. 10:653, 1982.

Dennison, P.H., and Lester, E.R.: An anesthetic technique for the repair of bronchopleural fistula. Br. J. Anaesth. 33:655, 1961.

Dumon, J.F., et al.: Principles for safety in application of neodymium-YAG laser in bronchology. Chest 86:163, 1984.

Edwards, E.M., and Hatch, D.J.: Experiences with double-lumen tubes. Anaesthesia 20:461, 1965.

Eisenman, T.S., and Ossoff, R.H.: Anesthesia for bronchoscopic laser surgery. Otolaryngology—Head and Neck Surgery 94:45, 1986.

El-Baz, N., et al.: One-lung high frequency positive pressure ventilation for sleeve pneumonectomy: an alternative technique. Anesth. Analg. 60:638, 1981.

El-Baz, N., et al.: One-lung high frequency ventilation for tracheoplasty and bronchoplasty: a new technique. Ann. Thorac. Surg. 34:564, 1982.

Eriksson, I., et al.: High frequency positive pressure ventilation during transthoracic resection of tracheal stenosis and during preoperative bronchoscopic examination. Acta Anaesth. Scand. 19(113):13, 1975.

Eriksson, I., and Sjöstrand, U.: High-frequency positive pressure ventilation and the pneumatic valve principle in bronchoscopy under general anesthesia. Acta. Anesth. Scand. (Suppl.) *64*:83, 1977.

Flacke, J.W., et al.: Influence of tidal volume and pulmonary artery occlusion on arterial oxygenation during endobronchial anesthesia. South Med. J. *69*:617, 1976.

Francis, J.G., and Smith, K.G.: An anesthetic technique for the repair of bronchopleural fistula. Br. J. Anaesth. *34*:817, 1962.

Furgang, F.A., and Saidman, L.J.: Bilateral tension pneumothorax associated with mediastinoscopy. J. Thorac. Cardiovasc. Surg. *63*:329, 1972.

Geffin, B., et al.: Anesthetic management of tracheal resection and reconstruction. Anesth. Analg. *48*:884, 1969.

Giesecke, A.H., and Egbert, L.D.: Perioperative fluid therapy: crystalloids. *In* Anesthesia, 2nd ed. Edited by R. D. Miller. New York, Churchill Livingstone, 1986, pp. 1313–1328.

Ginsberg, R.J.: New technique for one-lung anesthesia using an endobronchial blocker. J. Thorac. Cardiovasc. Surg. *82*:542, 1981.

Glenski, J.A., et al.: High frequency, small volume ventilation during thoracic surgery. Anesthesiology *64*:211, 1986.

Haugen, R.K., and Hill, G.E.: A large-scale autologous blood program in a community hospital: a contribution to the community's blood supply. JAMA *275*:1211, 1987.

Hermens, J.M., et al.: Anesthesia for laser surgery. Anesth. Analg. *62*:218, 1983.

Hildebrand, P.J., et al.: High frequency jet ventilation: a method for thoracic surgery. Anaesthesia *39*:1091, 1984.

Hogg, C.E., and Lorhan, P.H.: Pediatric bronchial blocking. Anesthesiology *33*:560, 1970.

Homi, J.: Conduct of anesthesia. *In* General Thoracic Surgery, 2nd Ed. Edited by T.S. Shields. Philadelphia, Lea & Febiger, 1983, pp. 254–266.

Hutchin, P., et al.: Pulmonary congestion following infusion of large fluid loads in thoracic surgical patients. Ann. Thorac. Surg. *8*:339, 1969.

Isonhower, N., and Cucchiara, R.F.: Anesthesia for vanishing lung syndrome: report of a case. Anesth. Analg. *55*:750, 1976.

Jenkins, V.A., and Clark, G.: Endobronchial anesthesia with the Carlens catheter. Br. J. Anaesth. *30*:13, 1958.

Katz, J.A., et al.: Pulmonary oxygen exchange during endobronchial anesthesia: effects of tidal volume and PEEP. Anesthesiology *56*:164, 1982.

Kerr, J.H., et al.: Observations during endobronchial anesthesia. I. Ventilation and carbon dioxide clearance. Br. J. Anaesth. *45*:159, 1973.

Kerr, J.H. et al.: Observations during endobronchial anaesthesia. II. Oxygenation. Br. J. Anaesth. *46*:84, 1974.

Khanam, T., and Branthwaite, M.A.: Arterial oxygenation during one-lung anaesthesia. Anaesthesia *28*:280, 1973.

Lee, J., and Salvatore, A.: Innominate artery compression simulating cardiac arrest during mediastinoscopy: a case report. Anesth. Analg. *55*:748, 1976.

Lee, P., and English, I.C.: Management of anesthesia during tracheal resection. Anaesthesia *29*:305, 1974.

Marshall, B.E., and Marshall, C.: Continuity of response to hypoxic pulmonary vasoconstriction. J. Appl. Physiol. *59*:189, 1980.

Mattox, K.L.: Comparison of techniques of autotransfusion. Surgery *84*:700, 1978.

McCarthy, G., et al.: High frequency jet ventilation for bilateral bullectomy. Anaesthesia *42*:411, 1987.

Moulaert, P., and Rolly, G.: High frequency jet ventilation for pulmonary resection. *In* Perspectives in High Frequency Ventilation. Edited by P.A. Sheck, N.H. Sjostrand, and R.B. Smith. Boston, Martinus-Nijhoff, 1983, pp. 227–32.

Neuman, G.G., et al.: High-frequency jet ventilation for tracheal resection in a child. Anesth. Analg. *63*:1039, 1984.

Normandate, J.P., and Feneck, R.O.: Bullous cystic lung disease: its anesthetic management using high frequency jet ventilation. Anaesthesia *40*:1182, 1985.

Oakes, D.D., et al.: Lateral thoracotomy and one-lung anesthesia in patients with morbid obesity. Ann. Thorac. Surg. *34*:572, 1982.

Ovassapian, A., et al.: Endobronchial intubation using flexible fiber-optic bronchoscope. Anesthesiology *59*:A501, 1983.

Ovassapian, A., and Schrader, S: Fiber-optic aided bronchial intubation. Semin. Anesthesia *6*:133, 1987.

Ovassapian, A.: A new fiber-optic intubating airway. Anesth. Analg. *66*:S132, 1987.

Parkhouse, J.: Anesthetic aspects of bronchial fistula. Br. J. Anaesth. *29*:217, 1957.

Rao, C.C., et al.: One-lung pediatric anesthesia. Anesth. Analg. *60*:450, 1981.

Read, R.C., et al.: Prospective study of the Robertshaw endobronchial catheter in thoracic surgery. Ann. Thorac. Surg. *24*:156, 1977.

Rees, D.I., and Wansbrough, S.R.: One-lung anesthesia: percent shunt and arterial oxygen tension during continuous insufflation of oxygen to the nonventilated lung. Anesth. Analg. *61*:507, 1982.

Rigg, D.: A comparison of the Robertshaw and Carlens-type double-lumen tubes for thoracic anesthesia. Anaesth. Intensive Care *8*:460, 1980.

Robertshaw, F.L.: Low resistance double-lumen endobronchial tubes. Br. J. Anaesth. *34*:576, 1962.

Rogers, R.C., et al.: High frequency jet ventilation for tracheal surgery. Anaesthesia *40*:32, 1985.

Rogers, S.N., and Benumof, J.L.: Halothane and isoflurane do not impair arterial oxygenation during one-lung ventilation in patients undergoing thoracotomy. Anesthesiology *59*:A532, 1983.

Rontal, M., et al.: Anesthetic management for tracheobronchial laser surgery. Ann. Otol. Rhinol. Laryngol. *95*:556, 1986.

Sanders, R.D.: Two ventilating attachments for bronchoscopes. Del. Med. J. *39*:170, 1967.

Satyanarayana, T., et al.: Bronchofiberscopic jet ventilation. Anesth. Analg. *59*:350, 1980.

Scamman, F.L., and Choi, W.W.: Low frequency jet ventilation for tracheal resection. Laryngoscope *96*:678, 1986.

Shinnick, J.P., and Freedman, A.P.: Bronchofiberoptic placement of a double-lumen endotracheal tube. Crit. Care Med. *10*:544, 1982.

Smith, R.B., et al.: High frequency ventilation during pulmonary lobectomy: three cases. Respiratory Care *26*:437, 1981.

Thornburn, J.R., et al.: Comparison of the effects of atropine and glycopyrrolate on pulmonary mechanics in patients undergoing fiber-optic bronchoscopy. Anesth. Analg. *65*:1285, 1986.

Ting, E.Y., et al.: Mechanical properties of pulmonary cysts and bullae. Am. Rev. Respir. Dis. *87*:538, 1963.

Torda, T.A., et al.: Pulmonary venous admixture during one-lung anesthesia. Anaesthesia *29*:272, 1974.

Twigley, A.J., and Hillman, K.M.: The end of the crystalloid era? Anaesthesia *40*:860, 1985.

Vale, R.: Selective bronchial blocking in a small child. Br. J. Anaesth. *41*:453, 1969.

Vourc'h, G., et al.: High frequency jet ventilation versus manual jet ventilation during bronchoscopy in patients with tracheo-bronchial stenosis. Br. J. Anaesth. *55*:969, 1983.

Weinrich, A., et al.: Continuous ketamine infusion for one-lung anesthesia. Can. Anaesth. Soc. J. *27*:485, 1980.

Wilks, D., et al.: Selective high frequency jet ventilation of the operative lung improves oxygenation during thoracic surgery. Anesthesiology *63*:A586, 1985.

Woods, F., et al.: Resection of the carina and mainstem bronchi with extracorporeal circulation. N. Engl. J. Med. *264*:492, 1961.

CHAPTER 23

JET VENTILATION

Nabil M. El-Baz

Jet ventilation is based on the intermittent delivery of a narrow stream of gases at high velocity into the trachea through a small catheter or a cannula. Jet ventilation was first used by Sanders (1967) to deliver large tidal volumes at slow respiratory rates to provide gas exchange during anesthesia and bronchoscopic surgery. Jet ventilation was later used by Heijman and associates (1972) at high respiratory rates and small tidal volumes to provide alveolar ventilation during anesthesia and routine surgery. Injector jet ventilation—IJV—and high frequency jet ventilation—HFJV—achieve adequate alveolar ventilation and oxygenation by generating different gas kinetics in the airways. Both techniques, however, use the basic principles of gas delivery for jet ventilation.

MECHANICS OF GAS DELIVERY

Jet ventilation is delivered through a noncompliant inspiratory tube and a narrow intratracheal catheter or special adaptor. Jet ventilation does not incorporate an expiratory tube, and gases are exhaled through the upper airway, which must be patent and open to the atmosphere.

Jet ventilation requires a source of gas at a relatively high pressure, such as the central oxygen supply, which is normally 50 to 60 psi. The pressure of the gas supply is regulated manually through a reducing valve and the selected pressure is referred to as the driving gas pressure—DGP. Gas flow through the inspiratory tube is interrupted by the ventilator's electromagnetic solenoid valve as shown in Figure 23–1. The function of this valve is controlled by an electric circuit, which is regulated manually through two dials to determine the number of valve openings—frequency, respiratory rate—and the duration of each opening—insufflation time, IT. The tidal volume insufflated with each valve opening is determined by the gas pressure selected—DGP—and by the duration of each opening—IT. The ventilator can deliver HFJV at a high respiratory rate and short inspiratory time or IJV at a low respiratory rate and long insufflation time. A spring-loaded valve, which is operated by hand

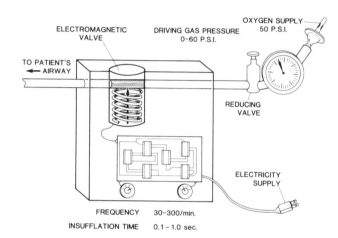

Fig. 23–1. High frequency ventilator. The reducing valve regulates the pressure of oxygen. Gas flow to the patient is interrupted by a solenoid electromagnetic valve.

for the delivery of injector jet ventilation, can be substituted for the electric circuit and solenoid valve.

GAS EXCHANGE

Injector jet ventilation delivers a large tidal volume—500 to 1500 ml—at a slow respiratory rate of 10 to 30 breaths/min. This method of jet ventilation achieves adequate gas exchange by convection—bulk flow—similar to conventional intermittent positive pressure ventilation—IPPV. Prolonged jet insufflation generates a negative pressure above the tip of the catheter, which causes the entrainment of air from the trachea and upper airways. As pointed out by Carden and associates (1973), this technique uses the Bernoulli principle, the venturi tube, and injector mechanics to entrain air and enlarge the insufflated tidal volume.

High frequency jet ventilation delivers a small tidal volume—50 to 250 ml—at a high respiratory rate of 60 to 600 breaths/min. Sjostrand (1977) noted that this method of ventilation achieves adequate gas exchange by a combination of convective flow and acceleration of gas diffusion. The repeated insufflations of small volumes at high velocity generates a turbulent flow of gases in the airways and a continuously positive airway pressure—CPAP. This increases FRC, improves gas mixing and distribution, and accelerates gas diffusion. Klain and Smith (1977) showed that the short periods of jet insufflation do not generate significant negative pressure and do not entrain air. CO_2 elimination during high frequency ventilation depends on the convective flow used—tidal volume. The exact mechanism by which HFV achieves gas exchange remains unknown.

JET VENTILATION FOR BRONCHOSCOPIC AND LASER SURGERY

Sanders (1967) and Eriksson (1975), Carden (1973), and Kwok (1984) and their associates reported the use of injector and high frequency jet ventilation through special bronchoscopic attachments to provide an unobstructed view of airway lesions and adequate alveolar ventilation during bronchoscopic examination and laser surgery. I and my colleagues reported in 1984 the use of one-lung and two-lung high frequency jet ventilation through a small catheter during laser vaporization of tracheobronchial lesions. Two-lung HFJV was used in 12 patients with subglottic and tracheal stenotic lesions. After induction of anesthesia, a 2 mm ID catheter was placed in the trachea distal to the stenotic lesion. The small catheter did not interfere with the placement of the bronchoscope in the trachea alongside the catheter. The catheter's position and the tracheal lumen's size near the lesion were examined during bronchoscopy to ensure an adequate lumen for gas exit. Two-lung HFJV achieved adequate gas exchange and the small catheter provided optimal surgical conditions. The parameters of HFV used and the blood gases obtained are shown in Figure 23–2. HFV was associated with continuous outflow of gases through the bronchoscope, which eliminated the smoke of tissue vaporization and prevented the contamination of the distal airways with blood and debris. HFV was used in these patients at F_{IO_2} of 0.21—air—which provided adequate oxygenation and eliminated the risk of catheter ignition by laser.

JET VENTILATION FOR AIRWAY SURGERY

The use of jet ventilation through a small catheter has been valuable during resection and reconstruction of the airways. The small size of the catheter provides optimal surgical access to the circumferences of the transected airways and facilitates the reconstruction of an airtight anastomosis. Lee and English (1974) reported that the use of IJV through a catheter during tracheal resection maintains adequate gas exchange and provides optimal surgical conditions. The use of injector jet ventilation during airway surgery, however, has been complicated, as noted by O'Sullivan and Healy (1985), by frequent displacement of the catheters and entrainment of air and blood into the airways. Chang and associates (1980) reported occasional barotrauma. Deslauriers and associates

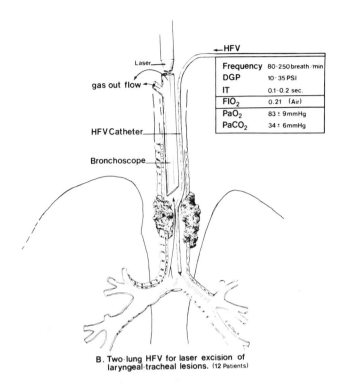

B. Two-lung HFV for laser excision of laryngeal-tracheal lesions. (12 Patients)

Fig. 23–2. The HFV catheter is positioned distal to the airway lesion. The bronchoscope is positioned alongside the catheter. The delivered HFV gases exit through the trachea and the bronchoscope. Top table shows the parameters of HFV and blood gases.

Frequency	80-250 breath/min
DGP	10-35 PSI
IT	0.1-0.2 sec.
FIO_2	0.21 (Air)
PaO_2	83 ± 9 mmHg
$PaCO_2$	34 ± 6 mmHg

(1979) minimized these problems by using apneic oxygen insufflation supplemented with occasional jet insufflation. Eriksson and associates (1975) reported that HFJV through a catheter during tracheal resection maintains adequate gas exchange and optimal surgical conditions. I and my co-workers showed in 1982 and 1983 that one-lung high frequency ventilation through a small catheter provides adequate gas exchange during tracheoplasty and bronchoplasty. We used one-lung HFV in six patients undergoing a right-sleeve pneumonectomy and tracheobronchial anastomosis. These patients initially received two-lung conventional ventilation through an endotracheal tube. After the transection of trachea and left main bronchus, a 2 mm ID catheter was advanced through the endotracheal tube and positioned inside the transected left main bronchus. Left lung HFV through the catheter was used during tracheobronchial anastomosis and maintained adequate gas exchange for periods of 1.5 to 3 hours. The parameters of HFV and blood gases obtained are shown in Figure 23–3. The small catheter provided optimal access and the small tidal volume of HFJV caused minimal movement of the catheter and the mediastinum. The continuous outflow of HFJV gases through the open bronchus prevented the contamination of the lung with the blood and debris. This technique of one-lung HFV through the small catheter, as reported by me and my colleagues (1983), was useful during the resection of tracheal and carinal lesions. We reported in 1983 that two-lung HFV provides adequate gas exchange

HFPPV	
Frequency	80–250 breath/min
DGP	15–25 PSI
IT%	40%
FIO₂	1.0
PaO₂	200–610 mmHg
PaCO₂	19–40 mmHg
6 Patients	

HFPPV CATHETER

ENDOTRACHEAL TUBE

LEFT LUNG HFPPV FOR RIGHT SLEEVE PNEUMONECTOMY

Fig. 23–3. The HFV catheter is passed through the endotracheal tube and the open trachea and then placed into the left main bronchus. HFV of the left lung achieved adequate gas exchange as shown in the top table. The delivered HFV gases exit through the open left main bronchus. After completion of the tracheobronchial anastomosis, the HFV catheter was removed and conventional ventilation was resumed through the endotracheal tube.

and operative conditions during tracheal reconstruction supported with a Montgomery tracheal T-tube.

JET VENTILATION DURING THORACIC SURGERY

Kittle (1986) reviewed the use of one-lung and two-lung high frequency jet ventilation during intrathoracic surgery. Two-lung high frequency ventilation was reported by Malina (1981) and Seki (1983) and their associates to maintain adequate gas exchange and cause minimal expansion and movement of the upper lung during thoracic surgery. These reports were contradicted by Glenski and colleagues (1986), who found that two-lung HFJV was associated with hyperinflation of the upper

lung and unacceptable surgical conditions. We reported in 1982 that one-lung high frequency ventilation provided adequate gas exchange and operative conditions in 26 patients undergoing intrathoracic surgery. These patients received conventional one-lung IPPV followed by a period of isolated one-lung HFJV and then a period of modified one-lung HFJV. The isolated one-lung HFJV was associated with improvement of oxygenation as a result of an improvement of ventilation and perfusion of the dependent lung. The deflation of the endobronchial tube cuff for modified—nonisolated—one-lung HFJV was associated with further improvement of oxygenation. Modified one-lung HFJV generates a continuous gas outflow at the carina that allows the participation of the upper lung in gas exchange and causes slight inflation of upper lung. The PaO₂, Qs/Qt, and gas flow obtained during the use of these three methods of ventilation are shown in Figure 23–4.

JET VENTILATION FOR TREATMENT OF BRONCHOPLEURAL FISTULA

Carlon (1981) and Turnbull (1981) and their associates reported that high frequency jet ventilation improves gas exchange in patients with broncho-pleural-cutaneous fistula. Carlon and Howland (1985) noted that high frequency jet ventilation is associated with low mean and peak airway pressures, which reduces trauma and gas flow through the fistula and facilitates the healing process.

PROBLEMS WITH JET VENTILATION

The clinical applications and value of jet ventilation have been limited because of the following problems: (1) the principle of gas delivery and the equipment for jet ventilation are completely different from those for conventional ventilation; (2) the circuits, adapters, ventilators, and catheters are prototypes and lack standardization and expert engineering; (3) jet ventilation requires

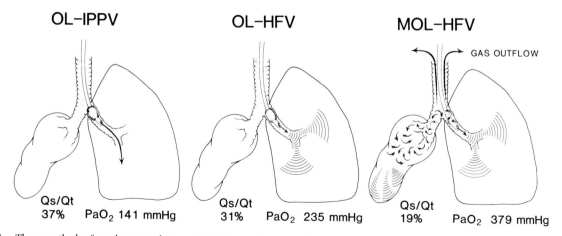

OL–IPPV	OL–HFV	MOL–HFV
		GAS OUTFLOW
Qs/Qt 37% PaO₂ 141 mmHg	Qs/Qt 31% PaO₂ 235 mmHg	Qs/Qt 19% PaO₂ 379 mmHg

Fig. 23–4. Three methods of one-lung ventilation. (OL-IPPV, one-lung intermittent positive pressure ventilation. MOL-HFV, modified one-lung high frequency ventilation. OL-HFV, one-lung high frequency ventilation.) Deflation of the tube cuff allows for gas exit and partial ventilation of the other lung. MOL-HFV is a differential two-lung ventilation and provides effective oxygenation. The use of these three techniques in the same patients achieved different gas kinetics, PaO₂, and Qs/Qt, as shown under each diagram.

a monitoring device and an alarm system to detect mechanical malfunctions and abnormal airway pressures; (4) jet ventilation precludes the use of inhalation anesthetics, and anesthesia has to be achieved intravenously, which is associated with high incidences of awareness and delayed recovery; and (5) jet ventilation is a medicolegal liability and its use has to be justified. Despite these problems, jet ventilation through a small catheter remains the method of choice for ventilation during anesthesia for airway surgery.

REFERENCES

Carden, E., et al.: A comparison of venturi and side-arm ventilation in anaesthesia for bronchoscopy. Can. Anaesth. Soc. J. 20:569, 1973.

Carlon, G.C., et al.: Clinical experience with high frequency jet ventilation. Crit. Care Med. 9:1, 1981.

Carlon, G.C., and Howland, W.S. (Eds.): High Frequency Ventilation in Intensive Care and During Surgery. New York, Marcel Dekker, Inc., 1985.

Chang, J.L., et al.: Unilateral pneumothorax following jet ventilation during general anesthesia. Anesthesiology 53:244, 1980.

Deslauriers, J., et al.: Sleeve pneumonectomy for bronchogenic carcinoma. Ann. Thorac. Surg. 28:465, 1979.

El-Baz, N., et al.: One-lung high frequency ventilation for tracheoplasty and bronchoplasty: a new technique. Ann. Thoracic. Surg. 34:564, 1982a.

El-Baz, N., et al.: One-lung high frequency ventilation through a small uncuffed tube for lung surgery. J. Cardiovasc. Surg. 84:823, 1982b.

El-Baz, N., et al.: High frequency positive pressure ventilation for tracheal reconstruction supported by tracheal T-tube. Anesth. Analg. 61:796, 1982c.

El-Baz, N., et al.: High frequency positive pressure ventilation for major airway surgery. *In* Perspectives in High Frequency Ventilation. Edited by P.A. Scheck, U.H. Sjostrand, and R.B. Smith. Boston, Martinus Nijhoff Publishers, 1983, p. 216.

El-Baz, N., et al.: High frequency ventilation through a small catheter for laser surgery of laryngotracheal and bronchial disorders. Ann. Otol. Rhinol. Laryngol. 94:483, 1985.

Eriksson, I., et al.: High frequency positive pressure ventilation (HFPPV) during transthoracic resection of tracheal stenosis and during preoperative bronchoscopic examination. Acata Anesthesiol. Scand. 19:13, 1975.

Heijman, K., et al.: High frequency positive pressure ventilation during anaesthesia and routine surgery in man. Acta Anaesthesiol. Scand. 16:176, 1972.

Kittle, C.F. (Ed.): Current Controversies in Thoracic Surgery. Philadelphia, W.B. Saunders Co., 1986, p. 183.

Klain, M., and Smith, R.B.: High frequency percutaneous transtracheal jet ventilation. Crit. Care Med. 5:280, 1977.

Kwok, L., et al.: Jet ventilation of one lung for laser resection of bronchial tumor. Anesth. Analg. 63:957, 1984.

Lee, P., and English, I.C.W.: Management of anaesthesia during tracheal resection. Anaesthesia 29:305, 1974.

Malina, J.R., et al.: Clinical evaluation of high frequency positive pressure ventilation (HFPPV) in patients scheduled for open chest surgery. Anesth. Analg. 60:324, 1981.

O'Sullivan, T.J., and Healy, G.B.: Complications of venturi jet ventilation during microlaryngeal surgery. Arch. Otolaryngol. 94:127, 1985.

Sanders, R.D.: Two ventilating attachments for bronchoscopes. Del. Med. J. 39:170, 1967.

Seki, S., et al.: Facilitation of intrathoracic operations by means of high frequency ventilation. J. Cardiovasc. Surg. 86:388, 1983.

Sjostrand, U.: Review of physiological rationale for and development of high frequency positive pressure ventilation (HFPPV). Acta Anaesthesiol. Scand. 64:7, 1977.

Turnbull, A.D., et al.: High frequency jet ventilation in major airway or pulmonary disruption. Ann. Thorac. Surg. 32:468, 1981.

Vourc'h, G., et al.: Manual jet ventilation. V. High frequency ventilation during laser resection of tracheobroncheal lesions. Br. J. Anaesth. 55:973, 1983.

CHAPTER 24

ANESTHESIA FOR PEDIATRIC THORACIC SURGERY

Babette J. Horn and Frank L. Sealeny

Conditions requiring thoracic surgery may affect children of any age. Anesthetic considerations in the older child and adolescent are similar to those in the adult patient. It is in the newborn that the pediatric anesthesiologist encounters the greatest challenge. Besides the technical problems created by the newborn's small size, unique anatomic, physiologic, and pharmacologic differences makes neonatal anesthesia a field unto itself.

PHYSIOLOGIC CONSIDERATIONS IN THE NEONATE

Cardiovascular Adaptation

The cardiovascular system undergoes several changes during the transition to extrauterine life. Closure of the ductus venosus and foramen ovale convert the circulatory system from a parallel circuit to a series circuit (Figs. 24–1, 24–2, and 24–3). Hypoxia, hypercarbia, sepsis, and hypothermia can cause undesirable right-to-left shunting of blood through the foramen ovale and ductus arteriosus, whose anatomic closure may not be complete until 2 weeks after birth. Pulmonary resistance, elevated during fetal life and immediately after birth, falls rapidly at first and attains adult values by 2 months of age (Fig. 24–4). During this time, however, the pulmonary vascular resistance is labile, and marked constriction and dilatation can result from physiologic, pharmacologic, and environmental manipulations. The syndrome of persistent pulmonary hypertension of the newborn—PPHN—characterized by refractory hypoxemia, hypercarbia, and acidosis, is common in patients with diaphragmatic hernias but can occur in virtually any stressed term infant.

Because it must work against increased resistance in utero, the right ventricle is hypertrophied and dominant in the newborn. Waugh and Johnson (1984) reported that both ventricles are noncompliant; their myocardial tissue has 30% fewer contractile elements than the adult's has.

Increases in preload cannot increase stroke volume because of the diminished contractility of the newborn myocardium (Fig. 24–5). Thornberg and Morton's (1983) study suggested that the infant is functioning on an unfavorable portion of the Starling curve, where only a modest rise in filling pressure can precipitate congestive heart failure. The anesthesiologist must scrupulously avoid overzealous administration of intravenous fluids.

The newborn's cardiac output, 180 to 240 cc/kg/min, is two to three times the adult value relative to size. This reflects the greater oxygen consumption and metabolic rate in this age group. Increases in cardiac output are achieved primarily by increases in heart rate—normal 120 to 160 bpm—because the infant's myocardial contractility is relatively fixed. Sympathetic innervation of the heart is incomplete, as Zaritsky and Chernow (1984) noted, further impairing the ability to increase stroke volume. Systemic blood pressure is low in the newborn period (Table 24–1). Awareness of normal values is essential for the appropriate diagnosis and treatment of hypotension.

Respiratory Adaptation

Sarnaik and Preston (1982) reported the anatomic, mechanical, and functional peculiarities of the newborn's respiratory system that increase the risk of arterial desaturation and hypoxemia. The trachea has an incompletely developed cartilaginous framework. Any extrathoracic obstruction, such as postextubation mucosal edema, causes tracheal collapse distally. Even a 1-mm ring of tracheal narrowing can cause severe respiratory distress because of the already small airway caliber (Fig. 24–6).

The infant has a highly compliant chest wall because of a horizontally oriented rib cage. In diseases of poor lung compliance—pulmonary edema, atelectasis—excessive lung recoil results in greater retraction of the soft chest wall and more loss of functional residual capacity

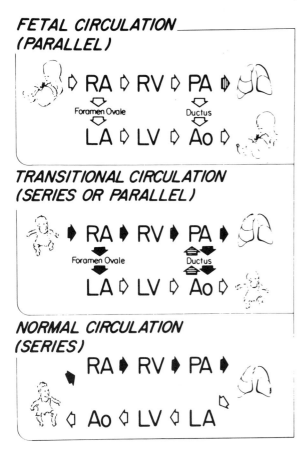

Fig. 24–1. Schematic representation of course of circulation during transition from fetal type circulatory pattern to adult type circulatory pattern. (Reproduced with permission from Ryan, J.F., et al. (Eds.): A Practice of Anesthesia for Infants and Children. Orlando, FL, Grune & Stratton, 1986, p. 176.)

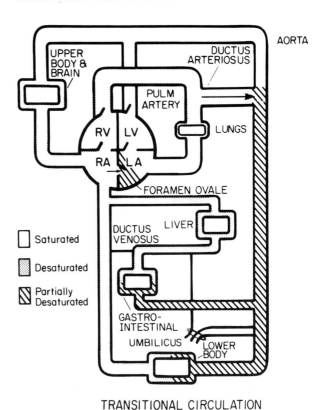

Fig. 24–2. Schematic diagram of transitional circulation of the neonate when pulmonary vascular resistance is high. Desaturated blood is shunted from the right atrium (RA) across the foramen ovale to partially desaturate the left atrial (LA) blood. (Reproduced with permission from Ryan, J.F., et al. (Eds): A Practice of Anesthesia for Infants and Children. Orlando, FL, Grune & Stratton, 1986, p. 117.)

than would occur in older children with stiffer chest walls.

In the supine position, the newborn's closing capacity impinges on tidal volume breathing. The resulting small airway collapse leads to atelectasis, ventilation/perfusion mismatch, and hypoxia. To prevent this from occurring intraoperatively, the anesthesiologist can use controlled ventilation and positive end-expiratory pressure—PEEP.

Because of their high oxygen consumption and increased work of breathing, infants breathe at rapid rates—30 to 50 breaths per minute. Cook (1981) reported that infants' diaphragms have a preponderance of fast-twitch muscle fibers that are prone to early fatigue. Conditions causing increased work of breathing are therefore not tolerated for long periods of time, and hypercarbia and respiratory failure occur.

Chemical and neural control of breathing are different in the newborn. The response to hypoxia is paradoxic, characterized by a brief period of hyperpnea, followed by apnea. The central chemoreceptors have a diminished sensitivity to PCO_2 compared with an adult's, i.e., a higher PCO_2 is needed to effect a similar increase in minute ventilation. Periodic breathing and apneic spells are common in the newborn, making close monitoring of respiratory function mandatory in the postoperative period.

Oxygen unloading at the tissue level is made more difficult by the high percentage of fetal hemoglobin in newborn erythrocytes. Because of its lower P_{50}, hemoglobin F "holds on" to oxygen more tenaciously than does adult hemoglobin. The generally high hemoglobin concentrations at birth—15 to 18 g/dl—is beneficial in increasing oxygen delivery to the cells (Fig. 24–7).

Metabolic Adaptation

Maintenance of normothermia is essential in the newborn. Adverse effects of hypothermia include apnea, hypoglycemia, metabolic acidosis, and increased oxygen consumption. Because of decreased subcutaneous tissue, a low surface area/volume ratio, and small body mass, the neonate has increased environmental heat losses. Nonshivering thermogenesis, mediated by catecholamine effects on brown fat deposits, is the primary heat-generating process in the newborn. This process increases oxygen consumption by as much as two hundred-fold. Methods of preventing heat loss intraoperatively include increasing ambient temperature and use of radiant warmers, heating blankets, and intravenous

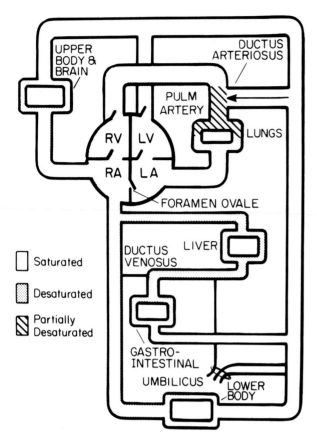

TRANSITIONAL CIRCULATION
LOW PULMONARY VASCULAR RESISTANCE

Fig. 24–3. Schematic diagram of the transitional circulation of the neonate when the pulmonary vascular resistance has fallen. Foramen ovale is closed and no intracardiac shunting can occur at that point. Left-to-right shunting of fully saturated blood from the aorta across the patent ductus arteriosus into the pulmonary artery arterializes blood flowing to the lungs. (Reproduced with permission from Ryan, J.F., et al. (Eds): A Practice of Anesthesia for Infants and Children. Orlando, FL, Grune & Stratton, 1986, p. 178.)

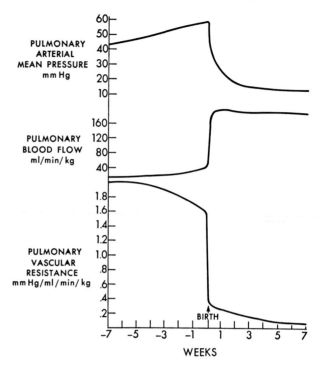

Fig. 24–4. The changes in pulmonary vascular resistance during the 7 weeks preceding birth, at birth, and in the 7 weeks postnatally. Prenatal data derived from lambs. (Reproduced with permission from Rudolph, A.M.: Congenital Diseases of the Heart. © 1974 by Year Book Medical Publishers, Inc., Chicago, p. 31.)

fluid warmers. Baumgart and associates (1987) showed that covering the head and extremities with plastic wrap effectively minimizes evaporative heat losses during surgery.

Hypoglycemia occurs frequently in this age group, especially in the premature, in the small-for-gestational-age infant, or in the infant of the diabetic mother. Causative factors in the development of neonatal hypoglycemia include diminished hepatic glycogen stores, decreased gluconeogenetic capabilities, and decreased response to glucagon secretion. Blood glucose values should be monitored frequently, and the intravenous dextrose concentration adjusted accordingly. Normal blood glucose values in the newborn are listed in Table 24–2.

PHARMACOLOGIC CONSIDERATIONS IN THE NEONATE

Virtually all drugs used in the practice of adult anesthesia have been safely used in pediatric anesthesia. Be-

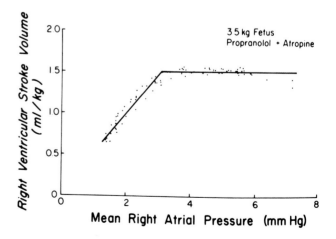

Fig. 24–5. Right ventricular stroke volume and right atrial pressure relationships in a sheep fetus. (Reproduced with permission from Ryan, J.F., et al. (Eds): A Practice of Anesthesia for Infants and Children. Orlando, FL, Grune & Stratton, 1986, p. 180.)

Table 24–1. The Relationship of Age to Blood Pressure

Age	Normal Blood Pressure (mm Hg)	
	Mean Systolic	Mean Diastolic
0–12 hour (Preterm)	50	35
0–12 hour (Full-term)	65	45
4 days	75	50
6 weeks	95	55
1 year	95	60
2 years	100	65
9 years	105	70
12 years	115	75

cause of the physiologic characteristics of the newborn, however, drug dosages must be altered and target organ responses carefully monitored.

Muscle relaxants such as succinylcholine and pancuronium supplement almost all newborn anesthetics. Goudsouzian (1986) noted that infants require a larger dose of succinylcholine calculated on a per kilogram basis because of their increased extracellular fluid compartment. Goudsouzian (1980) also pointed out that the newborn diaphragm fatigues easily, necessitating careful dosing of pancuronium.

Inhalation anesthetics such as nitrous oxide, halothane, and isoflurane are frequently used in pediatric thoracic surgery cases. Brett (1987), Friesen (1986), and Schieber (1986) and their associates reported that all these agents cause dose-dependent depression of cardiac function and Wear (1982) and Duncan (1987) and their colleagues noted that their use impaired baroreceptor

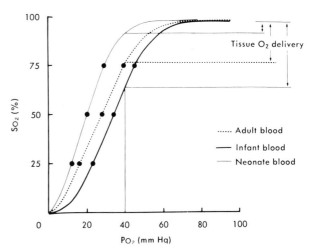

Fig. 24–7. Schematic representation of oxygen-hemoglobin dissociation curves with different oxygen affinities. In neonates with a lower P_{50} (20 mm Hg) and higher oxygen affinity, tissue oxygen unloading at the same tissue PO_2 is reduced. (Reproduced with permission from Motoyama, E.K., Cook, D.R.: Respiratory physiology. *In* Smith, R.M. (ed.): Anesthesia for Infants and Children. St. Louis, C.V. Mosby Co., 1980, p. 67.)

reflexes. Hypotension and bradycardia commonly occur when the potent inhalation agents are administered in high concentrations. Because halothane has a low therapeutic index in infants it must be used sparingly, with close attention paid to blood pressure and heart rate. Waugh and Johnson (1984) and Eisele and associates (1986) reported that nitrous oxide can increase pulmonary vascular resistance, which in theory is undesirable in neonates with the potential to develop persistent pulmonary hypertension of the newborn. Clinical studies reported by Hickey and co-workers (1986), however, have shown that nitrous oxide can be used in infants without significant increase in right-to-left shunting.

Fentanyl, a synthetic short-acting potent narcotic, has been used extensively in neonatal anesthesia. Hickey and associates (1985) noted that its popularity lies in its ability to attenuate the pulmonary vasoconstrictive response to tracheal stimulation. Schieber and colleagues (1985) and Robinson and Gregory (1981) reported that cardiovascular stability occurs with fentanyl analgesia as well. Administration of greater than 5 μg/kg of fentanyl, a modest dose, usually precludes tracheal extubation at the conclusion of surgery, because this agent is a potent respiratory depressant. The newer narcotics sufentanil and alfentanil have not yet been extensively evaluated in neonates, but appear equipotent to fentanyl in their respiratory depressant properties.

Barbiturates such as thiopental can be used as induction agents in newborns, but low doses should be used— 2 to 3 mg/kg. Both immaturity of the blood-brain barrier

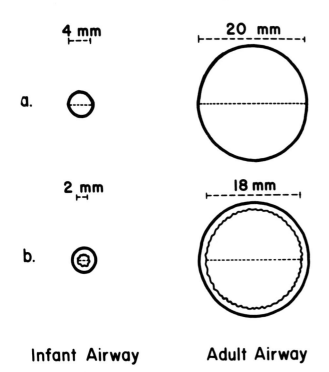

Fig. 24–6. Diagram of relative cross-sectional area of infant and adult trachea: (a) no tracheal edema, (b) 1 mm of edema encircling tracheal lumen.

Table 24–2. Normal Blood Glucose Values

Age	Blood Glucose (mg%)
Newborn (premature)	>30
Newborn (term)	>40
Adult	60–100

and a relatively high cerebral blood flow combine to deliver a large fraction of the injected drug to the brain, thus allowing a lower dose to be used with equal efficacy. In addition, the barbiturates are myocardial depressants, and unacceptable degrees of hypotension may result from use of larger doses.

Ketamine is a potent amnesic and analgesic agent that can be given intravenously—1 to 2 mg/kg— or intramuscularly—5 mg/kg—for the induction of general anesthesia. White and co-workers (1982) noted cardiovascular hemodynamics and spontaneous respirations are maintained because of sympathetic nervous system stimulation, accounting for the drug's popularity in pediatric anesthesia. Ketamine causes copious salivation, so prior or concurrent administration of an antisialogogue—atropine 20 μg/kg IM or 10 μg/kg IV—is necessary.

Atropine enjoys widespread use in pediatric anesthesia because of its anticholinergic properties. In the aforementioned dose range mentioned, it counteracts undesirable bradycardia associated with halothane and succinylcholine administration, vagal stimulation during laryngoscopy, and intraoperative visceral traction. Slow heart rates can lead to a drop in cardiac output because the newborn cannot compensate by increasing his stroke volume.

MONITORING

The purpose of monitoring any variable during surgery is to identify adverse trends before they become catastrophic events. Because of their diminished cardiopulmonary and metabolic reserves, infants require close intraoperative monitoring. Confounding the goal of vigilant invasive and noninvasive monitoring is the infant's small size, which can make even the simplest of procedures, such as applying electrocardiogram leads frustrating.

Standard Monitors

The following monitors are considered "standard of care" in pediatric anesthesia.

Temperature Probe. Rectal or esophageal temperatures most closely approximate core temperature, and are preferred over skin and axillary monitoring sites.

Electrocardiogram. Cardiac rate and rhythm are the primary data obtained from this monitor. Ischemia detection is not as important in this age group because coronary artery disease is uncommon. Smaller electrodes are available for placement on the trunk, as well as limb leads designed for use around the wrists and ankles.

Precordial or Esophageal Stethoscope. The thin chest wall of infants permits auscultation of both heart and breath sounds with a precordial stethoscope. According to Smith (1980) this is probably the most useful and important monitor in pediatric anesthesia.

Blood Pressure Cuff. Sizes to fit even the premature infant are now available. Usually the arm is not big enough to permit placement of a stethoscope, so only the systolic blood pressure is measured by looking for the "to-and-fro" movement of the sphygmomanometer needle.

Oxygen Analyzer. Inserted in the inspiratory limb of the anesthesia circuit. The American Academy of Pediatrics (1983), in its guidelines for perinatal care, and Lucey and Dangman (1984) emphasized that inspired oxygen concentrations must be carefully measured, because prolonged hyperoxia can lead to retinopathy in the infant whose postconceptual age is less than 46 weeks, in whom the retina has not completely matured.

Additional Monitors

Additional sophisticated monitoring devices are frequently used during pediatric thoracic surgery.

Indwelling Arterial Pressure Line. This is an invaluable intraoperative aid. Beat-to-beat display of the blood pressure facilitates early detection of hypotension, which can result from hypovolemia or decreased venous return secondary to great vessel compression. Samples for blood gas, hemoglobin, and glucose analyses are easily obtained from an indwelling arterial catheter. Several sites for cannulation exist, each with its own advantages and drawbacks. The right radial artery provides access to preductal blood, but insertion of even a 22-gauge catheter may be technically difficult in a newborn. Umbilical artery catheterization is relatively easy in the first 24 hours of life but carries with it the risks of lower extremity vasospasm and embolization of particulate matter to other major arterial vessels.

Doppler Ultrasonic Flow Detector. The Doppler device provides auscultatory confirmation of systolic pressures when placed over the radial or brachial artery and used in conjunction with a blood pressure cuff. Whyte and associates (1975) reported excellent agreement between Doppler readings and transduced blood pressure values.

Pulse Oximeter. The use of this monitor will almost certainly become "standard of care" in the operating room. It provides a continuous, real-time estimate of arterial oxygen saturation. The oxisensor is applied around a digit in the adult, and around a hand or foot in the infant. Light of a specific wavelength is transmitted through the skin and is absorbed by the hemoglobin in erythrocytes flowing in arterial vessels. Barker and Tremper (1987) reviewed the use of pulse oximetry. Oxy- and deoxyhemoglobins have different absorption patterns, and the oximeter detects the ratio of light absorption by these two substances and translates it into a saturation reading. In our hospital, use of the pulse oximeter during operations on newborns has resulted in fewer arterial cannulations and a decreased frequency of arterial blood gas sampling. With oximetry, Bautista and associates (1986) documented early detection of hypoxemia—and presumed improved patient care—in newborns having trachoesophageal fistula repair.

SPECIFIC PROBLEMS REQUIRING THORACOTOMY IN THE NEWBORN

Congenital Diaphragmatic Hernia

Although repair of a congenital diaphragmatic hernia is not accomplished via thoracotomy (see Chapter 53), it is included in any discussion of neonatal thoracic surgical emergencies. A substantial body of literature exists dealing with the many controversial aspects of this condition. Bohn and associates (1984, 1987) discussed the predictors of survival, Levin (1987) the timing of surgery, and Fox (1983), Ein (1980) and Drummond (1981) and their associates the operative pharmacologic and ventilatory strategies. Close examination of these reports fails to show any relationship between anesthetic agents used and survival. Both inhalation—halothane, isoflurane—and intravenous—fentanyl—analgesia, supplemented with muscle relaxants, have been used successfully for repair of these hernias. Nitrous oxide is avoided because it causes bowel distention and may necessitate use of 100% oxygen.

More important than the choice of anesthetic drugs is the preoperative and intraoperative airway management. Endotracheal intubation should be preceded by oxygenation with a bag and mask. Positive pressure ventilation is contraindicated because of the risk of increasing the infant's respiratory distress by distending the intrathoracic bowel. Once an artificial airway is established, vigorous hyperventilation—$PaCO_2$ 25 to 30 mm Hg—can be instituted. We prefer to use a high frequency infant ventilator brought to the operating room from the newborn ICU. Preductal blood gas tensions are measured and the ventilator settings adjusted accordingly. Only if preductal PaO_2 values exceed 100 mm Hg do we lower the inspirated FIO_2, and then only by increments of 2%. Vasoactive drug infusions such as dopamine or tolazoline are prepared preoperatively should their administration be necessary during operation. Because postoperative mechanical ventilation is the rule, the infant is transported from the operating room to the nursery with the endotracheal tube in place.

Tracheoesophageal Fistula

Three important problems must be addressed during the anesthetic evaluation of the infant born with a tracheoesophageal fistula. (1) Is the patient premature, and if so, is there evidence of hyaline membrane disease? (2) Are there coexisting cardiac or gastrointestinal malformations—VATER association*? (3) Is aspiration pneumonitis present?

The presence of any or all of these conditions may make intraoperative ventilatory management even more difficult than it usually is.

In addition to a complete blood count, a roentgenogram of the chest is a mandatory preoperative examination. The lung fields are examined closely, looking for infiltrates suggestive of aspiration pneumonia, or air bronchograms and reticular granular densities associated with hyaline membrane disease. In addition, the cardiac silhouette is inspected to see if cardiomegaly or a right-sided aortic arch is present. Our patients are evaluated

---

*The VATER association is a spectrum of associated anomalies in the newborn. These may consist of varying combinations of vertebral anomalies, anal malformations, tracheoesophageal fistula with esophageal atresia, renal anomalies and radial arm malformations.

by a neonatologist before surgery, and a cardiologist is consulted if evidence of congential heart disease exists.

Following placement of a gastrostomy using local anesthesia, general anesthesia is administered for repair of the tracheoesophageal fistula. The relative merits and drawbacks of various induction techniques are hotly debated by pediatric anesthesiologists. Awake endotracheal intubation has the advantage of maintaining spontaneous breathing. Should intubation prove difficult or impossible, the patient will still be able to ventilate spontaneously, and, it is hoped, will not become hypoxic. In the vigorous term infant, however, awake intubation can be difficult to perform. Other critics contend that the procedure is inhumane and that some anesthesia should be provided before manipulating the airway. Many advocate an intravenous rapid-sequence induction using muscle relaxants. Ideal intubating conditions exist because the patient is paralyzed. Should the endotracheal tube enter the fistula, however, oxygenation and ventilation will be impossible. Buchino and associates (1986) reported severe respiratory compromise and death from persistent wedging of the endotracheal tube in the fistula. A Storz pediatric bronchoscope can be passed through the endotracheal tube to verify proper placement. Proper tube placement is above the carina and below the fistula, a distance of only several millimeters in most patients. Deliberate endobronchial intubation—verified by loss of breath sounds over the left hemithorax—is done, following which the tube is withdrawn until bilateral breath sounds are detected. If the gastrostomy tube is placed under water and bubbles with respiration, then the tube lies above the fistula and has been withdrawn too far.

Maintenance of anesthesia is achieved with either low dose inhalational agents or intravenous narcotics. Intraoperative problems include hypotension from great vessel compression, hypoxia, and hypercarbia from lung retraction in the lateral position, and endotracheal tube obstruction from clotted blood. In the otherwise healthy term newborn without preoperative cardiopulmonary problems, extubation is usually possible at the conclusion of surgery. Premature infants, infants with serious associated anomalies, and those whose intraoperative courses have been complicated are usually brought back to the high risk nursery with the endotracheal tube still in place.

Congenital Lobar Emphysema

Although infants with congenital lobar emphysema—CLE—may develop respiratory distress immediately after birth, most children are diagnosed after 1 month of age. Tachypnea, cyanosis, and diminished breath sounds over the affected side are the usual presenting symptoms and signs. The degree of respiratory distress is occasionally so severe that endotracheal intubation is performed before arrival in the operating room. Regardless of where the intubation is done, it is important to begin any airway manipulation with several minutes of preoxygenation with bag and mask. Positive pressure ventilation further distends the hyperinflated lobe and should be avoided if at all possible.

Thoracotomy for removal of the emphysematous lobe is the usual surgical management of this problem. If the cardiopulmonary status allows, anesthesia is induced by having the infant breathe a mixture of halothane in 100% oxygen. Nitrous oxide and positive pressure ventilation are avoided to prevent further increases in size of the affected lobe. Clinically unstable or rapidly deteriorating infants are best managed by emergent awake intubation. If possible, anesthesia is maintained with halothane, oxygen, and spontaneous ventilation. Arterial blood gas analysis, however, often shows progressive hypoventilation and respiratory acidosis after the patient is placed in lateral position. In this case, it may be necessary to provide gentle manual positive pressure until the chest is opened and compression of the good lung relieved. At this point, pulmonary status improves markedly. Following lobectomy, most infants show complete return to normal of the arterial blood gases. Tracheal extubation at the conclusion of surgery is routine. Goto and associates (1987) stated that there may be a role for high-frequency jet ventilation in the intraoperative management of patients with congenital lobar emphysema.

REFERENCES

American Academy of Pediatrics and American College of Obstetrics and Gynecology: Guidelines for Perinatal Care. Evanston, IL, 1983, pp. 212–213.

Barker, S.J., and Tremper, K.K.: Pulse oximetry: applications and limitations. Int. Anesthesiol. Clin. 25:155, 1987.

Baumgart, S., et al.: Effect of heat shielding on convective and evaporative heat losses and on radiant heat transfer in the premature infant. J. Pediatr. 99:948, 1981.

Bautista, M.J., Kuwahara, B.S., and Henderson, C.U.: Transcutaneous oxygen monitoring in an infant undergoing tracheoesophageal fistula repair. Can. Anaesth. Soc. J. 33:505, 1986.

Bohn, D.J., James, I., and Filler, R.M.: The relationship between Pa_{CO_2} and ventilation parameters in predicting survival in congenital diaphragmatic hernia. J. Pediatr. Surg. 19:666, 1984.

Bohn, D., et al.: Ventilatory predictors of pulmonary hypoplasia in congenital diaphragmatic hernia, confirmed by morphologic assessment. J. Pediatr. 111:432, 1987.

Brett, C.M., et al.: The cardiovascular effects of isoflurane in lambs. Anesthesiology 67:60, 1987.

Buchino, J.J., et al.: Malpositioning of the endotracheal tube in infants with tracheoesophageal fistula. J. Pediatr. 109:524, 1986.

Cook, D.R.: Muscle relaxants in infants and children. Anesth. Analg. 60:335, 1981.

Drummond, W.H., et al.: The independent effects of hyperventilation, tolazoline, and dopamine on infants with persistent pulmonary hypertension. J. Pediatr. 98:603, 1981.

Duncan, P.G., Gregory, G.B., and Wade, J.G.: The effect of nitrous oxide on baroreceptor function in newborn and adult rabbits. Can. Anaesth. Soc. J. 28:339, 1987.

Ein, S.H., et al.: The pharmacologic treatment of newborn congenital diaphragmatic hernia—a 2-year evaluation. J. Pediatr. Surg. 15:384, 1980.

Eisele, J.H., Milstein, J.M., and Goetzmann, B.W.: Pulmonary vascular responses to nitrous oxide in newborn lambs. Anesth. Analg. 65:62, 1986.

Fox, W.W., and Duara, S.: Persistent pulmonary hypertension in the neonate: diagnosis and management. J. Pediatr. 103:505, 1983.

Friesen, R.H., and Henry, D.B.: Cardiovascular changes in preterm neonates recieving isoflurane, halothane, fentanyl and ketamine. Anesthesiology 64:238, 1986.

Goto, H., et al.: High-frequency jet ventilation for resection of congenital lobar emphysema. Anesth. Analg. 66:684, 1987.

Goudsouzian, N.G.: Maturation of neuromuscular transmission in the infant. Br. J. Anaesth. 52:205, 1980.

Goudsouzian, N.G.: Muscle relaxants in children. *In* A Practice of Anesthesia for Infants and Children. Edited by J.F. Ryan, et al.: Orlando, FL, Grune & Stratton, 1986, pp. 108–109.

Hickey, P.R., et al.: Blunting of stress responses in the pulmonary circulation of infants by fentanyl. Anesth. Analg. 64:1137, 1985.

Hickey, P.R., et al.: Pulmonary and systemic hemodynamic effects of nitrous oxide in infants with normal and elevated pulmonary vascular resistance. Anesthesiology 65:374, 1986.

Levin, D.L.: Congenital diaphragmatic hernia: a persistent problem. J. Pediatr. 111:390, 1987.

Lucey, J.F., and Dangman, B.: A re-examination of the role of oxygen in retrolental fibroplasia. Pediatrics 73:82, 1984.

Robinson, S., and Gregory, G.B.: Fentanyl-air-oxygen anesthesia for ligation of patient ductus arteriosus in preterm infants. Anesth. Analg. 60:331, 1981.

Sarnaik, B.P., and Preston, G.: Physiologic peculiarities of the respiratory system in neonates. Anesth. Rev. 9:31, 1982.

Schieber, R.B., Stiller, R.L., and Cook, D.R.: Cardiovascular and pharmacodynamic effects of high-dose fentanyl in newborn piglets. Anesthesiology 63:166, 1985.

Schieber, R.B., et al.: Hemodynamic effects of isoflurane in the newborn piglet: comparisons with halothane. Anesth. Analg. 65:633, 1986.

Smith, R.M.: Anesthesia for Infants and Children, 4th ed. St. Louis, C.V. Mosby Co., 1980, pp. 192–215.

Thornburg, K.L., and Morton, M.J.: Filling and arterial pressure as determinants of RV stroke volume in the sheep fetus. Am. J. Physiol. 244:H656, 1983.

Waugh, R., and Johnson, G.G.: Current considerations in neonatal anesthesia. Can. Anaesth. Soc. J. 31:700, 1984.

Wear, R., Robinson, S., and Gregory, G.B.: The effect of halothane on the baroresponses of adult and baby rabbits. Anesthesiology 56:188, 1982.

White, P.F., Way, W.L., and Trevor, B.J.: Ketamine: its pharmacology and therapeutic uses. Anesthesiology 56:119, 1982.

Whyte, R.K., et al.: Assessment of Doppler ultrasound to measure systolic and diastolic pressures in infants and young children. Arch. Dis. Child. 50:542, 1975

Zaritsky, B., and Chernow, B.: Use of catecholamines in pediatrics. J. Pediatr. 105:341, 1984.

Postoperative Management

CHAPTER 25

GENERAL PRINCIPLES OF POSTOPERATIVE CARE

Renee S. Hartz

The complexity and sophistication of perioperative care make thoracic surgery a uniquely challenging specialty. Surgeons must not only be thoroughly familiar with cardiac and respiratory physiology but also well-versed in current techniques of anesthetic management and intensive care technology.

Perioperative care of the thoracic surgical patient generally falls into one of four categories: (1) care of the cardiovascular system, (2) care of the respiratory system, (3) control of postoperative pain, and (4) drainage and obliteration of the pleural space.

CARE OF THE CARDIOVASCULAR SYSTEM

Ischemic Heart Disease

Arrhythmia, myocardial infarction, and heart failure are common complications during and after operations on the chest, any of which may potentially lead to the death of the patient. The incidence of these complications increases in older patients, who have a higher incidence of pre-existing cardiovascular and respiratory disease and are now candidates for thoracotomy.

The most important factor in determining the presence of silent cardiovascular disease is a high index of suspicion during the preoperative evaluation. Few patients volunteer a history of angina pectoris, and each must be questioned to determine whether he has symptoms that suggest ischemic heart disease. Whether or not the history is positive, the preoperative electrocardiogram may yield useful information. Patients with a history that suggests ischemia and those with electrocardiographic evidence of old infarction or ongoing ischemia should undergo exercise or thallium stress testing. If the stress test is positive, the patient should undergo cardiac catheterization and coronary arteriography before undergoing thoracotomy. An occasional patient requires myocardial revascularization. Since the introduction of balloon coronary angioplasty, it has been possible to relieve the ischemia with a less invasive procedure than coronary bypass.

In no instance should a patient with large areas of ischemic myocardium undergo elective thoracotomy, though select patients with chronic stage angina who have limited areas of ischemia may undergo thoracotomy without excessive risk. All high risk patients should be anesthetized by skilled anesthesiologists with full knowledge of hemodynamic monitoring. An arterial line and a Swan-Ganz catheter should be placed before the induction of anesthesia so that episodes of hypotension and hypertension can be quickly detected and corrected and cardiac filling pressures closely monitored. During the procedure, nitroglycerin should be administered intravenously and inotropic agents should be available. Ideally, such high risk patients should be operated on in institutions where an intra-aortic balloon pump is available and acute infarct intervention is practiced.

Myocardial Infarction

Arkins (1964), Driscoll (1961), and Tarhan (1972) and their associates estimated that 0.2 to 3.0% of patients undergoing thoracic surgical procedures sustain a myocardial infarction, and another 5 to 10% exhibit electrocardiographic changes. Obviously, the older the patient, the greater the likelihood of sustaining an infarct. Following perioperative infarction, the patient's prognosis may be serious. In a large Mayo Clinic series, published by Tarhan and colleagues (1978), only 0.13% of patients without a history of infarction suffered a perioperative infarct. In a classic study performed later at the same institution, however, Steen and co-workers (1978) reported that of 587 patients with a history of myocardial infarction who had anesthesia and surgery, 6.1% reinfarcted, and of those patients 69% died! When patients were operated on within three months of their previous infarction, 27% reinfarcted. Thus, determining not only whether but when a previous myocardial infarction occurred is crucially important.

Arrhythmia

According to Beck-Nielsen and associates (1973), arrhythmias occur in approximately 20% of noncardiac thoracic operations. The incidence increases with the patient's age and the magnitude of the procedure, especially with intrapericardial ligation of the pulmonary vessels, and is higher after pneumonectomy than after lobectomy. Such rhythm disturbances contribute significantly to mortality rates: Shields and Ujiki (1968), for example, noted a 14% mortality rate in patients with postoperative arrhythmia, compared to a 4% mortality rate in its abscence. Commonly occurring arrhythmias are sinus bradycardia, premature ventricular contractions—PVCs, junctional rhythm, and atrial fibrillation and flutter. As a rule, bradycardias are more difficult to treat than tachycardias. Whenever a patient develops postoperative rhythm disturbances, hypokalemia or arterial hypoxemia should be suspected; many arrhythmias are remedied simply by correcting these abnormalities. PVCs are ominous and should be aggressively treated with antiarrhythmic drugs even while waiting for laboratory values. Supraventricular rhythm disturbances such as atrial fibrillation, atrial flutter, and paroxysmal supraventricular tachycardia are common and are usually controlled with digitalis or with antiarrhythmic agents such as verapamil. The thoracic surgeon should be familiar with the dosages and adverse effects of all available antiarrhythmic agents and know how to institute temporary pacing for the treatment of bradycardia.

The issue of preoperative digitalis administration deserves consideration. Although the topic is controversial and the studies are not randomized, Shields and Ujiki (1968), Burman (1972), and Wheat and Buford (1961) noted that preoperative digitalis reduces the incidence of these complications. Some authors, such as Ellison (1979), have written that digitalis should be administered slowly over several days before the procedure and excluded when it is not considered until the night before surgery. Others, including Shields and Ujiki (1968), have written that digitalis is important enough to be administered the night before surgery, especially to patients over sixty years old and to those for whom pneumonectomy is a possibility.

Heart Failure

Heart failure is unusual in the absence of pre-existing heart disease but may occur with overzealous fluid administration. If intravascular volume overload develops, the surgeon should resort immediately to the use of the Swan-Ganz catheter to monitor the reduction of the fluid overload. Management of the heart failure per se should not be difficult for any thoracic surgeon. Kaplan (1983) developed a useful table to direct the treatment of heart failure appropriately (Fig. 25–1). An early and aggressive approach to such treatment should be kept in mind; when heart failure develops, the presence of ischemic heart disease should be considered and myocardial infarction ruled out with appropriate laboratory examinations and serial electrocardiograms.

Comment

The surgeon should maintain an aggressive approach to the diagnosis and treatment of underlying heart dis-

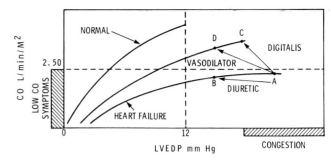

Fig. 25–1. Curves represent normal Frank-Starling mechanism, and therapeutic interventions are indicated when patients' hemodynamics fall outside the normal range. (Reprinted by permission from Churchill Livingstone from Kaplan, J.A., (Ed.): Complications of Thoracic Surgery. *In* Thoracic Anesthesia. New York, Churchill Livingstone, 1983, as modified by Mason, D.T.: Congestive Heart Failure: Mechanisms, Evaluation and Treatment. With permission of Yorke Medical Books, Technical Publishing, a division of Dun-Donnelly Publishing Corporation, a company of Dun & Bradstreet Corporation, 1976.)

ease before thoracotomy. The patients in our institution with suspected or proven ischemic heart disease who are to undergo thoracotomy are anesthetized with full monitoring—arterial lines, Swan-Ganz catheter, Foley catheter—and special attention is directed to minimizing myocardial oxygen consumption. Cardiac filling pressures, including central venous pressure and pulmonary capillary wedge pressure, are repeatedly measured, cardiac output determined, and peripheral vascular resistance calculated. To decrease myocardial oxygen demand, hypertension is avoided and the peripheral vascular resistance is maintained as near normal as possible. Nitroglycerin is administered continuously, and volume is given as needed to maintain the optimal filling pressures for that particular patient. The monitoring lines are kept in place for at least 24 hours postoperatively to facilitate patient management.

Routinely employing pacing wire in postoperative thoracotomy patients is not appropriate. Should bradycardia develop in the postoperative period, pacing can be instituted using the pacing port of a Swan-Ganz catheter. Digitalis should be given before major pulmonary resections, especially to patients over 60 years old. The benefits of digitalis administration far exceed its risks. If the patient is not on digitalis therapy, 0.5 to 1.0 mg of digoxin is administered in the 12 to 24-hour period before surgery. This dose of digoxin should not produce toxicity in a patient with normal renal function and greatly facilitates the management of postoperative supraventricular rhythm disturbances when they occur.

CARE OF THE RESPIRATORY SYSTEM

Before undertaking a pulmonary resection, the surgeon must be as confident as possible that the patient's pulmonary reserves are sufficient to tolerate the thoracotomy incision and the loss of lung volume. Once the surgeon has determined that the patient should tolerate the procedure (Table 25–1), the extent of pre-existing pulmonary disease and the extent of the resection dictate

Table 25–1. Pulmonary Function Test Criteria for Resection

Test	Unit	Normal	Pneumonectomy	Lobectomy	Biopsy or Segmental
MBC	Liters/min	>100	>70	40–70	40
MBC	Percent predicted		>55	40–70	35–40
FEV_1	Liters	>2	>2	>1	>0.6
FEV_1	Percent predicted		>55	40–70	≧40
FEV_{25-75}	Liters	2	>1.6	0.6–1.6	>0.6

Reprinted from Miller, J.I.: Thoracic surgery. *In* Kaplan, J.A., Thoracic Anesthesia. New York, Churchill Livingstone, 1983, p. 25. By permission of the publisher.

the amount of attention focused on the possibility of postoperative pulmonary complications. Dyspnea, when present, is a predictor of mortality, and its presence mandates full pulmonary function testing and blood gas determinations, as suggested by Meltman (1961). Smokers should be urged to stop smoking for as long as possible before the operation to restore bronchial ciliary action. Patients with chronic bronchitis should receive a suitable period of appropriate antibiotics—based on sputum culture results—before the planned procedure.

Preoperative education of the patient should include techniques of postoperative bronchial hygiene. *The patient must be able to generate an effective cough.* For those who cannot, instruction involves training in breathing techniques. Shapiro and colleagues (1979) recommended that the patient be taught to inspire and hold, forcefully contract the abdominal muscles, and then exhale. They also recommended teaching patients to cuddle a pillow to help their cough effort. Patients should also be taught to use an incentive spirometer during the postoperative period.

Other important factors in the postoperative care of the patient include proper positioning, chest physiotherapy, tracheal suctioning, control of pain, and possible prolonged intubation and ventilation. The role of intermittent positive pressure breathing—IPPB—remains controversial and transcatheter intratracheal injection of irritating solutions is practiced sporadically.

Proper positioning of the patient includes using gravity to assist in keeping the diaphragm depressed, the airways open, and pain at a minimum. Postural drainage is used in conjunction with positioning to assist the mucociliary action with gravity and is often accompanied with chest vibrations and percussion (Chapter 27). Tracheal suctioning should be integral to the care of any patient who is not able to mobilize secretions spontaneously. The managing physicians and nursing staff should be familiar with tracheal suctioning and use it frequently. If tracheal suctioning does not stimulate effective coughing and clearing of secretions, bronchoscopy may be necessary. Finally, prolonged intubation and ventilation, or reintubation, may be necessary. Many surgeons prefer to extubate thoracotomy patients immediately postoperatively. After long procedures in patients with impaired pulmonary function, abnormal blood gas values, or concomitant cardiac illness, however, mechanical ventilation should be instituted as soon as any signs of respiratory insufficiency develop (Chapter 26).

Atelectasis is always present after thoracotomy and occurs because of a decrease in functional residual capacity. The most significant cause of postoperative morbidity, it is promoted by decreased lung compliance, obstructive secretions in the airways, fluid accumulation within the operated hemithorax, and postoperative pain. Restoration of the FRC by the aforementioned measures should minimize the degree of atelectasis and prevent the development of consolidation in the atelectatic areas of the lung.

Comment

The philosophy is to encourage patient education for postoperative respiratory self-care and the implementation of such care by the thoracic surgery service. Respiratory therapy technicians are consulted liberally to assist in preoperative teaching and to administer postoperative treatments. Patients who are not believed to have pre-existing pulmonary disease can have simple screening pulmonary functions—FEV_1 and FVC—and room air blood gas sampling. Patients with resting or exertional dyspnea should undergo full pulmonary function testing with and without bronchodilators.

Our group uses a simple, inexpensive, incentive spirometer and teaches its use to all patients preoperatively. I believe that blow bottles are not useful and agree with Nunn and colleagues (1965), who present evidence that they may be deleterious. I advocate vigorous nasotracheal suctioning in patients who are not maintaining good bronchial hygiene on their own, and resort early to bedside bronchoscopy. Lastly, our threshold for instituting mechanical ventilation is low, both in the immediate postoperative period and in patients who develop signs of respiratory insufficiency later in their postoperative course.

DRAINAGE AND OBLITERATION OF THE PLEURAL SPACE

The unique physiology of the pleural space, with its normal negative pressure, separates thoracic surgery from other surgical disciplines. *All patients who undergo thoracotomy are left with some degree of pneumothorax and the potential for developing a residual pleural space.* Before closing the chest, the surgeon must seal all air leaks as well as possible. Large-bore thoracostomy tubes readily provide a means of evacuating air, accumulated blood, and other fluids. The types and positioning of tubes to drain the pleural space are myriad and depend on the surgeons' preferences. Both silicone and rubber catheters are commonly used after pulmonary resection and most surgeons use at least two tubes, one for air—placed at the apex of the lung—and one for fluid—placed posteroinferiorly. The pleural space is not drained following pneumonectomy unless excessive bleeding occurs or major fear of infection exists. Efforts are made to adjust the pressure in the operated hemithorax to be slightly negative, thus maintaining the mediastinum in a neutral position. Obliteration of the pleural space is normally accomplished by re-expansion of remaining lung tissue, shift of the mediastinum to the operated side, narrowing of the ipsilateral intercostal spaces, and elevation of the hemidiaphragm. Collections of air or fluid, or decreased compliance in the remaining lung tissue, may prevent the expansion necessary to obliterate the pleural space; adequate pleural drainage is therefore crucial.

Pleural drainage systems must include airtight seals to maintain an intrapleural vacuum, -3 to -5 mm Hg. The simplest form of chest drainage is the underwater seal system, which allows free egress of air and fluid from the intrapleural space. The staff must, however, be thoroughly familiar with the mechanics of the system to prevent catastrophes. The tubes should not normally be clamped—because doing so may result in tension pneumo- or hydrothorax, the fluid level in the water seal bottle must be maintained at all times, and the bottles must be kept below the level of the patient to prevent siphoning of water into the chest.

For those patients with large air leaks, and for those in whom a large amount of fluid must be drained from the chest, most surgeons prefer to maintain continuous negative pressure in the pleural space. The amount of suction is variable but must exceed the intrapleural vacuum developed by the patient during inspiration. When reversal of flow occurs in the tubing during inspiration, the amount of suction is insufficient to provide obliteration of the pleural space. If intermittent bubbling occurs while the patient is on water seal, suction should also be applied.

A widely used commercially available system for draining the pleural space is the Pleur-evac, a compact, nonbreakable, three-bottle chest drainage apparatus (Fig. 25–2). It can be used as a simple underwater seal system or attached to a vacuum line. The amount of suction is limited by the height of the column of water in the vacuum control chamber. The third component of the unit is a compartmentalized collection chamber.

Comment

The Pleur-evac drainage system is most commonly used, except when a large amount of bleeding is suspected, in which case an autotransfusion set-up is used. When more than 25 cm water suction is required to overcome an air leak, I and my associates convert to an Emerson three-bottle suction apparatus or put two centimeters of mercury in the bottom of the vacuum chamber of the Pleur-evac, delivering, in effect, about 50 cm water of suction. The nursing staff should be instructed

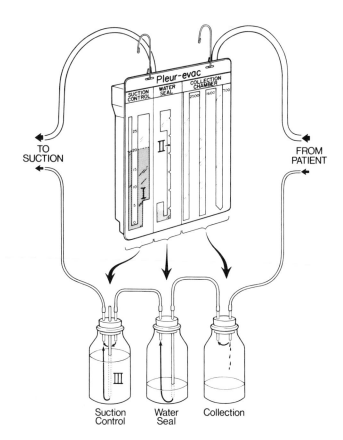

Fig. 25–2. The Pleur-evac is a compartmentalized, commercially available three-bottle suction apparatus. It can be used without suction as a simple water-seal device. The height of the column in the suction control chamber determines the amount of negative pressure applied to the pleural space (I). An additional feature of the Pleur-evac is the ability to measure the amount of negative pressure developed by the patient (II and III).

never to clamp chest tubes, but when a very slow air leak is suspected, tubes are clamped for a few hours with the patient under close supervision. For patient comfort, we place our chest tubes at or inferior to the anterior/superior iliac spine. For patients who are intubated, removal of chest tubes is accomplished using an "inflate and hold" technique. One person delivers a large inspiration to the patient and holds it while a second person removes the chest tube and places the dressing. For patients who are breathing normally when the tubes are removed, they are taught to inspire and hold or to breathe quietly while the chest tubes are removed. I do not advocate that patients force exhalation while the chest tubes are removed because a large, reflex, sudden, inspiratory effort may produce a pneumothorax.

CONTROL OF POSTOPERATIVE PAIN

Significant advances in controlling postoperative pain in thoracic surgical patients have been made. A heightened awareness exists that excessive pain contributes to most postoperative complications, and control of pain is approached in a highly scientific fashion. Pain increases atelectasis because of chest wall splinting and a resulting diminution in chest excursion. Pain increases sympathetic tone so that peripheral vascular resistance and myocardial oxygen consumption are correspondingly elevated. The increase in cardiac workload may provoke arrhythmias and previously masked cardiac ischemia. Pain, as noted by Cousins and Phillips (1984), also increases vagal tone, resulting in more nausea and vomiting and elevated hormonal tone so that water retention and hyperglycemia are initiated. Failure to control postoperative pain in the elderly patient who has had a thoracotomy may result in life-threatening cardiorespiratory complications.

The techniques of pain relief used depend largely on the medical and ancillary staff. The traditional method of injecting intramuscular narcotics every few hours has serious drawbacks: the patient experiences severe pain at low narcotic levels and possible confusion and agitation at high levels. An acceptable alternative to intermittent intramuscular narcotics is continuous intravenous infusion. This method can be safely practiced in all hospitals if the physician is aware of proper loading and maintenance doses. For meperidine, the doses are clearly established; for a 70 kg patient, a 100 mg loading dose should be administered over 30 to 60 minutes and a maintenance dose of 18 to 30 mg per hour can be continuously administered. Doses are based on the volume of distribution of the drug and on the desired analgesic blood level. As emphasized by Stapleton (1979) and Cousins (1984) and their colleagues, dosage should be reduced if liver function is abnormal, if vomiting occurs, or if respirations are depressed. Although the doses for morphine sulfate are not precisely established, the usual loading dose is 7.5 mg over an hour followed by 2.5 mg per hour by continuous infusion.

Angle intercostal nerve block for pain relief is fairly easy to implement once the catheters have been placed by the surgeon in the operating room. The catheters are placed at the posterior rib angles at the incision and two interspaces above and below the incision. Bupivacaine 0.5% with epinephrine 1:200,000 is infused intermittently. The usual dose is 3 to 5 ml every 6 to 18 hours per interspace. Signs of local anesthetic toxicity and inadvertent vascular injection must be carefully monitored.

Epidural blockade is a relatively new and highly effective method of achieving postoperative pain relief in the thoracotomy patient. Complications—nausea, vomiting, pruritus, urinary retention, and respiratory depression—have been markedly reduced by careful attention to administration and proper dosage. It is crucial that those who use epidural block are well-versed in catheter placement and aseptic technique, and that resuscitative equipment is readily available for patients with epidural catheters. The level of sensory block must be carefully ascertained—T10 umbilicus, T7 xiphoid, and T4–5 nipple. Subarachnoid injection may result in spinal anesthesia with hypotension, bradycardia, and apnea—motor block of T1 results in respiratory failure. In 40 postoperative thoracotomy patients treated with intermittent epidural morphine reported by Milvert and associates (1983), the mean interval between doses was 12

hours. Half of the patients required only one dose, and more than 24 hours of analgesia were produced in 13%. The authors noted a high incidence of urinary retention, but stated that most of their thoracotomy patients had urinary catheters for the procedure. Other authors prefer continuous epidural infusion of narcotics. El-Baz and colleagues (1982) compared intravenous morphine intermittent epidural morphine, and continuous epidural morphine at 0.18 mg per hour in the relief of post-thoracotomy pain in 60 patients. Patients who received continuous epidural morphine received additional bolus injections from the nursing staff as needed. Pain scores in the continuous epidural morphine group were significantly lower than those for the other two groups. Pain control did not differ between the other two groups, but those who received intermittent epidural morphine had a high incidence of central narcosis—four patients required naloxone, one required naloxone plus mechanical ventilation. The authors concluded that continuous morphine by the epidural route achieved "effective, segmental, and selective postoperative analgesia" (Fig. 25–3).

Brodsky and associates (1986) wrote that they prefer lumbar epidural narcotics and avoid the thoracic route to lower the complication rate. The catheter is placed before the operative procedure and used intraoperatively for injection of local anesthetics to reduce or eliminate the need for muscle relaxants. They start narcotics not

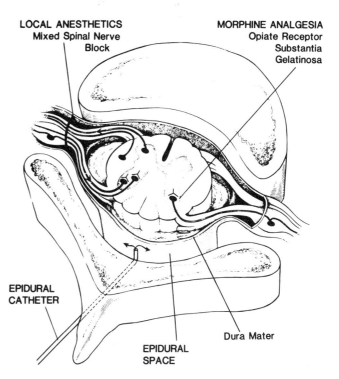

LOCAL ANESTHETICS
Mixed Spinal Nerve
Block

MORPHINE ANALGESIA
Opiate Receptor
Substantia
Gelatinosa

EPIDURAL
CATHETER

EPIDURAL
SPACE

Dura Mater

Fig. 25–3. Anatomic basis for narcotic analgesia and local anesthetic action. (Reprinted from El-Baz, N., and Ivankovich, A.D.: Management of postoperative thoracotomy pain: continuous epidural infusion of morphine. *In* Current Controversies in Thoracic Surgery, p. 219. Edited by C.F. Kittle. By permission of W.B. Saunders Co., Philadelphia, 1986.)

less than 45 minutes before the end of the operation so that "most patients awaken free of pain and are extubated in the operating room."

Comment

Our group uses epidural catheters for postoperative narcotic administration in patients who undergo major pulmonary resections and in those who are at high risk for pulmonary complications. We prefer fentanyl because its high lipid solubility lessens the possibility of ascending block and its onset of action is 15 minutes compared to approximately one hour for morphine. One to 1.5 μg/kg is given about 20 minutes before the incision is closed, followed by 0.5 μg/kg by continuous infusion. The catheter is left in place for five to seven days after the operative procedure, during which time our patients have received almost no parenteral analgesics. The patients ambulate sooner than with conventional pain relief techniques, and it is my impression that they are being discharged a day or so earlier than patients who were managed without this technique.

REFERENCES

Arkins, R., Smaessant, A.A., and Hicks, R.G.: Mortality and morbidity in surgical patients with coronary artery disease. J.A.M.A. *190*:458, 1964.

Beck-Nielsen, J., Sorensen, H.R., and Alstup, P.: Atrial fibrillation following thoracotomy for noncardiac diseases, in particular cancer of the lung. Acta Med. Scand. *193*:425, 1973.

Boysen, P.G., et al.: Prospective evaluation for pneumonectomy using the 99mTechnetium quantitative perfusion lung scan. Chest *72*:422, 1977.

Brodsky, J.B., Shulman, M.S., and Mark, B.D.: Management of postoperative thoracotomy pain: lumbar epidural narcotics. *In* Current Controversies in Thoracic Surgery. Edited by C.F. Kittle. Philadelphia, W.B. Saunders Co., 1986, pp. 228–232.

Burman, S.O.: The prophylactic use of digitalis before thoracotomy. Ann. Thorac. Surg. *14*:359, 1972.

Cousins, M.J., and Phillips, G.D.: Sleep, pain, and sedation. In The Society of Critical Care Medicine: Textbook of Critical Care. Edited by William Shoemaker et al. Philadelphia, W.B. Saunders Co., 1984, pp. 787–801.

Don, H.: Respiratory care. *In* Perioperative Management in Cardiothoracic Surgery. Edited by B.B. Roe. Boston, Little, Brown & Co., 1981, pp. 117–134.

Driscoll, A.C., et al.: Clinically unrecognized myocardial infarction following surgery. N. Engl. J. Med. *264*:633, 1961.

El-Baz, N., et al.: Continuous epidural morphine analgesia for pain relief after thoracic surgery. Anesthesiology 57:A205, 1982.

El-Baz, N., et al.: Continuous epidural morphine infusion for postoperative pain relief. Anesth. Analg. (Cleve.) *62*:258, 1983.

Ellison, R.G.: Cardiac complications of noncardiac intrathoracic surgery. *In* Complications of Intrathoracic Surgery. Boston, Little Brown & Co., 1979, pp. 93–100.

Melnert, J.H., Dupont, T.J., and Rose, D.H.: Intermittent epidural morphine installation for control of postoperative pain. Ann. Surg. *146*:145, 1983.

Meltman, C.: Assessment of operative risk in thoracic surgery. Am. Rev. Respir. Dis. *84*:197, 1961.

Nunn, J.F., et al.: Hypoxemia and atelectasis produced by forced expiration. Br. J. Anesth. *37*:3, 1965.

Olson, G.N., et al.: Pulmonary function evaluation of the lung resection candidate. Am. Rev. Respir. Dis., *111*:379, 1975.

Shapiro, B.A., Harrison, R.A., and Trout, C.A. (Eds.): Clinical Application of Respiratory Care, 2nd Ed. Chicago, Year Book Medical Publishers, Inc., 1979.

Shields, T.W., and Ujiki, G.T.: Digitalization for prevention of arrhythmias following pulmonary surgery. Surg. Gynecol. Obstet. *126*:713, 1968.

Stapleton, J.V., Austin, K.L., and Mather, L.E.: A pharmacokinetic approach to postoperative pain: continuous infusion of peltidine. Anaesth. Intensive Care 7:25, 1979.

Steen, P., Tinker, J., and Tarhan, S.: Myocardial reinfarction after anesthesia and surgery. J.A.M.A. *239*:2566, 1978.

Tarhan, S., et al.: Myocardial infarction after general anesthesia. J.A.M.A. *220*:1451, 1972.

Wheat, M.W., Jr., and Buford, T.H.: Digitalis in surgery: extension of classical indications. J. Thorac. Cardiovasc. Surg., *41*:162, 1961.

CHAPTER 26

VENTILATORY SUPPORT OF THE POSTOPERATIVE SURGICAL PATIENT

Thomas R. Todd and R. Keenan

PULMONARY PATHOPHYSIOLOGY

Pulmonary function and resultant gas exchange deteriorate following any major surgical procedure, particularly following pulmonary resections. Minute ventilation is well preserved, but its separate components are considerably altered. Vital capacity is reduced by 50 to 75% in the first 24 hours, as Churchill and McNeil (1927) reported. On average, tidal volume is diminished by 20% and functional residual capacity—FRC—by 35% in thoracic and upper abdominal procedures. There is normally a return to preoperative levels in 7 to 14 days. Despite the fall in tidal volume, minute ventilation is maintained by compensatory increases in respiratory rate.

Sighing, defined as a breath three times greater than tidal volume, normally occurs approximately ten times per hour and helps to maintain lung volume and pulmonary compliance. This effort is greatly diminished in the postoperative period because pain limits both chest wall and diaphragmatic excursion. In addition, narcotics alter central respiratory drive. Bendixen and associates (1964), Egbert and Bendixen (1964), and Zikria and co-workers (1974) consistently reported these findings. Atelectasis may result and is often aggravated by immobility, restricted ventilation caused by pain, and retained secretions. Pulmonary defense mechanisms such as coughing and mucociliarly clearance are compromised in the early postoperative period. Harris and associates (1975) reported a reduction of mucociliary clearance postoperatively from hypoxemia alone.

Latimer and associates (1971) found that the highest rates of pulmonary complications following surgery occurred with thoracic and upper abdominal procedures. Atelectasis occurs when the closing volume of the airways exceeds the expiratory reserve volume in the early postoperative period. At special risk are the elderly and smokers, whose closing volume is already elevated. In addition, obese patients already have a diminished expiratory reserve volume. Patients with chronic obstructive lung disease exhibit problems with both expiratory reserve volume and closing volume.

Several mechanisms eventually lead to decreased lung volume and resultant atelectasis. Complicating this process is a change in extravascular lung water. This results either from overtransfusion and left ventricular decompensation or from an alteration in the permeability of the pulmonary capillary membrane. The latter has been reported following shock, aspiration, and blood transfusion, all of which are common accompaniments of major surgery; it is called the adult respiratory distress syndrome—ARDS. In pulmonary surgery, the situation is aggravated on the ipsilateral side by pulmonary contusion secondary to surgical trauma and possibly on the contralateral side by intra- and postoperative increases in pulmonary artery pressure. This accumulation of extravascular water further affects regional ventilation. This and the atelectasis noted previously lead to significant alterations in ventilation and perfusion matching. Hypoxemia results. Characteristically, the postoperative patient demonstrates hypoxemia with hypercarbia, a late abnormality often signifying that the patient is tiring and will soon require mechanical assistance. Both arterial hypoxemia and a reduction in tidal volume increase respiratory rate, which initially leads to hypocarbia and a respiratory alkalosis. Prys-Roberts and colleagues (1967) reported an increased alveolar-arterial oxygen gradient with no evidence of abnormalities on chest roentgenogram. Several postoperative cardiovascular changes may alter ventilation-perfusion matching. We have already noted the problems associated with left ventricular overload. In addition, alterations in cardiac output from hypovolemia, sepsis, or increases in ventricular afterload may harm ventilation-perfusion matching.

Following thoracic surgical procedures, increases in right ventricular filling pressures caused by pulmonary hypertension may impair left ventricular function and result in hypotension. Increases in pulmonary artery pressure may lead to pulmonary edema because of the resultant increases in hydrostatic pressure within the fluid-exchanging vessels. These cardiopulmonary interactions, though obvious, are frequently overlooked in the management of these patients and will be emphasized further.

PREDICTING THE NEED

Despite the pathophysiologic alterations in pulmonary function, only a few patients require mechanical ventilatory support to maintain gas exchange postoperatively. The need for such support can often be predicted preoperatively. The same factors used to assess medical resectability can be applied to define a group of patients at high risk for postoperative respiratory failure. In addition, associated medical or surgical conditions may necessitate mechanical assistance even when minimal pulmonary dysfunction results from the operative procedure.

Arterial Blood Gases

Arterial hypoxemia—Pa_{O_2} less than 55 mm Hg on room air—by itself is insufficient to predict either resectability or postoperative dysfunction. Oxygenation depends on the ventilation-perfusion relationship in the remaining and the resected lung, as subsequently outlined. One should be more wary of a high arterial Pa_{O_2} in the face of an assessment that otherwise suggests significant obstructive or restrictive lung disease. A patient with poor pulmonary function cannot sustain a Pa_{O_2} greater than 80 torr unless his ventilation-perfusion inequalities have been maximized by obliteration of a significant portion of the pulmonary vascular bed, i.e., that portion with the lowest ventilation-perfusion ratios. Thus, a high Pa_{O_2}—greater than 80 torr—noted when pulmonary function studies show impairment should alert the surgeon to the possibility of pulmonary vascular hypertension. Hypercarbia, on the other hand—Pa_{CO_2} greater than 45 torr—is a direct indicator of advanced lung disease and minimal pulmonary reserve. These patients often require postoperative mechanical support even after nonpulmonary thoracic procedures.

Pulmonary Function Tests and Work of Breathing

These screening tests are frequently used to assess resectability. The forced expiratory volume in one second—FEV_1, the forced expiratory volume in one second expressed as a percentage of the forced vital capacity—FEV_1/FVC, and the maximum flow rate at 25, 50, and 75% of lung capacity are reduced by obstructive lung disease. Abnormalities in these values are correlated with increased surgical risk when the values recorded are less than 50% of the predicted norm. Mittman (1961) felt that a maximum voluntary ventilation—MVV—less than 50% of the expected value, even though this measurement is affected by patient cooperation and fatigue, indicates high risk.

Lockwood (1973), using a multifactorial analysis, defined a high risk group that included patients with a vital capacity less than 1.85 L, FEV_1 less than 1.2 L, $FEV_1/$ FVC less than 35%, and MVV less than 28 L/min. Shapiro and Walton (1982) suggested that patients in whom the percent predicted FVC plus the percent FEV_1/FVC was less than 100 had a 50% chance of developing acute ventilatory failure in the first 24 hours following a thoracic or upper abdominal procedure. This seems excessive. The only major area of agreement concerning the predictive accuracy of postoperative respiratory function is that a predicted postoperative FEV_1 less than 800 ml is incompatible with the tasks of daily living, as Kristersson (1972) and Olsen (1975) and their associates reported. Shapiro and co-workers (1977) described the relationship between work of breathing and minute ventilation. Oxygen consumption is exponentially related to tidal volume expressed as a percentage of vital capacity. Patients with reduced vital capacity are at risk for two reasons. First, their ability to improve ventilation by increasing tidal volume is severely limited. Second, the relative proportion of oxygen consumption spent on the work of breathing is high, and other organ systems are adversely affected postoperatively if the work of breathing must be increased. Viires and colleagues (1983) and Hussain and Roussos (1985) performed several elegant experiments that reveal the demand the work of breathing can make upon oxygen consumption and respiratory blood flow. Under maximal stress, respiratory muscle blood flow can account for 21% of cardiac output, compared to 3% at rest. Viires and colleagues' experiments were undertaken in animals with normal pulmonary reserve subjected to varieties of stress common in the postoperative period. That respiratory work could reach its limits in such situations suggests that patients with impaired respiratory function might reach threshold values of oxygen consumption and blood flow early. As Cherniak (1959) pointed out, increased airway resistance would exacerbate the situation.

Ventilation-Perfusion Studies

In assessing a patient for pulmonary resection, preoperative pulmonary function must be balanced against the function of the portion of lung to be removed. For example, the patient with a main stem bronchial obstruction and severe chronic obstructive lung disease can, from a respiratory standpoint, withstand removal of the involved lung, barring the development of other complications. The pneumonectomy is already established functionally, and removal of the lung may actually improve ventilation-perfusion matching. In other cases, the functional characteristics of the portion of the lung to be removed may be less obvious; in these circumstances, ventilation-perfusion scans may clarify the postoperative consequences of resection. Juhl and Frost (1975) devised a formula to predict postoperative FEV_1 where FEV_1 was equal to the preoperative FEV_1 times the percent perfusion to the uninvolved lung, assuming matched ventilation-perfusion in the contralateral lung.

When divided into lung zones, quantitative ventilation and perfusion studies can be used to predict the effect of resection on vital capacity and gas exchange. Tisi (1979) outlined four outcomes predictable from preoperative scans (Table 26–1). The need for mechanical ventilation is most likely under the third condition and somewhat less likely under the first.

Exercise

Exercise testing is a useful adjunct to the predictive tests. High risk patients may experience a fall in arterial saturation that can be assessed with pulse oximetry. Such an occurrence suggests the need for respiratory rehabilitation before surgery. Although stair-walking appears subjective and unscientific, it has remained the most tried and true method of preoperative evaluation. The addition of pulse oximetry has added some objectivity. Johnson and co-workers (1977) did correlate the ability to perform simple exercise—stair climbing—to postoperative mortality and morbidity. Miyoshi and associates (1987), in a prospective study, concluded that whereas pulmonary function studies—FEV_1, D_{CO}—determined postoperative complications, exercise-induced blood lactate thresholds determined mortality.

Pulmonary Artery Pressure

Elevated pulmonary artery pressure in patients with chronic obstructive lung disease signifies extensive disease and high risk. Right heart catheterization permits the use of a balloon to occlude flow to the diseased lung. Laros and Swierenga (1967) established a resting mean pulmonary artery pressure of 30 torr as their criterion for inoperability. Olsen (1975) and Karliner (1968) and their colleagues reported similar values. Increased pulmonary vascular resistance is also a measure of vascular compliance. Fee and co-workers (1978) defined a high risk category of pulmonary vascular resistance greater than or equal to 190 dynes/sec/cm⁵.

Summary

Several means are available to assess the risk of respiratory failure post thoracotomy. What tests should be routine, however, is often unclear. A preoperative FEV_1 of 900 ml or less in the absence of major airway obstruction virtually eliminates the patient from further consideration. All other patients should receive exercise oximetry on the stairs. A normal exercise test with no history of impaired exercise tolerance, a Pa_{O_2} between 55 and 80 torr, and a normal Pa_{CO_2} obviate further testing.

Table 26–1. Predicted Change in Postoperative Pulmonary Function Using Quantitative Ventilation and Perfusion Scans

Function of Resected Lung	Predicted Result
V/Q (resection) equals V/Q (rest of lung)	Decline in function proportional to extent of resection
V/Q (resection) = .0/0	"Autoresection"—No loss of function
V/Q (resection) >>> V/Q (rest of lung)	Decline in function >>> extent of resection
V/Q (resection) abnormal <<< V/Q (rest of lung)	Resection of dead space—improved function.

Adapted from Tisi, G.M.: State of the art: preoperative evaluation of pulmonary function. Am. Rev. Respir. Dis. *119*:293, 1979.

Desaturation with exercise testing, a Pa_{O_2} greater than 80 torr associated with a history of poor exercise tolerance, or a Pa_{CO_2} greater than 45 torr leads to further evaluation with ventilation-perfusion scanning and pulmonary artery pressure testing as indicated previously. Persistent uncertainty at any point in this evaluation process results in the recommendation of a 3- to 4-week period of respiratory rehabilitation with subsequent reassessment. Often, surprising improvement in vigor, exercise tolerance, and occasionally spirometry results from a period of abstinence from smoking and from graded exercise on a treadmill combined with intensive physiotherapy.

Concurrent Risk Factors

Serious medical or surgical problems may necessitate the use of postoperative ventilatory support independent of the degree of pulmonary dysfunction resulting from the surgical procedure.

Cardiac

The single most important associated medical condition is cardiac dysfunction. Cardiac risk factors devised by Goldman and associates (1977) include age, positive cardiac history or physical examination, and ECG abnormalities. Patients in the highest risk category have a 78% incidence of cardiac death or life-threatening complication. These patients should be prophylactically ventilated postoperatively to reduce the proportion of oxygen consumption consumed by the work of breathing. The type of anesthesia employed in such cases impairs respiratory drive for prolonged periods.

In the postoperative period, the ability to maintain oxygen consumption depends on adequate oxygen delivery to the tissues. From the Fick principle, oxygen consumption is determined by cardiac output—CO—and arterial-venous oxygen content difference $\dot{V}_{O_2} = CO(Ca_{O_2} - Cv_{O_2})$.

If cardiac dysfunction reduces cardiac output, then increased oxygen extraction must occur to maintain consumption. Even without a change in postoperative pulmonary function, the highly desaturated venous blood may lead to a relative arterial hypoxemia. Increases in respiratory rate then cause respiratory alkalosis and shift the oxyhemoglobin dissociation curve to the left, making oxygen uptake at the tissue level more difficult. As a result, these patients may require not only fluids or inotropes or both to improve cardiac output, but prophylactic ventilation to support gas exchange should be considered.

Multiorgan Dysfunction

Pontoppidan and associates (1972) noted that abnormalities in other organ systems increased the chance of ventilatory failure postoperatively. A careful assessment of renal and hepatic functions should be routine, and efforts should be made to maximize function preoperatively and to prevent further deterioration postoperatively.

Hemodynamic Instability

Alterations in capillary permeability occur during hypotension from any cause and exacerbate interstitial edema, resulting in a narrowing of terminal airways and alveolar collapse. Impaired cardiac output, either from inadequate filling pressures or from cardiac dysfunction, further reduces the transport of oxygen to the periphery. Sepsis, in which hypoxemia may occur early because of pulmonary artery hypertension and alterations in ventilation-perfusion ratios, is a particular problem.

Fluid therapy and the use of vasopressors lead to adverse changes in gas exchange. Pressor-induced increases in pulmonary vascular pressure increase the driving pressure for fluids across the capillary into the interstitium. Hemodilution from fluid therapy or blood loss or both combines with hypoxemia to result in a further reduction in arterial oxygen content.

Too often, the resuscitation of a patient who is septic or hypovolemic or in cardiogenic shock ignores gas exchange. The routine of assessing arterial blood gases during these events frequently reveals hypoxemia, which complicates attempts to restore hemodynamic stability. Thus, mechanical ventilatory assistance is often necessary to support gas exchange until hemodynamic stability is achieved and should be an immediate consideration during the resuscitative process of a hypotensive emergency.

Nature and Extent of Planned Surgery

Postoperative ventilatory support is a useful adjunct for certain thoracic procedures. If impaired compliance of the remaining lung on the operative side can be anticipated, postoperative ventilatory support should be considered. Spontaneous ventilation may lead to insufficient expansion and resultant pleural space problems, particularly following surgery for inflammatory or restrictive disease, e.g., tuberculosis and fibrosis. Patients with tuberculosis or those undergoing decortication should be considered for elective ventilatory support until postoperative compliance can be assessed.

Procedures such as esophagectomy are frequently accompanied by large third-space fluid losses and unpredictable changes in pulmonary capillary permeability. Intravenous fluid replacement may increase interstitial edema, with adverse effects in gas exchange. Additionally, these patients may have two or three incisions, with significant pain and an increased work of breathing. Anesthesia is prolonged and postoperative respiratory depression is frequent. Elective ventilatory support for the first 24 hours in these patients may prevent respiratory complications.

POSTOPERATIVE INDICATION FOR SUPPORT

The decision to initiate or continue mechanical ventilation postoperatively is based on the demonstration of impaired gas exchange. Inadequate reversal of anesthesia, particularly in combination with narcotic analgesics, depresses central respiratory drive and causes apnea.

Temporary support is all that is necessary. Patients who have been extubated in the operating room or recovery area and who require early reintubation usually have experienced ventilatory failure, reflected by an acute rise in Pa_{CO_2} and the development of acute respiratory acidosis. Shapiro and associates (1977) defined acute ventilatory failure as Pa_{CO_2} greater than 50 torr and pH less than 7.30. Table 26-2 lists other parameters. These criteria describe established ventilatory failure—therapy should have been started long before patients reached this point. Hypoxemic respiratory failure is an inability to maintain adequate arterial oxygenation. Intubation is usually required when the Pa_{O_2} is less than 60 torr or the AaD_{O_2} greater than 350 torr while breathing 100% oxygen by mask. Before this point is reached, and in contrast to those patients with inadequate ventilation, patients who are hypoxemic frequently respond to conservative management but may present a more protracted problem.

Nonventilatory Management

Supplemental oxygen by mask is often all that is necessary in cases of mild hypoxemia. When concentrations above 50% are required, a tandem-flow setup is necessary. As chest wall movement is frequently limited by pain, the judicious use of analgesics is essential. Regional hypoventilation caused by unilateral pain may result in ventilation-perfusion abnormalities. Intravenous narcotics tend to achieve adequate pain control with low dosage schedules, thus reducing the risk of impaired central respiratory drive. Epidural anagesia is an important adjunct, particularly in the high risk patient. The latter makes use of the specific opiate receptors on the dorsal columns. Opiate administration in this fashion may be given into the lumbar space via an indwelling line in doses that provide adequate to complete analgesia without any systemic side effects.

Changes in body position improve hypoxemia, especially in patients with unilateral pulmonary disease. By placing the noninvolved lung in a dependent position, gravity will ensure preferential flow of blood to that side. Rivera and associates (1984) demonstrated that changes from supine to the lateral decubitus position result in significant improvements in Pa_{O_2} in mechanically ventilated patients. Similar results can be obtained during spontaneous breathing. Experimentally, Albert and colleagues (1987) showed improvement in arterial oxygenation by the reduction of intrapulmonary shunt when oleic-acid lung-injured dogs were placed in a prone position.

Table 26–2. Criteria of Established Ventilatory Failure*

Respiratory rate	<4 or >35
Pa_{CO_2}	>50 mm Hg
Vd/Vt	>0.6
Vital capacity (VC)	<15 ml/kg
Negative inspiratory force (NIF)	< −20 ml H_2O

*Note that this says nothing concerning ventilation-perfusion inequalities.

Although no prospective randomized trials exist, aggressive chest physiotherapy, both pre- and postoperatively, doubtless improves gas exchange and reduces the incidence of pulmonary complications. Mobilization of secretions and the encouragement of cough and deep breathing maintain functional residual capacity—FRC—and improve patterns of breathing.

Frequently mentioned adjunctive therapies include intermittent positive pressure breathing—IPPB, incentive spirometry—IS, and continuous positive airway pressure—CPAP. The literature describing these techniques is conflicting. Neither Celli's group (1984) nor Ali and co-workers (1984) found any difference in pulmonary complications—atelectasis or pneumonia—among patients treated with IPPB, IS, or just deep breathing. In contrast, Stock and associates (1985) found that CPAP delivered by tight-fitting mask prompted a more rapid return of FRC and significantly reduced the incidence of atelectasis when compared with incentive spirometry or deep breathing. Patients whose hypoxemia was unresponsive to IS or routine chest physiotherapy experienced improved Pa_{O_2} and reduced AaD_{O_2} following the use of mask CPAP, as DeHaven and colleagues (1985) noted. One must, however, be cautious in employing mask CPAP in the early postoperative period because nausea and emesis may result in aspiration in patients who cannot remove the mask.

When upper airway obstruction secondary to glottic edema or tumor is suspected, a helium-oxygen mixture and racemic epinephrine can be used. At the commonly used concentration of 70% helium and 30% oxygen, the helium-oxygen mixture reduces the degree of turbulent flow in the central airways and improves laminar flow, allowing increased delivery of gas beyond the level of obstruction. At concentrations of oxygen above 40%, the advantages of the reduced density of helium are lost and the mixture becomes ineffective. Racemic epinephrine, administered as an aerosolized solution of 0.5 ml in 2.5 ml of saline every 4 hours, reduces inflammation and swelling of the laryngotracheal walls.

When to Reintubate

Clinical judgement rather than plain numbers determines when conservative methods of support are inadequate. Increased work of breathing is signalled by accessory-muscle recruitment. Progression to discoordinate breathing patterns in which abdominal—diaphragmatic—excursion is paradoxical to chest wall movement is a certain sign of impending failure. Tachypnea and a rising Pa_{CO_2} should prompt action before the levels shown in Table 26–2 are reached. Hypoxemia refractory to conservative therapy indicates continued loss of alveolar volume and FRC requiring positive pressure ventilation for correction. The combination of hypoxemia and hypercarbia should signal the need for immediate reintubation. The fatigued patient often presents the most difficult problem. When does one decide that it is time for mechanical support? Often the patient himself is the best guide. The lucid patient who can speak in sentences and report that he is the same or better provides a reliable index for continued conservatism. The onset of confusion, agitation, or the inability to speak in sentences in the previously lucid patient indicates that reintubation is now essential. As noted above, a combination of impending respiratory failure and hemodynamic instability can be lethal and warrants tracheal intubation and ventilatory support at an early stage.

Methods of Intubation

Reintubation for ventilatory or respiratory failure is best done with the patient awake but sedated. During awake intubation, patients must be subjected to minimal truama and stress. The act of intubation itself can initiate ventricular dysrhythmias, cause aspiration, and exacerbate hypoxemia. The procedure should be explained to the patient in a reassuring manner. Intravenous diazepam at a dose of 5 to 10 mg induces light sedation and relieves anxiety. A short-acting intravenous analgesic such as fentanyl—50 to 100 mg—may further reduce patient awareness. The mouth is suctioned to remove secretions and the back of the throat is sprayed with 1% lidocaine aerosol. The laryngoscope blade is inserted, and the vocal cords are visualized and sprayed with local anesthetic. All this takes time. The lidocaine should be applied to the pharynx and larynx intermittently, with 100% oxygen supplied by a tandem setup between applications. A pulse oximeter can assure that oxygen saturation is appropriate throughout the procedure.

Most patients can accommodate at least a 7.5-mm diameter endotracheal tube, but an 8- to 9-mm tube is preferable. Smaller tubes either do not accept a fiberoptic bronchoscope or do so only at the expense of severe limitation in air flow. Paralyzing agents are seldom required, but if used should be of the ultra-short-acting, nondepolarizing type such as atracurium. The equipment required for an emergency cricothyroidotomy or tracheostomy should be at the bedside if attempts at endotracheal intubation fail.

An alternate approach is nasotracheal intubation. The nares as well as the throat must be anesthetized with lidocaine spray. A 7.5- or 8-ml tube is usually well tolerated. Successful "blind intubation" requires practice, although with Magill forceps and laryngoscope, the tube can often be directly guided into the proper position.

Because flexible bronchoscopes are available, intubation should be neither blind nor difficult. Flexible bronchoscopy can be used for either oral or nasal routes. Pharmacologic management is the same as just described. The bronchoscope is passed through the endotracheal tube and then placed into the mouth or nostril. Once the vocal cords have been visualized, 2 to 3 ml of 1% lidocaine is flushed through the suction port to anesthetize the cords. The scope is then passed between the cords into the upper trachea and into either main stem bronchus. While in this position, the bronchoscope acts as a stent and the endotracheal tube is advanced into the airway. Proper position is confirmed by withdrawing the bronchoscope into the endotracheal tube and noting the distance of the latter above the tracheal carina. If flexible bronchoscopy is unavailable or is unsuccessful because of anatomy, rigid bronchoscopy may be attempted. The adaptor cap for attachment to the ventilator tubing should be removed from the endotracheal tube, as this piece limits the internal diameter. A 7-mm rigid bronchoscope passes through a 7.5-mm endotracheal tube. The principles of intubation are the same as for flexible bronchoscopy. Obviously, the nasal approach cannot be used. The rigid scope can be used like a laryngoscope to lever the tongue and epiglottis out of the way for better viewing of the vocal cords. Once the scope has been passed through the cords, ventilation can be initiated through the Venturi technique to relieve hypoxemia caused by intubation attempts. Once again, an oximeter, if available, should be used to monitor saturation during any reintubation attempt.

MECHANICAL VENTILATION

The following is designed to develop a pragmatic approach to ventilator management and reflects our personal bias; several means achieve this same end.

Ventilator Adjustments

Manipulation of ventilator controls are intended to improve oxygenation as assessed by Pa_{O_2} through changes in the fraction of inspired oxygen and positive end-expiratory pressure. Ventilation, as assessed by Pa_{CO_2}, is optimized by changes in respiratory rate, tidal volume, and inspiratory/expiratory ratio—I/E ratio.

Fraction of Inspired Oxygen—F_{IO_2}

Increases in oxygen concentration may increase arterial oxygen tensions but do nothing to improve pulmonary dysfunction. Higher inspired levels translate into higher values of Pa_{O_2} because of the fixed alveolar-arterial oxygen difference. Oxygen therapy is not, however, innocuous. Clinical experience and experimental data suggest that levels above 50% may produce irreversible lung injury within 24 hours. As Fisher and associates (1984) and Jackson (1985) described in their reviews, the current theory of oxygen-induced damage centers around the production of oxygen-derived free radicals such as superoxide anion, hydrogen peroxide, and hydroxyl radical. These molecules damage the alveolar epithelium, causing intracellular organelle disruption and producing interstitial and then alveolar edema. Organization of the exudative alveolar fluid results in hyaline membranes similar to those found in patients with ARDS. Although no hard data exist, subclinical damage may occur with concentrations of oxygen less than 50%. Thus, an important goal of mechanical ventilation is to achieve the lowest possible F_{IO_2}. A second adverse effect of high inspired concentrations of oxygen is absorption atelectasis. Normally, the nitrogen content of alveolar gas prevents alveolar collapse. With F_{IO_2} approaching 100%, however, persisting perfusion leads to continued oxygen absorption and alveolar collapse, with a resultant decrease in functional residual capacity—FRC. As McAslan and associates (1973) dem-

onstrated, a decrease in FRC usually results in an increase in intrapulmonary shunt.

Positive End-Expiratory Pressure—PEEP

At the end of expiration, airway pressure equals atmospheric pressure unless an intermediate resistance is provided. In spontaneously breathing man, this is normally provided by the closed glottis, resulting in a positive pressure at the end of expiration. Such a positive end-expiratory pressure—PEEP—maintains a higher end-expiratory lung volume or functional residual capacity. The maintenance of an appropriate FRC decreases the work required to achieve a specific tidal breath by moving the patient to a more advantageous position on the pressure-volume compliance curve (Fig. 26–1). PEEP improves arterial oxygenation by restoring FRC and by improving regional ventilation-perfusion disturbances. FRC may be increased either through alveolar recruitment or by increasing alveolar volume. As Tyler (1983) and Shapiro and colleagues (1984) outlined in excellent reviews, direct evidence for alveolar recruitment is lacking. Observations of immediate improvement in FRC with the application of PEEP, however, suggest that re-expansion of collapsed perfused alveoli plays a major role. Increases in alveolar volume have been documented at increasing levels of PEEP. Daly and associates (1973) demonstrated that alveolar diameters in normal rats increased linearly with up to 10 cm H_2O of PEEP. They also showed that although further increases in alveolar diameter could be measured above 10 cm H_2O of PEEP, changes in pressure, rather than volume, predominated.

As Hammon and colleagues (1976) showed, the addition of PEEP improves ventilation-perfusion abnor-

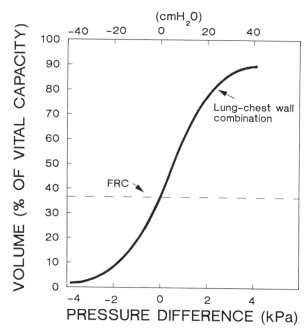

Fig. 26–1. Standard pressure-volume curve for the lungs. Note that when functional residual capacity (FRC) is reached, major increases in lung volume produce small changes in pressure or respiratory work.

malities, and thus intrapulmonary shunt, by increasing ventilation to areas characterized by low ventilation-perfusion—V/Q—ratios. Areas of low V/Q ratios are usually present in dependent lung zones. In dependent areas, perfusion is maximal because of the effect of gravity on the low pressure pulmonary circulation. Ventilation is impaired regionally by several factors, including retained secretions, decreased compliance—from extravascular lung water, pneumonitis—and increased pleural pressure. Hammon and colleagues (1976) demonstrated optimal levels of PEEP in normal and diseased lungs. Beyond these optimal levels, PEEP exerted a detrimental effect by overdistending nondependent alveoli and reducing perfusion to these areas, thereby contributing to increased dead space. Clinical studies by Downs (1973), Suter (1975), and Powers (1973) and their colleagues confirm improved oxygenation under PEEP ventilation, but as Powers and associates (1973) pointed out, increased levels of PEEP may cause reduced oxygen delivery through effects on cardiac output.

In contrast to its beneficial effects on pulmonary function, PEEP exerts a depressant action on the heart. Dorinski and Whitcomb (1983) summarized current thinking. The mechanisms responsible are not clear, but two have been proposed to explain the reduction in cardiac output seen with PEEP therapy.

Decreased Venous Return

Qvist and associates (1975) found that PEEP produced a diminished cardiac output in anesthetized, paralyzed dogs. The mechanism proposed was increased intrathoracic pressure sufficient to cause a fall in right atrial and thus right ventricular filling pressure. A fluid bolus restored cardiac output and raised transluminal right-sided filling pressures. In a study of patients with the adult respiratory distress syndrome, Potkin and associates (1987) used radionuclide angiography to demonstrate biventricular reductions in blood volume, caused primarily by reduced ventricular preload but also by changes in ventricular configuration.

Ventricular Dysfunction

Scharff and colleagues (1977) proposed that increases in right ventricular afterload with PEEP could lead to right ventricular dysfunction. Haynes (1980), using 2-D echocardiography, demonstrated a leftward shift of the intraventricular septum, resulting in decreased left ventricular area. This was restored by fluid re-expansion. They concluded that PEEP exerted a primary effect on the right ventricle with a secondary reduction in left ventricular function because of septal shifts. Jardin and associates (1981) supported their results. In contrast, Cassidy and Ramanathan (1984), using similar techniques, demonstrated that lateral wall restriction rather than septal movement produced the reduction in left ventricular filling and left ventricular volume. This study illustrated a direct impairment of left ventricular function caused by lung compression secondary to PEEP therapy.

Still others have cited the possibility of a neural or humoral depressant factor initiated by the application of PEEP. Liebman and colleagues (1978) found that 15 cm H_2O of PEEP produced significant decreases in cardiac output, but the tightening of pulmonary arterial bands did not produce equivalent pulmonary pressure changes. These authors conducted several experiments wherein a depression in cardiac output was observed even when the chest wall of animals had been removed and even in dogs who were cross-circulated with other animals supported with PEEP ventilation. On the contrary, Calvin and co-workers (1981) could not demonstrate any change in the contractile state of the left ventricle in patients with acute pulmonary edema. They concluded that decreased left ventricular preload alone accounted for the observed changes in cardiac output. As reported by Tittley and colleagues (1985), Weisel's group employed radionuclide angiography in postoperative coronary bypass patients to demonstrate a reduction in cardiac index with the application of 15 cm H_2O of PEEP. Their volume studies, however, showed no alteration in left or right ventricular performance. Metabolic studies undertaken in the same group of patients suggested only a minor role for myocardial ischemia in the cardiac response to PEEP.

Despite experimental evidence in animals that a neural or humoral depressant factor may exist, the overwhelming evidence to date in man suggests that the prime effect of PEEP on cardiac output is a reduction in left and right ventricular preload.

Monitoring PEEP

Numerous articles have described the various means of determining the best PEEP. The most accepted means are the calculation of oxygen transport and the determination of pulmonary compliance. Maximizing oxygen transport is the primary goal of PEEP therapy, as the following equation illustrates: oxygen delivery = $(1.39 \times Hgb \times Sa_{O_2} + 0.0031 \times Pa_{O_2}) \times (CO)$. The important contributors to oxygen delivery are oxyhemoglobin saturation and cardiac output. Pa_{O_2} plays a minor role in the equation. Management of PEEP therapy thus requires the insertion of a Swan-Ganz catheter to obtain cardiac output, and this should be routine when levels of PEEP above 10 cm H_2O are employed.

Suter and associates (1975) documented a high correlation between static compliance and oxygen transport measurements. The latter can be derived from the ventilator recordings themselves with the contribution of compliance to airway pressure determined by clamping the expiratory line at end inspiration. The fall in peak airway pressure during this maneuver determines the relative contribution to peak airway pressure of airway resistance and pulmonary compliance. The equalization pressure following the clamping of the expiratory line reflects the pressure generated from pulmonary compliance. An immediate impression of the efficacy of an incremental increase in PEEP can be obtained from an observation of the resultant increase in peak airway pressure. An increase in peak airway pressure greater than the increment in PEEP suggests that the results will be deleterious rather than efficacious. Hylkema and associates (1985) suggested optimizing the lung mechanical profile by plotting regression lines of pressure volume curves at various levels of PEEP. The value of PEEP achieving the greatest slope and smallest intersect volume was felt to represent the most efficient lung function obtainable. Despite these determinations, oxygen transport remains the standard in assessing the effectiveness of PEEP therapy.

In patients with unilateral lung disease, PEEP may prove deleterious. Kanarek and Shannon (1975) presented a case in which Pa_{O_2} decreased with the application of PEEP. They suggested that PEEP selectively increased lung volume on the normal side, secondarily raising the pulmonary vascular resistance and then shunting blood flow to the diseased lung. In an experimental study, Sanchez de Leon and colleagues (1985) showed an increased proportion of cardiac output to a collapsed lobe, thereby increasing shunt when PEEP was applied.

Adjuvant Means of Improving Oxygenation

Minimizing Lung Water

Respiratory failure is often precipitated by the accumulation of extravascular water because of permeability changes in the pulmonary capillaries, particularly following operative trauma but also in pneumonitis. The determinants of transcapillary fluid movement are permeability and pressure. The pressure gradient is the result of the net difference between oncotic and hydrostatic pressure across the membrane. Clinically, the only determinant that can be manipulated is intravascular hydrostatic pressure. In the lung this is best expressed by measurements of left ventricular preload or pulmonary capillary wedge pressure. A normal pulmonary capillary wedge pressure does not preclude diuresis when the pulmonary infiltrates are felt to be secondary to increased capillary permeability. As the amount of fluid entering the interstitium is directly proportional to the driving pressure, a lower wedge pressure is still desirable. Thus, in respiratory failure—particularly in cases of augmented permeability—the objectives should be to obtain the lowest possible wedge pressure compatible with adequate cardiac output and renal perfusion. If necessary, low dose dopamine—less than 5 μg/kg/min—can be employed to sustain urinary and cardiac output. Wedge pressure, however, may not always reflect left atrial filling pressures in patients with lung injury. The pulmonary circulation is a low pressure system. As such, the pressure in arterioles or venules may vary, depending on their position within the lung parenchyma. Thus, arterial pressure is low in nondependent areas above the level of the main pulmonary artery; and venous pressure is high in areas below the level of the left atrium. The converse is also true. Alveolar pressure, however, is relatively constant. West and colleagues (1964) described several lung zones that are defined by the relationships between pulmonary artery pressure, alveolar pressure, and left atrial pressure at various levels in the lung parenchyma (Fig. 26–2). As a result, measured wedge pres-

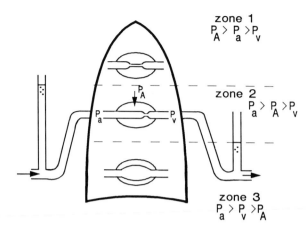

Fig. 26–2. The lung zones as defined by John West. In zone 1 alveolar pressure is greater than both arterial and venous pressure and there is little or no flow. In zone 2 the flow is determined by the gradient between arterial pressure and alveolar pressure, with a vascular waterfall existing between the alveolus and the pulmonary veins. In zone 3 both arterial and venous pressures are greater than alveolar pressure and flow is maximal. Reproduced with permission from Shapiro, B.A., et al.: Clinical Application of Respiratory Care, 3rd ed. Copyright © 1985 by Year Book Medical Publishers, Inc., Chicago.

sure varies depending on the zonal characteristics of the lung surrounding the catheter. One of us (T.R.T.) and associates (1978) showed that, depending on patient position, the level of PEEP, or the magnitude of left atrial pressure, catheter tips may lie in zone 2 or even in zone 1 areas. In such situations, the catheter-recorded pressures reflect alveolar and not venous pressure. Hasan and associates (1985) showed in cases of unilateral lung injury that catheters placed on the damaged side may actually better reflect left atrial pressure than catheters placed in the normal lung.

Postural Changes

Postural changes, as Rivara and colleagues (1984) illustrated, lead to significant improvements in oxygenation, particularly in unilateral lung disease. Frequent changes of position minimize the development of atelectasis in dependent portions.

Normalizing Pa_{CO_2}

Manipulations of tidal volume and respiratory rate are used to adjust levels of carbon dixode. The minute ventilation—rate × tidal volume—eventually determines arterial carbon dioxide tensions. An increase in either further reduces Pa_{CO_2}. Increases in tidal volume usually increase peak airway pressure, particularly when the lungs are damaged or noncompliant. Normalizing Pa_{CO_2} in patients who are hypocapnic can result in significant improvements in Pa_{O_2} and cardiac output, as Breivik and associates (1973) documented.

Airway Pressures

Improvement in gas exchange should not be made at the cost of barotrauma caused by high peak airway pressure. This is of particular concern in thoracic surgical patients with bronchial suture lines. Patients with high peak airway pressures should be closely monitored to rule out pneumothorax. Endotracheal tube patency must be assessed by bronchoscopy. The pleural spaces should be evacuated to allow full expansion of the lungs. Reducing the tidal volume reduces peak airway pressure. To maintain minute ventilation, respiratory rate must be increased to compensate for the lower tidal volume. Thus, when peak airway pressures are high because of incremental increases in PEEP or because of additional lung pathology, airway pressure may be reduced and Pa_{CO_2} maintained by supplying the same minute ventilation at lower tidal volumes and higher rates. The extreme example of this principle is high frequency jet ventilation—HFJV—which will be discussed subsequently.

Conventional Ventilators

Volume cycle ventilators are the mainstay of modern ventilatory therapy. These machines deliver a preset tidal volume at a specified respiratory rate. Generally, the inspiratory time is short—0.5 to 1.0 sec—and the gas is delivered in the sine wave pattern. Because the ventilator is designed to deliver constant volumes, high peak airway pressures may be generated during the inspiratory cycle if compliance of the lung-chest wall interface is poor. All machines have built-in pressure limits to prevent excessive barotrauma. Precise adjustments of F_{IO_2}, PEEP, I/E ratio, tidal volume, and respiratory rate can be made on all standard ventilators. An important hidden factor must be remembered when adjusting tidal volume. Although the machine delivers a constant preset volume to the system, the patient does not receive the entire amount. Changes in volume of the ventilator tubing—compression volume—account for the rest of the breath. Bartel and co-workers (1985) showed that up to 20% of the delivered tidal volume can be sequestered within the tubing in patients with low lung compliance. Most volume-cycle ventilators offer three modes of ventilatory support.

Control

In this mode, breaths initiated by the patient are not sensed by the machine. A preset tidal volume is delivered at a constant respiratory rate. This style of ventilation is generally reserved for patients who are apneic because of anesthesia, muscle relaxants, or head injury.

Assist Control

Preset respiratory rates and volumes are again delivered as in the control mode. The machine also senses the patient's respiratory effort and delivers the same preset volume for all patient-driven breaths. Minute ventilation, therefore, depends on the effort of the patient, but a lower limit is assured by the preset rate. The sensitivity of the machine to a patient-initiated breath can be altered. This most common mode of ventilation is used routinely in the postoperative period as well as for patients with prolonged respiratory failure.

Intermittent Mandatory Ventilation—IMV

The ventilator is set to deliver a specific tidal volume at a predetermined rate. In the IMV mode the ventilator also senses patient-initiated breaths as it does in the assist-control mode. Unlike the latter, however, the tidal volume delivered to the patient during these breaths depends entirely on the magnitude of the patient's respiratory effort. When the machine senses an inspiration, a fresh gas flow valve opens, allowing the patient to take a breath. No preset tidal volume is delivered during the patient-initiated breaths. In the IMV setting, minute ventilation is determined not only by the number of patient-initiated breaths, but also by their force. Once again, a minimum volume is assured by the preset IMV rate. Intermittent mandatory ventilation is frequently used postoperatively when extubation is expected within 24 hours and is also used as a weaning strategy in prolonged respiratory failure.

Ventilator Settings

In initiating ventilator therapy, respiratory rate, tidal volume, inspiratory time, PEEP, and F_{IO_2} are adjusted, based on the clinical knowledge about the patient. Subsequent adjustments are made by following serial arterial blood gases. Changes in oxygenation are made by adjusting F_{IO_2} or PEEP while Pa_{CO_2} is altered by varying respiratory rate or tidal volume. In making subsequent adjustments, one strives to achieve the lowest possible F_{IO_2} and the lowest possible peak airway pressure. In general, only one variable should be changed at a time to avoid unpredictable interactions.

High Frequency Ventilation—HFV

HFV offers an alternative when conventional ventilation fails and gas exchange is insufficient. It should also be considered when excessive F_{IO_2}—greater than 50%—or excessive peak airway pressures or both are required to achieve satisfactory Pa_{O_2} and Pa_{CO_2}. The delivery of small tidal volumes at high frequencies may improve alveolar mixing and alleviate the gas-exchange problem. Such is achieved with the maintenance of mean airway pressure but a reduction in peak airway pressure. There are several forms of high frequency ventilation.

High frequency positive pressure ventilation—HFPPV—refers to conventional ventilators set to deliver small tidal volumes at rates exceeding 40 per minute. The technique is useful for bronchoscopy and some open chest surgery, as Malina and colleagues (1981) showed. To avoid overdistention of the lung, sufficient time for exhalation must be allowed.

High frequency oscillation—HFO—delivers some volumes of fresh gas at rates of 900 to 3000 per min. The gas flow is rapidly interrupted by a piston or ball to produce oscillations. The mechanism for gas exchange is unclear. Molecular diffusion of gas in the airways may be enhanced by the turbulence generated by the oscillations.

During high frequency jet ventilation—HFJV—jets of gas at rates of 80 to 400 breaths per minute are delivered through a small cannula into the distal trachea. By the Venturi principle, additional gas is drawn into the airway—biased gas flow. Traditionally, these systems have been open, wherein the biased gas is drawn from atmosphere or from an oxygen source. As the degree of mixing of jet-stream gas and biased gas remained unknown, true F_{IO_2} was also uncertain. These systems have been particularly useful in the ventilatory management of patients with large bronchopleural fistulae. Table 26–3 displays the arterial blood gases on a standard volume cycle ventilator and then on HFJV in a patient with an iatrogenically created defect in the trachea and left main stem bronchus following complicated esophageal surgery reported by Panos and associates (1986). These systems have, however, been hampered by several difficulties. As noted, the mixing of biased gas and jet gas leads to an unknown F_{IO_2}. In addition, humidification of the biased gas is often difficult, resulting in drying of the airways. Importantly, these systems also lacked disconnect and high pressure alarms.

Although general agreement exists concerning the efficacy of HFJV in the management of bronchopleural fistula, controversy concerning its role in hypoxemic respiratory failure continues. McIntyre and colleagues (1986) failed to demonstrate any advantage of HFJV over conventional ventilators in their patients with respiratory failure of various causes. Carlon and associates (1981) documented their experience in 17 patients with various abnormalities causing hypoxemia that was refractory to conventional ventilation. Of the 17, 8 patients improved and survived on HFJV and none of the 17 patients experienced a deterioration when switched to the high frequency technique. Experimental work by Lucking and associates (1986) demonstrated an improvement in cardiac output and systemic hemodynamics with maintenance of gas exchange in dogs suffering from induced right ventricular dysfunction.

We developed a closed system of HFJV for such patients (Fig. 26–3). In this system the biased gas flow is supplied by a conventional ventilator set in an IMV mode—2 to 6 breaths per minute, tidal volume of 200 ml. This provides a constant F_{IO_2}, adequate humidification, the alarm systems of the conventional ventilator, and the ability to use PEEP. Heliou and colleagues (in preparation) compiled experience with 67 patients suffering from hypoxemic respiratory failure managed with this system. Figures 26–4 and 26–5 demonstrated the rapid improvement in Pa_{O_2} and the ability to decrease F_{IO_2} to acceptable levels within 24 hours. Of the 67

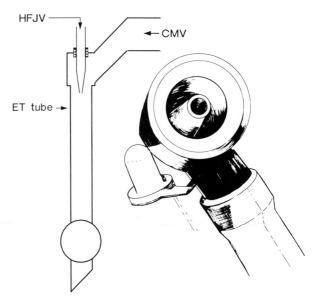

Fig. 26–3. A closed system of HFJV. A 3.5-mm cannula is inserted through the top of the swivel of the standard endotracheal tube (see insert). The biased or untrained gas flow comes from conventional mechanical ventilator (CMB) through the standard ventilatory tubing.

patients, 43 had significant improvements in Pa_{O_2} within hours of instituting HFJV.

Extracorporeal Membrane Oxygenation—ECMO

Occasionally, maximum ventilatory support including HFJV is insufficient to reverse hypoxemia, hypercarbia, or both. Extracorporeal membrane oxygenation may salvage a few of these patients in terminal respiratory failure. A multicenter National Institute of Health trial reported by Zapal and associates (1979) concluded that ECMO provided no survival advantage over continued conventional ventilatory support. The study has several intrinsic flaws, the most important of which is a large beta error; that is, the risk of not demonstrating a true benefit from the therapy was high, given the sample size. Several authors, including Solca (1985), Egan (in press), and Bartlett (1977) and their colleagues, reported their success with varying forms of ECMO. Our own experience with 17 patients has resulted in 4 survivors. The mean Pa_{O_2} before the institution of extracorporeal circulation was 32 torr.

A technique for the rapid institution of ECMO using percutaneous catheters and a Bio—medicus pump—the so called mini membrane—has been developed. Girotti and associates (1986) described the technique, and Rice and associates (1986) presented the results in 5 patients. Rapid percutaneous cannulation of the femoral veins provided venous drainage. Blood was returned through a cannula placed in the internal jugular vein. Oxygenation improved from 37 torr pre-ECMO to 186 torr post-ECMO. Carbon dioxide was normalized in all cases. Three of the five patients survived their pulmonary insult and were discharged from the hospital.

Gattinoni and colleagues (personal communication, 1987) have developed considerable experience with ex-

Table 26–3. Ventilatory Settings and Arterial Blood Gases in a Single Patient with a Large Bronchopleural Fistula*

Control-Mode Ventilation	High Frequency Jet Ventilation
Rate = 20	Rate = 20
V = 1000 ml	D/P = 10 psi
F_{IO_2} = 0.60	F_{IO_2} = 0.60
PEEP = 10	PEEP = 10
Arterial Blood Gases	
pH = 7.23	pH = 7.24
P_{CO_2} = 102	P_{CO_2} = 63
P_{O_2} = 57	P_{O_2} = 85

*Note the improvement in arterial carbon dioxide tension following the institution of high frequency jet ventilation.

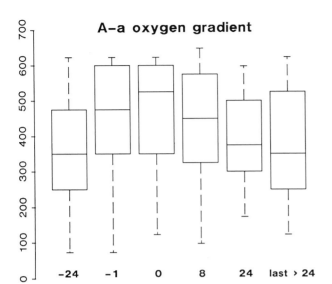

A–a oxygen gradient

Fig. 26–4. The alveolar-arterial oxygen gradient in 67 patients with hypoxemic respiratory failure subjected to high frequency jet ventilation. The values of AaDo$_2$ at minus 24, minus 1, and 0 represent the progressive increases in AaDo$_2$ before the institution of HFJV. Note the rapid improvement in AaDo$_2$ following the institution of HFJV at time 0.

tracorporeal circuitry designed to eliminate carbon dioxide in patients with chronic obstructive lung disease. Gattinoni noted that experimentation with heparin-impregnated materials suggests that the anticoagulation required for extracorporeal circulation may be significantly reduced or even eliminated in the future. Such developments and the ability to secure rapid cannulation as noted should lead to the increased use of ECMO in the future. The combination of ECMO and continuous flow ventilation has the potential of providing ultimate support when mechanical ventilation fails. Continuous-flow—apneic—ventilation appears capable of restoring

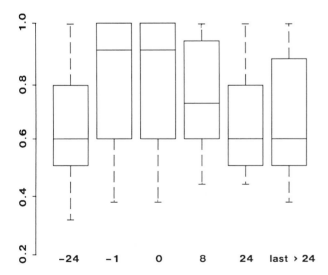

Fig. 26–5. The changes in the fraction of inspired oxygen (F$_{IO_2}$) following the institution of HFJV in patients with hypoxemic respiratory failure. Patients were subjected to HFJV at time 0. Within 24 hours the F$_{IO_2}$ has been lowered to less than 0.6.

Pa$_{O_2}$ in the severest forms of hypoxemic respiratory failure. The resultant hypercarbia caused by apneic ventilation should be handled by EMCO.

SPECIFIC PROBLEMS

Fighting the Ventilator

Patients and their ventilators are out of phase when the patients attempt to initiate an inspiration during the expiratory phase of the machine cycle. This struggling leads to increased oxygen consumption, increased intrathoracic pressures, and a reduction in alveolar ventilation. The stimulus may be inadequate ventilation or oxygenation, CNS disturbance, acidemia, or anxiety. Under such circumstances, one must first identify and correct acid-base and gas-exchange abnormalities. A switch to IMV ventilation may be all that is necessary. Pain and anxiety can be relieved by narcotics and sedatives. If struggling is secondary to CNS dysfunction, muscle relaxants may be required. Airway pressure should be assessed, and if it is increased, airway obstruction or pneumothorax should be suspected. If the patient is agitated this might be difficult to assess. Under such circumstances, and at any time the adequacy of ventilation is suspect, the patient should be disconnected from the machine and support provided by an ambu bag delivering 100% oxygen. Manual ventilation can be synchronized with the patient's efforts and airway resistance assessed. A chest roentgenogram is required to determine the presence or absence of a pneumothorax because auscultation in the ventilated patient is unreliable. Similarly, bronchospasm may not be fully appreciated if air entry is markedly diminished. Continued agitation in the presence of poor compliance and the absence of a pneumothorax demands bronchoscopic inspection of the endotracheal tube and distal airway.

At times, the physician may be unsure whether the high pressures required for ventilatory support are a function of poor pulmonary compliance or of increased airway resistance. This is particularly the case when bronchospasm is absent or minimal, for as noted previously, the presence of bronchospasm demands a certain minimal degree of airflow. A simple maneuver may settle the issue. At end inspiration, the expiratory line should be temporarily clamped. If the peak airway pressure falls dramatically, then the contribution of airway resistance to peak pressure is significant, because absence of flow eliminates the contribution of resistance to pressure. If clamping the expiratory line maintains peak airway pressure, a problem with pulmonary compliance exists.

Weaning and Extubation

Methods of weaning largely reflect individual bias, as there are few sound data to support anyone's system. The only viable principle is that no one system is perfect and that failure to wean by one means does not preclude success by another.

Electively Ventilated Patients

Patients electively ventilated for reasons other than respiratory failure can be weaned and extubated quickly.

The measurement of vital capacity—VC—and negative inspiratory force—NIF—are an important initial assessment. Both are easily obtained at the bedside with a standard respirometer—VC—and manometer—NIF. To evaluate VC, the patient is instructed to perform a maximal inspiration and then forcibly exhale into the respirometer. An estimate of NIF is obtained by a maximal inspiration against a closed airway. NIF reflects the ability to cough and clear secretions. Vital capacity indicates respiratory reserve and, because it is a voluntary maneuver, is a measure of patient alertness and cooperation. A forced vital capacity greater than 10 ml/kg body weight and an NIF of greater than -25 cm H_2O are prerequisites for extubation if no trial of spontaneous ventilation with an indwelling endotracheal tube is to be attempted. When measured VC and NIF are not appropriate, a trial of weaning is necessary. This can be achieved either by progressive decreases in intermittent mandatory ventilation—IMV—or by spontaneous breathing with continuous positive airway pressure—CPAP. The choice depends on the degree of impairment of VC and NIF and the experience and bias of the physician. Any weaning effort demands close monitoring of gas exchange, patient comfort, breathing pattern, and vital signs. Pulse oximetry provides constant monitoring of oxygen saturation.

Weaning Following Respiratory Failure

Those patients who required mechanical assistance for respiratory failure present a different challenge, as varying degrees of continued parenchymal disease, increased bronchoreactivity, respiratory muscle debility, and cardiovascular compromise demand a more cautious approach to weaning. The initial problem is to identify that weaning has become possible. This is usually signalled by F_{IO_2} less than 50%, PEEP less than or equal to 7 cm H_2O, and clearing on the chest roentgenogram. Further support for the initiation of the weaning effort can be obtained in the conscious patient by the ability to generate a forced vital capacity of at least 7 ml/kg body weight and a minimal NIF of -15 cm H_2O.

There are two basic methods of weaning, the classic—CPAP—and the IMV method. Although weaning via an open airway—T-piece method—has often been quoted as a variant of a classic wean, it possesses no distinct advantage. On the contrary, there are potential disadvantages in that the removal of end-expiratory pressure results over time in a progressive fall in functional residual capacity and the potentiation of ventilation-perfusion mismatching. Annest (1980) and Quan (1981) and their colleagues showed that this leads to increased work of breathing. The CPAP method places the entire ventilatory responsibility on the patient. It provides for intermittent stresses with periods of complete rest at high levels of assisted ventilation. Theoretically, this maximal stress followed by rest should provide beneficial respiratory muscle exercise. When using the classic technique, it is important to recognize that patients may initially tolerate CPAP for only a short time. It is common to start with 2 to 5 minutes of CPAP within a 4-hour rest period. Extending the interval should proceed slowly—

patients should not be stressed to the point of impending failure. Cohen and associates (1982) described the clinical signs of respiratory muscle fatigue. Increased respiratory rate is followed by alternation between rib-cage and abdominal breathing, which they termed respiratory alternans, then paradoxical abdominal movements during inspiration, and finally decreased Pa_{O_2} accompanied by a fall in minute ventilation, respiratory rate, and hypercarbia. Electromyographic recordings from their patients revealed high and low frequency discharges from the intercostal muscles. A fall in the ratio of high to low frequency power indicated fatiguing muscle and preceded the clinical signs of failure. Clinically, a simple guide to patient tolerance can be obtained by measurement of VC and NIF at the beginning and at the end of the CPAP wean. The wean period should not be extended unless the beginning and ending values are comparable. Pulse oximeters are a valuable adjunct in the monitoring of these patients.

During the IMV technique, a patient must constantly work and may fail if not able to sustain the effort. As noted, failure occurs when fatigue results in diminishing tidal volumes, which in turn reduce functional residual capacity through the collapse of alveoli and small airways. Gas exchange becomes increasingly impaired. In addition, the ventilator may itself impose an increased burden on the work of breathing. Marini and colleagues (1986) demonstrated higher work loads during patient-triggered ventilator breaths than during spontaneous breathing. Part of the explanation for this phenomenon lies in the resistance threshold of the ventilator itself. The resistance within the internal circuitry of respirators varies greatly. For this reason, when employing CPAP it is wise to use external circuits.

Nutrition

To be successfully weaned, a patient must be able to assume an ever increasing workload of breathing as assisted ventilation is reduced. Importantly, the work of breathing must be efficient and coordinated or fatigue will develop and reintubation will be required. As Roussos (1985) pointed out, respiratory muscles are normally continuously active and when put to rest atrophy quickly. These muscles must be rebuilt during weaning. For this reason, adequate nutritional support is crucial to supply protein for muscle development. If necessary, total parenteral nutrition—TPN—should be instituted to provide sufficient calories.

Most thoracic surgical patients can tolerate enteral feeds within 24 to 48 hours, so protein depletion is not usually a problem. Esophagectomy patients often have a jejunostomy feeding tube placed intraoperatively and can be started on alimentation quickly. TPN, however, should be instituted within 48 hours if attempts at enteral feeding fail. Nutritional requirements must be actively determined, as Dark and co-workers (1985) showed. Otherwise, increased carbohydrate calories will lead to increased CO_2 production, which can precipitate hypercapneic respiratory failure. Unless the patient is severely catabolic, 2000 to 2500 calories are given, 50% in the form of lipids. In addition, 1 g of protein/kg body weight per day should be supplied. Requirements in septic patients may be 30 to 50% higher. Fluid balance may be a problem in the thoracic surgical patient and in those with renal insufficiency. For these patients, monitoring of daily weights is a sensitive measure of fluid accumulation, allowing judicious use of diuretics or dialysis to maintain fluid balance. Hypophosphatemia is a well described cause of respiratory muscle fatigue and should be corrected.

The Decision to Extubate

Patients are ready for extubation when the criteria outlined in Table 26–4 are met and the patients are maintaining acceptable blood gases. Additionally, patients should be normotensive and should not have demonstrated dysrhythmias or tachycardia during the final weaning stages. Morganroth and colleagues (1984) quantitated these factors into ventilator and adverse factor scores. Failure to achieve the aforementioned criteria predicted an unsuccessful wean in their long-term ventilated patients. These criteria are conservative and, as DeHaven and associates (1986) pointed out, may underestimate the ability of some patients to tolerate extubation. The latter report advocated gas-exchange measurements of intrapulmonary shunt less than 15% or Pao_2/Fio_2 ratios greater than 300 on room air. Using these measures, 94% of patients were successfully extubated even though 48% did not meet the traditional standards. Many patients in this latter study, however, had not undergone prolonged ventilation. In the final analysis, the ability of the patient to sustain adequate ventilation and oxygenation with spontaneous ventilation over a fixed period of time warrants a trial of extubation. Unfortunately, no technique is fail-safe, nor does any system assess the ability to clear secretions with the endotracheal tube removed. Nonetheless, trials of extubation are appropriate when patients can maintain their own support over several hours.

Technique of Extubation

Before extubation it is imperative to ensure that the patient can protect his airway—gag reflex and cough—and that significant upper airway obstruction, especially glottic edema, is not present. To ensure that the airway is adequate, the cuff to the endotracheal tube is deflated, the patient is instructed to inspire, and then the endotracheal tube is occluded while the patient forcibly exhales. If the patient can exhale around the tube, glottic and subglottic edema are minimal. In the absence of such a leak, the glottis and upper airway should be examined using a flexible bronchoscope inserted transnasally. If the

Table 26–4. Criteria for Extubation

Fio_2	<50%
CPAP/PEEP	<7.5 cm H_2O
Respiratory rate	>8/min but <25/min
VC	10–15 ml/kg
NIF	> −20 cm H_2O

bronchoscope can be passed easily between the cords anteriorly, extubation may be attempted with caution. Postextubation stridor secondary to residual glottic edema usually responds to a helium-oxygen mixture—30% oxygen, 70% helium—and racemic epinephrine therapy. Failure to insert the bronchoscope between the cords and the tube should delay extubation for 24 to 48 hours so that edema might clear.

Tracheostomy

The timing of tracheostomy remains controversial. Historically, tracheostomy was performed after 48 hours of endotracheal intubation to prevent the tracheal damage caused by noncompliant cuffs. The development of compliant, low pressure cuffs has resulted in an extension of this time frame. In many centers, endotracheal intubation—particularly transnasal—is allowed to continue indefinitely. In North America, the tracheostomy is traditionally undertaken after two weeks. There is, however, little to support the arbitrary time period; yet a study by Stauffer and colleagues (1981) indicated a higher incidence of tracheal stenosis and laryngotracheal ulceration in patients undergoing tracheostomy more than 14 days after endotracheal intubation. The corollary was that no advantage was found to suggest that tracheostomy was better than prolonged endotracheal intubation. Of the many reasons given for performing tracheostomies, such as difficulty in suctioning, patient discomfort, laryngotracheal lesions, oral hygiene, and glottic edema, only the last two justify this approach. Stauffer and colleagues (1981) clearly showed that difficulty in suctioning and patient discomfort were minor problems and that tracheostomy may have a higher incidence of laryngotracheal complications. Difficulty in maintaining oral hygiene is, however, a common occurrence and leads to oral-pharyngeal infections, sialadenitis, and mucosal ulceration. As mentioned previously, extubation is contraindicated in the presence of glottic edema and tracheostomy maintains the airway and allows the edema to resolve. For these reasons, tracheostomy should be considered for patients intubated for 10 to 14 days and in whom it is expected that mechanical ventilatory support will be required for some time. It should be undertaken earlier when the reason for endotracheal intubation was a failure to clear secretions. When prolonged nasal or oral-tracheal intubation is considered, close monitoring of cuff pressures and of airway patency about the tube are essential.

The Difficult Wean

Failure to wean should prompt further investigations to reveal possible causes. A finding of a dead space to tidal volume ratio—Vd/Vt—of greater than 0.7 suggests an inability to wean, but this is a dynamic measurement and patients often show improvement over time. It becomes an accurate measure of subtle improvement in the long-term patient with a severe respiratory insult. In our experience, it may require up to 3 months of a stable respiratory situation before Vd/Vt improves and the criteria for weaning are reached.

Table 26–5. Systolic and Diastolic Pulmonary Artery Pressures Following Prolonged Mechanical Ventilatory Support*

Before Weaning	During Weaning	Day 1 Nitrates	Day 2 Weaned
60/29	80/12	47/24	35/17

*Note the major increase in systolic pressure observed during the weaning process. This was accompanied by pulmonary edema. Weaning proceeded smoothly in the face of nitrates.

Open lung biopsy sometimes reveals unsuspected and treatable disease. Ventilation-perfusion scanning may show areas of gross V/Q mismatch contributing to intrapulmonary shunt. Several patients fail weaning because of hemodynamic instability evident only during the weaning period. Insertion of a pulmonary artery catheter may uncover significant pulmonary arterial hypertension, which can be corrected with appropriate vasodilator therapy. Table 26–5 documents the results seen in a patient with left ventricular dysfunction and mitral valve replacement. The patient had failed numerous weaning attempts over several weeks. Once pulmonary artery pressures were controlled with sublingual nitrates, weaning proceeded rapidly and successfully.

Aubier and co-workers (1987) showed that digoxin improved diaphragmatic strength by 19.5% in ventilated patients with chronic obstructive lung disease. Its mechanism of action is unclear and its clinical significance is undergoing further evaluation.

Hemodynamic Monitoring

Patients undergoing pulmonary resection should be kept dry to reduce the parenchymal accumulation of fluid in the early postoperative period. This is especially important for those patients in respiratory failure. The desire for fluid restriction must be weighed against the need to maintain systemic perfusion. If necessary, low dose dopamine—less than 5 µg/kg/min—can be used to maintain renal perfusion, as evidenced by urine output greater than or equal to 35 ml/hr. In the face of a diminishing urine output or an increasing inotrope requirement, a Swan-Ganz catheter should be inserted to guide therapy. Table 26–6 outlines additional criteria for pulmonary arterial monitoring. Information obtained can be used to estimate left ventricular filling pressures by the pulmonary capillary wedge pressure. Determination of cardiac output is necessary to monitor oxygen delivery and may be adversely affected by increasing PEEP. The decision to infuse fluids, start inotropes, or institute vasodilator therapy is guided by the measurement of pul-

Table 26–6. Indications for Swan-Ganz Catheterization

Pulmonary edema with normal central venous pressure
Hypotension with normal or high central venous pressure
PEEP >10 cm H_2O
Recent myocardial ischemia or infarction
Previous failed wean
Significant inotrope requirements

monary arterial and systemic pressures and of cardiac output. When fluid infusion is required, colloids should be administered, especially if pulmonary capillary permeability is likely to be high. Crystalloid solutions are equally efficacious in raising filling pressures, but four times the volume of crystalloid is required when compared to colloid.

Following pneumonectomy, pulmonary pressures and pulmonary vascular resistance may rise considerably, because the entire cardiac output flows through the remaining lung. Pulmonary arterial hypertension may lead to right and then left ventricular failure. The use of vasodilators to modify left ventricular preload or afterload or both without sacrificing oxygen delivery or systemic perfusion requires the information obtainable with a pulmonary artery catheter.

Patients with a recent history of myocardial disease or with perioperative ischemic changes should be monitored to appreciate myocardial strain and work of breathing, particularly during the weaning process.

Complications of Swan-Ganz monitoring arise primarily during insertion of the catheters. Dysrhythmias such as premature ventricular beats and ventricular tachycardia are treated by withdrawal of the catheter with or without intravenous lidocaine—1 mg/kg. Recurrence of these rhythm disturbances on reinsertion demands intravenous antiarrhythmic drugs. Patients with left bundle-branch block should not be subjected to Swan-Ganz catheterization unless it is absolutely necessary. Establishment of a right bundle-branch block is a complication of catheter insertion and in these patients would result in complete heart block. If pulmonary arterial monitoring is required, a temporary transvenous pacemaker should be standing by before the catheter is placed.

The other major complication of these catheters is pulmonary artery disruption. This complication tends to occur in elderly patients with pulmonary artery hypertension. The commonest site is the origin of the right middle lobe artery. A traumatic bronchovascular fistula is created, leading to the endobronchial accumulation of blood. Important points of management are as follows. Firstly, the bleeding is from a low pressure system and usually stops spontaneously. Secondly, the immediate concern is protection of the airway—management includes vigorous suctioning, rigid bronchoscopy to clear blood and clots, and insertion of an endobronchial blocker to prevent further contamination. The immediate insertion of double-lumen tubes is to be condemned. Adequate suctioning is impossible, and asphyxia may result. As noted, a rigid bronchoscope provides ventilation and the ability to clear and control the airway. Thirdly, the pulmonary artery balloon should not be reinflated—it rarely tamponades the artery and probably leads to further tearing of the vessel wall. Fourthly, surgical resection may be necessary if a hemothorax develops or if an intraparenchymal hematoma is evident.

To minimize the risk of this complication, the catheter should only be advanced when the balloon is inflated. Between 1 and 1.5 ml of air should be necessary to occlude the vessel and produce a wedge tracing. The catheter should be withdrawn and reinserted if less than 1 ml of air occludes the artery.

COMPLICATIONS OF INTUBATION AND MECHANICAL VENTILATION

Airway

Stauffer and colleagues (1981) divided problems of achieving and maintaining an airway into those occurring early and late. Insertion of an endotracheal tube requires skill and practice. The incidence of failed attempts, inadvertent esophageal intubation, mouth or lip injury, and right main stem bronchus intubation is considerably higher in inexperienced hands. The commonest early complication is an inability to maintain the airway. In Stauffer and co-workers' (1981) report, 45% of early problems related to self-extubation, inability to seal the airway, or excessive cuff pressures required to maintain the seal. Early complications of tracheostomy include stomal infection and hemorrhage and the requirement for excessive cuff pressures.

All of these problems are easily overcome. Tubes should be well secured and patients constantly supervised. Inadvertent extubation requires a rapid reinsertion of the airway, providing high flow 100% oxygen while preparations are made. Tracheostomy tubes that fall out within 40 to 72 hours present a particular problem. Under such circumstances a fistulous track may not be established, suggesting that oral intubation may be safer and more expeditious. Any attempt to reinsert a tracheostomy tube should be undertaken with the patient in the operative position with neck extended and with support under the shoulders. The requirement for high cuff pressures to secure a seal is problematic. It suggests a capacious and dilated trachea. The insertion of a larger tube or the use of foam-cuff tubes usually solves the problem.

Late complications include tracheal stenosis either at the stoma site, cuff site, or the subglottic area. Late hemorrhage may be secondary to tracheal ulceration, pulmonary parenchymal pathology, or tracheo-innominate artery fistula. As the latter may present with a herald bleed, any hemorrhage in or around a tracheostomy tube deserves investigation. Fiber-optic bronchoscopy by way of the tube itself clears the airway and permits examination of the distal tracheobronchial tree and assessment of the extent of hemorrhage. If hemorrhage continues, the tracheostomy tube cuff should be hyperinflated and the tube tilted backwards, thus thrusting the cuff against the anterior tracheal wall. If the bleeding has stopped and no distal cause is apparent, the tracheostomy tube can be removed and bronchoscopy quickly conducted through the stoma to examine the anterior tracheal wall for ulceration. Continued hemorrhage may warrant intubation from above with an endotracheal tube or preferably with a rigid bronchoscope, removal of the tracheostomy tube, and digital control of the innominate artery, which is obtained by inserting the index finger into the airway and compressing the artery against the right sternoclavicular joint. Cooper (1977) described the procedure well.

Pulmonary Barotrauma

In the absence of direct thoracic trauma, bronchopleural fistulae result from high inspiratory pressures secondary to chest wall or parenchymal noncompliance. Tension pneumothorax is a surgical emergency requiring immediate decompression with a large-bore intravenous catheter followed by tube thoracostomy. Reviews by Shapiro and associates (1984) and Pierson and co-workers (1986) indicate a 2 to 7% incidence of clinical barotrauma in mechanically ventilated patients. Most can be managed by adjustment of conventional ventilators plus chest tube drainage. Jet ventilation may be required to manage large air leaks but has its own complications. Egol and associates (1985) described two cases of barotrauma and one case of hypotension secondary to use of jet ventilation. Our experience with 67 cases of ARDS employing high frequency jet ventilation noted pneumothoraces in 11 patients—16.4%.

Sepsis

Pulmonary sepsis is a major cause of postoperative morbidity and mortality. In a review of 327 ventilated patients by Gillespie and colleagues (1986), the mortality for patients with acute lung injury was 40% and rose to 81% when accompanied by multisystem failure. Aggressive pre- and postoperative physiotherapy is important in the high risk thoracic surgical patient. When pneumonia is suspect, accurate identification of infecting organisms is essential to guide antibiotic therapy. Cultures of tracheal aspirates, however, may represent contamination from the upper airway. Even washings obtained at bronchoscopy may be misleading. Protected brush specimens overcome these difficulties. The brush-containing cannula with its protective tip is advanced into a distal airway before the brush is extruded to collect the specimen. Immersing the brush in a standard volume of saline allows for quantification of the culture results. Presence of greater than 10^3 or 10^4 organisms/ml indicates a pathogenic organism. Johansen and colleagues (1988) reported that bronchoalveolar lavage and the protected brush specimen have reduced the need for open lung biopsy in the diagnosis of pulmonary infection, especially in the immunocompromised host. Candidal suprainfection is a devastating complication of prolonged antibiotic usage and is seen with increasing frequency in intensive care units. Frequent assessment of culture results and the reappraisal of antibiotic requirements reduce the incidence of this problem. Definition of the criteria of infection and the institution of appropriate therapy, as Soutter and one of the authors (T.R.T.) (1986) indicated, results in more reasonable success.

Other Complications

Lobar atelectasis can be improved by chest physiotherapy and bronchoscopy. Absorption atelectasis, oxygen toxicity, and positional hypoxemia were discussed previously. Gastrointestinal bleeding from stress ulceration is an uncommon complication but can be minimized by judicious use of antacids, sucralfate, or H_2 receptor antagonists. The role of gastric acidity and H_2 blockers in the upper respiratory colonization by gram-negative bacteria remains to be completely defined, but accumulating evidence, such as that of Dirks and associates (1987), suggests that cytoprotective agents such as sucralfate may avoid bacterial overgrowth and yet prevent gastrointestinal hemorrhage.

SPECIAL SITUATIONS

Flail Chest

Mechanical ventilation should not be considered a routine intervention in flail chest. Indications for mechanical support are the same as for any patient with respiratory failure and include arterial hypoxemia and hypercarbia unresponsive to conventional therapy. Experimentation by one of us (T.R.T.) and Shamji (1985) demonstrated that the unstable chest wall does lead to progressive hypoxemia even in the absence of pulmonary contusion. The ventilation-perfusion abnormality appears to be secondary to decreased pleural pressure on the ipsilateral side resulting in decreased regional ventilation. Considerable perfusion is maintained, resulting in hypoxemia. European authors, including Dor (1972), Eschapasse (1973) and Paris (1977) and their associates, reported large series of patients with flail chest managed by operative fixation of the unstable segment. The reports are anecdotal and uncontrolled, yet the observations are convincing. In practical terms, however, the indications for operative stabilization would include the inability to wean a patient from ventilatory support once the contusion has resolved and with maximal analgesia in the form of epidural narcotic administration. The requirement of a thoracotomy for other reasons should also lead one to stabilize the chest wall at the conclusion of the procedure.

Unilateral or Asymmetrical Lung Disease

Reduced compliance in one lung can lead to significant barotrauma on the uninvolved side as high airway pressures and PEEP are required to overcome the restriction on the diseased side. As discussed previously, application of PEEP in these circumstances can reduce arterial oxygenation through maldistribution of ventilation and perfusion. Siegel and associates (1985) promoted independent lung ventilation through a double-lumen endotracheal tube for patients with nonhomogeneous ARDS. Simultaneous independent ventilation reduced the intrapulmonary shunt and permitted a lowering of FIO_2 while maintaining an acceptable Pao_2. Each ventilator is separately programmed for tidal volume, PEEP, and I/E ratio. Modest hypoxemia can be corrected by positional changes. High frequency jet ventilation is also efficacious in these circumstances.

ARDS

There is nothing unique in the management of the adult respiratory distress syndrome. Corticosteroids have no benefit and may actually be deleterious (see Chapter 43).

Bronchopleural Fistula

Large volume bronchopleural fistulae are frequently worsened by conventional ventilation and, as discussed previously, are often amenable to closure when high frequency jet ventilation is employed. Where jet ventilation is not available or does not work, alternative techniques should be attempted. Increasing the volume of saline in the chest tube drainage bottle increases the pressure gradient against which the fistula must operate. Alternatively, ventilation to the affected segment can be eliminated by positioning a bronchial blocker into the appropriate orifice or by reverting to one-lung ventilation, isolating the affected side. In addition, despite large losses of administered tidal volume, the continued increase in tidal volume up to 2 L/breath helps re-expand the lung and provides adequate ventilatory support. Experience with tissue glue compounds to seal leaking airways is anecdotal but encouraging, as McCarthy and associates (1988) noted. In postpneumonectomy fistula, the pleural space can be opened and packed. In these situations, the patients should be transferred to an institution where jet ventilation is available.

REFERENCES

Albert, R.K., et al.: The prone position improves arterial oxygenation and reduces shunt in oleic-acid-induced acute lung injury. Am. Rev. Respir. Dis. 135:628, 1987.

Ali, J., et al.: Effect of postoperative intermittent positive pressure breathing on lung function. Chest 85:192, 1984.

Annest, S.J., et al.: Detrimental effects of removing end-expiratory pressure prior to extubation. Ann. Surg. 191:539, 1980.

Aubier, M., et al.: Effects of digoxin on diaphragmatic strength generation in patients with chronic obstructive pulmonary disease during acute respiratory failure. Am. Rev. Respir. Dis. 135:544, 1987.

Bartel, L.P., Bazik, J.R., and Powner, D.J.: Compression volume during mechanical ventilation: comparison of ventilators and tubing circuits. Crit. Care Med. 13:851, 1985.

Bartlett, R.H., et al.: Extracorporeal membrane oxygenation support for cardiopulmonary failure. J. Cardiovasc. Thorac. Surg. 73:375, 1977.

Bendixen, H.H., Smith, G.M., and Mead, J.: Pattern of ventilation in young adults. J. Appl. Physiol. 19:195, 1964.

Breivik, H., et al.: Normalizing low arterial CO_2 tension during mechanical ventilation. Chest 63:525, 1973.

Calvin, J.E., Driedger, A.A., and Sibbald, W.J.: Positive end-expiratory pressure (PEEP) does not depress left ventricular function in patients with pulmonary edema. Am. Rev. Respir. Dis. 124:121, 1981.

Carlon, G.C., et al.: Clinical experience with high frequency jet ventilation. Crit. Care Med. 9:1, 1981.

Cassidy, S.S., and Ramanathan, M.: Dimensional analysis of the left ventricle during PEEP: relative septal and lateral wall displacements. Am. J. Physiol. (Heart Circ. Physiol. 15) 246:H792, 1984.

Celli, B.R., Rodriguez, K.S., and Snider, G.L.: A controlled trial of intermittent positive pressure breathing, incentive spirometry and deep breathing exercise in preventing pulmonary complications after abdominal surgery. Am. Rev. Respir. Dis. 130:12, 1984.

Cherniak, R.: The oxygen consumption and efficiency of the respiratory muscles in health and emphysema. J. Clin. Invest. 38:494, 1959.

Churchill, E.D., and McNeil, D.: The reduction in vital capacity following operation. Surg. Gynecol. Obstet. 44:483, 1927.

Cohen, C.A., et al.: Clinical manifestations of inspiratory muscle fatigue. Am. J. Med. 73:308, 1982.

Cooper, J.D.: Tracheoinnominate artery fistula: successful management of 3 consecutive patients. Ann. Thorac. Surg. 24:439, 1977.

Daly, B.D.T., Edmonds, C.H., and Norman, J.C.: In vivo alveolar morphometrics with positive end expiratory pressure. Surg. Forum 24:217, 1973.

Dark, D.S., Pingleton, S.K., and Kerby, G.R.: Hypercapnia during weaning: a complication of nutritional support. Chest 88:141, 1985.

DeHaven, C.B., Hurst, J.M., and Branson, R.D.: Postextubation hypoxemia treated with a continuous positive airway pressure mask. Crit. Care Med. 13:46, 1985.

DeHaven, C.B., Hurst, J.M., and Branson, R.D.: Evaluation of two different extubation criteria: attributes contributing to success. Crit. Care Med. 14:92, 1986.

Dor, V., et al.: Les traumatismes graves du thorax, place de l'osteosynthese dans leur traitement—100 cas. Nouvelle Presse Medicale 1:519, 1972.

Dorinsky, P.M., and Whitcomb, M.E.: The effect of PEEP on cardiac output. Chest 84:210, 1983.

Downs, J.B., Klein, E.F., and Modell, J.H.: The effects of incremental PEEP on Pao$_2$ in patients with respiratory failure. Anesth. Analg. 52:210, 1973.

Driks, M.A., et al.: Nosocomial pneumonia in intubated patients given sucralfate as compared with antacids or histamine type 2 blockers: the role of gastric colonization. New Engl. J. Med. 317:1376, 1987.

Egan, T., et al.: Experience with ECMO for hypoxemic respiratory failure. Chest 94:681, 1988.

Egbert, L.D., and Bendixen, H.H.: Effect of morphine on breathing pattern: a possible factor in atelectasis. J.A.M.A. 188:485, 1964.

Egol, A., Culpepper, J.A., and Snyder, J.V.: Barotrauma and hypotension resulting from jet ventilation in critically ill patients. Chest 88:98, 1985.

Eschapasse, H., and Gaillard, J.: Volets thoraciques: principes de traitement. Ann. Chir. Thorac. Cardiovasc. 12:1, 1973.

Fee, H.J., et al.: Role of pulmonary vascular resistance measurements in preoperative evaluation of candidates for pulmonary resection. J. Thorac. Cardiovasc. Surg. 75:519, 1978.

Fisher, A.B., Forman, H.J., and Glass, M.: Mechanisms of pulmonary oxygen toxicity. Lung 162:255, 1984.

Gillespie, D.J., et al.: Clinical outcome of respiratory failure in patients requiring prolonged (>24 hours) mechanical ventilation. Chest 90:364, 1986.

Girotti, M.J., et al.: Simultaneous use of membrane oxygenation and high-frequency jet ventilation in acute pulmonary failure. Crit. Care Med. 14:511, 1986.

Goldman, L., et al.: Multifactorial index of cardiac risk in noncardiac surgical procedures. N. Engl. J. Med. 297:845, 1977.

Hammon, J.W., et al.: The effect of positive end-expiratory pressure on regional ventilation and perfusion in the normal and injured primate lung. J. Thorac. Cardiovasc. Surg. 72:680, 1976.

Harris, S.D., Johanson, W.G., Jr., and Pierce, A.K.: Bacterial lung clearance in hypoxic mice. Am Rev. Respir. Dis. 111:910, 1975.

Harwood, S.J.: Venovenous ECMO—a rapid percutaneous method for patients in severe respiratory distress. Transplant. Implant. Today 3:44, 1986.

Hasan, F.M., et al.: Influence of lung injury on pulmonary wedge-left atrial pressure correlation during positive end-expiratory pressure ventilation. Am. Rev. Respir. Dis. 131:246, 1985.

Haynes, J.B.: Positive end-expiratory pressure shifts left ventricular diastolic pressure-area curves. J. Appl. Physiol. (Respir. Environ. Exercise Physiol.) 48:670, 1980.

Hussain, S.N.A., and Roussos, C.: Distribution of respiratory muscle and organ blood flow during endotoxemic shock in dogs. J. Appl. Physiol. 59:1802, 1985.

Hylkema, B.S., et al.: Lung mechanical profiles in acute respiratory failure: diagnostic and prognostic value of compliance at different tidal volumes. Crit. Care Med. 13:637, 1985.

Jackson, R.M.: Pulmonary oxygen toxicity. Chest 88:900, 1985.

Jardin, F., et al.: Influence of positive end-expiratory pressure on left ventricular performance. N. Engl. J. Med. 304:387, 1981.

Johanson, W.G., Jr., et al.: Bacteriologic diagnosis of nosocomial pneumonia following prolonged mechanical ventilation. Am. Rev. Respir. Dis. 137:259, 1988.

Johnson, A.N., Cooper, D.F., and Edwards, R.H.: Exertion of stair-climbing in normal subjects and in patients with chronic obstructive bronchitis. Thorax 32:711, 1977.

Juhl, B., and Frost, N.: A comparison between measured and calculated changes in the lung function after operation for pulmonary cancer. Acta Anaesthesiol. Scand. 57(Suppl.):39, 1975.

Kanarek, D.J., and Shannon, D.C.: Adverse effect of positive end-expiratory pressure on pulmonary perfusion and arterial oxygenation. Am. Rev. Respir. Dis. 112:457, 1975.

Karliner, J.S., Coomaiaswamy, R., and Williams, M.H.: Relationship between preoperative pulmonary function studies and prognosis of patients undergoing pneumonectomy for carcinoma of the lung. Dis. Chest 54:32, 1968.

Kristersson, S., Lindell, S.E., and Svanberg, L.: Prediction of pulmonary function loss due to pneumonectomy using ^{133}Xe-radiospirometry. Chest 62:694, 1972.

Laros, C.D., and Swierenga, J.: Temporary unilateral pulmonary artery occlusion in the preoperative evaulation of patients with bronchial carcinoma. Med. Thorac. 24:269, 1967.

Latimer, R.G., et al.: Ventilatory patterns and pulmonary complications after upper abdominal surgery determined by preoperative and postoperative computerized spirometry and blood gas analysis. Am. J. Surg. 122:622, 1971.

Liebman, P.R., et al.: The mechanism of depressed cardiac output on positive end-expiratory pressure (PEEP). Surgery 83:594, 1978.

Lockwood, P.: The principles of predicting risk of post-thoracotomy function-related complications in bronchogenic carcinoma. Respiration 30:329, 1973.

Lores, M.E., et al.: Cardiovascular effects of positive end-expiratory pressure (PEEP) after pneumonectomy in dogs. Ann. Thorac. Surg. 40:464, 1985.

Lucking, S.E., et al.: High-frequency ventilation versus conventional ventilation in dogs with right ventricular dysfunction. Crit. Care Med. 14:798, 1986.

MacIntyre, N.R., et al.: Jet ventilation at 100 breaths per minute in adult respiratory failure. Am. Rev. Respir. Dis. 134:897, 1986.

Malina, J.R., et al.: Clinical evaluation of high-frequency positive pressure ventilation (HFPPV) in patients scheduled for open-chest surgery. Anesth. Analg. 60:324, 1981.

Marini, J.J., Rodriguez, M., and Lamb, V.: The inspiratory workload of patient-initiated mechanical ventilation. Am. Rev. Respir. Dis. 134:902, 1986.

McAslan, T.C., et al.: Influence of inhalation of 100% oxygen on intrapulmonary shunt in severely traumatized patients. J. Trauma 13:811, 1973.

McCarthy, P.M., et al.: The effectiveness of fibrin glue sealant for reducing experimental pulmonary air leak. Ann. Thorac. Surg. 45:203, 1988.

Mittman, C.: Assessment of operative risk in thoracic surgery. Am. Rev. Respir. Dis. 84:197, 1961.

Miyoshi, S., et al.: Exercise tolerance tests in lung cancer patients: the relationship between exercise capacity and post-thoracotomy hospital mortality. Ann. Thorac. Surg. 44:487, 1987.

Morganroth, M.L., et al.: Criteria for weaning from prolonged mechanical ventilation. Arch. Intern. Med. 144:1012, 1984.

Olsen, G.N., et al.: Pulmonary function evaluation of the lung resection candidate: a prospective study. Am. Rev. Respir. Dis. 111:379, 1975.

Panos, A., Demajo, W., and Todd, T.R.: High frequency jet ventilation in the management of bronchopleural fistula (BPF). Chest 89(Suppl.):521S, 1986.

Paris, F.: Surgical fixation of traumatic flail chest. *In* The fourth Coventry conference: Trauma of the chest. Edited by W.G. Williams and R.E. Smith. Wright. p. 20, 1977.

Pierson, D.J., Horton, C.A., and Bates, P.W.: Persistent bronchopleural air leak during mechanical ventilation: a review of 39 cases. Chest 90:321, 1986.

Pontoppidan, H., Geffin, B., and Lowenstein, E.: Medical progress: acute respiratory failure in the adult. N. Engl. J. Med. 287:743, 1972.

Potkin, R.T., et al.: Effect of positive end-expiratory pressure on right and left ventricular function in patients with the adult respiratory distress syndrome. Am. Rev. Respir. Dis. *135*:307, 1987.

Powers, S.R., et al.: Physiologic consequences of positive end-expiratory pressure (PEEP) ventilation. Ann. Surg. *178*:265, 1973.

Prys-Roberts, C., et al.: Radiographically undetectable pulmonary collapse in the supine position. Lancet *2*:399, 1967.

Quan, S.F., Falltrick, R.T., and Schlobohm, R.M.: Extubation from ambient or expiratory positive airway pressure in adults. Anesthesiology *55*:53, 1981.

Qvist, J., et al.: Hemodynamic responses to mechanical ventilation with PEEP. Anesthesiology *42*:45, 1975.

Rice, T.W., et al.: The mini-membrane—a new method of extracorporeal membrane oxygenation (ECMO) for profound acute respiratory failure. Clin. Invest. Med. *9*:A8, 1986.

Rivara, D., et al.: Positional hypoxemia during artificial ventilation. Crit. Care Med. *12*:436, 1984.

Roussos, C.: Ventilatory failure and respiratory muscles. *In* The Thorax, part B. Edited by C. Roussos and P.T. Macklem. New York, Marcel Dekker, 1985, p. 1253.

Sanchez de Leon, R., et al.: Positive end-expiratory pressure may decrease arterial oxygen tension in the presence of a collapsed lung region. Crit. Care Med. *13*:392, 1985.

Scharff, S.M., Caldini, P., and Ingram, R.H., Jr.: Cardiovascular effects of increasing airway pressure in the dog. Am. J. Physiol. *232*:H35, 1977.

Shapiro, B.A., and Walton, J.R.: Ventilatory support of the postoperative patient. *In* General Thoracic Surgery. Edited by T.W. Shields. Philadelphia, Lea & Febiger, 1982.

Shapiro, B.A., Cane, R.D., and Harrison, R.A.: Positive end-expiratory pressure therapy in adults with special reference to acute lung injury: a review of the literature and suggested clinical correlations. Crit. Care. Med. *12*:127, 1984.

Shapiro, B.A., Harrison, R.A., and Walton, J.R.: Clinical Application of Blood Gases, 2nd ed. Chicago, Year Book Medical Publishers, 1977.

Shapiro, B.A., et al.: Clinical Application of Respiratory Care, 3rd ed. Chicago, Year Book Medical Publishers, 1985.

Siegel, J.H., et al.: Quantification of asymmetric lung pathophysiology as a guide to the use of simultaneous independent lung ventilation in posttraumatic and septic adult respiratory distress syndrome. Ann. Surg. *202*:425, 1985.

Solca, M., et al.: Multidisciplinary approach to extracorporeal respiratory assist for acute pulmonary failure. Int. Surg. *70*:9, 1985.

Soutter, I., and Todd, T.R.J.: Systemic candidiasis in a surgical intensive care unit. Can. J. Surg. *29*:1997, 1986.

Stauffer, J.L., Olson, D.E., and Petty, T.L.: Complications and consequences of endotracheal intubation and tracheostomy: a prospective study of 150 critically ill adult patients. Am. J. Med. *70*:65, 1981.

Stock, M.C., et al.: Prevention of postoperative pulmonary complications with CPAP, incentive spirometry and conservative therapy. Chest *87*:151, 1985.

Suter, P.M., Fairley, H.B., and Isenberg, M.D.: Optimum end-expiratory airway pressure in patients with acute pulmonary failure. N. Engl. J. Med. *292*:284, 1975.

Tisi, G.M.: State of the art: preoperative evaluation of pulmonary function. Am. Rev. Respir. Dis. *119*:293, 1979.

Tittley, J.G., et al.: Hemodynamic and myocardial metabolic consequences of PEEP. Chest *88*:496, 1985.

Todd, T.R.J., Baile, E.M., and Hogg, J.C.: Pulmonary artery wedge pressure in hemorrhagic shock. Am. Rev. Respir. Dis. *118*:613, 1978.

Todd, T.R., and Shamji, F.: Pathophysiology of chest wall trauma. *In* The Thorax, part B. Edited by C. Roussos and P.T. Mackem. New York, Marcel Dekker, 1985, p. 979.

Tyler, D.C.: Positive end-expiratory pressure: a review. Crit. Care Med. *11*:300, 1983.

Viires, N., et al.: Regional blood flow distribution in dog during induced hypotension and low cardiac output. J. Clin. Invest. *72*:935, 1983.

West, J.B., Dollery, C.T., and Naimark, A.: Distribution of blood flow in isolated lung: relation to vascular and alveolar pressures. J. Appl. Physiol. *19*:713, 1964.

Zapal, W.M., et al.: Extracorporeal membrane oxygenation in severe acute respiratory failure: a randomized prospective study. J.A.M.A. *242*:2193, 1979.

Zikria, B.A., et al.: Alterations in ventilatory function and breathing patterns following surgical trauma. Ann. Surg. *179*:1, 1974.

CHAPTER 27

PHYSICAL THERAPY FOR THE THORACIC SURGICAL PATIENT

Ralph Braunschweig

Prevention of postoperative pulmonary complications after thoracic surgery is a team responsibility, and the physical therapist is an important member of that team. The goals of chest physical therapy are to: maintain or improve ventilation, prevent atelectasis, mobilize and drain secretions, maintain or regain full expansion of the lungs, maintain mobility of the spine and shoulder girdle, prevent postoperative venous thrombosis by mobilization of the lower extremities, and improve cardiopulmonary exercise tolerance. The range of services provided by a physical therapy department for the thoracic surgical patient include: preoperative assessment, preoperative patient education and training, postural drainage of secretions from the lungs, chest wall percussion and vibration, cough assistance, suctioning, deep breathing exercises, patient mobilization with special attention to the shoulder girdle, as well as a general fitness program to increase endurance in daily activities, and the application of transcutaneous electrical nerve stimulation—TENS—for control of pain.

Postoperative pulmonary complications are presumed to be caused by decreased lung volume. The classic studies by Beecher (1933a, 1933b) showed that following laparotomy tidal volume, inspiratory and expiratory reserves, residual volume, and functional residual capacity—FRC—all decreased. Many others have confirmed Beecher's findings, and Ali and colleagues (1974) showed that the decrease in FRC after thoracic surgery was less than that after upper abdominal operations. As summarized by Bartlett and his associates (1973), a lack of deep breaths is a basic causative mechanism of postoperative pulmonary complications.

CRITICAL EVALUATION OF PHYSICAL THERAPY

The precise value of physical therapy modalities to the patient is difficult to assess because other factors, such as the patient's preoperative pulmonary function, the surgeon's technique, the anesthetic management, and the intensity of nursing and surgical postoperative care, make simultaneous contributions toward the reduction in morbidity and mortality rates following a thoracic surgical procedure. Few data exist concerning the influence of physical therapy on the incidence of postoperative pulmonary complications following thoracic operations. Thoren (1954) documented a reduction in the incidence of postoperative pulmonary complications following upper abdominal operations from 42% to 12% when therapy included preoperative training; diaphragmatic, deep breathing; and coughing exercises with postural drainage. Wiklander and Norlin (1957) compared a group of patients receiving physical therapy with a group of controls. The incidence of moderate and severe collapse was cut in half in the treated group. Stein and Cassara (1970) reviewed the incidence of postoperative pulmonary complications in patients with normal and abnormal pulmonary function tests. They confirmed the low incidence of such complications in the group defined as "low risk." Among the "high risk" surgical patients, postoperative pulmonary complications developed in 5 of 23—22%—patients receiving physical therapy and 15 of 25—60%—controls, suggesting the effectiveness of the treatment.

Physical therapy can also be administered to patients receiving mechanical assistance to ventilation. Winning and associates (1975, 1977) reported a lower mean alveolar pressure and improved oxygenation after treatment, especially among patients with increased secretions. Mackenzie and associates (1980) demonstrated a significant increase in total lung/thorax compliance after postural drainage enhanced by percussion and vibration in mechanically ventilated patients. Ciesla and colleagues (1981) found dramatic improvement in oxygenation after bronchial drainage with percussion and vibration in patients with hypotension who were receiving mechanical ventilation with high levels of positive end-expiratory pressure—PEEP. In contrast, a decrease in the mean partial pressure of arterial oxygen during and immediately after chest physical therapy was found in studies by Newton and Stephenson (1978), Gormezano and Branthwaite (1972a, 1972b), and Holloway and co-workers (1966, 1969). This decrease was most often seen in critically ill patients or in patients following cardiac surgery with cardiovascular instability.

Because advanced age is an additional risk factor for postoperative pulmonary complications, Castillo and Haas (1985) studied, in patients over 65 years old, the effects of pre-and postoperative chest physical therapy treatment, including bronchodilation followed by modified postural drainage, percussion and vibration, breathing exercises, and incentive spirometry. They confirmed work by Thoren (1954), Stein and Cassara (1970), and others, who found that initiating chest physical therapy before patients are in pain, highly anxious, and dulled by medication helps them learn the procedures quickly and effectively, and that post-thoracotomy atelectasis was reduced from 59% to 0. The incidence of pneumonia was not significantly affected. In the preoperative period, patients should be encouraged to stop smoking, although no hard data exist on the required time of smoking cessation for adequate reduction in sputum production and improved mucociliary function.

Other investigators have examined the benefits of individual components of chest physical therapy. The effects of deep breathing on arterial oxygenation were studied by Ward and associates (1966) with coaching by a physical therapist with and without a 5-second hold and by Hedstrand and co-workers (1978) using the incentive spirometer and two other deep-breathing devices. They found that all produced about the same improvement in oxygenation. Grimby (1974) showed that breathing exercises given to the patient after surgery improve chest wall mobility. Vraciu and Vraciu (1977) studied the effect of adding breathing exercises taught by physical therapists to a regimen of incentive spirometry, ultrasonic nebulization, and routine instruction in deep breathing and coughing by nurses in postoperative cardiothoracic surgery patients. Although there was no significant difference in the incidence of postoperative pulmonary complications in the low risk groups, the high risk experimental group had an incidence of only 8% compared with 46% in the "routine" treatment group.

The effect of bronchoscopy in removing secretions from the airway and reducing atelectasis was summarized by Marini (1984). Mucus plugs of the central airways that can be visualized with the fiber-optic bronchoscope are rare to nonexistent in patients who are well hydrated and whose inspired gases during and after anesthesia are nearly saturated with humidity at body temperature. Bronchoscopy allows the instillation of 0.25% saline solution and extraction of central airway secretions; however, even when performed with supplemental ventilation through an endotracheal tube, it often produces bronchospasm, coughing, and arterial desaturation. In general, secretion retention should be treated with chest physical therapy of sufficient frequency and duration to mobilize the secretions, and bronchoscopy should be reserved for patients with persistent radiologic findings

of atelectasis after 12 to 16 hours of adequate physical therapy.

DEFINING THE TREATMENT PLAN

By consulting the physical therapy department several days before the planned procedure, the surgeon can obtain maximum benefit for his patients through preoperative assessment and training. The consultation request should contain the following information: the date and extent of the planned procedure, medical conditions that influence therapy, specific instructions that the surgeon may have given the patient that need to be reinforced by the therapist, e.g., smoking cessation, and the goals the surgeon seeks to achieve. To permit proper assessment, the medical record should contain a history of response to previous anesthesia and surgery, exercise tolerance, results of pulmonary function tests, chest roentgenograms, and arterial blood gases. If metastatic lesions are suspected, roentgenograms or bone scans of other areas of the body should also be available. The clinical evaluation by the physical therapist allows development of rapport between the patient and the therapist, formulation of a plan specific for that patient's condition, determination and treatment effectiveness, and patient education prior to surgery. After completing the assessment, the physical therapist enters the findings in the patient record and contacts the surgeon to discuss the plan for pre- and postoperative physical therapy, as well as the criteria for monitoring treatment effectiveness. At this point, the therapist may write the specific orders to be countersigned by the surgeon.

TREATMENT MODALITIES

Postural Drainage

Objectives

The aim of postural drainage is to use change of position and gravity to assist in mobilizing retained secretions and directing them toward the main bronchi and carina from which they may be coughed up or removed by suctioning. Knowledge of the anatomic ramifications and topographic relationships of the tracheobronchial tree (see Chapters 4 and 11) is mandatory to understand the appropriate positions for drainage of the various segments of the lung.

Technique

All the basal segments of the patient's lower lobes drain when the foot of the bed is raised; usually 18 inches is all that is required. Anterior basal segments drain when the patient is in the dorsal head-down position (Fig. 27–1). Lateral basal segments drain when the patient is in the lateral head-down position (Fig. 27–2). Posterior basal segments drain when the patient is lying prone with the head down (Fig. 27–3).

The medial basal segment of the right lower lobe drains when the patient is in the same position as that used for

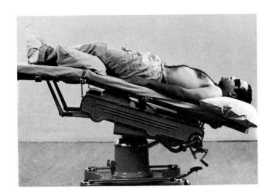

Fig. 27–1.   Position for draining the anterior segments of both lower lobes.

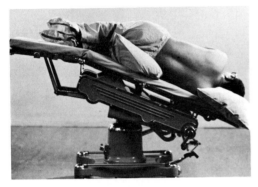

Fig. 27–2.   Position for draining the lateral segments of the left lower lobe.

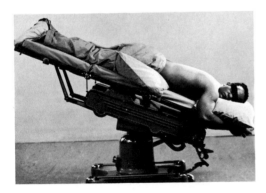

Fig. 27–3.   Position for draining the posterior segments of both lower lobes.

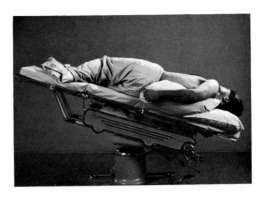

Fig. 27–4.   Position for draining the lingula.

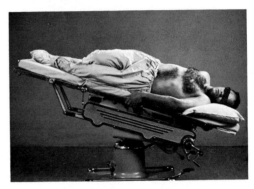

Fig. 27–5.   Position for draining the middle lobe.

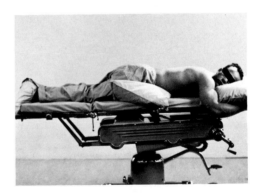

Fig. 27–6.   Position for draining the superior segments of both lower lobes.

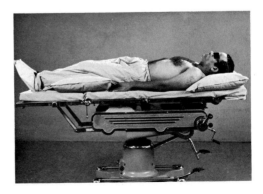

Fig. 27–7.   Position for draining the anterior segments of both upper lobes.

draining the lateral basal segment on the opposite side. The right middle lobe and lingula drain with the body rotated 45° about its long axis with the foot of the bed raised 18 inches. The lingula drains when the patient's left side is uppermost and the right middle lobe drains when the right side is uppermost. A pillow beneath one shoulder and hip helps hold the patient in position (Figs. 27–4, 27–5).

The superior segments of the lower lobes drain when the bed is horizontal and the patient is prone (Fig. 27–6). The anterior segments of both upper lobes drain when the patient lies supine with the bed horizontal (Fig. 27–7). To drain the left anterior segment, it is advantageous to raise the foot of the bed and turn the patient with slight rotation in the long axis of the body, because when the anterior segment has drained as far as the distal end of the left main stem bronchus, the secretions still must traverse 5 cm of this bronchus to reach the carina. If reflexes are intact, the patient will cough when secretions reach the distal end of the main stem bronchus, so raising the foot of the bed and turning the patient as described should rarely be needed. On the right side, the right main stem bronchus traverses only a short distance to the carina and the basic position thus needs no modification. The right apical segment drains while the patient is sitting (Fig. 27–8). The posterior segment of the right upper lobe drains with the patient turned 45° toward the prone position with the bed horizontal. The patient's left arm is placed behind the body and the upper hip is flexed with the knee bent. A pillow is used for support to prevent the patient from falling forward (Fig. 27–9). The left apical-posterior segment (Fig. 27–10) drains with the patient in the opposite position, but with the head of the bed raised so that the shoulder is elevated 14 inches. The right arm lies behind the body (Fig. 27–11).

Mechanical Stimulation of the Chest Wall

Objectives

After the patient has been placed in the appropriate postural drainage position, mechanical stimulation of the chest wall by percussion and vibration can help move secretions from the periphery toward the collecting seg-

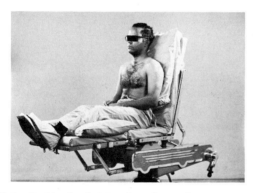

Fig. 27–8. Position for draining the right apical segment.

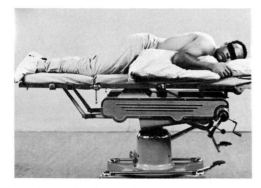

Fig. 27–9. Position for draining the posterior segment of the right upper lobe.

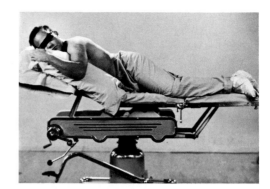

Fig. 27–10. Position for draining the apical posterior segment of the left upper lobe (view from front).

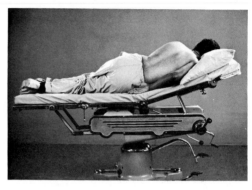

Fig. 27–11. Position for draining the apical-posterior segment of the left upper lobe (view from behind).

mental bronchi. Mackenzie and associates (1980) showed, in mechanically ventilated patients, that even in the absence of increased sputum production, atelectatic areas of the lung can be reinflated and total lung/ thorax compliance can be increased following percussion and vibration.

Techniques

The physical therapist places the patient in the appropriate postural drainage position and delivers rhythmical "clapping" strokes with cupped hands to the chest wall over the affected area of the lung. The air cushion between the cupped hand and the chest wall generates the typical hollow sound, transmits the energy to the underlying lung, and helps mobilize secretions. The strokes are performed rapidly during inspiration and expiration and should not be painful to the patient. After sufficient treatment time—3 to 5 minutes—over a given area, the physical therapist compresses the chest with vibratory movements during each expiration for several breaths and then attempts to make the patient cough or suctions the secretions derived from that area, before proceeding to the next.

Precautions

Before beginning the treatment, the therapist must ensure that ventilator tubing, endotracheal tubes, chest tubes, and other drains are secure and allow for movement without becoming dislodged. Unstable rib or thoracic spine fractures, or both, and coagulation defects, as well as increased intracranial pressure and lung abscess, are contraindications to mechanical stimulation, and the anticipated benefit must be weighed carefully against the risk of aggravating the underlying condition. Proper hand position is essential to the success of percussion and vibration. The patient's skin should be observed for evidence of erythema, soft tissue trauma, and petechiae.

Huffing and Coughing

Objectives

The rapid, forceful expulsion of air from the lungs helps remove secretions from the large airways. In coughing, the patient closes his glottis and builds up intrathoracic pressure before suddenly releasing the air. In huffing, air is expelled without closure of the glottis. Huffing is less likely to induce bronchospasm and may increase intracranial pressure less than repetitive coughing. Although huffing has not been studied in the postoperative patient, it seems to be almost as effective as coughing and less painful.

Technique

Adequate analgesia should be established before inducing a cough, and the physical therapist should support the patient's chest, especially in the area of the incision. The patient should be taught to support his own chest to allow effective coughing when the nurse or therapist is not at the bedside. The patient is instructed to take a deep breath, close his glottis, contract the muscles of expiration, and suddenly open his glottis to produce a cough. If the trachea is intubated, the patient will be unable to close his glottis, but rapid, forceful exhalation will help move secretions centrally so they can be removed by suctioning.

Precautions

Secretions must be kept thin and liquid; this can best be done by careful attention to the patient's hydration, as well as by heated humidification of inspired gases, especially for the patient with an artificial airway. Avoid repetitive coughing, as it may induce bronchospasm. If the patient cannot take an adequate breath, manual inflation with a bag-valve mask or mechanical ventilation can be used.

Suctioning

Objectives

There are two specific levels of suctioning: oropharyngeal, for patients who are unable to cough effectively to expectorate secretions, and tracheobronchial, to remove secretions from the larger airways of patients who are intubated. Some practitioners believe that even in the absence of an artificial airway passing a catheter into the trachea is a valuable technique, provided it is done carefully. Others believe it should not be used because of the risks of laryngeal irritation, laryngospasm, and

vagal stimulation. In any case, the only indication for suctioning is the presence of secretions in the airway.

Technique

Suctioning of secretions from the airway requires sterile technique and supplemental oxygen. After preoxygenating the patient by manually assisted ventilation with 100% oxygen, a sterile suction catheter is picked up with a sterile, gloved hand and attached to a vacuum source. The catheter is advanced, without suction being applied, until the tip is in proper position at the carina, then suction is applied by intermittently occluding the vent with a finger, and the catheter is withdrawn slowly with a rotating motion.

Precautions

Sterile technique must always be used to reduce the risk of infection. The suction catheter should be less than half the diameter of the artificial airway to allow enough space around the catheter for air to enter and to avoid applying suction to the lung itself. Hypoxemia can be prevented by preoxygenation, avoiding suction while advancing the catheter, limiting the force of suction to less than 120 mm Hg, limiting the duration of the total suctioning process to 20 seconds, and by re-expanding the lung with 100% oxygen following each procedure. For patients who become bradycardic during properly performed suctioning, a fiber-optic swivel adapter can be used to ventilate with supplemental oxygen and maintain PEEP during suctioning. During fiber-optic bronchoscopy, excessive use of the suction port to clear secretions from the tip can lead to hypoxemia. Monitoring of blood pressure and the electrocardiogram are recommended because hypotension and cardiac dysrhythmias may occur during or shortly after suctioning. They are usually caused by hypoxemia, hypercarbia, or vagal stimulation.

Breathing Exercises and Patient Mobilization

Objectives

Breathing exercises taught to patients in the preoperative period can reduce the effects of altered breathing patterns after thoracotomy and can help to obtain full expansion of the chest wall during spontaneous breathing. This is essential to help restore lung function and to prevent subsequent chest deformity. In addition, early upper and lower extremity exercises and early ambulation decrease the incidence of pulmonary embolism, and range-of-motion exercises and posture correction may prevent musculoskeletal dysfunction, especially frozen shoulder, following thoracotomy. Before the patient is discharged from the hospital, a program of graded exercises to regain a cardiorespiratory reserve should be taught.

Techniques

Relaxation Exercises. The patient is made comfortable in the supine position with pillows supporting the head, arms, and knees, with the neck and hips slightly flexed. The arms should be at the patient's sides with the palms down and the thumbs touching the body. The therapist demonstrates the difference between contraction and relaxation of individual muscles starting from the hand and working upward to the shoulders and neck. The patient should repeat these exercises many times.

Localized Breathing Exercises. Pressure is applied over the area resisting active muscular contraction to mobilize natural respiratory forces. This helps to fix the attention of the patient to the area, suggests the direction of effort, and tends to decrease activity in previously overworked parts of the chest. Practice before surgery improves the actions of the inspiratory muscles and helps the therapist determine precisely what the patient can do, so that after surgery, when certain parts of the chest move poorly, it is easy to recognize where assistance is needed before additional function is lost. Restoration of the proper movement is begun on one side before it is applied bilaterally.

The palms of the hands are used to apply pressure on all areas except over the upper lobes, where the fingers are used as well as the palms. The pressure should be firm but not so excessive as to make the patient give up and cause movement to begin elsewhere in the chest wall. The patient should think in terms of expanding against pressure rather than inspiration. The pressure is reduced only when full inspiration has been attained. During exhalation, the hands of the therapist are relaxed, but just before inspiration, the ribs are pressed slightly inward. The therapist then uses the patient's hands to press against the active chest movements. These exercises are given with the patient lying well supported by pillows in the same position as for relaxation. Later they can be performed in either the sitting or standing position. Diaphragmatic or lateral basal expansion is usually begun first, then posterior basal expansion, and finally apical pectoral expansion.

Lateral Basal Expansion. The palm of one hand is placed in the mid-axillary line over the lower ribs. Pressure is applied at the end of exhalation and continues through inspiration. The patient is told to expand the ribs in the direction of the hand on that side. Pressure is relaxed at the end of inspiration. The other side of the chest should be relaxed. When expansion has increased on one side, pressure is then applied to both sides of the chest.

Upper Lateral Expansion. The technique for upper lateral expansion is the same as that for lateral basal expansion except that the hands are placed immediately below the axilla.

Apical Pectoral Expansion. For apical pectoral expansion, pressure is applied with the fingertips above the clavicles and the hands on the pectoral muscles below the clavicles. The patient expands the chest forward and upward against the pressure of the therapist's hands.

Diaphragmatic Breathing Exercises. Diaphragmatic breathing is an important exercise for all thoracic surgical patients, because the diaphragm is the most powerful muscle of ventilation. It affects the expansion of the bases of the lungs, which are prone to infection after surgery. There are several variations of diaphragmatic exercises

for specific purposes, but the one described here is adapted best for patients having thoracic surgery.

The patient lies with knees bent and supported on pillows so that the hips are slightly flexed. The therapist's hands should rest lightly on the anterior rib cage so the therapist is aware of anterolateral movement. During expiration, the patient contracts the abdominal muscles. These are then relaxed for inspiration. Epigastric compression may be applied at the beginning of inspiration. The patient attempts to prolong each exhalation for periods of up to 15 seconds without losing control of the next inspiration. After thoracic surgery, the patient may breathe predominantly with the apices of the lungs. This should be pointed out to the patient and the therapist should demonstrate how the upper parts relax when the abdominal muscles are used during exhalation.

MODIFICATION IN PHYSICAL THERAPY TECHNIQUES FOR SPECIFIC THORACIC OPERATIONS

Empyema

Localized breathing exercises should not be used for patients in the acute stage of empyema. They may be used later to help the lung expand.

Pneumonectomy

Localized and diaphragmatic breathing exercises should be performed mainly on the normal side. Postural drainage is contraindicated postoperatively if the pericardium has been opened. These patients should be taught to "huff." Arm movements should be encouraged and the patients should be ambulatory within 24 hours following the operation.

Lobectomy or Thoracotomy

In lobectomy or thoracotomy, localized breathing exercises should be performed, particularly on the side of operation. When bronchiectasis is present, diaphragmatic breathing exercises, coughing, and postural drainage with percussion and vibration are especially valuable. Percussion should not be used when hemoptysis is present.

Decortication

Following decortication, lung expansion should be encouraged by having the patient perform the localized breathing exercises that were practiced before surgery. After surgery, these exercises should be performed as soon as the patient is able to cooperate. Percussion and vibration are contraindicated in the early postoperative period.

TRANSCUTANEOUS ELECTRICAL NERVE STIMULATION

Objectives

Transcutaneous electrical nerve stimulation—TENS—is the application of an electric current to peripheral nerves by externally applied electrodes to produce analgesia without respiratory depression or cardiovascular side effects. Warfield and associates (1985) delivered TENS by peri-incisional electrodes in the immediate postoperative period and demonstrated shorter recovery room stays and better tolerance of chest physical therapy for bronchial hygiene. Using similar techniques, Navarathnam and co-workers (1984) showed significant improvement in forced vital capacity among the patients receiving TENS, whereas Rooney and associates (1983) also confirmed decreased narcotic requirements in a similar group of patients following thoracotomy. Pain control with TENS also allows the patient to cooperate more fully with the therapist during deep breathing, coughing, and range-of-motion exercises.

Techniques

Sterile electrodes are applied in the operating room to the skin adjacent to the incision before the dressing is applied, and connecting cables are attached and secured. When the patient regains consciousness, the cables are attached to the stimulator and the pulse width, frequency, and amplitude are adjusted for maximum patient comfort.

Precautions

Although no clear contraindications to TENS have been established, use caution in applying electrical stimuli to patients who depend on a demand cardiac pacemaker. The pulse and electrocardiogram should be monitored when initiating treatment to determine if the output of the pacemaker is inhibited by the TENS unit.

REFERENCES

Ali, J., et al.: Consequences of postoperative alteration in respiratory mechanics. Am. J. Surg. *128*:376, 1974.
Bartlett, R., et al.: Respiratory maneuvers to prevent postoperative pulmonary complications: a critical review. J.A.M.A. *224*:7, 1973.
Beecher, H.K.: The measured effect of laparotomy on respiration. J. Clin. Invest. *12*:639, 1933a.
Beecher, H.K.: Effect of laparotomy on lung volume: demonstration of a new type of pulmonary collapse. J. Clin. Invest. *12*:651, 1933b.
Castillo, R., and Haas, A.: Chest physical therapy: comparative efficacy of preoperative and postoperative in the elderly. Arch. Phys. Med. Rehabil. *66*:376, 1985.
Ciesla, N., et al.: Chest physical therapy to the patient with multiple trauma: two case studies. Phys. Ther. *61*:202, 1981.
de la Rocha, A.G., and Chambers, K.: Pain amelioration after thoracotomy: a prospective, randomized study. Ann. Thorac. Surg. *37*:239, 1984.

Gormezano, J., and Branthwaite, M.A.: Pulmonary physiotherapy with assisted ventilation. Anaesthesia *27*:249, 1972a.
Gormezano, J., and Branthwaite, M.A.: Effects of physiotherapy during intermittent positive pressure ventilation. Anaesthesia *27*:258, 1972b.
Grimby, G.: Aspects of lung expansion in relation to pulmonary physiotherapy. Am. Rev. Respir. Dis. *110*:145, 1974.
Hedstrand, U., et al.: Effects of respiratory physiotherapy of arterial oxygen tension. Acta Anaesthesiol. Scand. *22*:349, 1978.
Holloway, R., et al.: The effect of chest physiotherapy on the arterial oxygenation of neonates during treatment of tetanus by intermittent positive-pressure respiration. S. Afr. Med. J. *40*:445, 1966.
Holloway, R., et al.: Effect of chest physiotherapy of blood gases of neonates treated by intermittent positive pressure respiration. Thorax *24*:421, 1969.
Mackenzie, C.F., et al.: Changes in total lung/thorax compliance following chest physiotherapy. Anesth. Analg. *59*:207, 1980.
Marini, J.J., et al.: Acute lobar atelectasis: a prospective comparison of fiberoptic bronchoscopy and respiratory therapy. Am. Rev. Respir. Dis. *54*:542, 1979.
Marini, J.J.: Postoperative atelectasis: pathophysiology, clinical importance, and principles of management. Resp. Care *29*:516, 1984.
Navarathnam, R.G., et al.: Evaluation of the transcutaneous electrical nerve stimulator for postoperative analgesia following cardiac surgery. Anaesth Intensive Care *12*:345, 1984.
Newton, D.A., and Stephenson, A.: Effect of physiotherapy on pulmonary functions: a laboratory study. Lancet *2*:228, 1978.
Rooney, S.M., et al.: Effect of transcutaneous nerve stimulation on postoperative pain after thoracotomy. Anesth. Analg. *62*:1010, 1983.
Stein, M., and Cassara, E.L.: Preoperative pulmonary evaluation and therapy for surgery patients. J.A.M.A. *211*:787, 1970.
Thoren, L.: Postoperative pulmonary complications: observations on their prevention by means of physiotherapy. Acta Chir. Scand. *107*:193, 1954.
Vraciu, J.K., and Vraciu, R.A.: Effectiveness of breathing exercises in preventing pulmonary complications following open heart surgery. Phys. Ther. *57*:1367, 1977.
Ward, R.H., et al.: An evaluation of postoperative respiratory maneuvers. Surg. Gynecol. Obstet. *123*:51, 1966.
Warfield, C.A., et al.: The effect of transcutaneous electrical nerve stimulation on pain after thoracotomy. Ann. Thorac. Surg. *39*:462, 1985.
Wiklander, O., and Norlin, U.: Effect of physiotherapy on postoperative pulmonary complications: a clinical and roentgenographic study of 200 cases. Acta Chir. Scand. *112*:246, 1957.
Winning, T.J., et al.: A simple clinical method of quantitating the effects of chest physiotherapy is mechanical ventilated patients. Anaesth. Intensive Care *3*:237, 1975.
Winning, T.J., et al.: Bronchodilators and physiotherapy during long-term mechanical ventilation of the lungs. Anaesth. Intensive Care *5*:48, 1977.

READING REFERENCES

Frownfelter, D.L.: Chest Physical Therapy and Pulmonary Rehabilitation. An Interdisciplinary Approach. 2nd Ed. Chicago, Year Book Medical Publishers, Inc., 1987.
Mackenzie, C.F., et al. (Ed): Chest Physiotherapy in the Intensive Care Unit. Baltimore, Williams & Wilkins, 1981.

Operative Procedures

CHAPTER 28

THORACIC INCISIONS

Willard A. Fry

The most versatile incision for general thoracic surgical operations is the posterolateral thoracotomy. Median sternotomy, the favorite of the cardiac surgeon, has been advocated by some groups for many general thoracic surgical procedures—especially for those on the anterior mediastinum and the lung. Some groups have suggested wider use of the axillary thoracotomy incision for many pulmonary operations.

When the patient is positioned for thoracotomy, especially in the lateral decubitus position, pad pressure points about the elbows with foam pads, place an axillary roll under the dependent axilla—to take pressure off of the brachial plexus, and place one or two pillows between the legs. Consider measures to discourage venous thrombosis in the lower extremities, such as tight elastic hose, sequential compression sleeves, or wrapping the legs with elastic bandages. These measures, if used, should be in effect at the beginning of the operation. Salzman (1985) and Scurr (1987) suggested that external pneumatic compression with sequential compression sleeves connected to a sequential compression device is the safest and most cost-effective prophylaxis against venous thromboembolic disease.

The use of prophylactic antibiotics for general thoracic surgical procedures remains controversial. Although the American College of Surgeons Committee on Preoperative and Postoperative Care (1983) recommended their use on a short-term basis, with the first dose being given parenterally prior to making the incision and with subsequent parenteral doses limited to the first 24 to 48 hours, Cameron (1981) and Ilves (1981) and their associates reported conflicting results in controlled trials the same year. In general, a first or second generation cephalosporin is used, and the main emphasis is on prophylaxis of the wound from *Staphylococcus aureus* infections.

POSTEROLATERAL THORACOTOMY

The posterolateral thoracotomy incision is made with the patient in the lateral decubitus position, with proper padding to the elbows, knees, and dependent axilla. Various maneuvers are available to hold the patient in an appropriate lateral position, including placing a sandbag under the operating table mattress, rolled sheets front and back, and bean bags. Two straps of 2″ adhesive tape are used as well. The dependent arm is flexed at the elbow. The superior arm can either be flexed similarly and appropriately padded—obtaining the so called "praying position," or it can be extended on a padded Mayo stand (Fig. 28–1A).

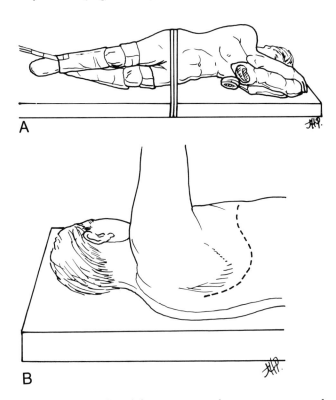

Fig. 28–1. Posterolateral thoracotomy. *A*, The patient is positioned in "praying position" with pillows between the knees and padding under the elbows. Wide adhesive tape secures the position. Note the axillary roll. *B*, The incision curves in an "S-shape" passing 4 cm under the tip of the scapula over in the fifth interspace anterior.

Only hairy portions of the skin that will be directly in the line of the incision or the chest tubes or their taping should be shaved, and if shaving is necessary, it should be done immediately prior to the operation, as recommended by Cruse and Foord (1973). My colleagues and I often find shaving is not necessary at all.

It is helpful to outline the proposed incision with a felt tipped marking pen. Most pulmonary operations are best performed through a fifth interspace incision.

As shown in Figure 28–1B, the incision starts in front of the anterior axillary line, curves 4 cm under the tip of the scapula, and then takes a vertical direction between the posterior midline over the vertebral column and the medial edge of the scapula. It is usually not necessary to go farther than the level of the spine of the scapula.

The electrosurgical unit is used for hemostasis and for musculofascial dissection. It is not recommended for incisions in the skin or subcutaneous tissues, based on the extensive wound healing studies of Cruse and Foord (1973). Glover and associates (1978) emphasized that use of the cutting current destroys less tissue than constant use of the coagulation current. The lower portion of the trapezius muscle is divided, and in the same plane more anteriorly the latissimus dorsi muscle is also divided. Next, the lower portion of the rhomboid muscle, if the thoracotomy is a high one, and the continuous plane with the serratus anterior muscle are divided.

The desired interspace is located by placing a large right-angle retractor beneath the scapula and passing the hand up paraspinally. Often the first rib is obscured to palpation, but attachments of the serratus posterior superior muscle to the second rib serve as an added guide.

Rib section at the costovertebral angle level is recommended for patients over 40 years of age to decrease the incidence of rib fracture (Fig. 28–2). Generally, small portions of the superior and inferior rib are excised subperiosteally to prevent the cut edges from overriding in the postoperative period. Although some recommend section over clips or ligatures of the neurovascular bundle, it is not necessary. It is unusual to resect a long segment of rib for a routine thoracotomy, although that was usually done in the past. For repeat thoracotomies, however, it is often advisable to resect a long rib segment subperiosteally and to approach the pleural space through the bed of the resected rib, as extensive adhesions are often encountered on such reoperations, and the wider entry into the pleural space through the bed of a resected rib can be beneficial (Fig. 28–3).

The intercostal muscle incision down to the parietal pleura is made carfully in the lower portion of the interspace to avoid injury to the neurovascular bundle. The surgeon pauses to see if the lung moves freely under the pleura. If it does move freely, then few adhesions in the area of the interspace can be expected. If the lung doesn't move freely, the surgeon must anticipate a significant number of adhesions and the need to divide them with care; particularly when the operation is a repeat thoracotomy. A large Finochietto-type rib spreader is inserted with attention to place the large superior blade behind the scapula. If desired, a smaller, Tuffier-type rib spreader can be placed more anteriorly to ensure a wide surgical field. The rib spreader is opened slowly and in stages to minimize the chance for rib fracture.

Closure of the incision is begun by inserting one or two chest tubes through a separate stab incision inferior to the skin incision in the anterior and midaxillary lines. The tract for the tube is tunneled for several centimeters to direct the tube—low and posterior for the back tube to drain fluid and high and anterior for the front tube to remove air. Tunneling the tube tract also reduces the chance for a pleurocutaneous fistula in the event that the tubes must remain in place for a long time, as when there is a prolonged postoperative air leak. Generally, two tubes are used if a significant resection has been performed, as the operator can expect both air and fluid accumulation. In selected cases such as a local excision of a lung lesion or an esophageal operation where the lung has not been cut, a single tube suffices. The size of the chest tube to be used depends upon the preference of the operating surgeon, the size of the patient, and the nature of the particular operation. In general, it is not necessary to use a posterior tube larger than 32F or an anterior tube larger than 28F. Tubes smaller than 24F tend to kink. Plastic tubes are preferred over rubber, as they are less likely to clot. The chest tubes should be secured, when inserted, with a heavy suture, our preference is for No. 1 nylon, to prevent slippage. The tubes are attached to a Y-tube connector, which is in turn affixed to an appropriate chest drainage system.

Many surgeons perform an intercostal nerve block with a long-acting local anesthetic such as 0.5% bupivacaine with epinephrine at the time of chest wall closure. Gallo and colleagues (1983) emphasized that an intercostal vascular injection must be avoided, as the intravascular injection of such compounds can have dire cardiovascular consequences. Generally, we block from the second to the seventh interspace. Inject at least 8 cm off the midline to avoid a subdural injection that would produce spinal anesthesia. If an epidural anesthetic technique is used (see Chapter 22) intraoperative intercostal nerve block is redundant.

Pericostal sutures, usually four, of heavy absorbable material such as No. 2 polyglycolic acid are then placed. Each of the two musculofascial planes is closed with running suture of a similar material, usually size 1 or 0, the subcutaneous tissues with a size 2–0 running suture of the same material and the skin with the surgeon's preferred material.

The main advantage of the posterolateral thoracotomy is the superb exposure for most general thoracic procedures. The main disadvantages are the time expended because of the length of the incision and the amount of muscle and soft tissue transected.

AXILLARY THORACOTOMY

The axillary thoracotomy was originally developed for operations on the upper thoracic sympathetic nerve system. It was modified for first rib resection for thoracic

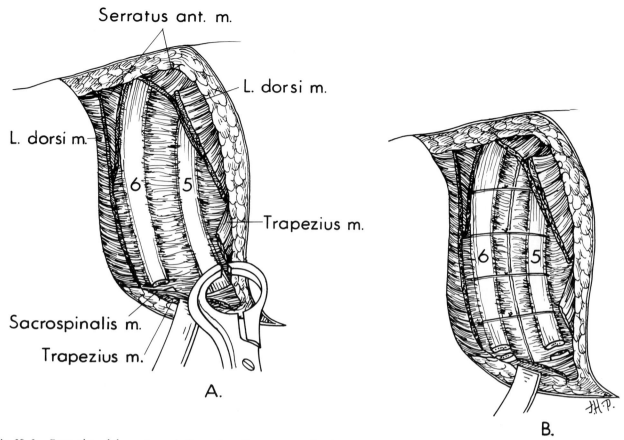

Fig. 28–2. Posterolateral thoracotomy. *A,* One or two ribs are sectioned at the costovertebral angle. A small portion of bone is removed to prevent overriding of the fragments at the time of closure. *B,* Four or more sutures of heavy absorbable suture are placed as pericostal sutures. The interspace distance is maintained. It is not necessary to suture the divided intercostal muscles except when a tight seal is desired for pneumonectomy.

outlet syndromes. Jensik (1987) used it preferentially for many years for pulmonary resections. Siegel and Steiger (1982) described how it has been rediscovered for more extensive general thoracic surgical procedures. Some groups refer to it as a lateral thoracotomy to avoid confusion with small, high axillary incisions for first rib resections or apical bleb resections. Other groups refer to it as a "mini-thoracotomy," but such nonspecific terminology should be discouraged. I prefer this incision for uncomplicated and straightforward pulmonary operations. It is not recommended for bulky tumors, for sleeve resections, for radical pneumonectomies, or for repeat thoracotomies. This incision is particularly useful when a double-lumen endotracheal tube can be used, as the controlled atelectasis combined with the ability of the anesthesiologist to elevate the mediastinum toward the operative field provides favorable operating conditions. The chief advantages are the speed of opening and closing, the reduced blood loss from minimal muscle transection, and the resulting reduced postoperative discomfort. As shown in Figure 28–4, the only muscle group that is actually transected is the intercostals.

Upper lobe lesions are best approached through the fourth interspace. Middle and lower lobe lesions are easily handled through the fifth interspace. The patient is placed in a lateral decubitus position with the arm abducted at 90° and positioned on an arm rest. Pad the antecubital fossa over the arm rest. The skin incision is made over the desired interspace, the latissimus dorsi muscle is elevated bluntly for a short distance and retracted posteriorly, and the serratus anterior muscle is split in the direction of its fibers. Avoid dividing the muscle too far posteriorly to avoid injuring the long thoracic nerve to serratus anterior muscle. The intercostal muscles are divided similarly to the way described for a posterolateral thoracotomy, and the pleural space is entered. The incision is so limited that wound towels and intercostal towels are not used. The intercostal muscle incision is carried forward to the anterior curve of the ribs and posteriorly to the level of the sacrospinalis muscle group. A Finochietto rib spreader is placed between the ribs, and a Tuffier rib spreader is placed in the opposite direction to retract the skin and latissimus dorsi muscle.

Closure of the axillary thoracotomy is accomplished with three pericostal sutures of No. 2 polyglycolic acid after the placement of one or two chest tubes and consideration of an intercostal nerve block. Generally, traction on the pericostal sutures suffices to close the chest wall, as it is difficult to use a ratchet-type rib approxi-

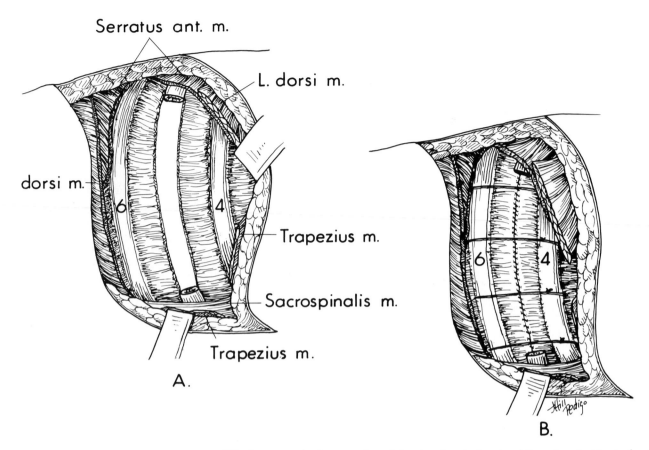

Fig. 28–3. Posterolateral thoracotomy. *A*, The fifth rib is resected subperiosteally and the pleural cavity is entered through an incision in the rib bed. Long rib resection is recommended for repeat thoracotomy. *B*, The rib bed is closed with running absorbable suture. The retained periosteum will regenerate rudimentary bone. The interspace distance is maintained.

mator through the small axillary thoracotomy incision. If there is a problem with rib approximation, a towel clip can be used to bring the ribs together. The serratus anterior muscle is closed with a running absorbable suture, as is the subcutaneous fascia layer. Skin closure is again at the surgeon's discretion.

The axillary thoracotomy is not recommended for the occasional thoracic surgeon or for a difficult operation, as the exposure is more limited than that of a posterolateral thoracotomy. In our opinion, however, it is a very useful incision that deserves wider application. My colleagues and I feel that there is less postoperative discomfort with the axillary thoracotomy than with either the posterolateral thoracotomy or the median sternotomy.

MEDIAN STERNOTOMY

The development of cardiac surgery has made median sternotomy the most common thoracic incision. It is the incision of choice for most cardiac operations and is used by preference by many thoracic surgeons for anterior mediastinal lesions, for bilateral procedures such as the surgical treatment of bilateral spontaneous pneumothorax, and for the resection of multiple pulmonary lesions.

Urschel and Razzuk (1986) wrote that they prefer it for many elective pulmonary resections, except for left lower lobe pulmonary resections. Cooper and colleagues (1978) demonstrated less alteration in pulmonary function by median sternotomy than by posterolateral thoracotomy. Median sternotomy was recommended by Baldwin and Mark (1985) and by Perelman (1987) for anterior transpericardial repair of postpneumonectomy bronchopleural fistula. Orringer (1984) described a partial median sternotomy for exposure of the lower cervical and upper thoracic esophagus.

The patient is positioned supine, with one or both arms extended, at the preference of the surgeon and the anesthesiologist. Both arms are often placed at the patient's side. The vertical skin incision is made from just below the suprasternal notch to a point between the xiphoid process and the umbilicus (Fig. 28–5). The pectoral fascia is divided and the periosteum scored with the electrosurgical unit. Take care when mobilizing tissues off of the area of the manubrium and dividing the tough interclavicular ligament. The tissues just to one side of the xiphoid process are mobilized and the sternum is divided with a power saw either from the top down or from the bottom up. The anesthesiologist should reduce ventilatory efforts as the sternum is being cut to lessen the

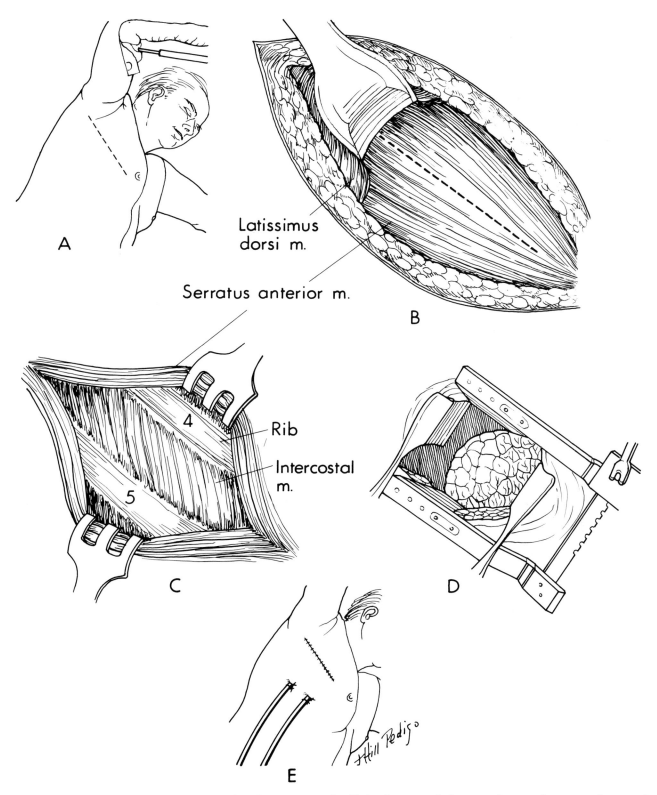

**Latissimus
dorsi m.**

Serratus anterior m.

Rib

**Intercostal
m.**

Fig. 28–4. Axillary thoracotomy. *A*, The arm is abducted 90° on a rest and padded with care. *B*, The latissimus dorsi muscle is retracted posteriorly. Incision in the serratus anterior muscle is made in the direction of its fibers and is extended back just short of the long thoracic nerve, taking care to preserve the nerve. *C*, The intercostal incision is extended posteriorly to the level of the sacrospinalis muscle and anteriorly to the curve in the ribs. *D*, Two rib spreaders facilitate exposure. *E*, Generally, two tubes are used and they are brought out near each other, so that a single maneuver will suffice at the time of tube removal.

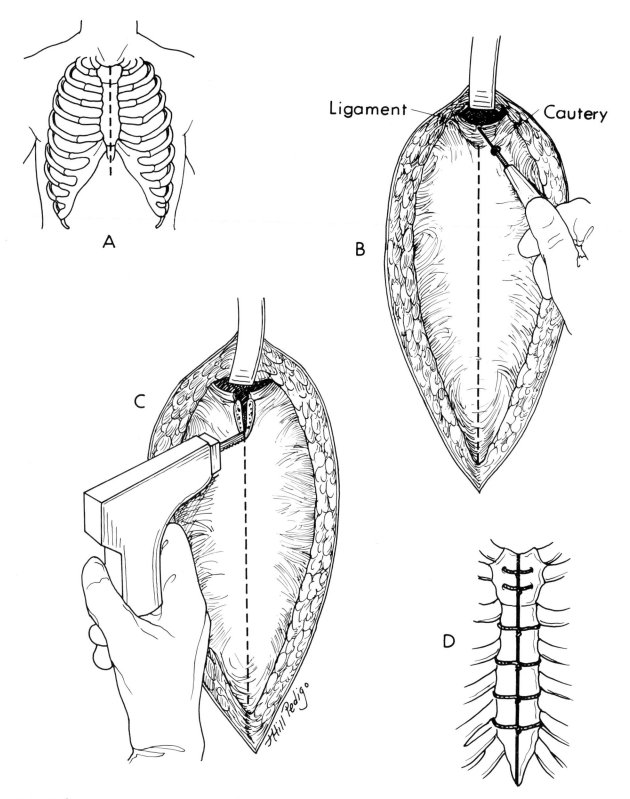

Fig. 28–5. Median sternotomy. *A*, Incision is made from suprasternal notch to a point between the xiphoid process and umbilicus. *B*, The interclavicular ligament is divided with care. *C*, The sternal saw can be used in either direction. The anesthesiologist should not ventilate the lungs while the sternum is being divided. *D*, The upper two wires of No. 5 monofilament steel are passed through the manubrium.

chance of injury to the lung. Once the sternum is split, the two edges are gently but firmly retracted, and periosteal bleeding points are controlled with the electrosurgical unit. Bone wax is often not necessary in general thoracic surgical procedures, because the patient is not anticoagulated, which patients undergoing cardiac procedures usually are. Robiscek and colleagues (1981) suggested that the foreign body effect of bone wax can have a deleterious effect on wound healing. A sternal spreader is placed low in the incision to minimize excessive traction on the upper ribs, with attendant occult fracture and neurologic insult, as described by Van der Salm (1980). The use of the Lebsche sternal blade should be familiar to the thoracic surgeon so that sternotomy can be performed if the power saw fails or is unavailable.

Chest tubes or mediastinal drains, if the pleural space has not been entered, are passed through separate stab incisions. Sternotomy closure is accomplished with four to seven parasternal sutures of No. 5 stainless steel wire, whose ends are securely twisted and buried in the sternal tissues. The pectoral fascia is closed with a running polyglycolic acid suture, as is the linea alba. The subcutaneous tissues are closed with running absorbable suture and the skin is closed with the surgeon's preferred material.

The usual vertical median sternotomy incision's scar is a source of concern to some patients, especially young females. Various alternatives have been proposed, and the transverse submammary skin incision used and described by Laks and Hammond (1980) appears to have definite cosmetic advantages for certain patients. Those authors do caution about skin flap viability for prolonged operations, as rather extensive undermining of the skin flaps is required.

The main advantages of median sternotomy for general thoracic surgical procedures are its speed in opening and closing, its familiarity to many surgeons, and its outstanding exposure for anterior mediastinal lesions. The major disadvantage is poor exposure of posterior hilar structures, especially those of the left lower lobe. My colleagues and I feel that a median sternotomy is more painful in the postoperative period than an axillary thoracotomy and that it is similar in postoperative discomfort to a posterolateral thoracotomy.

ANTERIOR THORACOTOMY

The anterior thoracotomy has the distinct advantage of allowing the patient to remain supine, with a resulting improvement in cardiopulmonary function. It has been used with decreasing frequency because of improvement of anesthetic techniques and management, the option of median sternotomy, and the development of mediastinal staging procedures such as mediastinoscopy and mediastinotomy. It remains the incision of choice of some surgeons for open lung biopsy. It is occasionally used in the Ivor Lewis procedure for carcinoma of the esophagus to eliminate the need for repositioning the patient after the intra-abdominal portion of the operation. Its main disadvantage is the limited exposure it provides.

The patient is positioned with a roll under the back and hips to elevate the operated side. The ipsilateral arm is placed under the back, on an elevated arm board, or on an overarm rest at the preference of the surgeon. An incision is made over the fourth or fifth interspace from the midaxillary line to curve parasternally (Fig. 28–6). In women, the incision is made in the inframammary crease. The pectoral muscles are divided with an electrosurgical unit, and the intercostal incision is made in the usual fashion. If a major resection is expected, one or two costal cartilages may be divided parasternally to facilitate exposure of the surgical field. If the cartilages are divided, the neurovascular bundles are divided over clamps and ligated to avoid tearing and excessive stretching of the blood vessels.

Closure of the anterior thoracotomy is similar to that of the other thoracotomy incisions. A heavy absorbable suture is placed through each end of the cartilage parasternally, if it has been divided.

THORACOABDOMINAL INCISION

The thoracoabdominal incision provides extended exposure, particularly for operations in the lower thorax and upper abdomen. It has been used less frequently in the 1980s and has been maligned more by hearsay perhaps than by actual fact. It can be particularly useful for difficult operations involving the lower esophagus. A seventh or eighth interspace incision is extended on the same oblique line into the upper quadrant over toward the midline. The costal margin is cut with a knife. Ginsberg (1987) recommended not excising a segment of cartilage and placing pericostal closure sutures securely on either side of the transected costal margin but not through the cartilage. He suggested that the incision results in a stable thorax with no significant increase in discomfort or dysfunction over a standard posterolateral thoracotomy. A curvilinear or radial incision can be made in the diaphragm to facilitate exposure. The diaphragm is closed with a running nonabsorbable suture such as No. 0 prolene. Costochondritis has been reported in some series. Its incidence is low, but if it occurs, it is a troublesome complication.

POSTERIOR THORACOTOMY

The posterior thoracotomy described by Overholt and Langer (1949) is mentioned here for completeness. Its advantages when first described were improved ventilation and lessened chance of spillage of secretions because of the prone position (Fig. 28–7). Improved anesthetic techniques, especially the development and increased use of the double-lumen endotracheal tube, have achieved those goals and eliminated the need to incur such disadvantages as the need for a special operating table, poor anterior hilar exposure, and poor access to the airway for the anesthetist.

Paulson (1987) recommended a posterior thoracotomy for certain bronchoplastic procedures. My colleagues and

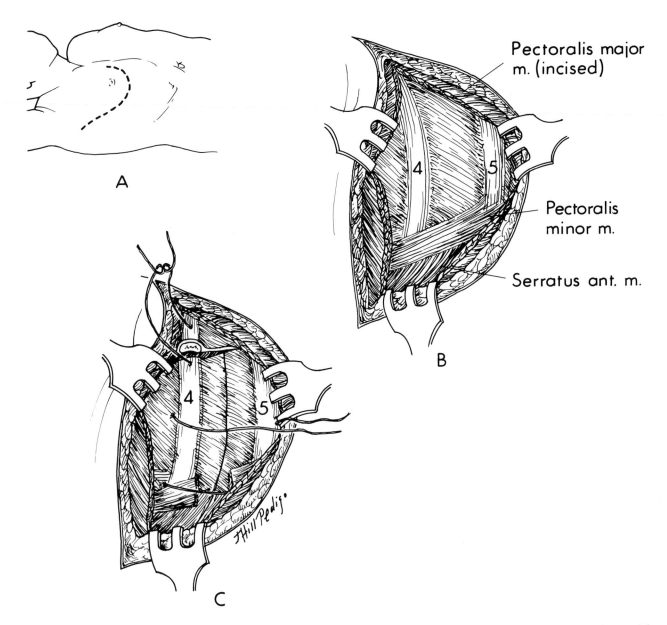

Fig. 28–6. Anterior thoracotomy. *A,* Outline of skin incision. *B,* Pectoralis major muscle divided over the fourth interspace. *C,* Closure of the intercostal incision by placement of pericostal sutures of heavy polyglycolic acid as well as sutures of the same material through the sectioned costal cartilage.

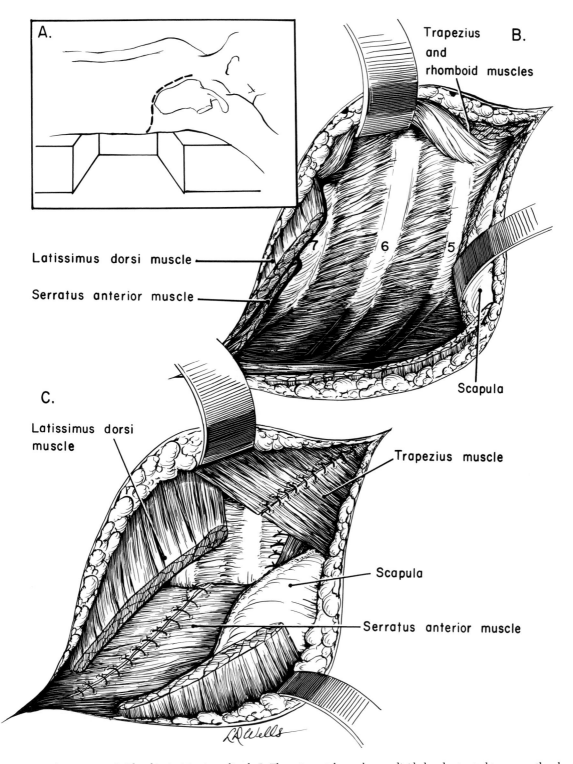

Fig. 28–7. Posterior thoracotomy. *A*, The skin incision is outlined. *B*, The extracostal muscles are divided and retracted to expose the chest wall. *C*, Closure shows the muscles being approximated in anatomic layers with careful apposition to reduce incisional bulge. (Redrawn from Johnson, J., MacVaugh, H, III, and Waldhausen, J.A.: Surgery of the Chest, Chicago, Year Book Medical Publishers, 1970.)

I feel that a high posterolateral thoracotomy through the third or fourth interspace provides the same advantages.

REFERENCES

American College of Surgeons Manual of Preoperative and Postoperative Care. Philadelphia, W.B. Saunders Co., 1983, pp. 365–6.

Baldwin, J.C., and Mark, J.B.D.: Treatment of bronchopleural fistula after pneumonectomy. J. Thorac. Cardiovasc. Surg. 90:813, 1985.

Cameron, J.L., et al.: Prospective clinical trial of antibiotics for pulmonary resections. Surg. Gynecol. Obstet. 152:156, 1981.

Cooper, J.D., Nelems, J.F., and Pearson, F.G.: Extended indications for median sternotomy in patients requiring pulmonary resection. Ann. Thorac. Surg. 26:413, 1978.

Cruse, P.J.E., and Foord, R.: A five-year prospective study of 23,649 surgical wounds. Arch. Surg. 107:206, 1973.

Gallo, J.A., Jr., et al.: Complications of intercostal nerve blocks performed under direct vision during thoracotomy J. Thorac. Cardiovasc. Surg., 86:628, 1983.

Ginsberg, R.: Personal communication, 1987.

Glover, J.L., Bendick, P.J., and Link, W.J.: The use of thermal knives in surgery: electrosurgery, lasers, plasma scalpel. Current Prob. Surg. 15(1):26, 1978.

Ilves, R., et al.: Prospective, randomized, double-blind study using prophylactic cephalothin for major, elective general thoracic operations. J. Thorac. Cardiovasc. Surg. 81:813, 1981.

Jensik, R.J.: Personal communication, 1987.

Laks, H., and Hammond, G.L.: A cosmetically acceptable incision for the median sternotomy. J. Thorac. Cardiovasc. Surg. 79:146, 1980.

Orringer, M.B.: Partial median sternotomy: anterior approach to the upper thoracic esophagus. J. Thorac. Cardiovasc. Surg., 87:124, 1984.

Overholt, R.L., and Langer, L.: The technique of pulmonary resection, Springfield, IL., Charles C Thomas, 1949.

Paulson, D.L.: Personal communication, 1987.

Perelman, M.I.: Late treatment of chronic bronchopleural fistula with long stump after pneumonectomy. International Trends in General Thoracic Surgery, vol. 2. Philadelphia, W.B. Saunders Co., 1987.

Robicsek, F., et al.: The embolization of bone was from sternotomy incision . Ann. Thorac. Surg. 31:357, 1981.

Salzman, E.W.: Physical techniques for prevention of venous thrombosis. In Surgery of the Veins. Edited by J.J. Bergan and J.S.T. Yao. Orlando, Grune & Stratton, Inc., 1985, pp. 519–528.

Scurr, J.H., Coleridge-Smith, P.D., and Hasty, J.H.: Regimen for improved effectiveness of intermittent pneumatic compression in deep venous thrombosis prophylaxis. Surgery 102:816, 1987.

Siegel, T., and Steiger, Z.: Axillary thoracotomy. Surg. Gynecol. Obstet. 155:725, 1982.

Urschel, H., and Razzuk, M.: Median Sternotomy as the standard approach for pulmonary resection. Ann. Thorac. Surg. 41:130, 1986.

Van der Salm, T.J., Cereda, J.M., and Cutler, B.S.: Brachial plexus injury following median sternotomy. J. Thorac. Cardiovasc. Surg. 80:447, 1980.

READING REFERENCES

Dart, C.H., Braitman, H.E., and Larab, S.: Supraclavicular thoracotomy for diagnosis of apical lung and superior mediastinal lesions. Ann. Thorac. Surg. 28:90, 1979.

Dartevelle, P., et al.: L'intérêt de la voie combinée cervicale et thoracique dans la chirurgie des syndromes de Pancoast et Tobias d'origine tumorale. Chirurgie 109:399, 1983.

Dartevelle, P., et al.: L'intérêt de la cervicotomie élargie dans les syndromes de Pancoast-Tobias. Ann. Chir. 38:80, 1984.

CHAPTER 29

PULMONARY RESECTIONS

Thomas W. Shields

PNEUMONECTOMY

Total removal of one lung is most often indicated for the treatment of bronchial carcinoma. Less frequent indications are extensive unilateral tuberculosis, extensive unilateral bronchiectasis, multiple lung abscesses, and the rare varieties of malignant tumors of the lung. Infrequently, other inflammatory lesions, such as fungal infections or metastatic lesions in the lung, require a pneumonectomy for their complete removal.

Operative Position

A pneumonectomy may be carried out in any one of the three standard thoracic positions: lateral, posterior, or anterior. A right pneumonectomy may be done without difficulty, as reported by Urschel and Razzuk (1986), through a median sternotomy incision. A left pneumonectomy is difficult and is not recommended through this approach because the left inferior pulmonary vein is difficult to mobilize and control because of the position of the heart.

The lateral position, in which a posterolateral incision with removal of the fifth rib is used, permits the best access to the hilus of the lung. The structures contained within the hilus may be approached from either the anterior or posterior aspect, and thus the operator is able to have a greater degree of control of the various structures than is afforded by the other approaches. The major disadvantage of the lateral position is that ventilation of the dependent lung is more difficult than in the posterior or anterior position. Note, however, that the perfusion of the dependent lung is increased as a result of the gravitational changes.

The posterior approach with the patient in the prone position has a major advantage in that the bronchial secretions will not flood the trachea because of the superior position of the main stem bronchus. Also, the main stem bronchus is the most accessible structure and may be isolated and divided as the initial stage in the dissection of the hilar structures. The major disadvantages are that the access to the entire hilus is initially limited and that

the vascular structures are the most distant from the operator.

The anterior approach with the patient in the supine position is the one least frequently used. Although fewer physiologic changes are incurred in the patient's cardiopulmonary function when this approach is used, the marked disadvantage of poor access to the hilus and its contained structures generally outweighs the physiologic considerations.

A right pneumonectomy may be done through a median sternotomy incision. As with the anterior thoracotomy approach, fewer adverse physiologic changes and less postoperative discomfort occur, as reported by Urschel and Razzuk (1986). Nevertheless the same disadvantage as recorded for the anterior approach is present: less ready access to the hilar structures.

Technique

When the pleural space is entered, the resectability of the lung is determined. This may require a greater or lesser freeing of adhesions of the lung to the chest wall and dissection of the hilar structures. Once resectability is determined, the pulmonary ligament is divided, and the pleura is incised as it reflects upon the hilus anteriorly, superiorly, and posteriorly. On the right, the azygos vein may be isolated and divided to give greater access to the hilus superiorly. Generally, the pulmonary artery is the first structure to be isolated and divided (Fig. 29-1).

Ligation of the veins as the initial step in a pneumonectomy for carcinoma has been advocated to lessen the possibility of spilling tumor cells into the circulation. The routine use of this maneuver, however, has not been shown to be beneficial, and the maneuver probably is not important. It has been suggested that initial ligation of the veins would lead to overfilling of the vascular bed with loss of an excessive amount of blood when the lung is removed, as well as resulting in an overdistended lung, which would be difficult to manipulate during the operative procedure. Miller and associates (1968) showed experimentally, however, that with initial ligation of the

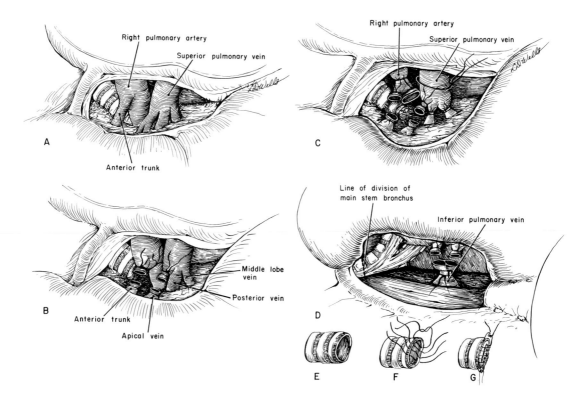

Fig. 29–1. *A–C*, Schematic illustrations of isolation, control, and division of vascular structures of the right lung during pneumonectomy. *D–G*, Division of main stem bronchus and its closure with the use of nonabsorbable sutures.

veins, reflex shunting of the blood from the lung occurs promptly, and thus distention of the vascular bed does not occur.

In mobilizing the artery, it is important to dissect down to the proper plane on the vessel to permit safe isolation of the structure from the surrounding tissues. Both sharp and blunt dissection should be used, and finger mobilization of the posterior aspect of the vessel is helpful. On occasion, on the right, the truncus anterior of the main stem pulmonary artery may be isolated and divided to obtain greater length of the main stem vessel. On the left, the artery may be isolated up to, or even proximal to, the ligamentum arteriosum, although one must guard against injury to the recurrent laryngeal nerve as it passes underneath the aortic arch from the front to the back at this point.

The ligation of the artery may be carried out in several ways. If it is long enough, the vessel may be doubly ligated with No. 00 or No. 0 nonabsorbable suture and the proximal end suture ligated to prevent rolling off of the proximal ligature. The vessel is then divided. If the vessel is too short to ligate safely in this manner, the artery may be held with two vascular clamps, divided, and the proximal cut end closed with a continuous suture of No. 4–0 or No. 5–0 nonabsorbable suture. Some surgeons prefer to treat the pulmonary artery in this manner as a routine procedure. A third method of controlling the vessel is the use of a mechanical stapling device such as a TA 30 instrument using 3.5 or V staples.

After control of the artery, the superior and then the inferior pulmonary veins are dissected, isolated, and di-

vided and the cut ends secured by one of the aforementined methods described for the pulmonary artery.

All the remaining tissue reflections are divided, and the main stem bronchus is freed up to its junction with the trachea. A bronchial clamp is placed just distal to this junction and the bronchus divided proximal to the clamp; a proximal as well as the distal clamp may be used, but this is not mandatory. The bronchial stump is then closed with interrupted, fine, nonabsorbable sutures. If one prefers, the mechanical stapling device also can be used to close the proximal end of the bronchial stump.

Takaro (1987) summarized the use and advantages of the mechanical stapler in bronchial closure. Hood (1985) recommended the TA 35 device with a staple size of 4.8 mm if a mechanical stapler is used. Both authors, among others, believe strongly that the use of the stapler has reduced the incidence of breakdown of the bronchial closure. This, however, is more likely the result of a different selection of patients being operated upon. In a discussion of Takaro's report, Vanetti and Bazelly (1987) reported better results with manual closure of the bronchial stump than with the use of a mechanical device. In fact, they were critical of the use of the new Premium TA 55 clip, with which Hakim and Milstein (1985) recorded an alarming 15% incidence of bronchial fistula.

Frequently one or two bronchial arteries need to be ligated after the bronchus has been divided. Bleeding must be controlled, for if not, these vessels may serve as a significant source of postoperative blood loss; the bronchial arterial system carries approximately 1% of the cardiac output.

After closure of its proximal end, the bronchial stump is covered with adjacent tissue, such as a pleural flap, the azygos vein, a pedicle graft of pericardial fat, or adjacent pericardium. This is done to provide the stump with a viable tissue cover to help prevent the possible development of a leak from the stump, which normally heals by secondary intention.

Special Techniques of Pneumonectomy

Under certain conditions, radical pneumonectomy with en bloc mediastinal dissection and intrapericardial ligation of the hilar vessels may be indicated. The technique of this procedure was described by Allison (1946) and Brock and Whytehead (1955–1956) in England, and Cahan (1951) and Gibbon (1955) and their associates in the United States. More often, rather than carrying out this procedure as a routine one, intrapericardial ligation of one or more of the hilar vessels is performed when the free extrapericardial portion of the vessel is too short or is involved with tumor, either of which would preclude a safe ligation of the vessel in question. The pericardium is opened anterior or posterior to the hilus, and the vessel or vessels are freed from the pericardial reflections, as described in Chapter 4. After removal of the lung, the pericardial defect, if small, is closed. If the opening is too large to close without compromise of the pericardial space, one of two maneuvers must be done to prevent postoperative herniation of the heart through the pericardial defect, with possible strangulation of the vessels and subsequent cardiac arrest. On the left, the pericardium is opened down to the diaphragm; whereas on the right, because this maneuver does not prevent herniation, the cut edges of the pericardium are tacked to the surface of the heart or the defect is closed with a prosthetic "soft-tissue" patch.

A supra-aortic pneumonectomy for resection of a lesion in the proximal left main bronchus was described by Abbey Smith and Nigam (1979). In this procedure, the transverse aortic arch is mobilized and the trachea and its divisions identified by dissection above the arch. The bronchus is mobilized, divided, and closed just distal to the tracheal carina. The pneumonectomy is then completed, usually by intrapericardial ligation of the vascular structures.

Tracheal-sleeve pneumonectomy also has been used to excise high lying carcinomas of either main stem bronchus. Jensik, (1972, 1982), Deslauriers (1985), and Dartevelle (1988) and their colleagues reported the technique and their experience with this highly selected procedure. Resection of the tracheal carina with the ipsilateral lung is carried out and the contralateral bronchus is then anastomosed to the distal end of the trachea. The technique of tracheal-sleeve pneumonectomy is described in Chapter 31.

When extensive pleural disease coexists with parenchymal disease that requires a pneumonectomy, a pleuropneumonectomy may be performed. This technique was described by Sarot and Gilbert (1949) in the man-

agement of extensive pleuropulmonary tuberculosis. Butchart (1976) and DeLaria (1978) and their colleagues and Faber (1986) describe the technique of extrapleural pneumonectomy and its use in patients with diffuse malignant mesothelioma. Essentially, a plane of cleavage is developed between the endothoracic fascia and the parietal pleura, and the pleura and lung are freed as one from the chest wall, diaphragm, and mediastinal structures down to the hilus. From this stage on, the vessels and bronchus are managed as in a standard pneumonectomy. Take care to prevent injury to the vessels of the chest wall and the structures of the mediastinum while developing the proper plane of dissection.

In patients with malignant mesothelioma, the adjacent pericardium and ipsilateral hemidiaphragm, and at times the lower portion of the chest wall, are excised. A prosthetic patch, which should be water-tight and strong, is used to replace the hemidiaphragm; Faber (1986) suggested using a Dacron velour patch. On the right, the excised pericardium must be replaced as well to prevent herniation of the heart.

Management of the Pleural Space

After removal of the specimen and adjacent lymph nodes as indicated, the pleural space is closed without drainage. If the development of an infection within the space is likely, a drainage tube may be placed in the space. The tube then is opened periodically to drain the accumulated fluid. Antibiotics may be instilled into the space at the time of closure.

After closure of the incision, the pressure within the space is adjusted as necessary to approximate a negative pressure of 2 to 4 cm of water on inspiration and a positive pressure of 2 to 4 cm of water on exhalation. Adjustment may be made simply by thoracentesis and removal of air until the trachea is in the midline at the sternal notch, or by the use of a manometer.

Some advocate that adjustment of the intrapleural pressure within the pneumonectomy space be made daily for 4 to 5 days after the pneumonectomy. When this is being done, antibiotics may be placed within the cavity. Others have found this procedure to be unnecessary and meddlesome, and check the pressure only if clinical signs indicate its need.

Fate of the Pleural Space

After pneumonectomy, elevation of the ipsilateral leaf of the diaphragm, shift of the mediastinum toward the side operated upon, and narrowing of the intercostal spaces of the ipsilateral side occur. In addition, serosanguineous fluid accumulates in the empty pleural space to fill the residual volume. The rate of accumulation of the fluid and the complete absorption of the air from the space are variable. Generally, the process is completed within 3 to 4 weeks, but may take as long as 7 months (Fig. 29–2).

In the past, the phrenic nerve on the side of the pneumonectomy was crushed to obtain a more prompt and higher elevation of the diaphragmatic leaf to reduce the residual volume of the postpneumonectomy space. The

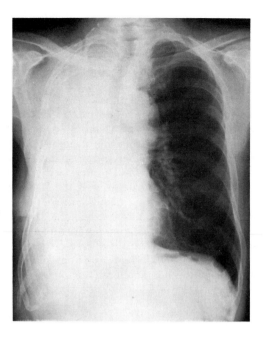

Fig. 29–2. Roentgenogram of chest 2 weeks after right pneumonectomy.

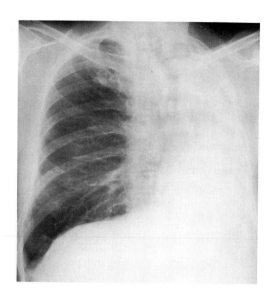

Fig. 29–3. Roentgenogram of chest 3 years after pneumonectomy.

resultant paralysis of the ipsilateral leaf of the diaphragm, however, permits paradoxic motion of this portion of the thoracic cage. Although this is of no real consequence during normal breathing, the paradoxic motion of this paralyzed leaf does interfere with the efficacy of the cough mechanism. Thus, it is not recommended as a routine procedure.

Also in the past, a thoracoplasty often was performed postoperatively to obliterate the residual pleural space. This was advised to prevent the overdistention of the remaining contralateral lung and to reduce the incidence of infection of the space. Overdistention of the contralateral lung, however, is in itself not detrimental to lung function, and a standard thoracoplasty does affect adversely the function of the contralateral lung. Gaensler and Strieder (1951) showed a loss of approximately 25 to 30% of the preoperative vital capacity and approximately 20% of the maximum voluntary ventilation in the contralateral lung after a standard thoracoplasty was performed over a nonfunctioning lung. A plombage type of thoracoplasty is followed by less functional loss, but the foreign body frequently becomes associated with infection and consequently its use is not advised.

The fluid within the pleural space is gradually absorbed so that only a potential space remains. As absorption takes place, the heart and mediastinum shift farther toward the ipsilateral side and the remaining lung herniates partially into the postpneumonectomy space to fill this residual thoracic volume (Fig. 29–3).

Complete absorption of the fluid is uncommon. Suarez and colleagues (1969) found that this occurred in only 10 of 37 patients who died at varying time intervals after pneumonectomy. In the other 27 individuals, variable amounts of air or fluid remained in simple or loculated spaces.

Physiologic Effects

After pneumonectomy, the pulmonary artery and right ventricular pressures rise temporarily and then, under normal circumstances, return to their previous level. Changes in cardiac output occur but are inconsistent. The ventilation of the remaining lung is increased by an increase in depth and rate of breathing. With the hyperventilation, the efficiency of oxygen uptake increases. An increase in the ratio of the tidal volume to the functional residual capacity occurs and leads to an improved mixing of the inspired gases. Compliance, however, is reduced, with subsequent increase in the work required to move the air in and out of the remaining lung. Diffusion capacity also is reduced after pneumonectomy.

As the remaining lung adjusts to the change in the thoracic volume available to it, it becomes hyperinflated. This results in an increase of 10 to 30% in its vital and total capacities.

The pulmonary artery pressure may be normal when the patient is at rest or performing light exercise because a normal lung is able to tolerate a doubling of its rate of blood flow. With moderate to marked exercise, when the cardiac output begins to exceed 7 L per min, however, the pulmonary artery pressure rises progressively.

The older the patient at the time of pneumonectomy or the greater the degree of pre-existent chronic obstructive airway disease in the remaining lung, the greater is the likelihood of functional incapacity. In evaluating the functional capacity, there appears to be a direct relationship to the pulmonary artery pressure; as the functional reserve decreases, the pulmonary artery pressure increases. The reduction in the functional capacity appears to be more directly related to the pulmonary artery pressure and pulmonary blood flow relationships in the remaining lung than to arterial saturation per se. The functional capacity appears to be governed and limited by the expansibility of the remaining vascular bed. When the limit of the bed is reached or exceeded, persistent pulmonary hypertension occurs and cor pulmonale results.

In children, the late functional loss after pneumonectomy is less than that observed in the adult. Gas exchange is normal when the child is at rest. The total lung capacity and vital capacity are increased well above that predicted for one lung, and the maximum voluntary ventilation—maximum breathing capacity—is generally normal. Diffusion capacity is normal if the pneumonectomy is performed prior to puberty; this is probably the result of growth of the remaining lung in the young child. If pneumonectomy is performed after puberty, reduction of the diffusion capacity occurs, as is noted in the adult. After pneumonectomy in children, pulmonary hypertension is not a significant development.

Morbidity

The morbidity rates after a pneumonectomy vary from almost zero to as high as 30%. Multiple factors influence the rates of occurrence and the types of nonfatal complications seen. Among these are the physical status of the patient, the nature of the pathologic process, the extent of the procedure, and the addition of various preoperative or postoperative adjuvant therapeutic modalities.

Nonfatal complications may be classified as those either unique to, or directly related to, the procedure: technical, pleural, pulmonary, cardiac, or septic, and as those related to the performance of any major operative procedure: cardiovascular, genitourinary, peripheral vascular, thromboembolic, hematologic, or others.

Of the complications related to the procedure per se, more than one etiologic factor, that is, technical, septic, or failure of healing, may play a role in the development of the complication. An example of this is the development of a bronchopleural fistula, which may occur in 3 to 5% of the patients undergoing pneumonectomy.

Early, 1 to 2 days postoperatively, a bronchopleural fistula may occur because of a technically poor closure of the bronchial stump. It is manifested by a massive air leak with the development of a progressive increase in clinically evident subcutaneous emphysema. A small amount of subcutaneous emphysema is normally seen as some of the air in the postpneumonectomy space at the time of closure is expelled out into the tissue of the chest wall with coughing or is forced out with a rapid accumulation of fluid within the space. Along with the development of the massive subcutaneous emphysema, patients may exhibit varying degress of respiratory insufficiency, because the bronchopleural fistula physiologically represents a modified open pneumothorax.

When the bronchial leak occurs later in the postoperative course, usually the eighth to the tenth postoperative day, it may be caused by failure of healing because of inadequate viable tissue coverage of the stump or infection of the fluid within the space and rupture of the empyema through the suture line of the bronchial stump. At this stage, the patient coughs up variable quantities of serosanguineous fluid from the respiratory tract. Danger of flooding of the remaining lung is present, and prompt, emergent drainage of the affected pleural space is indicated.

When a bronchopleural fistula occurs later than 2 weeks after pneumonectomy, it is most likely the result of rupture of a frank empyema through the bronchial stump, although at times, failure of healing of the bronchial stump may be the underlying cause. Clinically, the patient is most likely febrile and has a cough productive of purulent sputum. Hemoptysis may or may not be present.

Occult bronchopleural fistulas do occur. A significant fall of more than 1.5 cm in the height of the fluid level should alert suspicion. Whether or not the fluid escapes through the bronchus and is swallowed unnoticed by the patient or is lost by absorption through the parietal pleura as the result of the increased intrapleural pressure, which becomes potentially greater than atmospheric pressure, is unresolved. Nonetheless, confirmation of the diagnosis can be sought by instilling methylene blue into the postpneumonectomy space and watching for its appearance in the sputum. The management of an occult bronchopleural fistula poses a vexing clinical problem. When the patient remains asymptomatic and no signs of clinical infection are present, expectant treatment with systemic antibiotics and close observation is acceptable. More often than not there will be no further difficulty. If any finding of clinical infection occurs, however, prompt drainage of the pleural space is indicated.

The management of a clinically evident bronchopleural fistula depends on the time of its development postoperatively and its underlying cause. Early in the postoperative period, reoperation and repair of the bronchial stump occasionally may be indicated. Otherwise, initial evacuation of the fluid in the affected pleural space and institution of proper drainage are indicated. Jensen and Sharma (1985) suggested using fibrin glue to occlude the opening when the fistula is small. Moritz (personal communication, 1986) had success with this method for closing small bronchopleural fistulas that developed from a technical failure with the use of a mechanical stapling device. Glover and associates (1987) also reported successful use of this technique for closing small bronchopleural fistulas after similar suture line failures. In most situations, however, in the presence of a bronchopleural fistula, additional measures of closure of the fistula and control of the associated empyema are necessary. The various methods of drainage of the pleural space, obliteration of the pleural space, and ultimate closure of the fistula are covered in detail in Chapters 32 and 59. Transsternal division of a long bronchial stump, with closure of both the proximal and distal ends, has become popular. This technique was first suggested by Abruzzini (1961) and was reported by Maassen (1975), Bruni (1987), Perelman (1987) and Perelman and Ambatiello (1970) in Europe. In the United States, Baldwin and Marks (1985) and Cosgrove (1985) reported its use. Perelman, however reported in 1987 that he prefers to reamputate the stump with closure of the proximal end through a posterior approach with opening of the chronic empyema cavity.

Other significant complications primarily related to the procedure are empyema, hemothorax, respiratory insufficiency, and cardiac arrhythmias.

Empyema occurs less often than it once did, but still follows pneumonectomy in 1 to 3% of the patients. It may, or may not, be associated with a bronchopleural fistula. At operation, most surgeons instill antibiotic solutions into the pneumonectomy space, and systemic antibiotics are given postoperatively to lessen the likelihood of the development of this septic complication. If there is gross contamination at operation or if reoperation is necessary for control of the postoperative hemothorax or early bronchial leak, the risk of developing empyema increases. In these circumstances, the pleural space may be drained, as noted under management of the pleural space. When empyema does occur, the patient shows a greater or lesser degree of systemic toxicity, his white blood count is elevated, his appetite is poor, and general deterioration occurs. Drainage of the space is indicated, bacterial cultures and sensitivity studies of the fluid are obtained, and definitive management of the empyema is carried out as discussed in Chapter 59.

Postoperative hemothorax is an infrequent complication. The source of bleeding may be from an uncontrolled bronchial artery or from a vein or artery in the chest wall; slipping off of a ligature from a major vessel is fortunately rare and usually fatal. With the accumulation of blood in the pneumonectomy space, the patients show the systemic signs of continued internal bleeding as well as signs of shift of the mediastinum and heart toward the contralateral side with compression of the remaining lung and resultant respiratory insufficiency. Prompt recognition and control of the bleeding are necessary.

Respiratory insufficiency may be manifested clinically by dyspnea, tachypnea, rapid pulse, anxiety, and not infrequently, by mental confusion. The latter, particularly in the elderly, may be a prominent and early sign of hypoxia. Results of blood gas studies reveal a fall in both P_{O_2} and P_{CO_2} values, although if the situation deteriorates, P_{CO_2} may become elevated. A shift in the mediastinum toward the remaining lung, elevation of the left leaf of the diaphragm caused by gastric distention after a right pneumonectomy, retention of secretions with areas of atelectasis in the remaining lung, and restriction of chest wall movement because of severe postoperative pain are the major mechanical factors that may initiate the problem and should be corrected by appropriate therapeutic intervention.

The remaining lung itself may be the underlying element in the causation of respiratory insufficiency. The functional capacity of the residual lung tissue may be insufficient for adequate gas exchange. Impaired ventilatory function preoperatively as determined by the reduction of FEV_1 or MVV from the predicted normal suggests that respiratory insufficiency may occur postoperatively. Ali (1976) and his associates (1980) noted that when the FEV_1 is equal to 2.5 L or more, >85% of predicted normal, the patient can tolerate a pneumonectomy. When the FEV_1 is between 1 and 2.4 L, 40 to 80% of predicted normal, the patient has mild to moderate ventilatory impairment. When the FEV_1 is less than 1 L, <40% of predicted normal, severe impairment is present and pneumonectomy is contraindicated. When an MVV has been performed, a result of less than 45 to 50% of predicted normal contraindicates pneumonectomy.

In patients with borderline pulmonary function, Kristersson (1972), as well as Olsen (1974) and Boysen (1977) and their colleagues, reported that when the predicted postoperative FEV_1 determined by radionuclide studies (Chapter 15) exceeds 800 ml, the patient should tolerate a pneumonectomy. Nonetheless, the mortality in patients with such compromised pulmonary function exceeds 15%. Ali and his associates (1983) showed that patients with markedly reduced perfusion of the tumor-bearing lung—Q <33%, usually in the presence of large T2 or centrally located tumors—may tolerate a pneumonectomy. In 13 such patients, the 30-day postoperative mortality rate was 15%. Postoperatively reduced capacity may be exacerbated by varying degrees of inadequate ventilation, diffusion, or perfusion. Retained secretions, patchy areas of atelectasis, and pulmonary edema with resultant functional arteriovenous shunting may further contribute to the problem. Oxygen therapy, tracheobronchial toilet, tracheostomy, and assisted or controlled ventilation may be indicated to sustain the patient over the acute phase.

Cardiovascular complications may contribute to, and even initiate, the patient's respiratory difficulties. Myocardial infarction, heart failure, and cardiac arrhythmias are common causes.

Cardiac arrhythmias occur most frequently in patients over the age of 60 years and only rarely in anyone under the age of 50 years. The incidence following pneumonectomy in the older age group is approximately 20 to 30%. The arrhythmia may be sinus tachycardia, runs of premature ventricular contractions, a nodal rhythm, or auricular fibrillation or flutter or both. Auricular fibrillation and flutter are the most serious. Abnormal rhythms usually arise during the first postoperative week, the third and fourth days being the most common time. The duration is variable, and at times, the heart may spontaneously revert to a normal rhythm. Most patients, however, require therapy with antifibrillatory medication.

The cause of the abnormal rhythms is unknown, although mediastinal shift, hypoxia, and abnormal pH of the blood, as well as other factors, have been implicated but unproved. What is known is that the occurrence of an arrhythmia is more common with advanced age of the patient and a more extensive operative procedure, the incidence being highest after intrapericardial ligation of the pulmonary vessels. Previous cardiac arrhythmia, frequent premature atrial or ventricular contractions preoperatively, and a complete or incomplete right bundle branch block on the preoperative electrocardiogram have also been associated with increased incidence of this complication.

As a result of the high incidence and potential seriousness of postoperative arrhythmias, many use prophylactic digitalization in the older patient undergoing pneumonectomy. The potential danger of digitalis toxicity must be considered, but the advantages of prophylactic digitalization in reducing the incidence of arrhythmias, as shown by Wheat and Burford (1961) as well as by me and Ujiki (1968), seem to outweigh this possible danger. Our group uses this prophylaxis in all patients 60 years of age or older when a pulmonary resection is contemplated. When prophylactic digitalization has not been used and an atrial arrhythmia occurs postoperatively, intravenous administration of digoxin is begun promptly and repeated at four-hour intervals up to a loading dose of 1 mg. If this fails to convert the rhythm back to normal—normally 80% of the patients respond to this regimen—intravenous verapamil may be given. Electrical cardioversion is rarely necessary.

Mortality

The mortality rates after extensive operations should be computed on a 30-day basis. In some situations, as in pulmonary tuberculosis, this time should be extended to at least 60 days.

After pneumonectomy, the mortality rates vary from as low as 3% to as high as 30%. In patients undergoing a pneumonectomy for the treatment of tuberculosis, the average mortality rate is between 8 and 10%. In patients with carcinoma of the lung, the rates vary but are in the range of 5 to 15%; Ginsberg and his associates in the National Lung Cancer Study Group (1983) reported an overall 30-day postoperative mortality rate of only 6%. In patients over 70 years of age, the mortality rate may be as high as 30%; however, with proper preoperative selection and meticulous postopertive care, the mortality rate in patients over 70 may be kept as low as 6%, as reported by Ginsberg and associates (1983). In patients who have undergone an extended pneumonectomy—a pleuropneumonectomy or a tracheal-sleeve pneumonectomy—the 30-day postoperative mortality is higher than with a standard pneumonectomy. Rates as high as 25% have been recorded, but Faber (1986) recorded a rate of approximately 10% after pleuropneumonectomy and Dartevelle and associates (1988) recorded a rate of 10% after tracheal-sleeve pneumonectomy.

The major causes of death after a pneumonectomy are pulmonary insufficiency; septic complications, for example, empyema with or without an accompanying bronchopleural fistula; heart failure; and myocardial infarction.

Postpneumonectomy pulmonary edema is an unusual complication that is lethal when unrecognized. Peters (1987) reported that it usually follows a right pneumonectomy in a patient whose preoperative pulmonary function was good and whose first 12 to 24 hours postoperative were uneventful. Progressive dyspnea and apprehension occur first. Hypoxemia occurs, and when the condition is unrecognized and untreated, death occurs. Peters postulates from clinical observations and studies in the laboratory by Zeldin and associates (1984) that perioperative excessive fluid is the etiologic factor. The single remaining lung must remove a large fluid load, and the fluid filtered in the lung exceeds the capacity of the lymphatics. Fluid accumulates in the peribronchial spaces initially, which makes the lung stiffer, increasing the work of breathing. When the peribronchial space is filled, the alveoli fill rapidly with fluid, hypoxemia occurs, and death ensues. Treatment consists of morphine, diuretics and ventilatory support. The best treatment, of course, is prevention of fluid overload during and immediately following the procedure.

Another infrequent complication after pneumonectomy is embolization from pulmonary arterial stump thrombosis. Chuang and colleagues (1966) reported that this occurred in 1% of patients after a pneumonectomy. It is said to occur twice as often after a right than after a left pneumonectomy. Because a ligature of the arterial stump produces puckering and infolding of the vessel wall, which theoretically could increase the likelihood of thrombosis, vascular closure by suture technique or by the use of a stapler may lessen the minimal risk of this complication.

Pulmonary embolism from other sites also may cause death, as reported by Abbey Smith (1970). Massive gastrointestinal hemorrhage, cerebrovascular accidents, and technical accidents at operation account for a few deaths.

LOBECTOMY

Lobectomy is used primarily in the treatment of bronchial carcinoma. Less often, the complications of pulmonary tuberculosis, bronchiectasis, pulmonary infections, fungal diseases, and solitary metastatic tumors may also be indications for a lobectomy.

Operative Position

Any one of the three standard operative approaches, as well as a median sternotomy—except for doing a left lower lobectomy—can be used for lobectomy. As with a pneumonectomy, the lateral approach through a posterolateral incision is usually preferred. Entry into the pleural space is gained through the fifth intercostal space or the bed of the resected fifth rib.

Technique

After the pleural space is entered, the peripheral adhesions are divided by blunt or sharp dissection, or both, as indicated. The pulmonary ligament is divided, and the pleura is incised as it reflects upon the hilar structures. The oblique—major—fissure is then opened to expose the interlobar portion of the pulmonary artery. The arterial branches to the lobe to be resected are then isolated, double ligated, transfixed, and divided. Care must be exercised to identify and recognize any variations in the usual arterial pattern, as discussed in Chapter 4. After control of the arteries, the veins draining the lobe are identified and managed in a similar fashion. Either vessel may be secured by stapling (Fig. 29–4A). The lobar bronchus is then isolated and clamped distally to the proposed line of division. A noncrushing proximal clamp also can be used. After division of the bronchus, the proximal end of the stump is closed with interrupted, fine, nonabsorbable sutures or by a mechanical stapling

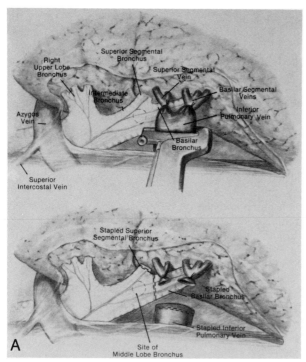

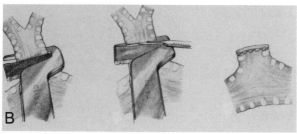

Fig. 29–4. Use of mechanical stapling device. *A*, Control of pulmonary vein. *B*, Closure of the bronchial stump. (Reproduced with permission from Hood, R.M.: Techniques in General Thoracic Surgery. Philadelphia, W.B. Saunders Co., 1985.)

device (Fig. 29–4B). Most thoracic surgeons cover the stump with adjacent tissue, although this usually is unnecessary because the remaining lung tissue generally will cover the stump effectively as it re-expands. Removal of the lobe is then completed by division of any remaining connections to the other lobe or lobes.

Special Techniques of Lobectomy

A radical lobectomy, as described by Cahan (1960), can be used in certain instances for treatment of carcinoma of the lung. In this procedure, the lymph nodes in the mediastinum are removed en bloc with the lobe. This is most easily and satisfactorily performed with the right upper lobe, although it can be done almost as well with the left one. Both right and left lower lobectomies are more difficult, and it is doubtful whether an adequate radical lymphatic dissection is possible in these anatomic locations.

Extension of the lobectomy on the right to include an adjacent lobe—a bilobectomy—is indicated on occasion. This is accomplished most often as a middle and right

lower bilobectomy, although at times a right upper and middle bilobectomy is performed. The technique is similar to that of a standard lobectomy. With the lower and middle bilobectomy, however, the bronchus is divided through the bronchus intermedius just distal to the take-off of the right upper lobe bronchus, so that a single stump remains; whereas with a middle and right upper bilobectomy, the two lobar bronchi must be dealt with separately.

A lobectomy may also include a sleeve resection of a portion of the main stem bronchus as initially performed by Allison and reported by Thomas (1956). This is indicated for the preservation of lung tissue in patients with benign disease or even with malignant disease. It may be accomplished with any lobe and adjacent main stem bronchus in benign disease—post-traumatic or inflammatory stenosis—or in the presence of a bronchial carcinoid. In patients with lung cancer, the procedure is performed mainly for lesions either in the right upper or left upper lobe bronchus and is less applicable for lesions in the other lobar bronchi. In patients with lung cancer, it can be done either as an elective or as a compromise procedure. Pulmonary function is preserved, as reported by Deslauriers (1986). The data published by Weisel and colleagues (1979) also suggest that this procedure is as adequate a cancer operation as pneumonectomy for patients with comparable stages of the disease and need not only be done as a compromise procedure for poor-risk patients with lung cancer. It may be extended to include an angioplastic procedure; however, as noted by Toomes and Vogt-Moykopf (1985), the mortality is almost double that of a bronchoplastic procedure alone, 17% versus 8.9%. The technique of the operation is discussed in detail in Chapter 30. Two unique postoperative complications are noted after bronchoplastic procedures. One is bronchial stenosis as the result of kinking or circular stenosis from scar contraction or granulomatous tissue formation. The second is fistula formation with the development of a pyopneumothorax or a fatal bronchovascular communication.

Management of the Pleural Space

After a lobectomy, the pleural space is routinely drained. Two thoracostomy tubes are used, one placed near the apex and one at the base, along the costal margin of the hemidiaphragm. These are connected to an underwater seal drainage system. Supplemental negative suction may be used according to the preference of the operator. The tubes are kept in the pleural space until no air leak is present and the drainage is less than 50 ml per 24 hours. Take care to maintain patency of the drainage system as long as the thoracostomy tubes are in place.

With the re-expansion of the remaining lung, elevation of the diaphragmatic leaf, and shift of the mediastinum toward the ipsilateral side, the pleural space is usually obliterated within several days to a week. An asymptomatic persistent air space, however, may remain for a longer period of time.

Physiologic Effects of Lobectomy

With resection of a lobe of the lung, a portion of the total alveolar, bronchial, and vascular masses is removed. There is an overinflation of the contralateral as well as the remaining ipsilateral lung tissue.

The remaining lung parenchyma is subjected to increased perfusion, though there is an absolute reduction in the diffusion surface. Although there is an increase in the ratio of the dead space to the total lung volume, a decrease of the dead space with respect to the tidal volume occurs. As a result, there is actually an improved ventilatory efficiency.

The late volumetric loss noted after a lobectomy is in proportion to the size of the lobe resected, although this loss is generally greater than the anatomic loss. A loss in diffusion capacity occurs, and early postoperatively, this is greater than the proportioned volume loss. The cause of the diffusion loss is unknown, but it may result from an alteration in the alveolocapillary membrane or an overventilation and the underperfusion of the remaining pulmonary tissue. The early disproportionate loss in diffusion capacity tends to be corrected slowly, and in 3 to 6 months the diffusion loss is generally directly proportional to the volumetric loss.

Note that the early functional loss after lobectomy is disproportionately greater than the pulmonary volume removed. As a consequence, early postoperative ventilatory insufficiency may occur in patients with compromised function, as judged by the preoperative FEV_1 or MVV. With time, function improves, and the late functional loss correlates with the number of segments removed during the lobectomy. The loss may vary markedly in the individual patient and is influenced by the degree of functional loss present preoperatively and the presence or absence of postoperative complications. The occurrence of hemorrhage, effusion, air leak, empyema, fibrothorax, or bronchopleural fistula exerts a serious adverse effect on postoperative pulmonary function.

Morbidity

The morbidity rates after lobectomy were once higher after resections for inflammatory disease processes than after resections for carcinoma. As reported by Keagy and colleagues (1985), however, postlobectomy morbidity is now more common in patients with carcinoma and more common in men than in women. The number of complications increases in the elderly and in extended resections involving radical lymphatic node dissections or bronchoplastic procedures.

As with pneumonectomy, the nonfatal complications may result from technical errors, may be common to any extensive operative procedure, or may be caused primarily by the removal of one of the lobes of the lung. In a series of 369 lobectomies reported by Keagy and associates (1985), 41% had nonfatal complications; 224 complications occurred in 151 patients. The respiratory system was involved in one third—50 patients required prolonged ventilation and 27 had atelectasis or excessive secretions. Cardiac complications also occurred in a third, with arrhythmias being the most common. In the remaining third, air leaks, pleural effusions, pneumothoraces, empyema—2.4%, postoperative hemorrhage, bronchial stump leaks—1.3%, pulmonary emboli, wound infections and one instance of gangrene occurred. Postoperative massive atelectasis (Fig. 29–5) and persistent residual air space (Fig. 29–6) present problems not seen after a pneumonectomy. Shallow breathing, reflex splinting of the chest wall, and impaired cough lead to retention of secretions in the ipsilateral lung. If the airway is not kept clear, atelectasis of the remaining lobe or lobes on the ipsilateral side occurs. If a massive atelectasis does develop, the patient becomes acutely short of breath and a variable degree of cyanosis ensues. Along with the tachypnea, a rapid pulse and a sharp temperature elevation occur. Physical findings and, if necessary, roentgenographic examination of the chest confirm the diagnosis. Prompt tracheobronchial suction, which may include bronchoscopic aspiration of the retained secretions, is indicated. If retention of secretions continues to be troublesome, a tracheostomy may be necessary.

A persistent residual air space frequently occurs after a lobectomy. It is more common in older persons and in those who have undergone resection for pulmonary tuberculosis than in other lobectomy patients. In the pulmonary tuberculosis group, the incidence is as high as 21%. Approximately two thirds to four fifths of these persistent spaces do not cause symptoms, and the clinical course of the patient is unaffected by their presence. An asymptomatic space gradually disappears over a period of months. This may occur either by absorption of the gases within the space and further expansion of the remaining lung or by the deposition of a pleural peel in the area. The other one fifth to one third of the air spaces, however, do cause symptoms and require surgical intervention of varying magnitude for their eventual control. The symptoms may consist of pain, dyspnea, hemoptysis, fever, or signs of continued air leak. The persistent air leak may be caused by seepage from the alveoli—a small peripheral parenchymal fistula—or from a frank bronchopleural fistula. With alveolar seepage, the composition of the gas in the space is the same as that of the gas in the alveolar spaces rather than the gas in the venous blood. Although it is impossible to maintain a negative pressure within the space because of this seepage, the space may remain sterile. In the presence of frank bronchopleural fistula, however, not only is a major air leak present, but also an empyema ultimately develops. Such a space is controlled by drainage and obliteration of the space, as discussed in Chapter 59.

As after pneumonectomy, empyema with or without a bronchopleural fistula is one of the major postoperative complications of lobectomy. It is more common after resections for inflammatory disease than after those for tumor. The initial treatment consists of adequate drainage. The space must be obliterated subsequently, but this is less of a problem than after pneumonectomy because lung tissue remains. Note, however, that pulmonary function on the involved side is generally markedly

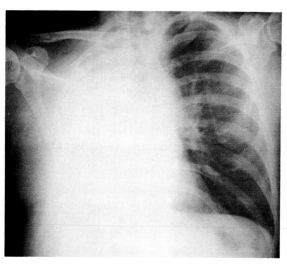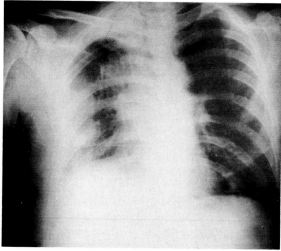

Fig. 29–5. *Left,* Roentgenogram of chest revealing massive atelectasis of remaining right lung 24 hours after right upper lobectomy. *Right,* Reexpansion of remaining right lung after bronchoscopy.

reduced by the development, and subsequent treatment, of the empyema.

Pulmonary insufficiency, although less common than after pneumonectomy, may occur after a lobectomy, even in the absence of other complications, and is most often related to the preoperative selection of the patients. Also, as after pneumonectomy, cardiac arrhythmias occur. These are primarily related to the age of the patient. In patients over 60 years of age, the incidence of cardiac arrhythmias may be as high as 15 to 20%. Preoperative digitalization reduces the incidence of this complication.

Mortality

The mortality rates are lower after lobectomy than after pneumonectomy. Patient selection and disease process are the major factors influencing the rates. In patients with pulmonary tuberculosis, the mortality rate is in the range of 1 to 2%; in patients with carcinoma of the lung, it may be as high as 8 to 10%, but as reported by Ginsberg (1983) and Keagy (1985) and their colleagues, it should be no greater than 3%.

The major causes of patient death after lobectomy are septic complications and cardiopulmonary insufficiency. Fatal pulmonary embolism occurs rarely. Fatal cardiac and other nonpulmonary complications occur infrequently.

SEGMENTECTOMY

The removal of one or more segments of the lung formerly was more often employed in the treatment of

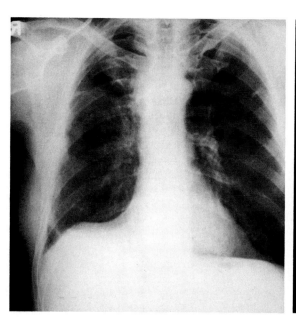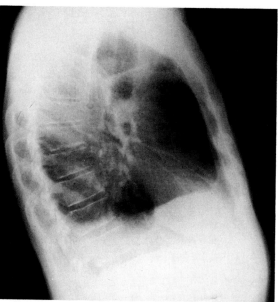

Fig. 29–6. Posteroanterior and lateral roentgenograms of the chest showing an asymptomatic residual air space 4 weeks after a right upper lobectomy for carcinoma of the lung.

pulmonary tuberculosis, bronchiectasis, and other suppurative lesions. These limited resections, however, are now being used mainly in the management of tumors of the lung, both benign and malignant. Not only are solitary metastatic tumors being resected in this manner, but also small peripheral primary lung tumors may be adequately removed by this procedure, as suggested by Jensik and colleagues (1973, 1979, 1986) as well as by me and Higgins (1974).

Operative Position and Technique

The lateral position is used by most surgeons, although the prone position is somtimes employed. The prone position is advantageous when a large quantity of bronchial secretions is present. The initial steps in a segmentectomy are carried out in the same manner as for lobectomy. Freeing of pleural adhesions, especially in patients with pulmonary tuberculosis, may be difficult and tedious. Often, extrapleural dissection is necessary. Avoid injuring the underlying vessels and nerves of the chest wall. Hemostasis must be complete to avoid postoperative bleeding.

After the hilar structures are exposed and the major fissure is opened, the pulmonary artery is identified, and the arterial branches to the segment or segments to be removed are identified, isolated, secured, and divided (Fig. 29–7). If the dissection is difficult, it is often a wise precautionary maneuver to free the main stem artery and place a tape about it. This ensures control of the vessel in the event of accidental injury to the structure during the dissection of the segmental branches. After control of the arterial supply, the segmental veins and then the bronchus are divided, although at times the order of these procedures may be reversed. Before dividing the bronchus, differential deflation and inflation of the segment to be removed should be done to help delineate the intersegmental planes. Remember that filling of the deflated segment may occur from the adjacent segments by means of collateral ventilation. Once the segmental planes are identified, the bronchus is divided and the proximal stump is closed with interrupted, fine, nonabsorbable sutures or with a mechanical stapler; additional coverage of the stump is not usually carried out.

Separation of the diseased segment is accomplished by blunt dissection. Vascular and small airway connections between the adjacent segments must be clamped, divided, and ligated. The removal of the segment is facilitated by applying traction distalward on the divided segmental hilar structures. The intersegmental position of the veins is a further guide to the intersegmental plane. The intersegmental vein is followed distally as the dissection is being completed; its branches to the subsegmental veins are ligated and divided as they are encountered.

After removal of the specimen, the raw surfaces of the adjacent segments are inspected, and any significant bleeding is controlled. A moist sponge is applied to the surface and the lung expanded. After 5 to 10 minutes, the sponge is removed and the lung surface inspected. If the dissection of the intersegmental plane has been done carefully, only small alveolar air leaks will be present. These tend to seal over promptly with re-expansion of the lung during the postoperative period. Any leaking from small bronchi, however, must be recognized and controlled; otherwise, the leak will persist and predispose to serious postoperative difficulties. Jensik (1986) advocated covering the raw surfaces with pleural flaps or reconstituting the lung by bringing the adjacent segments together. Such a step is generally unnecessary and may even lead to increased postoperative problems.

Management of the Pleural Space

Two thoracostomy tubes are placed into the space before the wound is closed, and these are connected to an underwater seal drainage system. Negative suction ranging from -10 to -20 cm water in the system is begun during closure as soon as the chest cage is reapproximated. Most believe this helps to re-expand the lung, which in turn helps to seal the raw surfaces of the pulmonary parenchyma. The subsequent management of the pleural tubes is the same as that described for lobectomy.

Physiologic Effects

The physiologic changes following a segmentectomy are the same as those noted following a lobectomy. The late functional loss is related to the number of segments removed as well as to the occurrence of postoperative complications. The functional gain by the preservation of a segment of lobe is generally less than expected from its volume. The parenchymal tissue saved, however, may play a valuable role in helping to fill the pleural space. Unfortunately, even this is relative, because the incidence of postoperative complications is greater after segmentectomy than after a lobectomy.

Morbidity

The nonfatal complications are similar to those occurring after a lobectomy. The major ones are prolonged air leak, either peripheral alveolar pleural fistula or true bronchopleural fistula, empyema, and persistent pleural air space. All are interrelated, and the incidence of any one alone, or in combination, varies most directly to the disease process and the difficulty experienced in the dissection of the intersegmental planes.

The incidence of peristent pleural air spaces is as high as 33% in patients with pulmonary tuberculosis (Fig. 29–8). Compared with the pleural air spaces occurring after a lobectomy, however, a smaller percentage of those after segmentectomy produce symptoms. When serious complications develop as a result of the space, they are most likely to be septic in nature. The empyema with or without a bronchopleural fistula must then be treated in the standard manner.

Mortality

Segmentectomy is essentially a benign procedure, and mortality rates of approximately 1% are reported when the procedure is done electively in patients with satisfactory pulmonary function and early stage disease. It

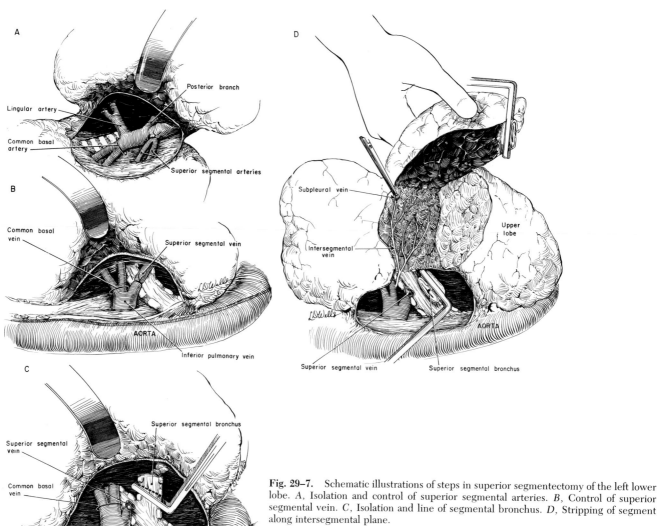

Fig. 29–7. Schematic illustrations of steps in superior segmentectomy of the left lower lobe. *A*, Isolation and control of superior segmental arteries. *B*, Control of superior segmental vein. *C*, Isolation and line of segmental bronchus. *D*, Stripping of segment along intersegmental plane.

may, however, be as high as 4 to 6% in patients with poor pulmonary function, more extensive tumor, or in those with a previous pulmonary resection, as reported by Jensik (1986) and Martini and associates (1986).

WEDGE AND LIMITED RESECTIONS

Peripheral granulomas, pulmonary blebs, benign tumors, and, on rare occasion, primary or metastatic carcinomas can be removed by a wedge or local resection of a portion of the lung. Limited resections are being increasingly employed for the resection of solitary or multiple metastatic, unilateral, or bilateral lesions. These procedures also are used for biopsy in diffuse lung disease.

Operative Position and Technique

A standard lateral or a supine position may be used. In the presence of bilateral metastatic disease, Takita

(1977) and Cooper (1978) and their colleagues reported that a median sternotomy incision can be used effectively to gain access to both hemithoraces simultaneously. This approach, however, is contraindicated if a previous thoracotomy has been done. Entry is made into the pleural space and any peripheral adhesions are freed. In a wedge resection, the area of the lung to be resected is identified, and a wedge clamp or clamps are applied so that a margin of surrounding normal lung parenchyma and the lesion are included. A basting, continuous No. 00 suture of either absorbable or nonabsorbable material is then placed beneath the clamp. The specimen is removed by cutting along the upper surface of the clamp. The clamp is removed and a continuous over-and-over suture of the same material as that used previously is placed for hemostasis.

Mechanical stapling devices such as the TA 55 stapler may be used to carry out the wedge resection (Fig. 29–9).

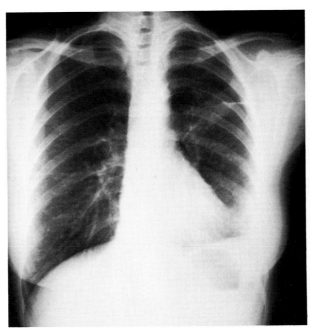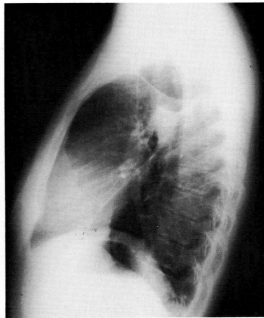

Fig. 29–8. Posteroanterior and lateral roentgenograms of the chest revealing an asymptomatic air space 6 weeks after a left apical posterior segmentectomy was performed for treatment of pulmonary tuberculosis.

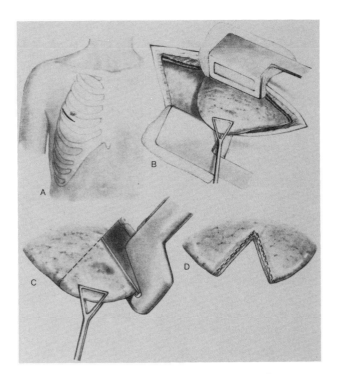

Fig. 29–9. Use of mechanical stapling device for a wedge resection of lung tissue. (Reproduced with permission from Hood, R.M.: Stapling techniques involving lung parenchyma. Surg. Clin. North Am. 3:474, 1984.)

In a limited or local resection, the visceral pleura is incised over the mass, and by sharp dissection the mass is removed, the blood vessels and minor bronchial structures being individually clamped and ligated. The visceral pleura is then reapproximated with several interrupted sutures or a continuous running suture.

Precision cautery excision of a small malignant tumor or other lesions not situated appropriately in the lung tissue for a wedge resection in a poor risk patient was described by Perelman (1983) and Cooper and associates (1986). This technique may facilitate a nonanatomical pulmonary resection. There is minimal to no air leakage from the charred surfaces of the lung. A similar result can be achieved as effectively by a standard cautery technique that has been used in the past, although late leaks may occur. The use of laser techniques for local lung excision is under investigation.

Drainage of the pleural space is then managed the same as for a lobectomy or a segmentectomy.

Physiologic Effects

The physiologic changes subsequent to a wedge resection in the absence of postoperative pleural complications are minimal. Those seen are more directly related to the thoracotomy incision than to the removal of the small portion of lung. Early in the postoperative period, the lung volume is restricted. Inspiratory capacity and the expiratory reserve volume are decreased. The end expiratory position is depressed as the result of pain in the chest wall. Alveolar hypoventilation with carbon dioxide retention and some degree of respiratory acidosis occurs. Oxyhemoglobin desaturation occurs and is most marked on the second and third postoperative days. This may persist for as long as 10 days. Compliance is reduced, resulting in an increased work of breathing. This is most marked the first few hours after operation and returns gradually to near normal within the first postoperative week.

Morbidity and Mortality

The morbidity rate after a wedge resection is minimal. When present, the complication is most often the result of either retention of secretions or pleural problems. Persistent air spaces occur, but with an incidence of less than 10%. Most of these spaces produce no symptoms and require no treatment.

The mortality rate for wedge resection is near zero for benign noninflammatory disease and likewise is low, 0.5%, even for patients with pulmonary tuberculosis.

COMPLETION LOBECTOMY OR PNEUMONECTOMY

Infrequently because of early, otherwise unresolvable postoperative complications—such as lobar infarction, bronchopleural fistula, or kinking of a bronchial anastomosis—a completion lobectomy, or more commonly a completion pneumonectomy is necessary to correct the problem. The dissection is often difficult because of inflammatory and fibrinous reactions about the vessels and the bronchus. The pulmonary vessels are best approached, when applicable, intrapericardially. The bronchial closure should be covered by a vascularized pedicle in most instances. The postoperative morbidity and mortality are generally increased above that which is seen after a comparable primary procedure, particularly when done for a bronchopleural fistula.

More often, although still not common, a completion lobectomy or pneumonectomy may become indicated remote from the original procedure because of a second primary bronchial carcinoma, locally recurrent tumor, or recurrent or new inflammatory disease in the residual ipsilateral lung. No series of completion lobectomies has been reported. McGovern and colleagues (1988), however, reported a series of 113 completion pneumonectomies; 64 were for the treatment of lung cancer, 20 for recurrent pulmonary metastases, and 29 were for benign but life-threatening processes. In this series, benign processes included 13 postoperative bronchial stump dehiscences for which a completion pneumonectomy was believed to be required.

In the entire series, the complication rate was 38.1% but was highest in those patients with benign processes—55.2%. The overall mortality was 12.4% but was zero percent for those with pulmonary metastases, 9.4% for those with lung cancer, and 27.6% for those with life-threatening benign disease. Operative mortality included 6 patients—42.8%—who died of intraoperative hemorrhage; 4 of these patients had received previous adjuvant radiation therapy. Multisystem failure was also a common cause of postoperative mortality.

Deslauriers (1988) emphasized the hazard of previous irradiation when a completion pneumonectomy is contemplated. He also noted that when the indication for the completion pneumonectomy is a benign process, especially a bronchial dehiscence, that other therapeutic options should be seriously considered whenever possible before resorting to a completion pneumonectomy because of its high morbidity and mortality rates in this situation.

The prognosis varies greatly after a successful completion pneumonectomy. In McGovern and associates' (1988) series, the overall 5-year actuarial survival was 28.4%. For those patients with lung cancer it was 26.4%; for those with pulmonary metastases it was 40.8%; and for those with benign conditions it was 27.2%.

REFERENCES

Abbey Smith, R.: Long-term follow-up after operation for lung carcinoma. Thorax 25:62, 1970.

Abbey Smith, R., and Nigam, B.K.: Resection of proximal left main bronchus carcinoma. Thorax 34:616, 1979.

Abruzzini, P.: Trattanento chirurgico della fistule del broncho principale consecutive a pneumonectomia per tubercolosi. Chir. Torac. 14:165, 1961.

Ali, M.K.: Preoperative pulmonary function evaluation for the lung cancer patient. In Cancer Patients Care at M.D. Anderson Hospital and Tumor Institute. Edited by R.L. Clark and C.D. Howe. Chicago, Year Book Medical Publishers, Inc., 1976.

Ali, M.K., et al.: Predicting loss of pulmonary function after pulmonary resection for bronchogenic carcinoma. Chest 77:337, 1980.

Ali, M.K., et al.: Regional and overall pulmonary function changes in lung cancer. J. Thorac. Cardiovasc. Surg. 86:1, 1986.

Allison, P.R.: Intrapericardial approach to the lung root in the treatment of bronchial carcinoma by dissection pneumonectomy. J. Thorac. Surg., 15:99, 1946.

Baldwin, J.C., and Mark, J.B.D.: Treatment of bronchopleural fistula after pneumonectomy. J. Thorac. Cardiovasc. Surg. 90:813, 1985.

Boysen, P.G., et al.: Prospective evaluation for pneumonectomy using the 99m technetium quantitative perfusion lung scan. Chest 72:422, 1977.

Brock, R., and Whytehead, L.L.: Radical pneumonectomy for bronchial carcinoma. Br. J. Surg. 43:8, 1955–1956.

Bruni, F.: Bronchopleural fistula: treatment of long stump after pneumonectomy. In International Trends in General Thoracic Surgery Vol. 2, Major Challenges. Edited by H. Eschapasse and H. Grillo. Philadelphia, W.B. Saunders Co., 1987.

Butchart, E.G., et al.: Pleuropneumonectomy in the management of diffuse malignant mesothelioma of the pleura. Thorax 31:15, 1976.

Cahan, G.C., Watson, W.L., and Pool, J.L.: Radical pneumonectomy. J. Thorac. Surg. 22:449, 1951.

Cahan, W.G.: Radical lobectomy. J. Thorac. Cardiovasc. Surg. 39:555, 1960.

Chuang, T.H., et al.: Pulmonary embolization from vascular stump thrombosis following pneumonectomy. Ann. Thorac. Surg. 2:290, 1966.

Cooper, J.D., Nelems, J.M., and Pearson, F.G.: Extended indications for median sternotomy in patients requiring pulmonary resection. Am. Thorac. Surg. 26:413, 1978.

Cooper, J.D., et al.: Precision cautery excision of pulmonary lesions. Ann. Thorac. Surg. 41:51, 1986.

Cosgrove, D.M., III: Closure of postpneumonectomy bronchopleural fistula. Presented at the Clinical Congress, American College of Surgeons, Thoracic Surgery Postgraduate Course, Chicago, October 14, 1985.

Dartevelle, P.G., et al.: Tracheal sleeve pneumonectomy for bronchogenic carcinoma: report of 55 cases. Ann. Thorac. Surg. 46:68, 1988.

DeLaria, G.A., et al.: Surgical management of malignant mesothelioma. Ann. Thorac. Surg. 34:4, 1978.

Deslauriers, J.: Involvement of the main carina. In International Trends in General Thoracic Surgery, Vol. 1, Lung cancer. Edited by by N.C. Delarue and H. Eschapasse. Philadelphia, W.B. Saunders Co., 1985.

Deslauriers, J.: Indications for completion pneumonectomy. Ann. Thorac. Surg. 46:133, 1988.

Deslauriers, J., et al.: Long-term clinical and functional results of sleeve lobectomy for primary cancer. J. Thorac. Cardiovasc. Surg. 92:871, 1986.

Faber, L.P.: Malignant pleural mesothelioma: operative treatment by extrapleural pneumonectomy. *In* Current Controversies in Thoracic Surgery. Edited by C.F. Kittle. Philadelphia, W.B Saunders, 1986.

Gaensler, E.A., and Strieder, J.W.: Progressive changes in pulmonary function after pneumonectomy. J. Thorac. Surg. 22:1, 1951.

Gibbon, J.H., Stokes, T.L., and McKeown, J.J., Jr.: The surgical treatment of carcinoma of the lung. Am. J. Surg. 89:484, 1985.

Ginsberg, R.J., et al.: Modern thirty-day operative mortality for surgical resections in lung cancer. J. Thorac. Cardiovasc. Surg. 86:654, 1983.

Glover, W., et al.: Fibrin glue applications through the fiberoptic bronchoscope: closure of bronchopleural fistulas. J. Thorac. Cardiovasc. Surg. 93:470, 1987.

Hakim, M., and Milstein, B.B.: Role of automatic staplers in the etiology of bronchopleural fistula. Thorax 40:27, 1985.

Hood, R.M.: Operations involving the lungs. *In* Techniques in General Thoracic Surgery. Edited by R.M. Hood. Philadelphia, W.B. Saunders Co., 1985.

Jensen, C., and Sharma, P.: Use of fibrin glue in thoracic surgery. Ann. Thorac. Surg., 39:521, 1985.

Jensik, R.J.: The extent of resection for localized lung cancer: segmental resection. *In* Current Controversies in Thoracic Surgery, Edited by C.F. Kittle. Philadelphia, W.B. Saunders Co., 1986.

Jensik, R.J., et al.: Segmental resection for lung cancer. A 15-year experience. J. Thorac. Cardiovasc. Surg. 66:563, 1973.

Jensik, R.J., et al.: Tracheal sleeve pneumonectomy for advanced carcinoma of the lung. Surg. Gynecol. Obstet. 134:231, 1972.

Jensik, R.J., Faber, L.P., and Kittle, C.F.: Segmental resection for bronchogenic carcinoma. Ann. Thorac. Surg. 28:475, 1979.

Jensik, R.J., et al.: Survival in patients undergoing tracheal sleeve pneumonectomy for bronchogenic carcinoma. J. Thorac. Cardiovasc. Surg., 84:489, 1982.

Keagy, B.A., et al.: Elective pulmonary lobectomy: factors associated with morbidity and operative mortality. Ann. Thorac. Surg. 40:349, 1985.

Kristersson, S., et al.: Prediction of pulmonary function loss due to pneumonectomy using I_{33} Xe-radiospirometry. Chest 62:649, 1972.

Maassen, W.: The transsternal and transpericardial approach for surgical treatment of fistulas of the main bronchus after pneumonectomy. Thoraxchirurgie 23:257, 1975.

Martini, N., et al.: The extent of resection for localized lung cancer: lobectomy. *In* Current Controversies in Thoracic Surgery. Edited by C.F. Kittle. Philadelphia, W.B. Saunders Co., 1986.

McGovern, E.M., et al.: Completion pneumonectomy: indications, complications, and results. Ann. Thorac. Surg. 46:141, 1988.

Miller, G.E., Aberg, T.H.J., and Gerbode, F.: Effect of pulmonary vein ligation on pulmonary artery flow in dogs. J. Thorac. Cardiovasc. Surg. 55:668, 1968.

Olsen, G.N., Block, A.J., and Tobias, L.A.: Prediction of postpneumonectomy function using quantitative macroaggregate lung scanning. Chest 66:13, 1974a.

Olsen, G.N., et al.: Pulmonary function evaluation of the lung resection candidate: a prospective study. Am. Rev. Respir. Dis. 111:379, 1974b.

Perelman, M.I.: Late treatment of chronic bronchopleural fistula with long stump after pneumonectomy. *In* International trends in General Thoracic Surgery, Vol. 2, Major Challenges. Edited by H. Eschapasse and H. Grillo. Philadelphia, W.B. Saunders Co., 1987.

Perelman, M.I.: Precision techniques for removal of pathologic structures from the lungs. Surgery 11:12, 1983.

Perelman, M.I., and Ambatiello, G.P.: Transpleuraler, transsternaler und kontralateraler Zugang bei Operationen wegen Bronchialfistel nach Pneumonecktomie. Thorax Chir. Vaskul. Chir. 18:45, 1970.

Perelman, M.I., Rymko, L.P., and Ambatiello, G.P.: Bronchopleural fistula: surgery after pneumonectomy. *In* International trends in General Thoracic Surgery, Vol. 2, Major Challenges. Edited by H. Eschapasse and H. Grillo. Philadelphia, W.B. Saunders Co., 1987.

Peters, R.M.: Postpneumonectomy pulmonary edema. *In* International Trends in General Thoracic Surgery, Vol. 2, Major Challenges. Edited by H.C. Grillo and H. Eschapasse. Philadelphia, W.B. Saunders Co., 1987.

Sarot, I.A., and Gilbert, L.: Extrapleural pneumonectomy and pleurectomy in pulmonary tuberculosis. Thorax 4:173, 1949.

Shields, T.W., and Higgins, G.A. Jr.: Minimal pulmonary resection. Arch. Surg. 108:420, 1974.

Shields, T.W., and Ujiki, G.: Digitalization for the prevention of cardiac arrhythmia following pulmonary surgery. Surg. Gynecol. Obstet. 126:743, 1968.

Suarez, J., Clagett, O.T., and Brown, A.L., Jr.: The postpneumonectomy space. J. Thorac. Cardiovasc. Surg. 57:539, 1969.

Takaro, T.: Use of staplers in bronchial closure. *In* International Trends in General Thoracic Surgery. Edited by H.C. Grillo and H. Eschapasse. Philadelphia, W.B. Saunders Co., 1987.

Takita, H., et al.: The surgical management of multiple lung metastases. Ann. Thorac. Surg. 24:359, 1977.

Thomas, C.P.: Conservative resection of bronchial tree. J.R. Coll. Surg. Edinb. 1:169, 1956.

Toomes, H., and Vogt-Moykopf, I.: Conservative resection for lung cancer. *In* International Trends in General Thoracic Surgery, Vol. 1, Lung Cancer. Edited by N.C. Delarue and H. Eschapasse. Philadelphia, W.B. Saunders Co., 1985.

Urschel, H.C., and Razzuk, M.A.: Median sternotomy as a standard approach for pulmonary resection. Ann. Thorac. Surg. 41:130, 1986.

Vanetti, A., and Bazelly, B.: Discussion of use of staples in bronchial closure. *In* International Trends in General Thoracic Surgery, Vol. 2, Major Challenges. Philadelphia, W.B. Saunders Co., 1987.

Weisel, R.D., et al.: Sleeve lobectomy for carcinoma of the lung. J. Thorac. Cardiovasc. Surg. 78:839, 1979.

Wheat, M.W., Jr., and Burford, T.H.: Digitalis in surgery. J. Thorac. Cardiovasc. Surg. 41:162, 1961.

Zeldin, R.A., et al.: Postpneumonectomy pulmonary edema. J. Thorac. Cardiovasc. Surg. 87:359, 1984.

CHAPTER 30

BRONCHIAL SLEEVE LOBECTOMY

Thomas W. Shields

A bronchial sleeve lobectomy is a modification of a standard lobectomy in which a portion of an adjacent bronchus—usually the main stem bronchus—is removed along with the resected lobe. The remaining distal bronchus—or bronchi—is anastomosed to the proximal bronchial stump to preserve the normal lung tissue distal to the resected lobe. Price Thomas (1956) reported that he performed the first sleeve lobectomy in 1947 in a patient with a bronchial adenoma, and Allison (1952) reported the first sleeve resection in a patient with bronchial carcinoma. Numerous investigators, including Paulson (1955, 1970), Johnston (1959), Jensik (1972), Naruke (1977), Bennett (1978), Weisel (1979), Rees (1970), Van den Bosch (1981), Vogt-Moykopf (1981), Ayabe (1982), Faber (1984), Toomes (1985), Fujimura (1985), and Deslauriers (1986) and their associates, have reported their experience with this procedure.

INDICATIONS

A bronchial sleeve lobectomy—or a sleeve resection of a bronchus alone–is indicated to preserve normally functioning lung distal to a pathologic process in or adjacent to a major bronchus. It is most often used to circumvent the necessity of a pneumonectomy in selected patients with bronchial carcinoma of the right upper lobe, less so in patients with carcinoma of the left upper lobe. Faber (1987) reported that his group used this procedure in 7% of their resections for lung cancer, although in most clinics the incidence of its use is much less. A sleeve resection may be extended to include other lobes or segments, as well as adjacent vascular structures; but these extended procedures are only infrequently indicated in patients with malignant disease (see Chapter 76). Deslauriers (1986) reported that proximal lobar or hilar node involvement does not preclude successful resection, but Faber (1987) noted that lymph node involvement in the region of the ipsilateral lymphatic sump (see Chapter 5) generally contraindicates a sleeve procedure.

Other indications for sleeve lobectomy are the presence of proximal—central—bronchial carcinoids and other rarer malignant tumors as well as benign endobronchial tumors without accompanying irreversible distal parenchymal damage. Infrequently, a benign bronchial stenosis from previous trauma or inflammatory process—such as severe tuberculous endobronchitis—may require a sleeve resection for its proper management.

OPERATIVE POSITION AND ANESTHETIC MANAGEMENT

Most sleeve lobectomies are done through a standard posterolateral thoracotomy incision, although some prefer the prone position. Urschel and Razzuk (1986) stated that a bronchoplastic procedure can be done without difficulty through a median sternotomy, but I would not recommend it.

The anesthetic management usually entails a double-lumen tube. For operations on the right, however, a long, single-lumen endotracheal tube can be advanced into the left main bronchus to ensure satisfactory ventilation of the left lung. When the procedure is on the left, high frequency jet ventilation (See Chapter 23) can be used, which obviates the use of a clamp on the proximal left bronchus and eliminates the need for a cuffed tube, the balloon of which might occlude the right upper lobe bronchus.

TECHNIQUE

The initial steps of a standard lobectomy with mobilization and division of the arterial and venous blood supply to the lobe to be resected are carried out. Care is taken to interfere as little as possible with the bronchial arterial supply in the mobilizing and freeing of any enlarged lymph nodes adjacent to the main stem bronchus. The main stem bronchus is then carefully dissected free from the surrounding tissues and adjacent pulmonary artery proximally. On the right, the azygos vein may need to be mobilized and divided to obtain adequate proximal exposure. Distal to the lobar takeoff, the bronchus is likewise mobilized to ensure adequate margins for the anastomosis. The bronchus must not be denuded of all adjacent tissue during the dissection. The bronchial arterial vessels to the bronchus must be preserved to ensure healing of the anastomosis. The bronchus is then divided proximally and distally beyond the gross tumor (Fig. 30–1). The bronchial divisions are made perpendicular to the bronchial wall, and tangential division should be avoided—the disparity of luminal size can be adjusted by crimping the membranous portion of the proximal cut end and stretching that of the distal end at the time of anastomosis. The cut margins should appear normal in color, and a tumor-free margin should be checked by frozen-section analysis of the proximal and distal bronchial margins of the specimen.

Reapproximation of the bronchial tree is accomplished by an end-to-end anastomosis. This is done with either 3-0 or 4-0 polyglycolic—Vicryl or Dexon—interrupted sutures. The sutures are placed into the cartilagenous portion of the bronchus first and the knots tied on the outside of the bronchus. When this is complete, the membranous portions are approximated and any size discrepancy corrected as necessary (Fig. 30–2). Oblique placement of the sutures through the cartilage should be avoided. Care is taken to prevent any angulation or kinking of the bronchial repair.

The anastomosis is then checked for any air leaks. Faber and associates (1984) recommended intraoperative flexible fiber-optic bronchoscopy to ensure that the lumen is not compromised and that the edges of the cut

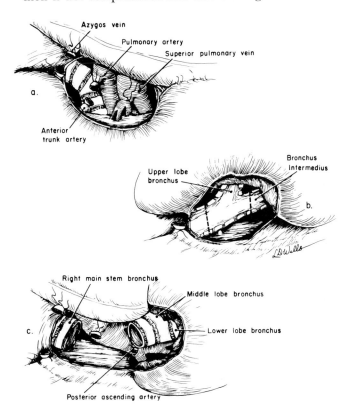

Fig. 30–1. Schematic illustration of steps of a right upper lobectomy and sleeve resection of the adjacent portion of the right main stem bronchus.

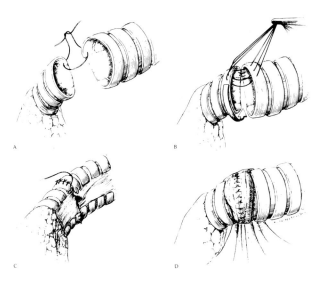

Fig. 30–2. Technique of bronchial anastomosis. *A,* Initial two or three sutures are placed in the cartilagenous portion of the bronchus just adjacent to the membraneous portion and tied. *B,* Cartilage-to-cartilage—mucosa-to-mucosa— approximation is obtained. *C,* Luminal disparity is corrected by tailoring the approximation of the membranous portions. *D,* A parietal pleural flap is placed circumferentially around the bronchus. (Reproduced with permission of Faber, L.P., et al.: Results of sleeve lobectomy for bronchogenic carcinoma in 110 patients. Ann. Thorac. Surg. 37:279, 1984.)

bronchi have been evenly approximated. The anastomosis is then covered circumferentially by a parietal pleural flap; if this is not available, the pericardial fat pad or a pericardial flap can be mobilized and brought up to cover the anastomosis. Any of these maneuvers is done to buttress the suture line and to possibly aid in the neovascularization of the anastomosis, both of which may serve to prevent the development of a bronchopleural fistula. Deslauriers and colleagues (1986) do not believe that coverage of the anastomosis is necessary.

Toomes and Vogt-Moykopf (1985) described extended sleeve resection of the bronchus to include more distal portions of the bronchial tree (Fig. 30–3 and 30–4). They

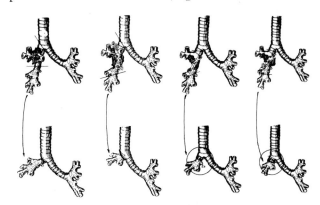

Fig. 30–3. Extended sleeve resection of the bronchus on the right side without and with simultaneous resection of middle lobe or the superior segment of the lower lobe. (Reproduced with permission of Toomes, H., and Vogt-Moykopf, I.: Conservation resection for lung cancer. *In* International Trends in General Thoracic Surgery, Vol. I. Lung Cancer. Edited by N.C. Delarue and H. Eschapasse. Philadelphia, W.B. Saunders Co., 1985, p. 88.)

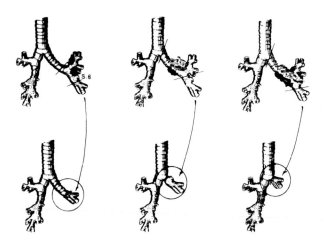

Fig. 30–4. Extended sleeve resection of the bronchus on the left side without and with simultaneous resection of the superior segmental bronchus—S.6—of the left lower lobe. (Reproduced with permission of Toomes, H., and Vogt-Moykopf, I.: Conservative resection for lung cancer. *In* International Trends in General Thoracic Surgery, Vol. I. Lung Cancer. Edited by N.C. Delarue and H. Eschapasse. Philadelphia, W.B. Saunders Co., 1985, p. 88.)

also described standard and extended sleeve resections of the pulmonary artery that can be done with or without a bronchoplastic procedure in some patients with more extensive but still localized and resectable carcinomas of the lung.

In resections of the pulmonary artery on the right, division of the azygos vein and mobilization and retraction of the superior vena cava medially gives greater access to the proximal portion of the artery. On the left, division of the ligamentum arteriosum—with care taken to avoid injury to the left recurrent nerve—and entrance into the left pulmonary recess and division of the fold of Marshall may be done to ensure greater length of the stem of the left pulmonary artery. Segmental resection of the involved portion of the vessel is then carried out after obtaining both proximal and distal control. Tangential resections should be avoided because the subsequent repair narrows the lumen of the vessel significantly. After resection, vascular continuity is reestablished by end-to-end anastomosis with a continuous suture of 5-0 or 6-0 nonabsorbable monofilament suture material. If a bronchial sleeve resection has been done at the same time—a combined bronchial sleeve resection and angioplasty—the bronchial anastomosis is always completed first and covered with a tissue flap before repair of the artery.

After completion of the procedure, the chest is drained and the incision closed in the standard manner.

POSTOPERATIVE CARE

Faber (1987) and his group recommended fiber-optic bronchoscopy the first postoperative day and as often as necessary thereafter. Many believe this is unnecessary as a routine and only carry out the procedure if the clinical or roentgenographic findings suggest retained secretions. Toomes and Vogt-Moykopf (1985) suggested the assessment of lung function by ventilation and perfusion scans before discharge, as well as bronchoscopic inspection of the suture line.

MORBIDITY

In addition to the complications that may occur after a standard lobectomy, several complications unique to a sleeve resection may occur: (1) kinking of the site of the bronchial anastomosis; (2) circumferential stenosis or granuloma formation, or both; (3) bronchial suture line dehiscence; and (4) kinking of the pulmonary artery. The first and last aforementioned complications should be avoided by proper technique and alignment of the structures at operation. When they do occur postoperatively, a completion pneumonectomy may be necessary because of sepsis or infarction of the remaining lung.

Stenosis and granulation tissue formation is rare with the use of absorbable suture material for the bronchial anastomosis, whereas granulation tissue formation was common with the use of nonabsorbable sutures—except monofilament wire. Late stenosis may result from an unrecognized asymptomatic anastomotic leak with localized infection, but such infections usually lead to erosion into the pulmonary artery with fatal hemorrhage from the bronchovascular communication.

Overt bronchial suture line disruption may also cause a bronchovascular fistula with fatal hemorrhage, but a bronchopleural fistula with empyema is the more common result of a major suture line dihiscence. The management of this complication is a completion pneumonectomy and control of the empyema by one of the appropriate methods outlined in Chapter 59.

In patients with carcinoma, Faber and associates (1984) reported that local recurrence may be observed as a late complication in approximately 9% of patients. These patients are rarely candidates for a completion pneumonectomy, and irradiation or chemotherapy or both may be indicated. Endobronchial laser techniques to relieve the obstructing tumor may be useful in this situation.

MORTALITY

Faber (1987) reported a mortality rate of 1.7%, and Deslauriers and colleagues (1986) as well as Naruke (1977) and Kawakami (1977) and their associates reported no mortality in their respective series of sleeve lobectomies, but Toomes and Vogt-Moykopf (1985) reported a mortality rate of 9% in patients undergoing a bronchoplastic procedure, one of 11% after angioplastic procedures, and a rate of 17% after a combined bronchoplastic and angioplastic procedure. These latter data undoubtedly reflect a more aggressive surgical approach to the treatment of lung carcinoma.

FUNCTIONAL RESULTS

The objective of a bronchial sleeve lobectomy is to preserve lung function that would be lost if a pneumonectomy were carried out. Toomes and Vogt-Moykopf (1985) evaluated 45 patients with perfusion/ventilation scans 3 weeks after sleeve lobectomy. The postoperative mean percentages of both for the operated side were preserved to just over half that determined preoperatively—22%/39% versus 39%/45%, respectively.

Deslauriers and colleagues (1986) presented data that showed that late—5 years postoperatively—pulmonary function studies revealed lower but not severely altered results respective to the percent of predicted values for the 19 patients studied. The FVC was 85.9% ± 17.5% and the FEV_1 was 74.9% ± 19.4%. Regional function determined by perfusion scans revealed ratios of 41.1% for the right lung to 58.9% for the left lung in 15 patients who had undergone a right sleeve lobectomy. In the 4 patients with left sleeve lobectomy, the ratio was 29.3% for the left lung and 51.7% for the right lung. Ventilation scans showed comparable results. Although the number of patients studied by both groups is small, the remaining ipsilateral lung tissue evidently contributes significantly to the overall remaining lung function. The procedure may be considered to be significantly valuable in preserving lung function that would be lost if a pneumonectomy had been carried out.

REFERENCES

Allison, P.R.: Course of Thoracic Surgery in Groningen 1954.

Ayabe, H., et al.: Bronchoplasty for bronchogenic carcinoma. World J. Surg. 6:433, 1982.

Bennett, F.W., and Smith, A.R.: A twenty-year analysis of the results of sleeve resection for primary bronchogenic carcinoma. J. Thorac. Cardiovasc. Surg. 76:840, 1978.

Deslauriers, J., et al.: Long-term clinical and functional results of sleeve lobectomy for primary lung cancer. J. Thorac. Cardiovasc. Surg. 92:871, 1986.

Faber, L.P.: Results of surgical treatment of stage III lung carcinoma with carinal proximity: the role of sleeve lobectomy versus pneumonectomy and the role of sleeve pneumonectomy. Surg. Clin. N. Am. 67:1001, 1987.

Faber, L.P., Jensik, R.J., and Kittle, C.F.: Results of sleeve lobectomy for bronchogenic carcinoma in 101 patients. Ann. Thorac. Surg. 37:279, 1984.

Fujimura, S., et al.: Prognostic evaluation of tracheobronchial reconstruction for bronchogenic carcinoma. J. Thorac. Cardiovasc. Surg. 90:161, 1985.

Jensik, R.J., et al.: Sleeve lobectomy for carcinoma, a ten-year experience. J. Thorac. Cardiovasc. Surg. 64:400, 1972.

Johnston, J.B., and Jones, P.H.: The treatment of bronchial carcinoma by lobectomy and sleeve resection of the main bronchus. Thorax 14:48, 1959.

Kawakami, M., et al.: Experience with bronchoplastic surgery—pre- and postoperative lung function. Sci. Rep. Res. Inst. Tohoku Univ. [Med.] 24:52, 1977.

Naruke, T., et al.: Bronchoplastic procedure for lung cancer. J. Thorac. Cardiovasc. Surg. 73:927, 1977.

Paulson, D.L., and Shaw, R.R.: Preservation of lung tissue by means of bronchoplastic procedures. Am. J. Surg. 89:347, 1955.

Paulson, D.L., et al.: Bronchoplastic procedures for bronchogenic carcinoma. J. Thorac. Cardiovasc. Surg. 59:38, 1970.

Price Thomas, C.: Conservative resection of the bronchial tree. J. R. Coll. Surg. Edinb. 1:169, 1956.

Rees, G.M., and Paneth, M.: Lobectomy with sleeve resection in the treatment of bronchial tumors. Thorax 25:160, 1970.

Toomes, H., and Vogt-Moykopf, I.: Conservative resection for lung cancer. In International Trends in General Thoracic Surgery, Vol. I. Lung Cancer. Edited by N.C. Delarue and H. Eschapasse. Philadelphia, W.B. Saunders Co., 1985, p. 88.

Urschel, H.C., Jr., Razzuk, M.A.: Median sternotomy as a standard approach for pulmonary resection. Ann. Thorac. Surg. 41:130, 1986.

Van Den Bosch, J.M.M., et al.: Lobectomy with sleeve resection in the treatment of tumors of the bronchus. Chest 80:154, 1981.

Vogt-Moykopf, I., et al.: Organsparende Operationsverfahren beim Bronchialkarzinom, Ergebnisse. Langenbecks Arch. Chir. 355:117, 1981.

Weisel, R.D., et al.: Sleeve lobectomy for carcinoma of the lung. J. Thorac. Cardiovasc. Surg. 78:839, 1979.

CHAPTER 31

TRACHEAL-SLEEVE PNEUMONECTOMY

Jean Deslauriers, Maurice Beaulieu, and André McClish

Most bronchial carcinomas involving the lower trachea are so extensive that curative resection is not possible. This involvement is often secondary to metastatic subcarinal nodes growing through the airway and into the tracheal lumen. Occasionally, however, tumors arising in the upper lobes or in the origin of either main bronchus are sufficiently localized to permit complete resection and reconstruction.

At present, surgical indications, techniques of resection, and even prospects for cure are unclear because very few institutions have significant experience with these procedures.

SELECTION FOR OPERATION

Tracheal-sleeve pneumonectomy is primarily indicated for patients whose lung cancer extends endobronchially to the lower trachea, the carina, or the medial wall of the opposite main bronchus. When this situation is suspected at bronchoscopy, random biopsies must be taken proximally, because a tension-free or tumor-free reconstruction is unlikely if the tumor extends more than 4 cm above the carina. Although tomography and CT scanning are useful to define the degree of extraluminal growth, the final decision to proceed with resection is nearly always based on operative findings—positive resection margin after pneumonectomy or gross extension to lower trachea.

Mediastinoscopy has an important role in preoperative staging because most, if not all, individuals with proven spread to superior mediastinal nodes are not candidates for tracheal-sleeve pneumonectomy. As for every case of presumably operable lung cancer, the presence of extrathoracic metastases must be ruled out before operation and the cardiopulmonary reserve carefully assessed.

Over a 20-year period, 1967 to 1987, 38 patients with primary lung cancer underwent sleeve pneumonectomy at our institution (Table 31–1). In 33 patients, the procedure was done concomitantly with right pneumonectomy, and in 3, it was done for a positive resection line

Table 31–1. Operative Procedure in 38 Patients with Tracheal-Sleeve Pneumonectomy for Primary Lung Cancer

Operative Procedure	Number of Patients
Right-sleeve pneumonectomy	33
Left-sleeve pneumonectomy (two stage)	3
Resection of stump recurrence	2
TOTAL	38

after proximal left pneumonectomy. Two additional patients had a stump recurrence 18 months and 6 years after previous left pneumonectomy.

OPERATIVE TECHNIQUE

Right Tracheal-Sleeve Pneumonectomy

The operation is done through a fifth interspace posterolateral thoracotomy. A thorough exploration with proper nodal staging must be done early so the extent of resection needed, if it is possible, is clearly defined. Preservation of distal lung by sleeve lobectomy should always be considered but is seldom feasible in those patients because of hilar or promixal pulmonary artery invasion—primary tumor or N1 nodes.

The pulmonary artery and veins are next ligated intrapericardially, and the azygos vein divided anteriorly and posteriorly so that its central portion is included in the resected specimen (Fig. 31–1A). The esophagus is freed from the carina and portions of its muscular layer can be excised with the tumor if necessary. The carina is then fully mobilized from its mediastinal bed and tapes passed around the lower trachea and left main bronchus.

Although some cases could be managed by limited excision of the lateral tracheal wall, a circumferential resection offers better tumor clearance. The trachea is transsected 1.0 cm proximal to the tumor—2.5 to 3.0 cm

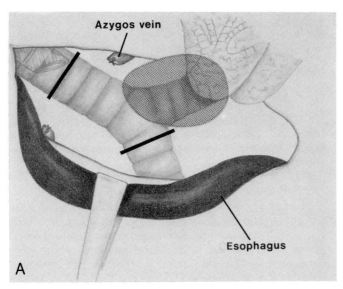

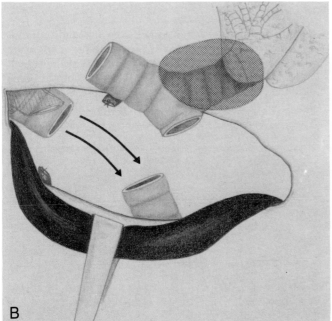

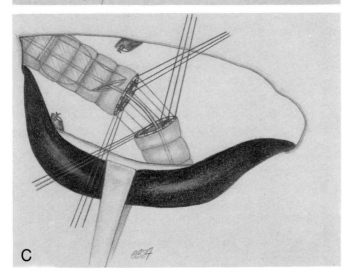

Fig. 31–1. Operative technique for right tracheal-sleeve pneumonectomy. *A*, Mobilization of the carina. *B*, Division of the trachea and left main bronchus. *C*, Circumferential anastomosis.

above the carina—and the left main bronchus near its orgin (Fig. 31–1*B*). Naef (1973) showed that when possible one should attempt to preserve extra tissue at the membranous portion—by creating a posterior flap. In the event of a positive resection margin by frozen section examination, the tracheal resection can be extended to a maximum length of 4.0 to 4.5 cm. Shields (1976) noted that residual tumor at the bronchial margin is not always a sign of unfavorable prognosis, so it may be wise on occasion to accept a positive resection line rather than doing an extensive procedure with compromised reconstruction.

Because of the relative fixity of the left main bronchus underneath the aorta, the trachea is pulled down (Fig. 31–1*C*) and the reconstruction done without tension—interrupted sutures through all layers. Maximum flexion of the neck will also reduce tension at the anastomosis. Size discrepancy between the lumens is corrected by stretching the smaller lumen to the size of the larger one by careful suture spacing. Synthetic absorbable sutures are used—Vicryl 3–0 for cartilage and 4–0 for membrane—because Gibbons (1981) presented good evidence that they induce less granulation tissue formation at the suture line. Once completed, the anastomosis should be checked for air leaks and the endotracheal tube pulled back to a sufficient distance above the suture line. Tissue flaps may be used to increase local vascular supply.

Figure 31–2 is a photograph of the proximal end of a resected specimen.

Left Tracheal-Sleeve Pneumonectomy

Carinal extension is exceedingly rare with left-sided lesions, and opinions differ about the operability of such tumors. Left tracheal-sleeve pneumonectomy (Fig. 31–3) is therefore carried out in a small number of cases and only as an alternative to conventional stump radiation therapy.

Abbott and associates (1955) and Grillo (1982a) described a one-stage operation—left posterolateral thoracotomy—but this approach is seldom used because properly exposing the carina underneath the aortic arch is difficult. We prefer a two-stage procedure. In the first stage, a left proximal pneumonectomy—subaortic or supra-aortic—is carried out, and 3 to 5 weeks later, the carina is resected from the right side. Because of the local inflammatory reaction and mediastinal shift that follows pneumonectomy, mobilization of the left main bronchial stump is potentially dangerous and one must be aware of the proximity of the left pulmonary artery stump and left recurrent nerve. Division of the trachea 1.5 cm above the bifurcation is sufficient for most tumors, but if necessary, it is possible to resect an additional length of distal trachea and elevate the right main bronchus for primary anastomosis.

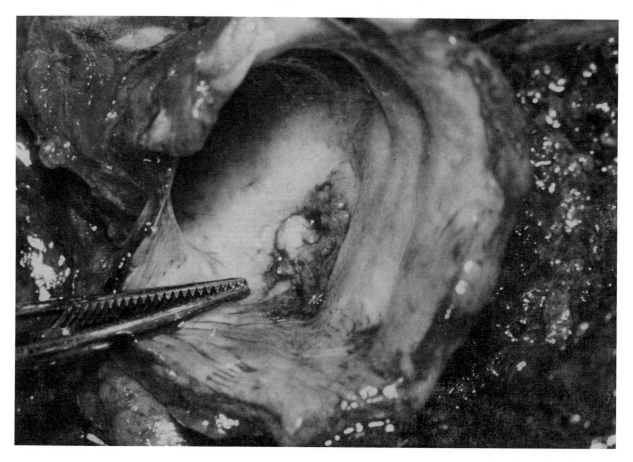

Fig. 31–2.   Resected specimen with right lung, carina, and proximal left main bronchus. Note the carcinoma in the proximal right main bronchus.

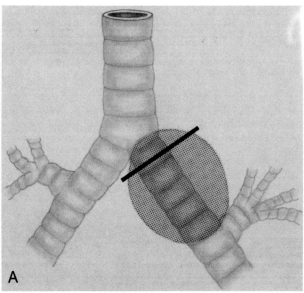

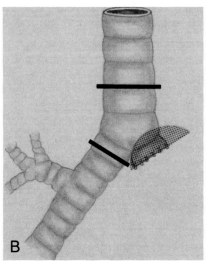

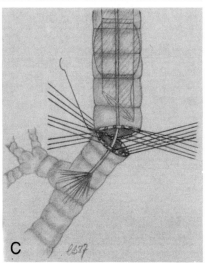

Fig. 31–3. Operative technique for left tracheal-sleeve pneumonectomy. *A,* Left proximal pneumonectomy. *B,* Division of trachea and right main bronchus. *C,* Circumferential anastomosis.

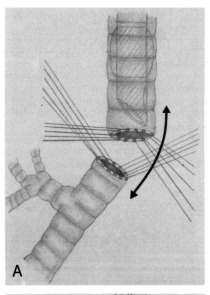

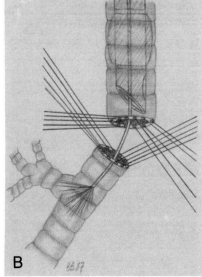

Fig. 31–4. Anesthetic techniques. *A,* Tube ventilation. *B,* High flow catheter ventilation.

MANAGEMENT OF ANESTHESIA

Catheter Ventilation

Despite improved anesthetic techniques, the problems associated with carinal reconstruction stem from the complexity of simultaneously controlling the airways, maintaining satisfactory anesthesia and gas exchange, and ensuring good surgical exposure of the trachea.

The tube ventilation system from above or across the operative field is the most conventional method, and Geffin and colleagues (1969) showed that it can be adapted to all carinal reconstructions (Fig. 31–4A). Oxygenation is maintained by positive-pressure ventilation alternating with periods of apnea, during which posterior sutures are inserted and tied. When two thirds of the anastomosis is done, the endotracheal tube is advanced across the suture line and the reconstruction completed.

Table 31–2. Results of Tracheal-Sleeve Pneumonectomy

Authors	Number of Cases	Operative Mortality (%)	Survival at 5 Years (%)
Mathey, et al. (1966)	2	0	—
Grillo (1982)	5	0	—
Jensik, et al. (1982)	34	29	15
Fujimara, et al. (1985)	7	0	—
Deslauriers, et al. (1987)	38	29	13

Table 31–3. Causes of Perioperative Death After Sleeve Pneumonectomy (11/38)

Cause	Number of Patients
Bronchopneumonia and respiratory failure	8
Pulmonary embolus	1
Bronchopleural fistula	1
Myocardial infarction (perioperative)	1
	11

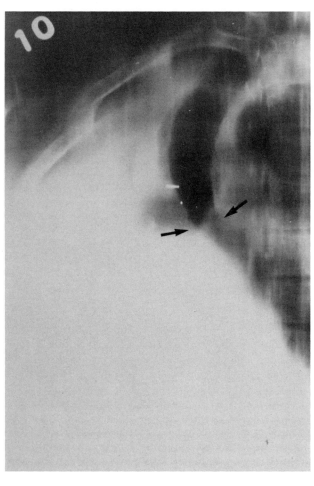

Fig. 31–5. Tracheal tomography demonstrating a normal anastomosis three years after sleeve pneumonectomy.

This system has the disadvantages of repeated tube manipulations with frequent interruptions in airway suturing. If the tube is across the operative field—armored tube into left main bronchus—it further restricts surgical access to the carina.

The technique of prolonged apneic oxygenations was described for carinal reconstructions. After hyperventilating the patient with 100% oxygen, Frumin (1959) and Heller (1964) and their associates showed that a period of 10 to 12 minutes of total apnea can often be tolerated. This technique is rarely used because the duration of safe apnea is unpredictable—cardiovascular response—in any individual patient.

Various methods involving high flow of gases have been recommended for anesthesia during bronchoscopy, laryngeal surgery, and tracheal reconstruction. All of these systems are described in Chapter 23.

The high frequency jet ventilation system that delivers a small tidal volume through an endotracheal catheter at a rate of 100 to 150 respirations/min has been used by El-Baz and colleagues (1981) for sleeve pneumonectomy. The absence of endotracheal tube in the operative field and the relative immobility of the lung facilitate surgical manipulations but the equipment and expertise are not yet available in most operating rooms.

The high-flow catheter technique described by McClish and co-workers (1985) for tracheobronchial reconstructions (Fig. 31–4B) has specific advantages with regard to simplicity of the equipment and anesthetic technique. It involves positive pressure ventilation with a high flow of gas and without air entrainment. Oxygen is supplied from a high pressure source capable of delivering at a pressure of 50 psi a flow of 100 L/min. Depending on airway resistance and lung compliance, the inflation flow can be adjusted—through a reducing valve—to generate an airway pressure of 25 to 40 cm H_2O.

To aspirate blood and mucus, remove necrotic debris, and check the reconstruction, fiber-optic bronchoscopy must be done before the patient leaves the operating room. Most patients are extubated within 4 to 5 hours of the completion of the operation.

MORBIDITY, MORTALITY, AND RESULTS

The postoperative period is often difficult, because all patients have transient but significant bronchorrhea probably related to lymphatic, autonomic nervous system, and ciliary epithelium interruption. Aggressive chest physiotherapy must be instituted early and endotracheal aspiration or bronchoscopy done at the earliest sign of secretion retention. Elective tracheotomy is avoided when possible. Antibiotics are given routinely, but steroids are not, although Naef (1973) described potential benefits, such as a decrease in the amount of secretions, local edema, or granulation tissue formation.

Table 31–2 records the results achieved in five series. Grillo (1982b) reported no operative deaths in 5 patients, but Jensik and associates (1982) had a 29% perioperative mortality. Most of the deaths followed bronchopleural fistula, possibly related to preoperative radiation—28 of 34 patients had 3200 to 5000 rads. In our series of sleeve pneumonectomies, the operative mortality was also 29%; the causes of death are listed in Table 31–3. All deaths followed right-sleeve pneumonectomy and most followed respiratory failure caused by infection in the remaining lung. This fatal complication was usually predictable, because symptoms appeared in the first 48 hours after operation: abundance of sputum, inability to cough, and increasing dyspnea. By the time secretions became purulent, infiltrations were noted on the roentgenogram and frank respiratory failure occurred.

Other major nonfatal complications included incapacitating bronchorrhea—3 patients, hemorrhage necessitating reoperation—2 patients, empyema—1 patient, and bronchopleural fistula—1 patient. Overall, close to 50% of patients had a major postoperative problem, as compared to 14% for standard resections.

Jensik and associates (1982) reported a 5-year survival rate of 15% in the 34 patients who underwent tracheal-sleeve pneumonectomy. In our series, the absolute survival rate is 47%—18 out of 38—at 1 year and 13%—4 out of 30—at 5 years. These small numbers of cases do not allow statistical analysis, but the long-term results indicate that the operation is beneficial to selected individuals (Fig. 31–5).

REFERENCES

Abbott, O.A., et al.: Experience with extending the indications for the use of tracheal and bronchial grafts. J. Thorac. Surg. *29*:217, 1955.

Deslauriers, J.: Involvement of the main carina. Int. Trends General Thoracic Surgery *1*:139, 1985.

Deslauriers, J., et al.: Sleeve pneumonectomy for bronchogenic carcinoma. Ann. Thorac. Surg. *28*:465, 1979.

El-Baz, N.M., et al.: One-lung high frequency positive-pressure ventilation for sleeve pneumonectomy: an alternative technique. Anesth. Analg. *60*:683, 1981.

Frumin, J.M., et al.: Apneic oxygenation in man. Anesthesiology *20*:789, 1959.

Fujimara, S., et al.: Prognostic evaluation of tracheobronchial reconstruction for bronchogenic carcinoma. J. Thorac. Cardiovasc. Surg. *90*:161, 1985.

Geffin, B., et al.: Anesthetic management of tracheal resection and reconstruction. Anesth. Analg. *48*:884, 1969.

Gibbons, J.A.: A comparison of synthetic absorbable suture with synthetic nonabsorbable suture for construction of tracheal anastomoses. Chest *79*:340, 1981.

Gilbert, A., Deslauriers, J., et al.: Tracheal sleeve pneumonectomy for carcinoma of the proximal left main bronchus. Can. J. Surg. *27*:583, 1984.

Grillo, H.C.: Carinal reconstruction. Ann. Thorac. Surg. *34*:356, 1982a.

Grillo, H.C.: Carcinoma of the lung: what can be done if the carina is involved. Am. J. Surg. *143*:694, 1982b.

Heller, M.L., et al.: Apneic oxygenation in man: polarographic arterial oxygen tension study. Anesthesiology *25*:25, 1964.

Jensik, R.J., et al.: Survival in patients undergoing tracheal sleeve pneumonectomy for bronchogenic carcinoma. J. Thorac. Cardiovasc. Surg. *84*:489, 1982.

Mathey, J., et al.: Tracheal and tracheobronchial resections. J. Thorac. Cardiovasc. Surg. *51*:1, 1966.

McClish, A., et al.: High-flow catheter ventilation during major tracheobronchial reconstruction. J. Thorac. Cardiovasc. Surg. *89*:508, 1985.

Naef, A.P.: Tracheobronchial reconstruction. Ann. Thorac. Surg. *15*:301, 1973.

Saunders, R.D.: Two ventilating attachments for bronchoscopy. Del. Med. J. *39*:170, 1967.

Shields, T.W.: The fate of patients after incomplete resection of bronchial carcinoma. Surg. Gynecol. Obstet. *139*:569, 1976.

CHAPTER 32

MEDIAN STERNOTOMY APPROACH TO THE LOWER TRACHEA AND MAIN STEM BRONCHI

Michail I. Perelman

The transmediastinal approach to the lower trachea and main stem bronchi is indicated chiefly for postpneumonectomy patients with bronchial fistulas. Other conditions for which this approach is indicated are rare and include a lung with multiple bronchial fistulas and empyema and pulmonary hemorrhage in a severely ill patient who has previously undergone pulmonary surgery. In the latter condition, preliminary transmediastinal transection and occlusion of the pulmonary artery and bronchus may be the first stage of a two-stage pneumonectomy. In patients with empyema, the advantage of transmediastinal approach over the conventional transpleural route is that it affords an aseptic access to the trachea and main bronchi through the mediastinal tissue and pericardium.

In 1960, Padhi and Lynn advocated the use of median sternotomy preceded by intrapericardial ligation of the pulmonary artery and superior pulmonary vein for operations to amputate a main bronchial stump that is closely adherent to pulmonary vessel stumps.

In 1963, I and Boguslavskaya reported the first two operations, performed in 1961, for fistulas of the right and left main bronchi, respectively, from a transsternal approach. On the right, a small incision of the pericardium was made over the right pulmonary artery stump, while on the left the transpericardial route of approach was used with ligation and transection of the left pulmonary artery stump; we also presented results of topographic studies undertaken to validate the use of transsternal access to bronchial fistulas. Also in 1963, Abruzzini described a technique of operation on main bronchial stumps from a transsternal approach without opening the pericardium. He recommended that, regardless of the side of intervention, access to the stump be gained through the space between the aorta and superior vena cava. Bogush and associates (1972) examined in detail various transsternal approaches to main bronchial stumps and recommended the transpericardial approach in all instances; this approach is now employed fairly often. These authors showed that the best spatial relations are created by approaching the right main bronchial stump through the aortocaval space and the left stump through the aortovenous space.

STERNOTOMY

I always performed a complete median sternotomy, as did other authors, until I found that dissection of the sternum longitudinally from the jugular notch to the level of the third intercostal space is sufficient in many patients with a long sternum. Dissecting the sternum transversely at this level and bringing the right and left halves of the dissected sternum apart with a single retractor provides an adequate operative field.

MEDIASTINAL APPROACH

Lower Trachea and Bronchi

The transitional pleural fold over the—usually—dilated left lung is dissected off to the left, and to the right of the ascending aorta a tetragonal space is entered, whose sides are the right margin of the ascending aorta and the initial portion of brachiocephalic trunk on the left, the superior vena cava on the right, the left brachiocephalic vein cranially, and the transitional pericardial fold—which corresponds to the margin of the right pulmonary artery—caudally. Once the superior vena cava and the ascending aorta with brachiocephalic trunk have been drawn apart, this tetragon is generally 5 to 7 cm in height and width. The trachea and its bifurcation are now palpable on the bottom of the space formed between the vessels and filled with fatty tissue and lymph nodes. The portion of the trachea above the bifurcation can be separated from the esophagus, after inserting a thick tube into the latter, and held on a rubber catheter or stay suture. The right main bronchus and the initial portion of the left main bronchus can also be mobilized.

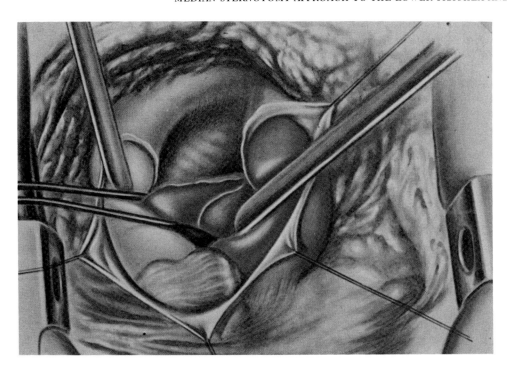

Fig. 32–1. Mediastinal-transpericardial approach to the lower trachea and right main bronchus. The aorta and superior vena cava have been drawn part. The dorsal pericardial wall has been dissected over the right pulmonary artery, which is held with a rubber catheter.

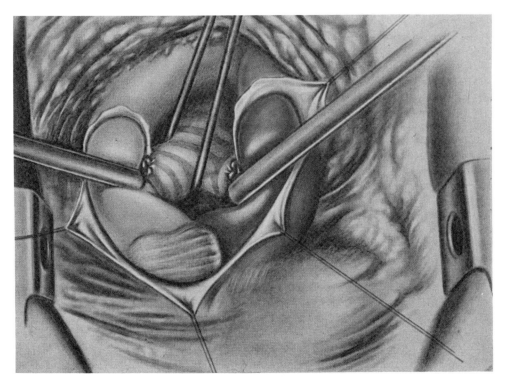

Fig. 32–2. The right pulmonary artery has been transected. The right main bronchus is held with a rubber catheter.

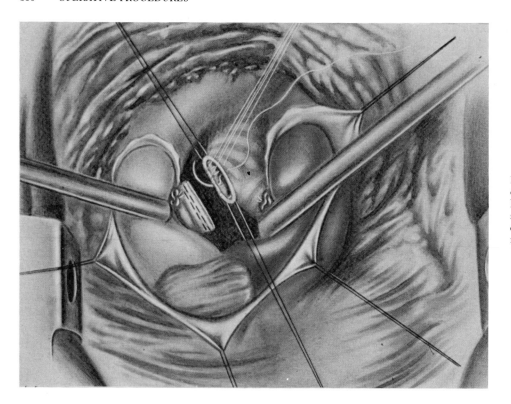

Fig. 32–3. The right main bronchial stump has been sutured with linear mechanical suture and dissected off from the trachea. The tracheal opening is closed with interrupted sutures.

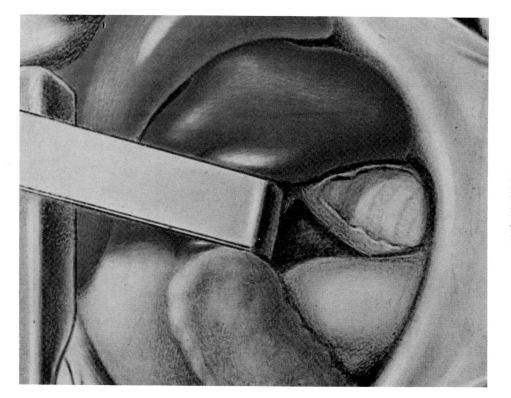

Fig. 32–4. Mediastinal-transpericardial approach to the left main bronchus. The pericardium has been opened and the dorsal pericardial wall dissected over the left main bronchus.

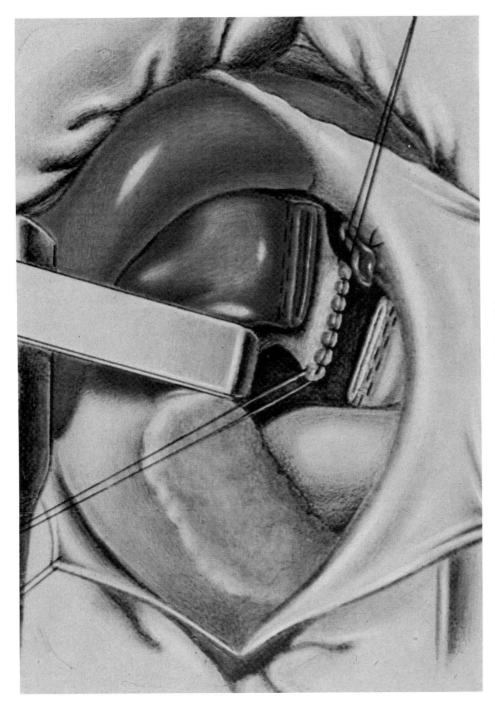

Fig. 32–5. The left pulmonary artery has been sutured with linear mechanical suture and transected, and a ligature has been applied to the distal end of the artery. The left main bronchial stump has been transected near the trachea. Interrupted sutures have been placed on the proximal end of the stump and a linear mechanical suture, on its distal end.

Such a purely mediastinal access to the trachea and main bronchi has limited exposure. It is therefore advisable, as a rule, to open the pericardium after sternotomy. The transpericardial approach affords a much broader scope for surgical manipulations.

MEDIASTINAL-TRANSPERICARDIAL APPROACH

Trachea and Right Main Bronchial Stump

After the sternotomy and after the transitional pleural fold has been moved to the left, the pericardium is opened by a vertical incision slightly to the right of the midline. The edges of the pericardium are sutured with stay sutures. The aorta and the superior vena cava are drawn apart. In right postpneumonectomy patients, the right pulmonary artery stump is ligated and transected for better operative exposure. For this, the dorsal pericardial wall is dissected over the artery, which is then held in place with a rubber catheter (Fig. 32–1). The proximal end of the artery is sutured with a linear mechanical suture using a stapler with branches 30 mm long, and a ligature is applied to the distal end. Distal to the applied stapler, the artery is divided and an additional

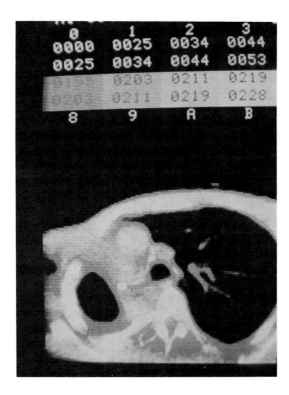

Fig. 32–6. Computer tomogram after left pneumonectomy. The mediastinum is grossly displaced to the left.

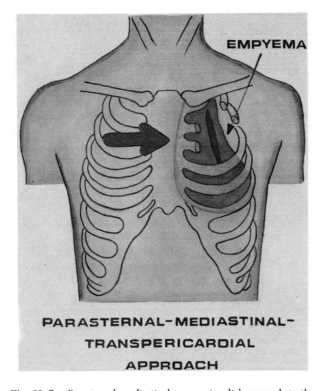

Fig. 32–7. Parasternal mediastinal-transpericardial approach to the left main bronchus after pneumonectomy, with resection of cartilages of the second and third ribs.

ligature is applied proximal to the staple line, bypassing the stapler. The opening in the dorsal pericardial wall is widened, thereby obtaining access to the lower trachea and the right main bronchus; only the proximal part of the left main bronchus is accessible (Figs. 32–2 and 32–3).

If a bronchopleural fistula is present, it is best to reamputate and remove the bronchial stump, if it is feasible. A linear mechanical suture—UO or TA stapler—is applied to the lateral tracheal wall, or the tracheal opening is closed with interrupted Vicryl 3–0 or 4–0 sutures. A bronchial stump that has been separated from the trachea and sutured may be the source of long-lasting mucous discharge into the residual pleural cavity or of a retention cyst. If removal of the stump is impractical or hazardous, it is advisable to destroy its mucosa chemically—with silver nitrate or trichloroacetic acid—or by electrocoagulation and then suture it with interrupted absorbable—Vicryl or PDS—sutures.

Left Main Bronchial Stump

After sternotomy, the transitional pleural fold is moved to the right and the pericardium is opened by a vertical incision 10 to 11 cm long to the left of the midline, 2 to 3 cm anterior to the left phrenic nerve. The pericardial edges are brought apart by stay sutures. The operating table is then tilted sideways and to the right, the heart is moved somewhat to the right, and the dorsal pericardial wall is opened (Fig. 32–4). As far proximally as possible, the left pulmonary artery stump and, in some cases, the superior pulmonary vein stump are ligated and transected. Bogush and colleagues (1972) considered that ligation and division of only the superior pulmonary vein are often sufficient. Vessels are mobilized after dissection of the dorsal pericardial wall, and their proximal ends are sutured with a linear mechanical suture and ligated additionally; the distal ends are ligated and sutured after transection. The opening in the dorsal pericardial wall is widened, gaining access to the left main bronchial stump (Fig. 32–5). In operations for bronchial fistula, the same procedure is followed as on the right.

PARASTERNAL MEDIASTINAL-TRANSPERICARDIAL APPROACH

Left Main Bronchial Stump

After a left pneumonectomy, the mediastinum usually shifts to the left; in many patients it is grossly displaced (Fig. 32–6). In such instances, I perform thoracotomy not transsternally but parasternally on the left, resecting cartilages of the second and third ribs (Fig. 32–7). Then, the—usually—thick and dense transitional pleural fold must be separated from the pericardium by sharp and blunt dissection and drawn to the left. This provides a more convenient access to the pericardium anterior to the left phrenic nerve than does a transsternal incision. The pericardium is now opened by a vertical incision and the operation is continued exactly as it is when using the previously described mediastinal-transpericardial approach to the left main bronchial stump.

MORBIDITY AND MORTALITY

Hemorrhage at the time of operation may occur in a significant number of patients—17% in the series of 39 operations I and my associates (1987) reported—but was controlled in all. Recanalization of the bronchus when the excluded stump is not removed may occur rarely. This complication is common, however, if the bronchus is only occluded and not actually divided.

The mortality rate is high—23%—with this approach, often because of the poor functional status of the patients operated upon. In our 1987 series, six patients died from cardiopulmonary insufficiency, two from thrombosis of the remaining sole pulmonary artery and one from recanalization of the bronchus.

PROGNOSIS

When the immediate operative procedure is successful, a 96% cure rate in the surviving patients can be expected. When postoperative deaths are included, however, only an overall 75% success rate is obtained.*

---

*Editor's footnote: One should be highly selective in using this procedure. It is perhaps best reserved for right-sided postpneumonectomy bronchial fistulas and is less often indicated for the management of left-sided bronchial fistulas. This is concurred in by the author.

REFERENCES

Abruzzini, P.: Chirurgische Behandlung der Fisteln des Hauptbronchus. Thoraxchir. Vask. Chir. *10*:259, 1963.
Bogush, L.K., Travin, A.A., and Semenenkov., Y.L.: Operatsii na glavnykh bronkhakh cherez polost' perikarda [Operations on the main bronchi via the pericardial cavity.] Moscow, Meditsina, 1972. (In Russian.)
Bruni, F., et al.: Traitement chirurgical des fistules après pneumonectomie: intervention modifiée d'Abruzzini. Ann. Chir. *39*:135, 1985.
Padhi, R., and Lynn, R.: The management of bronchopleural fistula. J. Thorac. Surg. *39*:385, 1960.
Perelman, M.I., and Boguslavskaya, T.B.: Operative approaches to tracheobronchial angles through the sternum and anterior mediastinum to close bronchial fistulas following pneumonectomy. *In* Aktual'nye voprosy tuberkulieza [*In* Current Problems of Tuberculosis.] No. 2. Moscow Central Institute for Advanced Medical Education Publication, 1963, p. 169. (In Russian.)
Perelman, M.I., Rymko, L.P., and Ambatiello, G.P.: Bronchopleural fistula: surgery after pneumonectomy. *In* International Trends in General Thoracic Surgery, Vol. 2, Major Challenges. Edited by H.C. Grillo and H. Eschapasse. Philadelphia, W.B. Saunders Co., 1987., p. 407.

READING REFERENCES

Bogush, L.K., Trawin, A.A., and Semenenkov, Y.L.: Transperikardiale Operationen an den Hauptbronchien und Lungengefässen. Stuttgart, Hippokrates Verlag, 1971.
Perelman, M.I., and Ambatiello, G.P.: Transsternaler und kontralateraler Zugang bei Operationen wegen Bronchialfistel nach Pneumonektomie. Thoraxchir. Vask. Chir. *18*:45, 1970.
Perelman, M.I., and Klimansky, V.A.: Operations on the Lungs. *In* Atlas of Thoracic Surgery, Vol. 1. St. Louis, C.V. Mosby Company, pp. 99–225, 1979.
Petrowskij, B.V., and Perelman, M.I.: Wiederherstellende und rekonstruktive Operationen am thorakalen Abschnitt von Trachen und Bronchien. Langenbecks Arch. Klin. Chir. *332*:859, 1968.

CHAPTER 33

EXTENDED RESECTION OF BRONCHIAL CARCINOMA IN THE SUPERIOR PULMONARY SULCUS

Donald L. Paulson

Tumors in the superior pulmonary sulcus are usually bronchial carcinomas that evoke a characteristic clinical syndrome because of their location at the extreme apex of the upper lobes of the lungs. Situated in the narrow confines of the thoracic inlet, these tumors extend locally to involve adjacent structures, including the lower roots of the brachial plexus, the intercostal nerves, the sympathetic chain, and the adjacent first and second ribs and vertebrae, causing constant and characteristic pain in the eighth cervical and first and second thoracic nerve root distribution and often causing a Horner's syndrome.

Other tumors that may produce a similar clinical syndrome by invasion of the thoracic inlet, such as more extensive carcinomas that extend to the inlet from another primary location in the remainder of the upper lobes, are excluded as apical chest tumors and are not pertinent to a discussion of the management of tumors in the superior pulmonary sulcus as described by Pancoast.

In the 1950s, tumors in the superior pulmonary sulcus were widely held to be resistant to irradiation and inaccessible to complete and curative resection. Average survival time of untreated patients after diagnosis was 10 to 14 months. Radiation therapy alone or following resection left few survivors after one year. Since the 1960s, results have been improving. Irradiation used alone has been reported to relieve pain, prolong survival, and in some instances effect a cure. The reports of irradiation combined with incomplete resection have been encouraging, although the results are not always comparable, because less extensive apical chest tumors are frequently confused with typical superior pulmonary sulcus tumors. Preoperative irradiation combined with extended resection has improved survival dramatically.

PRETREATMENT STUDIES

A tumor in the superior pulmonary sulcus is usually suggested by the characteristic history of pain in the shoulder and in the arm along dermatones corresponding to C8 and T1 nerve roots and by roentgenographic evidence of a small shadow at the extreme apex of the chest in the thoracic inlet. Planigraphy, bone scanning, and computed axial tomography are used to delineate the location of the tumor and the extent of involvement of the ribs, paraspinal region, and vertebrae. Magnetic resonance and vascular imaging may be indicated.

Cytohistologic proof of the tumor has been obtained in a small percentage of cases by sputum examination, flexible bronchoscopic aspirates, brush biopsies, and transbronchial needle biopsy. Percutaneous fine-needle biopsy through the posterior cervical triangle just anterior to the trapezius fold and the posterior portion of the first rib, using the CT scan and biplane fluoroscope for localization, is effective in obtaining cytohistologic proof in 95% of the patients for whom it has been used.

Open biopsy of the cupola of the pleura through a supraclavicular scalenotomy incision may be necessary for histologic diagnosis, particularly when the diagnosis is in doubt.

Mediastinoscopy and scalene node biopsy for palpable nodes are helpful for establishing the histologic diagnosis, for staging, and for determining the extent of involvement.

PREOPERATIVE IRRADIATION AND EXTENDED RESECTION

The results of preoperative irradiation combined with extended resection for proven carcinomas in the superior pulmonary sulcus, since the 1950s are significant in that 63% of the patients seen were considered operable and 98% of those were resected. Over 30% of all patients who completed combined treatment survived 5 years or longer, including 45% of those patients having T3N0 lesions—stage IIIa.

The purpose of preoperative irradiation is to limit the extent of the tumor so that it is better localized and, thus, more completely resectable. Using megavoltage equipment, a tumor dose of 3000 rads, given in 10 fractions over 12 days, is delivered over the tumor in the superior pulmonary sulcus, the chest wall, and the superior mediastinum beyond the midline.

The pathologic effects of irradiation of the tumor are related to the length of survival after extended resection. Those patients without nodal involvement who had no residual viable carcinoma in the chest wall or margins of resection did well and were long-term survivors. Those patients who had viable tumor in the chest wall, the margins of the resection, the perineural lymphatics, or the nerve roots at the intervertebral foramen, however, did poorly and died in less than 2 years, mainly from distant metastases, but also with local recurrence of carcinoma, regardless of postoperative external beam radiation therapy.

Clinical and experimental observations suggest that preoperative irradiation in doses not sufficient to cause gross regression of tumor decreases local recurrence, prevents growth of disseminated tumor cells, and increases survival when compared with irradiation or operation alone.

The theoretical advantages of preoperative over postoperative irradiation depend on the treatment being administered prior to surgical interference and its attendant risks of dissemination, implantation, or inflammation, together with violation of the vascular bed of the tumor, resulting in reduced oxygen tension and consequent diminished radiation sensitivity. Use of additional postoperative radiation in patients who have had preoperative radiation and resection raises the risk of radiation fibrosis and nerve entrapment of the brachial plexus caused by the increased cumulative dose exceeding the tolerance of normal tissues.

Contraindications for Surgical Resection

Extensive involvement of the brachial plexus, the paraspinal region—particularly the intervertebral foramina, and the bodies or laminae of the vertebrae; mediastinal perinodal involvement; and distant metastases, in addition to the usual cardiopulmonary limitations, are contraindications to surgical intervention. Venous obstruction, although not typical of a carcinoma in the superior pulmonary sulcus, is another contraindication to operation. In some instances, patients with ipsilateral involved mediastinal nodes have undergone resection for palliation of pain, but survival has been limited to 2 years. Similarly, resection of an extensively involved subclavian artery may rarely be necessary with grafting, although these patients usually do not survive 2 years.

Timing of Surgical Intervention

Two to three weeks after the completion of preoperative irradiation, a complete, extended en bloc resection is performed, usually including the entire first rib and the posterior portions of the second and third ribs; portions of the first three thoracic vertebrae—including the

transverse processes and portions of the bodies as indicated; the intercostal nerves, together with the eighth cervical nerve root—if involved, the lower trunk of the brachial plexus; and a portion of the stellate ganglion and dorsal sympathetic chain. The involved lung is resected by either lobectomy or segmentectomy, and a radical dissection of regional hilar and mediastinal lymph nodes is done.

Technique

The surgical technique may vary slightly with the location and extent of the lesion, but in general the approach is uniform.

The patient is placed in a lateral position with his arm extended over his head, exposing the axilla and the scapular area. A long, parascapular incision is made, starting just above the spine of the scapula and extending around the tip of the scapula ending at the anterior axillary line. It is not necessary to divide the upper portion of the trapezius and levator scapulae muscles, and it is important to the support of the shoulder girdle not to do so. The serratus anterior muscular attachments to the upper ribs, particularly the second rib, are divided, permitting good elevation of the scapula and shoulder to expose the apex of the thoracic cage. The serratus posterior superior muscle is divided at its insertion on the upper four ribs and preserved for later use in closing the thorax. The intrinsic dorsal musculature is separated by sharp dissection from the upper ribs and transverse processes to the laminae of the vertebrae.

The extended resection is performed in two phases: (1) anteriorly and (2) superiorly and posteriorly. The chest cavity is entered through an incision in the third interspace, avoiding the posterior portion until the extent of the tumor has been explored. Should the tumor extend to the third rib, the fourth interspace is entered and the fourth rib and intercostal muscle divided, allowing a wide margin anterior to the growth. The scapula is elevated by a rib spreader placed between the third and fourth ribs and the undersurface of the scapula. The third and second ribs and the intercostal muscles, nerves, and vessels are divided well anterior to the growth and attached lung. The first rib is separated at its costochondral junction. The end of the first rib is grasped and retracted inferiorly to put the cervical structures involved under tension. The subclavian artery and vein are identified and the scalenus anterior and medius muscles divided at their insertion on the first rib, or higher if indicated by the extent of the tumor (Fig. 33–1). The lower trunk of the brachial plexus is identified—and the extent of its involvement by the tumor determined—and divided distal to the point of invasion. If there is doubt concerning involvement of that portion contributed to by the eighth cervical nerve root, the division is deferred until the posterior portion of the resection is approached.

The posterior phase of the resection is begun inferiorly at the level of the lowermost divided rib and proceeds superiorly. The intrinsic dorsal musculature is retracted, and the transverse processes divided in sequence flush

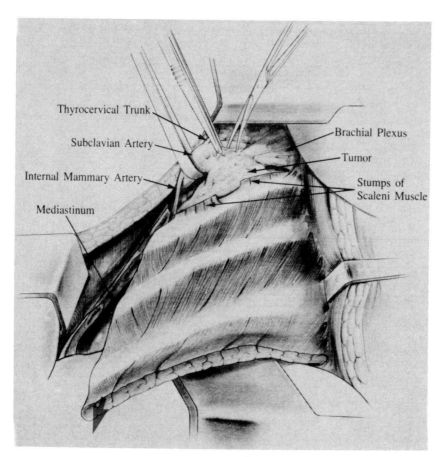

Thyrocervical Trunk

Subclavian Artery

Internal Mammary Artery

Mediastinum

Brachial Plexus

Tumor

Stumps of
Scaleni Muscle

Fig. 33–1. Division of scalenus anterior and medius muscle and identification of the subclavian artery and vein by retraction inferiorly of the first rib. (From Paulson, D.L.: Extended resection of bronchogenic carcinoma in the superior pulmonary sulcus. Surgical Rounds, 3:10, 1980.)

with the laminae, using bone shears. The heads of the ribs are then elevated by a periosteal elevator, and the intercostal nerve and vessels tensed, clipped, and divided (Fig. 33–2). The dorsal sympathetic chain is divided inferiorly. As the head of the first rib is approached, the posterior scalenus muscle and all musculotendinous attachments are divided superior to the first rib and transverse process down to the lamina. The head of the rib is elevated and the large first intercostal nerve divided. Vessels are clipped before division, but if uncontrolled bleeding or spinal fluid leak occurs at the intervertebral foramen, Surgicel or muscle may be lightly packed in the foramen. The involved eighth cervical nerve root is then divided, permitting downward traction on the first rib and underlying tumor mass.

The resection of the mass of involved structures superiorly is dictated by the extent of the tumor mass. If the lower trunk of the brachial plexus was not divided in the anterior dissection, it is now resected with the tumor mass. In case the eighth cervical nerve root is not involved—as suggested by the extent of pain to the elbow only—it is possible to preserve it and divide only that portion of the lower trunk contributed to by the first intercostal nerve. If there is any doubt, wider excision encompassing the eighth cervical nerve is preferable.

Dissection of the growth away from the subclavian artery may be tedious but can be accomplished through the adventitial plane. The wall of the artery usually is not invaded, and resection is rarely indicated. Branches

of the artery, including the internal mammary, the thyrocervical, and occasionally the vertebral, may have to be sacrificed.

Attention is then directed to the region of tumor attachment to the bodies of the vertebrae and, if possible, the tumor is elevated in the plane of its pseudocapsule. Marginal tissues are examined microscopically by rapid section as the dissection proceeds. Firm, bony attachments suggestive of tumor invasion are removed cleanly, using an osteotome. As much as one fourth of the bodies of involved vertebrae has been removed in this manner without disturbing spinal support. Gauze and Surgicel packs are used to control bleeding in soft tissues and cancellous bone.

The tumor mass with the involved dorsal sympathetic chain is now freed superiorly by sharp dissection to the stellate ganglion, and a portion of the sympathetic chain and ganglion resected according to the extent of growth.

The involved lung is resected as indicated. Pleural drainage is established by an upper anterior tube in the dome of the chest and a lower tube in the paravertebral gutter. The remaining lung is expanded and hemostasis carefully confirmed. The preserved serratus posterior superior muscle is used to aid closure of the defect posteriorly by suture to the intrinsic dorsal musculature and the remaining fourth rib. If portions of four ribs have been removed, the use of plastic mesh sutured to the margins of the defect under tension is helpful in mini-

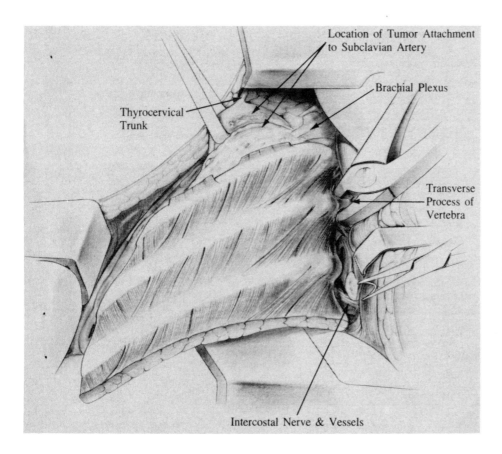

Fig. 33–2. Posterior approach to resection of the tumor by division of transverse processes of the vertebrae, elevation of the heads of the rib, and clipping of intercostal nerves and vessels at the intervertebral foramina prior to division. (From Paulson, D.L.: Extended resection of bronchogenic carcinoma in the superior pulmonary sulcus. Surgical Rounds, 3:10, 1980.)

mizing paradoxic motion. Usually, however, the remaining defect can be adequately covered by closure of the muscles of the shoulder girdle, chest wall, and skin.

Surgical Morbidity and Mortality

In addition to the expected postoperative development of atelectasis caused by pain and interruption of the chest wall, unique complications consist of persistence of spinal fluid leaks and pleural drainage, both of which eventually subside, as do parenchymal air leaks. In the event of a pneumothorax and spinal fluid leak, air may pass into the spinal canal, resulting in meningitis. If intraoperative bleeding or fluid leak occurs, avoid packing the foramen too deeply because it may produce pressure on the spinal cord and subsequent block.

Permanent neurologic deficits involving the ulnar nerve, resulting from resection of the lower trunk of the brachial plexus, are not incapacitating. If the extent of the tumor permits preservation of the eighth cervical nerve, the defect secondary to resection of the first and second nerve roots is not severe. Horner's syndrome, if

not present preoperatively, develops postoperatively secondary to resection of the dorsal sympathetic chain and at least a portion of the stellate ganglion. None of these defects are disabling, and all patients surviving over 3 years are relieved of their original pain. There have been no complications of irradiation following the doses recommended.

Operative mortality has been no more than 3%. The stage of nodal involvement, the local extent of the carcinoma, and the pathologic effects of irradiation at the chest wall level are the important factors in prognosis.

READING REFERENCES

Pancoast, H.K.: Superior pulmonary sulcus tumor: tumor characterized by pain, Horner's syndrome, destruction of bone, and atrophy of hand muscles. J.A.M.A. 99:1391, 1932.

Paulson, D.L., Weed, T.L., and Rian, R.L.: Cervical approach for percutaneous needle biopsy of Pancoast tumors. Ann. Thorac. Surg. 39:586, 1985.

Paulson, D.L.: Extended resection of bronchogenic carcinomas in the superior pulmonary sulcus. Surg. Rounds 3:10, 1980.

CHAPTER 34

THORACOPLASTY

Thomas W. Shields

The operative removal of the skeletal support of a portion of the chest is called a thoracoplasty. This procedure is accomplished by the subperiosteal removal of a varying number of rib segments. The removal of the skeletal support permits that portion of the chest wall to sink in toward the mediastinum and, thus, reduces the size of the hemithorax and permits partial collapse of the underlying lung. Extraperiosteal paravertebral thoracoplasty is the standard procedure.

At present this operation is used primarily in the treatment of chronic thoracic empyema when there is either insufficient or no remaining pulmonary tissue to obliterate the pleural space. Even for this purpose, it is used less than it once was, and many surgeons only use thoracoplasty as a procedure of last resort. It is never used in patients with pulmonary tuberculosis, except for the management of pleural and occasionally extensive combined pleuropulmonary disease.

Formerly a limited preresection "tailoring" thoracoplasty and the plombage type of thoracoplasty found selective use in certain patients.

In the former, a limited number of ribs of the upper portion of the chest were removed a week or so before thoracotomy when it was expected that the proposed resection would result in an insufficient amount of remaining lung tissue to fill the normal-sized thoracic cage. In the latter, an inert, foreign substance was placed in a space created beneath the rib cage by extraperiosteal stripping of the ribs of the upper portion of the chest.

Using a foreign substance to obtain collapse in the presence of underlying pleural infection is contraindicated. If the desired collapse cannot be obtained by a conventional thoracoplasty and a persistent infected space remains, a Schede thoracoplasty or one of its many modifications may be necessary. A modification of the standard thoracoplasty, described by Sawamura and reported by Iioka and associates (1985), may even reduce further the need for conventional thoracoplasty or the more deforming Schede procedure in patients with chronic pleural tuberculous or postpneumonic empyema.

OPERATIVE TECHNIQUE

Conventional Thoracoplasty

The standard procedure is that outlined by Alexander (1937). Now that the operation is used to control a chronic thoracic empyema, the procedure is accomplished in one stage. When it was employed in the treatment of pulmonary tuberculosis, it was done in two or more stages to circumvent adverse physiologic changes of paradoxic chest wall motion occurring in the postoperative period. The magnitude of the collapse procedure depends on the size of the empyema cavity. Ordinarily, seven ribs are resected. This allows the scapula and attached extracostal musculature to drop into the space and helps to maintain the collapse. Should fewer ribs be resected, the lower portion of the scapula may have to be excised, so that it does not impinge on the remaining ribs. This would prevent it from falling into the created space to help obtain optimal collapse.

With the patient in the lateral decubitus position, a parascapular incision is begun at the level of the spine of the scapula and extended inferiorly and laterally to the midaxillary line (Fig. 34–1). The subjacent extracostal muscles—trapezius, rhomboids, and latissimus dorsi—are incised to expose the rib cage and to allow the scapula to be retracted anteriorly and superiorly. Posteriorly, the attachments of the serratus posterior and erector spinae muscle groups are separated from the ribs of the upper half of the chest. Similarly, the insertions of the serratus anterior muscle are separated from the upper three or four ribs.

After exposure of the rib cage, the posterior half of the third rib is resected after incising and stripping off its periosteal investment. In patients with an empyema, the transverse process of the vertebral body generally need not be excised, but this can be done if necessary to achieve maximal collapse. This excision is facilitated by division of the costotransverse ligaments (Fig. 34–2). The rib is then resected further posteriorly to the level of the base of the transverse process. Some surgeons also prefer to excise the head of the rib as well, avulsing it

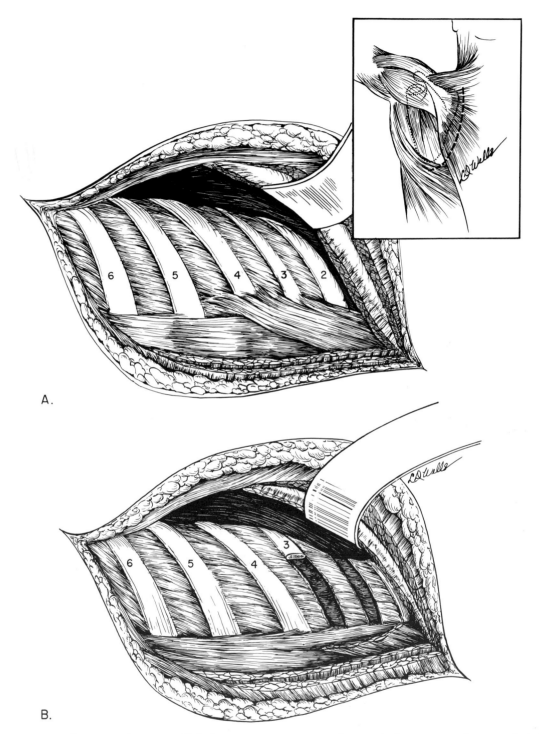

Fig. 34–1. *A*, Schematic illustration of exposure of left thoracic cage in preparation for a standard extraperiosteal paravertebral thoracoplasty. Inset shows the parascapular incision. *B*, Schematic illustration showing the resected posterior portion of the third rib, and the entire second rib prior to removal of the first rib.

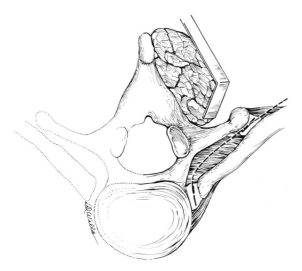

Fig. 34–2. Schematic illustration showing site of division of the costotransverse ligaments to facilitate removal of the head of the rib and the transverse process.

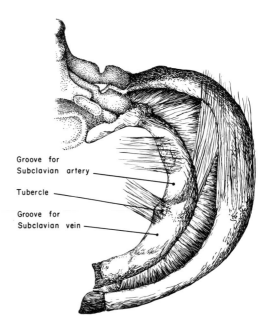

Groove for Subclavian artery

Tubercle

Groove for Subclavian vein

Fig. 34–3. Schematic illustration of first and second ribs. Scalene tubercle and adjacent important areas shown.

from its articulation with the vertebral body. Next, the second rib is resected subperiosteally from the costochondral junction to the vertebral body; the second transverse process may also be removed.

The first rib is removed if a limited thoracoplasty is done for obliteration of an apical empyema space that has occurred after a lobectomy. If the procedure is done for the collapse of a chronic postpneumonectomy empyema space, however, the first rib may not have to be removed and, in fact, Deslauriers (personal communication, 1987) believes it should always be left in place to preserve the structural integrity of the neck, shoulder girdle, and upper thorax. If there is any doubt of any apical residual space remaining, however, the first rib should be removed, as suggested by McMillan (1987). When this is indicated, the first rib is exposed and the periosteum incised on its lower edge. This usually is accomplished by scraping the edge with a periosteal elevator. The flat inferior surface is stripped of its periosteum. Starting far posteriorly, the outer or superior surface is stripped of its periosteum; care must be taken to protect the brachial plexus and subclavian vessels at this time. This is best accomplished by inserting a finger to retract the neurovascular structures away from the rib. Extreme caution is necessary at the scalene tubercle (Fig. 34–3). The rib then is divided at the level of the tip of the transverse process and avulsed from its costochondral junction anteriorly. The head of the first rib and the first transverse process are not resected. A portion of the remaining third rib and segments of the lower ribs are then resected subperiosteally to ensure complete obliteration of the empyema space.

Sawamura Modified Thoracoplasty

A posterolateral thoracotomy incision is made and all ribs overlying the empyema cavity are exposed. An incision is made through the intercostal bundle overlying the middle of the empyema and carried through the

parietal peel into the empyema cavity. All purulent and necrotic tissue is removed. The visceral peel overlying the collapsed lung is removed. Any bronchopleural fistula is closed. The parietal wall is partially decorticated to permit pliability and collapsed to obliterate the space. This is accomplished by stripping the ribs subperiosteally so that the parietal wall consists of parietal pleura, periosteum, and attached intercostal muscles. A percutaneous insertion of a chest tube into the empyema cavity is then carried out. This tube must be isolated from the newly developed extraperiosteal space. The incision in the collapsed parietal wall is closed so that it is airtight. The extraperiosteal space is cleansed and irrigated to prevent subsequent infection. The muscles and skin of the chest wall are then closed anatomically. After the procedure, the newly created extraperiosteal space fills with exudate, which exerts pressure on the parietal wall to keep it juxtaposed to the underlying lung. With time, this exudate is absorbed and the lung expands to obliterate the extraperiosteal space (Fig. 34–4).

Plombage Thoracoplasty

This modification of the conventional thoracoplasty was developed to overcome the adverse effects of decostalization of a portion of the chest wall. A foreign substance—paraffin, lucite spheres in a polyethylene bag, or fiberglass—was inserted in a space created between the ribs and the thoracic fascia and freed periosteal and intercostal musculature to maintain optimal collapse. Unfortunately, the use of a foreign body plomb is contraindicated in the management of a chronic empyema. Consequently, this procedure has been discarded.

Schede Thoracoplasty

The operation described by Schede (1890) for obliteration of a chronic empyema space is rarely, if ever,

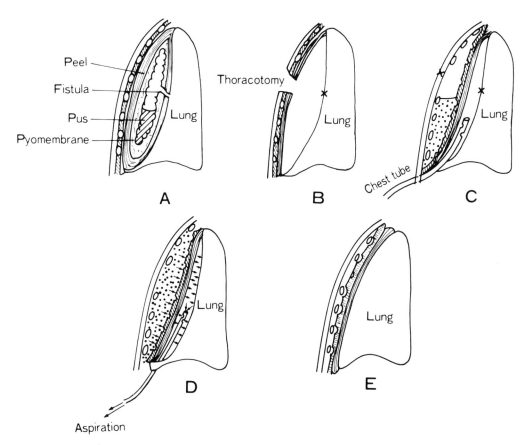

Fig. 34–4. Schematic illustration of technique of the Sawamura modified thoracoplasty. *A,* The empyema cavity with pulmonary fistulization is encapsulated by pyomembrane and thickened pleura. *B,* The empyema cavity is curetted and the visceral peel is decorticated. The pulmonary fistula is closed. *C,* The chest tube is inserted into the reducing empyema cavity and an exudate fills the extraperiosteal space. *D,* The empyema cavity is obliterated by compression of the exudate and by traction of the chest tube aspiration. *E,* The lung consequently expands by absorbing the exudate. (Reproduced with permission of Iioka, et al.: J. Thorac. Cardiovasc. Surg. *90:*179, 1985.)

performed at present, but has been widely modified by many surgeons. The Schede operation consists of radical unroofing of an empyema space by resecting the overlying ribs, intercostal bundles, and subjacent parietal pleural "peel." The extracostal muscles and skin are partially closed over gauze packing. As the packing is withdrawn a few days later, it is hoped that freshly granulating tissue sets up an obliterative healing process.

Grow (1946) and Kergin (1953) reported modifications of the Schede procedure that cause less blood loss and, thus, are less shocking to the patient. Also, the modifications provide better vascularity for the desired granulation tissue. All ribs are resected over the empyema space, but the intercostal bundles are left intact. By incisions through one or more of the exposed periosteal beds, a parietal decortication is accomplished. Superficial curettage of the underlying visceral pleural peel is executed. The intercostal muscle bundles, with their vascular supply intact, are allowed to fall across the visceral surface of the cavity. A bronchopleural fistula, if present, may be excised and closed by suturing a pedicled muscle graft over the opening. The incision is closed loosely over drains lying superficial to the muscle bundles. External pressure dressings are used to ensure apposition of the tissues.

PHYSIOLOGIC CHANGES AFTER THORACOPLASTY

The immediate physiologic sequelae of a standard extraperiosteal paravertebral thoracoplasty are related to the development of an area of paradoxic motion of the chest wall. The effort of breathing is increased as the result of the abnormal volume displacement and greater pleural pressure changes necessary to move air in and out of the lungs. If the mediastinum is mobile, mediastinal flutter occurs. *Pendelluft,* that is, air flow from one lung to the other during the ventilatory cycle, may theoretically occur. Maloney and his associates (1961), however, reported that, in the presence of a closed chest, the lung on the side of the paradoxic chest wall motion actually expands on the inspiration. Also, Gaensler (1965) showed, by using a pneumotachographic screen at the carina, that there is no air movement from one lung to the other after a thoracoplasty, as long as the proximal airway is patent.

Retained secretions, however, may cause partial airway obstruction. The cough mechanism is reduced in effectiveness as a result of the inability to generate a high positive pressure in the pleural space because of the unsupported portion of the chest wall. The postoperative problems attendant upon these changes are directly proportional to the number and length of the segments of rib resected.

The late physiologic changes after the operation are related not only to the extent of the rib resections and underlying lung collapse, but also to the late skeletal deformity that occurs. A greater or lesser degree of rotoscoliosis develops subsequent to the removal of the ribs and the transverse processes. This results in a diminution of function of the contralateral lung. Gaensler and Strieder (1951) found that when a thoracoplasty was done over a nonfunctioning lung, a permanent loss of approximately 27% of the preoperative vital capacity and 21% of maximal voluntary ventilation of the contralateral lung followed.

Iioka (1985) reported improvement in the percent vital capacity and FEV_1/predicted vital capacity after the Sawamura modified thoracoplasty. This was not as good as they obtained with decortication alone but was superior to the functional results after modified Elosser procedures.

The physiologic changes after a Schede thoracoplasty are related to the unstable chest wall and the degree of paradoxic motion that develops. In addition, sacrifice of the intercostal nerves results in paresis of the ipsilateral abdominal wall. In the modified procedure, the latter does not occur, since the nerves are left intact.

MORBIDITY

Postoperative morbidity after thoracoplasty is related not only to the type of procedure employed but also to the disease process present. The complications directly related to a conventional thoracoplasty are those caused by injury of the vessels or nerves during removal of the first rib or injury to the thoracic duct with resultant chylous effusion, retention of secretions with atelectasis, and septic complications.

Wound infection is uncommon, but infection of the apical or subscapular space may occur when the operation is performed for the treatment of a chronic empyema. This infection is particularly likely to occur if the empyema space is entered during the procedure.

MORTALITY

Death after a thoracoplasty is most often related to the underlying chronic disease process rather than to the operation per se. Hopkins and co-workers (1985) reported a 13% mortality rate in their entire series but noted a decline in this figure in the second half of their series. Iioka and associates (1985) reported only one death in 60 patients following a modified Sawamura procedure. Ideally, with modern management, a mortality rate of no more than 5% should occur.

RESULTS

The overall success rate of a thoracoplasty in eliminating intrathoracic space problems has improved over the years. Hopkins and co-workers (1985) reported a failure rate of 33% before 1976 but only 17% since then. Grégoire (1987) from Deslaurier's group reported no operative mortality and an early failure rate of only 12% in 17 patients with chronic postpneumonectomy empyema.

REFERENCES

Alexander, J.: Collapse Therapy of Pulmonary Tuberculosis. Springfield, IL, Charles C Thomas, 1937, p. 402.

Gaensler, E.A., and Strieder, J.W.: Progressive changes in pulmonary function after pneumonectomy: the influence of thoracoplasty, pneumothorax, oleothorax, plastic sponge plombage on the side of pneumonectomy. J. Thorac. Surg. 22:1, 1951.

Grégoire, R., et al.: Thoracoplasty: a forgotten role in the management of nontuberculous postpneumonectomy empyema. (To be published).

Grow, J.B.: Chronic pleural empyema. Dis. Chest 12:26, 1946.

Hopkins, R.H., et al.: The modern use of thoracoplasty. Ann. Thorac. Surg. 40:181, 1985.

Iioka, S., et al.: Surgical treatment of chronic empyema: a new one-stage operation. J. Thorac. Cardiovasc. Surg. 90:179, 1985.

Kergin, F.G.: An operation for chronic pleural empyema. J. Thorac. Surg. 26:430, 1953.

Maloney, J.V., Jr., Schmutzer, K.J., and Raschke, E.: Paradoxical respiration and "pendelluft." J. Thorac. Cardiovasc. Surg. 41:291, 1961.

McMillan, I.K.R.: Bronchopleural fistula: treatment by space reduction. In International Trends in General Thoracic Surgery, Vol. II, A Major Challenge. Edited by H.C. Grillo, and H. Eschapasse. Philadelphia, W.B. Saunders Co., 1987, p. 440.

Schede, M.: Die Behandlung der Empyeme. Verh. Cong. Innere Med., Wiesb. 9:41, 1890.

CHAPTER 35

DECORTICATION OF THE LUNG

Thomas W. Shields

Decortication of the lung consists of the removal of a restrictive, fibrous membrane or layer of tissue from the pleural surface of the lung. The layer also may be removed from the chest wall and diaphragm. The procedure is used in the treatment of fibrothorax resulting from either organized hemothorax or empyema. The empyema may be the result of an infected post-traumatic hemothorax, or may be postoperative or peripneumonic in origin. The empyema may be associated with a specific granulomatous disease process, such as tuberculosis.

The purpose of the procedure is to free the encased—"trapped"—lung and, as a result of the re-expansion of the lung, to obliterate the pleural space. If the operation is performed because of an organizing hemothorax, its objective is the preservation of pulmonary function and prevention of delayed suppurative complications. If done for empyema, the major goal is to free the lung for expansion, thereby obliterating the pleural space, eliminate much of the by-products of suppuration, expediting recovery and preserving lung function.

TECHNIQUE

Pulmonary decortication is best carried out through a standard posterolateral thoracotomy at the midchest level. The operation can be performed with or without rib resection. Rib resection provides the best visualization at the pleural level because the intercostal space is often narrowed by the pleural process.

If the entire pleural sac is to be excised, the extrapleural plane can be sought immediately and the parietal wall of the sac separated from it. Ultimately, the edge of the visceral peel is reached and care is to be exercised in turning these margins and beginning the separation of the visceral surface. Particular care should be taken in separating the pleural sac along the gutters of the mediastinum, along the pericardium, and, especially, at the diaphragmatic area where cleavage planes are often difficult to follow and avulsion of the diaphragm can occur with entry into the retroperitoneal area.

Although somewhat less than ideal from a theoretic

standpoint, a practical approach to the management of decortication is to incise through the parietal peel to gain entry into the space within the organized pleural mass. The content of this space is then evacuated, and appropriate cultures or samples are taken as required.

After the visceral coat is mechanically cleaned, an area over one of the lobes is selected for incision, avoiding a fissure if possible. With the use of a small scalpel, the peel is incised carefully down to the loose plane that lies immediately beneath the cicatricial coat and just above the visceral pleura (Fig. 35–1). Once this loose areolar plane is entered, the opening is enlarged and decortication is carried out mainly by blunt dissection, although sharp dissection is used at any point where intimate adherence exists between the visceral pleura and the peel. At the limits of the visceral investment, where it is met by the parietal portion of the pleural mass, the peel thins out and becomes merely a fibrous pleural symphysis obliterating the anatomic pleural space.

Thus, when the visceral coat has been decorticated, attention is directed to separation of the parietal coat, ultimately cutting the thinned-out pleural obliteration in the gutters. Separating the peel from over the diaphragm is usually less satisfactory because the cleavage plane is often much more difficult to follow.

The necessity of removing the parietal peel has been debated. It is true that, in uninfected hemothoraces and other sterile pleural processes, the complete re-expansion of the lung, so as to obliterate the pleural space, sets the stage for the resorption of even dense pleural coats. When dealing with an infection, a complete operation does indeed have a strong logical appeal.

During decortication, the anesthetist should expand the lung progressively, so that it is possible to recognize any areas of binding adhesions that still may be enfolding and distorting the lung and that would militate against the lung's assumption of increased or relatively normal volume. Such unfolding of the lung by severance or stripping of deforming symphyses has been termed "secondary decortication."

Injury to lung parenchyma must be repaired but

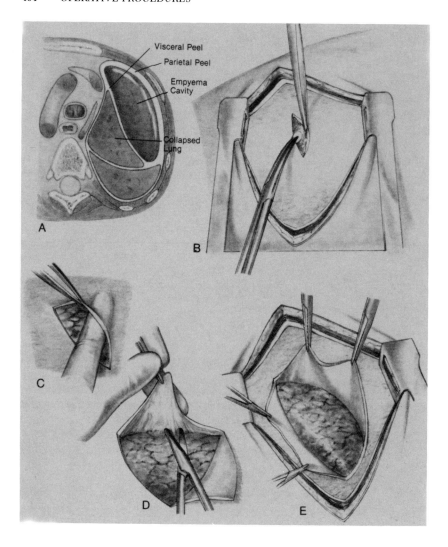

Fig. 35–1. Decortication of the pleura. *A*, Cross-sectional diagram of empyema cavity and relationship of chest wall and underlying lung. *B*, Incision of visceral peel with beginning dissection of peel. *C*, Finger dissection of peel. *D*, Sharp dissection as necessary. *E*, Progressive decortication with expansion of underlying lung. (Reproduced with permission of Hood, R.M.: Techniques in General Thoracic Surgery. Philadelphia, W.B. Saunders Co., 1985.)

should be minimal unless rather severe parenchymal disease or dense adhesions have been present between it and visceral peel. Adequate closed-tube drainage and the addition of suction to the closed drainage system promote prompt expansion of the lung in spite of leaks.

Objections may be voiced against making a direct opening into the pleural pocket, because this would offer the danger of contamination of the operative field by the content of the pleural mass. This hazard is probably not as great as might be presumed, because the operative area can be fairly well cleansed at the conclusion of the procedure by copious irrigation. Local tissue immunity, no doubt, plays a protecting role, and the expanded lung, which obliterates the pleural space, provides further protection. Appropriate antibiotics also are indicated in an attempt to avoid the development of postoperative suppuration.

ADDITIVE PROCEDURES

Necessary parenchymal resection for the removal of any underlying lung disease may be carried out following removal of the visceral peel. At times, if inadequate lung tissue remains to fill the pleural space, a concomitant

thoracoplasty may be advisable. Either parenchymal resection or thoracoplasty, however, definitely increases the risk of postoperative complications.

PHYSIOLOGIC RESULTS

In the presence of a significant fibrothorax, pulmonary function is markedly deranged. There is interference both in the mechanics of ventilation and in perfusion of the "captive" lung. Actually, perfusion is reduced to a greater extent than is ventilation.

The physiologic improvement obtained with successful decortication varies. The extent of disease of the underlying lung at the time of the development of the fibrothorax is the most important factor in determining the eventual outcome. The functional improvement may be good after decortication of a traumatic hemothorax, but may be only fair to poor after the procedure in patients with nontuberculous or tuberculous empyema. Iioka and his associates (1985) reported significant improvement in both percent VC and the FEV_1/predicted VC in 20 patients who underwent successful decortication of a chronic empyema. The duration of the presence of the fibrothorax appears not to be important, although it has been suggested that the shorter the duration of the pleural disease, the better is the eventual return of function.

In patients in whom the decortication proves successful, pulmonary function studies reveal an increase in the lung volumes, and improved ventilatory capacity, and an improved perfusion and oxygen uptake on the side operated upon. Improvement may continue for many months after the operation. Postoperative breathing exercises appear to be especially beneficial in these patients.

MORBIDITY AND MORTALITY

The incidence of nonfatal complications is approximately 10%. The major problems are related to sepsis, persistent air leak, and bleeding. Injury to lung or to vessels in the chest wall resulting in important hemorrhage postoperatively is rare but can defeat the purpose of the operation by recreating a second pleural clot, which may organize and again delay obliteration of the pleural space. Wound infection and empyema with or without a bronchopleural fistula are the most common septic complications. Persistent air leaks for 10 to 14 days, caused by injury of the underlying lung during the operation, are not uncommon, but with adequate drainage of the pleural space and re-expansion of the lung to obliterate the pleural space, serious septic complications do not occur.

The mortality rate after decortication should approach zero but has been reported to be as high as 8% by Benfield (1981). When death occurs, it is usually related to hemorrhage or to septic complications. Both hemorrhage and sepsis are more likely to occur when the procedure has been technically difficult or if a supplementary procedure has been carried out at the same time.

RESULTS

It is difficult to state categorically the results to be expected after a decortication for the management of a chronic empyema. Yeh and associates (1963) reported 25 successful results and no deaths after 27 decortications and Benfield (1981) reported 42 cures in 46 patients. Iioka and his colleagues (1985) reported a 100% success rate in a highly selected population of 20 patients. Therefore, a successful outcome of over 90% should be expected after decortication of a chronic empyema in selected patients. In patients with a clotted hemothorax, good results should exceed 95%.

REFERENCES

Benfield, G.F.A.: Recent trends in empyema thoracis. Br. J. Dis. Chest 75:358, 1981.
Iioka, S., et al.: Surgical treatment of chronic empyema. A new one-stage operation. J. Thorac. Cardiovasc. Surg. 90:179, 1985.
Yeh, T.J., Hall, D., and Ellison, R.G.: Empyema thoracis: a review of 110 cases. Am. Rev. Resp. Dis. 88:785, 1963.

READING REFERENCES

Barker, W.L., Neuhaus, H., and Langston, H.T.: Ventilatory improvement following decortication in pulmonary tuberculosis. Ann. Thorac. Surg. 1:532, 1965.
Burford, T.H.: Hemothorax and hemothoracic empyema. *In* Surgery World War II, Thoracic Surgery, Vol. 2. Washington, D.C., Office of the Surgeon General, Department of the Army, 1965. Chapter 6, p. 237.
Burford, T.H., Parker, E.F., and Samson, P.C.: Early pulmonary decortication in the treatment of post-traumatic empyema. Ann. Surg. 112:163, 1945.
Carroll, D., et al.: Pulmonary function following decortication of lung. Am. Rev. Tuberc. 63:231, 1951.
Cherniak, N.S., and Barker, W.L.: Cardiopulmonary function in tuberculosis. *In* Clinical Cardiopulmonary Physiology. Edited by B.L. Gordon. New York, Grune & Stratton, 1969, p. 600.
Gordon, J., and Welles, E.S.: Decortication in pulmonary tuberculosis including studies of respiratory physiology. J. Thorac. Surg. 18:337, 1949.
Hood, R.M.: Pleural decortication. *In* Surgical Diseases of the Pleura and Chest Wall. Edited by R.M. Hood. Philadelphia, W.B. Saunders Co., 1986.
Morton, J.R., Boushy, S.F., and Guinn, G.A.: Physiological evaluation of results of pulmonary decortication. Ann. Thorac. Surg. 9:321, 1970.
Patton, W.E., Watson, T.R., Jr., and Gaensler, E.A.: Pulmonary function before and at intervals after surgical decortication of the lung. Surg. Gynecol. Obstet. 95:477, 1952.
Samson, P.C.: Pleural complications of thoracic trauma. *In* Management of Thoracic Injuries. Edited by R.M. Hood. Springfield, IL, Charles C Thomas, 1969, p. 34.
Samson, P.C., and Burford, T.H.: Total pulmonary decortication. J. Thorac. Surg. 16:127, 1947.
Samson, P.C., et al.: Technical consideration in decortication for the pleural complications of pulmonary tuberculosis. J. Thorac. Surg. 36:431, 1958.
Rudstrom, P., and Thoren, L.: Decortication of lung. Acta Chir. Scand. 100:437, 1955.
Savage, T., and Fleming, H.A.: Decortication of lung in tuberculous disease. Thorax 10:293, 1955.
Siebens, A.A., et al.: The physiologic effects of fibrothorax and the functional results of surgical treatment. J. Thorac. Surg. 32:53, 1956.

CHAPTER 36

TRACHEAL ANATOMY AND SURGICAL APPROACHES

Hermes C. Grillo

ANATOMY

Functionally, the trachea serves principally as a conduit for ventilation. Viewed in this way, it would seem to be an ideal structure for replacement or reconstruction when involved by surgical disease. Anatomically, however, it presents several unique features that partially account for the difficulty in its surgical management. These are its unpaired nature, its unique structural rigidity, its short length, its relative lack of longitudinal elasticity, its proximity to major cardiovascular structures, and its blood supply.

My colleagues and I (1964) reported that the adult human trachea averages 11.8 cm in length—range: 10 to 13 cm—from the infracricoid level to the top of the carinal spur. There are usually from 18 to 22 cartilaginous rings within this length, approximately two rings per centimeter. Occasionally, rings are incomplete or bifid. In the adult, the internal diameter of the trachea measures about 2.3 cm laterally and 1.8 cm anteroposteriorly. These measurements vary roughly in proportion to the size of the individual. The cross-sectional shape in the adult is approximately elliptical.

The surgeon usually visualizes the trachea as he learned to see it in the "thyroidectomy" position, with the neck extended, as a structure that is half cervical and half thoracic. Mulliken and I (1968) pointed out that the trachea becomes almost entirely mediastinal when the neck is flexed, for the cricoid cartilage drops to the level of the thoracic inlet. This may be the permanent position in the aged because of cervical kyphosis. These simple observations contributed to the development of surgical reconstructive techniques that obviate the requirement for prostheses.

The trachea, when viewed laterally in the erect individual, courses backward and downward at an angle from a nearly subcutaneous position at the infracricoid level to rest against the esophagus and vertebral column at the carina. The larynx and the origin of the esophagus are intimately related anatomically at the cricopharyngeal level. Below this, the posterior membranous wall of the trachea maintains a close spatial relationship to the esophagus. A distinct, easily separable plane is present below the cricoid level, but a common blood supply is shared. Anteriorly, the thyroid isthmus passes over the trachea in the region of the second ring. The lateral lobes of the thyroid are closely applied to the trachea, and common blood supply is obtained from the branches of the inferior thyroid artery. Lying in the groove between trachea and esophagus are the recurrent nerves, coursing from beneath the arch of the aorta on the left and, therefore, having a longer course in proximity to the trachea there than on the right, where the nerve has looped around the subclavian artery and then approached the groove. A nonrecurrent nerve occasionally is present on the right. These nerves enter the larynx between the cricoid and thyroid cartilages just anterior to the inferior cornua of the thyroid cartilage.

The anterior pretracheal plane may be developed easily in the cervical region. Fibrofatty tissue, lymph nodes, and fine branches of the anterior jugular vein are present in front of this plane. The innominate vein lies anteriorly, away from the trachea. The innominate artery, however, crosses over the mid-trachea obliquely from its point of origin from the aortic arch to the right side of the neck. In children, the innominate artery is much higher and is encountered in the lower neck. In some adults, the artery is unusually high and crosses the trachea at the base of the neck when slight extension is present. Occasionally, a tiny branch of this artery may be encountered in the segment of the artery that crosses the trachea. At the level of the carina, the left main bronchus passes beneath the aortic arch, and the right beneath the azygos vein. The pulmonary artery lies just in front of the carina. On either side of the trachea lies fibrofatty tissue containing lymph nodes chains; a large packet of nodes lies just beneath the carina. (See Chapter 5.)

The course of the trachea from the anterior cervical position to the posterior mediastinal position with close relationships to major vascular structures makes access to the entire trachea through a single incision difficult. I (1969) emphasized that these anatomic facts demand precise definition of the extent and nature of the tracheal lesions in planning surgical procedures.

The cartilaginous rings give the human trachea its lateral rigidity. The rings extend approximately two thirds of the circumference. The posterior wall is membranous. The trachea is lined with respiratory mucosa, which is tightly applied to the inner surface of the cartilages, grossly. The normal epithelium is columnar and ciliated. The cilia clear particulate matter and secretions. Mucous glands are liberally present. In chronic smokers and in persons with other chronic irritation, squamous metaplasia frequently occurs; in extreme instances, few ciliated cells remain. Such individuals must clear secretions by coughing vigorously. This observation, plus the demonstrated feasibility of cutaneous reconstructions and occasional successes with prosthetic interpositions, makes it clear that ciliated epithelium, though highly desirable, is not essential for tracheal reconstruction. Between the cartilaginous rings and in the membranous wall, the submucosa is fibromuscular.

Considerable contraction of the muscular membranous wall can occur with coughing and with spasm. The tips of the cartilages are drawn inward during such contraction. Such transient narrowing of the airway may be observed fluoroscopically and during bronchoscopy in normal individuals. Some longitudinal flexibility exists; a degree of elasticity is present that appears to be greater in youth and to decrease with age. Calcification of the rings is seen most often with advancing age, although to lesser degree than in the cricoid cartilage. Local trauma or operation may lead to calcification. The normal trachea slides easily in its layer of fibrofatty areolar tissue from neck to mediastinum.

The blood supply of the human trachea is segmental, largely shared with the esophagus and derived principally from multiple branches of the inferior thyroid artery above and the bronchial arteries below. The arteries approach laterally and fine branches pass anteriorly to the trachea and posteriorly to the esophagus. Miura and I (1966) noted that the inferior thyroid artery nourishes the upper trachea, usually through a pattern of three principal branches with fine subdivisions and very fine collateral vessels but with many variations, as noted by Salassa and colleagues (1977). The bronchial vessels nourish the lower trachea. Sometimes the internal mammary artery contributes. Excessive circumferential dissection with division of the lateral pedicles during an operative procedure can easily devascularize the trachea.

METHODS OF RECONSTRUCTION OF THE TRACHEA

Surgical approach to the trachea has developed more slowly than other areas of thoracic surgery, because of the rarity of tracheal tumors, the anatomic complexities of reconstruction, and the biologic incompatibilities that met efforts at prosthetic reconstruction. Earlier hesita-

tions because of problems of physiologic management during reconstruction proved to be less formidable. The growth in frequency of postintubation benign lesions, as a result of the success of modern respiratory therapy, increased the urgency of developmental work.

The concept of direct end-to-end anastomosis of trachea to trachea was generally accepted as the ideal method of tracheal repair following reconstruction. It was long believed, however, as stated by Belsey (1950), that no more than 2 cm—about four tracheal rings—could be removed and anastomosis consistently made. As a result, lateral resection was done where possible with attempts made to patch the defect in various ways, using fascia, skin, pericardium, other tissues, and foreign materials. When such technique was applied to malignant neoplasms, inadequate removal of tumor resulted, with early recurrence. Failure of healing of such patches also occurred. Partial cicatrization was an additional factor. Attention was directed early to the development of an artificial trachea.

Prosthetic Replacement

Many materials have been used for prosthetic replacement of the trachea. Most of the work has been done in experimental animals, but a scattered experience in man has been reported. Replacements have consisted of tubes made of glass or metal; stainless steal mesh in either tubes or coils and tantalum mesh; lucite, polyethylene, and other plastic cylinders; tubes of Ivalon or Marlex mesh; Teflon with combinations of Ivalon or Dacron; and Silastic tubes, often with stainless steel wire or plastic rings to supply rigidity. Early prostheses were usually solid tubes that bridged defects between the two ends of the trachea. Their failure led to use of rigid meshwork cylinders that were intended to allow incorporation into the surrounding connective tissue. More recently, flexible meshwork has been supported by splinting plastic rings. These meshwork prostheses were based on the theory that they would be incorporated by connective tissue and that epithelium would then grow down over this bed of new connective tissue; the rigid rings would maintain an open airway. In most experiments, only short prosthetic bridges have been incorporated to any extent. Some of the longer prostheses have maintained an open airway, but firm healing with full tissue encasement and epithelialization has not occurred. This basically unhealed state might be acceptable as an airway, but these longer prostheses have been subject, in a high percentage of instances, to occlusion by formation of granulation tissue at the nonhealing ends, strictures at these ends, sepsis causing rejection of the prosthesis, or erosion of major vessels with fatal hemorrhage. An occasional long-term success has occurred, largely as an exception rather than as the rule. The problem is the biologic instability caused by placing a foreign body in a bed of connective tissue adjacent to an epithelium that necessarily is contaminated with bacteria. With a foreign body in place, a chronic abscess is presented to the mediastinum, with the described results. Borrie and Redshaw (1970) attempted to solve these problems by accepting a foreign tube as a permanent airway but making it with suturable cuffs that they hoped would become incorporated by connective tissue. Neville and his associates (1976) reported successes with a similar prosthesis. Vogt-Moykopf and Mickisch (1987) noted the many complications that occur.

Anatomic Mobilization

Perhaps most crucial to the evolution of mobilization techniques for tracheal reconstruction was recognition that the cervical trachea—as seen in the hyperextended surgical "thyroid" position—may be totally delivered into the mediastinum by cervical flexion. A few reports of clinical resections greater than 2 cm appeared, but few systematic studies of the anatomic potential are recorded. Michelson and associates (1961) noted that careful mobilization of the entire trachea in eight cadavers allowed for anastomosis with 1 pound of tension, after resection of 4 to 6 cm, with an additional 2.5 to 5.0 cm obtained by division of the left main bronchus.

Our detailed anatomic studies in cadavers attempted to answer the surgical questions of how much trachea could be resected and primary anastomosis made when the trachea was approached in progressive fashion from either a cervical or a transthoracic approach, depending on the location of the lesion. In one study, Mulliken and I (1968) mobilized the trachea through a cervico-mediastinal approach, carefully preserving the lateral tissue that bears the blood supply. Using a standard tension of 1000 to 1200 g for approximation, it was possible, with the neck in 15 to 35 degrees of flexion, to resect an average length of 4.5 cm—about 7 rings—and to increase this by 1.4 cm by entering the pleural space and mobilizing the right hilus (Fig. 36–1A). With greater degrees of cervical flexion, even longer resections are possible. Suprahyoid laryngeal release, described by Montgomery (1974), permits further resection, while minimizing the difficulties in swallowing that attended earlier techniques for release. Alternating lateral division of the intercartilaginous ligaments of the trachea to obtain extension has been proposed experimentally, but not applied clinically to any extent. This technique has the disadvantages of probable interference with tracheal blood supply and the need for extensive tracheal exposure to obtain a rather limited extension of length.

In approaching the lower half of the trachea, I and my colleagues (1964) accomplished mobilization progressively by first, freeing the hilus of the right lung and dividing the pulmonary ligament; second, freeing the pulmonary vessels from their pericardial attachments; and third, transplanting the left main bronchus, which is held in place by the arch of the aorta, to the bronchus intermedius. These earlier studies did not use cervical flexion but instead held the neck in the neutral position. At tensions under 1000 g, the first maneuver allowed for resection of 3 cm, the second for 0.9 cm additional, and the radical measure of bronchial implantation permitted an additional 2.7 cm (Fig. 36–1B). It has since become clear that cervical flexion combined with hilar and pericardial mobilization plus division of the pulmonary lig-

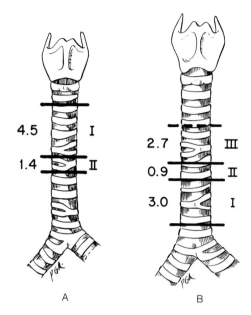

Fig. 36–1. Diagrams of the amounts of trachea that can be removed and yet permit primary anastomosis. *A,* Cervicomediastinal mobilization permitted removal of 4.5 cm under 1000 g tension, with cervical flexion. Intrathoracic dissection permitted removal of an additional 1.4 cm. *B,* Transthoracic hilar dissection and division of the pulmonary ligament, with the cervical spine in the neutral position, permitted removal of 3 cm, intrapericardial dissection an additional 0.9 cm, and division of the left main bronchus with reimplantation in the bronchus intermedius an additional 2.7 cm. The use of cervical flexion has demonstrated that the area designated I may be significantly greater than 3 cm. (From Grillo, H.C.: Surgical approaches to the trachea. Surg. Gynecol. Obstet. *129*:347, 1969.)

ament allows lengths of 5 to 6 cm to be removed by the transthoracic approach. Bronchial implantation has been reserved for carinal excision or similar complex maneuvers in order not to add another unnecessary risk to operation. Reimplantation of the left main bronchus into the bronchus intermedius was first used clinically by Barclay and his associates (1957).

The limits of safety with varying anastomotic tensions have not been established in man. Cantrell and Folse (1961) found in dogs that tensions below 1700 g permitted safety from disruption after anastomosis. In anatomic studies in the cadaver, we found that an average tension of 675 g only was required for approximation—maximum 1000 g—after a 7-cm resection. Such clinical measurements as we have made show tensions of about 600 g in resections of 4 to 5 cm in length.

Anatomic and clinical observations show that great attention must be paid to the lateral blood supply in tracheal mobilization. This fine segmental supply cannot be disrupted safely, particularly for anastomosis of a long distal segment to a short proximal segment; the distal segment must not be freed circumferentially.

Another peculiarity of tracheal reconstruction depends on the relative rigidity of the anterolateral walls. Transverse wedging of the anterior wall of the trachea may buckle the posterior wall into a partially obstructing valve. Circumferential resection—which may, however, be beveled—is most often preferable.

SURGERY OF THE TRACHEA

Anesthesia

The airway must be under full control at all times during reconstructive surgery of the trachea, so that hasty maneuvers are unnecessary and hypoxia does not occur. The patient should breathe spontaneously during the operation and at its conclusion so that ventilatory support will not be necessary. Cardiopulmonary bypass has been employed for tracheal surgery, but it is not necessary for relatively simple resection and, as noted by Geffin and colleagues (1969), presents real hazards for more complex procedures requiring extensive manipulation of the lung. Procedures are carefully explained to the patients before the operation. Induction is carried out slowly and gently, especially in a patient with a highly obstructed trachea. If a benign stenosis presents an airway diameter less than 5 mm, dilatation is performed and an endotracheal tube is passed beyond the lesion, to prevent arrhythmia caused by CO_2 buildup during the early stages of operation. Occasionally, a nearly obstructing tumor has required prompt bronchoscopy—with a ventilating bronchoscope—shortly after induction, with subsequent intubation. Frequent monitoring of blood gases and an electrocardiogram are essential. Bronchoscopic examination should be done by both the surgeon and the anesthetist who must deal with this airway until surgical access distal to the lesion has been obtained. If tracheostomy is already present, induction is simplified. Initial dissection is always done carefully to avoid increasing the degree of obstruction by roughness or pressure. The area below the obstruction is isolated first, so that a transection of the trachea can be performed at any point and an airway introduced across the operative field, should the degree of obstruction increase. Sterile anesthesia tubing, connectors, and endotracheal tubes are available in the operative field. I have not found it necessary to make distal incisions in the tracheobronchial tree for insertion of ventilatory catheters but, rather, have proceeded as described. If transthoracic resection is performed close to the carina, the endotracheal tube is passed into the left main bronchus and that lung alone is ventilated; if the P_{O_2} falls toward unsatisfactory levels, a previously isolated right pulmonary artery is temporarily clamped to eliminate the shunt through the right lung. Slow increase in shunting may occur during prolonged operation owing to low tidal ventilation, increasing atelectasis, and aspiration of secretions, and must be guarded against, as noted by Wilson (1987). El-Baz and associates (1982) reported that high frequency ventilation is a useful adjunct, especially in complex carinal reconstruction.

Surgical Approaches

Lesions in the *upper half of the trachea* that are known to be benign are best approached cervically (Fig. 36–2A). If a malignant lesion is present, be prepared for the cervicomediastinal and, possibly, thoracic approach. Placement of the cervical incision depends on the pathologic state, the presence of existing stomas, and the

possible need for sternotomy. If a postoperative temporary tracheostomy stoma may be required after a difficult laryngotracheal anastomosis, then the incision must be planned so that a stoma can be made away from the incision. If the initial dissection through the neck indicates need for further exposure, the upper sternum is split for a portion of its length; horizontal division of the sternum into an intercostal space is not necessary. Because the great vessels present anteriorly, division of more than the upper sternum is not helpful; division simply allows room to maneuver in managing the more distal trachea. Innominate vein division also adds nothing.

Rarely, this incision must be extended through the fourth intercostal space on the right to permit additional mobilization of the intrathoracic trachea by freeing the hilus of the right lung. Such an incision permits wide exposure of the entire trachea from cricoid to carina. This is almost never necessary in benign stenosis. If extirpative surgery and terminal tracheostomy are expected, the incision should avoid a vertical limb even if sternal division is needed. A large bipedicled flap is prepared through two horizontal incisions, as I suggested in 1966. A long-segment cutaneous tracheal replacement may also be so fashioned. Such circumstances are unusual but should be kept in mind in planning extensive procedures.

Lesions of the *lower half of the trachea* are most easily approached directly through a high right thoracotomy incision (Fig. 36–2B), although it is possible to excise even very low benign lesions from the anterior approach, when the medical status of the patient demands that thoracotomy be avoided. Cervical flexion devolves sufficient trachea into the mediastinum so that lower tracheal tumors are usually approachable completely through the right side of the chest without a sternal component. Fourth intercostal space or fourth rib resection is used. Median sternotomy to expose the trachea between the superior vena cava and aorta, after pericardial division, provides poor access for any but simple resections.

Reconstruction of the Upper Trachea

The upper flap is raised with or without circumcising an existing tracheostomy incision or including it in the original incision; individualization is required in each patient. Many existing tracheostomy stomas, even if they are to be allowed to close spontaneously later, will usually have to be remade in another opening in the skin because of changed postoperative relationships between trachea and overlying skin. If the lesion is high, benign, and short, only a limited field is required. Dissection is confined chiefly to the midline, the upper flap being raised to the level of the cricoid and the lower to the sternal notch to allow dissection in the pretracheal plane as needed. Dense scar is often present in association with benign stenosis and dissection is done close to the trachea to avoid damage to the recurrent nerves, especially near the cricoid. Isolation of the nerves is avoided because this would increase the danger of injury. Freeing the

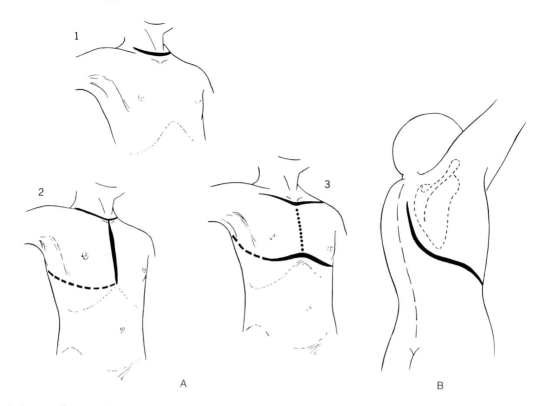

Fig. 36–2. *A,* Incisions for approach to the upper portion of the trachea. (1) Cervical incision allows access to upper trachea and to the mediastinum with somewhat limited exposure. (2) Median sternotomy, usually carried only through the upper two thirds of the sternum, allows more extended dissection into the mediastinum. Extension of the incision to the right fourth intercostal space (dotted line) allows exposure of the entire trachea from cricoid to carina and permits mobilization of the hilus. (3) Cervicomediastinal approach is here carried out beneath a bipedicled anterior skin flap. The flap is kept intact in case it is necessary to fashion a mediastinal tracheostomy. Such an incision is rarely needed. *B,* Incision for approach to the lower trachea and carina. The thorax is entered through the fourth intercostal space or the bed of the resected fourth rib. The high incision shown permits the scapula to be drawn out of the way. (From Grillo, H.C.: Surgical approaches to the trachea. Surg. Gynecol. Obstet. *129:347,* 1969.)

trachea below the lesion early allows easy establishment of airway control and expedites dissection of a cicatrized segment from the esophagus or prevertebral fascia. Mobilization is made as requred before and behind the trachea both proximally and distally. Tentative approximation with traction sutures, while the neck is flexed by the anesthetist, demonstrates whether approximation may be accomplished or whether further dissection is needed. A single layer of anastomotic sutures is placed in interrupted fashion so that the knots will be tied on the outside. Fine—No. 4–0—absorbable polymeric sutures are preferred. In many instances, the sutures will become inaccessible to direct vision during tying and must not break (Fig. 36–3A to E). The anterior approach may also be used for tumor, but in this situation, sternotomy is often required for adequate removal of paratracheal tissue. In this instance, the recurrent nerves are usually identified, and preserved if they are not involved by tumor.

When benign stenosis of the upper trachea also involves the subglottic larynx, one stage reconstruction is possible. As I (1982) reported, the technique is complex.

Reconstruction of the Lower Trachea

After confirmation of the extent of a tumor, anatomic mobilization is usually accomplished prior to severing

the trachea. If obstruction appears to be imminent during mobilization, the trachea is transected and distally intubated. If the line of transection is supracarinal, the left main bronchus is intubated. The need for elimination of an arterial shunt through the right lung has been discussed. Access to the subcarinal lymph nodes and lower paratracheal nodes is excellent. The recurrent nerves reach a point adjacent to the trachea promptly and should be sacrificed only deliberately as required. Cervical flexion by the anesthetist devolves a fair segment of trachea into the chest even in the lateral position and this, in combination with the mobilization maneuvers earlier noted, permits end-to-end anastomosis (Fig. 36–4A to C). Complex maneuvers may be necessary for excision and reconstruction of carinal lesions or lesions involving the right main bronchus or upper lobe bronchus (Fig. 36–5A to C). In general, my principle is to excise the tumor with a satisfactory margin and then use a suitable reconstruction for the specific situation. As I have described (1965, 1970), a second layer pedicled pleural flap is always placed around intrathoracic anastomoses. I described specific techniques of carinal reconstruction in detail. Laryngeal release is not helpful in carinal resection.

Tracheostomy is avoided after tracheal reconstruction to avoid drying of secretions or injury to the anastomosis.

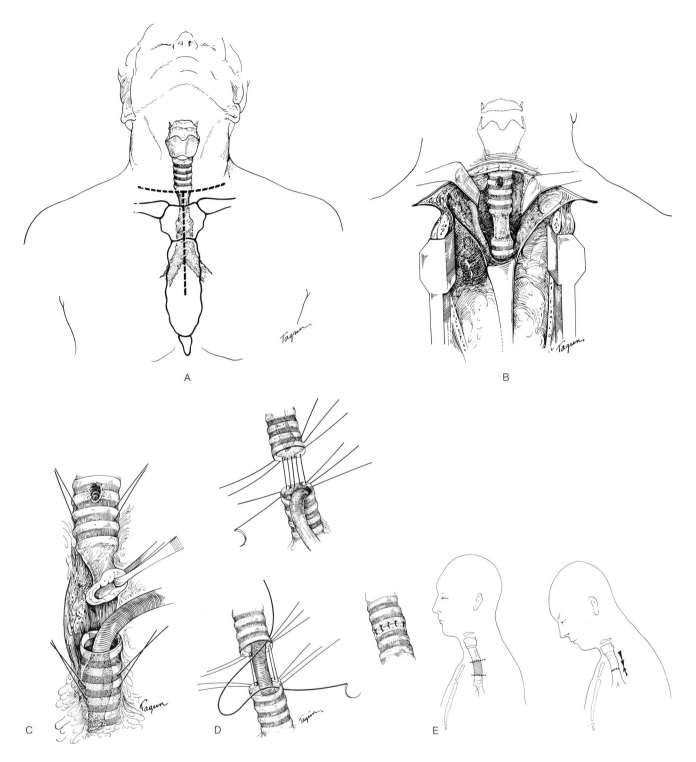

Fig. 36–3. Reconstruction of the upper trachea. *A,* The collar incision is often adequate for benign lesions in the upper and mid trachea. Partial division of sternum allows access to the mediastinum over the great vessels. *B,* The innominate vein is retracted but not divided because greater exposure will not be so obtained owing to the posterior position of the lower trachea. The pleura is intact. *C,* Direct intubation has been performed following division of the trachea below an adherent stenotic lesion. Dissection is now simplified. Traction sutures are shown and also the scar of the prior tracheostomy. *D,* Details of placement of sutures. Interrupted sutures passing through the cartilage and membranous wall are used. Knots are tied on the outside. *E,* Diagram to indicate that the majority of mobilization in the approach to the upper trachea is obtained by cervical flexion with downward devolvement of the trachea and a lesser amount by upward movement of the distal trachea. (A to D, From Grillo, H.C.: Surgery of the trachea. Curr. Probl. Surg. July 1970, p. 1.)

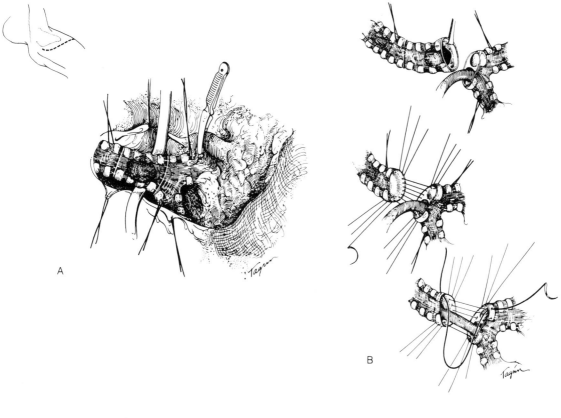

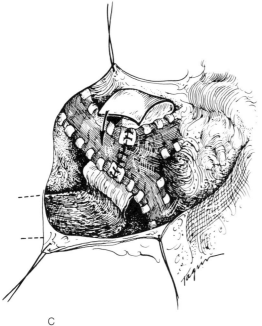

Fig. 36–4. Reconstruction of the lower trachea. *A*, Exposure through a thoracotomy. Hilar mobilization has been accomplished and also circumferential dissection of the trachea. When a tumor is present, paratracheal nodal tissue is excised with the specimen. Traction sutures have been placed proximally and distally. The lines of resection are shown. A clamp may be placed on the pulmonary artery later if the patient fails to maintain adequate oxygenation on intubation of the left main bronchus alone. This has been necessary in lesions close to the carina as well as in carinal resections. *B*, Details of management of resection and suturing. Intubation has been carried out across the operative field and the specimen is then removed. After placement of sutures on the anterior and lateral walls of the trachea, an elongated endotracheal tube is passed from above into the left main bronchus and the balance of the posterior sutures are placed prior to their being tied. *C*, Following completion of the anastomosis, which is facilitated by flexion of the patient's neck, a second layer of pedicled pleural flap is placed about the anastomosis (From Grillo, H.C.: Surgery of the trachea. Curr. Prob. Surg. July 1970, p. 1.)

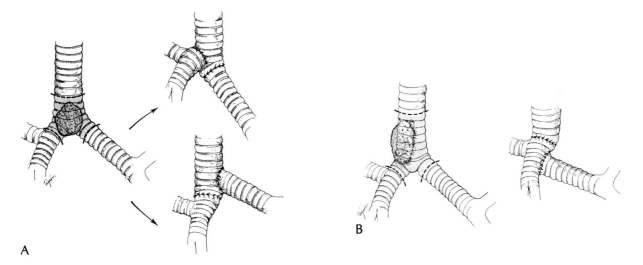

Fig. 36–5. Tracheal reconstruction following carinal resection. *A,* Following carinal resection without removal of a long segment of trachea, reconstruction is most frequently performed by implanting either the right or the left main bronchus into the stump of the devolved lower trachea. The corresponding right or left main bronchus is then implanted preferentially in a side opening fashioned in the lower portion of the trachea. Suture of the right main bronchus to the left main bronchus to fashion a new carina is conceptually attractive, but limits the ability to approximate the airway because of the tethering effect of the aorta on the left main bronchus. *B,* When a longer segment of trachea has been resected, most frequently it is necessary to mobilize the right lung and elevate the right main bronchus to reach the trachea, which has also been devolved as far distally as it will go. In such cases, the left main bronchus may have to be anastomosed to the bronchus intermedius. Preservation of some blood supply for all of these segments of airway is essential for the repair to heal successfully. (From Grillo, H.C.: Tracheal tumors: surgical management. Ann. Thorac. Surg. 26:112, 1978.)

It may, however, be necessary, temporarily, after laryngotracheal anastomosis.

Complex Methods

One sees few benign lesions or potentially curable malignant lesions that require resection of lengths of trachea and still leave a functional larynx, in which end-to-end reconstruction may not be done by present methods. In a rare instance I (1965) applied an extension of an earlier method developed experimentally and clinically for replacement of cervical trachea by fashioning an invaginated horizontally bipedicled tube of full-thickness skin supported by fully buried polypropylene rings. Results have been no more dependable than the use of prostheses. At present I believe both should be avoided. The alternatives are T-tubes for benign lesions and irradiation for malignant lesions nonresectable because of length.

Mediastinal Tracheostomy

Rarely, when a lesion involves a large portion of trachea and larynx but seems to be within possible bounds of cure, laryngotracheal resection may be indicated either for palliation in severe airway obstruction or for potential cure. The problems of mediastinal tracheostomy are not wholly solved. Attempts to pull the deeply situated distal tracheal stump to the surface placed excess tension on the suture line; attempts to carry complex skin tubes down to the trachea led to separation at the suture lines, sepsis, and osteomyelitis of the sternum. Massive hemorrhages from the innominate artery and aortic arch have been frequent complications of such methods. Muscle flaps have not fully protected these vessels. A technique that I devised (1966) attempted to

eliminate these problems by bringing the anterior skin *down* to the stump of the trachea by removing the heads of the clavicles, the upper portion of sternum, and the medial ends of the first two ribs (Fig. 36–6A, B). This procedure is done extrapleurally. Excellent blood supply is present in the flap, and the anastomosis is made to a circular opening in the middle point of the flap so that the suture line is a simple one. Hazards of bleeding do attend such procedures, however, if primary healing is not obtained. Elective division of the innominate artery, with appropriate preoperative angiography and intra-operative EEG monitoring, plus advancement of pedicled omental flaps to the upper mediastinum as recorded by Mathisen and associates (1987), have avoided such incidents.

TRACHEOSTOMY AND ITS PROBLEMS

Immediate complications of tracheostomy, such as intra- and early-postoperative hemorrhage, incorrect placement, injury to adjacent structures, and hypoxia during the procedure, have largely been eliminated by the deliberate performance of tracheostomy over an emergency airway established by endotracheal intubation or rigid bronchoscopy. Later complications, such as plugging of the tube, valve-like obstruction at the tip caused by dry secretions, slippage of cuffs or of the tube, and local sepsis, have been reduced in incidence by meticulous care of the tracheostomy, and their consequences minimized by early recognition and correction. In addition to the late obstructive complications to be discussed in Chapter 61, erosion of the innominate artery and tracheoesophageal fistula must be remembered, as pointed out by Mulder and Rubush (1969) as well as

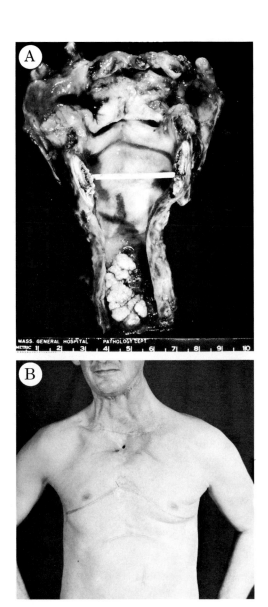

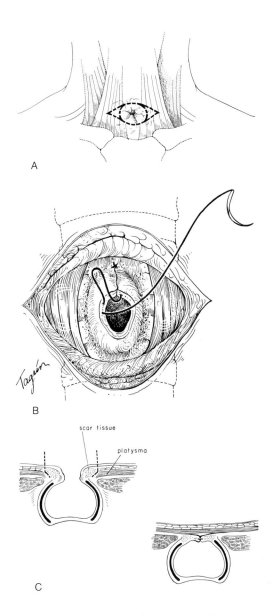

Fig. 36–6. Mediastinal tracheostomy. *A,* Laryngotracheal specimen to remove two obstructing lesions—mucoepidermoid carcinoma of the larynx and squamous cell carcinoma of the trachea, concurrently. Regional node dissections were done later. (From Grillo, H.C.: Surgery of the trachea. Curr. Probl. Surg. July 1970, p. 1.) *B,* Photograph of a patient 18 months after initial resection shows the anatomic features of a low mediastinal tracheostomy. The procedure was carried out between two horizontal incisions, one across the base of the neck and the other beneath the nipples. The upper chest wall defect is the result of the removal of the upper sternum and medial ends of clavicles and upper two ribs. The stoma sits just above the aortic arch. The short horizontal incision just below the stoma was necessary for control of bleeding in the innominate artery postoperatively. The horizontal incision below the xiphoid was initially placed as a relaxing incision to allow advancement of flaps upward.

Fig. 36–7. Technique for closure of persistent tracheal stoma. *A,* The skin around the margin of the stoma is elevated with a circumferential incision. The lateral extensions create an ellipse to provide access and permit plastic closure. *B,* After dissection of the skin and platysma above and below, and mobilization of the strap muscles laterally, the central circular flap is created, with great care not to destroy its basal blood supply. It is now being closed with a subcuticular suture. The epithelial surface faces the lumen. The strap muscles are next approximated and the skin and platysma are closed above in a horizontal layer. *C,* Cross-sectional view of closure. The line of circular incision is shown. The skin is turned inward and closed. In most instances the strap muscles are sutured together in midline to obtain a better cosmetic result. (From Lawson, D.W., and Grillo, H.C.: Closure of a persistent tracheal stoma. Surg. Gynecol. Obstet. *130*:995, 1970.)

others. I and my colleagues (1976) described a method for repair of postintubation tracheoesophageal fistula.

I prefer to perform a tracheostomy through a short horizontal incision about 1 cm below the cricoid and to identify the cricoid precisely so that the correct level of second and third rings may be selected. The thyroid isthmus usually must be divided. A vertical incision in the trachea is used. Extreme care should be exercised to avoid injuring the first ring, because subsequent erosion may damage the cricoid and produce a subglottic stricture that is extremely difficult to repair. If necessary, the tracheal opening should include the fourth ring also. A tube with an inner cannula is preferable. Initially, it is held not only by tapes but by skin sutures passed through the flanges and tied.

Another rare complication of tracheostomy is a persistent stoma that does not close even after many months. This usually results from a long, persistent tracheostomy, a large stoma caused by the operative procedure or sepsis, healing of skin to tracheal epithelium, and debilitating systemic states that depressed the healing response. Lawson and I (1970) devised a technique for closure that circumscribes the stoma, using the healed skin as a "first-stage" circular flap (Fig. 36–7A to C). When this skin is inverted with a subcuticular suture, a healed epithelial surface is presented to the tracheal lumen. The strap muscles are approximated and the skin and platysma are closed horizontally over this. Results of repair by this method have been excellent.

REFERENCES

Barclay, R.S., McSwan, N., and Welsh, T.M.: Tracheal reconstruction without the use of grafts. Thorax *12*:177, 1957.

Belsey, R.: Resection and reconstruction of the intrathroacic trachea. Br. J. Surg. *38*:200, 1950.

Borrie, J., and Redshaw, N.R.: Cervical tracheal reconstruction in sheep, using silastic prostheses with subterminal suture cuffs. Proc. Univ. Otago Med. School *48*:32, 1970.

Cantrell, J.R., and Folse, J.R.: The repair of circumferential defects of the trachea by direct anastomosis: experimental evaluation. J. Thorac. Cardiovasc. Surg. *42*:589, 1961.

El-Baz, N., et al.: One-lung high-frequency ventilation for tracheoplasty and bronchoplasty. Ann. Thorac. Surg. *34*:564, 1982.

Geffin, B., Bland, J., and Grillo, H.C.: Anesthetic management of tracheal resection and reconstruction. Anesth. Analg. *48*:884, 1969.

Grillo, H.C.: Circumferential resection and reconstruction of mediastinal and cervical trachea. Ann. Surg. *162*:374, 1965.

Grillo, H.C.: Terminal or mural tracheostomy in the anterior mediastinum. J. Thorac. Cardiovasc. Surg. *51*:422, 1966.

Grillo, H.C.: Surgical approaches to the trachea. Surg. Gynecol. Obstet. *129*:374, 1969.

Grillo, H.C.: Surgery of the trachea. Curr. Probl. Surg. July 1970, p. 1.

Grillo, H.C.: Primary reconstruction of airway resection of subglottic laryngeal and upper tracheal stenosis. Ann. Thorac. Surg. *33*:3, 1982a.

Grillo, H.C.: Carinal reconstruction. Ann. Thorac. Surg. *34*:356, 1982b.

Grillo, H.C., Dignan, E.F., and Miura, T.: Extensive resection and reconstruction of mediastinal trachea without prosthesis or graft: an anatomical study in man. J. Thorac. Cardiovasc. Surg. *48*:741, 1964.

Grillo, H.C., Moncure, A.C., and McEnany, M.T.: Repair of inflammatory tracheo-esophageal fistula. Ann. Thorac. Surg. *22*:112, 1976.

Lawson, D.W., and Grillo, H.C.: Closure of a persistent tracheal stoma. Surg. Gynecol. Obstet. *130*:995, 1970.

Mathisen, D.J., et al.: The omentum in the management of complicated cardiothoracic problems. J. Thorac. Cardiovasc. Surg. *95*:677, 1988.

Michelson, E., et al.: Experiments in tracheal reconstruction. J. Thorac. Cardiovasc. Surg. *41*:784, 1961.

Miura, T., and Grillo, H.C.: The contribution of the inferior thyroid artery to the blood supply of the human trachea. Surg. Gynecol. Obstet. *123*:99, 1966.

Montgomery, W.W.: Suprahyoid release for tracheal anastomosis. Arch. Otolaryngol. *99*:255, 1974.

Mulder, D.S., and Rubush, J.L.: Complications of tracheostomy: relationship to long-term ventilatory assistance. J. Trauma *9*:389, 1969.

Mulliken, J., and Grillo, H.C.: The limits of tracheal resection with primary anastomosis. Further anatomical studies in man. J. Thorac. Cardiovasc. Surg. *55*:418, 1968.

Neville, W.E., Bolandowski, P.J., and Soltanzadeh, H.: Prosthetic reconstruction of the trachea and cardia. J. Thorac. Cardiovasc. Surg. *72*:525, 1976.

Salassa, J.R., Pearson, B., and Payne, W.S.: Growth and microscopic blood supply of the trachea. Ann. Thorac. Surg. *23*:100, 1977.

Vogt-Moykopf, I., and Mickisch, G.H.: Prosthetic replacement of the trachea: discussion. *In* International Trends in General Thoracic Surgery, Vol. 2. Edited by H.C. Grillo and H. Eschapasse. Philadelphia, W.B. Saunders Co., 1987, p. 147.

Wilson, R.S.: Anesthetic management for tracheal reconstruction. *In* International Trends in General Thoracic Surgery, Vol. 2. Edited by H.C. Grillo and H. Eschapasse. Philadelphia, W.B. Saunders Co., 1987, p. 3.

CHAPTER 37

EXPOSURE OF THE CERVICAL ESOPHAGUS

Martin Rothberg and Thomas R. DeMeester

The first esophageal operations were performed on the cervical portion of the organ. In 1738, Goursand of France removed a foreign body from the cervical esophagus, and in 1877, Billroth and Czerny first successfully reconstructed the cervical esophagus following resection of a malignant tumor. Today, exposure of the cervical esophagus is commonly required for closure of endoscopic perforations, cricopharyngeal myotomy for motility disorders, suspension or resection of pharyngeal diverticula, and esophagoenteric anastomosis following esophageal resections.

SURGICAL APPROACH TO THE CERVICAL ESOPHAGUS

The cervical esophagus is approached through a left neck incision along the anterior border of the sternocleidomastoid muscle. The left side is chosen for two reasons. First, the esophagus in the neck extends to the left of the trachea, which facilitates dissection from this side. Second, the right recurrent laryngeal nerve lies farther from the wall than the left nerve, so it is less likely to be injured when encircling the esophagus from the left. The anatomic relationships of the esophagus in the neck are discussed in Chapter 6.

Patients who may have vocal cord paralysis should have the function of their cords evaluated before surgery. This is easily accomplished by passing a fiber-optic bronchoscope through the anesthetized nose and into the nasopharynx and observing the cord movement during speech.

The patient is placed on the operating table in the supine position. Once anesthetized, a rolled towel is placed transversely under the scapula to provide maximal hyperextension of the neck. The patient's neck is turned only slightly to the right to avoid distortion of the anatomy. The table is placed in a reversed Trendelenburg position to decrease venous congestion and soft-tissue edema, which may interfere with postoperative ventilation. A nasogastric tube is passed to facilitate palpation of the esophagus. The upper chest is incorporated into the operative field because enlargement of the thoracic inlet may be required (Fig. 37–1).

The incision along the anterior border of the sternocleidomastoid muscle extends from the superior aspect of the thyroid cartilage to the suprasternal notch. The platysma is sharply incised and hemostasis obtained. The sternocleidomastoid muscle is retracted laterally and the omohyoid muscle divided inferiorly as it courses anterior to the carotid sheath. The sternohyoid and sternothyroid muscles are divided at their sternal attachment. The middle thyroid vein is ligated as it enters the jugular vein. The carotid sheath and its contents are gently retracted laterally and the thyroid gland and trachea medially (Fig. 37–2). This exposes the deeper structures of the neck. The inferior thyroid artery is ligated as it enters the field posterior to the common carotid artery. The cervical esophagus lies along the vertebral bodies and longus colli muscle. The exposure, as seen by the surgeon, is shown in Fig. 37–3. Blunt dissection will separate the posterior esophagus from the prevertebral fascia. The left recurrent laryngeal nerve lies horizontally along the posterolateral wall of the trachea just above the tracheoesophageal groove. The esophagus is separated from the trachea by sharp dissection in the tracheoesophageal

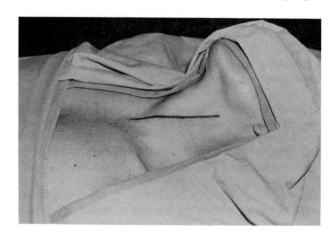

Fig. 37–1. Patient position for the left neck approach.

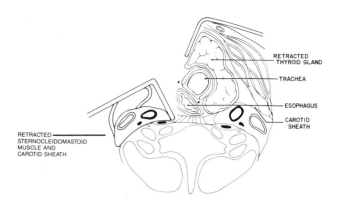

Fig. 37–2. Retraction to visualize the deep structures of the neck.

groove beneath the nerve. This dissection can be facilitated by grasping the esophagus with broad-tipped forceps and pulling it toward the surgeon. Fine-tipped forceps can damage the esophageal wall. With this maneuver, the right border of the esophagus can be visualized and a right-angled clamp passed around it (Fig. 37–4). Normally, there is sufficient space between the right recurrent laryngeal nerve and the right border of the esophagus to allow circumferential dissection without injury to this nerve. Failure to visualize the right border can result in damage to the esophageal wall or the right recurrent nerve when passing the clamp. The esophagus is encircled with a Penrose drain at a level just above the thoracic inlet to aid in its retraction (Fig. 37–5). The fibroareolar tissue between the esophagus and trachea is bluntly dissected down into the thoracic inlet as far as the finger will reach.

The cervical esophagus is lifted from its bed between the levels of the cricopharyngeus muscle and the thoracic inlet and retracted into the wound. Injury to the thoracic duct can occur where it courses along the left postero-

lateral esophageal wall; it arches laterally behind the carotid sheath, below the inferior thyroid artery, before it enters the venous system and, if necessary, ligation at this level may be performed without sequelae. Anterolateral retraction of the esophagus will bring the posterior junction between the cricopharyngeus and inferior pharyngeal constrictor muscles into view to perform a cricomyotomy, pharyngoesophageal suspension or diverticulectomy, esophagoenteric anastomosis, or esophagostomy.

EXPOSURE OF THE THORACIC INLET

The bony thoracic inlet measures 5 cm in the anteroposterior plane and 10 cm in the lateral plane. This can compromise the passage of an esophageal substitute into the neck and may necessitate widening of the thoracic inlet. To do so, the cervical skin incision is extended inferiorly over the sternal midline to the sternal angle, and the left pectoralis major muscle is reflected laterally to expose the bony thorax. The medial clavicular head, the anterior portion of the first rib—lateral to the internal mammary vessels and medial to the phrenic nerve, and the left half of the manubrium can be resected extrapleurally (Fig. 37–6). In this resection, the sternocleidomastoid and remnants of the strap muscles are reflected laterally, using the cautery to divide the muscular attachments at the bone. The clavicle is encircled with a right-angled clamp lateral to its junction with the first rib and divided with a Gigli saw. This maneuver must be done carefully to avoid damage to the subclavian vein. The intercostal muscles in the first interspace are divided along the superior border of the second rib, again with the cautery, from the medial border of the manubrium to the point of transection of the first rib. Avoid damaging the internal mammary vessels, which lie on the pleural

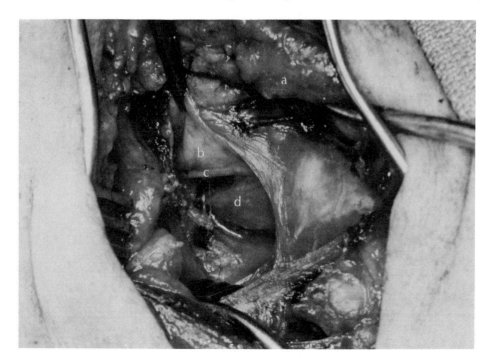

Fig. 37–3. Exposure as seen by the surgeon: thyroid gland (a), trachea (b), left recurrent laryngeal nerve (c), and esophagus (d).

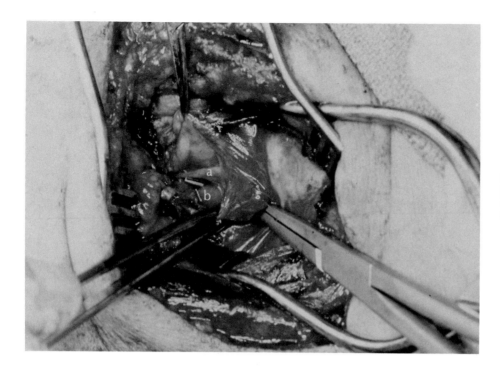

Fig. 37–4. Dissection of the right border of the esophagus: left recurrent laryngeal nerve (a), right-angled clamp around esophagus (b).

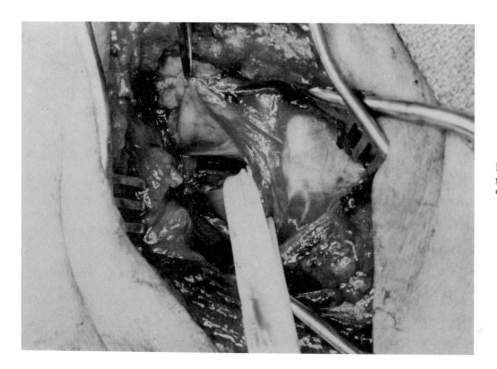

Fig. 37–5. Retraction of the esophagus into the wound with a Penrose drain.

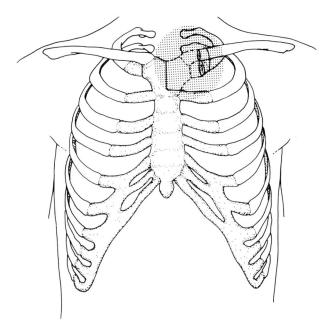

Fig. 37–6. Schematic diagram of the thoracic inlet area to be resected.

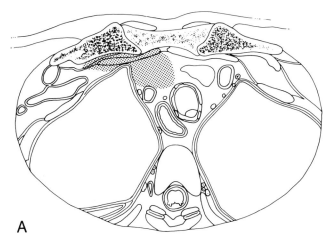
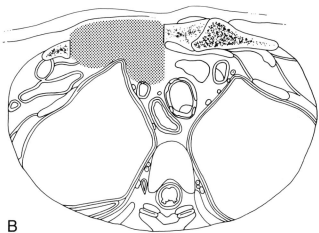

Fig. 37–7. Schematic diagram of the thoracic inlet as seen from above. *A*, Before resection. *B*, Widened thoracic inlet following resection.

surface. An L-shaped cut is made in the manubrium using the sternal saw along the line shown in Figure 37–6. The manubrium is then retracted laterally along with the attached medial segment of the clavicle. The first rib is divided laterally with a rib cutter and the whole left manubrioclavicular joint is removed. In addition to opening the thoracic inlet, this allows greater exposure of the esophagus (Fig. 37–7A,B). Before closure, the medial end of the remaining clavicle can be wired to the first rib if a cosmetic deformity appears likely.

For most procedures, this approach to the cervical esophagus affords adequate exposure and permits safe dissection while avoiding injury to the recurrent laryngeal nerves and related structures.

REFERENCES

Czerny, J.: Neue Operationen: vorläufige Mitteilung. Zentralbl. Chir. 4:443, 1877.
Goursand. Cited by Meade, R.H.: A History of Thoracic Surgery. Springfield, IL, Charles C Thomas, 1961, p. 567.

CHAPTER 38

RESECTION OF THE ESOPHAGUS

Thomas W. Shields

RESECTION OF THE CERVICAL ESOPHAGUS

Excision of the cervical esophagus is indicated in patients with primary carcinoma arising in this segment or, more rarely, in those with direct involvement by malignant lesions of the larynx or hypopharynx. In patients with carcinoma of the cervical esophagus, a concomitant laryngectomy is usually necessary. A radical neck dissection also may be indicated.

Technique

The technical steps of the laryngectomy and neck dissection are not discussed in this text. When there is a cooperative effort between the oncologic surgeon performing the resection and the thoracic surgeon performing the reconstruction, the procedure is most likely to be successful. Wookey (1948) stated that 10 cm of the thoracic portion of the esophagus can be removed through a neck incision and that a 3-cm margin below the tumor is adequate. In most instances of a primary tumor in the cervical esophagus, however, a greater portion of the thoracic esophagus should be removed with the operative specimen.

The standard approach in most institutions is a two-team approach with mobilization of the cervical tumor and upper thoracic esophagus through the neck incision by one team. The second mobilizes the lower esophagus through an abdominal transhiatal approach (page 426) and prepares either the stomach or colon, whichever is to be used to reconstitute pharyngogastrointestinal continuity. The thoracic esophagus is then removed from above and the substitute organ—preferably the stomach—is passed through the posterior mediastinum—the shortest route—or through a substernal route into the neck, where the anastomosis to the hypopharynx is done. This operation has been extensively carried out by Lam and associates (1981) in the Far East. Its use in England has been reported by Harrison (1969) and in America by Bains (1979), Spiro (1983), and Ujiki (1987) and their associates, as well as others. When the stomach is used it is unnecessary to resect the lesser curve, as suggested by Akiyama (1980) when the tumor is in the thoracic portion of the esophagus. The esophagus can simply be divided at the gastroesophageal junction. The esophagus can be divided during the abdominal phase, with the surgeon using a Penrose drain to guide the stomach into the neck, or after the stomach has been brought into the neck. The anastomosis to the hypopharynx is done at the highest point of the fundus. A nasogastric tube is placed through the anastomosis into the stomach and the neck incision is closed with a Penrose drain in place. At the time of closure of the abdomen, an optional jejunostomy tube can be placed. When the stomach is not suitable for replacement of the esophagus, the colon can be used, as initially advocated by Scanlon and Staley (1963). Wong (personal communication, 1986), stated that although he prefers to use the stomach, he finds no difficulty with using a portion of the colon under these circumstances. At times, neither the stomach nor the colon is available, and the jejunum must be used. The use of the jejunum represents the last choice, because in approximately 20% of persons the vascular arcade is inadequate to develop a loop long enough to reach high in the thorax or into the neck. Even when applicable, at least three or four jejunal vessels may have to be divided. When a long loop has been prepared, there is generally an excess of intestine relative to the mesentery. In almost every instance, Wong (personal communication, 1986) found it necessary to excise a segment in the middle of the jejunal loop to straighten the loop to avoid excessive length of the conduit and subsequent late complications. Kasai and Nishihira (1986), in most instances, used a pedicle jejunal segment to replace the esophagus after resection. They reported an overall mortality rate of 20%; however, no deaths have occurred in their last 19 patients. Nonetheless, a significant morbidity related to the transposed intestinal loop occurs and the procedure remains a last choice for most patients.

On occasion, the cervical esophagus is removed because of growth of tumor into it from an adjacent site. Reconstruction can be done as described, but at times a free intestinal graft, usually a jejunal segment or occasionally a colonic segment, can be used to restore local continuity. Peters (1971) and Flynn (1979) and their associates published early reports of this technique. Jurkiewicz (1984) and Hester and Jurkiewicz (1985), using microvascular techniques, had excellent results in over 90% of more than 75 patients when such grafts were used for local cervical esophageal replacement after postsurgical tumor extirpation or in the management of postirradiation or traumatic esophageal fistulas. Payne and associates at Mayo Clinic (Chapter 41) report similar good results after reconstruction with free intestinal grafts in these trying situations.

TRANSSTERNAL APPROACH TO UPPER THORACIC ESOPHAGUS

Occasionally a lesion in the superior mediastinal segment of the esophagus cannot be mobilized satisfactorily from the neck incision, and a transsternal approach is necessary for adequate exposure. This method was first reported by Waddell and Scannell (1957) and Cauchoix and Binet (1957). With this approach, the dissection of the esophagus can be carried out under direct vision to protect the left recurrent laryngeal nerve (Fig. 38–1). The remainder of the dissection is then carried out transhiatally. Ong (1978) and Wong (1981) and their colleagues and Orringer (1984) described their experiences with this approach.

EXCISION OF THE THORACIC ESOPHAGUS

Removal of the thoracic esophagus is most often used in the surgical treatment of squamous cell carcinoma of the thoracic esophagus and less frequently for excision of other malignant tumors of this structure. Less common indications for esophageal resection are extensive benign strictures or severe traumatic injury to the esophagus. Hemorrhage from esophagitis rarely requires esophageal resection, although bleeding from a penetrating Barrett's ulcer may.

Operative Approach

Many think that resection of the thoracic portion of the esophagus is best accomplished from the right side, although Sweet (1954), Ellis (1980), and Skinner (1983) recommended a left-sided approach, particularly for lesions in the lower third of the organ. Because the thoracic portion of the esophagus, except for its most distal part, is primarily on the right side of the visceral compartment of the mediastinum and the aortic arch lies over the esophagus on the left, the left-sided approach is less than ideal. Nonetheless, many variations in the operative approach have been described. Not only has a right or left thoracotomy been recommended, but many in the 1980s have advocated a transhiatal nonthoracotomy approach. Immediate or delayed reconstruction and the use of the stomach, colon, or jejunum to restore continuity, as well as other technical considerations, remain under debate. The stomach is used most often to restore continuity, with anastomosis in the chest, as suggested by Lewis (1946), or in the neck, as proposed by McKeown (1976). Akiyama (1980) along with his associates (1978, 1981, 1984) reported extensive experience with this latter procedure as a one-stage operation, placing the transposed stomach in a retrosternal position in its passage to the neck. Wong (1987a, b) placed the stomach in the posterior mediastium and performed the esophagogastric anastomosis either in the neck or in the apex of the chest. *When total esophagectomy is planned for the treatment of squamous cell carcinoma of the esophagus, regardless of the method and timing of reconstruction, exploration of the abdomen is indicated immediately preceding the thoracotomy.*

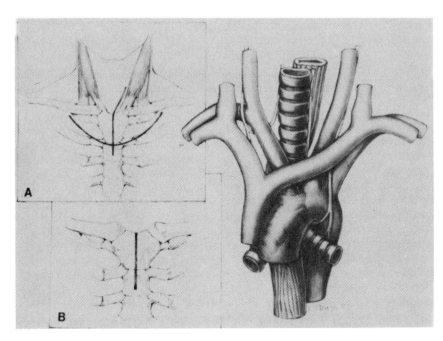

Fig. 38–1. Exposure of upper mediastinal structures, including the esophagus, obtained through a partial median sternotomy. An oblique left cervical incision with extension onto the midline of the chest in a curved anterior thoracic incision can be used to obtain exposure (Insert A). Partial median sternotomy through manubrium and extending across the angle of Louis to expose the upper mediastinum (Insert B). (Reproduced with permission from Orringer, M.B.: J. Thorac. Cardiovasc. Surg. 87:124, 1984.)

Right Thoracotomy Approach

Technique

When a right-sided transthoracic resection is contemplated, a modification of either the Lewis (1946) or McKeown (1976) technique is used. In the thoracic portion of the procedure, the patient is placed in the left lateral decubitus position or may be tilted at a 45° angle with the right side uppermost. The right pleural space is entered by a standard posterolateral incision with resection of the fifth rib or by an anterolateral incision. The pleural space is freed of adhesions, the pulmonary ligament divided from the diaphragm up to the right inferior pulmonary vein, the right lung retracted anteriorly, and the visceral mediastinal compartment exposed.

Resectability of the tumor is grossly evaluated and, if resection appears possible, the mediastinal pleura is opened above and below the esophageal lesion. The azygos vein may be divided at that time or later as indicated. The normal esophagus is freed from its bed above and below the lesion and Penrose rubber tapes are placed under the esophagus above and below the lesion. The mediastinal pleura over the lesion is incised so this portion can be removed with the tumor. Resectability is then determined by both blunt and sharp dissection, without sacrificing any of the segmental blood supply when possible, but in most instances one or more sets of the segmental arteries arising from the aorta or bronchial vessels have to be divided during this phase of the procedure. Once resection is decided upon, the tumor is freed from the adjacent structures. Care must be taken to protect the membranous portion of the trachea as well as the inferior pulmonary veins from injury (Fig. 38–2). Injury to the aorta is catastrophic, and although direct invasion of the wall by the carcinoma is infrequent, the desmoplastic reaction may make a safe plane of dissection difficult, if not at times impossible. When aortic bleeding occurs from direct injury of the wall of the aorta or attempted ligation of an intercostal or bronchial vessel too close to its origin from the aorta, direct repair by suturing may be successful in a few instances when the tear is small and the wall of the aorta is normal. When the laceration is large or the aortic wall abnormal, or both, however, control of the hemorrhage may be difficult, and fatal hemorrhage may occur. Attempts at closure with sutures tied over Teflon sponge pledgets may be useful. The initial placement of the clamp to control the bleeding or exposure of a laceration on the back wall of the vessels, however, may preclude this approach. Huang and Wu (1984) suggested that when the more simple measures are of no avail, the bleeding be controlled initially by finger pressure and the segment of aorta freed from its surrounding tissue and then wrapped with a tube of longitudinally incised vascular prosthesis. The wrapping is then closed by nonabsorbable sutures under slight tension to tamponade that portion of the aorta to control the bleeding.

Injury to the thoracic duct also should be avoided to prevent the postoperative development of a chylothorax.

Huang and Zhang (1965) pointed out the two most common sites of injury: the tumor bed of a midesophageal carcinoma invading the duct and the left superior mediastinum above the aortic arch where the duct crosses the left aspect of the esophagus upward and anteriorly to enter the root of the neck. Injury here can best be prevented by keeping the dissection closely applied to the esophageal wall. When an injury does occur and is recognized and the site identified, the duct can be ligated above and below the tear. When the site cannot be identified, the thoracic duct can be ligated above the diaphragm to control the leak (see Chapter 58). The adjacent lymph node-bearing tissue and lymph nodes are freed with the tumor as extensively as possible. Akiyama (1980), along with his associates (1981) is a strong proponent of extensive lymph node resection in patients with carcinoma of the esophagus. He reports as many as 20 to 30 identified lymph nodes in each operative specimen. The segmental vessels to the esophagus can be secured with silk ligatures, but metal clips are useful in this situation. One may, however, prefer to use clips only to mark residual tumor if complete resection is impossible. This practice provides an aid to the therapist for postoperative irradiation.

Once the lesion has been mobilized, attention is turned to either the distal or the proximal portion of the esophagus, depending on the preference of the surgeon. In mobilizing the proximal portion, it is necessary to incise the mediastinal pleura up to the thoracic inlet. The azygos vein, when not already divided, is double ligated and transfixed with No. 2-0 silk sutures and then divided. By gentle traction on the esophagus, the segmental arteries are identified, controlled, and divided from below upward to above the aortic arch. The right vagus nerve is divided high in the mediastinum, taking care not to injure the right recurrent nerve as it arises just below the level of the right subclavian artery. Likewise, during the lymph node dissection, avoid injuring the left recurrent nerve as it passes upward from the level of the aortic arch.

If the plan is immediate restoration of gastrointestinal continuity by bringing the stomach into the chest, a varying length of the proximal esophagus is dissected above the level of the azygos vein so the proximal blood supply is disturbed as little as possible. Opinions concerning an adequate margin above the tumor vary, but certainly 10 cm is minimal. The adequacy of the margin should be confirmed by frozen section examination. In mobilizing the distal portion of the esophagus below the tumor down to the esophageal hiatus, the left vagus nerve is usually divided and mobilized with the esophagus during this dissection, which is carried medially to the posterior wall of the pericardium and to the left pleura. The left pleural space may be opened, but is of no major consequence, although air or blood or both may occasionally have to be aspirated from the left pleural space. The esophagus is freed completely from the investments at the esophageal hiatus when this has not already been accomplished from below.

The technique of immediate gastric replacement is

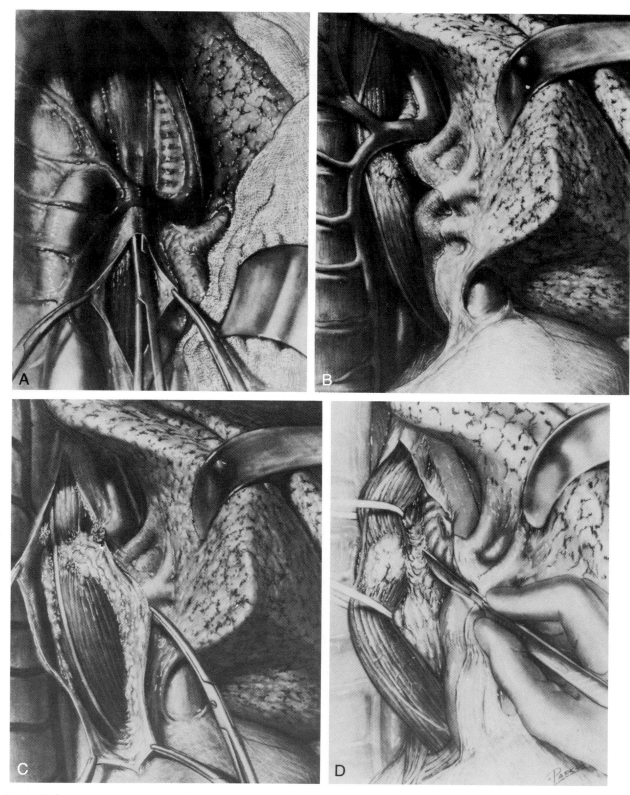

Fig. 38–2. Right transthoracic resection of the esophagus. *A*, Mediastinal pleura opened with mobilization of the azygos vein prior to its division for exposure of the esophagus. *B*, Right lung retracted forward to expose the tumor and entire length of esophagus. *C*, Division of the azygos vein to further expose the esophageal tumor. *D*, Dissection of the posterior wall of the trachea from the tumor under direct vision. (Reproduced with permission of Postlethwait, R.W.: Surgery of the Esophagus, 2nd ed. New York, Appleton-Century-Crofts, 1986.)

discussed in Chapter 39. Wong (1987a, b) suggested that the anastomosis between the proximal esophagus and gastric fundus be done as high as possible in the chest. The anastomosis may be done with either the EEA stapler (Fig. 38–3)—believed by many to result in a more secure anastomosis—or by individual suture technique.

If the resection has been done for benign disease, some form of antireflux modification, such as an inkwell type of anastomosis of the esophagus, is required, but for malignant disease this is not an important consideration, as survival is generally short.

If either an immediate gastric or colonic interposition between the cervical esophagus and the stomach is contemplated, the esophagus is freed to above the thoracic inlet. This procedure may be readily accomplished by blunt finger dissection about the esophagus and should progress as high as into the neck as possible. After the dissection is completed and proper hemostasis is ensured, two drainage tubes, which are subsequently connected to an underwater seal drainage system, are placed into the pleural space. The thoracic incision is then closed in the usual manner.

If the anastomosis is to be completed in the neck, the patient is then placed in the supine position of the abdomen either opened or re-opened through a high midline incision. The organ to be interposed—the stomach (Chapter 39), colon (Chapter 40), or even rarely a loop of jejunum—is mobilized and is made ready to pass up to the neck either through the posterior mediastinum or through a substernal tunnel. As pointed out by Ngan and Wong (1986), the posterior—orthotopic—route is the shortest. In infants and children, the entire stomach is not well tolerated in a thoracic position and should not be used to replace the esophagus. Either a gastric tube, described by Heimlich (1975), Gavriliu (1975), and An-

derson and her associates (1973, 1983), or a segment of colon or jejunum must be used.

The cervical incision, either on the left or on the right side, is made parallel to the anterior border of the sternocleidomastoid muscle. It should extend from well above the level of the midportion of the aforementioned muscle down to the sternal notch. The dissection is begun in the plane between the sternocleidomastoid muscle and the strap muscles, medial to the carotid sheath and lateral to the thyroid. The middle thyroid veins, as well as several small vessels from the internal jugular vein, may need to be divided. Division of the omohyoid muscle improves the exposure. The dissection is carried down to the prevertebral fascia and followed medially to the esophagus. The recurrent laryngeal nerve is protected. In the inferior part of the dissection, the mediastinum is entered.

The esophagus is freed from its bed; this is facilitated by having an indwelling nasogastric tube in place, and a Penrose rubber drain placed about the esophagus. Further mobilization of the esophagus to the level of the cricoid cartilage is accomplished as necessary. The esophagus is removed from the thorax and the stomach or colonic segment to be used as the interposition is brought into the neck by either of the aforementioned routes. As noted, the posterior route is the shorter of the two and, in my experience, there is less angulation of the cervical esophagus at the site of the esophagogastric anastomosis when the posterior route is used. The anastomosis is accomplished with two rows of sutures, an outer layer of interrupted 4-0 silk and an inner of interrupted or continuous 3-0 catgut. The nasogastric tube is placed through the anastomosis into the interposed stomach or colon, a Penrose rubber drain brought out through the incision, and the neck incision closed in a standard fashion. The abdominal incision is closed after placement of a temporary jejunostomy feeding tube.

Morbidity

The morbidity after thoracic esophagectomy is related to the underlying esophageal disease, the extent and radical nature of the dissection, the organ used to replace the esophagus, and the site of the anastomosis, i.e., in the thorax or in the neck. In addition, major morbid complications may occur in other organ systems, the cardiovascular and respiratory systems in particular.

Postoperative respiratory complications are common; at least 15 to 20% of patients experience such complications. Ventilatory failure with the need for tracheal intubation and controlled ventilation is frequent. Retention of secretions, as well as possible postoperative aspiration, must be avoided by careful postoperative management. Cardiac arrhythmias, myocardial infarction, and pulmonary embolism may occur.

Injury to one or both of the recurrent nerves, with paralysis of either vocal cord results in an increased possibility of aspiration in the early postoperative period. The injury may occur in the chest during the dissection, but the injury more commonly occurs in the neck as the result of traction on the trachea caused by the use of

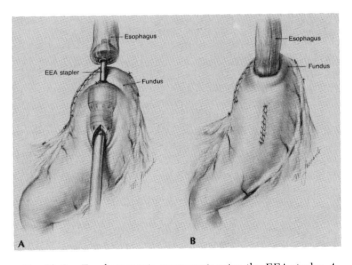

Fig. 38–3. Esophagogastric anastomosis using the EEA stapler. *A,* Staple is introduced through a gastrotomy, then brought out at a high point near the top of the fundus followed by introduction into the esophagus. *B,* Completed anastomosis and closure of gastrotomy. (Reproduced with permission of Postlethwait, R.W.: Surgery of the Esophagus, 2nd ed. New York, Appleton-Century-Crofts, 1986.)

metal retractors. Therefore, such retraction should be avoided. Identification of the nerve in the neck prior to complete mobilization of the cervical esophagus also lessens the incidence of injury. The incidence of palsy has been reported to be as high as 20% but Akiyama and associates (1981) reported a rate of 11.4%. Shahian and colleagues (1986) reported a rate of less than 4%. A rate of 5% certainly should be acceptable.

Anastomotic leak is the most feared complication when the anastomosis has been done in the chest. The incidence varies, but 1 to 2% as reported by Shahian and associates (1986), represents the ideal. Unfortunately, as reported by Postlethwait (1983), the rate frequently is as high as 10%. When the disruption occurs in the chest, it is associated with a 50% mortality rate, as reported by Xu and associates (1983) and others. Even when the patient survives, the prolonged morbidity is great.

Anastomotic disruption in the neck appears to occur more frequently. Shahian and associates (1986) noted an incidence of over 13%, but Orringer (1986) noted one of only 3%. An anastomotic leak in the neck, however, is much less significant. Death rarely results from the leak, and healing usually occurs spontaneously after appropriate drainage. Previous irradiation in the area, however, may delay or prevent closure of the esophageal-cutaneous fistula.

McCarthy and colleagues (1987) studied experimentally the use of fibrin glue to prevent esophagogastric anastomotic leaks. In their study, the leak rate from a poorly accomplished anastomosis in dogs was markedly reduced. Whether or not the use of fibrin glue in standard clinical situations will be helpful in preventing leaks from normally constructed anastomoses remains to be seen.

Stricture of the anastomosis may occur spontaneously, most often after the use of a small EEA stapler, as reported by Wong (1987b), but also after hand-sutured anastomosis. Most strictures, however, occur after an anastomotic leak.

Delayed emptying of the gastric or colonic conduit may occur because of angulation, rotation, or too great a length of the conduit. The role of a pyloromyotomy in decreasing delay of emptying of the stomach is unresolved, but most surgeons recommend its use.

Other complications may occur. The most common are sepsis, renal failure, neurologic complications, wound infection, chylothorax, and postoperative hemorrhage. All of these may be observed after any major procedure within the chest.

Mortality

With immediate reconstruction of the esophagogastrointestinal continuity by one of the aforementioned techniques, the 30-day postoperative mortality rate has been reported to be as low as 1.4% but also as high as 20%. Many factors enter into the reported mortality rates, such as the population under study, the underlying disease, the use of preoperative radiation therapy or chemotherapy, technical factors of reconstruction, and so forth. Akiyama and associates (1981), in a series of over 210 patients, reported a mortality rate of only 1.4%. Wang and Chien (1983) and Wu and associates (1982) reported rates of 5.3% and 3 to 5%, respectively, from their experiences in China. In America, Shahian (1986), Keagy (1984), and Griffith (1980) and their colleagues reported mortality rates of 6.2%, 6.7%, and 11.3%, respectively. Launois and associates (1983) in France reported a mortality rate of 17.8%. A rate under 5% is ideal, but one under 10% is acceptable.

When death does occur, it is often the result of disease in some other organ system, such as myocardial infarct, cerebrovascular accident, or a pulmonary infection. When it is related directly to the operative procedure, it is usually caused by an anastomotic leak in the thorax with subsequent pleural infection or an infection beneath the diaphragm. Technical accidents during operation, such as catastrophic injury to the aorta with resulting fatal hemorrhage, occur rarely.

Radical En Bloc Resection of the Esophagus

Skinner (1983) described a radical en bloc excision of the esophagus for patients with carcinoma. His approach is a modification of that proposed by Logan (1963), who unfortunately experienced a 21% mortality rate for the procedure. The objective of the en bloc resection is to remove 10 cm of normal esophagus on either end of the tumor along with complete excision of the immediately adjacent tissues, as well as the vascular supply and the lymphatic drainage areas of the esophagus. When the tumor is situated 10 cm or more below the aortic arch, operative approach is through the left chest. When the tumor is less than 10 cm below the arch, the procedure is carried out through a right thoracotomy with or without an accompanying upper midline abdominal incision.

Technique

The en bloc resection through a left thoracotomy approach is done through a standard left posterolateral incision with resection of the sixth rib. The left hemidiaphragm is opened by the aforementioned circumferential incision from the sternum to the hiatus (Chapter 8). The stomach, spleen, and greater omentum are mobilized, and the left gastric vessels are divided, as is the coronary vein. The adjacent tissues, along with a cuff of diaphragm surrounding the hiatus, are freed with the stomach down to the anterior surface of the vertebral bodies and aorta. The dissection is carried upward, ligating the thoracic duct and lumbar veins as they join the azygos. The mediastinal pleura is incised, and the dissection continues posteriorly on the surface of the aorta and vertebral bodies, the vascular structures being ligated as necessary up to 10 cm above the level of the tumor. Anteriorly, the pulmonary ligament is divided and the pericardium entered at the level of the inferior pulmonary vein. A segment of pericardium and right mediastinal pleura, including the right pulmonary ligament, is freed with the specimen. All lymph nodes in the area are also removed. The stomach is divided 10 cm distal to the tumor on both the greater and lesser curvature. If the lesion is a squamous cell carcinoma of the esophagus, the esophagus is freed underneath the aortic arch and mobilized up into the neck, where it is divided through a separate neck incision. If the lesion is an adenocarcinoma, the esophagus generally can be divided at the level of the arch within the chest. Gastrointestinal continuity is re-established either with the remaining stomach or with an interposed loop of colon.

The en bloc excision through a right thoracotomy entails the same principles. The pleura, right intercostal vessels, azygos system, thoracic duct, right posterolateral pericardium, and adjacent left mediastinal pleura are excised en bloc with the esophagus and the contained tumor down to the esophageal hiatus. Proximally, the esophagus is mobilized up into the neck. The stomach is mobilized through the hiatus if possible; if not, a separate abdominal incision is made and either the stomach or the colon is mobilized so it can be brought up to the neck for anastomosis with the cervical esophagus, again, through a separate cervical incision.

Morbidity

Respiratory problems are common, and prolonged ventilatory support is frequently necessary. Early complications were noted by Skinner (1983) to occur in over 50% of the patients. These consisted mainly of persistent pleural effusion, chylothorax, aspiration pneumonia, arrhythmias, anastomotic leaks, and wound infections.

Mortality

In Skinner's series (1983) there was an 11% 30-day operative mortality, more commonly observed in patients with midesophageal lesions. The mortality rate did not vary significantly with age.

Results

Early results suggest a 19% 5-year actuarial survival. Although these results appear impressive, the operative procedure has gained little popularity in the surgical community.

Esophagectomy Without Thoracotomy

Orringer and Sloan (1978) advocated blunt esophagectomy without thoracotomy—through abdominal transhiatal and cervical approaches—which has been used extensively for excision and reconstruction of cervical esophageal lesions (see pages 420 to 421) for the management of both benign and malignant thoracic esophageal lesions. Belsey (1978), Parker (1978), and Postlethwait (1979b), among others, criticized this approach, especially for the management of esophageal carcinoma. Many are still convinced that this is not a good "cancer" operation. Nevertheless, it has been accepted as a suitable procedure, as evidenced by the reports of Szentpetery (1979), Garvin (1980), Pinotti (1981), Steiger (1981), Yonezawa (1984), and Stewart (1985) and their associates. Although Shahian and co-workers (1986) wrote that it may be applicable for early lesions, they did not think it should be used for advanced stage III carcinoma of the esophagus. Its acceptance for management for extensive benign disease, however, has been almost universal. Orringer (1985) summarized his experience in 65 patients with benign disease in whom this procedure was used with good success.

Technique of Transhiatal Esophagectomy

The patient is placed in the supine position with the head turned to the right or left, depending on the preference of the operator, for exposing the cervical esophagus. Exposure on the left reduces the chance of injury to the recurrent nerves. The abdomen is opened through an upper midline incision. The stomach is mobilized and the right gastric and right gastroepiploic arteries and the gastroepiploic arcade are preserved. The short gastric vessels are individually ligated. The left gastric artery and vein are ligated at their origin. The entire anastomotic arcade along the lesser curvature of the stomach can be preserved, but many surgeons, such as Akiyama (1981, 1984) and Finley (1985) and their associates, advocate resection of most of this arcade along with the adjacent portion of the lesser curve of the stomach to ensure greater cleaning of the lymph node-bearing area along the distribution of the left gastric vessels in all patients with carcinoma. Essentially, this leaves a gastric tube including the fundus for transposition into the neck. The excision of the lesser curve is carried out with a stapling device. The cut margins can be oversewn with interrupted nonabsorbable sutures. A Kocher maneuver is used to mobilize the duodenum, and a pyloromyotomy or pyloroplasty is performed. The intra-abdominal esophagus is mobilized, and a Penrose drain is passed around the esophagogastric junction to provide traction. A mechanical "upper hand" retractor facilitates exposure during the dissection of the proximal stomach and esophagus. The esophageal hiatus is enlarged circumferentially by blunt stretching and can be incised laterally on the left side to allow insertion of the surgeon's entire hand into the mediastinum. Most esophageal vessels in the distal half of the esophagus can be ligated from the abdomen as necessary.

After the abdominal procedure is under way, the cervical dissection is begun. An incision is made along the interior border of either the right or left sternocleidomastoid muscle, as preferred. The esophagus is identified and freed posteriorly. This maneuver is facilitated by preoperative placement of an indwelling esophageal tube. The tracheoesophageal groove is developed, and the esophagus is encircled with a Penrose drain. Avoid injuring or traumatizing the recurrent laryngeal nerves. Exposure is obtained with retraction of the thyroid gland and trachea medially with finger and gauze, without the use of metal or self-retaining retractors, to prevent injury to the recurrent laryngeal nerve. The upper thoracic esophagus is exposed and freed under direct vision.

The upper third of the esophagus is mobilized from above—transcervically—and the middle and distal thirds from below—transabdominally—(Fig. 38–4). The posterior aspect of the esophagus is freed by finger dissection closely applied to the esophagus; this step is usually without problems because the plane is avascular. Next, the

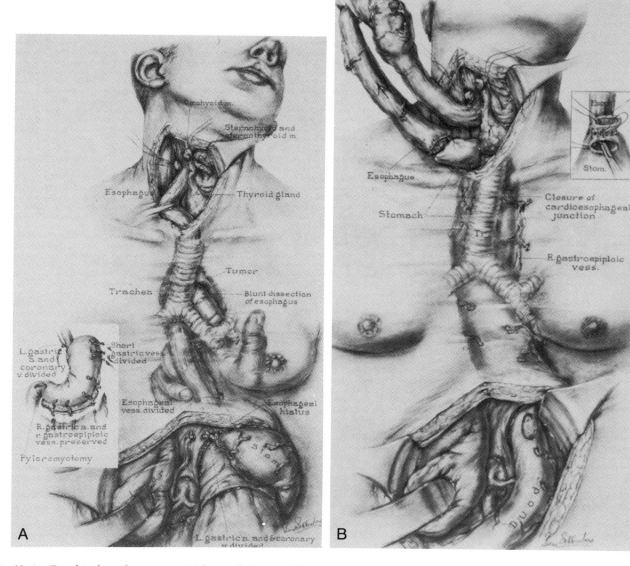

Fig. 38–4. Transhiatal esophagectomy. *A*, Blunt mobilization of thoracic esophagus from below. Insert shows gastric mobilization. *B*, Thoracic esophagus extracted through the neck incision and the stomach brought through the posterior mediastinum so that the highest point of the fundus lies in the neck. Insert shows details of a two-layer anastomosis. (Reproduced with permission of Stewart, J.R., et al.: Ann. Thorac. Surg. *40*:343, 1985.)

lateral attachments are pushed away from the esophagus, likewise by blunt finger dissection. Once the posterior and lateral aspects of the esophagus are free, the blunt dissection is continued around to the anterior surface. Injury of the main stem bronchi or the posterior tracheal membrane must be avoided. If the tumor extends through the esophageal wall, the tumor mass is fractured off the surrounding tissues. All these maneuvers are facilitated by the surgeon's simultaneously dissecting the esophagus from above with one hand and from below through the hiatus with the other. During the intrathoracic esophageal dissection, while the surgeon's entire hand is in the posterior mediastinum, the vena cava may be compressed; thus impeding venous return and caus-

ing poor cardiac output. Continuous monitoring of blood pressure is mandatory.

Once completely mobilized, the esophagus can be transected at the esophagogastric junction and oversewn securely, or the esophagus can be extracted into the neck incision, with the stomach being guided into the neck at the same time. The gastroesophageal junction can then be divided. If the gastroesophageal junction is divided in the abdomen, and if a GIA stapler is used, both staple lines should be oversewn. The cut end of the esophagus can be tacked to the fundus or to a large, rubber Penrose drain, which is then pulled through the posterior mediastinum into the neck, where the esophagus is extracted. When the drain has been used, the free end is tacked to the fundus of the stomach. Either one of these two maneuvers allows the stomach to be guided, not pulled, into the posterior mediastinum, using the esophagus or the Penrose drain as a traction guide. As the intrathoracic esophagus—with the tumor mass—is advanced out the cervical incision, the stomach is carefully advanced through the posterior mediastinum with a combination of manual guidance from below and gentle traction from above. In this fashion, the stomach, with proper axial alignment, is delivered through the posterior thoracic inlet into the neck under minimal tension. The stomach can be anchored posteriorly to the anterior longitudinal spinal ligament. The esophagogastrostomy is performed, usually by a two-layer, interrupted anastomosis. An indwelling nasogastric tube is placed through the anastomosis. A soft Penrose rubber drain is placed in the cervical incision and the incision is closed. A feeding jejunostomy is inserted before closure of the abdominal incision. If the stomach is unavailable for use, a loop of colon can be substituted to re-establish the pharyngogastric continuity (Chapter 40).

Morbidity

The complications following a transhiatal esophagectomy performed by those with experience with the procedure appear to be no greater than those occurring after a transthoracic esophagectomy. Stewart and associates (1985) reported an overall morbidity rate of 52%. Orringer and Orringer (1983) reported that in 143 operations— 100 for malignant disease processes and 43 for benign disease—the major complications were incidental splenectomy in 10%, pneumothorax in 51%, temporary recurrent nerve paresis in 37%, chylous fistulas in 4%, and intraoperative tracheal injury in 1.3%. Injury to the recurrent nerve can be reduced markedly by avoiding retraction of the thyroid and trachea with metal retractors in the neck. Shahian and colleagues (1986) report only a 3.6% incidence of this event. Intraoperative hemorrhage is infrequent and only rarely is thoracotomy required to control excessive bleeding. Respiratory problems are common, as seen with any esophageal resection. Likewise, anastomotic leak occurs in a variable number of patients. Orringer and Orringer (1983) reported a rate of 12%, Stewart and associates (1985) a leak rate of 13%, and Shahian and colleagues (1986) one of 15%. In 1986, Orringer reported a rate of only 3%.

Mortality

Like the morbidity rate, the mortality rate also varies. Rates as high as 13%, reported by Shahian and associates (1986), to as low as 4% and 2%, noted by Stewart (1985) and Finley (1985) and colleagues, respectively, have been recorded. In 125 patients with esophageal carcinoma, Orringer (1986) reported a 5% hospital mortality rate. These figures suggest that the procedure may be accomplished as safely as a transthoracic excision of the esophagus.

Functional Results

Late anastomotic stricture may occur. It usually can be managed readily with dilatation. Gastric emptying is generally satisfactory, although postoperative regurgitation may be seen in one fifth of the patients. Transient postvagotomy diarrhea also may occur.

DISTAL ESOPHAGECTOMY

Distal esophagectomy with proximal gastrectomy and esophagogastrostomy is an alternative method of treating squamous cell carcinoma of the lower third and at the level of the esophagogastric junction, adenocarcinoma of the proximal portion of the stomach that has infiltrated the distal esophagus, and some short benign strictures that cannot be dilated during an antireflux procedure (Chapter 82). In the patient with tumor, the major question to be considered is whether an adequate margin can be obtained proximal to the tumor and the anastomosis completed below the arch of the aorta without tension.

Operative Approach

The choices are two: a left posterolateral thoracotomy or a combined thoracoabdominal incision. The former has the advantages of rapid entry and closure plus exposure that is adequate but may be somewhat limited. This approach is usually satisfactory for squamous cell carcinoma and nearly always for stricture. The combined incision is more time-consuming and exposes the patient to risks such as costal chondritis. It provides, however, excellent exposure, particularly for lymph node dissection. The combined incision is preferred for adenocarcinoma of the cardia.

Technique

In the transthoracic approach, the patient is placed in the right lateral decubitus position. A left posterolateral thoracotomy is performed with resection of the seventh rib, the pulmonary ligament is divided, and the left lung is retracted anteriorly. The esophagus is identified above the tumor and freed from the surrounding tissues by blunt dissection. A rubber Penrose tape is placed about the esophagus. If a margin of normal esophagus is present below the lesion and above the diaphragm, a similar maneuver is carried out. Once the tissue planes have been established in normal areas, sharp dissection is carried to and then around the carcinoma. The pleura on the right is frequently opened. Dissection from the aorta may be difficult, and the esophageal arteries arising directly from the aorta must be secured, preferably by suture ligaments. The dissection cephalad should extend to near the arch of the aorta. Patients with a benign stricture may have marked panmural esophagitis with a severe, vascular connective tissue reaction around the esophagus requiring a prolonged, meticulous dissection.

The abdomen is entered by incising the phrenoesophageal ligament. The diaphragm is opened from the hiatus posteriorly to the chest wall. The incision is then carried forward as a circumferential incision at the periphery of the left hemidiaphragm 2 to 3 cm away from its attachment to the chest wall. The crural branch of the left phrenic nerve must be divided, but this is of little or no consequence relative to diaphragmatic function. The left hemidiaphragm is lifted like a trap door and provides excellent exposure to the left upper abdomen. At times, the performance of a Kocher maneuver and a pyloromyotomy may be difficult, but these steps are not always essential. The proximal portion of the stomach, the spleen, and at times the tail of the pancreas are mobilized. The left gastric and short gastric vessels are divided, and dissection is carried along the greater curvature for the necessary distance. All regional nodes, as well as the greater omentum—when the tumor is of gastric origin—are resected en bloc with the proximal portion of the stomach. The stomach is divided obliquely to ensure a greater length of the greater curve, and the distal stump is closed with two layers of sutures. A Kocher maneuver and pyloroplasty or myotomy complete the abdominal phase.

Additional proximal mobilization of the esophagus is carried out by division of its segmental vascular supply to about or above the level of the left main stem bronchus. The remaining portion of the stomach is brought into the chest, and a new opening in the anterior wall of the stomach is made for the esophagogastrostomy (Fig. 38–5). With the specimen and esophagus elevated superiorly, the posterior row of interrupted nonabsorbable sutures is placed between the esophagus and stomach about 2 cm above the proposed line of division of the esophagus and an equal distance above the opening in the stomach. The posterior wall of the esophagus is divided and the inner layer of interrupted, synthetic, absorbable sutures placed and tied, with attention to good apposition of the mucosa. The anterior wall of the esophagus is divided, the specimen removed, and the two anterior rows of sutures completed as an inkwell anastomosis. The anastomosis between the proximal cut end of the esophagus and remaining stomach also can be readily accomplished with the use of the EEA stapler (Fig. 38–3B). Many believe this affords an anastomosis that is less likely to leak. A frozen section examination of the proximal cut end should be obtained to ensure absence of submucosal lymphatic extension of the tumor at this site. The stomach should lie without tension. Anchoring sutures between the stomach wall and pleura or mediastinal tissues are placed to ensure the absence of tension on the anastomosis. If possible, the anastomosis should be inverted into the stomach by a modified antireflux maneuver to prevent regurgitation of gastric contents into the proximal esophagus. The diaphragmatic hiatus is then closed about the stomach with interrupted 2–0 silk sutures. The incision in the diaphragm is closed with interrupted sutures of No. 0 silk sutures. Drainage of the chest is provided and the chest incision is closed in the normal fashion.

In the thoracoabdominal approach, the patient is positioned with the left side elevated between 45° and 60°. A midline abdominal incision, an oblique incision on the left beginning halfway between xiphoid and umbilicus, or an upper transverse incision can be used. The abdomen is explored, and if the carcinoma appears to be resectable, the incision is extended over the seventh or eighth rib, to at least the posterior axillary line. The costal

arch is divided, the appropriate interspace opened, and the diaphragm incised to the hiatus. The diaphragmatic incision is extended backward and medially between the pericardial attachment of the diaphragm and the entrance of the left phrenic nerve into the left hemidiaphragm to the apex of the esophageal hiatus. The aforementioned circumferential diaphragmatic incision can be used as an alternative approach. The thoracic portion of the dissection is similar to that described, with one exception. With an adenocarcinoma of the cardia or with a squamous cell carcinoma that has extended to or through the hiatus, a circumferential cuff of diaphragm should be excised to remain with the specimen.

In the abdomen, the spleen, with the greater curvature of the stomach, is elevated and retracted to the right. The greater omentum is separated from the colon. The dissection is performed in a posterior plane, along the superior border of the pancreas to the celiac axis. The splenic vessels are secured at a convenient point; the left gastric artery at the celiac axis. This practice is for removal of the most frequently involved lymph nodes and, if necessary, a portion of the pancreas.

The stomach is then divided as described, but with removal of more of the fundus. A Kocher maneuver usually is done to allow the gastric remnant to extend high enough for the anastomosis. A pyloroplasty or pyloromyotomy is performed. The esophagogastric anastomosis is the same as previously described. Meticulous closure of the diaphragm and suturing of the appropriate margins to the stomach are done routinely (Fig. 38–5C). Chest drainage tubes are placed and the thoracoabdominal incision closed. Several centimeters of the costal arch should be resected to achieve a more satisfactory closure of the incision.

Morbidity

The morbidity rates after resection of the distal esophagus, proximal gastrectomy, esophagogastrostomy vary. The specific major complications are leak of the esophagogastric anastomosis, infradiaphragmatic infection, costochondritis—if a thoracoabdominal incision has been used, and postoperative dehiscence of the diaphragmatic incision with herniation of abdominal contents into the left pleural space. The incidence of each of these complications is related more to poor operative technique than to the poor general condition of most of these patients. Late complications related to regurgitation of gastric juice into the esophagus, stricture of the anastomosis, and the dumping syndrome may occur.

Mortality

The 30-day postoperative mortality rate in the past has been related most specifically to anastomotic leak with development of infection in the pleural or subphrenic space and occasionally to unrecognized evisceration of the abdominal contents into the chest because of breakdown of the diaphragmatic closure. Other fatalities, however, do occur as the result of other systemic complications, particularly pulmonary. The mortality rates reported from the various centers range between 5 and

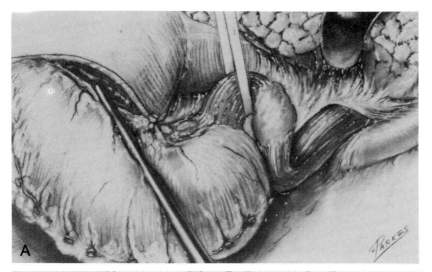

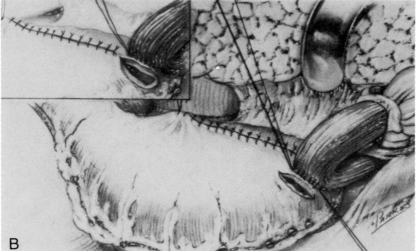

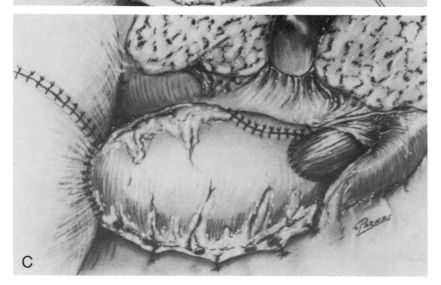

Fig. 38–5. Left transthoracic resection of tumor in lower third of the thoracic esophagus. *A,* Lower portion of the esophagus and upper third of the stomach mobilized with division of left gastric and short gastric vessels. *B,* Lower curvature has been closed and anastomosis below the arch of the aorta has been started. *C,* Completion of the anastomosis and closure of the diaphragm about the stomach. (Reproduced with permission of Postlethwait, R.W.: Surgery of the Esophagus, 2nd ed. New York, Appleton-Century-Crofts, 1986.)

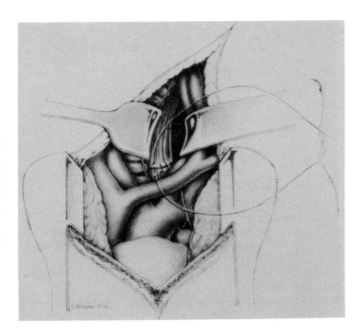

Fig. 38–6. Completion of segmental resection of upper esophagus through a transsternal approach. (Reproduced from Orringer, M.B.: J. Thorac. Cardiovasc. Surg. 87:124, 1984.)

10%. These rates may be improved by the prevention and management of anastomotic leaks, and by excellent pre- and postoperative care. Ellis and colleagues (1983) reported a mortality rate of less than 3% with this procedure.

SEGMENTAL RESECTION

Segmental resection of the esophagus is rarely carried out. It is difficult to mobilize a sufficient length of the esophagus without jeopardizing the blood supply essential to anastomotic healing. Short strictures, less than 5 cm long, have been resected in such a manner, and Davidson (1967) used this limited operation to resect small epidermoid carcinomas with fair results. The general application of such a technique, however, is severely restricted.

Orringer (1984) reported the use of a partial median sternotomy approach (Fig. 38–1) to the superior mediastinal esophagus in three patients for segmental resections of short—1.5 to 2 cm—benign strictures of the esophagus located 3 to 4 cm above the level of the tracheal carina in an otherwise normal esophagus. Primary end-to-end anastomosis was accomplished in all three with good results (Fig. 38–6).

REFERENCES

Akiyama, H.: Surgery for carcinoma of the esophagus. Curr. Probl. Surg. 17:53, 1980.

Akiyama, H., et al.: Use of the stomach as an esophageal substitute. Ann. Surg. 188:606, 1978.

Akiyama, H., et al.: Principles of surgical treatment for carcinoma of the esophagus. Ann. Surg. 194:436, 1981.

Akiyama, H., et al.: Development of surgery for carcinoma of the esophagus Am. J. Surg. 147:9, 1984.

Anderson, K.D.: Colon replacement of the esophagus. Editorial. Ann. Thorac. Surg. 36:622, 1983.

Anderson, K.D., and Randolph, J.G.: The gastric tube for esophageal replacement in children. J. Thorac. Cardiovasc. Surg. 66:333, 1973.

Bains, M.S., and Spriro, R.H.: Pharyngolaryngectomy, total extrathoracic esophagectomy and agastric transposition. Surg. Gynecol. Obstet. 139:693, 1979.

Belsey, R.: Discussion of Orringer, M.B., and Sloan, H.E.: Esophagectomy without thoracotomy. J. Thorac. Cardiovasc. Surg. 76:643, 1978.

Cauchoix, J., and Binet, J.P.: Anterior segmental approaches to the spine. Ann. R. Coll. Surg. Engl. 21:237, 1957.

Davidson, J.S.: Resection of squamous cell carcinoma of the esophagus with end-to-end oesophageal anastomosis. Br. J. Surg. 54:63, 1967.

Ellis, F.H., Jr.: Esophagogastrectomy for carcinoma: technical considerations based on anatomic location of lesion. Surg. Clin. North Am. 60:265, 1980.

Ellis, F.H., Jr., Gibb, S.P., and Watkins, E.J.: Esophagogastrectomy: a safe, widely applicable and expeditious form of palliation for patients with carcinoma of the esophagus. Ann. Surg. 198:531, 1983.

Finley, R.J., Grace, M., and Duff, J.H.: Esophagogastrectomy without thoracotomy for carcinoma of the cardia and lower part of the esophagus. Surg. Gynecol. Obstet. 160:49, 1985.

Flynn, M.B., and Acland, R.D.: Free intestinal autographs for reconstruction following pharyngolaryngoesophagectomy. Surg. Gynecol. Obstet. 149:858, 1979.

Garvin, P.J., and Kaminski, D.L.: Extrathoracic esophagectomy in the treatment of esophageal cancer. Am. J. Surg. 140:772, 1980.

Gavriliu, D.: Etat actuel du procédé de reconstruction de l'oesphage par tube gastrique. Ann. Clin. 19:219, 1965.

Gavriliu, D.: Aspects of esophageal surgery. Curr. Probl. Surg. 121:1, 1975.

Griffith, J.L., and Davis, T.: A twenty-year experience with surgical management of carcinoma of the esophagus and gastric cardia. J. Thorac. Cardiovasc. Surg. 79:447, 1980.

Harrison, D.F.N.: Surgical management of cancer of the hypopharynx and cervical esophagus. Br. J. Surg. 56:95, 1969.

Heimlich, H.J.: Reversed gastric tube (RGT) esophagoplasty for failure of colon, jejunum, and prosthetic interpositions. Ann. Surg. 182:154, 1975.

Hester, T.R., and Jurkiewicz, M.J.: Free intestinal grafts for reconstruction of pharynx and esophagus. Presented at 71st Annual Clinical Congress, American College of Surgeons, Chicago, Oct. 13, 1985.

Huang, G.J, and Wu, Y.K.: Operative technique for carcinoma of the esophagus. In Carcinoma of the Esophagus and Gastric Cardia. Edited by G.J. Huang and Y.K. Wu. Berlin, Springer-Verlag, 1984.

Huang, G.J., and Zhang, W.: Diagnosis and management of chylothorax following resection of carcinoma of the esophagus. Clin. J. Surg. 13:130, 1965. Quoted by Guo, J.H., and Wu, Y.K. (Eds): Carcinoma of the Esophagus and Gastric Cardia. Berlin, Springer-Verlag, 1984.

Jurkiewicz, M.J.: Reconstructive surgery of the cervical esophagus. J. Thorac. Cardiovasc. Surg. 88:893, 1984.

Kasai, M., and Nishihira, T.: Reconstruction using pedicled jejunal segments after reconstruction for carcinoma of the cervical esophagus. Surg. Gynecol. Obstet. 163:145, 1986.

Keagy, B.A., et al.: Esophagectomy as palliative treatment for esophageal carcinoma: results obtained in the setting of a thoracic surgery residency program. Ann. Thorac. Surg. 38:611, 1984.

Lam, K.H., et al.: Pharyngogastric anastomosis following pharyngolaryngoesophagectomy: analysis of 157 cases. World. J. Surg. 5:509, 1981.

Launois, B., Paul, J.L., and Lygidarkis, N.J.: Result of the surgical treatment of carcinoma of the esophagus. Surg. Gynecol. Obstet. 156:753, 1983.

Lewis, I.: The surgical treatment of carcinoma of the esophagus with special reference to a new operation for growths of the middle third. Br. J. Surg. *34*:18, 1946.

Logan, A.: The surgical treatment of carcinoma of the esophagus and cardia. J. Thorac. Cardiovasc. Surg. *46*:150, 1963.

McCarthy, P.M., et al.: Esophagogastric anastomoses: the value of fibrin glue in preventing leakage. J. Thorac. Cardiovasc. Surg. *93*:234, 1987.

McKeown, K.C.: Total three-stage oesophagectomy for cancer of the oesophagus. Br. J. Surg. *63*:259, 1976.

Ngan, S.Y.K., and Wong, J.: Lengths of different routes for esophageal replacement. J. Thorac. Cardiovasc. Surg. *91*:790, 1986.

Ong, B.B., et al.: Resection for carcinoma of the superior mediastinal segment of the esophagus. World. J. Surg. *2*:497, 1978.

Orringer, M.B.: Partial median sternotomy: Anterior approach to the upper thoracic esophagus. J. Thorac. Cardiovasc. Surg. *87*:124, 1984.

Orringer, M.B.: Transhiatal esophagectomy for benign disease. J. Thorac. Cardiovasc. Surg. *90*:649, 1985.

Orringer, M.B.: Discussion of Shakeran, O.M., et al.: Transthoracic versus extrathoracic esophagectomy: mortality, morbidity, and long-term survival. Ann. Thorac. Surg. *41*:237, 1986.

Orringer, M.B., and Orringer, J.S.: Esophagectomy without thoracotomy: a dangerous operation? J. Thorac. Cardiovasc. Surg. *85*:72, 1983.

Orringer, M.B., and Sloan, H.E.: Esophagectomy without thoracotomy. J. Thorac. Cardiovasc. Surg. *76*:643, 1978.

Parker, E.F.: Discussion of Orringer, M.B., and Sloan, H.E.: Esophagectomy without thoracotomy. J. Thorac. Cardiovasc. Surg. *76*:643, 1978.

Peters, C.R, McKee, D.M., and Berry, B.E.: Pharyngoesophageal reconstruction with revascularized jejunal transplants. Am. J. Surg. *121*:675, 1971.

Pinotti, H.W., et al.: Esophagectomy without thoracotomy. Surg. Gynecol. Obstet. *152*:344, 1981.

Postlethwait, R.W.: Technique for isoperistaltic gastric tube for esophageal bypass. Ann. Surg. *163*:395, 1979.

Postlethwait, R.W.: Esophagectomy without thoracotomy. Ann. Thorac. Surg. *27*:395, 1979.

Postlethwait, R.W.: Carcinoma of the thoracic esophagus. Surg. Clin North Am. *63*:933, 1983.

Scanlon, E.F., et al.: The treatment of carcinoma of the esophagus. Q. Bull. Northwest. Univ. Med. Sch. *30*:144, 1956.

Scanlon, E.F., and Staley, C.F.: Reconstruction of the cervical esophagus by use of colon transplants. Surg. Clin. North Am. *43*:3, 1963.

Shahian, D.M., et al.: Transthoracic versus extrathoracic esophagectomy: mortality, morbidity, and long-term survival. Ann. Thorac. Surg. *41*:237, 1986.

Skinner, D.B.: En bloc resection for neoplasms of the esophagus and cardia. J. Thorac. Cardiovasc. Surg. *85*:59, 1983.

Spiro, R.H., et al.: Gastric transposition in head and neck surgery. Am. J. Surg. *146*:483, 1983.

Steiger, Z., and Wilson, R.: Comparison of the results of esophagectomy with and without a thoracotomy. Surg. Gynecol. Obstet. *153*:653, 1981.

Stewart, J.R., et al.: Transhiatal (blunt) esophagectomy for malignant and benign esophageal disease: clinical experience and technique. Ann. Thorac. Surg. *40*:343, 1985.

Sweet, R.H.: Thoracic Surgery, 2nd ed. Philadelphia, W.B. Saunders Co., 1954.

Szentpetery, W., Wolfgang, T., and Lower, R.: Pull-through esophagectomy without thoracotomy for esophageal carcinoma. Ann. Thorac. Surg. *27*:399, 1979.

Ujiki, G.T., et al.: Mortality and morbidity of gastric 'pull-up' for replacement of the pharyngoesophagus. Arch. Surg. *122*:644, 1987.

Waddell, W.R., and Scannell, J.G.: Anterior approach to carcinoma of the superior mediastinal and cervical segments of the esophagus. J. Thorac. Surg. *33*:663, 1957.

Wang, P.Y., and Chien, K.Y.: Surgical treatment of carcinoma of the esophagus and cardia among the Chinese. Ann. Thorac. Surg. *35*:143, 1983.

Wong, J.: Techniques of esophageal replacement. Presented at General Thoracic Surgery Course, Faculty of Medicine, University of Toronto, May 29, 1986.

Wong, J.: Personal Communication, 1986.

Wong, J.: Esophageal resection for cancer. The rationale of current practice. Am. J. Surg. *153*:18, 1987a.

Wong, J.: Stapled esophagogastric anastomosis in the apex of the right chest after subtotal esophagectomy for carcinoma. Surg. Gynecol. Obstet. *164*:569, 1987b.

Wong, J., et al.: Surgical treatment of carcinoma of the upper third of the esophagus. *In* Medical and Surgical Problems of the Esophagus. Serono Symposia, Vol. 43, p. 324. Edited by S. Stepa, R.H.R. Belsey, and A. Moraldi. New York, Academic Press, 1981.

Wookey, H.: The surgical treatment of carcinoma of the hypopharynx and the oesophagus. Br. J. Surg. *35*:249, 1948.

Wu, W.K., et al.: Progress in the study and surgical treatment of cancer of the esophagus in China, 1940–1980. J. Thorac. Cardiovasc. Surg. *84*:325, 1982.

Xu, L.T., et al.: Surgical treatment of carcinoma of the esophagus and cardiac portion of the stomach in 850 patients. Ann. Thorac. Surg. *35*:542, 1983.

Yonezawa, T., et al.: Resection of cancer of the thoracic esophagus without thoracotomy. J. Thorac. Cardiovasc. Surg. *88*:146, 1984.

CHAPTER 39

REPLACEMENT OF THE ESOPHAGUS WITH THE STOMACH

Guo Jun Huang

The stomach is the most commonly adopted substitute for the resected esophagus, either for malignant or benign diseases. In my institution, where 1874 patients with carcinoma of the esophagus were treated surgically from 1958 through 1982, the stomach was used to replace the resected esophagus in 98.2% of the cases. Compared with other organs used for reconstruction of the resected esophagus, the stomach has the most ample and reliable blood supply, facilitating anastomosis with the esophagus at any level in the thorax or the neck, or even with the hypopharynx. The surgical procedure is simple and needs only one anastomosis, which saves time. In addition, there is no need for special preoperative preparation of the stomach besides an overnight fast. The distal remnant of the stomach is also frequently used to restore the continuity of the gastrointestinal tract after partial esophagogastrectomy for upper gastric or esophagogastric junctional diseases.

The drawbacks of using the stomach for reconstruction of the esophagus are its atonia and the dilatation and occupation of space involved when the intrapleural route of the transplantation is used. Dilatation of the intrapleural stomach is more marked in the early postoperative period and when oral intake is restarted, and may thus give rise to respiratory embarrassment. Impairment in function of the stomach after transplantation is often the chief cause of digestive and nutritional disorders. Furthermore, because the stomach is rich in intramural lymphatics that may be sites of metastases of esophageal carcinoma, its use as a substitute in such cases could result in incomplete eradication of cancer. Although postoperative gastric reflux can be prevented in most cases by an antireflux procedure added to the esophagogastric anastomosis, it remains a problem when the stomach is used as a substitute for total or subtotal esophagectomy with a high cervical esophagogastrostomy or hypopharyngogastrostromy.

When the stomach is used to replace the esophagus, reconstruction is frequently performed through the convenient intrapleural route, but can also be done through the posterior mediastinal route, i.e., the bed of the resected esophagus, with esophagogastric anastomosis above the aortic arch or in the neck. In cervical anastomosis, the intrapleural route is also the most commonly employed, but the posterior mediastinal and the retrosternal routes can also be used. The posterior mediastinal route involves the shortest distance for reconstruction and the most natural alignment with the remaining esophagus.

The use of a reversed gastric tube for reconstruction of the esophagus was strongly advocated and indeed practiced by Gavriliu (1975) and by Heimlich (1955, 1975). The tube consists of the greater curvature of the stomach with its base at the fundus, using the left gastroepiploic vessels for blood supply. The tube is turned in an antiperistaltic direction for anastomosis with the esophagus. An isoperistaltic gastric tube can also be made, using the right gastroepiploic vessels for blood supply (Fig. 39–1).

The advantage of using a gastric tube to replace the esophagus is that a considerable part of the stomach remains in situ, part of the gastric function thus being preserved. Even with the help of a stapler, however, the tedious and time-consuming tailoring and suturing, the considerable blood loss involved in fashioning the tube, and the higher risk of postoperative leakage from either the anastomotic or suture lines preclude routine use.

MOBILIZATION OF THE STOMACH

Lesions located at the middle and lower segments of the esophagus can usually be resected through a left thoracotomy approach. Except for resecting lesions at the lower end of the esophagus or at the esophagogastric junction, for which the incision can be made along the seventh rib, a posterolateral thoracotomy is made through the sixth interspace or through the sixth rib bed, with the patient in a right lateral position. The stomach can be mobilized through diaphragmatic incision, which

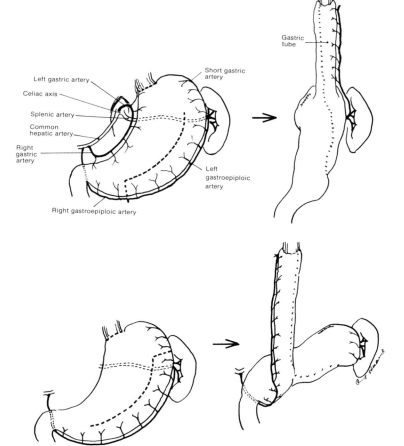

Fig. 39–1. Blood supply to the stomach and tailoring of a reverse gastric tube (above) and an isoperistaltic gastric tube (below), heavy broken lines indicating sites of division.

is made between the left lobe of the liver and the spleen, from the hiatus outward and anteriorly, making the medial flap of the incised diaphragm as wide as possible, with intact innervation by the phrenic nerve. A circumferential incision of the diaphragm can sometimes be used for maximal conservation of innervation, and therefore motor function, of the hemidiaphragm. The hiatus must not be opened until resection of the esophagus has been decided on. This approach provides excellent exposure to the lower thoracic esophagus, the esophagogastric junction, and the left upper abdominal cavity, facilitating mobilization of the stomach to replace the esophagus. If a wider exposure is needed, the thoracotomy incision can easily be extended across the costal arch, which is then divided, to form a combined thoracoabdominal incision.

If a right posterolateral thoracotomy approach is used for lesions of the esophagus behind or above the arch of the aorta, the stomach is usually mobilized through a separate upper midline or transverse abdominal incision. This necessitates repositioning the patient during the operation. The exposure of the fundus of the stomach through an abdominal incision, however, be it vertical oblique, or transverse, is usually not adequate, particularly in obese patients.

After intra-abdominal exploration, the stomach is mo-bilized by dividing the greater omentum and the short gastric vessels at a short distance from the greater curvature, with care to preserve the right gastroepiploic vessels, which together with the right gastric vessels constitute the sole blood supply to the mobilized stomach. The extent of mobilization of the greater curvature depends on the size of the stomach and the level of anastomosis. In general, it should reach the pyloric antrum, to free a sufficient length of the stomach for transplantation and release the connection between the stomach and the transverse colon, which otherwise would be under traction after the stomach is brought up to the chest. All divided vessels along the cut edges of the greater omentum and the gastrosplenic ligament should be securely ligated.

The esophagogastric junction is freed from the hiatus, and the lesser omentum and the gastrohepatic ligament are divided, the latter possibly containing a small artery that should be ligated with it. The next step is the ligation of the left gastric artery, which may be done by securing its major branches close to the stomach in cases of benign disease. In cases of malignant disease, all accessible celiac lymph nodes must be dissected and the left gastric vessels are freed to their proximal parts, where they are divided close to their origin between clamps and securely ligated.

Management of the left gastric vessels is one of the important points in resection of carcinoma of the esophagus and gastric cardia. Adequate exposure and careful manipulation are essential in the prevention of accidental bleeding from the vessels. The gastrohepatic ligament and the lesser omentum must be divided before division of the left gastric vessels, so that any bleeding from the vascular stump can be handled more easily, with the stomach retracted away frm the operative field.

Bleeding from the left gastric artery may occur in mobilization of the stomach for resection of carcinoma of the esophagus or gastric cardia, during dissection of enlarged metastatic lymph nodes, or as a result of crushing by clamps or slipping of ligatures, giving rise to copious hemorrhage. In managing such an accident, good exposure of the celiac region is crucial and must be provided by the assistant. Attempts to control the bleeding by massive tissue clamping or massive gauze packing must be avoided. Finger pressure is applied by the surgeon to the site of bleeding and the extravasated blood is swiftly removed by suction. In cases of severe bleeding, the lower part of the thoracic descending aorta can be temporarily occluded between the fingers of an assistant. When the site of bleeding has been located, it is gently and accurately grasped with two or three Allis forceps, applied one after the other, and then carefully transfixed.

In carcinoma of the lower esophagus, it is advisable also to resect part of the cardiac portion of the stomach to extirpate any intramural tumor infiltration and metastatic paracardiac lymph nodes. This can readily be done with a stapler.

In carcinoma of the midthoracic esophagus or of higher sites, the distal esophagus can be divided at the cardiac junction. The paracardiac adipose tissue, with its possibly metastatic lymph nodes, should be routinely removed along with the esophagus. The divided end of the esophagus is ligated with heavy silk and covered with a rubber sheath to avoid contamination. The cut end of the gastric cardia can be closed with two or three mattress sutures, which are then oversewn with Lembert sutures or a purse-string suture.

In bringing up the mobilized stomach to the supra-aortic or the cervical region for anastomosis, avoid a 360° rotation of the transplant, which may be concealed in the subdiaphragmatic region and which results in postoperative gastric obstruction. Likewise, in performing esophagogastrostomy, avoid twisting the esophageal stump, as a rotation of over 90° is likely to cause severe dysphagia.

Intrathoracic esophagogastrostomy is most frequently done at the supra-aortic region, the stomach being transplanted either intrapleurally or through the posterior mediastinal route, the latter being the rule when right thoracotomy approach is used. Intrapleural transplantation of the stomach has the advantage of affording easy anastomosis with the esophagus, but has the disadvantage of filling part of the space normally occupied by the lung, thus diminishing its ventilatory function.

The stomach can be transplanted through the posterior mediastinal route created by resection of the esophagus and anastomosed in the chest or in the cervical region with the remaining esophagus. This route has the advantages of not depriving the lung of any marked space and of having good alignment with the esophagus. A major shortcoming, however, is the inconvenience in performing the intrathoracic anastomosis when a left thoracotomy approach is used, especially in an elderly patient with an enlarged and elongated aortic arch. Furthermore, a large stomach with its plication at the anastomotic site may compress the membranous part of the trachea, possibly causing dyspnea. When the posterior mediastinal pleura is opened through the right thoracotomy approach, the greater curvature of the transplanted stomach, which is naturally facing the left side and more expansible than the lesser curvature, may be rotated to the right pleural cavity as a result of gastric distention or increased intrapleural negative pressure, or both, causing a 180° twisting at both the upper and lower ends of the transplanted intrathoracic stomach, with resulting mechanical obstruction. This can be prevented, however, by fixing the transplanted stomach to the mediastinal pleura with a few stitches.

After completion of the esophagogastrostomy or before closure of the thoracotomy incision, the diaphragm is closed around the gastric transplant with interrupted sutures spaced so as to admit only the fingertip between them. Any redundant part of the intrathoracic transplant is reduced into the abdomen to avoid or minimize postoperative suprahiatal gastric retention.

When the anastomosis is done in the neck, a cigarette drain or rubber tissue drain is inserted through a stab wound posterior to the neck incision, to be removed 48 hours later. Take precautions to keep air from entering the pleural cavity through the drainage wound.

CHOICE OF ANASTOMOTIC SITE

In selecting the site for anastomosis, a number of factors should be considered, such as malignant or benign nature of the lesion, completeness of resection in case of cancer, technical feasibility, and operative risk.

A high infra-aortic anastomosis is more difficult technically than a supra-aortic one when using the left thoracotomy approach, and an anastomosis done at the apex of either pleural cavity is not as easy as one performed in the neck. Leakage from an intrathoracic anastomosis is life-threatening, whereas a leak from a cervical anastomosis, as a rule, heals spontaneously after drainage.

In general, with the exception of benign lesions that justify local resection of the esophagus, reconstruction after resection of the esophagus for cancer must be by either supra-aortic—high intrathoracic—or cervical anastomosis, depending on the site of the lesion. In cases of midthoracic esophageal carcinoma in which the upper margin of the tumor reaches the level of the aortic arch or above, a subtotal esophagectomy must be done and the anastomosis should be made in the cervical region.

TECHNIQUE OF ANASTOMOSIS

Staplers for esophagogastric anastomosis have been widely used with broadly satisfactory results. The time required for anastomosis is shortened, and the incidence of postoperative leakage has been reduced, but there has been a higher incidence of anastomotic stricture and probably a higher incidence of postoperative reflux. In addition, it may not be possible to employ the stapling apparatus at certain sites with limited space, such as the cervical region. Therefore, manual anastomosis remains a fundamental technique.

As the esophagus does not hold sutures well, because of its lack of a serosa and the friability of its muscular coat, meticulous care and great skill are needed in performing anastomosis. The prevention of anastomotic leakage has been a subject of continuous study. Authors with different experiences have developed different techniques with different points of emphasis in esophageal anastomosis, and most of them have reported good results with their own methods. The consensus, however, is that the nature of suture material and the method of suturing are of relatively minor importance, whereas enhancement of, or at least minimal interference with, tissue healing is significant. Thus, such things as preservation of a good blood supply to the site of anastomosis; avoidance of undue tension; good apposition of tissue layers, especially for mucosal layers; avoidance of defects in the anastomotic line; minimization of tissue trauma and tissue strangulation from instrumentation, manipulation, or excessive suturing; prevention of infection at the anastomosis; and prevention and effective management of intrathoracic complications are stressed.

The stomach has an abundant intramural vascular network that allows mobilization of the whole organ and permits it to be brought up to the neck for anastomosis, provided the right gastric and right gastroepiploic vessels are well preserved. This makes the stomach the most commonly used organ for esophageal reconstruction. The blood supply to the site of anastomosis, however, must be meticulously preserved. In making the incision in the fundus for anastomosis, care must be taken that it is not too close to the sutured divided end of the stomach where the vascular network has been cut. In handling the stomach, exercise great gentleness to avoid contusion of the wall, which may result in focal ischemia. Damage to intramural venous channels is especially likely to occur if the stomach is not manipulated delicately. Postoperative gastric perforation, sometimes multiple, may result from focal necrosis caused by traumatic ischemia.

In manual esophagogastrostomy, I use a double-row suturing technique in which the first or inner row consists of single-layer, whole-thickness, interrupted sutures bringing together the esophageal and gastric stomas in accurate apposition and without tissue strangulation. Care is taken to approximate the mucosal layers precisely and intimately with no eversion or interposition. The second or outer row telescopes the anastomosis into the fundus of the stomach in much the same manner as fundoplication in Nissen's operation for hiatal hernia. This is accomplished by anchoring the gastric wall to the esophagus about 2.5 cm above the anastomotic line (Fig. 39–2). The telescoping serves to minimize tension on the anastomotic line from the weight of the transplant itself or from gastric distention and creates a valvular mechanism for the prevention of postoperative gastroesophageal reflux.

End-to-Side Esophagogastrostomy

If all or most of the stomach is available, an end-to-side esophagogastrostomy is usually preferred. The gastric stoma is made either at the highest point of the fundus or more conveniently on the anterior wall of the fundus 3 to 4 cm below, either by a linear incision or by a circular fenestration with a circumference approximating that of the esophageal stump. Excessive gastric mucosa can be trimmed off to prevent its eversion. Submucosal bleeders are carefully ligated with fine sutures.

In an end-to-side esophagogastrostomy, the fundus is usually wide enough to allow a snug fundoplication around the lower segment of the esophageal stump (Fig. 39–2). This is preferred to a purse-string type invagination of the anastomotic line, in which a dead space is created around the invaginated esophageal stump where fluid may collect and infection may occur (Fig. 39–3).

Good exposure of the esophagus is essential for laying sutures, especially for anastomosis in the narrow superior mediastinum, where the esophageal wall on the undersurface is hard to expose for this purpose. To overcome this difficulty, I have used a simple esophageal retractor made of malleable wire to lift the mobilized esophagus perpendicular to its bed so that sutures can easily be laid on the undersurface of the esophageal wall (Fig. 39–4).

When four or five anchoring sutures have been laid between the fundus of the stomach and the side of the esophageal wall, an opening is made on the wall of the fundus, 2.5 cm below the anchoring sutures, for anastomosis. The sutures are then tied and the esophageal retractor removed.

To facilitate anastomotic suturing, a soft, noncrushing auricular clamp or other suitable nontraumatizing clamp is applied to the esophagus just above the anchoring sutures. Ensure that the tip of the indwelling nasogastric tube has been withdrawn by the anesthetist to a short distance above this level to avoid the tube's being caught by the clamp. The application of this clamp prevents spillage of the esophageal contents and excessive bleeding from the esophageal stump, thus providing a bloodless field with minimal contamination (Fig. 39–2A). The esophagus is then divided at the level 2.5 cm below the anchoring sutures. In dividing the esophagus, avoid excessive traction on the esophagus to avoid undue retraction of the esophageal mucosa after division.

The esophagogastric anastomosis is made with single-layer, whole-thickness, interrupted sutures. The far half of the anastomosis is started by putting the first and the second stitches at the two ends. Gentle traction of these two stitches in opposite directions brings the edges of the stoma into alignment with good apposition of tissue layers. The third stitch is laid halfway between the first

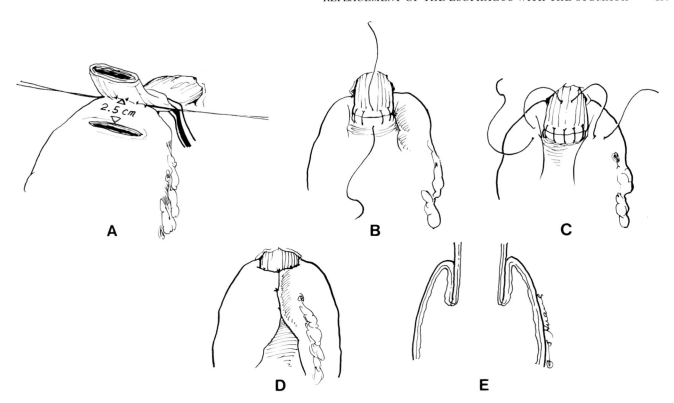

Fig. 39–2. Technique of end-to-side esophagogastrostomy. *A,* Placing of sutures to anchor the gastric fundus to the esophagus 2.5 cm above the line of resection. Note that a noncrushing clamp is applied to the esophagus for temporary hemostasis. *B,* Suturing the near half of the stoma, with knots tied outside the lumen. *C,* After completion of anastomosis, fundoplication is accomplished by placing external sutures in continuation with the anchoring sutures. *D,* Fundoplication completed. *E,* Longitudinal section of esophagogastrostomy and fundoplication.

two. The next two stitches are laid at the midpoints, followed by a further four laid in similar fashion to give a total of nine stitches evenly spaced out along the far half of the anastomotic line, with knots tied inside the lumen. Ensure good approximation of the mucosal and muscular layers (Fig. 39–5).

The near half of the anastomotic line is sutured from two ends inward, with knots tied preferably outside the lumen to avoid interposing them in the anastomotic line.

Before the completion of anastomotic suturing, the auricular clamp on the esophagus is removed and the nasogastric tube inserted before the operation is drawn out from the esophageal stump and connected to a gastric tube and a duodenal tube available at the operating table. The upper ends of these two tubes are then drawn out of the nostril by the anesthetist, using the original nasogastric tube as a guide, and the lower ends are inserted

into the gastric transplant. The gastric decompression tube is properly positioned and fixed at the nose by the anesthetist, whereas the duodenal feeding tube will be inserted into the duodenum after completion of the anastomosis (Fig. 39–6).

The suturing of the anastomosis is completed by adding a few final stitches to close the stoma (Fig. 39–2B). Fundoplication, which has been started by the anchoring sutures on the underside of the esophagus, is finished on the near side, as shown in Figure 39–2C, D.

The duodenal feeding tube is a fine Silastic or plastic tube about 1.5 mm in outer diameter and 1.2 m long with one or two side holes at the distal end, to which is attached a candy ball about 1.2 cm in diameter wrapped in a rubber glove finger. The ball serves as a pilot to bring the feeding tube into the duodenum when the surgeon, after having completed the anastomosis and put

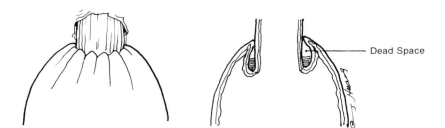

— Dead Space

Fig. 39–3. The dead space (right) after purse-string invagination of the anastomotic line (left) where fluid may collect and infection may arise.

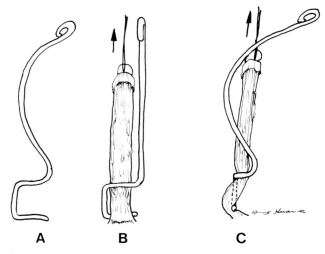

Fig. 39–4. A simple esophageal retractor that helps to expose the undersurface of the esophagus for laying of sutures. *A*, Oblique view. *B*, Front view. *C*, Lateral view. Arrows indicate direction of traction.

on clean gloves, pushes it from outside the stomach wall. Both tube and ball were previously disinfected by soaking in alcohol. A small cut is made in the rubber wrapping before the ball is inserted into the stomach, and subsequently the duodenum, to allow the candy to slowly dissolve.

End-to-End Esophagogastrostomy

Following partial esophagogastrostomy, such as in a case of resection of carcinoma of the gastric cardia, my current method of esophagogastrostomy is end-to-end anastomosis between the esophageal stump and the gastric tube, which is made from the greater curvature of the stomach, most conveniently by a stapler. The cut line is oversewn by a row of nonabsorbable Lembert sutures. After placing several anchoring stitches between the esophageal stump and the gastric tube as in end-to-side esophagogastrostomy, the upper tip of the gastric tube is amputated to leave an opening about equal in size to that of the esophageal stump so that the mucosal edges of the esophageal and gastric stomas can be approximated by a single layer of whole-thickness interrupted sutures. It is advisable in doing the anastomosis to rotate the gastric stump 90° clockwise so that the sutured lesser curvature comes to the midpoint of the far half of the anastomotic line. In this way, the suture line of the gastric tube and the anastomotic line are both in clear view so that tissue approximation and suturing in this critical area can be optimal (Fig. 39–7).

The technical details of end-to-end esophagogastrostomy are essentially the same as end-to-side anastomosis. After putting in the first row of anchoring sutures for invagination of the anastomotic line and before dividing the esophagus, a soft, noncrushing auricular clamp is applied just proximal to them to control spilling and bleeding from the esophageal stump during anastomosis.

Just before completion of anastomosis, the gastric decompression tube and the duodenal feeding tube are

inserted in the same manner as in end-to-side anastomosis.

After completion of anastomosis, invagination sutures are laid in such a way that the anastomotic line is telescoped into the gastric tube for a distance of about 2.5 cm (Fig. 39–7D, E). The anastomosed esophagus and gastric tube are then placed in the original esophageal bed in the posterior mediastinum.

PYLOROPLASTY

Severe postoperative gastric retention occurs only occasionally after intrathoracic or cervical esophagogastrostomy. The causes are usually mechanical obstruction of the outlet of the transplanted stomach caused by rotation or adhesion compression of the prepylorus. Although the vagi are invariably resected along with carcinoma of the esophagus or gastric cardia, postoperative pylorospasm occurs only rarely. Su (1978), in his extensive roentgenologic studies of gastrointestinal function at different periods after resection of carcinoma of the esophagus or gastric cardia without pyloroplasty, reported that in the majority of patients there was hyperperistalsis of the abdominal stomach and rapid passage of barium through the pylorus. A comparative study of gastric function following use of the stomach as a substitute after resection of carcinoma of the esophagus with or without concomitant pyloroplasty as reported by me and my colleagues (1985) showed that in both groups the interval between the ingestion of barium and the first passage of barium through the pylorus was significantly shorter postoperatively than preoperatively, postoperative gastric emptying times were no different, there was no reflux of barium from the thoracic stomach to the esophagus in recumbent positions, and postoperative gastric free acids were markedly decreased. Clinical evaluation and grading of postoperative symptomatology also showed no significant difference between the two groups.

In the vast majority of hospitals in China, resection of carcinoma of the esophagus or gastric cardia using stomach as a substitute has been performed without pyloroplasty. In over 3000 such operations at my institution during the past 29 years, concomitant pyloroplasty was done in only a few cases. Clinical observations of this large series of cases showed that in about 10% of patients there was a sensation of fullness after meals during the early postoperative period, probably a result of delayed gastric emptying, and in about 20% a typical dumping syndrome after meals, indicating rapid gastric emptying. In the remaining 70%, however, there was no marked postprandial discomfort attributable to pyloric dysfunction. Postoperative gastroesophageal reflux or reflux esophagitis has not been a problem in our experience with this series of patients. This may be attributable at least in part to the preventive effect of a fundoplication incorporated into the esophagogastric anastomosis. Secondary pyloroplasty has only been necessary in two patients in this series, both of whom came back over a year after resection of esophageal carcinoma with acute non-

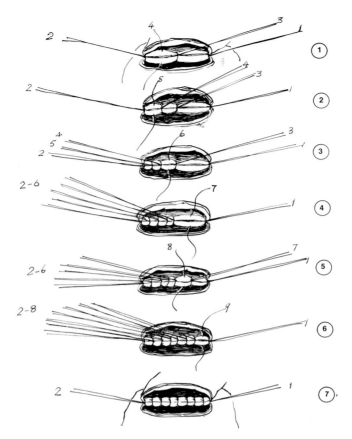

Fig. 39–5. Order of laying sutures on the far half of the anastomotic stoma, leaving knots inside the lumen.

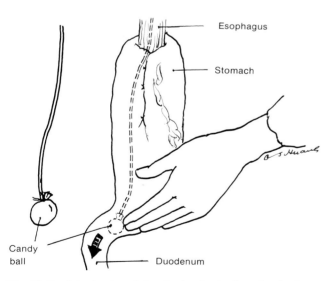

Fig. 39–6. Introduction of the duodenal tube into the duodenum from outside the gastric wall. Note that a small cut is made in the rubber wrapping of the ball to allow the candy to dissolve.

organic pylorospasm. Based on wide clinical experience, including the study mentioned above, it may be concluded that routine pyloroplasty is not necessary in the resection of carcinoma and other lesions of the esophagus and gastric cardia using stomach as a substitute. When adequate exposure is provided by an abdominal approach, and the stomach is long enough to replace the esophagus, however, pyloroplasty, being a simple procedure, may be justified.

SPECIFIC COMPLICATIONS*

Anastomotic

Anastomotic complications, i.e., an anastomotic leak, a fistula to the aorta with subsequent bleeding, or a stricture, are serious problems after esophagogastrostomy. The first constitutes one of the major causes of operative mortality.

Anastomotic Leak

I reported in 1963 that among 1503 esophagogastrostomies in nine leading hospitals in China there was an incidence of an anastomotic leak of 4.8%, with mortality

*This section appeared previously in Huang, G.J.: Preoperative and postoperative care and management of postoperative complications. *In* Carcinoma of the Esophagus and Gastric Cardia. Edited by Huang, G.J., and Wu, K.Y. Berlin, Springer-Verlag, 1984.

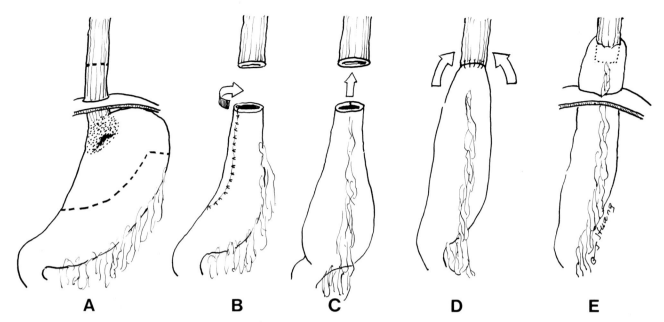

Fig. 39–7. Technique of end-to-end esophagogastrostomy. *A,* Extent of partial esophagogastrectomy (broken lines). *B,* Clockwise rotation of the gastric tube through 90°. *C,* Bringing up the gastric tube for anastomosis with the esophagus. *D,* Single-layer esophagogastrostomy completed. *E,* Telescoping the anastomotic line about 2.5 cm into the gastric tube.

of 57.5%. More recent statistics show that the incidence of anastomotic leak is still 3% to 5%.

A small number of leaks are missed because of difficulty in diagnosis. An anastomotic leak may be misdiagnosed as acute empyema or mediastinal abscess. On the other hand, perforation of the transplanted intrathoracic stomach and occasionally the esophageal stump may well be mistaken for anastomotic leak if additional evidence is lacking. A small, encapsulated anastomotic leak may escape notice altogether in the absence of obvious symptoms and signs.

In my series of 1373 resections for carcinoma of the esophagus during the period of 1958 to 1979, an esophagogastric anastomotic leak occurred in 52 patients, an incidence of 3.9% (1984). Twenty-two deaths occurred in this group, a mortality rate of 42.3%. The incidence of leakage in relation to the site of esophagogastric anastomosis is shown in Table 39–1.

Most anastomotic leaks occur between 2 and 7 days after operation, with an average of 4.5 days. Zhang and I (1980) judged the time of occurrence of the anastomotic leak clinically in 61 cases and found that in 80.3% it was

between 2 and 8 days after operation, with a peak at 5 to 6 days.

Early leaks—developing within 3 days of operation—are probably caused by technical defects, whereas late leaks—over 7 days after operation—are most likely caused by healing defects. The earlier the leak, the more severe is the problem, and hence the poorer the prognosis.

Clinical manifestations vary according to the site of anastomosis. Small leaks from cervical anastomoses usually cause only local inflammation and tenderness, with or without subcutaneous crepitation but without constitutional symptoms, and may be difficult to differentiate from localized wound infection. Diagnosis can be verified, however, on incision of the wound, and spontaneous healing usually takes place after drainage. With a more extensive leak, marked local infection occurs and the patient may have low grade or moderate fever with leukocytosis. There may be spontaneous rupture of the wound with discharge of foul, purulent material, possibly containing saliva or gastric or intestinal fluid.

An intrathoracic leak during the early postoperative

Table 39–1. Incidence of Esophagogastric Anastomotic Leakage Following Resection for Carcinoma of the Esophagus According to the Site of Anastomosis (1958–1979)

Site of Anastomosis	Resections	Leaks	Incidence (%)
Cervical	43	6	14.0
Intrathoracic supra-aortic	1056	36	3.4
Intrathoracic infra-aortic	249	10	4.0
Total	1348	52	3.9

Huang, G.J.: Preoperative and postoperative care and management of postoperative complications. *In* Carcinoma of the Esophagus and Gastric Cardia. Edited by Huang, G.J. and Wu, Y.K. Berlin, Springer-Verlag, 1984, p. 285.

period may cause an acute tension pyopneumothorax, high fever, dyspnea, or even shock and death, whereas a leak developing after 4 to 5 days usually gives rise to a more localized empyema or pyopneumothorax. The patient may have chest pain followed quickly by fever, tachycardia, and general constitutional symptoms. Roentgenograms of the chest usually show pleural effusion, with one or more fluid levels, usually confined to the ipsilateral side but occasionally may appear on the opposite side, if the contralateral mediastinal pleura was opened during the operation. Thoracentesis usually yields turbid, foul fluid.

A late-developing or very small leak may resemble an encapsulated intrapleural or mediastinal abscess close to the site of anastomosis. The patient may have persistently high or moderate fever, aching in the chest or back, and some degree of dysphagia. Roentgenograms of the chest may show encapsulated effusion with or without fluid level close to the site of anastomosis, or what appears to be a localized pleural reaction. A barium swallow may or may not show a small, fistulous tract leading from the anastomosis to the encapsulated cavity; once the cavity is drained or aspirated, however, the fistula is usually obvious on barium examination. The possibility of localized anastomotic leak must be kept in mind in cases of persistent fever and general weakness after the operation or of an unexplained pleural reaction or encapsulated effusion with or without fluid level. Leak from a low mediastinal anastomosis may give rise to symptoms and signs of peritonitis, which are usually confined to the upper abdomen. The infection arises when the fluid leaking from the anastomosis in the posterior mediastinum drains into the peritoneal cavity.

The diagnosis of leak is usually straightforward in cervical anastomoses, but may be quite difficult in intrathoracic anastomoses. Among the 1373 resections for esophageal carcinoma, only about one third of the intrathoracic leaks were promptly recognized by typical symptoms and signs.

When deciding on the form of treatment, the time of occurrence of the intrathoracic leak, the site of the anastomosis, the size of the leak, and the general condition of the patient must all be taken into consideration. In small or late-developing leaks, there is generally a good chance of success with conservative treatment, i.e., drainage, antibiotics, and nutritional support, but in larger or early-developing leaks, conservative treatment is likely to fail. On thoracic re-exploration, the leak is occasionally found to involve one third or more of the circumference of the anastomosis, with everting mucosal margins, a situation that precludes spontaneous healing.

As mentioned, small cervical leaks usually heal spontaneously after incision and drainage of the wound. In the case of extensive necrosis of the transplanted stomach, however, excision of the necrotic wall and subsequent reconstruction to establish alimentary continuity are necessary.

For promptly recognized early intrathoracic anastomotic leaks, the choice of treatment I recommended (1984) may be between: (1) Immediate thoracic re-ex-

ploration with excision of the primary anastomosis and construction of a new one. This offers an excellent chance of success if pleural infection is not yet established and if adequate lengths of both esophagus and stomach remain to allow reanastomosis without tension. At my institution, about two thirds of a limited number of patients so treated recovered smoothly after the second operation. (2) Immediate thoracic re-exploration with excision of the primary anastomosis, exteriorization of the esophageal stump in the neck, closure of the gastric stoma and reduction of the stomach back into the abdomen, and constuction of a feeding gastrostomy or jejunostomy. A subcutaneous or retrosternal colon interposition is performed later to re-establish alimentary continuity. (3) Conservative treatment if the patient's condition does not allow reoperation. In such cases adequate, efficient, closed-chest drainage of the pyopneumothorax is important. Pleural infection is treated by antibiotic coverage. Adequate nutrition is maintained. If all these measures go smoothly and the leak is reasonably small, the chance of spontaneous healing of both the fistula and the empyema is good, although the process usually takes about 1.5 to 3 months. Unfortunately in many such situations this does not occur and the patient dies.

In patients in whom the leak occurs or is first recognized late in the postoperative period, secondary thoracotomy is not advisable because of active infection and pleural adhesions. For such cases, conservative management is indicated; the success rate varies.

Aortoanastomotic Fistula

On rare occasions, a leak at the anastomosis or perforation of an intrathoracic gastric ulcer results in erosion of the adjacent adherent aorta, forming a fistula and leading to fatal hemorrhage. This usually occurs about 2 to 3 weeks after operation. Prodromal symptoms such as discomfort or pain in the chest and low grade fever may be present for a short time before massive fatal hematemesis occurs. Sometimes bleeding is temporarily halted by formation of a clot at the fistula; intermittent hematemeses may then persist for 2 to 3 days, only to be followed by dislodgement of the clot and fatal hemorrhage.

The avoidance of aortoanastomotic fistula depends on the prevention of leakage from the anastomosis and ulcer formation in the transplanted stomach, which may result from operative trauma. It is advisable not to have the anastomosis in direct contact with the aorta. An anastomosis at the level of or below the aortic arch should be separated from the aorta by a pedicle of omentum, usually available on the wall of the stomach.

Stricture

The reported incidence of stricture of the anastomosis varies with different authors and different techniques. In my institution (1984), stricture of the esophagogastrostomy stoma occurred in 0.9% of the cases of carcinoma of the esophagus.

Dysphagia within a month or so after operation is often caused at least in part by swelling or congestion of the anastomosis as a result of general hypoproteinemia or inflammation, and will therefore slowly improve as these conditions subside.

An occasional patient may have severe obstruction at the anastomosis in the early postoperative period as a result of errors in surgery.

Anastomotic stenosis appearing late after surgery is often caused by recurrence of tumor, but in the majority of cases it is cicatricial and benign in nature. In rare instances, a second primary carcinoma of the remaining segment of the esophagus may be the cause.

Use of excessive sutures at the anastomosis, poor approximation of muscosal layers, local infection, granulation formation, and reflux esophagitis are some of many causes of cicatricial stricture. The causes of late cicatricial stenosis are not always certain; it is my impression that reflux esophagitis is not a common factor. The use of certain staplers for anastomosis may lead to eventual cicatricial stenosis through excessive crush injury of both esophageal and gastric walls at the anastomosis.

Stricture of the anastomosis should be examined by barium swallow. The contour and distensibility of the esophageal wall above the anastomosis as shown on roentgenograms may help differentiate cicatricial from cancerous stenosis. Esophagoscopy and biopsy are usually needed to determine the precise nature of the stricture.

Benign cicatricial strictures are usually treated by endoscopic dilatation, repeated at intervals until a reasonable improvement of dysphagia is obtained, but can also be dealt with by dilatation and intubation, the tube then serving both as a passage for food and as an indwelling dilator. Benign strictures of cervical anastomoses can sometimes be treated by local plastic operations to enlarge the lumen or by the interposition of a free jejunal graft (Chapter 41).

In strictures caused by local recurrence of cancer, dilatation can only afford a temporary improvement of dysphagia. Local irradiation may offer some palliation as the tumor tissue recedes, but in some cases, subsequent scar formation may further aggravate the stenosis. In some cases with no evidence of metastasis, a secondary operation with esophageal reconstruction may be carried out.

Prepyloric Obstruction Caused by Torsion of Transplanted Stomach

As I pointed out (1984), postoperative prepyloric obstruction caused by torsion of the transplanted stomach is a rare but serious complication that is entirely preventable. It occurs mostly in high esophagogastrostomies and is a result of inadvertent rotation of the stomach through 360° counterclockwise as viewed from below. The twisting takes place in the prepyloric segment. This twisting inevitably causes obstruction and retention, but apparently does not interfere with the stomach's blood supply. This complication cannot occur if the surgeon is aware of the risk and places the transplanted stomach carefully in the correct position before constructing the anastomosis.

REFERENCES

Gavriliu, D.: Aspects of esophageal surgery. Curr. Probl. Surg. 12:1, 1975.

Heimlich, H.J.: Reverse gastric tube (RGT) esophagoplasty for failure of colon, jejunum, and prosthetic interpositions. Ann. Surg. 182:154, 1975.

Heimlich, H.J., and Winfield, J.M.: Use of gastric tube to replace or bypass esophagus. Surgery 37:549, 1955.

Huang, G.J.: Leakage of esophagogastric anastomosis following resection of carcinoma of the esophagus and gastric cardia (in Chinese). Chin. J. Surg. 11:859, 1963.

Huang, G.J., et al.: Surgery of esophageal carcinoma. Semin. Surg. Oncol. 1:74, 1985.

Huang, G.J.: Preoperative and postoperative care and management of postoperative complications. In Carcinoma of the Esophagus and Gastric Cardia. Edited by Huang, G.J. and Wu, Y.K. Berlin, Springer-Verlag, 1984, p. 285.

Huang, G.J., Zhang, D.C., and Zhang, D.W.: A comparative study of resection of carcinoma of the esophagus with and without pyloroplasty. In Esophageal Disorders: Pathophysiology and Therapy. Edited by T.R. DeMeester and D.B. Skinner. New York, Raven Press, 1985, p. 383.

Su, J.H.: Roentgenological study of gastrointestinal function following resection of carcinoma of the esophagus and gastric cardia (in Chinese). Cancer Res. Prev. Treat. 1:9, 1978.

Zhang, D.W., Huang, G.J., and Zhang, R.G.: Early secondary thoracotomy in the treatment of anastomotic leakage following resection for carcinoma of the esophagus and gastric cardia: a report of 7 cases (in Chinese). Chin. J. Oncol. 2:231, 1980.

CHAPTER 40

REPLACEMENT OF THE ESOPHAGUS WITH COLON

Ronald H.R. Belsey

INDICATIONS

The use of colon for esophageal replacement is indicated when long-term survival of the patient can confidently be expected: (1) in cases of type IB—long-gap—and type II congenital atresia; (2) following resection of benign strictures or tumors; (3) for advanced functional disorders; (4) following numerous previous failed antireflux procedures; and (5) in certain cases of malignant obstruction with an apparently good prognosis following radical surgery. The right or left colon is available for replacement. Left colon is preferable to right for the following reasons: (1) its smaller diameter; (2) the more constant and reliable blood supply from the left colic artery; (3) its adequate length for total esophageal replacement; and (4) its better ability to propel a solid bolus.

Right colon can be used when left colon is debarred by intrinsic disease or previous surgery. Incorporation of terminal ileum in the transplant has been advocated, but inclusion of the ileocecal valve may hinder progression of the swallowed bolus. Ventemiglia and colleagues (1977) investigated preoperative angiography and found a marginal artery in only 6 to 20 studies on the right colon—30%—but in all twenty—100%—of the left colons studied. Nicks (1967) demonstrated by autopsy injection studies frequent anomalies in the venous drainage from the right colon that might jeopardize the survival of the transplant.

Why colon? The frequently employed alternative organ is the stomach, entire or tubed. The advantages of the stomach as an esophageal substitute are its reliable blood supply and the simple technique, involving a single anastomosis. Disadvantages include high morbidity from anastomotic failures, a tendency to dilatation and defective propulsion, and frequent late complications such as recurrent esophagitis and stenosis, gastric ulceration, and hemorrhage.

The observed advantages of colon, especially left colon, are: the fewer lethal anastomotic problems—leaks can heal spontaneously, the progressive improvement in propulsive functional capacity, and its suitability for use in children. These advantages outweigh the disadvantages of the more complicated operative technique, which involves three anastomoses.

Contraindications to colon interposition consist of: (1) Intrinsic colonic pathology. In practice, mild degrees of diverticulosis with no previous history of infection have not proved to be a significant contraindication. (2) Mesenteric endarteritis. The endarteritis is commonly associated with systemic hypertension. Routine preoperative angiography is not recommended. The condition of the left colic artery and the vascular supply to the left colon can be more accurately assessed at operation. (3) In 15% of cases, colonic propulsive motility is subnormal. Preoperative detection of this defect is currently difficult. The history of bowel activity may be significant. Roentgenologic evidence on the rapidity or frequency of bowel evacuation is not a reliable guide. When perfected, motility studies on colonic function may provide essential information.

Jejunal interposition can be used for limited replacements, but variations in the vascular anatomy frequently debar it from extensive reconstructions.

In planning the reconstruction, the following features must be observed: (1) An isoperistaltic interposition is mandatory. (2) Protection of vascular pedicle from mechanical obstruction by torsion, kinking, or tension is vital to the success of the technique. (3) Three routes for the reconstruction are available: mediastinal, transpleural, and retrosternal. The menace to the integrity of the pedicle is least in the more direct mediastinal route and greatest in the more tortuous retrosternal route. (4) A cologastric anastomosis incorporating an antireflux principle is essential to prevent peptic colitis. (5) The tailoring of the transplant should prevent any intrathoracic redundancy, which can lead to mechanical obstruction by kinking. Moderate redundancy of the intra-abdominal segment of the transplant is well tolerated. (6)

The preferred anastomotic technique is by a single inverting layer of interrupted sutures of monofilament stainless steel wire or other nonirritant material. The advantages of wire are the complete lack of tissue reaction and the insignificant size and the security of the knots.

PREOPERATIVE PREPARATION

The general measures necessary in the preparation of a patient for major thoracic surgery are universally accepted and need not be repeated. Less generally recognized is the importance of eliminating all oronasal foci of infection. The mouth is probably the most heavily contaminated cavity in the body. Every esophageal resection incurs a risk of mediastinal infection. Following the extraction of septic teeth, the gums should be allowed to heal before the operation. In the present context, the major concern is the preparation of the colon as a transplant for esophageal replacement. The aim is an empty, dry colon to reduce the risk of peritoneal, pleural, or mediastinal contamination during the interposition procedure. Time should be allowed for a full standard colon prep in every case for which a resection and replacement might prove to be indicated at thoracotomy. The need for preoperative antibiotic therapy is debatable. Neomycin has caused severe enteritis because of changes in bowel flora. In my experience, no increase in peritoneal or pleural infection has been observed following the omission of preoperative antibiotic therapy.

RECONSTRUCTION WITH LEFT COLON

Operative Technique

Exposure

The extended left sixth interspace thoracotomy incision, with division of the costal margin at the anterior limit of the sixth interspace, peripheral detachment of the diaphragm from its origin on the chest wall, and extension of the incision through the oblique muscles as far as the lateral margin of the rectus sheath, affords adequate exposure of the entire left hemithorax and the upper abdomen with access to the organs available for reconstruction: the stomach, left colon, or jejunum. In those patients who have not had previous abdominal surgery, it may not be necessary to carry the incision across the costal margin. The spleen recedes beneath the posterior part of the diaphragm and is protected from injury.

Exploration

The position and extent of the esophageal lesion is determined by the preoperative studies. Exploration of the mediastinum is deferred until later in the procedure. The first step is the examination of the splenic flexure of the left colon: the adequacy of its preparation, the condition of the left colic and middle colic arteries by palpation of pulsation and compressibility, and the visible pulsation of the marginal artery and branches (Fig.

40–1). The marginal artery distal to its origin from the left colic artery, the main trunk of the middle colic artery, and the marginal artery to the right of the connections of the middle colic are all temporarily occluded by atraumatic vascular clamps to isolate the supply from the left colic vessels. Further inspection confirms the adequacy of the blood supply. The clamps are promptly removed.

Mobilization of the Left Colonic Transplant

This step is done before the mediastinum is explored. Postponing mediastinal dissection and mobilization of the esophagus prevents considerable blood loss from periesophageal vascular adhesions during the abdominal phase of the procedure. The greater omentum is detached from the colon from the splenic flexure to a point well to the right of the middle colic artery. The descending colon is mobilized by division of the peritoneal reflection along the lateral margin as far down as the junction of the descending with the sigmoid colon, where the colon is anchored to the posterior abdominal wall by a condensation of peritoneal tissue. With determined retraction of the abdominal wall, this band can be divided under direct vision. Mobilization of the splenic flexure and transverse colon, with its mesocolon, from the posterior abdominal wall necessitates division of the various ill-defined and irregular bands of vascular areolar tissue. The major vessels are contained in the mesocolon.

Isolation of the Blood Supply to the Transplant

Following complete mobilization, the vascular anatomy of the left colon can be accurately determined. The continuity of the marginal artery in the region of the splenic flexure is confirmed. The mesocolon is divided above and below the left colic vessels. The division is extended to the right as far as the left branch of the middle colic artery, maintaining a 1- to 2-cm fringe of mesocolon to protect the marginal artery. The left colic artery, arising from the inferior mesenteric, usually supplies two branches to the marginal artery. The marginal artery is divided distal to or below both branches of the left colic. The division of the right-hand end of the marginal artery, or the left branch of the middle colic, is deferred until the esophagus is liberated from the mediastinum and the extent of the resection and length of transplant necessary for replacement are determined.

Pyloromyotomy

At this stage of the operation, a pyloromyotomy is performed. In the absence of a gastrostomy or abdominal wall adhesions resulting from previous gastric surgery, the myotomy is performed on the anterior aspect of the pylorus. In the presence of a gastrostomy or extensive adhesions, a myotomy can be performed with equal effectiveness on the posterior aspect of the sphincter through the lesser sac, which is extensively opened during the mobilization of the colon. A pyloromyotomy is a satisfactory gastric drainage procedure and does not incur the risk of duodenal reflux that may follow a pyloroplasty.

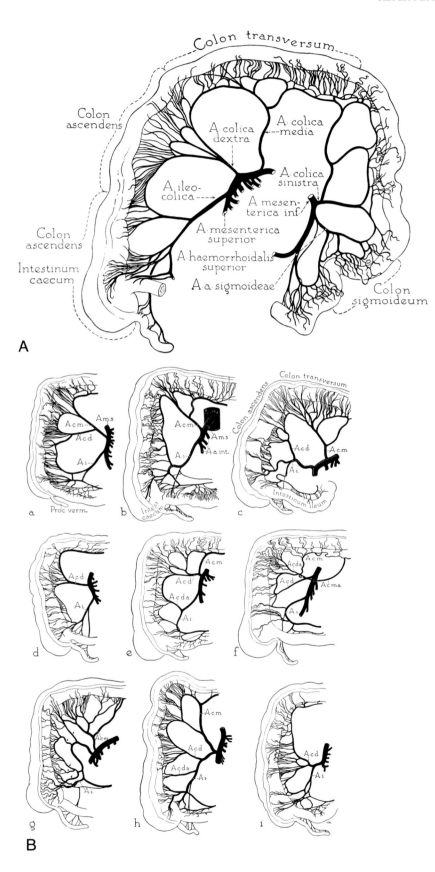

Fig. 40–1. Arterial supply of the colon. *A*, The commonest pattern of arterial source of the main colic arteries. *B*, Variations in origin of the ileocolic, right colic, and middle colic arteries encountered in 125 specimens, arranged in the order of decreasing frequency. (Reproduced with permission from Anson, B.J.: Atlas of Human Anatomy. Philadelphia, W.B. Saunders Co., 1950.)

Mobilization of the Esophagus

The preliminary intra-abdominal maneuvers having been completed, attention can return to the mediastinum. Mobilization of the esophagus for the excision of benign lesions is easily achieved through the left thoracotomy incision. Most malignant lesions are equally accessible, except those directly involving the aortic arch. In the latter case, a right thoracotomy, combined with a separate laparotomy incision, may be preferable. The single incision approach has obvious advantages. In the management of benign lesions by left colon replacement, only the diseased segment will be excised, followed by an intrathoracic esophagocolic anastomosis. Subsequent anastomotic problems are less menacing and can be managed conservatively.

Many bypass procedures with colon usually call for a long segment of transplant capable of reaching the cervical esophagus, or even the pharynx in some cases. At this stage, the probable length of the transplant necessary for replacement or bypass can be estimated. An excessively long transplant can be tailored to a suitable length; if it is too short, tension on the anastomoses may promote complications.

Closure of the Cardia

The esophagogastric junction is divided. The stomach is repaired with two rows of inverting sutures. The cardia will not be used for the subsequent cologastric anastomosis. The lower esophagus is ligated to prevent contamination of the mediastinum and pleura. If a bypass procedure is planned with the esophagus left in situ, the cardia is not divided, as it is important to maintain drainage of the lower segment between the stricture and the cardia to avoid creation of a closed loop of obstructed esophagus and the potential risk of a blowout.

Division of the Colon and Isolation of the Transplant

The point of division of the marginal artery and transverse colon at the proximal end of the planned transplant can now be selected. For a short segment transplant, this is just to the left of or distal to the point where the left branch of the middle colic joins the marginal artery. A single ligature is placed on the marginal artery, and the vessel is divided on the transplant side of the ligature. The divided vessel is allowed to bleed momentarily, as this affords the most graphic demonstration of the adequacy of the blood supply to the transplant from the left colic artery, a more reliable indication than that afforded by the use of any form of flow meter. The vessel is picked up and ligated.

Preparation of the long segment transplant for total replacement involves a different procedure. The marginal artery between the two branches of the middle colic is carefully examined and assessed. If the marginal artery is well developed and continuous, the left branch of the middle colic is divided near its origin from the main trunk of the middle colic, the intervening mesocolon is divided, and the marginal artery is ligated close to the point where the right branch of the middle colic joins the marginal artery. Selection at this point results in a transplant long enough to reach the pharynx, if necessary, with retention of the right branch of the middle colic. The marginal artery is allowed to bleed momentarily, as previously described, to confirm the adequacy of the blood supply. Rarely, the marginal artery between the two branches of the middle colic may be defective, or replaced by a plexus of vessels, the adequacy of which in terms of blood supply to the proximal end of the transplant may prove difficult to assess. In this situation, the two branches of the middle colic are retained to substitute for the defective margin. The main trunk of the middle colic is cleared and divided well proximal to the point of division into the two main branches. The continuity of the supply to the colon is maintained through the juncture of the two branches of the middle colic.

Any palpable residual colonic contents are milked from the segment destined for transplantation and into the descending colon below the level where it will be divided. The length of transplant having been determined, the colon is now divided at the appropriate sites between two pairs of Pott's aortic clamps. The descending colon is divided below both branches of the left colic artery. The advantages of Pott's aortic clamps are the narrow blades and the minimal trauma to the colonic tissue.

Colocolic Anastomosis

The continuity of the colon is restored by end-to-end anastomosis of the transverse colon to the descending colon. The divided ends of the bowel are approximated and held in this position by a seromuscular suture placed through the mesenteric border of the two segments. The Pott's clamps are removed and any residual fecal matter carefully mopped out of the now open bowel segments. Pledgets of gel-foam may be inserted into the proximal transverse and descending colon to absorb any residual liquid fecal matter and reduce the risk of contamination during the anastomosis. These pledgets pass naturally when bowel function returns. Specimens are taken for culture as a guide to postoperative antibiotic therapy if necessary. The blood supply to the bowel segment is checked, especially for any evidence of venous engorgement, suggesting interference with the venous drainage caused by tension or rotation. An end-to-end, single-layer, inverting anastomosis is achieved by interrupted sutures of 5–0 or 6–0 monofilament stainless steel wire with the reef knots tied on the luminal side, commencing at the mesenteric border approximated by the initial suture, and working around each side alternately until finally the anastomosis is completed by two or three sutures placed on the antimesenteric margins from the outside, with careful inversion of the colonic mucosa.

Cologastric Anastomosis

During the colocolic anastomosis, the transplant is wrapped in warm, moist gauze with the divided ends occluded by the clamps and with the vascular pedicle protected from tension or rotation.

The design of the cologastric anastomosis is an essential feature of the procedure and creates an effective antireflux mechanism to prevent peptic colitis. The anastomosis is performed on the posterior aspect of the stomach, near the greater curve, at a point one third of the length of the fundopyloric distance distal to the fundus. An 8- to 12-cm segment of the transplant is retained in the infradiaphragmatic high pressure region and creates an antireflux device similar in principle to the Mark IV antireflux operation for correction of an incompetent cardia; it is not necessary to perform any type of fundoplication around the intra-abdominal colonic segment to achieve this objective. The lower posterior cologastric anastomosis also protects the vascular pedicle against tension or angulation. The low posterior anastomosis is advocated even when a retrosternal colonic bypass is performed.

The stomach is rotated on its long axis toward the right and maintained in this position by two traction sutures placed near the greater curve. The distal end of the transplant is approximated to the selected point by a seromuscular suture, and a transverse full-thickness incision is made into the lumen of the stomach between this point and the greater curve. The Pott's clamp is removed from the distal end of the transplant, and end-to-side cologastric anastomosis is performed using the technique previously described, with interrupted inverting sutures of monofilament stainless steel wire. Care is taken not to rotate the pedicle or the transplant. Hemostasis of the gastric incision is best achieved by closer spacing of the full-thickness anastomotic sutures rather than by cautery. Larger vessels may need ligation. Following completion of the cologastric anastomosis, the stomach is allowed to fall back into its anatomical position and the two stay sutures are removed.

Placement of the Transplant

Three routes for the transplant are available: (1) transhiatal and posterior mediastinal, following esophageal resection; (2) transhiatal and transpleural or through an additional opening in the diaphragm for a bypass procedure; and (3) retrosternal. The choice of route is influenced by one overriding consideration, the avoidance of tension, rotation, kinking, or other forms of mechanical obstruction of the vascular pedicle to the transplant. Loss of the transplant because of ischemic necrosis can usually be assigned to this cause. Obstruction of the venous drainage from the transplant can prove as dangerous as embarrassment of the arterial inflow. The more direct and linear the path of the transplant, the lower the risk of vascular obstruction. The route that approaches this ideal most closely is the transhiatal posterior mediastinal route adopted for the majority of replacements following resection of benign lesions.

Transhiatal and Posterior Mediastinal Route. The proximal end of the transplant is closed temporarily by a running suture, after removal of the Pott's clamp, to reduce soiling during the placing of the transplant. A tunnel is created digitally through the lesser sac behind the fundus up to the hiatus. The cardia is already mobilized and the peritoneal reflection and phrenoesophageal membrane are divided during the resection of the

eosphagus and closure of the cardia. The end of the transplant is passed up through this tunnel, through the hiatus, and into the mediastinum without rotation. The pedicle lies medial to the transplant against the right pleura. Any venous engorgement of the transplant indicates rotation or kinking. If the hiatus is not available when a bypass procedure is planned, the left lobe of the liver is mobilized by division of the triangular ligament, and a separate opening is made in the central tendon of the diaphragm. A circle of tendinous tissue is excised to prevent contraction of the opening. The transplant is passed up behind the fundus and into the left pleural cavity.

If a long segment interposition for total replacement is indicated, the esophageal resection has already vacated the mediastinal tunnel up to the apex of the thorax. The end of the transplant is threaded up deep to the aortic arch and anchored to the stump of the esophagus or the side of the mobilized esophagus near the apex of the thorax with two stout sutures. Sutures of different colors can be used to confirm the absence of rotation when the transplant is delivered into the neck. The cervical esophagus is mobilized as high as possible from within the thorax because of the greater ease of identifying the appropriate tissue planes.

The Transpleural Route. This route is the second choice. If a colonic bypass procedure by the transpleural route is planned, a tunnel is established through the superior thoracic outlet to accommodate the transplant. The pleura and deep cervical fascia are incised transversely posterior to the inner ends of the first rib and clavicle. The internal mammary artery and vein can be divided. The lateral margin of the costoclavicular ligament is incised. The anterior jugular vein is gently dissected posteriorly by digital and blunt dissection until an adequate tunnel is created and the dissecting finger reaches the skin in the posterior triangle of the neck just above the clavicle and posterior to the sternocleidomastoid muscle. Two stout sutures loaded on large, curved, cutting needles are passed through the end of the transplant, up through the tunnel created, and out through the skin of the neck. The end of the transplant is drawn up into the tunnel and approximated to the skin by the anesthetist, who then ties two sutures over a bridge of skin to retain the transplant until the cervical incision is made.

Retrosternal Route. This route pursues a more tortuous, and consequently more hazardous, course. The danger areas are the region of the xiphoid, where the transplant takes a right-angle bend upwards; in the retrosternal tunnel, where rotation may inadvertently occur; and at the narrow superior thoracic outlet. The low posterior cologastric anastomosis previously described is advocated to avoid mechanical embarrassment of the pedicle at its orgin if an anterior anastomosis is attempted. The transplant is passed through the lesser sac, behind the stomach, through the gastrohepatic omentum, to the xiphoid region. The retrosternal tunnel must be large enough to accommodate the transplant without compression. The anterior margin of the diaphragm is incised backward, or detached from its costal origin sufficiently to reduce the sharp angulation of the transplant around the anterior margin. The superior thoracic outlet at the upper limit of the tunnel must be dissected and enlarged under direct vision from the cervical incision to avoid any constriction at this point. A flat strip of metal, with two perforations at its lower end, is passed down through the tunnel. The closed end of the transplant is sutured to these perforations and drawn up through the tunnel. In this manner, rotation of the transplant in the tunnel can be avoided. It is never necessary to perform a median sternotomy to ensure correct placement of the transplant in the retrosternal tunnel. An infected sternotomy wound is one of the most dreaded of all postthoracotomy complications.

Once the transplant reaches the cervical incision, a critical inspection of the blood supply is essential. Any evidence of venous engorgement is a danger signal indicating mechanical interference with the vascular pedicle. The whole course of the transplant from its origin must be reviewed until the cause of the problem is determined and corrected by readjusting the lie of the transplant or by eliminating the offending anatomical factor. Obstruction of venous drainage can lead to loss of the transplant, or progressive fibrosis of the proximal end of the transplant and recurrent obstruction, leaks from the esophagocolic anastomosis and salivary fistulae, or strictures of this anastomosis. Complications at the esophagocolic anastomosis occur more commonly following the use of the retrosternal route.

Intrathoracic Esophagocolic Anastomosis

Following resection of the lower esophagus, an end-to-end esophagocolic anastomosis is performed by the standard one-layer wire suture technique. The divided end of the esophagus is held open by four stay sutures to maintain the mucosa in apposition to the muscle layer, to expose the diameter of the lumen, and to facilitate the tailoring of the anastomosis in the event of any discrepancy in the size of the two lumina. The closed end of the transplant is excised and the blood supply checked. An inverting end-to-end anastomosis is accomplished by a single row of closely spaced full-thickness interrupted wire sutures with the knots tied on the luminal surface, except for the last two or three sutures.

Prevention of Intrathoracic Colic Redundancy

Any redundant transplant must be excluded from the thorax, as kinking may result in obstruction, necessitating further surgery. On completion of the esophagocolic anastomosis, the transplant, which usually contracts during manipulation, is gently stretched manually to its normal length. Any redundant transplant is pulled gently downward into the abdominal cavity. The transplant is anchored to the margin of the hiatus by running or interrupted nonabsorbable seromuscular sutures around two thirds of the circumference, avoiding the area of the vascular pedicle. Before closure, the management of the defect in the transverse mesocolon must be considered. Attempts to suture the defect result in several small defects, with an enhanced risk of small bowel obstruction and strangulation. Our practice is to leave the defect wide open, with the assumption that a large defect is less likely to lead to strangulation than multiple small defects. The greater omentum is wrapped around the colocolic anastomosis and plugged into the mesocolon defect to discourage small bowel herniation. The diaphragm is reattached to its costal origins, and the incision is closed with catheter drainage of the pleural cavity.

Cervical Esophagocolic Anastomosis

When a cervical anastomosis is planned, the colon is anchored to the margin of the hiatus without any tension of the intra-abdominal portion of the vascular pedicle. Any intrathoracic redundancy can be corrected by gentle upward traction on the transplant at the time of the cervical anastomosis. Excess colon is trimmed back prior to the anastomosis. With the patient turned in the supine position, an incision is made along the anterior border of the left sternocleidomastoid muscle. After division of the middle thyroid veins and the inferior thyroid artery, the thyroid gland is retracted medially and the carotid sheath posteriorly.

If the cervical esophagus is freed adequately from within the thorax, it is simple to deliver the organ from the mediastinum with the closed proximal end of the transplant attached. The esophagus is trimmed back to the level just distal to the cricopharyngeal sphincter, which is preserved as a major structure for protecting the air passages against reflux and aspiration.

The closed end of the transplant is excised and the blood supply inspected for any evidence of venous engorgement or arterial ischemia. When first opened, the bleeding may appear to be mainly venous, suggesting some obstruction to the venous drainage. After allowing free hemorrhage for a few minutes, the bleeding becomes progressively more arterial, the colonic mucosa pinks up and loses the cyanotic appearance, suggesting venous obstruction. Persistence of cyanosis and venous engorgement indicates a serious obstruction at a lower level and may call for reopening of the thoracotomy wound. It is an error of judgement to proceed with the anastomosis if there is any persisting doubt about the adequacy of the colonic blood supply.

An end-to-end esophagocolic anastomosis is accomplished as for an intrathoracic anastomosis. The cervical incision is closed without drainage, because it communicates freely with the left pleura and insertion of a drain may result in a persisting pneumothorax as well as increased risk of anastomosis leakage. Cervical tissue planes are adequately drained internally by the intercostal catheter.

Cervical Bypass Anastomosis

With the patient supine, an oblique incision is made along the anterior margin of the left sternocleidomastoid or a transverse collar incision is made and the skin flaps elevated. With the sternocleidomastoid retracted laterally, the proximal end of the transplant is located in the tunnel created from within the thorax behind the inner ends of the first rib and clavicle. After obtaining a firm grip on the transplant with Babcock forceps to prevent retraction back into the thorax, the transplant is liberated by dividing the sutures anchoring it to the skin of the posterior triangle. The transplant is drawn out of the thorax as far as possible with gentle traction and a constant watch on the blood supply, to eliminate any intrathoracic redundancy. Any excess length of the transplant is trimmed back as necessary. The cervical esophagus is exposed as previously described. A vertical incision is made in the lateral wall of the esophagus and the edges distracted by two stay sutures. The closed end of the transplant is excised and the blood supply observed. The length of the esophagotomy incision is tailored to the diameter of the transplant. A side-to-end esophagocolic anastomosis is effected by the single-layer wire technique. The cervical incision is closed without drainage.

Retrosternal Route

If the retrosternal route has been employed, the cervical incision was made during the creation of the retrosternal tunnel. The proximal end of the transplant has already been placed through the tunnel into the cervical incision. To establish the bypass, a side-to-end esophagocolic anastomosis is performed as described in the previous section. When bypassing an unresectable esophageal obstruction, drainage of the esophagus must be maintained both above and below the obstruction. Division of the cervical esophagus for an end-to-end esophagocolostomy and dropping the closed lower esophageal stump back into the mediastinum creates a closed loop, with an ulcerated and infected stricture at the lower end and a suture line at the upper limit. Secretion from the glands in the esophageal mucosa may result in progressive distention of the closed loop; formation of a mediastinal cyst, causing pressure effects on the adjacent mediastinal structures such as the trachea or superior vena cava; and ultimately rupture through the suture line, leading to a fatal mediastinitis. The pseudodiverticulum created in the upper esophagus by this technique has not been found to cause any complications.

RECONSTRUCTION WITH RIGHT COLON

Mobilization of the right colon requires a separate laparotomy incision. A right fifth or sixth interspace thoracotomy follows if an esophageal resection and replacement are planned. Alternatively, if a bypass procedure is intended, the retrosternal route can be developed from the laparotomy incision and an additional cervical incision. The first step is inspection of the vascular anatomy of the right colon with confirmation of the presence of the normal middle colic artery and an adequate, well developed marginal artery. A critical area is the ileocecal junction. It is common practice to include the terminal ileum and ileocecal valve in the transplant, but this is only feasible when the marginal artery is obviously continuous in this region and the blood supply is adequate. The possible disadvantages of including the ileocecal valve have already been discussed.

The right colon and transverse colon are mobilized in a similar fashion to that already described for the left colon. The appendix is excised. The greater omentum is detached from the hepatic flexure and transverse colon to a point well to the left of the middle colic artery. The right colic and ileocecal arteries are sacrificed close to their origins from the superior mesentery artery to maintain continuity of the marginal artery. The middle colic artery with both branches intact forms the vascular pedicle of the transplant. The vascular anatomy of the right colon is more variable than that of the left and may limit its use for esophageal substitution. The length of the transplant necessary having been determined, the colon segment is mobilized in a similar fashion to that described for the left colon. The marginal artery is divided to the left of both branches of the middle colic. Following division of the transverse colon and the terminal ileum, an end-to-end ileocolic anastomosis is performed if there is no gross dissimilarity in the lumina of the two viscera. Alternatively, the divided end of the transverse colon can be closed and an end-to-side ileocolostomy performed. The same anastomotic technique is employed as in the case of the left colon interposition.

The pedicle from the middle colic artery dictates an anterior cologastric anastomosis. Retention of a segment of transplant within the abdomen discourages reflux but is not as effective in preventing reflux as the posterior cologastric anastomosis.

If esophageal resection and replacement are indicated, the cardia is mobilized from the hiatus together with the lower third of the esophagus and then divided. The stomach is closed. The lower end of the esophagus is ligated. The closed end of the ileum is attached to the lower end of the esophagus with two stout sutures of different colors to diminish the risk of rotation. The laparotomy incision may be closed at this stage. Alternatively, with the patient positioned on the table in the oblique rather than a full left lateral position, the chest is opened through the anterior right fifth or sixth interspace and the esophagus is mobilized from the mediastinum. The synchronous exposure of thorax and abdomen permits the inspection of the vascular pedicle as the transplant is transferred to the thoracic cavity and reduces the risk of inadvertent rotation. It is common practice for two surgical teams to work synchronously on the mobilization of the transplant and the esophageal resection. When the retrosternal route is preferred for a bypass procedure, the tunnel is developed from the laparotomy and an additional cervical incision. The precautions necessary to prevent mechanical interference with the pedicle are the same as in the previously described routes. In the event of a bypass, the cardia is left in continuity to maintain drainage of the lower esophageal segment below the obstructing lesion.

Both the intrathoracic and cervical anastomoses following resection are accomplished by the previously described technique. The esophagoileal anastomosis is facilitated by the correspondence in size of the two lumina. For a bypass procedure, the side-to-end esophagoileal anastomosis is advocated to maintain drainage of the segment of esophagus between the anastomosis and the stricture.

Reconstruction with colon, preferably left, following a transhiatal esophagectomy is accomplished in the same manner when performed through an extended left thoracotomy incision. The use of the flat metal strip to draw the proximal end of the transplant up to the cervical incision reduces the risk of rotation of the transplant or its pedicle and subsequent ischemic necrosis.

POSTOPERATIVE CARE

Management of the patient follows along the same lines as after any major thoracic operation. Oral alimentation is restored as soon as a barium esophagogram indicates healing of the anastomoses. If the described anastomotic technique with monofilament wire is employed, it is safe to start the patient on fluids on the third postoperative day, progressing rapidly to soft solids. Ice cream is always acceptable to the patient following any major esophageal procedure.

POSTOPERATIVE COMPLICATIONS

Necrosis of Transplant

The common cause is technical mismanagement of vascular pedicle caused by: inadequate exposure; excessive handling of the transplant; prolonged use of vascular clamps; torsion, tension, or kinking of the pedicle during placement of the transplant; or an anterior colon gastric anastomosis. Other causes of necrosis are failure to observe mesenteric endarteritis, anomalies of the vascular anatomy, or signs of obstruction to the venous drainage.

Signs of transplant necrosis include: septic toxemia, fetor, and regurgitation of foul-smelling secretions. Endoscopy confirms the diagnosis, but opaque swallows and roentgenography may fail to reveal the complication until ischemic dissolution of the transplant occurs. Once the diagnosis is confirmed, the transplant is excised, probably through the original incision. The stomach and esophageal stump are closed; a cervical esophagostomy is performed, either a lateral esophagostomy if the intrathoracic remnant is to be retained or an end esophagostomy if the remainder of the esophagus is exteriorized and abandoned. A feeding gastrostomy or jejunostomy, depending upon which organ will ultimately be used for subsequent reconstruction, is performed. Any further attempt at reconstruction is delayed for 3 to 6 months and will probably consist of a cervical esophagogastrostomy.

Anastomotic Fistulae

The highest recorded incidence of leaks has been at the esophagocolic anastomosis. These leaks can be observed in postoperative esophagograms in asymptomatic patients. Fortunately, these fistulae usually run a benign course and heal spontaneously, because of the nonerosive nature of the colonic secretion. Operative repair is seldom necessary. An important advantage of colon

over gastric interposition is the lower morbidity associated with anastomotic problems.

Anastomotic Strictures

The incidence of strictures has been largely eliminated by the routine employment of the anastomotic technique described in the text. The essential features of this technique are tissue apposition without tissue strangulation and the avoidance of excessive quantities of suture material.

Wound Infection

Wound infection is an uncommon complication in spite of the theoretical risks of contamination from encroachment of the lumina of both esophagus and colon.

Paracolic Hiatal Herniation

Herniation of small bowel through the hiatus alongside the colon transplant can only occur if a circumferential suture of the seromuscular layer of the transplant to the margins of the hiatus is omitted or incorrectly sited.

Herniation of Small Intestine Through the Mesocolon

This complication has been largely eliminated by the technique of inserting the greater omentum into the defect in the mesocolon before closure of the extended thoracotomy incision.

Progressive Fibrostenosis in the Proximal End of the Transplant

This late complication has been reported. The probable explanation is a reaction to chronic venous engorgement secondary to mechanical embarrassment of the vascular pedicle. Management is by prevention. If the stenosis cannot be controlled adequately by repeated dilatation when necessary, the esophagocolic anastomosis along with the stenotic segment of the transplant is excised and followed by reanastomosis.

Redundancy of the Transplant

A major complication is redundancy of the transplant within the thorax, and intermittent obstruction caused by mechanical kinking. The complication is avoidable by intraoperative tailoring of the length of the transplant and by replacing any redundant transplant below the diaphragm after completion of the anastomosis and before anchoring the transplant to the margin of the hiatus. If upward prolapse occurs, resulting in kinking and obstruction of a redundant loop, the original incision is reopened and the loop freed and returned to the abdomen. Redundant colon below the diaphragm is well tolerated and rarely causes obstructive symptoms.

Sluggish Colon

Another major long-term complication is a functionally inadequate transplant caused by the use of a segment of inherently sluggish colon for reconstruction. If reliable tests for assessing colonic function before surgery can be developed, the sluggish colon can be detected and rejected as an unsuitable organ for esophageal substitution and replaced by stomach or jejunum.

Gastrocolic Reflux and Peptic Colitis

This complication was described by Malcolm (1986). In all instances, the cologastric anastomosis was performed at the cardia, at the apex of the fundus of the stomach, or on the anterior surface of the stomach. This late complication has been eliminated by the routine employment of the antireflux cologastric anastomosis described in the text.

POSTOPERATIVE MORTALITY

Postlethwait (1983) reviewed the published data on colonic interposition in 474 patients operated upon between 1971 and 1981 in 12 different centers, indicating no extensive experience in any one group of surgeons. The operative mortality rate was 4.9%, the same as in my experience. The general consensus is that the operative mortality should be under 5% in cases in which the interposition was performed for benign disease. The mortality rate probably approaches 10% in cases of malignant obstruction treated by this technique.

LONG-TERM FUNCTIONAL RESULTS

Benages (1981), Corazziari (1977), and Jones (1973) and associates investigated a small series of adult patients by pH and manometric studies following the technique of colon interposition described here. All three reports had similar conclusions: (1) The resting pH in the colon transplant remains neutral with no evidence of reflux. (2) Rapid clearing by stimulated peristalsis is observed following the installation of 0.1 N HCl. (3) Peristaltic contractions occur spontaneously in approxiamtely one third of the patients studied and in response to an acid bolus in all patients. The functional results tend to improve with the passage of time. When employed for reconstruction in infants and children, the colon transplant has been observed to grow at the same rate as the child when followed into adult life.

REFERENCES

Benages, A., et al.: Motor activity after colon replacement of esophagus. J. Thorac. Cardiovasc. Surg. 82:335, 1981.

Corazziari, E., et al.: Functional evaluation of colon transplants used in esophageal reconstruction. Amer. J. Dig. Dis. 22:7, 1977.

Jones, E.L., et al.: Response of the interposed human colonic segment to an acid challenge. Ann. Surg. 117:75, 1973.

Malcolm, J.A.: Occurrence of peptic ulcer in colon used for esophageal replacement. J. Thorac. Cardiovasc. Surg. 55:763, 1968.

Nicks, R.: Colonic replacement of the oesophagus: some observations on infarction and wound leakage. Br. J. Surg. 54:124, 1967.

Postlethwait, R.W.: Colonic interposition for esophageal substitution: collective review. Surg. Gynecol. Obstet. 156:377, 1983.

Ventemiglia, R., et al.: The role of preoperative mesenteric arteriography in colon interposition. J. Thorac. Cardiovasc. Surg. 74:98, 1977.

CHAPTER 41

FREE INTESTINAL TRANSFER AND MICROVASCULAR TECHNIQUES IN RECONSTRUCTION OF THE ESOPHAGUS

W. Spencer Payne, Victor F. Trastek, and Jack Fisher

Standard techniques for esophageal reconstruction, as described by DeSanto and Carpenter (1980), entail the interposition of pedicled cutaneous or myocutaneous skin-lined tubes or mobilization and interposition of appropriate lengths of stomach or intestine perfused through pedicles of normal anatomic vascular channels.

The feasibility of free intestinal transfer to the neck was first demonstrated by Carrel (1907). Except for sporadic but important clinical and laboratory reports from the late 1940s through the 1970s by Androsov (1960), Hiebert (1961), Hopkins 1963), McKee (1978), Nakayama (1964), Peters (1971), Roberts (1961), and Seidenberg (1959) and their associates, and Jurkiewicz (1965, 1984), and Longmire (1947), microvascular technology did not reach general clinical application until the early 1970s. As patency rates for small-vessel anastomoses began to exceed 95%, microvascular surgery found application in many areas of surgery. The operative microscope and specially designed microvascular instruments significantly improved success rates for microvascular anastomoses. Success rates with free intestinal transfer for reconstruction of the hypopharynx and cervical esophagus improved, as Chang (1980), Fisher (1984), Gluckman (1982), Hester (1980), Katsaros (1982), and McKee (1978) and their colleagues reported.

At the Mayo Clinic in 1981, two of us (W.S.P., J.F.) (1988) began using microvascular surgery effectively in the reconstruction of esophageal continuity in four specific clinical circumstances: (1) elective free jejunal transfer for reconstruction of the pharynx and cervical esophagus at the time of radical resection for cancer; (2) free jejunal transfer for reconstruction of benign, often traumatic, pharyngeal and cervical esophageal strictures, in which the larynx is usually preserved; (3) salvage of partially failed substernal gastric or colonic interposition by free jejunal transfer to bridge defects between hypopharynx or cervical esophagus and the remaining upper

thoracic gastric or colonic interposition, in which the larynx is often preserved; and (4) microvascular circulatory augmentation of the oral end of standard pedicled isoperistaltic colonic interposition in patients with complex laryngopharyngeal or tracheoesophageal defects with or without an intact larynx.

RECONSTRUCTION AFTER LARYNGOPHARYNGECTOMY

Free jejunal transfer for reconstruction of the pharynx and cervical esophagus after ablative surgery for cancer is an established technique (Fig. 41–1). DeSanto and associates (1983) noted that it has several advantages over previous reconstructive techniques. It allows for a single-stage reconstruction at the time of the ablative procedure and is particularly useful for patients who have experienced failure of previous reconstruction. It is applicable to patients who have had previous irradiation or who are candidates for postreconstruction irradiation. The revascularized segment of bowel actually enhances local tissue healing and supports split-thickness skin grafts applied directly to it. Mobilization of the jejunal segment for transfer is considerably simpler than that of colon, stomach, or regional myocutaneous or cutaneous flaps. Finally, with highly predictable local healing, duration of hospitalizations is reduced and rehabilitations are improved. Unfortunately, many patients treated with this procedure have limited survival from the underlying malignant disease, which is unaffected by the method of reconstruction. According to DeSanto and colleagues (1983), whether the level of palliation of free jejunal transfer will continue to justify its use over other techniques available is yet to be determined.

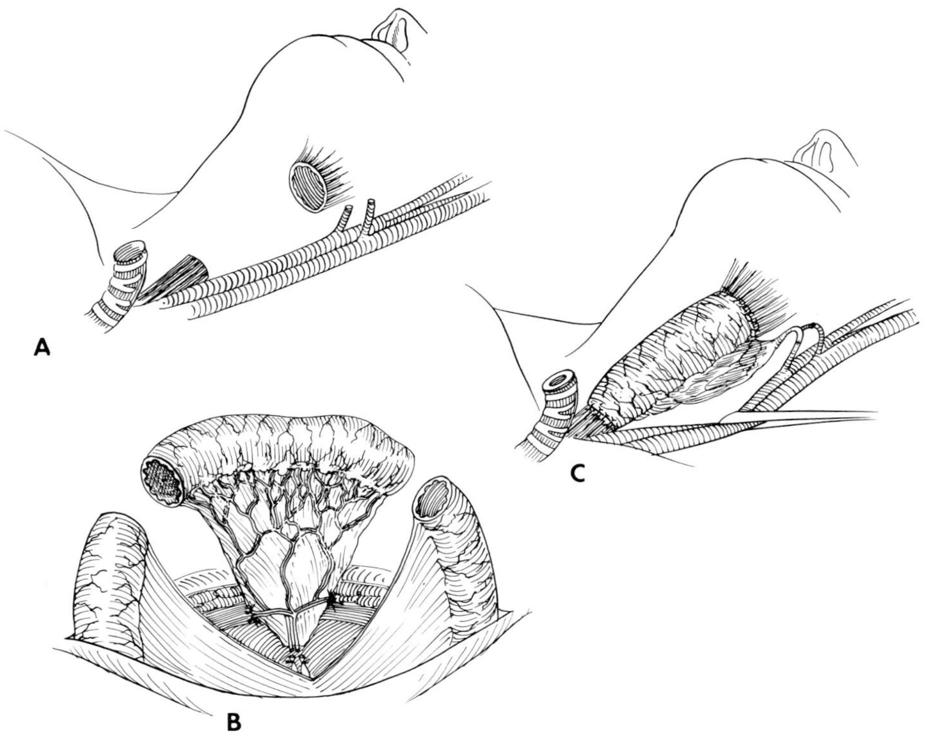

Fig. 41–1. Free jejunal transfer at time of laryngopharyngectomy: *A,* Circumferential defect of pharynx and cervical esophagus. *B,* Jejunal segment isolated with vascular pedicle, and *C,* Jejunopharyngeal and jejunoesophageal anastomoses and arterial and venous microvascular anastomoses completed. (From DeSanto, L.W., Pearson, B.W., and Fisher, J.: Reconstruction of the pharynx and cervical esophagus. *In* Otolaryngology, Vol. 4. Edited by G.M. English. Philadelphia, Harper & Row, Publishers, 1983, p. 1.)

Technique

Jejunal Procurement

Simultaneously with the cervical laryngopharyngectomy procedure, a second surgical team performs laparotomy and identifies a suitable segment of jejunum approximately 40 cm distal to the ligament of Treitz (Fig. 41–1*B*). This point is selected on the basis of both a suitable caliber of bowel and an adequate length of mesenteric vessels for subsequent anastomosis. The isolated segment of jejunum to be used for reconstruction is allowed to perfuse on a single vascular pedicle of mesenteric artery and vein until the time of transfer to minimize the warm ischemic period. Small bowel continuity can be immediately restored by end-to-end jejunostomy, and the mesenteric defect is closed after the isolated jejunum is transferred.

Jejunal Transfer and Microvascular Anastomosis

After the defect in the pharyngeal or esophageal continuity is well defined and sites for proximal and distal bowel anastomosis are well exposed, suitable recipient vessels in the neck are prepared. If the transfer is low in the neck, the preferred arterial recipient vessel is the transverse cervical artery. In the midneck, the external carotid or one of its branches is used (Fig. 41–1*C*) or, in some cases, an end-to-side microvascular anastomosis is made to the common carotid artery. In the upper neck area, the external carotid system is used. An end-to-side venous anastomosis between the mesenteric vein and the internal jugular vein is usually preferred.

After the sites for proposed bowel and vascular anastomoses are prepared, the jejunal segment is transferred to the neck by division of the mesenteric vascular pedicle in the abdomen. Care must be taken to maintain an isoperistaltic orientation of the jejunal segment to be transferred. The proximal bowel anastomosis in the neck is created first, because it is the more difficult one and tends to stabilize the jejunum and permit orientation of the vascular pedicle for subsequent microvascular anastomosis without tension or angulation. The bowel anastomosis in the neck is formed with a single circumferential layer of multiple interrupted 3–0 polyglactin 910—Vicryl—sutures. Warm ischemia is well tolerated by the jejunum for up to 3 hours, more than enough time to effect microvascular anastomosis and reperfusion. The vascular anastomoses are all made by standard microvascular technique with 8–0 to 10–0 nylon monofilament sutures, depending on vessel size. Systemic anticoagulation, hypothermia, and vascular flushing are not used. After the vascular anastomoses have been created, occluding microvascular clamps are released, and the jejunal segment is allowed to be reperfused. The distal jejunal bowel anastomosis is then effected in the same manner as the proximal one (Fig. 41–1*C*).

PHARYNGOESOPHAGEAL RECONSTRUCTION WITH INTACT LARYNX

Absence of the larynx and pharynx greatly facilitates the technique of free jejunal transfer, but this situation does not exist when a functioning larynx is to be preserved. The larynx can usually be preserved when free jejunal transfer is used in the repair of benign traumatic cervical esophageal or pharyngeal stenoses or for longer, more distal reconstructions in which a microvascular anastomosis procedure is performed in the neck.

Our basic method is to approach the pharynx and cervical esophagus through an oblique left cervical incision parallel to the anterior border of the sternocleidomastoid muscle. With retraction of the carotid sheath laterally, the retropharyngeal-prevertebral space is entered just cephalad to the omohyoid. The larynx is rotated medially, and the site of stenosis is identified by passing a rubber bougie down the esophagus from the mouth. With the site of the stricture identified, the cervical esophagus or pharynx is incised, and the stricture is removed circumferentially.

If the site of resection is low in the neck or if the site of distal jejunal anastomosis is in the upper chest, exposure is enhanced by division of the strap muscles—omohyoid, sternohyoid, and sternothyroid—and interruption of ipsilateral thyroid vessels.

To gain access for still lower intrathoracic anastomoses, one can disconnect the sternocleidomastoid muscle from its sternoclavicular origin, divide the manubrium in the midline, and remove its ipsilateral half en bloc with the medial two thirds of the clavicle and anterior end of the first rib. This technique of exposure, as we (J.F., W.S.P.) and associates (1984) described, permits easy access to the upper end of a partially sloughed substernal colon; also, the upper end of the native esophagus can be dependably exposed for anastomosis as low as the T4 level

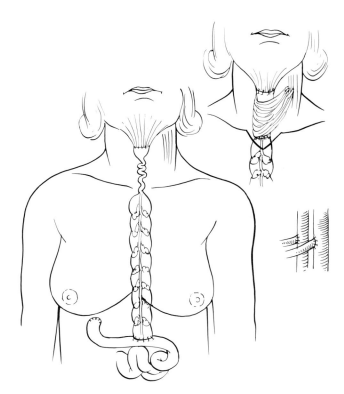

Fig. 41–3. A 68-year-old woman with previous total esophagogastrectomy reconstructed with colon sustained ischemic necrosis of the cephalad end of the colon. Esophageal continuity was reconstructed with free jejunal transfer. Recipient vessels were the common carotid and internal jugular. (From Payne, W.S., and Fisher, J., 1988. By permission of W.B. Saunders Co.)

if the ipsilateral internal mammary vessels are also divided.

Experience suggests that full-length median sternotomy is not a desirable incision for exposure of substernal colon or gastric remnant or for the placement of free jejunum transfer, because sternal closure is difficult under these circumstances. The technique for free jejunal transfer is as previously described.

PREOPERATIVE EVALUATION FOR COMPLEX RECONSTRUCTIONS

Examples of some of our more complex applications of free jejunal transfer or microvascular augmentation of pedicled colonic interposition are shown in Figures 41–2 through 41–6. Figure 41–7 shows the use of the technique after a partial failure of reversed gastric tube. Thorough preoperative evaluation of these patients, who have complex reconstruction problems, is essential. Although we have gained confidence in the reliability of microvascular techniques in preserving or augmenting the blood supply of interposed bowel, we believe it is important to define potential alternative methods of reconstruction preoperatively. Such planning is especially important for patients who have undergone multiple operations and in whom preconceived strategies may

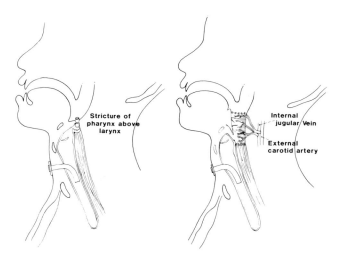

Fig. 41–2. An 18-year-old man sustained a mandibular fracture and neck injury in a vehicle accident and required tracheotomy and repair of the fracture. Subsequently, inability to swallow or phonate developed, and he became dependent on tracheostomy for airway and gastrostomy for feeding. Examination revealed almost complete stenosis of the pharynx at the level of the epiglottis. At cervical exploration, retrograde passage of a bougie up the esophagus from the gastrostomy established the site of stricture. The stricture and a portion of pharynx, supraglottic larynx, and epiglottis were excised. The defect was repaired with free jejunal transfer. (From McCaffrey, T.V., and Fisher, J.: Repair of traumatic cervical esophageal stenosis using microvascular free jejunum transfer. Ann. Otol. Rhinol. Laryngol. 93:512, 1984. By permission of Annals Publishing Company.)

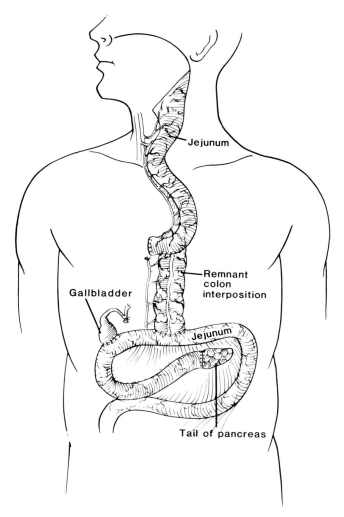

Fig. 41–4. A 55-year-old man with a self-inflicted severe lye burn required emergency esophagectomy, gastrectomy, and pancreaticoduodenectomy. Six months later, substernal colonic interposition was carried out with ischemic slough of the upper half. The pharyngocolonic defect was reconstructed with free transfer of a 25-cm segment of jejunum. (From Payne, W.S., and Fisher, J., 1988. By permission of W.B. Saunders Co.)

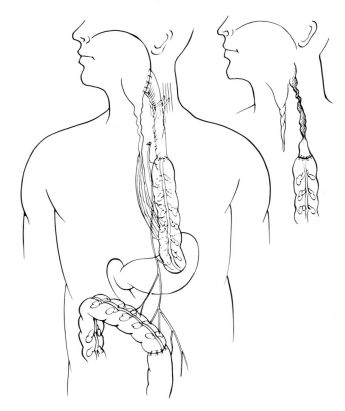

Fig. 41–5. A 44-year-old man who accidentally ingested nitric acid sustained severe strictures at the cricopharyngeus and throughout the cervical esophagus. Subsequent colonic interposition sloughed the cervical and pharyngeal portions. Attempts at tubed deltopectoral flap reconstruction also necrosed. Free jejunal transfer successfully restored the pharyngocolonic defect. (From Payne, W.S., and Fisher, J., 1988. By permission of W.B. Saunders Co.)

prove to be infeasible at the time of exploration. Thus, we thoroughly evaluate the entire gastrointestinal tract before operation, using contrast radiographic and endoscopic techniques to explore all sinuses, fistulas, and stomas as well as normal enteric orifices. Occasionally, we use selective angiography if the integrity of critical visceral vessels is in question because of previous operation or disease. Additionally, mechanical and antibiotic preparation of the large bowel is often desirable before operation, even though it is not required for jejunal transfer per se.

The basic precept must be maintained that the patient is to have successful reconstruction; the specific method to be used is of little consequence to the patient so long as it is effective. In this context, free jejunal transfer and microvascular circulatory augmentation have become important, but not exclusive, methods of reconstruction.

A major consideration is the maintenance of airway and speech. Many of our patients had part or all of the larynx intact, and problems with aspiration and airway, access during operation, and wound closure were taken into consideration preoperatively.

Preoperative evaluation also includes oculoplethysmography with sequential bilateral carotid occlusion to determine the adequacy of cross-circulation if use of the common carotid as the recipient vessel is a possibility. Impaired cross-circulation is a contraindication to the use of the common carotid artery. Even though good collateral circulation has been demonstrated preoperatively, intraoperative electroencephalographic monitoring is used when the common carotid is to be occluded for microvascular anastomosis.

RESULTS

Among 40 patients who underwent esophageal reconstruction with microvascular techniques, only two deaths occurred, one related to inta-abdominal sepsis and the other to cerebral edema in a patient with previous irradiation and bilateral neck dissections in whom the internal jugular veins had been sacrificed bilaterally. Mi-

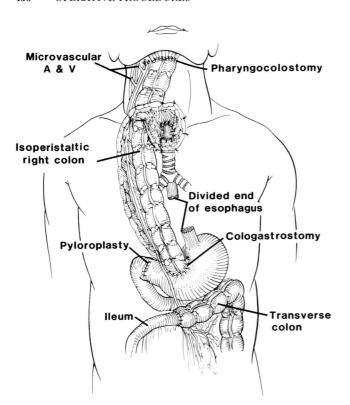

Fig. 41–6. A 43-year-old man sustained severe radiation injury to the neck during treatment of a lymphoma. Larynx, pharynx, cervical esophagus, and overlying skin were sloughed. In addition, there was a long, continuous fistulous communication between the thoracic esophagus and the full length of membranous trachea. The esophagus was reconstructed by a subcutaneously placed isoperistaltic right colonic segment between the base of the tongue and the stomach. To prevent gastric reflux aspiration through a large tracheo-esophageal fistula, the esophagogastric junction was interrupted. Because pedicled colon was to be anastomosed to heavily irradiated pharyngeal tissues, the ileocecal artery and vein were anastomosed to common carotid and internal jugular vessels to augment perfusion of middle colonic vessels. Additionally, this maneuver permitted application of split-thickness skin graft to cover the cervical portion of the colon. The introitus of the tracheo-esophageal stoma was lined with pedicled omentum with split-thickness skin graft to effect complete epithelial coverage of the stoma. (From Payne, W.S., and Fisher, J., 1988. By permission of W.B. Saunders Co.)

crovascular anastomoses remained patent in all but two patients, both of whom had pre-existing postirradiation changes in the neck that made vascular anastomoses particularly difficult to create and that caused thrombosis and loss of graft. In both of these patients, alternative reconstructions were effected. When the common carotid artery was used as the site for arterial microvascular anastomosis, cerebral complications did not occur. Of the 38 surviving patients, all but one resumed a normal oral diet. The single exception was a patient who was being nutritionally supported by a jejunostomy feeding tube at the time of the report. Although the continuity of his alimentary tract had been restored, extensive oral, lingual, and oropharyngeal scarring from caustic injury prevented initiation of swallowing.

Microvascular surgical techniques have been most ap-

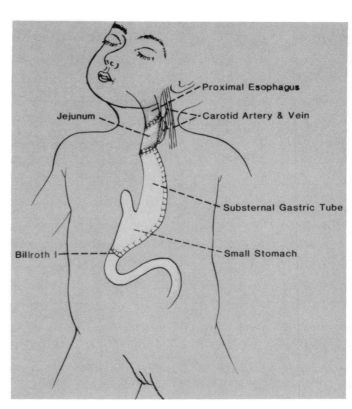

Fig. 41–7. An infant with esophageal agenesis underwent esophageal reconstruction in which the reversed gastric tube procedure of Gavriliu was done. Because of subsequent ischemic stenosis at the cervical esophagogastrostomy site, the patient required free jejunal transfer to the neck to restore continuity and swallowing. (From Fisher, J., et al.: Microvascular surgery in esophageal reconstruction. Plast. Reconstr. Surg. In press. By permission of the American Society of Plastic and Reconstructive Surgeons.)

plicable in esophageal reconstruction for patients with complex reconstruction problems. Sixteen of 17 patients so managed have had complete and successful restoration of swallowing under circumstances in which multiple previous standard techniques had failed.

We believe that successful management of complex reconstruction problems requires a multidisciplinary approach that includes not only the thoracic surgeon and the microvascular surgeon but also often a laryngologist.

Although we have gained confidence in the reliability of microvascular techniques, we believe that the final goal should always be successful reconstruction. Thus, alternative strategies need to be considered for the individual patient, and preparation for them should be made before the operation, because operative findings occasionally preclude preconceived plans. The goal is always restoration of anatomic continuity and functional swallowing. Microvascular techniques merely provide an added, but important, means to that end.

REFERENCES

Androsov, P.E., et al.: Cited by Chang T.-S., Hwang, O.-L., and Wang-Wei: Reconstruction of esophageal defects with microsurgically revascularized jejunal segments: a report of 13 cases. J. Microsurg. 2:83, 1980.

Carrel, A.: The surgery of blood vessels, etc. Johns Hopkins Hosp. Bull. 18:18, 1907.

Chang, T.-S., Hwang, O.-L., and Wang-Wei: Reconstruction of esophageal defects with microsurgically revascularized jejunal segments: a report of 13 cases. J. Microsurg. 2:83, 1980.

DeSanto, L.W., and Carpenter, R.J.: Reconstruction of the pharynx and upper esophagus after resection for cancer. Head Neck Surg. 2:369, 1980.

DeSanto, L.W., Pearson, B.W., and Fisher, J.: Reconstruction of the pharynx and cervical esophagus. In Otolaryngology. Vol. 4, Chapt. 43. Edited by G.M. English. Philadelphia, Harper & Row, Publishers, 1983, p. 1.

Fisher, J., Payne, W.S., and Irons, G.B., Jr.: Salvage of a failed colon interposition in the esophagus with a free jejunal graft. Mayo Clin. Proc. 59:197, 1984.

Gluckman, J.L., and McDonough, J., Donegan, J.O.: The role of the free jejunal graft in reconstruction of the pharynx and cervical esophagus. Head Neck Surg. 4:360, 1982.

Hester, T.R., Jr., et al.: Reconstruction of cervical esophagus, hypopharynx, and oral cavity using free jejunal transfer. Am. J. Surg. 140:487, 1980.

Hiebert, C.A., and Cummings, G.O., Jr.: Successful replacement of the cervical esophagus by transplantation and revascularization of a free graft of gastric antrum. Ann. Surg. 154:103, 1961.

Hopkins, D.M., and Bernatz, P.E.: Experimental replacement of the cervical esophagus. Arch. Surg. 87:265, 1963.

Jurkiewicz, M.J.: Vascularized intestinal graft for reconstruction of the cervical esophagus and pharynx. Plast. Reconstr. Surg. 36:509, 1965.

Jurkiewicz, M.J.: Reconstructive surgery of the cervical esophagus. J. Thorac. Cardiovasc. Surg. 88:893, 1984.

Katsaros, J., and Tan, E.: Free bowel transfer for pharyngoesophageal reconstruction: an experimental and clinical study. Br. J. Plast. Surg. 35:268, 1982.

Longmire, W.P., Jr.: A modification of the Roux technique for antethoracic esophageal reconstruction: anastomosis of the mesenteric and internal mammary blood vessels. Surgery 22:94, 1974.

McKee, D.M., and Peters, C.R.: Reconstruction of the hypopharynx and cervical esophagus with microvascular jejunal transplant. Clin. Plast. Surg. 5:305, April 1978.

Nakayama, K., et al.: Experience with free autografts of the bowel with a new venous anastomosis apparatus. Surgery 55:796, 1964.

Payne, W.S., and Fisher, J.: Esophageal reconstruction: free jejunal transfer or circulatory augmentation of pedicled intestinal interpositions using microvascular surgery. In International Trends in General Thoracic Surgery, Vol. 4. Malignant Esophageal Disease. Edited by E.W. Wilkins, Jr. and Wong, J. Philadelphia, W.B. Saunders Co., 1988, p. 250.

Peters, C.R., McKee, D.M., and Berry, B.E.: Pharyngoesophageal reconstruction with revascularized jejunal transplants. Am. J. Surg. 121:675, 1971.

Roberts, R.E., and Douglass, F.M.: Replacement of the cervical esophagus and hypopharynx by a revascularized free jejunal autograft: report of a case successfully treated. N. Engl. J. Med. 264:342, 1961.

Seidenberg, B., et al.: Immediate reconstruction of the cervical esophagus by a revascularized isolated jejunal segment. Ann. Surg. 149:162, 1959.

Thoracic Trauma

CHAPTER 42

TRAUMA TO CHEST WALL, PLEURA, AND THORACIC VISCERA

Jeffrey Swanson and Donald D. Trunkey

CHEST WALL TRAUMA

Fractures

Chest wall trauma, the most common chest injury, occurs in about 40% of all patients admitted with torso injuries. Most of these patients have minor injuries, such as rib fractures, costochondral separation, fracture of the clavicle, and fracture of the sternum. In some instances rib fractures, particularly in the older individual, can be life-threatening. Older patients with rib fractures often splint, hypoventilate, and develop atelectasis that progresses to bronchopneumonia and death. For all of these reasons we are liberal in our criteria for admitting patients with chest trauma to the hospital, particularly older patients.

Fractures of the clavicle are common and rarely cause major pathophysiologic changes. Although painful, they usually do not embarrass ventilation and only rarely are associated with major vessel lacerations. Fractures of the sternum are being reported with increasing frequency and constitute 5 to 10% of all thoracic injuries. Part of this increased incidence may be caused by better recognition and physician awareness of the close association of fractured sternum with steering column trauma. Isolated sternal fractures do not usually cause major problems except pain. Because of the painful sequelae, they may require operative management, but isolated sternal fractures are uncommon and are usually associated with other significant chest wall trauma, including flail chest. The most common associated visceral injury is myocardial contusion, which can lead to significant arrhythmias and hemodynamic instability.

The scapula is uncommonly fractured. It is protected by a thick coat of muscle and lies in a protected position. Therefore, fractures of the scapula are associated with a significant amount of kinetic energy imparted to that portion of the body and should make the clinician suspicious of significant associated injuries. Fractures in-volving the glenoid fossa and acromion, however, may have significant pathophysiologic orthopedic consequences.

The one thing common to almost all injuries involving the bony thorax is pain. Pain, in and by itself, can lead to decreased ventilation, decreased vital capacity, inability to clear secretions, and retention of carbon dioxide. As more ribs are fractured, there is a progression of pathophysiologic findings, including ventilation/perfusion abnormalities, increase of respiratory work, hypoxemia, and a decrease in the functional residual capacity. These are especially common when multiple rib fractures result in flail chest; the bellows action of the chest wall muscles reduces, leading to further abnormalities in ventilation. If the flail segment is large enough, this segment may collapse during inspiration, shifting the mediastinum toward the contralateral side on inspiration, with a concomitant obstruction to venous return to the heart. Negative intrathoracic pressure is reduced, contributing to decreased ventilation.

Schall (1979) and Landercasper (1984) and their associates pointed out the significance of associated injuries and chest wall trauma. Some investigators believe that these may be the primary pathophysiology. Clearly, they do contribute, but we believe that they are not necessarily primary. The most common associated injury is pulmonary contusion, which is associated with ventilation/perfusion abnormalities, but Craven and colleagues (1979) reported that this may be less than previously appreciated. There is an associated atelectasis and shunting of blood in the larger contusions, either of the chest wall or the lung. Compliance decreases and airway resistance increases; the associated decrease in pulmonary diffusion and increase in respiratory work is additive to that contributed by the chest wall defect. Ultimately, the combination of the pain, the decrease in ventilation, and the sequelae of the associated injuries lead to retention of carbon dioxide, hypoxemia, and respiratory insufficiency.

The history can be crucial in diagnosing chest wall injury, even in the unconscious patient. The paramedics should be questioned about the mechanism of injury and the character of the patient's breathing during transport. If the patient was extricated from behind the steering wheel, a strong suspicion of chest wall injury should be entertained. The paramedics' observations and treatment should be carefully noted and often direct the resuscitating surgeon to life-threatening airway and chest wall injuries.

In the conscious patient, the hallmark of chest wall injury is pain, which is often aggravated by coughing, deep breathing, and change of body position. Signs of minor chest wall injuries include localized palpable tenderness and compression pain. In addition, crepitation may be either palpated or auscultated.

In moderate and severe chest wall injuries, in addition to the pain, ventilatory insufficiency is common. Specific signs of ventilatory insufficiency include air hunger, cyanosis, use of the accessory muscles of ventilation, and a ventilatory rate faster than 25 per minute. Less specific manifestations include those of a generalized symphathetic discharge; anxiety, fear, agitation, tachycardia, and cold, clammy skin. If the injury is severe, there may be a flail chest either laterally or anteriorly. Observation usually confirms the presence of paradoxic motion of the chest wall with inspiration and expiration. Many patients with flail chest do not manifest the problem initially, underscoring the need for repeated examinations of those patients with chest wall pain.

Chest roentgenograms have limited value and use in the diagnosis of chest wall injury. In our experience, up to 50% of rib fractures are not evident on plain roentgenograms. Their routine use is advocated primarily to identify associated injuries, particularly intrathoracic visceral complications. Other laboratory tests may be valuable, particularly if there are signs of ventilatory insufficiency. We advocate routine blood gas determinations. A carbon dioxide tension >40 mm Hg in an acutely injured patient who does not have a documented chronic hypercapnia must be taken as absolute evidence of ventilatory insufficiency. Hypoxemia usually indicates associated lung injury. Vital capacity and inspiratory force are also useful measurements in the patient with chest wall injury, but are not usually performed in the emergency room. Parenchymal lung function can be assessed by computed tomography, oxygen tension to fractional inspired oxygen ratio, shunt fraction, and compliance, but most of these require invasive monitoring and are performed in the intensive care unit.

Open Chest Wound

The diagnosis of open chest wound should be obvious. In addition to the local wound pain, there may be signs of ventilatory insufficiency if the patient has an associated pneumothorax. The larger the pneumothorax, the more significant ventilatory insufficiency is. If the open pneumothorax is large, there is often associated hissing noise with inspiratory and expiratory movement. A bloody froth is characteristic of air escaping from the open wound during expiration.

Tension Pneumothorax

The diagnosis of tension pneumothorax can be difficult in a noisy emergency room. The classic signs are decreased breath sounds and percussion tympany on the ipsilateral side and tracheal shift to the contralateral side. Confirmation is by chest roentgenogram. In the patient who appears dead or dying, we do not hesitate to insert chest tubes bilaterally. Tube thoracostomy is a benign procedure that can be life-saving when the diagnosis of a tension pneumothorax is inconclusive.

Hemothorax

The diagnosis of massive hemothorax is invariably made by the presence of shock, ventilatory embarrassment, and contralateral shift of the mediastinum. Roentgenograms of the chest confirm the extensive blood loss, but most of the time tube thoracostomy has been done immediately to relieve the threat of ventilatory embarrassment. If a gush of blood is obtained when the chest tube is placed, the tube should be clamped immediately and autotransfusion considered. The simple devices for this should be in all major trauma resuscitation centers. The only contraindication to autotransfusion is suspected associated hollow viscus injury. Lesser degrees of hemothorax are usually diagnosed by routine chest roentgenograms. We recommend tube thoracostomy for any patient who has roentgenographic evidence of fluid in the chest after trauma.

Airway Disruption

Hemoptysis, airway obstruction, progressive mediastinal air, subcutaneous emphysema, tension pneumothorax, and persistent, massive air leak after placement of a chest tube suggest disruption of the tracheobronchial tree. Bronchoscopy is mandatory in all cases of suspected tracheobronchial injury, not only to confirm the diagnosis but also to direct the surgeon to the proper hemithorax for surgical treatment.

Pulmonary Contusion

The diagnosis of pulmonary contusion can be difficult because the standard chest roentgenograms miss approximately one third of the injuries. They may become evident later in the patient's course or may be diagnosed earlier by CT scan. We have been impressed with the efficacy of CT scan for abdominal injuries, and in so doing have found several patients with unsuspected pulmonary contusions and even traumatic pneumatoceles. We do not, however, advocate routine CT scan for the diagnosis of pulmonary contusion.

Air Embolism

Thomas (1973), Yee (1983) and Paris (1975) and their associates reported that air embolism often follows penetrating and blunt chest injury. In our experience it occurs in 4% of all major thoracic trauma cases. Sixty-five percent of cases result from penetrating injuries to the chest and 35% of cases from blunt chest trauma, almost invariably because of lacerations of the lung secondary to rib fractures. Between 1975 and 1988 we treated over 100 cases of air embolism.

The key to diagnosis is to have a high index of suspicion. The pathophysiology is a fistula between a bronchus and the pulmonary vein. Those patients who are breathing spontaneously have a pressure differential from the pulmonary vein to the bronchus that causes approximately 22% of patients to have hemoptysis on presentation. If, however, the patient has a Valsalva-type respiration, grunts, or is intubated with positive pressure in the bronchus, the pressure differential is from the bronchus to the pulmonary vein, causing systemic air embolism. These patients present in one of three ways: focal or lateralizing neurologic signs, sudden cardiovascular collapse, and froth when the initial arterial blood specimen is obtained. Any patient who has obvious chest injury but does not have obvious head injury, and yet has focal or lateralizing neurologic findings, should be assumed to have air embolism. Confirmation can be obtained by fundoscopic examination showing air in the retinal vessels. Patients who are intubated and have a sudden unexplained cardiovascular collapse with absence of vital signs should immediately be assumed to have air embolism to the coronary vessels. Finally, those patients who have a frothy blood sample drawn for an initial blood gas determination have air embolism. When a patient comes into the emergency room in extremis and an emergency thoracotomy is carried out, air should always be looked for in the coronary vessels. If this is found, the hilum of the offending lung should be immediately clamped to reduce the ingress of air into the vessels.

TREATMENT OF SPECIFIC INJURIES

Chest Wall Injuries

The treatment of chest wall and associated injuries depends on a stepwise prioritization of the patient's problems. The first prioritization takes place immediately on seeing the patient. Within a few seconds, it can be determined whether the patient is hemodynamically stable or unstable, conscious or unconscious, and whether or not the patient has ventilatory insufficiency. In general, the unconscious patient or the patient who is hemodynamically unstable requires almost immediate airway intubation and the establishment of ventilation. The timing depends on the severity and the cause of the injuries. Once the airway is established and ventilation ensured, other emergency treatment should be carried out. Open pneumothoraces should be closed with occlusive dressings. Flail segments of the chest wall should be stabilized by endotracheal intubation or mechanical ventilation or temporarily by placing sandbags next to the flail segment or by turning the patient so that the flail segment is against the mattress. Chest tubes should be inserted to evacuate pneumothoraces and massive hemothoraces. If the patient becomes unstable, further

treatment is best carried out in the operating room. If, on the other hand, the patient is stabilized, further diagnostic studies can be undertaken and treatment planned accordingly.

In the conscious hemodynamically stable patient, prioritization of treatment is based on pain, the absence or presence of ventilatory insufficiency, and associated injuries. In general, most patients with rib fractures require hospitalization for control of the pain and a period of observation to rule out associated injuries and complications of the pain.

There is no simple approach to treatment of patients with chest wall injuries. In general, we direct our attention to the treatment of pain, the presence or absence of ventilatory insufficiency, and the chest wall defect. The patient may have one or all of these problems, and therefore treatment must be individually tailored.

In general, strapping of the chest is not advocated, because it may promote atelectasis and reduce vital capacity. At times it may reduce pain and aid the patient in coughing sufficiently so that the benefit outweighs the theoretical disadvantages. Occasionally, patients with single rib fractures are managed effectively with oral analgesics, but again caution should be exercised, because most narcotics may adversely affect ventilation and clearing of secretions. Most patients with pain as their primary problem should be managed with intercostal nerve blocks or other regional analgesia. Administration of 0.5 to 1.0% lidocaine with 1:100,000 epinephrine around the intercostal nerve to the involved segment is advised. Usually the intercostal nerve above and below the injury should be injected. An alternative is to use bupivacaine hydrochloride, which can provide longer relief. Repeated injections may be necessary to achieve adequate ventilation and cough. In more severe injuries, continuous epidural analgesia has been useful. An alternative is to use epidural morphine, but both of these procedures usually require constant monitoring in a critical care unit.

Occasionally, operative treatment is indicated for minor to moderate chest wall injuries. Examples would include separation of the costochondral junction and sternal fractures. Costochondral separation may not heal because of poor blood supply. In such instances, excision of the cartilage may give dramatic relief of the pain. Sternal fractures are also associated with significant pain and may be unstable. In both instances an operative approach and wiring of the fracture reduces morbidity.

Operative management of chest wall injuries falls into two categories: treatment for open pneumothorax and for rib and sternal fractures. The treatment of open chest wounds depends on the extent and wounding agent. In general, stab wounds and low velocity gunshot wounds usually require simple skin debridement and irrigation, allowing the wound to heal secondarily or to do delayed primary closure on the fifth postinjury day. More extensive wounds, particularly those from shotgun blasts, require major debridement and removal of foreign bodies, bone fragments, and wadding from the shell. If the wound is extensive enough that closure is impossible, a myocutaneous flap may be valuable. Pectoralis muscle, latissimus dorsi, and rectus abdominis flaps all lend themselves to covering chest wall defects (see Chapter 51). Synthetic materials, such as Marlex, are not used as commonly as they once were because of the advent of the more satisfactory myocutaneous flaps.

Operative stabilization of rib fractures is not a new technique, but Paris (1975), Schmit-Neuerburg (1982) and Thomas (1978) and their co-workers suggested that its use be reinstituted in an effort to reduce morbidity or mortality in severe flail chest injuries. It is used most advantageously when thoracotomy is required to treat associated injuries. There are many techniques for stabilizing rib fractures, including Kirschner wires and the use of wire suture and steel plates. Besson and Saegesser (1983) reported the use of staples to stabilize the fractures. Our own experience has been confined primarily to plates that have been placed across flail segments. We have had no experience with the Russian UKL staple or the Judet staples. Our technique is to use plates on every other rib and to secure the adjacent rib to the strutted rib with a polyglycolate suture. Soft tissue consisting of muscle and subcutaneous tissue is then closed over the plate using monofilament sutures. The wounds are irrigated with antibiotic solutions—kanamycin and bacitracin. In our experience, operative stabilization has minimized the duration of mechanical ventilation and the consequent complications. The rationale is to minimize ventilator time when a chest wall injury is the primary reason for its use. It will not be of major benefit when the primary indication for mechanical ventilation is the parenchymal lung injury or associated neurologic injuries.

Ventilatory insufficiency can be categorized as minor, moderate, or severe. Most importantly from a treatment standpoint, we can divide treatment into ventilatory and nonventilatory support. The indications for ventilatory management are shown in Table 42–1. If at all possible, it is best to avoid ventilator therapy, because chronic intubation and the use of ventilators sets the stage for major complications, primarily pulmonary sepsis. If the patient meets the criteria outlined in Table 42–1, however, there is often no other recourse. Aggressive conservative management, on the other hand, may prevent the patient with moderate ventilatory insufficiency from falling into the severe category. This treatment includes adequate relief of pain, nasotracheal suction, incentive respirometers, chest physiotherapy, and supplemental oxygen to maintain the oxen tension above 60 mm Hg.

Trinkle and associates (1975) discussed some controversial adjunctive measures in treating ventilatory insufficiency, including restriction of intravenous fluids, steroids, diuretics, and salt-poor albumin. None of these adjuctive measures is necessary. The resuscitation of the trauma patient should be based on maintaining flow to the critical organs, and this is best determined by keeping atrial filling pressures as near normal as possible, maintaining adequate urinary output—>0.5 ml/kg/hr, and reversing the clinical signs of shock. Once the patient has been resuscitated, fluid management should be based on replacing sensible and insensible losses. Keeping the patient "dry" does not selectively reduce edema in the chest wall or in parenchymal lung injuries. The efficacy of diuretics in treating chest wall injuries and underlying pulmonary contusions is unproved. It is unrealistic to think that contusions of the chest wall or the lung can be selectively "dehydrated." The injudicious use of diuretics may give the patient volume depletion and embarrass renal function. The administration of salt-poor albumin is equally controversial and Lucas and colleagues (1980), in one randomized study, showed that its use adversely affects mortality and morbidity. Steroid use is controversial; not a single randomized study demonstrates its efficacy. Most studies show detrimental side effects of the steroids, including increased infection rates and impaired wound healing.

Tension Pneumothorax

The treatment of tension pneumothorax is tube thoracostomy. After the initial chest tube has been placed it is prudent to obtain an immediate chest film to assess the adequate removal of air and the position of the tube. Persistent air leak should alert the surgeon that there may be significant visceral injury that requires operative intervention.

Hemothorax

The treatment of hemothorax is to restore blood volume and evacuate the hemothorax by closed-tube thoracostomy. If for any reason blood accumulates after initial

Table 42–1. Indications for Mechanical Ventilation

	Normal	Ventilator Indicated
Ventilatory		
Respirations	12–20	>35
Carbon dioxide tension	35–40 torr	>50 torr
Vital capacity	65–70 ml/kg	<10–15 ml/kg
Maximum inspiratory force	−75 to 100 cm H_2O	<−25 cm H_2O
Parenchymal		
Alveolar to arterial oxygen tension difference	50–75 torr	>350 torr
Shunt	<5%	>15%
Wasted ventilation (Vd/Vt)	0.4–0.4	>0.6
Compliance	40–50 ml/cm H_2O	<30 ml/cm H_2O

chest tube placement and cannot be removed, another chest tube is inserted. Using this technique we had to perform only 3 decortications between 1977 and 1987.

In the presence of a massive hemothorax, essentially all such patients require emergent thoracotomy. Our indications for thoracotomy are an initial blood loss of >1000 ml or a blood loss of 250 ml/hr for 3 hours, or more than 1500 ml over a 24-hour period. In approximately 85% of patients with massive hemothorax, a systemic vessel such as an intercostal artery or an internal mammary artery has been injured. The hilum of the lung or the myocardium may be injured. In about 15% of instances, the bleeding is from deep pulmonary lacerations resulting either from fractured ribs or penetration by missiles; these injuries are treated by oversewing the lesion or in some instances resecting a segment or lobe.

Air Embolism

The treatment of air embolism is immediate thoracotomy, preferably in the operating room. Many of these patients have emergency-room thoracotomies. In most cases we open the left chest, because the diagnosis has usually not been made and we are simply attempting resuscitation. If the patient has an obvious right chest injury such as flail chest or penetration, it is appropriate to open that hemithorax first if air embolism is suspected and the patient is in extremis. If the left chest is open, air is found in the coronary vessels, and there is no obvious left lung injury, the sternum is transected and the right chest opened and the hilum of the right lung clamped. Definitive treatment is to oversew the lacerations of the lung, and in some instances a lobectomy and rarely a pneumonectomy may be required. Other resuscitative measures in patients who have had cardiac arrest from air embolism include internal cardiac massage and reaching up and holding the ascending aorta with the thumb and index finger for one or two beats—this tends to push air out of the coronary vessels and thus reestablishes perfusion. One milliliter of 1:1000 epinephrine can be injected intravenously or down the endotracheal tube to provide an alpha-adrenergic effect, driving air out of the systemic microcirculation. It is prudent to vent the left atrium and ventricle as well as the ascending aorta to remove all residual air once the hilum of the injured lung has been clamped. This prevents further air embolism when the patient is moved. Using aggressive diagnosis and treatment a 55% salvage can be achieved in patients with air embolism secondary to penetrating trauma and 20% salvage in patients with air embolism from blunt trauma.

Tracheobronchial Tree Lacerations

Treatment for tracheal bronchial injuries is straightforward. An airway must be established. After broncho-scopic confirmation, the appropriate posterior lateral thoracotomy is performed.*

INJURIES TO THE HEART

The spectrum of traumatic injury of the heart runs from the inconsequential to the immediately catastrophic.

Blunt cardiac injury is thought to occur by one of several mechanisms, including a direct blow to the precordium, compression between the sternum and the vertebral column, differential deceleration, or indirectly by a rapid increase in chamber hydrostatic pressure related to abdominal and lower extremity compression. Blunt cardiac trauma only became frequent with the advent of high speed motor vehicles. In fact, Lasky (1963) reported that 17% of "moderate" motor vehicle accident traumas result in injury to the heart, and Sigler (1945) noted that this figure reaches 76% of those "severely" injured.

In Parmley's (1958c) series of 546 patients with fatal blunt cardiac injury, 64% had suffered rupture of one or more chambers and 50% had associated multiple organ injuries. Dow (1982) reported associated aortic disrup-

---

*Editor's footnote: Deslauriers (1987) stated that 80% of traumatic tracheobronchial tears occur within 2.5 cm of the tracheal carina; lobar or segmental bronchi are seldom affected. Unless the tear or complete disruption is distal in the left bronchial tree, all these injuries, including those of the left main stem bronchus—within 2 to 2.5 cm of the tracheal carina—are best repaired through the right chest because this affords the maximum exposure of the tracheal carina and the proximal portion of the left main stem bronchus as well as the right main stem bronchus. Anesthesia can be conducted through a double-lumen endotracheal tube, a long tube into the left bronchus for one-lung anesthesia when the injury is in the right bronchial tree or even at times more appropriately when available by high frequency jet ventilation.

The chest is entered through a standard posterolateral thoracotomy, and the superior mediastinum and posterior hilar area are opened after ligature and division of the azygos vein. The tears or total bronchial disruption are identified and the edges of the margins of the injury debrided as necessary. Repair of the laceration or anastomosis of a completely divided bronchus is done by mucosal apposition with interrupted sutures of 0-3 or 0-4 Vicryl (see Chapter 30). The suture line is covered with adjacent tissue. A pleural flap, the mobilized pericardial fat pad, a percardial flap, or even a pedicled intercostal muscle flap can be used. When a distal bronchial repair cannot be done safely or is accompanied by a major vascular injury, resection is sometimes necessary.

Although the diagnosis of these injuries should be made shortly after the traumatic event, some of these injuries are missed initially and only recognized later by persistence of atelectasis of the ipsilateral lung (Fig. 42–1) or lobe or the development of pulmonary sepsis. Partial disruptions are more likely to lead to incomplete obstruction of the bronchial tree distal to the injury. This partial obstruction is prone to lead to recurrent or persistent infection with eventual destruction of the associated lung parenchyma. When this occurs, resection is almost always necessary.

Complete disruption most often results in total obstruction of the distal bronchial tree. Under these circumstances, infection rarely occurs and the distal, obstructed bronchial tree becomes filled with a clear, thick, tenacious mucoid material. This can be readily aspirated at the time of a late repair. Any late repairs may be technically difficult because of associated dense scar tissue in the area of injury. Excellent ventilatory function can be expected to return if the bronchial stenosis is resected and the continuity is re-established within a few weeks up to 6 months after the initial injury. Later repair may result in restoration of expansion of the involved lung, but its ventilatory functional status may be only partially recovered.

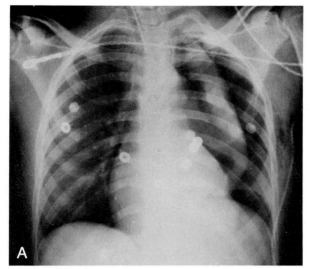

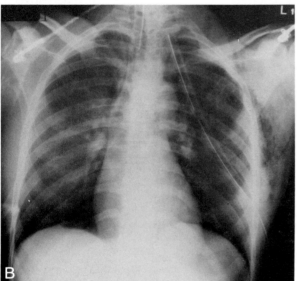

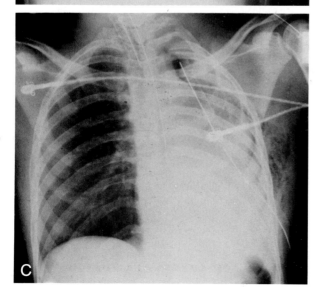

Fig. 42–1. *A*, Initial PA chest roentgenogram after severe blunt trauma; left pneumothorax and fractures of the first and second ribs posteriorly. *B*, Re-expansion of lung after closed tube thoracostomy with no air leak after first 6 hours. *C*, Subsequent complete collapse of left lung 48 hours later. Failure to expand; bronchoscopy subsequently revealed complete stenosis of left main stem bronchus. Thoracotomy revealed complete disruption of left main bronchus just proximal to upper lobe orifice. Primary repair of complete bronchial disruption 2 weeks after initial injury resulted in complete re-expansion and normal function of the left lung.

tion in 25% of patients with myocardial rupture. Sutherland (1983) and Harley (1983) and their colleagues showed that if they are systematically sought using sensitive radionuclide angiography, segmental wall motion abnormalities can be detected in 55 to 74% of patients sustaining multisystem trauma with blunt chest injury.

Whereas blunt injury from motor vehicle accidents is the most frequent cause of cardiac trauma in suburban and rural areas, urban populations are more susceptible to penetrating injury of the heart. Symbas (1976), Evans (1979), Trinkle (1974) and Sugg (1968) and their associates noted that although gunshot wounds are increasing in frequency, their immediate mortality is high and stab wounds are, therefore, still seen more frequently in the emergency room. Symbas (1976) and Evans (1979) and their associates pointed out that although all chambers of the heart may be injured, the relative frequency of involvement is related to their relative area of exposure to the anterior chest wall—ventricles more frequently injured than atria and right-sided chambers more frequently than left. As one would expect, gunshot wounds involve more than one chamber of the heart and have associated thoracic and intra-abdominal organ injuries more commonly than stab wounds. Evans (1979) and Richardson (1981) and their colleagues reported that gunshot wounds that traverse the mediastinum involve the heart in from 28% to 85% of cases.

The specific lesions suffered by the heart vary greatly depending on the wounding agent and the amount of energy imparted. Myocardial contusion is the most frequent result of blunt trauma to the heart. The incidence of this problem varies with the criteria used to make the diagnosis, but Jones (1975) and Saunders (1977) and their co-workers found an incidence of about 20% using electrocardiography in patients with blunt chest trauma. Harley (1983) and associates reported an incidence up to 74% with more sensitive evaluations of wall motion. Pathologically the contusion consists of patchy myocardial hemorrhage and cellular necrosis. Saunders and Doty (1977) stated that this differs from ischemic myocardial infarction by a more abrupt transition from normal to abnormal tissue and evolution toward more complete myocardial repair owing to normal coronary circulation. Utley and colleagues (1976) demonstrated experimentally a decrease in cardiac output that was directly proportional to the amount of contused myocardium. In addition to reducing hemodynamic performance, myocardial contusion can induce various arrhythmias that are usually atrial but may include ventricular arrhythmias. Conduction defects may also occur, but Sims and Geddes (1969) noted that high grade atrioventricular block appears to be rare.

Myocardial contusion usually heals, but with severe injury or underlying coronary compromise, transmural necrosis can occur. In these cases, the involved region can progress to secondary rupture or the formation of akinetic scar tissue or dyskinetic ventricular aneurysm.

Primary myocardial rupture is usually fatal. Sigler (1945) reported, however, that 10 to 30% of these patients survive at least 30 minutes, and Martin and as-sociates (1984) reported that in their series, cardiac rupture made up 0.5% of patients admitted with blunt injury. Dow (1982) pointed out that multiple chamber rupture occurs in 30% and disruption of the cardiac septa was present in 10% of the patients in Parmley and associates' (1958c) series. Most of the ventricular septal defects were located near the apex. Experimental evidence of Inkley and Barry (1985) indicated that ventricular ruptures occur predominantly when these chambers are compressed while maximally distended during end diastole. Kirsh and Sloan (1977) stated that atrial ruptures are thought to occur during systole with deep inspiration, but Martin and colleagues (1984) believe that tears at the cavoatrial or pulmonary venoatrial junction are more likely to be caused by differential deceleration.

Coronary artery injury is most frequent with penetrating trauma, but can occur in blunt accidents. Espada and associates (1975) noted that because of their anterior anatomic position, the anterior descending and the proximal right coronary arteries are the most frequently involved. The mechanism of blunt injury probably involves intimal disruption and secondary thrombosis. Laceration of a coronary artery is associated with intrapericardial bleeding and tamponade.

Distal infarction is the obvious sequel to coronary artery division, with the magnitude of the infarction related to the presence or absence of collateral circulation and how far proximally the artery is injured. Haas (1986) and Forker (1971) and their colleagues reported coronary artery fistula as a complication in survivors of both penetrating and blunt trauma.

Valvular incompetence can also complicate blunt and penetrating cardiac injury and may be overlooked in the presence of more serious wounds. In Parmley and associates' (1958c) autopsy series of 546 cases of nonpenetrating cardiac injury, 6% had valvular damage. Most of these had other, more serious, associated injuries. According to Kirsh and Sloan (1977) left-sided valves appear to be injured most frequently, and lesions consist of either leaflet tears or disruption of a portion of the subvalvular apparatus. The resulting heart failure is proportional to the degree of regurgitation and associated myocardial injury. Hurley and Mayfield (1986) and Cuadros and associates (1984) noted that tricuspid regurgitation is better tolerated than left-sided incompetence.

Kissane and Rose (1961) reported traumatic pericarditis may occur as an isolated injury and present with a typical friction rub and repolarization changes. This can produce a pericardial effusion that may be bloody. Tabatznik and Isaacs (1961) noted that it can evolve toward a Dressler's syndrome and Goldstein (1965) reported the occurrence of constrictive pericarditis. Similarly, the pericardium may be disrupted, especially along the left pleural surface. Hurley and Mayfield (1986) described herniation of the heart under these circumstances. More frequently, the pericardium assumes significance in trauma victims while remaining intact with underlying cardiac injury. Hemodynamic compromise from pericardial tamponade is common in this case, and although this is usually related to accumulation of blood around the heart, Cummings (1984) and Robinson (1985) and their associates have described the development of tension pneumopericardium. This latter phenomenon is most frequently related to an associated disruption of the tracheobronchial tree and is explained by persistence or re-establishment of perivascular, pleuropericardial communication.

Diagnosis

Survivors of serious cardiac injury frequently present with acute hemodynamic compromise related to hemorrhage, tamponade, or both. The predominance of one or the other is dictated by the relative integrity of the pericardium and the wounding agent. Exsanguination is the major presentation in 34% of gunshot wounds of the heart but only 9% of cardiac stab wounds. Penetrating wounds in any area that could involve the heart must be assumed to have done so. Blunt cardiac injury is less obvious and evidence of precordial trauma may be absent. This diagnosis must be considered in all steering wheel trauma and patients with a pattern of injury suggesting high energy attenuation. Physical examination in the acutely compromised patient may reveal limited ventilation related to traumatic hemothorax or distended neck veins and elevated central venous pressure—CVP—with tamponade. Subtle signs such as Beck's triad are rarely appreciated in the emergency setting.

In these patients a chest roentgenogram can help identify associated injury and verify the position of tubes and lines placed for resuscitation. The classic "water bottle" appearance of pericardial effusion is lacking. Transfer to the operating room should supersede any other diagnostic evaluation in these critical patients. If the diagnosis of tamponade is unclear, or if the patient's condition deteriorates, pericardiocentesis may be performed and a plastic IV catheter left in the pericardial space for diagnostic and temporary therapeutic purposes. In experienced hands a small, subxiphoid pericardiotomy can be performed as expeditiously as a pericardiocentesis and avoids the high percentage of false negative or false positive results seen with pericardiocentesis that Trinkle and associates (1974) reported. The use of pericardiocentesis for definitive treatment, as proposed by Blalock and Ravitch (1943), is currently of historic interest only.

Patients with more stable hemodynamics may have a more thorough evaluation. Electrocardiography may demonstrate repolarization changes, conduction abnormalities, or arrhythmias associated with myocardial contusion, but these changes may not be present for 12 to 24 hours after the injury and serial ECGs are therefore imperative. Similarly, the serum creatine kinase myocardial band—CK MB—is frequently elevated with myocardial injury, but the elevation of the enzyme may be delayed. Unfortunately, the CK MB fraction is not as specific to myocardium as was once thought, and Potkin and colleagues (1982) reported that these criteria are not perfectly reliable.

Two-dimensional echocardiography is an excellent means of evaluating patients with blunt cardiac trauma. Miller (1982) and King (1983) and their associates reported that this modality allows examination of wall motion and valve function, detection of pericardial fluid, and estimation of ejection fraction. The addition of Doppler technique can reveal regurgitant flow.

Scintigraphic techniques have also been employed in the evaluation of cardiac trauma. Technetium pyrophosphate scans are used to label intracellular hydroxyapatite in injured myocardial cells. Unfortunately, Brantigan and colleagues (1978), as well as Ridriguez and Shatney (1982) reported that the sensitivity of this test appears to be low. Sutherland (1983) and Harley (1983) and associates noted, on the contrary, that first-pass and multigated radionuclide angiography appears to be a sensitive means for determining focal wall-motion abnormalities and decreased right and left ventricular ejection fractions. These studies suggest that myocardial injury, particularly of the anteriorly situated right ventricle, is much more frequent than is recognized with other diagnostic tests. This modality also allows sequential examination to evaluate the extent of functional recovery with healing.

Further precision in monitoring the trauma victim's hemodynamic equilibrium can be obtained with a pulmonary artery catheter. A Swan-Ganz catheter should be considered for any patient with unexplained instability despite apparently adequate fluid resuscitation, particularly if there is any other reason to suspect cardiac injury. This device provides continuous evaluation of cardiac function at different right- and left-sided filling pressures, and Flanchbarm and co-workers (1986) stated that it is particularly useful in the patient with traumatic myocardial injury who must undergo emergency surgery for associated injuries. Traumatic left-right shunts can also be diagnosed if an oxygen saturation step-up is detected between the right atrium and the pulmonary artery.

Finally, cardiac catheterization with coronary angiography should be considered for patients with new heart murmurs, progressive heart failure, or unexpectedly compromised hemodynamics. This is particularly important if electrocardiographic evidence suggests coronary injury.

Management

In general, patients with severe chest trauma and possible cardiac injury should be managed in hospitals with facilities for autotransfusion and cardiopulmonary bypass and by personnel sophisticated in the surgery of the heart. Acutely unstable patients with cardiac injury should undergo immediate thoracotomy, ideally in the operating room. Those who present with exsanguination are generally explored through an anterolateral thoracotomy on the side of greatest bleeding. If intrapericardial injury is confirmed, this incision can be extended across the sternum into an opposite side interspace for better exposure of the heart. If, however, the presentation is one of acute pericardial tamponade, a median sternotomy incision is preferred for its better exposure of the arch vessels and superior postoperative ventilatory mechanics. In this latter situation a preliminary pericardiocentesis or subxiphoid pericardial window is frequently performed to allow temporary hemodynamic improvement for safer transport to the operating room and anesthetic induction. When the median sternotomy incision is chosen, both pleural spaces should be explored unless the wounding agent could not possibly have entered them.

Cardiac Wounds

Control of hemorrhage is the immediate goal and can frequently be achieved with simple digital compression of ventricular wounds. Atrial wounds may be less easily compressed and are sometimes better managed by application of a side-biting vascular clamp. If hemorrhage cannot be controlled because of the nature or location of the injury, cardiopulmonary bypass is mandatory, though the implications of systemic heparinization must be weighed heavily in the face of multiple associated injuries. In rare circumstances, inflow occlusion of both cavae with cardiac fibrillation provides dry conditions for a 2- to 3-minute repair.

The technique of repair of free-wall cardiac wounds is straightforward. Ventricular wounds are closed with 2-0 or 3-0 Dacron horizontal mattress sutures over felt pledgets. If the wound is near a coronary artery, the mattress suture should take purchase on the far side of the coronary and pass under the vessel to avoid compromise of the lumen. Atrial wounds are best closed with continuous 3-0 or 4-0 polypropylene.

Coronary Artery Injury

Laceration or division of a major coronary artery is most ideally managed with maintenance of distal circulation. Simple, anterior injuries can sometimes be managed by direct repair using magnification and carefully placed 7-0 polypropylene sutures. If this is not possible and the injury involves the proximal two thirds of a significant vessel, then proximal and distal ligation with distal coronary artery bypass grafting is the procedure of choice. Evans and colleagues (1979) stated that small or distal coronary artery branches may be suture ligated.

Intracardiac Injuries

Valvular injuries and traumatic septal defects are usually better tolerated and can be deferred for subacute management. Massive left-sided regurgitation or a large left-right shunt can, however, sometimes mandate urgent repair because of precipitous heart failure. These lesions are managed using standard cardiopulmonary bypass. Although prosthetic valves are frequently placed in these patients, conservative techniques of repair are ideally suited to these otherwise normal tissues and Cuadros and associates (1984) suggested that these should be considered whenever possible. Significant septal defects are closed according to the same principles that govern the management of congenital or postinfarction defects.

Myocardial Contusion

The ideal management of the patient with myocardial contusion is expectant and parallels that of myocardial infarction. Continuous monitoring for at least 24 hours is important because the primary cause of mortality in these patients is dysrhythmia. Sequential ECGs and serum CK MB determination during this period can provide a sense of the extent and evolution of the myocardial injury and provide a basis for judgment regarding discontinuation of monitoring. Ventricular ectopy should be treated aggressively, and lidocaine is the first-line choice. Echocardiography or radionuclide angiography should be considered for diagnostic and prognostic guidance. If heart failure develops, a pulmonary artery catheter should be placed and appropriate inotropic support initiated. Intra-aortic balloon counterpulsation may become necessary.

INJURY TO THE THORACIC AORTA

Penetrating Injuries

Pentrating wounds most frequently involve the ascending aorta, and Symbas and Sehdeva (1970), as well as Parmley and colleagues (1958a), emphasized that early exsanguination is the rule. Small wounds from knives or small caliber firearms may allow long enough survival to permit repair. Dshanelidze (1922) reported the first successful treatment of any aortic injury, a small penetrating wound of the ascending aorta. Peripheral bullet embolism may be seen with any vascular injury, and Mattox and associates (1979) reported that it is frequently seen with gunshot wounds of the thoracic aorta.

Clinical Presentation

Penetrating aortic injury is usually obvious, with the patient in shock and a wound near or with possible involvement of a major vascular structure. Aortography is of no benefit in these patients, who belong in the operating room.

Management

Penetrating wounds of the aorta that are compatible with life are invariably small and can be managed with lateral repair.

Blunt Injuries

Blunt injury of the thoracic aorta is more frequent, but also most frequently lethal. Parmley's and colleagues' (1985b) autopsy review of thoracic aortic disruption revealed that 85% of these patients died before reaching a hospital. Injuries involving the ascending aorta were almost uniformly fatal. Of those patients who survived the first half hour, 21% died in the following 6 hours, 32% within 24 hours, and 60% were dead in one week. The frequency of this injury is underlined by Greendyke's (1966) series showing a 16% incidence of aortic rupture in fatal motor vehicle accidents.

Mechanism

The mechanism of blunt aortic disruption is most commonly thought to involve differential deceleration of adjacent segments of aorta. This is believed to explain the fact that 85% of these injuries occur at the aortic isthmus, which represents the junction between the relatively "fixed" distal aortic arch and the more mobile descending thoracic aorta. Shearing stress develops at this point during high speed deceleration injury and results in a transverse, linear transection. With complete transection the patient exsanguinates rapidly but, in a lucky few, some continuity is maintained in the adventitia or mediastinal pleura, or both. An unstable false aneurysm is thereby created, with evolution usually toward second rupture and, rarely, to the formation of a chronic, calcified pseudoaneurysm, which Bennett and Cherry (1967) and Fleming and Green (1974) showed is anatomically unstable with eventual enlargement and rupture.

Cammack and colleagues (1959) reported that, although horizontal deceleration tends to produce lesions of the descending thoracic aorta, the ascending aorta and arch are injured by vertical deceleration. Arch aortic tears most frequently involve the origin of the brachiocephalic artery. Parmley and associates (1958b) and Greendyke (1966) described multiple tears in 20% of these patients.

Clinical Presentation

Blunt trauma to the aorta is more subtle and one third to one half of patients, as Kirsh and colleagues (1976) reported, have no external evidence of thoracic injury at the time of initial physical examination. Clinicians must, therefore, be highly suspicious of all trauma where the mechanism of injury suggests significant deceleration.

Hypotension and shock may be present, but overly ambitious resuscitation may hasten secondary rupture. In this regard, Mattox and co-workers (1986) showed that the use of pneumatic antishock garments in these patients is without benefit and is perhaps even detrimental.

Conscious patients may complain of retrosternal or interscapular pain. Specific clinical signs are infrequent, but Malm and Deterling (1960) reported that the "acute coarctation syndrome"—upper extremity hypertension and decreased femoral artery pulses may be present. Upper extremity hypertension was seen in 31% of Symbas and colleagues' (1973) collected series of 2000 patients. A systolic murmur was also noted in 26% of the patients in this series.

Diagnosis

The chest roentgenograms nearly always show some abnormality. Widening of the superior mediastinum is the most frequent finding (Fig. 42–2) but is not specific because insignificant mediastinal bleeding from rib or sternal fractures or small vessels can enlarge the mediastinum. Technique is important and Schwab (1984) and Shaikh (1988) and their associates reported that fewer false positive images are obtained with upright than with supine roentgenograms of the chest.

Other radiographic changes include distortion of the aortic knob with obscuration of the aortic outline, left apical cap, deviation to the right of the trachea or esophagus—NG tube, depression of the left main stem bronchus, widening of the paravertebral stripe, or left hemothorax. Indirect signs of high energy injury such as

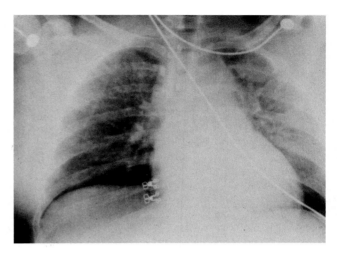

Fig. 42–2. Widened mediastinal shadow following blunt trauma. Aortic rupture suspected and confirmed by aortography.

fracture of the first two ribs, multiple rib fractures, sternal fracture, or pulmonary contusion should raise the possibility of aortic injury.

The definitive confirmation of aortic disruption is made with aortography (Fig. 42–3). This study demonstrates the location of the pseudoaneurysm or intimal tear. A ductus diverticulum can present a problem of interpretation in younger patients but is distinguished from a pseudoaneurysm by its smooth junction with the aorta and its strict localization to the inferomedial aspect of the aorta. Computed tomography and other diagnostic studies are not as reliable as arteriography.

Management

The treatment of blunt injuries can be complex. For the stable patient with angiographic documentation of

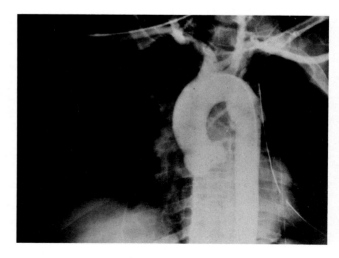

Fig. 42–3. Aortogram showing complete initial disruption of aorta following blunt trauma in patient shown in Figure 42–2. Successful repair carried out without complication.

aortic disruption at the level of the isthmus, the best approach is through a fourth interspace, posterolateral thoracotomy. Ideally, a double-lumen endotracheal tube is placed, because one-lung anesthesia provides better exposure and protects the left lung from excessive intraoperative manipulation.

Controversy exists regarding the necessity or desirability of providing some form of distal aortic perfusion during the period of aortic cross-clamping necessary for repair. Katz (1981) and Wadouh (1984) and their associates presented clinical and experimental evidence indicating that, among other factors, the probability of developing paraplegia is related to the duration of aortic cross-clamping. Furthermore, Katz (1981) and Laschinger (1982, 1983) and their colleagues showed that distal aortic perfusion restores spinal cord blood flow and reduces the incidence of paraplegia. Other authors, such as Mattox and colleagues (1985) and Antunes (1987), believe that paraplegia is more likely, because of the segmental nature of the cord blood supply, and is, therefore, influenced by proximity of the clamp to the injury and the number of intercostals sacrificed. The aforementioned surgeons demonstrated that, in their hands, a simple clamp and repair technique without distal aortic perfusion is a safe method for managing this injury and does not increase the incidence of paraplegia. These studies support the notion that cross-clamp time is, perhaps, not the most important factor in the development of this dreaded complication.

In circumstances when some form of distal aortic perfusion is thought desirable, three options exist. The first of these is standard cardiopulmonary bypass by either the femoro-femoral or atrio-femoral route. The obvious disadvantage to this technique is the necessity for systemic anticoagulation in the face of possible associated injuries.

A second possibility is the use of a heparin-bonded—Gott—shunt, which Crawford (1973), Wakabayashi (1975) and Akins (1981) and their co-workers prefer. Flow through these shunts is not always predictable, however, and the surgeon should be skilled in aortic cannulation techniques. Complications of shunt placement include bleeding and dissection at the cannulation site.

Olivier and associates (1984) suggested that the aorta can be cannulated above and below the injury, with distal perfusion assured using a centrifugal pump and obviating the necessity of systemic heparinization. Promising methods of spinal cord protection currently being investigated include monitoring of somatosensory evoked potentials to define safe limits of ischemia, by Laschinger (1983) and Mattox (1985) and their colleagues, and techniques of localized spinal cord cooling to protect the cord from ischemic injury, by Coles (1983) and Colon (1987) and their associates.

Most authors recommend the use of an interposition graft for vascular repair in this situation, particularly in the frequent circumstance of a circumferential disruption with distraction of the two ends. Primary repair is usually reserved for partial aortic tears. Although McBride and colleagues (1987) suggested that, with adequate mobilization, a direct anastomosis is feasible in most patients, we prefer to avoid the additional dissection this requires and favor the use of an interposition graft.

Injury to the ascending aorta is approached through a median sternotomy with full preparation for standard cardiopulmonary bypass. The femoral vessels are exposed, the patient is heparinized, and either femoro-femoral or right atrio-femoral bypass is initiated before approaching the aorta. The injury is isolated between cross-clamps—with the distal clamp usually placed proximal to the origin of the brachiocephalic artery—and cold cardioplegic solution is delivered to the heart. Repair usually necessitates an interposition graft.

Approximately 5% of aortic disruptions occur at the level of the diaphragmatic hiatus. Adequate exposure of this injury usually requires a thoracoabdominal incision, usually through the ninth intercostal space. The proximity of this particular injury to the artery of Adamkiewicz dictates special care in the preservation of intercostal and lumbar branches at this level.

Occasionally a patient is not considered a candidate for operative repair of an aortic injury because of associated severe head injury, extensive body surface burns, or pre-existing pathology. In these patients, Akins and associates (1981) reported that elective delay of operation—in some cases indefinitely—can be achieved with beta blockade and antihypertensive therapy.

Morbidity and Mortality

Complications of thoracic aortic injury, other than paraplegia, include rebleeding and false aneurysm formation.

In a collected series of 387 patients undergoing repair of an acute blunt injury to the thoracic aorta, Mattox and associates (1985) reported paraplegia postoperatively in 6.9% of the surviving patients. The operative mortality in this collected series was 20.7%. Most postoperative and in-hospital deaths resulted from complications arising from associated injuries occurring at the time of the original trauma rather than to the aortic repair.

REFERENCES

Akins, C.W., et al.: Acute traumatic disruption of the thoracic aorta: a ten-year experience. Ann. Thorac. Surg. *31*:305, 1981.

Antunes, M.J.: Acute traumatic rupture of the aorta: repair by simple aortic cross-clamping. Ann. Thorac. Surg. *44*:257, 1987.

Bennett, D.E., and Cherry, J.K.: The natural history of traumatic aneurysms of the aorta. Surgery *61*:516, 1967.

Besson, A., and Saegesser, F.: Color atlas of chest trauma and associated injuries, Vol. 1. Medical Economic Books, Oradell, NJ, 1983.

Blalock, A., and Ravitch, M.M.: A consideration of the nonoperative treatment of cardiac tamponade resulting from wounds of the heart. Surgery *14*:157, 1943.

Brantigan, C.O., et al.: Evaluation of technetium scanning for myocardial contusion. J. Trauma *18*:460, 1978.

Cammack, K., Rapport, R.L., and Paul, J.: Deceleration injuries of the thoracic aorta. Arch. Surg. *79*:244, 1959.

Coles, J.G., et al.: Intraoperative management of thoracic aortic aneurysm: experimental evaluation of perfusion cooling of the spinal cord. J. Thorac. Cardiovasc. Surg. *85*:292, 1983.

Colon, R., et al.: Hypothermic regional perfusion for protection of the spinal cord during periods of ischemia. Ann. Thorac. Surg. 43:639, 1987.

Craven, K.D., Oppenhemier, L., and Wood, L.D.H.: Effects of contusion and flail chest on pulmonary perfusion and oxygen exchange. J. Appl. Physiol. 47:729, 1979.

Crawford, E.S., and Rubio, P.A.: Reappraisal of adjuncts to avoid ischemia in the treatment of aneurysms of descending thoracic aorta. J. Thorac. Cardiovasc. Surg. 66:693, 1973.

Cuadros, C.L., Hutchinson, J.E., and Mogtades, A.H.: Laceration of a mitral papillary muscle and the aortic root as a result of blunt trauma to the chest. J. Thorac. Cardiovas. Surg. 88:134, 1984.

Cummings, R.G., et al.: Pneumopericardium resulting in cardiac tamponade. Am. J. Thorac. Surg. 37:511, 1984.

Deslauriers, J.: Major injuries: bronchial rupture. In International Trends in General Thoracic Surgery, Vol. 2, Major Challenges. Edited by H.C. Grillo and H. Eschapasse. Philadelphia, W.B. Saunders, p. 246, 1987.

Dow, R.W.: Myocardial rupture caused by trauma. Surgery 91:246, 1982.

Dshanelidze, I.I.: Manuscript, Petrograd, 1922. Cited by Lilienthal, H.: Thoracic Surgery: The Surgical Treatment of Thoracic Diseases. Philadelphia, W.B. Saunders Co., 1926, p. 489.

Espada, R., et al.: Surgical management of penetrating injuries to the coronary arteries. Surgery 78:755, 1975.

Evans, J., et al.: Principles for the management of penetrating cardiac wounds. Ann. Surg. 189:777, 1979.

Flanchbarm, L., Wright, J., and Siegel, J.H.: Emergency surgery in patients with post-traumatic myocardial contusion. J. Trauma 26:795, 1968.

Fleming, A.W., and Green, D.C.: Traumatic aneurysms of the thoracic aorta. Ann. Thorac. Surg. 18:91, 1974.

Forker, A.D., and Morgan, J.R.: Acquired coronary artery fistula from nonpenetrating chest injury. JAMA 215:289, 1971.

Goldstein, S.: Constrictive pericarditis after blunt chest trauma. Am. Heart J. 69:544, 1965.

Greendyke, R.M.: Traumatic rupture of the aorta: special reference to automobile accidents. JAMA 195:119, 1966.

Haas, G.E., et al.: Traumatic coronary artery fistula. J. Trauma 26:854, 1986.

Harley, D.P., et al.: Myocardial dysfunction following blunt chest trauma. Arch. Surg. 118:1384, 1983.

Hurley, E.J., and Mayfield, W.: Cardiac injuries. In Trauma Management, Vol. III. Cervicothoracic Trauma. Edited by F.W. Blaisdell and D.D. Trunkey. New York, Thieme Inc., 1986, pp. 192–222.

Inkley, S.R., and Barry, F.M.: Traumatic rupture of interventricular septum proved by cardiac catheterization. Circulation 18:916, 1958.

Jones, J.J., Hewitt, R.L., and Drapanan, T.: Cardiac contusion: a capricious syndrome. Ann. Surg. 181:567, 1975.

Katz, N.M., et al.: Incremental risk factors for spinal cord injury following operation for acute traumatic aortic transection. J. Thorac. Cardiovasc. Surg. 81:669, 1981.

King, R.M., et al.: Cardiac contusion: a new diagnostic approach utilizing two-dimensional echocardiography. J. Trauma 23:610, 1983.

Kirsh, M.M., and Sloan, H.: Blunt Chest Trauma—General Principles of Management. Boston, Little, Brown, Co., 1977, p. 157.

Kirsh, M.M., et al.: The treatment of acute traumatic rupture of the aorta: a ten-year experience. Ann. Surg. 184:308, 1976.

Kissane, R.W., and Rose, S.M.: Traumatic pericarditis. Am. J. Cardiol. 7:97, 1961.

Landercasper, J., Cogbil, T.H., and Lindesmith, L.A.: Long-term disability after flail chest injury. J. Trauma 24:410, 1984.

Laschinger, J.C., et al.: Detection and prevention of intraoperative spinal and ischemia after cross-clamping of the thoracic aorta: use of somatosensory evoked potentials. Surgery 92:1109, 1982.

Laschinger, J.C., et al.: Experimental and clinical assessment of the adequacy of partial bypass in maintenance of spinal cord blood flow during operation on the thoracic aorta. Ann. Thorac. Surg. 36:417, 1983.

Lasky, I.I.: Traumatic nonpenetrating heart disease: a review. Med. Times 91:917, 1963.

Lucas, C.E., et al.: Impaired pulmonary function after albumin resuscitation from shock. J. Trauma 20:446, 1980.

Malm, J.R., and Deterling, R.A.: Traumatic aneurysm of the thoracic aorta simulating coarctation. J. Thorac. Cardiovas. Surg. 40:271, 1960.

Martin, T.D., et al.: Blunt cardiac rupture. J. Trauma 24:287, 1984.

Mattox, K.L., et al.: Intravascular migratory bullets. Am. J. Surg. 137:192, 1979.

Mattox, K.L., et al.: Clamp/repair: a safe technique for treatment of blunt injury to the descending thoracic arota. Ann. Thorac. Surg. 40:456, 1985.

Mattox, K.L., et al.: Prospective randomized evaluation of antishock MAST in post-traumatic hypotension. J. Trauma 26:779, 1986.

McBride, L.R., et al.: Primary repair of traumatic aortic disruption. Ann. Thorac. Surg. 43:65, 1987.

Miller, F.A., et al.: Two-dimensional echocardiographic findings in cardiac trauma. Am. J. Cardiol. 50:1022, 1982.

Olivier, H.F., et al.: Use of the BioMedicus centrifugal pump in traumatic tears of the thoracic aorta. Ann. Thorac. Surg. 38:586, 1984.

Paris, F., et al.: Surgical stabilization of traumatic flail chest. Thorax 30:521, 1975.

Parmley, L.F., Mattingly, T.W., and Manion, W.C.: Penetrating wounds of the heart and aorta. Circulation 17:953, 1958a.

Parmley, L.F., et al.: Nonpenetrating traumatic injury of the aorta. Circulation 17:1086, 1958b.

Parmley, L.F., Manion, W.C., and Mattingly, T.W.: Nonpenetrating traumatic injury of the heart. Circulation 18:371, 1958c.

Potkin, R.T., et al.: Evaluation of noninvasive tests of cardiac damage in suspected cardiac contusion. Circulation 66:627, 1982.

Robinson, M.D., and Markovchick, V.J.: Traumatic pneumopericardium: a case report and literature review. J. Emerg. Med. 2:409, 1985.

Richardson, J.D., et al.: Management of transmediastinal gunshot wounds. Surgery 90:671, 1981.

Ridriguez, A., and Shatney, C.: The value of technetium pyrophosphate scanning in the diagnosis of myocardial contusion. Ann. Surg. 48:472, 1982.

Saunders, C.R., and Doty, D.B.: Myocardial contusion. Surg. Gynecol. Obstet. 144:595, 1977.

Schall, M.A., Fischer, R.P., and Perry, J.F.: The unchanged mortality of flail chest injuries. J. Trauma 19:492, 1979.

Schmit-Neuerburg, K.P., Weiss, H., and Labitzke, R.: Indications for thoracotomy in chest wall stabilization. Injury 14:26, 1982.

Schwab, C.W., et al.: Aortic injury: comparison of supine and upright portable chest films to evaluate the widened mediastinum. Ann. Emerg. Med. 13:896, 1984.

Shaikh, K.A., Schwab, C.W., and Camishion, R.C.: Aortic rupture in blunt trauma. Am. Surg. 52:47, 1986.

Sigler, L.H.: Traumatic injury of the heart: incidence of its occurrence in 42 cases of severe accidental bodily injury. Am. Heart. J. 30:459, 1945.

Sims, B.A., and Geddes, J.S.: Traumatic heart block. Br. Heart J. 31:140, 1969.

Sugg, W.L., et al.: Penetrating wounds of the heart. J. Thorac. Cardiovasc. 56:531, 1968.

Sutherland, G.R., et al.: Frequency of myocardial injury after blunt chest trauma as evaluated by radionuclide angiography. Am. J. Cardiol. 52:1099, 1983.

Symbas, P.N., and Sehdeva, J.S.: Penetrating wounds of the thoracic aorta. Ann. Surg. 171:441, 1970.

Symbas, P.N., et al.: Traumatic rupture of the aorta. Ann. Surg. 178:6, 1973.

Symbas, P.N., Harlaftis, N., and Waldo, W.J.: Penetrating cardiac wounds: a comparison of different therapeutic methods. Ann. Surg. 183:377, 1976.

Tabatznik, B., and Isaacs, J.P.: Postpericardiotomy syndrome following traumatic hemopericardium. Am. J. Cardiol. 7:83, 1961.

Thomas, A.H., and Roe, B.B.: Air embolism following penetrating lung injuries. J. Thorac. Cardiovasc. Surg. 66:533, 1973.

Thomas, A.N., et al.: Operative stabilization for flail chest after blunt trauma. J. Thorac. Cardiovasc. Surg. 75:793, 1978.

Trinkle, J.K., et al.: Management of the wounded heart. Ann. Thorac. Surg. 17:230, 1974.

Trinkle, J.K., et al.: Management of flail chest without mechanical ventilation. Ann. Thorac. Surg. 19:355, 1975.

Utley, J.R., et al.: Cardiac output, coronary flow, ventricular fibrillation, and survival following varying degrees of myocardial contusion. J. Surg. Res. *20*:539, 1976.

Wadouh, F., et al.: The arteria radicularis magna anterior as a decisive factor influencing spinal cord damage during aortic occlusion. J. Thorac. Cardiovasc. Surg. *88*:1, 1984.

Wakabayashi, A., et al.: Herparinless left heart bypass for resection of thoracic aortic aneurysms. Am. J. Surg. *130*:212, 1975.

Yee, F.S., Thomas, A.N., and Wilson, R.: Management of air embolism in blunt and penetrating thoracic trauma. J. Thorac. Cardiovasc. Surg. *85*:661, 1983.

READING REFERENCES

Deslauriers, J., et al.: Diagnosis and long-term follow-up of major bronchial disruptions due to nonpenetrating trauma. Ann. Thorac. Surg. *33*:32, 1982.

Logeais, Y., et al.: Traumatic rupture of the right main bronchus in an 8-year-old child successfully repaired 8 years after injury. Ann. Surg. *172*:1039, 1970.

Nonoyama, A., et al.: Total rupture of the left main bronchus successfully repaired 9 years after injury. Ann. Thorac. Surg. *21*:445, 1976.

CHAPTER 43

ADULT RESPIRATORY DISTRESS SYNDROME

Timothy E. Baldwin, Charles L. Rice, and C. James Carrico

Adult respiratory distress syndrome—ARDS—is a common form of acute respiratory failure that is caused by a wide variety of conditions. Conditions associated with the development of ARDS include forms of direct and indirect injury to the lung (Table 43–1) that result in diffuse injury to the alveolar capillary endothelium. Such injury leads to increased permeability and non-hydrostatic pulmonary edema, which is further characterized by: (1) hypoxemia resistant to oxygen supplementation, (2) decreased lung compliance, and (3) diffuse bilateral pulmonary infiltrates.

In 1972, the Lung Program of the National Heart, Lung, and Blood Institute estimated that the incidence of ARDS in the United States was about 150,000 cases per year. Today, the incidence is probably higher, because of our increased ability to treat other catastrophic illnesses.

Despite advances in critical care, the mortality rate of patients who develop ARDS remains greater than 50% in most studies, such as those of the National Heart, Lung, and Blood Institute (1979), Divertio (1982), and Fowler and associates (1983). Fein (1983) and Montgomery (1985) and their colleagues noted that when ARDS is accompanied by other organ system failures or sepsis, mortality rates increase. In the National Heart, Lung, and Blood Institute's multicenter study (1979), the mortality rate increased incrementally from 45% with ARDS alone to 56%, 72%, 84%, and 100%, respectively, with failure of one, two, three, or four other systems in addition to ARDS. Kaplan and co-workers (1979) reported that in patients with sepsis and ARDS, the mortality rate is as high as 90%. In patients with ARDS and renal failure, a mortality rate of 85% has been reported.

PATHOPHYSIOLOGY

In normal lung tissue, the alveolar surface is composed of type I and type II pneumocytes. These epithelial cells are supported by a basement membrane. The type I pneumocyte is a highly differentiated, flattened squamous cell that cannot replicate. Type I pneumocytes are thin and have a large surface area. Bachofen and Weibel (1982) reported that these cells cover about 95% of the alveolar surface (Fig. 43–1).

The type II pneumocyte is a cuboidal cell with microvilli on the alveolar surface (Fig. 43–2). Petty and Cherniack (1983) demonstrated that surfactant is produced and secreted by type II pneumocytes. These cells are more resistant to injury than type I cells. Type II pneumocytes can replicate and differentiate to form type I pneumocytes. The alveolar epithelial cells are joined by tight junctions that are normally impermeable to water.

Alveolar capillaries are situated in alveolar walls between adjacent alveoli. Capillary endothelial cells also lie on a basement membrane (Fig. 43–3). In some areas, the capillary and epithelial basement membranes fuse to form a thin membrane that faciliates gas exchange. In other areas, the membranes are separated by the interstitial space, which contains connective tissue elements, fibroblasts, and fluid. Capillary endothelial cells are joined by loose junctions that allow small amounts of fluid and nutrients into the interstitium. Excess interstitial fluid is drained by the pulmonary lymphatics.

The most accepted current description of the pathophysiology of ARDS is based on the concept of capillary endothelial injury. This injury to the capillary endothelium causes increased gap formation between the endothelial cells, which leads to increased permeability with leakage of fluid, protein, and cells into the interstitium. When the capacity of the lymphatics that drain the interstitium is exceeded, fluid begins to accumulate. This fluid in the interstitium collects first around the bronchi and large pulmonary vessels, which results in the characteristic roentgenographic appearance of interstitial pulmonary edema. Edema then spreads to involve the areas around the alveolar capillaries.

When the capacity of the interstitial space is exceeded, alveolar flooding occurs. Sensitive type I cells are damaged and sloughed, leaving behind a denuded basement membrane. The alveoli are filled with protein-rich fluid that contains erythrocytes, leukocytes, debris from type

Table 43–1. Some Conditions Associated with Adult Respiratory Distress Syndrome

Conditions Associated with Direct Lung Injury
Pneumonia
    Viral
    Bacterial
    Myocoplasma
    Fungal
    Legionnaire's
Aspiration
    Gastric contents
    Near-drowning with water aspiration
Toxic Inhalation
    Smoke
    Chemical fumes
    Oxygen toxicity
Pulmonary Contusion
Radiation Pneumonitis
Conditions Associated with Indirect Lung Injury
Shock
    Septic
    Anaphylactic
    Cardiogenic*
    Hemorrhagic†
Embolism
    Fat
    Air
    Amniotic fluid
Disseminated Intravascular Coagulation
Trauma
    Extrathoracic
    Head
    Burns
Metabolic
    Diabetic ketoacidosis
    Uremia
Pancreatitis
Post Cardiopulmonary Bypass
Drugs
    Narcotics—heroin, methadone, darvon, codeine
    Barbiturates
    Salicylates
    Ethchlorvynol
    Thiazides
    Propoxyphene
    Colchicine
    Paraquat

*See Edelman, N.H., et al.: Experimental cardiogenic shock: pulmonary performance after acute myocardial infarction. Am. J. Physiol. *219*:1723, 1970.

†See Buckberg, G.D., et al.: Pulmonary changes following hemorrhagic shock and resuscitation in baboons. J. Thorac. Cardiovasc. Surg. *59*:450, 1970.

I cells, and fibrin strands. This material may form sheets that adhere to the denuded basement membrane, forming hyaline membranes. The roentgenographic pattern is that of diffuse alveolar infiltrates.

Before alveolar flooding, the gas-exchange surfaces remain intact. Iliff and associates (1972) reported a decrease in compliance that results in some increase in the work of breathing, and leads to tachypnea. Ralph and colleagues (1985) documented that when alveoli are flooded, air spaces are lost and areas of low V/Q are increased. Said and associates (1965) noted that flooding also inactivates surfactant, leading to premature airway closure. The results are a decrease in functional residual capacity, decreased static and dynamic compliance, an increase in low-V/Q alveoli and an increase in shunting—Qs/Qt. These changes cause a hypoxemia that is relatively unresponsive to increases in inspired oxygen concentration—FIO_2. Glauser and co-workers (1979) pointed out that when the initial insult causes direct damage to the alveolar epithelium, not the capillary endothelium, direct alveolar flooding or hemorrhage can occur without interstitial edema. In most instances of primary alveolar epithelial injury, however, capillary endothelial injury occurs simultaneously or follows shortly, leading to the aforementioned changes in pulmonary physiology.

The events described up to this point represent the early or exudative phase of ARDS. A few days after initial injury, this exudative phase gives rise to a proliferative phase. Type II pneumocytes proliferate to replace the sloughed type I cells. These type II cells are about ten times thicker than the type I cells they replace, thus, as Bachofen and Wiebel (1977) pointed out, diffusion distance is increased. Fibroblasts in the interstitium show cytologic features consistent with an activated state. Zapol and associates (1983) suggested that such breaks in the alveolar basement membrane may allow these activated fibroblasts into the alveolus. Zapol and colleagues (1979) noted that total lung collagen content greatly increases as fibrosis obliterates the interstitium, alveoli, and alveolar ducts. Zapol (1977) and Jones (1985) and their co-workers also pointed out that alveolar capillaries are also destroyed, contributing to an increased pulmonary vascular resistance—PVR. Also, Harlan and associates (1983) showed that increases in circulating thromboxane in patients with ARDS contributes to the increase in PVR.

As pulmonary fibrosis and vascular obliteration advance, the normal pulmonary architecture becomes severely deranged. A separation between the air spaces and vasculature develops, resulting in increased dead space and shunting. Fibrosis also greatly decreases pulmonary compliance, necessitating mechanical ventilation with high airway pressures. Lamy and colleagues (1976) reported that these high airway pressures can cause overdistention of the terminal airways, which can lead to the formation of cavities. Areas of ischemic necrosis and autolysis can also result in the formation of cavities. These areas contribute to increased VD/VT. Zapol and associates (1983) noted that these cavities can also rupture from high ventilatory pressures, leading to pneumothorax,

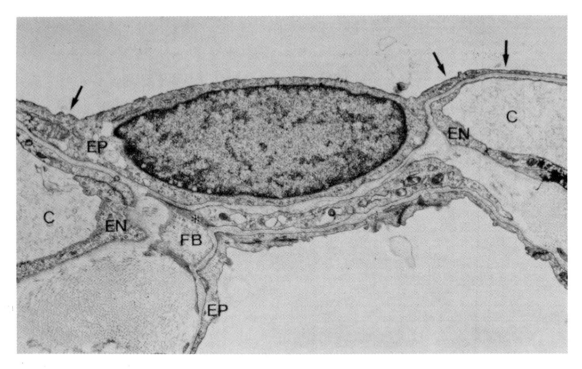

Fig. 43–1. Type I alveolar cell with thin cytoplasmic extensions (arrows). C=alveolar capillary; EP=Type I pneumocyte; EN=endothelial cell lining of capillary; FB=fibroblast process with an intracytoplasmic bundle of contractile filaments (*). × 8600.

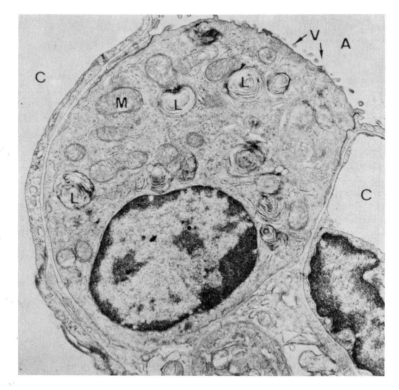

Fig. 43–2. Type II alveolar cell with osmiophilic lamellated bodies (L) and mitochrondria (M) in cytoplasm, and short microvilli (V) at surface toward alveolus (A). Note type I cell in vicinity. × 8600.

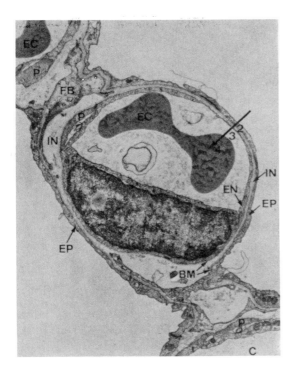

Fig. 43–3. Electron micrograph of alveolar capillary (C) from monkey lung with erythrocyte (EC). Note endothelial cell lining of capillary (EN), processes of pericytes (P) and the thin extensions of squamous alveolar epithelial cells (EP) covering the alveolar surface. The interstitial space (IN) is bounded by two basement membranes (BM) and contains some fibroblast processes (FB) as well as a few connective tissue fibrils. This lung was fixed by instillation of fixative into airways, which resulted in a loss of the surface lining layer; hence only parts 2 (tissue barrier), 3 (blood plasma), and 4 (erythrocyte) of the gas exchange pathway are preserved. × 8600. (Reproduced with permission from Weibel, E.R.: Morphometric estimation of pulmonary diffusion capacity. I. Model and method. Respir. Physiol. *11*:54, 1970/71.)

tension pneumothorax, or the formation of a bronchopleural fistula.

Not all patients with ARDS pass through this sequence of progressive destruction of the pulmonary system. Even with significant pulmonary fibrosis, recovery can occur. In patients who recover, type II pneumocytes differentiate into type I pneumocytes to regenerate the alveolar epithelium. Much of the interstitial fibrosis then resolves: The follow-up studies of Lakshminarayan (1976), Klein (1976), Yahav (1978), and Elliott (1981) and their associates, as well as the study of Douglas and Downs (1977) demonstrated remarkable recovery of pulmonary function. Lung mechanics and volumes usually recovered or were only mildly reduced within 6 to 12 months. Patients who did not have pre-existing lung disease returned to normal physical activity.

MECHANISMS OF PULMONARY ENDOTHELIAL INJURY

As previously noted, the final common pathway to ARDS includes the development of increased alveolar capillary permeability. Therefore, a great deal of effort

has been devoted to defining the mechanisms of endothelial injury and the mediators involved in the injury process. Because of the diversity of the conditions that are associated with the development of ARDS (Table 43–1), Maunder (1986) and Winn (1987) and their colleagues suggested that there are multiple mechanisms of injury.

Growing evidence suggests that one mechanism of injury involves the activation of granulocytes, which aggregate and adhere to the capillary endothelium. Bachofen and Weibel (1977) and Hasleton (1983) reported that pathologic examinations of lungs from patients with early ARDS have demonstrated large numbers of neutrophils sequestered in the pulmonary vasculature and interstitium. Weiland and colleagues (1986) noted that bronchoalveolar lavage in early ARDS has also shown an increase in neutrophils. Hammerschmidt (1980) and MacDonnell (1987) and their associates, as well as Zapol and Falke (1985), noted that endotoxemia, trauma, burns, immune complexes, pancreatitis, and sepsis can lead to complement activation. Becker and Ward (1980) reported that other factors, including prostaglandins, leukotrienes, and lymphokines, can cause neutrophil migration.

Neutrophils can release proteases, toxic oxygen radicals, toxic products of arachidonic acid metabolism and platelet-activating factor. Sacks (1978), Weiss (1981) and Martin (1981) and their co-workers showed that superoxide, peroxide, and other toxic oxygen radicals released by activated neutrophils can damage endothelial cells, parenchymal cells, membranes, and enzymes. Bruce and associates (1981) and Carp and Janoff (1980) noted that oxygen radicals inactivate alpha-proteinase inhibitor, which normally protects the lung from damage by proteolytic enzymes.

Neutrophil-derived proteases include elastase and collagenase. Janoff and colleagues (1979) reported that these substances can digest structural proteins, including collagen and elastin, thus destroying interstitial architecture. Janoff (1983) also reported that the proteases can also activate complement and cleave fibrinogen and Hageman factor, thus leading to amplification of inflammation and lung injury.

Hechtman and associates (1984) showed that platelet-activating factor can also be synthesized and released by activated neutrophils. This can lead to platelet aggregation and embolization. Greene and co-workers (1981) demonstrated angiographic evidence of pulmonary thrombosis in 48% of patients with ARDS, and Bone and colleagues (1976) reported disseminated intravascular coagulation in 23%. Manwaring and associates (1978) found that fibrin-degradation products also alter microvascular permeability. The role of platelet aggregation, coagulation, and fibrinolysis in ARDS is unclear. Moreover, Binder and co-workers (1980) reported that the use of anticoagulants is not efficacious.

Neutrophils also increase the production of arachidonic acid metabolites, including prostaglandins—PG, thromboxane—Tx—and leukotrienes. Harlan (1983) and Winn (1983) and their associates reported that prostaglandin H_2—PGH_2—and thromboxane A_2—TxA_2—are potent pulmonary vasoconstrictors and can cause pulmonary hypertension and an increase in lymph flow. TxA_2 also causes platelet aggregation and bronchoconstriction.

Bernard and Brigham (1986) and Nunn (1987) reported that leukotrienes B_4 and C_4 can cause chemotaxis, bronchoconstriction, and increased pulmonary endothelial permeability. The role of these factors in the pathogenesis of ARDS is still unclear, but they may play a part in pulmonary vasoconstriction and pulmonary hypertension.

Although this evidence implicates the neutrophil in the pathogenesis of at least some forms of ARDS, other pathways must also be capable of initiating injury and causing ARDS, because Ognibene (1986) and Winn (1987) and their colleagues reported that this syndrome can occur in patients who are severely neutropenic. Direct damage to the alveolar capillary interface can occur with acid aspiration, toxic inhalation, and fat embolization. Probably, other mechanisms of injury are yet to be delineated and may include other cellular or chemical mediators. Andreadis and Petty (1985) noted that the pathogenic mechanisms that cause alterations in the pulmonary vasculature that lead to lung injury in ARDS may also have damaging effects on other organ systems.

CLINICAL CHARACTERISTICS

The development of ARDS starts with the initial, predisposing acute injury or illness. At first, the clinical findings are those associated with only the acute injury or disease process. Petty and Ashbaugh (1971) noted that the signs of progressive respiratory failure and ARDS itself usually begin to appear after 12 to 24 hours. Pepe and colleagues (1982) noted that within 72 hours, this initial tachypnea and tachycardia progress to dyspnea and hypoxemia as interstitial edema and alveolar flooding occur. The edema and alveolar flooding result in severe hypoxemia; decreased static and dynamic compliance; diffuse bilateral infiltrates—interstitial first, then alveolar; pulmonary hypertension; and a decrease in functional residual capacity (Fig. 43–4).

In early stages, dead space is only moderately increased. If the patient progresses to severe pulmonary fibrosis with widespread destruction of normal pulmonary architecture, dead space is markedly elevated, compliance markedly reduced, and diffusion capacity significantly decreased. Early changes in ventilatory mechanics are caused by alveolar edema with airway closure. Suter (1985) reported that the later changes are related to parenchymal consolidation, fibrosis, and increased surface tension.

TREATMENT

Although ARDS was first described by Ashbaugh and colleagues in 1967, treatment is still mainly supportive, although agents that may interrupt some of the pathogenic processes in ARDS are being developed and tested. In addition to the provision of supportive care,

efforts must be made to identify and treat the underlying cause. Unless this can be accomplished, a continued assault on the lung with progression of respiratory and other organ system failure is likely. Vigilance in preventing and treating infections and other organ system dysfunctions that frequently occur in patients with ARDS is crucial, because concurrent sepsis or multisystem failure greatly increases mortality. This is especially true of secondary respiratory infection.

The goals of supportive care for patients with ARDS are to ensure adequate tissue oxygen delivery and adequate patient comfort and to minimize the risks of further damage to the lungs or other organ systems.

Support of Gas Exchange

Patients with severe respiratory failure require some form of support of gas exchange to assure adequate ventilation and oxygenation. Patients with ARDS may have an increased work of breathing secondary to decreased compliance or increased dead space, or both. Patients who cannot overcome this increase in ventilatory work become hypercarbic and require mechanical support to provide adequate ventilation. The main reason that patients with ARDS require mechanical support, however, is to overcome ARDS-induced hypoxemia, which is relatively resistant to increases in inspired oxygen concentration. When adequate oxygenation—$Po_2 \geq 60$ and $Sao_2 \geq 90$ mmHg— cannot be maintained with a nontoxic level of inspired oxygen—$Fio_2 \leq 0.50$—measures to increase lung volume and functional residual capacity are required to improve oxygenation by decreasing shunt—Qs/Qt—and ventilation/perfusion—V/Q—mismatching. Possible therapeutic modes include continuous positive airway pressure—CPAP, positive end-expiratory pressure—PEEP—and mechanical ventilatory support.

In early ARDS, alveolar flooding and airway closure cause decreased compliance and functional residual capacity—FRC, an increase in shunting, and hypoxemia. PEEP and CPAP increase FRC by shifting tidal ventilation to above the critical closing pressure, thus opening previously closed or partially closed airway units. Suter (1985) reported that this opening results in markedly improved static and dynamic compliance, a decrease in low–ventilation-to-perfusion—V/Q—areas and decreased shunting—Qs/Qt, which results in improved oxygenation. PEEP does not decrease alveolar edema, but rather as Malo and associates (1980) stated, it spreads the fluid over the greater surface area of an open alveolus, thus decreasing diffusion distance. In addition to improved ventilation-perfusion matching, this decreased diffusion distance may contribute to improved gas exchange.

PEEP increases intrathoracic pressure, which can cause barotrauma and can interfere with cardiac filling, thus causing a decrease in cardiac output. The hemodynamic effects can usually be overcome by fluid administration. PEEP must therefore be carefully titrated to allow adequate arterial oxygenation with an $Fio_2 \leq 0.50$, while still allowing sufficient cardiac output for adequate tissue perfusion and minimizing the risk of bar-

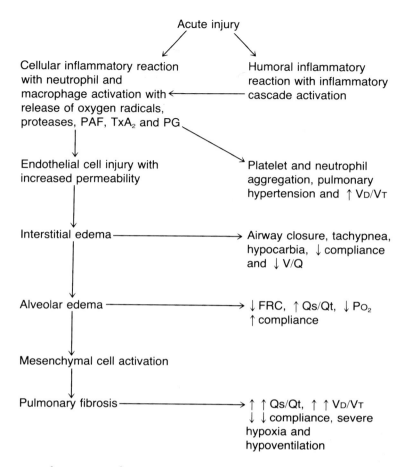

Fig. 43–4. Clinical characteristics and progression of ARDS.

otrauma. Pepe and colleagues (1984), however, noted that the use of PEEP in patients at risk to develop ARDS is not beneficial and has some risk of morbidity.

Suter (1985) reported that as parenchymal consolidation, fibrosis, and severe derangements of the pulmonary architecture occur in the later stages of ARDS, PEEP may be less effective and may not alter the severely decreased static and dynamic compliances. The hemodynamic effects of PEEP at this stage may be small as pressure is transmitted less well through such stiffened lungs.

High-frequency ventilation has been studied as a mode of ventilation in patients with severe ARDS. Carlon and co-workers (1983) conducted a randomized prospective study of 309 patients and found that although it was safe, it had no benefit over conventional mechanical ventilation.

Nonspecific Supportive Therapies

Fluid replacement therapy in ARDS has long been controversial, with some advocating crystalloids and others, colloids. Advocates of colloids argue that plasma oncotic pressure is increased with the use of colloids, thus minimizing fluid movement out of the capillary. With ARDS, however, the capillary endothelium loses integrity, and allows proteins to move out of the vas-

culature. Therefore, colloid molecules quickly equilibrate across the membrane. Sibbald (1983) and Metildi (1984) and their associates reported that any increase in plasma oncotic pressure rapidly disappears. Furthermore, as Lowe and colleagues (1977) pointed out, the accumlation of colloid molecules in the pulmonary interstitium and alveoli may actually increase edema. Because of the lack of demonstrated benefit and the high cost of colloid solutions, crystalloid therapy is preferred.

The goal of fluid therapy in patients with ARDS is to ensure adequate cardiac output and tissue perfusion, while keeping filling pressures as low as possible to minimize any hydrostatic component of pulmonary edema. The pulmonary artery catheter can provide useful guidance by providing measurements of cardiac output and filling pressures, and by allowing measurement of mixed venous oxygenation to help assess the adequacy of tissue perfusion. The clinician must balance the benefit of increased cardiac output—with the risk of increased filling pressures—against the possibility of resultant increased pulmonary edema. In the setting of increased cardiac output and pulmonary capillary wedge pressure, the judicious use of diuretics may be useful in maintaining optimal hemodynamics.

In patients with severe hypoxemia, it may be necessary to take measures that minimize oxygen consumption. For example, elevations in body temperature should be treated, as fever increases metabolism. Sedation, and in extreme cases neuromuscular paralysis, may be necessary to minimize nonessential oxygen consumption. In addition, as desaturation becomes more severe, and is refractory to other lung-directed support, maintenance of adequate oxygen delivery by increasing hemoglobin concentration may be necessary. Typically, such therapy is warranted when oxygen extraction ratio—arterial oxygen content minus mixed venous oxygen content divided by the arterial oxygen content—exceeds 40%. Any decision to give red blood cells for this purpose must be balanced against the potential infections and immunosuppressive hazards of homologous blood transfusion. In our experience, increasing the hemoglobin concentration to greater than 12 g/dl, is rarely valuable.

Potential New Supportive Therapy

The National Heart, Lung and Blood Institute (1979) conducted a multicenter, randomized, prospective study using extracorporeal membrane oxygenation—ECMO—which demonstrated that ECMO could correct hypoxemia and remove carbon dioxide, but did not improve survival in patients with severe ARDS. This study has been widely criticized because the strict entry criteria resulted in selection of only patients with far-advanced ARDS, which resulted in greater than 90% mortality in both the ECMO and control groups.

Gattinoni and co-workers (1980, 1986) reported significantly improved survival rates using a technique known as low-frequency positive-pressure ventilation and extracorporeal removal of carbon dioxide. This technique employs a partial venous bypass to effect removal of carbon dioxide and supply a portion of oxygen requirements, while ventilating the patient with three to four breaths per minute. These results are promising but await further verification.

General Patient Support

As previously discussed, concurrent infection or multiorgan system failure greatly increases the morbidity and mortality associated with ARDS. The clinician must therefore be vigilant in efforts to protect other organ systems and to prevent infection. For example, prophylaxis against stress-related gastric bleeding by use of antacids, H_2 blocking agents, or sucralfate is strongly indicated. In addition, strict adherence to sterile technique and constant surveillance for possible sites of infection are crucial. Any infection that is detected should be aggressively treated with appropriate antimicrobial therapy.

Attention must also be given to ensure adequate nutritional support, as starvation impairs respiratory function and healing. Nutrition can be administered either enterally or intravenously, but, when possible, enteral feeding is preferred as Border and colleagues (1987) noted, as it decreases the risk of gastrointestinal hemorrhage and of abdominal sepsis. With parenteral nutrition, it must be remembered that the administration of excess carbohydrates can lead to fat synthesis and cause increased carbon dioxide production. Parenteral nutrition should therefore be used with care, because it may contribute to hypercarbia in ARDS patients, who already have a predisposition to carbon dioxide retention because of greatly elevated dead space. Such a condition could lead to ineffective ventilation and decreased carbon dioxide elimination.

Therapy Directed at Interrupting the Injury Process

Several approaches have emerged that attempt to interrupt the process of injury in the lung. These therapies are primarily aimed at the interruption of the inflammatory processes. These therapies include the use of steroids, nonsteroidal anti-inflammatory drugs—NSAID—and prostaglandins—primarily PGE_1.

Although steroids have been widely used in treating ARDS, the efficacy of this therapy has not been proved in rigorous clinical trials. Theoretically, benefits include: (1) stabilization of lysosomal membranes as Clermont and associates (1974) pointed out, thus decreasing protease release; (2) decreased neutrophil chemotaxis; (3) decreased complement activation as Hammerschmidt and co-workers (1979) noted; (4) decreased availability of arachidonic acid, thus decreasing production of TxA_2, leukotrienes, and PGH_2; and (5) preservation of endothelial integrity which Appel and Shoemaker (1984) suggested. Despite these theoretical benefits, Weigelt and colleagues (1985) were unable to show that steroid therapy in patients with early respiratory failure improved pulmonary function. Ashbaugh and Mair (1985), however, suggested that in patients with ARDS who develop idiopathic pulmonary fibrosis, steroid therapy may be beneficial and improve survival. Steroid therapy also carries many hazards, including impaired healing, increased susceptibility to infection, and stress gastritis.

Nunn (1987) noted that nonsteroidal anti-inflammatory agents inhibit cyclo-oxygenase, thus interfering with TxA_2 and prostaglandin synthesis. Bernard and Brigham reported that they can also modulate granulocyte margination and activity. Also, Price and associates (1986) showed that they block the development of pulmonary hypertension induced by Escherichia coli infusion in goats. The role of these agents, if any, in the treatment of ARDS will be determined in experimental trials.

The agent that has shown the greatest promise to date is PGE_1. Craddock (1978) reported that unlike PGH_2, which causes pulmonary vasoconstriction and pulmonary hypertension, other prostaglandins such as PGE_1 can cause pulmonary vasodilation and may actually modulate the inflammatory response. Early studies using PGE_1 have yielded promising results. Riukin and colleagues (1975) demonstrated that PGE_1 can suppress neutrophil chemotaxis; Zurier and co-workers (1974) reported that it can block lysosomal enzyme release; and Lehmeyer and Johnston (1978) showed that it suppresses superoxide production. In a double-blind study of 50 patients with ARDS, Holcroft and associates, in unpublished data, reported that the infusion of 30 ng/kg/minute of PGE_1 for a period of up to 7 days resulted in a reduction in mortality from 70.8% in controls to 34.6% in the treatment group. Right ventricular dysfunction has been demonstrated by Eddy and colleagues (1988) in multiply injured patients and has been associated with increased mortality. By decreasing pulmonary vascular resistance, PGE_1 may improve right ventricular function, and this might contribute to decreased mortality. Further studies are needed to confirm these results.

PREVENTION

Many clinical, physiologic, and laboratory parameters have been studied in attempts to identify patients likely to develop ARDS. To date, identification by predisposing clinical events, as Maunder (1985) suggested, has been the most useful technique. Pepe and co-workers (1982) identified high-risk events, which include: sepsis syndrome, aspiration of gastric contents, multiple blood transfusions, pulmonary contusion, and multiple major fractures. Pepe and colleagues (1982, 1983) showed that having multiple risk events increases the chances of developing ARDS. Where possible, it is important to prevent the development of sepsis, to avoid airway contamination—which may lead to sepsis—or aspiration, and to perform early fracture fixation when possible.

The most useful laboratory test in the selection of patients at risk for developing ARDS remains sequential arterial blood gas analysis. Weigelt and associates (1981) reported that decreasing arterial oxygen tension necessitating increases in inspired oxygen concentration may indicate pulmonary deterioration. Several substances have been proposed as markers or mediators of lung injury, including lactoferrin, phospholipase A_2, and factor VIII antigen. Maunder (1985) suggested that laboratory analyses for these or other similar substances may one day be useful in predicting patients at risk to develop ARDS. Although the use of PEEP is an important therapeutic modality in patients with ARDS, Pepe and co-workers (1984) demonstrated that the prophylactic use of PEEP does not prevent the development of ARDS.

SUMMARY

The high mortality rate associated with ARDS has changed little since 1967, when ARDS was first described. Currently, therapy remains primarily supportive. As our understanding of the many cellular and humoral factors involved in the pulmonary injury process increases, however, hope for specific therapeutic strategies to prevent or interrupt this process increases.

REFERENCES

Andreadis, N., and Petty, T.L.: Adult respiratory distress syndrome: problems and progress. Am. Rev. Respir. Dis. *132*:1344, 1985.

Appel, P.J., and Shoemaker, W.C.: Hemodynamic and oxygen transport effects of prostaglandin E1 in patients with adult respiratory distress syndrome. Crit. Care Med. *12*:528, 1984.

Ashbaugh, D.G., and Maier, R.V.: Idiopathic pulmonary fibrosis in adult respiratory distress syndrome: diagnosis and treatment. Arch. Surg. *120*:350, 1985.

Ashbaugh, D.G., et al.: Acute respiratory distress in adults. Lancet *2*:319, 1967.

Bachofen, M., and Weibel, E.R.: Alterations of the gas exchange apparatus in adult respiratory insufficiency associated with septicemia. Am. Rev. Respir. Dis. *116*:589, 1977.

Bachofen, M., and Weibel, E.R.: Structural alterations of lung parenchyma in the adult respiratory distress syndrome. Am. J. Surg. *144*:124, 1982.

Becker, E.L., and Ward, P.A.: Chemotaxis. *In* Clinical Immunology. Edited by C.W. Parker. Philadelphia, W.B. Saunders Co., 1980, pp. 272–297.

Bernard, G.R., and Brigham, K.L.: Pulmonary edema: pathophysiologic mechanisms and new approaches to therapy. Chest *89*:594, 1986.

Binder, A.S., et al.: Effect of heparin on fibrinogen depletion on lung fluid balance in sheep after emboli. J. Appl. Physiol. *48*:414, 1980.

Bone, R.C., Francis, P.B., and Pierce, A.K.: Intravascular coagulation associated with the adult respiratory distress syndrome. Am. J. Med. *61*:585, 1976.

Border, J.R., et al.: The gut-origin septic states in blunt multiple trauma (ISS-40) in the ICU. Ann. Surg. *206*:427, 1987.

Bruce, M.C., et al.: Inactivation of alpha₁-proteinase inhibitor in infants exposed to high concentrations of oxygen (Abstract). Am. Rev. Respir. Dis. *123*(Suppl.):166, 1981.

Carolon, G.C., et al.: High frequency jet ventilation: a prospective randomized evaluation. Chest *84*:551, 1983.

Carp, H., and Janoff, A.: Potential mediator of inflammation: phagocyte-derived oxidants suppress the elastase-inhibitory capacity of alpha₁-proteinase inhibitor in vitro. J. Clin. Invest. *66*:987, 1980.

Clermont, H.G., Williams, J.S., and Adams, J.T.: Steroid effect on the release of the lysosomal enzyme acid phosphatase in shock. Ann. Surg. *179*:917, 1974.

Craddock, P.R.: Corticosteroid-induced lymphopenia, immunosuppression, and body defense. Ann. Intern. Med. *88*:564, 1978.

Divertie, M.B.: The adult respiratory distress syndrome. Mayo Clin. Proc. *57*:371, 1982.

Douglas, M.E., and Downs, J.B.: Pulmonary function following severe acute respiratory failure and high levels of positive end-expiratory pressure. Chest *71*:18, 1977.

Eddy, C.A., Rice, C.L., and Amardi, D.M.: Right ventricular dysfunction in multiple trauma victims. Am. J. Surg. (in press).

Elliott, C.G., Morris, A.H., and Cengiz, M.: Pulmonary function and exercise gas exchange in survivors of adult respiratory distress syndrome. Am. Rev. Respir. Dis. *123*:492, 1981.

Fein, A.M., et al.: The risk factors, incidence, and prognosis of the adult respiratory distress syndrome following septicemia. Chest *83*:40, 1983.

Fowler, A.A., et al.: Adult respiratory distress syndrome: Risk with common predispositions. Ann. Intern. Med. *98*:593, 1983.

Gattinoni, L., et al.: Treatment of acute respiratory failure, with low-frequency positive-pressure ventilation and extracorporeal removal of CO_2. Lancet *2*:292, 1980.

Gattinoni, L., et al.: Low-frequency positive pressure ventilation with extracorporeal CO_2 removal in severe acute respiratory failure. JAMA *256*:881, 1986.

Glauser, F.L., Millen, J.E., and Falls, R.: Effects of acid aspiration on pulmonary alveolar epithelial membrane permeability. Chest *76*:201, 1979.

Greene, R., et al.: Early bedside detection of pulmonary vascular occlusion during acute respiratory failure. Am. Rev. Respir. Dis. *124*:593, 1981.

Hammerschmidt, D.E., et al.: Corticosteroids inhibit complement-induced granulocyte aggregation: a possible mechanism for their efficacy in shock states. J. Clin. Invest. *63*:798, 1979.

Hammerschmidt, E.E., et al.: Association of complement activation and elevated plasma C_5 with adult respiratory distress syndrome. Lancet *1*:947, 1980.

Harlan, J., et al.: Selective inhibition of thromboxane synthesis during experimental endotoxemia in the goat: effects on pulmonary hemodynamics and lung lymph flow. Br. J. Clin. Pharmacol. *1*:1235, 1983.

Hasleton, P.S.: Adult respiratory distress syndrome—a review. Histopathology *7*:307, 1983.

Hechtman, H.B., Valeri, C.R., and Shepro, D.: Role of hormonal mediators in adult respiratory distress syndrome. Chest 86:623, 1984.

Holcroft, J.W., et al.: Increased survival of patients with acute respiratory failure (ARDS) resulting from shock, trauma, or sepsis treated with prostin VR sterile solution (PGE 1; Alprostadil). Unpublished. Investigation data: University of California and The Upjohn Company.

Iliff, L.D., Greene, R.E., and Hughes, I.M.B.: Effects of interstitial edema on distribution of ventilation and perfusion in isolated lung. J. Appl. Physiol. 33:462, 1972.

Janoff, A., et al.: Lung injury induced by leukocytic proteases. Am. J. Pathol. 97:111, 1979.

Janoff, A.: Proteases and lung injury, state of the art mini-review. Chest 83:548, 1983.

Jones, R., et al.: Pulmonary vascular pathology. In Acute Respiratory Failure, Edited by W.M. Zapol, and K.J. Falke. New York, Marcel Dekker, 1985, pp. 23–160.

Kaplan, R.L., Sahn, S.A., and Petty, T.L.: Incidence and outcome of the respiratory distress syndrome in gram-negative sepsis. Arch. Intern. Med. 139:867, 1979.

Klein, J.J., et al.: Pulmonary function after recovery from adult respiratory distress syndrome. Chest 69:350, 1976.

Lakshminarayan, S., Stanford, R.L, and Petty, T.L.: Prognosis after recovery from adult respiratory distress syndrome. Am. Rev. Respir. Dis. 113:7, 1976.

Lamy, M., et al.: Pathologic features and mechanisms of hypoxemia in adult respiratory distress syndrome. Am. Rev. Respir. Dis. 114:267, 1976.

Lehmeyer, J.E., and Johnston, R.B., Jr.: Effect of anti-inflammatory drugs and agents that elevate intracellular ABP on the release of toxic oxygen metabolites by phagocytes: studies in a model of tissue-bound I$_a$G. Clin. Immunol. Immunopathol. 9:482–490, 1978.

Lowe, R.J., et al.: Crystalloid vs. colloid in the etiology of pulmonary failure after trauma: a randomized trial in man. Surgery 81:676, 1977.

Lung Program, National Heart and Lung Institute. Respiratory Diseases: Task Force on Problems, Research Approaches, Needs. Bethesda, MD, National Institute of Health, 1972.

MacDonnell, K.F., Fahey, P.J., and Segal, M.S. (eds.): Respiratory Intensive Care. Boston, Little, Brown, & Co., 1987, p. 423.

Malo, J., et al.: How does PEEP reduce Qs/QT in pulmonary edema? Fed. Proc. 39:280, 1980.

Manwaring, D., Thorning, D., and Curreri, P.W.: Mechanisms of acute pulmonary dysfunction induced by fibrinogen degradation product D. Surgery 84:45, 1978.

Martin, W.J., et al.: Oxidant injury of lung parenchymal cells. J. Clin. Invest. 68:1277, 1981.

Maunder, R.J.: Clinical prediction of the adult respiratory distress syndrome. Clin. Chest Med. 6:413, 1985.

Maunder, R.J., et al.: Occurrence of the adult respiratory distress syndrome in neutropenic patients. Am. Rev. Respir. Dis. 133:3113, 1986.

Metildi, L.A., et al.: Crystalloid versus colloid in fluid resuscitation of patients with severe pulmonary insufficiency. Surg. Gynecol. Obstet. 158:207, 1984.

Meyrick, B.O.: Pathology of pulmonary edema. In Petty, T.L., and Cherniack, R.M. (eds): Semin. Respir. Med. 4:267, 1983.

Montgomery, A.B., et al.: Causes of mortality in patients with the adult respiratory distress syndrome. Am. Rev. Respir. Dis. 132:485, 1985.

National Heart, Lung, and Blood Institute, Division of Lung Diseases: Extracorporeal Support for Respiratory Insufficiency. Bethesda, MD: National Institutes of Health, 1979, pp. 243–5.

Nunn, J.F.: Applied Respiratory Physiology. Boston, Butterworths; 1987; pp 290–291 and 450–459.

Ognibene, F.P., et al.: Adult respiratory distress syndrome in patients with severe neutropenia. N. Engl. J. Med. 315:548, 1986.

Pepe, P.E., Hudson, L.D., and Carrico, C.J.: Early application of positive end-expiratory pressure in patients at risk for the adult respiratory distress syndrome. N. Engl. J. Med. 311:281, 1984.

Pepe, P.E., et al.: Clinical predictors of the adult respiratory distress syndrome. Am. J. Surg. 144:124, 1982.

Pepe, P.E., et al.: Early prediction of the adult respiratory distress syndrome by a simple scoring method. Ann. Emerg. Med. 12:749, 1983.

Petty, T.L., and Ashbaugh, D.G.: The adult respiratory distress syndrome. Chest 60:233, 1971.

Price, S., et al.: Indomethacin, dazoxiben and extravascular lung water after E. coli infusion. J. Surg. Res. 41:189, 1986.

Ralph, D.D., et al.: Distribution of ventilation and perfusion during positive end-expiratory pressure in the adult respiratory distress syndrome. Am. Rev. Respir. Dis. 131:54, 1985.

Riukin, I., Rosenblatt, J., and Becker, E.: The role of cyclic ABP in the chemotactic responsiveness and spontaneous mobility of rabbit neutrophil. J. Immunol. 115:1126, 1975.

Sacks, T., et al.: Oxygen radicals mediate endothelial cell damage by complement-stimulated granulocytes: an in vitro model of immune vascular damage. J. Clin. Invest. 61:1161, 1978.

Said, S., et al.: Pulmonary surface activity in induced pulmonary edema. J. Clin. Invest. 44:458, 1965.

Suter, P.M.: Assessment of respiratory mechanics in ARDS. In: Acute Respiratory Failure. Edited by W.M. Zapol and K.J. Falke. New York, Marcel Dekker, 1985, pp. 507–520.

Sibbald, W.J., et al.: The short-term effects of increasing plasma colloid osmotic pressure in patients with noncardiac pulmonary edema. Surgery 93:620, 1983.

Weigelt, J.A., Synder, W.H., III, and Mitchell, R.A.: Early identification of patients prone to develop adult respiratory distress syndrome. Am. J. Surg. 142:687, 1981.

Weigelt, J.A., et al.: Early steroid therapy for respiratory failure. Arch. Surg. 120:536, 1985.

Weiland, J.E., et al.: Lung neutrophils in the adult respiratory distress syndrome: clinical and pathophysiologic significance. Am. Rev. Respir. Dis. 133:218, 1986.

Winn, R., et al.: Thromboxane A$_2$ mediates lung vasoconstriction but not permeability after endotoxin. J. Clin. Invest. 72:911, 1983.

Winn, R., et al.: Neutrophil depletion does not prevent lung edema after endotoxin infusion in goats. J. Appl. Physiol. 62:116, 1987.

Weiss, S.J., et al.: Role of hydrogen peroxide in neutrophil-mediated destruction of cultured endothelial cells. J. Clin. Invest. 68:714, 1981.

Yahav, J., Liberman, P., and Molho, M.: Pulmonary function following the adult respiratory distress syndrome. Chest 74:457, 1978.

Zapol, W.M., and Falke, K.J. (eds): Acute Respiratory Failure, Vol. 24, New York, Marcel Dekker, 1985, p. 423.

Zapol, W.M., et al.: Vascular obstruction causes pulmonary hypertension in severe acute respiratory failure. Chest 71:307, 1977.

Zapol, W.M., et al.: Pulmonary fibrosis in severe acute respiratory failure. Am. Rev. Respir. Dis. 119:547, 1979.

Zapol, W.M., et al.: Pathophysiologic pathways of the adult respiratory distress syndrome. In Care of the Critically Ill Patient, Edited by J. Tinker and M. Rapin. New York, Springer Verlag, 1983, pp. 341–358.

Zurier, R.B., et al.: Mechanisms of lysosomal enzyme release from human leukocytes. J. Clin. Invest. 53:297, 1974.

READING REFERENCES

Edelman, N.H., et al.: Experimental cardiogenic shock: pulmonary performance after acute myocardial infarction. Am. J. Physiol. 219:1723, 1970.

Buckberg, G.D., et al.: Pulmonary changes following hemorrhagic shock and resuscitation in baboons. J. Thorac. Cardiovasc. Surg. 59:450, 1970.

Pleet, A.B.: "Shock Lung" syndrome following diabetic ketoacidosis; treatment with heparin. Chest 63:434, 1973.

CHAPTER 44

MANAGEMENT OF FOREIGN BODIES OF THE UPPER AERODIGESTIVE TRACT

Lauren D. Holinger and Anita King Bowes

Techniques of endoscopic manipulation and extraction of foreign objects and preoccupation with technical expertise have often overshadowed the broader clinical aspects of foreign body management. The collection of recovered foreign bodies at the Children's Memorial Hospital in Chicago, Department of Bronchology, while it was under the direction of Paul H. Holinger, M.D., accumulated over 5000 objects. This is indeed impressive but is perhaps placed in a more realistic perspective if one realizes that this collection was amassed over a period of more than 35 years. The National Safety Council tells us that each year in the United States there are approximately 1000 deaths from ingestion of foreign bodies. The discrepancy, of course, lies in the fact that those foreign bodies that cause death usually do so quickly. Often such patients are examined by no physician other than the coroner or medical examiner.

ETIOLOGY

The propensity of small children to put whatever comes into their grasp into their mouths is well known. To this may be added their tendency to imitate adults. The parent who holds pins, screws, or nails in his mouth should not be surprised when an infant puts such an object in his own mouth at the first opportunity.

Foreign body ingestion may be encouraged by failure of the patient's protective mechanisms in several ways. Most common of these is probably the loss of tactile sense in the hard palate when the patient wears a full upper denture. Diminution of perception and reflex action when the person is in a state of alcoholic intoxication, epileptic seizure, deep sleep, or unconsciousness is also a contributing cause.

Carelessness may contribute to foreign body ingestion in many ways: improper preparation of food, hasty eating and drinking, permitting children to play while eating, talking with food in the mouth, giving food such as peanuts to children who do not have the molar teeth to chew

them, and improper supervision of small children playing near infants. Small children have been seen to deliberately feed an object they knew to be dangerous—such as a safety pin—to an infant sibling. Such primitive solutions to the problem of sibling rivalry can be eliminated only by careful supervision.

A well known cause of foreign body ingestion is the inappropriate reuse of food containers. The most dangerous container is the Coca-Cola bottle. Many children throughout the world have been conditioned to believe that anything that comes from a soft drink bottle is to be consumed with relish. Children are poisoned every day by substances that were inappropriately stored in the ever-handy beverage bottle.

Some foreign bodies are made to resemble objects that would normally be put in or near the mouth and are physically easy to ingest, such as light, slippery, plastic imitation lipsticks and doll bottle caps. The plastic tip from a Bic pen can be aspirated by older children and even by adults.

Marketing trends also affect the type of foreign body ingested. Rarely today does one see safety pins as foreign bodies because of the popularity of disposable diapers. Disc battery ingestion has been reported since the mid 1970s because of the increased use of calculators, cameras, watches, and hearing aids. This is one of the few true foreign body emergencies, because, as Maves and associates (1984) noted, esophageal perforation can occur within 8 to 12 hours of the ingestion. Jacks have been replaced by attractively colored Lite Brite pegs and other nonradiopaque plastic toys that now challenge the endoscopist.

ROENTGENOGRAPHIC AIDS

Roentgenographic studies provide valuable assistance to the endoscopist, not only in documenting presence of a foreign body but also as an aid in extraction. Incomplete studies may lead to errors in diagnosis. An ingested object may lodge anywhere from the base of the skull to the floor of the perineum. Although many foreign bodies are radiolucent, special techniques such as inspiration-expiration films and fluoroscopy—with or without contrast material—may help to establish the diagnosis.

Appropriate study and proper technique are needed to accurately locate the foreign body. The relationship of the foreign object to surrounding structures must be understood and visualized in the widest plane to properly plan the endoscopic procedure.

The lateral soft tissue film of the neck is one of the most useful single studies available to the endoscopist. Even without supplementary contrast material, the caliber of the airway is often readily appreciated. Holinger (1962) suggested an "endoscopic" lateral film, in which the arms and shoulders are held backward and downward. A profile of the air column in the larynx and trachea is thus visible in a single film (Fig. 44–1). Holinger (1972) also advocated the use of the lateral neck xeroradiogram in the evaluation of patients with suspected foreign body

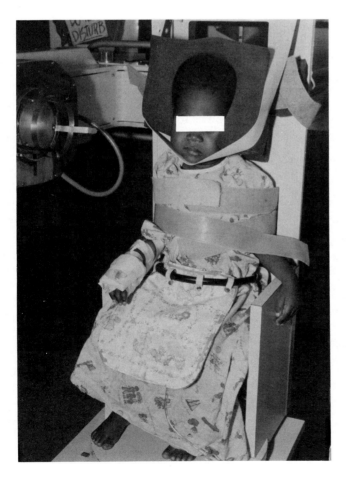

Fig. 44–1. Specially built chair used at the Children's Memorial Hospital in Chicago for soft tissue lateral films of the neck and airway. The chin is held up, the shoulders down for consistently high quality studies.

ingestion. The technique amplifies small differences in soft tissue densities.

In addition to the anteroposterior and lateral films of the chest normally taken during inhalation (Fig. 44–2A), similar films taken at the end of exhalation are helpful (Fig. 44–2B). Such studies are especially useful in delineating obstructive emphysema because the trapping of air behind the foreign object—and the failure of the trapped air to empty on exhalation—is most apparent on this film. Some radiologists prefer lateral decubitus films. A dynamic demonstration of this phenomenon can be obtained by fluoroscopy, during which the motion of the chest throughout the entire respiratory cycle can be continuously observed.

Contrast material such as barium is used with great caution and only after plain films have been inadequate to delineate the specific problem. An object such as a chicken or pork bone may be apparent in the lateral soft tissue film of the neck. Administration of contrast material in such a situation necessitates delay of the endoscopic procedure until the material has passed beyond the stomach. Contrast material retained above an obstructive foreign body not only complicates the removal of the foreign object but also might be aspirated into the respiratory tract.

Bronchography has occasionally been useful to demonstrate the relationship of a foreign object to the bronchial tree or to localize a radiolucent plastic foreign object. If contrast material must be used, Lipiodol is preferable because it is translucent and less likely to obscure the object during endoscopy.

LARYNGEAL FOREIGN BODY

Laryngeal foreign bodies that cause complete obstruction result in sudden death unless removed immediately at the scene of the incident. Objects that are only partially obstructive may cause hoarseness, aphonia, croupy cough, odynophagia, hemoptysis, wheezing, and varying degrees of dyspnea. These symptoms may be caused by the foreign body itself or by a residual laryngeal reaction from a foreign body that has migrated to the trachea. Such symptoms can also be caused by attempts at removal. If the foreign body is in fact lodged in the esophagus, there may still be sufficient periesophageal reaction and obstruction to cause secretions to overflow into the larynx and cause the laryngeal symptoms as secondary manifestations of the presence of a foreign body.

TRACHEAL FOREIGN BODY

Signs of tracheal foreign bodies include: audible slap, palpatory thud, and asthmatoid wheeze. The diagnosis is made by roentgenographic studies, auscultation, palpation, and bronchoscopy. The audible slap is best heard at the open mouth during cough. The asthmatoid wheeze is best heard with the ear at the patient's open mouth. This sign is especially significant if there is a history of initial choking, gagging, and wheezing.

BRONCHIAL FOREIGN BODY

The most common symptoms of bronchial foreign bodies are coughing and wheezing. There may be a history

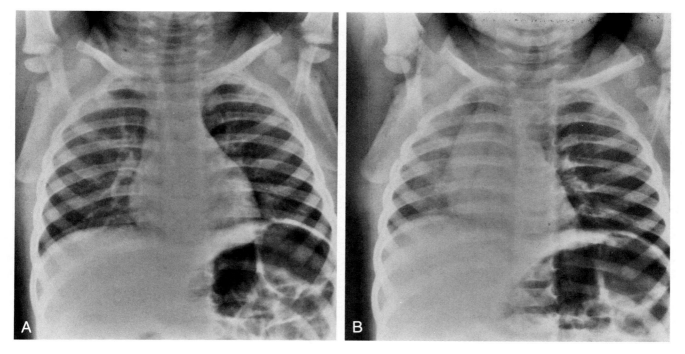

Fig. 44–2. *A*, Anteroposterior film of the chest during inspiration. *B*, Anteroposterior film of the chest during expiration. Note the trapping of air in the left lung field caused by a peanut in the left main stem bronchus.

of aspiration or of tooth extraction. Obstructive foreign bodies cause emphysema, atelectasis, pulmonary edema, and eventually, pulmonary abscess. Organic materials are more apt to cause a relatively violent reaction, with the symptoms of laryngotracheal bronchitis, cough, and irregular fever. Any of these late manifestations may be obscured by prior treatment with antibiotics or steroids.

The physical signs of bronchial foreign bodies vary. Co-existing pathology, tracheobronchial anatomy, and type and location of the foreign body vary from one patient to another. Secretions, whether normal or pathological, may shift from one location to another. The foreign body itself may shift position and cause, from time to time, a variation in the aeration distal to the foreign object. Jackson divided such obstruction into four types. Figure 44–3 demonstrates the relatively fixed location of the foreign object in one bronchus. Foreign bodies in the lower trachea, however, may give rise to a variety of signs and symptoms localized in either or both lungs as the foreign body shifts its position in the region of the tracheal carina.

Roentgenographic examination should be made in conjunction with a careful physical examination. Obstructive emphysema, which may be apparent only on a good expiratory roentgenogram, sometimes can be discerned more readily by watching the patient's chest rise and fall with respiration and noting the lag in emptying on the obstructed side. Localization of the site of lodgement on the chest film depends upon an accurate knowledge of the segments of the lung and the orifices of the segmental bronchi. The current medical practice of treating "asthmatic" or croupy children with antibiotics and steroids

can obscure signs and symptoms that would normally be expected with a retained foreign object. Clearing of symptoms with these agents cannot always be assumed to be diagnostic of a specific disease process. The fact that a wheeze disappears or that a pneumonic process clears may merely mean that a patient's reaction to the presence of the foreign object has been temporarily controlled. The recurrence of "asthma" after the withdrawal of therapy should heighten the physician's suspicion of a foreign object as the possible underlying cause of distress.

TREATMENT

Heimlich Maneuver

Complete airway obstruction by a foreign body can be recognized in the conscious victim when a person who has been eating or has had a foreign body in his mouth is suddenly unable to speak or cough, even when asked, "can you speak?" Reflexively, or as a result of training, the victim may use the "distress signal of choking," which is the gesture of clutching the neck between the thumb and open palm. The Heimlich maneuver is indicated.

Finger Probing

Foreign objects that do not immediately cause complete obstruction but present with gagging, coughing, sputtering, wheezing, and so forth, place the physician in a position in which he may inadvertently make the patient worse. In such situations, probing the hypopharynx with the finger may impact a foreign body that

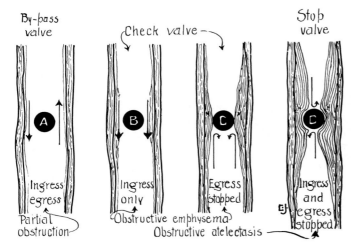

Fig. 44–3. Schematic illustration of the three types of bronchial obstruction encountered clinically.

Type 1, By-pass valve obstruction. The foreign body, *A,* permits the by-passage of air in and out on inspiration and expiration, so that no collapse or emphysema occurs in the tributary lung.

Type 2, Check valve obstruction. *B* and *C* represent the same foreign body in different phases of the respiratory cycle. *B,* The swollen mucosa has retreated because of enlargement of the bronchial lumen on inspiration. At the beginning of expiration, the bronchial wall contracts sufficiently to bring the swollen mucosa into contact with the foreign body, *C,* This valve-like closure traps the air in the subjacent lung or portion of lung, which becomes emphysematous from repetition of the valvular action at each respiratory cycle. This is obstructive emphysema.

Type 3, Stop-valve obstruction. A foreign body, *D,* is embedded in swollen mucosa, completely obstructing a bronchus at all stages of respiration. Absorption of the air results in collapse of the subjacent lung. This condition is obstructive atelectasis. If a main bronchus is obstructed, massive collapse of the corresponding lung occurs.

Type 4, A fourth type was omitted from the schema for clearness. In check-valve obstruction, the reverse of type 2, air is forced out on expiration, especially the forced expiration of cough, but ingress is checked by the ball-valve action of the foreign body. This hastens atelectasis, and this type quickly merges into type 3. (From Jackson, C., and Jackson, C.L.: Distress of the Air and Food Passages of Foreign Body Origin. Philadelphia, W.B. Saunders Co., 1936.)

is loose in the hypopharynx tightly into the larynx, thus transforming partial obstruction into complete obstruction; force the foreign body into the esophagus, where it may compress the trachea against the upper sternum, causing an obstruction that cannot be relieved even by tracheotomy; or—as the physician originally intended—remove the foreign body through the mouth or allow it to be carried harmlessly through the alimentary tract (Fig. 44–4).

Inhalation-Postural Drainage Technique

Burrington and Cotton (1972) introduced a controversial alternative to bronchoscopic extraction, consisting of inhalation of bronchodilator followed by postural drainage and percussion. This technique was continued up to 4 days before resorting to bronchoscopy.

Law and Kosloske (1976), however, found this technique had only a 25% success rate, compared to an 89% success rate with bronchoscopy. They reported an episode of cardiopulmonary arrest secondary to migration

of the foreign body from the bronchus to the trachea. This technique has been abandoned because of the greater risk of complication.

Flexible Bronchoscopy

Open-tube—rigid—bronchoscopy is the method of choice for removal of most foreign bodies from the tracheobronchial tree. Flexible fiber-optic bronchoscopy has no application in infants because there is no channel for ventilation, suction, or instrumentation. Thorburn and colleagues (1986) recommend flexible fiber-optic bronchoscopy in certain circumstances, including head and neck injury, patients with tracheotomy, and cases of peripheral foreign bodies.

Open-Tube—Rigid—Endoscopy

The open-tube bronchoscope is the instrument of choice for foreign body extractions. All other techniques should be discouraged unless the circumstances leave the physician no other choice.

The suspicion of the presence of a "foreign body" carries with it the unreasoning connotation that haste is always necessary. Deliberate speed is, of course, desirable in emergent situations. A properly trained endoscopic team with a full selection of instruments to meet the mechanical problems is of inestimable value in rising to the challenge presented by the true acute emergency. The experienced endoscopist also appreciates the value of careful preparation of himself, the patient, the instruments and the team before starting the procedure, because minimal morbidity and mortality depend upon adequate preparation. If 2 hours are spent in such preparation, the safe endoscopic removal of the foreign body may take only 2 minutes. But if only 2 minutes are taken for preparation, the endoscopist may find himself attempting ineffective, makeshift procedures for the next frustrating 2 hours, as Holinger (1962) pointed out.

Following an unsuccessful attempt, for whatever reason, repeated instrumentation is not to be undertaken for several days, especially because the trauma of a second procedure might cause more edema, necessitating postoperative intubation. Such an interval might be used for steroid and antibiotic coverage to lessen laryngeal and bronchial reaction. Steroids should be withheld if there seems to be danger of esophageal perforation.

Time is also required to permit the stomach to empty of residual barium or food. Ideally, endoscopic procedures should be undertaken in the morning, when the team is at its best and a full range of ancillary services—anesthesia and radiology—is available. Children, especially, should be treated early in the day so that any untoward laryngeal reaction can be diagnosed and treated quickly.

Hospitals large enough to generate sufficient endoscopic treatment experience should concentrate this experience in the hands of those who are to handle foreign body problems. To request a doctor to remove foreign bodies but deny him the full range of endoscopic practice is a disservice to the patient. Even in the most specialized clinics, ingested foreign bodies constitute less than 10%

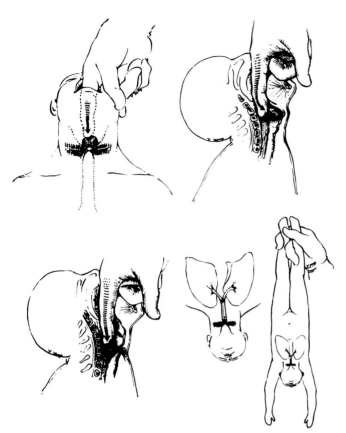

Fig. 44–4. Possible methods of impaction of a foreign body by ill-advised first aid. (From Tucker, G.F., Jr., Trans. Am. Bronchoesoph. Assoc., *49*:181, 1969.)

of the overall endoscopic experience. Those hospitals that presume to offer this service to the patient must have available not only an experienced endoscopist but also a full team of nurse assistants, anesthesiologists, and radiologists, fully equipped to meet not only the apparent problems but also the unplanned complications.

Preliminary Study

The first step in the solution of the mechanical problem presented by the presence of any foreign body is the study of roentgenograms made in at least three planes: anteroposterior, lateral, and that corresponding to the greatest plane of the foreign body. The next step is to put a duplicate of the foreign body into a lung model and simulate the position shown by the roentgenograms to get an idea of the probable presentation. Because shifting may change the presentation, the duplicate foreign body is turned into as many different positions as possible to educate the eye in comprehending the possible presentations that may be encountered at bronchoscopy. For each presentation, a method of disimpaction, disengagement, disentanglement, or version and seizure should be worked out, as Jackson and Jackson (1936, 1959) emphasized.

Selection and Use of Forceps

Preliminary selection and test of forceps with a duplicate of the foreign body should be made in every case.

It is sad to see a child arrive very ill or moribund from prolonged efforts elsewhere to remove a foreign body with forceps, the utter uselessness of which could have been determined in a moment by testing on a duplicate. In some cases, different forceps must be ready for different presentations. Forceps jaws must expand sufficiently to encompass the foreign body, if not in every diameter, at least in the diameter of the selected presentation.

Prepared by this practice and the roentgenograms, the endoscopist introduces the bronchoscope. The location of the foreign body is approached slowly and carefully to avoid overriding or displacement. A study of the presentation is as necessary for the bronchoscopist as for the obstetrician. The bronchoscopist should try to determine: the relation of the presenting part to the surrounding tissues and the probable position of the unseen portion, as determined by the appearance of the presenting part combined with the knowledge obtained by the roentgenographic studies.

The standard forward-grasping forceps has a powerful grip and is used on dense foreign bodies that require a very firm grip to prevent the forceps from slipping off. For more delicate manipulation, and particularly for friable foreign bodies, a lighter forceps, such as a fenestrated peanut forceps, is best. Forceps should be held in the right hand, the thumb in one ring and the third finger in the other ring. These fingers are used to open

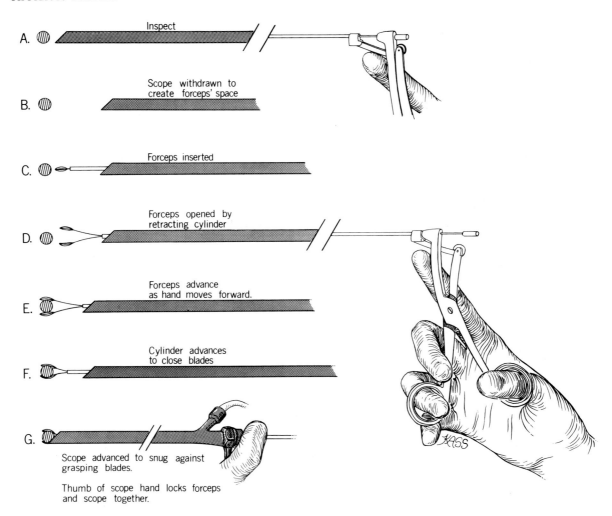

A. Inspect

B. Scope withdrawn to create forceps' space

C. Forceps inserted

D. Forceps opened by retracting cylinder

E. Forceps advance as hand moves forward.

F. Cylinder advances to close blades

G. Scope advanced to snug against grasping blades.

Thumb of scope hand locks forceps and scope together.

Fig. 44–5. Proper grasp of forceps. The right thumb and third finger are inserted into the rings and the right index finger is placed high on the handle. All traction is made with the index finger, the ring finger being used only to open and close the forceps. If any pushing is deemed safe, it may be done by placing the index finger behind the thumbnut on the eyelet. (From Jackson, C., and Jackson, C.L.: Diseases of the Air and Food Passages of Foreign Body Origin. Philadelphia, W.B. Saunders Co., 1936.)

and close the forceps; all traction and pulsion is achieved by the right index finger, which is positioned on the forceps handle near the stylet (Fig. 44–5).

The bronchoscopist must resist the impulse to seize the foreign body as soon as he discovers it and must carefully study its size, shape, position, and relation to surrounding structures before making any attempt at extraction. When the most favorable point and position for grasping have been ascertained, the closed forceps is inserted through the bronchoscope. The forceps is advanced until it lightly touches the foreign body then is allowed to expand. It is advanced far enough to grasp the object. If there are no sharp points on the foreign body, it is held and the tube mouth is advanced against it. If it is too large to come out through the tube, it is held against the tube mouth, the grasp of the forceps being firmly maintained by the fingers on the right hand while all traction for withdrawal is made by the left hand, which firmly clamps forceps and bronchoscope as one

piece. Thus the three units are brought out as one, the endoscope keeping the vocal cords apart until the foreign body has entered the glottis.

Pins, needles, and similar pointed objects fall into two groups: (1) bendable pins, and (2) breakable pins and needles. It is often desirable to bend a pin but less desirable to break it. When searching for pointed or sharp objects, special care must be taken not to override them. Pins are almost always found point upward.

Jackson's dictum states: "look not for the foreign body; look for the point." If the point is free, it should be worked into the lumen of the bronchoscope by manipulation with forceps and the lip of the tube. It then may be seized with the forceps and withdrawn. Should the pin be grasped by the shaft, it is almost certain to turn across the tube mouth, where one pull may cause perforation, enormously increasing the difficulties of removal and perhaps resulting in serious trauma (Fig. 44–6).

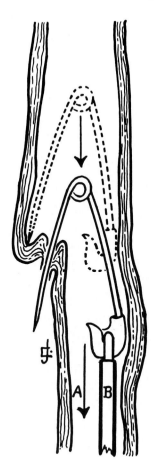

Fig. 44–6. Schematic drawing of what will happen if the dictum "Advancing points perforate: trailing points do not" is ignored. (From Jackson, C., and Jackson, C.L.: Diseases of the Air and Food Passages of Foreign Body Origin. W.B. Saunders Co. Philadelphia, 1936.)

Extraction of pointed, radiopaque foreign bodies in the lung periphery are attempted only under simultaneous biplane fluoroscopic guidance.

The sheathing and protective methods for the removal of pins apply also to the removal of tacks and other double-pointed objects. Tacks and staples are best managed with a special stable bronchoscope and forceps.

Hollow metallic objects are best held with one of the forceps jaws inside and one outside, or removed with hollow object—internal expansion—forceps. Hard, smooth, globular objects like ball-bearings are best held with the ball-bearing forceps.

ESOPHAGEAL FOREIGN BODIES

The esophagus is a vulnerable site for retention of swallowed materials because of weak peristalsis and multiple narrowings. The incidence is higher in children and edentulous adults, but is declining because of better public education and public safety measures. Chaikhouni and colleagues (1985) noted a high correlation with underlying esophageal abnormalities and esophageal foreign bodies. These include stricture, hiatal hernia, reflux, mental disease, neurologic disease, repaired congenital tracheoesophageal fistula, and recurrent spasm. Five physiologic constrictions are well described, the most common being the cricopharyngeal narrowing at C6, followed by the hiatal narrowing at T10/T11, the thoracic

inlet at T1, the aortic arch at T4, and the tracheal bifurcation at T6.

Signs and symptoms of esophageal foreign body most commonly include dysphagia, pain, sensation of foreign body, wheezing, increased salivation, and tracheal aspiration secondary to esophageal obstruction. Rarely, a patient may be totally asymptomatic. Foreign bodies most associated with perforation are bones, pins, dental appliances, jacks, safety pins, wooden sticks, and coins.

Treatment

Enzyme Digestion

Enzymes used consist of caroid, chymotrypsin, and papain. This method was first described by Richardson (1945). Contraindications include: impaction longer than 36 hours, known or suspected perforation, and a foreign body that is sharp or has bony fragments. Death caused by perforation, mediastinitis, and major vessel rupture has been reported with this method.

Glucagon

Trenkner and associates (1983) stated that although the success rate is relatively low, the risk for adults is minimal and justifiable. With a success rate of approximately 37%, it is accepted as a safe and worthwhile step in the treatment of distal esophageal foreign bodies. Trenkner recommends a Gastrografin study initially to confirm the

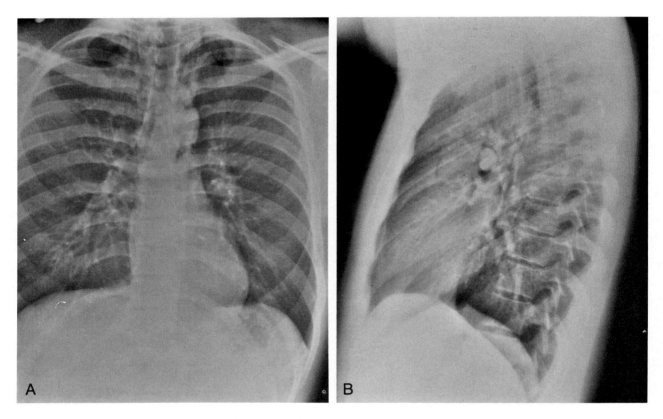

Fig. 44–7. *A*, Anteroposterior roentgenogram with pneumomediastinum secondary to perforation of the esophagus. *B*, Lateral roentgenogram demonstrating the pulmonary artery outlined by pneumomediastinum.

presence of the nonradiopaque foreign body and to determine its location. Glucagon is then given IV in the upright position, 0.5 mg to 2.0 mg, followed by ingestion of water. This procedure may be repeated in 10 to 15 minutes. A repeat Gastrografin study is then done to determine if the foreign body has passed. In doses greater than 20 μg, glucagon causes a significant decrease in lower esophageal sphincter pressure with no apparent changes in esophageal peristalsis of the esophageal body.

A known complication is vomiting, especially with rapid IV administration, which may cause aspiration or esophageal rupture if the bolus is sharp or contains bony fragments. Absolute contraindications include pheochromocytoma or insulinoma.

Foley Catheter Extraction

McGuirt (1982) recommended the use of a Foley catheter in the removal of esophageal foreign body. He stated the advantages are cost effectiveness and less emotional trauma to the patient. The disadvantages include: underlying or associated diseases will be missed, and unidentified foreign body may be left behind, and blind manipulation of a rough foreign body may perforate the esophagus. Additional disadvantages include prolonged radiation exposure under fluoroscopy, the possible aspiration of the foreign body, as Bigler (1966) noted, and the emotional trauma of a prolonged, frightening, uncomfortable procedure without anesthesia.

Contraindications to this technique are airway compromise or total esophageal obstruction. Advocates of the technique recommended it only with a smooth, inert, radiopaque foreign body that has been lodged less than 48 to 72 hours. A preoperative contrast study must be negative for total obstruction, multiple foreign bodies, and any underlying esophageal pathology. An endoscopist should be standing by and have available airway maintenance equipment, endoscopic grasping instruments, and endoscopes!

Fiber-Optic Esophagoscopy

Advocates of this instrument state that the main advantage is that general anesthesia is not required. Bendig (1986) noted that the advantages also include built-in suction, air insufflation, magnification, and the ability to examine the stomach and duodenum. Disadvantages include possible aspiration, airway obstruction associated with uncontrolled removal, and inadvertent esophageal trauma with blind manipulation or a rough or sharp object.

Contraindications, proposed by Bendig (1986), include: impaction longer than 2 weeks, acute symptoms and ingested batteries or nonsmooth foreign bodies. As with the technique of Foley catheter extraction, an experienced endoscopist should be standing by!

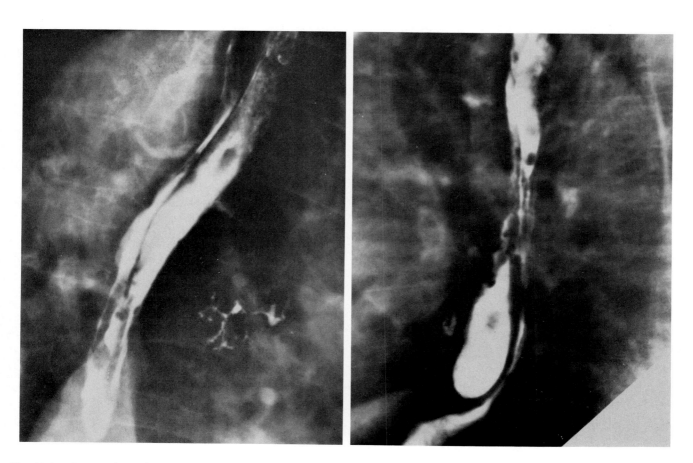

Fig. 44–8. Gastrografin study demonstrating an upper esophageal perforation.

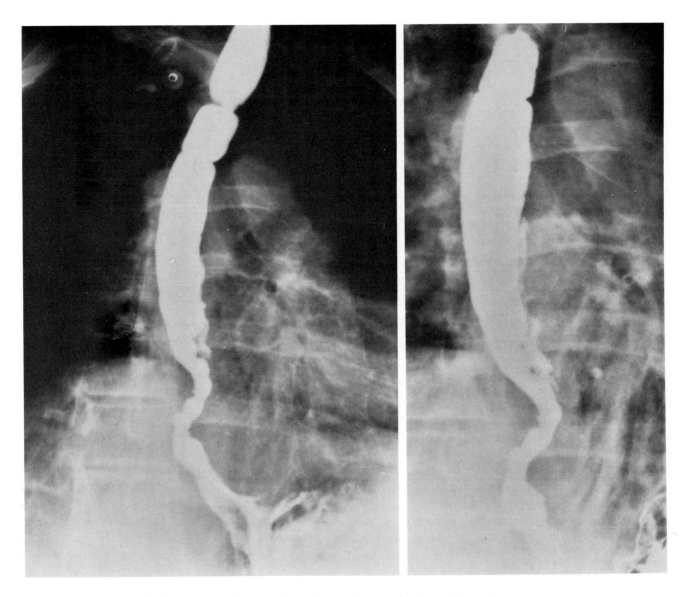

Fig. 44–9. Gastrografin study demonstrating a lower esophageal perforation secondary to meat impaction.

Open-Tube Esophagoscopy

As with bronchial foreign bodies, open-tube esophagoscopy is the preferred technique. General endotracheal anesthesia allows orderly removal of foreign bodies while minimizing the risk of aspiration.

Many instruments have been developed for manipulation of foreign bodies of virtually any size, configuration, or position. Special note should be made of pointed objects such as safety pins. They can be dealt with by any of 16 described methods. The most frequently used are (1) endogastric version, (2) endogastric straightening, (3) point sheathing, and (4) closing methods.

Complications and Pitfalls

Most complications are caused by inexperience in introducing the esophagoscope or traction on the presenting part of a foreign body without first determining the possible result of such traction. The esophagus is exceedingly intolerant of trauma, much more so than any other viscus.

Esophageal injury varies from a minimal mucosal tear to major rupture involving adjacent structures. Symptoms and signs of perforation include tachypnea, odynophagia, dysphagia, vomiting, and chest or back pain. Physical signs of perforation include cervical emphysema, fever, tachycardia, limitation of cervical movement, and the crunch sign, as described by Hamman (1937). Goligher (1948), Barrett (1956), and Colman (1958) recognized and reported that mediastinitis may not be apparent for up to 48 hours after perforation during endoscopy.

If a perforation is suspected, the chest roentgenogram may show mediastinal or cervical emphysema (Fig. 44–7), mediastinal widening, fluid levels, or widening of the prevertebral space from edema or abscess. A soft tissue film of the neck is most sensitive, demonstrating emphysema in 95% of perforations. When perforation is highly suspect, a Gastrografin swallow is the preferred initial study (Figs. 44–8 and 44–9). It readily demonstrates a large perforation, causes little tissue reaction, and is rapidly absorbed if a leak is present. Furthermore, Gastrografin does not obstruct visualization at endoscopy. If the Gastrografin swallow is negative, barium is used. It is more sensitive and defines even small tears.

Donnelly and Deverall (1968) and Shockley and associates (1985) outlined the following indications for surgery: (1) to remove a foreign body that cannot be removed at endoscopy, (2) to close primarily a large perforation—if within 48 hours, and (3) to drain a mediastinal abscess. Seybold (1950) and Paulson (1960) and associates reported a 40 to 70% incidence of mortality in esophageal perforation treated with antibiotics alone. Foster and colleagues (1965) and Dawes (1964) arrived at similar conclusions. In some cases, a compromise approach is advocated: antibiotics and drainage of the wound by placement of a chest tube at or close to the site of perforation.

The treatment of choice for perforations depends upon whether the injury is more or less than 48 hours old. If less than 48 hours, minor anterior and lateral cervical tears can be treated by intravenous antibiotics alone. If the site of injury can be identified with contrast or endoscopy, exploration of the neck or chest with primary closure is accomplished and drains are placed at the perforation site. If the perforation is older than 48 hours, drainage alone is unsatisfactory, for at this stage the patient is most likely to have diffuse mediastinitis. Large doses of antibiotics and gastric and pleural drainage are needed. Total parenteral nutrition is also recommended (see Chapter 45).

REFERENCES

Barrett, N.R.: Discussion on unusual aspects of eosphageal disease. Proc. R. Soc. Med. *49*:529, 1956.

Bendig, D.W.: Removal of blunt esophageal foreign bodies by flexible endoscopy without general anesthesia. Am. J. Dis. Child. *140*:789, 1986.

Bigler, F.C.: The use of a Foley catheter for removal of blunt foreign bodies from the esophagus. J. Thorac. Cardiovasc. Surg. *51*:759, 1966.

Burrington, J.D., and Cotton, E.K.: Removal of foreign bodies from the tracheobronchial tree. J. Pediatr. Surg. *7*:119, 1972.

Chaikhouni, A., Kratz, J.M., and Crawford, F.A.: Foreign bodies of the esophagus. Am. Surg. *51*:173, 1985.

Colman, B.H.: Perforation of the hypopharynx and cervical esophagus. J. Laryngol. Otol. *72*:790, 1958.

Dawes, J.D.K.: Traumatic perforation of the pharynx and esophagus. J. Laryngol. Otol. *78*:18, 1964.

Donnelly, R.J., and Deverall, P.B.: The management of esophageal foreign bodies and their complications. Postgrad. Med. J. *44*:830, 1968.

Foster, J.H., et al.: Esophageal perforation: diagnosis and treatment. Ann. Surg. *161*:701, 1965.

Goligher, J.C.: Postcricoid pharyngo-esophageal perforation due to endoscopy treated by immediate suture. Lancet *i*:985, 1948.

Hamman, L.: Spontaneous interstitial emphysema of the lungs. Trans. Assoc. Amer. Physicians *52*:311, 1937.

Holinger, P.H.: Foreign bodies in the air and food passages. Trans. Amer. Acad. Ophthalmol. Otolaryngol. *66*:193, 1962.

Holinger, P.H., et al.: Xeroradiography of the larynx. Ann. Otol. *81*:806, 1972.

Jackson, C., and Jackson, C.L.: Diseases of the air and food passages of foreign body origin. Philadelphia, W.B. Saunders Co., 1936.

Jackson, C., and Jackson, C.L.: Diseases of the nose, throat, and ear. 2nd ed. Philadelphia, W.B. Saunders Co., 1959.

Law, D.K., and Kosloske, A.M.: Management of tracheobronchial foreign bodies in children: a re-evaluation of postural drainage and bronchoscopy. Pediatrics *58*:362, 1976.

Maves, M.D., Carithers, J.S., and Birck, H.G.: Esophageal burns secondary to disc battery ingestion. Ann. Otol. Rhinol. Laryngol. *93*:364, 1984.

McGuirt, W.F.: Use of Foley catheter for removal of esophageal foreign bodies. Ann. Otol. Rhinol. Laryngol. *91*:599, 1982.

Paulson, D.L., and Shaw, P.R., and Kee, J.L.: Recognition and treatment of esophageal perforations. Ann. Surg. *152*:13, 1960.

Richardson, J.R.: New treatment for esophageal obstruction due to meat impaction. Ann. Otol. Rhinol. Laryngol. *54*:328, 1945.

Seybold, W.D., Johnson, M.A., and Leary, W.V.: Perforation of the esophagus. Surg. Clin. N. Amer. *30*:1155, 1950.

Shockley, W.W., Tate, J.L., and Stucker, F.J.: Management of perforations of the hypopharynx and cervical esophagus. Laryngoscope *95*:939, 1985.

Thorburn, J.R., et al.: A technique for foreign body removal from the airway. Endoscopy *18*:71, 1986.

Trenkner, S.W., et al.: Esophageal food impaction: treatment with glucagon. Radiology *149*(2):401, 1983.

Tucker, G.F., Jr.: Laryngeal and tracheobronchial foreign bodies. Trans. Pa. Acad. Ophthalmol. Otolaryngol. *19*(1):12, 1966.

CHAPTER 45

TRAUMA TO THE ESOPHAGUS

Thomas W. Shields and Robert M. Vanecko

The esophagus is subject to various forms of accidental trauma, which may be penetrating, operative, blunt, or chemical. The incidence of each varies with the patient population under observation.

PENETRATING TRAUMA

Penetrating trauma can be classified as arising either internally—intraluminal—or externally—extraluminal. Intraluminal injuries result from instrumentation, ingestion of a foreign body, or a rapid increase of intraluminal pressure; extraluminal injuries arise from gunshot or stab wounds of the neck or chest and, infrequently, blunt trauma. The associated injuries frequently present with external trauma often obscure the esophageal injury and prevent its early recognition unless a high index of suspicion is maintained by those treating such injuries.

Intraluminal Injuries

Internal penetrating injuries are conveniently separated into three categories: instrumental injuries, foreign body injuries, and noninstrumental injuries, i.e., those caused by sudden changes in intraluminal pressure.

Instrumental Injuries

These injuries may occur during diagnostic or therapeutic procedures involving the esophagus. They are more common secondary to rigid than to flexible esophagoscopy. In the former, Wychulis and associates (1969) reported the incidence to be approximately 0.4% in routine diagnostic examination. Meyers and Ghahremani (1975) noted, however, that the actual number of perforations may be increasing because of more frequent use of the flexible esophagoscope.

The more common sites of perforation are at two of the normal anatomic sites of narrowing of the esophagus: the level of the junction of the interior constrictor and the cricopharyngeus muscles in the neck and the distal end of the esophagus as it reaches the diaphragm to join the stomach. The third area of narrowing, at the level of

the aortic arch and left main bronchus, is seldom involved.

When a pathologic process is present, examination with biopsy or therapeutic dilatation may lead to rupture at the involved site. An incidence of 4.9% following pneumatic dilatation was reported by Bennett and Hendrix (1970). Rarely rupture may occur with improper placement and inflation of the gastric balloon of a Sengstaken-Blakemore tube to control bleeding esophageal varices (Fig. 45–1). Perforation during the placement of an indwelling tube for palliation of a malignant stricture is not an uncommon event. Shemesh and Bat (1986) reported that endoscopic injection sclerotherapy for esophageal varices has resulted in esophageal perforations. Also, O'Neill and associates (1984) pointed out that esophageal perforation may occur during attempted endotracheal intubation.

The clinical features and management of perforation from any of the aforementioned sources depend on the location and the nature of the injury. The extent of the injury as well as the time of recognition also play important roles in this regard.

Cervical Perforation. Partial disruption of the cervical esophagus with mucosal tear may occur more frequently

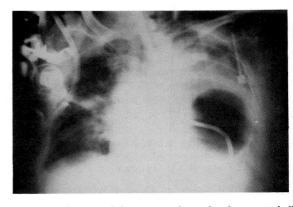

Fig. 45–1. Perforation of thoracic esophagus by the gastric balloon of a Sengstaken-Blakemore tube.

494

than recognized but may be potentially serious if an intramural abscess develops. A perforation of all layers of the esophagus, however, is much more common. Usually, the endoscopist may suspect injury because of unusual difficulty or the occurrence of bleeding during the procedure. With a complete perforation of the wall, oropharyngeal secretions with their contained aerobic and anaerobic microorganisms are free to contaminate the visceral compartment within the neck. As air and secretions are forced out of the esophagus on swallowing, contamination and air extend into the other fascial compartments of the neck and may descend into the mediastinum.

Clinically, within several hours of the injury, the patient complains of pain and stiffness in the neck, dysphagia, and at times respiratory distress. On examination, the patient is febrile and has varying degrees of dysphonia—usually a nasal twang to the voice—and cervical tenderness. Crepitance caused by subcutaneous air may be found on palpation of the neck.

Roentgenographic examination of the neck may reveal air in the fascial planes, widening of the retroesophageal space, and obliteration of the normal cervical vertebral curvature (Fig. 45–2). In some neglected patients, a retroesophageal abscess with an air-fluid level may be present.

In most patients with instrumental perforation of the cervical esophagus, neither roentgenographic examination of the esophagus with the use of a contrast medium nor esophagoscopy is indicated. In fact, such examinations may be misleading because they frequently fail to identify the site of perforation; therefore, they are not recommended.

The management of these injuries is adequate drainage of the visceral compartment of the neck and prevention of continued contamination of the area. These goals are best achieved by an anterior cervical mediastinotomy, repair of the laceration, and drainage of the area. The technique of cervical mediastinotomy is described in

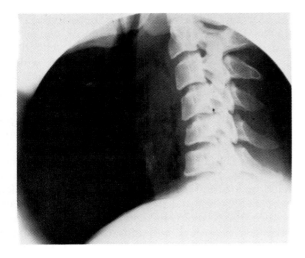

Fig. 45–2. Lateral roentgenogram of the neck revealing widening of and free air in retroesophageal space after perforation of the esophagus in the neck.

Chapter 89. Repair of the perforation is best performed with interrupted, nonabsorbable, fine sutures. At times, owing to either the degree of inflammation or the duration of time between the injury and its recognition— approximately 12 hours or more—or both, no attempt at direct repair of the laceration is indicated. In such a situation, one must rely on adequate drainage, cessation of swallowing, and aspiration of oropharyngeal secretions. Appropriate antibiotics to control the mircroorganisms in the oropharyngeal secretions are indicated in all patients.

Occasionally, when the injury is recognized immediately and is thought to be minor or when there is a question about the presence of a perforation through all layers of the esophagus, expectant treatment can be employed. This therapy consists of cessation of swallowing, aspiration of oropharyngeal secretions, rest, and antibiotics. With such a regimen, a successful response may be obtained; however, acute cervical mediastinal suppuration may occur, so the patient must be observed carefully. Berry and Ochsner (1973) reported that two thirds of their patients managed expectantly required subsequent drainage.

The morbidity of instrumental injury to the cervical esophagus is minimal when recognized early and appropriately treated. Death is rare and, when it does occur, is related to spread of the infection into the mediastinum and failure to recognize the underlying problem.

Thoracic Perforation. Although perforation of the wall of the thoracic esophagus may lead initially only to contamination of the visceral compartment of the mediastinum, most often the mediastinal pleural layer is perforated as well, and this perforation leads to prompt contamination of either of the pleural spaces. The left pleural space is usually involved when the injury is in the most distal portion of the esophagus; the right when the perforation is more proximal. Because of the necrotizing inflammatory process that accompanies these injuries, the infection may spread and involve other structures in the mediastinum. Reflux of gastric juice frequently occurs and further adds to the severity of the inflammatory process.

These injuries to the thoracic esophagus are associated with pain, fever, dysphagia, and, frequently, marked respiratory distress. The pain may be thoracic, precordial, or even epigastric. Radiation of the pain may occur to the intrascapular region. With contamination of the pleural space, there may be severe unilateral pleural pain that is aggravated by breathing. Fever is present and tachycardia is frequently disproportionate to the degree of temperature elevation. Dysphagia is present and may be localized by the patient to the vicinity of perforation. The degree of respiratory distress varies with the severity of the pleural contamination, the amount of hydropneumothorax, and at times the presence of airway compression.

Physical examination may reveal the patient to be toxic, with grunting, guarded respirations. Subcutaneous air may be palpated in the neck, and varying degrees of a hydropneumothorax may be elicited.

Roentgenographic examination of the chest may reveal a widened mediastinal shadow, mediastinal air, and varying amounts of air or fluid, or both, in either pleural space (Fig. 45–3). Evaluation of the lumen of the esophagus and demonstration of the site of the leak may be accomplished by fluoroscopy and ingestion of a suitable contrast medium. A water-soluble contrast medium can be used, but better results can be obtained with water-suspended barium sulfate. As in injuries of the cervical esophagus, esophagoscopy is of little or no value in suspected instrumental perforations of the thoracic esophagus.

As Mayer and associates (1977) emphasized, the management of these injuries is based on four principles: (1) elimination of the source of soilage, (2) provision of adequate drainage, (3) augmentation of host defenses by antibiotics, and (4) maintenance of adequate nutrition. The techniques to achieve these four desired goals vary with the initial status of the esophagus—normal or diseased, benign or malignant; the time of recognition and institution of therapy after the occurrence of injury; the extent of contamination of the mediastinum, the pleural space, or both; and the underlying nutritional status of the patient.

Ideally, when the injury is recognized promptly and the esophagus was initialy normal, a Levin tube is placed for continuous aspiration of the oropharyngeal secretions, and appropriate antibiotics are started; immediate thoracotomy with closure of the esophageal perforation and drainage of the mediastinum and pleural space is carried out. Buttressing of the closure of the esophageal laceration with a pleural flap is recommended as a routine when possible. Continued aspiration of oropharyngeal and gastric secretions is indicated postoperatively. Nutrition is maintained by intravenous fluid administration until normal swallowing is resumed, usually in 5 to 7 days.

When the injury has occurred in or above an obstructing lesion or when institution of treatment has been delayed, direct repair of the esophageal injury may be contraindicated. Continued soilage must be prevented by diversion of oropharyngeal and gastric secretions from the area of esophageal injury and adequate drainage of the mediastinal and pleural space instituted.

The prevention of continued soilage is a perplexing problem. Numerous methods have been proposed, from the simple use of multiple indwelling nasogastric tubes with or without a decompressing gastrostomy to complex surgical procedures to close the perforation or to isolate the thoracic esophagus or even the emergency resection of the organ. Inherent, of course, is the adequate drainage of the pleural and mediastinal spaces.

The major problem is generally the reluctance of the surgeon to adopt an aggressive policy in the management of these injuries, and frequently it is a story of too little, too late. Most recommend that once the patient's condition is stabilized by fluid replacement and other necessary resuscitative measures, most patients should undergo exploratory thoracotomy with mobilization of the esophagus and closure of the perforation. The closure should be buttressed—or even accomplished—with a pleural flap, as suggested by Grillo and Wilkins (1975) (Fig. 45–4). or an appropriate transposed vascularized pedicled muscular flap. A fundic patch, as described by Thal and associates (1965), may be appropriate at times. Any organic or functional disease of the esophagus distal to the perforation should be corrected when possible. Decortication and debridement of any empyema pockets should be done and adequate drainage of the mediastinal and pleural space ensured.

If closure of the perforation cannot be accomplished with a reasonable chance for success, an esophageal exclusion should be carried out. Many techniques have been suggested, but the most suitable should be one, such as the modified esophageal exclusion, suggested by Urschel and associates (1974), in which pharyngoesophagogastric continuity can be restored without major surgical intervention. Triggiani and Belsey (1977), however, as well as DeMeester (1986), do not hesitate to totally exclude the esophagus with subsequent restoration of pharyngogastric continuity with an interposed organ at a later date. Urschel (personal communication, 1987), described using, in his technique for incontinuity exclusion, a sheet of silastic, artifical dura or a piece of pericardium wrapped around the esophagus—usually the abdominal portion—below the perforation over which a heavy suture—No. 2 Prolene—is placed and the suture then doubled through a polyethylene Rumell tourniquet. This is brought out through the abdominal wall in the left upper quadrant near a concurrently performed gastrostomy. The suture is tightened to occlude the esophagus and held in place with a clamp at the end of the polyethylene Rumell tourniquet. The pleural and mediastinal spaces are drained. The proximal esophagus is excluded by a lateral cervical esophagostomy that effectively occludes the distal thoracic portion of the esophagus. After 3 to 6 weeks, healing is determined by contrast studies. If no leak is demonstrated, the clamp is removed from the tourniquet and the polyethylene tube and Prolene suture removed by simply withdrawing them from the abdomen. Occasionally, some stricturing is noted at the site of occlusion, but this may be readily

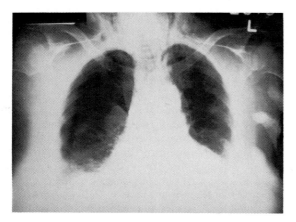

Fig. 45–3. Perforation of thoracic esophagus with right pneumothorax and mediastinal and cervical emphysema.

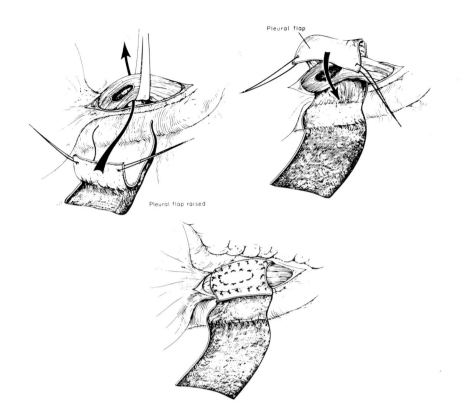

Fig. 45–4. Use of a pedicled flap of parietal pleura to seal perforation of the thoracic esophagus. (Reproduced with permission of Grillo, H.G., and Wilkins, E.W., Jr.: Esophageal repair following late diagnosis of intrathoracic penetration. Ann. Thorac. Surg. 29:387, 1975.)

corrected by esophageal dilatation. With this technique, Urschel reported excellent results, with only three deaths in over 90 patients.

In patients with carcinoma or other serious accompanying esophageal disease, surgical resection may be attempted, as Mayer and colleagues (1977) suggested; however, appreciable mortality rates may be expected. Occasionally, a patient with irradiated, nonresectable carcinomas suffers a perforation during an attempted peroral dilatation. This may result in a chronic, contained perforation, as Cameron and associates (1979) described. When the perforation is contained within the mediastinum, and drains readily back into the esophagus and there are minimal symptoms and no clinical signs of sepsis, the patient may be treated expectantly with antibiotics, nothing by mouth, and nasogastric suction. Hyperalimentation may or may not be necessary. We have managed several such patients successfully, and Wesdrop and colleagues (1984) treat all such perforations of esophageal tumors in this conservative manner and report over a 90% success rate. Other investigators, such as Sandrasagra and associates (1978) have recommended the insertion of an esophageal tube as a stent in such situations.

Except under these circumstances, most believe that the expectant approach of simple pleural drainage in the management of esophageal perforation is less than ideal and is followed by frequent failure. Santos and Frater (1986), however, reported success with drainage only when this was accompanied by copious irrigation of the esophagus and pleural space by peroral intake of large volumes of fluid. We have had one success with such management through a serendipitous chain of events. Antibiotic coverage should be guided by culture of the drainage. Nutritional support may require intravenous hyperalimentation. Management of each patient must be individualized, but the four goals remain unchanged.

The morbidity and mortality rates vary markedly with instrumental injury to the esophagus. Prompt recognition and institution of treatment within 24 hours—preferably less than 12 hours—lessen the incidence and severity of the morbid complications. Bladergroen and colleagues (1986) reported an 80% survival after iatrogenic perforations. The initial status of the injured esophagus, however, plays a significant role. Once persistent leakage and infection are established, the outlook for a satisfactory result is diminished and death is more likely to occur. Likewise, the extremes of age play an adverse role.

Abdominal Perforation. Instrumental injury to the abdominal portion of the esophagus is infrequent, as Walsh (1979) noted. With the injury in this location, contamination of the peritoneal space may occur, with the development of signs and symptoms of an acute abdominal catastrophe. One must remember, however, that perforation of the distal thoracic esophagus may mimic such an event. Roentgenographic examination of the chest and abdomen, as well as of the esophagus, with contrast material should resolve the actual site of the perforation. At times, the injury may be confined to the retroperitoneal space and a more indolent course may be observed. The aforementioned therapeutic goals enumerated for the management of injuries located in the thoracic esophagus obtain in the abdominal area as well. The surgical approach for drainage and possible repair in this situation is transabdominal rather than transthoracic.

Foreign Body Injuries

In review of the literature, Barber and associates (1984) mentioned a great variety of objects and materials that were inappropriately ingested, especially by children, by mentally disturbed or deranged persons, and occasionally by individuals with upper and lower dentures. Many such objects pass into the stomach; others lodge in the esophagus and require removal by endoscopic manipulation. In some instances, sharp or jagged foreign bodies lacerate the wall partially or completely. Most commonly, such laceration occurs in the cervical esophagus, but any point of normal narrowing in the thoracic esophagus or at a diseased area may be the site of perforation. The more common offenders are bones, especially chicken or pork bones—fish bones more commonly lodge in the hypopharynx; bits of shellfish shells; partial dentures; plastic eating utensils—frequently in the mentally disturbed; and metal objects such as open safety pins or metal beverage can openers. Perforation of the wall may occur spontaneously or during the extraction of the foreign body. Although a patient may become acutely ill from peforation by such objects, an indolent course with late abscess formation or pyopneumothorax is common (Fig. 45–5). These complications tend to occur especially in a child or a mentally troubled individual who does not recognize the ingestion of the foreign body. Foreign bodies placed externally to the esophagus also may cause perforation. Albin and associates (1985) reported perforation of the thoracic esophagus with the Angelchick antireflux prosthesis.

The diagnosis of foreign body perforation may be suggested by the history and physical examination and a high index of suspicion in the various patient groups. Roentgenographic examinations may reveal the foreign body but frequently may be negative, owing to the low density of many of the foreign bodies. The use of soft tissue techniques, as noted by Love and Berkow (1978), permits visualization of about 75% of ingested bones, and this may be further improved with the use of xeroradiography. The other roentgenographic features depend on the degree and the extent of the inflammatory process external to the esophageal wall. When an unexplained hydropneumothorax is evident, thoracentesis confirms the pyogenic nature of the process.

Endoscopy with removal of the foreign body is indicated, along with appropriate drainage of the involved area. Esophagotomy is necessary for removal of any foreign body that cannot be removed by endoscopic manipulation. In the neck, this procedure is accomplished via a cervical mediastinotomy, whereas in the chest either a posterior mediastinotomy, as described in Chapter 89, or a thoracotomy approach is indicated, depending on the extent of the disease process. The morbidity and mortality of foreign body perforation vary with its time

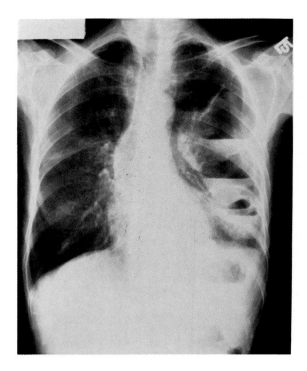

Fig. 45–5. Loculated pyopneumothorax following erosion of nonopaque foreign body through the wall of the distal end of the thoracic esophagus.

of recognition and the appropriateness of the therapy. Bladergroen and associates (1986) reported a 94% survival in this group of patients.

Noninstrumental Injuries

Rapid increase of the intraluminal pressure within the esophagus may result in partial or complete rupture of the esophageal wall. This rupture is usually the result of internal changes in pressure accompanying vomiting, but may occur with defecation, convulsions, lifting, and even labor of childbirth. It may also be a remote effect of blunt abdominal trauma. Rarely, it may be the result of the exposure to compressed air. Twelve accidental pneumatic ruptures of the esophagus were reported by Gelfand and associates (1977). Common sources were accidents involving compressed air hoses and tanks or explosion of an inflated tire when a young child bit a bulge on an inner tube that protruded through a defect in the wall of a tire. Conlan and associates (1984) reported several cases that occurred in children who had been playing with carbonated beverages.

In contrast to the rare accidental pneumatic rupture, postemetic rupture—the so-called spontaneous perforation or Boerhaave syndrome—is seen frequently. Rupture during a vomiting episode is thought to occur as a result of the contractions of the cricopharyngeus muscle, which converts the flaccid esophagus into a high pressure chamber, as gastric air and contents are forced into the esophagus through a relaxed cardia. Hardy and Wallace (1977) noted that a force of 0.5 to 1.5 kg (mVsec²) of pressure is necessary to rupture the normal esophagus, but less may be required when a disease process is present. Most often, the injury is located in the distal portion of the esophagus—terminal 6 to 8 cm—and extends through all layers of the posterolateral wall on the left. This may be the result of the distribution of smooth muscle at this location. In this region of the esophagus, the longitudinal fibers taper out as they pass onto the stomach wall, resulting in a weakened area at this site.

On occasion, a partial disruption occurs. Rarely, extensive dissection of the air within the intramural layers of the esophagus occurs, as described by Borrie (1970), Kelley (1972), and Berliner (1982) and their associates. A partial laceration of the wall may extend into the proximal stomach and cause major upper gastrointestinal bleeding, the Mallory-Weiss syndrome (1929). In this situation, the problem is control of the bleeding. If bleeding does not stop with expectant, supportive management, surgical intervention is required. This operative procedure is best accomplished by an abdominal approach, gastrotomy, and suture ligation of the bleeding point.

Massive bleeding with complete rupture of the esophageal wall is rare; however, varying amounts of bleeding were recorded in 55% of the patients seen by Abbott and colleagues (1970), but this high incidence has not been confirmed by other authors.

"Spontaneous Rupture"—Boerhaave's Syndrome

Classically, patients with so-called spontaneous rupture of the esophagus present with severe chest pain and dyspnea after an episode of vomiting. Shoulder pain may be present, but some patients complain only of abdominal pain that can be more specifically located in the epigastrium. Marked thirst is occasionally observed. In many patients—the unconscious or unreliable alcoholic patient—the history is unobtainable, and the diagnosis must be established by the physical examination, roentgenographic findings, and at times thoracentesis. Unfortunately, a major delay in time of diagnosis relative to the occurrence of the event is common in many cases of "spontaneous rupture."

The physical findings vary with the duration of the disease and the involvement of either pleural space. Subcutaneous emphysema is present in most patients, and cyanosis may be observed. The abdominal findings may vary from epigastric tenderness to marked upper abdominal distention. Bowel sounds frequently are decreased to absent.

Roentgenographic examination of the chest and abdomen reveals, in varying degrees, mediastinal emphysema, pleural effusion, hydropneumothorax, and rarely pneumoperitoneum. Early, and particularly helpful in patients with abdominal complaints, a patchy, irregular density may be visible behind the left cardiac silhouette. This feature has been termed the "V" sign by Naclerio (1957). Fluoroscopy with contrast media opacification of the esophagus is helpful in localizing the injury and is especially helpful when the clinical features are obscure.

When patients have a hydropneumothorax and the history and other features do not suggest the underlying cause, a thoracentesis is most helpful. In adults, when thoracentesis reveals a pyopneumothorax, the diagnosis of a perforating injury of the esophagus must be considered the most likely possibility until proved otherwise.

Once the diagnosis is established, a multiple-faceted therapeutic approach is indicated to achieve the four aforementioned goals in the management of the esophageal injuries. Direct surgical repair, when instituted from 6 to 12 hours after injury in an otherwise healthy individual, leads to the least morbidity and mortality. When this approach is used indiscriminately in patients whose injury is of longer duration, however, complications, as noted by Keighley and associates (1972), are frequent—84%—and a protracted course is to be expected. Most complications—development of an empyema, persistent fistulas, and late abscess formation—are related to leakage from the site of repair. When the anatomic situation is less than ideal and direct repair is attempted, support of the suture line by coverage with adjacent tissue is indicated. Functional and, at times, actual surgical isolation of the esophagus from the gastrointestinal tract, as well as adequate drainage, is indicated. These latter two steps are required when no direct surgical repair of the rupture site is feasible. Antibiotics and hyperalimentation are essential adjuncts in the management of these patients.

Mortality rates in patients with spontaneous rupture depend on the time interval from injury to recognition, the underlying physical status of the patient, and the aggressiveness and appropriate individualization of therapy. Abbott and colleagues (1970) reported a mortality of 51.4% in 35 treated patients; all 12 untreated patients died. Keighley and associates (1972) reported only an 8% mortality in a smaller number of patients; the norm is probably somewhere in between.

Extraluminal Injuries

External penetrating injuries of the esophagus are seldom encountered. As reported by Conn and associates (1963), these injuries represent less than 1% of the intrathoracic injuries caused by penetrating trauma and, as noted by Sheely and colleagues (1975), the cervical esophagus is injured in only about 0.5% of penetrating neck injuries.

Cervical Esophagus

Although the cervical esophagus is in a protected location, Yap and associates (1984) pointed out that it is more vulnerable to external penetrating injuries than the thoracic esophagus. Gunshot wounds are the most common cause of injury, but injury from stab wounds also occurs (Fig. 45–6).

The diagnosis of penetrating injury is greatly facilitated by awareness of its possible existence. These wounds are frequently associated with an injury to the trachea, the large vessels of the neck, or the spinal cord, or a combination of these. Occasionally, an isolated injury of the esophagus may occur, particularly with stab wounds by a thin-bladed instrument.

Clinically, dysphagia or spitting of blood, or both, may

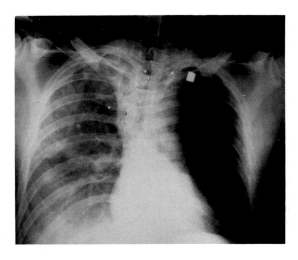

Fig. 45–6. Gunshot wound of neck with perforation of wall of the cervical segment of the esophagus.

be present and should increase suspicion of possible esophageal injury. Subcutaneous emphysema from an isolated injury of the esophagus occurs only in about a third of such instances. When crepitus is palpable, a combined injury of the trachea and esophagus must be considered. Though not essential, retropharyngeal air or subcutaneous air, or both, may be seen in roentgenograms of the neck. Occasionally, roentgenograms of the chest may reveal a pneumomediastinum, but this finding almost always indicates concomitant airway injury.

An esophagram, although not recommended, may be obtained to confirm the suspicion of esophageal injury, but this examination, of necessity obtained under emergency conditions, may fail to disclose the injury. The same is true for esophagoscopy, and this latter examination usually is not indicated.

Penetrating injuries of the neck should be exposed through an incision along the anterior border of the sternocleidomastoid muscle. The esophagus can be mobilized and repaired from either side of the neck, so the side selected depends primarily on the site of the penetration and the possibility of associated injury to one or more of the vascular structures. Occasionally, both sides of the neck must be explored through separate incisions. The injury of the esophagus is repaired in two layers using interrupted nonabsorbable sutures. Adequate drainage of the neck is essential. If the upper mediastinum is contaminated, this should be drained as well. Drains should be left in place until oral feedings have been instituted—5 to 7 days—and there is no evidence of an esophagocutaneous fistula. Aspiration of the oropharyngeal secretions, as well as appropriate antibiotics, should be used in all these injuries. If the trachea and esophagus were injured simultaneously, Feliciano and associates (1985) recommended rotation of a flap of viable muscle between the repair of the esophagus and that of the trachea.

The morbidity and mortality rates related to esophageal injury should be minimal when the problem is rec-

ognized promptly. Major complications and death are more often related to associated injuries, especially those of the cervical spinal cord.

Thoracic Injuries

Penetrating injuries of the thoracic esophagus are caused almost exclusively by gunshot wounds in either a civilian or military setting, or by explosive fragments encountered almost exclusively in military operations. The central anatomic location of the esophagus, the protection afforded by the vertebral bodies, heart and aorta, and the relatively small, compact size of the esophagus all diminish its susceptibility to injury.

The diagnosis of penetrating injuries of the thoracic esophagus is difficult. Most often, these injuries occur as part of a complex injury involving at the least the thoracic wall and lung; however, one or more of the following structures may be involved: the heart, great vessels, diaphragm or even one or more intra-abdominal structures.

Although a variety of symptoms and findings are present in penetrating injuries of the esophagus, most of these may be just as easily attributed to concomitant involvement of other thoracic structures. Dysphagia strongly suggests the possibility of esophageal injury, but is not commonly present. Pneumomediastinum is frequently present when the esophagus is injured, but is more commonly caused by tracheal or bronchial injury.

The path of bullets through the body frequently may be fairly accurately predicted by observing the wound entrance and exit or by noting the wound of entrance and determining the location of the bullet within the body by roentgenographic studies. The path of the missile may be erratic, however, so that any combination of injuries must be considered in each individual patient. The anatomic structures involved may be influenced by the position of the victim at the time of injury and, as noted, the path of the missile may be somewhat zig-zag or the missile may have ricocheted off bony structures.

Careful review of the roentgenograms of the chest frequently reveals small fragments of the bullet outlining the tract of injury. When these observations indicate the possibility of esophageal injury, exploration should be considered. An esophagogram may be attempted to demonstrate the location of the injury, but this study may appear normal and should not cloud the clinical impression, especially when done with Gastrografin; a water suspension of barium sulfate is a better constrast material in these situations. Esophagoscopy is not particularly helpful. Although these examinations may further reinforce the clinical suspicion of esophageal injury, it is still easy to miss the perforation despite such diligent time-consuming examinations.

The treatment of penetrating injuries is based on early recognition, primary repair, and adequate drainage, as noted in the management of intraluminal injuries. The associated injuries to other vital structures in the thorax lead to early exploration in many of these patients. The esophageal injury usually is discovered by systematic exploration of the path of the missile. The repair of the esophagus is part of a complicated surgical procedure requiring attention to other injured structures. Most of the esophageal injuries are through-and-through perforations, in which there should always be an even number of rents in the esophagus. Occasionally, a lateral tear occurs, resulting in one large laceration. As noted by Symbas and colleagues (1972), extensive debridement may be necessary because of diffuse hemorrhage, acute coagulation necrosis, or acute inflammation in the adjacent wall of the esophagus.

Ideally, when early diagnosis and exploration occur, the esophageal defect should be repaired primarily. At times only a minimum of debridement is necessary and the edges of the wound may be approximated by interrupted sutures of nonabsorbable material placed into the full thickness of the esophageal wall. This closure may be reinforced with a second muscular layer suture line. The adjacent mediastinal pleura is widely incised to ensure adequate drainage into the pleural space, which in turn is drained in the appropriate manner.

When operative exploration has been delayed because injury of the esophagus was unsuspected or when the esophageal wall has been extensively damaged, serious complications frequently ensue. Primary repair is no longer desirable; the treatment goals in these situations center around the adequate drainage, diversion or exclusion of the esophagus, antibiotics, and hyperalimentation, as Popovsky and associates (1976) emphasized. Fistulization in these situations is common and, to achieve a satisfactory outcome, the ingenuity and resourcefulness of the surgeon are severely tested.

The morbidity and mortality rates of thoracic injuries are increased by the presence of an esophageal injury. It is difficult, however, if not impossible, to quantitate its exact role.

OPERATIVE TRAUMA

Exclusive of direct esophageal procedures, operative injury to the esophagus occurs infrequently. Laceration of the cervical esophagus during thyroidectomy or laryngectomy has been reported. The thoracic esophagus may be injured during a vagotomy or hiatal hernia repair. Esophageal injury may occur during a pneumonectomy, most often for inflammatory disease, as Takaro and colleagues (1960) noted; Shama and Odell (1985) reported an incidence of 0.5% in a series of 869 pneumonectomies for inflammatory disease. It may also occur during a resection for carcinoma of the lung, as Benjamin and associates (1969) reported.

When injury to the esophagus is recognized during the aforementioned procedures, direct primary repair is almost always successful. When the injury is unrecognized, all the complications common to any esophageal rupture may occur. Accordingly, the treatment must be directed to alleviate the resulting problems on an individual basis.

BLUNT TRAUMA

Blunt trauma to the esophagus is infrequent but may be sustained during deceleration injuries to the chest, such as hitting the steering wheel during high-speed collisions. The esophageal wall may be ruptured simultaneously with the adjacent membranous tracheal wall, or its blood supply compromised so that necrosis and subsequent perforation into the trachea occur. This injury may occur when the esophagus and trachea are compressed between the sternum and thoracic vertebral bodies. Hughes and Fox (1954) estimated that approximately one third of the acquired benign tracheoesophageal fistulas have this mechanism of development; the remainder are caused by an inflammatory process. Infrequently, an acute rupture results from a rapid increase in intraluminal pressure. Tomasyek (1984) and Purvis (1981) and their associates mentioned esophageal rupture occurring with fractures of the cervical spine. Rarely, a necrotizing injury of the esophageal wall occurs if the esophagus is torn away from its blood supply by severe blunt injury. Necrosis of a greater or lesser length of the esophagus may result from such an injury.

In the compressive injury of the esophagus and trachea, despite the usual presence of subcutaneous air, the frequent association of multiple system trauma delays the recognition of the esophagotracheal injury. The presence of the fistula is evidenced usually sometime after the third day by spasms of coughing on eating or drinking. Aspiration of oropharyngeal secretions into the lungs occurs, with the development of pulmonary infection. Once the fistula is suspected, the diagnosis should be confirmed by endoscopic and roentgenographic studies. When the condition of the patient is stabilized, direct repair of the fistula is indicated. Chapman and Braun (1970) recommended that the repair be done as soon as possible, preferably via a right thoracotomy. Division of the azygos vein is done to permit wide exposure of the esophagus and trachea. Dissection, isolation, and division of the fistula is carried out without compromising the lumen of either structure. The fistulous openings of each organ are closed with interrupted, fine, nonabsorbable sutures or with fine sutures of Vicryl. A flap of adjacent tissue, usually pleura or, when this is unavailable, a vascularized pedicled flap of intercostal muscle, should be interposed between the two closures. A tracheostomy, if not already present, has been suggested to protect the tracheal suture line.

When a free perforation occurs from blunt trauma, the injury should be managed as described in the discussion of spontaneous perforation.

When extensive necrosis occurs with dissolution of the esophagus, emergency esophagectomy or surgical exclusion of the esophagus from the gastrointestinal tract with appropriate mediastinal and pleural drainage may be lifesaving for the patient. Subsequent reconstitution of gastrointestinal tract continuity may be accomplished later by a gastric or a colon interposition.

CHEMICAL TRAUMA

Chemical burns of the esophagus result from the ingestion of caustic substances, either a strong acid or alkali. The latter is the more common offender and is found in many household cleaning agents, usually as sodium or potassium hydroxide. Most of the injuries occur from accidental ingestion by young children, usually under 5 years of age. Occasionally, adults may ingest one of these agents, usually in an attempted suicide.

Pathologically, the site of caustic injury of the esophagus may be located almost equally in any one of its anatomic subdivisions or may be widespread throughout. Normally, the greater period of contact is in the lower esophagus; hence, more extensive injury usually occurs in this area.

The burn injury to the esophagus has been divided into three phases. Inflammation, edema, and necrosis occur during the initial few days after injury. Sloughing of esophageal tissue with mucosal ulceration, and the appearance of soft, red, moist granulation tissue occur in the second phase. The esophageal wall is weakest during this period, which may last 3 to 4 weeks. In the third phase, cicatrization and stricture formation may progress for many weeks as the destroyed esophageal submucosa and muscularis are replaced with scar tissue.

The signs and symptoms of the initial injury are related to the strength and amount of the substance swallowed. Increased salivation and dysphagia are common. Burns of the mouth and pharynx are easily observed. Respiratory distress occurs when the burn extends into the epiglottis or larynx. In severe instances, shock and life-threatening respiratory distress may occur within an hour of injury. When the offending agent happens to be in a very dilute solution, symptoms may be minimal and there may be no evidence of oral burns.

The injury to the esophagus occurs almost simultaneously with the contact of the caustic agent with the esophageal mucosa. Treatment, therefore, is designed to minimize the extent of scarring and subsequent stricture formation. Early esophagoscopy, within the first 2 days, is recommended. The esophagoscope is passed until the first area of burn is observed. No attempt is made to pass beyond this area. Webb and associates (1970) have outlined useful criteria for making a rough estimate of the severity of the burn, and these criteria may be correlated roughly with the incidence of subsequent stricture formation.

Further examination of the esophagus usually is not necessary for 3 to 4 weeks. At this time, the indicated examination is a roentgenographic evaluation of the esophagus by a barium swallow. The number and length of any strictures usually are well delineated by this study. Interval roentgenographic studies then may be used to evaluate the progression of healing or stricture formation and the effects of treatment.

As Borja (1969) and Haller (1971) and their associates noted, a 3- to 6-week course of corticosteroids and antibiotics is recommended in the acute phase of the injury in an attempt to diminish the frequency and the degree of stricture formation. Subsequent bougienage is recommended in those patients with a definite stricture of the esophagus. This procedure is started during the early phase of cicatrix formation, which begins the third or fourth week after injury. Danger of instrumental per-foration, however, is present, and a string guide is essential to avoid this risk. Bougienage is repeated at varying intervals dictated in part by the initial severity of the burn and serial roentgenographic studies. The most important factor, however, is the ability of the patient to swallow and to maintain nutrition. Recurrent or increasing dysphagia indicates the need for additional mechanical dilatation.

Surgical intervention is seldom necessary in the acute phase of caustic injuries to the esophagus. Gago and colleagues (1972), however, reported emergency resection of a necrotic esophagus within hours of severe caustic injury in an adult and a delayed resection in an infant. Burrington and Raffensperger (1978) reported several acute tracheoesophageal fistulas resulting from caustic ingestion in small children. In these unusually severe injuries, tracheostomy, cervical esophagostomy, and gastrostomy with isolation—blind-ending—of the thoracic esophagus are required. Several months later, it is then necessary to create a substitute esophagus using a reversed gastric tube or colon interposition.

Estrera and associates (1986) recommended an aggressive approach for second or third degree burns of the esophagus (Table 45–1) rather than the aforementioned standard treatment of antibiotics, steroids, and subsequent dilatation as required. In patients with second degree burns, they suggest intraesophageal stenting through a celiotomy approach (Fig. 45–7), and the stent is left in place for at least 21 days. Antibiotics and steroids also are given. In patients with third degree burns without full-thickness involvement, a stent is likewise used, but in those with extensive full-thickness necrosis, urgent radical total esophagogastrectomy is carried out along with a temporary cervical esophagostomy and jejunostomy. Reconstruction is performed at a later date. In such patients with third degree burns treated with a delayed resection, the mortality was 100%; with the aggressive urgent approach, the mortality was zero in their report. When an esophagectomy is indicated in such a situation, Hwang and colleagues (1987) suggested that the esophagectomy is best done by the transhiatal route.

Surgical intervention may also be considered in longstanding strictures when it becomes difficult or impossible to maintain an adequate lumen despite repeated dilatation. In these situations, it becomes necessary to create a substitute esophagus using either a reversed gastric tube or a substernal colon interposition, as described in Chapters 39 and 40. Although an increased risk for the development of carcinoma in residual, strictured esophagus has been suggested, Marchand (1955) was unable to find a documented esophageal carcinoma in the long-term follow-up of 133 patients with such injury. The risk of resecting the diseased esophagus may be greater than the risk of developing an esophageal carcinoma; therefore, it appears reasonable to leave the diseased esophagus in situ under such circumstances.

The danger of developing an esophageal mucocele, as reported in patients with an isolated—blind loop—esophagus by Kamath and colleagues (1987), is probably near zero, because generally no functioning mucosa is

Table 45–1. Endoscopic Grading of Corrosive Burns of Esophagus and Stomach*

Grade	Pathological Condition	Endoscopic Findings
First degree	Superficial involvement of mucosa	Mucosal hyperemia and edema (occasionally superficial mucosal desquamation)
Second degree	Transmucosal involvement, with or without involvement of muscularis	Sloughing of mucosa
	No extension into the periesophageal or perigastric tissue	Hemorrhages, exudates, and ulceration, pseudomembrane formation and granulation tissue if examined late
Third degree	Full-thickness injuries with extension into periesophageal or perigastric tissues	Sloughing of tissues with deep ulcerations
	Mediastinal or intraperitoneal organs may be involved	Complete obliteration of esophageal lumen by massive edema; charring and eschar formation; full-thickness necrosis with perforation

*This grading system was adopted and modified from the classification of thermal injury of the skin.
Reproduced with permission of Estrera, A., et al.: Corrosive burns of the esophagus and stomach: a recommendation for an aggressive surgical approach. Ann. Thorac. Surg., *41*:276, 1986.

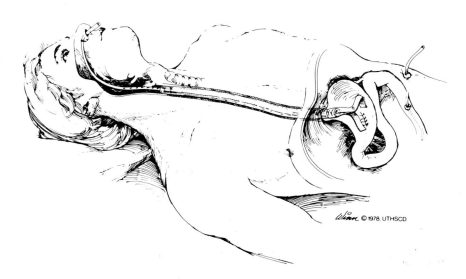

Fig. 45–7. Technique of intraluminal esophageal stenting for corrosive esophagogastric injury. Reproduced with permission of Estrera, A., et al.: Corrosive burns of the esophagus and stomach: a recommendation for an aggressive surgical approach. Ann. Thorac. Surg. *41*:276, 1986.

present in patients with caustic burns, in contrast to those with achalasia or other benign conditions that may necessitated bypass.

REFERENCES

Abbott, O.A., et al.: Atraumatic so-called "spontaneous" rupture of the esophagus: a review of 47 personal cases with comments on a new method of surgical therapy. J. Thorac. Cardiovasc. Surg. 59:67, 1970.

Albin, J., Allan, T., and Khalil, K.G.: Intrathoracic esophageal perforation with the Angelchick anti-reflux prosthesis: report of a new complication. Gastrointest. Radiol. 10:330, 1985.

Barber, G., et al.: Esophageal foreign body perforation: report of an unusual case and review of the literature. Am. J. Gastroenterol. 79:509, 1984.

Benjamin, I., Olsen, A.M., and Ellis, F.H., Jr.: Esophagopleural fistula: a rare postpneumonectomy complication. Ann. Thorac. Surg. 7:139, 1969.

Bennett, J.R., and Hendrix, T.R.: Treatment of achalasia with pneumatic dilatation. Mod. Treatment 7:1217, 1970.

Berliner, L., Redmond, P., and Pachter, H.L.: Spontaneous intramural perforation of the esophagus: case report and review of the literature. Am. J. Gastroenterol. 77:355, 1982.

Berry, B.E., and Ochsner, J.L.: Perforation of the esophagus. J. Thorac. Cardiovasc. Surg. 65:1, 1973.

Bladergroen, M.R., Lowe, J.E., and Postlethwait, R.W.: Diagnosis and recommended management of esophageal perforation and rupture. Ann. Thorac. Surg. 42:235, 1986.

Borja, A.R., et al.: Lye injuries of esophagus: analysis of ninety cases of lye ingestion. J. Thorac. Cardiovasc. Surg. 57:533, 1969.

Borrie, J., and Sheat, J.: Spontaneous oesophageal perforation. Thorax 25:294, 1970.

Burrington, J.D., and Raffensperger, J.G.: Surgical management of tracheoesophageal fistula complicating caustic ingestion. Surgery 84:329, 1978.

Cameron, J.L., et al.: Selective nonoperative management of contained intrathoracic esophageal disruptions. Ann. Thorac. Surg. 27:404, 1979.

Chapman, N.D., and Braun, R.A.: The management of traumatic tracheoesophageal fistula caused by blunt chest trauma. Arch. Surg. 100:681, 1970.

Conlan, A., et al.: Pharyngoesophageal barotrauma in children: a report of six cases. J. Thorac. Cardiovasc. Surg. 88:452, 1984.

Conn, J.H., et al.: Thoracic trauma: analysis of 1022 cases. J. Trauma 3:22, 1963.

DeMeester, T.R.: Perforation of the esophagus (editorial). Ann. Thorac. Surg. 42:231, 1986.

Estrera, A., et al.: Corrosive burns of the esophagus and stomach: a recommendation for an aggressive surgical approach. Ann. Thorac. Surg. 41:276, 1986.

Feliciano, D.V., et al.: Combined tracheoesophageal injuries. Am. J. Surg. *150*:710, 1985.

Gago, O., et al.: Aggressive surgical treatment for caustic injury of the esophagus and stomach. Ann. Thorac. Surg. *13*:243, 1972.

Gelfand, E.T., Fisk, R.L., and Callaghan, J.C.: Accidental pneumatic rupture of the esophagus. J. Thorac. Cardiovasc. Surg. *74*:142, 1977.

Grillo, H.G., and Wilkins, E.W., Jr.: Esophageal repair following late diagnosis of intrathoracic perforation. Ann. Thorac. Surg. *29*:387, 1975.

Haller, J.A., Jr., et al.: Pathophysiology and management of acute corrosive burns of the esophagus: results of treatment in 285 children. J. Pediatr. Surg. *6*:578, 1971.

Hardy, J.D., and Wallace, W.H.: Spontaneous rupture of the esophagus. *In* Rhoads Textbook of Surgery, Principles and Practice. Edited by J.D. Hardy. Philadelphia, J.B. Lippincott Co., 1977.

Hughes, F.A., and Fox, J.R.: Acquired non-malignant esophagotracheobronchial fistula. J. Thorac. Surg. *27*:384, 1954.

Hwang, T.L., Shen-Chen, S.M., and Chen, M.F.: Nonthoracotomy esophagectomy for corrosive esophagitis with gastric perforation. Surg. Gynecol. Obstet. *164*:537, 1987.

Kamath, M.V., et al.: Esophageal mucocele: a complication of blind loop esophagus. Ann. Thorac. Surg. *43*:263, 1987.

Keighley, M.R.B., et al.: Morbidity and mortality of oesophageal perforation. Thorax *27*:353, 1972.

Kelley, D.L., Nengebauer, N.K., and Fosburg, R.G.: Spontaneous intramural esophageal perforation. J. Thorac. Cardiovasc. Surg. *63*:504, 1972.

Love, L., and Berkow, A.E.: Trauma to the esophagus. Gastrointest. Radiol. *2*:305, 1978.

Mallory, G.K., and Weiss, S.: Hemorrhage from lacerations of the cardiac orifice of the stomach due to vomiting. Am. J. Med. Sci. *178*:506, 1929.

Marchand, P.: Caustic strictures of the esophagus. Thorax *10*:171, 1955.

Mayer, J.E., Jr., Murray, C.A., III, and Varco, R.L.: The treatment of esophageal perforation with delayed recognition and continuing sepsis. Ann. Thorac. Surg. *23*:586, 1977.

Meyers, M.A., and Ghahremani, G.G.: Complications of fiberoptic endoscopy. Radiology *115*:293, 1975.

Naclerio, E.A.: The "V-sign" in the diagnosis of spontaneous rupture of the esophagus. An early roentgen clue. Am. J. Surg. *93*:291, 1957.

O'Neill, J. Griffin, J., and Cottrell, J.: Pharyngeal and esophageal perforation following endotracheal intubation. Anesthesiology *60*:487, 1984.

Popovsky, J., Lee, Y.C., and Berk, J.L.: Gunshot wounds of the esophagus. J. Thorac. Cardiovasc. Surg. *72*:609, 1976.

Purvis, J.M., Apple, D., and Murray, H.: Esophageal and hypopharyngeal injury in patients with cervical spine trauma. Ann. Otol. Rhinol. Laryngol. *90*:323, 1981.

Sandrasagra, F.A., English, T.A.H., and Milstein, B.B.: Esophageal intubation in the management of perforated esophagus with stricture. Ann. Thorac. Surg. *25*:399, 1978.

Santos, G.H., and Frater, R.W.M.: Transesophageal irrigation for the treatment of mediastinitis produced by esophageal rupture. J. Thorac. Cardiovasc. Surg. *91*:57, 1986.

Shama, D.M., and Odell, J.A.: Esophagopleural fistula after pneumonectomy for inflammatory disease. J. Thorac. Cardiovasc. Surg. *89*:77, 1985.

Sheely, C.H., et al.: Penetrating wounds of the cervical esophagus. Am. J. Surg. *139*:707, 1975.

Shemesh, E., and Bat, L.: Esophageal perforation after fiberoptic endoscopic injection sclerotherapy for esophageal varices. Arch. Surg. *121*:243, 1986.

Symbas, P.N., Tyras, D.H., and Hatcher, C.R., Jr.: Penetrating wounds of the esophagus. Ann. Thorac. Surg. *13*:552, 1972.

Takaro, T. Walkup, H.E., and Okano, T.: Esophagopleural fistula as a complication of thoracic surgery: a collective review. J. Thorac. Cardiovasc. Surg. *40*:179, 1960.

Thal, A.P., Hatafuku, T., and Kurtzman, R.: New operation for distal esophageal stricture. Arch. Surg. *90*:464, 1965.

Tomasyek, D., and Rosner, M.: Occult esophageal perforation associated with cervical spine fracture. Neurosurgery *14*:492, 1984.

Triggiani, E., and Belsey, R.: Oesophageal trauma: incidence, diagnosis, and management. Thorax *32*:241, 1977.

Urschel, H.C., Jr., et al.: Improved management of esophageal perforations: exclusion and diversion in continuity. Ann. Surg. *179*:587, 1974.

Walsh, P.: Rupture of the abdominal esophagus. Br. J. Surg. *66*:601, 1979.

Webb, W.R., et al.: An evaluation of steroids and antibiotics in caustic burns of the esophagus. Ann. Thorac. Surg. *9*:95, 1970.

Wesdrop, I.C.E., et al.: Treatment of instrumental oesophageal perforation. Gut *25*:398, 1984.

Wychulis, A.R., Fontana, R.S., and Payne, W.S.: Instrumental perforations of the esophagus. Chest *55*:184, 1969.

Yap, R., et al.: Traumatic esophageal injuries: 12-year experience at Henry Ford Hospital. J. Trauma *24*:623, 1984.

READING REFERENCES

Brewer, L., et al.: Options in the management of perforation of the esophagus. Am. J. Surg. *152*:62, 1986.

Michel, L., Grillo, H., and Malt, R.A.: Esophageal perforation. Ann. Thorac. Surg. *33*:203, 1982.

Richardson, J., et al.: Unifying concepts in treatment of esophageal leaks. Am. J. Surg. *149*:157, 1985.

Symbas, P.N., Hatcher, C.R., and Vlasis, S.E.: Esophageal gunshot injuries. Ann. Surg. *191*:703, 1980.

CHAPTER 46

DIAPHRAGMATIC INJURIES

Panagiotis N. Symbas and Thomas W. Shields

Diaphragmatic lacerations may result from penetrating or blunt trauma to this musculotendinous structure that separates the thoracic and abdominal cavities. If the laceration is unrecognized and not promptly repaired, one or more of the abdominal viscera will herniate into the thoracic cavity, with resulting early or late compromise of ventilatory or gastrointestinal function. Immediate herniation is most often associated with a large tear in one of the diaphragmatic leaves, but the symptoms of the herniation may be obscured by the symptoms of other associated injured organs or structures. Small rents such as those caused by stab wounds rarely are symptomatic early, but if they are unrepaired, progressive abdominal visceral herniation occurs because of the pressure gradient between the thoracic and peritoneal cavities. As the traumatic diaphragmatic hernia enlarges, the likelihood of ventilatory compromise or of mechanical obstruction, with or without strangulation, of a portion of the contained gastrointestinal tract increases.

Diaphragmatic injuries can be separated into two categories: those that are recognized at the time of initial hospitalization for the evaluation of an episode of trauma and those that are missed initially and recognized at some time remote from the first hospitalization.

RECOGNITION DURING INITIAL HOSPITALIZATION

The mechanism, symptoms, and other features of blunt and penetrating injuries are dissimilar. Therefore, the initial recognition and the management of these two types of injury are best discussed separately.

Blunt Diaphragmatic Trauma

Rupture of a portion of the diaphragm usually results from decelerating injuries suffered in motor vehicle accidents or from falls from great heights. Other crushing injuries to the lower chest or upper abdomen may also result in laceration of the diaphragm. Beal and McKennan (1988) reported an incidence of a ruptured diaphragm of 3% in those patients suffering severe blunt

trauma who survived long enough to be admitted to the hospital.

The rupture most commonly occurs in the left leaf. Contrary to common belief, the right hemidiaphragm is not immune from injury. In the series reported by Estrera and colleagues (1985), right-sided injury was observed in 34% of the patients sustaining recognized blunt injury to the diaphragm. Brown and Richardson (1985) and Beal and McKennan (1988) also noted a similar incidence, as well as the occasional occurrence of bilateral rupture. Injuries on the right side are usually posterolateral to the central tendon. The pericardial or central portion of the diaphragm also may be ruptured, and avulsion of the diaphragm from the rib cage infrequently occurs.

Pathology

On the left side, the organs most commonly herniated into the chest are the stomach, spleen, large bowel, liver, small intestine, and omentum. On the right, when herniation occurs the liver is always present and the colon is occasionally herniated as Brown and Richardson (1985) reported. Vascular injuries—tears of the juxtahepatic vena cava and hepatic vein injuries—as well as lacerations of the liver are frequently associated with rupture of the right hemidiaphragm.

Symptomatology

Symptoms and signs of diaphragmatic rupture—respiratory distress, cardiac disturbances, deviated trachea, and bowel sounds in the chest—are present in the minority of patients initially seen after the blunt injury; most symptoms present are related to other organ system injuries or to the presence of hypovolemic shock.

Roentgenographic Examinations

The routine roentgenogram of the chest is the most efficient study when the patient is stable enough to have the procedure done. It is abnormal in almost all and is diagnostic of rupture in over half of the patients. The abnormal roentgenogram of the chest shows an elevated,

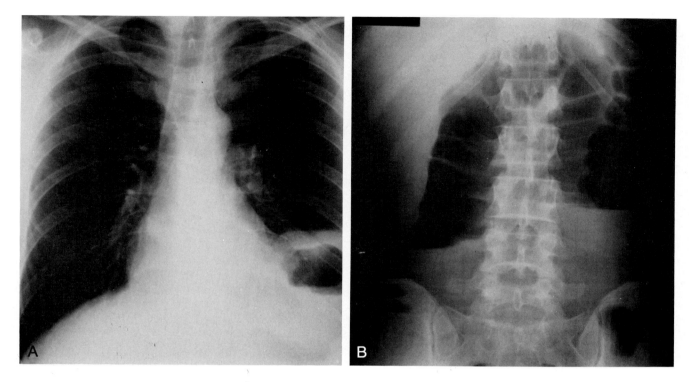

Fig. 46–1. Roentgenograms of a 30-year-old man following a vehicular accident. *A*, Frontal view of the chest shows abnormal diaphragmatic silhouette. *B*, Plain roentgenogram of the abdomen reveals upward displacement of the transverse colon. (Reproduced with permission from Symbas, P.N., Vlasis, S.E., and Hatcher, C., Jr.: Blunt and penetrating diaphragmatic injuries with or without herniation of organs into the chest. Ann. Thorac. Surg. *42*:158, 1986.)

obscured, or irregular diaphragmatic dome on the side of the visceral herniation. The costophrenic angle is almost always blunted because of contained fluid. With lacerations on the left, one or more air-fluid levels and radioluceny in the lower lung field, with or without shifting of the mediastinum away from the side of the hernia, appear (Fig. 46–1). Occasionally, the nasogastric tube can be seen to turn upward into the chest (Fig. 46–2). With right-sided injuries, the right leaf is markedly elevated with or without an associated fluid collection; air fluid levels are less frequently observed. Occasionally, a rounded shadow protruding above the leaf appears on the lateral film; this is highly diagnostic for right-sided rupture (Fig. 46–3). Nondiagnostic findings of a pneumothorax or hydrothorax—hemothorax—or both, are also frequently present.

Diagnosis

The roentgenogram of the chest may be diagnostic, as noted. In those patients too ill to be moved, Ammann and colleagues (1983) suggested using bedside real-time sonographic examination. In patients not requiring emergency operation, the diagnosis may be confirmed with barium contrast studies of either the upper or lower gastrointestinal tract. Computed tomography, as Heiberg (1980) and Toombs (1981) and their associates reported, can likewise be used to demonstrate the herniation. When right-sided injury is suspected and conditions permit, fluoroscopic examination and radio-

nuclide liver scan, as well as ultrasonography and computed tomography, can be done to delineate the herniated portion of the liver. The use of diagnostic pneumoperitoneum is rarely indicated. In patients requiring emergency operation for control of bleeding or correction of other life-threatening injuries, the diagnosis must be made at operation. Both leaves of the diaphragm must, therefore, be adequately inspected in all patients with severe blunt chest and upper abdominal injuries who are operated upon.

Treatment

Because of the danger of development of respiratory and even circulatory embarrassment or visceral obstruction, with incarceration or strangulation of the involved portion of the gastrointestinal tract, diaphragmatic injury should be repaired surgically as soon as possible after the diagnosis is established and when the patient's clinical condition permits. Although a diaphragmatic leaf may be best exposed through the chest, the approach chosen should be based on the clinical findings in each patient. Because the major source of massive bleeding is usually a lacerated abdominal viscus, Beal and Mc-Kennan (1988) prefer the abdominal approach. When the hernia is discovered shortly after the accident, however, a transthoracic approach can be used when bleeding is not the major problem.

Tears of the left hemidiaphragm are most often repaired through the abdomen because of frequently as-

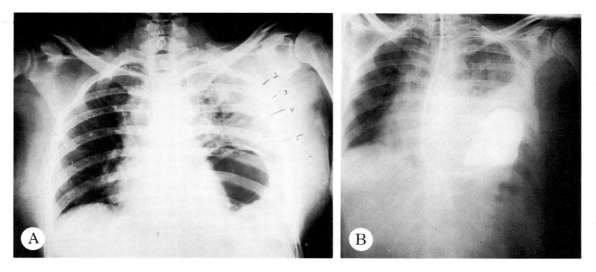

Fig. 46–2. *A,* Roentgenogram of chest made 12 hours after severe trauma, showing multiple rib fractures and a large gas bubble in the lower portion of the left side of the chest. *B,* Barium study revealed the large gas shadow to be the stomach, which had herniated through the ruptured diaphragm.

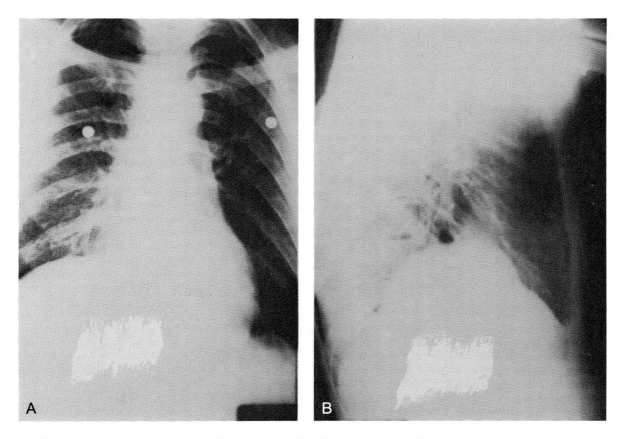

Fig. 46–3. Chest roentgenograms of a patient with ruptured right hemidiaphragm and partial herniation of the liver. *A,* Posteroanterior view suggested only minimal elevation of the right hemidiaphragm. *B,* Lateral view was fairly impressive. (Reproduced with permission of Estrera, A., et al.: Blunt traumatic rupture of the right hemidiaphragm: experience in 12 patients. Ann. Thorac. Surg. 39:525, 1985.)

sociated injuries to intra-abdominal organs, although in the absence of any symptoms suggesting such injury, a left thoracotomy is adequate. Tears of the right hemi-diaphragm, when recognized preoperatively, are best repaired through a right thoracotomy, as Estrera and associates described in 1979. In 1985, however, these authors recommended that the approach be individualized, depending primarily upon which cavity—thorax or abdomen—shows continued evidence of bleeding. When injury to the retrohepatic vena cava or hepatic veins is encountered during an abdominal approach, Estrera and associates (1985) extend the incision by a median sternotomy to place a temporary vena caval shunt to control the bleeding.

After control and repair of other associated visceral injuries, the diaphragmatic tear is closed with interrupted figure-of-eight No. 0 nonabsorbable sutures. Prosthetic material is rarely needed in acute blunt trauma injuries. Disruption of the repaired diaphragmatic leaf is rare.

Mortality

The mortality rates may be high in these patients, not as the result of the diaphragmatic injury per se but as the consequence of other severe visceral trauma. One of us (PNS) and associates (1986) reported a 22% mortality rate in this group of patients. Brooks (1978) and Brown and Richardson (1985) reported rates of 14% and 17%, respectively. Beal and McKennan (1988) reported a mortality rate of 40.5%. Ninety-seven percent of their patients had associated injuries and 87% of those who died were in severe hypovolemic shock when admitted to the hospital.

Penetrating Diaphragmatic Injuries

These injuries usually result from stab wounds or gunshot wounds of the lower chest—below the nipples; the upper abdomen—epigastrium; the flanks; or the back; although no site of entrance of a wound of the trunk is exempt. Injury to either diaphragmatic leaf occurs with almost equal frequency.

Pathology

The diaphragmatic injury is generally small, and herniation of the abdominal viscera into the chest is usually absent early. Only if the injury is missed does late herniation occur because of the different pressures in the two cavities.

Symptomatology

The history and physical exam per se do not indicate diaphragmatic injury. The presence of abdominal complaints or findings in a patient who has sustained a chest wound, however, is diagnostic of diaphragmatic injury, as is the presence of chest findings in one in whom the site of entrance of the wound is in the abdomen or flank. Many patients, however, have only findings associated with the cavity of entrance, and the diaphragmatic injury remains unsuspected until the time of exploration or, unfortunately, is occasionally missed entirely when ex-

ploration of either the chest or abdomen was thought not indicated. This latter event most often occurs with stab wounds, because patients with gunshot wounds of the trunk usually undergo either emergency abdominal or thoracic exploration.

Roentgenographic Findings

In 93 instances of penetrating injuries of the diaphragm, Miller and associates (1984) reported the roentgenogram of the chest to have been normal in 43% and abnormal in 57%. The abnormalities were a hemothorax or a pneumothorax, or both, in 96% and herniated abdominal contents or pneumoperitoneum in 2% each. One of us (PNS) and associates (1986) found the roentgenogram to be normal in one third of 185 patients with this type of injury.

Diagnosis

A high index of suspicion of the presence of a diaphragmatic injury must be present in all penetrating injuries of the trunk from the nipple line to the umbilicus. Miller and associates (1984), among others, have suggested that all such penetrating injuries, symptomatic or not, should be explored and complete inspection of both leaves of the diaphragm be carried out. In their series, 13% of the patients had no associated injuries. We concur with this policy for any gunshot wound, but at times a more conservative approach can be used in the management of stab wounds; most of which will, of course, be explored because of associated symptomatology. In the absence of any findings or suggestion of injury to the diaphragm or any visceral injury, however, exploration may not be mandatory. A few stab-wound injuries to the diaphragm will undoubtedly be missed with this approach, possibly as high as 13% according to Miller and associates' (1984) report. Unfortunately, pneumoperitoneum, abdominal paracentesis, and barium studies generally are of no aid in identifying these missed injuries early. Ultrasonography or CT examination prior to the patient's dismissal from the hospital may lead to the discovery of some of these missed injuries. Elective barium studies should be recommended in a 4- to 6-week period after the patient's discharge when routine exploration has not been done.

Treatment

In the absence of intrathoracic organ injury or major intrapleural bleeding, the abdominal approach is always preferred because it permits detection and treatment of nonevident intra-abdominal injury and enables the surgeon to examine both diaphragmatic leaflets, which is not possible through a transthoracic approach. Any injury to the diaphragm can be repaired readily with No. 0 nonabsorbable interrupted sutures.

Mortality

Diaphragmatic injury should not cause death. Associated organ injury, however, results in a variable number of deaths. In a series by one of us (P.N.S.) of 185

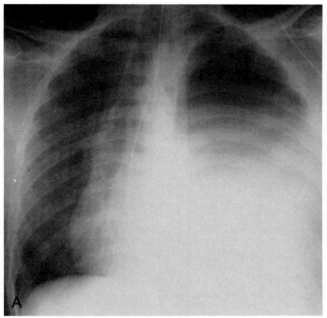

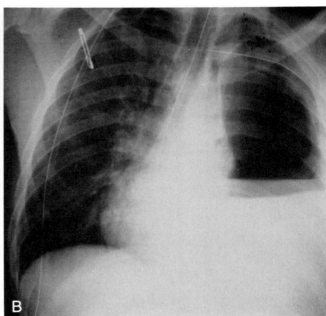

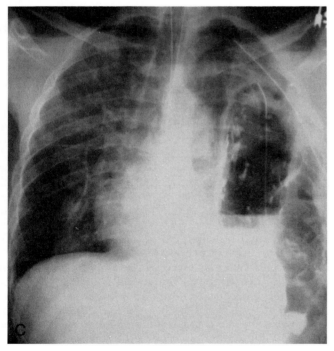

Fig. 46–4. Chest roentgenograms of a 46-year-old man who was involved in a car accident 6 years earlier. *A,* Supine chest roentgenogram shows radiodensity of the lower left lung field and radiolucency of the upper left field with displacement of the mediastinum. *B,* Erect frontal view shows two air-fluid levels. *C,* Upper gastrointestinal series and barium enema demonstrate both the stomach and large bowels in the left chest. (Reproduced with permission from Symbas, P.N., Vlasis, S.E., and Hatcher, C., Jr.: Blunt and penetrating diaphragmatic injuries with or without herniation of organs into the chest. Ann. Thorac. Surg. *42*:158, 1986.)

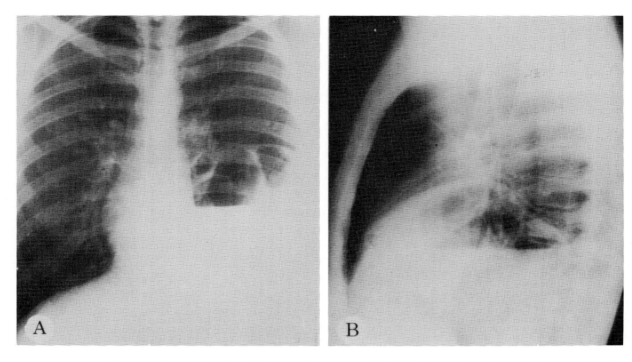

Fig. 46–5. Traumatic diaphragmatic hernia through the left paracardiac portion of the left hemidiaphragm discovered 15 years after the initial injury. *A*, PA roentgenogram of chest showing multiple air-fluid spaces in the lower half of the left chest. *B*, Lateral roentgenogram made with the patient in the upright position.

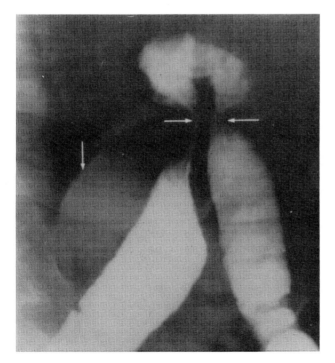

Fig. 46–6. Counter-incision breakdown after hiatal hernia repair. Nonobstructive hernia. The medial portion of the diaphragm is visible (vertical arrow). The lovebird sign is well shown. (Reproduced with permission of Felson, B.: Chest Roentgenology. Philadelphia, W.B. Saunders Co., 1973, pp. 421–449.

penetrating injuries, there were four deaths, a mortality rate of 2.2%.

LATE RECOGNITION

The initial injury to the diaphragm, from either blunt or penetrating trauma, may be undetected during the patient's first hospitalization and may only become manifest because of symptoms or signs related to a hernia of one or more abdominal viscera into the chest. Although no large body of data is available, it is most likely that more late diaphragmatic hernias result from missed stab wound injuries than from blunt trauma. In a small series reported by Hegarty and colleagues (1978), 22 of 25 late hernias were from previous stab wounds. Nonetheless, many examples of herniation caused by blunt injuries have been observed (Figs. 46–4 and 46–5).

These hernias may be recognized any time from a few weeks to over three or four decades after the original injury. The hernias resulting from blunt trauma tend to be larger, especially those involving the left hemidiaphragm, and to contain multiple abdominal viscera, whereas those from penetrating trauma tend to contain only colon or a portion of the stomach, or both.

Symptomatology

The larger hernias are more likely to produce ventilatory signs and symptoms caused by the reduction of the lung volume on the side of the hernia. Gastrointestinal problems caused by interference of the normal functioning of the contained viscera may also occur. The

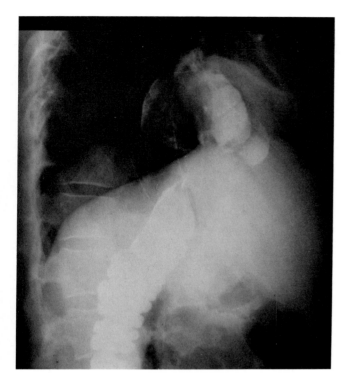

Fig. 46–7. Barium enema showing apposition of loops of large bowel herniating into thorax through a previous stab wound of the diaphragm. (Reproduced with permission from Symbas, P.N., Vlasis, S.E., and Hatcher, C., Jr.: Blunt and penetrating diaphragmatic injuries with or without herniation of organs into the chest. Ann. Thorac. Surg. 42:158, 1986.)

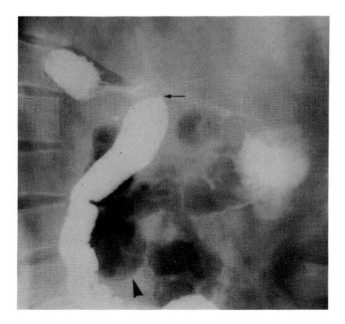

Fig. 46–8. Obstruction of the distal segment. Lateral view. Note the single beak (arrow). The stomach, outlined with barium, is not herniated. The proximal colon shows moderate gaseous distention (arrowhead). (Reproduced with permission of Felson, B.: Chest Roentgenology, Philadelphia, W.B. Saunders Co., 1973, pp. 421–449.)

smaller hernias that contain only a loop of large bowel or stomach become symptomatic because of partial, and at times of complete, obstruction of the contained segment. When complete obstruction occurs, strangulation of the herniated visceral segment may develop and is an ominous complication.

Diagnosis

Roentgenographic examination of the chest reveals an abnormality of the involved diaphragmatic leaf but does not differentiate it from various other causes of elevation of the diaphragm. The most important studies are either barium by mouth or a barium enema, as Felson (1973) pointed out. He noted that whichever of the organs is herniated—stomach or colon—the point of entry and exit through the torn diaphragmatic leaf is most often through a small single defect. Moreover, the edges of the defect are closely applied to the herniated viscus. Thus, the points of entry and exit are closely applied and constricted. This results in a side-by-side, beak-like narrowing of the barium column (Figs. 46–6 and 46–7). Carter and associates (1951) recorded that if the herniated bowel becomes obstructed, the number of beaks will be reduced to one; and dilatation proximal to the site of constriction will be observed (Fig. 46–8). The obstruction within the hernia is often of the closed-loop type, so distention of the loop within the hernia may be great. These authors also noted that the combination of a high left hemidiaphragm and the presence of splenic flexure obstruction is almost diagnostic of a traumatic diaphragmatic hernia.

Other diagnostic studies such as pneumoperitoneum, pneumothorax, and angiography are less rewarding than the barium studies. Ultrasonography and CT studies may be helpful at times but probably less so than they potentially are in the evaluation of patients thought to have acute injury of the diaphragm.

Treatment

Once the hernia is recognized, reduction of the hernia and repair of the diaphragmatic defect through the transthoracic route is indicated. The frequent presence of marked adhesions between the herniated viscus and thoracic contents necessitate this route. In the presence of obstruction with or without strangulation of the contained viscus, the incarcerated diaphragmatic hernia must be approached by the transthoracic route. After mobilization of the obstructed or strangulated viscus, the abdomen may need to be entered through an abdominal incision to complete the necessary operative repair or resection and diversion of the involved viscus. Repair of the diaphragmatic defect is accomplished by direct suture repair in almost all instances. Only rarely in the presence of large tears from original blunt trauma is a prosthetic graft necessary.

Morbidity and Mortality

The morbidity following repair of a diaphragmatic hernia that was recognized late is that seen after any major thoracotomy. The mortality, however, may vary greatly depending upon the status of the hernia at the time of its repair. When the procedure is done electively, the mortality rate should approach zero. In marked contrast, however, is the excessive mortality rate experienced in those patients who present with a strangulated, gangrenous viscus in the hernia. In such instances, the mortality may be as high as 80%, as Hegarty and associates (1978) reported. These missed hernias must therefore be recognized and repaired before obstruction and gangrene of the contained visceral segment occur.

REFERENCES

Ammann, A.M., et al.: Traumatic rupture of the diaphragm: real time sonographic diagnosis. AJR *140*:915, 1983.

Beal, S.L., and McKennan, M.: Blunt diaphragm rupture: a morbid injury. Arch Surg. *123*:828, 1988.

Brooks, J.W.: Blunt traumatic rupture of the diaphgragm. Ann. Thorac. Surg. *26*:199, 1978.

Brown, G.L., and Richardson, J.D.: Traumatic diaphragmatic hernia: a continuing challenge. Ann. Thorac. Surg. *39*:170, 1985.

Carter, B.N., Giuseffi, J., and Felson, B.: Traumatic diaphragmatic hernia. AJR *65*:56, 1951.

Estrera, A.S., Platt, M.R., and Mills, L.J.: Traumatic injuries of the diaphragm. Chest *75*:306, 1979.

Estrera, A.S., Landay, M.J., and McClelland, R.N.: Blunt traumatic rupture of the right hemidiaphragm: experience in 12 patients. Ann. Thorac. Surg. *39*:525, 1985.

Felson, B.: Chest Roentgenology. Philadelphia, W.B. Saunders Co., 1973, p. 437.

Hegarty, M.M., et al.: Delayed presentation of traumatic diaphragmatic hernia. Ann. Surg. *188*:229, 1978.

Heiberg, E., et al.: CT recognition of traumatic rupture of the diaphragm. AJR *135*:369, 1980.

Miller, L.W., et al.: Management of penetrating and blunt diaphragmatic injury. J. Trauma *24*:403, 1984.

Symbas, P.N., Vlasis, S.E., and Hatcher, C.R., Jr.: Blunt and penetrating diaphragmatic injuries with or without herniation of organs into the chest. Ann. Thorac. Surg. *42*:158, 1986.

Toombs, B.D., Sandler, C.M., and Lester, R.G.: Computed tomography of chest trauma. Radiology *140*:733, 1981.

READING REFERENCES

Clay, R.C., and Hanlon, C.R.: Pneumoperitoneum in the differential diagnosis of diaphragmatic hernia. J. Thorac. Cardiovasc. Surg. *21*:57, 1951.

Ebert, P.A., Gaertner, R.A., and Zuidema, G.D.: Traumatic diaphragmatic hernia. Surg. Gynecol. Obstet. *125*:59, 1967.

Fagan, C.J., et al.: Traumatic diaphragmatic hernia into the pericardium: verification of diagnosis by computed tomography. J. Comp. Asst. Tomogr. *3*:405, 1979.

Hood, R.M.: Traumatic diaphragmatic hernia (collective review). Ann. Thorac. Surg. *12*:311, 1971.

Lucido, J.L., and Wall, C.A.: Rupture of the diaphragm due to blunt trauma. Arch. Surg. *86*:989, 1963.

Mansour, K.A., et al.: Diaphragmatic hernia caused by trauma: experience with 35 cases. Am. Surg. *41*:97, 1975.

Nelson, J.B., Jr., et al.: Diaphragmatic injuries and posttraumatic hernia. J. Trauma *2*:36, 1960.

Sutton, J.P., Carlisle, R.B., and Stephenson, S.E., Jr.: Traumatic diaphragmatic hernia: a review of 25 cases. Ann. Thorac. Surg. *3*:136, 1967.

Symbas, P.N.: Blunt traumatic rupture of the diaphragm. Ann. Thorac. Surg. *26*:193, 1978.

The Chest Wall

CHAPTER 47

CHEST WALL DEFORMITIES

Kenneth J. Welch and Robert C. Shamberger

Congenital and acquried anterior thoracic deformities can be conveniently arranged into four groups: (1) pectus excavatum; (2) pectus carinatum; (3) sternal clefts, including ectopia cordis; and (4) miscellaneous conditions, including vertebral and rib anomalies, Jeune's disease—asphyxiating thoracic dystrophy—and manubrial and rib dysplasia. Total experience with the surgical treatment of these conditions at the Children's Hospital, Boston, from 1952 to 1987 is seen in Table 47–1.

PECTUS EXCAVATUM

Pectus excavatum—funnel chest or trichterburst—presents as a depression of the sternum and the lower costal cartilages, and in older patients it involves the most anterior portion of the ribs. The extent of sternal and cartilaginous deformity is variable, and numerous methods of grading and defining these deformities have been proposed, such as those by Hümmer and Willital (1984) and Oelsnitz (1981) and by one of us (K.J.W., 1980), but none has been universally accepted. Asymmetry is frequently present but may be unappreciated until the time of surgical correction. The right side is often more depressed than the left, with a variable degree of sternal obliquity.

Pectus excavatum is usually present from birth. Occasional de novo cases—<5%—appear at adolescence.

Table 47–1. Surgical Correction of Congenital Chest Wall Deformities: The Children's Hospital, Boston Experience

Type of Deformity	Number of Cases
Pectus excavatum	1234
Pectus carinatum	203
Poland's syndrome	10
Vertebral and rib anomalies	7
Thoracoabdominal ectopic cordis	9
Thoracic ectopia cordis	4
Cleft sternum	4
Total	1471

Family history of some type of anterior thoracic deformity is present in 37% of patients, as we noted in 1988. The first and second ribs, corresponding costal cartilages, and manubrium are usually normal. In response to some unknown stimulus, the lower costal cartilages grow too rapidly, the sternebral segments are forced inward, and a concave deformity ensues. Rib length, angle of declination, and contour are normal in young children. The spine is usually straight. This depression deformity reduces the prevertebral space with obligatory left cardiac displacement and axial rotation. Uncorrected, the deformity usually worsens at adolescence. Self-limited deformities are either gone or vastly improved by age 3 years. Transient deformity with paradoxic breathing is common in infants, and for this reason correction of pectus excavatum should never be performed before 2 years of age. With the infant crying, observation of the chest during full inspiration and forced expiration reveals any persisting fixed or rigid deformity. Surgery is recommended for children with fixed and worsening deformity greater than 5 on a scale of 1 to 10, as defined by my (K.J.W., 1980) previously published index. (Fig. 47–1 and 47–2).

A broad, thin chest is gradually acquired in most children with uncorrected pectus excavatum. This appearance, with dorsal lordosis, hook shoulder deformity, and costal flaring, is caused by increased costal cartilage length and caudal declination of the ribs off the horizontal plane. Rib deformity is seldom seen before the age of 5 years, when the disease is limited to costal cartilage overgrowth. The ideal age for operation is between 2 and 5 years, for boys and girls meeting the aforementioned criteria.

Waters and associates (1988) identified scoliosis in 26% of 508 patients with pectus excavatum. Full spine films, taken from chin to pelvis, shoes off, should be obtained in all patients with pectus excavatum and with scoliosis greater than 10° observed in chest roentgenograms. Though initially mild, thoracolumbar curves in boys and girls can rapidly worsen well before adolescence. Asymmetric pectus excavatum with a deep right gutter and

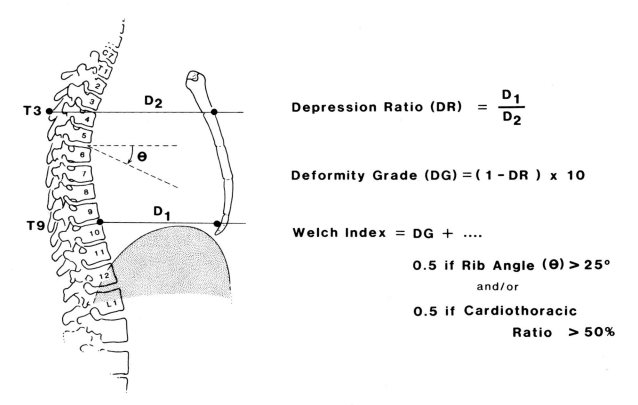

Fig. 47–1. Welch Index for determining the severity of pectus excavatum deformities.

sternal obliquity often is accompanied by more serious right thoracic and left lumbar scoliosis. Early correction of the associated pectus excavatum may improve the curve, make it easier to manage by exercises or bracing, and in some patients avoid the need for spine fusion. In a review of 132 patients with scoliosis and associated anterior chest wall deformity by Waters and associates (1988), 99 patients had pectus excavatum, 28 had pectus carinatum and 5 had "mixed" deformities. The mean lateral deformity for the primary curve at the time of evaluation of their pectus excavatum deformity was 15.2°—range 6° to 78°. At the most recent follow-up visits—mean 46.9 months, range 9 to 107 months—the postoperative spinal deformity was 16.9°—range 3° to 47°. Eighteen patients underwent therapeutic intervention for their scoliosis. Eleven patients were treated with bracing, but three had significant progression despite bracing and required operative intervention. Three patients with a deformity greater than 40° at presentation required early operative fusion without bracing. Twenty-eight patients had scoliosis associated with carinate deformities, and five patients had both pre- and postoperative studies available. The mean preoperative curve was 9.4° and the mean postoperative curve was 8.4°.

Etiology and Incidence

Ravitch (1977) reported that funnel chest may be as common as 1 in 300 to 1 in 400 live births. The condition is most likely multifactorial and clearly has an increased familial incidence. In our 1988 review, 37% of 704 patients had a family history of chest wall deformity. Three of four siblings were involved in one family. Patients with Marfan's syndrome have a high incidence of chest wall deformities, which are often in the most severe form and usually accompanied by scoliosis. Patients with abdominal musculature deficiency syndrome—prune belly syndrome—commonly have pectus excavatum, 8 of 43 patients in my (K.J.W.) and Kearney's (1974) experience. It also occurs with Werdnig-Hoffmann paralysis and other myopathies. A few patients have broad chromosomal defects, such as Turner's syndrome. These and other associations are seen in Table 47–2. The disorder is congenital in that it is nearly always present at birth or within the first year of life—86%—and has been observed in full form in a 32-mm stillborn embryo.

The resected cartilages are bizarrely deformed, rotated, and in various V or L configurations. Light microscopy reveals areas of aseptic perichondritis with spotty obliteration of the perichondrial sheath, vacuolization, disorderly arrangement of cartilage cell columns, areas of aseptic necrosis, and other features of an active process in cartilage. Although the sternal depression appears to be caused by overgrowth of costal cartilages, the etiology of this deformity is unknown. Early investigators such as Lester (1957) attributed its development to an abnormality of the diaphragm, but there has been little evidence to support this theory.

Congenital heart disease was identified in 1.5% of our patients who underwent chest wall correction (Table 47–3). Among all patients with congenital heart disease

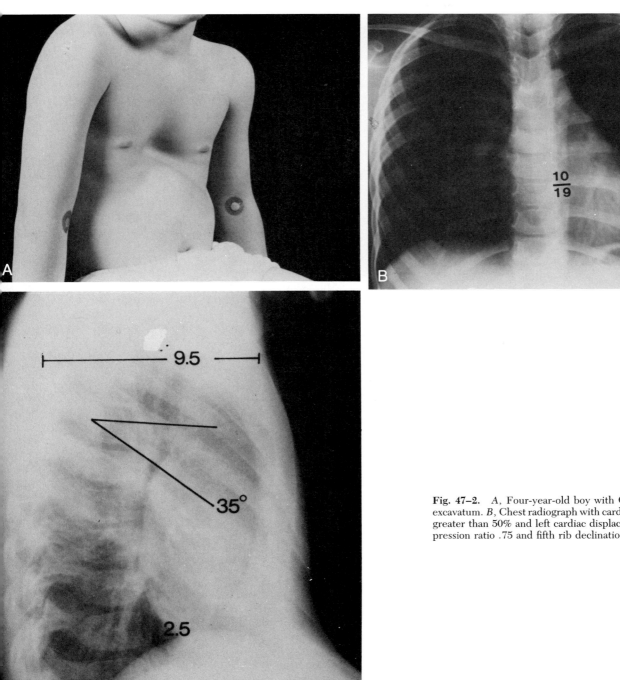

Fig. 47–2. *A*, Four-year-old boy with Grade 8 pectus excavatum. *B*, Chest radiograph with cardiothoracic ratio greater than 50% and left cardiac displacement. *C*, Depression ratio .75 and fifth rib declination of 35°.

Table 47–2. Musculoskeletal Abnormalities Identified in 133 of 704 Cases of Pectus Excavatum

Scoliosis	107
Kyphosis	4
Myopathy	3
Poland's syndrome	3
Marfan's syndrome	2
Pierre-Robin syndrome	2
Prune belly syndrome	2
Neurofibromatosis	3
Cerebral palsy	4
Tuberous sclerosis	1
Congenital diaphragmatic hernia	2

evaluated at our institution, 0.17% had anterior chest wall deformities. We perform chest wall surgery prior to correction of the cardiac lesion, particularly in those patients who require a Fontan procedure or other retrosternal conduit.

Asthma is frequently identified in patients with pectus excavatum and carinatum. In a review of 694 consecutive cases, a subgroup of 35 patients was identified with asthma—5.2%—comparable to the occurrence in a general pediatric population. These patients must have adequate serum levels of bronchodilators prior to and at the onset of their anesthesia. To avoid episodes of bronchospasm during induction of anesthesia, we obtain preoperative pulmonary function tests on admission in children older than five to confirm the adequacy of the bronchodilator therapy as well as to determine appropriate serum theophylline levels. In patients with severe asthma or past steroid requirement, we use perioperative prednisone for a 24-hour period.

Symptoms

Pectus excavatum is well tolerated in infancy, except for increased frequency of upper respiratory infections that tend to be frequent and lingering, progressing to bronchitis, bronchiolitis, and croup. A history of recurring pneumonia is common; usually the left lower lobe or right middle lobe is involved. Stridor is rare. Chronic

Table 47–3. Congenital Heart Disease Associated with Pectus Excavatum and Carinatum

Aortic ring	1
Aortic regurgitation	1
ASD primum	2
ASD secundum	3
Complete atrioventricular canal	3
Dextrocardia	3
Ebstein malformation	1
Idiopathic hypertrophic subaortic stenosis	2
Patent ductus arteriosus	1
Pulmonic stenosis	1
Total anomalous pulmonary venous return	1
Transposition of great arteries	6
Tetralogy of Fallot	3
Tricuspid atresia	1
Truncus arteriosus	1
Ventricular septal defect	6

upper airway obstruction caused by tonsillar and adenoidal hypertrophy may be potentiating but is not causative. Older children complain of pain in the area of the deformed cartilages or of precordial pain after sustained exercise. A few patients have palpitations or syncope, presumably caused by transient atrial arrhythmias. These patients may have mitral valve prolapse, which is associated with atrial arrhythmias and which we (1987) identified in patients with pectus excavatum.

Pathophysiology

Some authors contend, as do Haller and colleagues (1970), that there is no cardiovascular or pulmonary impairment resulting from a pectus excavatum deformity. This contrasts, however, with the general clinical impression that many patients following surgical repair have increased stamina or level of activity that is spontaneously reported by their parents. These findings date back to the surgical repair performed by Sauerbruch in 1913 (1920). His patient was an 18-year-old boy who developed dyspnea and palpitations with limited exercise. Three years after the operative repair he could work 12 to 14 hours a day without tiring and without palpitations. Anecdotal reports during the next three decades confirmed this observation. Over the years, we and others have looked for some physiologic abnormality or combination of abnormalities that could explain clinical and symptomatic improvement following surgery. The problem has been that early physiologic measurements of cardiac and pulmonary function were crude and did not in general yield convincing evidence of a cardiopulmonary deficit. Many early results fell within the broad range of normal values, though often at the lower limit of the range.

A systolic ejection murmur grade II-III/IV is frequently identified in patients with pectus excavatum and is magnified with a short interval of exercise. It was reported in 57 to 100% of patients by Schaub and Wegmann (1954) and Evans (1946) and, in our 1987 review, was identified in 92% of 704 patients. It is attributed to the close proximity of or contact between the posterior sternal cortex and the pulmonary artery, which results in direct increased transmission of a flow murmur.

Electrocardiographic abnormalities are common and are attributed to the abnormal configuration of the chest wall and the displacement and rotation of the heart into the left thoracic cavity. Preoperative findings in a study group of 32 patients are shown in Table 47–4. Most significant are the cases of conduction blocks or frank arrhythmias. Patients with a history of palpitations should have a 24-hour Holter study as well as an echocardiogram to exclude the possibility of mitral valve prolapse. Resolution of these supraventricular arrhythmias has been anecdotally reported following correction of a pectus excavatum deformity.

Deformity of the chest wall led many authors to attribute the symptomatic improvement in patients following surgery to initial impairment in pulmonary function. This was difficult to prove, however, with the wide range of cardiopulmonary function that exists from individual

Table 47–4. Electrocardiographic Findings in a Group of 32 Patients with Pectus Excavatum

Abnormality	Number of Patients
Right axis deviation	15
Depressed ST-T segments (2, 3, AVF)	11
Tall P waves	7
Right bundle branch block	5
Combined block	3
Left ventricular hypertrophy	4
Left atrial hypertrophy	1
Paroxysmal atrial tachycardia	1

From Welch, K.J.: Chest wall deformities. *In* Pediatric Surgery, Edited by T.M. Holder and K.W. Ashcraft. Philadelphia, W.B. Saunders Co., 1980.

to individual, and depends heavily on physical training and body habitus.

Pulmonary Function Studies

As early as 1951, Brown and Cook performed respiratory studies on patients before and after surgical repair and demonstrated that although vital capacity was normal in these patients, the maximum breathing capacity was diminished—50% or more—in 9 of 11 cases and that it was increased an average of 31% following the surgical repair. Weg and associates (1967) evaluated 25 Air Force recruits with pectus excavatum and compared them with 50 unselected basic trainees. Although the lung compartments of both groups were equal, as were the vital capacities, the maximum voluntary ventilation showed a significant decrease compared with the control population. Castile and colleagues (1982) evaluated seven patients with pectus excavatum, five of whom were symptomatic with exercise. The mean total lung capacity as a percentage of predicted in the excavatum patients was 79%. Flow volume configurations all appeared to be normal and did not suggest airway obstruction. Workload tests were performed and a normal response to exercise of dead space to tidal volume ratio and alveolar-arterial oxygen difference did not suggest a significant ventilation/perfusion abnormality in the symptomatic patients. The measured oxygen uptake increasingly exceeded predicted values as the workloads approached maximum, whereas in the normal subjects a linear response was seen. The mean oxygen uptake at maximal effort exceeded the predicted values by 25.4% in the symptomatic patients. The two asymptomatic patients, on the other hand, demonstrated normal linear oxygen uptake during exercise. This increased oxygen uptake suggests an increased work of breathing in these patients, although the vital capacities were only mildly reduced or normal.

Cahill and co-workers (1984) performed pre- and postoperative studies in 19 patients with pectus carinatum—5 patients—and excavatum—14 patients. No abnormalities were demonstrated in the pectus carinatum patients. The excavatum patients demonstrated low-normal vital capacities, which were unchanged by operation, but a small improvement in the total lung capacity and

a significant improvement in the maximal voluntary ventilation was seen. Exercise tolerance also improved in patients following surgery, as determined both by total exercise time and the maximal oxygen consumption. Mead and associates (1985) attempted to demonstrate a decrease in rib-cage mobility by assessing intra-abdominal pressure, but was unable to define any increased abdominal pressure swings that would have been predicted.

Blickman and colleagues (1985) assessed pulmonary function by xenon perfusion and ventilation scintigraphy before and after surgery in 17 patients. Ventilation studies were abnormal in 12 patients before surgery and improved in 7 following surgery; perfusion scans were abnormal in 10 patients before surgery and improved following operation in 6. The ventilation/perfusion ratios were abnormal in 10 of the 17 patients preoperatively and returned to normal following surgery in 6 (Fig. 47–3).

Cardiovascular Studies

Posterior displacement of the sternum can produce a deformity of the heart, particularly of the right ventricle, with anterior indentation, as Howard (1959) demonstrated, and this is relieved by surgical repair. Garusi and D'Ettorre (1964) also demonstrated by angiography that the heart is displaced to the left, often with a sternal imprint on the anterior wall of the ventricle. Elevated

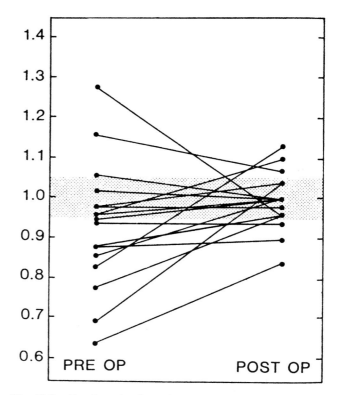

Fig. 47–3. Ventilation/perfusion lung scans and pre- and postoperative studies in 17 patients (from Blickman, et al.: Pectus excavatum in children: pulmonary scintigraphy before and after corrective surgery. Radiology 156:781, 1985.)

right heart pressures have been reported by some authors, as have pressure curves similar to those seen in constrictive pericarditis. Bevegård in 1962 studied 16 patients with pectus excavatum by right heart catheterization and workload studies. The physical work capacity at a given heart rate was significantly lower in the sitting than in the supine position for patients with the pectus excavatum. The group of patients with 20% or greater decline in the physical work capacity from the supine to the sitting position had a shorter sternovertebral distance than patients with less decrease in the physical work capacity. The measured stroke volume at rest decreased from supine to sitting positions a mean of 40.3%, similar to normal subjects. In the supine position, the stroke volume increased 13.2% with exercise. In the sitting position, the increase in stroke volume from rest to exercise was 18.5%, significantly lower—p <0.001—than the 51% increase seen in normal subjects. Thus, with limitations of the stroke volume with a heavier work load, the increased cardiac output could be achieved only by increased heart rate. Intracardiac pressures measured at rest and with exercise were normal in all subjects despite this apparent limitation of ventricular volume. Gattiker and Bühlmann (1967) confirmed this limitation of the stroke volume in a study of 19 patients. In the upright position at a pulse of 170, the physical work capacity was lower than in the supine position—mean 18% decrease—because of the decrease in stroke volume. Beiser and associates (1972) performed cardiac catheterization in six patients with moderate degrees of pectus excavatum. Normal pressures were obtained at rest in the supine position. The cardiac index was normal at rest in the supine position, and the response to moderate exercise was within the normal range. The response to upright exercise was below the predicted normal in two patients and at the lower limit of normal in three. The cardiac index was 6.8 ± 0.8 L/min/m² while it was 8.9 ± 0.3 L/min/m² in a group of 16 normal controls—p <0.01. The difference in these two groups again seemed to be caused primarily by a difference in stroke volume. Stroke volume was 31% lower and cardiac output 28% lower during upright as compared with supine exercise. Postoperative studies were performed in three patients and two achieved a higher level of exercise tolerance following surgery. The cardiac index was increased by 38%. The heart rates were unchanged, and the increase resulted from an enhanced stroke volume following surgery.

Radionuclide angiography and workload studies were performed by Peterson and associates (1985) in 13 patients with pectus excavatum. Ten of the thirteen patients were able to reach the target heart rate before surgical repair, four without symptoms. After operation, all but 1 patient reached the target heart rate during the exercise protocol and 9 of 13 patients reached the target without becoming symptomatic. The left and right ventricular end diastolic volumes were consistently increased after repair at rest, and the mean stroke volume was increased 19% after repair. The ventricular volume changes demonstrated previously by catheterization were substantiated by the radionuclide technique, although an increase in the cardiac index was not demonstrated.

Echocardiographic Studies

Bon Tempo (1975), Salomon (1975), and Schutte (1981) and their associates reported mitral valve prolapse in patients with narrow anterior-posterior chest diameters, anterior chest wall deformities, and scoliosis. One prospective study in adults, published by Udoshi and colleagues (1979), demonstrated mitral valve prolapse by echocardiogram in 6 of 33 patients—18%—with pectus excavatum, and a French study by Saint-Mezard and associates (1986) identified mitral valve prolapse in 11 of 17 patients—65%—with pectus excavatum. Anterior compression of the heart against the vertebral column by the depressed sternum, with resulting deformity of the mitral annulus or the ventricular chamber, has been proposed as the cause of mitral valve prolapse in these patients. As we reported in 1987, among our patients were 23 with pectus excavatum and mitral valve prolapse confirmed preoperatively by echocardiogram; postoperative studies failed to demonstrate mitral valve prolapse in 10 patients—43%.

Surgical Repair

The first surgical treatments of pectus excavatum were reported by Meyer in 1911 and Sauerbruch in 1920. In 1939, Ochsner and DeBakey summarized early experience with surgical repair using various techniques. Ravitch in 1949 reported a technique that included excision of all deformed costal cartilages with the perichondrium, division of the xiphoid from the sternum, division of the intercostal bundles from the sternum, and a transverse sternal osteotomy overcorrecting the sternum anteriorly with Kirschner wire fixation in the first two patients and silk suture fixation in later patients. Others, such as Rehbein and Wernicke (1957), have used internal fixation with Kirschner wires or metallic struts, but no evidence has been presented to determine that such methods provide better long-term results than those achieved without metal fixation. The complication rate is certainly greater with their use. Oelsnitz (1981) and Hecker and associates (1981) reached the same conclusion in their large series of patients, in which satisfactory repairs were achieved in 90 to 95% of patients. In 1954 and 1956 the "sternal turnover" was proposed by the Judets (1954) and Jung (1956) in the French literature. Wada and colleagues (1970) reported a large series from Japan that used this technique, which is essentially a free graft of sternum, but it appears to be a radical approach and has been associated with major complications if infection occurs. A final approach, suggested by Allen and Douglas (1979), that must be mentioned is the implantation of silastic molds into the subcutaneous space to fill the deformity. Although this approach may improve the contour of the chest, extrusion has occurred, and it does nothing to increase the thoracic cavity volume, improve respiratory mechanics, or relieve pressure on the heart. It is most frequently used in adults who have long passed the ideal age for repair. In 1958, we reported a technique for the satisfactory and safe correction of pectus excavatum that emphasized total preservation of the perichondrial sheaths of the costal cartilage, preservation of the upper intercostal bundles, and anterior fixation of the sternum with silk sutures. The technique we use today remains unchanged more than 700 cases later. The technique uses the best features of operations described by Lester (1946), Garnier (1934), and Ravitch (1949), adding instrumentation for meticulous resection of costal cartilages and the use of electrosurgery.

Operative Technique

Our operative technique is illustrated in Figure 47–4 A through J. The technique provides for precise resection of costal cartilages with preservation of perichondrial sheaths, without injury to mediastinal structures, and without pleural or pericardial entry. Special instruments were designed for the dissection of the perichondrial sheaths from the costal cartilages. Rib resection instru-

ments are of little value in resecting the soft cartilage in young children. Electrocautery has reduced operating time to 1½ to 2 hours in patients to age 5, 2 to 3 hours in early adolescents, and 4 hours in patients at full growth, including adults. Blood loss is well below transfusion requirement in patients of all ages. This technique was reviewed at our institution in 704 patients with no deaths and with few and minor complications—4.4%. Safe and effective repair is possible at any age and with the most severe deformities, but the most favorable results are obtained in the younger patients. Our oldest patient was 43 years old. Hemovac drainage is used for 48 hours or until drainage for an eight-hour shift is less than 15 ml. No type of brace, bar, or external traction is used. In early cases, patients with Marfan's syndrome, those requiring reoperation, and adults with severe asymmetric deformity, a short-segment, ⁵⁄₃₂-inch Steinmann pin was used for internal fixation and drilled transsternally and then through a longitudinal sleeve of resected cartilage and on into the intramedually cavity of

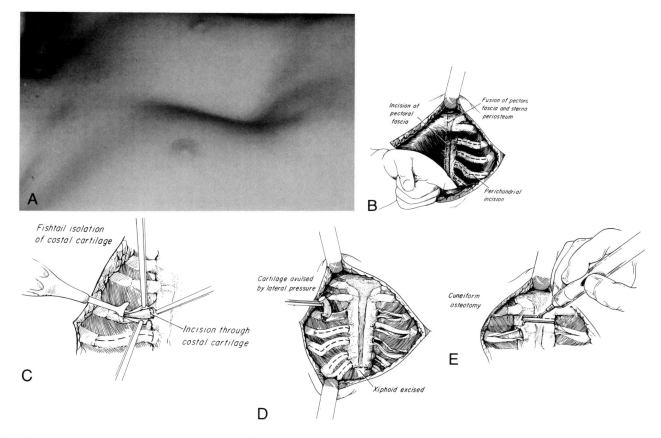

Fig. 47–4. *A,* Same patient as in Figure 47–2*A* anesthetized for pectus excavatum repair. Note deep symmetrical depression unchanged in the supine position. *B,* A short transverse incision is made well within the nipple lines at the level of the fifth interspace. Superior and inferior flaps are developed to the angle of Louis and to the tip of the xiphoid. A vertical incision is made at the junction of pectoral muscle and fascia. The cartilaginous deformity is exposed to the junction of the rib and cartilage by dissecting away elements of the pectoralis serratus and rectus muscles. *C,* Cartilage elevator is used to open the perichondrium from the sternum to the costochondral junction. The cartilage is completely isolated, preserving perichondrium divided at the medial end. *D,* The third costal cartilage is removed by lateral avulsion at the costochondral junction. Subsequently, the fourth and fifth cartilages are completely removed; then segments of the sixth and seventh cartilages approximately 5 cm long are removed, preserving the costal arch. In all cases the third to seventh costal cartilages are removed bilaterally. The xiphoid then is removed from the apex of the rectus flap. *E,* A transverse cuneiform osteotomy is made at the angle of Louis between the second and third costal cartilages. The posterior cortex of the sternum remains intact.

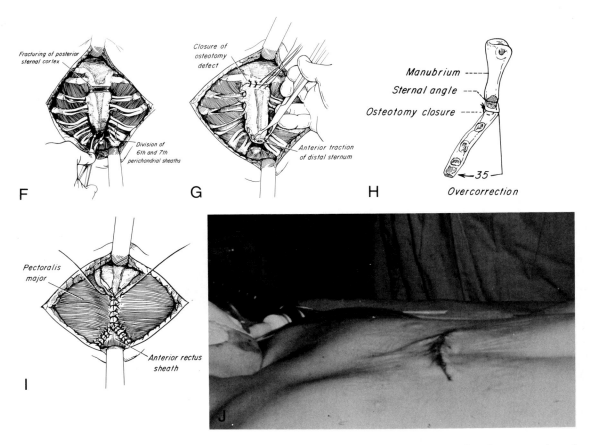

Fig. 47–4 Continued. *F,* The perichondrial sheaths of the sixth, and seventh costal cartilages are detached at their point of attachment to the sternum. The retrosternal space is not disturbed. The pleural and pericardial cavities are not entered. The sternum can now be brought forward into overcorrection of about 35°. *G,* The osteotomy is completely closed using three to four No. 1 silk sutures placed through the drill holes in bone. *H,* Overcorrection of 35° is accomplished on closing the osteotomy defect. *I,* Closure involves suturing pectoral muscles to the retained midline strip of pectoral fascia and periosteum. The apex of the rectus flap is drawn up into the corresponding pectoral defect to provide a watertight inverted Y suture closure. *J,* Completed repair with normal contour. Flail chest has not been a problem. (Reproduced with permission from Welch, K.J.: Chest wall deformities. *In* Pediatric Surgery, Edited by T.M. Holder and K.W. Ashcraft. Philadelphia, W.B. Saunders Co., 1980.)

the right fourth or fifth rib, selecting the highest point. This method is no longer used because of its significant complication rate—21%, 6 of 28 cases; versus 3.5%, 24 of 676—in the remainder of the series. In one patient, the pin migrated into the left thorax, caused a pericardial effusion, and was removed by anterior thoracotomy. A second patient had a pulmonary contusion and hemoptysis following trauma to the chest in a basketball game. Two pins were broken in motor vehicle accidents. There appears to be no completely satisfactory method of internal fixation. Death has resulted from use of a retrosternal metal bar through erosion of the left ventricle.

Complications

Complications of pectus excavatum repair in 704 patients (Table 47–5) are few and relatively unimportant, except for major recurrence in 17 of our patients (1988). In 2% of patients, a limited pneumothorax required aspiration or was simply observed. Tube thoracostomy has not been required since 1978 and was required in only four patients in this series. Wound infection has been rare with use of perioperative antibiotic coverage.

The most distressing complication following surgical correction of pectus excavatum is major recurrence of the deformity years after the original repair. Such patients often seem to have a broad connective tissue disorder with hypotonia, poor muscular development, and an asthenic or "marfanoid habitus." It is difficult to predict which unfortunate patients will have a major recurrence, but these patients are certainly at greater risk. True Marfan's patients eventually have mitral and tri-

Table 47–5. Complications of Pectus Excavatum Repair: 47 Cases in 704 Patients

Pneumothorax*	11
Wound infection	5
Wound hematoma	3
Wound dehiscence	5
Pneumonia	3
Seroma	1
Hemoptysis	1
Hemopericardium	1
Major recurrence	17

*Four patients required chest tube placement.

cuspid valve involvement, a widened aortic root, and ocular findings of dislocated lens. They have poor osseous and cartilaginous matrix. Many develop severe scoliosis in addition to the most severe forms of pectus deformities. There are no biochemical or genetic markers for this disease, so diagnosis must be made on clinical findings. Pulmonary reserve gradually diminishes, and repair of the pectus excavatum in combination with spine fusion is necessary though its results are often poor.

Sanger and associates (1968) reported on surgical correction of recurrent pectus excavatum. They resected the regenerated fibrocartilage plate, repeated the osteotomy, and closed the pectoral muscles behind the sternum. Ten patients had an early good result. Our experience with 12 patients led to a consistent finding. Although recurrences appear to be symmetric, they are in fact right-sided with a deep right parasternal gutter and sternal obliquity. The third, fourth, and fifth rib ends migrate medially and are in contact with the right edge of the sternum. Resection of segments of the third to fifth ribs is necessary to unlock the deformity. After clearing the tip of the sternum, resection of the left fibrocartilage plate to the level of the third perichondrial sheath allows the sternum to be brought forward and rotated to an acceptable horizontal plane. Ten of twelve repeat operations were accomplished without pleural cavity entry. Follow-up patients who were reoperated on ranged from 10 to 17 years. Eight have acceptable thoracic contour; two have a broad, shallow depression with cartilage angularity; and two have frank recurrence. Patients are followed to full growth, age 16 for girls and 19 for boys (Figs. 47–5 to 7). Use of clinical and Moiré photography, as used by Shochat and colleagues (1981), for initial evaluation and follow-up studies leads to improved clinical assessment of results and obviates the need for multiple radiographic examinations. We have performed no secondary repairs since 1980, although our patients may have gone elsewhere (Table 47–6).

Table 47–6. **Results of Surgical Repair of Pectus Excavatum**

Satisfactory repair	664
Mild recurrence	23
Major recurrence	17 (2.7%)

PECTUS CARINATUM

Pectus carinatum is the most common and accepted term to describe anterior protrusion deformities of the chest. It is much less frequent in our experience than depression deformities—16.7%—and consists of a spectrum of abnormal thoracic development. It is often divided into four types (Table 47–7). The most frequent form consists of anterior displacement of the sternum with symmetric concavity of the costal cartilages, termed chondrogladiolar by Brodkin (1949). Howard (1958) wrote that it looks as if a giant hand had pinched the chest from the front, forcing the sternum forward and the lower costal cartilages and the ribs inward lateral to the sternum. Asymmetric deformities with anterior displacement of costal cartilages on one side and normally positioned or oblique sternum and normal cartilages on the contralateral side are much less common. Mixed lesions have a carinate deformity on one side and a depression or excavatum deformity on the contralateral side, often with sternal obliquity. These are classified by some authors as a variant of the excavatum deformities. Most unusual are the upper or chondromanubrial deformities, the "pouter pigeon" deformity, with protrusion of the manubrium and second and third costal cartilages and relative depression of the gladiolus or body of the sternum.

Etiology

The etiology of pectus carinatum is no better understood than that of pectus excavatum. It appears as an overgrowth of the costal cartilages with forward buckling

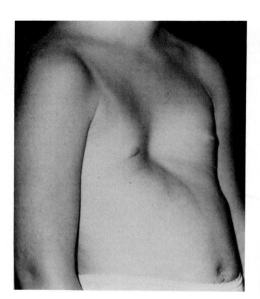 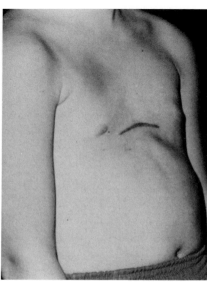

Fig. 47–5. Pectus excavatum repair: preoperative and 6 weeks postoperative photographs of a 6-year-old girl.

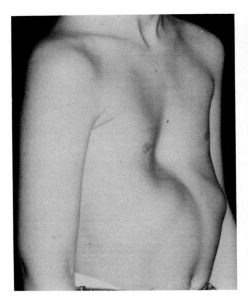

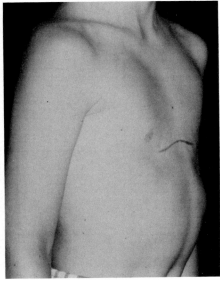

Fig. 47–6. Pectus excavatum repair: preoperative and 6 weeks postoperative photographs of a 7-year-old boy.

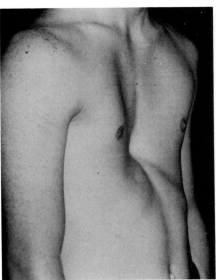

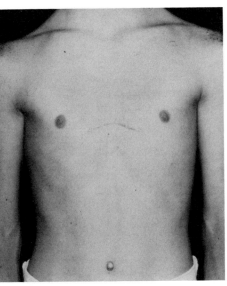

Fig. 47–7. Pectus excavatum repair: preoperative and 6 weeks postoperative photograph of a 14-year-old boy.

and anterior displacement of the sternum. Again, there is a clear-cut family incidence, suggesting a genetic basis. In our 1987 review of 152 patients, 26% had a family history of chest wall deformity. A family history of scoliosis was obtained in 12% of the patients. It is much more frequent in boys—119 patients—than in girls—33 patients. Associated musculoskeletal anomalies are listed in Table 47–8. Scoliosis and other deformities of the spine are most common.

Pectus carinatum usually appears in childhood, and in almost half of the patients, the deformity was not identified until after the eleventh birthday. The deformity may appear in mild form at birth, and often progresses, particularly during the period of rapid growth at puberty. The chondromanubrial deformity is often noted at birth and is associated with a short, truncated sternum with absent sternal segmentation or premature obliteration of sternal sutures. Since it was described by Currarino and

Table 47–7. Frequency of Pectus Carinatum Deformities

Chondrogladiolar	
Symmetric	89
Asymmetric	49
Mixed Carinatum/Excavatum	14
Chondromanubrial	3

Table 47–8. Musculoskeletal Abnormalities Identified in 34 of 152 Cases of Pectus Carinatum

Scoliosis	23
Poland's syndrome	4
Neurofibromatosis	2
Morquio's disease	2
Vertebral anomalies	1
Hyperlordosis	1
Kyphosis	1

Silverman in 1958, it has been linked with an increased risk of congenital heart disease. In a prospective review by Lees and Caldicott (1975), 135 patients with sternal fusion anomalies were identified, and 18% of these had documented congenital heart disease.

Surgical Repair

Surgical repair of carinate deformities has had a colorful history, starting with the first reported case of correction by Ravitch, in 1952, of the upper or chondromanubrial deformity. He resected multiple costal cartilages and performed a double sternal osteotomy. Lester (1953) reported two methods of repair for chondrogladiolar deformity. The first method, involving resection of the anterior portion of the sternum, was abandoned because of excessive blood loss and unsatisfactory results. The next, although no less radical a technique, used subperiosteal resection of the entire sternum. Chin (1957) and later Brodkin (1958) advanced the transected xiphoid and attached rectus muscles to a higher site on the sternum—the xiphosternopexy. This produced posterior displacement of the sternum in young patients with a flexible chest wall. Howard (1958) combined this method with subperichondrial costal cartilage resection and a sternal osteotomy. Ravitch (1960) reported repair of the chondrogladiolar deformity by resection of costal cartilage in a one- or two-stage procedure and use of reefing sutures to shorten and displace the perichondrium anteriorly. A sternal osteotomy was used in one of three cases. Robicsek and associates (1963) reported subperichondrial resection of costal cartilages, transverse sternal osteotomy and displacement, and resection of the protruding lower portion of the sternum. Xiphoid and rectus muscles were reattached to the new lower margin of the sternum, pulling it posteriorly. In 1973 we reported in 26 patients an approach to these deformities that we continue to use (Fig. 47–8A through E).

Operative Technique

In females, we prefer to place the incision within the inframammary fold, thus avoiding the complications of breast deformity and development described by Hougaard and Arendrup (1983). Subperichondrial resection of the costal cartilages is performed with specially designed Welch Pectus Elevators (Codman and Shurtleff, Randolph, MA). The third cartilage is broad and flat, the fourth and fifth are circular, and the sixth and seventh are narrow and deep. Sternal osteotomies through the anterior cortex are created with the Hall drill (Zimmer USA, Inc., Warsaw, IN); occasionally, a second osteotomy is required.

The upper or chondromanubrial deformity must be managed in a special manner, which we have described (Fig. 47–9A and B). In this situation, the costal cartilages must be resected from the second cartilage inferiorly. A generous wedge osteotomy is performed at the point of maximal protrusion of the sternum. The superior segment of the sternum can then be displaced posteriorly as the osteotomy is closed, advancing the inferior segment anteriorly. A single-limb medium Hemovac drain

(Snyder Laboratories, Inc., New Philadelphia, OH) is brought through the inferior skin flap, as with the excavatum patients, with the suction ports in a parasternal position to the level of the highest costal cartilage resection. The pectoralis muscle flaps are joined in the midline and anchored to the sternal periosteum, advancing the flaps inferiorly to cover the often bare sternum. The xiphoid is removed from the U-shaped rectus muscle flap, which is then joined to the caudal end of the sternum centrally and to the pectoral muscle flaps laterally to completely close the mediastinum. Nonabsorbable 2–0 silk sutures are used for the muscle closure and 3–0 inverted silk sutures for the combined subcuticular and superficial fascial layers. Perioperative antibiotics are used, giving one dose of cefazolin immediately prior to surgery and three postoperative doses. All patients are warned to avoid aspirin-containing compounds for 2 weeks prior to surgery to avoid abnormalities of platelet adhesion and function.

Operative Results

Results are overwhelmingly successful in these patients (Figs. 47–10A, and B and 47–11A and B). In our 1987 review of 152 cases, postoperative recovery was generally uneventful. Blood transfusions are rarely required, and none have been given in the last 5 years. There is a 3.9% complication rate (Table 47–9). Only three patients required revision, each having additional lower costal cartilages resected for persistent unilateral malformation of the costal arch.

POLAND'S SYNDROME

Poland (1841) described congenital absence of the pectoralis major and minor muscles, associated with syndactyly. Since then it has become apparent that this entity is a spectrum, often involving chest wall and breast deformity as well. The extent of thoracic involvement may range from hypoplasia of the sternal head of the pectoralis major and minor muscles with normal underlying ribs to complete absence of the anterior portions of the second to fourth ribs and cartilages, often called the second to fourth rib syndrome (Fig. 47–12). Breast involvement is frequent in females, ranging from varying degrees of breast hypoplasia to complete absence of the breast—amastia—and nipple—athelia. Minimal subcutaneous fat and an absence of axillary hair are often found on the involved side. Hand deformities are frequent and occurred in the patient described by Poland. They may include hypoplasia—brachydactyly, fused fingers—syndactyly—and mitten or claw deformity—ectromelia—

Table 47–9. Complications of Pectus Carinatum Repair: 7 Cases in 152 Patients

Pneumothorax*	4
Atelectasis	1
Wound infection	1
Local tissue necrosis	1

*Two patients required chest tube placement

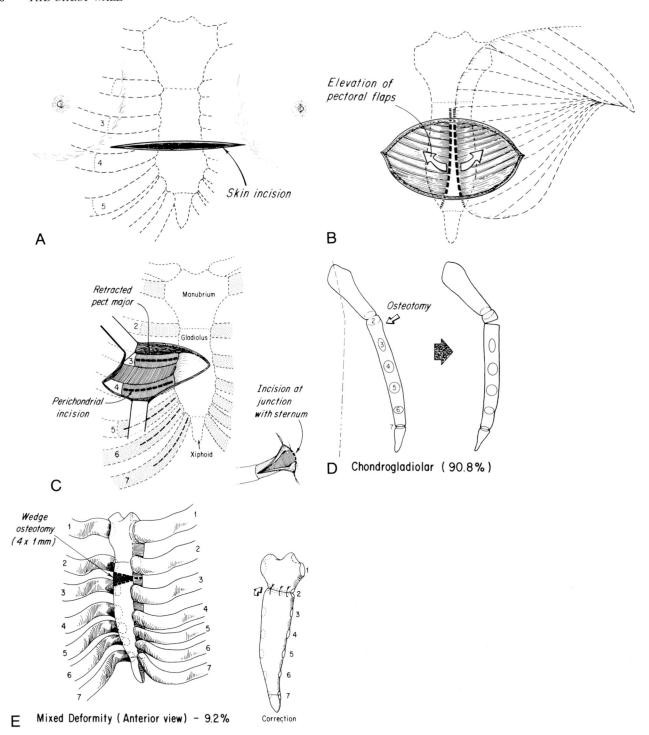

Fig. 47–8. Surgical repair of symmetrical chondrogladiolar pectus carinatum. *A*, A transverse incision is placed below and well within the nipple lines at the site of the future inframammary crease. *B*, The pectoralis major muscle is elevated from the sternum along with portions of the pectoralis minor and serratus anterior muscles. Anterior distraction of the muscles during this dissection facilitates identification of the avascular areolar plane just anterior to the costal cartilages and the intercostal muscle bundles. *C*, Subperichondrial resection of the costal cartilages is achieved by incising the perichondrium anteriorly. It is then dissected away from the costal cartilages in the bloodless plane between perichondrium and costal cartilage. Cutting back the perichondrium to 180° at its junction with the sternum (inset) facilitates visualization of the back wall and encirclement of the costal cartilages. *D*, With the chondrogladiolar deformity, a single or double osteotomy after resection of the costal cartilages allows posterior displacement of the sternum to an orthotopic position. *E*, The mixed pectus deformity is corrected by full and symmetrical resection of the third to seventh costal cartilages followed by transverse offset (0° to 10°) wedge-shaped sternal osteotomy. Closure of this defect permits both anterior displacement and rotation of the sternum. (Reproduced with permission from Shamberger, R.C., and Welch, K.J.: Surgical correction of pectus carinatum (pigeon breast). J. Pediatr. Surg. 22:48, 1987.)

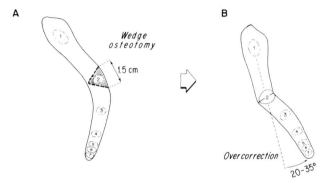

Chondromanubrial (very rare)

Fig. 47–9. *A,* The chondromanubrial type of deformity is depicted with a broad wedge-shaped sternal osteotomy placed through the anterior cortex at the obliterated sternomanubrial junction. *B,* Closure of the osteotomy after fracture of the posterior cortex achieves posterior displacement of the superior portion of the sternum, which is secured only by its attachment to the first rib. The lower portion of the sternum is over corrected 20 to 30°. (Reproduced with permission from Shamberger, R.C., and Welch, K.J.: J. Pediatr. Surg. 1988.)

which have been reported by Clarkson (1962) and Walker and colleagues (1969). Poland's syndrome may also occur in combination with Sprengel's deformity, an anomaly of the scapula with elevation, winging, and decreased size.

This condition is present from birth and Freire-Maia (1973) and McGillivray (1977) and their associates estimated an incidence of 1/30,000 to 1/32,000. Abnormalities in the breast can be defined at birth by absence of the underlying breast bud and the hypoplastic, often superiorly displaced, nipple. The etiology is unknown. Hypoplasia of the ipsilateral subclavian artery has been proposed by Bouvet and colleagues (1978) as the origin of this malformation but David (1979) believes the decreased blood flow to the extremity may rather be the consequence of decreased muscle mass of the hypoplastic limb. Although some forms of syndactyly have been de-

scribed as autosomal dominant traits, a similar pattern has not been demonstrated in patients with chest wall deformities, which appear to be sporadic in their occurrence. Reports, such as those of David (1982) and Sujansky and associates (1977), of multiple cases within a family are rare. Poland's syndrome is associated with a second rare syndrome, the Möbius syndrome, involving bilateral or unilateral facial palsy and abducens ocular palsy. Fontaine and Ovlaque (1984) identified nineteen such cases, but a unifying etiology is lacking. An unusual association between Poland's syndrome and childhood leukemia has been reported by Boaz and co-authors (1971).

In our experience with 41 patients with Poland's syndrome evaluated from 1970 to 1987, 21 were boys. The lesion was right-sided in 23 patients, left-sided in 17 patients and bilateral in 1. Hand anomalies were noted in 23 patients—56%—and breast anomalies in 25. In ten patients, the underlying rib cage required reconstruction, and in three cases rib or cartilage grafts were needed for complete repair.

Operative Repair

Assessment of the extent of involvement of the various musculoskeletal components is critical for optimal reconstruction. If involvement is limited to absence or hypoplasia of the sternal component of the pectoralis major and minor muscles, there is little functional deficit and repair is not necessary except for breast augmentation in women at full growth (Fig. 47–13A and B). If the underlying costal cartilages are depressed or absent, then repair must be considered to minimize the concavity, to eliminate the paradoxic motion of the chest wall if ribs are absent, and in girls to provide an optimal base for breast reconstruction. Ravitch (1966) reported correction of posteriorly displaced costal cartilages by unilateral resection of the cartilages, a wedge osteotomy of the sternum allowing derotation of the sternum and fixation with Rehbein struts and Steinmann pins. We found that suitable repair can be achieved with bilateral costal cartilage

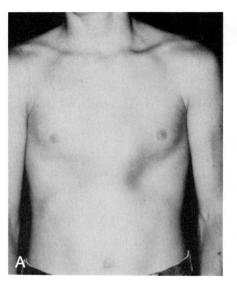
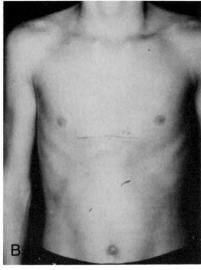

Fig. 47–10. *A,* Preoperative photograph of a 15-year-old boy with symmetric chondrogladiolar pectus carinatum. Note the upper keel-shaped protrusion and the lower depressed runnels lateral to the sternum. *B,* Postoperative photograph shows correction of both components of the deformity.

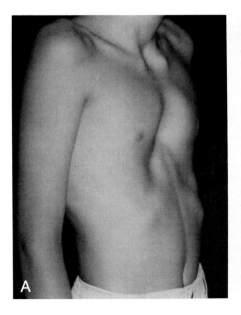

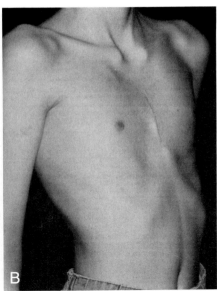

Fig. 47–11. *A,* A 15-year-old male with the chondromanubrial deformity. Note the posterior depression of the lower sternum accentuated by the anterior bowing of the costal cartilages. *B,* Following repair, the sternal contour is improved and costal cartilages reform in a more appropriate fashion. (Reproduced with permission from Shamberger, R.C., and Welch, K.J.: J Pediatr. Surg. 1988.)

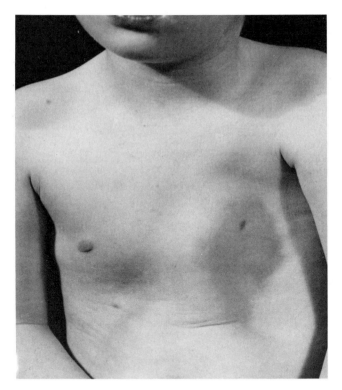

Fig. 47–12. A 3-year-old boy with Poland's syndrome. The pectoralis major and minor muscles and the serratus to the level of the fifth rib are absent. There is sternal obliquity away from this side. The second to fourth ribs were deficient and short, ending in points. The corresponding cartilages were absent. The endothoracic fascia lies beneath a thin layer of subcutaneous tissue. Note the hypoplastic nipple.

resection and an oblique osteotomy, as in the patients with the mixed pectus carinatum/excavatum deformity, which allows correction of the rotational deformity. The sternum is then displaced anteriorly, which allows correction of the posteriorly displaced costal cartilages. An unappreciated carinate deformity is often present on the contralateral side, which accentuates the ipsilateral concavity.

Absence of the medial portion of the ribs can be managed with split rib grafts taken from the contralateral side. These must be secured to the sternum medially and the "dagger pointed" hypoplastic rib ends laterally. The grafts can be covered with prosthetic mesh if needed for further support. Remember that in these cases there is little tissue present between the endothoracic fascia and the fascial remnants of the pectoral muscles. Coverage of the area can also be augmented with transfer of a latissimus dorsi muscle flap, particularly helpful in those girls who will require breast augmentation, as suggested by Ohmori (1980) and Haller (1984) and their associates. It is seldom if ever required in boys and has the disadvantage of adding a second and posterior thoracic scar.

STERNAL CLEFTS

Several entities involving failure of ventral fusion of the thoracic wall can be divided into three groups: (1) thoracic ectopia cordis, (2) thoracoabdominal ectopia cordis, and (3) cleft sternum without ectopia cordis. The combined Children's Hospital of Boston experience and the total available literature provides 118 cases with live births (Table 47–10). The various anatomical disorders will be discussed under their separate headings.

Cleft Sternum

Cleft sternum with an orthotopic heart may be complete or incomplete and results from failure of ventral

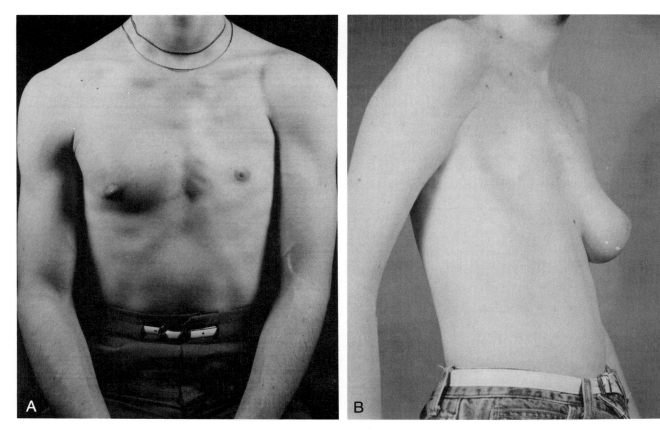

Fig. 47–13. *A,* Muscular 15-year-old boy with loss of left axillary fold, orthotopic sternum and normal cartilages. He compensates adequately for loss of the pectoralis major and minor muscles. Surgery is not indicated in males with these findings, similar to the original case reported by Poland. *B,* Fourteen-year-old girl with Poland's disease. Note the high position of the right nipple, right amastia, right sternal rotation and depressed right anterior chest. The second to fourth ribs and cartilages were missing, reconstructed with rib grafts. Breast augmentation will be required at full growth.

fusion of the sternal bars at or about the eighth week of gestation. In such cases, although there is sternal separation, there is skin coverage of the midline defect, an intact pericardium, and intact pleural envelopes with a normal diaphragm. Omphaloceles do not occur in this group, and the condition causes few difficulties other than dramatic increase in the deformity with crying or Valsalva maneuver. The total available experience consists of 41 reported cases. Of these, eight patients had complete sternal separation and none had intrinsic con-

genital heart disease. Most authors now recommend treatment in the newborn period when all such malformations can be dealt with by simple direct closure without the use of prosthetic materials. Repair was successful whether deformities were complete or incomplete in 38 of 41 patients. One death was caused by progressive hydrocephalus, another by endobronchial hemorrhage caused by the vascular association of airway hemangiomas, and a third, apparently by sepsis in a patient who did have coarctation of the aorta.

Table 47–10. Cleft Sternum, Thoracic Ectopia Cordis, and Thoracoabdominal Ectopia Cordis—Cantrell's Pentalogy*

	Number of Patients	Alive	Dead
Thoracic ectopia cordis Separate omphalocele, 8 patients	34 (4)	4	30 (4)
Thoracoabdominal ectopia cordis Cantrell's pentalogy, 34 patients	43 (9)	18 (4)	25 (5)
Cleft sternum Normal heart, 41 patients	41 (4)	38 (4)	3
TOTALS	118 (17)	60 (8)	58 (9)

*Numbers in parentheses represent patients from Children's Hospital, Boston.

Cleft sternum and the vascular association was reported by Leiber (1982) and by Hersh (1985) and Kaplan (1985a) and their colleagues. This was a chance finding in reviewing the total literature. The association consists of cleft sternum and capillary hemangioma in a cervicofacial distribution. Ten such cases can be identified in the various reports and were overlooked. Except for one patient with airway involvement, none had hemangioma involvement of major viscera. Treatment, as with all such cutaneous lesions of the infantile hemangioendothelioma type, is patient observation.

Surgical Repair

From the first report by Lannelongue (1888) to that by Schieken and associates (1987) there have been 41 cases. Brown and Patterson (1977), Daum and Heiss (1970), Lambrecht (1975), and Meissner (1964) reported two or more cases.

Operation in the perinatal period is recommended for all cases, because direct approximation and suture closure is possible and effective without compressive cardiac problems and with no recurrences or delayed healing. (Fig. 47–14A and B) Klassen (1949) and Bernhardt (1968), Salley (1985), Samarrai (1985), and Firmin (1980) and their colleagues all recommended neonatal repair of complete or incomplete clefts.

Direct approximation and suture closure with partial transverse division of sternal bands was recommended by Maier and Bortone (1949) and Longino and Jewett (1955). This maneuver is no longer considered necessary.

Reconstruction of the anterior chest wall using multiple oblique chondrotomies and medial sliding was reported by Sabiston (1958) and subsequently by Ando (1977) and Keeley (1960) and their associates. The technique is still useful in older infants with a less flexible thoracic cage and a widening defect. Autologous grafts, including costal cartilages, split ribs and resection of the costal arch complex, were reported by Burton (1947), Asp and Sulama (1961), Ravitch (1977), and by one of us (K.J.W., 1980) (Fig. 47–15).

Hofmann (1965) and Ravitch (1977) reported closure employing Marlex or Teflon mesh as prosthetic materials. An acrylic prosthesis was recommended by Verska (1975) and Krontiris and Tsironis (1963) in a 30-year-old patient and by Daoud and colleagues (1980) in an older child (Fig. 47–15).

Ectopia Cordis

Although the problem of isolated cleft sternum without visceral involvement appears to be satisfactorily resolved, surgical treatment of the two remaining groups continues to be met with frustration in most reports. The lethal cardiac factor in ectopia cordis, the so-called naked heart, and in patients with the Cantrell pentalogy noted by Cantrell and associates (1958) was first identified by Stensen (1671), who reported the high incidence of associated major intrinsic congenital heart disease. The cardiac lesions encountered in the two groups combined are listed in Table 47–11.

Etiology

The etiology of thoracic ectopia cordis and thoracoabdominal ectopia cordis—Cantrell's pentalogy—is much debated. Rather than being a simple delay of ventral fusion of the sternal bars beyond 8 or 9 weeks gestation, as in the case of sternal clefts, the etiology of the other two conditions is far more complex. Higginbottom (1979), Hersh (1982), Opitz (1985), and Kaplan and associates (1985b) considered them to be caused by disruption of amnion and possibly disruption of the chorionic layer or yolk sac as well. This occurs during the third or fourth week of gestation, at a time when cardiac chamber formation is occurring rapidly, and interferes with normal development through lack of compression by an intact anterior abdominal and thoracic wall. The obligatory oligohydramnios might be responsible for some degree of reduced thoracic volume and pulmonary hypoplasia. Disrupted bands, in addition to producing cardiac anomalies, also cause finger or extremity amputations, facial clefts, and abdominal visceral abnormalities. VonPraagh (1983) had the intriguing notion, based upon embryologic studies by Patton (1946) and Bremer (1939), that there is acute hyperflexion of the craniocervical segment of the embryo, which pins the heart down in the extrathoracic position with the submental cardiac apex. The abnormal fetal configuration caused by oligohydramnios may persist to delivery and oppose traction by the gubernaculum cordis, which normally pulls the cardiac apex into caudal alignment, tying it to the supraumbilical raphe. Chromosome abnormalities have been reported by Say and Wilsey (1978), King (1980), and Stoll (1986). Stoll (1986) also commented on the supraumbilical raphe and gubernaculum cordis. Teratogenic factors have been reported by Beaudoin (1982) and by Kalter and Warkany (1959) but do not seem to generally apply.

Thoracic Ectopia Cordis

Thoracic ectopia cordis was first reported by Stensen (1671). Thirty-three intervening cases in live births can be identified, four from our institution. Including Stensen's patient, 30 are dead and 4 are alive. Stensen's report was translated by Willius (1948). Stenson identified the four components of the tetralogy of Fallot in a patient with thoracic ectopia cordis; such is the fate of eponyms. Thoracic ectopia cordis is one of the most dramatic presentations in surgery (Fig. 47–16A). The naked and beating heart is indeed external to the thorax, usually at the upper to mid thoracic level. Clearly visible are the auricular appendages, chamber orientation, coronary vasculature and cephalic orientation of the cardiac apex. The gubernaculum cordis initially extends to the supraumbilical raphe, and is often inadvertently divided along with the umbilical cord, which is somewhat high but otherwise normal. Cardiac anomalies are unusually frequent in this group—31 of 34 cases. The first successful repair of thoracic ectopia cordis was accomplished by Koop (1975), as reported by Saxena, and published by VonPraagh (1983). Fortunately, this infant had a nor-

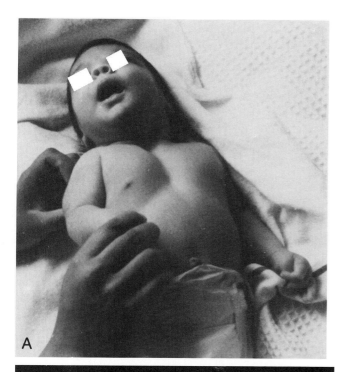

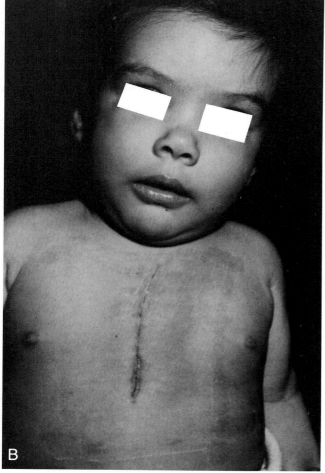

Fig. 47–14. *A,* Nearly complete sternal cleft in a 4-month-old girl. The heart was normal, there was no respiratory paradox but marked forward bulging of the central depressed area with crying. *B,* Postoperative photograph at six weeks shows normal chest contour with solid healing of the sternal bars.

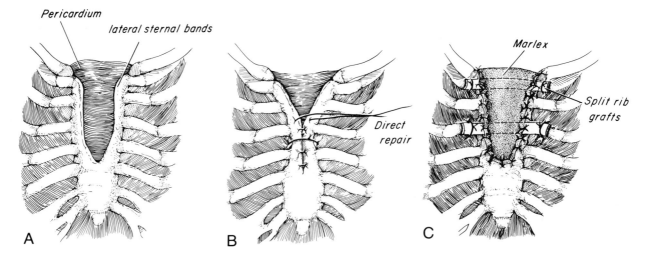

Fig. 47–15. *A*, Drawing of an upper sternal cleft shows the lateral sternal bands, absence of sternal segmentation, the exposed pericardium, and clavicular separation. *B*, Simple closure of most sternal clefts is possible, preferably in the neonatal period, by freshening the medial edges of the sternal bars and drawing them together with No. 2 Tevdek sutures. *C*, Broad defects and those encountered after the neonatal period require innovative complex reconstruction. Split rib grafts overlaid with Marlex mesh provided secure closure for this patient. (Reproduced with permission from Welch, K.J.: Chest wall deformities. *In* Pediatric Surgery, Edited by T.M. Holder and K.W. Ashcraft. Philadephia, W.B. Saunders Co., 1980.)

mal heart. The sternal bands were 2 inches—5 cm—apart and could not be approximated without cardiac compromise. The first operation consisted of skin flap coverage only at age 5 hours. The second operation, at 7 months, involved insertion of an acrylic resin to widen the sternal cleft. The sternal cleft was subsequently closed with a Dacron/Marlex patch at age 5 years. VonPraagh (1987) indicated that the child was entirely well at age 12. Success in two other patients include that by Dobell (1982) and Yada (1980) and their colleagues. Yada's patient had a double-outlet left ventricle successfully repaired plus parietal reconstruction. Smith and

Table 47–11. Cardiac Lesions in 77 Patients with Thoracic and Thoracoabdominal Ectopia Cordis

Pulmonic stenosis	19
Ventricular septal defect	18
Tetralogy of Fallot	18
Atrial septal defect	15
Diverticulum left ventricle	13
Single 11	
Double 2	
Persisting left superior vena cava	11
Double outlet left ventricle	6
Transposition of great vessels	4
Hypoplastic left heart	3
Common atrium	3
Common truncus	3
Cleft mitral valve	3
Patent ductus arteriosus	3
Absent ductus arteriosus	3
Total anomalous pulmonary venous drainage	2
Tricuspid atresia	2
Mitral atresia	2
Coarctation	2
Aortic stenosis	2
Common atrioventricular canal	1

associates (1987) collected 31 patients with ectopia cordis. Eleven had complete but separate omphalocele. In 15 cases, an attempt was made to reposition the heart in the chest; all died. Four patients had temporary silo construction; two survived with normal hearts. Ten patients had skin coverage only with no positional change; two survived with normal hearts. Twenty-five of the thirty-one patients had major intrinsic congenital heart disease.

We encountered four patients with thoracic ectopia cordis in our institution; three had no treatment; all died. One had skin coverage of the heart and repair of a large and separate omphalocele; he died of fungal sepsis. We are stimulated by recent reports, especially that of Yada (1980), who recommended early operation on such patients. Prenatal uterine sonography provides the diagnosis. A two-dimensional echocardiogram is of no value because of air interference. Cardiac catheterization is urgent and mandatory. Our one patient so studied had a hypoplastic left ventricle; further treatment was withheld. Following catheterization, direct transport to the operating room is recommended, with total repair of the cardiac defect. Following this, some type of cardiac enclosure must be provided. The incidence of sepsis is high with the use of prosthetic materials, but they may play a role by allowing time for circumferential ingrowth of fibrovascular tissue, reducing the eventration and allowing secondary skin closure of a much smaller area. One appealing idea is the use of Op Site, reported by Ein and Shandling (1978). This is an adhesive plastic sheet used successfully in omphalocele closure. It has not been used to date for thoracic ectopia cordis.

Dobell and associates' case (1982) is interesting in that there was adequate intrathoracic space to accommodate the naked heart, which was held forward by a thin pericardial sling. Parietal and skin closure was accomplished

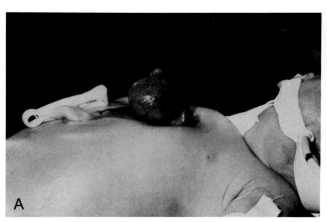
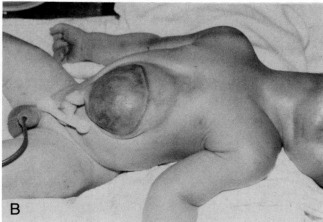

Fig. 47–16. *A,* Thoracic ectopia cordis in a high central position. The cardiac apex is cephalad; any movement of the heart resulted in bradycardiac arrest. The patient had severe aortic overriding and complex tetralogy of Fallot. No treatment was attempted. *B,* Newborn male with Cantrell's pentalogy. Note flaring of the lower sternal area merging with a large epigastric omphalocele. The septum transversum and the inferior portion of the pericardium were absent. The patient died shortly after closure of the omphalocele without cardiac intervention.

in the one-stage operation. Brock's case (1950) reported by Scott (1955) was also successful.

Thoracoabdominal Ectopia Cordis—Cantrell's Pentalogy

Of the 43 patients reported to date, of whom about half lived and half died, we have encountered 9 patients. The essential features of the Cantrell pentalogy are a cleft lower sternum, a half-moon anterior diaphragmatic defect caused by failure of development of the septum transversum, absence of the parietal pericardium, as-

sociated adjacent or completely separate omphalocele, and in most patients a major form of congenital heart disease, the most common being tetralogy of Fallot (Fig. 47–16*B*). The condition was described first by Holt (1897). The first successful repair in a patient with a normal heart was performed by Brock (1950) and reported by Scott (1955). Cantrell and colleagues described three cases in 1958 with a review of the literature. Five patients in their series had both thoracic ectopia cordis and a separate omphalocele with an intervening bridge of normal skin. None of the five patients or others in the

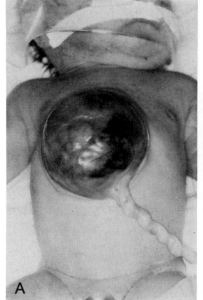
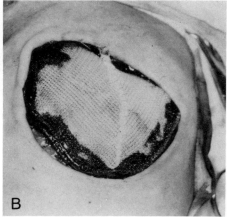
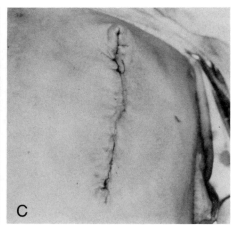

Fig. 47–17. Cantrell's pentalogy with very high thoracoabdominal ectopia cordis; only the manubrium is intact. The large spherical omphalocele contains abdominal and thoracic viscera. *B,* Immediate closure of the omphalocele was accomplished with Teflon mesh. *C,* Complete skin healing at age 6 days without herniation. The patient remained ventilator bound in intractable failure to death at one week. Once again, the classical features of tetralogy of Fallot as with Stensen's case. (Courtesy of M. Curci)

literature survived, including our most recent patient, reported by Smith and associates (1987). Of our nine patients with Cantrell's pentalogy, five survived. Two with tetralogy of Fallot diagnosed by cardiac catheterization had an early systemic pulmonary artery shunt followed by complete surgical repair of the cardiac lesions under hypothermia arrest and parietal reconstruction. One was completely corrected at age 4 months and one at 7 months. Immediate neonatal intervention is required in patients with a large upper omphalocele and lower sternal cleft, often requiring the use of Teflon mesh or other prosthetic material (Fig. 47–17A through C and Fig. 47–18A through C). When patients have an omphalocele and complete but separate thoracic ectopia cordis, there is not enough skin to cover both areas. Escharotics have been valuable in this situation. Of the 43 Cantrell patients in the literature, 18 survived and 25 died, usually because of the severity of the underlying cardiac lesion, but at times because of delay in cardiac intervention. A more aggressive approach should be taken with this group if salvage is to be improved. Review of the literature was carried out by Ravitch (1977), to whom we are indebted for much of our understanding of these three apparently separate entities. Toyama (1972) found five Cantrell patients without congenital heart disease. Currently there appear to be eight such cases. Thirteen patients reported by Shapinker (1951), Mulder and associates (1960), and Murphy (1968) had a single or double diverticulum of the left ventricle without other cardiac lesions.

The absence of parietal compression, in both thoracic and abdominal thoracic ectopia cordis, provides evidence that parietal abdominal and thoracic resistance is essential for the formation, rotation, and ultimate descent of the heart with a caudally directed apex.

MISCELLANEOUS CONDITIONS

Asphyxiating Thoracic Dystrophy of the Newborn—Jeune's Disease

Jeune (1954) described a newborn condition charaterized by a narrow and rigid chest with multiple cartilage anomalies. The patient died early in the perinatal period because of respiratory insufficiency. Oberklaid (1977) reported ten such children and characterized their skeletal abnormalities, including broad, short, horizontal ribs terminating in the axilla, and no visible sternebrae (Fig. 47–19). This is part of a generalized chondrodystrophy. Surgical intervention, as reported by Barnes (1972), Karjoo (1973) and attempted by Mustard (1980), has been unsuccessful. It is now apparent that this is a spectrum of conditions. In the lethal form, in addition to pulmonary insufficiency, patients had microcystic degeneration of the kidneys, liver, and pancreas. Some died of pure renal failure, although some with the minor form, except for vulnerability to recurring pulmonary infections, survived, with one 32-year-old man reported by Friedman (1975). Our three patients had progressive respiratory insufficiency and died without surgical intervention. One

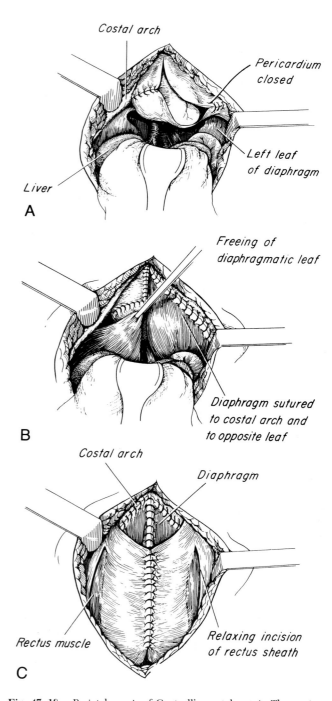

Fig. 47–18. Parietal repair of Cantrell's pentalogy. *A*, The pericardium is closed after appropriate lateral and inferior dissection to the vena cava. The right and left widely separated dorsal leaves of the diaphragm are identified. The liver is retracted inferiorly after division of the falciform ligament. *B*, Pedicles of diaphragm are developed from each side, then transposed medially. They are sutured together and to each costal arch. *C*, After diaphragmatic closure, the falciform ligament is reconstructed. Closure continues by advancement of the anterior sheath of the rectus muscle to the midline. Lateral relaxing incisions are required. Parietal repair can be accomplished at the time of complete cardiac correction under deep hypothermia. (Reproduced with permission from Welsh, K.J.: Chest wall deformities. *In* Pediatric Surgery. Edited by T.M. Holder and K.W. Ashcraft. Philadelphia, W.B. Saunders Co., 1980.)

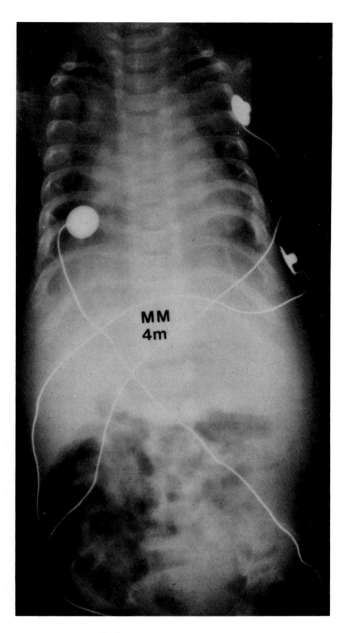

Fig. 47–19. Jeune's disease—asphyxiating thoracic dystrophy. Radiograph showing the short horizontal ribs and extreme narrowing of the chest above the level of D8. The patient died of progressive respiratory insufficiency at one month of age. There was no surgical intervention. Postmortem examination revealed alveolar hypoplasia and cystic tubular disease.

autopsied patient, however, had normal lungs that had grown appropriately to age 6 months. There is some overlap with patients who have short rib polydactyly syndrome and a narrow thorax, reported by Bidot-Lopez (1978), also with short-limbed dwarfism of the Majewski (1971) type, the Saldino/Noonan (1972) type, and the Naumoff (1977) type.

Prenatal diagnosis of this condition is now possible, as Elejalde (1985) and Skiptunas and Weiner (1987) reported. In one family, a sibling had died of Jeune's disease at 6 months. With diagnosis of the same condition in a later pregnancy, an abortion was elected. Schinzell and associates (1985) reported another instance of prenatal sonographic diagnosis and elective abortion at 17 weeks of fetal age. Todd and colleagues (1986) take an optimistic view of Jeune's dystrophy, recommending an expansion technique to increase thoracic volume, using a plate of methyl methacrylate—acrylic—sewn to the edges of a split sternum. Progressive deterioration of respiratory function is considered an indication for the procedure, and late follow-up is needed. Kaufman and Kirkpatrick (1974) considered Jeune's thoracic dysplasia as a spectrum of disorders and provided identifying osteoskeletal changes.

Absent and Fused Ribs

Many older children or young adults present with apical thoracic deformities. Carefully obtained upper thoracic radiographs reveal posterior fusion of the first and second ribs or, in some, anterior fusion with a spanning cartilage plate involving two or more cartilages. This results in a forward bowing of the clavicles, outward displacement of the manubrium and prominence of the first, second, and third costal cartilages. The anterior fusions are readily dealt with because they are cartilaginous in nature. The posterior fusions usually do not cause symptoms, and no patient has presented with thoracic outlet syndrome. The difficulty of completely resecting the fused first and second ribs has lead us to not

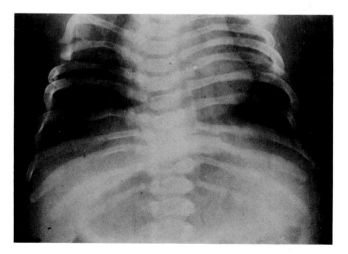

Fig. 47–20. Chest radiograph of a 6-month-old patient with rib gap syndrome and mandibular hypoplasia. Ribs 5 to 8 are hypoplastic and widely separated. Lung hernia was not present.

intervene surgically, because of adjacent neurovascular hazards. Ravitch (1977) mentioned a group of children who have absent portions of the ribs, hemivertebrae, and infantile scoliosis. Such patients may develop a lung hernia anterior to the medial border of the latissimus dorsi and below the angle of the scapula. Rickham (1959) and Ravitch (1977) reported lung hernias. Reconstruction depends upon anatomical findings and usually involves split-rib grafts harvested from the opposite side. Most require unilateral staged fusion and rod fixation. Control of respiratory paradox in the young infant may require a temporary acrylic prosthetic garment with Velcro straps, but all will ultimately require an anatomical correction. LeRoux and Stemmler (1971) reported the use of methyl methacrylate molded at the table and formed into a Marlex sandwich or pocket. The method has been used extensively following resection of chest wall malignancies.

Miller (1972) and Nicholls (1973) and their colleagues described a group of infants with rib gaps, cleft palate, and Pierre-Robin mandibular defects with micrognathia (Fig. 47–20). A small group of patients have combined rib and spinal defects. There may be complete or partial absence of ribs, rib and cartilage fusions, pseudoarthroses, hemivertebrae, and collapsed vertebrae (Fig. 47–20). Most develop severe structural scoliosis requiring staged fusion and rod fixation.

REFERENCES

Pectus Excavatum

Allen, R.G., and Douglas, M.: Cosmetic improvement of thoracic wall defects using a rapid setting silastic mold: a special technique. J. Pediatr. Surg. 14:745, 1979.

Beiser, G.D., et al.: Impairment of cardiac function in patients with pectus excavatum, with improvement after operative correction. N. Engl. J. Med. 287:267, 1972.

Bevegård, S.: Postural circulatory changes at rest and during exercise in patients with funnel chest, with special reference to factors affecting the stroke volume. Acta Med. Scand. 171:695, 1972.

Blickman, J.G., et al.: Pectus excavatum in children: Pulmonary scintigraphy before and after corrective surgery. Radiology 156:781, 1985.

Bon Tempo, C.P., et al.: Radiographic appearance of the thorax in systolic click–late systolic murmur syndrome. Am. J. Cardiol. 236:27, 1975.

Brown, A.L., and Cook, O.: Cardio-respiratory studies in pre- and postoperative funnel chest (pectus excavatum). Dis. Chest 20:378, 1951.

Cahill, J.L., Lees, G.M., and Robertson, H.T.: A summary of preoperative and postoperative cardiorespiratory performance in patients undergoing pectus excavatum and carinatum repair. J. Pediatr. Surg. 19:430, 1984.

Castile, R.G, Staats, B.A, and Westbrook, P.R.: Symptomatic pectus deformities of the chest. Am. Rev. Respir. Dis. 126:564, 1982.

Evans, W.: The heart in sternal depression. Br. Heart J. 8:162, 1946.

Garnier, C.: Traitement chirurgical du thorax en entonnoir. Rev. Orthop. 21:385, 1934.

Garusi, G.F., and D'Ettorre, A.: Angiocardiographic patterns in funnel-chest. Cardiologia 45:312, 1964.

Gattiker, H., and Bühlmann, A.: Cardiopulmonary function and exercise tolerance in supine and sitting position in patients with pectus excavatum. Helv. Med. Acta 33:122, 1967.

Haller, J.A., et al.: Pectus excavatum: A 20 year surgical experience. J. Thorac. Cardiovasc. Surg. 60:375, 1970.

Hecker, W.C., Procher, G., and Dietz, H.G.: Results of operative correction of pigeon and funnel chest following a modified procedure of Ravitch and Haller. Z. Kinderchir. 34:220, 1981.

Howard, R.: Funnel chest: its effect on cardiac function. Arch. Dis. Child. 32:5, 1959.

Hümmer, H.P., and Willital, G.H.: Morphologic findings of chest deformities in children corresponding to the Willital-Hümmer classification. J. Pediatr. Surg. 19:562, 1984.

Judet, J., and Judet, R.: Thorax en entonnoir. Un procédé opératoire. Rev. Orthop. 40:248, 1954.

Jung, A.: Le traitement du thorax en entonnoir par le "retournement pédiculé" de la cuvette sterno-chondrale. Mém. Acad. Chir. 82:242, 1956.

Lester, C.W.: The surgical treatment of funnel chest. Ann. Surg. 123:1003, 1946.

Lester, C.W.: The etiology and pathogenesis of funnel chest, pigeon breast, and related deformities of the anterior chest wall. J. Thorac. Surg. 34:1, 1957.

Mead, J., et al.: Rib cage mobility in pectus excavatum. Am. Rep. Respir. Dis. 132:1223, 1985.

Meyer, L.: Zur chirurgischen Behandlung der angeborenen Trichterbrust. Verh. Berl. Med. Ges. 42:364, 1911.

Ochsner, A., and DeBakey, M.: Chone-chondrosternon: report of a case and review of the literature. J. Thorac. Surg. 8:469, 1939.

Oelsnitz, G.: Fehlbildungen des Brustkorbes. Z. Kinderchir. 33:229, 1981.

Peterson, R.J., et al.: Noninvasive assessment of exercise cardiac function before and after pectus excavatum repair. J. Thorac. Cardiovasc. Surg. 90:251, 1985.

Ravitch, M.M.: The operative treatment of pectus excavatum. Ann. Surg. 129:429, 1949.

Ravitch, M.M.: Congenital Deformities of the Chest Wall and Their Operative Correction. Philadelphia, W.B. Saunders Co., 1977.

Rehbein, F., and Wernicke, H.H.: The operative treatment of the funnel chest. Arch. Dis. Child. 32:5, 1957.

Saint-Mezard, G., et al.: Prolapsus valvulaire mitral et pectus excavatum: Association fortuite ou groupement syndromique? La Presse Médicale 15:439, 1986.

Salomon, J., Shah, P.M., and Heinle, R.A.: Thoracic skeletal abnormalities in idiopathic mitral valve prolapse. Am. J. Cardiol. 36:32, 1975.

Sanger, P.W., Robicsek, F., and Daugherty, H.K.: The repair of recurrent pectus excavatum. J. Thorac. Cardiovasc. Surg. 56:141, 1968.

Sauerbruch, F.: Die Chirurgie der Brustorgane, Berlin, J. Springer, 1920, p. 437.

Schaub, V.F., and Wegmann, T.: Elektrokardiographische Veränderungen bei Trichterburst. Cardiologia 24:39, 1954.

Shochat, S.J., et al.: Moiré phototopography in the evaluation of anterior chest wall deformities. J. Pediatr. Surg. 16:353, 1981.

Schutte, J.E., et al.: Distinctive anthropometric characteristics of women with mitral valve prolapse. Am. J. Med. 71:533, 1981.

Shamberger, R.C., Welch, K.J., and Sanders, S.P.: Mitral valve prolapse associated with pectus excavatum. J. Pediatr. 111:104, 1987.

Shamberger, R.C., and Welch, K.J.: Surgical correction of pectus excavatum. J. Pediatr. Surg. 23:615, 1988.

Udoshi, M.B., et al.: Incidence of mitral valve prolapse in subjects with thoracic skeletal abnormalities: prospective study. Am. Heart J. 97:303, 1979.

Wada, J., et al.: Results of 271 funnel chest operations. Ann. Thorac. Surg. 10:526, 1970.

Waters, P.M., et al.: Scoliosis in children with pectus excavatum and pectus carinatum. J. Orthoped. Surg. 8:491, 1988.

Weg, J.G., Krumholz, R.A., and Harkleroad, L.E.: Pulmonary dysfunction in pectus excavatum. Am. Rev. Respir. Dis. 96:936, 1967.

Welsh, K.J.: Satisfactory surgical correction of pectus excavatum deformity in childhood: a limited opportunity. J. Thorac. Surg. 36:697, 1958.

Welch, K.J., and Kearney, G.P.: Abdominal musculature deficiency syndrome: prune belly. J. Urol. 111:693, 1974.

Welch, K.J.: Chest wall deformities. In Pediatric Surgery, Edited by T.M. Holder and K.W. Ashcraft. Philadelphia, W.B. Saunders Co., 1980.

Pectus Carinatum

Brodkin, H.A.: Congenital chondrosternal prominence (pigeon breast): a new interpretation. Pediatrics 3:286, 1949.

Brodkin, H.A.: Pigeon breast: congenital chondrosternal prominence. Arch. Surg. 77:261, 1958.

Chin, E.F.: Surgery of funnel chest and congenital sternal prominence. Br. J. Surg. 44:360, 1957.

Currarino, G., and Silverman, F.N.: Premature obliteration of the sternal sutures and pigeon-breast deformity. Radiology 70:532, 1958.

Hougaard, K., and Arendrup, H.: Deformities of the female breasts after surgery for funnel chest. Scand. J. Thorac. Cardiovasc. Surg. 17:171, 1983.

Howard, R.: Pigeon chest (protrusion deformity of the sternum). Med. J. Aust. 2:664, 1958.

Lees, R.F., and Caldicott, W.J.H.: Sternal anomalies and congenital heart disease. AJR 124:423, 1975.

Lester, C.W.: Pigeon breast (pectus carinatum) and other protrusion deformities of the chest of developmental origin. Ann. Surg. 137:482, 1953.

Ravitch, M.M.: Unusual sternal deformity with cardiac symptoms: operative correction. J. Thorac. Surg. 23:138, 1952.

Ravitch, M.M.: The operative correction of pectus carinatum (pigeon breast). Ann. Surg. 151:705, 1960.

Robicsek, F., Sanger, P.W., Taylor, F.H., and Thomas, M.J.: The surgical treatment of chondrosternal prominence (pectus carinatum). J. Thorac. Cardiovasc. Surg. 45:691, 1963.

Shamberger, R.C., and Welch, K.J.: Surgical correction of pectus carinatum. J. Pediatr. Surg. 22:48, 1987.

Welch, K.J., and Vos, A.: Surgical correction of pectus carinatum (pigeon breast). J. Pediatr. Surg. 8:659, 1973.

Poland's Syndrome

Boaz, D., Mace, J.W., and Gotlin, R.W.: Poland's syndrome and leukaemia. Lancet 1:349, 1971.

Bouvet, J.-P., et al.: Vascular origin of Poland syndrome? A comparative rheographic study of the vascularisation of the arms in eight patients. Eur. J. Pediatr. 128:17, 1978.

Clarkson, P.: Poland's syndactyly. Guy's Hosp. Rep. 111:335, 1962.

David, T.J.: Vascular origin of Poland syndrome? Eur. J. Pediatr. 130:299, 1979.

David, T.J.: Familial Poland anomaly. J. Med. Genet. 19:293, 1982.

Fontaine, G., and Ovlaque, S.: Le syndrome de Poland-Möbius. Arch. Fr. Pediatr. 41:351, 1984.

Freire-Maia, N., et al.: The Poland Syndrome: clinical and geneological data, dermatoglyphic analysis, and incidence. Hum. Hered. 23:97, 1973.

Haller, J.A., Jr., et al.: Early reconstruction of Poland's syndrome using autologous rib grafts combined with a latissimus muscle flap. J. Pediatr. Surg. 19:423, 1984.

McGillivray, B.C., and Lowry, R.B.: Poland syndrome in British Columbia: incidence and reproductive experience of affected persons. Am. J. Med. Genet. 1:65, 1977.

Ohmori, K., and Takada, H.: Correction of Poland's pectoralis major muscle anomaly with latissimus dorsi musculocutaneous flaps. Plast. Reconstr. Surg. 65:400, 1980.

Poland, A.: Deficiency of the pectoralis muscles. Guy's Hosp. Rep. 6:191, 1841.

Ravitch, M.M.: Atypical deformities of the chest wall: absence and deformities of the ribs and costal cartilages. Surgery 59:438, 1966.

Sujansky, E., Riccardi, V.M., and Matthew, A.L.: The familial occurrence of Poland syndrome. Birth Defects 13:117, 1977.

Walker, J.C., Meijer, R., and Aranda, D.: Syndactylism with deformity of the pectoralis muscle: Poland's syndrome. J. Pediatr. Surg. 4:569, 1969.

Sternal Clefts

Ando, T., et al.: Surgical repair of sternal cleft with special reference to a surgical case of total sternal cleft in a newborn infant. J. Jpn. Assoc. Thorac. Surg. 25:306, 1977.

Asp, K., and Sulamaa, M.: Ectopia cordis. Acta Chir. Scand. 283:52, 1961.

Bernhardt, L., Meyer, T., and Young, W.P.: Bifid sternum. J. Thorac. Cardiovasc. Surg. 55:758, 1968.

Brown, J.H., and Patterson, D.: Surgical repair of a large incomplete cleft sternum. Aust. N.Z. J. Surg. 47:232, 1977.

Burton, J.F.: Method of correction of ectopia cordis. Arch. Surg. 54:79, 1947.

Daoud, S., et al.: Sternal cleft. Correction by silastic prosthesis. Chir. Pediatr. 21:415, 1980.

Daum, R., and Heiss, W.: Zur operativen Korrektur angeborener Sternumspalten. Thoraxchirurgie Vaskulare Chirurgie 17–18:432, 1969–1970.

Firmin, R.K., Fragomeni, L.S., Lennox, S.C.: Complete cleft sternum. Thorax 35:303, 1980.

Hersh, J.H., et al.: Sternal malformation/vascular dysplasia association. Am. J. Med. Genet. 21:177, 1985.

Hofmann, S.: Obere Sternumspalte. Dtsche Med. Wochenschr. 90:2198, 1965.

Jewett, T.C., Jr., Butsch, W.L., and Hug, H.R.: Congenital bifid sternum. Surgery 52:932, 1962.

Kaplan, L.C., Kurnit, D.M., and Welch, K.J.: Anterior midline defects: association with ectopia cordis or vascular dysplasia defines two distinct entities. Am. J. Med. Genet. 21:203, 1985a.

Kaplan, L.C., et al.: Ectopia cordis and cleft sternum: evidence for mechanical teratogenesis following rupture of the chorion or yolk sac. Am. J. Med. Genet. 21:187, 1985b.

Keeley, J.L., Schairer, A.E., and Brosnan, J.J.: Failure of sternal fusion. Bifid sternum. Arch. Surg. 81:641, 1960.

Klassen, K.: Discussion of Maier and Bortone. J. Thorac. Surg. 18:851, 1949.

Krontiris, A., and Tsironis, A.: Bifid sternum: successful repair by use of an acrylic plaque: report of a case. J. Int. Coll. Surg. 41:301, 1964.

Lambrecht, W.: Zur Operation angeborener Sternumspalten. Z. Kinderchir. Grenzgeb. 17:128, 1975.

Lannelongue: De l'ectocardie et de sa cure par l'autoplastie. Ann. Med. Chir. 4:101, 1888.

Leiber, B.: Angeborene supraumbilikale Mittelbauchraphe (SMBR) und kavernose Gesichtshämangiomatose—ein neues Syndrom? Med. Kinderheilkd. 130:84, 1982.

Longino, L.A., and Jewett, T.C., Jr.: Congenital bifid sternum. Surgery 38:610, 1955.

Maier, H.C., and Bortone, F.: Complete failure of sternal fusion with herniation of pericardium. Thorac. Surg. 18:851, 1949.

Meissner, F.: Fissura sterni congenita. Zentralbl. Chir. 48:1832, 1964.

Ravitch, M.M.: Spectacular problems in surgery: congenital absence of sternum. Surg. Gynecol. Obstet. 116:1963.

Ravitch, M.M.: Congenital deformities of the chest wall and their operative correction. Philadelphia, W.B. Saunders Co., 1977.

Sabiston, D.C., Jr.: The surgical management of congenital bifid sternum with partial ectopia cordis. J. Thorac. Surg. 35:118, 1958.

Salley, R.K., and Stewart, S.: Superior sternal cleft: repair in the newborn. Ann. Thorac. Surg. 39:582, 1985.

Samarrai, A.A., Charmockly, H.A, and Attra, A.A.: Complete cleft sternum: Classification and surgical repair. Int. Surg. 70:71, 1985.

Schieken, L.S., et al.: Aneurysm of the ascending aorta associated with sternal cleft, cutaneous hemangioma, and occlusion of the right innominate artery in a neonate. Am. Heart J. 113:202, 1987.

Verska, J.J.: Surgical repair of total cleft sternum. J. Thorac. Cardiovasc. Surg. 69:301, 1975.

Welch, K.J.: Chest wall deformities, In Pediatric Surgery. Edited by T. Holder and K. Ashcraft. Philadelphia, W.B. Saunders Co., 1980, pp. 162–182.

Ectopia Cordis

Beaudoin, A.R.: Teratogenic action of platinum thymine blue. Life Sciences 31:757, 1982.

Bremer, L.: Textbook of Embryology. Philadelphia, W.B. Saunders Co., 1939.

Cantrell, J.R., Haller, J.A., and Ravitch, M.M.: A syndrome of congenital defects involving the abdominal wall, sternum, diaphragm, pericardium, and heart. Surg. Gynecol. Obstet. 107:602:1958.

Dobell, A.R.C., Williams, H.B., and Long, R.W.: Staged repair of ectopia cordis. J. Pediatr. Surg. 17:353, 1982.

Ein, S.H., and Shandling, B.: A new nonoperative treatment of large omphaloceles with a polymer membrane. J. Pediatr. Surg. *13*:255, 1978.

Hersh, J.H., et al.: Sternal malformation/vascular dysplasia association. Am. J. Med. Genet. *21*:177, 1985.

Higginbottom, M.C.: The amniotic ban disruption complex: timing of amniotic rupture and variable spectra of consequent defects. Pediatrics *95*:544, 1979.

Kalter, H., and Warkany, J.: Experimental production of congenital malformations in mammals by metabolic procedure. Physiol. Rev. *39*:69, 1959.

King, C.R.: Ectopia cordis and chromosomal errors. Pediatrics *66*:328, 1980.

Opitz, J.M.: Editorial comment following paper by Hersh, J.H., et al. and Kaplan, L.C., et al. on sternal cleft. Am. J. Med. Genet. *21*:201, 1985.

Patten, B.M.: Human Embryology. Toronto, Blakiston Co. 1946.

Say, B., and Wilsey, C.E.: Chromosome aberration in ectopia cordis (46, xx, 17 qt). Am. Heart. J. *95*:274, 1978.

Scott, G.W.: Ectopia cordis: report of a case successfully treated by operation. Guys Hosp. Rep. *104*:55, 1955.

Smith, S., et al.: The naked heart (complete extrathoracic ectopia cordis) manifestation of the amniotic band disruption. Complex case report and review of the literature. Cited in VonPraagh, R., et al.: Malpositions of the heart. *In* Heart Disease in Infants, Children, and Adolescents. Edited by A.J. Moss, F.H. Adams, and G.C. Emmanouilides. Baltimore: Williams & Wilkins, 1988.

Stensen, N.: An unusually early description of the so-called tetralogy of Fallot. *In* Acta Medica et Philosophica Hafnienca, Vol. 1. Edited by T. Bartholin, 1671–1672, p. 202. Translated into English by F.A. Willius. Proc. Staff Meet. Mayo Clin. 23:316, 1948.

Stoll, S.C.: A supraumbilical midline raphe with sternal cleft in a 47xxx woman. (Letter to the editor.) Genetics, Sept. 1986.

VonPraagh, R., et al.: Malpositions of the heart. *In* Heart Disease in Infants, Children, and Adolescents. Edited by A.J. Moss, F.H. Adams, and G.C. Emmanouilides. Baltimore: Williams & Wilkins, 1983.

Yada, I., et al.: Successful surgical treatment for ectopia cordis using silon. Thorac. Surg. *80*:848, 1980.

Thoracoabdominal Ectopia Cordis—Cantrell's Pentalogy

Holt, L.E.: A remarkable case of ectocardia with displacement: the heart beating in the abdominal cavity. Medical News *71*:769, 1897.

Mulder, D.G., Crittenden, I.H., and Adams, F.H.: Complete repair of a syndrome of congenital defects involving the abdominal wall, sternum, diaphragm, pericardium and heart. Excision of left ventricular diverticulum. Ann. Surg. *151*:113, 1960.

Murphy, D.A.: The surgical treatment of a syndrome consisting of thoracoabdominal wall; diaphragmatic, pericardial, and ventricular septal defects; and a left ventricular diverticulum. Ann. Thorac. Surg. *6*:528, 1968.

Ravitch, M.M.: Congenital Deformities of the Chest Wall and Their Operative Correction. Philadelphia, W.B. Saunders Co., pp. 53–70, 1977.

Shapinker, S.: Diverticulum of the left ventricle of the heart: review of the literature and report of a successful removal of the diverticulum. Arch. Surg. *63*:629, 1951.

Toyama, W.M.: Combined congenital defects of the anterior abdominal wall, sternum, diaphragm, pericardium, and heart: a case report and review of the syndrome. Pediatrics *50*:778, 1972.

Miscellaneous Conditions

Barnes, N.D.: Chest reconstruction in thoracic dystrophy. Arch. Dis. Child. *46*:833, 1971.

Bidot-Lopez, P.: A case of short rib polydactyly. Pediatrics *3*:427, 1978.

Elejalde, B.R., Mercedes de Elejade, M., and Bilman, M: Analysis of the human fetal skeleton and organs with xeroradiography. Am. J. Obstet. Gynecol. *151*:666, 1985.

Friedman, J.M.: Thoracic skeletal abnormalities in idiopathic mitral valve prolapse. Am. J. Cardiol. *36*:32, 1975.

Jeune, M.: Polychondrodystrophie avec blocage thoracique d'evolution fatale. Pediatrie *9*:390, 1954.

Karjoo, M.: Pancreatic exocrine enzyme deficiency associated with asphyxiating thoracic dystrophy. Arch. Dis. Child. *48*:143, 1973.

Kaufman, H.J., and Kirkpatrick, J.A.: Jeune's thoracic dysplasia, a spectrum of disorders. *In* Skeletal Dysplasias. Edited by D. Bergsma. New York, Stratton Intercontinental Medical Book Corporation, 1974.

LeRoux, B.T., and Stemmler, P.: Maintenance of chest wall stability: a further report. Thorax *26*:424, 1971.

Majewski, F.: Polysyndactyly, short limbs, and genital malformations—a new syndrome? Z. Kinderheilkd. *111*:118, 1971.

Miller, K.E., Allen, R.P., and Davis, W.S.: Rib gap defects with micrognathia. The cerebro-costomandibular syndrome—a Pierre Robin-like syndrome with rib dysplasia. Am. J. Roentgenol. Radium Ther. Nucl. Med. *114*:253, 1972.

Naumoff, P.: Short rib-polydactyly syndrome type 3. Radiology *122*:443, 1977.

Nicholls, S.J., and Fletcher, E.W.L.: Congenital rib defects with the Pierre Robin syndrome. Pediatr. Radiol. *1*:246, 1973.

Oberklaid, F.: Asphyxiating thoracic dysplasia, clinical, radiological and pathological information on 10 patients. Arch. Dis. Child. *52*:758, 1977.

Ravitch, M.M.: Congenital Deformities of the Chest Wall and Their Operative Correction. Philadelphia, W.B. Saunders Co., pp. 272–284, 1977.

Rickham, P.P.: Lung hernia secondary to congenital absence of the ribs. Arch. Dis. Child. *34*:14, 1959.

Saldino, R.M., and Noonan, C.D.: Severe thoracic dystrophy with striking micromelia, abnormal osseous development, including the spine, and multiple visceral anomalies. Am. J. Roentgenol. Radium. Ther. Nucl. Med. *11*:257, 1972.

Schinzel, A., et al.: Prenatal sonographic diagnosis of Jeune syndrome. Radiology *154*:777, 1985.

Skiptunas, S.M., and Weiner, S.: Early prenatal diagnosis of asphyxiating thoracic dysplasia (Jeune's syndrome). Value of fetal thoracic measurement. J. Ultrasound Med. *6*:41, 1987.

Todd, D.W., Tinguely, S.J., and Norberg, W.J.: A thoracic expansion technique for Jeune's asphyxiating thoracic dystrophy. J. Pediatr. Surg. *21*:161, 1986.

CHAPTER 48

INFECTIONS OF THE CHEST WALL

Joseph LoCicero, III, and Lawrence L. Michaelis

Chest wall infections can be either primary problems arising spontaneously or secondary infections caused by previous procedures or pre-existing disease states. The result is the same, with equally devastating potential complications. Management of such infections may be as simple as administering routine antibiotic therapy or may require multiple and prolonged drainage procedures and complex reconstructive operations. Prompt intervention is essential to minimize serious morbidity.

SKIN AND SOFT TISSUE

The thorax accounts for one fifth of the total body surface area and thus can be afflicted with many common nonspecific soft tissue infections. Furuncles and boils common to any hair-bearing surface frequently occur. Superficial infections often develop in minor injuries and burns of the chest as they do elsewhere in the body.

Abscesses

Two potentially serious infections specific to the chest wall and involving large potential spaces are subpectoral and subscapular abscesses. These occasionally present as primary infections, but more often are secondary to a chronically infected thoracotomy incision. They are characterized by local pain, with or without swelling, combined with fever and leukocytosis. Prompt drainage and appropriate antibiotic therapy usually lead to successful resolution. Suction catheters are rarely required because these spaces are obliterated once drained.

Gangrene

Necrotizing soft tissue infections may occur as a complication of empyema or trauma. These infections frequently begin when the pleural material is drained through the soft tissues either by chest tube or thoracotomy. Pingleton and Jeter (1983) reported extensive synergistic gangrene of the chest wall with *Bacteroides melaninogenicus* and *Streptococcus viridans* following tube thoracostomy for empyema. Delay in recognition led to the patient's demise. I (J.L.) and Vanecko (1985)

reported loss of the pectoralis major and serratus muscles caused by clostridial myonecrosis at the site of a tube thoracostomy in a patient with Boerhaave's syndrome. Radical debridement and daily dressing changes under general anesthesia eventually led to a successful outcome. Early recognition, radical debridement of all involved necrotic tissue, and treatment with high dose antibiotic therapy—usually penicillin—are all necessary for a good chance for cure.

Empyema Necessitatis

Infrequently seen today, this soft tissue infection is caused by an undrained underlying pleural infection. An untreated empyema may eventually burrow through the chest wall and into the subcutaneous tissue of the chest. Suspicion of this entity should be raised by the patient's history and confirmed by physical and roentgenographic examination of the chest. The soft tissue component may require separate drainage, but often resolves with appropriate drainage of the empyema.

Mondor's Disease

This benign condition is a localized thrombophlebitis occurring in the superficial veins of the breast and anterior chest wall. The true incidence of this entity is unknown. Reports have been infrequent. Because the condition produces few symptoms and signs, most examples are probably not referred to informed examiners for study.

The earliest description was by Fagge (1869). Williams (1931) attributed the disease to thrombophlebitis, and later so did Mondor (1939), for whom the condition is named. Most cases occur in women, and frequently no antecedent cause can be found. Radical mastectomy may predispose to the development of this disease, as Herrman (1966) proposed, whereas benign conditions such as fibrocystic disease have no association with this entity. In a few instances, in which a biopsy was performed, Farrow (1955) described a sclerosing endophlebitis with complete or partial obliteration of the lumen.

Clinically, the disease presents as a cord-like structure

in the subcutaneous tissue of the axilla, chest, or abdomen. Its greatest significance may be the possible confusion with inflammatory carcinoma of the breast. It does not tend to recur or lead to thromboembolism. In most subjects no specific therapy is indicated because it regresses spontaneously.

Miscellaneous

Several other conditions may present as infections of the chest wall. Golladay and associates (1985) noted three benign conditions in 24 children who presented with chest wall masses. These included trichinosis, nodular fasciitis, and myositis ossificans, all confirmed by excisional biopsy.

CARTILAGE AND BONY STRUCTURES

Tietze's Syndrome

Painful, nonsuppurative swelling of the costal cartilages without abnormal histologic change is referred to as Tietze's syndrome. This condition, which is not a disease, was described in two patients by Tietze (1921), who attributed the changes to tuberculosis. This has never been confirmed. Following his publication, case reports have been sporadic. Kayser (1956), who reviewed the world literature, could find only 156 cases. The true frequency of this condition is not known, but the symptom complex appears to be common. Peyton (1983) described 76 women in his office practice and 156 men and women visiting an emergency room who complained of this syndrome. Symptoms include chest pain and swelling of the costochondral junction. The junction, usually the second, is usually prominent and is tender to deep palpation. He noted that emotional tension is frequently associated with this symptom complex. Rarely are further tests necessary to confirm this diagnosis, but Edelstein and colleagues (1985) pointed out that computed tomography of the chest is helpful to exclude chest wall masses in these patients.

As might be expected for a condition as vague as this, several invasive treatments have been advocated, from hydrocortisone infiltration to surgical removal of the involved area. The latter hardly seems justified. In most patients, reassurance and symptomatic treatment with compounds containing ibuprofen are sufficient.

Costochondritis

Infections of the costal cartilage cause great debility. They are chronic beyond all expectation and thus demoralizing to the patient and the surgeon alike. When recognized and treated properly, response is rapid, but the required treatment is unseemingly radical for what appears to be such a minor problem. This often leads to delay in appropriate management. Recognizing the basic problem, Moschowitz (1918) pointed out that the chronicity was due less to the type of infecting organism and more to the avascular nature of the cartilage. He urged removal of the cartilage for cure.

Before 1940, most chondritis was spontaneous, usually caused by tuberculosis. Some cases were caused by typhoid or paratyphoid fever. In contrast, today most infections are surgical complications. Most follow median sternotomy performed for cardiac procedures. Some follow thoracotomy, tube thoracostomy, or chest wall trauma. Occasionally, fungal infections may burrow through the chest wall to cause chondritis.

Because the fifth to the ninth costal cartilages are fused, infections involving any one of these segments dictate a major resection for cure. The xiphoid is partially a cartilagenous structure, and thus may promote bilateral spread of the infection. This avascular hyaline cartilage behaves like a foreign body once infected. When free of perichondrium, it begins to take on a moth-eaten appearance in the depths of a draining wound. The disintegration of the cartilage, however, occurs slowly but the cartilage is never completely reabsorbed. Sequestra characteristic of chronic osteomyelitis do not classically form in chondritis. The cartilage remains exposed and unmoved in the depths of the narrow, granulating wound.

Many organisms have been cultured from costochondritis. The primary infecting organisms include: *Escherichia coli*, *Streptococcus pneumoniae*, *Pseudomonas aeruginosa*, *Mycobacterium tuberculosis*, staphylococci, streptococci, and Nocardia. Once the wound is opened and drained, subsequent cultures may grow a variety of organisms, depending upon the environment and the antibiotic regimen the patient is receiving.

Usually, the disease manifests itself as a drainage sinus in the region of the cartilages. Local pain and tenderness are present. As with any other chronic infection, general debility and, perhaps, low grade fever accompany an elevated white cell count. In most patients, the diagnosis is confirmed by tenderness over the cartilages and infection in the vicinity.

The preferred therapy is radical excision, as Murphy (1916) and Moschowitz (1918) advocated. Any involved cartilage should be removed completely (Fig. 48–1). If the lower ribs are involved, all fused segments must be excised. No bare cartilage should remain in the infected wound. The more conservative approach is to pack the wound and reconstruct it later, as Lewis (1967) and Ta-

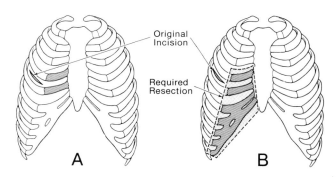

Fig. 48–1. Diagram illustrating cartilage resection necessary for proper treatment of costochondritis. *A*, Initial incision and costal involvement. *B*, Delay may lead to secondary costal arch involvement necessitating arch removal.

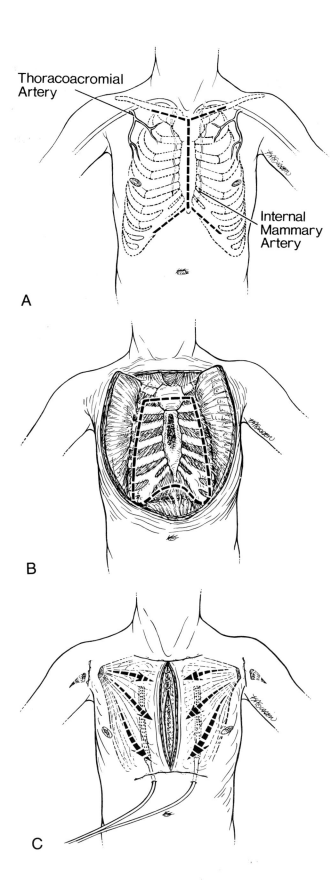

Thoracoacromial
Artery

Internal
Mammary
Artery

A

B

C

Fig. 48–2. Depiction of one-stage operation for chronic sternal osteomyelitis. *A*, The H-shaped incision used to expose the sternum and costal cartilages. *B*, Bilateral pectoralis major myocutaneous flaps have been raised. The extent of the planned resection is shown. *C*, Humeral detachment of the pectoralis muscles with advancement and closure over suction drains. (From Johnson, P., et al.: Management of chronic sternal osteomyelitis. Ann. Thor. Surg. *40*:69, 1985.)

lucci and Webb (1983) advocated. Others, such as Hines and Lee (1983) and Arnold and Pairolero (1984) have shown that the defect may be closed in one stage with a minimal morbidity. Techniques of reconstruction will be discussed subsequently.

Osteomyelitis

Although spontaneously appearing osteomyelitis of the sternum or ribs did occur when tuberculosis was prevalent, it is rare today. Even when tuberculosis was more common, osteomyelitis of the sternum was uncommon. In a series of over 1000 patients with bone and joint tuberculosis reported by Wassersug (1941), the sternum was involved in only 1.1%. Today, primary sternal osteomyelitis occurs in heroin addicts. More often, secondary infections, usually following cardiac surgical procedures, are the etiologic factors; Ochsner and associates (1972) noted a 1.5% infection rate with an overall 10% mortality. The factors that have been implicated in the development of postoperative sternal infections, enumerated by Talamonti and associates (1987), include: diabetes, low cardiac output, use of bilateral internal mammary artery grafts, and most significantly, reoperation for excessive postoperative bleeding. Patients reported by Talamonti and associates (1987) who were explored within 7 hours did not become infected, whereas all patients who were explored after prolonged—>13 hrs—bleeding became infected.

Manifestations of this condition are similar to those of chondritis. When osteomyelitis involves the sternum, there may be an associated chondritis, which can be mistaken for the principal cause of chronicity. The first sign of postoperative sternal osteomyelitis may be an unstable sternum or serosanguineous discharge.

In case of chronic sternal osteomyelitis, the most successful results have been achieved by extensive sternal and chondral removal followed by myocutaneous reconstruction. The most commonly used reconstruction is bilateral pectoralis major flap advancement, as described by Johnson and associates (1985). A modified "H" incision is used to mobilize the pectoralis major muscles with the blood supply based upon the thoracoacromial artery (Fig. 48–2A). This also allows adequate exposure of the sternum, which is then excised (Fig. 48–2B). If possible, the upper manubrium with the clavicular attachments is left intact. Next, the humeral heads of the pectoralis major muscles are transected and the flaps advanced over drains to close the defect (Fig. 48–2C). This gives a good cosmetic result with preservation of pulmonary function.

Diagnosis of osteomyelitis of the ribs is usually made because of local inflammatory signs and symptoms or because of a persistently draining sinus. When the infection is secondary to open drainage of an empyema, it can be one cause of a slowly healing wound. Sequestration from ribs affected by osteomyelitis has been reported. The sequestrum may even pass into the lungs, as Roe and Benioff (1955) noted. Confirmation is usually made by chest roentgenography. Although computed tomography of the chest is usually not necessary for con-

firmation of the diagnosis, it may help in evaluating possible underlying associated intrathoracic pathology.

Excision of all diseased bone usually provides adequate treatment for osteomyelitis of the ribs. To prevent the problem following empyema drainage, Churchill (1929) recommended a clean division of the ribs, leaving no rib exposed or unprotected by periosteum. Occasionally, extensive excision may be required. In patients in whom the infection is overwhelming and an extensive excision is required, mechanical ventilation may be necessary until the infection is obliterated and reconstruction can be safely attempted.

Osteoradionecrosis

One of the most difficult problems encountered by the thoracic surgeon is a large necrotic ulcer of the chest wall following radiation therapy for carcinoma of the breast or other condition. Often, more infection and necrosis exist than are visible externally. Prosthetic materials usually cannot be used in the infected field, and transfer of viable flaps has been difficult. Despite all of precautions taken by radiotherapists, these infections do occasionally arise. Treatment requires close cooperation between the thoracic surgeon and the plastic and reconstructive surgeon.

The foremost principle in the treatment of a radionecrotic ulcer is wide surgical excision and primary coverage of the defect, as Arnold and Pairolero (1984) described. Biopsies of the affected area should be sent for pathologic analysis when radiation was performed for a local malignancy to ensure that there is no residual tumor.

Provisions for covering the expected defect with viable tissue must be carefully considered before the surgical procedure. Understanding and employment of myocutaneous flaps have advanced. Jurkiewicz and colleagues

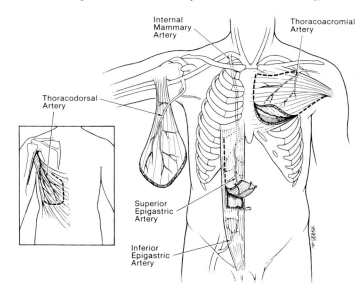

Fig. 48–3. Representation of the most common myocutaneous muscle flaps with their individual blood supply used for chest wall reconstruction.

(1980) described a variety of flaps, including pectoralis major, rectus abdominis and latissimus dorsi flaps (Fig. 48–3). This last flap was first described by Tansini (1906) but was rediscovered by McCraw and colleagues (1978). Hines and Lee (1983) used this flap in five patients and noted that even if the primary blood supply, the thoracodorsal artery, was cut at the time of initial mastectomy, collateral blood supply appeared adequate. They also pointed out that the muscle, albeit smaller and thinner when the thoracodorsal nerve has been resected, remains usable.

In most instances, foreign material should be avoided when infection is present. Usually, the resulting paradoxic movement of the chest wall in these patients is minimally debilitating and not worth the risk of secondary infection. Myocutaneous flaps have been beneficial in those situations in which a large portion of the chest wall or sternum must be removed (see Chapter 51).

REFERENCES

Arnold, P.G., and Pairolero, P.C.: Chest wall reconstruction: experience with 100 consecutive patients. Ann. Surg. *199*:725, 1984.

Churchill, E.: The technic of rib resection and osteomyelitis of the rib ends. J.A.M.A. *92*:644, 1929.

Edelstein, G., et al.: CT observation of rib abnormalities: spectrum of findings. J. Comput. Assist. Tomogr. *9*:65, 1985.

Fagge, C.H.: Remarks on certain cutaneous affections: with cases. Guy's Hosp. Rep. 15 (3rd series):259, 1869.

Farrow, J.H.: Thrombophlebitis of the superficial veins of the breast and anterior chest wall (Mondor's Disease). Surg. Gynecol. Obstet. *101*:63, 1955.

Golladay, E.S., et al.: Chest wall masses in children. South. Med. J. *78*:292, 1985.

Herrman, J.B.: Thrombophlebitis of breast and contiguous thoracoabdominal wall (Mondor's disease). NY State J. Med. *66*:3146, 1966.

Hines, G.L., and Lee, G.: Osteoradionecrosis of the chest wall: management of post resection defects using Marlex mesh and a rotated latissimus dorsi: myocutaneous flap. Am. Surg. *49*:608, 1983.

Johnson, P., et al.: Management of chronic sternal osteomyelitis. Ann. Thor. Surg. *40*:69, 1985.

Jurkiewicz, M.J., et al.: Infected median sternotomy wound: successful treatment by muscle flaps. Ann. Surg. *191*:738, 1980.

Kayser, H.L.: Tietze's syndrome: a review of the literature. Am. J. Med. *21*:982, 1956.

Lewis, F.J.: Chondritis as a postoperative complication. Lancet 87:247, 1967.

LoCicero, J., and Vanecko, R.M.: Clostridial myonecrosis of the chest wall complicating spontaneous esophageal rupture. Ann. Thor. Surg. *40*:396, 1985.

McCraw, J.B., Penix, J.O., and Baker, J.W.: Repair of major defects of chest wall and spine with a latissimus dorsi myocutaneous flap. Plast. Reconstr. Surg. *62*:197, 1978.

Mondor, M.H.: Tronculite Sou-cutane Subaigue de la Paroi Thoracique Anteo-Laterale. MEM. ACAD. CHIR. *65*:1271, 1939.

Moschowitz, A.: The treatment of diseases of the costal cartilages. Ann. Surg. *68*:168, 1918.

Murphy, J.B.: Bone and joint diseases in relation to typhoid fever. Surg. Gynecol. Obstet. *23*:119, 1916.

Ochsner, J.L., Mills, N.L., and Woolverton, W.C.: Disruption and infection of the median sternotomy incision. J. Cardiovasc. Surg. *13*:394, 1972.

Peyton, F.W.: Unexpected frequency of idiopathic costochondral pain. Obstet. Gynecol. *62*:605, 1983.

Pingleton, S.K., and Jeter, J.: Necrotizing fasciitis as a complication of tube thoracostomy. Chest *83*:925, 1983.

Roe, B.B., and Benioff, M.A.: Late hemoptysis from rib sequestrum thirty-four years following empyema drainage. Surgery *38*:764, 1955.

Talamonti, M.S., et al.: Early re-exploration for excessive postoperative hemorrhage lowers wound complication rates in open heart surgery. Am. J. Surg. *53*: 102, 1987.

Talucci, R.C., and Webb, W.R.: Costal chondritis of the costal arch Ann. Thor. Surg. *35*:318, 1983.

Tansini, I.: Sopra il mio nuovo processo di amputazione dell mammella. Riforma Medica (Palermo) *12*:757, 1906.

Tietze, A: Ueber eine eigenartige Haufung von Fallen mit Dystrophie der Rippenknorpel. Beri. Klin. Wochenschr. *58*:829, 1921.

Wassersug, J.D.: Tuberculosis of the sternum. N. Engl. J. Med. *225*:445, 1941.

Williams, G.A.: Thoraco-epigastric phlebitis producing dyspnea. J.A.M.A. *96*:2196, 1931.

READING REFERENCES

Culliford, A.T., et al.: Sternal and costochondral infections following open heart surgery. J. Thorac. Cardiovasc. Surg. *72*:714, 1976.

CHAPTER 49

THORACIC OUTLET SYNDROME

Harold C. Urschel, Jr.

Thoracic outlet syndrome refers to compression of the subclavian vessels and brachial plexus at the superior aperture of the thorax. It was previously designated according to presumable etiologies, such as scalenus anticus, costoclavicular, hyperabduction, cervical rib, and first rib syndromes. The various syndromes are similar, and the specific compression mechanism is often difficult to identify; however, the first rib seems to be a common denominator against which most compressive factors operate.

The symptoms are either neurologic, vascular, or mixed, depending on which component is compressed. Occasionally, the pain is atypical in distribution and severity and experienced predominantly in the chest wall and parascapular area, simulating angina pectoris, as I and my colleagues (1973) noted.

Diagnosis of the nerve compression group, as I and my associates (1971) noted, can be objectively substantiated by determining the ulnar nerve conduction velocity. In the vascular compression group, diagnosis is usually established clinically, rarely requiring the use of angiography.

The ulnar nerve conduction velocity test—UNCV—as described by Jebsen (1967) and Caldwell and associates (1971) has widened the clinical recognition of this syndrome and has improved diagnosis, selection of treatment, and assessment of therapeutic results.

Physiotherapy to improve posture, strengthen shoulder girdle muscles, and stretch neck muscles is employed initially in most cases of thoracic oulet syndrome and is often successful in cases of mild compression. Surgical treatment involves extirpation of the first rib, usually through the transaxillary approach, and is reserved, as I and Razzuk (1972) emphasized, for cases of severe compression that have not responded to medical therapy.

ANATOMIC CONSIDERATIONS

The subclavian vessels and brachial plexus traverse the cervicoaxillary canal to reach the upper extremity. The outer border of the first rib divides this canal into a proximal division composed of the scalene triangle and the space bounded by the clavicle and the first rib—the costoclavicular space. The distal division comprises the axilla. The proximal division is the most critical for neurovascular compression. It is bounded superiorly by the clavicle and the subclavius muscle; inferiorly by the first rib; anteromedially by the border of the sternum, the clavipectoral fascia, and the costocoracoid ligament; and posterolaterally by the scalenus medius muscle and the long thoracic nerve. The scalenus anticus, inserting on the scalene tubercle of the first rib, divides the costoclavicular space into two compartments: an anterior compartment containing the subclavian vein, and a posterior compartment containing the subclavian artery and brachial plexus. The axilla, which is the outer division of the cervicoaxillary canal, with its underlying structures including the pectoralis minor muscle, the coracoid process, and the head of the humerus, is also an area of potential compression.

Compression Factors

A multiplicity of factors may cause compression of the neurovascular bundle at the thoracic outlet. The basic factor, which was pointed out by Rosati and Lord (1961), is deranged anatomy to which congenital, traumatic, and atherosclerotic factors may contribute (Table 49–1).

Bony abnormalities are present in approximately 30% of patients, either as cervical rib, bifid first rib, fusion of first and second ribs, clavicular deformities, or previous thoracoplasty.

Pathologic changes in the configuration of the cervicoaxillary canal alter the normal functional dynamics and serve as the basis of the clinical maneuvers used in the diagnosis of the thoracic outlet syndrome.

Adson or Scalene Test. This maneuver described by Adson in 1951, tightens the anterior and middle scalene muscles, thus decreasing the interscalene space and magnifying any pre-existing compression of the subclavian artery and brachial plexus. The patient is instructed to: (1) take and hold a deep breath, (2) extend his neck fully,

Table 49–1. Etiologic Factors in Thoracic Outlet Syndrome

Anatomic
  Potential sites of neurovascular compression
    interscalene triangle
    costoclavicular space
    subcoracoid area
Congenital
  Cervical rib and its fascial remnants
  Rudimentary first thoracic rib
  Scaleni muscles
    anterior
    middle
    minimus
  Adventitious fibrous bands
  Bifid clavicle
  Exostosis of first thoracic rib
  Enlarged transverse process of C7
  Omohyoid muscle
  Anomalous course of transverse cervical artery
  Brachial plexus postfixed
  Flat clavicle
Traumatic
  Fracture of clavicle
  Dislocation of head of humerus
  Crushing injury to upper thorax
  Sudden, unaccustomed muscular efforts involving shoulder girdle
    muscles
  Cervical spondylosis and injuries to cervical spine
Atherosclerosis

and (3) turn his face toward the side. Obliteration or diminution in the radial pulse suggests compression.

Costoclavicular Test—Military Position. The shoulders are drawn downward and backward. This maneuver narrows the costoclavicular space by approximating the clavicle to the first rib, thus tending to compress the neurovascular bundle. Changes in the radial pulse with production of symptoms indicate compresssion.

Hyperabduction Test. When the arm is hyperabducted to 180°, the components of the neurovascular bundle are pulled around the pectoralis minor tendon, the coracoid process, and the head of the humerus. If the radial pulse is decreased, compression should be suspected.

Arm Claudication Test. The shoulders are drawn upward and backward. The arms are raised to the horizontal position with the elbows flexed 90°. With exercises of the hands, numbness or pain is experienced in the hands and forearms if compression is present.

SIGNS AND SYMPTOMS

The symptoms of thoracic outlet syndrome depend on whether the nerves or blood vessels, or both, are compressed at the thoracic outlet.

I and my associates (1971, 1972) observed that symptoms of nerve compression, occur most frequently, pain and paresthesia being present in about 95% of patients, and motor weakness in approximately 10%. Pain and paresthesia are segmental in 75% of cases, 90% occurring in the ulnar nerve distribution. Pain is usually insidious in onset and commonly involves the neck, shoulder, arm and hand. In some patients, the pain is atypical, involving the anterior chest wall or the parascapular area, and is termed pseudoangina because it simulates angina pectoris. As I and my associates (1973) reported, these patients have normal coronary arteriograms and markedly decreased ulnar nerve conduction velocities, strongly suggesting the diagnosis of thoracic outlet syndrome. The usual shoulder, arm, and hand symptoms that might have provided the clue for the diagnosis of thoracic outlet syndrome are initially either absent or minimal compared to the severity of the chest pain. Without a high index of suspicion, the diagnosis of thoracic outlet syndrome is frequently overlooked, and many of these patients become "cardiac cripples" without an appropriate diagnosis or develop severe psychologic depression when told that their coronary arteries are normal and that they have no significant cause for their pain.

There are two distinct groups of patients with pseudoangina. Group I patients have symptoms and clinical findings suggesting angina pectoris, but have normal coronary arteriograms and significant depression of ulnar nerve conduction velocity. Group II patients have both significant coronary artery disease, as evidenced by 75% or greater stenosis in one or more of the major coronary arteries on coronary arteriography, and thoracic outlet syndrome, as evidenced by depression of the ulnar nerve conduction velocity. A high index of suspicion of thoracic outlet disease in such individuals must be maintained so that the appropriate methods of diagnosis and management can be exercised. Objective laboratory tests that are important for differentiating these two groups of patients include ECG, exercise stress tests, coronary arteriogram, EMG, UNCV, cine esophagogram and roentgenogram of the chest.

To understand the symptomatic overlap between coronary artery disease and this atypical manifestation of the thoracic outlet syndrome, that is, pseudoangina, it is necessary to review the neuroanatomy, innervation, and pain pathways of the arm, chest wall, and heart.

At least two types of pain pathways are present in the arm—the commonly acknowledged C5 to T1 cutaneous "more superficial" fibers, and the T2 to T5 afferent spinal fibers, which travel with the sympathetic nerves and transmit "deeper" painful stimuli from the ulnar median and parascapular distribution, as reported by Kuntz (1951). The cell bodies of the two types of afferent neurons are situated in the dorsal root ganglia of the corresponding spinal segments. They synapse in the dorsal gray matter of the spinal cord and the axons of the second order neurons, cross the midline, and ascend in the spinothalamic tract to the brain.

Compression of the "superficial" C8 to T1 cutaneous afferent fibers elicits stimuli that are transmitted to the brain and recognized as integumentary pain or paresthesias in the ulnar nerve distribution. In contrast, compression of the predominantly "deeper" sensory fibers elicits impulses that are interpreted by the brain as deep pain originating in the arm or referred to the chest wall.

The pseudoangina experienced in thoracic outlet compression shares with angina pectoris the same dermatomal distribution in that the heart, arm, and chest wall have afferent fibers convergent on T2 to T5 spinal cord segments and cell bodies that are located in the corresponding dorsal root ganglia. Referred pain to the chest wall is a component in both pseudoangina and angina pectoris. Because somatic pain is more common than visceral pain, the brain interprets activity arriving in a given pathway as a pain stimulus in a particular somatic area.

Two theories attempt to explain the mechanism of referred pain from the heart or arm stimuli to chest wall. The convergence theory holds that somatic and visceral afferents converge on the same spinothalamic neurons; when the same pathway is stimulated by activity in visceral afferents, the signal reaching the brain is the same and the pain is projected to the somatic area. The facilitation effect theory holds that because of subliminal fringe effects, incoming impulses from visceral structures, such as the heart, lower the threshold of spinothalamic neurons receiving afferents from somatic areas, so that minor activity in the pain pathways from the somatic areas—activity that would normally die out in the spinal cord—passes on to the brain and is interpreted as somatic pain rather than pain in the viscera, where the stimulus was initiated.

Symptoms of vascular compression in thoracic outlet syndrome, much less common than those of neurologic compression, include coldness, weakness, easy fatigability of the arm and hand, and pain that is usually more diffuse in distribution. Raynaud's phenomenon is occasionally noted. Venous compression is recognized by edema, venous distention, and discoloration of the arm and hand. Thrombosis of the subclavian vein—"effort thrombosis" or Paget-Schroetter syndrome—is infrequently noted but was described by Lang (1962).

Objective physical findings, in contrast, are more common in patients with primarily vascular rather than neural compression. Loss or diminution of radial pulse and reproduction of symptoms can be elicited with Adson's test, costoclavicular—military position, and hyperabduction maneuvers in most patients with vascular compression. Other possible findings are venous distention and edema, trophic changes, Rayaund's phenomenon, temperature changes, subclavian vein thrombosis, and even arterial occlusion and claudication. In cases of neural compression, the objective neurologic findings, which occur less frequently, consists of hypoesthesia, anesthesia, and occasional muscular weakness or atrophy.

DIAGNOSIS

The basic diagnostic considerations of the thoracic outlet syndrome include the history and physical examination, roentgenograms of chest and cervical spine, neurologic consultation, electromyogram, and ulnar nerve conduction velocity. On occasion, a cervical myelogram, coronary angiogram, and venograms may be necessary to elicit the diagnosis.

Cardinal for the establishment of the thoracic outlet diagnosis in pseudoangina is the elimination of the possibility of significant coronary artery disease by submaximal exercise stress testing and coronary arteriography where indicated. Subsequently, after excluding pulmonary, esophageal, and chest wall causes, the diagnosis of thoracic outlet syndrome must be entertained and established by the appropriate clinical evaluation and the slowing of the ulnar nerve conduction velocity.

Nerve Conduction Velocity

Motor conduction velocities of the ulnar, median, radial, and musculocutaneous nerves can be reliably measured, as described by Jebsen (1967). Caldwell and associates (1971) have improved and adapted to clinical use the technique of measuring UNCV in evaluating patients with thoracic outlet compression. Conduction velocities over proximal and distal segments of the ulnar nerve are determined by recording the action potentials generated in the hypothenar or first dorsal interosseous muscles. The points of stimulation are the supraclavicular fossa, mid-upper arm, area below the elbow, and wrist. The Meditron 201-AD or the TECA B-3 electromyograph, including the coaxial cable with three-needle or surface electrodes, can be used for this examination. The normal average UNCV values are 72 m/sec across the thoracic outlet, 55 m/sec around the elbow, 59 m/sec in the forearm, and 2.5 to 3.5 m/sec at the wrist. In patients with the thoracic outlet syndrome, I and my colleagues (1971) found that the average UNCV value is reduced to 53 m/sec across the outlet, with a range of 32 to 65 m/sec.

Angiography

Simple clinical observations usually suffice to determine the degree of vascular impairment in the upper extremity and, as Lang (1962) noted, peripheral angiography is rarely needed. Bruits in the supra- or infraclavicular spaces suggest stenoses, and absence of pulse denotes total obstruction. In these instances, retrograde or antegrade arteriograms of the subclavian and brachial arterial systems are indicated to demonstrate localized pathologic changes. To employ arteriography or phlebography routinely for demonstrating temporary occlusion of the vessels in different arm positions would seem redundant to an adequate clinical examination in most patients, and is associated with some morbidity—unnecessary although minimal. The UNCV is usually depressed in patients with vascular compression as well as nerve compression, and serves to satisfy the physician and patient with regard to objective testing; moreover, it is less expensive and safer. In instances of venous stenosis or obstruction, as in the Paget-Schroetter syndrome, phlebograms are indicated to discern the extent of thrombosis to determine the status of collateral venous circulation.

Differential Diagnosis

Thoracic outlet syndrome should be differentiated from a variety of neurologic, vascular, pulmonary, and esophageal lesions. It is necessary to differentiate it from

Table 49–2. Differential Diagnosis of Nerve Compression

Cervical spine
    Ruptured intervertebral disc
    Degenerative disease
    Osteoarthritis
    Spinal cord tumors
Brachial plexus
    Superior sulcus tumors
    Trauma—postural palsy
Peripheral nerves
    Entrapment neuropathy
        carpal tunnel—median nerve
        ulnar nerve—elbow
        radial nerve
        suprascapular nerve
Medical neuropathies
Trauma
Tumor

lesion of the cervical spine, brachial plexus, and peripheral nerves (Table 49–2).

Several arterial and venous phenomena (Table 49–3) can be confused with thoracic outlet syndrome; however, the differentiation can often be made clinically.

In patients with atypical presentations such as chest pain, a high index of suspicion of thoracic outlet in addition to angina pectoris must be maintained.

THERAPY

Patients with the thoracic outlet syndrome usually should receive physiotherapy before operative intervention. Such therapy must be properly performed because many of these patients receive the same treatment as persons with "cervical syndrome," which often exaggerates the symptoms of thoracic outlet compression. Proper physiotherapy for thoracic outlet compression includes heat massages, active neck exercises, scalenus anticus muscle stretching, strengthening of the upper trapezius muscle, and posture instruction. Since sagging of the shoulder girdle, common among the middle aged, is a major etiologic factor in this syndrome, many of the pa-

Table 49–3. Differential Diagnosis of Vascular Compression

Arterial
    Arteriosclerosis
        aneurysm
        occlusive disease
    Thromboangiitis obliterans
    Embolism
    Functional
        Raynaud's disease
        reflex vasomotor dystrophy
        causalgia
        vasculitis, collagen disease, panniculitis
Venous
    Thrombophlebitis
    Mediastinal venous obstruction
        malignant
        benign

tients with less severe disease are improved by strengthening the shoulder girdle and improving posture. More than half of the patients seen in consultation required no surgical procedure but were improved significantly with conservative management.

Most patients with a UNCV above 60 m/sec improve with conservative management; however, most patients with a UNCV below 60 m/sec require surgical resection of the first rib and correction of other bony abnormalities.

As Roos (1966) and Roos and Owens (1966) suggested, resection of the first rib, with cervical rib when present, is best performed through the transaxillary approach for complete removal, with decompression of the seventh and eighth cervical and first thoracic nerve roots. It can be accomplished without major muscle division, as in the posterior approach advocated by Clagett (1962) or retraction of the brachial plexus, as in the anterior supraclavicular approach suggested by Falconer and Li (1962). The infraclavicular approach does not allow complete removal of the first rib. The transaxillary approach shortens the postoperative disability and provides better cosmetic results when compared with both the anterior and posterior approaches, particularly because 80% of patients are females.

Technique of Transaxillary Resection of First Rib

The patient is placed in the lateral position with the involved extremity abducted to 90° by traction straps wrapped carefully around the forearm and attached to an overhead pulley. An appropriate amount of weight, usually 1 to 2 pounds, depending on the build of the patient, is used to maintain this position without undue traction. Traction can be increased intermittently by the anesthesiologist for exposure. The axilla and forearm are prepared and draped. A transverse incision is made below the hairline between the pectoralis major and the latissimus dorsi muscles and deepened to the external intercostal fascia. Care should be taken to prevent injury to the intercostobrachial cutaneous nerve, which passes from the chest wall to the subcutaneous tissue in the center of the operative field. The dissection is extended cephalad next to the external intercostal fascia up to the first rib. With gentle dissection, the neurovascular bundle is identified and its relation to the first rib and both scalene muscles clearly outlined to avoid injury to these structures. The insertion of the scalenus anticus muscle on the first rib is dissected and the muscle divided. The first rib is dissected subperiosteally with a periosteal elevator and carefully separated from the underlying pleura to avoid pneumothorax. The rib is then divided at its middle portion. With use of an alligator forceps, the anterior portion of the rib is pulled away from the vein, and the costoclavicular ligament is cut and the rib divided at its sternal attachment. The anterior venous compartment is thus decompressed. The posterior segment of the rib is then grasped with alligator forceps and retracted away from its bed to facilitate its dissection and separation from the subclavian artery and brachial plexus posteriorly. The scalenus medius muscle *should not* be cut from the rib but rather stripped with a periosteal elevator to avoid injuring the long thoracic nerve that lies on its posterior margin. The dissection of this rib segment is carried to its articulation with the transverse process of the vertebra and divided. If the dissection is kept in the subperiosteal plane, no damage occurs to the first thoracic nerve root, which lies immediately under the rib. Complete removal of the neck and head of the first rib is achieved by a long, special double-action pituitary rongeur. The eighth cervical and first thoracic nerve roots can be visualized clearly at this point. If a cervical rib is present, it is removed at this time and the seventh cervical nerve root can be observed. Only the subcutaneous tissues and skin require closure, because no large muscles have been divided. Only occasional, intermittent firm traction is required for exposure, and no evidence of brachial plexus stretching or neuritis has been observed when this technique is used. The patient is encouraged to use his arm normally and can be discharged from the hospital between 2 and 3 days following the surgical procedure.

It is preferable to remove the entire first rib, including its head and neck, to avoid future irritation of the plexus, because a residual portion, particularly if it is long, may cause recurrence of symptoms. The periosteum should be fragmented and destroyed to prevent callus formation and "regeneration" of the rib.

Removal of incompletely resected or "regenerated" rib can best be accomplished through the posterior approach. For lysis of adhesions of the brachial plexus in symptomatic patients with decreased ulnar nerve conduction velocity following previous complete resection of the first rib, the anterior supraclavicular approach is used.

Results of Therapy

The clinical results of first rib resections in properly selected patients are good in 85%, fair in 10%, and poor in 5%. A good result is indicated by complete relief of symptoms, a fair result by improvement with some residual or recurrent mild symptoms, and a poor result by no change from the preoperative status.

Uniform improvement of symptoms is usually obtained in patients with primarily vascular compression. In patients with predominantly nerve compression, however, two groups with different rates of improvement are observed. The first group includes patients with the classic manifestations of ulnar neuralgia and elicitation of pulse diminution, in whom an average preoperative UNCV is reduced to 53 m/sec. Ninety-five precent of this group are improved by first rib resection. In the second group are patients with atypical pain distribution who may or may not have shown pulse changes by compression tests, and in whom the average preoperative ulnar nerve conduction velocity was only reduced to 60 m/sec. Surgical intervention is carried out in such patients as a therapeutic trial after prolonged conservative therapy has failed. Although, as I and my associates (1971) observed, many patients in the second group are improved, the fair and poor results all occur in these patients.

UNCV and clinical status are highly correlated. Patients with good postoperative results have a preoperative average UNCV of 51 m/sec and show return to a normal average of 72 m/sec after operation. In those who have fair results, the preoperative UNCV averages 60 m/sec and increases to an average of only 63 m/sec after operation. In the poor result group, there is no appreciable change in the postoperative from the preoperative values; in fact, the average conduction time was only 58 m/sec.

No hospital mortality has been directly related to this procedure. Postoperative morbidity after the transaxillary approach includes clinically inconsequential pneumothorax in 15%, hematoma in 1%, and infection in 1%.

RECURRENT THORACIC OUTLET SYNDROME

Extirpation of the first rib offers relief of symptoms in patients with thoracic outlet syndrome not improved by physiotherapy. Ten percent of the surgically treated patients develop variable degrees of shoulder, arm, and hand pain and paresthesias that are usually mild and short lasting, and that usually respond well to a brief course of physiotherapy and muscle relaxants. In 1.6% of patients, however, symptoms persist, become progressively more severe, and often involve a wider area of distribution because of entrapment of the intermediate trunk in addition to the lower trunk and C8 and T1 nerve roots. Symptoms may recur from 1 month to 10 years following initial rib resection, but as I and my colleagues (1976) noted, in most instances recurrence is within the first 3 months. Symptoms consist of aching or burning pain, often associated with paresthesia, involving the neck, shoulder, parascapular area, anterior chest wall, arm, and hand. Vascular lesions are uncommon and consist of causalgia minor and infected false aneurysms.

I (1987) identified two distinct groups of patients requiring reoperation. Pseudorecurrence occurs in patients who never had relief of symptoms following the initial operation. Cases can be separated etiologically as follows: cases in which (1) the second rib was mistakenly resected instead of the first; (2) the first rib was resected, leaving a cervical rib; (3) a cervical rib was resected, leaving an abnormal first rib; or (4) a second rib was resected, leaving a rudimentary first rib. The second group, in whom true recurrence takes place, includes those patients whose symptoms were relieved after the initial operation but who developed recurrence with a significant piece of the first rib remaining and a second group who had complete resection of the first rib but demonstrated excessive scar formation on the brachial plexus.

Physiotherapy should be instituted in all patients with symptoms of neurovascular compression following first rib resection. If symptoms persist and conduction velocity remains below normal, reoperation is indicated.

Reoperation for recurrent thoracic outlet syndrome is always performed through the posterior thoracoplasty approach to provide better exposure of the nerve roots and brachial plexus, thereby reducing the danger of injury to these structures as well as providing adequate exposure of the subclavian artery and vein. It also provides a wider field for easy resection of any bony abnormalities or fibrous bands and allows extensive neurolysis of the nerve roots and brachial plexus, not always accessible through the limited exposure of the transaxillary approach. The anterior or supraclavicular approach is inadequate for reoperation.

The basic elements of reoperation include: (1) resection of persistent or recurrent bony remnants of either a cervical or the first rib, (2) neurolysis of the brachial plexus and nerve roots, and (3) dorsal sympathectomy. Sympathectomy removes the T1, T2, and T3 thoracic ganglia. Avoid damaging the C8 ganglion—upper aspect of the stellate ganglion—which produces Horner's syndrome. This provides relief of major and minor causalgia and alleviates the paresthesias in the supraclavicular and intraclavicular areas. The incidence of the "postsympathetic" syndrome has been negligible in this group of patients. The use of a nerve stimulator to differentiate scar from nerve root is cardinal to avoid damage in reoperation in these patients.

The technique of the operation includes a high thoracoplasty incision, extending from 3 cm above the angle of the scapula, halfway between the angle of the scapula and the spinous processes, and caudad 5 cm from the angle of the scapula. The trapezius and rhomboid muscles are divided the length of the incision. The scapula is retracted from the chest wall by incising the latissimus dorsi over the fourth rib. The posterior superior serratus muscle is divided and the sacrospinalis muscle retracted medially. The first rib remnant and cervical rib remnant, if present, are located and removed subperiosteally. After the rib remnants have been resected, the regenerated periosteum is extirpated. In my experience, most regenerated ribs occur from the end of an unresected segment of rib rather than from periosteum, although the latter is possible. Because of this, at the initial operation it is important to remove the first rib totally to reduce the incidence of bony regeneration in all patients with primarily nerve compression and pain symptoms.

After removal of any bony rib remnant, if there is excessive scar it may be prudent to perform the sympathectomy initially. This involves resection of a 1-inch—2.5 cm—segment of the second rib posteriorly to locate the sympathetic ganglion. In that way, the first thoracic nerve may be easier to locate beneath rather than through the scar.

Neurolysis of the nerve root and brachial plexus is performed, using a nerve stimulator. Neurolysis is carried down to but not into the nerve sheath. It is extended peripherally over the brachial plexus as far as any scar persists. Excessive neurolysis is not indicated, and opening of the nerve sheath produces more scar than it relieves. To minimize excessive scar, efforts in the initial operation for thoracic outlet should include complete extirpation of the first rib, avoidance of hematomas by adequate drainage either by catheter or by opening the pleura, and avoidance of infection.

The subclavian artery and vein are released if symptoms mediate. Debridement of the scalenus medius muscle is carried out. The dorsal sympathectomy is completed via extrapleural dissection. Meticulous hemostasis is effected, and a large, round Jackson-Pratt catheter drain is placed in the area of the brachial plexus, although not touching it. This drain is brought out through the subscapular space through a stab wound into the axilla. Methylprednisolone acetate—Depo-Medrol—80 mg is left in the area of the nerve plexus, although the patient is not given systemic steroids unless keloid formation has previously been manifested. The wound is closed in layers with interrupted heavy Vicryl sutures to provide adequate strength, and the arm is kept in a sling to be used gently for the first 3 months. Range-of-motion exercises are carried out to prevent shoulder limitation; however, overactivity is contraindicated to minimize excessive scar formation.

When the problem is vascular, involving false or mycotic aneurysms, special techniques for reoperation are employed. A bypass graft is interposed from the innominate or carotid artery proximally, through a separate tunnel distally, to the brachial artery. This is usually performed with saphenous vein, although other conduits may be employed. The arteries feeding and leaving the infected aneurysm are ligated. At a subsequent stage, the aneurysm is resected through a transaxillary approach with no fear of bleeding or ischemia of the arm.

Special instruments have been devised to provide adequate resection through the transaxillary or posterior route. These include a modified strengthened pituitary rongeur and a modified Leksell double-action rongeur for first rib removal without danger to the nerve root.

The sympathectomy relieves chest wall pain that mimics angina pectoris, esophageal disease, or even a lung tumor by denervating the deep fibers that travel with the arteries and bone.

Results of reoperation have been excellent if an accurate diagnosis was established and proper procedure executed. Follow-up of over 400 patients has ranged from 6 months to 15 years. All patients improved initially following reoperation; in 79% improvement was maintained for more than 5 years. Symptoms easily managed with physiotherapy developed in 14%; 7% required a second reoperation, in every instance because of rescarring. There were no deaths in the series and only one case of significant infection requiring drainage.

REFERENCES

Adson, A.W.: Cervical ribs: symptoms, differential diagnosis for section of the scalenus anticus muscle. J. Int. Coll. Surg. 16:546, 1951.

Caldwell, J.W., Crane, C.R., and Krusen, U.L.: Nerve conduction studies in the diagnosis of the thoracic outlet syndrome. South Med. J. 64:210, 1971.

Clagett, O.T.: Presidential address: research and prosearch. J. Thorac. Cardiovasc. Surg. 44:153, 1962.

Falconer, M.A., and Li, F.W.P.: Resection of the first rib in costoclavicular compression of the brachial plexus. Lancet 1:59, 1962.

Jebsen, R.H.: Motor conduction velocities in the median and ulnar nerves. Arch. Phys. Med. 48:185, 1967.

Kuntz, A.: Afferent innervation of peripheral blood vessels through sympathetic trunks. South Med. J. 44:673, 1951.

Lang, E.K.: Roentgenographic diagnosis of the neurovascular compression syndromes. Radiology 79:58, 1962.

Roos, D.B.: Transaxillary approach for first rib resection to relieve thoracic outlet syndrome. Ann. Surg. *163*:354, 1966.

Roos, D.B., and Owens, J.C.: Thoracic outlet syndrome. Arch. Surg. *93*:71, 1966.

Rosati, L.M., and Lord, J.W.: Neurovascular Compression Syndromes of the Shoulder Girdle. Modern Surgical Monographs. New York, Grune & Stratton, 1961, p. 168.

Urschel, H.C., Jr., and Razzuk, M.A.: Current concepts: management of the thoracic outlet syndrome. N. Engl. J. Med. *286*:1140, 1972.

Urschel, H.C., Jr., et al.: Objective diagnosis (ulnar nerve conduction velocity) and current therapy of the thoracic outlet syndrome. Ann. Thorac. Surg. *12*:608, 1971.

Urschel, H.C., Jr., et al.: Thoracic outlet syndrome masquerading as coronary artery disease. Ann. Thorac. Surg. *16*:239, 1973.

Urschel, H.C., Jr., et al.: Reoperation for recurrent thoracic outlet syndrome. Ann. Thorac. Surg. *21*:19, 1976.

Urschel, H.C., Jr.: Thoracic outlet syndrome: reoperation. *In* International Trends in General Thoracic Surgery, Major Challenges, Vol. 2, p. 374. Edited by H.C. Grillo and H. Eschapasse. Philadelphia, W.B. Saunders Co., 1987.

READING REFERENCES

Adson, A.W., and Coffey, I.R.: Cervical rig: a method of anterior approach for relief of symptoms by division of the scalenus anticus. Ann. Surg. *85*:839, 1927.

Rob, C.G., and Standover, A.: Arterial occlusion complicating thoracic outlet compression syndrome. Br. Med. J. *2*:709, 1958.

Roos, D.B.: Experience with first rib resection for thoracic outlet syndrome. Ann. Surg. *173*:429, 1971.

Telford, E.D. and Mottershead, S.: Pressure at the cervicobrachial junction. J. Bone Joint Surg. (Am.) *30*:249, 1948.

Urschel, H.C., Jr., Paulson, D.L., and McNamara, J.J.: Thoracic outlet syndrome. Ann. Thorac. Surg. *61*:1, 1968.

Urschel, H.C., Jr., and Razzuk, M.: The failed operation for thoracic outlet syndrome: the difficulty of diagnosis and management. Ann. Thorac. Surg. *42*:523, 1986.

CHAPTER 50

CHEST WALL TUMORS

Peter C. Pairolero

Chest wall tumors encompass a kaleidoscopic panorama of bone and soft tissue disease. Included among these tumors are primary neoplasms—both benign and malignant—of the bony skeleton, chest wall metastases, neoplasms that invade the chest wall from the lung, pleura, mediastinum, muscle, and breast, and benign non-neoplastic conditions (Table 50–1). Nearly all of these disorders have at one time or another been irradiated either as the treatment of choice or in combination with chest wall resection, and it is common to have patients present with a postradiation necrotic chest wall tumor. The thoracic surgeon is frequently asked to evaluate all of these patients; most to establish a diagnosis, some to treat for cure, and a few to manage necrotic, foul-smelling chest wall ulcers. All are a diagnostic and therapeutic challenge. Surgical extirpation in many of these patients is frequently the only remaining modality of treatment, and this may be compromised by incorrect diagnosis or an inability to reconstruct large chest wall defects. From a practical standpoint, however, treatment for cure is most often limited to resection of primary chest wall tumors.

INCIDENCE

Primary tumors of the chest wall are uncommon, and few series have been reported. Most reports such as

those by Pascuzzi (1957), Groff (1967) and Stelzer (1980) and their associates, excluded patients with soft tissue tumors and included only patients with primary bone tumors. When combined, however, the soft tissues become a major source of chest wall tumors as Graeber (1982), Pairolero (1985), and King (1986) and their associates noted. Indeed, soft tissues are the most common source of primary chest wall malignancy, accounting for nearly 50% of these tumors treated surgically. Altogether, primary tumors of the chest wall, including both bony and soft tissue tumor, comprise approximately 2% of all primary tumors found in the body. The reported incidence of malignancy in these tumors varies from approximately 50% to 80%, with the higher malignancy rate found in those series including soft tissue tumors. Malignant fibrous histiocytoma, chondrosarcoma, and rhabdomyosarcoma are the most common primary malignant neoplasms that the thoracic surgeon is asked to manage, and cartilaginous tumors, desmoid, and fibrous dysplasia are the most common primary benign tumors (Table 50–2).

BASIC PRINCIPLES

Signs and Symptoms

Chest wall tumors generally present as slowly enlarging masses. Most are initially asymptomatic, but with continued growth, pain invariably occurs. At first the pain is frequently generalized, and the patient is often treated for a neuritis or musculoskeletal complaint. Nearly all malignant tumors are likely to become painful, as compared to only two thirds of benign tumors. In some instances of rib tumors, a mass may not be apparent on physical examination, but instead is detected on roentgenogram of the chest. On occasion, fever, leukocytosis, and eosinophila accompany some of these tumors.

Diagnosis

The diagnostic evaluation of patients with suspected chest wall tumors should include a careful history and

Table 50–1. Classification of Chest Wall Tumors

Primary Neoplasms of Chest Wall
  Malignant
  Benign

Metastatic Neoplasms to Chest Wall
  Sarcoma
  Carcinoma

Adjacent Neoplasms with Local Invasion
  Lung
  Breast
  Pleura

Non-neoplastic Disease
  Cyst
  Inflammation

Table 50–2. Primary Chest Wall Tumor

Malignant
  Myeloma
  Malignant Fibrous Histiocytoma
  Chondrosarcoma
  Rhabdomyosarcoma
  Ewing's Sarcoma
  Liposarcoma
  Neurofibrosarcoma
  Osteogenic Sarcoma
  Hemangiosarcoma
  Leiomyosarcoma
  Lymphoma

Benign
  Osteochondroma
  Chondroma
  Desmoid
  Fibrous Dysplasia
  Lipoma
  Fibroma
  Neurilemoma

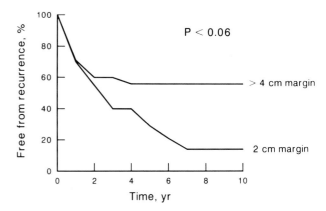

Fig. 50–1. Percentage of patients with malignant chest wall neoplasms remaining free from recurrent cancer by extent of resection margin. Zero time on abscissa represents day of chest wall resection. (Reproduced from King, R.M., et al.: Primary chest wall tumors: factors affecting survival. Ann. Thorac. Surg. *41*:597, June 1986, with permission of the publisher.)

physical and laboratory examination followed by conventional plain and tomographic chest roentgenography. Previous roentgenograms of the chest are important in determining growth rate. Computed tomography should be used to delineate soft tissue, pleural, mediastinal, and pulmonary involvement. The role of magnetic resonance imaging is not yet fully known, but preliminary evaluation indicates still further delineation of tissue pathology.

Chest wall tumors that are clinically suspected of being primary neoplasms—either benign or malignant—should be diagnosed by excisional rather than incisional or needle biopsy. Likewise, necrotic tumor should be diagnosed by excision. If there is a history of known primary neoplasm elsewhere and the chest wall mass is suspected of being a metastasis, however, then needle or incisional biopsy to establish diagnosis of dissemination is reasonable. If the mass presenting on the chest wall might be empyema necessitans or a tuberculous lesion, aspiration may be helpful in making the diagnosis.

Treatment

Wide resection of primary malignant chest wall neoplasm is essential to successful management. The extent of resection should not be compromised because of an inability to close the chest wall defect. Consequently, the mandatory ingredients for successful management of these neoplasms are wide resection and dependable reconstruction as I and Arnold (1985, 1986) and Arnold and I (1979, 1984) pointed out.

Opinions about what constitutes wide resection do differ. King and associates (1986) analyzed the effect of extent of resection on long-term survival in patients with primary malignant chest wall neoplasm. The percentage of patients with a 4-cm or greater margin of resection remaining free from cancer at 5 years was 56% compared to only 29% for patients with a 2-cm margin (Fig. 50–1). Many surgeons consider a margin of resection free of

tumor of several centimeters to be adequate. Although this may be adequate for chest wall metastases, benign tumor, and certain low grade malignant primary bone neoplasms such as chondrosarcoma, a 2-cm resection margin is inadequate for more malignant neoplasms, such as malignant fibrous histiocytoma and osteogenic sarcoma, that can spread within the marrow cavity or along such tissue planes as the periosteum or parietal pleura. Consequently all primary malignant neoplasms initially diagnosed by excisional biopsy should have further resection to include at least a 4-cm margin of normal tissue on all sides. High grade malignancies should also have the entire involved bone resected. For neoplasms of the rib cage, this includes removal of the involved ribs, the corresponding anterior costal arches if the tumor is located anteriorly, and several partial ribs above and below the neoplasm. For tumors of the sternum and manubrium, resection of the entire involved bone and corresponding costal arches bilaterally is indicated. Any attached structures, such as lung, thymus, pericardium, or chest wall muscles, should also be excised.

The role of resection for chest wall metastases and recurrent breast cancer is controversial. Nonetheless, most thoracic surgeons would agree that tumor ulceration is an indication for excision. For these patients, wound hygiene is crucial and surgical excision is frequently the only treatment option available. The goal in treating patients with necrotic tumor should be a healed wound following local excision. Although the length of survival is not increased after resection, the quality of life is certainly improved.

SPECIFIC TUMORS

Primary Bone Tumors

Primary chest wall tumors historically have included both neoplasms and such non-neoplastic conditions as cysts, infections, and fibromatosis. Although these tumors represent an array of different causes, it is still prudent to combine them because most present similarly and many have common roentgenographic features. Primary bone neoplasms constitute the majority of these tumors.

Primary bone neoplasms involving the chest wall are uncommon. In the Mayo Clinic's series of 6034 bone tumors reported by Dahlin and Unni (1986) 355—5.9%—occurred in either the ribs—85%—or the sternum—15%. Overall, 89% were malignant and only 11% benign. Sternal tumors were slighly more likely to be malignant—96% versus 88%. The most common benign bone neoplasms were cartilaginous in origin—osteochondroma and chondroma. The most common malignant neoplasms were myeloma, chondrosarcoma, malignant lymphoma, and Ewing's sarcoma.

Benign Rib Tumors

Osteochondroma. This is the most common benign bone neoplasm, constituting nearly 50% of all benign rib tumors. The incidence, however, may actually be higher, because most patients are asymptomatic, and the tumors are often not removed. Men are affected three times more frequently than women. The neoplasm begins in childhood and continues to grow until skeletal maturity is reached. The onset of pain in a previously asymptomatic tumor may indicate malignant degeneration.

Osteochondromas arise from the metaphyseal region of the rib and present as a stalked bony protuberance with a cartilaginous cap. A rim of calcification may be present at the periphery of the tumor, and there is often stippled calcification within the tumor (Fig. 50–2). Microscopically, bony proliferation occurs to varying degrees, and the thickness of the cartilaginous cap also varies.

All osteochondromas occurring in children after puberty or in adults should be resected. Asymptomatic osteochondromas may occur before puberty, but if pain or increase in size occurs, the tumor should be resected.

Chondroma. Chrondromas constitute 15% of all benign neoplasms of the rib cage. Most occur anteriorly at the costochondral junction. Both sexes are affected equally, and the tumor can occur at any age. These neoplasms usually present as a slowly enlarging mass that may be nontender or slightly painful. Roentgenographically, chondroma is an expansile lesion causing thinning of the cortex. The differentiation between a chondroma and a chondrosarcoma is impossible on clinical and roentgenographic examination. Grossly, chondroma presents as a lobulated mass. Microscopically, the tumor is characterized by lobules of hyaline cartilage. The microscopic differentiation between a chondroma and a low grade chondrosarcoma can be extremely difficult. All chondromas must be considered malignant and should be treated by wide excision. Although this resection may seem extensive for what may turn out to be a benign tumor, modern reconstructive techniques make the risk negligible, and long-term results are excellent.

Fibrous Dysplasia. This is a cystic non-neoplastic lesion and is probably a developmental abnormality characterized by fibrous replacement of the medullary cavity

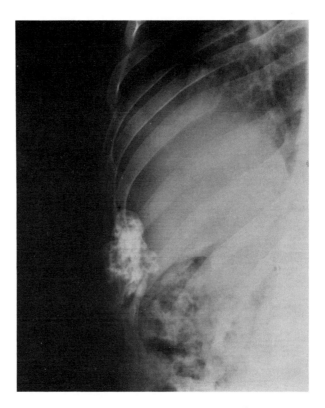

Fig. 50–2. Fifty-two-year-old male with osteochondroma arising in anterior right ninth rib. Note intact cortex and stippled calcification within tumor.

of the rib. Most cases present as solitary lesions, and when multiple lesions are encountered, Albright's syndrome—multiple bone cysts, skin pigmentation, and precocious sexual maturity in girls—should be suspected.

Fibrous dysplasia is usually manifested by a slowly enlarging, nonpainful mass in the posterolateral rib cage. Both sexes are affected equally. The disease begins in childhood, often in infancy, but is not detected until routine screening chest roentgenography in young adulthood. Roentgenographically, there is a characteristic appearance, consisting of expansion and thinning of the bony cortex with a central "ground-glass" appearance (Fig. 50–3). Microscopically, some degree of calcification with bony trabeculation and fibrous formation appears. Treatment should be conservative. Many lesions stop growing at puberty. Local excision is indicated for painful, enlarging lesions.

Histiocytosis X. This is not a neoplasm, but is a part of the spectrum of disease involving the reticuloendothelial system, including eosinophilic granuloma, Letterer-Siewe disease, and Hand-Schüller-Christian disease. Microscopically, all three components are similar and consist of a mixed inflammatory infiltrate of eosinophils and histiocytes.

Eosinophilic granuloma is limited to only bone involvement, whereas Hand-Schüller-Christian disease and Letterer-Siwe disease may have systemic signs and symptoms such as fever, malaise, weight loss, lymph-

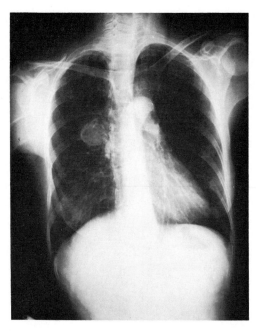

Fig. 50–3. Fibrous dysplasia involving the posterior ribs. Resection necessitated excision of the lateral portion of the adjacent vertebral body.

adenopathy, and splenomegaly; leukocytosis, eosinophilia, and anemia are also often present with these two diseases. Most patients with eosinophilic granuloma present with pain limited to the area of skeletal involvement. Histiocytosis X occurs in persons under 50 years of age. Letterer-Siewe disease typically occurs in infants, Hand-Schüller-Christian disease in children, and eosinophilic granuloma in young to middle-aged adults.

Bone lesions occur in all three clinical variants of histiocytosis X. The skull is most commonly involved, but 10 to 20% of patients have rib lesions. The roentgenographic appearance is similar for all three forms of the disease. The lesion presents as an expansile lesion in the ribs, with periosteal new bone formation and uneven destruction of the cortex producing endosteal scalloping. Confusion with osteomyelitis may occur because of accompanying fever, malaise, and elevated white blood cell count.

Because of the expansile nature of histiocytosis X, excisional biopsy is required to establish the diagnosis. In patients with eosinophilic granuloma, excision alone should result in cure if the lesion is solitary. For patients with multiple lesions of eosinophilic granuloma, low-dose radiation therapy—300 to 600 rads—to each lesion has been helpful. Characteristically, the other two variants of the disease run a chronic course requiring corticosteroids and chemotherapy.

Malignant Rib Tumors

Myeloma. This is the most common primary malignant rib neoplasm, accounting for one third of all tumors in the Mayo Clinic series reported by Dahlin and Unni (1986). Most myelomas involving the chest wall occur as a manifestation of systemic multiple myeloma, and a patient with a myeloma of the rib cage will almost inevitably develop the manifestations of the systemic disease. Solitary myeloma involving the rib is secondary only to solitary vertebral involvement. Myeloma is most common in the fifth through seventh decades of life and is rare under the age of 30. Two thirds of the patients are men. Pain is the most common symptom and often occurs without a palpable mass. Most patients are anemic, with an increase in the erythrocyte sedimentation rate. Abnormal protein electrophoresis is present in 85% of patients, and up to 50% have hypercalcemia and Bence Jones protein in their urine.

Roentgenographically, myeloma presents as a punched-out, osteolytic lesion with cortical thinning. Pathologic fracture is common. Grossly, the tumor is typically gray and friable. Microscopically, sheets of closely packed cells with abundant cytoplasm is observed. Mitosis is rare, but hyperchromatism and multinuclear cells are present.

Whether the rib changes are solitary or multiple, local excision is done to confirm the diagnosis, and radiation therapy is the treatment of choice for solitary and both irradiation and chemotherapy for multiple lesions. Five-year survival is approximately 20%.

Chondrosarcoma. Accounting for nearly 30% of all primary malignant bone neoplasms, chondrosarcoma is most frequently a neoplasm of the anterior chest wall, with 75% arising in either the costochrondral arches or the sternum. The tumor most commonly occurs in the third and fourth decades of life and is relatively uncommon in persons under the age of 20. Chondrosarcoma is more frequent in men. Nearly all patients present with a slowly enlarging mass, which has usually been painful for many months. Grossly, chondrosarcoma is a lobulated neoplasm that may grow to massive proportions and consequently may extend internally into the pleural space or outwardly into the muscle and adipose tissue of the chest wall (Fig. 50–4). Microscopically, the findings range from normal cartilage to obvious malignant changes. Lichtenstein and Jaffe (1943) described the characteristic findings of plump, atypical, and multiple nuclei, which may be more apparent in the peripheral areas of a growing tumor (Fig. 50–5). Differentiation from chondroma may be extremely difficult. From a practical standpoint, all tumors arising in the costal cartilages should be considered to be malignant and should be treated by wide resection.

The cause of chondrosarcoma is unknown. Although malignant degeneration of benign cartilaginous tumors—secondary chondrosarcoma—has been reported, most chondrosarcomas arise de nova. Lichtenstein (1977) was the first to suggest an association between trauma and chondrosarcoma. McAfee and associates (1985) subsequently reported that 12.5% of their patients had sustained severe crushing injury to the ipsilateral chest wall.

Roentgenographically, chondrosarcoma has a characteristic appearance. The tumor appears as a lobulated mass arising in the medullary portion of the bone (Fig. 50–6). The cortex is often destroyed and the margins of the tumor are poorly defined (Fig. 50–7). Mineralization

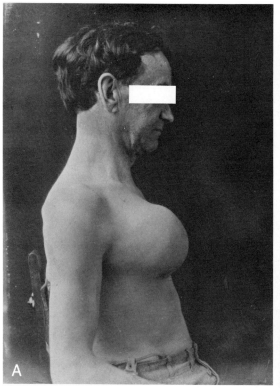

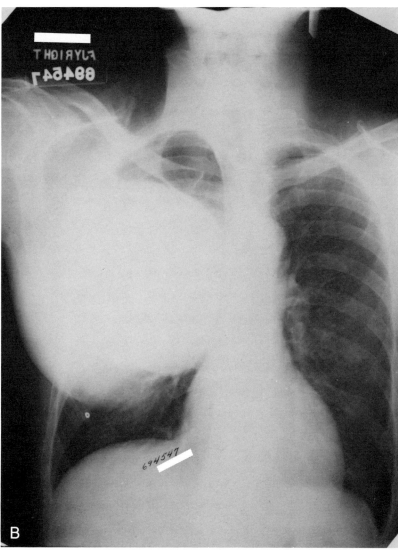

Fig. 50–4. *A,* Fifty-six-year-old white male with huge chondrosarcoma arising from right anterior third costochrondral arch. *B,* Chest roentgenogram of the same patient.

of the tumor matrix is common, producing a mottled type of calcification. Pathologic fracture is uncommon. Computed tomography can be helpful in determining the extent of the neoplasms (Fig. 50–8).

Definitive diagnosis of chondrosarcoma can only be made pathologically. Histological confirmation, however, is sometimes difficult, because most chondrosarcomas are well differentiated. This tendency to be well differentiated may result in misdiagnosis of chondroma and subsequent undertreatment, leading to local recurrences. Generous sampling in the pathology laboratory of different areas within the tumor may facilitate histologic diagnosis. For this reason, excisional biopsy rather than incisional or needle biopsy of all chest wall masses suspected of being chondrosarcoma is indicated.

Chest wall chondrosarcoma typically grows slowly and recurs locally. If it is left untreated, metastases occur late. Prompt, complete control of the primary neoplasm is the main determinant of survival; the objective of the first operation should be resection wide enough to prevent local recurrence. This involves resection of a 4-cm margin of normal tissue on all sides. Wide resection results in cure in nearly all patients (Fig. 50–9), with 10-year survival approaching 97%, as McAfee and associates (1985) reported.

Ewing's Sarcoma. Ewing's sarcoma involving the rib cage accounts for 12% of all primary malignant neoplasms of the bony thorax. Two thirds of all cases of Ewing's sarcoma occur in persons younger than 20, but young infants rarely develop this tumor. Boys are affected twice as often as girls. Signs and symptoms are common. A painful, enlarging mass is common. Fever, malaise, anemia, leukocytosis, and an increased sedimentation rate may be present. Roentgenographically, mottled destruction containing both lytic and blastic areas appears. An "onion-skin" appearance of the surface of the bone, caused by elevation of the periosteum and multiple layers of subperiosteal new bone formation, may be seen, but

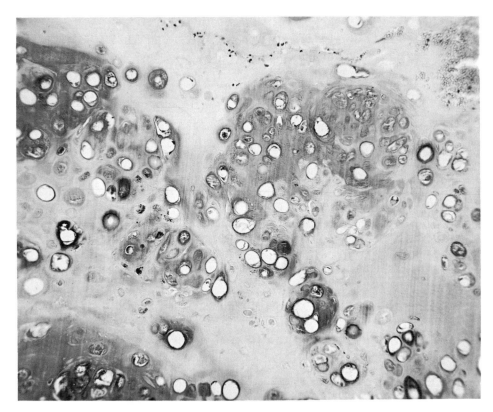

Fig. 50–5. Photomicrograph demonstrating typical cellular changes of chondrosarcoma.

this feature is not pathognomic because it may be found in other bone tumors, both benign and malignant. Radiating spicules may also be present on the surface of the bone, which makes the lesion indistinguishable from osteogenic sarcoma. Pathologic fractures are rare. The roentgenographic appearance is also similar to that of osteomyelitis. This similarity, combined with fever, leukocytosis, and an increase in sedimentation rate, may lead to the erroneous diagnosis of osteomyelitis.

Ewing's sarcoma tends to be whitish-gray and is soft and not encapsulated. Histologically, the tumor is cellular, and there may be difficulty in distinguishing Ewing's sarcoma from lymphoma. Early spread to the lungs and to other bones is common and occurs in 30 to 75% of patients.

Adequate biopsy is necessary for correct diagnosis. Ewing's sarcoma is radiosensitive, so irradiation is the treatment of choice. Adjuvant chemotherapy is also used. Five-year survival is 40 to 50%.

Osteogenic Sarcoma. Osteosarcoma of the bony thorax is less common than chondrosarcoma and constitutes 6% of all primary malignant bone neoplasms. Unfortunately, it is more malignant and, hence, carries a much less favorable prognosis. Osteogenic sarcoma generally occurs in teenagers and young adults and commonly affects more young men than women. Most patients present with a rapidly enlarging tumor that is often painful. Serum alkaline phosphatase levels are frequently elevated. Roentgenographically, bone destruction with indistinct borders that gradually merge into adjacent normal bone

appears. Calcification characteristically occurs at right angles to the cortex, producing a "sunburst" appearance. Pathologic fractures are rare. Grossly, the tumor is large and lobulated, with extension through cortical bone and into adjacent soft tissue. Microscopically, the predominant component may be bony, cartilaginous, or fibrous.

The treatment of osteogenic sarcoma consists of wide resection of the tumor, including the entire involved bone—rib or sternum—and adjacent soft tissues—lung or muscle. Radiation therapy has not been valuable in managing this neoplasm, and the role of chemotherapy remains controversial. In general, the prognosis is poor; the 5-year survival rate is 20%.

Tumors of the Manubrium, Sternum, Scapula, and Clavicle

Dahlin and Unni (1986) reported that primary neoplasms of the manubrium and sternum constitute 15% of all primary chest wall bone tumors. Nearly all—96%—are malignant. The majority are chondrosarcomas, myeloma, malignant lymphoma, and osteogenic sarcomas. In addition, the sternum is a frequent site of metastatic neoplasms, such as carcinomas originating in the breast, thyroid gland, or kidney; the last two often present as pulsating tumors. Benign tumors such as chondromas, hemangiomas, and bone cysts have been reported.

The scapula as Dahlin and Unni (1986) noted, is a common site for primary bone neoplasms, having an incidence of 2.8%, approximately half those of the ribs and sternum combined—5.9%. Although it is an infrequent

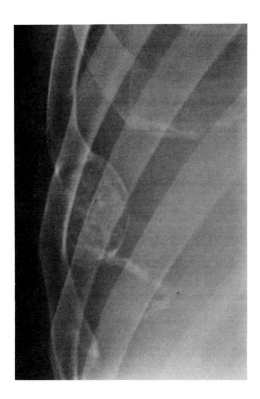

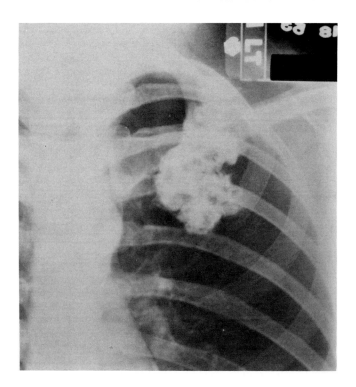

Fig. 50–6. Fifty-three-year-old man with chondrosarcoma of right anterior sixth rib. Mass had been present 18 months without pain. (Reproduced from McAfee, M.K., et al.: Chondrosarcoma of the chest wall: factors affecting survival. Ann. Thorac. Surg. *40*:535, 1985, with permission of the publisher.)

Fig. 50–7. Thirty-two-year-old woman with chondrosarcoma of left anterior first rib. Both supraclavicular pain and a mass had been present for two months. (Reproduced from McAfee, et al.: Chondrosarcoma of the chest wall: factors affecting survival. Ann. Thorac. Surg. *40*:535, 1985, with permission of the publisher.)

site for metastatic tumors, the same kinds of primary bone neoplasms occur in the scapula as in the rib cage. The malignant tumors include myeloma, Ewing's sarcoma, chondrosarcoma, osteogenic sarcoma, and lymphoma.

Primary neoplasms of the clavicle are uncommon, accounting for less than 1% of all primary bone tumors. Ninety percent are malignant. Over two thirds of the malignant tumors are radiosensitive, being either myelomas—43%—or Ewing's sarcoma—22%. The clavicle is more likely to be a site of metastatic disease than of primary tumors.

Arnold and I (1978) emphasized that primary malignant neoplasms of the manubrium, sternum, scapula, and clavicle should be treated by wide resection, including all of the involved bone and a 4-cm margin.

Primary Soft Tissue Tumors

Primary soft tissue tumors may arise from any component of the thoracic cage, and a variety have been reported, based upon a histologic diagnosis of the predominant cell type. Preoperative differentiation between these neoplasms is difficult. Pain often is present. Progressive enlargement is usually apparent by both physical and roentgenographic examination. Wide resection of the tumor and adjacent structures is the treatment of choice.

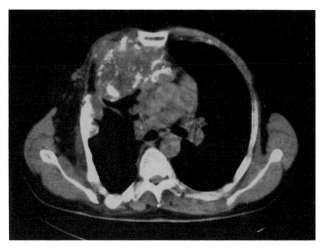

Fig. 50–8. Computerized tomography of a 59-year-old male with chondroscarcoma arising in the right anterior chest wall. Note destruction of cortex and stippling within neoplasm.

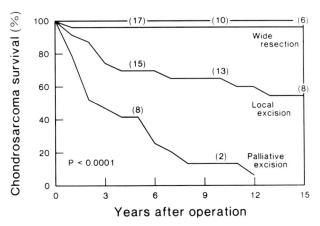

Fig. 50–9. Survival of patients with chest wall chondrosarcoma by extent of operation. Zero time on abscissa represents day of operation. (Reproduced from McAfee, et al.: Chondrosarcoma of the chest wall: factors affecting survival. Ann. Thorac. Surg. *40*:535, 1985, with permission of the publisher.)

Benign Soft Tissue Tumors

Various benign tumors involving all chest wall structures has been reported. Predominant among these are fibromas, lipomas, giant cell tumors, neurogenic tumors, vascular tumors, such as hemangiomas with or without arteriovenous fistulas, and less commonly, benign tumors of connective tissue. Malignant degeneration is uncommon, and all should be treated by local excision.

Desmoid. Desmoid tumor deserves special consideration. Forty percent of all desmoids occur in the shoulder and chest wall. Encapsulation of the brachial plexus and the vessels of the arm and neck is common. The tumor often extends into the pleural cavity, markedly displacing mediastinal structures (Fig. 50–10). Initially, the tumor presents as a poorly circumscribed mass with little or no pain. Paresthesias, hyperesthesia, and motor weakness occur later, following neural encasement. Veins or arteries are rarely occluded. Desmoid occurs most commonly between puberty and 40 years of age and is rarely observed in infants or the very old. Men and women are affected equally.

Grossly, the tumor originates in muscle and fascia and frequently extends along tissue planes. Microscopically, a monotonous pattern of elongated spindle-shaped

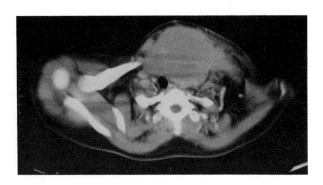

Fig. 50–10. Computerized tomogram of 35-year-old female with desmoid tumor arising in the left axilla. Note marked intrathoracic component displacing trachea and brachiocephalic vessels to left.

cells infiltrating the surrounding tissue is invariably seen. Most pathologists consider desmoid to be a form of benign fibromatosis as do Goellner and Soule (1980) and Hayry and associates (1982). Because these tumors invade adjacent structures, however, and because Soule and Scanlon (1962) reported malignant degeneration, some, including Hajdu (1979), consider it to be a low grade fibrosarcoma. Whatever the cause, the tumor tends to be recurrent if inadequately excised and should be treated with wide resection, like primary malignant chest wall neoplasms. Encapsulation of thoracic outlet structures presents a special problem in management. Enucleation of the tumor from these structures followed by radiation therapy is current practice.

Malignant Soft Tissue Tumors

Malignant Fibrous Histiocytoma. As I and Arnold (1985) and King and associates (1986) pointed out, malignant fibrous histiocytoma is the most common primary chest wall neoplasm the thoracic surgeon is asked to evaluate. The tumor characteristically occurs in late adult life, with the majority of cases occurring between the ages of 50 and 70. These neoplasms are rare in childhood, and approximately two thirds occur in men. Malignant fibrous histiocytoma often presents as a painless, slowly enlarging mass. Pregnancy, however, may accelerate the growth rate, resulting in pain. Weiss and Enzinger (1978) reported that fever and leukocytosis with neutropenia or eosinophilia are occasionally present. Excellent circumstantial evidence suggests that some chest wall malignant fibrous histiocytomas are radiation-induced; Weiss and Enzinger (1978) reported the development of this tumor within the irradiated area following therapy for breast cancer, Hodgkins' lymphoma, and myeloma.

Grossly malignant fibrous histiocytoma tends to be lobulated and to spread for considerable distances along fascial planes or between muscle fibers, which accounts for its high recurrence rate following resection. Histologically, the tumor has a highly variable morphologic pattern, ranging from well differentiated, elongated spindle cells to highly anaplastic pleomorphic histiocyte-like cells. The neoplasm is unresponsive to both irradiation and chemotherapy and should be treated by wide resection. Five-year survival is approximately 38% (Fig. 50–11).

Rhabdomyosarcoma. This is the second most common chest wall soft tissue malignant neoplasm and occurs most frequently in children and young adults. These tumors are rare after the age of 45, and men are affected only slightly more often than women. Rhabdomyosarcomas present as a rapidly enlarging mass that is usually deep-seated and is intimately associated with striated muscle tissue. Generally, the tumor is neither painful nor tender, despite evidence of rapid growth. Both grossly and microscopically it has few neoplastic characteristics. As with most rapidly growing tumors, the overall appearance reflects the degree of cellularity and the extent of secondary changes such as hemorrhage and necrosis.

Modern therapy had profoundly altered the clinical course of this disease. Wide resection followed by irra-

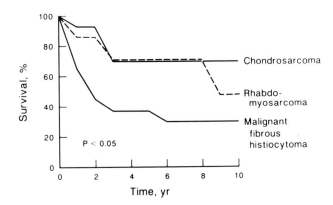

Fig. 50–11. Overall survival of patients with chest wall malignant neoplasms following resection. Zero time on abscissa represents day of chest wall resection. (Reproduced from King, et al.: Primary chest wall tumors: factors affecting survival. Ann. Thorac. Surg. *41*:597, 1986, with permission of the publisher.)

diation and multidrug chemotherapy has resulted in 5-year survivals of 70% (Fig. 50–11). Inadequately treated, the tumor rapidly recurs both locally and metastatically.

Liposarcoma. This is primarily a neoplasm of adult life, with the peak incidence between the ages of 40 and 60 years. It rarely occurs in infants and small children. Most patients are men. Malignant degeneration of a pre-existing lipoma is rare. Association with antecedent trauma has been reported.

Grossly, liposarcomas are well encapsulated and lobulated. Microscopically, abundant anaplastic lipoblasts are common. Treatment is with wide excision. Five-year survival is approximately 60%, and recurrence is usually local, reflecting incomplete excision. Radiation therapy and chemotherapy have little to offer.

Neurofibrosarcoma. Chest wall neurofibrosarcoma frequently occurs along the intercostal nerve and is typically a disease of adult life, occurring in persons between 20 and 50 years of age. Three fourths of these neoplasms occur in men, and approximatley half are associated with von Recklinghausen's disease. Grossly, the tumor is encapsulated. Microscopically, there is a monotonous pattern of elongated spindle-like cells that spread for considerable distances along the nerve sheath. Treatment is by wide excision.

Leiomyosarcoma. These are primarily neoplasms of adult life but occur less frequently than malignant fibrous histiocytoma and liposarcoma. Approximately two-thirds of patients are women. Children rarely develop these tumors. Most neoplasms present as a slowly enlarging mass that may be painful.

Grossly, leiomyosarcomas are whitish-gray and lobulated, with foci of hemorrhage and necrosis. Cyst for-

mation is often present. Microscopically, the tumor appears as swirling, elongated, spindle-like cells. Treatment is with wide excision. Recurrence is both local and metastatic.

CONCLUSIONS

The key to successful treatment of all chest wall tumors is still early diagnosis with aggressive surgical resection and adequate chest wall reconstruction. This procedure can generally be performed in one operation, with minimal respiratory insufficiency and with low operative mortality. Most importantly, current techniques allow potential long-term survival for all patients with primary chest wall tumor.

REFERENCES

Arnold, P.G., and Pairolero, P.C.: Chondrosarcoma of the manubrium. Resection and reconstruction with pectoralis major muscle. Mayo Clin. Proc. 53:54, 1978.
Arnold, P.G., and Pairolero, P.C.: Use of pectoralis major muscle flaps to repair defects of anterior chest wall. Plast. Reconstr. Surg. 63:205, 1979.
Arnold, P.G., and Pairolero, P.C.: Chest wall reconstruction: experience with 100 consecutive patients. Ann. Surg. 199:725, 1984.
Dahlin, D.C., and Unni, K.K.: Bone tumors: general aspects and data on 8,542 cases. Springfield, IL, Charles C. Thomas, 1986.
Goellner, J.R., and Soule, E.H.: Desmoid tumors: an ultrastructural study of eight cases. Hum. Pathol. 11:43, 1980.
Graeber, G.M., et al.: Initial and long-term results in the management of primary chest wall neoplasms. Ann. Thorac. Surg. 34:664, 1982.
Groff, D.B., and Adkins, P.C.: Chest wall tumors. Ann. Thorac. Surg. 4:260, 1967.
Hajdu, S.I.: Pathology of soft tissue tumors. Philadelphia, Lea & Febiger, 1979, pp. 122–135.
Hayry, P., et al: The desmoid tumor. II. Analysis of factors possibly contributing to the etiology and growth behavior. Am. J. Clin. Pathol. 77:674, 1982.
King, R.M., et al.: Primary chest wall tumors: factors affecting survival. Ann. Thorac. Surg. 41:597, 1986.
Lichtenstein, L., and Jaffe, H.L.: Chondrosarcoma of bone. Am. J. Pathol. 19:553, 1943.
Lichtenstein, L.: Bone Tumors, 5th ed. St. Louis, C.V. Mosby Co., 1977, p. 186.
McAfee, M.K., et al.: Chondrosarcoma of the chest wall: factors affecting survival. Ann. Thorac. Surg. 40:535, 1985.
Pairolero, P.C., and Arnold, P.G.: Chest wall tumors: experience with 100 consecutive patients. J. Thorac. Cardiovasc. Surg. 90:367, 1985.
Pairolero, P.C., and Arnold, P.G.: Thoracic wall defects: surgical management of 205 consecutive patients. Mayo Clin. Proc. 61:557, 1986.
Pascuzzi, C.A., Dahlin, D.C., and Clagett, O.T.: Primary tumors of the ribs and sternum. Surg. Gynecol. Obstet. 104:390, 1957.
Soule, E.G., and Scanlon, P.W.: Fibrosarcoma arising in an extra-abdominal desmoid tumor: report of a case. Mayo Clin. Proc. 37:443, 1962.
Stelzer, P., and Gay, W.A. Jr.: Tumors of the chest wall. Surg. Clin North Am. 60:779, 1980.
Weiss, S.W., and Enzinger, F.M.: Malignant fibrous histiocytoma: an analysis of 200 cases. Cancer 41:2250, 1978.

CHAPTER 51

CHEST WALL RECONSTRUCTION

Peter C. Pairolero

Reconstruction of chest wall defects has been a constant challenge to the surgeon. Since 1970, numerous authors have made significant contributions to reconstruction of the thorax. Muscle and musculocutaneous flaps of the latissimus dorsi, pectoralis major, serratus anterior, rectus abdominis, and external oblique muscles have been used most frequently. The clarification of the functional anatomy and blood supply of these muscles has resulted in more aggressive resections in the treatment of chest wall tumors and in the surgical amelioration of the ravages of radiation therapy. Reports by McCormack (1981), Larson (1982), Arnold (1986), and their colleagues and by me and Arnold (1985, 1986 a,b) confirmed that aggressive resection of the chest wall with immediate, dependable reconstruction is reasonable for managing these problems.

ETIOLOGY

Defects of the chest wall occur almost always as a result of neoplasm, irradiation, or infection (Table 51–1). The chest wall defect produced by resection of most neoplasms involves loss of the skeleton and frequently the overlying soft tissues as well. Infection, radiation necrosis, and trauma produce partial or full-thickness defects, depending upon their severity.

Table 51–1. Etiology of Chest Wall Defects

Neoplasm
  Primary chest wall
  Metastatic chest wall
  Contiguous lung cancer
  Contiguous breast cancer

Infection
  Median sternotomy wound
  Lateral thoracotomy wound
  Osteomyelitis
  Costochondritis

Radiation Necrosis

Trauma

CONSIDERATION FOR RECONSTRUCTION

The ability to close large chest wall defects is the main consideration in the surgical treatment of most chest wall afflictions. Excision should not be undertaken if the surgeon does not have the confidence and ability to close the defect. The critical questions of whether or not the reconstructed thorax will support respiration and protect the underlying organs must be answered when considering both the extent of resection and the method of reconstruction. This is true whether the thorax is involved with a neoplasm, an infection, or radiation necrosis. Adequate resection and dependable reconstruction are the mandatory ingredients for successful treatment. These two important items are accomplished most safely, as Arnold and I (1984) noted, by the joint efforts of a thoracic surgeon and a plastic surgeon.

Reconstruction of chest wall defects involves consideration of many factors (Table 51–2). The location and size are of utmost importance, but the past medical his-

Table 51–2. Considerations for Reconstruction of Chest Wall Defects

Location

Size

Depth
  Partial thickness
  Full thickness

Duration

Condition of Local Tissue
  Irradiation
  Infection
  Residual tumor
  Scarring

General Condition of Patient
  Chemotherapy
  Corticosteroid
  Chronic infection

Life Style and Type of Work

Prognosis

tory and local conditions of the wound may drastically alter a reconstructive choice. Primary closure remains the best option available when possible. If the defect is partial thickness and will accept and support a skin graft, reconstruction in this manner is quite reasonable. If a partial thickness defect will not reliably accept a skin graft, a situation that frequently occurs with radiation necrosis, omental transposition with skin grafting is used. If full-thickness reconstruction is required, both the structural stability of the thorax and soft tissue coverage must be considered.

SKELETAL RECONSTRUCTION

Reconstruction of the bony thorax is controversial. Differences of opinion exist about who should be reconstructed and what type of reconstruction should be done. In general, all full-thickness skeletal defects that have the potential for paradox should be reconstructed. The decision not to reconstruct the skeleton depends on the size and location of the defect. Defects less than 5 cm in greatest diameter anywhere on the thorax are usually not reconstructed. Posterior defects less than 10 cm likewise do not require reconstruction because the overlying scapula provides support. Larger defects, however, should be reconstructed, and autogenous tissue such as fascia lata or ribs and prosthetic material such as the various meshes, metals, or methyl methacrylate has been used.

Stabilization of the bony thorax is best accomplished with prosthetic material such as Prolene mesh (Ethicon, Inc., Somerville, NJ) or 2 mm polytetrafluoroethylene (Gore-tex) soft tissue patch (W.L. Gore and Associates, Inc., Elkton, MD). Placing either of these materials under tension improves the rigidity of the prosthesis in all directions. The soft tissue patch is superior because it prevents movement of fluid and air across the reconstructed chest wall. Marlex mesh (Daval, Inc., Providence, RI) is used less frequently because when placed under tension, it is rigid in one direction only. Reconstruction with rigid material such as methyl methacrylate impregnated meshes is not necessary.

Full-thickness skeletal defects resulting from excision of tumors of both the sternum and lateral chest wall should be reconstructed if the wound is not contaminated. If the wound is contaminated from previous radiation necrosis or necrotic neoplasm, reconstruction with prosthetic material is not advised, as the prosthesis may subsequently become infected, resulting in obligatory removal. In this situation, reconstruction with a musculocutaneous flap alone is preferred. Similarly, resection of the bony thorax in a patient who has been previously irradiated may not require skeletal reconstruction as the lung frequently adheres to the underlying parietal pleura and paradox does not occur. Covering radiation skin necrosis with soft tissue is frequently adequate.

SOFT TISSUE RECONSTRUCTION

Both muscle and omental transposition can be used to reconstruct soft tissue chest wall defects (Table 51–3).

Table 51–3. Autogenous Tissue Available for Chest Wall Reconstruction

Muscle
Latissimus dorsi
Pectoralis major
Rectus abdominis
Serratus anterior
External oblique
Trapezius
Omentum

Muscle is the tissue of choice for soft tissue coverage of full-thickness defects where skeletal reconstruction is not required. Muscle can be transposed as muscle alone or as a musculocutaneous flap. The omentum should be reserved for partial-thickness reconstruction or as a back-up procedure for muscle transposition that has failed in full-thickness defects.

Muscle Transpositon

Latissimus Dorsi

The latissimus dorsi muscle is the largest flat muscle in the thorax. Its dominant thoracodorsal neurovascular leash has an arc of rotation that allows coverage of the lateral and central back as well as the anterolateral and central front of the thorax as Campbell (1950) and Bostwick and associates (1979) pointed out. Its dependable musculocutaneous vascular connections also make it a reliable musculocutaneous flap. This muscle flap can cover huge chest wall defects because virtually one-half of the back can be elevated on the blood supply of a single latissimus dorsi muscle in the uninjured, nonirradiated patient (Fig. 51–1). The donor site may need skin grafts when large musculocutaneous flaps are elevated, but this represents a small disadvantage when considering that large, robust flaps can be transposed to either the anterior or posterior chest for full-thickness reconstruction. If the dominant blood supply has been compromised from previous trauma or surgery, Fisher and colleagues (1983) showed the muscle can still dependably be transposed on the branch of the adjacent serratus anterior muscle.

Pectoralis Major

The pectoralis major muscle is the second largest flat muscle on the chest wall and in many respects is the mirror image of the latissimus dorsi muscle. As Arnold and I (1979) reported, its dominant thoracoacromial neurovascular leash, which enters posteriorly about midclavicle, allows both elevation of the muscle, either as a muscle or musculocutaneous flap, and rotation centrally for chest wall reconstruction. The pectoralis major muscle is equally as reliable as the latissimus dorsi flap. I and Arnold (1984, 1986b) showed that it is beneficial in reconstructing anterior chest wall defects such as those resulting from sternal tumor excisions and infected median sternotomy wounds (Fig. 51–2). Generally, only the muscle is transposed, and the skin can be closed pri-

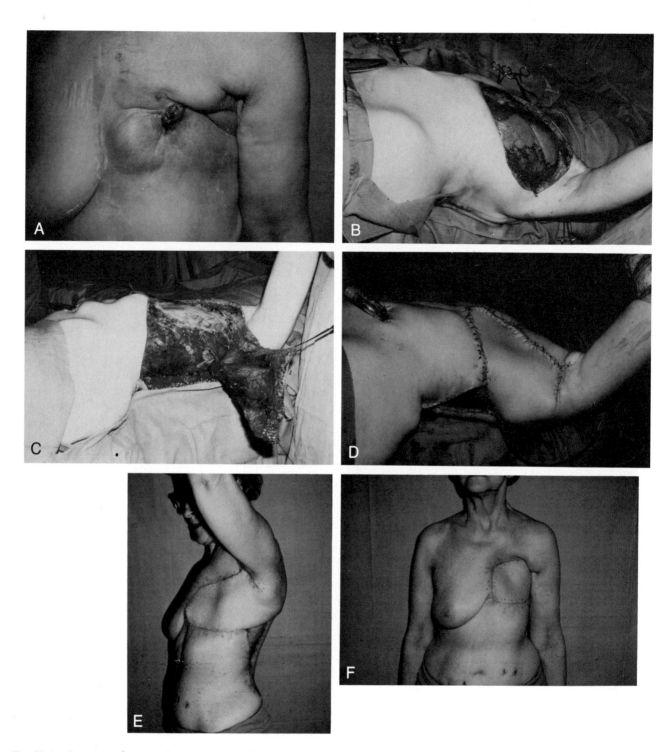

Fig. 51–1. Latissimus dorsi muscle. *A*, Sixty-year-old woman 4 years after mastectomy with recurrent tumor involving full-thickness chest wall. *B*, Intraoperative view at the time of full-thickness chest wall resection. *C*, The thoracic skeleton has been replaced with Prolene mesh and a large left latissimus dorsi musculocutaneous flap elevated. *D*, The musculocutaneous flap has been rotated into place and a portion of the donor site skin grafted. *E* and *F*, Appearance of the chest wall 3 months following resection. (Reproduced from Arnold, P.G., and Pairolero, P.C.: Chest wall reconstruction: experience with 100 consecutive patients. Pairolero, P.C.: Ann. Surg. *199*:725, 1984, with permission of the publisher.)

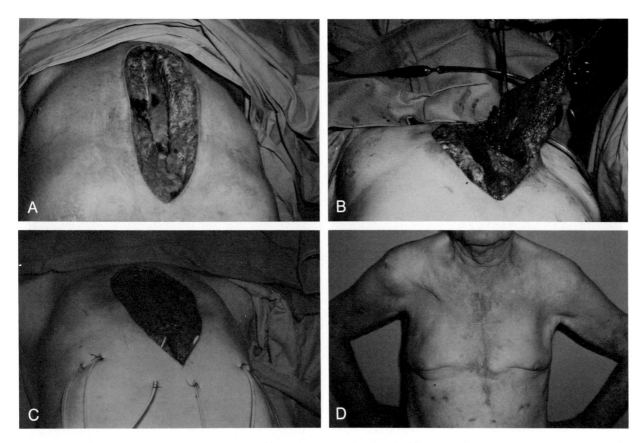

Fig. 51–2.   Pectoralis major muscle. *A,* Seventy-two-year-old male approximately 3 months following median sternotomy for coronary artery bypass graft for coronary artery disease. This is the appearance after multiple debridements that removed essentially the central portion of the sternum. *B,* At the time of closure the left pectoralis major muscle is totally mobilized and separated from the humeral attachment. The right pectoralis major muscle is mobilized over the midaxillary line but not separated from its humeral attachment. *C,* The two muscles are sutured together in the midline and a large portion of the left pectoralis major muscle is draped into the defect in the central sternal area. *D,* Appearance approximately 3 months following closure. (Reproduced from Arnold, P.G., and Pairolero, P.C.: Chest wall reconstruction: experience with 100 consecutive patients. Ann. Surg. *199:*725, 1984, with permission of the publisher.)

marily, thereby avoiding the distortion created by centralizing the breast. Reconstruction in this manner is more symmetrical and aesthetically acceptable. If central skin must be excised, symmetry of the breast can still be maintained, because the transposed muscle readily accepts and supports an overlying skin graft. If necessary, the muscle can also be transposed on its secondary blood supply through the perforators from the internal mammary vessels.

Rectus Abdominis

Use of the rectus abdominis muscle for chest wall reconstruction is based on the internal mammary neurovascular leash. The inferior epigastric vessels must be divided to allow rotation to the chest wall. This muscle can be mobilized and moved either as a muscle or as a musculocutaneous flap (Fig. 51–3) with the skin component oriented either horizontally or vertically or both. The vertical skin flap, however, is more reliable because it is oriented along the long axis of the muscle and thus maintains more musculocutaneous perforators. The donor site is usually closed primarily.

I and Arnold (1985) believe the rectus abdominis muscle is most useful in reconstruction of lower sternal

wounds. Either muscle can be used, as their arcs of rotation are identical. The muscle that has patent and uninjured internal mammary vessels must be chosen. Angiographic demonstration of vessel patency may help determine which musculocutaneous unit would be most reliable, particularly in previously irradiated patients or in patients with infected sternotomy wounds. Also, in many infected sternotomy wounds the internal mammary artery may have previously been used for coronary artery bypass.

Serratus Anterior

The serratus anterior muscle is a small flat muscle located in the midaxillary line between the latissimus dorsi and pectoralis major muscles. Its blood supply comes from the serratus branch of the thoracodorsal vessels and from the long thoracic artery and vein. This muscle can be used alone or as an adjunctive muscle with the pectoralis major or the latissimus dorsi muscles. As Arnold and colleagues (1984) pointed out, the muscle also augments the skin-carrying ability of either adjacent muscle. I and my colleagues (1983) found that this muscle is particularly useful as an intrathoracic muscle flap.

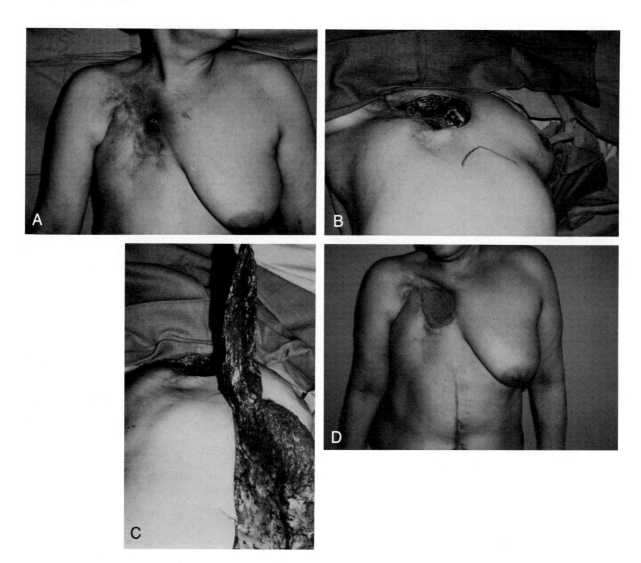

Fig. 5–3. Rectus abdominis muscle. *A,* Forty-nine-year-old woman 5 years following mastectomy and radiation therapy with radionecrotic area on the right chest. *B,* The wound is excised, including a portion of the right sternum and the right anterior chest wall. *C,* Contralateral (left) rectus abdominis muscle is elevated for transposition into the defect. *D,* Four months after closure with split-thickness skin graft over the transposed rectus abdominis muscle. (Reproduced from Arnold, P.G. and Pairolero, P.C.: Chest wall reconstruction: experience with 100 consecutive patients. Ann. Surg. *199*:725, 1984, with permission of the publisher.)

External Oblique

The external oblique muscle can also be transposed as a muscle or musculocutaneous flap (Fig. 51–4), and it is most useful in closing defects of the upper abdomen and lower thorax. It reaches the inframammary fold without tension but, as Hodgkinson and Arnold (1980) noted, does not readily extend higher. The primary blood supply is from the lower thoracic intercostal vessels as Lund (1913), Hedblom (1921), Harrington (1927), Zinninger (1930), Maier (1947), Watson and James (1947) and Bisgard and Swensen (1948) demonstrated. With this muscle, lower chest wall defects can be closed without distorting the breast.

Trapezius Muscle

The trapezius muscle has been useful to close defects at the base of the neck or the thoracic outlet but is not consistently useful for other chest wall reconstructions. Its primary blood supply is the dorsal scapular vessels.

Omental Transposition

Omental transposition, as Jurkiewicz and Arnold (1977) noted has been most useful in reconstructing partial-thickness chest wall defects, particularly in radiation necrosis that does not involve tumor (Fig. 51–5). In this situation, the skin and soft tissue are debrided down to what remains of the thoracic skeleton, which may be either bone or cartilage but frequently is only irradiated ischemic scar. The transposed omentum with its excellent blood supply from the gastroepiploic vessels adheres to the irradiated wound and readily accepts and supports an overlying skin graft. Because the omentum has no structural stability of its own, it is not particularly useful

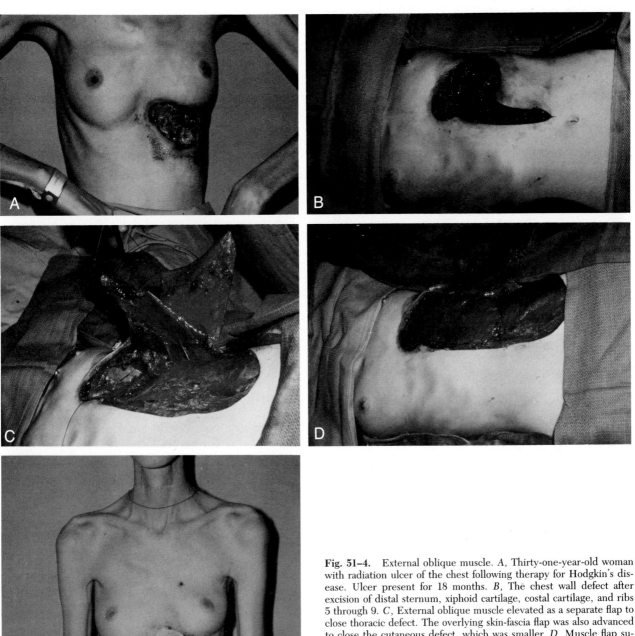

Fig. 51–4. External oblique muscle. *A*, Thirty-one-year-old woman with radiation ulcer of the chest following therapy for Hodgkin's disease. Ulcer present for 18 months. *B*, The chest wall defect after excision of distal sternum, xiphoid cartilage, costal cartilage, and ribs 5 through 9. *C*, External oblique muscle elevated as a separate flap to close thoracic defect. The overlying skin-fascia flap was also advanced to close the cutaneous defect, which was smaller. *D*, Muscle flap sutured into position to close the chest wall defect. *E*, Four months postoperatively. (Reproduced from Hodgkinson, D.J. and Arnold, P.G.: Chest wall reconstruction using the external oblique muscle. Br. J. Plast. Surg. 33:216, 1980, with permission of the publisher.)

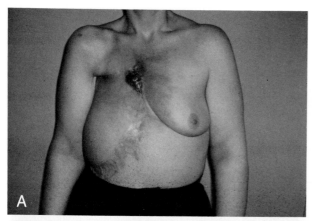

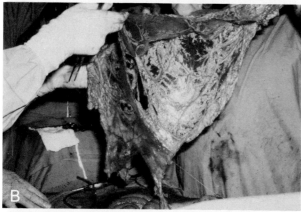

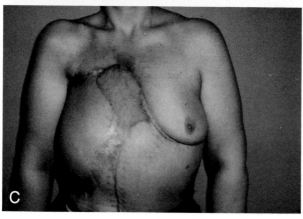

Fig. 51–5. Omentum. *A,* Forty-four-year-old woman after modified mastectomy with radiation. Radiation necrosis previously treated by rotation of large cutaneous flap based on the right. Wound breakdown developed, and the present problem required excision of skin and soft tissue only; there was no evidence of recurrent tumor; *B,* Greater omentum was mobilized on right gastroepiploic vessels in preparation for transposition into defect. *C,* Appearance of chest 6 months after closure, with a stable split-thickness skin graft. (Reproduced from Arnold, P.G and Pairolero, P.C.: Chest wall reconstruction: experience with 100 consecutive patients. Ann. Surg. *199:*725, 1984, with permission of the publisher.)

in full-thickness defects because additional support, such as fascia lata, bone, or prosthetic material, is necessary.

Omental transposition is helpful when planned muscle flaps have failed with partial necrosis. Generally, this results in only a soft tissue defect, and pleural seal with respiratory stability is not required, thus allowing a most threatening situation to be salvaged.

Infected Median Sternotomy Wounds

Infected median sternotomy wounds present a special problem as I and Arnold (1984) noted. Left untreated, these infections can extend to aortic and cardiac suture lines, prosthetic grafts, and intracardiac prostheses. In addition, septic thrombosis may develop in aortocoronary grafts. Early recognition of sternal wound infection is crucial for successful management.

The pectoralis major muscle is ideal for closing infected sternotomy wounds. Mobilizing this muscle allows an arc of rotation that reaches the entire anterior thoracic wall except the lower sternum. If the sternum has been resected, the muscle is mobilized from the nondominant side of the patient by completely dividing the humeral attachments and transposing the muscle into the sternal defect to obliterate the mediastinal space. The contralateral muscle is then transposed without humeral division to cover the deeper muscle, and the wound is closed. If the sternum has not been resected, mobilization of one or both muscles without division of humeral attachments is generally sufficient for closing upper sternotomy wounds.

Infections of the lower sternum are best treated with either a rectus abdominis muscle flap or an omental transposition. The rectus abdominis muscle is preferred for small wounds because laparotomy and potential peritoneal contamination are avoided. The blood supply to this muscle, however, is based on the distal aspect of the internal mammary artery, which may have been interrupted previously either by use of this artery for coronary revascularization or by ligation with sternal resection. If the internal mammary artery is not intact or if the wound is large, omental transposition is performed, followed by split-thickness skin grafting 48 hours later.

CLINICAL EXPERIENCE

Arnold and I (1984) and I and Arnold (1986a) reported over 200 consecutive chest wall reconstructions performed at the Mayo Clinic during the past 10 years; 114 patients had chest wall tumor, 56 had radiation necrosis, 56 had infected median sternotomy wounds, 8 had costochrondritis, and 29 patients had a combination of these. Ages ranged from 12 to 85 years, with a mean of 53.4 years. One hundred seventy-eight patients underwent skeletal resection of the chest wall. An average of 5.4 ribs was resected. Total or partial sternectomies were performed in 60 patients. Skeletal defects were closed with prosthetic material in 66 patients and with autogenous ribs in 12. One hundred sixty-eight patients underwent 244 muscle transpositions including 56 latissimus dorsi, 49 pectoralis major, 14 rectus abdominis, 13 serratus anterior, 8 external oblique, and 2 trapezius transpositions, and 2 advancements of the diaphragm. The omentum was transposed in 20 patients.

The mean number of operations per patient was 1.9. Most of the multiple procedures were debridements in patients with infected wounds. Hospitalization averaged 16.5 days. There was one perioperative death. Four patients required tracheostomy. Most other patients, as Meadows and associates (1985) reported, had only minor changes in pulmonary function.

Follow-up averaged 32.4 months. There were 49 late deaths, predominantly from pulmonary or distant metastases. No late deaths related to either resection or reconstruction of the chest wall occurred. All patients who were alive 30 days after operation had excellent results at the time of the last follow-up or at death.

CONCLUSION

Reconstruction of many chest wall defects can be performed in one operation, with minimal respiratory insufficiency, a short hospitalization, and low operative mortality. The key ingredients for successful management are accomplished most safely by the joint efforts of a thoracic and a plastic surgeon.

REFERENCES

Arnold, P.G., and Pairolero, P.C.: Use of pectoralis major muscle flaps to repair defects of the anterior chest wall. Plast. Reconstr. Surg. 63:205, 1979.

Arnold, P.G., Pairolero, P.C., and Waldorf, J.C.: The serratus anterior muscle: intrathoracic and extrathoracic utilization. Plast. Reconstr. Surg. 73:240, 1984.

Arnold, P.G., and Pairolero, P.C.: Chest wall reconstruction: experience with 100 consecutive patients. Ann. Surg. 199:725, 1984.

Arnold, P.G., and Pairolero, P.C.: Surgical management of the radiated chest wall. Plast. Reconstr. Surg 77:605, 1986.

Bisgard, J.D., and Swenson, S.A., Jr.: Tumors of the sternum: report of a case with special operative technic. Arch. Surg. 56:570, 1948.

Blades, B., and Paul, J.S.: Chest wall tumors. Ann. Surg. 131:976, 1950.

Bostwick, J., III, et al: Sixty latissimus dorsi flaps. Plast. Reconstr. Surg. 63:31, 1979.

Campbell, D.A.: Reconstruction of the anterior thoracic wall. J. Thorac. Surg. 19:456, 1950.

Fisher, J., Bostwick, J., and Powell, R.W.: Latissimus dorsi blood supply after thoracodorsal vessel division: the serratus collateral. Plast. Reconstr. Surg. 72:502, 1983.

Harrington, S.W.: Surgical treatment of intrathoracic tumors and tumors of the chest wall. Arch. Surg. 14:406, 1927.

Hedblom, C.A.: Tumors of the bony chest wall. Arch. Surg. 3:56, 1921.

Hodgkinson, D.J., and Arnold, P.G.: Chest-wall reconstruction using the external oblique muscle. Br. J. Plast. Surg. 33:216, 1980.

Jurkiewicz, M.J., and Arnold, P.G.: The omentum: an account of its use in the reconstruction of the chest wall. Ann. Surg. 185:548, 1977.

Larson, D.L., et al: Major chest wall reconstruction after chest wall irradiation. Cancer 49:1286, 1982.

Lund, F.B.: Sarcoma of the chest wall. Ann. Surg. 58:206, 1913.

Maier, H.C.: Surgical management of large defects of the thoracic wall. Surgery 22:169, 1947.

McCormack, P., et al: New trends in skeletal reconstruction after resection of chest wall tumors. Ann. Thorac. Surg. 31:45, 1981.

Meadows, J.A., III, et al.: Effect of resection of the sternum and manubrium in conjunction with muscle transposition on pulmonary function. Mayo Clin. Proc. 60:604, 1985.

Pairolero, P.C., and Arnold, P.G.: Management of recalcitrant median sternotomy wounds. J. Thorax. Cardiovasc. Surg. 88:357, 1984.

Pairolero, P.C., and Arnold, P.G.: Chest wall tumors: Experience with 100 consecutive patients. J. Thorac. Cardiovasc. Surg. 90:367, 1985.

Pairolero, P.C., and Arnold, P.G.: Thoracic wall defects: surgical management of 205 consecutive patients. Mayo Clin. Proc. 61:557, 1986a.

Pairolero, P.C., and Arnold, P.G.: Primary tumors of the anterior chest wall. Surgical Rounds 9:19, 1986b.

Pairolero, P.C., Arnold, P.G., and Piehler, J.M.: Intrathoracic transposition of extrathoracic skeletal muscle. J. Thorac. Cardiovasc. Surg. 86:809, 1983.

Watson, W.L., and James, A.G.: Fascia lata grafts for chest wall defects. J. Thorac. Surg. 16:399, 1947.

Zinninger, M.M.: Tumors of the wall of the thorax. Ann. Surg. 92:1043, 1930.

READING REFERENCES

Blades, B., and Paul, J.S.: Chest wall tumors. Ann Surg. 131:976, 1950.

Boyd, A.D., et al.: Immediate reconstruction of full-thickness chest wall defects. Ann. Thorac. Surg. 32:337, 1981.

Brown, R.G., Fleming, W.H., and Jurkiewicz, M.J.: An island flap of the pectoralis major muscle. Br. J. Plast. Surg. 30:161, 1977.

Burnard, R.J., Martini, N., and Beattie, E.J., Jr.: The value of resection in tumors involving the chest wall. J. Thorac. Cardiovasc. Surg. 68:530, 1974.

Converse, J.M., Campbell, R.M., and Watson, W.L.: Repair of large radiation ulcers situated over the heart and the brain. Ann. Surg. 133:95, 1951.

Fell, G.E.: Forced respiration. J.A.M.A. 16:325, 1891.

Graham E.A., and Singer, J.J.: Successful removal of an entire lung for carcinoma of the bronchus. J.A.M.A. 101:1371, 1933.

Irons, G.B., et al: Use of the omental free flap for soft-tissue reconstruction. Ann. Plast. Surg. 11:501, 1983.

Jurkiewicz, M.J., et al.: Infected median sternotomy wound: successful treatment by muscle flaps. Ann. Surg. 191:738, 1980.

Kiricuta, I.: L'emploi du grand epiploon dans la chirurgie du sein cancereux. Presse Med 71:15, 1963.

Le Roux, B.T.: Maintenance of chest wall stability. Thorax 19:397, 1964.

Martini, N., Starzynski, T.E., and Beattie, E.J., Jr.: Problems in chest wall resection. Surg. Clin. North Am. 49:313, 1969.

McGraw, J.B., Penix, J.O., and Baker, J.W.: Repair of major defects of the chest wall and spine with the latissimus dorsi myocutaneouus flap. Plast. Reconstr. Surg. 62:197, 1978.

Myre, T.T., Kirklin, JW.: Resection of tumors of the sternum. Ann. Surg. 144:1023, 1956.

O'Dwyer, J.: Fifty cases of croup in private practice treated by intubation of the larynx with a description of the method and of the dangers incident thereto. Med. Rec. 32:557, 1887.

Parham, F.W.: Thoracic resection for tumors growing from the bony wall of the chest. Trans. South. Surg. Gynecol. Assoc. 11:223, 1898.

Pickrell, K.L., Kelley, J.W., and Marzoni, F.A.: The surgical treatment of recurrent carcinoma of the breast and chest wall. Plast. Reconstr. Surg. 3:156, 1948.

Ramming, K.P., et al.: Surgical management and reconstruction of extensive chest wall malignancies. Am. J. Surg. 144:146, 1982.

Rees, TD., and Converse, J.M.: Surgical reconstruction of defects of the thoracic wall. Surg. Gynecol. Obstet. 121:1066, 1965.

Starzynski, T.E., Snyderman, R.K., and Beattie, E.J., Jr.: Problems of major chest wall reconstruction. Plast. Reconstr. Surg. 44:525, 1969.

The Diaphragm

CHAPTER 52

PARALYSIS AND OTHER PATHOLOGIC CONDITIONS OF THE DIAPHRAGM

Thomas W. Shields

Although the major anatomic function of the diaphragm is the separation of the thoracic and abdominal cavities, its major physiologic function is its role in ventilation. The movement of this musculotendinous structure is responsible for the largest fraction of air moved during inspiration. With quiet breathing, this accounts for approximately 75 to 80% of the total amount of air brought into the lungs.

Primarily, the diaphragm is a muscle of inspiration, and the downward descent of the central tendon results from a coordinated contraction of all its muscle fibers. The resultant vertical movement is approximately 1 to 2 cm during quiet breathing, but may be as great as 6 to 7 cm with deep, forced breathing. It is estimated that each centimeter of vertical movement contributes an intake of approximately 300 to 400 ml of air during normal breathing.

Some muscular activity of the diaphragm, however, does occur during exhalation. Contraction of the diaphragmatic muscle fibers does not cease abruptly at the onset of expiration but gradually declines during the initial portion of expiration and reaches zero at about the midpoint of expiration. Persistent diaphragmatic activity during the early phase of expiration provides precise regulation of the shift in air flow from inspiration to expiration. During vigorous breathing efforts, activity of the diaphragm also occurs toward the end of maximum expiratory efforts. The muscular activity at this time, as Agostoni and Torri (1962) reported, limits the degree to which the lungs collapse.

Either the right or left hemidiaphragm may be paralyzed without significant respiratory embarrassment in the normal person. Although ventilation on the paralyzed side is maintained by transmission of the cyclic pressure changes produced by the functioning hemidiaphragm across the mediastinum, initially, a 20 to 30% reduction occurs in the vital capacity and the total lung capacity. Fackler and co-workers (1967) reported the return of these lung volumes to normal after 6 months. Bilateral diaphragmatic paralysis may be tolerated by normal persons, but as McCredie and associates (1962) noted, a marked reduction of vital capacity and expiratory flow rates results, particularly while the individual is in the supine position.

PARALYSIS OF THE DIAPHRAGM

Paralysis of the hemidiaphragm may be suggested by an elevated leaf of the diaphragm on a roentgenogram of the chest, but may be identified positively only by the fluoroscopic observation of paradoxic movement of the paralyzed hemidiaphragm. This movement is best demonstrated by the classic "sniff" test. The sudden inspiratory movement causes the normal hemidiaphragm to descend, whereas the paralyzed hemidiaphragm will move in the opposite direction.

Paralysis may result from tumor invasion of the phrenic nerve or involvement of the nerve trunk or its motor nerve cells in the spinal cord by infection or trauma. The paralysis may be temporary or permanent. Unexplained paralysis frequently is a result of a viral infection, and bilateral paralysis may occur. Piehler and co-workers (1982) reviewed the records of 142 patients with unexplained diaphragmatic paralysis. Less than half were symptomatic. Subsequent improvement was better in those who had pain or cough than in those with dyspnea. Only 3.5% had an underlying malignancy and only one patient—0.7%—had progressive atrophy. The diaphragm returned to a normal position in less than 10%.

Therapeutic temporary paralysis of a phrenic nerve has been used in the past for treatment of pulmonary tuberculosis. This procedure can be used to elevate the hemidiaphragm to help obliterate the pleural space after the removal of a portion of the lung. Temporary paralysis can be obtained postoperatively by percutaneous infiltration of the nerve trunk in the neck with a local anesthetic solution, or at times, direct exposure of the nerve in the neck will be required. Mechanical injury to the nerve at the time of thoracotomy and pulmonary resection is best avoided as a routine measure, even if a residual pleural space is anticipated, because the paradoxic movement of the diaphragmatic leaf interferes with an effective cough mechanism.

INFECTIONS INVOLVING THE DIAPHRAGM

Temporary hemidiaphragmatic elevation, fixation, and even paralysis commonly result from infection above or below the diaphragm. Treatment by appropriate drainage of the infected area usually solves most of the problems. On rare occasions, however, such infections may result in perforation of the diaphragm and produce a diaphragmatic defect, which may require repair.

DIAPHRAGMATIC HERNIAS

Although herniation through the diaphragm may occur, but rarely, through defects resulting from infection, most hernias occur through the normal apertures or congenital defects (Fig. 52–1). The normal apertures of the diaphragm, through which pass the esophagus, aorta, and inferior vena cava, are tightly sealed with an investing layer of pleura above and a layer of peritoneum below. This thick layer of tissue continues over the structures passing through the diaphragm and forms a tight seal. If this investing layer of tissue is interrupted either above or below the diaphragm, a hernia may form. The communication that develops may result from congenital absence of part of the diaphragm, incomplete formation of the various layers of the diaphragm, incomplete migration of the foregut, or faulty formation of vascular structures. Hernias may also follow trauma or stress or, on occasion, may be iatrogenic.

Diaphragmatic hernias can be divided into the congenital and acquired hernias, but this division is artificial, because congenital weakness may be a contributing factor in the formation of acquired hernias. The various diaphragmatic hernias are discussed in detail in other chapters: traumatic hernias in Chapter 46, congenital posterolateral diaphragmatic hernias—Bochdalek hernias—in Chapter 53, parasternal hernia—foramen of Morgagni—and other congenital hernias in Chapter 54, paraesophageal hernias in Chapter 55 and sliding esophageal hiatal hernias in Chapter 82.

EVENTRATION OF THE DIAPHRAGM

Eventration of the diaphragm is a rare anomaly, the cause of which still is to be understood completely. In general, congenital eventration of the diaphragm or the eventration occurring in newborn infants is probably a true congenital defect acquired during the fetal period. Severe cardiorespiratory symptoms in the newborn or neonate with a large unilateral eventration may be present because of secondary hypoplasia of the lung on the involved side. The appropriate resuscitative measures are required to correct acid-base balance, ventilatory insufficiency, and poor systemic perfusions as in the neonate with a symptomatic congenital posterolateral diaphragmatic hernia (Chapter 53). Once the condition of the newborn is stabilized, surgical correction of the eventration is indicated.

The repair of the defect is an emergency procedure in newborns or neonates with respiratory distress. It usually is accomplished through a thoracic approach. An incision is made in the circumference of the diaphragm, a few centimeters from the costal margin. The thinned-out diaphragm then is put on a stretch and reattached to the costal margin.

Eventration that occurs in children and adults is

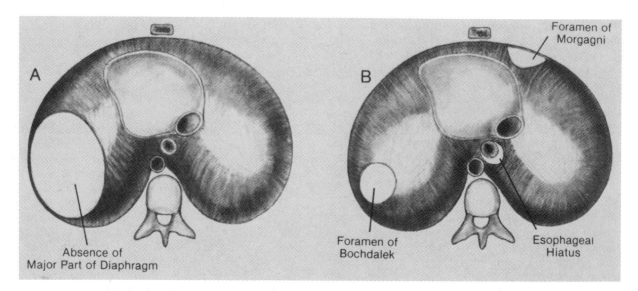

Fig. 51–1. Congenital defects of the diaphragm. *A,* Congenital absence of a major portion of the left hemidiaphragmatic leaf. *B,* Parasternal—foramen of Morgagni—defect, posterolateral—foramen of Bochdalek—defect in the left, and congenital enlargement of the esophageal hiatus. (Reproduced with permission of Hood, M.: Techniques in General Thoracic Surgery, Philadelphia, W.B. Saunders Co., 1985.)

thought to be caused by an acquired complete or incomplete paralysis of the diaphragmatic leaf. In infants, acquired eventration may result from birth trauma or operative injury for correction or palliation of congenital cardiac lesions. Smith and associates (1986) found that Blalock-Taussig shunts caused most of the acquired eventrations. They also found that plication was a safe procedure that could be performed either through a thoracic or an abdominal approach. Failure to achieve extubation within a week was a poor prognostic sign. When this occurred in infants, the overall mortality—67%—was high, particularly in the presence of major associated conditions. More often than not, localized eventration, which usually occurs on the right, with protrusion of liver through the defect, does not require surgical treatment. The older patient may have cardiorespiratory or gastrointestinal symptoms, or both, secondary to the eventration. Operative repair is indicated for the older patient who has symptoms. A transthoracic approach is preferred. Entry into the pleural space is made through the bed of the eighth rib or the eighth intercostal space. After any adhesions that may be present are freed, the thinned-out diaphragmatic leaf is incised. Repair is then carried out by imbricating one layer over the other with interrupted sutures of No. 00 or No. 0 silk or other nonabsorbable suture material (Fig. 52–2). This repair is usually attended with low mortality and morbidity rates. A second method of repair is by plication, illustrated in Figure 52–3. Wright and associates (1985) achieved excellent relief of exertional dyspnea and orthopnea following transthoracic diaphragmatic plication of unilateral, nonmalignant diaphragmatic paralysis. There was a significant increase in arterial oxygen tension and all lung volumes except residual volume in their patients.

Agenesis of the diaphragm and the presence of an accessory diaphragm have been reported by Nazarian (1971) and Geisler (1977) and their colleagues. A syndrome described by Spitz and associates (1975) consists of midline supraumbilical abdominal wall defects, defects of the lower sternum, deficiency of the anterior diaphragm and diaphragmatic pericardium, and congenital cardiac defects—Cantrell's pentalogy (Chapter 47).

TUMORS OF THE DIAPHRAGM

Primary tumors of the diaphragm are rare. They are mainly of a mesenchymal origin, because almost all of the diaphragmatic structure is derived from mesenchyme; however, neurogenic tumors do occur. In series reported in the literature and those from the Ohio State University Hospital, the incidence of benign tumors is slightly higher than that of malignant tumors (Table 52–1).

The clinical manifestations of diaphragmatic tumors are not specific, but in general, the patients complain of pain with breathing. The first evidence of any problem may be a nondescript feeling of fullness in the subcostal area. Half of the reported neurogenic tumors of the diaphragm, Trivedi (1958) noted, were associated with hy-

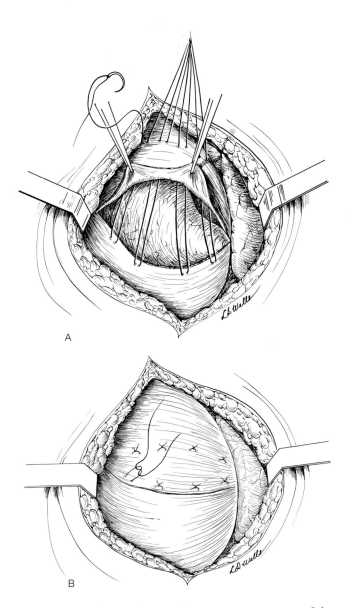

Fig. 52–2. Technique of repair of symptomatic eventration of the diaphragm. (Shields, T.W.: The diaphragm. *In* Operative Surgery: Principles and Techniques, Chapter 16. Edited by P. Nora. Philadelphia, Lea & Febiger, 1972.)

pertrophic pulmonary osteoarthropathy. Most benign tumors, however, are symptomless and are discovered only on routine roentgenograms of the chest. The usual roentgenographic examinations are generally insufficient for positive identification of a diaphragmatic tumor, and special studies, such as pneumoperitoneum (Fig. 52–4) and arteriography (Fig. 52–5), may be needed to identify such tumors. Pneumoperitoneum is useful, especially in differentiating diaphragmatic tumors located on the right from tumors of the liver.

Surgical removal, when possible, is indicated for all tumors of the diaphragm. If the tumor is located in the periphery of the diaphragm, the adjacent portion of the diaphragm and part of the chest wall may be removed in continuity. In certain selected instances, enough nor-

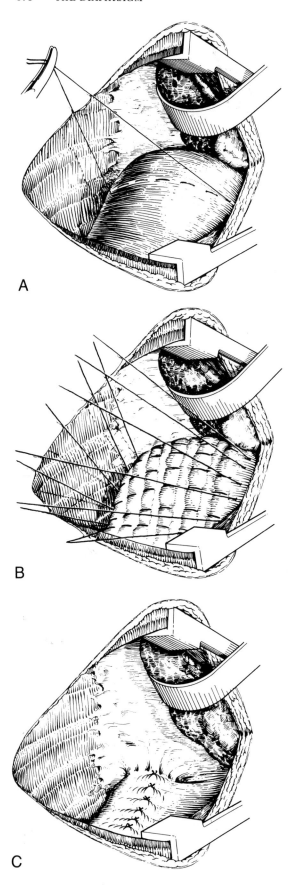

A

B

C

Fig. 52–3. Techniques of plication of an eventration of a diaphragmatic leaf. *A*, Four to six rows of 00 or 000 nonabsorbable sutures are inserted into the hemidiaphragm in an anterolateral to a posteromedial direction. Each row consists of five to six pleats. The branches of the phrenic nerve are avoided when the nerve is still functional. *B*, The sutures are left untied until all rows are in place. *C*, Sutures tied to plicate and shorten the nonfunctioning leaf. (Reproduced with permission of Spitz, L.: Rob and Smith's Operative Surgery: Thoracic Surgery, 4th Ed. Edited by J.W. Jackson and D.K.C. Cooper. London, Butterworths, p. 7.)

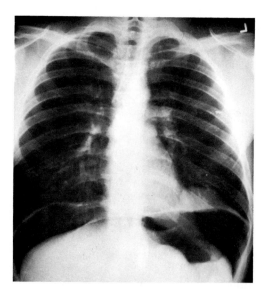

Fig. 52–4. The diagnosis of a diaphragmatic tumor was easily confirmed by a pneumoperitoneum. This tumor was excised and found to be a fibrosarcoma.

Table 52–1. Primary Tumors of the Diaphragm*

Benign	Number	Malignant	Number
Angiofibroma	3	Chondrosarcoma	1
Adenomas	2	Fibroangioendothelioma	1
Chondroma	1	Fibromyosarcoma	2
Cysts	12	Fibrosarcoma	9
Fibroma	3	Hemangioendothelioma	1
Fibrolymphangioma	1	Hemangiopericytoma	1
Fibromyoma	1	Leiomyosarcoma	1
Hamartoma	1	Mesothelioma	2
Lymphangioma	1	Myosarcoma	2
Leiomyoma	1	Neurofibrosarcoma	2
Lipoma	11	Rhabdomyosarcoma	3
Neurofibroma	4	Sarcoma, various cell types	7
Rhabdomyofibroma	1	Synovioma	1
TOTALS	42		33

*Collected from the literature, including six diaphragmatic tumors seen at Ohio State University Hospitals, Columbus, Ohio.

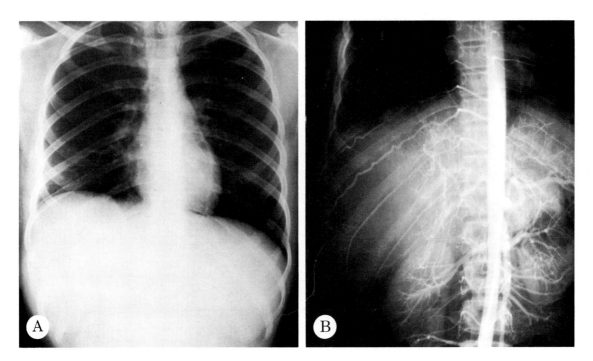

Fig. 52–5. *A,* PA roentgenogram of the chest revealing an elevated hemidiaphragm. Suggestion of the presence of a mass occupying the lateral three fourths of the right diaphragmatic leaf is noted. *B,* Aortogram of the same patient shown in *A,* demonstrating displacement of the normal vascular structures in the liver by a large neurofibroma of the diaphragm. Hypertrophy of the intercostal vessels is visualized clearly on this aortogram.

mal diaphragm may be left after the tumor has been removed to permit advancement of the remaining segment up the chest wall for reattachment to the rib cage. In general, with an aggressive approach and with removal of as wide a margin of normal tissue as possible, insufficient tissue for closure will remain. Marlex mesh or a Gore–Tex soft tissue patch is an adequate substitute for replacing large portions of the diaphragm that have been removed during excision of the tumor. Postoperative radiation therapy may be indicated, depending on the histologic type of the tumor.

The morbidity and mortality rates after excision of diaphragmatic tumors are minimal. Ventilatory loss on the side of the resection is noted, but the magnitude of such losses has not been documented.

The prognosis after resection of benign tumors, as would be expected, is excellent. However, after excision of most, if not all, of the malignant lesions, the prognosis is poor. Recurrence of a malignant lesion is common and death is the usual result.

REFERENCES

Agostoni, E., and Torri, G.: Diaphragm contraction as a limit to maximum expiration. J. Appl. Physiol. *17*:427, 1962.
Fackler, C.D., Perret, G.E., and Bedell, G.N.: Effect of unilateral

phrenic nerve section on lung function. J. Appl. Physiol. *23*:923, 1967.

Geisler, F., Gottlieb, A., and Fried, D.: Agenesis of the right diaphragm repaired with Marlex. J. Pediatr. Surg. *12*:587, 1977.

McCredie, M., Lovejoy, F.W., Jr., and Kalfreider, N.L.: Pulmonary function in diaphragmatic paralysis. Thorax. *17*:213, 1962.

Nazarian, M., et al.: Accessory diaphragm: report of a case with complete physiological evaluation and surgical correction. J. Thorac. Cardiovasc. Surg. *61*:293, 1971.

Piehler, J.M., et al.: Unexplained diaphragmatic paralysis: a harbinger of malignant disease? J. Thorac. Cardiovasc. Surg. *84*:861, 1982.

Smith, C.D., et al.: Diaphragmatic paralysis and eventration in infants. J. Thorac. Cardiovasc. Surg. *91*:490, 1986.

Spitz, L., et al.: Combined anterior abdominal wall, sternal, diaphragmatic, pericardial and intracardiac defects: a report of five cases and their management. J. Pediatr. Surg *10*:491, 1975.

Trivedi, S.A.: Neurilemmoma of the diaphragm causing severe hypertrophic pulmonary osteoarthropathy. Br. J. Tuberc. *52*:214, 1958.

Wright, C.D., et al.: Results of diaphragmatic plication for unilateral diaphragmatic paralysis. J. Thorac. Cardiovasc. Surg. *90*:195, 1985.

READING REFERENCES

Campbell, E.J.M.: The Respiratory Muscles and the Mechanics of Breathing. London, Lloyd-Luke, 1958.

Clagett, O.T., and Johnson, M.A., III: Tumors of the diaphragm. Am. J. Surg. *78*:526, 1949.

Easton, P.A., et al.: Respiratory function after paralysis of the right hemidiaphragm. Am. Rev. Respir. Dis. *127*:125, 1983.

Haller, J.A., et al.: Management of diaphragmatic paralysis in infants with special emphasis on selection of patients for operative plication. J. Pediatr. Surg. *14*:779, 1979.

Keltz, H., Kaplan, S., and Stone, D.J.: Effect of quadriplegia and hemidiaphragmatic paralysis on the thoraco-abdominal pressure during respiration. Am. J. Phys. Med. *48*:109, 1969.

Koontz, A.R., and Levin, M.B.: Agenesis of the right half of the diaphragm. Am. Surg. *34*:657, 1968.

McNamara, J.J., et al.: Eventration of the diaphragm. Surgery *64*:1013, 1968.

Olafson, G., Ransling, A., and Olen, O.: Primary tumors of the diaphragm. Chest *59*:568, 1971.

Sbokes, C.G., et al.: Fibrosarcoma of the diaphragm. Br. J. Dis. Chest *71*:99, 1977.

Thomas, T.V.: Congenital eventration of the diaphragm. Ann. Thorac. Surg. *10*:180, 1970.

Wiener, M.F., and Chou, W.H.: Primary tumors of the diaphragm. Arch. Surg. *90*:143, 1965.

CHAPTER 53

CONGENITAL POSTEROLATERAL DIAPHRAGMATIC HERNIA

Marleta Reynolds

Infants with a congenital diaphragmatic hernia diagnosed at birth have a poor prognosis despite major advances in prenatal diagnosis, neonatal transport systems, and ventilatory support. A better understanding of the pulmonary pathology and pathophysiology associated with the diaphragmatic defect have led to changes in therapy but minimal improvement in survival. Investigations into in-utero correction and manipulations of prostanoid homeostasis are on the forefront of experimental study to reduce the seemingly fixed mortality rates of infants with congenital diaphragmatic hernia.

EMBRYOLOGY

The classic congenital diaphragmatic hernia of Bochdalek is a posterolateral defect in the diaphragm caused by a failure of the pleuroperitoneal canal to close at eight weeks gestation (Fig. 53–1). Eighty percent occur on the left side, and they occasionally are bilateral. The defect ranges from a small circular hole—the characteristic Bochdalek hernia—to total absence of the hemidiaphragm. In moderate-sized defects a small rim of muscle exists posteriorly.

When the intestines return to the abdomen from the yolk sac at 10 weeks gestation, the intestines and other abdominal viscera may herniate into the chest and alter growth of the ipsilateral lung. If the mediastinum is pushed to the contralateral side of the chest by the abdominal viscera, the contralateral lung may fail to grow. Autopsy studies by me and my associates (1984), and by Nguyen (1983) and Geggel (1985) and their associates, of newborns with congenital diaphragmatic hernia demonstrated pulmonary hypoplasia in both lungs. The ipsilateral lung's weight may be 20 to 50% below normal. Geggel and colleagues (1985) reported that the contralateral lung's volume is 12 to 42% below normal. The pulmonary hypoplasia consists of a decrease in the number of bronchioles and arterioles and in the number and

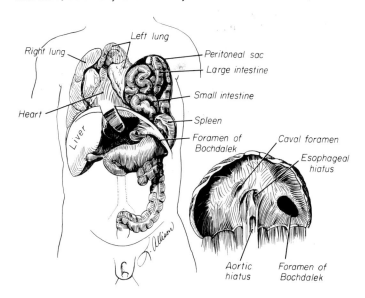

Fig. 53–1. Congenital diaphragmatic hernia of Bochdalek. (Reproduced with permission of Shields, T.W.: The diaphragm. *In* Operative Surgery: Principles and Techniques. Edited by P. Nora. Philadelphia, Lea & Febiger, 1972.

577

size of the alveoli. In addition, the muscularization of the arterioles is abnormal.

Geggel and colleagues (1985) documented a correlation between the extent of arteriolar muscularization and the clinical course of infants with congenital diaphragmatic hernia. Those infants with involvement of only the preacinar arteries exhibited a "honeymoon" period during the postoperative course. Those infants with muscularization extending further out into the interacinar arterioles did not. During the "honeymoon" period, the first 6 to 24 postoperative hours, adequate oxygenation is possible. A sudden deterioration coincident with a marked rise in pulmonary vascular resistance and return to fetal circulation follows. Profound hypoxemia, acidosis, and hypercarbia result from the underlying pulmonary hypoplasia. With the return to fetal circulation, blood is shunted right to left across the foramen ovale and patent ductus arteriosus. Further hypoxemia and acidosis result, and a vicious cycle is established that leads to the infant's death from hypoxia and acidosis (Fig. 53–2).

Nakayama and associates (1985) and I and my associates (1984), among others, noted that major associated anomalies exist in at least 22 to 40% of infants treated for congenital diaphragmatic hernia. Puri and Gorman (1984) reported that the incidence increases to 56% if stillborns are included. These anomalies include major chromosomal abnormalities, congenital heart disease, genitourinary anomalies, and other conditions. Anomalies of rotation and fixation of the intestines are always present.

Prenatal diagnosis of congenital diaphragmatic hernia is being made with increasing frequency and accuracy. Berk and Grundy (1982) reported low amniotic fluid lecithin/sphingomyelin ratios in mothers carrying fetuses with congenital diaphragmatic hernia. Ultrasound findings that suggest diaphragmatic hernia include herniated abdominal viscera, abnormal upper abdominal anatomy, and mediastinal shift away from the side of herniation, as Adzick and colleagues (1985a) described. Polyhydramnios was present in 76% of the cases they reported and was a predictor of poor prognosis. Both Adzick (1985a) and Nakayama (1985) and their associates reported that the accuracy in prenatal diagnosis ranges from 50 to 97%, but this may be improved by amniography and single-section computed tomography. Other anomalies can often be identified by ultrasound as noted by Adzick and

colleagues (1985a). Prenatal diagnosis allows parental counseling and maternal transport for delivery. Unfortunately, as Nakayama and associates (1985) noted, early diagnosis has made little alteration in survival rates.

PRESENTATION

A congenital diaphragmatic hernia may cause symptoms in the first hours or days of life or later in infancy or childhood. The diaphragmatic defect may also be identified on a roentgenogram obtained for unrelated reasons in an asymptomatic patient of any age. The newborn infant may develop life-threatening respiratory distress. An older infant or child may present with respiratory symptoms or feeding intolerance. The morbidity and mortality associated with a congenital diaphragmatic hernia is directly related to the age of the patient at presentation (Table 53–1).

Some babies with congenital diaphragmatic hernia become symptomatic in the delivery room. The diagnosis is suspected if the abdomen is scaphoid and there are heart sounds in the right chest. Roentgenograms of the chest demonstrate gas-filled loops of intestines in the chest (Fig. 53–3). An oral-gastric tube placed into the stomach to decompress the intestines may appear in the chest and an abdominal film reveals a paucity of gas (Fig. 53–4).

Any baby with respiratory distress at birth who is suspected of having a diaphragmatic hernia should be quickly intubated and ventilated. Mask bagging only increases the distention of the herniated stomach and intestines and further compromises ventilation.

Mechanical ventilation with 100% FIO_2 and low airway pressures—<25 mmHg with 5 of PEEP—should be used. Vascular access using an umbilical artery catheter is adequate for arterial blood gas sampling and fluid and drug administration. The baby should be rapidly transported to a center with a surgeon and neonatal intensive care unit equipped to care for such an infant. Profound respiratory acidosis is typically found with the first arterial blood gas. High frequency ventilation to rates up to 100 to 150 breaths per minute helps create a respiratory alkalosis. Sodium bicarbonate infusion is begun to further induce alkalosis. Prolonged hypoxemia, acidosis, and hypercarbia produce pulmonary vasoconstriction and persistent fetal circulation. Myocardial dysfunction

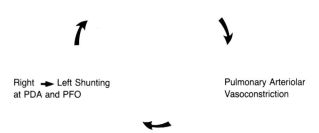

Hypoxemia, Acidosis, Hypercarbia

Right → Left Shunting at PDA and PFO

Pulmonary Arteriolar Vasoconstriction

Fig. 53–2. Persistent fetal circulation.

Table 53–1. Infants with Congenital Diaphragmatic Hernia, 1962–1983

Onset and Severity of Symptoms	Number	Mortality
<6 hours "Critical"	44	33–83%
<6 hours "Noncritical"	53	6–11%
6–24 hours	15	0%
>24 hours	32	0%
	144	

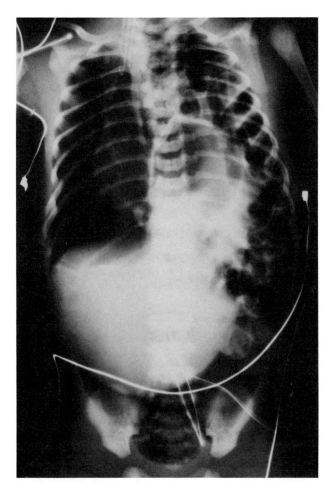

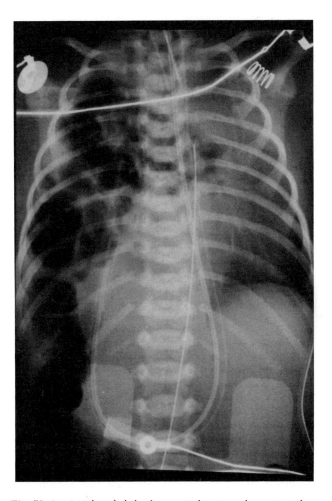

Fig. 53–3. This "baby-gram" demonstrates multiple loops of intestine in the left chest and few loops in the abdomen. The mediastinum is shifted to the contralateral side.

Fig. 53–4. A right-sided diaphragmatic hernia is demonstrated on this roentgenogram. The orogastric tube is seen in the right chest, identifying the location of the stomach.

may necessitate support with dobutamine and renal perfusion with low dose dopamine. Because dopamine in higher doses may constrict the pulmonary vasculature, it is used only in low doses. Five percent albumin can be used to treat systemic hypotension in boluses of 10 to 15 ml. Vasodilating drugs should probably be reserved for the postoperative period.

A congenital diaphragmatic hernia may be found incidentally in an older infant or child. Newman and his colleagues (1986) found that the older infant or child with a diaphragmatic hernia may also present with respiratory or gastrointestinal symptoms. Diagnosis is made with chest roentgenograms or barium studies of the gastrointestinal tract. The hernia should be repaired at the time of diagnosis. The lungs of these children are not hypoplastic and the operative mortality should be 0%.

OPERATIVE CORRECTION

The high frequency neonatal ventilator is moved from the neonatal intensive care unit to the operating room for use during the operation. Any sudden deterioration of vital signs during transport, in the operating room, or

during the postoperative period usually indicates a pneumothorax on the contralateral side. Gibson and Fonkalsrud (1983) and Srouji and associates (1981) reported that a contralateral pneumothorax or a pneumomediastinum is associated with an increase in mortality and should be prevented with the use of low airway pressures. A tube thoracostomy with a No. 10 French chest tube should be rapidly placed if a pneumothorax is suspected.

The correction of a congenital diaphragmatic hernia is performed through a paramedian incision. The abdominal viscera are returned to the abdomen from the chest, and the hernia sac, if present, is excised. Extralobar pulmonary sequestrations, often an associated malformation in infants with congenital diaphragmatic hernia, are resected at the time of hernia repair. A small diaphragmatic defect is closed with permanent suture and Teflon pledgets. Larger defects can be closed with an abdominal wall muscle flap or a polytetrafluoroethylene—PTFE—membrane. When the hemidiaphragm is completely absent, a PTFE membrane can be sutured to the ribs both anteriorly and posterolaterally. The medial portion of the membrane can be sutured to the contralateral diaphragmatic leaf and the adventitia overlying the aorta and esophagus. A chest tube is placed in the ipsilateral thorax and attached to a three-way stopcock and closed.

Controversy continues regarding the best method of thoracic drainage. Suggestions have included no chest tube, bilateral prophylactic chest tubes, underwater seal, and tubes exposed to atmospheric pressure. Tyson and associates (1985) recommended "balanced thoracic drainage" to maintain normal intrathoracic pressure. The ipsilateral chest tube attached to a three-way stopcock allows removal of air or fluid, depending on the clinical picture and the findings on roentgenograms of the chest. I prefer this method.

Associated intra-abdominal anomalies should be corrected at the time of hernia repair if the baby's condition is stable. If fascial closure causes compromise of respiratory excursion, a ventral hernia can be created by closing the skin only. Occasionally, even the skin cannot be closed and a "silo" of silastic sheeting can be used to temporarily contain the abdominal viscera.

POSTOPERATIVE MANAGEMENT

The postoperative management combines all available means to reduce pulmonary vascular resistance and improve oxygenation. Manual hyperventilation, as Fong and Pemberton (1985) advocated, or ventilator rates of 100 to 150 breaths per minute, as Sawyer (1986) and Vacanti (1984) and their colleagues suggested, produces respiratory alkalosis. Karl and colleagues (1983) reported that high frequency oscillation with frequencies from 375 to 1800 cycles per minute produced a temporary respiratory alkalosis when other methods failed in four infants with congenital diaphragmatic hernia; they combined hyperventilation with airway pressures not exceeding 25 mm Hg. A sodium bicarbonate infusion is used to treat the acidosis that is present shortly after delivery, which generally persists into the postoperative period. Vacanti and colleagues (1984) recommended pancuronium—0.1 mg/kg/hour—and fentanyl—1 μg/kg/hour—to control ventilation and reduce pulmonary vascular reactivity. Intravenous fluids are kept to a minimum because the need for multiple drugs quickly exceeds maintenance requirements.

Frequent arterial blood gas determinations coupled with continuous pulse oximetry or transcutaneous Po_2 and Pco_2 monitoring provide a constant assessment of ventilatory status. Fio_2 should be decreased only gradually—2% at a time—and only cautiously. Even these small changes in Fio_2 may reverse the progress made (Fig. 53–5).

Vasodilators and inotropic drugs are reserved for those infants who do not respond to hyperventilation. Bloss and colleagues (1980) reported that tolazoline is useful. I have used sodium nitroprusside and nitroglycerine with some success in some infants. Drummond and associates (1981) reported that the response to some of these drugs is unpredictable and seldom long-lasting. Positive ino-

tropic drugs may be needed to maintain blood pressure when vasodilators are used.

Stolar and associates (1985) found abnormal prostanoid homeostasis in an infant with congenital diaphragmatic hernia. Advances in pharmacologic manipulations of the prostaglandins may provide new drugs to lower pulmonary vascular resistance.

Extracorporeal membrane oxygenation—ECMO—has been successfully used in over 25 centers in the United States to treat reversible respiratory failure in newborn infants. Hardesty (1981), Bartlett (1986), Weber (1987), Redmond (1987), and Langham (1987) and their colleagues reported survival rates among infants with congenital diaphragmatic hernia treated with ECMO ranging from 38 to 77%. This wide range in survival rates probably reflects differences in selection criteria and the experience of the particular center. Some centers place all infants with congenital diaphragmatic hernia who fail medical management on ECMO. Standard criteria have not been established, but in general include alveolar-arterial oxygen gradient—$AaDo_2$—<600 for 12 hours; acute deterioration—pH <7.15 or Pao_2<55 mm Hg—for two consecutive hours; failure of conventional management; and progressive barotrauma. Contraindications to the use of ECMO as described by Bartlett and associates (1986) include pre-existing intraventricular hemorrhage; weight less than 2000 g; and congenital or neurologic abnormalities incompatible with normal life. Another contraindication is pulmonary hypoplasia so severe that survival would be impossible despite successful ECMO. Bartlett and associates (1986) suggested that the lack of a "honeymoon period"—a Po_2 >60—indicates the most severe pulmonary hypoplasia. The infants who will not survive despite ECMO cannot be accurately identified. Most centers accept all infants with congenital diaphragmatic hernia as ECMO candidates. Trento and associates (1986) noted that once placed on ECMO, infants with congenital diaphragmatic hernia are at greater risk than other infants for fatal bleeding complications.

FACTORS IN SURVIVAL

Several methods have been used to predict survival in infants with congenital diaphragmatic hernia. Boix-Ochoa and colleagues (1974) reported that an arterial blood pH <7.0 with a Pco_2 >100 is an early predictor for a poor outcome. Touloukian and Markowitz (1984) devised a scoring system based on pre-operative roentgenographic findings. The roentgenographic findings include the side of the diaphragmatic hernia, location of the stomach, presence of pneumothorax, and relative volume of aerated ipsilateral and contralateral lung. A total score can be derived for each patient and identifies the high risk patient.

Alveolar-arterial oxygen tension differences—$AaDo_2$—are used more frequently to predict survival. Harrington (1982) and Manthei (1983) and their associates reported that preoperative and postoperative $AaDo_2$ >500 mm Hg correlated with little chance of survival. Manthei and colleagues (1983) also noted that initial post-

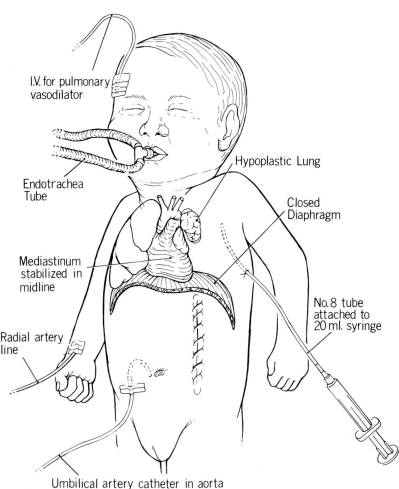

I.V. for pulmonary vasodilator

Endotrachea Tube

Mediastinum stabilized in midline

Radial artery line

Umbilical artery catheter in aorta distal to the ductus

Hypoplastic Lung

Closed Diaphragm

No.8 tube attached to 20 ml. syringe

Fig. 53–5. Illustration of the total postoperative management of a poor-risk infant. The mediastinum is stabilized with the pleural catheter, blood gases are monitored above and below the ductus arteriosus, and the intravenous lines are used for the administration of vasodilator drugs. (Reproduced with permission of Ramenofsky, M.L. and Luck, S.R.: Diaphragmatic anomalies. *In* Swenson's Pediatric Surgery, 4th ed. Edited by J.G. Raffensperger. East Norwalk, CT, Appleton-Century-Crofts, 1980, p. 675.

operative improvement, as evidenced by a transient decrease in AaDo$_2$, was followed by a sudden rise in AaDo$_2$. Expecting this deterioration allows prompt institution of aggressive measures to prevent and treat the decline in oxygenation. Extracorporeal membrane oxygenation should be considered in infants with demonstrable "honeymoon" period.

FUTURE PROSPECTS

Because the degree of pulmonary hypoplasia determines survival in infants with congenital diaphragmatic hernia, investigations of in-utero correction began. Harrison (1980a) and Adzick (1985b) developed a model for congenital diaphragmatic hernia in the fetal lamb and observed that changes identical to those found in man occurred in the fetal lamb. Harrison and colleagues (1980b) reported that the in-utero correction of the defect in fetal lambs allowed sufficient lung growth for survival. Similar trials are expected in man. The optimal time predicted for in-utero intervention in man is between 22 and 28 weeks gestation. As Harrison and co-workers (1985) pointed out, the accurate diagnosis and assessment of other anomalies by ultrasound and chromosomal analysis is a prerequisite for maternal intervention.

In-utero repair may save those infants who could not otherwise survive because of the severity of the pulmonary hypoplasia and the restructuring of the pulmonary arterioles. Based on the morphometric studies of pathologic specimens and clinical correlation, two types of infants with congenital diaphragmatic hernia become symptomatic at birth. In those infants who do not have a "honeymoon" period in the postoperative course and never demonstrate adequate lung function, as evidenced by a Po$_2$ of <60 mm Hg, the muscularization of the arterioles extends into the interacinar arterioles. These infants have the largest diaphragmatic defects and the smallest lungs. Survival in this group is doubtful. Identification of this group of infants in early gestation may allow correction of the defect and improvement in the pulmonary hypoplasia. The other group of infants has a "honeymoon period" and a Po$_2$ of >60 mm Hg in the postoperative period. The pulmonary hypoplasia is not as severe in these infants and the muscularization of the arterioles extends only into the preacinar arterioles. I believe that ECMO should be available in the postoperative period for this group of infants because they can probably survive with this form of aggressive management.

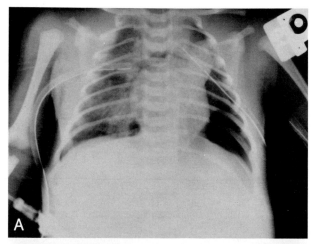

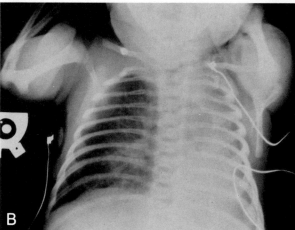

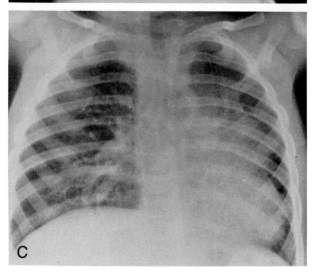

Fig. 53–6. *A,* Early post-operative roentgenogram shows a small left lung. *B,* One month later there is hyperinflation of the contralateral lung and the mediastinum has shifted into the ipsilateral chest. *C,* Even 2 years following repair of the diaphragmatic hernia, the contralateral lung and mediastinum are still in the ipsilateral chest. The child was asymptomatic at the time.

LONG-TERM FOLLOW-UP

The evaluations of lung function in infants surviving repair of congenital diaphragmatic hernia reported by Chatrath (1971), Wurnig (1980), and Freyschuss (1984) and their associates provided some conflicting results. Fifteen-year follow-up in the review by Wurnig and colleagues (1980) identified reduced pulmonary function represented by restrictive or obstructive changes or both. Freyschuss and associates (1984) evaluated 20 patients at 6 to 22 years of age. Most of these patients required operation at less than 48 hours of age. In these patients, perfusion of the ipsilateral lung was reduced, as was the fractional ventilation. Total lung capacity, FEV_1, and FEV% were normal. Residual volume and FRC were increased. No functional impairment was identified in any patient. This report supports the work of both Wohl and colleagues (1977) and Reid and Hutcherson (1976), who demonstrated decreased blood flow to the ipsilateral lung in similar series of patients. As the number of survivors with congenital diaphragmatic hernia increases, the fate of the most severely hypoplastic lungs becomes evident (Fig. 53–6). Long-term follow-up should extend to the fourth and fifth decade of life to more accurately predict the eventual outcome.

REFERENCES

Adzick, N.S., et al.: Diaphragmatic hernia in the fetus: prenatal diagnosis and outcome in 94 cases. J. Pediatr. Surg. *20*:357, 1985a.

Adzick, N.S., et al.: Correction of congenital diaphragmatic hernia in utero. IV. An early gestational fetal lamb model for pulmonary vascular morphometric analysis. J. Pediatr. Surg. *20*:673, 1985b.

Bartlett, R.H., et al.: Extracorporeal membrane oxygenation (ECMO) in neonatal respiratory failure. Ann. Surg. *204*:236, 1986.

Berk, C., and Grundy, M.: "High risk" lecithin/sphingomyelin ratios associated with neonatal diaphragmatic hernia. Br. J. Obstet. Gynecol. *89*:250, 1982.

Bloss, R.S., et al.: Tolazoline therapy for persistent pulmonary hypertension after congenital diaphragmatic hernia repair. J. Pediatr. *97*:984, 1980.

Boix-Ochoa, J., et al.: The important influence of arterial blood gases on the prognosis of congenital diaphragmatic hernia. World J. Surg. *1*:783, 1977.

Chatrath, R.R., El Shafie, M., and Jones, R.S.: Fate of hypoplastic lungs after repair of congenital diaphragmatic hernia. Arch. Dis. Child. *46*:633, 1971.

Drummond, W.H., et al.: The independent effects of hyperventilation, tolazoline, and dopamine on infants with persistent pulmonary hypertension. J. Pediatr. *98*:603, 1981.

Fong, L.V., and Pemberton, P.J.: Congenital diaphragmatic hernia and the management of persistent fetal circulation. Anaesth. Intens. Care *13*:375, 1985.

Freyschuss, U., Lannergren, K., and Frenckner, B.: Lung function after repair of congenital diaphragmatic hernia. Acta Pediatr. Scand. *73*:589, 1984.

Geggel, R.L. et al.: Congenital diaphragmatic hernia: arterial structural changes and persistent pulmonary hypertension after surgical repair. J. Pediatr. *107*:457, 1985.

Gibson, C., and Fonkalsrud, E.W.: Iatrogenic pneumothorax and mortality in congenital diaphragmatic hernia. J. Pediatr. Surg. *18*:555, 1983.

Hardesty, R.L., et al.: Extracorporeal membrane oxygenation: successful treatment of persistent fetal circulation following repair of congenital diaphragmatic hernia. J. Thorac. Cardiovasc. Surg. *81*:556, 1981.

Harrington, J., Raphaely, R.C., and Downes, J.J.: Relationship of alveolar-arterial oxygen tension difference in diaphragmatic hernia of the newborn. Anesth. 56:473, 1982.

Harrison, M.R., Jester, J.A., and Ross, N.A.: Correction of congenital diaphragmatic hernia in utero. I. The model: intrathoracic balloon produces fatal pulmonary hypoplasia. Surgery 88:174, 1980a.

Harrison, M.R., et al.: Correction of congenital diaphragmatic hernia in utero. II. Simulated correction permits fetal lung growth with survival at birth. Surgery 88:260, 1980b.

Harrison, M.R., et al.: Fetal diaphragmatic hernia: fatal but fixable. Semin. Perinatol. 9:103, 1985.

Karl, S.R., Ballantine, T.V.N., and Snider, M.T.: High-frequency ventilation at rates of 375 to 1800 cycles per minute in four neonates with congenital diaphragmatic hernia. J. Pediatr. Surg. 18:822, 1983.

Langham, M.R., Jr., et al.: Extracorporeal membrane oxygenation following repair of congenital diaphragmatic hernias. Ann. Thorac. Surg. 44:247, 1987.

Manthei, V., Vaucher, Y., and Crowe, C.P.: Congenital diaphragmatic hernia: immediate preoperative and postoperative oxygen gradients identify patients requiring prolonged respiratory support. Surgery 93:83, 1983.

Nakayama, D.K., et al.: Prenatal diagnosis and natural history of the fetus with a congenital diaphragmatic hernia: initial clinical experience. J. Pediatr. Surg. 20:118, 1985.

Newman, B.M., et al.: Presentation of Congenital Diaphragmatic Hernia Past the Newborn Period. Arch. Surg. 121:813, 1986.

Nguyen, L., et al.: The mortality of congenital diaphragmatic hernia: is total pulmonary mass inadequate, no matter what? Ann. Surg. 198:766, 1983.

Puri, P., and Gorman, F.: Lethal nonpulmonary anomalies associated with congenital diaphragmatic hernia: implications for early intrauterine surgery. J. Pediatr. Surg. 19:29, 1984.

Redmond, C.R., et al.: Extracorporeal membrane oxygenation for respiratory and cardiac failure in infants and children. J. Thorac. Cardiovasc. Surg. 93:199, 1987.

Reid, I.S., and Hutcherson, R.J.: Long-term follow-up of patients with congenital diaphragmatic hernia. J. Pediatr. Surg. 11:939, 1976.

Reynolds, M., Luck, S.R., and Lappen, R.: The "critical" neonate with diaphragmatic hernia: a 21-year perspective. J. Pediatr. Surg. 19:364, 1984.

Sawyer, S., et al.: Improving survival in the treatment of congenital diaphragmatic hernia. Ann. Thorac. Surg. 41:75, 1986.

Srouji, M.N., Buck, B., and Downes, J.J.: Congenital diaphragmatic hernia: deleterious effects of pulmonary interstitial emphysema and tension extrapulmonary air. J. Pediatr. Surg. 16:45, 1981.

Stolar, C.J.H., Dillon, P.W., and Stalcup, S.A.: Extracorporeal membrane oxygenation and congenital diaphragmatic hernia: modification of the pulmonary vasoactive profile. J. Pediatr. Surg. 20:681, 1985.

Touloukian, R.J., and Markowitz, R.I.: A preoperative X-ray scoring system for risk assessment of newborns with congenital diaphragmatic hernia. J. Pediatr. Surg. 19:252, 1984.

Trento, A., Griffith, B.P., and Hardesty, R.L.: Extracorporeal membrane oxygenation experience at the University of Pittsburgh. Ann. Thorac. Surg. 42:56, 1986.

Tyson, K.R.T., Schwartz, M.Z., and Marr, C.C.: "Balanced" thoracic drainage is the method of choice to control intrathoracic pressure following repair of diaphragmatic hernia. J. Pediatr. Surg. 20:415, 1985.

Vacanti, J.P., et al.: The pulmonary hemodynamic response to perioperative anesthesia in the treatment of high-risk infants with congenital diaphragmatic hernia. J. Pediatr. Surg. 19:672, 1984.

Weber, T.R., et al.: Neonatal diaphragmatic hernia: An improving outlook with extracorporeal membrane oxygenation. Arch. Surg. 122:615, 1987.

Wohl, M.E.B., et al.: Repair of congenital diaphragmatic hernia. J. Pediatr. 90:405, 1977.

Wurnig, P., Balogh, A., and Hopfgartner, L.: Fifteen years of surgical therapy for congenital diaphragmatic hernia: results and follow-up. Z. Kinderchir. 29:134, 1980.

CHAPTER 54

FORAMEN OF MORGAGNI HERNIA, MISCELLANEOUS CONGENITAL DIAPHRAGMATIC HERNIAS, AND CARDIAL INCOMPETENCE

Thomas W. Shields

FORAMEN OF MORGAGNI HERNIA

Anatomy

On each side of the sternum is a potential space, known as the foramen of Morgagni, or the space of Larrey, through which passes the internal mammary artery to become the superior epigastric artery.

This triangular space is between the muscular fibers originating from the xiphisternum and the costal margin that insert on the central tendon of the diaphragm. The left space is less likely to develop a hernia because it is protected by the pericardial sac. The ligamentum teres defines the medial border of the hernia through either space.

Most often, a foramen of Morgagni hernia contains only a piece of omentum that is caught up in the defect and then enlarges as the person grows and produces the mass within the hernial sac. At times, the hernia contains colon and, occasionally, small intestine or other abdominal viscera (Fig. 54–1).

Incidence

Hernias through the foramen of Morgagni are uncommon at any age but are even more rare in the child than in the adult (Fig. 54–2). They are more common on the right side than on the left and usually contain a sac. Chin and Duchesne (1955) found 30 examples of retrosternal hernias in a mass roentgenographic survey of the chest. In the past, these hernias probably were frequently unrecognized on routine roentgenograms of the chest, because the densities in the right cardiophrenic angle produced by them were interpreted as caused by the pericardial fat pad or a pleuropericardial cyst (Fig. 54–3).

Symptoms

A foramen of Morgagni hernia usually does not cause symptoms in childhood but is often symptomatic in the adult. Women are affected more often than men are and the obese more often than the thin. The patient with a foramen of Morgagni hernia may complain of dull pain in the right subcostal area. Intermittent, partial intestinal obstruction may occur, but complete intestinal obstruction is uncommon.

Diagnosis

Roentgenographic studies of the chest reveal a density, either solid or containing air, adjacent to the right or left side of the heart. In small hernias, Lanuza (1971) described the so-called sign of the cane that refers to a curvilunar accumulation of fat continuous with the properitoneal fat line of the anterior abdominal wall. This sign suggests that a small anterior cardiophrenic mass may be a foramen of Morgagni hernia. A CT examination of an anterior cardiophrenic mass may reveal the presence of bowel (Fig. 54–4), thus confirming the diagnosis. Contrast studies of the large intestine and often the upper gastrointestinal tract are indicated in the evaluation of some patients. At times, if the diagnosis remains doubtful, a diagnostic pneumoperitoneum may be carried out. If a communication is present between the hernial sac and the peritoneum, air enters the sac and confirms the diagnosis.

Surgical Repair

The abdominal approach for surgical repair of this hernia is chosen if the diagnosis is known preoperatively. A subcostal incision or a right epigastric paramedian incision may be used. With the latter incision, the rectus muscle is retracted laterally to expose the posterior rectus and transversalis fascia. After the abdomen has been opened, the contents of the hernia are reduced into the peritoneal cavity and the margins of the hernial sac are identified. As noted, the ligamentum teres defines the medial border of the hernia. The repair is made with

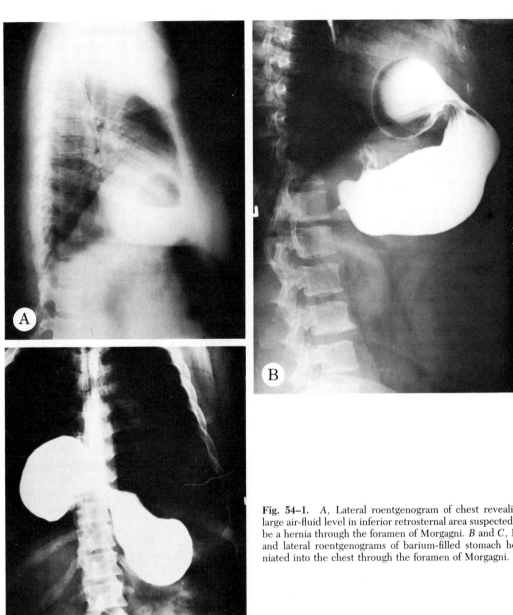

Fig. 54–1. *A*, Lateral roentgenogram of chest revealing large air-fluid level in inferior retrosternal area suspected to be a hernia through the foramen of Morgagni. *B* and *C*, PA and lateral roentgenograms of barium-filled stomach herniated into the chest through the foramen of Morgagni.

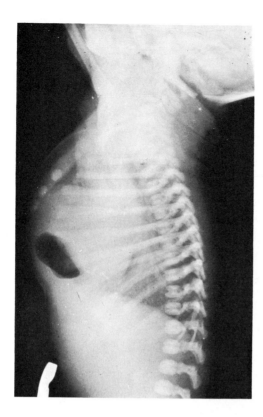

Fig. 54–2.   Roentgenogram of the chest made in the lateral position in an infant with a congenital foramen of Morgagni hernia that was found to contain most of the stomach at the time of repair.

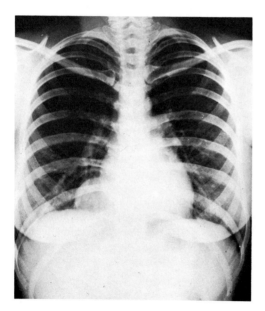 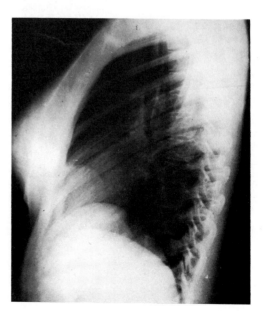

Fig. 54–3.   PA and lateral roentgenograms of the chest of a patient with a foramen of Morgagni hernia that was shown to contain omentum and small bowel.

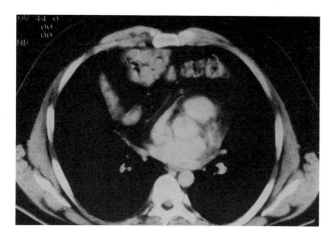

Fig. 54–4. CT of chest revealing the presence of bowel anterior to the heart in a hernia arising through a foramen of Morgagni. (Used with permission of Denise Aberle, M.D., University of California at Los Angeles School of Medicine.)

interrupted mattress sutures, and usually it is necessary to pull the diaphragm up to the posterior part of the sternum and to the posterior rectus sheath (Fig. 54–5). After repair, the abdomen is closed and, in most patients, it is not necessary to enter into the chest or to drain the pleural space.

Frequently, a foramen of Morgagni hernia is encountered while the anterior mediastinum is being explored for an undiagnosed mediastinal mass in either anterior cardiophrenic angle. As soon as the mass has been identified as a foramen of Morgagni hernia, the sac is opened and explored, and the contents are reduced into the peritoneal cavity. The repair is then accomplished in a manner similar to that just described, and in this instance it is also best to suture the diaphragm to the posterior part of the sternum and the rectus sheath. Frequently, repair is best accomplished by passing the sutures around a rib anteriorly or through the chest wall. On occasion, because of the size of the defect and a deficiency of available tissue, it is necessary to sew in a small piece of plastic mesh or a soft tissue Gore–Tex patch.

MISCELLANEOUS CONGENITAL DIAPHRAGMATIC HERNIAS

Hernias may occur through the central portion of the diaphragm, and frequently the eventration is partial or localized, with marked thinning out of the tissues of the diaphragm to form a ring and a hernial sac. When such a hernia occurs on the right side, a mushroom-like projection of liver that has grown through the opening in the right diaphragmatic leaf may be found. On the roentgenogram of the chest, this projection is occasionally misinterpreted as a diaphragmatic tumor. Differentiation may be made by instituting a pneumoperitoneum, following which air appears to surround the liver protrusion. Repair of this type of hernia is unnecessary if clear identification can be made by the pneumoperitoneum. If not, exploration is required to rule out the possibility of a primary tumor of the diaphragm.

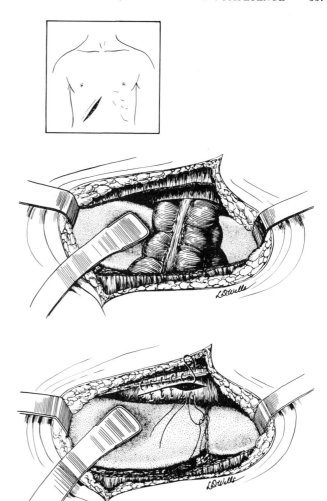

Fig. 54–5. Schematic illustration of technique of closure of foramen of Morgagni hernia by the transabdominal approach. (Shields, T.W.: The diaphragm. *In* Operative Surgery: Principles and Techniques, Chapter 16. Edited by P. Nora. Philadelphia, Lea & Febiger, 1972.)

If the hernia is on the left side, the stomach is occasionally herniated through the central portion of the diaphragm; it usually is identified as an air-containing cyst on the top of the diaphragm. The hernia may be associated with a partial absence of the pericardium, and the stomach and small intestine may herniate into the pericardial sac and cause cardiac symptoms. In general, when such defects occur through the central portion of the left hemidiaphragm or into the pericardium, they should be repaired as soon as they are discovered. In infants and children, the repair usually is accomplished through an abdominal approach, similar to that described for the repair of the foramen of Bochdalek hernia. In contrast, in the older child and adult, repair is accomplished through a thoracic approach.

CARDIAL INCOMPETENCE AND HIATAL HERNIA

Cardial incompetence with or without a hernia through the esophageal hiatus is a common abnormality in infants and children, whose symptoms differ from those of adults. The infant with an esophageal hiatal hernia usually has a history of vomiting, failure to thrive, respiratory complications, and anemia. If a hernia is suspected, careful study of esophageal mobility by cinefluoroscopy and barium meal is indicated to confirm the diagnosis.

Medical therapy consisting of proper positioning of the infant has been successful in most of these young patients. Formerly this was accomplished by placing the infant in a special chair that maintained the child in a 60° upright angle. Studies of Meyers and Herbst (1982) and Orenstein and associates (1983), however, showed that placing the infant in the prone position with the head elevated at an approximately 30° angle is more beneficial in preventing reflux than the previously recommended infant seat. Frequent, small, thickened feedings are a helpful part of the therapy. Surgical treatment is indicated only in those patients who do not respond to conservative medical management. Such patients continue to demonstrate esophagitis, bleeding, anemia, recurrent aspiration with respiratory symptoms and, on occasion, stricture formation.

Approximately 15% of these infants require surgical intervention. The incidence of neurologic disorders is high in this subset of patients; Fonkalsrud and colleagues (1985) reported them in 32% of their series of infants and children who required surgical correction of the esophageal reflex. The preferred procedure is a transabdominal Nissen fundoplication or one of its modifications. Good results may be expected in approximately 95% of the patients. Recurrent reflux and late development of a paraesophageal hernia are two of the more common causes of the occasional failure of the surgical procedure. Late deaths caused by unrelated pre-existing anomalies may be observed, as St. Cyr and associates (1986) pointed out, but this is obviously a function of the selection of the patients for surgical intervention.

SHORT ESOPHAGUS

A congenital short esophagus occurs when the descent of the stomach into the abdominal cavity is not complete at birth. It also may occur when the development of the right crus of the diaphragm is incomplete. Infants and children with this defect usually have the same findings as those described for patients with congenital hiatal hernias. However, operative repair is almost always indicated, and, unfortunately, the repair is frequently difficult because of the amount of stomach that is in the chest and the short length of the contracted esophagus. Often, the problem of the congenital short esophagus remains unless one of the varieties of visceral interposition is used to replace the cardioesophageal junction.

REFERENCES

Chin, E.F., and Duchesne, E.R.: The parasternal defect. Thorax 10:214, 1955.

Fonkalsrud, E.W., Ament, M.E., and Berquist, W.: Surgical management of the gastroesophageal reflux syndrome in childhood. Surgery 97:42, 1985.

Lanuza, A.: The sign of the cane: a new radiological sign for the diagnosis of small Morgagni hernias. Radiology 101:293, 1971.

Meyers, W.F., and Herbst, J.J.: Effectiveness of positioning therapy for gastroesophageal reflux. Pediatrics 69:768, 1982.

Orenstein, S.R, Whitington, P.J., and Orenstein, D.M.: The infant seat as treatment for gastroesophageal reflux. N. Engl. J. Med. 309:760, 1983.

St. Cyr, J.A., et al.: Nissen fundoplication for gastrointestinal reflux in infants. J. Thorac. Cardiovasc. Surg. 92:661, 1986.

READING REFERENCES

Baran, E.M., Houston, H.E., and Lynn, H.B.: Foramen of Morgagni hernias in children. Surgery 62:1076, 1967.

Bently, G., and Lister, J.: Retrosternal hernia. Surgery 57:567, 1965.

CHAPTER 55

PARAESOPHAGEAL HIATAL HERNIA

Arthur E. Baue and Keith S. Naunheim

CLASSIFICATION

Hiatal hernias are generally classified into four types, the most common of which is the sliding or type I hiatal hernia. A type I hernia develops because of circumferential weakening of the phrenoesophageal ligament. This ligament is formed by the fusion of endothoracic and endoabdominal fascia at the diaphragmatic hiatus (Fig. 55–1). The distal esophagus normally resides within the abdomen and is held there by the phrenoesophageal ligament. If this structure becomes attenuated, the distal esophagus and cardia can slip through the hiatus and into the thoracic cavity. This is frequently accompanied by loss of tone and competence in the lower esophageal sphincter—LES—which may result in acid reflux and esophagitis.

Paraesophageal, or type II, hiatal hernia is an uncommon disorder that is distinctly different from sliding hiatal hernia. In a paraesophageal hernia the phrenoesophageal membrane is not diffusely weakened, but focally weakened, anterior or lateral to the esophagus. The gastric cardia and lower esophagus remain below the diaphragm and the gastric fundus protrudes or rolls through the defect into the mediastinum (Fig. 55–1). Paraesophageal hiatal hernia is by far the less common of these two defects and Hill (1968) and Ozdemir (1973) and their colleagues and Sandereed (1967) reported it to account for only 3 to 6% of all patients undergoing surgical repair of hiatal hernias. Because most patients with hiatal hernias do not undergo operative correction, probably only 1 to 2% of all hiatal hernias are type II defects.

A type III or "mixed" hiatal hernia is a combination of types I and II—a sliding and rolling hernia. If a type I hiatal hernia enlarges, the attenuated phrenoesophageal membrane may also focally weaken anteriorly, allowing protrusion of the gastric fundus. Rotation of the stomach may result in the body or fundus obtaining a higher position within the chest than the cardia, a situation usually found only in type II hernias. Pearson and colleagues (1983) suggested that true type II hernias are rare; they suggested that most are, in fact, misdiagnosed type III defects with a supradiaphragmatic lower esophageal sphincter. There has been, however, little support in the literature for this controversial viewpoint. How often a type II—paraesophageal—hernia becomes a type III hernia is not known. Frequently, however, when a patient has a large paraesophageal hernia with rotation of the body and fundus of the stomach into the chest, the esophagogastric junction is in a location higher than the hiatus of the diaphragm. In such circumstances, however, the esophagogastric junction is in the posterior aspect of the hiatus and the patient does not usually have symptoms of an attenuated intrinsic sphincter with esophagitis.

A type III defect is frequently present when a type II hernia has been present for many years. The mechanism for this seems to be gradual enlargement of the hiatus so that the esophagogastric junction no longer lies within or below the hiatus. The attachments of the esophagogastric junction remain intact posteriorly. Evidence increasingly suggests that a type I—sliding—hernia is caused by esophageal contraction abnormalities with a pull on the esophagogastric junction; patients with significant or severe esophagitis rarely have a paraesophageal herniation, and patients with a large paraesophageal herniation seldom have significant esophagitis despite a supradiaphragmatic esophagogastric junction.

Progressive enlargement of the diaphragmatic opening can eventually lead to herniation of other organs, including colon and omentum—a type IV hiatal hernia.

The term parahiatal hernia has been used in the past, but this type of defect seems to be nonexistent. We have never seen a defect in the diaphragm alongside the hiatus with protrusion of stomach into the chest with identifiable crural or diaphragmatic fibers between the hernia orifice and the esophageal hiatus.

ANATOMY AND PATHOPHYSIOLOGY

In a true paraesophageal hiatal hernia, the lower esophagus and cardia remain fixed below the diaphragm in the posterior aspect of the diaphragmatic hiatus. A focal weakening of the phrenoesophageal membrane oc-

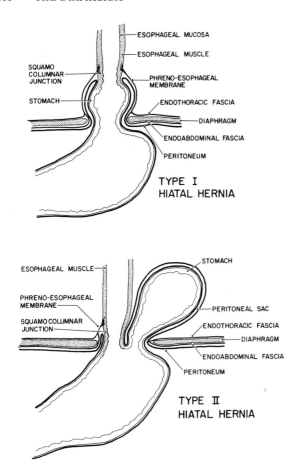

Fig. 55–1. Diagram demonstrating the two types of hiatal hernia. The type I hiatal hernia is not a true hernia in that the endoabdominal fascial lining of the abdomen remains intact. In the type II hernia, a defect in the fascia allows a peritoneal sac to pass through the opening in the hiatus and enter the pleural cavity.

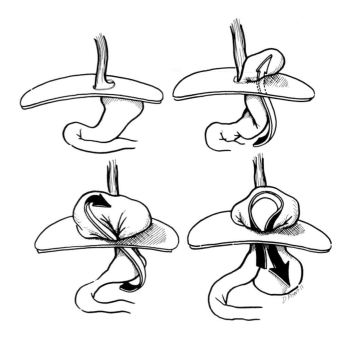

Fig. 55–2. Mechanics of incarceration and strangulation with paraesophageal hernia. Note that fundus may prolapse back into abdomen. (Reproduced with permission from Postlethwait, R.W., (Ed.): Surgery of the Esophagus, 2nd ed. East Norwalk, CT, Appleton-Century-Crofts, 1986.)

curs anterior or lateral to the esophagus, and the combination of negative intrathoracic and positive intra-abdominal pressure pushes the abdominal viscera through the defect. The protruding organs are circumferentially covered by a layer of peritoneum that forms a true hernia sac, unlike the type I or sliding hernia, in which the stomach forms the posterior wall of the hernia sac. The intrathoracic migration of stomach evolves by the so called organoaxial rotation (Fig. 55–2). The lesser gastric curve is anchored within the abdomen by the posterior attachments of the lower esophagus, the left gastric artery, and the retroperitoneal fixation of the pylorus and duodenum. These three points define the long axis of the stomach, and they remain relatively fixed in the abdomen in a type II hernia. The greater curvature, however, is relatively mobile and rotates about the "long axis" by moving first anteriorly and then upward, as the hernia evolves. The fundus is the first part of the stomach to protrude upward through the anterior hernia sac. As the hiatal defect enlarges, the body and antrum continue the axial rotation and migrate into the thorax, leaving the cardia and pylorus within the abdomen. The stomach then resides "upside down" within the chest, with the

greater curvature pointing cephalad and the cardia remaining below the diaphragm (Fig. 55–3). The stomach may initially occupy a retrocardiac position, but as the hernia enlarges, rotation occurs into the right chest. With huge hernias, most of the stomach lies within the right hemithorax with the greater curvature of the stomach pointing toward the right shoulder. This rotation places an upward tension on the omentum and is why the transverse colon may also herniate into the sac.

As with any true anatomic hernia, possible complications include bleeding, incarceration, volvulus, obstruction, strangulation, and perforation.

Gastritis and ulceration have been endoscopically visualized in as many as 30% of the patients who have type II hiatal hernias. Wichterman and associates (1979) suggested that these ulcers are the result of poor gastric emptying and torsion of the gastric wall, particularly after repeat incarcerations, which may impair the blood supply and lymphatic drainage. Although brisk bleeding can occur, these ulcers more frequently cause a slow, chronic blood loss with resultant anemia.

The most serious complication of the type II hernia is gastric volvulus associated with incarceration and strangulation. Hill (1968), Ozdemir (1973), and Wichterman (1979) and their colleagues reported that approximately 30% of paraesophageal hernias present with this problem. After a meal, the fundus may prolapse down from the hernia sac and back into the abdomen (Fig. 55–2). This twists and angulates the stomach in its midportion just proximal to the antrum, resulting in partial or complete obstruction. Distention of the intrathoracic stomach and further rotation of the fundus can result in obstruction at the gastroesophageal junction. Further

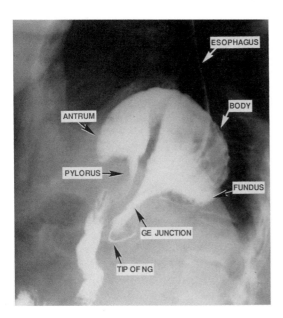

Fig. 55–3. Barium study of the stomach that demonstrates the "upside down" appearance of the stomach within the thoracic cavity. Note the NG tube extending through the length of the esophagus with the tip at the GE junction below the hiatus. The fundus, body, and antrum are above the diaphragm.

twisting may lead to pyloric obstruction, which results in an incarcerated gastric segment and closed-loop obstruction. If unchecked, this ultimately leads to strangulation, necrosis, and perforation. Unless this process is recognized and corrected, the resulting mediastinitis and shock are fatal.

As was mentioned earlier, a type III defect is frequently present when a type II hernia has been present for many years. The mechanism for this seems to be gradual enlargement of the hiatus so that the esophagogastric junction no longer lies within or below the hiatus. The attachment of the esophagogastric junction remains intact posteriorly.

SYMPTOMS

Many type II hernias cause few or no symptoms and remain undiagnosed for years until recognized on a routine roentgenogram of the chest. Chronic bleeding from gastritis or ulceration of the intrathoracic gastric segment may lead to iron deficiency anemia with resultant fatigue and exertional dyspnea. Most patients, however, present with complaints of postprandial discomfort, caused by an intrathoracic gastric segment that becomes dilated by food and swallowed air. Frequently, these complaints have been present for many years. Patients usually describe sensations of substernal fullness or pressure, and this is often mistaken for angina. Often, this discomfort is accompanied by nausea and is somewhat relieved by belching or regurgitation. Most of the aforementioned authors, as well as Ellis and colleagues (1986), noted that symptoms of gastroesophageal reflux were distinctly uncommon in their patients with type II hiatal hernias. Although Pearson and associates (1983) noted that most

of their patients had severe symptoms, it is probably because of the high percentage of combined—type III—hernias in their patient population. True dysphagia is also uncommon. Lastly, a large type III or IV hernia may occupy a portion of the thoracic cavity and result in postprandial respiratory symptoms of breathlessness with a sense of suffocation. Symptoms may be mild despite a huge hernia. Patients seem to get used to or tolerate these gas-bloat symptoms well.

When gastric volvulus and obstruction occur, patients present in extreme distress. Most such patients give a long history of complaints, such as those outlined previously, but have never sought medical advice. The chief complaints at the time of presentation are severe pain and pressure in the chest or the epigastric region. It is usually accompanied by nausea and may be misdiagnosed as a myocardial infarction. Vomiting may occur, but more frequently the patient complains of retching and an inability to regurgitate. The patient may also complain of the inability to swallow saliva. If the volvulus is allowed to progress, strangulation of the intrathoracic portion of stomach occurs resulting in a toxic clinical picture including fever, "third spacing" of fluid, and hypovolemic shock. Acute hemorrhagic pancreatitis has also been reported in cases of gastric volvulus and is felt to be caused by distortion of the pancreatic duct with impaired drainage.

DIAGNOSIS

The diagnosis of paraesophageal hiatal hernia is usually first suspected because of an abnormal roentgenogram of the chest. The most frequent finding is a retrocardiac

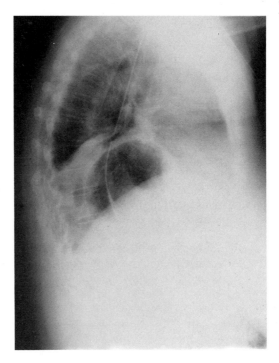

Fig. 55–4. Retrocardiac air bubble and type II hiatal hernia. Note wedge of atelectatic lung compressed by large hernia sac.

air bubble with or without an air-fluid level (Fig. 55–4). In a giant paraesophageal hernia, the sac and its contents occasionally protrude into the right thoracic cavity. The differential diagnosis includes mediastinal cyst or abscess and dilated obstructed esophagus as in end-stage achalasia. A barium study of the upper gastrointestinal tract is the diagnostic study of choice. The pathognomonic finding is an "upside down" stomach within the chest (Fig. 55–3). The radiologist must pay careful attention to the position of the cardia; this not only confirms the diagnosis of type II defect, but may be important in deciding whether an antireflux procedure should be performed at the same time as an anatomic repair. A barium enema may help determine if any portion of colon is involved.

After the presence of the hernia has been established roentgenographically, one must determine whether it has a functional effect on the competence of the lower esophageal sphincter. This is best accomplished by endoscopy and esophageal function testing.

Although symptoms of gastroesophageal reflux are rare in patients with a pure type II hiatal hernia, they are occasionally present and may indicate pathologic peptic esophagitis. Preoperative esophageal testing may help confirm or refute this suspicion. Esophageal manometry is useful in determining the location of lower esophageal sphincter—LES—which marks the gastroesophageal junction, an area that can be difficult to locate on barium study. An LES at a supradiaphragmatic level suggests a huge paraesophageal hernia or a type III—"mixed"—paraesophageal and sliding hiatal hernia, which is more likely to have a component of reflux and esophagitis. Ambulatory esophageal pH testing can help diagnose gastroesophageal reflux, which is best treated by a fundoplication procedure at the time of surgical correction (Chapter 82).

These test results must, however, be considered in the context of the enitre clinical picture. Although Walther and associates (1984) found pH evidence for pathologic reflux in 9 of 15 patients—60%—in their paraesophageal hernia series, at endoscopy only 2 patients—13%—were found to have mild—grade I—esophagitis, which was of questionable clinical significance.

Upper endoscopy can play an important role in the diagnostic workup of these patients. Reports from the literature citing endoscopic results conflict. Pearson and associates (1983) endoscoped all 51 patients with primary incarcerated giant hiatal hernias and found that 30% had grade I esophagitis and an additional 30% had grade II–IV esophagitis, but virtually all these patients had type III or combined hernias. Ellis and colleagues (1986) reported a series that included 39 patients with primary type II defects and found only 5 patients—13%—with endoscopic evidence of mild to moderate esophagitis, an incidence identical to Walther and associates (1984).

Apparently, pure type II hiatal hernias are infrequently associated with an incompetent lower esophageal sphincter or significant gastroesophageal reflux, which probably occur more frequently in type III defects. Preoperative endoscopy and esophageal motility studies can help establish the location of gastroesophageal junction and LES with relation to the diaphragm. The combination of esophageal pH testing and endoscopy determine whether significant acid reflux exists and whether pathologic esophagitis is present. These tests should be employed before elective operation for any type II hernia patient with symptoms of acid reflux. They should also be routinely used for any patient with known or suspected type III hernia with a supradiaphragmatic LES.

THERAPY

No acceptable medical treatment regimen exists for patients with paraesophageal hiatal hernia. Patients followed expectantly are at great risk, as noted by Skinner and Belsey (1967) who found a 29% mortality in 21 patients treated medically. Because of the serious and life-threatening nature of complications in this disorder, the presence of the defect is, in itself, a surgical indication.

When a patient with a type II hernia presents with gastric volvulus and obstruction, decompression with a nasogastric tube must be promptly performed. In the absence of signs of toxicity, an operation can then be scheduled at the earliest convenience. The inability to decompress a gastric volvulus in this situation constitutes a surgical emergency and mandates immediate operative intervention, whether or not signs of toxicity exist.

Although the necessity for operation is universally recognized, controversy exists regarding what operation should be done and through what approach. The repair can be easily performed through either an abdominal or thoracic approach, and strong proponents for both exist. No matter what the approach, the operative principles for hernia repair apply: reduction of the hernia, resection of the sac, and closure of the defect.

Those who endorse the thoracic approach emphasize the ease of intrathoracic dissection of the hernia contents and sac. In type III defects, the thoracic approach allows the thorough dissection of the esophagus in cases of moderate to severe esophageal shortening; this may allow reduction of a fundoplication beneath the hiatus without the need for a lengthening procedure. The proponents of a transthoracic repair, however, usually neglect to note the increased morbidity and discomfort attendant to the thoracotomy approach. In addition, a transthoracic repair may allow the stomach to rotate organoaxially after it is pushed back into the peritoneal cavity. This then produces a volvulus of the body of the stomach in which the greater curvature adheres to the liver. We are aware of two patients in whom this occurred, and these patients required a laparotomy postoperatively to correct the volvulus; these patients were reported by Wichterman and associates, including one of us (A.E.B.) (1979).

Those who suggest an abdominal approach point out that the procedure is easily performed through the abdomen and that concomitant abdominal procedures can be undertaken simultaneously. In addition, it allows placement of a gastrostomy tube, which obviates the need for a postoperative nasogastric tube and which may also decrease the risk of recurrent volvulus. The only patient in whom this approach might prove difficult is one with a proven type III or "mixed" lesion with known reflux and a foreshortened esophagus. In this case, the thoracic approach could be a better alternative. Familiarity with the dissection of the esophagus as done with a transhiatal esophagectomy, however, allows mobilization of most of the esophagus through an enlarged diaphragmatic hiatus.

The second controversial point deals with the indications for an antireflux operation at the time the anatomic hernia is corrected. Many authors, including Pearson (1983) and Ozdemir (1973) and their associates, have written that they routinely perform an antireflux procedure on all patients regardless of the presence or absence of reflux symptoms. Hill and Tobias (1968) espoused simple anatomic repair alone and had excellent results with no recurrences and no postoperative reflux in 19 patients. Perhaps Ellis and colleagues' (1986) approach is the most enlightened—patients with type II hiatal hernia should undergo preoperative endoscopy, manometry, and pH testing, and only those patients with symptoms or objective evidence of gastroesophageal reflux should be considered for an antireflux repair, usually a Belsey mark IV operation or a loose Nissen wrap. Most patients with a pure paraesophageal hiatal hernia do not have reflux and are well served with a simple hernia reduction and diaphragmatic hiatal repair.

OPERATIVE TECHNIQUE

We prefer and recommend the abdominal approach through an upper midline incision. The left lobe of the liver is mobilized and retracted to the right. The contents of the hernia sac are reduced back into the peritoneal cavity by gentle traction. If resistance is encountered while the hernia contents are being reduced, a small rubber catheter inserted in the hernia sac allows entry of air as downward tension is placed on the contents of the sac. This decreases the suction effect that holds the viscera within the chest. Occasionally in cases of a tight incarceration, the hiatal ring itself may have to be incised to allow return of the organs to the abdominal cavity. This can be done safely on the left side of the crus posteriorly along the side of the aorta.

The hernia sac is dissected free from the thoracic cavity and resected. Once this has been accomplished, the dead space in the mediastinum disappears as the lungs expand. No drainage of this space is necessary. The large diaphragmatic defect is located anterior to the lower esophagus, which usually remains bound to the posterior aspect of the hiatus by fibrous attachments. Care is taken during an ensuing dissection not to damage these posterior attachments, which hold the lower esophagus and its sphincter in an intra-abdominal position. The crural defect is closed beginning anteriorly with a stout 0 interrupted nonabsorbable suture. The closure is continued in a posterior direction until the hiatus just admits the tip of the forefinger beside the esophagus.

If the patient had objective evidence of significant reflux esophagitis preoperatively, an antireflux procedure

is now performed. If the posterior attachments of the lower esophagus are taken down during dissection, then it is likely that the LES has been disturbed and will be incompetent. In these patients we also perform an antireflux procedure at this time, and our procedure of choice is a loose Nissen fundoplication. If there is doubt about whether the esophagogastric junction is below the hiatus, it is best to mobilize the junction and the lower esophagus. Sufficient mobilization allows the junction to be brought 4 to 5 cm below the hiatus. The hiatus can then be narrowed or repaired by approximating the crura, beginning posteriorly over the aorta and behind the esophagus. This displaces the esophagus anteriorly into its normal position as it passes through the hiatus.

The stomach is now fixed within the peritoneal cavity by using two methods. The first is a modified Hill suture plication in which three interrupted nonabsorbable sutures are placed between the lesser curvature of the stomach and the preaortic fascia (Fig. 55–5). These sutures hold the gastroesophageal junction within the abdominal cavity and prevent the development of a type I—sliding—hernia postoperatively. If the esophagus has been mobilized during the repair, then these sutures can be attached to the crural repair posteriorly. The second maneuver is the performance of a Stamm gastrostomy, which serves two functions. First, it removes the need for a nasogastric tube placement. Many patients with incarcerated type II hernias have a prolonged period of postoperative gastric stasis, and a gastrostomy allows continued drainage without the discomfort or complications of an indwelling nasogastric catheter. Secondly, the gastrostomy fixes the stomach to the anterior wall, thus

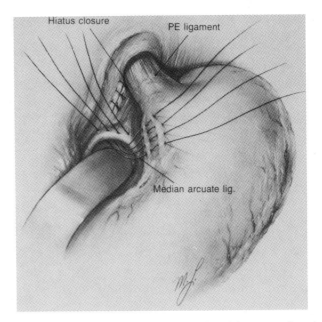

Fig. 55–5. Hill suture plication after reduction of the paraesophageal hernia and repair of the hiatal defect to maintain the position of the gastroesophageal junction within the abdominal cavity. (Reproduced with permission from Postlethwait, R.W. (Ed.): Surgery of the Esophagus, 2nd ed. East Norwalk, CT, Appleton-Century-Crofts, 1986, p. 245.)

maintaining its position within the abdominal cavity and preventing an intra-abdominal gastric volvulus, a reported complication of transthoracic repairs. The gastrostomy tube can be removed 8 to 12 days after the operation.

If gangrene or perforation is found at the time of operation, all devascularized tissue must be resected and all infected tissue debrided. Broad-spectrum antibiotics that incude anaerobic coverage are strongly advised in this setting because of the possibility of perforation and mediastinal contamination by salivary leakage.

MORBIDITY AND MORTALITY

Elective surgical repair of paraesophageal hernias is safe. A collective review of 163 such patients (Table 55–1) reveals that the operative mortality was less than 1%, a figure similar to that quoted for repair of sliding hiatal hernias. Emergency procedures in cases of gastric volvulus, however, carry a much higher mortality, appproximately 17% (Table 55–1). This 17-fold increase in operative risk underscores the need for elective repair at the time of initial diagnosis.

Operative complications are the same as for antireflux procedures, with two additions. In patients with gastric volvulus and obstruction, pulmonary complications apparently increase, probably because of episodes of regurgitation and aspiration. Also, prolonged gastric stasis may persist for a period of 7 to 10 days after operative repair because of lingering inflammation and edema in the released gastric segment.

RESULTS

Long-term results are generally excellent, regardless of whether or not an antireflux procedure is done in addition to simple repair. Hill and Tobias (1968) performed simple repair and had no recurrence or reflux in 22 patients over a 15-year follow-up. Wichterman and colleagues (1979), who routinely performed concomitant antireflux procedures, noted identical results. Recurrent type I hernias with reflux, however, have been reported by Ozdemir (1973)—10%, Pearson (1983)—8%, and their colleagues and Sanderud (1967)—8%—despite fundoplication at the time of initial repair. Simultaneous fundoplication is therefore apparently ineffective prophylaxis against recurrent herniation with resultant reflux. Fundoplication could be more appropriately used selectively in those patients with documented reflux.

Table 55–1. Operative Mortality for Paraesophageal Hernia Repair

Author	Elective (%)	Emergency (%)
Beardsley (1964)	—	3/10 (30)
Sanderud (1967)	0/14 (0)	1/7 (14)
Hill (1968)	0/19 (0)	2/10 (20)
Ozdemir (1973)	0/19 (0)	2/12 (16)
Wichterman (1979)	0/16 (0)	1/6 (16)
Carter (1980)	—	1/14 (7)
Pearson (1983)	0/47 (0)	1/4 (25)
Walther (1984)	0/15 (0)	—
Ellis (1986)	1/39 (2)	—
Total	1/169 (0.6)	11/63 (17.4)

Operative mortality reported as number of deaths divided by number of operated patients. Emergency defined as gastric volvulus.

REFERENCES

Beardsley, J.M., and Thompson, W.R.: Acutely obstructed hiatal hernia. Ann. Surg. 159:49, 1964.

Carter, R., Brewer, L.A., and Hinshaw, D.B.: Acute gastric volvulus: a study of 25 cases. Am. J. Surg. 140:99, 1980.

Ellis, F.H., Crozier, R.E., and Shea, J.A.: Paraesophageal hiatus hernia. Arch. Surg. 121:416, 1986.

Hill, L.D. and Tobias, J.A.: Paraesophageal hernia. Arch. Surg. 96:735, 1968.

Ozdemir, I.A., Burke, W.A., and Ikins, P.M.: Paraesophageal hernia: a life-threatening disease. Ann. Thorac. Surg. 16:547, 1973.

Pearson, F.G., et al.: Massive hiatal hernia with incarceration: a report of 53 cases. Ann. Thorac. Surg. 35:45, 1983.

Sanderud, A.: Surgical treatment for the complications of hiatal hernia. Acta Chir. Scand. 133:223, 1967.

Skinner, D.B., and Belsey, R.H.R.: Surgical management of esophageal reflux and hiatus hernia: long-term results with 1030 patients. J. Thorac. Cardiovasc. Surg. 53:33, 1967.

Walther, B., et al.: Effect of paraesophageal hernia on sphincter function and its implication on surgical therapy. Am. J. Surg. 147:111, 1984.

Wichterman, K., et al.: Giant paraesophageal hiatal hernia with intrathoracic stomach and colon: the case for early repair. Surgery 86:497, 1979.

CHAPTER 56

PACING THE DIAPHRAGM IN CHRONIC VENTILATORY INSUFFICIENCY

William W. L. Glenn and Hiroyuki Koda

Since its introduction into clinical use in 1964, diaphragm pacing has been employed to treat chronic hypoventilation in about 700 patients in many clinics, some for as long as 15 to 18 years. The technique, which uses electrical stimulation of the phrenic nerves, is applicable to selected cases of chronic ventilatory insufficiency resulting from malfunction of the respiratory control centers or secondary to a lesion in the upper motoneurons of the phrenic nerves.

CLINICAL APPLICATION

Selection of Patients

Diaphragm pacing is not indicated if the ventilatory condition is improving spontaneously, nor is it intended for temporary use, in drug poisoning for instance, or in other states of hypoventilation for which conventional means of artificial respiration suffice. It is not warranted in chronic hypoventilation if noninvasive methods of ventilatory support can conveniently meet the patient's needs. Positive-pressure ventilation through the nose by a tight-fitting face mask, for administration during sleep, that Kerby and associates (1987) mentioned and Braun (1987) discussed, may, if extended experience proves it effective, supplant diaphragm pacing in cases of chronic hypoventilation treatable by part-time pacing, for periods of time limited to the patient's tolerance of the mask.

Before a commitment is made to implant a diaphragm pacemaker in patients referred with chronic ventilatory insufficiency, certain perioperative matters must be considered, such as what will be their postoperative and subsequent care. Ventilatory insufficiency is usually only one of several disabilities present. Most patients are unable to care for themselves, apart from coping with their ventilatory problem. Should they be institutionalized for a long period, they may be neglected and, despite adequate ventilation, suffer deterioration. What aids are available to each one in terms of professional and family care and of housing, whether home or institution, must be explored and all possible support sought and, hopefully, assured to provide the paced patient the maximal opportunity for a meaningful existence. If the patient has no chance of achieving a cognitive state or is suffering from another life-threatening disease, diaphragm pacing is ill advised. Concern over possible iatrogenic injury to the phrenic nerve or diaphragm is not cause for denying treatment by pacing: safe techniques for implanting the electrodes are easily learned and the stimulation can be applied without harming phrenic nerves or diaphragm by strictly monitoring all aspects of it and heeding specified caveats (see Table 56–1). Several techniques for peripheral nerve stimulation are included in a review of diaphragm pacing by me and Phelps (1985). With the intention of avoiding manipulation of or contact with the phrenic nerves, Peterson (1986), Jammes (1986) and Ishii (1986) and their associates developed techniques modified from earlier ones for stimulating the diaphragm intramuscularly, transcutaneously, and transvenously. The clinical application of these techniques has been limited.

Indications for Diaphragm Pacing

Chronic Hypoventilation Syndromes

Idiopathic Central Alveolar Hypoventilation. In the absence of an identifiable organic lesion of the respiratory centers, the exact cause of hypoventilation may go undetermined. Weese-Mayer and associates (1988), using magnetic resonance imaging—MRI—and computed tomography—CT, failed to identify a specific lesion in the brain stem of infants with congenital central alveolar hypoventilation, but provided evidence for a more diffuse CNS process. Hypoventilation at birth or a history of apnea, like that accompanying near-miss episodes in sudden infant death syndrome—SIDS, suggested to Guilleminault and associates (1982) congenitally defective

Table 56–1.   Caveats in Diaphragm Pacing

Concern	Caveat
Selection of patients for diaphragm pacing	Structures to be affected by electrical stimulation must be adequate.
Operative technique	Iatrogenic injury to the phrenic nerve is the most common cause of failure to pace a normal nerve. Infection of any of the implantable components usually requires removal of all.
Use of pacemaker	Lack of complete understanding of proper settings of electronic parameters can lead to inadequate pacing or irreparable damage to the phrenic nerve and diaphragm.
Pacing schedule	The pacing schedule must be individualized for each patient's particular problem. Patients who require full-time pacing, particularly small children, need day-to-day supervision for first 6 to 8 months of pacing.
Pacemaker apparatus	Pacemaker failure in a quadriplegic can be disastrous. A fail-safe alarm system must be available for patients to activate with head or tongue. Failure of the pacemaker apparatus is most commonly caused by battery failure, broken antenna wire or connector, component failure in implanted radio receiver, circuit failure in exterior transmitter, and electrode wire breakage (which is the least likely cause of failure). Failure to pace or pace properly may be also an indication of injury to the nerve.
Upper airway obstruction and tracheal aspiration	Airway obstruction from several causes may interfere with ventilation. A clear airway during pacing is essential.
Sedatives, tranquilizers, narcotics	*Any respiratory depressant is contraindicated.* Pacing alone does not support ventilation in the sedated patient.
Major operations or disease, respiratory complications	Pacing may not provide sufficient ventilatory support in disorders that stimulate or depress general body metabolism.
Fatigue of diaphragm	Fatigue of the diaphragm results in inadequate ventilation and, if persistent, irreparable damage to the nerve and diaphragm. The diaphragm must be rested by providing passive ventilation should fatigue occur and the pacemaker parameters and schedule adjusted.

(Reproduced with permission from Glenn, W.W.L., Hogan, J.F., and Phelps, M.L.: Ventilatory support of the quadriplegic patient with respiratory paralysis by diaphragm pacing. Surg. Clin. North Am. *60*:1076, 1980.)

respiratory center control. In the older patient, the history may reveal a prior attack of encephalitis or an undiagnosed febrile illness, yet there is no residual organic deficit. Cases of associated disorders reported by Brouillette and colleagues (1986) included congenital rubella, hypothalamic dysfunction, Hirschsprung's disease, and ganglioneuromas. Clinical findings are chronic hypercapnia and hypoxemia. Hypoventilation is most severe during sleep and almost always present to some degree. When I and my associates (1978b) monitored blood gases, we found arterial oxygen tension typically decreased during sleep—Pa_{O_2} <70 mm Hg—and carbon dioxide tension increased—Pa_{CO_2} >60 mm Hg. Malfunction of respiratory center control was evidenced, according to Farmer and colleagues (1978), by loss of normal ventilatory response to hypercapnia or hypoxemia, or both, but the voluntary control of ventilation is not impaired. Bradley and associates (1984) reported an unusual case in which nocturnal hypoventilation was associated with a normal ventilatory response to hypoxia and hypercapnia; ventilatory failure, treated successfully by diaphragm pacing, was caused by generation of a pattern of rapid, shallow breathing.

Organic Lesions of the Brain Stem or Above. Brain stem lesions associated with hypoventilation with or without apnea are most commonly of vascular origin, including arteriovenous malformations, hemorrhage, and infarction. Other space-occupying lesions that interfere with respiratory control are, most notably, tumors. Brain stem lesions usually involve also some of the cranial nerve nuclei and the long motor and sensory tracts. The clinical picture in cases I and my associates (1980a) reviewed is of: (1) central alveolar hypoventilation, which may or may not be accompanied by paralysis of some respiratory muscles; (2) dysphagia and aspiration—the latter a common and serious complication that may necessitate closure of the larynx—caused by involvement by the lesion of the cranial nerve nuclei supplying the pharyngeal muscles; and (3) nonrespiratory skeletal muscle involvement, manifested by partial or complete hemi- or quadriplegia. Patients without respiratory muscle paralysis are usually able to ventilate adequately unassisted during the waking hours, but develop hypoventilation with or without periodic apnea during sleep. Voluntary control of respiration is usually not impaired.

Lesions of the Cervical Cord. Respiratory paralysis caused by a lesion of the cervical cord above C3—most often caused by motor vehicle and sports accidents and usually accompanied by quadriplegia—we found amenable to diaphragm pacing, provided the lower motoneurons of the phrenic nerves are functionally intact (1980b, 1984).

To prevent unnecessary implantation of a diaphragm

pacemaker following trauma to the central nervous system, pacing is not offered until *the patient's total neurologic status has been stable for a minimum of three months.*

Chronic Obstructive Pulmonary Disease—COPD

Most patients with COPD do not require diaphragm pacing, because they are either in stable condition or can be safely oxygenated. As I and my colleagues pointed out (1978b), the primary indication for pacing in COPD is the patient's inability to maintain oxygenation despite well controlled oxygen therapy. There are, however, definite limits to the efficacy of pacing. These limits may be imposed by diaphragm flattening, diminished elastic recoil, high airway resistance, and a degree of lung hyperinflation that approaches the limits of the inspiratory movement of the thoracic cage.

Several conditions must be met for diaphragm pacing to be helpful to patients with COPD. First, significant, hemodynamically compromising hypoxia is a prerequisite, because safe oxygenation rather than the elimination of carbon dioxide retention is the major therapeutic objective. Second, even well controlled oxygen therapy must fail or present high risks before more complex approaches such as pacing are tried. Third, expiratory flow must be adequate, because in COPD the latter is always more rate-limiting than inspiratory flow. Fourth, because pacing affects only one inspiratory muscle, the diaphragm, adequate function of this muscle must be demonstrated.

Experience suggests that pacing is particularly useful at night, when the most severe respiratory failure occurs. Therefore, it can be used primarily as a device for the safe maintenance of adequate respiration and blood gases while full oxygenation is provided—"pacing protected oxygenation."

Screening Tests

A basic requirement for successful diaphragm pacing is normal or near-normal function of phrenic nerves, lungs, diaphragm, and thoracic skeleton. Preoperative screening tests are carried out on all candidates for the procedure. Such tests are listed in Table 56–2. Five of these tests, one in each of the groups listed, are particularly important for determining the suitability of pacing.

Percutaneous Stimulation of the Phrenic Nerves in the Neck

Shaw and colleagues (1975, 1980) described the test of the phrenic nerves' functional integrity before operation: After placing an indifferent electrode behind the neck in contact with the skin, an electrode probe—usually available from the physiotherapist as part of the neural stimulation equipment, set to deliver 5 to 10 mamp for 1 msec at a repetition rate of 1/sec—is directed behind the lateral border of the sternocleidomastoid muscle and moved up and down along the body of the anterior scalene muscle (Fig. 56–A). The phrenic nerve is found by first identifying the brachial plexus lying lateral to the scalene muscle border; the phrenic nerve is found lying

Table 56–2. Screening Tests for Candidates for Diaphragm Pacing

Functional status of components of respiration

Phrenic nerves
  Viability: Diaphragm response to
    percutaneous stimulation of phrenic nerves in neck
    transvenous stimulation of phrenic nerves in thorax
    direct stimulation of phrenic nerves at operation
  Impulse conduction: time and muscle action potential

Respiratory center
  Ventilatory response to normocapnic hypoxia, hypercapnic hyperoxia, and hypercapnic hypoxia
  Ventilatory response to airway occlusion 0.1 sec after onset of inspiration
  Arterial blood gas levels at rest and during sleep
  Urinary phosphoryltransferase enzyme levels (for Leigh's disease)

Lung
  Routine pulmonary function test
  Xenon-133 perfusion and ventilation scan
  Arterial blood gas levels at rest and during maximum hyperventilation
  Flow volume curves

Diaphragm
  Voluntary excursions measured at fluoroscopy (supine)
  Transdiaphragmatic pressures (Pdi) at maximum inspiration

Upper airway
  For presence of obstruction, air flow rates; polysomnographic study

Adapted from Glenn, W.W.L.: Diaphragm pacing: present status. PACE *1*:357, 1978.

medial to the plexus. A forceful contraction of the diaphragm signifies normal or near-normal diaphragm function, whereas a weak contraction may signify either failure to locate all of the phrenic nerve fibers with the stimulating probe or, more likely, viability of just a few neurons or subnormal function of the diaphragm muscle. The potentially maximal descent cannot be determined, because it cannot be known whether all the phrenic nerve fibers are being stimulated. Therefore, the quality of the response is taken as a measure of nerve viability. Shaw and associates (1980) wrote that the absence of contraction when the anatomic location of the nerve is stimulated nearly always means nonviability of the nerve. If there is doubt that the probe has located the nerve, direct exploration is planned. Should a viable nerve be found, the neck wound is closed and a monopolar electrode implanted on the thoracic portion of the nerve at a subsequent operation (see Thoracic Approach p. 599). Phrenic nerve conduction time—PNCT—and muscle action potential—MAP—should be determined if visible contraction of the diaphragm is diminished. To detect the onset of diaphragm contraction, two electrodes are placed on the skin over the eighth interspace in the anterior and posterior axillary lines. A third electrode—ground—is placed in the region of the xiphoid process. A stimulus is then applied to the phrenic nerve in the neck, and the time required for the impulse to pass along the phrenic nerve to the diaphragm is recorded (Fig. 56–1B). Shaw and associates (1980) found the PNCT in

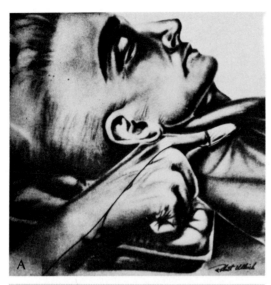

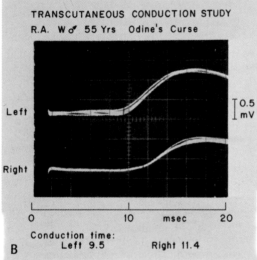

TRANSCUTANEOUS CONDUCTION STUDY
R.A. W ♂ 55 Yrs   Odine's Curse

Left

Right

0.5 mV

0   10   msec   20

Conduction time:
   Left 9.5   Right 11.4

Fig. 56–1. *A*, Technique of percutaneous phrenic nerve stimulation (see text). (Glenn, W.W.L., et al.: Long-term ventilatory support by diaphragm pacing in quadriplegia. Ann. Surg. *183*:566, 1976.)

B, Percutaneous phrenic nerve stimulation prior to implantation of a pacemaker. Top: Left phrenic nerve, conduction time 9.5 milliseconds. Bottom: Right phrenic nerve, conduction time 11.4 milliseconds. It may be significant that the patient was a mail carrier who carried the mail bag over his right shoulder for many years.

normal adult volunteers to be 8.40 msec ± 0.78 msec SD, range 7.5 to 10 msec. Prolongation beyond 14 msec usually is an indication of serious local or systemic disease. The normal range of the MAP is 0.2 to 0.7 mv. Brouillette and associates reported in 1983 that infants and small children, because of their small size, had a shorter PNCT, 6.5 msec ± 1.2 msec SD.

Induction of Hypercapnia and Hypoxia

In patients with hypoventilation of central origin, the ventilatory response to hypercapnia and hypoxia has been either subnormal or absent, as Farmer and associates (1978) reported.

Blood Gas and pH Levels

In samples of arterial blood during quiet breathing and maximum voluntary hyperventilation both blood gas and pH levels must be determined. This indication of pulmonary competence reflects the functional state of the lungs, phrenic nerves, and diaphragm and is a particularly useful test if phrenic nerve and diaphragm function is believed normal but lung function is subnormal because of parenchymal disease. Patients whose arterial blood gases are subnormal on quiet breathing and do not become normal or near normal with hyperventilation cannot be improved by diaphragm pacing. Other tests of pulmonary function, as listed in Table 56–2, should be carried out in these patients to determine the nature and extent of the underlying disorder.

Transdiaphragmatic Pressure Gradient—Pdi

Using the technique developed by Milic-Emili and associates (1964) and Roussos and Macklem (1977) for measuring Pdi to assess functional status of the diaphragm, Newsom Davis (1976) found no change in Pdi in paralyzed diaphragms during voluntary inspiration. I and my associates, likewise measuring Pdi pressure, elicited a subnormal response in the diaphragms paralyzed by a high cervical cord lesion when applying maximal electrical stimulation to the phrenic nerve. This was true at the time of initial testing in all patients who later were paced, probably because the diaphragm had atrophied following their accident.

Sleep Study

O_2 saturation and CO_2 retention are monitored to determine the presence and severity of sleep apnea. These findings are correlated with airflow in the trachea, movement of the chest wall, or changes in pressure in the esophagus. All are correlated with the stage of sleep. Periods of hypoventilation or apnea caused by upper airway obstruction—UAO—as well as those due to central apnea may be present and must be identified as I and my associates (1978b) recommended.

STIMULATING APPARATUS

The diaphragm pacemaker consists of four main parts: a radiofrequency generator and transmitter, an external coil antenna, a radiofrequency receiver, and a monopolar platinum ribbon electrode. I prefer the monopolar electrode designed for phrenic nerve stimulation (Fig. 56–2) to the bipolar electrode used earlier, as less dissection is required for its implantation and, because it does not encircle the nerve, compression injury is less likely (Fig. 56–3). The bipolar electrode is indicated if another electrical stimulator, such as a cardiac pacemaker, is already in place. Programmed radiofrequency pulses are transmitted by the antenna through the intact skin to the subcutaneously placed radio receiver, where they are converted to electrical pulses and delivered by electrodes to the phrenic nerves. I and my associates (1972, 1980b) described the electronic apparatus and the

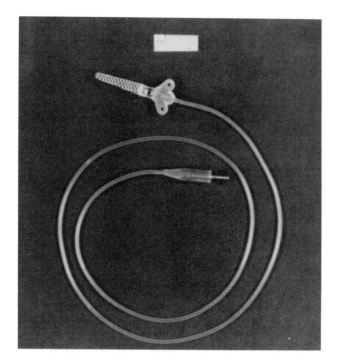

Fig. 56–2. Detail of platinum ribbon monopolar neural electrode designed for phrenic nerve stimulation.

method of its application in detail. Depending on whether the diaphragm is to be paced unilaterally or bilaterally, the external components are supplied as single or double units. Avery Laboratories provided instructions for the operation, maintenance, and trouble-shooting of the electronic apparatus.

A totally implantable stimulator, using a lithium battery for its power source, that can be integrated and programmed from the exterior, was constructed in the laboratory to enable my colleagues and me to carry out long-term stimulation experiments in animals, as Hogan (1976) and Oda (1979) and their colleagues reported. We also constructed a prototype of a clinical, totally implantable, programmable stimulator and tested it on animals,

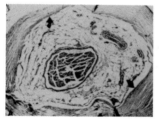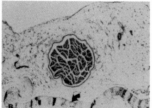

Fig. 56–3. *A,* Section of left phrenic nerve at electrode level after stimulation with a bipolar electrode for 126 days at 26 Hz. Epineural fibroadipose layer is completely surrounded by a thick fibrous capsule (arrows), but nerve fascicle itself is histologically unremarkable. *B,* Section of right phrenic nerve at electrode level after stimulation with a monopolar electrode of 154 days at 27 Hz. A band of fibrous tissue (arrow) has developed at the lower margin facing the electrode. The nerve fascicle is histologically unremarkable. Hematoxylin and eosin stain, × 39. (From Kim, J.H., et al.: Light and electron microscopic studies of phrenic nerves after long-term electrical stimulation. J. Neurosurg. 58:85, 1980.)

as Hogan and associates (in press) reported; this stimulator meets all the requirements for controlled diaphragm pacing. The stimulator is more convenient than the radiofrequency one; among other attributes, it eliminates the need for an external transmitter and antennas.

PACEMAKER IMPLANTATION

Preoperative Preparation

The electronic pacemaker parts to be implanted in the body are sterilized as follows: the neural electrode, metal plate anode electrode, and plastic envelope to contain the electrode junctions by *autoclave* just before use; the radio receiver by ethylene oxide gas at least 48 hours before use. The manufacturer states that the receiver may be autoclaved, but we use gas sterilization to prevent any possibility of injury to the electronic components by the high temperatures of the autoclave.

Routine antiseptic precautions are taken, with the addition of the double glove/double mask technique, including frequent changing of the outer gloves during the procedure. Antibiotics, which should be continued postoperatively, are administered prophylactically 3 hours before the operation. Infection must be assiduously guarded against. Infection, if it involves the neural electrode, is a serious event, requiring removal of the receiver-electrode assembly and maintenance of a prolonged period without pacing. Not until the infection has been cured is it safe to install a new electrode.

Cervical Approach

The cervical approach for implanting the electrodes on the phrenic nerves has largely been abandoned because of its failure to enable inclusion within the electrode cuff of the lowest component of the nerve, the so-called accessory branch, or "nebenphrenicus" (Fig. 56–4). This branch arises from the fifth cervical segment of the spinal cord and joins the other phrenic nerve components from C3 and C4 at or below the level of the clavicle. Cervical implantation of the neural electrodes is now reserved for those patients who have extensive thoracic deformity or parenchymal lung disease. The cervical approach was described in the second edition of this text and in an article by me and my associates in 1980(b).

Thoracic Approach

The portion of the phrenic nerve that lies above the heart is approached by entering the chest anteriorly through the second interspace. A 15-cm skin incision is made at the second interspace, from the lateral border of the sternum to just beyond the anterior axillary line. The pectoralis major and minor muscles are split in the direction of their fibers, and the chest is entered through the second interspace. The incision is extended through the pleura laterally for better exposure when needed. The internal mammary artery and vein are divided for better exposure, and the ribs are spread apart. Division of the internal mammary vessels, which may be required

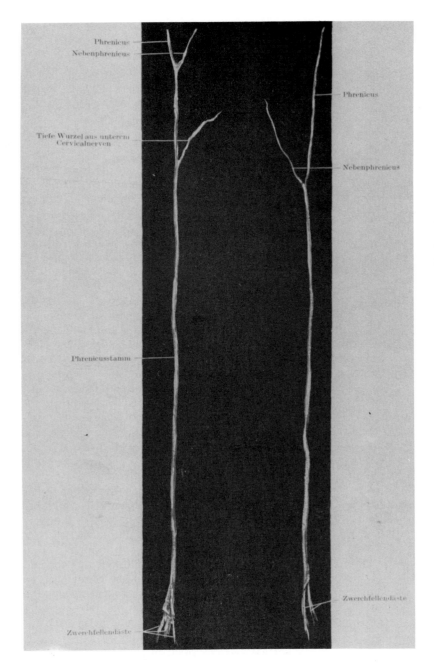

Phrenicus
Nebenphrenicus

Tiefe Wurzel aus unterem
Cervicalnerven

Phrenicusstamm

Zwerchfellendäste

Phrenicus

Nebenphrenicus

Zwerchfellendäste

Fig. 56–4. Phrenic nerves removed by the operation of exeresis. This was practiced in the early twentieth century in the treatment of apical tuberculosis. To completely paralyze the diaphragm, surgeons found it necessary to remove all branches of the phrenic nerve. This they accomplished by avulsing the nerves in the neck. The "Nebenphrenicus" is probably the branch of the 5th cervical, the so-called accessory branch, shown here joining the other branches at a high level on the right side and a low level on the left. On the left side, such a branch would probably not be stimulated by an electrode placed in the usual cervical location. The specimen from the right side illustrates, in addition, a branch from the lower cervical cord joining the main trunk. This branch certainly would be missed by stimulation from the cervical location. (Glenn, W.W.L., and Sairenji, H.: Diaphragm pacing in the treatment of chronic ventilatory insufficiency. *In* The Thorax, Part B. Edited by C. Roussos and P.T. Macklem. New York, Marcel Dekker, 1985, pp. 1434–1436.)

for myocardial revascularization later, can be avoided by extending the second interspace incision laterally or by entering the chest through the third interspace anterolaterally. A midsternal approach has been advocated to approach both nerves at the same operation. The exposure of the nerves for the accurate placement of the electrodes using these alternative approaches may be more difficult than using the preferred approach through the second interspace anteriorly. The patient is rotated to the contralateral side, the lung is retracted, and the phrenic nerve is identified as it passes superficially under the pleura. A site for placement of the electrode is selected 5 to 10 cm above the heart, which allows the electrode to lie flat against the mediastinum (Fig. 56–5). Parallel incisions 1.5 cm long are made through the

pleura on each side of the nerve, with preservation of the perineural blood vessels. A 4-0 monofilament suture is inserted over and over into the mediastinal tissues parallel to the ventral incision in the pleura. Care must be taken not to puncture the underlying vascular structures. The ends of the suture, with needles attached, are held loosely in bulldog clamps. A right-angled clamp is passed behind the nerve and its jaws spread to create a tunnel to accommodate the electrode cuff, the toe of which is then passed from ventral to dorsal behind the nerve and vascular bundles. The silicone rubber heel of the electrode is then fixed firmly in position to the tissues on the ventral side of the nerve by passing the previously placed monofilament suture in the mediastinal tissue over and over through the apertures in the heel and

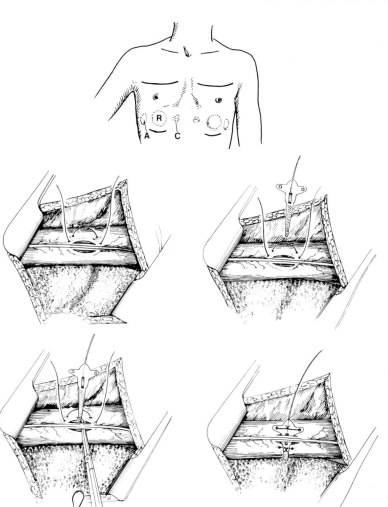

Fig. 56–5. Transthoracic approach to the phrenic nerves. *Top;* Above nipples: incisions in second interspace to expose phrenic nerves. At costal margin: incisions to implant RF receivers (*R*), anode electric plate (*A*), and electrode connectors (*C*). *Middle and Bottom;* Technique of implanting neural monopolar electrode behind phrenic nerve. (Modified from Glenn, W.W.L.: The diaphragm. *In* Thoracic and Cardiovascular Surgery, 4th ed. Edited by W.W.L. Glenn. East Norwalk, CT, Appleton-Century-Crofts, 1983, p. 363.)

underlying tissues and then tying it firmly on top of the heel. The toe is likewise fixed to the tissues on the dorsal side of the nerve using a single mattress suture to prevent torsion on or a twisting of the electrode.

A second skin incision about 5 cm long is made transversely at the costal margin in the anterior axillary line. A subcutaneous pocket about 10 cm deep and 5 cm wide is created to accommodate the radio receiver. The upper extent of the pocket should be about 2 to 4 cm below the inframammary fold. The electrode wire and connector attached to the phrenic nerve is passed from within the thorax through the third or fourth interspace anteriorly into the subcutaneous pocket and out through the subpectoral incision. Passage of the electrode is facilitated by first pulling a No. 28 plastic tube from the thoracic cavity into the subcutaneous pocket, using this tube as the carrier for the electrode and connector, which are compartmentalized within it by a suture. A segment of the wire is retained in the thorax to be looped and laid on the anterior surface of the lung to prevent tension on the neural electrode.

The anode electrode from the receiver, marked by a red thread embedded in the silicone rubber collar, is then connected to the wire attached to the anode plate,

and the cathode electrode to the wire attached to the electrode cuff. The receiver is inserted through the incision and into the subcutaneous pocket cephalad to the incision, where it is advanced to the upper end of the pocket and fixed firmly with interrupted 3–0 plain catgut sutures placed in the tissue close to its lower border. Then cathode and anode electrode junctions are enclosed in a Teflon plastic bag, which is fixed in place in the subcutaneous pocket alongside and medial to the receiver pocket. The anode plate and attached wire are placed in the subcutaneous pocket lateral to the receiver pocket. Both the copper coil of the receiver and the metal plate of the anode must face *outwards*, toward the undersurface of the skin. All incisions are closed snugly to obliterate dead space and to immobilize the receiver capsule. A chest tube for drainage is inserted in the posterior axillary line, with care taken to avoid entanglement with the implanted electronic components, to remain for 48 hours.

Prior to closure of the chest, the integrity of the pacemaker system is tested. A sterile antenna attached to an off-table transmitter is held directly over the implanted radio receiver and stimulation is applied. If a good response is obtained, the threshold to stimulation is noted.

It should be in the range of 1.0 to 2.0 mamp. A higher threshold may signal displacement of the electrode or interposition of tissue between electrode and nerve. After a final inspection of the neural electrode implantation site, the redundant loop of wire is laid on the surface of the expanded upper lobe and the thoracotomy wound is closed. Pacemaker function is again assessed before leaving the operating room.

For bilateral pacing, the operation to implant on the contralateral side is delayed for about two weeks.

Antibiotics, which were started preoperatively, are continued intravenously after each of the two procedures q 6 h for 48 hours then by mouth for a week.

The scheduled pacing regimen is not begun for 12 to 14 days postoperatively. To test for early malfunction of the pacemaker, however, two or three electrically-induced inspirations are attempted on the day following the operation and several times thereafter. Pacing for longer periods at this time could induce a pleural effusion. Should the trial fail to activate the diaphragm, the external unit is carefully checked for malfunction. If the external unit is in good order, the implanted components are examined. The receiver with its electrode attachment in the subcutaneous pocket is exposed first. If no fault is found there but pacing is still not effected, the neural electrode on the phrenic nerve is exposed and examined for displacement, which could be a cause of pressure on or of loss of contact with the nerve. Shaw and colleagues (1980) found that if the phrenic nerve was damaged by pressure or infection, the return of function may take many months.

CONDUCT OF PACING

About two weeks after implantation of the pacemaker, the current level and respiration rate at which pacing is to be instituted are established. The other electrical parameters, namely the inspiration duration and stimulus frequency, have been preset in the transmitter at optimum levels derived from results in patients following studies in our laboratory conducted by me (1980b) and Oda (1981) and our associates. They can be altered by the physician whenever necessary. Details for regulating the parameters for the several available types of transmitters are supplied by the manufacturer. A fluoroscopic study and base-line measurements are made of diaphragm excursions and of that current which initiates contraction of a hemidiaphragm—threshold—and that which produces maximum contraction. The current eliciting the first visible contraction of the diaphragm is recorded. Alternatively, albeit less accurately, threshold can be determined at the bedside; it is that current eliciting the first observed flicker of diaphragm muscle contraction at the costal margin.

At fluoroscopy, diaphragm contractions are measured, and the results recorded, during attempted voluntary and electrically-stimulated respiration, with the patient in the supine position. The examination is done easily using a scale attached to the fluoroscope screen. The scale is made by sticking lead numerals, numbers 1 through 12, 1 cm apart onto a strip of paper tape and securing them with another strip. With the scale attached to the center of its undersurface, the screen is mobilized exactly 30 cm above the x-ray table with the numeral 1 positioned parallel to the dome of the hemidiaphragm. Measurement of diaphragm descent by this means can easily be accurately repeated for comparison whenever desired.

In normal young adults, diaphragm descent on voluntary inspiration is 8 to 10 cm, somewhat less in young children and older adults, and is greater on the left side than on the right. In paced patients, provided the stimulating electrode has been implanted in the thorax, ensuring inclusion of all phrenic nerve fibers within its cuff, application of stimulation at maximal parameters causes greater descent than does voluntary inspiration. Thus, at fluoroscopy, if diaphragm contractions on stimulation are shallower than expected, and certainly if on stimulation less than 5 cm, one must assume neuromuscular system malfunction. If the electrode implantation is in the neck, one should suspect a lack of stimulation of all motoneurons. Whatever the exact cause for the small diaphragm descent, optimal benefit will not be derived from the pacing regimen.

The current for pacing is that, or very slightly more, that effects just maximal descent of the diaphragm regardless of the other pacing parameters. Because it essentially corresponds to the maximal tidal volume during pacing, the maximal current can be determined at the bedside, although less accurately. Threshold and maximal levels are reassessed, preferably at fluoroscopy, one month after operation, then as necessary until stable parameters are reached. Minor variations in current requirements are to be expected after six months, but major variations occur when the system malfunctions. The following day pacing is instituted for a trial period. The respiratory rate and, if necessary, the stimulus frequency, are adjusted according to the pacing mode selected (Table 56–3). A change in preset inspiration duration—1.3 sec—is rarely necessary for pacing older children and adults. During the trial on pacing V_T is determined and the adequacy of ventilation is measured by E_{TCO_2} and or S_{AO_2}.

Pacing in Adults and Older Children

The goal of pacing, provision of ventilatory assistance commensurate with the patient's ventilatory deficit, is reached by employing stimulus parameters that experimental and clinical experience has shown keep the diaphragm as free from fatigue as possible: low current level, slow respiration rate, low stimulus frequency and short inspiration duration, in brief, the electric charge that will mimimize the duty cycle of the contracting muscle (Table 56–3).

Unilateral Pacing

If part-time pacing will fulfill the patient's needs, one hemidiaphragm alone is paced. The pulse interval—PI—is set at 50 to 40 msec—20 to 25 Hz—and the respiration rate—rpm—at 12 to 14. A schedule of 8 to a maximum

Table 56–3. Pacing Schedules for Older Children and Adults

Side(s) Paced	Status of Diaphragm	Time Paced	Time Paced hr/24 hr	Respiratory Rate (rpm)	Pulse Frequency (msec)
Unilateral	Unparalyzed or paralyzed	Part-time	12	12–14	40–50 (25–20 Hz)
Bilateral simultaneously	Paralyzed	Part-time	8–20	8–16	50–90 (20–11 Hz)
Bilateral alternate sides	Unparalyzed or paralyzed	Full-time	12 each side	12–14	40–50 (25–20 Hz)
Bilateral simultaneously	Unparalyzed or paralyzed	Full-time	24	6–10	120–140 (8.33–7.16 Hz)

The pacing schedule is individualized according to the specific ventilatory assistance required and the capacity of the pacing system to provide it. In general, the lowest respiratory rate and pulse frequency are employed. The current delivered to the nerve is always adjusted to just maximal tidal volume. If ventilatory assistance is needed only during sleep, pacing of one hemidiaphragm for 10–12 hours/day may be sufficient. In this case conditioning of the diaphragm is not necessary and pacing is started two weeks after implantation of the stimulator at a respiratory rate of 12 to 14 and a pulse frequency of 25 to 20 Hz. If, on the other hand, ventilatory support is to be full time, the diaphragm muscle must first be conditioned to low-frequency stimulation at a slow rate. Both hemidiaphragms are paced simultaneously beginning two weeks after implantation of the second unit. Pacing is applied for 15 min/hour, at 10 rpm and a pulse frequency of 10 or 11 Hz. The time on pacing is gradually increased, the respiratory rate is decreased and the frequency lowered until full-time pacing without fatigue is possible 4 to 6 months later. The effectiveness of pacing is monitored hourly by end-tidal CO_2 measurements (acceptable range 30–45 mm Hg) or tidal and minute volumes (for basal requirements refer to Radford nomogram) (Glenn and associates, 1984). A pacing schedule for infants and small children is described by Brouillette and associates (1988).

Adapted from Glenn, W.W.L., et al.: Twenty years of experience in phrenic nerve stimulation to pace the diaphragm. PACE 9:780, 1986.

of 12 hours on pacing per 24 hours followed by at least 12 hours off pacing is started about 2 weeks after implantation of the pacemaker. A baseline sleep study off and on pacing is done to demonstrate the immediate efficacy of this regimen and reveal any induction of upper airway obstruction. If obstruction is present, and it nearly always is when pacing is done during sleep, a tracheostoma is made to bypass it, after which the patient can be discharged from the hospital, to be followed at three-month intervals for the first year and six-month intervals thereafter.

Bilateral Pacing

When pacing of one side alone does not move enough air, both hemidiaphragms are paced. Stimulation is applied alternately, either for specified periods or on alternate breaths—rarely used, or simultaneously for specified periods up to a maximum of 12 hours daily or continuously for 24. Except in the simultaneous application, bilateral stimulation employs the same electrical parameters as unilateral (Table 56–3). Pacing is initiated 2 weeks after installation of the second stimulator, on completion of tests similar to those done preparatory to unilateral pacing. Because the threshold and maximal current for pacing is never the same in both hemidiaphragms, each side is tested individually.

For full-time ventilatory support, continuous simultaneous bilateral pacing is desired. It is applicable to most older children and adults with respiratory muscle paralysis who qualify for pacing, and in selected patients with severe central hypoventilation in whom pacing of one hemidiaphragm is not enough assistance.

A prerequisite to carrying out simultaneous continuous full-time pacing is conditioning of the diaphragm muscle.

Leith (1976) and Gross (1980) with their associates reported studies in which skeletal muscle was strengthened and endurance increased through appropriate exercise, voluntary or electrically induced. Salmons and Vrbová (1969) showed that electrical stimulation of skeletal muscle at a *low frequency* over time converts the fast-twitch muscle fibers, which fatigue rapidly with exercise or stimulation, to slow-twitch ones that resist fatigue. This is the rationale Oda and colleagues (1981) and I and my colleagues (1984) used for applying low-frequency stimulation intermittently for an extended time as the first stage in the conduct of diaphragm pacing for full-time ventilatory assistance. Pathophysiological studies on the paced diaphragm show minimal morphologic changes in diaphragm muscle fibers stimulated for long periods at low frequency, in contrast to marked changes in fiber structure, as revealed on gross and microscopic studies in muscle stimulated at high frequency, as Ciesielski and associates (1983) reported (Fig. 56–6).

Conditioning of Diaphragm Muscle

Three adjustable pacing parameters are manipulated to achieve a fatigue-resistant diaphragm muscle: electrical pulse frequency—pulse interval, respiration rate, and time on pacing. The stimulus frequency is initially set at 90 or 100 msec PI—11.1 or 10 Hz, the rpm at 9 or 10. Pacing is applied about 15 minutes per hour when awake.

During conditioning, ventilation is monitored hourly, or as often as necessary, by measurement of end-tidal CO_2, transcutaneous O_2 saturation, or tidal volume at the beginning and end of each pacing period. Measurement of end tidal CO_2 using a capnometer is the simplest and most reliable method.*

*Hewlett Packard Corp., Waltham, MA 02154

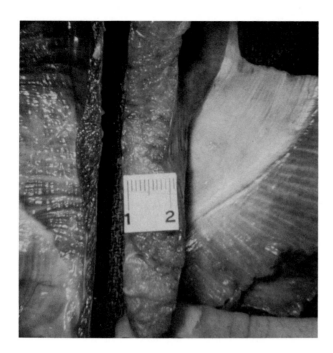

Fig. 56–6. Influence of stimulus frequency on muscle structure. Experiment 17009. The thickened pale hemidiaphragm (right) stimulated at high frequency (27 Hz) compared with the darker, thinner hemidiaphragm (left) of the unstimulated contralateral hemidiaphragm. Microscopic study revealed increased diameter of the stimulated fibers. The animal underwent alternating 6-week periods of stimulation and rest for approximately 1 year. When compared with muscle stimulated for a similar period at low frequency (11 Hz), the gross appearance of the stimulated and nonstimulated muscle was the same and there was only slight increase in muscle fiber diameter. (From Ciesielski, T.E., et al.: Response of the diaphragm muscle to electrical stimulation of the phrenic nerve: a histochemical and ultrastructural study. J. Neurosurg. 58:92, 1983.)

After 4 to 6 weeks of such stimulation, the PI is widened by 10 msec, and thereafter by 10 msec about every 4 to 6 weeks up to 130 msec—7.69 Hz; in patients with a small ventilatory capacity relative to their body size, it may not be possible to widen it to more than 120 msec and still maintain adequate ventilatory support, although in those with large ventilatory capacity it can be widened safely to 140 msec—7.14 Hz. Initially at 90 msec—11.1 Hz—the upper abdominal wall vibrates because of the widely spaced diaphragm contractions. The vibrations, which are measured in acceleration units, become greater as the PI is widened, but lessen when contractions fuse as the muscle becomes conditioned to the lower stimulus frequency (Fig. 56–7). The indication to widen the PI further is the lessening of the intensity of the vibration while VT remains at least the same or is increasing; no attempt is made to widen it more rapidly than the patient can comfortably tolerate. In the older child or adult, stimulation at 120 to 130 msec will usually provide sufficient ventilation by the third or fourth month following initiation of pacing.

The respiration rate is decreased by 1/min after 4 to 6 weeks and again after 4 to 6 weeks. When a schedule of 24 hours of continuous pacing has been reached in the older child or adult, a rate of 7 to 9 should be sufficient

for the supine position. I and my associates in 1972 advised that in the paralyzed patient the rpm should be increased by 1 for the sitting position to compensate for a fall in VT; in addition, to enhance VT with this change in position, they fit the patient with a snug abdominal binder. Elastic stockings from toes to groin are applied if postural hypotension is a problem. Mead and colleagues (1984) provided the physiologic basis for the change in VT as related to posture in the paralyzed patient during pacing.

The time on pacing is restricted initially to 15 minutes during each waking hour. The pacing periods can usually be lengthened by 15 minutes every week, with each pacing period followed by a similarly long period on the positive pressure ventilator. Pacing during sleep is started when a 3-hour on/off waking-hour schedule has been reached; then the same schedule is employed as for the waking hours. If after several weeks there are no signs of diaphragm fatigue from 3 hours of pacing, the time on pacing is increased to 4 to 6 hours, followed by a like period off. Over the next 6 to 8 weeks the periods on pacing are gradually lengthened and those on the ventilator shortened. The point at which a patient can be paced full time—24 hours continuously— should coincide with the optimal PI and rpm—130 msec (7.69 Hz) and 7 to 9, respectively.

Upon evidence of diaphragm fatigue, the mechanical ventilator is immediately substituted. The pacemaking apparatus is checked for malfunction and the pacing parameters reviewed. The pacing periods may have to be shortened temporarily. The stimulus frequency should not be increased, because stimulating at a higher frequency would eventually necessitate reconditioning the diaphragm muscle to low-frequency pacing.

Conditioning the diaphragm to withstand continuously applied low-frequency stimulation takes at least 4 to 6 months using the preceding schedule under circumstances that are ideal. When function of each component of the respiratory system has not been optimal I and my associates (1984) found it may not be possible to achieve full-time pacing, or at least achievement may take longer.

Because low-frequency stimulation causes minimal alteration of muscle fiber structure, it would appear that one could employ it in all cases of pacing. I and my associates (1980b) found, however, that unless the diaphragm has been conditioned and the two hemidiaphragms are paced simultaneously, VT accompanying low-frequency stimulation is inadequate to meet ventilatory needs (Fig. 56–8).

Patients who have respiratory paralysis and need continuous ventilatory support through pacing alone and those who have severe central alveolar hypoventilation—CAH—who need it as a supplement to spontaneous respiration, if they were started on pacing—either unilateral or bilateral in the alternate breath or alternate side method—at a high frequency—40 to 50 msec PI; 25 to 20 Hz—and a respiration rate of 12 to 14/min, they will first have to be conditioned to continuous, low frequency stimulation. An effective method for this is initially pacing the two hemidiaphragms simultaneously at 90 to 100

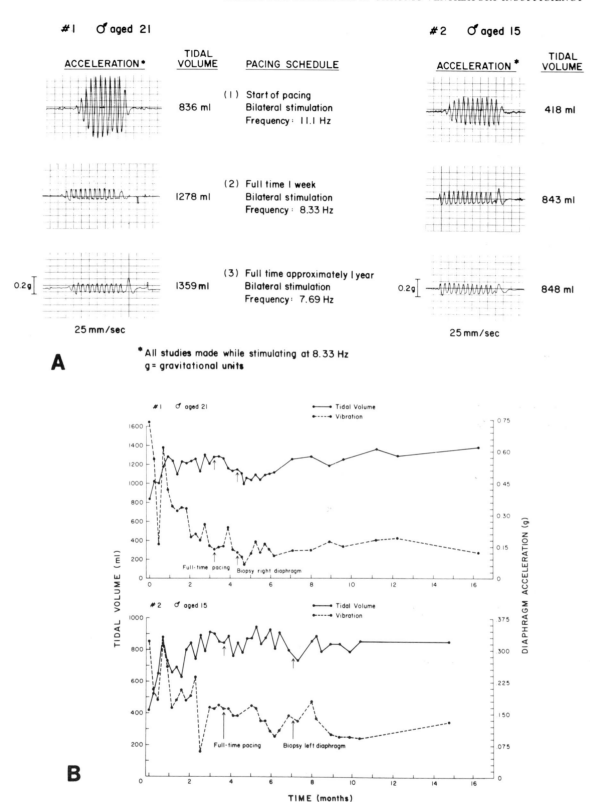

Fig. 56–7. Diaphragm pacing by electrical stimulation of the phrenic nerve. *A,* Muscle contraction acceleration and tidal volume studies in 2 quadriplegic, respirator-dependent patients: (1) soon after the initiation of bilateral simultaneous diaphragm pacing, (2) when full-time ventilatory support was achieved, and (3) after approximately 1 year of such support. The gradual fusion of individual pulses is indicative of conditioning of muscle to low-frequency stimulation. *B,* Acceleration and tidal volume are charted for the entire study period in cases 1 and 2. All studies were made after a rest period of at least 2 hours on a mechanical ventilator. The greatest changes in acceleration and tidal volume took place during the first 3 to 4 months after pacing was instituted. (From Glenn, W.W.L., and Phelps, M.L.: Diaphragm pacing by electrical stimulation of the phrenic nerve. Neurosurgery *17:*974, 1985.)

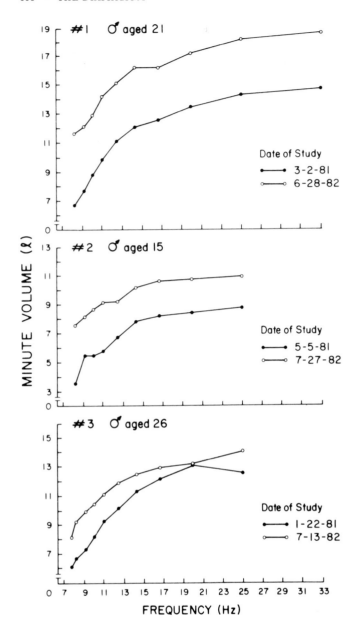

Fig. 56–8. Minute volume of ventilation during pacing of diaphragm at various pulse intervals in three patients. (Electrical frequency was measured as the pulse interval in milliseconds and, for convenience of reporting, converted to pulse frequency in Hertz [Hz]). The study performed at the beginning of pacing is compared with one performed about one year after full-time ventilatory support was achieved. There was an increase in minute volume at all stimulation frequencies that was proportionately greater at the lower frequencies. (Glenn, W.W.L., et al.: Ventilatory support by pacing of the conditioned diaphragm in quadriplegia. N. Engl. J. Med. *310*:1150, 1984.)

msec—11.1 to 10 Hz—for 12 hours, followed by 12 hours on a mechanical ventilator. The time on pacing is gradually extended as the PI and rpm are adjusted, as mentioned before. Conditioning these hemidiaphragms to withstand continuous simultaneous stimulation at a PI adjusted to 130 msec—7.69 Hz—and rpm to 7 to 9, is likely to take about 3 to 4 months. It is preferably carried out on an inpatient basis for more careful monitoring of the conditioning process.

To assure the optimal operation of the pacemaker, movement of the diaphragm should be observed under the fluoroscope with the pacemaker on and off at biweekly intervals during the first month postoperatively and, if the diaphragm is being conditioned, every 4 to 6 weeks therafter until the patient is discharged, to make whatever adjustment in the stimulating parameters that is required. A sudden or progressive rise in the threshold is cause for alarm. If the phrenic nerve conduction was

normal preoperatively, prolongation beyond 12 msec indicates nerve damage, and if pacing is ineffective, the cuff electrode is removed. At the operation to remove the cuff, the viability of the nerve is tested by direct stimulation above and below the cuff. After the first 6 months of stimulation, threshold and maximum levels usually remain about the same, rising or falling slightly over many years.

Pacing in Infants and Young Children

Pacing in this age group presents special problems. Because of immaturity of the lungs, chest wall, and diaphragm and a high metabolic rate, both hemidiaphragms must be paced simultaneously to gain sufficient ventilation. (Fig. 56–9). When Hunt and associates (1978) and others applied it in this age group, bilateral pacing was done with the same stimulus parameter levels as noncontinuous pacing in adults. Pacing at these pa-

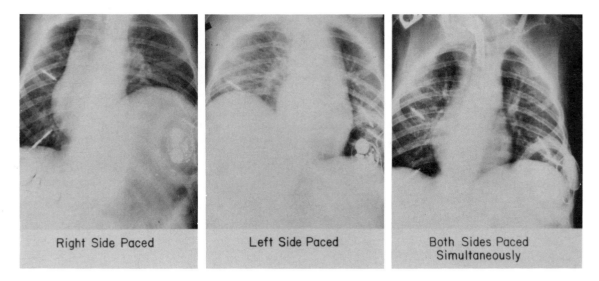

Right Side Paced   Left Side Paced   Both Sides Paced
Simultaneously

Fig. 56–9. Roentgenograms demonstrating effect of diaphragm pacing on mediastinal motion in childhood. Pacing of only one side failed to provide adequate ventilatory assistance because of instability of the mediastinum and paradoxical motion of the unstimulated hemidiaphragm. (From Glenn, W.W.L., and Sairenji, H.: Diaphragm pacing in the treatment of chronic ventilatory insufficiency. *In* The Thorax, Part B. Edited by C. Roussos and P.T. Macklem. New York, Marcel Dekker, 1985, pp. 1434–1436.)

rameters over a prolonged period, however, causes hypertrophy and shortening of the diaphragm muscle fibers (Fig. 56–6). Brouillette and associates (1988) revised the stimulus parameters for pacing the diaphragm in the infant and small child. By appropriately shortening the inspiration duration, they made pacing more efficient and by lowering the stimulus frequency during pacing conditioned the muscle to resist fatigue and allow extension of the time the diaphragm can be paced safely. Despite this, full-time pacing in the ventilator-dependent infant or small child has as yet not been possible. In these patients it is prudent to pace no more than 12 hours consecutively even though they appear to tolerate a few hours more. In the child 8 to 10 years old, if indicated, full-time pacing may be attempted using the aforementioned method of simultaneous continuous pacing described for older individuals. In my group's (1984) experience, conditioning has taken longer and required a slightly higher frequency stimulation at a slightly higher respiratory rate.

TRACHEOSTOMY

Early in my group's experience (1978b, 1980b) with diaphragm pacing we recognized that a permanent tracheostoma was necessary to maintain a clear and unobstructed airway. When positive pressure ventilation is used, a cuffed tracheostomy tube is employed, except in the infant and small child in whom the tracheostomy tube fills the tracheal lumen. The balloon is inflated fully only during measurement of tidal and minute volume. When underinflated, a small amount of air can escape around the cuff, permitting the patient to talk and relieving some of the pressure of the cuff on the trachea. Once the patient is on partial or full-time pacing, patency of the tracheostoma is maintained with a short plastic tube, preferably custom-made to fit it. When the patient

is awake the tube is plugged to enable talking but opened during sleep to ensure an unobstructed airway (Fig. 56–10).

EMERGENCY EQUIPMENT

For ventilator-dependent patients, provision must be made for clearing the airway and instituting an alternative method of artificial respiration. If diaphragm pacing or any method of ventilatory support fails, the following equipment must be readily available: Ambu bag, portable ventilator,* portable suction, tracheostomy tubes of

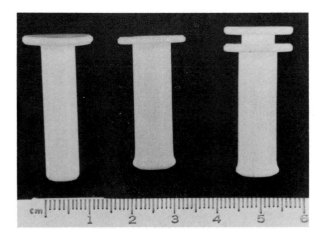

Fig. 56–10. Teflon tracheostomy button used to plug the tracheostoma in patients requiring permanent tracheostomy. The tube is not inserted until the stoma is well established. The buttons can be custom milled in a machine shop in sizes corresponding to the length of the tracheostoma tract from skin level to just inside the tracheal lumen and the diameter of the tracheostomy tube it replaces. (From Glenn, W.W.L., et al.: Long-term ventilatory support by diaphragm pacing in quadriplegia. Ann. Surg 183:566, 1976.)

*Puritan-Bennett Corp., Lenexa, KS 66215

appropriate size, portable oxygen tank, and an alarm system the patient can activate.

REHABILITATION

For patients with muscular paralysis, rehabilitation is begun at the start of pacing and is continued at a rehabilitation unit specializing in the care of paralyzed patients. I recommend the book by Phillips and associates (1987) on the subject of spinal cord injuries. In the rehabilitation unit patients are provided with an electric wheelchair and other self-operable environmental control systems to enable them to live outside the hospital or other institutional environment. No special rehabilitation program is needed by patients with central alveolar hypoventilation who do not have paralysis of respiratory or skeletal muscles. But because these patients are apt to be forgetful, there should always be someone nearby to clean and change the tracheostomy tube and to remind them when to attend to their pacemaker—battery check, proper application of antennas to the skin, starting and stopping pacing.

PRECAUTIONS FOR DIAPHRAGM PACING

A common misconception is that, once implanted, the diaphragm pacemaker needs no more attention or adjustment than a cardiac pacemaker. This is *not* the case. In contrast to the cardiac pacemaker, which delivers a single impulse of electric charge far greater than that required to initiate a maximum contraction of the heart muscle, the diaphragm pacemaker delivers electrical charge to the phrenic nerve in a series of impulses of gradually increasing intensity that must be carefully adjusted to obtain a smooth contraction of the diaphragm. Less current delivered to the nerve than will effect contraction of each individual diaphragm muscle fiber may result in an inadequate tidal volume, whereas an excess of current over that required to effect maximum contraction of the diaphragm will not only fail to increase V_T but it may cause irreparable damage to the stimulated muscle and possibly the phrenic nerve.

Table 56–1 lists warnings to physicians regarding all aspects of treating patients with diaphragm pacing. They are based on our experience with 84 diaphragm pacemaker patients treated over the past 22 years (1986), with reinforcement from the experience of others as derived from data garnered from a review of the case records of approximately 400 patients. The most obvious problems have been as follows: those related to poor selection of patients, that is, selection of individuals who could not appreciably benefit from pacing; operative complications—especially iatrogenic nerve injury—usually related to lack of experience with the new technique; equipment failure; inappropriate pacing schedules—overpacing and underpacing; inadequacy of supervision of the pacing program following hospital discharge; and lack of family support and patient cooperation.

RESULTS

The achievement of total ventilatory support in patients with respiratory paralysis caused by lesions of the spinal cord and brain stem demonstrates conclusively the effectiveness of diaphragm pacing as a method of long-term artificial respiration. The first such patient to undergo total ventilatory support by pacing, a 26-year-old quadriplegic male with a C1–C2 fracture dislocation, was begun on alternate-side pacing for 12 hours each side in 1970 and continued thus uninterruptedly, except when the ventilator was substituted for performance of an emergency procedure, until 1986 when he died from renal failure complicating multiple renal calculi. The second such patient, an 18-year-old female who became quadriplegic as a result of a C1–C2 fracture dislocation, was begun on bilateral pacing with sides paced alternately for about 16 hours daily and simultaneously for about 8 hours when sitting. She has been pacing without interruption since 1971, a total of 17 years as of 1988, meanwhile completing college and law school and taking up the practice of law, thus achieving her goal of "a meaningful independence." Stimulation in both of these patients, the first two quadriplegics to undergo treatment by diaphragm pacing, was at a high frequency, and for most of the time was applied to both sides alternately. In subsequent patients, stimulation was applied simultaneously and continuously, which was necessary for a variety of reasons, and at high frequencies has caused fatigue and the need to revert to part-time pacing or to discontinue pacing. No patient has survived for long periods on high-frequency stimulation administered simultaneously to both sides.

Only since 1980, when I and my associates (1984) introduced the technique of continuous simultaneous bilateral stimulation using low frequency and slow respiration rate has the simultaneous and continuous pacing of both hemidiaphragms, providing full-time ventilatory support, been possible almost consistently. The overall results of the Yale series of 84 patients are listed in Table 56–4. More than 90% of the patients have benefited from diaphragm pacing. In 38 patients—45.24%—the ventilatory goal was achieved. Partial success, meaning that significant benefit was gained from pacing but another method of ventilatory support was also required, was obtained in 40 patients—46.62%; two of whom were being conditioned for full-time pacing at the time of the report.

Forty-six of our series of 84 patients died since 1966, when the procedure was used for the first time in a patient with chronic alveolar hypoventilation. Pacing-related complications, overpacing, underpacing, and iatrogenic injury to the phrenic nerve were observed in eight of the 84. Such complications could now be avoided. In several patients with central alveolar hypoventilation, either idiopathic or secondary to a lesion of the brainstem, who were treated initially with unilateral pacing, a stimulator was implanted on the contralateral side to improve ventilation. With still more improvement needed, the patients who were started on alternate-

Table 56–4. Diaphragm Pacing: Results of Treatment. Yale Series—84 Patients

Diagnosis	Success	Partial Success	Failure	Never Paced
Lesion of brain stem or above	17	14*	2	0
Lesion of upper cervical cord	13	17*	2	1
Idiopathic CAH	8	8	0	0
Lesion of peripheral components of respiration	0	1	1	0
Total	38	40	5	1
Frequency (%)	45.24	47.62	5.95	1.19

*2 patients conditioning at the time of the report.

side stimulation for 12 hours each side were changed to either simultaneous bilateral stimulation for 12 hours, at a medium frequency and respiration rate, with mechanical ventilation provided the remaining time, or they were converted to low-frequency—PI 130 msec; 7.6 Hz—stimulation at a low rpm—7 to 8, as used in quadriplegic patients, and paced bilaterally continuously. Competition of the pacing rhythm did not interrupt the patient's own, intrinsic rhythm. Mechanical supplementation was the only recourse in patients in whom pacing on the contralateral side was not possible for various reasons. Conversion from high to low frequency was accomplished as described on p. 604.

Investigators from several other clinics, including Carter (1987), McMichan (1979), and Oakes (1980) and their associates, and Fodstad (1987) and Vanderlinden (personal communication, 1985) reported results of pacing in older children and adults similar to our own. The Children's Memorial Hospital in Chicago has the largest experience with diaphragm pacing in the treatment of chronic hypoventilation in infants and small children. Central alveolar hypoventilation was the principal diagnosis in the cases reported by Brouillette (personal communication, 1987). Hunt and associates (in press) stated that since 1976 they have implanted diaphragm pacemakers in 32 patients who were either partially or totally ventilator dependent, including some older children. Pacing was bilateral and simultaneous for no more than 12 consecutive hours. A mechanical ventilator was supplemented when necessary. In some cases, cor pulmonale and prior lung infection compromised pacing's effectiveness. Seven patients in their series died. All but one of the survivors, a patient whom they were unable to pace, have been rehabilitated by pacing and are cared for at home.

A report from Carter and associates (1987) at the Texas Institute for Rehabilitation and Research compares their experience over the past 17 years in treating ventilator dependent spinal cord injury patients. Thirty-seven patients were treated by either mechanical ventilation—19 patients—or diaphragm pacing—18 patients. Data on the mode of pacing and the pacing schedules is not given, though presumably patients who had pacemakers implanted before 1980, when low-frequency pacing and conditioning of the diaphragm was introduced, were paced with high-frequency stimulation. There was no significant difference in the mortality between the me-

chanically ventilated—32%—and the diaphragm paced—39%—groups, although the former died sooner after the spinal cord injury—13 months—than the latter—46 months. It will be interesting to compare these methods of ventilatory support in ventilator dependent patients who are suitable candidates for diaphragm pacing using low frequency pacing techniques.

The future of diaphragm pacing depends on: (1) the acceptance of the responsibility by the physicians for the total care of their patients for as long as is required; (2) the support of the patients by the family until they are ready to seek "meaningful independence"; (3) the improvement of pacemaker technology, including the commerical production of a totally implantable diaphragm pacemaker programmable from the exterior; (4) a better definition of the indications for the use of this physiological method of ventilatory support based on knowledge of the pathophysiological changes in the respiratory components, especially the diaphragm and phrenic nerve but also the thoracic cage and pulmonary parenchyma, that result from continuous phrenic nerve stimulation over many years.

REFERENCES

Bradley, T.D., et al.: Chronic ventilatory failure caused by abnormal respiratory pattern generation during sleep. Am. Rev. Respir. Dis. *130*:678, 1984.

Braun, N.M.T.: Nocturnal ventilation: a new method. Am. Rev. Respir. Dis. *135*:523, 1987.

Brouillette, R.T., Ilbawi, M.N., and Hunt, C.E.: Phrenic nerve pacing in infants and children: a review of experience and report on the usefulness of phrenic nerve stimulation studies. J. Pediatr. *102*:32, 1983.

Brouillette, R.T., et al.: Obstructive sleep apnea and central hypoventilation syndrome: two pediatric sleep-related breathing disorders. The Child's Doctor *3*:22, 1986.

Brouillette, R.T., et al.: Stimulus parameters for phrenic nerve pacing in infants and children. Pediatr. Pulmonol. *4*:33, 1988.

Carter, R.E., et al.: Comparative study of electrophrenic nerve stimulation and mechanical ventilatory support in traumatic spinal cord injury. Paraplegia *25*:86, 1987.

Ciesielski, T.E., et al.: Response of the diaphragm muscle to electrical stimulation of the phrenic nerve: a histochemical and ultrastructural study. J. Neurosurg. *58*:92, 1983.

Farmer, W.C., Glenn, W.W.L., and Gee, J.B.L.: Alveolar hypoventilation syndrome: studies of ventilatory control in patients selected for diaphragm pacing. Am. J. Med. *64*:39, 1978.

Fodstad, H.: The Swedish experience in phrenic nerve stimulation. PACE *10*:246, 1987.

Glenn, W.W.L., et al.: Total ventilatory support in a quadriplegic patient with radiofrequency electrophrenic respiration. N. Engl. J. Med. *286*:513, 1972.

Glenn, W.W.L., Gee, J.B.L., and Schachter, E.N.: Diaphragm pacing: application to a patient with chronic obstructive pulmonary disease. J. Thorac. Cardiovasc. Surg. *75*:273, 1978a.

Glenn, W.W.L., et al.: Combined central alveolar hypoventilation and upper airway obstruction: treatment by tracheostomy and diaphragm pacing. Am. J. Med *64*:50, 1978b.

Glenn, W.W.L., et al.: Characteristics and surgical management of respiratory complications accompanying pathologic lesions of the brain stem. Ann. Surg. *191*:655, 1980a.

Glenn, W.W.L., Hogan, J.F., and Phelps, M.L.: Ventilatory support of the quadriplegic patient with respiratory paralysis by diaphragm pacing. Surg. Clin. North Am. *60*:1055, 1980b.

Glenn, W.W.L., et al.: Ventilatory support by pacing of the conditioned diaphragm in quadriplegia. N. Engl. J. Med. *310*:1150, 1984.

Glenn, W.W.L., and Phelps, M.L.: Diaphragm pacing by electrical stimulation of the phrenic nerve. Neurosurgery *17*:974, 1985.

Glenn, W.W.L., et al.: Twenty years of experience in phrenic nerve stimulation to pace the diaphragm. PACE *9*:780, 1986.

Gross, D., et al.: The effect of training on strength and endurance of the diaphragm in quadriplegia. Am. J. Med. *68*:27, 1980.

Guilleminault, C., et al.: Congenital central alveolar hypoventilation syndrome in six infants. Pediatr. *70*:684, 1982.

Hogan, J.F., Holcomb, W.G., and Glenn, W.W.L.: A programmable, totally implantable, battery-powered diaphragm pacemaker: design characteristics. *In* Proceedings of the Fourth New England Bioengineering Conference, Edited by S. Saha, pp. 221–223. Elmsford, NY, Pergamon, 1976.

Hogan, J.F., Glenn, W.W.L., and Koda, H.: Electrical techniques for stimulation of the phrenic nerve to pace the diaphragm: inductive coupling and battery-powered total implant in asynchronous and demand modes. Submitted for publication.

Hunt, C.E., et al.: Central hypoventilation syndrome: experience with bilateral phrenic nerve pacing in 3 neonates. Am. Rev. Respir. Dis. *118*:23, 1978.

Hunt, C.E., et al: Diaphragm pacing in infants and children. (in press).

Ishii, K., et al.: Effects on hemodynamics and ventilation of transvenous electrophrenic respiration in postoperative cardiac patients: experimental and clinical studies. Nippon Kyobu Geka Gakkai Zasshi. *34*:948, 1986.

Jammes, Y., et al.: Essai d'une nouvelle technique d'electrostimulation diaphragmatique transcutanee chez l'homme. Presse Med. *15*:467, 1986.

Kerby, G.R., Mayer, L.S., and Pingleton, S.K.: Nocturnal positive pressure ventilation via nasal mask. Am. Rev. Respir. Dis. *135*:738, 1987.

Leith, D.E., and Bradley, M.: Ventilatory muscle strength and endurance training. J. Appl. Physiol. *41*:508, 1976.

McMichan, J.C., et al.: Electrophrenic respiration. Mayo Clin. Proc. *54*:662, 1979.

Mead, J., et al.: Effect of posture on upper and lower rib cage motion on tidal volume during diaphragm pacing. Am. Rev. Respir. Dis. *130*:32, 1984.

Milic-Emili, J., et al.: Improved technique for estimated pleural pressure from esophageal balloons. J. Appl. Physiol. *19*:207, 1964.

Newsom Davis, J., et al.: Diaphragm function and alveolar hypoventilation. Q.J. Med. *45*:87, 1976.

Oakes, D.D., et al.: Neurogenic respiratory failure: a 5-year experience using implantable phrenic nerve stimulators. Ann. Thorac. Surg. *30*:118, 1980.

Oda, T., et al.: A totally implantable diaphragm pacemaker for experimental studies: effect of stimulating current level on diaphragm fatigue. Trans. Internat. Soc. Artif. Organs. (Suppl.) *3*:484, 1979.

Oda, T., et al.: Evaluation of electrical parameters for diaphragm pacing: an experimental study. J. Surg. Res. *30*:142, 1981.

Peterson, D.K., et al.: Intramuscular electronic activation of the phrenic nerve. IEEE Trans. Biochem. Eng. *33*:342, 1986.

Phillips, L., et al.: Spinal Cord Injury: A Guide for Patient and Family. New York, Raven Press, 1987.

Roussos, C.S., and Macklem, P.T.: Diaphragmatic fatigue in man. J. Appl. Physiol. *43*:189, 1977.

Salmons, S., and Vrbová, G.: The influence of activity on some contractile characteristics of mammalian fast and slow muscles. J. Physiol. (Lond.) *201*:535, 1969.

Shaw, R.K., Glenn, W.W.L., and Holcomb, W.G.: Phrenic nerve conduction studies in patients with diaphragm pacing. Surg. Forum *22*:195, 1975.

Shaw, R.K., et al.: Electrophysiological evaluation of phrenic nerve function in candidates for diaphragm pacing. J. Neurosurg. *53*:345, 1980.

Weese-Mayer, D.E., et al.: Am. Rev. Respir. Dis. *137*:393, 1988.

The Pleura

CHAPTER 57

BENIGN AND MALIGNANT PLEURAL EFFUSIONS

Steven A. Sahn

Pleural effusion provides the clinician an opportunity to diagnose, at least presumptively, the underlying disease. A pleural effusion is usually caused by lung disease but also may reflect systemic disease involving the gastrointestinal tract, heart, kidney, or reticuloendothelial system. An important consideration is whether the effusion is caused by a benign or malignant process. A systematic approach to the patient with a pleural effusion enables the most effective differentiation of nonmalignant effusion, which resolves with appropriate therapy, from malignant pleural effusion, which signifies a short survival, is crucial.

PLEURAL SPACE PHYSIOLOGY

The pleural space normally contains a small amount of fluid. Yamada (1933) recorded that this amount is generally less than 1 ml. Black (1972) summarized the available data and noted that the equilibrium between the movement of fluid into and out of the space resulted in less than 3 ml of fluid normally within the space.

Evidence presented by Broaddus and Staub (1987) suggests that in normal man, the entrance and exit rates of pleural liquid and protein are slow. A low protein—< 1.4 g/dl—filtrate enters the pleural space from the parietal pleura and exits by parietal pleural lymphatics through stomas situated between mesothelial cells. The lymphatic system has an extensive capacity for accomodating increased pleural fluid formation; and hence, some defect in lymphatic drainage most likely occurs in large pleural effusions. Some fluid may also enter from the systemic vessels of the visceral pleura.

In pleural or systemic disease, the normal equilibrium may be upset. The entrance rate may increase, the removal rate may decrease, or both. An efflux block apparently predominates in malignancy and chronic rheumatoid pleurisy, whereas parapneumonic effusions tend to have increased rates of formation. Hydrostatic or oncotic pressures, or both, may be primarily affected, as in congestive heart failure or nephrotic syndrome. Increased permeability pleural effusions occur in inflam-

matory and malignant diseases of the pleurae. Lymphatic obstruction with impaired removal of normally produced fluid or liquid of high protein content occurs with carcinoma and lymphoma involving the mediastinal lymph nodes and pleural surface.

When air enters a closed space, such as in a pneumothorax—alveolar gas, analysis of its component gases shows that the oxygen tension is lower and the carbon dioxide tension higher than in the air obtained from a pleural space that communicates directly with an open bronchus. The gas content of the latter approximates the values of ambient air.

Magnussen and associates (1974) demonstrated that reabsorption of pneumothorax gas takes days to weeks because once the oxygen and carbon dioxide tensions in the pleural space approximate values in the surrounding tissue and venous blood, the absorption rate is limited by nitrogen, a gas with poor diffusion properties.

THORACENTESIS

Indications

When a pleural effusion is suspected on physical examination and confirmed by a roentgenogram of the chest, a diagnostic thoracentesis should be performed to establish the cause. Exceptions to this are when the clinical diagnosis is secure and only a small volume of pleural fluid is present, as in viral pleurisy, or in a patient with uncomplicated congestive heart failure—consistent clinical history, afebrile, Pa_{O_2} appropriate, and bilateral pleural effusions of approximately equal size with a large cardiac silhouette. Continued observation of the aforementioned situations may be warranted; thoracentesis should be performed if the situation changes adversely.

There are no absolute contraindications to performing a diagnostic thoracentesis. If the clinician believes that the information obtained by pleural fluid analysis will help in patient management, thoracentesis should be done. Relative contraindications include a bleeding diathesis, anticoagulation, a small volume of pleural fluid, patients on mechanical ventialtion, and a low benefit-to-risk ratio.

Diagnostic Value

Analysis of pleural fluid provides a definitive diagnosis in approximately 20% of patients and a presumptive diagnosis in 50% but is of no further diagnostic help in the remainder. A substantial number of the remaining patients, however, have infection eliminated as a potential cause of the pleural effusion, and therefore thoracentesis is clinically valuable. Thus, as discussed by Collins and me (1987), in about 75% of patients the cause of the effusion can be established, and in 9 of 10 patients, the information gained by fluid analysis helps in clinical decision-making.

I emphasized (1987b) that only a few diagnoses can be established definitively by thoracentesis. These include: malignancy, empyema, tuberculosis, fungal infection, lupus pleuritis, chylothorax, urinothorax, esophageal rupture, and hemothorax (Table 57–1). A putrid odor establishes the diagnosis of an anaerobic empyema. The probability of finding lupus erythematosus cells in the pleural fluid of a patient with lupus pleuritis is enhanced by allowing the fluid to stand at room temperature for several hours before staining, as Reda and Baigelman (1980) suggested. Acid fast bacillus—AFB—stain of pleural fluid in tuberculous pleurisy yields less than 10%, but culture of the fluid provides a diagnosis in up to 50% of the infections. I (1985c) noted that a low pH—around 6.00—and a high amylase is found only in pleural fluid from esophageal rupture. A chylomicron layer appears at the top of the centrifuged specimen from a patient with a chylothorax. Stark and associates (1982) reported that a pleural-fluid-to-serum creatinine ratio of > 1 establishes the diagnosis of urinothorax. A pleural-fluid-to-blood hematocrit ratio of > 0.5 establishes the diagnosis of hemothorax and has therapeutic implications.

Complications

Collins and I (1987) recorded such complications as site pain, bleeding—local, intrapleural, and intra-abdominal, pneumothorax, empyema, and spleen and liver puncture after thoracentesis. In addition, hypoxemia and unilateral pulmonary edema can occur with therapeutic thoracentesis. Brandstetter and Cohen (1979) documented a substantial decrease in the Pa_{O_2} following therapeutic thoracentesis despite relief of dyspnea, suggesting that factors other than the oxygen chemosensors are responsible for dyspnea associated with a large pleural effusion. Estenne and colleagues (1983) suggested that relief of dyspnea in this setting is related to the ability of the inspiratory muscles of the thoracic cage to operate in a more advantageous portion of their length-tension relationship. Unilateral pulmonary edema is most likely to occur when a large alveolar-pleural pressure gradient is created following the removal of a large volume of fluid; this most commonly occurs in endobronchial malignancy with atelectasis or when the visceral pleura is trapped by tumor or fibrosis which permits the creation of markedly negative pleural pressures.

Pleural Fluid Analysis

A complete pleural fluid analysis requires 35 to 50 ml of pleural fluid. An entire battery of routine pleural fluid tests is neither clinically necessary nor cost-effective. The tests requested should be based on the clinical presentation. The following tests are probably cost-effective for all patients who have a diagnostic thoracentesis: total protein, lactic dehydrogenase—LDH—white blood cell count and differential, and either glucose or pH. Concomitant serum total protein, LDH, and glucose should be measured; arterial pH should be measured if the pleural fluid pH is < 7.30 and acidemia is suspected. The aforementioned tests allow categorization to a transudate or an exudate, narrow the differential diagnosis of the exudate, determine the degree of pleural inflammation, and provide information on the acuteness of the pleural injury. Gram and AFB stains and pleural fluid cultures should be obtained when infection is suspected. Pleural fluid cytology should be requested when malignancy or an undiagnosed exudate is suspected; fluid can be stored in the refrigerator with heparin added until preliminary

Table 57–1. Diagnoses That Can Be Established by Thoracentesis

Diagnosis	Diagnostic Pleural Fluid Tests	Usual Time Course
Empyema	Observation (pus, putrid odor), stain, or culture	immediately to 48 hours
Malignancy	Cytology	24–48 hours
Lupus pleuritis	Lupus erythematosus cells present	hours
Tuberculous pleurisy	Stain, culture	minutes to 3 weeks
Esophageal rupture	Amylase, pH	a few hours
Fungal pleurisy	Stain, culture	minutes to days
Chylothorax	Centrifugation, triglycerides, lipoprotein electrophoresis	minutes to 48 hours
Hemothorax	Centrifugation	minutes
Urinothorax	Creatinine (PF & S)	hours

(Reproduced with permission from Sahn, S.A.: Pleural fluid analysis: narrowing the differential diagnosis. Semin. Respir. Med. 9:22, 1987.)

results are available. Lipid studies should be ordered when there is a milky supernatant and immunologic studies ordered for suspected rheumatoid or lupus pleuritis. A pleural fluid amylase should only be requested when pancreatitis, pancreatic pseudocyst, or esophageal rupture is considered or there is an undiagnosed left pleural effusion.

Observation

The color, odor, and character of the pleural fluid can suggest diagnostic possibilities (Table 57–2). A grossly bloody effusion in the absence of trauma is most likely caused by malignancy, but Stelzner and associates (1983) noted it occurs in postcardiac injury syndrome, and Bynum and Wilson (1976) noted it in pulmonary infarction. A whitish pleural effusion is caused by chyle, cholesterol, or a large number of leukocytes. Brownish-colored fluid results when an amebic liver abscess has ruptured into the pleural space, as Daniels and Childress (1956) reported. Metzger and colleagues (1984) stated that a black pleural fluid suggests aspergillus invasion of the pleura. Miller and associates (1985) noted that pleural fluid the color of enteral tube feeding suggests that a narrow-bore feeding tube has penetrated the pleura. A putrid odor is diagnostic of anaerobic empyema, as Bartlett and Finegold (1974) emphasized, and an ammonia smell suggests urinothorax. A viscous effusion, according to Rassmussen and Faber (1967), suggests malignant mesothelioma because of increased levels of hyaluronic acid.

Categorization of Pleural Fluids

Classifying the pleural effusion into a transudate or an exudate is an important deductive step; which is why total protein and LDH should be ordered routinely. The diagnosis of a transudate limits the diagnostic possibilities that are usually discernible from the clinical presentation (Table 57–3). Transudates are caused by imbalances in

hydrostatic and oncotic pressures or result from movement of fluid from the peritoneal to the pleural space by diaphragmatic lymphatics or defects caused by a pressure gradient across the diaphragm. Transudative effusions are noninflammatory effusions with few mononuclear cells.

In contrast, the differential diagnosis of the exudative effusion is more extensive (Table 57–4). Exudates are caused by inflammation—infectious, immunologic, or neoplastic—of the pleura and by impaired lymphatic drainage of the pleural space—malignancy—and are associated with either a capillary protein leak or decreased protein removal from the pleural space. Acute exudates have elevated leukocyte counts with mostly polymorphonuclear—PMN—leukocytes. In the subacute or chronic states, these effusions may have low cell counts with mostly mononuclear cells.

Light and colleagues (1972) stated that exudates meet at least one and transudates none of the following pleural fluid criteria:(1) pleural-fluid-to-serum total protein ratio > 0.5; (2) pleural-fluid-to-serum LDH ratio > 0.6; and (3) pleural fluid LDH > two thirds of the upper limits of the normal serum value. When only LDH meets the exudate criteria, malignancy or parapneumonic effusion should be suspected.

Cellular Content

The total leukocyte count in pleural fluid is virtually never diagnostic; however, counts > 50,000/μl usually are found only in parapneumonic effusions. Transudates usually have < 1,000 leukocytes/μl and chronic exudates, such as in malignancy and tuberculous pleurisy, usually have < 5,000 leukocytes/μl. Pleural fluid leukocyte counts > 10,000/μl indicate substantial pleural inflammation and are most commonly seen with parapneumonic effusions but also can be observed with pancreatitis, postcardiac injury syndrome, and pulmonary infarction. With a grossly purulent effusion, the leuko-

Table 57–2. Diagnostic Hints From Observation of Pleural Fluid

	Suspected Diagnosis
Pleural Fluid Color	
Yellow-white	Empyema
Red (frank blood)	Malignancy, trauma, PCIS*, PE†
White	Chylothorax, cholesterol effusion, empyema
Brown (anchovy)	Amebic liver abscess with rupture
Black	Aspergillus
Same as enteral tube feeding	Penetration of visceral pleura by enteral feeding tube
Yellow-green	Rheumatoid pleurisy
Pleural Fluid Odor	
Putrid	Anaerobic empyema
Ammonia	Urinothorax
Character	
Purulent	Empyema
Viscous	Mesothelioma
Debris	Rheumatoid pleurisy
Food particles	Esophageal rupture

*PCIS—Postcardiac injury syndrome
†PE—Pulmonary embolism

Table 57–3.   Transudative Pleural Effusions

Cause	Comment
Congestive heart failure	Usually biventricular failure clinically
Cirrhosis	Rare without clinical ascites
Nephrotic syndrome	Frequently subpulmonic and bilateral
Peritoneal dialysis	Usually within 48 hours of initiating dialysis
Hypoalbuminemia	Edema fluid never isolated to pleural space
Constrictive pericarditis	Due to systemic venous hypertension
Malignancy	<10% transudates
Atelectasis	Increased intrapleural negative pressure
Urinothorax	Smells like ammonia

Reproduced with permission from: Sahn, S.A.: Pleural fluid analysis: measuring the differential diagnosis. Semin. Respir. Med. 9:22, 1987.

Table 57–4.   Causes of Exudative Pleural Effusions by Mechanism

Infectious

  Parapneumonic (usual pyogens)
  Tuberculous pleurisy
  Parasites (amebiasis, paragonimiasis, echinococcosis)
  Fungal disease
  Atypical pneumonias (virus, mycoplasma, Q fever, Legionella)
  Nocardia, Actinomyces
  Subphrenic abscess
  Hepatic abscess
  Splenic abscess
  Hepatitis
  Spontaneous esophageal rupture

Malignancy

  Carcinoma
  Lymphoma
  Mesothelioma
  Leukemia
  Chylothorax

Immunologic

  Lupus pleuritis
  Rheumatoid pleurisy
  Mixed connective tissue disease
  Post-cardiac injury syndrome
  Sarcoidosis

Other Inflammatory

  Pancreatitis
  Spontaneous esophageal rupture
  Asbestos
  Pulmonary embolism
  Radiation therapy
  Uremic pleurisy

Iatrogenic

  Drug-induced
  Esophageal perforation
  Esophageal sclerotherapy
  Subclavian catheter misplacement
  Enteral feeding tube placed into pleural space

Lymphatic Abnormalities

  Malignancy
  Yellow nail syndrome
  Lymphangiomyomatosis

Chronic Negative Increased Intrapleural Pressure

  Trapped lung
  Atelectasis
  Cholesterol effusion

Movement of Fluid From Abdomen to Pleural Space

  Pancreatitis
  Pancreatic pseudocyst
  Meigs' syndrome
  Carcinoma
  Chylothorax from chylous ascites
  Urinothorax

Reproduced with permission from: Sahn, S.A.: Pleural fluid analysis: narrowing the differential diagnosis. Semin. Respir. Med. 9:22, 1987.

cyte count often is less than anticipated as many of the PMNs have undergone lysis and the debris from these cells accounts for the turbidity and purulence of the fluid.

As I pointed out (1987c), the timing of thoracentesis in relation to the acute pleural injury determines the predominant cell type in the exudate. Therefore, all acute exudative pleural effusions are PMN leukocyte predominant. As the time from the acute insult lengthens, the number of mononuclear cells increases if pleural injury is not persistent. Patients with pneumonia, pulmonary embolism, and pancreatitis usually have PMN predominant effusions as these patients tend to present shortly after the onset of symptoms; a prominent symptom usually is pleuritic pain.

Yam (1967) reported that pleural fluid lymphocytosis suggests tuberculous pleurisy, lymphoma, or carcinoma, and Chusid and Siltzbach (1974) pointed out that it may suggest sarcoidosis. Yam (1967) emphasized that when lymphocytes represent 85 to 95% of the total cellular population, tuberculous pleurisy should be strongly considered. An undiagnosed lymphocyte-predominant exudate is an indication for percutaneous pleural biopsy, because diseases associated with this cellular profile can be diagnosed by sampling pleural tissue. Approximately one third of patients with transudative pleural effusions have a lymphocyte predominance; this finding, however, is not clinically important and does not indicate a need for pleural biopsy.

Pleural fluid eosinophilia—> 10% of total cells being esoinophils—suggests, according to Campbell and Webb (1964), a benign, self-limited pleural effusion associated with air or blood in the pleural space. Therefore, it frequently is seen following hemothorax, pulmonary infarction, pneumothorax, or repeat thoracentesis. Other causes include parasitic disease, fungal infection, drug-induced pleurisy, and benign asbestos pleurisy. Pleural fluid eosinophilia is rare with tuberculous pleurisy, as Spriggs and Boddington (1968) pointed out.

The presence of blood-tinged pleural fluid has little diagnostic importance, because only a few drops of blood result in a liter of pleural fluid appearing serosanguineous. The finding of more than 100,000 red cells/μl, as Stelzner and associates (1983) noted, narrows the differential diagnosis of the exudate to trauma, malignancy, pulmonary embolism, and post-cardiac injury syndrome. A frequent question, however, is whether the bloody effusion is real or caused by a traumatic thoracentesis. A nonuniform color during aspiration, clotting of the fluid within several minutes, and the absence of hemosiderin-laden macrophages suggest a traumatic thoracentesis.

Biochemistry

Good and colleagues (1980) stated that a low pleural fluid glucose—< 60 mg/dl or a pleural-fluid-to-serum ratio of < 0.5—and a low pleural fluid pH—< 7.30 with a normal blood pH—narrows the differential diagnosis of the exudate to rheumatoid pleurisy, empyema, malignant effusion, tuberculous pleurisy, lupus pleuritis, and esophageal rupture. The observation that a low pleural fluid glucose and pH occurred concomitantly sug-

gested to Potts and co-workers (1978) that the processes responsible for these phenomena were interrelated. I reported (1985b) that a low pleural fluid glucose results from decreased transport of glucose from blood to pleural fluid together with increased glucose utilization by constituents of pleural fluid such as PMNs, bacteria, and malignant cells. The mechanisms I (1985c) noted that are responsible for pleural fluid acidosis include increased acid production by pleural fluid cells and bacteria and decreased acid efflux from the pleural space, usually caused by pleuritis, tumor, or fibrosis. Light and associates (1980) suggested that parapneumonic effusion, a pleural fluid pH of < 7.10, usually in association with a glucose of < 40 mg/dl and an LDH > 1000 U/L, indicates the need for chest tube drainage. Moreover, as I observed (1987a), a low pleural fluid pH in malignancy has prognostic, diagnostic, and therapeutic implications—as will be explained subsequently.

Light and Ball (1973) noted that an increased pleural fluid amylase—above the upper limits of normal of the serum or a pleural-fluid-to-serum ratio greater than 1—indicates one of four diagnoses: acute pancreatitis, pancreatic pseudocyst, esophageal rupture, or malignancy. Kaye (1968) reported that approximately 10% of patients with acute pancreatitis who have pleural effusions usually have high amylase levels. These effusions resolve over several days to weeks as the acute pancreatitis subsides. As Lorch and I (1987) noted, a pancreatic pseudocyst, a sequela of severe pancreatitis, may be associated with pleural effusions because of fistulous tracts between the pseudocyst and the pleural space. The patient may be asymptomatic or present with dyspnea; these effusions characteristically have high amylase levels, frequently > 100,000 U/L. Maulitz and associates (1979) reported that patients with esophageal rupture develop high pleural fluid amylase levels—of salivary origin—within several hours following the acute event.

TREATMENT OF BENIGN EFFUSIONS

Treatment of benign pleural effusions is directed at the underlying disease, with the exception of a parapneumonic effusion, for which pleural space drainage may be indicated. If the underlying disease is treated appropriately, the pleural effusion resolves in days—pancreatitis, uncomplicated parapneumonic effusion—to weeks—tuberculous pleurisy, rhematoid pleurisy.

Pleural space drainage may be indicated in complicated parapneumonic effusion or empyema, and for the patient with a large, symptomatic, malignant pleural effusion, which will be discussed subsequently. When a parapneumonic effusion is discovered, an immediate thoracentesis must be performed to determine the need for chest tube drainage. If the effusion is not purulent, the Gram stain is negative, the pleural fluid pH is > 7.30, and glucose is > 60 mg/dl, chest tube drainage is not indicated as long as appropriate antibiotic therapy is instituted. Definite indications for immediate tube thoracostomy are: (1) aspiration of pus; (2) positive Gram stain signifying a large organism load in the pleural space;

and (3) positive pleural fluid culture. As Light (1980) and Potts (1976) and their associates pointed out, when the thoracentesis fluid is not purulent but has a biochemical profile of pH < 7.10, glucose < 40 mg/dl, and LDH of > 1000 U/L, the pleural fluid has a high likelihood of loculating in the pleural space and behaving clinically as a classic empyema. These effusions must be drained immediately with tube thoracostomy but still may progress to multiple loculations, requiring a thoracotomy for ultimate resolution. Free-flowing, nonpurulent effusions with biochemical characteristics in the indeterminate zone—pH 7.10 to 7.30, glucose 40 to 60 mg/dl, LDH < 1000 U/L—need to be reassessed by thoracentesis in 8 to 12 hours while the clinical response on appropriate antibiotic therapy is observed. If the clinical course is satisfactory and the biochemical markers have stabilized or improved, observation is warranted. If the pH falls or the patient's condition worsens, tube drainage should be instituted. If the patient does not respond to tube thoracostomy within 48 hours, then an "empyemectomy" and decortication, as described in Chapter 59, is usually necessary.

When a parapneumonic effusion is suspected, a thoracentesis must be performed immediately so that pleural space drainage can be instituted as soon as possible, if necessary. If delay occurs, "fibrogenic" pleural fluid remains in the space and fibrogenesis with fibroblast migration and collagen formation proceeds rapidly, making spontaneous resolution unlikely and resulting in morbidity and mortality.

MALIGNANT PLEURAL EFFUSIONS

Definition and Incidence

Malignant pleural effusions are diagnosed by finding malignant cells in the pleural fluid or pleural tissue by closed needle biopsy, by biopsy through thoracoscopy or thoracotomy, or at autopsy. In some cases of documented malignancy with pleural effusion, malignant cells cannot be demonstrated in either pleural fluid or pleural tissue and probably are not present at the time of the diagnostic procedure. I (1987a) believe these effusions are best termed paramalignant because they are associated with and caused by the malignancy but do not result from pleural invasion. Paramalignant effusions can be caused by a direct local effect of the tumor, by systemic manifestations of the malignancy, or by therapy (Table 57–5). Impaired pleural space lymphatic drainage is the most important mechanism responsible for both paramalignant and malignant pleural effusions.

As I (1987b) noted, lymphomas account for approximately 10% of all malignant pleural effusions and are the most common cause of chylothorax. Both Hodgkin's disease and non-Hodgkin's lymphoma have been associated with pleural effusions with variable incidences, probably through different mechanisms. Pleural effusions seem to result more commonly from impaired lymphatic drainage of the pleural space in Hodgkin's disease, whereas direct pleural involvement tends to be more common in non-

Hodgkin's lymphoma. These observations were recorded by Weick (1973), Jenkins (1981), and Xaubet (1985) and their associates.

Diffuse malignant mesothelioma arises from mesothelial cells or possibly from a precursor cell that is situated in the submesothelial connective tissue. The association of asbestos exposure and malignant mesothelioma was established in 1960 by the report of Wagner and colleagues. McDonald and co-workers (1970) recorded that the incidence of malignant mesothelioma is approximately one per million per year in the general population that is not exposed to asbestos. Emonot and associates (1979) reported that the incidence can rise 20-fold in certain populations and is even higher in shipyard communities.

Virtually all cancers metastasize to the pleura. Lung cancer is the most common to involve the pleura because of its proximity to the pleural surface and, as Meyer (1966) suggested, its propensity to invade the pulmonary arteries and embolize to the visceral pleura. Breast cancer also frequently metastasizes to the pleura, causing approximately 25% of malignant pleural effusions. Ovarian carcinoma and gastric cancer are next in frequency, and each represents < 5% of malignant pleural effusions. Approximately 7% of patients with malignant pleural effusions, however, have an unknown primary site at the time of the initial diagnosis of the malignant effusion.

Pathogenesis

Impaired lymphatic drainage of the pleural space is the most important mechanism responsible for accumulation of large amounts of pleural fluid in malignancy. The lymphatic system can be blocked at any point from the stoma of the parietal pleura to the mediastinal and parasternal—internal mammary—lymph nodes. The autopsy studies of Meyer (1966) and Chernow and me (1977) clearly demonstrated the association of mediastinal lymph node involvement and the presence of substantial pleural fluid. Conversely, these studies showed evidence of pleural involvement with tumor in the absence of pleural effusions, lending support to this mechanism. Furthermore, as Meyer (1966) noted, pleural effusions usually do not occur when the pleura is involved by sarcoma because of the absence of lymphatic metastasis. Weick and associates (1973) noted that Hodgkin's disease tends to cause pleural effusions by lymphatic obstruction, and Xaubet and associates (1985) noted that non-Hodgkin's lymphoma tends to produce effusions by both lymphatic obstruction and direct pleural invasion.

The inflammatory response to pleural tumor invasion results in increased microvascular permeability and produces small volumes of pleural effusion. Chretien and Jaubert (1985) suggested that oxygen radicals, arachidonic acid metabolites, proteases, lymphocytes, and immune complexes are probably causative.

Pleural effusion is an early manifestation of a malignant mesothelioma and probably results from a combination of increased capillary permeability from direct pleural invasion and impaired lymphatic drainage of the pleural

Table 57–5. **Causes of Paramalignant Pleural Effusions**

Cause	Comment
Local Effect of Tumor	
Lymphatic obstruction	Predominant mechanisms of pleural fluid accumulation
Bronchial obstruction with pneumonia	Parapneumonic effusion; does not rule out operability in lung cancer
Bronchial obstruction with atelectasis	Transudate; does not rule out operability in lung cancer
Chylothorax	Disruption of thoracic duct; chyle in pleural space; lymphoma most common cause
Superior vena cava obstruction	Transudate; due to increased systemic venous pressure
Systemic Effect of Tumor	
Pulmonary embolism	Hypercoagulable state
Low plasma oncotic pressure	Serum albumin <1.5 g/dl; associated with anasarca
Results of Therapy	
Radiation therapy	6 weeks to 6 months—radiation pleuritis
	Late—mediastinal fibrosis, SVC obstruction, constrictive pericarditis
Drug reactions	
Methotrexate	Pleuritis, pleural thickening or effusion occurs with low or high dose therapy
Procarbazine	Blood eosinophilia; hypersensitivity reaction
Cyclophosphamide	Pleuropericarditis
Mitomycin	Aggregates of lymphocytes and eosinophils in pleura; prompt relief of symptoms with drug withdrawal
Bleomycin	Resolves in weeks to months

Reproduced with permission from: Sahn, S.A.: Malignant pleural effusions. Semin. Respir. Med. 9:43, 1987.

space. As the tumor progresses and the visceral and parietal pleura fuse, the fluid diminishes or disappears.

Autopsy series have shown that in patients with carcinoma of the lung, pleural metastasis is almost always found on both the visceral and parietal pleural surfaces. Meyer (1966) noted that rarely is only the visceral pleural surface involved, and isolated parietal pleural metastases were never identified. Visceral pleural metastasis in lung cancer appears to be either through contiguous spread or through pulmonary arterial invasion and embolization. Once seeded with tumor, these malignant cells migrate from the visceral to parietal pleural surface by either preformed or tumor-induced pleural adhesions. Alternatively, free tumor cells shed from the visceral pleural surface can adhere to the parietal pleura and multiply. Chernow and I (1977) reported that adenocarcinoma of the lung is the most common cell type to involve the pleura, because of its peripheral location. When bilateral pleural metastases occur in lung cancer, hepatic spread and parenchymal invasion in the contralateral lung also usually occur. Once contralateral lung metastasis occurs, pulmonary artery invasion and embolization follow, as in the ipsilateral lesion. The data concerning the laterality of the pleural effusion in relation to the primary lesion support this mechanism. Chernow and I (1977) pointed out that in lung cancer, pleural effusions occur either ipsilaterally or bilaterally and virtually never occur solely in the contralateral pleural space. With other cancers, pleural involvement is usually from tertiary spread from established liver metastases with no predilection for side. Fentiman and associates (1981) summarized the conflicting data in breast carcinoma, with some studies showing

a high incidence of ipsilateral pleural effusion and others no predilection for side. Probably two mechanisms are operative: chest wall lymphatic invasion resulting in ipsilateral effusion, and hepatic spread with bilateral or contralateral hematogenous spread.

Clinical Presentation

The most common presenting symptom of patients with carcinoma or lymphoma of the pleura and a large pleural effusion is dyspnea on exertion. In diffuse pleural mesothelioma, patients generally present with the insidious onset of either dyspnea or chest pain. Taryle and colleagues (1976) noted that almost all patients with a malignant mesothelioma present with some symptoms whereas Weick and associates (1973) reported that up to 25% of patients with carcinoma or lymphoma of the pleura may be relatively asymptomatic when the pleural effusion is discovered on a routine chest roentgenogram.

Because malignant involvement of the pleura signals advanced disease, these patients frequently have weight loss and appear chronically ill. Chernow and I (1977) found that pleural effusion provided the initial diagnosis of cancer in almost 50% of these patients.

Patients with carcinoma of the pleura may have chest pain caused by involvement of the parietal pleura, ribs, or chest wall. Elmes and Simpson (1976) emphasized, however, that the chest pain associated with malignant mesothelioma is more common and impressive but is nonpleuritic and frequently referred to the upper abdomen or shoulder.

Physical examination may show cachexia and lymphadenopathy in cancer and lymphoma but may be unremarkable in malignant mesothelioma, except for the findings of a moderate to large pleural effusion.

Roentgenograms of the Chest

The pleural effusion associated with lung cancer is ipsilateral to the primary lesion. This may be because of direct pleural involvement, mediastinal lymph node infiltration, or an endobronchial lesion with pneumonia or atelectasis. With other primary sites, with the possible exception of breast cancer, there appears to be no ipsilateral predilection and bilateral effusions are common, and as Chernow and I (1977) pointed out, are usually the result of mediastinal lymph node metastasis.

Patients with carcinomatous pleurisy usually present with a moderate to large effusion—500 to 2000 ml; 10% have effusions < 500 ml and a similar number have massive pleural effusion—complete opacification of the hemithorax. Malignancy is the most common cause of a massive pleural effusion; in a series by Maher and Berger (1972), 67% of 46 massive pleural effusions were caused by malignancy. The roentgenographic finding of bilateral effusions with a normal heart size suggests malignancy, most commonly carcinoma, which Rabin and Blackman (1957) noted. Benign effusions associated with this roentgenographic finding include lupus pleuritis, esophageal rupture, cirrhosis with ascites, nephrotic syndrome, and constrictive pericarditis.

When an apparently large pleural effusion is present—1500 ml—with an absence of contralateral mediastinal shift, malignancy is almost always the cause and the patient has a poor prognosis. The following diagnoses should be considered in this context: (1) carcinoma of the ipsilateral main stem bronchus causing atelectasis; (2) a fixed mediastinum caused by malignant lymph nodes; (3) malignant mesothelioma—the density represents mostly tumor with a small effusion; and (4) extensive tumor infiltration of the ipsilteral lung roentgenographically mimicking a large effusion.

As Whitcomb and associates (1972) and MacDonald (1977) described, in Hodgkin's disease, patients with pleural effusions usually have associated lymphadenopathy and parenchymal infiltrates. In contrast, Jenkins and colleagues (1981) reported that in non-Hodgkin's lymphoma, intrathoracic lymphadenopathy occurs in few of the cases associated with either pulmonary disease or pleural effusions.

Heller and colleagues (1970) noted that in malignant mesothelioma the initial roentgenogram usually shows a moderate to large unilateral pleural effusion. Following therapeutic thoracentesis, the pleura may show thickening or nodularity. Evidence of asbestos exposure, such as interstitial lung disease or pleural plaques, may be identified in the contralateral lung and pleura. Roentgenographic clues suggesting that the large effusion may be caused by mesothelioma rather than carcinoma are pleural nodularity; absence of contralateral mediastinal shift with an apparent large effusion; and a tendency for loculation.

Pleural Fluid Characteristics

Malignant pleural effusions may be serous, serosanguineous, or grossly bloody. A grossly bloody effusion suggests direct pleural involvement, whereas a serous effusion results from either lymphatic obstruction or an endobronchial lesion with atelectasis. Light and co-workers (1973) suggested that when the red blood cell count in the pleural fluid is > 100,000/μl in the absence of trauma, malignancy is the most likely diagnosis. Most of the nonred blood cells—2500 to 4000/μl—in pleural fluid, as Yam (1967) noted, are lymphocytes, macrophages, and mesothelial cells; more than 50% of the cellular population are lymphocytes in about one half of the cases. The percentage of PMNs is usually < 25% of the cell population, but on rare occasions, when there is intense pleural inflammation, the PMN may predominante. Deresinski (1978) reported that pleural fluid eosinophilia is inexplicably rare—approximately 5%—in bloody, malignant pleural effusions.

Carcinomatous pleural effusions usually are exudates, with a protein concentration of about 4 g/dl; Chernow and I (1977) and Light and associates (1972), however, reported protein concentrations from 1.5 to 8 g/dl. Approximately 5 to 10% of malignant pleural effusions are transudates. These transudative malignant effusions are caused by early stages of lymphatic obstruction, atelectasis from bronchial obstruction, or concomitant congestive heart failure. When an effusion meets exudative criteria by LDH but not protein, Light and associates (1972) emphasized that malignancy should be suspected. Good and colleagues (1980) stated that approximately one third of patients with malignant pleural effusions have a low pleural fluid pH—< 7.30, range of 6.95 to 7.29—and a low glucose concentration—< 60 mg/dl or pleural-fluid-to-serum ratio of < 0.5—at presentation. These effusions usually have been present for several months and are associated with a large tumor burden and fibrosis of the pleural surface. Good and colleagues (1985) suggested that the abnormal pleural membrane reduces glucose entry into the pleural space and impairs glucose end product efflux, resulting in a local acidosis. Furthermore, Good and associates (1978) noted that low pH-low glucose malignant effusions are associated with short survival, ease of diagnosis by cytology and pleural biopsy, and a poor response to intrapleural sclerosing agents.

Pleural effusions caused by lymphoma have characteristics similar to those of carcinoma of the pleura. These effusions, however, tend to be less hemorrhagic and less likley to result in pleural fluid acidosis and low glucose concentrations. I (1985a) pointed out that a pleural effusion in malignant mesothelioma is more likely to have a low pH and low glucose content and greater protein and LDH concentrations than effusions from carcinoma of the pleura. Because of an overlap of values in an individual patient, however, these data are not helpful in separating carcinoma from mesothelioma.

Diagnosis

From my (1988) compilation of several large series totaling over 500 cases of malignancy, pleural fluid cytology had a diagnostic yield of 66% and percutaneous pleural biopsy 46%. When both procedures were performed, a positive diagnosis was obtained in 73%. Several observations can be made from these data: (1) pleural fluid cytology is more sensitive than pleural biopsy; (2) the tests are complementary, but pleural biopsy adds little to cytologic examination; (3) the lower yield from pleural biopsy results from sampling error and possibly operator technique; and (4) the wide range of incidence of positive results with both tests probably relates to imprecise handling of specimens, expertise of the cytopathologist, and the possibility that the pleural effusion was paramalignant at the time of the procedure. Repeat cytologic examination and pleural biopsy may be diagnostic, and Salyer (1975) and Boutin (1981) and their colleagues urged that a second procedure be done if suspicion for malignancy is high. Repeat thoracentesis for cytology a few days following the first procedure provides freshly shed cells and less degenerative mesothelial cells. Repeat pleural biopsy provides a greater sampling area. From the thoracoscopy data of Canto (1985), the yield of pleural biopsy probably could be increased by performing the procedure as close to the diaphragm and midline as possible because pleural metastases tend to originate near the diaphragm and spread cephalad toward the costal pleura.

Some patients with exudative pleural effusions remain without a diagnosis following repeat cytologic examination and pleural biopsy. Options at this time include observation, thoracoscopy, or open pleural biopsy. Recommending an invasive procedure is easier psychologically for the physician but creates morbidity for the patient. Thoracoscopy, as Boutin and associates (1985) reported, has a high yield—80 to 97%—in malignant pleural disease when multiple biopsies are taken, frozen sections of each biopsy are examined, and the visceral pleura is also biopsied. Open pleural biopsy requires a thoracotomy with associated morbidity, a low incidence of mortality, and economic burden. Treatable causes of exudative effusions such as tuberculosis, pleurisy, and pulmonary embolism must be excluded before invasive procedures are performed. Patients with a positive tuberculin skin test and a leukocyte-predominant exudate should be treated with antituberculous drugs, because approximately 5 to 10% of patients with tuberculous pleurisy are not diagnosed bacteriologically following pleural fluid and tissue culture and pleural histologic examination. Bronchoscopy should be done before thoracoscopy or open pleural biopsy if there is absence of contralateral shift with a large effusion, evidence of ipsilateral volume loss, or a pulmonary lesion in addition to the pleural effusion. According to Feinsilver and associates (1986), the value of bronchoscopy in an undiagnosed pleural effusion without the aforementioned factors is limited.

An alternate approach is observation with repeat cytology and pleural biopsy at a later time if the effusion has not regressed. Malignant pleural effusions almost never resolve spontaneously; an increase in the size of the pleural effusion heightens the suspicion of malig-

nancy. Furthermore, if the clinician "misses" a malignant pleural effusion for several weeks, in almost no situation has a disservice been done to the patient who has widespread, incurable disease. The diagnosis of a malignancy that characteristically is responsive to therapy, such as breast, prostate, thyroid, small cell, and germ cell cancer and lymphoma, however, must be considered carefully. Screening tests such as mammography, serum acid phosphatase, and thyroid scan should be done as appropriate.

Measurements of carcinoembryonic antigen, hyaluronic acid, and LDH isoenzymes have no diagnostic value. Chromosomal analysis of pleural fluid is expensive and not available in all laboratories, but may be helpful in the diagnosis of lymphoma, leukemia, and mesothelioma.

The antemortem diagnosis of malignant mesothelioma requires both clinical and histologic observations. Diagnosis from exfoliative cytology is difficult, and Whitaker (1978) questions its value. Even when malignancy is diagnosed, it may be impossible to differentiate metastatic adenocarcinoma from a malignant mesothelioma. Percutaneous needle biopsy does not consistently yield a definitive diagnosis and frequently prompts a misleading diagnosis of adenocarcinoma. High levels of hyaluronic acid are reported to establish the diagnosis of mesothelioma; however, Rasmussen and Faber (1967) observed that most patients with mesothelioma have intermediate levels, frequently seen in metastatic carcinoma and other inflammatory diseases. Thoracoscopy has been recommended, but the pathologist may be unable to reach a diagnosis; usually thoracotomy is required to obtain adequate tissue for examination. Mesotheliomas, as Edge and Choudhury (1978) noted, tend to invade surgical sites. Prophylactic irradiation should be given postoperatively. On occasion, even after adequate tissue has been examined from the thoracotomy, diagnosis remains uncertain. The subsequent course or biopsy from a tumor implant at the surgical site often provides the diagnosis.

Most pathologists can confidently diagnose a sarcomatous or mixed histologic variant but have difficulty in differentiating the epithelial form of mesothelioma from the more common metastatic adenocarcinoma. Special tissue stains, newer immunologic techniques, and electron microscopy aid in the antemortem diagnosis of patients with the epithelial variety of mesothelioma (see Chapter 60).

Prognosis

Establishing the diagnosis of a malignant pleural effusion portends a poor prognosis. Patients with carcinoma of the lung, stomach, and ovary generally survive only a few months from the time of diagnosis of the malignant effusion, whereas patients with breast cancer may survive several months to years, depending upon the response to chemotherapy. Patients with lymphomatous pleural effusions tend to have a survival intermediate between breast cancer and other carcinomas.

I (1985a) observed that patients with low pH-low glucose malignant effusions survive only a few months, whereas those with a normal pH and glucose survive for about 1 year. Thus, the biochemical findings in the pleural fluid provide the clinician with information that is helpful in deciding on a rational plan of palliative treatment.

Even though a pleural effusion is an ominous sign in lung cancer, usually ruling out operability, Decker and colleagues (1978) reported that approximately 5% of these patients have a paramalignant effusion or effusion from another cause and may be operative candidates. The burden falls to the clinician to diagnose the cause of the pleural effusion before making a decision about possible curative surgery. Circumstances suggesting that the pleural effusion in lung cancer is paramalignant and that the patient may still be cured by resection are squamous cell type, roentgenographic volume loss, serous effusion, transudate, and parapneumonic effusion.

Treatment

When the pleural effusion has been documented to be malignant or paramalignant and the patient is not a surgical candidate, the clinician must make a decision concerning palliative therapy. Factors that must be considered in this decision are the patient's general condition, symptoms, and expected survival. Management options range from observation in the asymptomatic patient to thoracotomy with pleurectomy and pleural abrasion. Some asymptomatic patients develop progressive pleural effusions, producing dyspnea that requires therapy, but others reach a new steady state of pleural fluid formation and absorption and do not progress to a symptomatic stage requiring therapy. In the debilitated patient with a short expected survival, based on the extent of disease, general status, and the biochemical characteristics of the fluid, it is more prudent to perform a therapeutic thoracentesis periodically on an outpatient basis than to recommend hospitalization and tube thoracostomy with instillation of a sclerosing agent, with its associated morbidity.

Pleurectomy and pleural abrasion are virtually completely effective in obliterating the pleural space and controlling recurrence of the effusion. Pleural abrasion should be carried out in most patients who undergo thoracotomy for an undiagnosed pleural effusion and are found to have malignancy, because this prevents the subsequent development of a symptomatic pleural effusion. Pleurectomy, however, even when indicated, as Martini and colleagues (1975) discussed, is a major surgical procedure associated with substantial morbidity and some mortality. Thus, this procedure should be reserved for patients with an expected survival of several months, who are in relatively good condition, who have a trapped lung, or who have failed a sclerosing-agent procedure.

Technique of Pleurectomy*

Beattie (1963) described pleurectomy well. The thorax is entered by a posterolateral incision, with entrance into the pleural space preferably by an intercostal incision in

---

*Addendum by the Editor, T.W. Shields

the fifth or sixth interspace. The extrapleural dissection is begun in the plane between the parietal pleura and the extrathoracic fascia at the margins of the intercostal incision before the rib spreader is inserted. The parietal pleura is then stripped circumferentially to the mediastinum; more tumor tends to be present at the diaphragmatic costopleural junction than at the apical pleura, and it is recommended that the upper half of the pleural dissection be completed first. Care must be taken in continuing the pleural dissection over the mediastinal surface to avoid injury to the phrenic, recurrent laryngeal, or sympathetic nerves or stellate ganglion. Damage to the vascular structures of the mediastinum likewise must be avoided. Dissection is continued down from the apex to the pulmonary hilus, which completes the initial phase of the procedure. The inferior portion of the parietal pleura is then dissected free. Care must be taken at the costophrenic sulcus not to remove the diaphragmatic attachment to the chest wall. It is unnecessary, as well as often impossible, to remove the diaphragmatic pleura, but the reflection of the pleura posteriorly on the lower mediastinal surface in association with the pulmonary ligament should be freed to the inferior border of the hilus. Dissection of the mediastinal pleura from pericardium is difficult and should not even be attempted in the region of the phrenic nerve. If the lung is free and ventilates well, no visceral pleural dissection is indicated. If, on the other hand, the lung is bound down with fibrin, a standard decortication is necessary. After hemostasis is obtained satisfactorily, pleural drainage and closure are completed in the standard manner.

The procedure is applicable only to a highly selected group of patients in good general condition whose malignant pleural effusion has failed to respond to other local therapy. Best results are obtained when the primary lesion is a carcinoma of the breast or, occasionally, a melanoma. Results vary, but are more often poor in patients with carcinoma of the lung. Complications are frequent, as high as 23%, and mortality rates are significant, 10 to 18%. When decortication of the lung is necessary in conjunction with the pleurectomy, the mortality rate is significantly increased.

Chemotherapy or Irradiation

In general, systemic chemotherapy is disappointing for the control of malignant pleural effusions. Nonetheless, patients with lymphoma, according to Weick (1973) and Xaubet (1985) and their associates; breast cancer, from the reports of Fentiman (1981) and Jones (1975) and their colleagues; or small cell carcinoma of the lung, as Livingston and co-workers (1982) noted may respond well to chemotherapy. Information about steroid receptors obtained from malignant pleural fluid in patients with breast cancer can provide a source for determining potential response to hormonal manipulation. In general, radiation therapy is of limited value in controlling carcinomatous malignant pleural effusions. Roy and associates (1967) suggested, however, that when there is predominantly mediastinal node involvement, irradiation may be valuable for patients with lymphoma or small cell carcinoma of the lung or when the effusion is a chylothorax.

Use of a Sclerosing Agent

For most patients, the most effective method, short of pleurectomy or pleural abrasion, for controlling the malignant pleural effusion is chest tube drainage with instillation of a sclerosing agent. Currently, tetracycline hydrochloride is the sclerosing agent of choice because it has resulted in a high success rate with minimum toxicity. The major adverse effect has been chest pain, which can be ameliorated, at times, with parenteral narcotics. The effectiveness of tetracycline depends primarily on its fibrogenicity rather than its antineoplastic activity. In an experimental model, I and Good (1981) showed that tetracycline produces extensive pleural fibrosis and symphysis in a dose-dependent manner.

If the clinician has documented that therapeutic thoracentesis results in relief from dyspnea and the rate of recurrence and the return of symptoms is rapid, instillation of tetracycline should be considered. If expected survival is several months, the patient is not debilitated, and the pleural fluid pH is > 7.30, the patient is a good candidate for pleurodesis. Attempting pleurodesis is useless if the lungs cannot be expanded fully; this would occur in main stem bronchial obstruction with atelectasis or a trapped lung. The documentation of a low pleural fluid pH—< 7.30—not only suggests a limited survival but a poor response to sclerosing agents. The large tumor bulk and the fibrosis involving the pleural surfaces in low pH effusions apparently diminish the effectiveness of tetracycline in producing pleural symphysis.

The technique of tetracycline instillation is critical for a good result in the properly selected patient (Table 57–6). The pleural surfaces must be in close contact at the time inflammation is induced with tetracycline; this is best accomplished with chest tube drainage of the pleural effusion. If the effusion is large, the fluid should be drained slowly over the first several hours with intermittent clamping of the tube to diminish the likelihood of unilateral pulmonary edema. This complication is most likely to occur when there is an endobronchial obstruction or trapped lung that does not allow the lung

to expand to the chest wall and that results in a precipitous drop in intrapleural pressure. Furthermore, this procedure should not be attempted in the aforementioned situations because it likely will not be successful.

Tetracycline in a dose of 20 mg/kg should be instilled into the pleural space when the pleural effusion is absent or minimal and the lung is expanded fully. Studies in my laboratory suggest that the patient need not be rotated through various positions following tetracycline instillation. This is often uncomfortable and difficult for the patient and requires additional personnel time. Radiolabeling of tetracycline has demonstrated that following intrapleural instillation, the tetracycline is distributed completely throughout the pleural space within seconds and the distribution is not enhanced by rotating the patient. The only exception may be in an individual with multiple pleural loculations, for whom rotation may be beneficial. The chest tube should be removed when drainage is < 150 ml of fluid per day. With proper patient selection and good technique, the malignant effusion should be controlled in 80 to 85% of cases. Success does not depend on producing complete pleural symphysis but on diminishing the amount of accumulation of pleural fluid so that dyspnea is relieved. Wooten and associates (1987) noted that both tetracycline and lidocaine—used by some clinicians in an attempt to ameliorate chest pain—are absorbed systemically and reach therapeutic levels by 30 to 60 minutes; thus, a history of allergic reactions to either drug is a contraindication to its use. The dose of lidocaine should not exceed 150 mg or 3 mg/kg, whichever is less.

The management of malignant mesothelioma is discussed in Chapter 60. Judgment in management of these patients is the keynote of appropriate care.

REFERENCES

Bartlett, J.G., and Finegold, S.M.: Anaerobic infections of the lung and pleural space. Am. Rev. Respir. Dis. *110*:56, 1974.
Beattie, E.J., Jr.: The treatment of malignant pleural effusions by partial pleurectomy. Surg. Clin. North Am. *43*:99, 1963.
Black, L.F.: The pleural space and pleural fluid. Mayo Clin. Proc. *47*:493, 1972.
Boutin, C., Cargnino, P., and Viallat, J.R.: Thoracoscopy in malignant effusion. Am. Rev. Respir. Dis. *124*:588, 1981.
Boutin, C., et al.: Thoracoscopy. In The Pleura in Health and Disease. Edited by J. Chretien, J. Bignon, and A. Hirsch. New York, Marcel Dekker, 1985, p. 587.
Brandstetter, R.D., and Cohen, R.P.: Hypoxemia after thoracentesis: a predictable and treatable condition. J.A.M.A. *242*:1060, 1979.
Broaddus, C., and Staub, N.C.: Pleural liquid and protein turnover in health and disease. Semin. Respir. Med. *9*:7, 1987.
Bynum, L.J., and Wilson, J.E., III: Characteristics of pleural effusions associated with pulmonary embolism. Arch. Intern. Med. *136*:159, 1976.
Campbell, G.D., and Webb, W.R.: Eosinophilic pleural effusion. Am. Rev. Respir. Dis. *90*:194, 1964.
Canto, A., et al.: Points to consider when choosing a biopsy method in cases of pleurisy of unknown origin. Chest *84*:176, 1983.
Chernow, B., and Sahn, S.A.: Carcinomatous involvement of the pleura: an analysis of 96 patients. Am. J. Med. *63*:695, 1977.
Chretien, J., and Jaubert, F.: Pleural responses in malignant metastatic tumors. In The Pleura in Health and Disease. Edited by J. Chretien, J. Bignon, and A. Hirsch. New York, Marcel Dekker, 1985, p. 489.
Chusid, E.L., and Siltzbach, L.E.: Sarcoidosis of the pleura. Ann. Intern. Med. *81*:190, 1974.

Table 57–6. Procedure for Pleurodesis

1. Place chest tube in midaxillary line directed toward diaphragm.
2. Remove fluid in controlled manner under water seal.
3. Assess tube position on radiograph to position patient for optimal drainage.
4. Connect chest tube to suction (-20 cm H_2O).
5. Demonstrate minimal tube drainage at bedside and lung expansion and small or absent effusion on roentgenograph.
6. Give morphine sulfate IV.

With patient supine:

7. Instill lidocaine HCl 150 mg or 3 mg/kg (whichever is less) in 50 ml of saline through chest tube and clamp tube for 5 minutes.
8. Instill tetracycline HCl (20 mg/kg) in 50 ml of saline through chest tube and clamp for one hour.
9. Connect chest tube to suction (-20 cm H_2O).
10. Remove chest tube when dainage <150 ml/day.

Clarkson, B.: Relationship between cell type, glucose concentration, and response to treatment in neoplastic effusions. Cancer *17*:914, 1964.

Collins, T.R., and Sahn, S.A.: Thoracentesis: complications, patient experience, and diagnostic value. Chest *91*:817, 1987.

Daniels, A.C., and Childress, M.E.: Pleuropulmonary amebiasis. Calif. Med. *85*:369, 1956.

Decker, D.A., et al.: The significance of a cytologically negative pleural effusion in bronchogenic carcinoma. Chest *74*:640, 1978.

Deresinski, S.C.: Eosinophils, pleural effusions, and malignancy. Ann. Intern. Med. *89*:424, 1978.

Edge, J.R., and Choudhury, S.L.: Malignant mesothelioma of the pleura in Barrow-in-Furness. Thorax *33*:26, 1978.

Elmes, P.C., and Simpson, M.J.C.: The clinical aspects of mesothelioma. Q. J. Med. *45*:427, 1976.

Emont, et al.: Epidemiology of primary malignant mesothelial tumors in Canada. Cancer *26*:914, 1970.

Estenne, M., Yernault, J-C, and Detryer, A.: Mechanism of relief of dyspnea after thoracocentesis in patients with larger pleural effusions. Am. J. Med. *74*:813, 1983.

Feinsilver, S.H., Barrows, A.A., and Braman, S.B.: Fiberoptic bronchoscopy and pleural effusion of unknown origin. Chest *90*:516, 1986.

Fentiman, I.S., et al.: Pleural effusion in breast cancer: a review of 105 cases. Cancer *47*:2087, 1981.

Good, J.T. Jr., Taryle, D.A., and Sahn, S.A.: Pleural fluid pH in malignant effusions: pathophysiologic and prognostic implications. Chest *74*:338, 1978.

Good, J.T. Jr., et al.: The diagnostic value of pleural fluid pH. Chest *78*:55, 1980.

Good, J.T. Jr., Taryle, D.A., and Sahn, S.A.: The pathogenesis of low glucose, low pH malignant effusions. Am. Rev. Respir. Dis. *131*:737, 1985.

Heller, R.M., Janower, M.L., and Weber, A.L.: The radiological manifestations of malignant pleural mesothelioma. Am. J. Roentgenol. *108*:53, 1970.

Jenkins, P.F., et al.: Non-Hodgkin's lymphoma, chronic lymphatic leukemia, and the lung. Br. J. Dis. Chest *75*:22, 1981.

Jones, S.E., Durie, B.G.M., and Salmon, S.E.: Combination chemotherapy with adriamycin and cyclophosphamide for advanced breast cancer. Cancer *36*:90, 1975.

Kaye, M.D.: Pleuropulmonary complications of pancreatitis. Thorax *23*:297, 1968.

Light, R.W., et al.: Pleural effusions: the diagnostic separation of transudates and exudates. Ann. Intern. Med. *77*:507, 1972.

Light, R.W., and Ball, W.C., Jr.: Glucose and amylase in pleural effusions. J.A.M.A. *225*:257, 1973a.

Light, R.W., Erozan, Y.S., and Ball, W.C.: Cells in pleural fluid: their value in differential diagnosis. Arch. Intern. Med. *132*:854, 1973b.

Light, R.W., et al.: Parapneumonic effusions. Am. J. Med. *69*:507, 1980.

Livingston, R.B., et al.: Isolated pleural effusion in small cell lung carcinoma: favorable prognosis. Chest *81*:208, 1982.

Lorch, D.G., and Sahn, S.A.: Pleural effusions due to diseases below the diaphragm. Semin. Respir. Med. *9*:227, 1987.

MacDonald, J.B.: Lung involvement in Hodgkin's disease. Thorax *32*:664, 1977.

MacDonald, J.B., et al.: Epidemiology of primary malignant mesothelial tumors in Canada. Cancer *26*:914, 1970.

Magnussen, H., et al.: Transpleural diffusion of inert gases in excised lung lobes of the dog. Respir. Physiol. *20*:1, 1974.

Maher, G.G., and Berger, H.W.: Massive pleural effusions: malignant and non-malignant causes in 46 patients. Am. Rev. Respir. Dis. *105*:458, 1972.

Martini, N., Bains, M.S., and Beattie, E.J., Jr.: Indications for pleurectomy in malignant effusion. Cancer *35*:734, 1975.

Maulitz, R.M., et al.: The pleuropulmonary consequences of esophageal rupture: an experimental model. Am. Rev. Respir. Dis. *120*:363, 1979.

Metzger, J.B., Garagusi, V.F., and Kermin, D.M.: Pulmonary oxalosis caused by *Aspergillus niger*. Am. Rev. Respir. Dis. *129*:501, 1984.

Meyer, P.C.: Metastatic carcinoma of the pleura. Thorax *21*:437, 1966.

Miller, K.S., Tomlinson, J.R., and Sahn, S.A.: Pleuropulmonary complications of enteral tube feedings: two reports, review of the literature, and recommendations. Chest *88*:230, 1985.

Potts, D.E., Levin, D.C., and Sahn, S.A.: Pleural fluid pH in parapneumonic effusions. Chest *70*:328, 1976.

Potts, D.E., et al.: The acidosis of low glucose effusions. Am. Rev. Respir. Dis. *117*:665, 1978.

Rabin, C.B., and Blackman, N.S.: Bilateral pleural effusion. Its significance in association with a heart of normal size. J. Mt. Sinai Hosp. *24*:45, 1957.

Rasmussen, K.N., and Faber, V.: Hyaluronic acid in 247 pleural fluids. Scand. J. Respir. Dis. *48*:366, 1967.

Reda, M.G., and Baigelman, W.: Pleural effusion in systemic lupus erythematosus. Acta Cytol. *24*:553, 1980.

Roy, P.H., Carr, D.T., and Payne, W.S.: The problem of chylothorax. Mayo Clin. Proc. *42*:457, 1967.

Sahn, S.A., and Good, J.T., Jr.: The effect of common sclerosing agents on the rabbit pleural space. Am. Rev. Respir. Dis. *124*:65, 1981.

Sahn, S.A.: Malignant pleural effusions. Clin. Chest Med. *6*:113, 1985a.

Sahn, S.A.: Pathogenesis and clinical features of diseases associated with a low pleural fluid glucose. *In* The Pleura in Health and Disease. Edited by J. Chretien, J. Bignon, and A. Hirsch. New York, Marcel Dekker, 1985b, p. 267.

Sahn, S.A.: Pleural fluid pH in the normal state and in diseases affecting the pleural space. *In* The Pleura in Health and Disease. Edited by J. Chretien, J. Bignon, and A. Hirsch. New York, Marcel Dekker, 1985c, p. 253.

Sahn, S.A.: Malignant pleural effusions. Semin. Respir. Med. *9*:43, 1987a.

Sahn, S.A.: Malignant pleural effusions. *In* Pulmonary Diseases and Disorders, 2nd ed. Edited by A.P. Fishman. New York, McGraw-Hill Book Co., 1988.

Sahn, S.A.: Pleural fluid analysis: narrowing the differential diagnosis. Semin. Respir. Med. *9*:22, 1987b.

Salyer, W.R., Eggleston, J.C., and Erozan, Y.S.: Efficacy of pleural needle biopsy and pleural fluid cytopathology in the diagnosis of malignant neoplasm involving the pleura. Chest *67*:536, 1975.

Spriggs, A.I., and Boddington, M.M.: Absence of mesothelial cells from tuberculous pleural effusions. Thorax *15*:169, 1968.

Stark, D.D., et al.: Biochemical features of urinothorax. Arch. Intern. Med. *142*:1509, 1982.

Stelzner, T.J., et al.: The pleuropulmonary manifestations of the postcardiac injury syndrome. Chest *84*:383, 1983.

Taryle, D.A., Lakshminarayan, S., and Sahn, S.A.: Pleural mesotheliomas. An analysis of 18 cases and review of the literature. Medicine (Baltimore) *55*:153, 1976.

Wagner, J.C., Sleggs, C.A., and Marchand, P.: Diffuse pleural mesothelioma and asbestos exposure in the North Western Cape Province. Br. J. Ind. Med. *17*:260, 1960.

Weick, J.K., et al.: Pleural effusion in lymphoma. Cancer *31*:848, 1973.

Whitaker, D.: The cytology of malignant mesothelioma in Western Australia. Acta Cytol. *22*:67, 1978.

Whitcomb, M.E., et al.: Hodgkin's disease of the lung. Am. Rev. Respir. Dis. *106*:79, 1972.

Wooten, S.A., et al.: Pharmacokinetics of tetracycline and lidocaine following intrapleural installation. Am. Rev. Respir. Dis. *135*:A245, 1987.

Xaubet, A., et al.: Characteristics and prognostic value of pleural effusions in non-Hodgkin's lymphomas. Eur. J. Respir. Dis. *66*:d135, 1985.

Yam, L.T.: Diagnostic significance of lymphocytes in pleural effusions. Ann. Intern. Med. *66*:972, 1967.

Yamada, S.: Über die serose Flüssigkeit in der Pleurahöhle der gesunder Menschen. Z. Gesamte Exp. Med. *90*:342, 1933.

READING REFERENCES

Antman, K.H.: Multimodality treatment for malignant mesothelioma based on a study of natural history. Am. J. Med. *68*:356, 1980.

Hillerdal, G.: Malignant mesothelioma 1982: review of 4710 published cases. Br. J. Dis. Chest *77*:321, 1983.

Schienger, M., et al.: Mesotheliomes pleuraux malins. Bull. Cancer (Paris) *56*:265, 1969.

CHAPTER 58

CHYLOTHORAX AND ANATOMY OF THE THORACIC DUCT

Joseph I. Miller, Jr.

CHYLOTHORAX

Chylothorax is the presence of lymphatic fluid in the pleural space resulting from a leak of the thoracic duct or one of its major divisions. This condition is being recognized more frequently, after both cardiac and general thoracic surgery. Increased understanding of the physiology, pathogenesis, diagnosis, and management of chylothorax have decreased the initial 50% mortality to a mortality of 10% in major medical centers.

ANATOMY OF THE THORACIC DUCT

A sound knowledge of the anatomy of the thoracic duct is required to appreciate the etiology and, subsequently, surgical management of chylothorax. Davis (1915) and Nix and associates (1957) reported that the anatomy of the thoracic duct was constant only in its variability. Embryologically, it is a bilateral structure and has the potential of having many varied anatomic patterns. The pattern and anatomy of the thoracic duct is considered to be normal, as reported by Davis (1915), in only 65% of humans. Many anatomical variations occur in lymphatic and lymphaticovenous anastomosis.

The usual anatomic pattern of the thoracic duct is shown in Fig. 58–1. The thoracic duct is the left main collecting vessel of the lymphatic system and is far larger than the right terminal lymphatic duct. Most commonly, the thoracic duct originates from the cisterna chyli in the midline at the level of the second lumbar vertebra. The cisterna chyli is 3 to 4 cm long and 2 to 3 cm in diameter. It is generally found along the vertebral column at the level of L2, but may be found anywhere between T10 and L3, generally on the right side of the aorta.

From the cisterna chyli, the thoracic duct ascends to enter the chest through the aortic hiatus at the level of T10 to T12, just to the right of the aorta. Above the diaphragm, the duct lies on the anterior surface of the vertebral column behind the esophagus and between the aorta and the azygos vein. The duct usually lies in front of the right intercostal arteries with the nerves close by. The duct continues upward on the right side of the vertebral column to approximately the level of the fifth or sixth thoracic vertebra, where it crosses behind the aorta and aortic arch into the left posterior mediastinum. From there, it passes superiorly in close approximation to the left side of the esophagus and the pleural reflection into the neck. Before exiting the mediastinum, the duct receives tributaries from the bronchomediastinal trunk of the right lymphatic duct. As it leaves the thorax, the thoracic duct ascends in the neck about 4 cm above the clavicle and turns laterally behind the carotid sheath and in front of the inferior thyroid and vertebral arteries. At the medial margin of the anterior scalene muscle it drops down to enter the angle of union of the internal jugular and subclavian veins. The anatomic manner in which the thoracic duct ends varies. It may enter the jugular vein as a single trunk or as multiple trunks. Near its opening, it usually is joined by the collecting lymphatic trunks from the left upper extremity and the left side of the head and neck.

The only thing constant about the anatomy of the thoracic duct is the numerous anatomical variations. Davis (1915) reported nine major variations, and Anson (1950) listed 12 different anatomic variations of the lower portion of the thoracic duct. In 1922, Lee reported a detailed study of the collateral circulation of the lymphatic system in the mediastinum. He identified various connections between the thoracic duct and the azygos vein, as well as other connections between intercostal veins and the thoracic duct within the chest. The thoracic duct contains valves in various locations throughout its entire course.

Lymph from the right side of the head, neck, and chest wall, as well as from the right lung and the lower half of the left lung, through the bronchomediastinal trunk, drains into the right lymphatic duct. This duct also carries lymph from the heart and the dome of the liver, and from the right diaphragm. The right lymphatic duct is

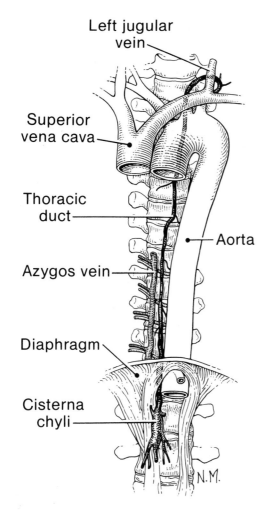

Left jugular
vein

Superior
vena cava

Thoracic
duct

Aorta

Azygos vein

Diaphragm

Cisterna
chyli

N.M.

Fig. 58–1. Anatomy of the thoracic duct.

Table 58–1. Composition of Chyle

Component	Amount (per 100 ml)
Total Fat	0.4–5 g
Total cholesterol	65–220 mg
Total Protein	2.21–5.9 g
Albumin	1.2–4.1 g
Globulin	1.1–3.6 g
Fibrinogen	16–24 g
Sugar	48–200 g
Electrolytes	Similar to plasma
	Amount
Cellular Elements	
Lymphocytes	400–6800/mm³
Erythrocytes	50–600/mm³
Antithrombin globulin	>25% plasma concentrate
Prothrombin	>25% plasma concentrate
Fibrinogen	>25% plasma concentrate

small and is rarely visualized, as Bessone and colleagues (1971) pointed out.

COMPOSITION OF CHYLE

The term "chyle" comes from the Latin "chylus," meaning juice. It is the lymph that originates in the intestine. The fat contained in the intestinal lymph gives chyle its characteristic appeerence. Thoracic duct lymph is not pure chyle, but a mixture of lymphs originating in the intestine, liver, abdominal wall, and lower extremities. Ninety-five percent of the volume of the thoracic duct lymph originates in the liver and the intestinal tract. Under normal circumstances, the amount of lymph originating in the extremities is negligible.

The primary function of the thoracic duct is the transport of digestive fat to the venous system. Monk and Rosenstein (1891) observed a thoracic duct fistula and recognized that the thoracic duct lymph was clear during fasting, but became milky following a fatty meal. About 60 to 70% of the ingested fat is absorbed by the intestinal lymphatic system and conveyed to the blood stream by the thoracic duct. The composition of chyle is listed in Table 58–1. The main component of chyle is fat. Thoracic

duct lymph contains from 0.4 to 5 g of fat per 100 ml and 50 to 70% of absorbed fat is conveyed to the blood stream by way of the thoracic duct. This is made up of neutral fat, free fatty acids, sphingomyelin, phospholipids, cholesterol, and cholesterol esters. The total amount of cholesterol ranges from 65 to 220 mg/100 ml.

Those fatty acids with less than 10 carbon atoms in the chain are absorbed directly by the portal venous system. This particular fact forms the basis for the use of medium-chain triglycerides as an oral diet in the conservative management of chylothorax. Neutral fat, as Ross (1961) noted, is found in the lymph in the form of minute globules that are less than 0.5 mm in diameter. Ingested fat passes from the intestine to the systemic circulation in about 1.5 hours, with a peak absorption at 6 hours after ingestion.

Ross (1961) and Roy and associates (1967) reported that the total protein content of thoracic duct lymph ranges from 2.2 to 5.9 g/ml and is approximately half of that found in the plasma. Thoracic duct lymph contains as much as 4% protein, consisting of albumin, globulin, fibrinogen, and prothrombin, with an albumin ratio of 3 to 1. Sugar concentration in thoracic duct lymph ranges from 40 to 200 g/100 ml. The electrolyte composition is similar to that found in plasma, with sodium, potassium, chloride, calcium, and inorganic phosphorus being the predominant electrolyte components.

Antithrombin globulin, prothrombin, and fibrinogen are all present in human thoracic duct lymph in concentrations greater than 25% of plasma levels. Stuttman and associates (1965) reported that factors V and VIII are present in concentrations of approximately 8.9% and 4.5%, respectively, in thoracic lymph.

The main cellular elements of thoracic duct lymph are lymphocytes. They range from 400 to 6800 cells/mm³. As Hyde and colleagues (1974) noted, most of these lymphocytes are T-lymphocytes. Thoracic duct lymphocytes differ qualitatively and quantitatively from peripheral blood lymphocytes in their reactivity to antigenic stimulation.

In clear lymph, there are approximately 50 red cells/

mm³, whereas in the postabsorptive states, as Shafiroff and Kau (1959) reported, the number may increase to 600 red cells/mm³ of thoracic duct lymph. In addition, fat soluble vitamins, antibodies, enzymes—including pancreatic lipase, alkaline phosphatase, SGOT, and SGPT—and urea nitrogen are also present in thoracic duct lymph. Because of the numerous constituents of thoracic duct lymph, it is readily apparent why the persistent loss of this fluid can interfere with nutrition and immunity.

PHYSIOLOGY OF THE THORACIC DUCT

The function of the thoracic duct is the transport of ingested fat to the venous sytem. Volume and weight of flow of lymph have been estimated to be 1.38 ml/kg of body weight/hour. Crandall and associates (1943) found that the rate of flow increases following ingestion of food and water, and also during abdominal massage, with a maximum flow of 3.9 ml/min and a minimum flow of 0.38 ml/min. Hepatic lymph increases by 150% following meals, whereas intestinal lymph increases to up to 10 times the basal flow following fatty meals. Starvation and complete rest decrease the flow of thoracic duct lymph.

The forward flow of chyle from the cisterna chyli to the entrance into the left subclavian-internal jugular vein junction is influenced by several factors: (1) The inflow of chyle into the lacteal system creates a vis a tergo, which is in turn produced by the intake of food and liquid into the intestine and is augmented by intestinal movement. (2) Negative intrathoracic pressure on inspiration and the resultant gradient between this negative pressure and positive intra-abdominal pressure helps the upward flow of chyle. (3) Muscular contractions of the thoracic duct wall are probably the most important factor. Contractions of the duct wall occur every 10 to 15 seconds independent of respiratory movements. The intraductal pressure ranges from 10 to 25 cm H$_2$O, and with obstruction, as Shafiroff and Kau (1959) observed, it may rise to 50 cm H$_2$O. These rhythmic contractions cause the duct to empty into the subclavian vein. The thoracic duct valves, located throughout its course but which are mostly in the upper portion, permit only upward unidirectional flow.

The flow of chyle varies greatly with the content of the meal and is particularly increased when the fat content of the food is high. Volumes up to 2500 ml of chyle in 24 hours have been collected from the cannulated human thoracic duct. Most of the body's lymphocytes are transported through the thoracic duct system back to the venous system.

The lymph circulation performs the vital function of collecting and transporting excess tissue fluid, extravasated plasma protein, absorbed lipids, and other large molecules from the interstitial spaces back to the blood stream.

ETIOLOGY OF CHYLOTHORAX

There have been numerous classifications of chylothorax. Most have been based upon information obtained at postmortem examination. In 1971, Bessone and colleagues suggested classifying chylothorax into (1) congenital chylothorax; (2) postoperative traumatic chylothorax; (3) nonsurgical traumatic chylothorax; and (4) nontraumatic chylothorax. DeMeester (1983), however, has published a more thorough classification (Table 58–2).

Congenital Chylothorax

Chylothorax in the neonate, although rare, is the leading cause of pleural effusion in this age group. In most cases, the exact cause cannot be ascertained. Birth trauma or congenital defects in the duct wall or both may be precipitating factors. Increased venous pressure in birth trauma, causing thoracic duct rupture, has been suggested as a possible cause. In rare incidences, malformations of the lymphatic system, particularly in the thoracic duct itself, have been shown to be the cause of congenital chylothorax. The thoracic duct may be absent or atretic, and in occasional instances, multiple dilated lymphatic channels with abnormal communications have been noted, as well as multiple fistulae between the thoracic duct and pleural space.

Traumatic Chylothorax

The second major cause of chylothorax is traumatic chylothorax, which may occur with either blunt or penetrating trauma or after a surgical procedure. The most common form of nonpenetrating injury to the thoracic duct is produced by a sudden hyperextension of the spine with rupture of the duct just above the diaphragm. Sudden stretching over the vertebral bodies may be enough in itself to tear the duct, but usually the duct has been

Table 58–2.   Etiology of Chylothorax

Congenital
   Atresia of thoracic duct
   Thoracic duct-pleural fistula space
   Birth trauma
Traumatic
   Blunt
   Penetrating
   Surgical
      Cervical
         Excision of lymph nodes
         Radical neck dissection
      Thoracic
         Ligation of patent ductus arteriosus
         Excision of coarctation
         Esophagectomy
         Resection of thoracic aortic aneurysm
         Resection of mediastinal tumor
         Left pneumonectomy
      Abdominal
         Sympathectomy
         Radical lymph node dissection
   Diagnostic procedures
      Lumbar arteriography
      Subclavian vein catheterization
Neoplasms
Miscellaneous

fixed as a result of prior disease or malignancy. This may be secondary to a blast or blunt trauma. Episodes of vomiting or a violent bout of coughing can also result in tearing of the thoracic duct. Biet and Connolly (1951) believe this is generally caused by a shearing of the thoracic duct by the right crus of the diaphragm. These are the most commonly mentioned causes of chylothorax resulting from nonpenetrating injuries to the chest. Penetrating injury from a gunshot or a stab wound to the thoracic duct is unusual, and is apt to be overshadowed by damage to other structures of more immediate importance.

Operative Injuries

Injury at operation is fairly common. Chylothorax has been reported following almost every known thoracic surgical procedure, including operations on the aorta, esophagus, heart, lungs, and sympathetic nervous system. Injury has also been reported following surgery in the neck, after such operations as radical neck resection and scalene node biopsy. It has also been reported following abdominal operations of sympathectomy and radical lymph node dissection. In addition, it has been reported with translumbar aortography and subclavian venous catheterization. An occasional instance has been reported after an attempt to introduce a cannula into the left internal jugular vein.

Often a latent interval of 2 to 10 days passes between the time of injury and the development of a chylothorax that becomes clinically evident. This is because of the accumulation of lymph in the posterior mediastinum until the mediastinal pleura ruptures, usually on the right side at the base of the pulmonary ligament. Once established, the thoracic duct pleural fistula does not tend to close, in contrast to the dictum that in the absence of obstruction a fistula will close. Spontaneous sealing of a fistula after a closed injury may be expected in only approximately 50% of patients, and death generally ensues in the remaining patients unless the fistula is surgically closed.

Intraoperatively, the duct is most vulnerable to damage in the upper part of the left chest, particularly, as Higgins and Molder (1971) noted, with procedures involving mobilization of the aortic arch, the left subclavian artery, or the esophagus. The classically described course of the duct explains why damage to it below the level of the fifth or sixth thoracic vertebra usually results in a right-sided chylous effusion, and why damage above this level usually results in effusion on the left side.

Neoplastic Chylothorax

Ross (1961) stated that the thoracic duct can be involved in both benign and malignant disease by direct lymphatic permeation in continuity with the primary growth, by direct invasion of the duct by the primary growth, or by tumor embolus in the main duct. The chylothorax may be either unilateral or bilateral. DeMeester (1983) reported that the predominant mechanism of the leak is by rupture of distended tributaries because of back pressure from the neoplastic obstruction or actual erosion of the duct itself. It has been most frequently reported following lymphosarcoma, retroperitoneal lymphoma, or primary carcinoma of the lung. Rarely, malignant chylous leaks may fill the pericardial sac with chyle and produce signs and symptoms of cardiac tamponade.

Miscellaneous Causes

Infections, filariasis, pancreatic pseudocysts, thrombosis of the jugular and subclavian veins, cirrhosis of the liver, and tuberculosis can all cause chylothorax.

Benign lymphangiomas arising in the thoracic duct may also produce single or multiple cyst-like spaces filled with chyle.

Pulmonary lymphangiomatosis, reported by Cunn (1973) and Silverstein (1974) and their associates, is a rare cause of chylothorax. This condition is seen in women of reproductive age who have shortness of breath as the major complaint. Pneumothorax and hemoptysis can be seen in addition to chylothorax, and these women usually die of pulmonary insufficiency within 10 years of presentation.

PATHOLOGIC PHYSIOLOGY

Chylothorax can cause cardiopulmonary abnormalities, as well as serious metabolic and immunologic deficiencies. The accumulation of chyle in the chest can result in compression of the underlying lung, with a reduction of vital capacity and mediastinal shift, resulting in shortness of breath, and occasionally, symptoms of marked respiratory distress. In general, the development is insidious, and symptoms occur gradually. In contrast, with rapid accumulation, shock, tachypnea, tachycardia and hypotension can occur. Chyle is thought to be bacteriostatic because of its lecithin and fatty acid content, and therefore is usually sterile. Because it is nonirritating, chyle does not tend to form a peel that can result in a trapped lung.

The loss of protein, fat-soluble vitamins, and fat contained in chyle can lead to serious metabolic defects and death in patients with chylothorax. Shafiroff and Kau (1959) emphasized that the loss of lymphocytes and antibodies can also interfere with the immunological status of a patient with chylothorax.

DIAGNOSIS

The diagnosis of a chylothorax is suggested by the presence of a nonclotting milky fluid, which is obtained from the pleural space at thoracentesis or chest tube insertion. The diagnosis is confirmed by the finding of free microscopic fat and fat content of the fluid higher than that of the plasma. In traumatic chylothorax, the chyle may initially appear blood-stained, and this may be misleading. On microscopic examination, the presence of fat globules that clear with alkali and ether, or stain with Sudan-3, is diagnostic. Lymphocytes are the predominant cells found in chyle, while in traumatic chylus effusion, red blood cells are at least initially present. Chylous effusions must be distinguished from pseudochyle and cholesterol pleural effusions. Boyd (1986) noted that pseudochyle occurs with malignant tumors or infection and is milky in appearance because of the presence of lecithin-globulin complex. Pseudochyle contains only a trace of fat, and fat globules cannot be seen with Sudan-3 stain smears. Milky pleural effusions also can be seen secondary to tuberculosis, and Bower (1968) reported it to occur in rheumatoid arthritis. Cholesterol pleural effusions that are seen in these two disease entities acquire their milky appearance from a high concentration of cholesterol crystals. If it is still difficult to distinguish chyle from pseudochyle or cholesterol pleural fluid, a test consisting of feeding a patient a fat stained with green No. 6 dye, which will stain the chylous effusion approximately one hour after ingestion of the dye, is a helpful diagnostic test. Obtaining cholesterol and triglyceride levels of the fluid can help because most chylous effusions have a cholesterol/triglyceride ratio of less than 1, whereas nonchylous effusions have a ratio greater than 1. In addition, if the fluid has a triglyceride level of more than 110 mg/100 ml, there is a 99% chance that the fluid is chyle. If the triglyceride level is less than 50 mg/100 ml, Staats and colleagues (1980) noted that there is only a 5% chance that the fluid is chyle.

Another helpful index in determining if a leak is related to a chylous leak is the rate of fluid accumulation in the chest. The rate of accumulation in the chest from a chylous fistula exceeds 400 to 500 ml per day, and is an average of approximately 700 to 1200 ml per day in a 70-kg adult. The flow rate is obviously proportionally less in infants and children, depending on the body surface area. A detailed analysis of the effusion should produce values similar to those listed in Table 58–1 if the effusion is indeed a chylous effusion. Once a chylothorax is diagnosed, a complete history and physical examination should be performed to discern the etiology. Chylothorax in a postoperative period generally develops 7 to 14 days postoperatively. Surgery in the region of the aorta, esophagus, or posterior mediastinum should suggest the presence or the possibility of a chylothorax. Blunt trauma 2 to 6 weeks earlier should also suggest the presence of a potential chylothorax.

In nontraumatic chylothorax, an extensive search for the cause of the pleural effusion must be undertaken. Computerized tomography and lymphangiography are diagnostic techniques that are helpful in the study of chylothorax. Occasionally, lymphangiography details the exact site of leakage and also the anatomical abnormalities of the thoracic duct. A CT examination of the chest is a good way to demonstrate the presence of mediastinal disease that could cause a chylothorax. A mediastinal mass or enlarged mediastinal nodes, as well as primary lung cancer, could easily be demonstrated by this technique.

MANAGEMENT

The ideal management of the patient with chylothorax is unknown. The disease occurs in various situations, and

Table 58–3. Modalities Used in Treatment of Chylothorax

Conservative
  Nothing by mouth
  Medium-chain triglycerides
  Central hyperalimentation
  Drainage of pleural space
    Thoracentesis
    Closed chest tube thoracostomy
  Complete expansion of lung
Operative
  Direct ligation of thoracic duct
  Mass ligation of thoracic duct tissue
  Pleuroperitoneal shunting
  Pleurectomy
  Fibrin glue
Radiation therapy

opinion about which types of chylothorax should be treated operatively is diverse: the postsurgical or post-traumatic types only, or the nontraumatic types as well. Whether young children should undergo surgery is also controversial. The development of a lymphatic leak in the thorax certainly necessitates decisive management if considerable morbidity and mortality are to be avoided. Well standardized guidelines have emerged that have enhanced the understanding and treatment of this difficult clinical problem.

Table 58–3 lists the various modalities used in the treatment of chylothorax. They can be divided into conservative therapy, operative therapy, and radiation therapy.

Current treatment of chylothorax is thoracic duct ligation, introduced by Lampson and associates (1948). They showed that the mortality rate from chylothorax decreased from 50% to 15%. Before this report of successful control of traumatic chylothorax by direct ligation of the thoracic duct, the mortality rate for this condition was 45%; nontraumatic chylothorax had a mortality rate of 100%. Treatment of the condition before 1948 consisted of thoracentesis or closed chest tube thoracostomy and a low fat diet. Today the crucial decision in the management of these patients is when to advocate surgical intervention. There is no unanimous opinion on whether to operate or, if surgery is not undertaken initially, on how long conservative management should be used before resorting to surgical intervention.

Conservative therapy consists of maintaining effective thoracostomy tube drainage with good expansion of the lung. The most important aspect is to maintain adequate nutrition, as loss of chylous fluid causes electrolyte imbalance and increases nutritional needs. Central hyperalimentation is routinely used while keeping the patient NPO. Any oral feedings increase output through the fistula. There is no standard of how long conservative therapy should be tried before considering operative intervention. Williams and Burford (1964) as well as Selle and associates (1971) recommended that 14 days is a maximum limit for conservative therapy before surgical intervention. In approximately 50% of patients, the thoracic duct leak closes spontaneously, and the other 50%

require surgical intervention. When chest tube drainage is consistently greater than 500 ml per day for two weeks, surgical intervention is definitely indicated, except for those patients for whom thoracotomy is contraindicated, such as those with vertebral fractures or with nonresectable tumors. If a lung is entrapped and pleural synthesis cannot be achieved with re-expansion by closed chest tube thoracostomy, then early surgical intervention is indicated. If chylous drainage is still present after a period of carefully supervised nonoperative conservative therapy, patients with congenital, traumatic, or postoperative chylothorax should undergo surgical treatment.

OPERATIVE THERAPY OF A CHYLOUS FISTULA

Several techniques may be used to control a chylous fistula, singly or in a combination: direct ligation of the thoracic duct, mass ligation of the thoracic duct, pleuroperitoneal shunting, and pleurectomy. Occasionally, decortication may be required when the lung is entrapped. Stenzel and colleagues (1983) suggested that fibrin glue be applied in some instances.

In unilateral chylothorax, the chest should be opened on the side of the effusion. When the effusion is bilateral, it is more prudent to explore the right side first, with ligation of the duct low in the right chest. Exploration of the left side is done later, if necessary. Ross (1961) stated that the easiest way to find the duct and the leakage point is to give the patient 100 to 200 ml of olive oil through a nasogastric tube 2 to 3 hours before the operation—what remains in the stomach at the time of anesthetic induction can be removed by the same nasogastric tube. This causes filling of the duct with milky chyle, which is readily recognized throughout the course of the operation. An alternative method is to inject a 1% aqueous solution of Evans blue dye into the leg. This causes staining of the thoracic duct within 5 minutes that lasts up to 12 minutes. The disadvantage of the dye is that the adjacent tissues are also stained when there is free escape of chyle.

Ligation of the thoracic duct just above the diaphragm throughout the right chest is currently favored by most authors, including Selle (1971), Patterson (1981), and Milson (1985) and associates, regardless of the site of the chylous leak. As noted, the thoracic duct is a single structure from T12 to T8 in over 75% of all patients.

The three techniques used to control the leak of chyle are: direct closure of the fistula, suture of the leaking mediastinal pleura, and supradiaphragmatic ligation of the duct. The best method is to find the actual point of leakage and to close it with nonabsorbable sutures with the use of Teflon pledgets, compressing the leakage point in the adjacent tissue between the two pledgets, and, if possible, allowing the main portion of the duct to remain patent. Either of the first two techniques, and particularly the second, should be combined with supradiaphragmatic ligation of the duct. This alone is entirely effective in instances in which no attempt has been made

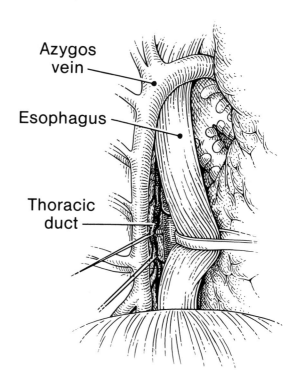

Fig. 58–2. Surgical anatomy of the thoracic duct in the right suprahepatic location.

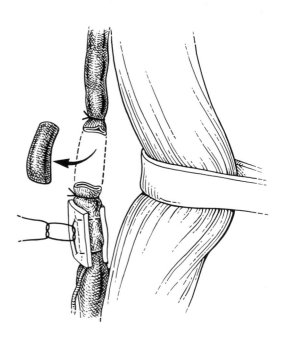

Fig. 58–3. Mass ligation of the thoracic duct using Teflon pledgets with nonabsorbable suture.

Table 58–4. Management of Chylothorax

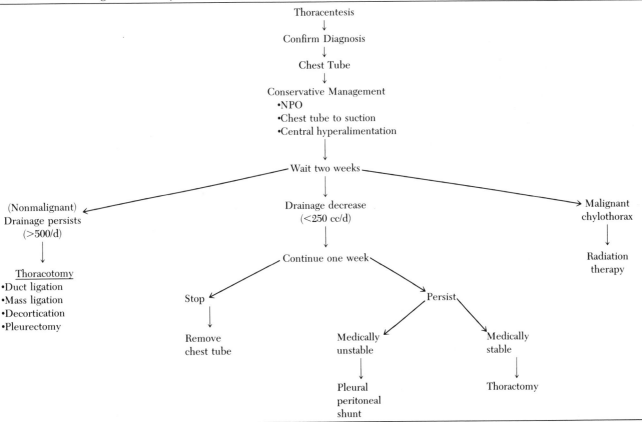

---

to directly close the fistula. The most favorable site for elective ligation is low in the right chest just above the right crus of the diaphragm where the duct lies on the vertebral column between the aorta and the azygos vein (Fig. 58–2).

If a definite source of leak cannot be identified when the right chest is explored, despite use of the previously described ingestion of fat—milk or cream—or olive oil before surgery, then supradiaphragmatic ligation of the duct should be performed. This method was originally described by Murphy and Piper (1977) and subsequently championed by Patterson and colleagues (1981).

Supradiaphragmatic Ligation of the Thoracic Duct

A standard posterolateral thoracotomy incision is made, going through the bed of the resected right sixth rib. Generally, the pleura has a shaggy appearance because of fibrin deposits. After these deposits are cleaned off, the pulmonary ligament is divided between clamps and the pulmonary ligament swept upwards to the level of the inferior pulmonary vein. The retropleural area is often thickened up to 1 to 2 cm and should be biopsied, if this is the case. It is best to ligate the duct en masse by going around the duct, taking a generous bite of tissue around the duct, and going close to the vertebral bodies, but avoiding the esophagus, aorta, and azygos vein. This suture should be tied with large pledgeted sutures on either end, as shown in Fig. 58–3. This effects a mass

ligature in the area between the azygos vein and the aorta just above the diaphragm. One must take care not to enter the wall of the esophagus. In effect, all tissue between the azygos vein and the aorta is ligated in the mass ligature.

A parietal pleurectomy is performed to achieve pleural synthesis. At the same time, if the underlying lung is trapped, it is decorticated. Two chest tube catheters are placed into the thoracic cavity and the chest closed in the usual fashion. In general, the chest tubes can be removed in 5 to 7 days, and recovery is rapid.

Other Techniques to Control Chylothorax

Milson and associates (1985) and Weese and Schouten (1984) reported the successful use of pleuroperitoneal shunting with the double-valve Denver peritoneal shunt in the treatment of chylothorax. I have used this method in three patients, with success in all three.

Stenzel and colleagues (1983) reported the successful use of fibrin glue in one case of postsurgical chylothorax after an extrapleural ligation of the patent ductus arteriosus.

In nontraumatic chylothorax, the cause must be determined, and if neoplasm or infection is the cause, it must be treated specifically with radiation therapy, chemotherapy, or antibiotic therapy. If chylous drainage persists in these situations, pleural synthesis by catheter drainage of the pleura with instillation of nitrogen mustard or other irritants can be tried. In some cases, even though not desirable, thoracic duct ligation or pleurectomy may be needed to control the chylothorax. Radiation therapy has been successful in managing chylothorax in patients with mediastinal lymphoma and carcinoma. Irradiation of the pleural lymphatics to 2000 rads causes closure of the thoracic duct leak in most cases. I have observed four patients with nontraumatic chylothorax in whom no malignancy could be found who recieved radiation to the pleural lymphatics to 2000 rads with success in all cases.

GUIDELINES FOR MANAGEMENT

In an excellent review of the indications for surgery, Selle and others (1971) established the following guidelines: (1) idiopathic cases in the neonate usually respond well to thoracentesis. (2) Nontraumatic chylothorax, exlusive of the neonatal group, usually suggests a widespread fatal illness, and operative intervention is usually ineffective and should, therefore, be avoided. (3) In cases resulting from trauma, an initial trial of nonoperative therapy is indicated. Transthoracic ligation of the duct is indicated when the average daily chyle loss has exceeded 1500 ml a day in adults for more than 5 days. (4) If the chyle flow has not diminished within 14 days or if nutritional complications appear imminent, surgery is indicated. Table 58–4 lists my approach in the management of chylothorax. Thoracentesis is performed to confirm the diagnosis. Once the diagnosis of chylothorax has been established, a chest tube is inserted by closed chest tube thoracostomy. The patient is kept NPO and nutritional replacement is begun, using central hyperalimentation. Rarely is the patient allowed to drink, and if so, a medium-chain triglyceride diet is used. This method is continued for two weeks. If drainage greater than 500 ml per day persists, and the underlying cause is nonmalignant, the patient is taken to the operating room for surgical control of the leak in the aforementioned manner. A success rate of greater than 90% may be expected with surgical intervention. Moreover, the mortality rate should be zero.

If the drainage is less than 250 ml per day, and appears to be decreasing, I may continue to try conservative therapy for one more week. If the leakage stops, the chest tube is removed. If this is to be done, one should give a trial of a high fat diet before removing the chest tube. If leakage persists at this time, pleuroperitoneal shunting could be performed if the patient is a medically compromised candidate, or thoracotomy and the previously mentioned procedures can be performed. If conservative therapy fails to control the chylothorax after two weeks and the underlying condition is a malignancy, then irradiation is administered. Generally, radiation therapy to the amount of 2000 rads controls most cases of this variety of chylothoraces.

REFERENCES

Anson, B.J.: An Atlas of Anatomy. Philadelphia, W.B. Saunders Co., 1950.

Bessone, L.N., Ferguson, T.B., Burford, T.H.: Chylothorax: a collective review. Ann. Thorac. Surg. 12:527, 1971.
Biet, A.B., and Connolly, N.K.: Traumatic chylothorax: a report of a case and a survey of the literature. Br. J. Surg. 39:564, 1951.
Bower, B.C.: Chyliform pleural effusion in rheumatoid arthritis. Am. Rev. Respir. Dis. 47:4515, 1968.
Boyd, A.: Chylothorax. In Surgical Disease of the Pleura and Chest Wall. Edited by R.M. Hood, et al.: Philadelphia, W.B. Saunders Co., 1986.
Crandall, L., Jr., Barker, S.B., and Graham, D.C.: A study of the lymph from a patient with thoracic duct fistula. Gastroenterology 1:1040, 1943.
Cunn, B., Liebow, A.A., and Friedman, P.J.: Pulmonary lymphangiomatosis: a review. Am. J. Pathol. 79:398, 1973.
Davis, M.K.: A statistical study of the thoracic duct in man. Am. J. Anat. 171:212, 1915.
DeMeester, T.R.: The pleura. In Surgery of the Chest, 4th Ed. Edited by D.C. Sabiston and E.C. Spencer. Philadelphia, W.B. Saunders Co., 1983.
Higgins, C.B., and Molder, D.G.: Chylothorax after surgery for congenital heart disease. J. Thorac. Cardiovasc. Surg. 61:411, 1971.
Hyde, P.V., Jerky, J., and Gishen, P.: Traumatic chylothorax. S. Afr. J. Surg. 12:57, 1974.
Lampson, R.S., et al.: Traumatic chylothorax: a review of the literature and report of a case treated by mediastinal ligation of the thoracic duct. J. Thorac. Surg. 17:778, 1948.
Lee, F.C.: The establishment of collateral circulation following ligation of the thoracic duct. Johns Hopkins Hosp. Bull. 33:21, 1922.
Milson, J.W., et al.: Chylothorax: an assessment of current surgical management. J. Thorac. Cardiovasc. Surg. 89:221, 1985.
Munk, I., and Rosenstein, A.: Zur Lehre von der Resorption in Darm nach Untersuchungen an einer Lymph(chylus)fistel beim Menschen. Virchuis Arch. Path. Anat. 123:484, 1891.
Murphy, T.O., and Piper, C.A.: Surgical management of chylothorax. Ann. Surg. 43:719, 1977.
Nix, J.T., et al.: Chylothorax and chylous acites: a study of 302 selected cases. Am. J. Gastroenterol. 28:40, 1957.
Patterson, G.A., et al.: Supradiaphragmatic ligation of the thoracic duct in intractable chylous fistula. Ann. Thorac. Surg. 32:44, 1981.
Ross, J.K.: A review of surgery of the thoracic duct. Thorax 16:12, 1961.
Roy, P.H., Carr, D.T., and Payne, W.S.: The problem of chylothorax. Mayo Clin. Proc. 42:457, 1967.
Selle, J.G., Synder, W.A., and Schreiber, J.T.: Chylothorax. Ann. Surg. 177:245, 1971.
Shafiroff, G.P., and Kau, Q.Y.: Cannulation of the human thoracic lymph duct. Surgery 45:814, 1959.
Silverstein, E.F., et al.: Pulmonary lymphangiomyomatosis. Am. J. Roentgenol. Radium Ther. Nucl. Med. 120:832, 1974.
Staats, R.A., et al.: The lipoprotein profile of chylous and unchylous pleural effusion. Mayo Clin. Proc. 55:700, 1980.
Stenzel, W., et al.: Treatment of post surgical chylothorax with fibrin glue. J. Thorac. Cardiovasc. Surg. 31:35, 1983.
Stuttman, L.J., Dumont, A.E., and Shinowara, G.: Coagulation factors in human lymph and plasma. Am. J. Med. Sci. 250:292, 1965.
Weese, J.L., and Schouten, J.T.: Internal drainage of intractable malignant pleural effusions. Wis. Med. J. 83:21, 1984.
Williams, K.R., and Burford, T.H.: The management of chylothorax. Ann. Surg. 160:131, 1964.

READING REFERENCES

Blalock, A., Cunningham, R.S., and Robinson, C.S.: Experimental production of chylothorax by occlusions of the superior vena cava. Ann. Surg. 104:359, 1936.
Donini, I., and Batteggati, M.: The lymphatic system. London, Piccin Medical Books, 1972, p. II–26.
Goorwitch, J.: Traumatic chylothorax and thoracic duct ligation. J. Thoracic. Surg. 29:467, 1955.
Klepser, R.G., and Berny, J.F.: The diagnosis and surgical management of chylothorax with the aid of lipophilic dyes. Dis. Chest 25:409, 1954.

CHAPTER 59

INFECTIONS OF THE PLEURA

Joseph I. Miller, Jr.

It is important to consider the diagnosis and management of infections of the pleural space from the perspective of the thoracic surgeon. Table 59–1 is an outline of surgical problems of the pleural space. This discussion focuses on empyema thoracis resulting from operative and nonoperative causes.

EMPYEMA THORACIS

The term empyema refers to a collection of pus in a natural body cavity. Pleural empyema is the accumulation of pus within the pleural space, and is referred to as empyema thoracis.

Empyema thoracis must be considered a surgical disease. The success in treating it is proportional to the

Table 59–1. Surgical Diseases of the Pleura and Pleural Space

Nonoperative
  Empyema thoracis
    Postpneumonic
    Iatrogenic
    Post-traumatic
    Infectious
  Lung entrapment
  Pleural tumors
    Benign
      Asbestosis
      Mesothelioma
    Malignant
      Mesothelioma
      Metastasis
Operative
  Resectional space problem associated with infection
    Post open lung biopsy or wedge resection
    Postlobectomy
    Postpneumonectomy
  Infections secondary to thoracic surgical procedures
    Esophageal procedures
    Cardiac procedures
    Pulmonary procedures
  Benign air spaces

promptness of the treatment, and prevention and treatment have the same goal. The pleural empyema may be unilateral or bilateral, may be localized or diffuse, and may be acute or chronic. The distinction between acute and chronic empyema is a matter of time, and is largely arbitrary. In general, chronicity may be determined by the nature of the causative organism, but usually implies a failure of diagnosis and management in the acute stage.

The infected fluid may be thick or watery, odorless or putrid, clear or cloudy, unilateral or bilateral, localized and loculated, or diffuse and involving an entire pleural space.

Laboratory values are useful in defining an empyema when the fluid is yellow and clear. Weese and associates (1973) defined an empyema thoracis as a pleural fluid with a specific gravity greater than 1.018, a white blood cell count greater than 500 cells/mm^3, or a protein level greater than 2.5 g/dl. Vianna (1971) defined an empyema as a pleural fluid with positive bacterial cultures or white blood cell count greater than 15,000 cells/mm^3 and a protein level greater than 3 g/dl. When the pleural fluid pH is less than 7, pleural fluid glucose below 40 mg/dl, and the pleural fluid LDH is greater than 1000 U/L, combined with a positive Gram stain of the pleural fluid, the fluid is an empyema.

The distinction between acute and chronic empyema is made, in general, between 4 to 6 weeks. Some individuals consider an empyema chronic if it fails to respond to treatment within a reasonable period of time; others define chronicity in terms of pathologic changes in the pleural space surrounding tissues, that is, when the walls become thick and fibrous. The time at which a firm pleural symphysis can be postulated is reached when the sediment in the pleural fluid represents 75 to 80% of the total.

PATHOGENESIS OF EMPYEMA

The American Thoracic Society in 1962 classified empyema into three phases based on the natural history of the disease. These three stages are not sharply defined, but gradually merge together. The first is the exudative or acute phase, which is characterized by the outpouring of sterile pleural fluid in the pleural space in response to inflammation of the pleura. The pleural fluid has low viscosity and a low cellular content, and the visceral pleura and related lung are mobile. Pleural fluid in this stage is characterized by a low white blood cell count, a low LDH level, and a normal glucose level and pH.

The fibrinopurulent or transitional phase is characterized by the appearance of more turbid fluid because of an increase in polymorphonuclear leukocytes. Fibrin is deposited on both pleural surfaces, forming a limiting peel that prevents extension of the empyema but also begins to trap and fix the lung. Pleural fluid becomes increasingly more turbid and the lung progressively less expandable with time. Fibrin is deposited in a continuous sheet, covering both the visceral and parietal pleura in the involved area. As this stage progresses, the tendency is to loculation and the formation of limiting membranes. At this stage, the pleural fluid, pH, and glucose levels become progressively lower, and the LDH level progressively higher.

The organizing or chronic phase is characterized by the organization of the pleural peel, with ingrowth of capillaries and fibroblasts. The pleural fluid is viscous, consisting of 75% sediment on standing. This organization can occur as early as 7 to 10 days after the onset of disease, and usually by 4 to 6 weeks, the process has entered the chronic phase. In this phase, the pleural fluid pH is frequently less than 7.0, and the sugar is less than 40 mg/dl.

Etiology of Empyema

Table 59–2 is a classification of empyema according to disease process. Despite antibiotics, more than 50% of all empyemas are secondary to complications of a primary pneumonic process in the lungs. Before the antibiotic era, most empyema fluids grew *Streptococcus pneumoniae*. Then between 1955 and 1965, *Staphylococcus aureus* was the most common causative organism. According to Bartlett and associates (1974), anaerobic or-

ganisms are the most commonly isolated bacteria. The route by which the primary pulmonic process enters the pleural space is conjectural. Direct spread of the infection through the visceral pleura is probably the most common route. Lymphangitic and hematogenous routes are possible. Chronic pulmonary infection, which damages bronchi sufficiently to make this recognizable by bronchography, is sometimes complicated by empyema. An empyema may complicate pulmonary infection distal to any lesion obstructing the bronchus.

Empyema occurs in approximately 1 to 3% of lung abscesses because of rupture of the lung abscess into the free pleural space. A tension pyopneumothorax may develop. Empyema may occur because of generalized sepsis in a small percentage of patients. Patients particularly prone to empyema from generalized sepsis are trauma victims, cardiac surgical patients, and patients with immunosuppression. As LeRoux and associates (1986) noted, empyema occurs in about 1% of patients with pulmonary tuberculosis and myocotic infections, and as a post-traumatic event in 3 to 5% of patients; blood in the pleural space is associated with incomplete lung expansion and is an invitation to infection.

The second largest etiologic category of empyema is the post-surgical development of infection in the pleural space following surgery of the esophagus, lungs, or mediastinum. Light (1983) reported that the procedure most frequently implicated is pneumonectomy; the complication occurs in 2 to 12% of patients after this procedure.

According to LeRoux and co-workers (1986), in approximately 8 to 11% of patients, the preceding lesion causing an empyema thoracis is an unrecognized subphrenic abscess in the patient who has undergone an abdominal, urologic, or pelvic operation. Silent pericolic abscess, which is a complication of either diverticulitis or colonic carcinoma, may erode through the diaphragm into the pleural space and come to clinical attention as an apparently spontaneous empyema.

Empyema may likewise occur secondary to a spontaneous pneumothorax with a persistent bronchopleural fistula; it may occur following parasitic infections, secondary to retained foreign bodies in the bronchial tree, or from several other miscellaneous causes.

The etiology in two reported series of empyema in 215 patients is given in Table 59–3.

Microbiology

Before the development of effective antibiotic treatment, pneumococcus and streptococcus were the most frequent causative organisms of empyema. Staphylococcus is the most frequent causative organism, particularly in children under the age of 2. Radvitch and Fein (1961) reported that it was cultured in 92% of patients in this age group. Gram-negative organisms, such as pseudomonas, *Klebsiella pneumoniae*, *Escherichia coli*, *Aerobacter aerogenes*, proteus, and salmonella are the next most common organisms. As anaerobic culture techniques have improved, these organisms have been recognized with increasing frequency.

Bartlett and colleagues (1974) reviewed the pleural

Table 59–2. Etiology of Empyema According to Disease Process

Cause	Percent
Pyogenic pneumonia	50
Lung abscess rupture	1–3
Secondary to generalized sepsis	1–3
Pulmonary tuberculosis	1
Pulmonary mycotic infection	1
Post-traumatic	3–5
Postsurgical (esophagus, lungs, mediastinum)	25
Extension from subphrenic abscess	8–11
Secondary to bronchopleural fistula of spontaneous pneumothorax	<1
Secondary to parasitic infestation	<1
Retained foreign bodies in bronchial tree	<1
Miscellaneous	1

Table 59–3. Etiology of Empyema in 215 Patients

Event or State	Patients	
	Number	Percent
Pulmonary infection	122	57
Following surgical procedures	42	20
Following trauma	13	6
Spontaneous pneumothorax	7	3
Esophageal perforation	5	2
Following thoracentesis	4	2
Subdiaphragmatic infection	4	2
Undetermined	18	8
Total	215	100

Compiled from Snider, G.L., and Saleb, S.S.: Empyema of thorax in adults: review of 105 cases. Chest 54:12, 1968; and Hall, D.P., and Elkin, R.G.: Empyema thoracis: a review of 110 cases. ARRD 88:785, 1963.

fluid's bacteriologic features in 83 patients from medical wards who had not undergone a thoracic operation, and who had not received antibiotics before thoracentesis. They reported that 35% of their patients had only anaerobic organisms, whereas an additional 41% had both anaerobic and aerobic organisms, and only 24% had exclusively aerobic organisms. Most patients—72%—had more than one species of organism cultured from their pleural fluid, with an average of 2.3 species per patient. Sullivan (1973) and Varky (1981) and their associates also reported that anaerobic bacteria recovered from the pleural fluid were the most common causes of adult pleural empyema. Among the anaerobic bacteria, the bacteroides species are the most commonly isolated, followed by the Fusobacterium species, and the Peptococcus species.

Aerobic bacteria still infect the pleural space. Streptococcus, however, accounts for only a small percentage of aerobic isolates. *Staphylococcus aureus* and streptococcus species other than *Streptococcus pneumoniae* account for most gram-positive isolates. Of the aerobic gram-negative bacteria, pseudomonas species and Escherichia coli account for over two thirds of aerobic gram-negative pleural empyemas. Each of these is associated with a parapneumonia effusion in 40 to 50% of patients, as Tillotson and Lerner (1967, 1968) noted.

CLINICAL SYMPTOMATOLOGY

It may be difficult to distinguish symptoms of empyema from those of the primary causative process, such as a pneumonia, mediastinitis, subphrenic abscess or post-traumatic hemothorax. The patient's presentation varies depending on the causal organisms, the volume of pus in the pleural space, and the state of the host defense mechanisms, so there is a wide range, from absence of symptoms to severe illness with toxemia. The early treatment of pulmonary infections with antibiotics without an established diagnosis in a patient with the general features of an inflammatory or probable respiratory illness often masks many symptoms of empyema.

The signs and symptoms of empyema are not specific, but reflect the underlying pulmonary process. The patient frequently complains of a pleuritic-type chest pain, with a feeling of heaviness on the involved side of the thorax. The patient may cough and bring up purulent sputum; usually fever, shortness of breath, and sometimes tachycardia may be present. Physical examination reveals decreased breath sounds on the involved side of the chest. The involved hemithorax is contracted, respiratory excursions are limited, the percussion note is dull, and breath sounds are decreased in the area of involvement. There may be clubbing of the fingers, and at times even pulmonary osteoarthropathy may be present.

An empyema that has been present for 4 to 6 weeks is in the chronic phase, and may severely restrict the involved hemithorax in its movements. This usually results in a delay in recognizing the development of an empyema, while treating a pneumonic inflammatory process.

An empyema that evolves into the chronic phase may develop any number of complications, such as empyema necessitans, chondritis and osteomyelitis of ribs, bronchopleural fistula, pericarditis, mediastinal abscess, and disseminated infections.

Factors that promote the development of a chronic empyema are listed in Table 59–4.

DIAGNOSIS OF EMPYEMA

The diagnosis of acute and chronic empyema can often be made on history and physical examination alone. Other modalities helpful in establishing the diagnosis of a pleural empyema are the PA and lateral chest roentgenograms, computed tomography, and thoracentesis with analysis of the pleural fluid.

The most important modalities in the diagnosis of pleural empyema are routine PA and lateral chest roentgenograms. DeMeester (1983) noted that these provide more information regarding intrathoracic condition than any other form of physical examination or test. Both the PA and lateral view are essential for accurate localization of the pleural abnormality. The initial chest roentgenogram may show a pneumonia or pneumonitis with a large pleural effusion, or even potential total opacification of one hemithorax. The chest roentgenogram may show multiple loculations and air-fluid levels with areas of atelectasis in the lung. Tracheal or mediastinal shift toward the unaffected side evidences significant pleural fluid. A

Table 59–4. Factors That Promote Development of Chronic Empyema

Delay in diagnosis
Improper choice of antibiotics
Loculation or encapsulation by a dense inflammatory reaction
Presence of bronchopleural fistula
Foreign body in the empyema space
Chronic infection
Irreversible chronic lung infection
Entrapment of lung by thick visceral peel
Inadequate previous drainage or premature removal of tube

few patients develop cardiopulmonary dysfunction. Parapneumonic empyemas are nearly always posterior and lateral and extend inferiorly as far as the diaphragm. A localized empyema of any size in the typical situation, as LeRoux and Dodds (1964) pointed out, is one of the common causes of a posteriorly situated D-shaped roentgenographic opacity. A large empyema may occupy most of the pleural space, but the aerated lung remains translucent and is usually visible anteriorly. In occasional cases, it may be difficult on roentgenogram alone to distinguish between lung abscess and empyema. The presence of a fluid level is not helpful, as an empyema may contain air from gas-forming organisms, a previous pneumothorax, a broncopleural fistula, or thoracentesis. In these situations, bronchoscopy, bronchography, and CT scanning may be useful diagnostic adjuncts.

A CT scan is useful in the diagnosis and management of multiloculated empyemas. The CT scan can define the areas of loculation and extent of involvement precisely, and estimate the involvement of the hemithorax.

Thoracentesis is the sine qua non in establishing the diagnosis of a pleural empyema. Based on history and physical examination and the PA and lateral chest roentgenograms, a needle thoracentesis should be performed in all patients with suspected pleural empyema. The aspiration of pus clearly establishes the diagnosis of empyema and helps in determining future management. Thoracentesis fluid obtained should undergo microbiotic examination with a Gram stain, and culture and sensitivity studies for the appropriate antibiotic therapy should be instituted. The pleural fluid should also be tested for pH, cell count with differential, sugar, protein, and LDH. If malignancy is suspected, a specimen should also be sent for cytologic examination.

With antibiotic use, pleural fluid may be only slightly cloudy, and in approximately 50% of patients, cultures fail to grow any specific organism. An infection may exist despite the lack of growth on culture because of the masking effect of the antibiotics or the failure to obtain anaerobic cultures. A simultaneous sputum culture can be helpful, because the dominant organism responsible for the pneumonia is frequently the cause of the empyema.

Potts (1976) and Light (1980) and their associates showed that the pH of the pleural fluid indicates the need for drainage in parapneumonic effusions.

The pH of the liquid may fall before organisms are shown by Gram stain. A pleural-fluid pH below 7.0 is an indication for chest tube drainage of an empyema. Turbid effusions that are microscopically negative, a pleural glucose content below 40 ml/dl, and an LDH greater than 1000 IU/dl suggest empyema, and drainage should be instituted.

Bronchoscopy should be performed on all patients with spontaneous empyema to exclude endobronchial or endotracheal tumor or an inhaled foreign body. A patent bronchial airway is one of the conditions necessary for the lung to re-expand following intercostal drainage of the infected pleural fluid or removal of the pleural peel by decortication or empyemectomy.

PARAPNEUMONIC EMPYEMA

Table 59–5 presents an algorithm for managing parapneumonic empyema or nonoperative empyema. Pleural fluid secondary to a bacterial pneumonia may range from a sterile serous fluid to bacterially contaminated fluid to thick pus. Once the presence of an empyema has been established by thoracentesis and pyogenic organisms have been recovered, an initial decision must be made to management. The thickness of the exudate, the duration of the empyema before treatment, the organism, and the patient's condition all affect the decision-making process. If not managed in the acute exudative phase, an empyema leaves a space that is not readily obliterated by a combination of surrounding tissue and tends to persist, bound by the rigid chest wall and a thickened, immobile visceral pleura.

The objectives of treatment for chronic empyema that LeRoux (1986), DeMeester (1983) and Cohn (1978) and their associates noted are elimination of the underlying disease process, control of the infection, removal of the purulent material, sterilization of the empyema cavity, obliteration of the pleural space, and restoration of normal movement to the lung. Thoracentesis, intercostal tube drainage, rib resection-tube drainage, open-rib drainage, decortication, excision exenteration—empyemectomy, sterilization, thoracoplasty, and muscle flap closure are used in the treatment of thoracic empyema.

Thoracentesis is the initial step in establishing a diagnosis in any patient with suspected empyema thoracis and should be performed whenever a pleural effusion is detected during a pneumonic process or other pathologic condition that may cause empyema. Guided by PA and lateral chest roentgenograms and CT scan surveillance, a thoracentesis is performed in the lowest intercostal space that is at the dependent portion of the fluid-containing space. On the right side, the thoracentesis should not be performed below the tenth or eleventh intercostal space because of the recess of the diaphragm and the potential for injury to the liver or inferior vena cava. On the left side, thoracentesis should rarely extend below the tenth intercostal space because of the potential for damage to the spleen, left lobe of the liver, or aorta. Rarely it may be difficult to locate an effusion that has loculated, and in this situation, ultrasound of the chest may help in determining the exact location in which to insert the needle. The needle's bore must be large enough for the removal of debris. If, on thoracentesis, the fluid is clear, watery, or only slightly turbid—what has been called thin pus—then specimens should be sent to the laboratory for culture and sensitivity studies for bacterial, acid-fast organisms, and fungi and for studies of the fluid's pH, cell count, and sugar protein and LDH content. If the culture is positive or the Gram stain is positive, one then may attempt to remove all fluid by thoracentesis alone or procede with insertion of a chest tube. If the pH is less than 7.0, the sugar content less than 40 mg/dl or the LDH greater than 1000 U/dl, chest tube thoracostomy is indicated to evacuate all fluid in the early exudative phase of the process.

Table 59–5.   Management of Empyema

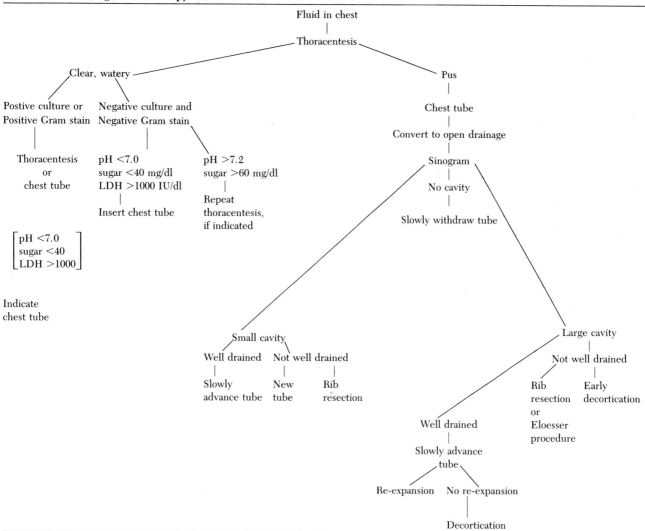

In performing a chest tube thoracostomy, a No. 32 to 36 French tube with multiple holes should be inserted into the most dependent portion of the empyema cavity through the appropriate intercostal space. Caution should be exercised in inserting the intercostal catheter because tube placement is to some extent a blind maneuver, and in an attempt to place the catheter at a completely dependent site, the diaphragm is occasionally punctured or the intercostal vessels injured.

If the pleural fluid is clear, watery, or slightly turbid but culture and Gram stain are negative, the following guidelines apply: If the pH is greater than 7.2, repeat thoracentesis is generally all that is indicated. If the pH is less than 7.0, the sugar is less than 40 mg/dl, the LDH greater than 1000 IU/dl, and the fluid is free-floating, it is probably safer, however, to insert a large-bore chest tube to completely remove the fluid. It is better to remove all the pleural fluid than to leave some fluid, which may form a loculated empyema.

Any patient with clear, watery, or slightly turbid em-

pyema can generally be managed with evacuation of the pleural fluid by either thoracentesis or closed chest tube thoracostomy in an early stage of the disease process. If complete re-expansion is maintained and clinical evidence of infection subsides, this is generally all that is indicated.

If thoracentesis reveals gross pus, a chest tube should be inserted immediately in the lowest dependent portion of the empyema cavity. A large-bore No. 32 or No. 36 chest tube should be inserted whenever gross pus is present. The surgical and medical staff should be taught that it is preferable not to remove all the pus by thoracentesis, but to leave some so that it will be easy to find the correct location to insert the dependent chest tube. Drainage of the pus will result in either obliteration of the pleural space and cure, or persistence of the pleural space. Closed drainage is unsatisfactory if there is persistent toxicity and no change in roentgenographic evidence of empyema. Following 48 to 72 hours of chest tube drainage, a repeat chest roentgenogram may indicate complete evacuation of all pleural fluid. If multiple loculations persist and there is inadequate drainage of the pleural space, a repeat CT scan of the chest may indicate the extent of involvement. Creek (1953) and Bergh (1977) and colleagues recommended using fibrinolytic enyzmes, that is, streptokinase and streptodornase, in the presence of thick pus and fibrin to improve drainage. Instillation of these fibrinolytic enzymes into the pleural space may improve drainage and breakup of fibrinopurulent deposits. A dose of 25,000 units of streptokinase in 50 cc of saline may be injected on one or two successive days, followed by clamping of the chest tube for 4 hours to further break up the loculated deposits, and then opening of the chest tube to closed drainage.

In 10 to 12 days, the closed drainage is converted to an open system. At this time, complete synthesis between the visceral and parietal pleura should have been accomplished. A sinogram, using propyliodone or Gastrografin, can then be performed to assess the presence of an empyema space, its size, and its location. The findings on sinography determine further management of the patient with a gross putrid empyema. Three potential findings are obtained on sinography: (1) no cavity is present; (2) a small cavity; or (3) a large cavity. If no cavity is present, the chest tube can be slowly withdrawn over 4 to 6 weeks, allowing the empyema tube tract to heal from the inside out. If a small, well drained cavity is present, the same method of slowly withdrawing the empyema tube can be performed. If a small, poorly drained cavity is present, a new tube can be inserted in a more dependent portion, or open rib resection may be performed.

If a large, well drained cavity is present, one may slowly withdraw the tube. If re-expansion occurs, the process is completed with synthesis of the visceral and parietal pleura. If the lung does not re-expand, decortication can be peformed at 6 weeks to 2 months. If a large, poorly drained cavity remains, either early decortication or a simple open rib resection or Eloesser procedure should be performed.

The chronic phase of the empyema begins around 6 weeks after the onset of the acute illness. The modality of treatment used for chronic empyema depends upon the general condition of the patient, the size of the cavity, the status of the underlying lung, and the presence or absence of a bronchopleural fistula. The initial management of all patients consists of open drainage with a chest tube and good cleansing of the cavity. Initial cleansing can be performed with sterile half-strength Dakin's solution—0.5% aqueous sodium hypochlorite—to remove the fibrinous exudate, leaving a healthy, red, granulating surface on the visceral and parietal pleura. Following cleansing of the cavity, sterile saline can be used to irrigate the cavity. If the cavity has been well managed by the chest tube, and is well drained, the tube can be slowly withdrawn at 10 to 14 day intervals, allowing the cavity to slowly obliterate as the tube is pulled out, while still maintaining adequate drainage. If the cavity is not completely closed at 6 weeks and the patient is a suitable medical candidate, decortication is generally indicated.

If not, chest tube thoracostomy is converted to either an open rib resection or an Eloesser flap.

For the patient who has a large, persistent cavity—the pleural space is not obliterated—and who is not considered a candidate for decortication, open drainage of the empyema space is indicated. Open rib resection drainage remains the standard by which all other means of drainage must be judged in the treatment of empyema. It can be performed under general or local anesthesia with minimal discomfort to the patient. The advantages of this approach are obvious. It allows the empyema cavity to be visualized and obvious fibrinous exudates to be debrided. Loculations can be broken down. The drainage site must drain the empyema cavity completely. The surgeon can directly evaluate the thickness and extent of the pleural peel and the degree of lung entrapment so that the necessity for decortication can be determined. The tube can be placed at an ideal dependent site so that drainage is maximally effective.

Mayo and McElvein (1966) recommend early thoracotomy for all patients as an extension of this procedure. Other authors, including Hoover and associates (1986), have advocated early thoracotomy in the management of all patients with empyema thoracis who are medically suitable candidates and in whom multiple loculations are still present as early as 7 to 10 days after institution of closed chest tube thoracostomy.

Decortication is the procedure of choice if effective drainage was not established early, expansion failed to occur, or there is significant entrapment of the lung. A decision for decortication should be based upon the pulmonary function impairment, physical examination, evaluation of the patient's general medical status, and careful review of all roentgenograms and CT examinations. Assuming the patient is a suitable medical candidate for surgery, the operative decision can be based upon the thickness of the pleural peel, and the amount of collapsed, nonfunctioning lung. If one fourth to one third of the involved lung is entrapped, decortication should generally be considered.

Contraindications to decortication include the poor general condition of the patient, continuing sepsis, and significant parenchymal disease in the lung to be decorticated. A bronchial fistula usually implies the necessity of a concomitant pulmonary resection and may deter operation.

Thoracoplasty is rarely indicated in the management of chronic parapneumonic empyema. In those patients who have a persistent space, despite decortication, muscle flap transposition procedures can easily obliterate any remaining empyema space.

The principles of empyema management are easily followed by the experienced thoracic surgeon, but are applied inconsistently by others. Early diagnosis and effective management are important factors for successful management.

Surgical Procedures

Open Drainage

This method can be employed when closed chest tube drainage of the pleural space is inadequate. Two different types of procedures can be performed.

The first involves simple rib resection, in which segments of one to three ribs overlying the lowest part of the empyema cavity are resected and a large-bore chest tube is inserted into the empyema cavity, connected to the appropriate underwater seal drainage apparatus, and later converted to open drainage. When this technique is used, the pocket to be drained must be accurately located roentgenographically and by thoracentesis before the operation. In general, the tube should be placed dependently and back no further than the posterior axillary line. If the tube is not dependent, the next lower rib is easily removed.

The second method is the open flap procedure, as Eloesser originally described in 1935 and reported in 1969, which provides better drainage in that it creates a skin-lined fistula that provides drainage without tubes. This procedure is usually elected after closed tube thoracostomy drainage or simple rib resection when long-term open drainage is necessary. It can also be used to drain a postpneumonectomy empyema, with or without a bronchopleural fistula, and when open tube drainage would be uncomfortable, such as when the tube is located high in the axilla or the paravertebral area. Symbas and colleagues (1971) modified the Eloesser procedure, and made a significant advance in converting the original U-shaped flap to an inverted U-shaped flap.

In performing the open flap drainage procedure, the incision must be planned carefully to be effective. An inverted U-shaped flap of skin 6 to 7 cm long with a base 6 to 8 cm wide. The base of the flap is placed parallel to the most dependent portion of the empyema cavity. The top of the inverted U-shaped flap is placed two to three intercostal spaces or ribs above the base of the cavity. The inverted U is performed by incising down through skin, subcutaneous tissue, and all muscle fascia to the rib cage. Three inches of two to three ribs are totally resected. The tongue of the flap is completely debrided of all tissue, except underlying subcutaneous tissue. The underlying tongue is tacked down to the bottom of the empyemata space, using 0 polydioxane suture. The margins of the flap are approximated with interrupted polydioxane suture to close over the exposed rib ends.

Open flap drainage is easier to care for, and generally cleaner than open tube drainage. The cavity is packed daily, depending on the rate of soilage. Pseudomonas frequently develops, and the use of packing soaked in 1% acetic acid provides good control of the growth.

Decortication

The success of pulmonary decortication depends primarily on three factors: (1) the pleural irritation or inflammation results in a fibroelastic "peel" which traps the lung; (2) the visceral pleura remains relatively normal; and (3) the lung must be expansile so that the space can be obliterated by pulmonary re-expansion when decortication is complete. The technique of decortication is described in Chapter 35. On entering the chest, the decision is made whether both parietal and visceral pleural layers need to be removed, or whether decortication can be limited to the visceral pleura. In general, only

the visceral pleura must be removed in the early phases of chronic empyema. If a rigid, thickened parietal pleura restricts the mobility of the thoracic cage, it should be removed. This generally entails an extrapleural dissection. If both the parietal pleura and the visceral pleura are to be removed, an attempt can be made to excise the whole empyema sac without opening it. This empyemectomy, as Samson (1971) noted, has the theoretical advantage of reducing the possibility of contamination of the wound and the remaining pleural cavity. The more practical approach is to open the empyema cavity, evacuate the contents, define its limits, and then decorticate the lung.

When a chronic pathologic process is present or the underlying lung disease prevents re-expansion, complete obliteration of the pleural space by decortication cannot be accomplished without combining the decortication with a small modified thoracoplasty or a muscle flap transposition. In this situation, a small modified two- or three-rib extraperiosteal thoracoplasty can be performed. I prefer, however, to close the remaining pleural space with a muscle flap transposition of serratus anterior or latissimus dorsi.

Thoracoplasty

Thoracoplasty in the treatment of empyema is discussed briefly for the sake of completeness, and the technique is described in Chapter 34. I believe that a thoracoplasty should not be performed unless it is absolutely necessary, because space obliteration by muscle flap transposition makes this procedure obsolete. Previously, patients with empyematous spaces unresponsive to decortication underwent a standard thoracoplasty, either an extrapleural operation or one of the Schede type. In the latter procedure, all underlying ribs and intercostal structures and the parietal pleura and peel are removed to allow the space to fill in with granulation tissue.

EMPYEMA AFTER RESECTION

Empyema that complicates pulmonary resection must be considered separately from empyema that occurs spontaneously or after trauma. When empyema complicates a pulmonary resection that is short of pneumonectomy, the ability of the remaining lung to fill the pleural space after management of the empyema by drainage or decortication, and thereby to obliterate the pleural space, depends on the state of the remaining lung and its location, apical or basal. Empyema after upper lobectomy nearly always requires more than simple drainage, which nearly always suffices after lower lobectomy. After pneumonectomy, the empyema space is inevitably large, and nearly always permanent. In these circumstances, alternative methods of treatment include sterilization, permanent drainage, thoracoplasty, and obliteration of the space by muscle flap transposition.

The incidence of empyema after pulmonary resection varies with the indications for the resection—inflammatory or neoplastic disease, with or without preoperative radiation. With resection for pulmonary tuberculosis, sputum conversion having been achieved, the incidence of bronchopleural fistula with empyema in the series Lynn (1958) reported was 6.7% after lobectomy. When sputum was still positive for acid-fast organisms, Teixera (1968) reported it was 10%.

With pneumonectomy, as opposed to lesser resections, LeRoux and associates (1986) reported that the incidence of empyema varies between 2 to 13%. When pneumonectomy is completed through an empyema, the incidence of continued pleural infection is 45%.

Although empyema may occur at any time postoperatively, even years later, most empyemas develop in the early postoperative period. The pleural space may be contaminated at the time of pulmonary resection, with the development of a bronchopleural or esophagopleural fistula, or from blood-borne sources. After pulmonary resection, less than a pneumonectomy, empyema occurs more often when the pleural space is incompletely filled by expansion of the remaining lung, mediastinal shift, and elevation of the diaphragm. Symptoms and signs vary, and if resection was performed for neoplastic disease, they may be difficult to distinguish from those caused by dissemination of tumor. The possibility of empyema must be considered in any patient with clinical features of infection after pulmonary resection. Expectoration of serosanguineous liquid and purulent discharge from the wound or the drain sites is almost diagnostic. On chest roentgenogram, there is usually a pleural opacity, with or without a fluid level, when resection has been less than a pneumonectomy. After pneumonectomy, a fall in the fluid level early postoperatively, or the appearance of a new fluid level when the pneumonectomy site was uniformly opaque, strongly suggests an infected pleural space with bronchopleural fistula. The timing of surgical intervention and the type of operative procedure undertaken are tailored to the individual patient. An algorithm for the management of postresectional empyema is given in Table 59–6.

General Principles of Treatment

When the diagnosis of postresectional empyema, with or without a bronchopleural fistula, is made, surgical drainage by closed chest tube thoracostomy and institution of appropriate antibiotic therapy is crucial. Once adequate drainage has been established and the patient stabilized—usually in 10 to 14 days, the course of management can be determined. If a bronchopleural fistula is present, the fistula should be closed by a myoplasty or omentoplasty, followed by single-stage muscle flap closure of the remaining space. If the patient is medically unstable, the closed chest tube thoracostomy can be converted to open drainage by an Eloesser procedure.

If the patient has only an empyema space without a bronchopleural fistula, the cavity is sterilized by irrigation with the appropriate antibiotic solution, as determined by the antibiotic sensitivities of the chest tube drainage, and a single-stage muscle flap closure of the remaining cavity is performed. A complete discussion of muscle flap closure is given on pp. 641–643. If the patient is medically unstable, closed chest tube thoracostomy can be converted to an open Eloesser flap.

Postpneumonectomy Empyema

Postpneumonectomy empyema remains a problem. It is associated with a bronchopleural fistula in approximately 40% of patients, and in only 20% of patients does the bronchopleural fistula close spontaneously. One of the most important advances in the treatment of this complication was the report by Clagett and Geraci (1963) in which they described rib resection with antibiotic irrigation and closure of the space in 6 to 8 weeks. Stafford and Clagett (1972) reported a success rate of 75 to 88% in using this method in sterilization of the empyema and permanent closure. My own experience with this method has not achieved that success rate. When the offending organism is *Staphylococcus aureus*, there is a fair chance of success, but when multiple bacterial organisms are present, the rate of success is only about 20%.

Table 59–7 presents an algorithm for treatment of the postpneumonectomy empyema space. Once the diagnosis of postpneumonectomy empyema, with or without bronchopleural fistula, has been established, prompt

Table 59–6. Postresectional Empyema

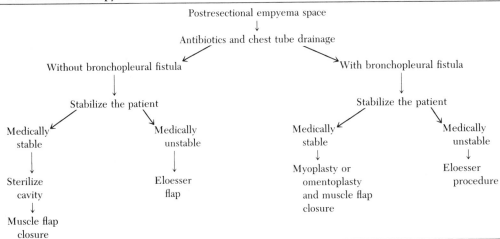

Table 59–7. Postpneumonectomy Empyema Space

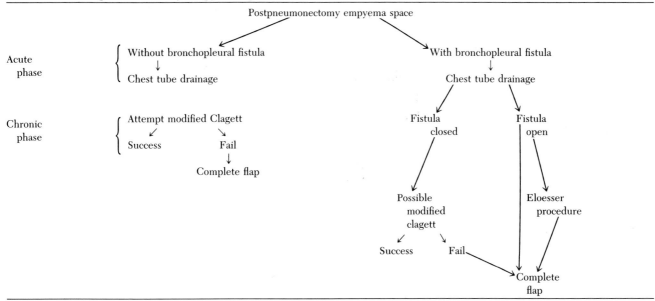

pleural drainage by closed chest tube thoracostomy is mandatory. Chest tube thoracostomy is continued until the mediastinum becomes stabilized, generally requiring approximately 2 weeks. Thereafter, open drainage or another modality of therapy for the empyema space can be undertaken safely without shift of the mediastinum. Once the patient is medically stable and has entered into the chronic phase at 3 to 4 weeks, if no bronchopleural fistula is present, a modified Clagett procedure is performed. A second small chest tube is inserted into the second intercostal space, and a continuous inflow-outflow irrigation system is established through the pleural cavity. The irrigant is based on antibiotic sensitivities to the pleural drainage. This is generally 2 g of cephalosporin in 500 cc of D_5W, running at a rate of 50 cc an hour through the inflow catheter, with continuous drainage through the outflow catheter. Occasionally, if gram-negative organisms are present, I use 0.25% neomycin as the irrigant. This method achieves sterilization of the space in approximately 50% of patients. If the method is successful and the return irrigant is negative on 3 consecutive days after 2 weeks of irrigation, the chest tubes can be removed, and pleural fluid is allowed to reaccumulate to fill the remaining space. If the modified Clagett technique fails, a complete muscle flap closure of the pneumonectomy space can be performed.

If a patient with a postpneumonectomy empyema has a bronchopleural fistula, it is likewise treated during the acute phase with closed chest tube thoracostomy, with conversion to open drainage at the appropriate time when mediastinal stabilization has occurred. If the fistula closes, one can attempt the aforementioned modified Clagett sterilization of the cavity. In the patient in whom the bronchopleural fistula persists, the fistula and space are then managed by transposition of muscle flaps into

the empyema space, as I and my associates (1984) reported.

Muscle Flap Closure of the Postpneumonectomy Empyema Space

I believe that the best way to treat a postpneumonectomy space is single-stage muscle flap closure, completely obliterating the pneumonectomy space by the transposition of the thoracic skeletal muscles.

Abrashanoff (1911) reported extrathoracic muscle transposition for closure of a bronchopleural fistula. Since then, muscle flaps have been used to obliterate spaces, close a bronchopleural fistula, and reinforce tracheobronchial and esophageal anastomosis. In the late 1970s, our group used extrathoracic muscle flaps to close bronchopleural fistula and postlobectomy empyema cavities, but not until 1980 did we attempt to fill an entire pneumonectomy space with muscle flaps.

Because of their excellent blood supply and ability by pedicle flap to reach almost any location in the pleural space, muscle flaps are ideal tissue to fill a contaminated space. The extrathoracic muscle flaps used in various combinations in our (1984) patients in order of frequency are the latissimus dorsi, the serratus anterior, the pectoralis major, the omentum, and the rectus abdominis. The percentage of flap coverage of normal pneumonectomy space in the adult by each flap is: latissimus dorsi—30 to 40%; serratus anterior—10 to 15%; pectoralis major—20 to 30%; pectoralis minor—0 to 2%; omentum—5 to 15%; and the rectus abdominis—5 to 15%. These figures are based on clinical estimation of coverage at the time of operation and cadaver studies.

Extrathoracic muscle flaps require a route of entry when transposed into the thoracic cavity. Segments of rib, determined by the blood supply of the muscles (Fig. 59–1), are resected, to prevent kinking and constriction

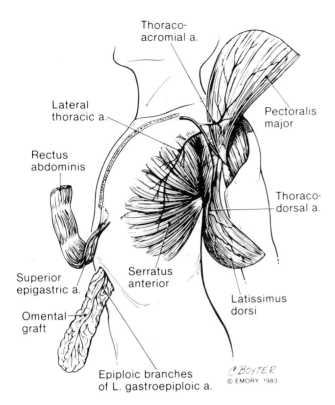

Fig. 59–1. Extrathoracic muscle flaps that can be used in closure of a postpneumonectomy empyema cavity. (a = artery). (Reproduced with permission of Miller, J.I., et al.: Single-stage complete muscle flap closure of the postpneumonectomy empyema space: a new method and possible solution to a disturbing complication. Ann. Thorac. Surg. 38(3):227, 1984.)

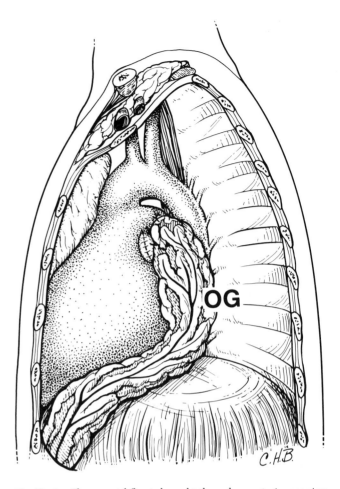

Fig. 59–2. The omental flap is brought through an anterior opening in the diaphragm and placed over the bronchial stump. (OG = omental graft). (Reproduced with permission of Miller, J.I., et al.: Single-stage complete muscle flap closure of the postpneumonectomy empyema space: a new method and possible solution to a disturbing complication. Ann. Thorac. Surg. 38(3):227, 1984.)

and consequent swelling and ischemia of the muscle when the muscle is transposed into the pleural space.

Specific Muscle Flaps and Omentum

Omentum. The omentum can be brought into the pleural space as a flap or a free graft. It is the flap of choice to cover an open bronchial stump because of the excellent vascular supply. Neovascularization is evident in the stump within 48 hours after placement of an omental flap around a closed stump. The omental flap is usually brought up through a separate anterior opening in the diaphragm, and is laid over the bronchial stump; tacking sutures are placed around the flap (Fig. 59–2). Normally, I do not use this flap unless an open bronchial stump is present or there is not enough muscle available to fill the space.

Pectoralis Major. The pectoralis major flap is one of the two most commonly used extrathoracic muscle flaps. It has a dual blood supply from the predominant thoracoacromial artery to the major pedicle, and from the internal mammary to the major pedicle and secondary pedicles. It can be used as a reverse turn-over flap or placed directly into the wound. It requires a 5-cm rib resection for entry into the chest. It is the flap of choice for sternal infections and ranks after the latissimus dorsi and serratus anterior for the pleural space.

Latissimus dorsi. The latissimus dorsi flap is the most commonly used flap for thoracic defects. Its predominant blood supply is from the thoracodorsal artery. It can be used as a turn-over flap or placed directly into the wound. It may be brought through the incision or through a separate small rib resection.

Serratous Anterior. This is my second choice of flap for filling a pneumonectomy space, and is particularly good for filling a small space. The entrance into the chest is through the primary chest incision.

Rectus Abdominis. In general, the rectus abdominis is used for closure of the lowest third of sternal defects. It is held in reserve for problems involving the pleural space in case a residual space remains. It is generally the last flap applied.

Surgical Technique of Single-Stage Complete Muscle Flap Closure

Single-stage muscle flap closure is performed for a persistent postpneumonectomy empyema space at approximately 3 months for benign disease and 6 months to one year for malignant disease. The six basic steps for complete flap closure are: (1) appropriate antibiotics are given, based on the sensitivities of the pleural drainage; (2) the original incision is re-opened; (3) the cavity is debrided widely so that good granulation tissue is present; (4) a bronchopleural fistula is identified, and if present, the edges are freshened, and the fistula is closed, if technically possible. An omental flap is brought up through the anterior diaphragmatic incision (Fig. 59–2) and tacked around the fistula with 3-0 Prolene sutures; (5) appropriate muscle flaps are then swung to fill the pleural space; and (6) the procedure is begun with a latissimus dorsi flap and followed with any necessary flaps to fill the entire space, depending upon the anatomical location and size of the space. The filling of the entire pleural space is shown in Fig. 59–3. Mathes and Nahai (1982) discussed in detail the technique of flap mobilization in their excellent work on muscle and musculocutaneous flaps.

All extrathoracic muscle flaps require a route of entry into the chest. The location of the opening is usually determined by the blood supply of the muscle and should be placed so that the blood supply is under no tension after transposition. Generally, 4 to 5 cm of the appropriate rib is all that must be resected to allow for flap entry. Figure 59–4 shows the typical site of entry for the pectoralis major and latissimus dorsi flaps. The sine qua non for success with single-stage complete muscle flap closure is that the entire space must be filled. If a space is left, it is usually just beneath the fifth or sixth rib in the midaxillary line and can be closed by a short resection of the ribs over it without cosmetic deformity. Following transposition of the muscle flaps, the wound is closed primarily and chest tubes are connected to Pleuro Vac suction for 7 to 10 days. Appropriate antibiotics are given.

The two predominant points in this surgical technique are that no residual space can be left and that a sufficient number of flaps must be available so that any intrathoracic space can be filled. To date, I have used this technique in over 14 patients, with only two failures.

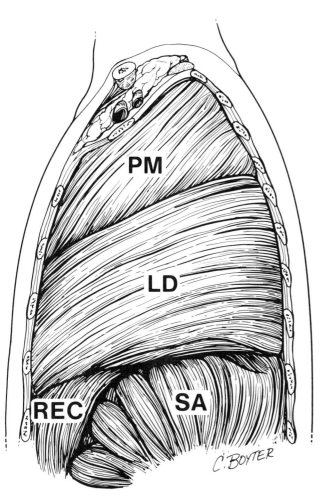

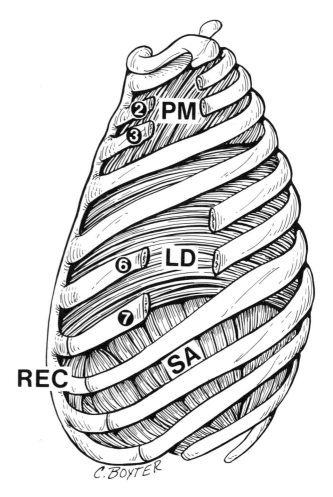

Fig. 59–3. An entire pleural space filled with muscle flaps and their usual anatomical location. (PM = pectoralis major; LD = latissimus dorsi; REC = rectus abdominis; SA = serratus anterior). (Reproduced with permission of Miller, J.I., et al.: Single-stage complete muscle flap closure of the postpneumonectomy empyema space: a new method and possible solution to a disturbing complication. Ann. Thorac. Surg. 38(3):227, 1984.)

Fig. 59–4. Usual sites of rib resection for entrance of the pectoralis major (PM) and latissimus dorsi (LD) flaps into the pleural spaces. (REC = rectus abdominis; SA = serratus anterior). (Reproduced with permission of Miller, J.I., et al.: Single-stage complete muscle flap closure of the postpneumonectomy empyema space: a new method and possible solution to a disturbing complication. Ann. Thorac. Surg. 38(3):227, 1984.)

Postresectional Lobectomy Empyema

Our group's algorithm for the treatment of the post-resectional empyema space following lobectomy is given in Table 59–8. The basic principles that apply to the pneumonectomy space apply to the management of the empyema space following resectional lobectomy. In general, a persistent lower lobectomy space (Fig. 59–5) can be easily closed and filled by application of the serratus anterior and latissimus dorsi flap. This is illustrated in Fig. 59–6. If a bronchopleural fistula is present, this is closed by myoplasty, using a pedicled intercostal muscle flap, followed by obliteration of the space with the latissimus dorsi and serratus anterior muscles. If an upper lobe space persists following lobectomy, with or without bronchopleural fistula, the fistula is closed with a pedicle intercostal muscle flap, followed by a reverse pectoralis major turn-over flap into the superior space through the second intercostal space.

TUBERCULOSIS OF THE PLEURA

According to Hood (1965), tuberculosis of the pleura and tuberculous effusions are rare, accounting for approximately 1 to 3 of exudative pleural effusions. When a tuberculous pleural effusion does exist, it generally is thought to be a sequel to a primary infection occurring 3 to 6 months previously. The pleura becomes infected with tuberculosis by extension of parenchymal disease to the visceral pleura with rupture of the subpleural foci into the pleural space, or, as DeMeester (1983) noted, from shedding of the bacilli into the pleural space from involved hilar nodes. Delayed hypersensitivity appears to play an important role in the pathogenesis of tuberculous pleural effusions and in determining which clinical pattern the disease process will take. Tuberculous pleurisy is the most common type of the extrapulmonary tuberculosis.

Once the pleura becomes infected, various clinical patterns may develop, not all of which become a frank empyema. These range from a thin, relatively transient effusion to a pleural space filled with thick, contaminated pyogenic organisms from an associated bronchopleural fistula. In general, as Hood (1965) described, the clinical patterns can be divided into three types: a thin, watery, sterile pleural effusion; frank tuberculous empyema; and mixed tuberculous pyogenic empyema, with or without bronchopleural fistula. Tuberculous pleuritis generally manifests clinically as an acute illness. Symptoms arise abruptly in approximately two thirds of the patients and last from 1 week to 1 month. In the other third, the symptoms are chronic, lasting more than a month before diagnosis. The symptoms most often mimic an acute bacterial pneumonia. Eighty percent of patients have a nonproductive cough, and 75% have pleuritic chest pain. If both cough and pleuritic chest pain are present, the pain usually precedes the cough. Most patients have a low grade fever with temperatures to 100 to 101°F—37.8 to 38.3°C.

Pleural effusions secondary to tuberculosis are almost

Table 59–8. Postlobectomy Empyema

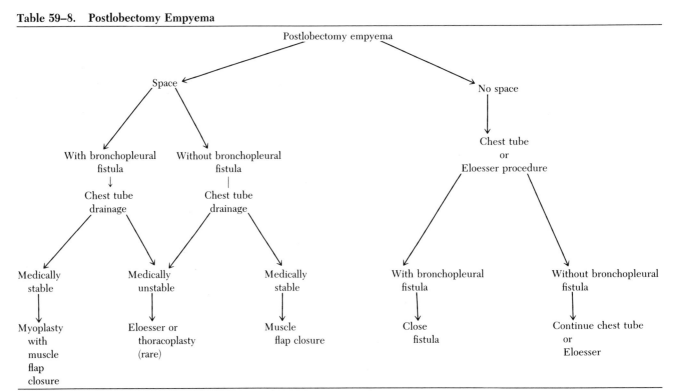

(Reproduced with permission from Miller, J.I., et al.: Ann. Thorac. Surg. 38(3):227, 1984.)

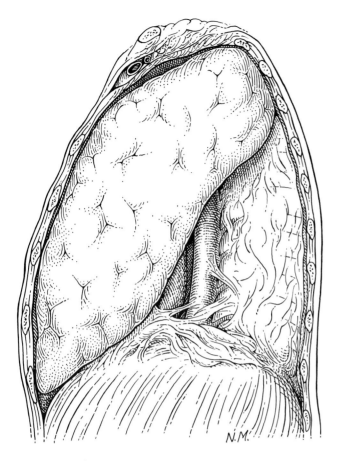

Fig. 59–5. Schematic diagram showing a residual empyema cavity after a lower lobectomy.

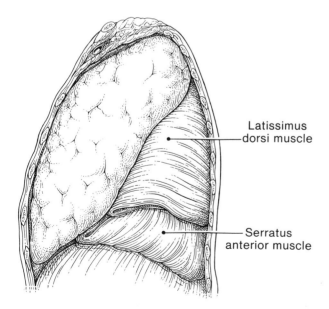

Latissimus dorsi muscle

Serratus anterior muscle

Fig. 59–6. Diagram showing flap closure of a lower lobectomy empyema cavity with the latissimus dorsi and serratus anterior muscles.

always unilateral, and are usually small to moderate in size. Laboratory examination of the peripheral white cell count is usually normal. Light (1983) reported that the chest roentgenogram may show only a small pleural effusion, with or without parenchymal lesions, or advanced parenchymal disease with dense pleural thickening between the lung and the chest wall that is frequently calcified. The diagnosis is etiologically confirmed by one or more of the following specific findings: identification of acid-fast bacilli on smear of sputum or gastric contents; tuberculous bacilli cultured from the pleural fluid; or tuberculous granuloma in the pleural biopsy.

A tuberculin skin test should be performed on all patients with an exudative pleural effusion. DeMeester (1983) reported that the tuberculin skin test is positive in 60 to 80% of patients with tuberculous pleuritis. A negative skin test, however, does not rule out tuberculous pleuritis. In a series of 36 patients with tuberculous pleuritis, 31% had a negative intermediate PPD. Although the pleuritis is thought to be caused at least in part by delayed hypersensitivity, circulating adherent cells in the acute phase of the disease suppress the specifically sensitive T-lymphocytes in the peripheral blood and in the skin, but not in the pleural fluid as Ellner (1978) pointed out. If the patient is not anergic, the intermediate PPD almost always becomes positive within 2 months of the development of symptoms. If the patient has not converted to a positive skin test after 3 months, it is rare that the cause of the exudative effusion is tuberculosis.

Culture and analysis of the pleural fluid is important in the diagnostic evaluation of the exudative pleural effusion in a patient with suspected tuberculous pleuritis. Fluid is almost always an exudate, with the protein level generally above 3.5 g/dl, and frequently above 5 g/dl. In most patients, as Light (1983) emphasized, the pleural fluid differential white cell count reveals more than 50% lymphocytes. Light (1983) also stated that if more than 10% of the pleural fluid cells are eosinophils, one can exclude the diagnosis of tuberculous pleuritis. The pleural fluid glucose may be reduced in cases of tuberculous pleuritis, but this is a nonspecific finding. The most useful study for ruling out tuberculosis is analysis of the fluid for mesothelial cells. Several series, including those of Hurwitz (1980) and Light (1973), have confirmed that pleural fluid from patients with tuberculosis rarely contains more than 5% mesothelial cells. Cultures of the pleural fluid as DeMeester (1983) noted, reveal tuberculous bacilli in 30 to 60% of patients. The percentage of positive yield can be increased by centifuging volumes of pleural fluid or by performing multiple cultures. Cultures from the sputum or gastric analysis frequently yield tubercular bacilli and should be performed unless there are roentgenographic lesions present on chest roentgenogram.

Pleural biopsy is one of the best methods for establishing the diagnosis of tuberculous pleuritis. The demonstration of granuloma in the parietal pleura suggests tuberculous pleuritis; caseous necrosis and acid-fast bacilli need not be demonstrated. More than 95% of patients with granulomatous pleuritis have tuberculosis. Light (1983) reported that needle biopsy of the pleura was positive in 60 to 80% of patients with tuberculous pleurisy. A biopsy demonstrating caseating or noncaseating granulomata is usually accepted as indicative of tuberculosis, although only identification by culture of tuberculous bacilli from the specimen is completely diagnostic.

Clinical Presentation

Tuberculous involvement of the pleura may be seen in three clinical presentations: a self-limited tuberculous pleuritis of short duration, generally 6 to 8 weeks, that leaves the patient with a variable amount of fibrosis; a frank tuberculous empyema, with or without concomitant parenchymal disease, that results in a degree of pleural scarring fibrosis and potential entrapment of the lung; a frank mixed tuberculous pyogenic empyema, with or without a bronchopleural fistula that may or may not be associated with significant parenchymal disease.

In the first clinical setting, the pleural effusion is generally in a young person, with a newly acquired positive tuberculin skin test. Usually a small subpleural focus of infection has ruptured into the pleural space. The pleural effusion is rarely positive for tuberculous bacilli, and protein levels may be slightly increased. Cytologic examination of the fluid in this situation generally reveals a preponderance of lymphocytes, and as Hood (1965) noted, only 20% of this group of patients have a positive culture for *Mycobacterium tuberculosis*. In this situation, a positive skin test, despite a negative culture report, indicates that emperic treatment with isoniazid and rifampin should be instituted. The therapy should be continued for at least 6 months. If the PPD skin test is negative but the lymphocyte count in the pleural fluid is more than 50% and fewer than 5% of the cells are mesothelial cells, emperic therapy with isoniazid and rifampin for 2 months and then a repeat skin test are indicated. If the repeat skin test is positive, treatment should be continued for a total of at least 6 months. If the tuberculin skin test is negative at 2 months, treatment should be discontinued. The treatment of tuberculous pleuritis is intended to prevent the development of active tuberculosis, to relieve the patient's symptoms, and to prevent the development of a fibrothorax.

Frank tuberculous empyema caused by rupture of the tubercular bacilli through the visceral pleural surface into the pleural space produces a range of symptoms, from no symptoms to severe systemic symptoms of toxicity and fever. Once the diagnosis is suspected and established by analysis of the pleural fluid or the finding of tuberculous bacilli, therapy with antituberculous drugs should be instituted immediately. In general one should avoid draining the pleural space unless, as Hood (1965) outlined, there is minimal parenchymal disease, and the drainage can be considered therapeutic for an empyema not responding to antibiotic therapy; there is little or no possibility of resection, and the need for decortication can be prevented by drainage; drainage could terminate the disease problem months before expected resectional

surgery; or a bronchopleural fistula develops. Prompt re-expansion should be accomplished. Drainage of a chronic empyema space before definitive surgery is generally contraindicated. Drainage should be avoided, if possible, in the management of pure tuberculous empyema, especially when a major surgical procedure appears to be necessary.

The third clinical presentation of tuberculous disease is a mixed infection of tuberculosis and pyogenic empyema. The mixed infection usually results from contamination from a repeated thoracentesis, ill-advised chest tube insertion, a bronchopleural fistula acquired from rupture of a tuberculous cavity into the pleural space, or a tuberculous empyema that has eroded into the lung, establishing a fistula. Diagnosis is established by an air-fluid level on the chest roentgenogram and by culture of a pyogenic organism from the pleural fluid, in addition to tuberculous bacilli. Appropriate antibacterial and antituberculosis therapy should be instituted immediately. This requires close cooperation between the pulmonologist and thoracic surgeon in dictating management and timing of intervention. Maximum control of the infection must be obtained. In general, therapy should be continued for a minimum of 3 to 6 months before any major surgical intervention. Analysis of pulmonary function studies, chest roentgenography, CT scan, and bronchoscopy are imperative before deciding to undertake a major operative procedure.

Thoracentesis is used to relieve symptoms of dyspnea by decreasing the size of the pleural effusion as quickly and completely as possible. Tube drainage should be discouraged unless necessitated by bronchopleural fistula or superimposed bacterial infection.

Table 59–9 presents an algorithm for the management of patients with pleural tuberculosis. Open drainage of a mixed pyogenic tuberculous empyema, with or without a bronchopleural fistula, is indicated when management cannot be handled by a chest tube or the patient is medically unstable and not considered a potential surgical candidate for other procedures. In these cases, the open pleural flap, as described by Eloesser, is a useful modality in the surgical management of these patients.

If the residual disease is limited exclusively to the pleura, decortication is indicated when evidence of clinical toxicity is no longer present and further thoracentesis fails to yield fluid, or if the fluid obtained still leaves the lung with a complete entrapment. The extent of pleural involvement should be equal to 25 to 30% of an involved hemithorax before decortication is performed. If involvement is less than this, little lung function is lost by leaving this alone. Hood (1965) stated that patients should be treated with antituberculous therapy for a minimum of 6 months before any decortication procedure.

If pulmonary resection is contemplated at the time of decortication or pleurectomy, all disease must be removed, with prompt re-expansion of the remaining lung. If a space is left following resection, except in the case of pleuropneumonectomy, the chance of a tuberculous empyema recurring is high. If a space remains after resection, it must be closed by thoracoplasty or muscle flap

Table 59–9. Management of Pleural Tuberculosis with Pleural Effusion

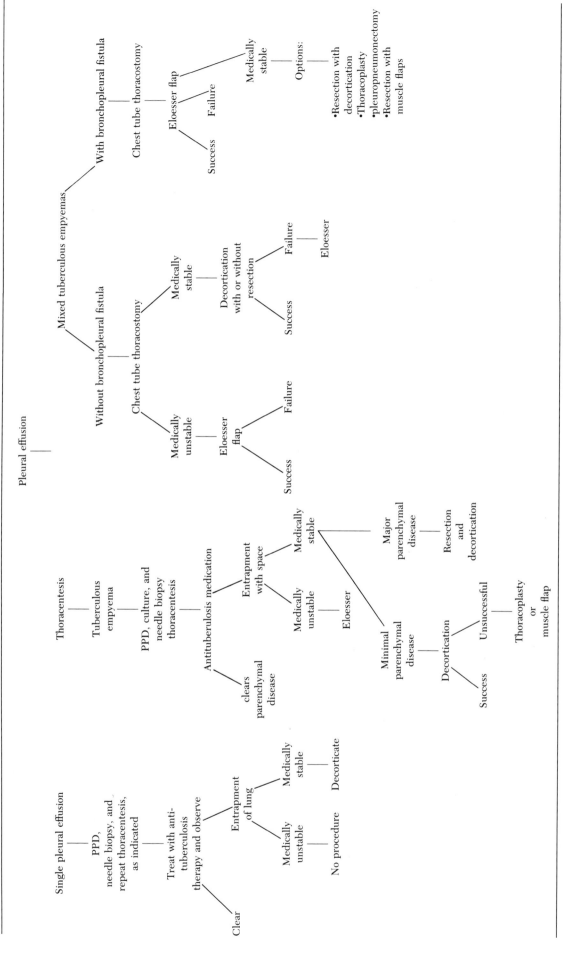

transposition procedures. Pleuropneumonectomy is performed only as a last resort, as the morbidity and mortality for this procedure are high. The reported mortality rates of 20 to 40% are probably related to patient selection. This technically difficult procedure is described in Chapter 29.

DeMeester (1983) pointed out that when surgical intervention is required for pleural disease only, the mortality is low, and the chances of serious complication, such as empyema or bronchopleural fistula, are minimal. Mortality and morbidity rates rise in proportion to the extent of the disease, as expressed by the complexity of the surgical procedure required to eradicate or control it, and can be as high as 20 to 40%. Postoperative complications of empyema and bronchopleural fistula are highest in patients undergoing pleuropneumonectomy. In those patients who have disease that necessitates pleuropneumonectomy, postoperative complications can be lessened by appropriate preoperative antibiotic and antituberculous therapy, high amputation of the appropriate bronchial stump, and adequate coverage by pleural or pericardial flaps. Balanced drainage of the pneumonectomy space, as I and my associates (1975) suggested, for 2 to 3 weeks in the presence of a preoperatively contaminated space is a useful modality for these patients. The space can then be sterilized by an inflow-outflow catheter irrigation system with infusion of antibiotic therapy for 2 weeks, followed by removal of the tubes.

FUNGAL DISEASE OF THE PLEURA

Light and associates (1973) reported that fungal disease accounts for approximately 1% of all pleural effusions, and generally results secondary to underlying established parenchymal disease with involvement of the pleural space. Management of primary fungal disease is discussed in Chapter 69. Pleural involvement is seen occasionally in aspergillosis with rupture of the cavity into the pleural space. Herring and Pecora (1976) found that only 24 cases of pleural aspergillosis were reported between 1958 and 1970. Approximately 20% of patients with coccidioidomycosis have blunting of the pleural angle on routine chest roentgenography. The pleural effusion varies in size, but is generally unilateral. Rarely is a pleural effusion seen in the patient with *Cryptococcus neoformans* infection. Young and associates (1980) found reports of only 30 cryptococcal pleural effusions in a review of the literature. When it occurs, the effusion is generally unilateral and involves more than 50% of the affected hemithorax. Pleural involvement secondary to histoplasmosis, actinomycosis, nocardia, and sarcoidosis is rare. Diagnosis and management are based on analysis of pleural fluid with appropriate cultures and biopsies of the pleura. Therapy is directed toward the underlying parenchymal disease, with appropriate antifungal drugs, such as amphotericin B, myostatin and penicillin. In general, open drainage should be avoided. If a mixed fungal pyogenic empyema is present and the patient is toxic, open drainage of the empyema in conjunction with the appropriate antibiotics and antifungal drug is necessary. The objectives in the treatment of fungal disease of the pleura are to avoid secondary pyogenic contamination and to obviate subsequent surgical resections of underlying involved lung, which have high morbidity and mortality rates.

REFERENCES

Abrashanoff: Plastische Methode der Schliessung von Fistelgangen, welche von inneren Organen kommen. Zentralbl. Cir. 38:186, 1911.

American Thoracic Society: Management of nontuberculous empyema. Am. Rev. Resp. Dis. 85:93, 1962.

Bartlett, K.M., et al.: Bacteriology of empyema. Lancet 1:338, 1974.

Bergh, N.P., et al.: Intrapleural streptokinase in the treatment of hemothorax and empyema. Scand. J. Thorac. Cardiovasc. Surg. 11:265, 1977.

Clagett, O.T., and Geraci, J.E.: A procedure for the management of postpneumonectomy empyema. J. Thorac. Cardiovasc. Surg. 45:141, 1963.

Cohn, L.H., and Blaisdell, E.W.: Surgical treatment of nontuberculous empyema. Arch. Surg. 100:376, 1970.

Creech, O. Jr., et al.: The intrathoracic use of streptokinase-streptodornase. Am. Surg. 19:128, 1953.

DeMeester, T.R.: The pleura. In Textbook of Thoracic Surgery. Edited by D. Sabiston. Philadelphia, W.B. Saunders Co., 1983.

Ellner, J.J.: Pleural fluid and periphral blood lymphocytes function in tuberculosis. Ann. Intern. Med. 89:932, 1978.

Eloesser, L.: An operation for tuberculous empyema. Surg. Gynecol. Obstet. 60:1096, 1935.

Eloesser, L.: Of an operation for tuberculous empyema. Ann. Thorac. Surg. 5:355, 1969.

Herring, M., and Pecora, D.: Pleural aspergillosis: a case report. Ann. Surg. 42:300, 1976.

Hood, R.M.: Tuberculosis of the pleura. In Surgical Diseases of the Pleura and Chest Wall. Springfield, IL, Charles C Thomas, 1965.

Hoover, E.L., et al.: Reappraisal of empyema thoracis. Chest 90:511, 1986.

Hurwitz, S., Leiman, G., and Shapiro, C.: Mesothelial cells in pleural fluid: TB or not TB? S. Afr. Med. J. 57:937, 1980.

LeRoux, B.T., and Dodds, T.C.: A Portfolio of Chest Radiographs. Edinburgh, E. and S. Livingston, 1964.

LeRoux, B.T., et al.: Suppurative diseases of the lung and pleural space. Part 1. Empyema thoracis and lung abscess. Curr. Probl. Surg. 23:6, 1986.

Light, R.W.: Parapneumonic effusion and infection of the pleural space. In Pleural Diseases. Edited by R.W. Light. Philadelphia, Lea & Febiger, 1983.

Light, R.W.: Tuberculous pleural effusions. In Pleural Diseases. Edited by R.W. Light. Philadelphia, Lea & Febiger, 1983.

Light, R.W., Erozan, Y.S., and Ball, W.C.: Cells in pleural fluid: their value in differential diagnosis. Arch Intern. Med. 132:854, 1973.

Light, R.W., et al.: Parapneumonic effusions. Am. J. Med. 69:507, 1980.

Lynn, R.B.: The bronchial stump. J. Thorac. Surg. 36:70, 1958.

Mathes, S.J., and Nahai, F.: Clinical Applications for Muscle and Musculocutaneous Flaps. St. Louis, C.V. Mosby, 1982.

Mayo, P., and McElvein, R.B.: Early thoracotomy for pyogenic empyema. Ann. Thorac. Surg. 2:649, 1966.

Miller, J.I., Fleming, W.H., and Hatcher, C.R., Jr.: Balanced drainage of the contaminated pneumonectomy space. Ann. Thorac. Surg. 19:585, 1975.

Miller, J.I., et al.: Single-stage complete muscle flap closure of the postpneumonectomy empyema space: a new method and possible solution to a disturbing complication. Ann. Thorac. Surg. 38:227, 1984.

Potts, D.E., Levin, D.S., and Sohn, S.A.: Pleural pH in parapneumonic effusions. Chest 70:238, 1976.

Radvitch, M.M., and Fein, R.: The changing picture of pneumonia and empyema in infants and children. JAMA 175:1039, 1961.

Samson, P.C.: Empyema thoracis: essentials of present day management. Ann. Thorac. Surg. *11*:210, 1971.

Stafford, E.G., and Clagett, O.T.: Postpneumonectomy empyema: neomycin instillation and definitive closure. J. Thorac. Cardiovasc. Surg. *63*:771, 1972.

Sullivan, K.K., et al.: Anaerobic empyema thoracis. Arch. Intern. Med. *131*:521, 1973.

Symbas, P.N., et al.: Nontuberculous pleural empyema in adults. Ann. Thorac. Surg. *12*:69, 1971.

Teixera, J.: The present status of thoracic surgery in tuberculosis. Dis. Chest *53*:19, 1968.

Tillotson, J.R., and Lerner, A.M.: Characteristics of pneumonia caused by *Escherichia coli*. N. Engl. J. Med. *277*:115, 1967.

Tillotson, J.R., and Lerner, A.M.: Characteristics of nonbacteremic pseudomonas pneumonia. Ann. Intern. Med. *69*:295, 1968.

Varkey, B., et al.: Empyema thoracis during a 10-year period. Arch. Intern. Med. *191*:1771, 1981.

Vianna, N.J.: Nontuberculous bacterial empyema in patients with and without underlying diseases. JAMA *215*:69, 1971.

Weese, W.C., et al.: Empyema of the thorax then and now. Arch. Intern. Med. *131*:516, 1973.

Young, E.J., et al.: Pleural effusions due to *Cryptococcus neoformans*: a review of the literature and report of two cases with cryptococcal antigen determinatus. Ann. Rev. Respir. Dis. *121*:743, 1980.

READING REFERENCES

Beck, C.: Thoracoplasty in America and visceral pleurectomy with report of a case. J.A.M.A. *28*:58, 1897.

Bowditch, H.I.: Paracentesis thoracis: an analysis of 25 cases of pleuritic effusion. Am. Med. Monthly, 1853, p.3.

Eggers, C.: Radical operation for chronic empyema. Ann. Surg. *77*:327, 1923

Fowler, G.R.: A case of thoracoplasty for the removal of a large cicatricial fibrous growth from the interior of the chest, the result of an old empyema. Med. Record *44*:938, 1893.

Graham, E.A., and Bell, R.D.: Open pneumothorax: its relation to the treatment of acute empyema. Am. J. Med. Sci. *156*:939, 1918.

Hewitt, C.: Drainage for empyema. Br. Med. J. *1*:317, 1876.

Hippocrates. *In* Major Classic Descriptions of Disease. Springfield, IL, Charles C Thomas, 1965.

Hood, R.M.: History of empyema management. *In* Surgical Diseases of the Pleura and Chest. Edited by R.M. Hood. Philadelphia, W.B. Saunders Co., 1986.

Lawrence, G.H.: Empyema. *In* Problems of the Pleural Space. Edited by G.H. Lawrence. Philadelphia, W.B. Saunders Co., 1983.

Trousseau, A.: Lectures on Clinical Medicine Delivered at the Hotel-Dieu, Paris. Translated by J.R. McCormick. London, The New Sydenham Society *3*:198, 1870.

CHAPTER 60

PRIMARY TUMORS OF THE PLEURA

Thomas W. Shields

Neoplastic involvement of the pleura occurs frequently. Most of these tumors are metastatic from other primary sites—breast, lung, ovary, kidney, and stomach to name some of the more common primary sites—and only a few arise de novo from the pleural tissues. The few that do are mostly malignant and can easily be confused with secondary deposits. Some pathologists still do not classify a tumor as a mesothelioma without having performed a careful autopsy to rule out the possibility of a primary lesion elsewhere. Although no reasonable doubt exists concerning the existence of mesotheliomas, a definitive diagnosis based on histologic criteria alone is difficult.

The embryology of the pleura explains the difficulties of diagnoses by histologic structure alone. The pleura is derived from mesoderm, which forms two lamellae. The parietal lamella fuses with the ectoderm, forming the somatopleura. The visceral lamella fuses with the entoderm, forming the splanchnopleura. Hence all three germ layers are involved in formation of the pleura, and this is reflected in the histologic types of primary neoplasia of the pleura. The pathology of mesotheliomas consists of epithelial and mesenchymal elements of either a pure or mixed form in variable stages of benignity or malignancy. Mesotheliomas by definition arise from mesothelial cells, yet these cells have the neoplastic potential of all three embryologic germ cell layers.

PLEURAL MESOTHELIOMA

Epidemiology

Oncologists have become increasingly interested in the epidemiology of pleural mesotheliomas. Wagner and his associates (1960) reported 40 pleural mesotheliomas in patients who lived in the Northwest Cape Province of South Africa, which contains large asbestos mines. Selikoff and his colleagues (1965) reported the incidence of mesothelioma to be 1 in 55 autopsy subjects among the members of Asbestos Workers Union in New York and New Jersey. Whitwell and Rawcliffe (1971) reported

that 80% of their patients with mesothelioma had a history of industrial exposure to asbestos, the men in shipyards and the women in sackware repairing. Basal asbestosis was present in 17% of these patients, and excessive asbestos bodies were found in the rest. Whitwell and associates (1977) found that of 88 patients with pleural mesothelioma who had been exposed to asbestos, the lung tissue of 73 contained over 100,000 asbestos fibers per gram of dried lung; in 26 patients with histologic asbestosis, the lung tissue contained over 3 million fibers. In 100 control lungs from necropsy of patients without lung cancer or any history of industrial exposure, there were less than 10,000 fibers per gram of dried lung in 57% of the specimens and less than 20,000 fibers in 71%; no specimen had more than 50,000 fibers. Selikoff and Hammond (1978), in reviewing reports of mesothelioma in France, Great Britain, the Netherlands and elsewhere, as well as in their studies, noted that most of the instances could be traced to prior asbestos exposure. Characteristically, a long latent period between the time of exposure and the development of the tumor elapses. An increased risk can be identified 20 years after the first exposure and, as Selikoff (1977) reported, the incidence continues to rise after 35 to 40 years. Peto and his associates (1981a, 1981b) pointed out that the cumulative lifetime risk of developing mesothelioma increases as a constant times the third or fourth power of time since exposure; that is, risk = K (time since first exposure). Dose and duration of exposure are reflected in the constant part of the equation. Therefore, as Antman and associates (1986) noted, the younger the age of first exposure, the higher the cumulative lifetime risk.

Even though among asbestos workers 6 to 7% of all deaths are caused by pleural or peritoneal mesothelioma, approximately 20% of the deaths are caused by carcinoma of the lung. Interestingly, there is also more than the expected number of deaths caused by primary tumors of other organ systems (Table 60–1). Although the most important etiologic factor is exposure to asbestos, chronic severe pulmonary disease, radiation, and zeolite contact have been associated with the development of malignant

Table 60–1. Deaths Among 17,800 Asbestos Insulation Workers in the United States and Canada January 1, 1967–January 1, 1977

	Expected*	Observed
Number of men	17,800	
Man-years of observation	166,855	
Total deaths, all causes	1,660.96	2,270.00
Total cancer, all sites	319.90	994.00
Lung cancer	105.97	483.00
Pleural mesothelioma	†	66.00
Peritoneal mesothelioma	†	109.00
Cancer of esophagus	7.01	18.00
Cancer of stomach	14.23	22.00
Cancer of colon-rectum	37.86	59.00
All other cancer	154.83	235.00
Asbestosis	†	162.00
All other causes	1,351.06	1,114.00

*Expected deaths are based upon white male age-specific mortality data of the U.S. National Center for Health Statistics for 1967–1975 and extrapolation to 1976.

†These are rare causes of death in the general population.

The membership of the International Association of Heat and Frost Insulators and Asbestos Workers, AFL-CIO, CLC, was enrolled on January 1, 1967, and has been observed since.

Selikoff, I.J. and Hammond, E.C.: Asbestos-associated disease in United States shipyards. *In* CA—A Cancer Journal for Clinicians 28:88, 1978.

mesothelioma. Moreover, as Antman (1981) pointed out in patients with malignant mesothelioma, the incidence of a history of asbestos exposure may vary from 0 to over 80%. Of course, asbestosis exposure may be manifested by benign disease processes such as asbestosis, pleural plaques, and benign pleural effusion (Table 60–2).

Experimentally, the pleural cavity is sensitive to carcinogenic agents, and numerous agents can produce tumor, including pure silicon dioxide. The yield of malignant mesotheliomas is high when asbestos is injected into the pleural cavity of hamsters.

Both the experimental and epidemiologic studies are impressive, but the mechanism of relationship between asbestos and mesotheliomas remains clouded. There are two families of asbestos fibers based on crystalline structure: serpentine—chrysotile—and amphibole. The latter includes amosite, tremolite, crocidolite, and anthophyllite. Crocidolite—blue asbestos—is the most harmful, although mesotheliomas have been observed in patients after exposure to amosite and even only to chrysotile, which is believed to be the least harmful type of asbestos fiber (Fig. 60–1). The quantitative relationship is nebulous; there does not appear to be a direct correlation with the degree of exposure, and mesotheliomas have been reported even in housewives exposed to the clothing of an asbestos worker.

Classification

The most widely accepted classification of mesotheliomas is an anatomic one that divides them into the diffuse and localized types. From a diagnostic viewpoint it would be simple if all localized lesions were benign and all diffuse lesions malignant. For practical purposes diffuse lesions can be assumed to be malignant; a significant number of localized lesions, however, are also malignant (Fig. 60–2). Stout and Himardi (1951) reported a 30% incidence of malignancy in solitary mesotheliomas. Okike and his associates (1978) reviewed 60 patients with localized mesothelioma seen at the Mayo Clinic. Eight—13.3%—of the lesions were considered to be malignant by histologic criteria, and all but one patient with a localized malignant mesothelioma was dead within 2 years. In contrast, only 2 of the 52 patients who were judged to have benign lesions developed a recurrent lesion.

LOCALIZED BENIGN MESOTHELIOMA

Benign pleural mesotheliomas, which are always localized, usually arise from the visceral pleura on a stalk, and project into the pleural space in a pedunculated manner. Adhesive bands may form to the parietal or other portions of the visceral pleura. Sessile attachment to the pleura also occurs. The tumor may arise, however, from the mediastinal, diaphragmatic, or chest wall portions of the parietal pleura. Size and shape can vary from a small nodule to a huge mass that may completely fill the hemithorax. Solitary mesotheliomas also may be contained within the lung parenchyma so that grossly they are indistinguishable from a primary bronchial lesion.

Gross Features

Localized mesotheliomas are smooth-walled and composed of dense, whorled fibrous tissue that may soften in areas to form cysts filled with viscid fluid resembling synovial fluid. They are usually avascular growths that may become partially calcified. A solitary mesothelioma associated with pleural effusion usually resembles a cau-

Table 60–2. Thoracic Surgical Procedure in 1577 Persons Exposed to Asbestos*

Condition	Total Number	Operation	Number	Percent
Asbestosis	101	Lung biopsy	26	26
Plaques	168	Exploration	24	14
Benign effusions	68	Decortication or biopsy	15	22
Mesotheliomas	41	Resection or biopsy	29	71
Bronchial carcinomas	23	Resection or biopsy	19	83

Adapted from Gaensler, E.A., et al.: Thoracic surgical problems in asbestos-related disorders. Ann. Thorac. Surg. *40*:82, 1985.

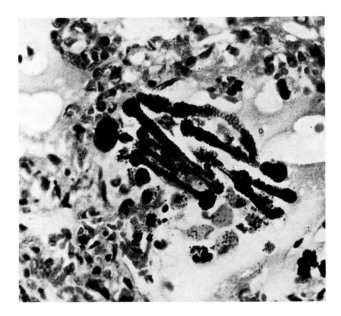

Fig. 60–1. Photomicrograph of asbestos bodies in the lung. (Spencer, H.: Pathology of the Lung. Oxford, Pergamon Press, 1962.)

liflower mass arising from either the parietal or visceral pleura by a narrow pedicle and projecting into the pleural cavity. Such lesions may often produce a bloody pleural effusion—a point to bear in mind because bloody pleural effusion associated with intrathoracic neoplasm usually connotes malignant spread and hence inoperability. In this instance, however, a completely resectable and curable lesion may be associated with a bloody pleural effusion.

Histologic Features

The tumor is characterized by uniform elongated cells and varied amounts of collagen and reticulum fibers in bundles of many sizes. The spindle cell contains an oval, slightly indented nucleus with slightly acidophilic cytoplasm. Occasional mitotic figures appear in cellular zones of a given tumor, but pleomorphism and nuclear anaplasia are absent. Depending on the area sampled, three histologic patterns can be distinguished: fibrous or acellular, cellular, and mixed (Fig. 60–3).

Clinical Features

Solitary mesotheliomas frequently are asymptomatic and are discovered incidentally on roentgenograms of the chest. They tend to grow slowly. In one instance, serial roentgenograms over 15 years showed only a modest increase in size. Chest pain is unusual unless the lesion arises from the parietal pleura. Occasionally, solitary mesotheliomas attain tremendous size and produce symptoms of bronchial compression and atelectasis. Cough, heaviness of the chest, and shortness of breath may result. Pleural effusion may occur with solitary mesotheliomas and produces the usual signs and symptoms. A benign localized mesothelioma is often accompanied by hypertrophic pulmonary osteoarthropathy. Okike and his associates (1978) noted this combination in 20% of

Table 60–3. Symptoms of Localized Benign Mesothelioma of the Pleura

Symptom	Benign (52 patients)
Asymptomatic	28
Chronic cough	17
Chest pain	12
Dyspnea	10
Fever	9
Hypertrophic pulmonary arthropathy and digital clubbing	10
Pleurisy	3
Loss of weight	3
Hemoptysis	1
Pneumonitis	1

Okike, N., Bernatz, P.E., and Woolner, L.B.: Localized mesothelioma of the pleura. Benign and malignant variants. J. Thorac. Cardiovasc. Surg. 75:363, 1978.

their patients (Table 60–3) and usually with lesions larger than 7 cm. Rarely, a large tumor has associated symptoms of severe hypoglycemia.

Hypertrophic Pulmonary Osteoarthropathy

This symptom complex occurs in association with many intrathoracic disease processes. Clagett and his colleagues (1952) reported that hypertrophic pulmonary osteoarthropathy occurred in 66% of cases of localized mesothelioma, although more recent data reveal this association in only 20% of instances. Nonetheless, this pattern contrasts markedly with the overall 5% incidence of hypertrophic pulmonary osteoarthropathy in bronchial carcinoma, as reported in one of the lead articles in Lancet (1959). I observed the incidence to be only 2 to 3% in the latter disease.

Clubbing of the fingers and toes occurs in association with a wide variety of lung disorders. Hypertrophic pulmonary osteoarthropathy may be associated with clubbing of the fingers and toes, although the latter is not actually part of the syndrome.

Clubbing is the enlargement of the distal phalanges, usually of both the hands and feet. Diner (1962) described periosteal new growth with lymphocytic and plasma cell infiltration of connective tissue around the nail beds, resulting in increased fibrous tissue between nail bed and phalanx. Van Hazel (1940) reported the digital arteries to be enlarged and elongated 10 to 15 times normal. Also, Cudkowicz and Armstrong (1953) noted the presence of arteriovenous anastomosis in the distal finger segments near the junction of the dermis and the subcutaneous tissue.

Clinically, the distal phalanx is enlarged—especially widened—with a loss of the obtuse angle that the nail bed normally forms with the plane of the proximal skin surface. A spongy sensation upon depression of the proximal nail bed is characteristic. It has been impressive that the patients themselves are rarely aware of the anatomic changes in their fingers, no matter how dramatic the appearance, even though a spouse or other member of the family may have noted them.

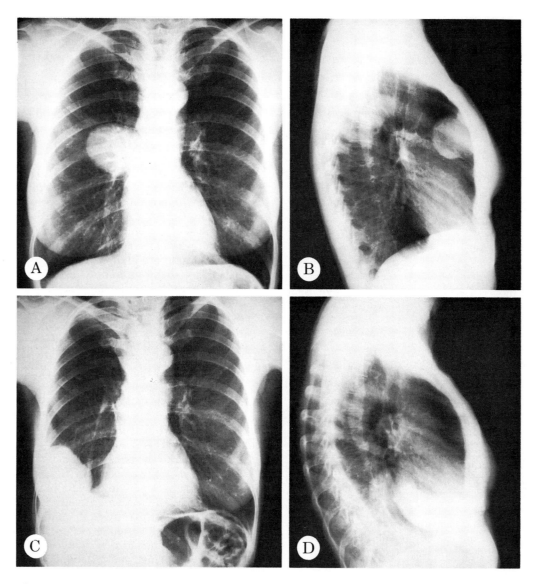

Fig. 60–2. *A* and *B*, PA and lateral roentgenograms of the chest showing a large, solitary mass that was diagnosed as a "benign" mesothelioma following a right upper lobectomy. *C* and *D*, PA and lateral roentgenograms of a recurrent intrapleural mass 6 months later. The mass was removed by a completion pneumonectomy. The patient succumbed from recurrent diffuse, malignant mesothelioma several months later.

No common denominator appears to be present in the various processes associated with clubbing. The processes can be broadly classified into pulmonary, cardiac, and extrathoracic.

Neoplastic lesions of the lung causing clubbing are generally associated with hypertrophic pulmonary osteoarthropathy, whereas the congenital structural and inflammatory pulmonary lesions associated with clubbing rarely show signs of arthropathy. Non-neoplastic pulmonary disorders seen with clubbing include pulmonary arteriovenous fistula, lung abscess, bronchiectasis, empyema, pulmonary infarction, emphysema, chronic bronchitis, chronic inflammation of the lung, sarcoidosis, idiopathic pulmonary fibrosis, diffuse interstitial fibrosis, primary pulmonary hypertension, pneumoconioses, and atelectasis.

Among the cardiac lesions associated with clubbing,

cyanotic heart disease is classic. In cardiac processes, hypertrophic pulmonary osteoarthropathy rarely occurs in combination with clubbing. Trevor (1952) could find only three examples of periostitis in over 3000 patients with congenital cyanotic heart disease. Other disorders in this category are: mitral stenosis, subacute bacterial endocarditis, aortic aneurysms, and even a dilated esophagus. Cross and Wilson (1950) reported an interesting example of unilateral clubbing, occurring in the extremity distal to an axillary arteriovenous aneurysm.

Extrathoracic disease processes seen with clubbing include: cirrhosis of the liver, ulcerative colitis, myelogenous leukemia, Hodgkin's disease, carcinoma of the nasopharynx, and syringomyelia.

Clubbing of the fingers without primary disease occurs on a familial basis and is usually associated with thickening of the skin of the face. Camp and Scanlon (1948)

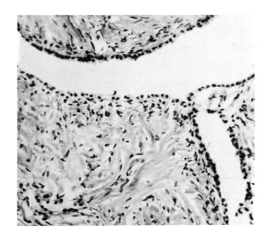

Fig. 60–3. Photomicrograph of a benign fibrous mesothelioma.

described yet another group, usually adolescent boys, with hypertrophic pulmonary osteoarthropathy unaccompanied by obvious primary disease that they regarded as being distinct from the hereditary form of clubbing.

Osteoarthropathy means disease of the bones and joints. Its frequent associations and simultaneous occurrence with clubbing of the fingers suggest that a single causative factor exists; however, hypertrophic pulmonary osteoarthropathy may be present without clubbing. Gynecomastia is similarly seen with hypertrophic pulmonary osteoarthropathy, yet also occurs as a solitary extrathoracic manifestation of an intrathoracic neoplasm.

Clinical symptoms vary from minimally detectable stiffness of the wrists to systemic toxicity. Some of the systemic manifestations seem to be related to one or more endocrine, collagen, or immunologic mechanisms of the body that are not directly related to the osteoarthropathy. Chills and spiking temperature, markedly elevated sedimentation rate, and malaise with obvious systemic toxicity may be present.

The classic findings in hypertrophic pulmonary osteoarthropathy include stiffness of the joints, edema over the ankles and occasionally of the hands, arthralgia of the long bones—especially the tibia—and generalized malaise. At times, the joint and bone pain is severe.

The involvement is usually bilateral. The distal ends of the ulna and radius are most frequently involved, and roentgenographic evidence of the periosteal thickening is most commonly seen here. The bones of the hands, ankles, knees, elbows, and shoulders are involved in that approximate order. Finger pressure on the anterior surface of the distal tibia often elicits pain in advance of roentgenographic changes.

The etiologic basis of hypertrophic pulmonary osteoarthropathy and clubbing remains an enigma. A single cause for these two frequently associated yet distinct phenomena seems unlikely. Flavell (1956) reported relief from the pain of hypertrophic osteoarthropathy following division of the vagus nerve at the hilus of the lung in patients with inoperable pulmonary neoplasms. Diner (1962) described dramatic relief of symptoms following

cervical or thoracic vagotomy. Ginsburg (1958) found that blood flows in the hand and foot were similar in a control group and in patients with hypertrophic pulmonary osteoarthropathy. Lovell (1950), however, demonstrated increased blood flow in patients with clubbing secondary to congenital cyanotic heart disease. These patients had dilated venous plexuses in the skin of the nail-bed area, accompanied by increased caliber in the digital arteries and abnormal arteriovenous communications.

Two threads of information may be drawn from the many investigations and observations. First, clubbing of the fingers has some connection with arteriovenous shunting. Whether these abnormal arteriovenous communications permit a substance that is normally altered or detoxified in the lung to appear in the systemic circulation or whether small emboli that are usually filtered out by the lung are allowed to appear there is highly debatable. Cudkowicz and Armstrong (1953) demonstrated precapillary bronchopulmonary anastomosis in patients with clubbing. Desaturation of the blood per se seems an unlikely explanation because the incidence of clubbing in severely emphysematous patients is so low. Second, a significant bit of circumstantial evidence is the relationship of hypertrophic pulmonary osteoarthropathy to involvement of the pleura. This aspect is borne out by the examples of pleural mesotheliomas and peripheral bronchial carcinomas. A neoplastic process involving the pleura, the embryologic origin of which is pluripotential, may elaborate a substance that elicits osseous and articular responses. This same neoplastic process might also create an arteriovenous fistula, producing clubbing.

The clinical significance of hypertrophic pulmonary osteoarthropathy is perhaps greater in its diagnostic than its therapeutic implications. Removal of the pulmonary lesion for the most part gives dramatic remission of the arthralgia and peripheral edema. In the series reported by Okike and his associates (1978), eight of ten patients with localized benign mesothelioma experienced complete relief of the symptom complex after operative removal of the tumor. Osseous roentgenographic changes regress much more slowly. Recurrence of the pulmonary neoplasm does not necessarily mean return of the symptoms of osteoarthropathy, particularly when the pulmonary lesion is a bronchial carcinoma. Recurrence of a mesothelioma, on the other hand, is usually heralded by a return of the symptoms present with the original osteoarthropathy. The presence of the extrathoracic manifestations is an added impetus to remove the pulmonary pathologic process. Irradiation and chemotherapy are much less effective in ablating the symptoms. Division of the posterior plexus of nerves at the pulmonary hilus should be considered if the lesion is unresectable, in light of the experience of Flavell (1956). It is difficult to understand how cervical vagotomy would relieve symptoms of osteoarthropathy, as Diner (1962) reported, because the vagus nerve constitutes only a portion of the innervation to the lung.

Hypoglycemia

A fascinating association of hypoglycemia and mesenchymal tumors has piqued the curiosity of clinicians.

Devroede and Tirol (1968) noted that 99 examples of hypoglycemia secondary to a mesenchymal tumor had been reported since 1929. Nineteen of the neoplasms were intrathoracic mesenchymal tumors. Doubtless there have been many more such patients that were either unrecognized or not reported.

Most intrathoracic lesions producing endocrine, neurologic, or osteoarthritic changes in the body do so without regard to the size of the intrathoracic lesion. In contrast, mesotheliomas causing hypoglycemia are usually large and, as such, would seem to bear some relation to the cause. As in instances of hypoglycemia from other causes, the patient may present with central nervous system symptoms of syncope, convulsions, or coma; death may result from the effect of hypoglycemia on the central nervous system.

Nelson and co-workers (1975) reviewed the numerous theories to explain the mechanism of hypoglycemia. Among these are increased glucose consumption by the tumor; a defect in glucose regulators, that is, adrenocorticotropic hormone, growth hormone, or glucagon; ectopic secretion of insulin by the tumor, the presence of a stimulator of insulin release, or a potentiator of circulating insulin; the inhibition of glycogenolysis; the inhibition of lipolysis and hepatic gluconeogenesis; and the presence of a nonsuppressible insulin-like activity.

Most of these theories have been disproved, and Nelson and co-workers (1975) suggested that increased glucose utilization by the tumor is probably a partial explanation. They suggest that the major factor is probably the release of metabolites, notably L-tryptophan, by the tumor. These metabolites would exhibit insulin-like activity through the inhibition of gluconeogenesis.

The clinical significance of hypoglycemia is that coma or convulsions in a patient with a chest mass may represent a remedial situation rather than hopeless cerebral metastasis. With removal of the tumor, correction of the hypoglycemia occurs in almost all instances. Recurrence of the lesion is sometimes accompanied by a return of the hypoglycemic state.

Roentgenographic Features

The appearance of a localized mesothelioma is for the most part indistinguishable from that of other nodules of the lung (Fig. 60–4). A circumscribed pulmonary mass of varying size usually is located in the lung periphery or in the projection of an interlobar fissure. The larger neoplasms may have irregular shapes, although the margins are usually sharply defined. Localized mesotheliomas statistically arise more often from the visceral pleura than from the parietal pleura; occasionally, movement of the mass may be demonstrated with changes in position when the tumor is on a stalk. As noted, infrequently a pleural effusion may be present.

Diagnosis

The nature of the solitary lesion is established most often at the time of thoracotomy and subsequent histologic examination. It is doubtful that tissue obtained by percutaneous transthoracic needle biopsy would be sufficient for precise diagnosis.

Treatment

Localized mesotheliomas are usually amenable to surgical resection (Fig. 60–5). Tumors that are considered benign on the basis of being localized may, however, be malignant both histologically and clinically, so adequate removal of the original lesion must be ensured. Nothing in my experience suggests that lobectomy is preferable to local resection of a pedunculated solitary mesothelioma. If the lesion is within the lung parenchyma, however, resection of the lobe may be advisable. A segmentectomy is occasionally sufficient, but even a bilobectomy may be necessary. Localized mesotheliomas of the mediastinal, diaphragmatic, and remaining parietal pleura should be excised as widely as can be accomplished satisfactorily.

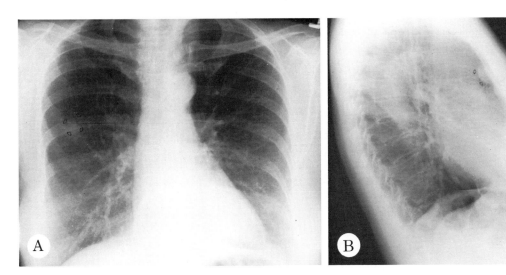

Fig. 60–4. PA and lateral roentgenograms of the chest of a 68-year-old woman revealing a small peripheral mass that was found upon removal to be a benign fibrous mesothelioma.

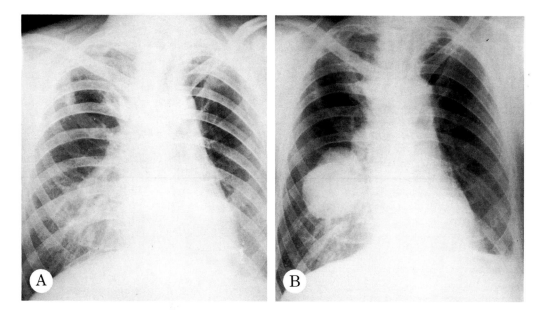

Fig. 60–5. *A*, Roentgenogram of the chest of patient with bilateral apical tuberculosis and an asymptomatic mass located at the level of the anterior end of the fourth rib on the right. *B*, Roentgenogram of the patient 10 years later revealing marked, but still localized, growth of previously found on mass on the right. Upon removal, the lesion was proven to be a benign fibrous mesothelioma.

Results

After adequate resection, patients with benign localized mesothelioma have the same life expectancy as the general population. Rarely, a benign lesion recurs, and at times such a recurrence represents a malignant change in the tumor.

LOCALIZED MALIGNANT MESOTHELIOMA

Pathologic Features

The localized malignant mesothelioma, like the benign variety, is generally a firm, encapsulated tumor. In contrast, however, it frequently exhibits a homogeneous, soft, smooth consistency on cut section, with occasional areas of necrosis and hemorrhage. Histologically, three groups of malignant mesothelioma can be distinguished: tubulopapillary, fibrous, and bimorphic. The tubulopapillary lesion possesses acinar and papillary formations. Interspaced in the sparse but bizarre stroma are elongated spindle cells of varied sizes, with the vesicular nuclei, prominent nucleoli, and esoinophilic cytoplasm. Areas of infarction with necrosis are present in some of the tumors. The fibrous malignant mesothelioma contains elongated spindling cells and fibrous stroma resembling fibrosarcoma. The bimorphic lesion displays varied mixtures of the cellular and fibrous components. Martini and his associates (1987) believe that almost all localized malignant mesotheliomas are in fact fibrosarcomas and should be managed as such.

Clinical Features

Most of these patients, in contrast to those with localized benign mesotheliomas, have symptoms. Chest pain, cough, dyspnea, and fever are the most common.

Osteoarthropathy rarely, if ever, occurs with the localized malignant lesion.

Roentgenographic Features

The findings in patients with these lesions are similar to those seen in patients with the benign variety. Occasionally, rib erosion may occur as the result of invasion of the chest wall.

Diagnosis

In most instances, the diagnosis is not apparent until histologic examination of the resected specimen. Invasion of the chest wall or other adjacent structures within the chest should alert one to the malignant nature of the lesion.

Treatment

Wide local excision, including pulmonary and pleural resections, is carried out as indicated. Resection of a lesion arising from the parietal pleura should include the adjacent chest wall. Recurrences frequently are found on the diaphragmatic surface of the pleura, which suggests drop metastasis or seeding from surgical manipulations. Therefore, the lesion should be handled carefully at the time of operation. When complete resection is possible, postoperative adjuvant therapy—irradiation or chemotherapy—is not indicated. When the resection is incomplete, however, radiation therapy, both internal—brachytherapy—and external should be used, according to Martini and associates (1987). Localized recurrence of a solitary benign or malignant mesothelioma should be evaluated for possible resection.

Results

With complete resection, Martini and colleagues (1987) reported 10 patients who survived 1 to 10 years after resection. In contrast, those in whom only an incomplete resection could be accomplished died of their disease within 1 to 20 months after diagnosis. The median survival time was 7 months.

DIFFUSE MALIGNANT MESOTHELIOMA

Gross Findings

This tumor arises from the pleura and grows selectively along the pleural surfaces. Any portion of the parietal, visceral, or mediastinal pleura may be the site of origin. This description includes interlobar fissures, which may give an unusual roentgenographic appearance. The involved lung may become completely encased (Fig. 60–6). The underlying lung parenchyma is usually affected more by compression than by tumor replacement. Clinically, diffuse mesotheliomas tend, curiously, to arise from the lower aspects of the pleural cavity.

Typically, the diffuse mesothelioma appears as sheets of tumor tissue or as multiple flat nodules lining the visceral and parietal pleura. The pleura over the lower lobes and diaphragm is usually more extensively affected. It is ivory with areas of yellow because of local necrosis. The involved tissue is firm. Direct extension over the pericardial surfaces across to the pleura of the contralateral lung occurs. At autopsy the tumor may be seen to have spread through the diaphragm and to have infiltrated the peritoneal surfaces. Frequently the tumor may grow out the site of a chest tube tract, thoracentesis site, or thoracotomy incision. Invasion into the lung parenchyma is usually superficial, and infiltration into the ribs and intercostal muscle occurs less frequently than one might expect.

The metastatic propensity of the mesothelioma was once thought to be low and distant metastases rare. Contiguous spread to adjacent structures and regional lymph nodes was held to be the pattern. It is now apparent that distant metastases, as well as lymphatic metastases, do occur frequently. Several authors, including Semb (1963), Urschel and Paulson (1965), and Wanebo and associates (1976) pointed this out in their series of patients with these tumors. At autopsy, thoracic lymph node metastases are present in as many as 67% of specimens. Hematogenous spread is reported in from one third to over two thirds of the autopsy examinations; the liver, lung, brain, and adrenal gland are the chief sites of metastatic deposits.

Histologic Features

As previously noted, all three germ layers are involved in the formation of the pleura; hence neoplastic mesothelial cells have the potential for great variation in histologic pattern. In fact, one of the most characteristic features of mesothelioma is the presence of several distinct histologic patterns in different areas of the tumor. A frozen section from one area may show epithelial cells, whereas another area shows stromal elements with malignant features.

Diffuse mesotheliomas are usually of mixed fibrous and epithelial elements. Whitwell and Rawcliffe (1971) described four varieties: tubulopapillary, sarcomatous, undifferentiated polygonal-celled, and mixed type. Kannerstein and associates (1978), however, divided them simply into three types: epithelial, sarcomatoid—fibrous, or mixed—biphasic cell types. This is the more commonly used classification.

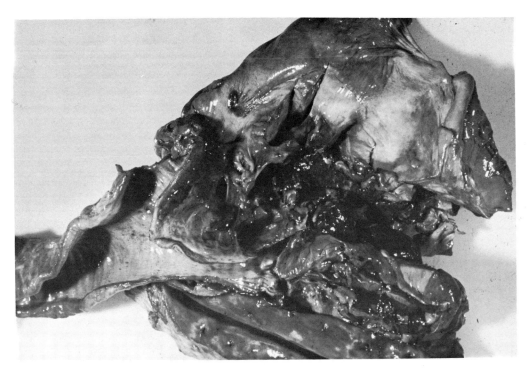

Fig. 60–6. Autopsy specimen on left lung encased by a diffuse mesothelioma.

The epithelial ones resemble adenocarcinoma and consist of complex acinar spaces lined by mesothelial cells. These mesotheliomas form papillary fronds that project into the lumen of dilated cystic spaces. The undifferentiated polygonal-cell type resembles an alveolar-cell lung cancer or a metastatic adenocarcinoma of the pleura (Fig. 60–8). Tumors nests or sheets of epithelial-like cells are surrounded by a fibrous stroma.

In the sarcomatous tumors, a few mesothelium-lined clefts are present and the lesion is almost a pure sarcoma (Fig. 60–7). They may resemble a myxofibrosarcoma or a densely fibrotic fibrosarcoma, or the pattern may have features of both types of tumor.

The mixed variety is mainly a variable mixture of the two aforementioned types. Approximately 50 to 60% of the tumors are epithelial, but the percentage of mixed lesions increases with the amount of tumor tissue examined per specimen.

Laboratory Findings

At times it is difficult to establish the tissue diagnosis by histological means alone. Additional studies—histochemical, immunochemical and electron microscopy—are necessary under these circumstances.

Histochemical Features

Malignant mesothelioma cells may produce hyaluronic acid. Histochemically, colloidal iron or Alcian blue stains with or without hyaluronidase digestion have been used to demonstrate the presence of the material. Other lesions such as bronchial carcinoma, mesenchymal tumors, and inflammatory lesions also may produce hyaluronic acid, but Suzuki (1981) found more stromal hyaluronic in mesothelomia than in the aforementioned conditions. Hyaluronic acid in pleural effusions, however, is not diagnostic because it occurs in significant quantities in effusions from other causes (see Chapter 57).

The exclusion of intracellular mucin, which is often seen in adenocarcinomas of the lung, is necessary, because this is not normally produced by mesothelioma cells. Periodic acid-Schiff stain with or without diastase digestion or mucicarmine stains may be used to identify mucin.

Immunopathologic Diagnosis

Numerous techniques of immunohistochemistry using diverse antigenic substances have been studied to determine their value in the differential diagnosis of adenocarcinoma from mesothelioma. Unfortunately, the results have been controversial with the use of CEA and keratin antibodies. Battifora and Kopinski (1985) reported that the reactions of monoclonal antibody MFG-2 to MFGRA may help differentiate these two types of tumors. Chung (1985) suggested using vimentin staining as a possible adjunct in the differential evaluation. Continued investigation, however, is necessary in this entire field.

Electron Microscopy

The epithelial form has long, abundant microvilli and cell membranes, which may be continuous or discontin-

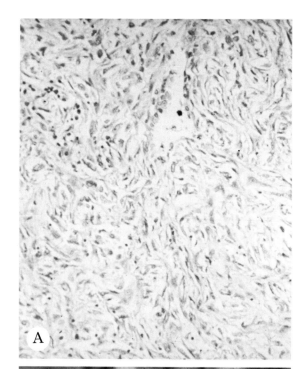

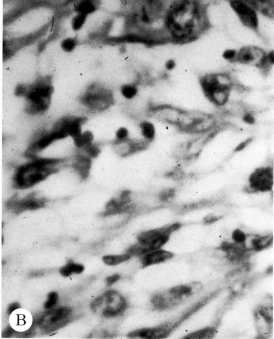

Fig. 60–7. Photomicrograph of a malignant mesothelioma of the sarcomatous variety.

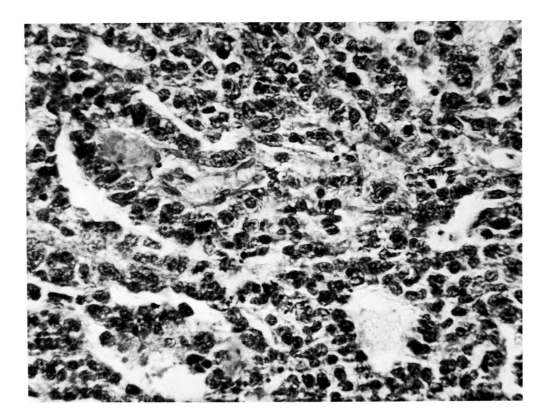

Fig. 60–8. Photomicrograph of epithelial type of malignant mesothelioma.

uous. Glycogen granules may be present and tonofilaments appear. Cilia and mucinous secretory granules are absent. Large mitochondria, cell junctions, and occasionally microvilli within intracytoplasmic vacuoles appear. In the biphasic form, epithelial cells, intermediate cells—with less distinct features than the epithelial cells have—and mesenchymal cells appear. In the fibrous—sarcomatous—type the cells are rich in rough-surfaced endoplasmic reticulum, and direct cell-to-cell contact is frequent. The cells look like fibroblasts.

Antman and colleagues (1986) stated that unless the pattern is unequivocally pathognomic of mesothelioma, the findings of at least two of the three supplemental methods must be characteristic to establish the diagnosis of malignant mesothelioma versus adenocarcinoma.

Clinical Features

Most series show a peak incidence of occurrence of mesotheliomas in the sixth and seventh decades of life, although a quarter of the patients are under 50. There is a ratio of men to women of 2:1 to 5:1.

The most common symptoms of diffuse malignant mesothelioma are chest pain—frequently severe, dyspnea, cough, and weight loss. Fever may occur and on occasion may mask the underlying nature of the thoracic disease. Fatigue also occurs occasionally. A pleural effusion of greater or lesser extent is present in most patients and local chest wall changes may be evident—retraction of the interspaces and even a chest wall mass. Palpable

metastatically involved lymph nodes may be present in the neck in 10% of the patients.

Roentgenographic Features

Pleural effusion is present in over 75% of the patients. The effusion may be massive on occasion (Fig. 60–9) but generally does not fill the entire hemithorax. It may be associated with an intrathoracic mass in about three-fourths of the instances. A mass without accompanying effusion is less frequent than an effusion alone. The mediastinum is only infrequently widened.

Computed tomography of the chest may suggest the possibility of mesothelioma and is important in defining its extent, as Grant and associates (1983) noted, when the diagnosis is known. In pleural effusion, in at least one third of instances, CT reveals pleural plaques, especially in the contralateral hemithorax. The fissure, particularly toward the basal region, become markedly thickened. The fissure may also appear nodular when tumor infiltration occurs. Pleural thickening, often irregular and nodular, appears on the internal margin. This may be recognized on the mediastinal surfaces as well. The ipsilateral hemithorax is often contracted (Fig. 60–10). Alexander and co-workers (1981), among others, noted that the ipsilateral lung volume decreased in mesothelioma before the hemithorax contracts. Pulmonary nodules may be identified, and irregular calcifications within the tumor nodules may appear. Plaques of dense calcification as well as minimal linear calcifications along the edge of the tumor and thoracic wall may be present.

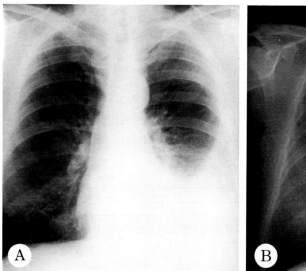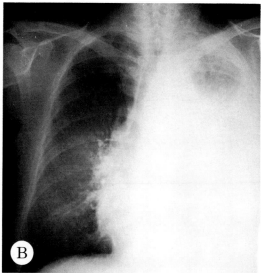

Fig. 60–9. *A*, Roentgenogram of chest of patient with malignant mesothelioma and small pleural effusion. *B*, Several months later, after diagnostic thoracotomy, the roentgenogram of the chest revealed a massive recurrent effusion.

Lastly, rib destruction and a soft tissue mass may be demonstrated by CT when there is extension outside the thoracic cage.

Diagnosis

Most believe that pleural biopsy with thoracentesis yields the highest diagnostic return. Ratzer and his associates (1967) reported that 75% of patients with diffuse mesotheliomas had malignant cells in the pleural fluid; by contrast, none had malignant cells on cytologic examinations of the sputa. Even when the cytologic examination of the pleural fluid is positive, however, definitive classification of the lesion as a mesothelioma is difficult. Wanebo and his colleagues (1976) were able to do so in only one third of the patients with this finding.

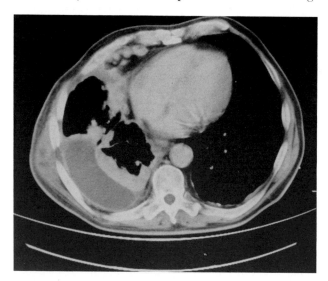

Fig. 60–10. CT of the chest of a patient with a mesothelioma of the right hemithorax. Tumor in the major fissure, pleural effusion posteriorly, and marked contraction of involved hemithorax are evident.

Because cytologic examination is probably much less frequently positive than Ratzer (1967) noted and even more difficult to interpret in this disease, needle biopsy is most often resorted to at the present time, and Lewis (1986) reported relying on this examination as the primary diagnostic approach; whereas formerly his group (1976, 1981) most often used thoracoscopy. With thoracoscopy, they established the diagnosis in over half of their 46 patients with the disease, but now they perform this procedure only when percutaneous needle biopsy is negative.

Small tissue samples, however, are difficult to interpret and frequent seeding of the needle tract also has been observed, as Shearin and Jackson (1976) emphasized.

A diagnostic thoracotomy, preferably limited, with resection of a segment of a rib to get adequate exposure, may be necessary to establish the nature of the disease. Occasionally, biopsy of an enlarged, palpable lymph node yields the diagnosis. Bronchoscopy may show distortion of the bronchi because of compression, but rarely provides a tissue diagnosis.

After establishing the diagnosis and defining the extent of the disease, the disease process may be categorized into one of four stages (Table 60–4), as Butchart and associates (1976) suggested. This is simple and, as Pom-

Table 60–4. Staging of Malignant Mesothelioma

Stage	Structures Involved by Tumor
I	Ipsilateral pleura and lung
II	Chest wall, mediastinum, pericardium, or contralateral pleura
III	Thorax and abdomen, or lymph nodes outside the chest
IV	Distant hematogenous metastases

fret and colleagues (1984) reported, predicts survival with statistical significance. It also permits planning of the appropriate therapeutic approach.

Therapy

The treatment of diffuse mesothelioma has been unsuccessful in most instances. Ratzer and associates (1967), however, reported a few 6- to 7-year survivals without treatment, which makes the evaluation of palliative therapeutic measures difficult to assess. Nevertheless, few patients survive longer than 2 years, and the average survival is about 10 to 14 months. Irradiation and chemotherapy have not consistently prolonged life, or, for that matter, contributed significantly to palliation.

The role of surgical intervention is difficult to define. Other than advising thoracotomy to establish the diagnosis, many surgeons question the role of any surgical therapy in patients with a diffuse mesothelioma for several reasons. First, the anatomic-pathologic state does not usually permit surgical removal with a tumor-free margin because the parietal pleura characteristically is involved. Second, one of the most striking pathologic features of diffuse malignant mesotheliomas, as noted, is the phenomenon of seeding. A patient with a diffuse malignant mesothelioma who has undergone thoracotomy may return in a few weeks with tumor growing out of the previous incision. This phenomenon is all the more striking when one considers the relative infrequency of implants in the wound after thoracotomies for highly undifferentiated bronchial carcinomas.

Surgical Intervention

Many, including Lewis (1986), believe that the role of surgery in malignant mesothelioma is only to establish the diagnosis and that this should be done by the procedure of the least possible magnitude. Others, however, suggest a more aggressive approach and advocate either a thoracotomy with pleurectomy or a radical extrapleural pneumonectomy. McCormack (1982, 1986) and Martini (1987) and their associates advocate pleurectomy for the epithelial variety of mesothelioma and complete excision when possible for the fibrosarcomatous type. In patients undergoing pleurectomy, internal radiation therapy by the most appropriate method—implanted radiation sources, brachytherapy—is used in areas of residual tumor. External irradiation is then given 4 to 6 weeks postoperatively. When the latter is completed, the patient is given chemotherapy. No postoperative deaths occurred in their group of patients, and they recorded a morbidity of only 12%. In their series of 33 patients, 20 patients had a median survival of 21 months and 13 patients were still alive from 10 to 53 months after the pleurectomy.

Worn (1974) and Faber (1986) and Butchart (1976, 1981) and DeLaria (1978) and their associates advocate radical pleuropneumonectomy in selected patients with the disease. The procedure should be reserved for patients with stage I disease who are in good medical condition. Butchart and associates (1976) suggested a schema (Fig. 60–11) that can be used to select potential candidates, although Faber (1986) believes it to be a little

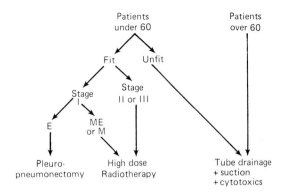

Fig. 60–11. Schematic representation of the management of diffuse malignant mesothelioma of the pleura. E = epithelial type; ME = mixed epithelial and mesenchymal type; M = mesenchymal type. (Butchart, E.G., et al.: Pleuropneumonectomy in the management of diffuse malignant mesothelioma of the pleura. Thorax *31*:22, 1976.)

restrictive. When the procedure is contemplated, prethoracotomy biopsies should be avoided when possible. The technique of the procedure is discussed in Chapter 29. The postoperative mortality rates have been high except in Faber's 1986 series, in which the rate was just under 10% (Table 60–5). Two-year survival rates have been 10 to 35% but five-year survival is much less (Table 60–5). Effective palliation of symptoms may, however, be observed in approximately 25% of the patients.

Whether this more extensive procedure is better than the lesser one of pleurectomy alone remains unanswered. The trend, however, appears to favor the less radical approach, especially because both are essentially palliative rather than curative.

Radiation Therapy

Although radiation therapy has been used extensively, both as the primary modality or as an adjuvant measure, little evidence supports its effectiveness, as Antman and associates (1986) noted. Some patients may, however, experience palliation of pain. Irradiation is frequently used after surgical decortication, and its combination with chemotherapy may eventually be fruitful.

Chemotherapy

Aisner and Wiernik (1981) reviewed the results of single-agent chemotherapy, combination chemotherapy, and combined modality therapy. They found that single-agent therapy was of little or no value. Combination chemotherapy with doxorubicin was more effective than combinations without it. Zidar and associates (1983) reported that a combination of cisplatin and doxorubicin may have synergistic effects. Combination chemotherapy alone, however, has not been as successful as hoped for. Combined modality therapy with "surgical debulking," chemotherapy, and irradiation is currently the treatment plan for most investigational studies.

Prognosis

The prognosis for patients with diffuse mesothelioma is poor. The median survival despite various types of therapeutic intervention is 10 to 15 months.

Table 60–5. Results of Pleuropneumonectomy

Author	Year	No. of Cases	Postop. Deaths (Percent)	2-Year Survival (Percent)	5-Year Survival (Percent)
Worn	1974	62	Not Stated	37	10
Butchart	1976	29	31.0	10	3.5
Bamler	1974	17	23.0	35	—
Faber	1986	32	9.4	25	—

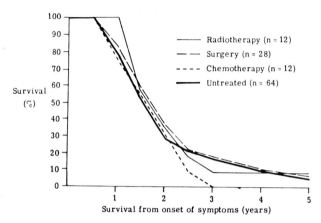

Fig. 60–12. Actuarial survival curves of patients treated by surgery, radiotherapy, and chemotherapy and of untreated patients. (Reproduced with the permission of Law, M.R.: Malignant mesothelioma: a study of 52 treated and 64 untreated patients. Thorax 39:255, 1984.)

Law and colleagues (1985) reported the survival of 52 treated and 64 untreated patients with malignant mesothelioma of the pleura. In the treatment and nontreatment groups the median survival was essentially the same—18 to 20 months—regardless of the therapy employed—decortication, chemotherapy, or irradiation—(Fig. 60–12) or the cell type present—epithelial, sarcomatous, or mixed cell types. Approximately one third of the patients in this series, as in others mentioned in the text, survived 2 years. An occasional 5-year survivor was observed regardless of the treatment rendered.

REFERENCES

Aisner, J., and Wiernik, P.H.: Chemotherapy in the treatment of malignant mesothelioma. Semin. Oncol. 8:355, 1981.

Alexander, E., et al.: CT of malignant pleural mesothelioma. Am. J. Radiol. 137:287, 1981.

Antman, K.H.: Clinical presentation and natural history of benign and malignant mesothelioma. Semin. Oncol. 8:313, 1981.

Antman, K.H., Shemin, R.J., and Carson, J.M.: Malignant pleural mesothelioma: a combined mortality approach. *In* Current Controversies in Thoracic Surgery. Edited by C.F. Kittle. Philadelphia, W.B Saunders Co., 1986.

Bamler, K.J., and Maassen, W.: Über die Verteilung der benignen und malignen Pleuratumoren im Krankengut einer lungenchirurgischen Klinik mit besonderer Berücksichtigung des malignen Pleuramesothelioms und seiner radikalen Behandlung einschliesslich der Ergebnisse des Zwerchfellensatzes mit Konservierter Dura mater. Thoraxchirurgie 22:386, 1974.

Battifora, H., and Kopinski, M.I.: Distinction of mesothelioma from adenocarcinoma: an immunohistochemical approach. Cancer 55:1679, 1985.

Butchart, E.G., et al.: Pleuropneumonectomy in the management of diffuse malignant mesothelioma of the pleura. Experience with 29 patients. Thorax 31:15, 1976.

Butchart, E.G., et al.: The role of surgery in diffuse malignant mesothelioma of the pleura. Semin. Oncol. 8:321, 1981.

Camp, J.D., and Scanlon, R.L.: Chronic idiopathic hypertrophic osteoarthropathy. Radiology 50:581, 1948.

Churg, A.: Immunohistochemical staining for vimentin and keratin in malignant mesothelioma. Am. J. Surg. Pathol. 9:360, 1985.

Churg, J., and Selikoff, I.J.: Chapter 19. *In* Geographic Pathology of Pleural Mesothelioma in the Lung. Edited by A.A. Liebow and D.E. Smith. Baltimore, Williams & Wilkins, 1968.

Clagett, O.T., McDonald, J.R., and Schmidt, H.W.: Localized fibrous mesothelioma of the pleura. J. Thorac. Surg. 24:213, 1952.

Cross, W.K., and Wilson, C.M.: The circulating changes associated with aneurysm of the axillary artery and clubbing of the fingers. Clin. Sci. 9:59, 1950.

Cudkowicz, L., and Armstrong, J.B.: Finger clubbing and changes in the bronchial circulation. Br. J. Tuberc. Dis. Chest 47:277, 1953.

DeLaria, G.A., et al.: Surgical management of malignant mesothelioma. Ann. Thorac. Surg. 26:375, 1978.

Devroede, J., and Tirol, A.F.: Giant pleural mesothelioma associated with hypoglycemia and hyperthyroidism. Am. J. Surg. 116:130, 1968.

Diner, W.C.: Hypertrophic osteoarthropathy. J.A.M.A. 181:555, 1962.

Faber, L.P.: Malignant pleural mesothelioma: operative treatment by extrapleural pneumonectomy. *In* Current Controversies in Thoracic Surgery. Edited by C.F. Kittle. Philadelphia, W.B. Saunders Co., 1986.

Flavell, G.: Reversal of pulmonary hypertrophic osteoarthropathy by vagotomy. Lancet 1:260, 1956.

Gaensler, E.A., McLoud, T.C., and Carrington, C.B.: Thoracic surgical problems in asbestos-related disorders. Ann. Thorac. Surg. 40:82, 1985.

Ginsburg, J.: Observations on the peripheral circulation in hypertrophic pulmonary osteoarthropathy. Q.J. Med. 27:335, 1958.

Grant, D.C., et al.: Computed tomography of malignant pleural mesothelioma. J. Comp. Assist. Tomogr. 7:626, 1983.

Kannerstein, M., Churg, C., and McCaughey, W.T.E.: Asbestos and mesothelioma: a review. Pathol. Ann. 13:81, 1978.

Law, M.R., et al.: Malignant mesothelioma of the pleura: a study of 52 treated and 64 untreated patients. Thorax 39:255, 1984. Churg, A.: Immunohistochemical staining for vimentin and keratin in malignant mesothelioma. Am. J. Surg. Pathol. 9:360, 1985.

Lead article: Lancet 2:389, 1959.

Lewis, et al.: Direct diagnostic thoracoscopy. Ann. Thorac. Surg. 21:536, 1976.

Lewis, R.J.: Malignant pleural mesothelioma: a nonsurgical problem. *In* Current Controversies in Thoracic Surgery. Edited by C.F. Kittle. Philadelphia, W.B. Saunders Co., 1986.

Lewis, R.J., Sisler, G.E., and MacKenzie, J.W.: Diffuse, mixed malignant pleural mesothelioma. Ann. Thorac. Surg. 31:53, 1981.

Lovell, R.R.H.: Observations on the structure of clubbed figures. Clin. Sci. 9:299, 1950.

Martini, N., et al.: Pleural mesothelioma. Ann. Thorac. Surg. 43:113, 1987.

McCormack, P., et al.: Surgical treatment of pleural mesothelioma. J. Thorac. Cardiovasc. Surg. 84:834, 1982.

McCormack, P.M., and Martini, N.: Malignant pleural mesothelioma:

operative treatment by pleurectomy. *In* Current Controversies in Thoracic Surgery. Edited by C.F. Kittle. Philadelphia, W.B. Saunders Co., 1986.

Nelson, R., et al.: Hypoglycemic coma associated with benign pleural mesothelioma. J. Thorac. Cardiovasc. Surg. *69*:306, 1975.

Okike, N., Bernatz, P.E., and Woolner, L.B.: Localized mesothelioma of the pleura. Benign and malignant variants. J. Thorac. Cardiovasc. Surg. *75*:363, 1978.

Peto, J., Seidman, H., and Selikoff, I.J.: Mesothelioma mortality in asbestos workers: implication for models of carcinogenesis and risk assessment. Brit. J. Cancer *44*:001, 1981b.

Peto, J., Henderson, B.E., and Pike, M.C.: Trends in mesothelioma incidence in the United States and the forecast epidemic due to asbestos exposure during World War II. *In* Quantification of Occupational Cancer. Banbury Report. Vol. 9. Edited by R. Peto and Schneiderman. New York, Cold Springs Harbor Laboratory, 1981a.

Pomfret, E., et al.: Intensive treatment of patients with malignant mesothelioma. Proc. Am. Assoc. Cancer Res. *24*:156, 1984.

Ratzer, E., Pool, J., and Melamed, M.: Pleural mesotheliomas. Am. J. Roentgenol. *99*:863, 1967.

Selikoff, I.J.: Cancer risk of asbestos exposure. *In* Origins of Human Cancer. New York, Cold Spring Harbor Laboratory, 1977, pp. 1764.

Selikoff, I.J., Churg, J., and Hammond, E.C.: Relation between exposure to asbestos and mesothelioma. N. Engl. J. Med. *272*:560, 1965.

Selikoff, I.J., and Hammond, E.C.: Asbestos-associated disease in United States shipyards. CA—A Cancer Journal for Clinicians *28*:87, 1978.

Semb, G.: Diffuse malignant pleural mesothelioma: a clinicopathologic study of 10 fatal cases. Acta Chir. Scand. *126*:78, 1963.

Shearin, J.C., Jr., and Jackson, D.: Malignant pleural mesothelioma. Report of 19 cases. J. Thorac. Cardiovasc. Surg. *71*:621, 1976.

Stout, A.P., and Himardi, G.M.: Solitary (localized) mesothelioma of the pleura. Ann. Surg. *133*:50, 1951.

Suzuki, Y.: Pathology of human malignant mesothelioma. Semin. Oncol. *8*:268, 1981.

Trevor, R.W.: Hypertrophic osteoarthropathy in association with congenital cyanotic heart disease—a report of two cases. Ann. Intern. Med. *48*:660, 1952.

Urschel, H.C., and Paulson, D.L.: Mesotheliomas of the pleura. Ann. Thorac. Surg. *1*:559, 1965.

Van Hazel, W.: Joint manifestations associated with intrathoracic tumors. J. Thorac. Surg. *9*:495, 1940.

Wagner, J.C., Sleggs, C.A., and Marchand, P.: Diffuse pleural mesothelioma and asbestos exposure in the North Western Cape Province. Br. J. Ind. Med. *17*:260, 1960.

Wanebo, H.J., et al.: Pleural mesothelioma. Cancer *38*:248, 1976.

Whitwell, F., Scott, J., and Grimshaw, M.: Relationship between occupations and asbestos-fiber content of the lungs in patients with pleural mesothelioma, lung cancer, and other diseases. Thorax *32*:377, 1977.

Whitwell, F., and Rawcliffe, R.M.: Diffuse malignant pleural mesothelioma and asbestos exposure. Thorax *26*:6, 1971.

Worn, H.: Möglichkeiten und Ergebnisse der chirurgischen Behandlung des malignen Pleuramesothelioms. Thoraxchirurgie *22*:391, 1974.

Zidar, B., et al.: Treatment of six cases of mesothelioma with doxorubicin and cisplatinum. Proc. A.S.C.O. *2*:225, 1983.

READING REFERENCES

Arkless, D., Goranow, I., and Krastinow, G.: Hypoglycemia in an intrathoracic fibroma. Med. Bull. Veterans Admin. *19*:225, 1942.

Arrigoni, M.C., et al.: Benign tumors of the lung: A ten-year surgical experience. J. Thorac. Cardiovasc. Surg. *60*:589, 1970.

Barclay, N., Ogbeide, M., and Grillo, A.: Gross hypertrophic pulmonary osteoarthropathy in a 7-year-old child. Thorax *25*:484, 1970.

Barrett, N.R.: The pleura. Thorax *25*:515, 1970.

Brown, W.J., and Johnson, L.C.: Post inflammatory "tumors" of the pleura: three cases of pleural fibroma of the interlobar fissure. Milit. Surgeon *109*:415, 1951.

Cudkowicz, L., and Wraith, D.C.: A method of study of the pulmonary circulation in finger clubbing. Thorax *12*:313, 1957.

Ehrenhaft, J.L., Sensenig, D.M., and Lawrence, M.D.: Mesotheliomas of the pleura. J. Thorac. Cardiovasc. Surg. *40*:393, 1960.

Godwin, M.C.: Diffuse mesotheliomas with comment on their relation to localized fibrous mesotheliomas. Cancer *10*:298, 1957.

Jensik, R., et al.: Pleurectomy in treatment of pleural effusion due to metastatic malignancy. J. Thorac. Cardiovasc. Surg. *46*:322, 1963.

Kauffman, S.L., and Stout, A.P.: Mesothelioma in children. Cancer *17*:539, 1964.

Maier, H.C., and Barr, D.: Intrathoracic tumors associated with hypoglycemia. J. Thorac. Cardiovasc. Surg. *44*:321, 1962.

Marie, P.: De l'oste-arthropathic hypertrophiante pneumonique. Rev. Med. Paris *10*:1, 1890.

Ozello, L., and Speer, F.D.: Malignant diffuse mesothelioma of the pleura. Cancer *10*:1015, 1957.

Porter, J.M., and Cheek, J.M.: Pleural mesothelioma. J. Thorac. Cardiovasc. Surg. *55*:882, 1968.

Roberts, G.H.: Asbestos bodies in lungs at necropsy. Clin. Pathol. *20*:570, 1967.

Spry, C.J., Williamson, D.H., and James, M.L.: Pleuromesothelioma and hypoglycemia. Proc. R. Soc. Med. *61*:1105, 1968.

Sternon, I., Paramentier, G., and Rutsaert, J.: Comas hypoglycemiques et mesotheliome pleural benin. Acta. Clin. Belg. *26*:44, 1971.

Von Bamberger, E.: Ueber Knochenveränderungen bei chronischen Lungen- und Herzkrankheiten. Z. Klin. Med. *18*:193, 1890.

Webster, I.: Mesotheliomatous tumors in South Africa—pathology and experimental pathology. Ann. N.Y. Acad. Sci. *132*:623, 1966.

Wierman, H., Clagett, O.T., and McDonald, J.R.: Articular manifestations in pulmonary diseases. J.A.M.A. *155*:1459, 1954.

Yacoub, M.A.: Relation between the histology of bronchial carcinoma and hypertrophic pulmonary osteoarthropathy. Thorax *20*:537, 1965.

The Trachea

CHAPTER 61

BENIGN AND MALIGNANT DISEASES OF THE TRACHEA

Hermes C. Grillo

Primarily medical problems of the trachea, such as tracheobronchitis, and problems of airway management in respiratory failure will not be considered. The latter is discussed in Chapter 26.

TUMORS OF THE TRACHEA

Primary Neoplasms

Patients with primary tumors of the trachea present with symptoms and signs of upper airway obstruction, hemoptysis, or recurrent pneumonia (Fig. 61–1). The patient with an obstructive lesion of the upper airway may complain first of dyspnea on exertion. Stridor appears initially on forced respiration and eventually during breathing at rest. In extreme instances, dyspnea may progress until the patient becomes desperately short of breath on the most minimal effort and may even be unable to complete full sentences. Episodes of intermittent airway, obstruction may occur when secretions occlude a narrowed airway. These symptoms may then be relieved partially by vigorous coughing or suctioning. Patients reach such extreme clinical situations without diagnosis because roentgenograms of the chest most often show normal lung fields. Close examination of the tracheal air shadow is rarely made in routine roentgenograms of the chest. Persistent cough is another symptom of tracheal tumor. Hemoptysis occurs variably in the presence of primary tumors and usually instigates more exhaustive diagnostic study. Some patients with primary tumors manifest their disease with recurrent bilateral pneumonia. These episodes may clear with appropriate antibiotic and physiotherapeutic treatment, only to reappear. Unilateral pneumonia has been associated with a lesion low in the trachea, primarily lateralized.

Ninety patients with primary tumors of the trachea—exclusive of larynx and main bronchi—seen at the Massachusetts General Hospital over a 38-year period were reported by me (1978). Squamous cell carcinoma was present in 42 patients and 29 patients had adenoid cystic carcinoma. The term formerly used—"cylindroma"—implies an unjustified benignity. The remaining patients had various tumors, including chondrosarcoma, carcinoid adenoma, carcinosarcoma, pseudosarcoma, spindle cell sarcoma, adenosquamous carcinoma, adenocarcinoma, mucoepidermoid carcinoma, squamous papilloma, fibroma, hemangioma, chondroma, chondroblastoma, granular cell tumor, and monocytic leukemia. Chondromas occur often at the cricoid level. This general order of frequency has been borne out in other collected series. Thus, in a series reported by Houston and his associates (1969), of 53 malignant tumors of the trachea seen at the Mayo Clinic over 30 years, 24 patients had squamous cell carcinoma and 19 had adenoid cystic carcinoma. One patient had mucoepidermoid carcinoma. Hajdu and his associates (1970) reported 41 patients with primary tracheal carcinoma seen at the Memorial Hospital in New York over a period of 33 years; the tumors were distributed as follows: squamous cell carcinoma, 30; adenoid cystic carcinoma, 7; and mucus-secreting carcinoma, 4.

Squamous Cell Carcinoma

These tumors may be single, well localized lesions, relatively diffuse, or multiple lesions (Fig. 61–2). They may be exophytic or present as an ulcerative lesion with indistinct margins. Approximately one third of the subjects have extensive mediastinal spread or pulmonary metastases when first seen. The disease apparently spreads first to the regional lymph nodes and then by direct extension to the mediastinal structures. Upper tracheal lesions may also involve the larynx. Occasionally, it is not possible to tell whether a lesion of the lower larynx has extended to the trachea or the reverse. Such indeterminate patients were omitted from the figures mentioned.

Adenoid Cystic Carcinoma

These tumors may extend for a greater distance in the tracheal wall than is grossly evident (Fig. 61–3). At-

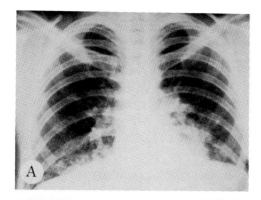

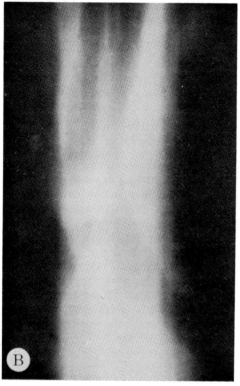

Fig. 61–1. *A*, Roentgenogram of the chest showing bilateral pneumonia that recurred in a young man without prior lung disease. *B*, Demonstration of a supracarinal tracheal tumor by laminography. *C*, The resected specimen showing a view that is essentially that seen by bronchoscopy. The tumor was carcinoid. (*C* from Grillo, H.C.: Surgery of the trachea. *In* Current Problems in Surgery. Chicago, Year Book Medical Publishers, 1970.)

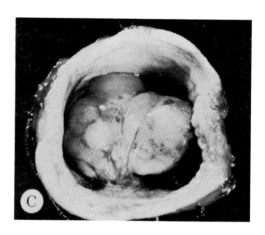

tempts at surgical extirpation therefore require wide tracheal margins with examination of frozen sections of the margins during operation. Only a portion of the tumor may present intratracheally. Such lesions, when first seen, frequently have not invaded mediastinal structures, even when the tumor is large, but have displaced these structures. Metastasis may occur to regional nodes, to the lungs and less commonly to bone.

Retrospective study of the course of primary carcinoma of the trachea showed that numerous patients succumbed to local obstructive problems or surgical attempts at removal of the tumors rather than from the metastatic or invasive disease. These facts instigated a more aggressive surgical approach. Although cases are few, many of the patients treated by excision of squamous cell carcinoma, and most receiving postoperative irradiation, are disease-free after many years. A few have had later resections of squamous lung cancer. The course of adenoid cystic carcinoma is long, but even patients with microscopically positive resection margins or locally involved nodes, all subjected to irradiation, remain disease-free after many years.

Secondary Neoplasms

The trachea is sometimes involved by carcinoma of the esophagus, lung, thyroid gland, or larynx. Carcinoma of the cervical or upper thoracic esophagus often invades the trachea because of the proximity of the membranous tracheal and the esophageal walls. Evaluation of an upper esophageal carcinoma endoscopically requires concomitant bronchoscopy. Tracheoesophageal fistula is a frequent and dire complication of these lesions; fistula also may occur during or after radition treatment. Carcinoma of the lung involves the trachea either by proximal extension from the main bronchus or by extrinsic compression and invasion from disease in the paratracheal lymph nodes. Most often, esophageal or pulmonary carcinoma involving the trachea is clearly beyond surgical cure. In rare, selected patients in whom preresectional

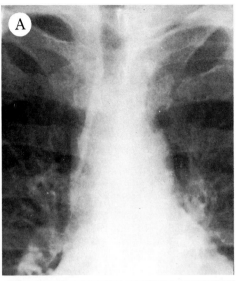

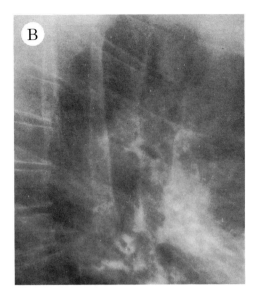

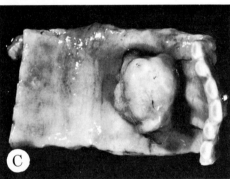

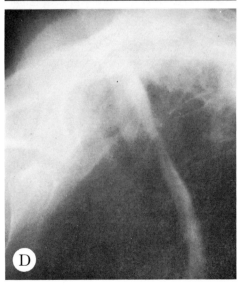

Fig. 61–2. *A* and *B*, Roentgenograms of an exophytic squamous cell carcinoma of the lower trachea. *A*, PA view showing the lesion, which had caused dyspnea, stridor, and hemoptysis. *B*, Detail of lateral roentgenogram showing the lesion a short distance above the carina. *C*, Surgical specimen of the lesion. This tumor did not recur, and a subsequent squamous cell carcinoma of the right upper lobe was also successfully removed. (*C* from Grillo, H.C.: Circumferential resection and reconstruction of the cervical and mediastinal trachea. Ann. Surg. *162*:374, 1965.) *D*, Detail of an oblique view of a barium study of the trachea and the esophagus, showing a lengthy tracheal lesion compromising the airway and thickening the septum between the trachea and esophagus. This primary squamous cell carcinoma of the trachea was removed by 10½ ring excision with primary anastomosis. No recurrence was evident at 12-year follow-up.

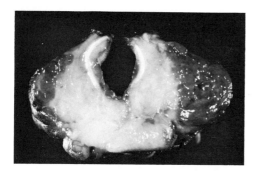

Fig. 61–3. Cross-sectional view of adenoid cystic carcinoma of the trachea invading the adjacent thyroid gland. The large bulk of tumor posteriorly displaces the esophagus. The anterolateral muscular wall of the esophagus was included with the specimen. The patient had airway obstruction that had been relieved by bronchoscopic removal of some of the obstructing tissue. Because of involvement of the base of the larynx, laryngotracheothyroidectomy, with mediastinal tracheostomy was required.

irradiation has confined a lesion of the esophagus that has involved the trachea by direct extension, and in whom no other metastases are evident, combined tracheoesophageal resection and reconstruction is justified. Deslauriers (1985), among others, believes that carinal pneumonectomy or lobectomy is indicated when N2 lymph nodes are negative.

Follicular and even papillary carcinoma of the thyroid may invade the trachea in a localized area (Fig. 61–4). Sometimes these lesions cause symptoms of an intratracheal lesion. Involvement may also be predicted by imaging and bronchoscopic studies. Most often, invasion is discovered during operation. If the tumor is otherwise potentially curable surgically, concurrent resection of the involved segment of trachea with primary repair is indicated, now that dependable reconstructive techniques are available. The more invasive, undifferentiated tumors of the thyroid, as I and Zannini (1986) noted, justify tracheal resection only if the prognosis after radical extirpation is otherwise hopeful—an uncommon situation.

Recurrences of laryngeal carcinoma in the cervical stoma following laryngectomy for extrinsic primary cancer of the larynx may well represent recurrence in the paratracheal lymphatics. Experience with radical removal of these lesions is poor. The trachea may also be compressed or invaded by miscellaneous tumors that occur in the neck and mediastinum. These tumors include carcinoma of the head and neck metastatic to lymph nodes, malignant thymoma, and lymphoma.

OTHER COMPRESSING LESIONS

Goiter

Large goiters may cause airway compression that occasionally is severe enough to cause symptoms. Massive goiters are now rare in the United States. The slow growth of goiters may lead to deformity of the cartilaginous rings without their complete destruction. Thus, following removal of such a goiter, the trachea may remain distorted in shape and narrowed, but significant

airway obstruction is not present. If enough tracheal chondromalacia has occurred, removal of the supporting mass of thyroid tissue allows the trachea to collapse with respiratory efforts. Several methods of managing this problem have evolved, including temporary tracheostomy, supporting traction sutures tied over external buttons, and tracheal buttressing with plastic rings.

An anterior substernal goiter usually does not exert compression on the trachea because of its position in front of the great vessels. Katlic and associates (1985) reported that the trachea is occasionally compressed in association with a posterior descending goiter that enters the upper thoracic strait lateral to esophagus and trachea.

Vascular Compression

Symptoms of tracheal compression may be produced by congenital vascular rings or by aneurysms of the innominate artery or of an anomalous subclavian artery that passes behind the trachea and esophagus. Distortion of the trachea by an enlarged, somewhat tortuous but nonaneurysmal innominate artery is seen occasionaly as a roentgenographic finding but is rarely clinically significant.

INFLAMMATORY DISEASES

Postinfectious Strictures

Strictures of the trachea are rare following endotracheal tuberculosis. When these lesions do occur, they can be extensive, involving the trachea subtotally and causing significant airway obstruction. Main bronchi may also be involved. The fibrosis is submucosal. Strictures following diphtheria were reported but are not seen now. Sclerosing mediastinitis, often attributed to histoplasmosis, may produce sometimes unmanageable tracheobronchial stenosis.

Post-Traumatic Stenosis

Acute trauma to the trachea is discussed in Chapter 42. Simple lesions such as lacerations inflicted with a clean blade do not present late problems if properly repaired initially. Complex lacerations of the trachea often produce late stenosis. The trachea may be totally separated from the larynx by the injury, with obliteration of this portion of the airway as cicatricial healing progresses. For survival, such patients have had a tracheostomy tube inserted either at the point of separation or below. Frequently, temporary or permanent paralysis of one or both vocal cords also has occurred. In addition, the larynx has suffered injury of varying degrees in many of these patients.

Post-traumatic tracheal stenosis must be carefully evaluated for the possibility of reconstruction. In particular, the state of the larynx must be accurately determined; as I have noted (1969, 1979), its reconstruction must precede tracheal rebuilding. If permanent cord palsy exists, it may be necessary to reposition the cords to provide an adequate airway and voice prior to tracheal repair. The surgeon must remember that "esophageal"

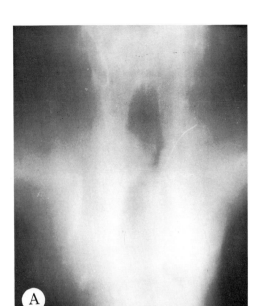

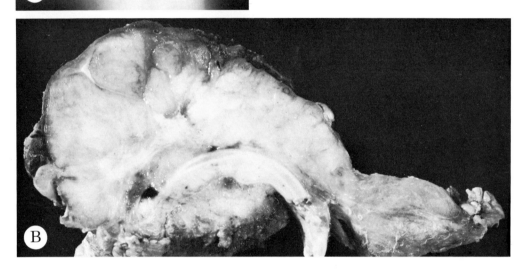

Fig. 61–4. Tracheal invasion by thyroid carcinoma. *A,* Detail of laminogram of the upper trachea showing luminal encroachment by recurrent, well-differentiated carcinoma of the trachea. Thyroidectomy had been performed 4 years earlier. Upper tracheal resection was performed with removal of part of the cricoidal cartilage and reimplantation of the trachea into the larynx. The patient died years later from osseous metastases without airway recurrence. *B,* Specimen of mixed papillary and follicular carcinoma of the thyroid invading and obstructing the trachea. (*B* from Grillo, H.C.: Circumferential resection and reconstruction of the cervical and mediastinal trachea. Ann. Surg. *162*:374, 1965.)

voice is really pharyngeal voice with an air bolus delivered through the esophagus. Such speech is much more effective when the air is delivered from the respiratory tract, even if both cords are paralyzed. A lengthy post-traumatic tracheal stenosis may be more apparent than real if complete separation with retraction occurred originally. Ocassionally, as Mathisen and I (1987) pointed out, concurrent pharyngoesophageal separation may present an unusually difficult reconstructive problem.

Postintubation Damage

Intubation either with oral or nasal endotracheal tubes or with tracheostomy tubes has been used increasingly to deliver mechanical ventilatory support in respiratory failure. Assistance supplied through cuffed tubes has thus far proved to be the only practicable method of management for adults with poor pulmonary or chest wall compliance. High flow respirators with uncuffed tubes, electrophrenic respirators, and negative pressure tank respirators have not proved to be satisfactory for managing these severe problems. High frequency ventilation

for long-term use remains developmental. A whole spectrum of tracheal lesions resulting from such treatment has been discerned by Andrews and Pearson (1971) as well as by me (1969, 1970) (Fig. 61–5). The most common lesions, and those most amenable to definitive treatment, are those responsible for the various forms of airway obstruction. Because a single patient may have more than one lesion and because the treatment of these lesions differs, precise definition of the pathologic state is essential in planning treatment. Lindholm (1970) showed that endotracheal tubes may cause obstruction at the laryngeal level even after only 48 hours of intubation, glottic edema, vocal cord granulomas, erosions particularly over the arytenoids, formation of granulation tissue, polypoid obstructions, and actual stenosis, particularly at the subglottic intralaryngeal level. Subglottic injury is also produced by cricothyroidotomy and by cricoid erosion caused by high tracheostomy or the kyphosis of age. Montgomery (1968) noted that subglottic stenosis may be difficult to correct.

At the tracheostomy site, granulomas that can obstruct

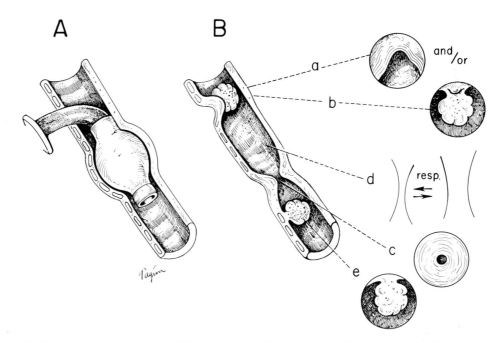

Fig. 61–5. Diagram of inflammatory lesions related to cuffed tracheostomy tubes. *A*, Location of the stoma and the distorting effect of a conventional cuff. *B*, Lesions developing at corresponding sites of injury. At the stoma an anterior stricture (a) or a granuloma (b) may occur, or there may be a combination of both. At the cuff site (c), circumferential stricture occurs. Between the stoma and such a stricture varying degrees of tracheal malacia may result with functional occlusion (d). At the site of erosion by the tip of the tube (e) a granuloma may occur. Innominate erosion and a tracheoesophageal fistula are seen at both cuff level and tip level.

the airway may form during healing. If the tracheostomy stoma has been made too large by turning a large flap or excising a large segment in the initial tracheostomy, or if erosion is caused by sepsis and heavy prying equipment, cicatricial healing may produce an anterior A-shaped stenosis that can severely compromise the airway. The posterior wall of the trachea may be relatively intact in these patients. At the level of the inflatable cuff, whether placed on a tracheostomy tube or an endotracheal tube, circumferential erosion of the tracheal wall may occur. If this erosion is deep enough, all the anatomic layers of the trachea may be destroyed, so that cicatricial repair results in a tight circumferential stenosis (Fig. 61–6). Malacia may also result. Below this level at the point where the tip of the tube may pry against the tracheal wall, additional erosion may occur with formation of granuloma, especially in children, for whom uncuffed tubes are used. In the segment between the stomal and cuff level, varying degrees of chondromalacia with resulting tracheomalacia may occur. Here the cartilages are not totally destroyed but only thinned. Bacterial infection in this segment of the trachea during the period of ventilatory support probably contributes to this process.

The etiologic basis of the cuff stenosis has been variously attributed to pressure necrosis by the cuff, irritative quality of materials in rubber and plastic cuffs and tubes, irritant materials produced by a gas sterilization, hypotension, and bacterial infection. Careful studies by Cooper and me (1969a), as well as by Florange and his colleagues (1965), of autopsy specimens of patients who have

been on ventilators with inflated cuffs (Fig. 61–7), prospective studies of similar patients by Andrews and Pearson (1971), and analysis of surgically removed lesions caused by cuffs and experimental reproduction of these lesions under controlled conditions by Cooper and me (1969a, 1969b) point to pressure necrosis as the principal etiologic agent. As my associates and I (1971) showed, if standard Rusch cuffs are inflated just to provide a seal at ventilatory pressures of about 25 cm H_2O, intracuff pressures are 180 to 250 mm Hg. Carroll and associates (1969) noted that although these pressures are not exactly those exerted on the tracheal mucous membrane, high pressures are indeed exerted. The trachea has an ellip-

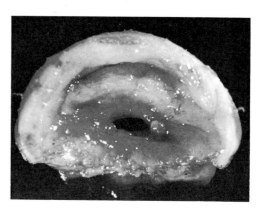

Fig. 61–6. Circumferential stenosis at cuff level. This surgical specimen shows the narrow size to which the lumen may be reduced before recognition of symptoms.

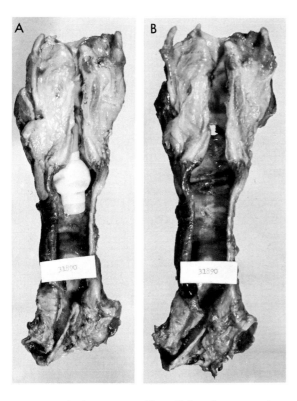

Fig. 61–7. Tracheal injury caused by cuffed tracheostomy tube. Autopsy specimen of larynx and trachea. *A*, Portex tracheostomy tube had been in place for 19 days. Not the dilatation of the trachea where the cuff had been inflated. *B*, Inflammatory erosive changes have bared multiple cartilages. There is also a distal erosion caused by the tip of the tube. Similar injuries occur with metal or rubber tubes. (Grillo, H.C.: Surgery of the trachea. *In* Current Problems in Surgery. Chicago, Year Book Medical Publishers, 1970.)

tical form, so it becomes deformed at the point where a seal is obtained. If perfusion pressures in the patient are lower than normal, necrosis can occur even more easily.

The mucosa overlying the cartilages is initially destroyed. The bared cartilages become necrotic and ultimately slough. Attempts at repair following full-thickness damage to the tracheal wall lead only to scar formation. Even further erosive damage can lead to tracheoesophageal fistula posteriorly or to perforation of the innominate artery anteriorly. Because the erosion is circumferential, the resultant strictures are also.

Patients with the aforementioned lesions develop symptoms and signs of airway obstruction consisting of dyspnea on exertion, stridor, cough, and obstructive episodes. Hemoptysis does not occur. In a few patients, pneumonia, sometimes bilateral, has been noted. On occasion, a patient while still intubated begins to develop obstruction from formation of granulations around the tip of the tube. In most instances, the obstruction appears only after extubation, because the tube splints a cuff stenosis or potential stomal stenosis as long as it remains in place. Any patient who develops symptoms of airway obstruction who has been intubated for 48 hours or more within the previous 2 years must be considered to have organic obstruction until proved otherwise. Many such patients have been treated for varying lengths of time

with the incorrect diagnosis of asthma. Such errors resulted from lack of awareness of these lesions and the fact that in most patients routine roentgenograms of the chest show normal lung fields.

Symptoms occurred in a few patients within 2 days of extubation; most demonstrated symptoms between 10 and 42 days after extubation, and few at greater intervals, usually within a few months. If a patient remains moderately sedentary while recovering from his original disease, the airway may shrink to a critical diameter of 4 to 5 mm before symptoms become obvious. At this aperture, fatal obstruction may occur at any time.

Although general improvement has occurred with design of large-volume cuffs, most of these cuffs can still produce tracheal injury if slightly overinflated beyond their resting maximal volume, because of their relatively inextensible materials. Stomal injuries continue to occur for the reasons described. Cricothyroidotomy may lead to severe subglottic injury.

DIAGNOSTIC STUDIES

Tracheal lesions often are recognized late despite a prolonged period of symptoms. As physicians become aware of the possibility of tracheal lesions, they will be increasingly suspicious of the diagnosis of adult-onset asthma. Appropriate roentgenographic examinations will be used increasingly to rule out the possibility of a tracheal lesion in any patient who has obstructive airway symptoms with roentgenographic demonstration of normal lung fields. Rarely, even specialized techniques will fail to reveal an unusual lesion, and bronchoscopic examination will be required.

Roentgenographic Examination of the Trachea

Roentgenographic studies of the trachea are used not only to rule in or out the presence of a tracheal lesion but also to define the location, extent, and sometimes the character of the lesion (Fig. 61–8). Further, these studies demonstrate the involvement ·of paratracheal structures by neoplastic lesions. I (1970) have found the following roentgenograms to be helpful.

Lateral films of the neck with the chin raised demonstrate most lesions of the upper half of the trachea. Careful technique shows the cartilaginous structures of the larynx as well as the trachea and the relationship of the trachea to the vertebral column posteriorly. If the patient has an existing tracheostomy stoma or has a tracheostomy scar, a radiopaque marker placed on the skin at this level helps to identifiy its relationship to inflammatory post-tracheostomy lesions. If a neoplastic lesion is present, a swallow of barium helps indicate any deformity of the tracheoesophageal septum or of the esophagus itself.

Anteroposterior views of the airway from larynx to carina, using a copper filter, provide a useful overall assessment.

Oblique views throw the tracheal air column into relief.

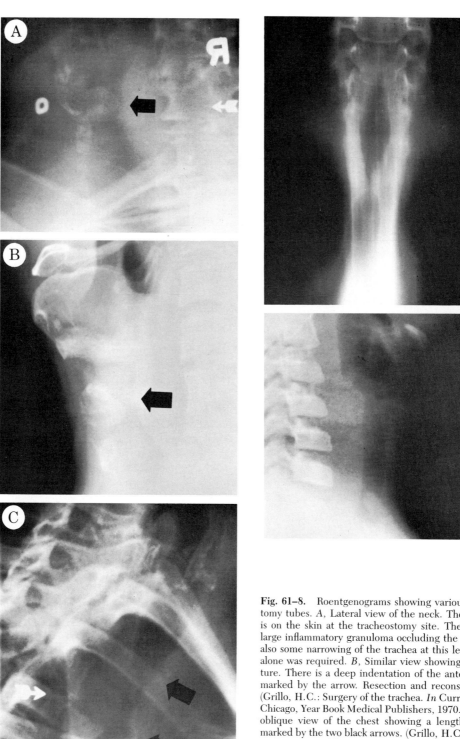

Fig. 61–8. Roentgenograms showing various injuries from tracheostomy tubes. *A,* Lateral view of the neck. The circular opaque marker is on the skin at the tracheostomy site. The black arrow points to a large inflammatory granuloma occluding the tracheal lumen. There is also some narrowing of the trachea at this level. Endoscopic removal alone was required. *B,* Similar view showing an anterior stomal stricture. There is a deep indentation of the anterior trachea at the level marked by the arrow. Resection and reconstruction were necessary. (Grillo, H.C.: Surgery of the trachea. *In* Current Problems in Surgery. Chicago, Year Book Medical Publishers, 1970.) *C,* Detail of left anterior oblique view of the chest showing a lengthy mid-tracheal stenosis marked by the two black arrows. (Grillo, H.C.: Surgery of the trachea. *In* Current Problems in Surgery. Chicago, Year Book Medical Publishers, 1970.) *D,* Laminogram showing the stenosis in Figure 61–8C. The upper narrowing is at the laryngeal level and is normal. *E,* Lateral neck view with hyperextension to demonstrate granuloma in a child's trachea at the level of the tube's tip. Ventilatory support without a cuff had been given following a cardiac operation in this child.

Fluoroscopy helps demonstrate malacia and clarify vocal cord function.

Tracheal laminograms help give precise measurement of the extent of lesions and their relative distances from landmarks such as the vocal cords and the carina. A magnifying effect occurs in the roentgenograms, but at the same time the trachea is somewhat foreshortened because of its oblique passage through the chest. It should be noted in viewing all roentgenograms, as well as during bronchoscopy, that the level of the vocal cords is not that of the lowermost portion of the larynx. There is approximately 1.5 to 2 cm of larynx between the vocal cords and the inferior border of the cricoid cartilage. Planning of operative procedures must take this into account.

Contrast studies of the trachea add little information except with tracheoesophageal fistula.

Computed tomography is valuable only in showing the mediastinal extent of a tumor. It is of little use in assessing benign stenosis.

If a patient with tracheal stenosis still has a tracheostomy tube in place, it must be removed during the roentgenographic examination to obtain useful information. Even if a tube has been in place for many months, it should be removed cautiously, with provision made for its immediate reinsertion. Emergency equipment including suctioning devices and a range of replacement tubes should be available. The physician must be competent to perform such intubation under slight difficulty. The airway often becomes nearly totally obstructed within 20 to 40 minutes following removal of such a tube. Occasionally, considerable force is required for reinsertion of an airway. Weber and I (1978a,b) described the roentgenographic findings in tracheal tumors and stenosis.

Bronchoscopy

Bronchoscopic examination is required, sooner or later, in all of these patients. When a lesion is known to be present, whether it is neoplastic or inflammatory, and when all else points to its surgical correctability, bronchoscopy is best deferred until preparations have been made for definitive treatment of the lesion. The trauma of bronchoscopy in a patient who is subtotally obstructed may precipitate complete obstruction. Little is lost by delaying the bronchoscopy until the time of definitive operation. Frozen sections are obtained for histologic diagnosis. In the presence of most obstructive lesions, the requirements for resection are clear at the outset. The bronchoscopy is done with the patient under general anesthesia, permitting unhurried, atraumatic examination and manipulation. Bronchoscopic examination and removal are all that is required in patients with polypoid granulomas at the stomal site or at the site of the tube tip. Esophagoscopy is also performed when neoplasms are examined. Rigid bronchoscopy, under general inhalation anesthesia, using pediatric bronchoscopes serially, is used to dilate severe stenosis for emergency relief. Urgent operation is almost never required. Obstructing tumors may similarly be relieved in an emergency situation or if time is needed to assess a patient, by "coring out" tumor tissue with the tip of the bronchoscope assisted with biopsy forceps. In thirty years I have never encountered dangerous bleeding or obstruction. The use of laser has been unnecessary.

Other Diagnostic Studies

Pulmonary function studies in patients with obstructing lesions of the trachea confirm a high degree of airway obstruction. Measurements are sometimes useful in clarifying the presence of parenchymal disease, and may alter the extent of the operative approach. Obstructing lesions generally require surgical relief.

Bacteriologic cultures are made of tracheal secretions and of tracheostomy wounds. Antibiotic sensitivities guide the prophylactic program for intraoperative protection. In the presence of neoplasms, the usual clinical and roentgenographic evidence of possible distant metastases is sought.

OPERATIVE VERSUS NONOPERATIVE TREATMENT

The goals of surgical treatment of tracheal lesions vary greatly in neoplastic and inflammatory lesions. With malignant neoplasm, the goal of surgical intervention is not only the relief from the obstruction but also possible cure. Irradiation alone usually results in recurrence of squamous cell carcinoma in 1 to 2 years and of adenoid cystic in 3 to 5 years. When it is used post resection where microscopic disease alone is present, numerous cases have apparently been cured. Laser therapy is only palliative in almost every case because the depth of tumor base would require full-thickness removal of the tracheal wall for cure. Because of the magnitude of surgical effort involved, I usually reserve resection of neoplasms for those patients who seem to have potentially curable lesions. This criterion excludes patients with massive involvement of the mediastinum or with distant metastases. Because of the long clinical course of adenoid cystic carcinoma, resection of an obstructing tracheal lesion may be justified in the presence of limited pulmonary metastases.

Such cases are few and, unfortunately, treatment is so widely diffused that prospective study is difficult to accomplish in statistically meaningful terms, except very slowly. If the lesion is frankly out of bounds, I have used palliative irradiation. Both squamous cell and adenoid cystic carcinomas may respond. In a few situations in which the obstructive element was severe and the lesion extensive, although not necessarily incurable, radical destructive surgery rather than reconstructive surgery has been applied. Thus, when the larynx is also involved, a laryngotrachectomy is performed, sometimes with partial esophageal removal.

The perferred treatment of benign obstruction of the trachea is resection and reconstruction when the patient can tolerate it. With careful evaluation, planning, and execution, most patients with lesions such as tracheal stenosis can be successfully treated operatively when they have recovered from the primary disease that led to the stenosis. Nonoperative methods of temporizing are, however, available. When the disease is not malignant, undue risks must not be taken. Rarely, the medical condition may not permit even the relatively benign procedure required. If the patient has serious neurologic or psychiatric deficits that will prevent cooperation in the postoperative phase, reconstruction is best deferred. The patient and his anesthesia must be selected to avoid the need for ventilatory support postoperatively. If ventilatory support is needed postoperatively in a shortened trachea, the cuff will probably rest against the anastomosis and may lead to dehiscence.

The temporizing methods available are repetitive bronchoscopic dilatation of a stenosis or reinstitution of a tracheostomy, dilatation of the stricture, and passage of a tracheostomy tube or a silicone T-tube through the lesion to splint the airway. Lesions in the immediate supracarinal position are not easily managed in this way. A tube long enough to remain seated often causes episodes of obstruction when it is near the carina, and a T-Y tube may lead to bronchial granulations.

Repeated dilatation and splinting have been proposed as definitive methods for treating tracheal stenosis. In most severe lesions in which the whole thickness of the tracheal wall has been converted to scar tissue, even prolonged stenting for many years will not lead to permanent recovery. Numerous patients have been treated this way. Despite repeated trials, it has been impossible, with only rare exceptions, to remove the splinting tube. When lesser degrees of damage have occurred, either in the completeness of a stricture of the circumference of the trachea or in the depth of the trachea, a period of prolonged splinting, on occasion, may result in an adequate airway after removal of the splint. Such a result has been reported in children. Toty (1987) pointed out that laser treatment can only lead to cure in granuloma—also easily removed by bronchoscopy—and thin, web-like stenosis. Such lesions are rare. In the usual postintubation stenosis, definitive opening would lead to tracheal perforation. The principal effect of the laser in these lesions has been to delay definitive treatment.

Prevention of Tracheal Stenosis

The incidence of stenosis at the stomal level can be reduced by careful placement of the stoma, avoidance of large apertures, elimination of heavy and prying ventilatory connecting equipment, and meticulous care of the tracheostomy.

Many proposals have been made to reduce the heretofore inevitable occurrence of some stenoses at the cuff level. These methods have included use of double-cuff tubes, changes in materials and sterilization techniques, attempts to avoid cuffs altogether, use of disc and sponge seals instead of cuffs, use of spacers to relocate the cuff level periodically, and prestretching of plastic cuffs. The only promising methods, accepting the present need for cuffs in management of adult patients in severe respiratory failure, have been intermittent inflation of cuffs cycled to the respirator, described by Arens and his col-

leagues (1969), and the development of large-volume, low pressure cuffs that conform to the shape of the trachea rather than deforming it, suggested by Cooper and me (1969b) and by me and my co-workers (1971) (Fig. 61–9). Such a cuff provided a seal at intracuff pressures of 33 mm Hg compared with 270 mm Hg in a comparative Rusch standard cuff. Thus, in a series of 45 patients in whom such a cuff was compared, on a randomized basis, with standard cuffs, 25 patiens with the soft cuff showed half as much damage—scaled on the basis of endoscopic observations at the time of deflation of the cuff—as 20 patients with standard cuffs. All severe damage was in the standard group. Incidence of cuff stenosis has dropped markedly as equipment has improved but low pressure cuffs must be inflated carefully to avoid converting them to high pressure cuffs.

I believe that cricothyroidostomy should be avoided. Although laryngeal injury is rare, it may not be correctible when it occurs. Tracheal injuries—also rare—are reparable when they *first* occur. Inappropriate treatment has served to make some incorrectible.

RESULTS OF TREATMENT

Most of the reported results of tracheal surgery in both benign and malignant disease are of isolated patients or of small groups of patients. This applies as much to nonprosthetic approaches as to use of prostheses. With the development of improved techniques of anatomic mobilization and direct anastomosis, and with the increasing incidence of benign disease consequent to current respiratory therapy, greater numbers of patients are being treated surgically for tracheal lesions.

Non-Neoplastic Disease

I reported (1979) 208 patients who underwent reconstruction for postintubation tracheal injury between 1965 and early 1979. Reconstruction was done for the following additional conditions: post-traumatic stenosis, ten; postsurgical stenosis, four; congenital, two; postburn stenosis, two; tuberculosis, two; stenosis caused by foreign body, one; and idiopathic stenosis, two. In seven patients, a cuffed tube was inserted to prevent aspiration and respirators were not used. Thirty-three of the referred patients had undergone prior reconstructive attempts or other previous major tracheal procedures.

One hundred thirteen had postintubation stenoses at the site of an inflatable cuff—twenty-three of whom had had only an endotracheal tube without subsequent tracheostomy. There were 78 stomal stenoses and 13 stomal and cuff stenoses, and in 4 the origin was uncertain.

Nine patients with tracheoesophageal fistula were corrected by the technique I reported with Moncure and McEnany (1976). One presented with tracheoinnominate cuff fistula. Corrective reconstructive surgery was effected through the cervical route alone in 126 of these patients, with the addition of an upper sternotomy in 83, through the transthoracic route in 6 and a skin tube replacement was constructed in one patient—a total of 216 operations in 208 patients.

A

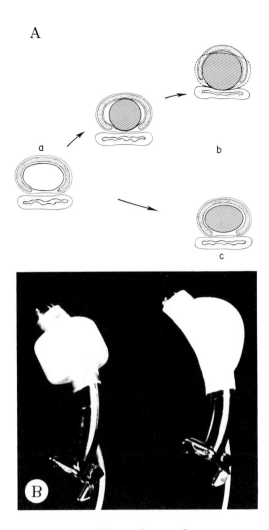

B

Fig. 61–9. *A,* Diagram of the mechanism of pressure necrosis by a tracheostomy cuff and its avoidance. (a) Normal elliptical shape of the trachea. When a conventional cuff is inflated, it may expand in circular fashion in its widest diameter but at this point fails to occlude the basically irregularly elliptical shape of the trachea. In (b) further distention has been required to effect a seal. At this point the trachea is deformed by the cuff and much of the considerable intracuff tension is transmitted to the tracheal wall. In (c) a large-volume low-pressure cuff has been inflated with a minimal amount of air. The cuff conforms to the irregular shape of the lumen and provides a seal at low intracuff pressures. Correspondingly low pressure are transmitted to the tracheal wall. *B,* Comparison of a standard cuff and a large-volume low-pressure cuff. On the left the large-volume cuff is shown spontaneously filled with air. No stretch has been placed on the rubber of the cuff wall at this point. The volume is sufficient to occlude most adult tracheas. On the right a Rusch cuff has been distended with 8 ml of air. It is tense and eccentric. The stretching of the rubber has created a hard structure that exerts considerable pressure on the trachea, which it must deform to provide a seal. (Grillo, H.C., et al.: J. Thorac. Cardiovasc. Surg. 62:898, 1971.)

In 168 of 203 patients followed, the results were good or excellent. An "excellent" result denotes an anatomically and functionally normal airway. The patient suffers no limitation whatsoever because of his airway, and on either roentgenographic or bronchoscopic examination, or both, essentially no narrowing is demonstrated at the anastomotic site. Patients classified as "good" have no functional difficulty whatsoever but may have a minimal anatomic narrowing that is definable on either roentgenographic study or bronchoscopic examination.

The results in 21 patients were classified as "satisfactory." These patients are able to carry out all of their normal daily activities but do have enough narrowing of their airway to limit major physical effort.

In nine patients the outcomes were listed as failures. Causes of failure included inadequate appreciation of existing neurologic dysphagia, cardiac decompensation requiring postoperative ventilation, unappreciated severe laryngeal dysfunction, and restenosis. Five deaths occurred. In four of the patients who died, reconstruction was contraindicated but undertaken because no therapeutic alternative existed. The other developed bilateral pneumonia and could not be weaned from postoperative need for respiratory support. I and my colleagues (1986) described the complications of tracheal surgery for both benign stenosis and neoplasms in detail.

Pre-existing laryngeal injuries, as I (1982) noted, demand careful evaluation and variations in technique of repair—48 patients required partial removal of the lower border of the cricoid for impinging stomal stenosis. In 18 the anterior subglottic larynx was resected and a plastic repair performed on the thyroid cartilage.

Pearson and Andrews (1971) reported 60 patients with tracheal stenosis seen at the Toronto General Hospital—in 34 the stenosis was at the stomal and in 26 at the cuff level. Thirty-seven segmental resections were performed. In 33 of the patients the results were good, in 1 fair. There was one failure and two operative deaths. Six of the patients developed significant restenosis, and reresection was performed with good results in all but one of the group. Laryngeal release was used as an adjunctive procedure in five of these patients.

Congenital stenosis of the trachea is seen as a "web" at the cricoid tracheal level or as a more extensive area of stenosis of the trachea between the cricoid and carina, involving a portion, a segment, or, on rare occasions, all of the trachea. It may take various forms such as a funnel beginning in the upper trachea with the narrowest point somewhere in midtrachea. Below this the trachea may be normal. A similar funnel may occur in the lower trachea. A segmental collar-like stenosis may involve a third or more of the trachea. This condition occurs in the lower trachea in association with a "pulmonary artery sling" in which the left pulmonary artery passes to the right of the trachea and then posterior to it before turning left.

In many of these anomalies, the tracheal cartilages may appear as completely circular rings at the points of stenosis. When such a segmental stenosis has formed developmentally in association with a pulmonary artery sling, division of the sling alone will not correct the stenosis. Only when the sling is exerting pressure on an otherwise normal trachea to produce a malacic compression will correction of the arterial anomaly lead to airway relief. In the presence of an accompanying stenosis, correction of the trachea should take precedence. Dilatation is not useful when circular rings are present because dilatation can lead only to splitting of these rings. In some instances, disorganization of the cartilages with various types of defects and branching is seen along with a tendency for these deformed rings to collapse. The presence of completely circular rings can be identified in most instances by careful observation with a magnifying bronchoscopic telescope. The mucosa may also occasionally be in valve-like folds with a stenotic segment. On rare occasions total agenesis of the trachea occurs in a living infant.

Infants with congenital tracheal stenosis are best managed conservatively, if possible. Ultimately surgical correction may be done with greater degrees of safey as the size of the airway and child increase. In acute situations a carefully placed tracheostomy may be the best option as I and Zannini (1984) suggested. Idriss and his colleagues (1984) described the use of a pericardial "gusset" for lengthy congenital stenosis.

Congenital tracheal malacia has often been alluded to but rarely documented.

Neoplasms

Primary tracheal tumors are rare. About one third are clearly beyond cure or surgical palliation when seen. In most instances, the reasons for incurability were either mediastinal invasion or pulmonary metastases. These patients were subjected to radiation therapy with variable results. If responsive, patients with squamous cell carcinoma obtained relief for 6 to 24 months. Prolonged palliation has resulted in patients with adenoid cystic carcinoma, but no true "cures."

I reported (1978) on 36 patients who underwent tracheal resection with primary reconstruction for tumor through 1977—34 had cylindrical or carinal reconstruction; 2 had "window" resections. Ten had squamous cell carcinoma, nine had adenoid cystic carcinoma, nine had other primary tracheal tumors, and eight had secondary tumors. Ten carinal resections were done with a variety of reconstructive techniques. In four patients laryngeal release proved useful. Five deaths occurred, three following carinal resection. Five patients with squamous cell carcinoma survived without disease—10 months to 13½ years. Six with adenoid cystic carcinoma were living from 1 to 15 years after resection. Postoperative irradiation was used in selected patients. Eight other patients were alive without known disease. Patients with secondary tumors, especially thyroid carcinoma, gained good palliation, and I and Zannini (1986) recorded a few probable cures.

Pearson and associates (1984) reported 9 of 12 patients who had complete resections for adenoid cystic carcinoma were alive from 1 to 20 years afterward and 4 of 6 with squamous cell carcinoma were alive. Eschapasse (1974) collected case histories of 152 patients with primary tracheal tumors treated by French and Soviet groups. Fifty resections with anastomosis were noted. Perelman and Koroleva (1987) reported 75 sleeve or carinal resections for primary tumors, with 5-year survival of 13% for squamous cell and 66% for adenoid cystic carcinoma.

The results of surgical extirpation and reconstruction of benign tracheal lesions make it clear that the techniques are safe and effective when carried out with extreme care. Late stenosis, a former *bête noir* of this type of surgical procedure, has not proved to be a problem. The rarity and dispersion of tracheal tumors make it impossible to delineate a therapeutic program cartegorically. However, the preceding data suggest the following: first, at least one third of primary tracheal cancers are resectable with potential for extirpation of the disease when the patient is first seen. All benign tumors should be removed. Second, reoperation when an initial procedure has been too conservative does not often lead to cure of a malignant tumor. Third, primary irradiation alone is unlikely to effect many cures. Postoperative irradiation, however, may well control microscopic residual disease. Fourth, there is a place for tracheal resection in selected patients with bronchial carcinoma (see Chapter 31) and thyroid cancer.

REFERENCES

Andrews, M.J., and Pearson, F.G.: The incidence and pathogenesis of tracheal injury following cuffed tube tracheostomy with assisted ventilation: an analysis of a two-year prospective study. Ann. Surg. *173*:249, 1971.

Arens, J.F., Ochsner, J.L., and Gee, G.: Volume-limited intermittent cuff inflation for long-term respiratory assistance. J. Thorac. Cardiovasc. Surg. *58*:837, 1969.

Carroll, R., Hedden, M., and Safar, P.: Intratracheal cuffs: performance characteristics. Anesthesia *31*:275, 1969.

Cooper, J.D., and Grillo, H.C.: The evolution of tracheal injury due to ventilatory assistance through cuffed tubes: a pathologic study. Ann. Surg. *169*:334, 1969a.

Cooper, J.D., and Grillo, H.C.: Experimental production and prevention of injury due to cuffed tracheal tubes. Surg. Gynecol. Obstet.*129*:1235, 1969b.

Deslauriers, J.: Involvement of the main carina. *In* International Trends in General Thoracic Surgery, Vol. 1. Edited by N. Delarue and H. Eschapasse. Philadelphia, W.B. Saunders Co., 1985, p. 139.

Eschapasse, H.: Les tumeurs trachéales primitives. Traitement Chirurgicale. Rev. Mal. Respir. *2*:425, 1974.

Florange, W., Muller, J., and Forster, E.: Morphologie de la nécrose trachéale après trachéotomie et ultilisation d'une prosthése respiratoire. Anesth. Analg. *22*:693, 1965.

Grillo, H.C.: The management of tracheal stenosis following assisted respiration. J. Thorac. Cardiovasc. Surg. *57*:52, 1969.

Grillo, H.C.: Surgery of the trachea. *In* Current Problems in Surgery. Chicago, Year Book Medical Publishers, 1970.

Grillo, H.C.: Tracheal tumors: surgical management. Ann. Thorac. Surg. *26*:112, 1978.

Grillo, H.C.: Surgical treatment of post-intubation tracheal injuries. J. Thorac. Cardiovasc. Surg. *78*:860, 1979.

Grillo, H.C.: Primary reconstruction of airway after resection of subglottic laryngeal and upper tracheal stenosis. Ann. Thorac. Surg. *33*:3, 1982.

Grillo, H.C., and Zannini, P.: Management of obstructive tracheal disease in children. J. Pediatr. Surg. *19*:414, 1984.

Grillo, H.C., and Zannini, P.: Resectional management of airway invasion by thyroid carcinoma. Ann. Thorac. Surg. *42*:287, 1986.

Grillo, H.C., et al.: A low pressure cuff for tracheostomy tubes to minimize tracheal injury: a comparative clinical trial. J. Thorac. Cardiovasc. Surg. 62:898, 1971.

Grillo, H.C., Moncure, A.C., and McEnany, M.T.: Repair of inflammatory tracheo-esophageal fistula. Ann. Thorac. Surg. 22:112, 1976.

Grillo, H.C., Zannini, P., and Michelassi, F.: Complications of tracheal reconstruction. J. Thorac. Cardiovasc. Surg. 91:322, 1986.

Hajdu, S.I., et al.: Carcinoma of the trachea. Clinicopathological study of 41 cases. Cancer 25:1448, 1970.

Houston, H.E., et al.: Primary cancers of the trachea. Arch. Surg. 99:132, 1969.

Idriss, F.S., et al.: Tracheoplasty with pericardial patch for extensive tracheal stenosis in infants and children. J. Thorac. Cardiovasc. Surg. 88:527, 1984.

Katlic, M.R., Grillo, H.C., and Wang, C.A.: Substernal goiter: analysis of 80 Massachusetts General Hospital cases. Am. J. Surg. 149:283, 1985.

Lindholm, C.E.: Prolonged endotracheal intubation. Acta Anaesth. Scand. 33(Suppl):1, 1970.

Mathisen, D.J., and Grillo, H.C.: Laryngotracheal trauma. Ann. Thorac. Surg. 43:254, 1987.

Montgomery, W.W.: The surgical management of supraglottic and subglottic stenosis. Ann. Otol. 77:534, 1968.

Pearson, F.G., and Andrews, M.J.: Detection and management of tracheal stenosis following cuffed tube tracheostomy. Ann. Thorac. Surg. 12:359, 1971.

Pearson, F.G., Todd, T.R.J., and Cooper, J.D.: Experience with primary neoplasms of the trachea and carina. J. Thorac. Cardiovasc. Surg. 88:511, 1984.

Perelman, M.I., and Koroleva, N.S.: Primary tumors of the trachea. In International Trends in General Thoracic Surgery, Vol. 2. Edited by H.C. Grillo and H. Eschapasse. Philadelphia, W.B. Saunders Co., 1987, p. 91.

Toty, L., et al.: Laser treatment of postintubation lesions. In International Trends in General Thoracic Surgery, Vol. 2. Edited by H.C. Grillo and H. Eschapasse. Philadelphia, W.B. Saunders Co., 1987, p. 31.

Weber, A.L., and Grillo, H.C.: Tracheal tumors: A radiological, clinical and pathological evaluation of 84 cases. Radiol. Clin. North Am. 16:227, 1978a.

Weber, A.L., and Grillo, H.C.: Tracheal stenosis: An analysis of 151 cases. Radiol. Clin. North Am. 16:291, 1978b.

SECTION 14

The Lung

CHAPTER 62

CONGENITAL LESIONS OF THE LUNG

Marleta Reynolds

Most congenital lesions of the lung are recognized when respiratory symptoms develop in the newborn or infant. Some are identified in the asymptomatic child on an incidental roentgenogram of the chest. The remainder are diagnosed in the older child during evaluation for a respiratory infection. In an infant with severe respiratory distress, knowledge of the pathology and the ability to make a quick and accurate diagnosis based on a roentgenogram of the chest may be critical. In the past, arteriography and bronchography were the additional diagnostic studies of choice when time permitted, but now ultrasound and computed tomography allow greater diagnostic accuracy.

TRACHEAL AGENESIS AND ATRESIA

Tracheal agenesis or atresia leads to fatal respiratory distress at birth. Maternal polyhydramnios is often associated, and the birth may be premature. Babies with tracheal atresia have an audible cry, and the larynx is normal at laryngoscopy. Intubation beyond the vocal cords is impossible and immediate tracheostomy is lifesaving. Two of three babies with tracheal atresia reported by Sankran and associates (1983) were alive at 15 months of age. Each baby had a normal-sized lower trachea and normal bronchi, an esophageal atresia, and distal tracheoesophageal fistula.

Complete tracheal agenesis has been reported in more than 50 infants. There are usually multiple associated anomalies, especially of the remainder of the tracheobronchial tree. Cyanotic at birth, infants with tracheal agenesis improve with bag and mask ventilation. At laryngoscopy the larynx is normal, but intubation is not possible. Esophageal intubation and ventilation provide temporary airway access through a communication between the bronchi and the esophagus. No long-term survivors have been reported although a wide variety of procedures have been attempted. Evans (1985) and Milstein (1985) and their associates reviewed the available literature and categorized the associated malformations.

BRONCHIAL ANOMALIES

Abnormal bronchial development may result in complete bronchial atresia, an aberrant origin of a main stem or segmental bronchus from the trachea, or the abnormal communication of the bronchus with another foregut derivative. Structural abnormalities of a bronchus may lead to lobar emphysema (Fig. 62–1).

Tracheal Bronchus and Diverticulum

A tracheal diverticulum may arise from the cervical or thoracic portion of the trachea and end blindly or in a rudimentary lung. The diverticulum resembles a bronchus. If the bronchial structure connects to a normal

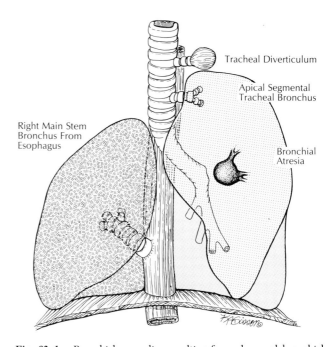

Fig. 62–1. Bronchial anomalies resulting from abnormal bronchial development. Symptoms result from bronchial obstruction and pulmonary infection. From Luck, S.R., et al.: Congenital bronchopulmonary malformations. Curr. Probl. Surg. 23:251, 1986. Used by permission.

segment or lobe of lung, it is referred to as a tracheal bronchus. The accessory lung has normal pulmonary arterial and venous supply. Symptoms may result from stenosis of the tracheal bronchus or from other associated pulmonary anomalies. A roentgenogram of the chest obtained because of recurrent pneumonia, stridor, or newborn respiratory distress reveals the portion of lung involved (Fig. 62–2). At bronchoscopy, the tracheal bronchus can be seen and a bronchogram demonstrates any intrinsic pathology of the tracheal bronchus. Surgical resection of the tracheal bronchus and adjoining lung tissue is only necessary when it is clinically indicated (Fig. 62–3). McLaughlin and colleagues (1985) reported 18 children with treacheal bronchi who presented with recurrent pneumonia and other respiratory symptoms. Bronchography revealed bronchial stenosis and bronchiectasis of the involved lung segment in five. Their symptoms were relieved by surgical resection.

Bronchial Atresia

An atretic bronchus ends blindly in lung tissue. At birth the portion of lung adjacent to the atretic bronchus is fluid-filled. The fluid is soon reabsorbed and replaced by air from the adjacent lung tissue through the pores of Kohn. Eventually, retained secretions result in a mucocele. Compression of adjacent normal bronchial structures leads to emphysematous change in the lung. Symptoms of wheezing and stridor may develop, and there is significant risk of pulmonary infection. A roentgenogram of the chest shows a hilar mass with radiating solid channels surrounded by hyperaerated lung. Computed tomography can differentiate the centrally placed cystic mucocele characteristic of bronchial atresia from a bronchogenic cyst or lobar emphysema. Resection is indicated to prevent pulmonary sepsis. Haller and colleagues (1980) observed for nine years a child with mild symptoms who had bronchial atresia and the associated lobar emphysema. Progressive respiratory symptoms even-

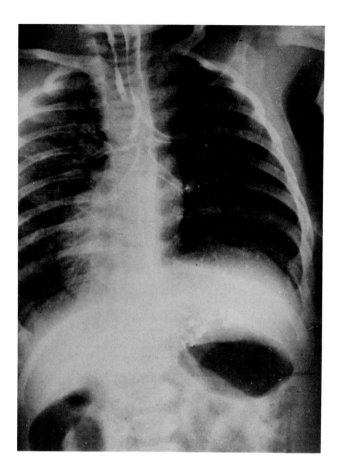

Fig. 62–3. Bilateral tracheal bronchi in a child being evaluated for chronic cough. Conservative treatment was recommended. From Holinger, P.H.: Abnormalities of the larynx and tracheobronchial tree. Swenson's Pediatric Surgery, 3rd ed. Edited by O. Swenson. New York, Appleton-Century-Crofts, 1969, p. 297. Used by permission.

tually prompted resection of the involved segment. The report documents the natural history of the lesion and further supports timely resection.

Anomalous Bronchi

The most common communication between the trachea or bronchus and another foregut derivative is a tracheoesophageal fistula. Other anomalous connections are rare. Since 1950, three infants from my institution who had an esophageal bronchus were reported by Gans and Potts (1951) and by Nikaidoh and Swenson (1971). All presented with respiratory distress and pneumonia and were found by esophagogram to have a portion of lung communicating with the esophagus through a bronchial structure.

The anomalous origin of a lobar or segmental bronchus from the esophagus—"esophageal bronchus"—may be right- or left-sided and may involve the upper or lower lobes. The vascular supply to the involved lobe varies; some lobes have a normal pulmonary vascular pattern and others a systemic supply. Extralobar and intralobar sequestrations—identified by the anomalous blood supply and absence of bronchial communication—occasionally communicate with the esophagus or other foregut

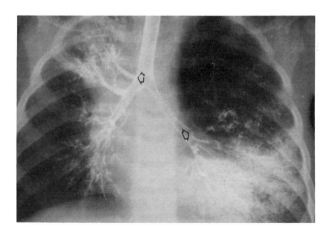

Fig. 62–2. Incidental tracheal bronchus. The patient, a 3-year-old with a history of wheezing, also had an obstructed left upper lobe apical bronchus and emphysema of the left upper lobe. Left upper lobectomy was curative. Congenital malformations of the lung. From Swenson's Pediatric Surgery, 4th ed. Edited by J.G. Raffensperger. New York, Appleton-Century-Crofts, 1980, p. 700. Used by permission.

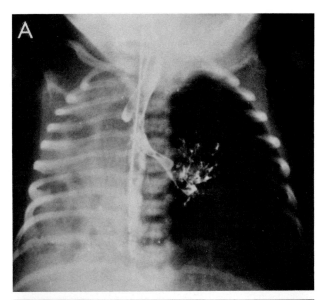

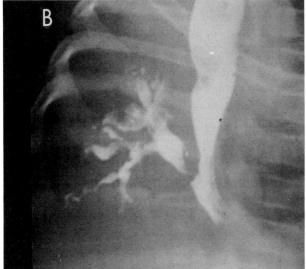

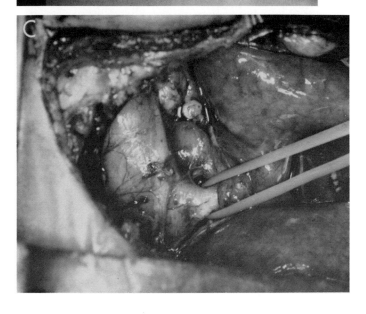

Fig. 62–4. *A*, Atretic right bronchus in a 1-month-old girl who presented with respiratory distress, cough, and fever. *B*, The esophagogram outlines the right bronchus and lung. *C*, At surgery the right esophageal bronchus is identified. A right pneumonectomy was performed. She has had significant morbidity in the four years since surgery. Congenital malformations of the lung. From Swenson's Pediatric Surgery, 4rd ed. Edited by J.G. Raffensperger. New York, Appleton-Century-Crofts, 1980, p. 702. Used by permission.

derivatives. Confusion over terminology has prompted some authors to refer to all of these anomalies as congenital bronchopulmonary foregut malformations.

A persistent or recurrent pneumonia in an infant or child may be caused by the bronchial communication with the esophagus. An esophagogram outlines the esophageal bronchus (Fig. 62–4). Resection of the chronically infected portion of the lung is indicated.

Bronchial Stenosis

A true congenital bronchial stenosis is rare. Bronchial stenosis is seen most often in the right main stem bronchus secondary to inflammatory changes following improper and frequent suctioning of an infant on prolonged ventilatory support. Granulation tissue builds up at the main stem orifice. The lung distal to the obstruction becomes chronically infected or emphysematous (Fig. 62–5). Repeated bronchial dilatations may be necessary to restore normal lung function and treat the infection. Bronchoplastic procedures may reduce the need for pulmonary resection when the chronic infection does not resolve following attempts at bronchial dilatation.

Bronchobiliary Fistula

The most uncommon bronchopulmonary malformation is the bronchobiliary fistula. The six cases reported in the world literature were reviewed by Sane and his colleagues (1971). All infants presented with respiratory distress. Bile-stained sputum led to bronchoscopy and bronchography. The fistula usually joined the right main stem bronchi near the carina. Division of the fistula should be curative.

CONGENITAL LOBAR EMPHYSEMA

Congenital lobar emphysema refers to the isolated hyperinflation of a lobe in the absence of an extrinsic bronchial obstruction. The left upper lobe is involved most often, followed in incidence by involvement of the right middle lobe. Boland and colleagues (1956) found hypoplastic cartilage in the bronchus of two of seven patients with lobar emphysema. Lincoln and associates (1971) described hypoplastic or absent cartilage in 22 of 28 examples reviewed. A series collected by Scarpelli and Auld (1978) reported a 25% incidence of dysplasia of the bronchial cartilage. Stovin (1959) reported abnormal orientation and distribution of the bronchial cartilage in his series of patients.

A subset of lobar emphysema is the "polyalveolar lobe" first described by Hislop and Reid (1970). In an infant with classic congenital lobar emphysema they found an increase in the number of alveoli within the affected lobe. A subsequent report by Tapper and associates (1980) reevaluated a group of infants with congenital lobar emphysema and found that 6 of 16 had the abnormal characteristics of the polyalveolar lobe.

Lobar emphysema produces symptoms in infancy. There is often a history of tachypnea, retraction of the chest wall, and wheezing since birth. An upper respiratory infection may complicate the condition and precipitate severe respiratory distress. Most children with lobar emphysema present before 6 months of age. Some infants develop symptoms in the first few days of life and require urgent intervention. Physical examination reveals a shift of the trachea and mediastinum to the contralateral hemithorax. Breath sounds are decreased on the affected side, with associated hyperresonance. Roentgenograms of the chest show hyperaeration of the affected lobe with atelectasis of the adjacent lobes and a mediastinal shift (Fig. 62–6). Careful inspection of vascular markings reduces the risk of misdiagnosis of this lesion as a tension pneumothorax.

In a newborn with severe respiratory distress, a roentgenogram of the chest is the only preoperative study that is indicated. In an infant with moderate respiratory distress, computed tomography helps rule out a perihilar bronchogenic cyst. A subcarinal mass usually affects an entire lung rather than a single lobe which is affected in congenital emphysema.

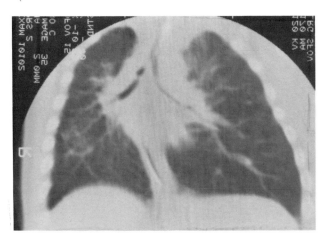

Fig. 62–5. Recurrent right upper lobe and entire right lung atelectasis in an infant with hyaline membrane disease who required prolonged intubation and ventilation. The right main stem bronchus was stenotic. Repeated dilatations have been palliative. This CT scan was obtained to clarify distal anatomy or identify other pathology. There are two areas of significant stenosis in the right main stem bronchus.

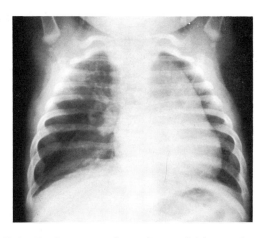

Fig. 62–6. Roentgenogram of a newborn with lobar emphysema involving the right middle lobe. Note the compressed right lower lobe and mediastinal shift.

At operation, the chest is opened as soon as possible after induction of anesthesia. Positive pressure ventilation causes further overinflation of the involved lobe and increases the risk of cardiovascular compromise. The abnormal lobe usually herniates through the thoracotomy incision. The lobe feels like sponge rubber, does not deflate, and bounces back into shape after it is compressed. Its edges are rounded and poorly defined. The remaining lung is atelectatic. Before resection, the mediastinum must be carefully examined for lesions that could have obstructed the bronchus. After lobectomy, the remaining lung expands to fill the chest. The emphysematous lobe characteristically does not deflate, even after it is removed from the chest.

Infants with hyaline membrane disease who require prolonged mechanical ventilation may develop acquired lobar emphysema (Fig. 62–7). The right lower lobe is most frequently affected. Suction trauma may cause squamous metaplasia of the bronchial orifice, and repeated barotrauma contributes to the ruptured alveoli and emphysematous changes. Radionucleotide scans demonstrate poor perfusion of the affected lobe. Cooney and colleagues (1977) recommended lobectomy when the infant cannot be weaned from the ventilator because of the acquired emphysematous lobe.

In older infants with a history of respiratory problems, computed tomography may help identify other causes of acquired lobar emphysema such as extrinsic bronchial compression from enlarged lymph nodes, a bronchogenic cyst, or anomalous blood vessels. In an older child with an acute onset of symptoms, bronchoscopy is indicated to rule out an aspirated foreign body or an endobronchial mass. The bronchoscopy should be planned to immediately precede thoracotomy. Oxygen, antibiotics, and humidity are administered prophylactically.

PULMONARY DYSPLASIA

Pulmonary Agenesis and Aplasia

Unilateral pulmonary agenesis results from lack of development of a single lung bud. Lung parenchyma and pulmonary vessels are lacking. Sbokes and McMillan (1977) reported a 50% incidence of associated cardiac disease, especially when the agenesis was on the right side.

A newborn with unilateral pulmonary agenesis may be asymptomatic or present with tachypnea, dyspnea, and cyanosis. Older infants or children may present with wheezing that suggests asthma or bronchitis. On physical examination, the trachea and mediastinal structures are shifted to the involved side. The overall shape of the chest is normal. Signs of airway obstruction and poor bronchial drainage may be recognizable. A roentgenogram of the chest reveals absence of lung markings and mediastinal shift to the ipsilateral side (Fig. 62–8). The differential diagnosis includes total lung atelectasis, total lung sequestration, or lung with an esophageal bronchus. The normal position of the diaphragm and normal intercostal spaces precludes atelectasis. An esophagogram

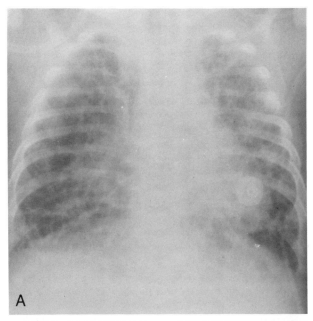

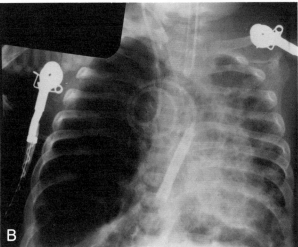

Fig. 62–7. *A,* Roentgenogram of the chest of a 2-month-old infant with bronchopulmonary dysplasia. *B,* Within three months lobar emphysema developed in his right lower lobe. Further mediastinal shift and increasing ventilator requirements prompted lobectomy.

and computed tomography exclude the other possibilities. Echocardiography helps in diagnosing the associated cardiac lesions. There is no particular treatment for pulmonary agenesis, but correction of the cardiac anomaly may relieve some of the symptoms. Massuni and associates (1966) reported that 30% of infants with agenesis die in the first year of life and 50% within the first 5 years. The mortality was higher with right-sided agenesis. Maltz and Nadas (1968) reviewed the world literature and found 164 cases of pulmonary agenesis. Of the 36 patients reported by 1954, 24 were alive in 1968.

Bilateral pulmonary agenesis is incompatible with life although Claireaux and Ferreira (1958) reported one infant who survived 15 minutes. The trachea ends blindly

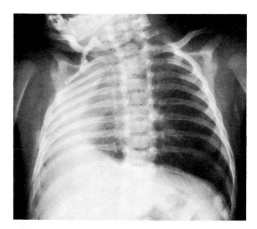

Fig. 62–8. Roentgenogram of the chest of a newborn with respiratory distress and agenesis of the right lung. There is marked mediastinal shift to the ipsilateral side.

or into primitive lung tissue. The incidence of associated anomalies is high.

Pulmonary aplasia is similar to pulmonary agenesis in that pulmonary parenchyma and vessels are absent. The blind bronchial stump may serve as a source of repeated infection in the normal contralateral lung. The stump may be identified by bronchoscopy or computed tomography. Once recognized, the chronically infected stump should be resected (Fig. 62–9).

Primary Pulmonary Hypoplasia

Pulmonary hypoplasia can be identified pathologically by the radial alveolar count and the lung-weight-to-body-weight ratio. Pulmonary hypoplasia is primary if no obvious cause for the hypoplasia can be found. Swischuk and associates (1979) reported that four of eight infants with primary pulmonary hypoplasia had mean radial alveolar counts lower than normal and thickening of the pulmonary arteriolar wall. The hypertrophy of the muscular layer of the pulmonary arteriole develops in response to fetal stress. This hypertrophy is frequently found in infants with pulmonary hypoplsia and other causes for pulmonary hypertension. Haworth and Hislop (1981) suggested that the normal postnatal regression of the pulmonary arteriolar muscle does not occur.

Primary pulmonary hypoplasia produces symptoms immediately after birth. An infant develops severe respiratory distress often unresponsive to supplemental oxygen. A roentgenogram of the chest demonstrates small lungs and the absence of other causes for respiratory distress. The thickened pulmonary arterioles predispose the infant to an exaggerated response to hypoxemia, acidosis, and hypercarbia. Therapy is aimed at lowering the pulmonary vascular resistance and reversing the inevitable persistent fetal circulation. Right-to-left shunting of blood occurs at three levels: across the patent foramen ovale, across the patent ductus arteriosus, and within the pulmonary capillary bed. Six of the eight infants reported by Swischuk and associates (1979) died despite aggressive management.

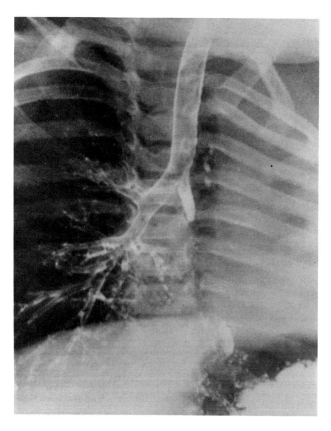

Fig. 62–9. The blind bronchial stump of pulmonary aplasia. Retained secretions in the stump lead to recurrent pulmonary infections. In this setting, bronchography has been replaced by computed tomography and bronchoscopy. From Holinger, P.H.: Abnormalities of the larynx and tracheobronchial tree. Swenson's Pediatric Surgery, 3rd ed. Edited by O. Swenson. New York, Appleton-Century-Crofts, 1969, p. 298. Used by permission.

Secondary Pulmonary Hypoplasia

Secondary pulmonary hypoplasia is associated with various fetal and maternal abnormalities (Table 62–1). One of the most common is Potter's syndrome, in which bilateral renal agenesis results in oligohydramnios and compression of the developing fetus by the uterus. The fetus's face is distorted and the chest is bell-shaped. The lungs' volume is smaller with a decrease in the number of airway generations and alveoli (Fig. 62–10). The alveoli and pulmonary aterioles are smaller than normal. Other conditions that result in oligohydramnios—amniotic fluid leaks and renal dysplasias—are also associated with pulmonary hypoplasia.

Neurologic or musculoskeletal conditions that depress fetal respiratory movements are associated with hypoplastic lungs. Vilos and associates (1984) observed the fetus of a woman with myotonic dystrophy with ultrasound; the fetus had no respiratory movements, and the lungs were hypoplastic at birth. Wigglesworth and Desai (1979) reported that in experimental animals, the in-utero transection of the spinal cord and the resulting inability of the animal to make respiratory movements result in significant pulmonary hypoplasia.

Infants who have congenital bony dysplasias may also

Table 62–1. Conditions Associated With Secondary Pulmonary Hypoplasia

Oligohydramnios
   Potter's syndrome (bilateral renal agenesis)
   Renal dysplasias
   Amniotic fluid leak

Bone dysplasias with a small or rigid chest wall
   Achondroplasia
   Chrondrodystrophia fetalis calcificans
   Spondyloepiphyseal dysplasia
   Osteogenesis imperfecta
   Thanatophoric dwarfism
   Neonatal hypophosphatemia

Decreased fetal respiratory movements
   Congenital arthrogryposis multiplex congenita
   Camptodactyly and multiple ankylosis syndrome
   Congenital myotonic dystrophy
   Asphyxiating thoracic dystrophy

Diaphragmatic elevation
   Membranous diaphragm
   Abdominal mass or ascites
   Phrenic nerve agenesis

Intrathoracic space-occupying lesions
   Congenital diaphragmatic hernia
   Congenital cystic adenomatoid malformation
   Mediastinal neoplasms and cystic hygroma
   Enteric cysts (esophageal duplication)

Pulmonary vascular anomalies
   Pulmonary artery agenesis
   Scimitar syndrome

Miscellaneous
   Omphalocele
   Down's syndrome
   Rhesus isoimmunization of the fetus

Reproduced with permission from Luck, S.R., et al.: Congenital bronchopulmonary malformations. Curr. Probl. Surg. 23:251, 1986.

have small and rigid chests and associated hypoplastic lungs; thanatophoric dwarfism is a good example. Most of these infants die from respiratory problems (Fig. 62–11). Jeune's syndrome, a familial chondrodystrophy, is also called asphyxiating thoracic dystrophy. These infants' chests are small and rigid and the lungs hypoplastic (Fig. 62–12). Futile attempts at chest reconstruction have been made, but survival has not been reported.

The developing lungs can also be affected by the abnormal development or function of the diaphragm. Phrenic nerve agenesis results in poor diaphragmatic muscle development and pulmonary hypoplasia. Infants with large abdominal masses or ascites have restricted lung development because of the elevation of the diaphragm. Hershenson and associates (1985) evaluated the chest size in infants with giant omphaloceles and found them significantly decreased compared to controls. Many of the infants in their series had prolonged respiratory insufficiency, and autopsy study of one infant confirmed the presence of pulmonary hypoplasia.

The most common cause of secondary pulmonary hypoplasia is a congenital diaphragmatic hernia (see Chapter 53). The herniated viscera physically restricts lung growth on the ipsilateral side. In addition, shift of me-

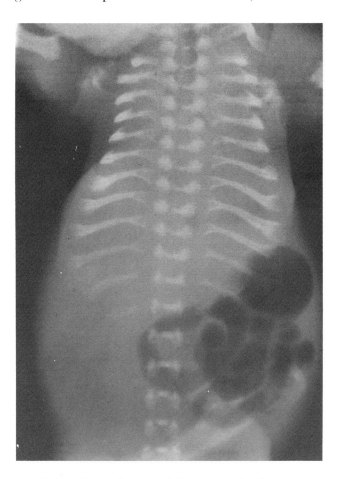

Fig. 62–11. Thanatophoric dwarf. Normal lung development is restricted by the size of the chest. From Luck, S.R., et al.: Congenital bronchopulmonary malformations. Curr. Probl. Surg. 23:251, 1986. Used by permission.

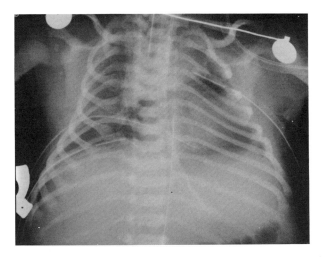

Fig. 62–10. Potter's syndrome with secondary pulmonary hypoplasia. The chest is bell-shaped. Chest tubes have been inserted to manage pneumothoraces resulting from barotrauma. From Luck, S.R., et al.: Congenital bronchopulmonary malformations. Curr. Probl. Surg. 23:251, 1986. Used by permission.

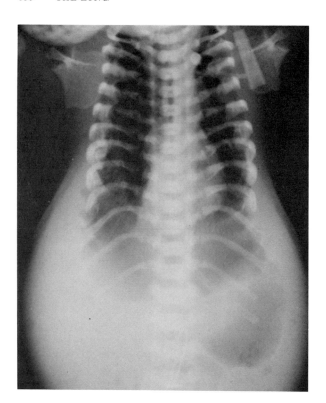

Fig. 62–12. Jeune's syndrome or asphyxiating thoracic dystrophy. The size and shape of the chest precludes normal lung development. From Luck, S.R., et al.: Congenital bronchopulmonary malformations. Curr. Probl. Surg. *23*:251, 1986. Used by permission.

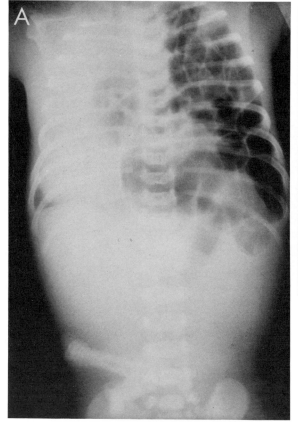

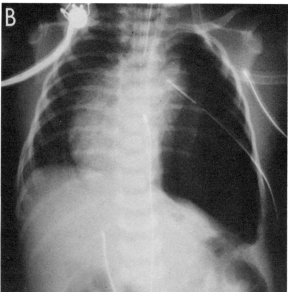

Fig. 62–13. Congenital diaphragmatic hernia. *A*, The left chest is filled with intestines and the mediastinum is shifted to the contralateral side. The abdomen lacks normal intestinal gas pattern. *B*, After surgical repair of the hernia, the severely hypoplastic ipsilateral lung is identified. The contralateral lung is also hypoplastic. From Luck, S.R., et al.: Congenital bronchopulmonary malformations. Curr. Probl. Surg. *23*:251, 1986. Used by permission.

diastinal structures results in contralateral pulmonary hypoplasia (Fig. 62–13). Kitagawa and associates (1971) reported that the lungs in infants with congenital diaphragmatic hernia had fewer airway generations, alveoli, and pulmonary arterioles. Clinical correlation with the autopsy findings demonstrates that the most severe respiratory failure was present in those infants in whom the muscularization of the pulmonary arterioles extended out from the preacinar arterioles into the interacinar arterioles. The high mortality rate associated with congenital diaphragmatic hernia is directly related to the pulmonary hypoplasia. High pulmonary vascular resistance and persistent fetal circulation are treated with high frequency ventilation, 100% oxygen, sedation, alkalinization, and vasodilators. Extracorporeal membrane oxygenation has been used successfully to save 50% of infants with congenital diaphragmatic hernia who would otherwise have succumbed to respiratory failure.

Some cases of secondary pulmonary hypoplasia cannot be readily explained. For instance, Cooney and Thurlbeck (1982) reported that Down's syndrome is associated with pulmonary hypoplasia. The autopsy study of seven children with Down's syndrome revealed hypoplastic lungs in six without evidence of congenital heart disease or other pulmonary anomalies. Chamberlain and colleagues (1977) found that infants with rhesus isoimmunization have associated pulmonary hypoplasia. Respiratory insufficiency is a frequent cause of death in these infants. The etiology and pathophysiology of the associated pulmonary hypoplasia is unknown.

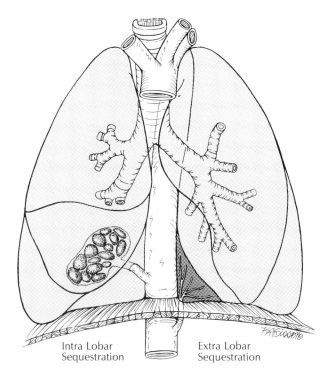

Intra Lobar
Sequestration

Extra Lobar
Sequestration

Fig. 62–14. Pulmonary sequestrations may be intralobar or extralobar. There are no bronchial communications and the arterial supply to the segment or lobe is systemic. From Luck, S.R., et al.: Congenital bronchopulmonary malformations. Curr. Probl. Surg. 23:251, 1986. Used by permission.

SEQUESTRATION

A pulmonary sequestration is a segment or lobe of lung tissue that has no bronchial communication with the normal tracheobronchial tree. The arterial blood supply is from a systemic vessel. The vessel often arises from the abdominal aorta and travels upward and penetrates the diaphragm to supply the sequestration. The venous return is usually through the pulmonary veins but may be to the systemic venous system. An extralobar sequestration is separate from the normal lung and has its own visceral pleura. An intralobar sequestration is situated within normal lung parenchyma (Fig. 62–14).

A sequestration probably arises from a lung bud that is pinched off from the caudal foregut with its own blood supply. Boyden (1958) proposed this theory after reviewing data collected from embryos. Further study by Iwai and associates (1973) corroborated these findings.

Extralobar Sequestration

An extralobar sequestration is triangular and usually located adjacent to the aorta or esophagus in the posterior costophrenic angle. It also may occur in other locations, such as the upper portion of the visceral compartment of the mediastinum. It is most often asymptomatic and found on an incidental roentgenogram of the chest. The inferiorly located ones may be associated with a congenital diaphragmatic hernia. Angiography used to be the diagnostic study of choice, but in most instances ultrasound and computed tomography can correctly identify this lesion (Fig. 62–15).

Intralobar Sequestration

Savic and associates (1979) reviewed a large series of sequestrations, and of 391 intralobar sequestrations 164 were in the right lower lobe and 227 were located in the left lower lobe. Only nine instances of sequestration occurred in the upper or middle lobes. In 96% of the sequestrations in this series, the venous return was to the pulmonary venous system.

Communication through the pores of Kohn may lead to chronic infection in the sequestered lobe. Children and young adults with recurrent left lower lobe pneumonia should be suspected of having an intralobar sequestration (Fig. 62–16). Infection can also lead to abscess formation and further cloud the diagnostic picture. In some children and adults, degenerative arteriosclerotic changes in the systemic artery supplying the sequestration may lead to hemoptysis. One of my patients presented with hemoptysis and an expanding lung mass. The systemic artery leading to the sequestration had become atherosclerotic and developed a false aneurysm within the sequestered lobe (Fig. 62–17). In the newborn, high flow through the systemic artery with normal pulmonary venous return may result in congestive heart failure.

Diagnosis in the newborn can often be made by ultrasound and in the child and young adult by computed tomography. Occasionally, angiography is indicated if a question exists regarding the exact diagnosis or the lo-

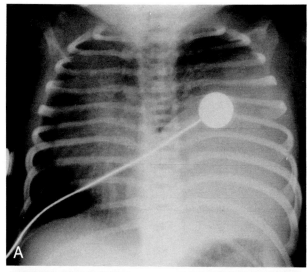

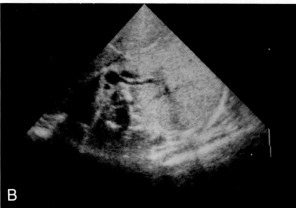

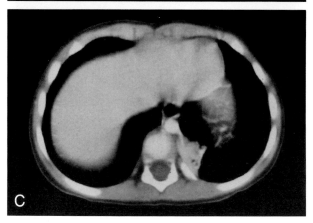

Fig. 62–15. *A*, Abnormal roentgenogram of the chest of a newborn with respiratory distress. *B*, Ultrasound identified the anomalous vessel coursing through the diaphragm and entering the sequestration. *C*, This CT scan clearly demonstrates the anomalous artery arising from the thoracic aorta and entering the sequestered lung.

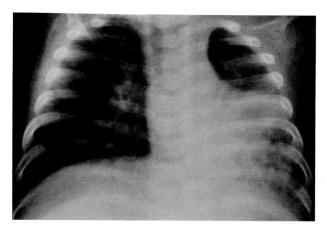

Fig. 62–16. A recurrent left lower pneumonia should suggest the possibility of an intralobar sequestration. From Luck, S.R., et al.: Congenital bronchopulmonary malformations. Curr. Probl. Surg. 23:251, 1986. Used by permission.

cation of the anomalous arterial or venous blood supply (Fig. 62–18). Bronchoscopy is not indicated.

Treatment consists of a segmental resection of the sequestration or at times a lobectomy when inflammatory changes prevent resection of the sequestered segment alone. Careful identification of the arterial supply and suture ligation is necessary. Harris and Lewis (1940) reported an attempted lobectomy in a 5-year-old that ended in exsanguinating hemorrhage when the systemic arterial supply was not recognized and divided before control was obtained. The venous return must also be identified before resection. Thilenius (1983) and Alivazatos (1985) and their colleagues reported pulmonary infarction following inadvertent ligation of the total venous return of the right lung during resection of a right lower lobe sequestration. Shermeta (personal communication, 1985) identified a similar anomaly and successfully re-anastomosed the pulmonary veins of the upper and middle lobe to the left atrium. Anomalous venous drainage of a single lobe or lobes of the right lung to the inferior vena cava below the diaphragm or to the right atrium is referred to as the "scimitar syndrome." This anomaly is discussed further in Chapter 64.

PARENCHYMAL PULMONARY LESIONS

Congenital parenchymal pulmonary lesions include isolated cystic lesions or diffuse cystic disease. Primary lymphangiectasia usually presents as diffuse cystic disease in infancy and is fatal. Other diffuse cystic disease is associated with various syndromes or diseases—Marfan's syndrome, interstitial fibrosis, histiocytosis, and Ehlers-Danlos syndrome. Surgical therapy is not indicated.

An isolated cystic lesion may be congenital or acquired, and differentiation between the two may be difficult. Careful review of all chest roentgenograms made since birth helps make the differentiation. Computed tomography is excellent at differentiating and identifying

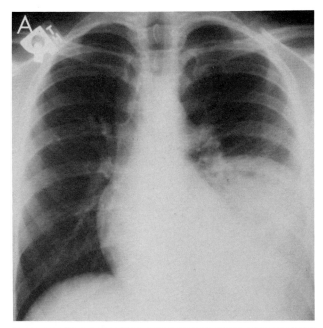

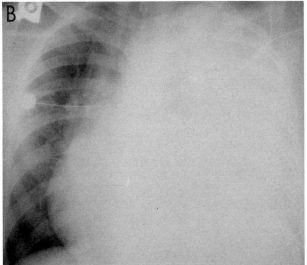

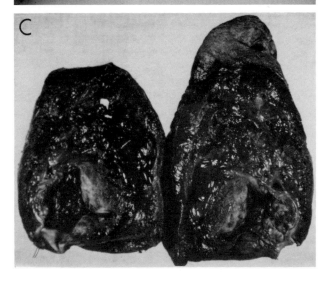

Fig. 62–17. *A*, This boy had had repeated right lower lobe pneumonia and presented at age 12 with hemoptysis and a consolidated right lower lobe. *B*, Rupture of the sequestration produced a massive hemothorax and shock. Emergency left lower lobectomy was performed. *C*, The pathologic specimen reveals an aneurysm of the atherosclerotic vessel arising from the aorta. From Luck, S.R., et al.: Congenital bronchopulmonary malformations. Curr. Probl. Surg. 23:251, 1986. Used by permission.

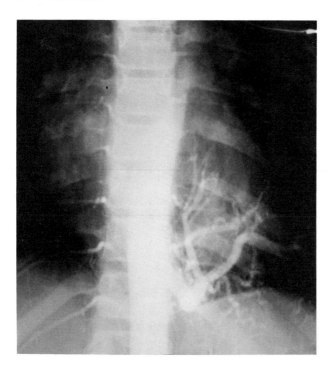

Fig. 62–18. This aortogram demonstrates the systemic arterial supply of an intralobar sequestration. Angiography is indicated if cumputed tomography does not accurately identify the lesion or if concomitant congenital heart disease is suspected. From Congenital malformations of the lung. Swenson's Pediatric Surgery, 4th ed. Edited by J.G. Raffensperger. New York, Appleton-Century-Crofts, 1980, p. 703. Used by permission.

a bronchogenic cyst or congenital cystic adenomatoid malformation from an isolated pulmonary cyst.

BRONCHOGENIC CYSTS

Bronchogenic cysts can be found in the hilum of the lung, the mediastinum (see Chapter 90), and the posterior sulcus and within the pulmonary parenchyma (Fig. 62–19). The cysts are lined with ciliated columnar or cuboidal epithelium on a fibromuscular base. Squamous metaplasia may replace the epithelial lining and when secondarily infected, the epithelium may be destroyed. The cyst walls are thin and may contain cartilage and bronchial glands. The cysts are usually single, but may be multilocular or multiple. The lower lobes are most commonly involved with parenchymal bronchogenic cysts, and the cysts frequently communicate with the tracheobronchial tree. Parenchymal cysts usually present with signs of pulmonary sepsis. Mediastinal bronchogenic cysts may compress the airway, and the presenting signs represent airway obstruction or pulmonary sepsis.

An air-filled bronchogenic cyst on chest roentgenogram is sharply defined and round (Fig. 62–20). The cyst can expand rapidly, and if it ruptures it may produce a tension pneumothorax. Needle aspiration may temporize, but prompt surgical resection is necessary.

A cystic lesion that communicates with the airways and that contains secretions or pus has an air-fluid level on a decubitus or upright chest roentgenogram (Fig.

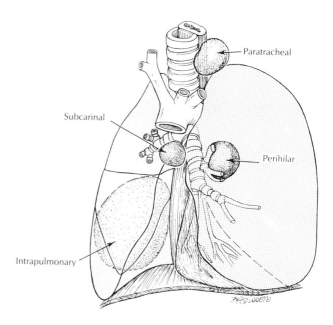

Fig. 62–19. Bronchogenic cysts are formed by abnormal budding of the respiratory tract and may be found in a variety of locations. From Luck, S.R., et al.: Congenital bronchopulmonary malformations. Curr. Probl. Surg. 23:288, 1986. Used by permission.

62–21). The infected cyst often has a surrounding pneumonia. Sometimes the infected cysts are difficult to differentiate from an empyema or solid pulmonary lesion (Fig. 62–22). A triangular shadow on the roentgenogram usually indicates an empyema. Computed tomography may differentiate between a solid and cystic lesion (Fig. 62–23).

Surgical resection is indicated for all bronchogenic cysts. Mediastinal bronchogenic cysts are best treated by simple excision. Parenchymal cysts require segmental or lobar resection.

CONGENITAL CYSTIC ADENOMATOID MALFORMATION

A spectrum of cystic and solid lesions of the lung can be identified histologically as congenital cystic adenomatoid malformations. In all varieties there is an overgrowth of terminal bronchiolar-type tubular structures and a lack of mature alveoli (Fig. 62–24). Luck and associates (1986) summarized the histologic appearance of congenital cystic adenomatoid malformations as follows: (1) There is an adenomatoid increase of terminal respiratory bronchiolar-like structures lined by ciliated columnar epithelium. Interspersed cysts may resemble immature alveoli. Connective tissue stroma contains disorganized elastic tissue and smooth muscle. (2) The mucosa of cysts lined with bronchial-type epithelium may show polypoid overgrowth projecting into the lumen of the cysts. (3) Bronchial mucoserous glands and cartilaginous plates are absent throughout the cystic parenchyma. (4) Occasional groups of alveolar cysts may be lined with mucus-secreting cells that resemble intestinal mucosa and do not resemble normal bronchial cells.

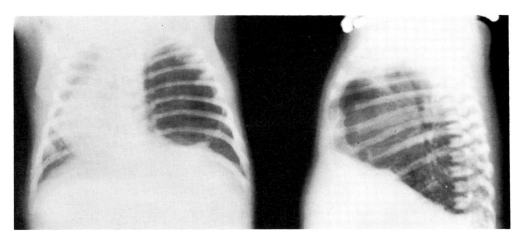

Fig. 62–20. This roentgenogram of the chest demonstrates a bronchogenic cyst of the left upper lobe.

Stocker and associates (1977) and Bale (1979) outlined the classification of these lesions based on the clinical presentation and pathologic picture (Table 62–2). A predominantly solid lung mass is usually found in the stillborn or premature infant and is associated with fetal anasarca, ascites, and maternal polyhydramnios (Fig. 62–25). The combined solid-cystic lesion may produce respiratory distress in the near-term infant at birth. The primarily cystic lesion is usually found in the older infant, child, or adult because of an associated unresolving or recurrent pneumonia.

A diagnosis based on the roentgenogram of the chest is often difficult. A multicystic lesion may resemble a congenital diphragmatic hernia with bowel loops in the chest (Fig. 62–26)—a roentgenogram that includes the abdomen and shows a paucity of abdominal bowel gas indicates a congenital diaphragmatic hernia. A single cyst may resemble congenital lobar emphysema. Computed

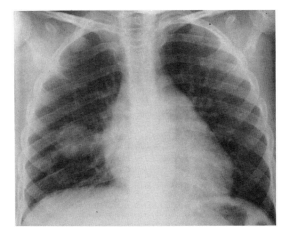

Fig. 62–22. This intrapulmonary bronchogenic cyst resembles a solid pulmonary lesion. This 4-year-old patient had presented with hemoptysis. From Luck, S.R., et al.: Congenital bronchopulmonary malformations. Curr. Probl. Surg. 23:251, 1986. Used by permission.

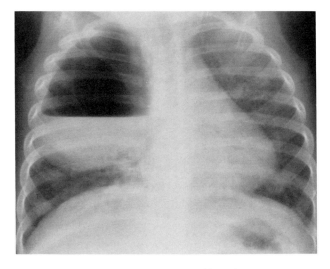

Fig. 62–21. An air-fluid level in an infected bronchogenic cyst is seen in this roentgenogram. This 10-month-old girl presented with a four day history of fever and cough. From Luck, S.R., et al.: Congenital bronchopulmonary malformations. Curr. Probl. Surg. 23:251, 1986. Used by permission.

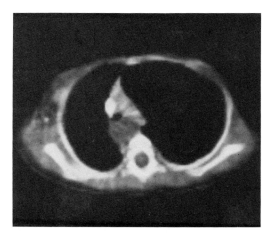

Fig. 62–23. Mediastinal bronchogenic cyst. From Luck, S.R., et al.: Congenital bronchopulmonary malformations. Curr. Probl. Surg. 23:251, 1986. Used by permission.

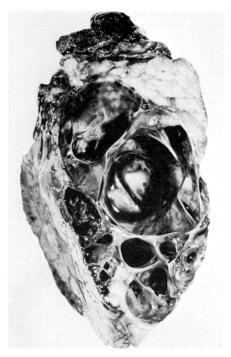

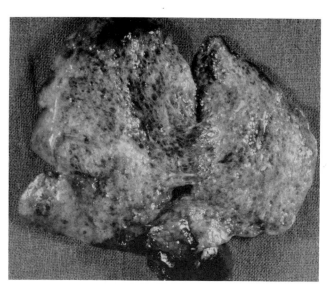

Fig. 62–25. This solid type of cystic adenomatoid malformation was found at autopsy in an infant who died shortly after birth. From Luck, S.R., et al.: Congenital bronchopulmonary malformations. Curr. Probl. Surg. 23:294, 1986. Used by permission.

Fig. 62–24. Specimen removed from an infant with cystic adenomatoid malformation. Microscopically, there was marked proliferation of terminal bronchioles, and cartilage was lacking.

Table 62–2. Classification of Congenital Cystic Adenomatoid Malformations

Clinical Presentation (Bale)*	Cystic Lesion†	Intermediate Lesion†	Solid (Adenomatoid) Lesion†
Age Fetal anasarca/ascites	Term newborn or older	Infant	Stillborn or premature
Maternal polyhydramnios	None	±	Occasional
Other anomalies	Rare	Rare	Common
Gross appearance	Cystic; sometimes solid areas	Either or both	Solid; sometimes cystic areas
Histopathology			
Bronchiolar proliferation	+	Varying degrees	+ + +
Alveolar appearance	Mature; separating bronchiolar-type cysts		Immature
Mucoid epithelium/cartilage	Occasional	Occasional	Common
Prognosis	Good	Good	Poor

Clinical Presentation (Stocker)‡	Type I Lesion	Type II	Type III
Age Fetal anasarca/maternal poly- hydramnios	Term, occasional stillborn Rare	Stillborn or Premature Common	Common
Other anomalies	Rare	Common	None reported
Gross appearance	Single or multiple large cysts 2 cm diameter	Multiple, evenly spaced cysts; 1 cm diameter	Large mass, no or tiny cysts
Histopathology			
Bronchiolar proliferation	+	+ +	+ + +
Mucoid epithelium/cartilage Cyst wall	Mucoid cells in ⅓ of cases; rare cartilage prominent bands of smooth muscle and elastic tissue	None Striated muscle in 5/16 cases	None
Prognosis	Good	Poor	Poor

*Based on 21 cases with only 9 neonates; 4 autopsies.

† + to + + + indicates increasing proportion.

‡Based on 38 stillborn or newborn cases; 26 autopsies.

Reproduced with permission from Luck, S.R., et al.: Congenital bronchopulmonary malformations. Curr. Probl. Surg. 23:251, 1986.

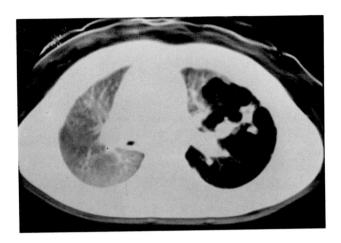

Fig. 62-27. Computed tomography can differentiate these cystic-solid lesions from pneumonia or bronchiectasis. From Luck, S.R., et al.: Congenital bronchopulmonary malformations. Curr. Probl. Surg. 23:297, 1986. Used by permission.

tomography is often necessary to make the diagnosis correctly in the older infant and child (Fig. 62–27).

Surgical resection is indicated to treat the presenting symptoms. The newborn with a large congenital cystic adenomatoid malformation presents with severe respiratory distress secondary to the space-occupying mass, the compression of the contralateral lung, and the inadequate volume of functioning lung tissue at the time of presentation. The contralateral lung may also be hypoplastic. Emergency thoracotomy and lobectomy is often life-saving. In the older child or adult, surgical resection is required to remove the source of recurrent pneumonia. Hartman and Schochat (1983) reported malignancy within the congenital cystic adenomatoid. Luck and associates (1986) summarized the reports of malignant tumors in 10 children with cystic lung disease and advocated lobectomy for the treatment of all congenital cystic adenomatoid malformations, symptomatic or not.

REFERENCES

Alivazatos, P., et al.: Pulmonary sequestration complicated by anomalies of pulmonary venous return. J. Pediatr. Surg. 20:76, 1985.

Bale, R.M.:Congenital cystic malformation of the lung. Am. J. Clin. Pathol. 71:411, 1979.

Boland, R.B., Schneider, A.F., and Boggs, J.: Infantile lobar emphysema. AMA Arch. Pathol. 61:289, 1956.

Boyden, E.A.: Bronchogenic cysts and the theory of intralobar sequestration; new embryonic data. J. Thorac. Cardiovasc. Surg. 33:604, 1958.

Chamberlain, D., et al.: Pulmonary hypoplasia in babies with severe rhesus isoimmunisation: a quantitative study. J. Pathol. 122:43, 1977.

Claireaux, A., and Ferriera, H.P.: Bilateral pulmonary agenesis. Arch. Dis. Child. 33:364, 1958.

Cohen, A.M., Solomon, E.H., and Alfidi, R.J.: Computed tomography in bronchial atresia. Am. J. Radiol. 135:1097, 1980.

Cooney, P.R., Menke, J.A., and Allen, J.E.: "Acquired" lobar emphysema: a complication of respiratory distress in premature infants. J. Pediatr. Surg. 12:897, 1977.

Cooney, T.P., and Thurlbeck, W.M.: Pulmonary hypoplasia in Down's syndrome. N. Engl. J. Med. 307:1170, 1982.

Evans, J.A., Reggin, J., and Greenberg, C.: Tracheal agenesis and associated malformations: a comparison with tracheoesophageal

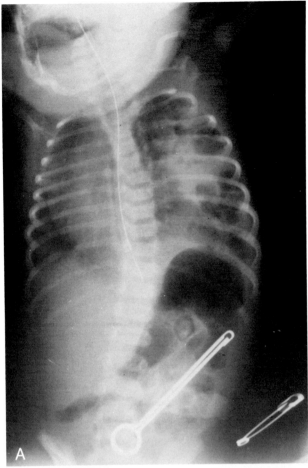

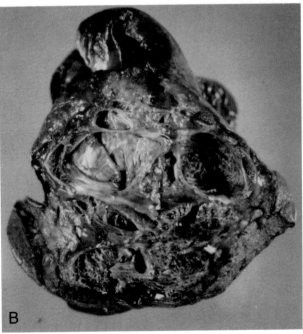

Fig. 62–26. A, This "babygram" demonstrates what appears to be multiple air-filled spaces in the left chest. The normal appearance of the gas in the abdomen suggests a cystic adenomatoid malformation in the chest rather than a congenital diaphragmatic hernia. B, A left upper lobectomy was performed. The specimen reveals both solid and cystic elements of the malformation. From Luck, S.R., et al.: Congenital bronchopulmonary malformations. Curr. Probl. Surg. 23:295, 1986. Used by permission.

fistula and the VACTERL association. Am. J. Med. Genet. *21*:21, 1985.

Gans, S.L., and Potts, W.J.: Anomalous lobe of lung arising from the esophagus. J. Thorac. Surg. *21*:313, 1951.

Haller, J.A., et al.: The natural history of bronchial atresia: serial observation of a case from birth to operative correction. J. Thorac. Cardiovasc. Surg. *79*:868, 1980.

Harris, H.A., and Lewis, I.: Anomalies of the lungs with special reference to the danger of abnormal vessels in lobectomy. J. Thorac. Cardiovasc. Surg. *9*:666, 1940.

Hartman, G.E., and Shochat, S.J.: Primary pulmonary neoplasias of childhood: a review. Ann. Thorac. Surg. *36*:108, 1983.

Haworth, S., and Hislop, A.: Normal structural and functional adaptation to extrauterine life. J. Pediatr. *98*:915, 1981.

Hershenson, M.B., et al.: Respiratory insufficiency in newborns with abdominal wall defects. J. Pediatr. Surg. *20*:348, 1985.

Hislop, A., and Reid, L.: New pathological findings in emphysema in childhood: polyalveolar lobe with emphysema. Thorax *25*:282, 1970.

Iwai, K., et al.: Intralobar pulmonary sequestration, with special reference to developmental pathology. Ann. Rev. Resp. Dis. *107*:911, 1973.

Kitigawa, M., et al.: Lung hypoplasia in congenital diaphragmatic hernia: a quantitative study of airway, artery, and alveolar development. Br. J. Surg. *58*:342, 1971.

Lincoln, J.C.R., et al.: Congenital lobar emphysema. Ann. Surg. *173*:55, 1971.

Luck, S.R., Reynolds, M., and Raffensperger, J.G.: Congenital bronchopulmonary malformations. Curr. Probl. Surg. *23*:251, 1986.

Maltz, D.L., and Nadas, A.: Agenesis of the lung: presentation of 8 cases and review of the literature. Pediatrics *42*:175, 1968.

Massuni, R., Taleghani, M., and Ellis, I.: Cardiorespiratory studies in congenital absence of one lung. J. Thorac. Cardiovasc. Surg. *51*:561, 1966.

McLaughlin, F.J., et al.: Tracheal bronchus: association with respiratory morbidity in children. J. Pediatr. *106*:751, 1985.

Milstein, J.M., Lau, M., and Bickers, R.G.: Tracheal agenesis in infants with VATER association. Am. J. Dis. Child. *139*:77, 1985.

Nikaidoh, H., and Swenson, O.: The ectopic origin of the right main bronchus from the esophagus. J. Thorac. Cardiovasc. Surg. *62*:151, 1971.

Sane, S.M., Sieber, W.K., and Girdany, B.R.: Congenital bronchobiliary fistula. Surgery *69*:599, 1971.

Sankaran, K., et al.: Tracheal atresia, proximal esophageal atresia, and distal tracheoesophageal fistula: report of two cases and review of literature. Pediatrics *71*:821, 1983.

Savic, B., et al.: Lung sequestration: report of seven cases and review of 540 published cases. Thorax *34*:96, 1979.

Say, B., et al.: Agenesis of the lung associated with a chromosomal abnormality (46,XX,2p?). J. Med. Genet. *17*:477, 1980.

Sbokes, C.G., and McMillan, I.K.: Agenesis of the lung. Br. J. Dis. Chest. *77*:183, 1977.

Scarpelli, E.A., and Auld, P.: Pulmonary Disease of the Fetus, Newborn, and Child. Philadelphia, Lea & Febiger, 1978, pp. 194–196.

Shermeta, D., Personal communication, 1985.

Stocker, J.T., Madewell, J.E., and Drake, R.M.: Congenital cystic adenomatoid malformation of the lung. Hum. Pathol. *8*:155, 1977.

Stovin, P.: Congenital lobar emphysema. Thorax *14*:254, 1959.

Swischuk, L.E., et al.: Primary Pulmonary Hypoplasia and the Neonate. J. Pediatr. *95*:573, 1979.

Tapper, D., et al.: Polyalveolar lobe: anatomic and physiologic parameters and their relationship to congenital lobar emphysema. J. Pediatr. Surg. *15*:931, 1980.

Thilenius, O.G., et al.: Spectrum of pulmonary sequestration: association with anomalous pulmonary venous drainage in infants. Pediatr. Cardiol. *4*:97, 1983.

Vilos, G.A., et al.: Absence or impaired response of fetal breathing to intravenous glucose is associated with pulmonary hypoplasia in congenital myotonic dystrophy. Am. J. Obstet. Gynecol. *148*:558, 1984.

Wigglesworth, J.S., and Desai, R.: Effects on lung growth of cervical cord section in the rabbit fetus. Early Hum. Dev. *3*:51, 1979.

CHAPTER 63

PULMONARY COMPLICATIONS OF CYSTIC FIBROSIS

Susan R. Luck

PULMONARY COMPLICATIONS OF CYSTIC FIBROSIS

Cystic fibrosis—CF—is an inherited disease of the exocrine glands and is associated with multiple organ dysfunction that results from ductal obstruction by thick mucus secretions. It is the most common lethal genetic disease in white children and is inherited as an autosomal recessive trait. The estimated incidence in the white population is 1 in every 2000 live births; in blacks in the United States, it is 1 in every 17,000 live births. The disease is virtually unknown in orientals. Although the frequency is approximately equal in boys and girls, girls succumb at younger ages, especially after the age of 16 years. The cystic fibrosis locus has been mapped to the long arm of chromosome 7 and is adjacent to DNA markers that facilitate identification. Beaudet and Buffone (1987) and Ostrer and Hejtmancik (1988) summarized the advances in prenatal diagnosis and in heterozygote identification among relatives of cystic fibrosis patients. Eventually, elucidation of the molecular basis of the disease may permit specific therapy.

The levels of sodium and chloride in the eccrine sweat of patients with CF are almost always elevated to three to six times normal, usually greater than 60 to 80 mEq/L. This abnormality is present from birth and persists without any relationship to the severity of pancreatic or pulmonary disease. The diagnosis of CF is confirmed by the demonstration of an elevated sweat chloride concentration in a patient with typical chronic pulmonary disease or pancreatic insufficiency or both. Unusual variants of the disease have been reported, and the diagnosis cannot depend upon one criterion alone. Bijman and Quinton (1984) demonstrated a defect in chloride ion transport in human sweat gland preparations both in vitro and in vivo. Decreased reabsorption of chloride, and to a lesser extent of sodium, probably is caused by an abnormally low permeability of the cells of the sweat tubule to the re-entry of chloride ions from the lumen of the gland. Chloride impermeability may underlie the clinical malfunction of all other eccrine glands. Hyponatremic collapse can occur after heat exposure and excessive sweating.

A wide spectrum in the extent and severity of all clinical manifestations is presumably secondary to individual variation in the basic disease mechanism. The major clinical sequelae and their approximate incidence are: (1) pancreatic insufficiency with malabsorption of fat and fat-soluble vitamins—85%; (2) chronic pulmonary disease with bronchiolar obstruction and recurrent infection—eventually 100%; (3) atrophy of the Wolffian duct structures with absence of the vas deferens and fibrosis of the epididymus, resulting in azoospermia—virtually in all older boys; and (4) neonatal bowel obstruction from inspissated meconium—meconium ileus—10%. Related conditions include poor weight gain and delayed maturation, pancreatitis, and glucose intolerance; an increased incidence of pneumothorax and bronchiectasis; and recurrent abdominal pain and bowel obstruction from hard, impacted stool—meconium ileus equivalent. Finkelstein and colleagues (1988) reported insulin-dependent diabetes mellitus in 7% of adults with cystic fibrosis who survived to 20 years of age. This complication is associated with accelerated clinical deterioration. Biliary tract abnormalities include an increased incidence of cholelithiasis—as high as 25%; focal biliary cirrhosis and portal hypertension—symptomatic in 5 to 10%. Also seen are rectal prolapse, absent or delayed menarche, and reduced fertility in women. Sinusitis and nasal polyps are common. Hypertrophic pulmonary osteoarthropathy and inappropriate antidiuretic hormone—ADH—secretion may occur in cystic fibrosis as in other types of chronic pulmonary disease.

Although the initial description by Andersen (1938) was that of a fatal disease of infancy, the symptoms may not be recognized until the patient is an adolescent or an adult. Thoracic surgeons must include cystic fibrosis in the differential diagnosis of chronic interstitial lung disease and bronchiectasis. Several groups, including

Shwachman (1977), Huang (1987), MacLusky (1985), and Penketh (1987) and their associates, detailed the progression and treatment of this disease in adults.

PATHOPHYSIOLOGY OF PULMONARY DISEASE

Pulmonary infection and disease are the most significant clinical components of cystic fibrosis. The basic pathologic processes of distal airway obstruction and infection are self-perpetuating; once established, they ultimately lead to cardiorespiratory failure. Esterly and Oppenheimer (1968) noted that the earliest histologic changes appear in the tracheobronchial exocrine submucosal glands, which become obstructed and dilated. Thereafter, thick mucus obstructs bronchioles and bronchi in a scattered fashion throughout the lungs. Bacterial colonization and mucosal infection follow. Ciliated cells are destroyed as bronchial epithelium undergoes metaplasia; the submucosa is infiltrated by inflammatory cells; and adjacent lymphoid tissue proliferates. Microabscess formation and peribronchial fibrosis weaken the bronchial walls, and the incidence of bronchiectasis rises steadily. Bronchiolar stenosis and dilatation are irreversible. Areas of alveolar overinflation intermingle with microatelectasis and diffuse fibrosis, but true emphysematous changes appear much later. Destructive emphysema is uncommon. Ventilation and pulmonary perfusion decrease in a scattered fashion throughout the lungs. Cor pulmonale is the end result of chronic hypoxia.

Staphylococcus aureus and *Hemophilus influenzae* infect the lungs of young children with the disease. *Pseudomonas aeruginosa* is isolated most frequently in older patients and in those with severe lung disease. Vasil (1985) and Thomassen and co-workers (1987) reviewed the properties of this organism and its unique interaction with the human host. Mucoid strains predominate, and they are protected from antibiotics and host defenses by a polysaccharide matrix—alginate. Frequently, these organisms are resistant to multiple antibiotics. The presence of stagnant secretions and chronic mucosal infection alone, however, cannot explain the inevitable destructive bronchopulmonary disease. Evidence supports the role of a poorly controlled inflammatory and immunologic response to *Pseudomonas* infection. Complex interactions occur between antibodies, immunoglobulins, phagocytic cells, lymphocytes, and the toxic products of the bacteria. Alveolar macrophages become ineffective phagocytes, and neutrophils release tissue-destructive proteases. Antigen–antibody complexes may cause both local and systemic tissue damage. Hypergammaglobulinemia and increased numbers of circulating and sputum immune complexes correlate with progressively severe lung disease and clinical deterioration. Although the reduction of inflammatory products within the airway by chest physiotherapy and antibiotics undoubtedly allow local defenses to regain control, modulation of the immune response by vaccines or monoclonal antibodies may play an increasing role in supportive care and therapy. Auer-

bach and associates (1985) demonstrated a clinical benefit to children receiving low-dose steroids on alternate days.

Goldmann and Klinger (1986) reviewed the colonization by *Pseudomonas cepacia* of patients in several cystic fibrosis centers. Earlier clinical deterioration and death occur in those patients who also have moderate or advanced lung disease. A few have died with fulminant pneumonia and bacteremia. This pathogen is resistant to most antibiotics, including the aminoglycosides. Ceftazidime improves the clinical course in some patients.

PULMONARY FUNCTION STUDIES

There is a wide spectrum in the degree of pulmonary dysfunction among different patients. The rapidity of deterioration varies not only among individuals but also at different times in the same person. Wessel (1983) reviewed those measurements of lung volumes and pulmonary mechanics that provide an objective basis for long-term follow-up and assessment of the efficacy of specific treatment. Pulmonary function studies are performed at regular intervals in all CF centers. Most children can cooperate by the age of 5 to 6 years. The early and scattered obstruction of peripheral airways causes measurable and predictable abnormalities in arterial oxygenation, pulmonary volumes and capacities, and airflow mechanics. The uneven apportionment of inspired gases and blood flow to the alveoli results in an increase in the alveolar–arterial PO_2 gradient. Arterial hypoxemia is the first sign of impaired lung function, but measurement of arterial PO_2 may be unreliable in children who cry or are excited after a needle puncture. The normally ventilated areas of lung continue to maintain a normal carbon dioxide tension. An increase in PCO_2 is a preterminal finding associated with cor pulmonale.

Clinically useful information is provided by volume displacement spirometry. Even minimal degrees of scattered airway obstruction can produce measurable evidence of increased dead space ventilation and air-trapping. The most sensitive indicators of abnormal lung volumes are increases in residual volume—RV, functional residual capacity—FRC, and RV/TLC—total lung capacity. Vital capacity—VC—and TLC are decreased only in patients with moderate to advanced lung involvement; those who are suffering the restrictive effects of lung destruction and fibrosis. Because early disease is confined to the small airways, maximum expiratory airflows are decreased initially only at small lung volumes. Therefore, the $Vmax_{75}$—the maximum expiratory airflow after expiration of 75% of the VC—and the MEF—the average maximum expiratory flow during the middle 50% of VC—are much more sensitive than the FEV—forced expiratory volume—and the forced expiratory volume at one second—FEV_1.

Longstanding hypoxia and lung infection eventually result in pulmonary vasoconstriction and fibrosis with a chronic increase in right ventricular afterload. The physical signs of right-heart failure are overshadowed by those of extreme pulmonary disease. Edema and hepatomegaly are late findings. Moss (1965) outlined the diagnostic criteria for cor pulmonale in CF: (1) an S-K clinical score* of 40 or less; (2) VC less than 60% of predicted normal; and (3) the inability to raise arterial PO_2 to 300 torr after breathing 100% oxygen for 10 minutes. Because the hyperinflated lungs surround the heart, the findings of cardiomegaly and right ventricular hypertrophy are absent or underestimated on the chest roentgenograph and electrocardiogram. Lester (1980) correlated the echocardiographic abnormalities with the progression of cardiac decompensation and also with the S-K score.

ROENTGENOGRAPHIC FINDINGS

The earliest roentgenographic abnormalities are evidence of hyperinflation with flattening of the diaphragmatic domes and an increased anteroposterior diameter. Bronchovascular markings are prominent, especially in the upper lobes. Atelectasis of the right upper lobe, right middle lobe, or left lower lobe in infants and young children should suggest the diagnosis of cystic fibrosis. The chest roentgenogram of a patient with well established disease reveals a diffuse cystic interstitial process with maximum involvement of the upper lung fields (Fig. 63–1). Schwartz and Holsclaw (1974) suggested that the differential diagnosis in an older patient with undiagnosed disease should include chronic bronchitis, sarcoidosis, histiocytosis X, tuberculosis or other granulomatous infection, and connective tissue disease. Brasfield and colleagues (1980) reported that the most frequently occurring abnormalities include hyperinflation, usually of the upper lobes; patchy linear and nodular densities, probably representing bronchiectasis or small peribronchial abscesses; and lobar segmental atelectasis (Fig. 63–2). Fellows and associates (1979) suggested that increasingly prominent densities may represent dilated bronchial artery collaterals. Apical blebs appear in older patients. The impression of microcardia, seen late in the course of the disease, is secondary to extensive pulmonary overinflation. A normal or small heart size does not rule out cor pulmonale. Computed tomography—CT—can specifically delineate radiopaque lesions, particularly the extent and severity of bronchiectasis.

COMPREHENSIVE TREATMENT

Antibiotics have prolonged survival but have failed to halt the progressive course of the disease in children. Intensive therapeutic and prophylactic regimes initiated in the late 1950s were targeted to control pulmonary secretions, treat and prevent pulmonary infection, and

to ameliorate the multiple medical problems unique to these patients. Although scientific documentation of efficacy is lacking for many of these measures, such efforts have greatly prolonged life expectancy, from 4 years in the 1950s to 19 years in 1976. Early and compulsive care can retard pulmonary damage for lengthy periods. Even when irreversible disease is established at the time of diagnosis, a better quality of life can be sustained for years.

The mainstay of therapy is to encourage deep breathing and coughing, which efficiently mobilize secretions. Hofmeyer and colleagues (1986) reported that segmental postural drainage, chest percussion or vibration, breathing exercises, and active aerobic exercise when feasible, all contribute to this goal. Mist or nebulization therapy thin the thick sputum and provoke coughing. Chest physiotherapy can be more effective if preceded by aerosol inhalation of a bronchodilator such as albuterol. Room humidification, especially at night, is recommended. Aerosol treatments with the mucolytic agent N-acetyl-L-cysteine or with antibiotics are frequently recommended but without firm evidence to support routine use. Bronchoscopy and bronchial lavage have been used to clean out accumulations of tenacious secretions in failing patients. No one has demonstrated sustained improvement. Stern and associates (1978b) believe the technique is indicated only for persistent lobar or segmental atelectasis. Associated respiratory-tract lesions—sinusitis, nasal polyps, and hypertrophied tonsils and adenoids—should be treated as indicated.

The prescription of "suppressive" oral antibiotics is controversial. Rubio (1986) reviewed the specific antibiotic therapy for exacerbations of pulmonary infection. The most useful drugs include dicloxacillin, erythromycin, the tetracyclines, trimethoprim-sulfamethoxazole, and the second-generation cephalosporins. Chloramphenicol has been used in many patients when sputum cultures show insensitivity to the other available oral medications. Patients who fail to improve with oral therapy or who have advanced disease must receive systemic antibiotics. Ceftazadime, a third-generation cephalosporin, or the combination of a semisynthetic penicillin and an aminoglycoside are the most effective antibiotics against *Pseudomonas aeruginosa*. The renal clearance of aminoglycosides is increased in CF patients, and these drugs must be administered more frequently. When frequent or prolonged courses are necessary, the drugs can be administered at home through a temporary peripheral catheter, a central venous catheter, or a subcutaneous port.

Many cystic fibrosis patients have positive skin tests to inhalant allergens. The efficacy of an aerosolized bronchodilator, such as albuterol, for patients with allergies can be substantiated and should be prescribed for patients in whom pulmonary function improves after a treatment. The empiric administration of steroids must rest on the impression of a good clinical response. *Aspergillus fumigatus* frequently colonizes the respiratory mucosa of patients with cystic fibrosis. Laufer and associates (1984) believed that allergic bronchopulmonary

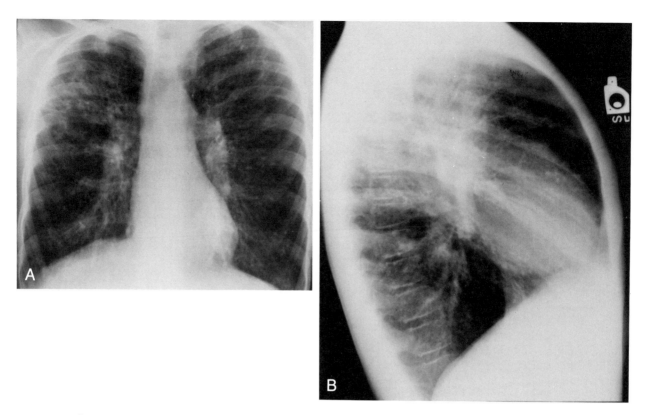

Fig. 63–1. *A* and *B*, The roentgenograms of a 12-year-old boy show hyperexpansion of the chest wall and depressed diaphragms from overinflated lungs. Linear and patchy densities are concentrated in a contracted right upper lobe. Note the normal heart size and the prominent pulmonary arteries. The vertebral column is osteoporotic.

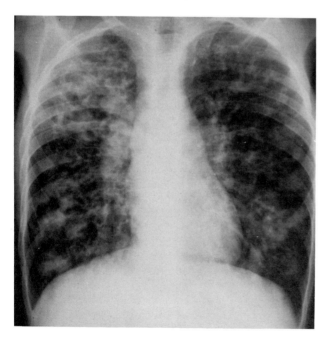

Fig. 63–2. Nodular cystic changes—bronchiectasis and scarring—and linear densities are prominent in the roentgenogram of a 16-year-old with more severe disease.

aspergillosis—ABPA—probably plays a role in destructive pulmonary disease that steroid therapy could prevent. ABPA should be suspected in those patients with asthma symptoms and progressive disease or recurrent exacerbations despite otherwise adequate therapy. Affected patients may expectorate brown mucus plugs. A presumptive diagnosis rests on the demonstration of elevated levels of IgE and precipitation of *Aspergillus* antibodies, positive skin reaction to *Aspergillus,* and eosinophilia.

Pancreatic exocrine insufficiency prevents the normal absorption of long-chain fats and fat-soluble vitamins. An increased caloric intake is indispensable for normal growth. The diet should be high in protein, with fat intake adjusted to individual tolerance. All patients should receive increased doses of multivitamins and water-soluble preparations of vitamin E. Vitamin K is given in the first year of life and thereafter for specific indications. Additional salt and fluid are advised during warm weather. Vaisman and associates (1987) showed that the resting expenditure of energy in these patients is higher than normal even when pulmonary function is at baseline. Those with less pancreatic involvement obviously can be expected to exhibit better growth, less pulmonary disease, and prolonged longevity. The malnourished patient who is in a constant state of catabolism cannot control recurrent infection even with maximal medical treatment. The importance of supplemental nutrition to the maintenance and recovery of pulmonary function in this group has received increasing attention. Both Shepherd (1980) and Levy (1985) and their colleagues reported that long-term enteral supplementation through a nasogastric tube, gastrostomy, or jejunostomy can produce a statistically significant improvement in pulmonary function. Mansell and associates (1984) suggested that a short-term course of parenteral nutrition can improve the strength of respiratory muscles and some parameters of pulmonary function, although the effect is transient unless better nutrition is sustained.

SURGICAL EVALUATION AND INTERVENTION

Di Sant'Agnese (1953) recorded in the 1940s and 1950s that 10% of young children with CF developed lobar atelectasis and bronchiectasis, and some died as a result. Persistent lesions were resected. Andersen (1958) and Holsclaw (1970) and Taussig (1974) and their colleagues reported that pyopneumothorax, empyema, and lung abscesses complicated staphylococcal pneumonia in these young patients. The focus of thoracic surgery, however, has shifted in adolescents and adults. Pneumothorax and hemoptysis are the major problems. Symptomatic bronchiectasis is localized and suitable for resection in only a few patients. Hodson and Bathen (1988) and Jones and associates (1988) reported successful heart-lung transplantation, which will be a therapeutic option for some cystic fibrosis patients with end-stage lung disease.

A large pulmonary abscess is uncommon. Holsclaw (1970) and Lester and colleagues (1983) noted that most respond to prolonged antibiotic therapy and bronchoscopic aspiration (Fig. 63–3). Otherwise, pulmonary resection is indicated. Fungal disease and tuberculosis are

rare. Katznelsen and co-workers (1964) reported seven children with extensive suppurative and granulomatous inflammation of lung tissue and hilar lymph nodes seen between 1954 and 1964. The extent of this process of botryomycosis varied but included the mediastinum, chest wall, pericardium, extradural space, and vertebral bodies. Five of the seven died. Although the etiology was unclear at that time, the lesion probably resulted from uncontrolled staphylococcal and *Pseudomonas* infection.

Preoperative Preparation

A systematic evaluation of all involved organ systems is obtained. The results of previous pulmonary function and clinical scoring are vital for estimation of operative risks and prognosis of long-term outcome. This retrospective information and an echocardiogram are crucial in the care of the extremely and chronically ill patient with an acute complication. Previously unsuspected portal hypertension, diabetes mellitus, gastroesophageal reflux, or cholelithiasis can complicate recovery, and their occurrence must be recognized. Specific preoperative measures include vigorous chest physiotherapy, systemic antibiotics based on current sputum cultures, correction of any coagulation deficits, and relief of stool impaction. Immediate and maximal caloric support should be guaranteed by peripheral or central parenteral nutrition or enteral formula supplements.

Anesthetic Considerations

Most postoperative complications are respiratory, and these can be limited with appropriate care. Lamberty and Rubin (1985) reviewed 77 patients who underwent

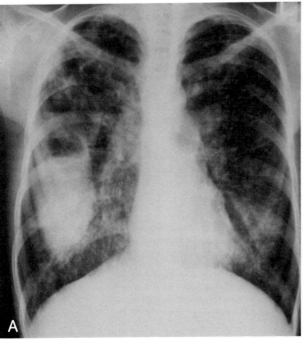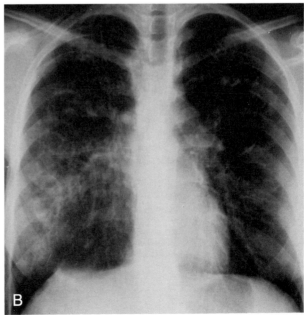

Fig. 63–3. *A* and *B*, Roentgenograms of a 17-year-old girl who developed a multiloculated abscess after a prolonged pulmonary exacerbation of infection. *B*, The abscess had cleared with scarring 2 months later after antibiotic therapy.

general anesthesia for various procedures. The long-term decline of pulmonary function was comparable with that expected in other patients at similar ages. Anesthetic techniques must allow for the pathophysiology of this disease.

The ventilation–perfusion imbalance and pulmonary fibrosis are responsible for the slow diffusion of inhaled gases, including oxygen. These defects result in oxygen desaturation and in prolonged anesthetic induction and emergence time with inhalant agents. Therefore, intravenous induction should be used in all cases.

Spontaneous respiration in some patients depends upon a hypoxic respiratory drive. Tidal volumes decrease if spontaneous respiration is allowed under anesthesia. Ventilation must be supported through a cuffed endotracheal tube with assisted or controlled ventilation. Light non-narcotic preoperative sedation and awake extubation are mandatory. Hyperventilation and hypocarbia must be avoided.

Bronchial hyperreactivity is common. Many patients are prone to develop laryngospasm, bronchospasm, and paroxysmal attacks of coughing.

Increased secretions continue to accumulate during the operation. Frequent endotracheal suctioning must be accomplished. Ketamine produces bronchorrhea, and this agent is contraindicated. Inspired air and gases must be humidified during and after the operation.

A pulse oximeter, an end-tidal carbon dioxide monitor, an airway pressure monitor, and an arterial catheter can provide useful data during, and sometimes after, the operation. Intravenous atropine is given at the time of induction. Nasal polyps must be excluded before passing a nasotracheal tube. Single-lung ventilation and fluid overload should be avoided. Nitrous oxide is contraindicated in the presence of a pneumothorax or large bullae. Hypoalbuminemia and aminoglycoside therapy may prolong the action of nondepolarizing muscle relaxants. At the conclusion of the procedure, all narcotics and muscle relaxants must be completely reversed. The patient should be thoroughly suctioned, awake, and coughing before extubation. Both Schuster and Fellows (1977) and Rich and associates (1978) found that prompt extubation was feasible in many cases. Robinson and Branthwaite (1984) electively ventilated all those in whom a delay in adequate spontaneous respiration was expected. Those patients who are extremely ill from malnutrition or liver disease are easily oversedated and have decreased tolerance of local anesthetics. Humidified oxygen is provided postoperatively. Chest physiotherapy should be resumed immediately. Regional analgesia can be instituted by intercostal or epidural block with bupivacaine or fentanyl.

PNEUMOTHORAX

Pneumothorax is the most common surgical complication of pulmonary disease in cystic fibrosis. A pneumothorax probably follows the rupture of subpleural air cysts through pleura weakened by the effects of chronic inflammation. Tomashefski and associates (1985b) iden-

tified three different pathologic types of air cysts in older patients with cystic fibrosis who were dying of pulmonary disease. All cysts occur more frequently in the upper lobes. Bronchiectatic cysts are the only ones large enough to be well defined on chest roentgenograms, but their thick collagenous walls would seem to prevent rupture. Smaller subpleural emphysematous cysts, which give the lung surface a bubbly appearance, are the likely site of pleural rupture. Interstitial air cysts located adjacent to interlobular septa may cause interstitial air dissection with pneumomediastinum.

Di Sant'Agnese and Vidaurreta (1960), Lifshitz and associates (1968), and Holsclaw (1970) described pneumomediastinum and subcutaneous emphysema with and without pneumothorax in a few patients. Tomashefski and colleagues (1985a) reported that examination of visceral pleura obtained from cystic fibrosis patients during pleurectomy for pneumothorax or at autopsy shows little difference from that of patients with spontaneous pneumothorax of other cause. Pleural elastic fibers overlying air cysts are disrupted and degenerated. The uninhibited elastase released by bacteria and inflammatory cells may contribute to the disruption of these fibers.

Pneumothorax commonly occurs in adolescents and adults with advanced pulmonary disease and severe airflow obstruction. By 1970, several groups had recognized the increased frequency and the attendant morbidity and mortality of this complication (Table 63–1). As older groups of patients are followed for longer periods of time, the incidence of pneumothorax increases: from 12% of children older than 10 years to over 20% of adults older than 20 years. McLaughlin and colleagues (1982) reported, however, that the occurrence of pneumothorax correlates better with clinical scoring and increasing pulmonary disease than with age. A small pneumothorax may be asymptomatic, but most patients cough and complain of chest pain, increased dyspnea and on occasion mild hemoptysis. Chest roentgenograms often reveal bullous disease in the upper lobes and evidence of tension within the pleural space (Fig. 63–4).

Pneumothorax is more common in boys and young men, perhaps because of their longer life expectancy. Regardless of age, boys and men are likely to have higher clinical scores than girls and women who present with a pneumothorax at the same age, and are more likely to survive the acute episode. There is no predilection as to the side of occurrence. Thirty to fifty percent of all affected patients eventually develop a pneumothorax on both sides. A potentially lethal tension pneumothorax may occur in up to 40% of cases. Almost every reported series describes a few patients who died with a tension or concomitant bilateral pneumothorax before treatment could be instituted. Associated mortality is high even in the patient who survives initial treatment. Thirteen percent of 72 patients with pneumothorax followed by Schuster (1983) from 1969 to 1982 died during hospitalization for management of the initial episode even though the pneumothorax was under control at the time of death. Penketh and associates (1987) reported that 25% of 61

Table 63–1.   Incidence of Pneumothorax in Patients with Cystic Fibrosis

Institution	No. of Patients Followed	No. of Patients with Pneumothorax (%)	Average or Median Age at First Pneumothorax (years)	No. of Episodes of Pneumothorax	No. of Patients with Bilateral Pneumothorax (%)
Babies' Hospital, New York Lifschitz, 1953–1967	710	20 + (3)	14	36 +	6 (30)
Rainbow Babies' & Children's Hospital, Cleveland Stowe, 1957–1974	666	29 (4)	—	47	9 (30)
Children's Memorial Hospital, Chicago Luck, 1971–1976	280 total 144 ≥ 10 yrs	18 (12)	15	40	6 (33)
University of Minnesota Hospitals Rich, 1963–1977	440 total 245 ≥ 10 yrs	28 (6) 27 (11)	— 15½	— 52	— 13 (48)
Brompton Hospital, London Mitchell-Hegge, 1964–1969	49	7 (14)	16	10	3 (49)
Penketh (1982), 1965–1981	243	46 (19)	17	106	—
Penketh (1987), 1965–1983	316	61 (19)	—	133	—
Children's Hospital Medical Center, Boston Holsclaw, 1950–1970	~2200	51 (2)	15	93	—
Schuster (1983), 1969–1982	—	72	18	180	27 (39)

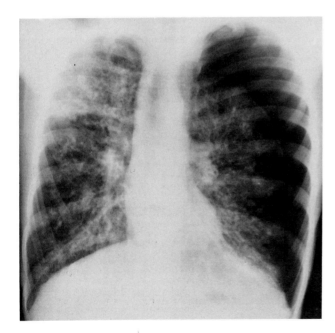

Fig. 63–4.   This roentgenogram is of the same patient as in Figure 63–1, now 14 years of age. There is a left tension pneumothorax with hyperexpansion of the left hemithorax and mediastinal shift to the right. He was treated by pleural abrasion after emergency tube thoracostomy. A right pneumothorax occurred 1 year later, and a right abrasive pleurodesis was performed.

patients followed at the Brompton Hospital, London, from 1965 to 1983, died with a pneumothorax.

Observation, needle aspiration, and closed-tube thoracostomy were the methods of treatment initially employed. Disappointing results have been reported (Table 63–2). Fifty to eighty percent of all episodes of pneumothorax observed or aspirated either fail to resolve or recur. The rate of failure or recurrence after closed-tube thoracostomy is 30 to 75%. Full pulmonary expansion may require more than one chest tube. Even the insertion of multiple tubes does not guarantee sufficient pleural reaction to prevent a subsequent large simple pneumothorax or tension pneumothorax (Fig. 63–5). Autopsy studies of Boat (1969), Schuster (1983), and Tomashefski (1985a) and their associates have been unable to correlate the numbers of chest tubes placed with the degree of pleural scarring.

Complications of lung laceration, chest wall bleeding, and the development of bronchopleural fistulae have been reported. Prolonged and multiple-tube thoracostomy decompression is painful, restricts ambulation, and impedes chest physiotherapy. Children who have a persistent air leak are confined to bed, retain secretions, eat poorly, and pursue a rapidly deteriorating course. As resolution of the pneumothorax is delayed, the patient faces increasing anesthetic and operative risks.

The high rate of failure of the aforementioned management has prompted more aggressive attempts to ensure the prompt formation of a diffuse pleural symphysis. Chemical sclerosis with aqueous solutions of quinicrine, silver nitrate, and tetracycline have been employed in a small percentage of the cases in most series. The random

Table 63–2. Treatment of Pneumothorax by Observation, Needle Aspiration, or Tube Thoracostomy

Institution	No. of Episodes of Pneumothorax	Observation or Aspiration		Closed Tube Thoracostomy	
		No. Treated	No. Failed or Recurred (%)	No. Treated	No. Failed or Recurred (%)
Babies' Hospital, New York Lifshitz, 1953–1967	35	14	7 (50)	21	7 (30)
Rainbow Babies' and Children's Hospital, Cleveland Stow, 1957–1974	47	14	6 (43)	20	14 (70)
Children's Memorial Hospital, Chicago Luck, 1971–1976	44	18	14 (78)	25	14 (56)
University of Minnesota Hospitals Rich, 1963–1977	52	8	6 (75)	19	14 (74)
Brompton Hospital, London Penketh (1982), 1965–1981	81	31	17 (55)	43	27 (63)
Children's Hospital Medical Center, Boston Schuster (1983), 1969–1982	180	77	61 (80)	94	70 (74)

instillation of variable amounts of sclerosant has produced inconsistent results, although each drug can create diffuse pleural adhesions when used in sufficient amounts. Quinicrine has been used in more patients with cystic fibrosis than the other drugs have, but has been unavailable in a convenient sterile form since 1977. Schuster and co-workers (1983) recommended instilling 100 mg as a 2% solution in isotonic saline. The chest tube is clamped for 1 to 2 hours while the patient is turned in various positions to coat all pleural surfaces. This procedure can be repeated over several days. In

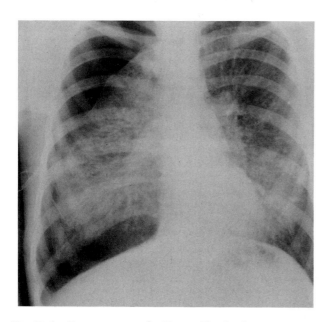

Fig. 63–5. Roentgenogram of a 15-year-old girl with recurrent right pneumothorax after the treatment of four previous episodes of pneumothorax by tube thoracostomy. Localized pleural adhesions have not prevented a tension effect with flattening of the right diaphragm.

the reports of Boat (1969), Cattaneo (1973), Kattwinkel (1973), Stowe (1975), and Schuster (1983) and their colleagues, as well as that of Jones and Giammona (1976), 20 of 22 patients had been treated successfully, although at least 5 had severe toxic reactions. Even when the dose of drug is restricted to 100 mg or less, low-grade fever and transient chest pain are common.

Silver nitrate has been abandoned because of severe pain with instillation and the common occurrence of large pleural effusions. Effective chemical sclerosis with tetracycline appears to depend upon the total dose of the instilled drug. Sahn and Potts (1978) showed that a solution of 35 mg/kg body weight consistently produced complete obliteration of the pleural cavity in rabbits, as opposed to a solution of 7 mg/kg, which produced early fibrinous adhesions but not long-term symphysis. This dose-related response may explain the recurrence of pneumothorax in six of seven patients reported by Schuster and colleagues in 1983 because they used small doses of the drug. Although it is readily available in all hospitals, tetracycline's clinical acceptance as a sclerosant is limited by immediate and severe chest pain.

Tribble and associates (1986) treated five patients with cystic fibrosis and pneumothorax by talc—dry USP pure talc—insufflation combined with thoracoscopy and division of all pleural adhesions. This minimally invasive procedure was uncomplicated and without recurrence after 6 months to 4 years. Under general or regional anesthesia, two trocars are introduced through a single intercostal space; one, for the introduction of a straight-rod lens telescope; and the other, to carry the forceps and the cannula for insufflation. After all adhesions are lysed with the biopsy forceps, approximately 2 g of sterile talc powder are insufflated under direct vision, coating the entire pleural surface. A chest tube is brought out through the same interspace. Although this technique is not widely reported, it combines a high rate of pleural symphysis with minimal risks of patient discomfort or complications.

Direct surgical intervention offers a prompt and definitive solution while affording the opportunity to eliminate the commonly present apical bullae. Lifshitz and co-workers (1968) first reported thoracotomy for pleural abrasion and apical bleb resection in children with cystic fibrosis. Extensive experience with both pleurectomy and pleural abrasion has accumulated since 1970 (Table 63–3). Morbidity and mortality are low, considering these patients' depressed physical status. Even staged bilateral procedures have been performed successfully by most groups. The best results are seen when the operation is performed early after stabilization, which may include emergency placement of a chest tube. Operative mortality increases when the operation is delayed or when pulmonary function is severely depressed. Patients with severe airflow obstruction or with cor pulmonale may survive the procedure, but Boat and associates (1969), Mitchell-Heggs and Batten (1970), and I and my associates (1977) reported that the mortality in 6 months is high. Preoperative preparation, as previously described, should be instituted immediately after admission. The operative approach should include a limited incision that preserves the major chest-wall muscles. An anterior thoracotomy that divides only the intercostal muscles, reflecting the pectoralis major, provides adequate exposure for apical pleurectomy and oversewing or resection of apical bullae. Rich and colleagues (1978) believe that a stapled resection is contraindicated because the noncompliant lung prevents adequate closure. Abrasive pleurodesis can be accomplished through a small axillary incision using a dry gauze, a cautery tip cleaner, or any sterile scouring pad directed with a ring forceps. Chest tubes are removed after the air leak has ceased and the lung is well expanded.

Immediate operative and anesthetic complications are uncommon. Pleurectomy appears to carry a higher risk of hemorrhage than does abrasive pleurodesis. Atelectasis and recurrent pneumothorax were particularly devastating in Penketh and associates' (1987) series; five of six patients with these complications died within 6 months. Stowe and colleagues (1975) found that the three-year survival of 15 patients who underwent thoracotomy from 1957 to 1974 was similar to that of 14 others treated without operation. Such data are not reported in the other series listed in Table 63–3. McLaughlin (1982), Rich (1978), Stowe (1975) and their associates and Robinson and Branthwaite (1984) reported postoperative assessment of pulmonary function in limited numbers of patients. There is a minimal long-term decline over that expected on the basis of progression of the underlying lung disease.

Late sequelae of a pneumothorax or a specific treatment modality are impossible to predict precisely in a patient with cystic fibrosis. Any complication may precipitate a further decline in precarious pulmonary reserve, culminating in death a few months later from cardiorespiratory failure. Ideal treatment would ensure a rapid resolution of the pneumothorax, eliminate the possibility of recurrence, and incur the least morbidity and mortality. Current recommendations are based on experience with relatively small numbers of patients, often accumulated over long years that bridge various advances in medical therapeutics. Operative treatment is not randomized or prospectively determined in any report; long-term follow-up, so important in these chronically ill patients, is not always available. Nevertheless, the following conclusions are warranted: (1) Pneumothorax occurs in patients with longstanding pulmonary infection and with severe and progressive airflow obstruction. (2) Any form of treatment is palliative and no improvement in baseline status can be expected. (3) A patient presenting with a pneumothorax should be considered as a

Table 63–3. Treatment of Pneumothorax by Pleurectomy, or Abrasive Pleurodesis

Institution	No. of Patients Treated	No. of Episodes Treated	No. Failed or Recurred	Complications	Deaths
Rainbow Babies' and Children's Hospital, Cleveland					
Stowe, 1957–1974	15	17	2	2 hemorrhage 1 deep wound infection	2 within 6 months
Olsen, 1970–1985	28	30	2	—	—
University of Minnesota Hospital					
Rich, 1963–1977	20	31	1	2 hemorrhage, atelectasis	1 with severe malnutrition
Brompton Hospital, London					
Robinson, 1966–1982	18	25	5	2 hemorrhage 3 air leak, subcutaneous emphysema 1 atelectasis	5 within 6 months (1 at 1 week)
Children's Hospital Medical Center, Boston					
Schuster (1983), 1969–1982	20	20	0	1 empyema (Pseudomonas)	2 within 4 months

candidate for some form of pleurodesis. Assessment and treatment of any general physical impairment is urgent. (4) Closed-tube thoracostomy and chemical sclerosis are apparently appropriate primary therapy, with talc poudrage being the most effective with the least complications. (5) Bilateral occurrence of pneumothorax is high. Consideration should be given to concomitant contralateral chemical pleurodesis, particularly if a general anesthetic is required for primary treatment. (6) Heart-lung transplantation, as Hodson and Bathen (1988) noted, is contraindicated in the presence of diffuse adhesions. Only localized, apical adhesions should be encouraged in a patient who may become a transplant candidate.

HEMOPTYSIS

Hemoptysis, like pneumothorax, occurs in older patients with well established lung disease. Enlarged bronchial arteries supply multiple bronchopulmonary anastomoses in areas of bronchiectasis or abscess, usually in the upper lobes. The frequently immediate arrest of hemoptysis by bronchial artery embolization confirms this source of bleeding. Initial massive hemoptysis—greater than 300 ml of blood loss per 24 hours—is first seen at an average age of 15 years and occurs in at least 8% of those patients surviving beyond the age of 15. Blood streaking of the sputum can be seen for several years earlier. The most common precipitating event is an exacerbation in pulmonary infection, although such episodes may be difficult to distinguish from advancing pulmonary disease. Coagulopathy is uncommon. The natural history of untreated hemoptysis in cystic fibrosis has been documented at two large centers, but with differing conclusions and therapeutic recommendations. Holsclaw and associates (1979) described 19 patients treated between 1959 and 1969. Their patients had severe pulmonary disease with a S-K score of 55 or less in 15—79%—and an associated pneumothorax in 5. In six patients, the initial attack was terminal. Five died within one month; and two others, within 6 months. These authors concluded that this ominous complication with a 6-month mortality of 68% should be treated by early lung resection whenever feasible. On the other hand, all of the 38 patients reviewed by Stern and colleagues (1978a) stopped bleeding within 4 days and survived the acute episodes. Only five required blood transfusion. Without specific intervention, 14—37%—survived longer than 5 years; one, for 20 years. However, 17 had recurrence of massive hemoptysis. The S-K score was the most accurate prognostic finding: all with a score less than 35 died—5 patients; whereas 15 with scores greater than 60 survived.

As a group, patients with massive hemoptysis do not appear to have a worse prognosis than those with a similar degree of lung disease who never bleed. Nevertheless, the dramatic onset of profuse bleeding, with the potential of asphyxiation and exsanguination, inspires a sense of urgency for definitive treatment. Emergency bronchial artery ligation and pulmonary resection were reported by Levitsky and associates (1970) and by Keen (1971).

Some patients with poor pulmonary function may even improve because much of the bleeding and resected lung tissue is nonfunctional and has acted as a source of continuing sepsis. Obviously, as Porter (1983) and Trento (1985) and their colleagues pointed out, an operative approach should be reserved for those with localized parenchymal disease and a reasonable clinical status. Schuster and Fellows (1977) recommended bronchoscopy as a highly sensitive routine to localize the site of bleeding. Stern and colleagues (1978a), however, found bronchoscopy technically difficult and unreliable. The placement of a double-lumen endotracheal tube or bronchial balloon tamponade may facilitate stabilization and subsequent resection during an acute hemorrhage. Swersky and co-workers (1979) tamponaded the bronchial bleeding with Fogarty balloons placed through a bronchoscope, but this cumbersome technique cannot prevent recurrence.

Fellows (1979), Remy (177), and Uflacker (1985) and their associates, among others, have used selective bronchial artery embolization (see Chapter 68) as an alternative to expectant medical therapy or to operative resection for hemoptysis of varying causes, including cystic fibrosis (Fig. 63–6). Long-term control of bleeding with minimal complication has been reported by experienced angiographers. Angiography and embolization can be performed in virtually every patient with local anesthesia and mild sedation. An angiographic catheter is advanced percutaneously through a femoral artery. The bronchial arteries may arise from the aorta at a sharp angle, and subintimal dissection by the catheter must be avoided. Numerous patterns of bronchial artery anatomy are seen. Retrograde aortic flushing is minimized by the hand injection of small volumes of contrast media through a catheter tip well seated 2 to 3 cm within the bronchial artery trunk. Contrast shunted through anastomoses with the pulmonary circulation may highlight the pulmonary veins. The contrast medium rarely extravasates at the bleeding point. Nonionic contrast media are less toxic to the spinal cord, and the use of these agents should minimize the dangers of transverse myelitis. The visualization of spinal radicular branches is not an absolute contraindication to embolization, as the rare demonstration of the artery of Adamkiewicz certainly would be. Pieces of absorbable gelatin sponge—Gelfoam—1 to 3 mm in diameter are aspirated into a tuberculin syringe and slowly injected through the wedged catheter. The smaller emboli are injected first to occlude the most peripheral branches. Twenty to one hundred fragments per artery are necessary for near-complete embolization. Blood is aspirated frequently between injections, confirming catheter position within the lumen. The embolization of each artery is concluded when approximately 90% of the peripheral runoff has been blocked. At this point, forward arterial flow is so slow that further injection may flush retrograde into the aorta. In some cases, multiple vessels must be embolized to control recurrent hemorrhage, a time-consuming procedure. Revascularization and recannulation may occur. Embolization should be repeated if hemorrhage recurs. The value of

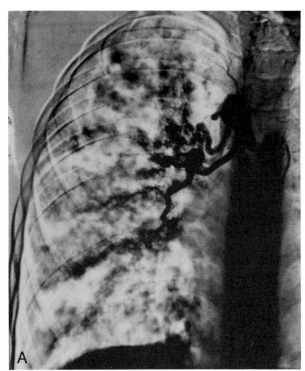
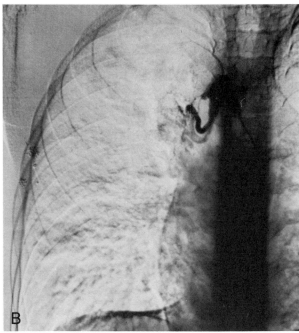

Fig. 63–6. Roentgenograms of the patient shown in Figure 63–2 who was admitted with hemoptysis of over 500 ml of blood and a recent history of increasing pulmonary disability. *A,* A selective injection of the right upper lobe bronchial artery shows marked dilatation and tortuosity of the vessel. The site of hemorrhage was not identified. *B,* After embolization of the artery with absorbable gelatin sponge—Gelfoam—a repeat bronchial injection shows near-complete occlusion of the artery. The bleeding stopped after the procedure.

preangiographic bronchoscopy to guide specific bronchial artery embolization is doubtful because (1) most patients can determine the side of hemorrhage; (2) most bleeding comes from the upper lobes, from the right more often than from the left; and (3) regardless of the actual site of bleeding, multiple vessel embolization is probably indicated whenever possible.

This technique stops acute hemorrhage in 80 to 100% of all patients. Long-lasting control can be expected in 75 to 80%. All patients appear to be good candidates for embolization, and this approach should not be reserved for those with the poorest pulmonary function. Morbidity and hospitalization time can be decreased in all. Lung tissue is preserved, and the procedure can be repeated without difficulty. Immediate side effects include transient fever and chest pain. Distal aortic embolization has caused small intestinal gangrene and transient cerebral and extremity ischemia. Dysphagia and esophagobronchial fistula have been reported.

ATELECTASIS AND BRONCHIECTASIS

Mearns (1972) and Schuster (1964) and their colleagues reviewed their respective series of children who underwent resection for bronchiectasis between 1947 and 1967. The clinical findings and outcome were remarkably similar. The ages of their combined 44 patients varied from 6 months to 15 years, with a median of 6 years. Most had localized involvement of the right upper lobe (Fig. 63–7). The lower lobe and lingula were the sites

involved on the left. The diagnosis and localization of the bronchiectatic lesion was based on plain chest roentgenograms correlated with the clinical findings. Preoperative bronchography was poorly tolerated, and this technique was abandoned. *Staphylococcus aureus* was the predominant organism. Patients who were selected for operation had frequent febrile exacerbations and limitation of activity. Even severe illness and respiratory impairment were not absolute contraindications to resection of localized disease. The operative mortality was 10%, but most survivors did experience an improvement in clinical status. Some lived for many years. Marmon and associates (1983) described nine older children operated upon between 1969 and 1981. There were no operative complications or deaths.

Symptomatic localized bronchiectasis is seen less frequently than previously. Lobar atelectasis and bronchiectasis are avoided or treated expeditiously in most patients. The disease seen in older adolescents usually involves more than one lobe. Computed tomography provides a noninvasive technique to evaluate the entire lung field for extent and severity of disease (Fig. 63–8). If operation is elected, intensive preoperative chest physiotherapy and appropriate antibiotics are prescribed in the hospital.

CONCLUSIONS

Five decades of persistent medical care and investigation have expanded the horizons of each child and adult

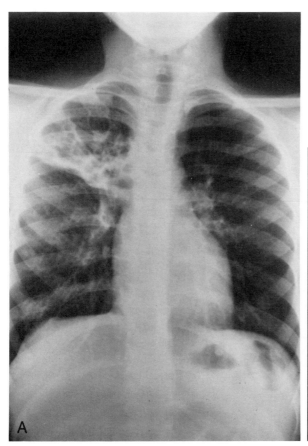

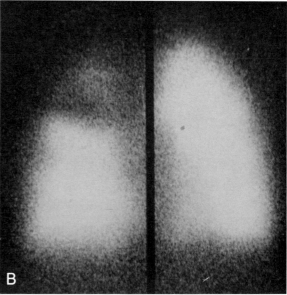

Fig. 63–7. Roentgenogram and perfusion scan of a 9-year-old girl who had a persistently productive cough despite intensive treatment. *A*, The right upper lobe has remained contracted with extensive cystic changes for 4 years. Peribronchial abscesses contain air-fluid levels. *B*, An anterior projection pulmonary perfusion scintigram performed with ⁹⁹ᵐTc albumin microspheres confirms the poorly perfused status of this bronchiectatic lobe.

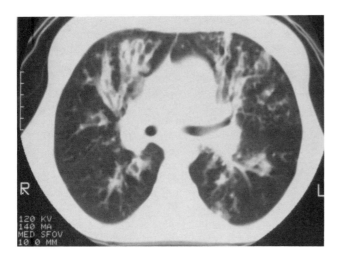

Fig. 63–8. Computed tomography demonstrates bilateral saccular bronchiectasis in multiple lung segments, worse in the lingula and right middle lobe, of a 17-year-old girl with increasing and now nocturnal cough—productive of purulent secretions. The bronchi are surrounded by edema and inflammation. The hilar lymph nodes are enlarged.

with cystic fibrosis. Survival is possible for many, although the emotional and financial consequences of lifelong therapy are formidable. As the genetic and cellular basis of the disease becomes clear, specific rather than palliative treatment may become possible. Pulmonary complications usually occur when the effects of the disease are escalating, and the patient is ill-served by procrastination of definitive management. Heart-lung transplantation is not likely to become commonly available. The thoracic surgeon must be prepared to recommend an appropriate and well defined approach to operative and angiographic intervention. Mearns and colleagues (1972) stated the goal of the thoracic surgeon in treating cystic fibrosis: the aim of surgical treatment is to slow down the progression of the disease; to prolong life; and most important to improve the quality of that life.

REFERENCES

Andersen, D.H.: Cystic fibrosis of the pancreas and its relation to celiac disease: a clinical and pathologic study. Am. J. Dis. Child. 56:344, 1938.

Andersen, D.H.: Cystic fibrosis of the pancreas: a review. J. Chronic Dis. 7:58, 1958.

Auerbach, H.S., et al.: Alternate-day prednisone reduces morbidity and improves pulmonary function in cystic fibrosis. Lancet 2:686, 1985.

Beaudet, A.L., and Buffone, G.J.: Prenatal diagnosis of cystic fibrosis. J. Pediatr. *111*:630, 1987.

Bijman, J., and Quinton, P.M.: Influence of abnormal CF impermeability and sweating in cystic fibrosis. Am. J. Physiol. *247*:C3, 1984.

Boat, T.F., et al.: Pneumothorax in cystic fibrosis. JAMA *209*:1498, 1969.

Brasfield, D., et al.: Evaluation of scoring system. Am. J. Roentgenol. *134*:1195, 1980.

Cattaneo, S.M., Sirak, H.D., and Klassen, K.P.: Recurrent spontaneous pneumothorax in the high-risk patient. J. Cardiovasc. Surg. *66*:467, 1973.

di Sant'Agnese, P.A.: Bronchial obstruction with lobar atelectasis and emphysema in cystic fibrosis of the pancreas. J. Pediatr. *12*:178, 1953.

di Sant'Agnese, P.A., and Davis, P.B.: Cystic fibrosis in adults. Am. J. Med. *66*:121, 1973.

di Sant'Agnese, P.A., and Vidaurreta, A.M.: Cystic fibrosis of the pancreas. JAMA *172*:2065, 1960.

Esterly, J.R., and Oppenheimer, E.H.: Observations in cystic fibrosis of the pancreas. III. Pulmonary lesions. Johns Hopkins Med. Bull. *122*:94, 1968.

Fellows, K.E., et al.: Selective bronchial arteriography in patients with cystic fibrosis and massive hemoptysis. Radiology *114*:551, 1979.

Finkelstein, S.M., et al.: Diabetes mellitus associated with cystic fibrosis. J. Pediatr. *112*:373, 1988.

Goldmann, D.A., and Klinger, J.P.: *Pseudomonas cepacia*: biology, mechanisms of virulence, epidemiology. J. Pediatr. *108*:806, 1986.

Hodson, M.E., and Bathen, J.C.: Heart-lung transplantation for cystic fibrosis. Excerpta Med. Asia Pac. Congr. Ser. *74*:195, 1988.

Hofmeyer, J.L., Webber, B.A., and Hodson, M.E.: Evaluation of positive expiratory pressure as an adjunct to chest physiotherapy in the treatment of cystic fibrosis. Thorax *41*:951, 1986.

Holsclaw, D.S.: Common pulmonary complications of cystic fibrosis. Clin. Pediatr. *9*:346, 1970.

Holsclaw, D.S., Grand, R.J., and Schwachman, H.: Massive hemoptysis in cystic fibrosis. J. Pediatr. *76*:829, 1970.

Huang, N.N., et al.: Clinical features, survival rate, and prognostic factors in young adults with cystic fibrosis. Am. J. Med. *82*:871, 1987.

Jones, R.E., and Giammona, S.T.: Intrapleural quinicrine for pneumothorax in a child with cystic fibrosis. Am. J. Dis. Child. *130*:777, 1976.

Jones, K., Higenbottam, T., and Wallwork, J.: Successful heart-lung transplantation for cystic fibrosis. Chest *93*:644, 1988.

Kattwinkel, J., et al.: Intrapleural instillation of quinicrine for recurrent pneumothorax. JAMA *226*:557, 1973.

Katznelsen, D., et al.: Botryomycosis, a complication in cystic fibrosis. J. Pediatr. *65*:525, 1964.

Keen, G.: Hemoptysis in cystic fibrosis (Correspondence). Br. Med. J. *1*:110, 1971.

Lamberty, J.M., and Rubin, B.K.: The management of anaesthesia for patients with cystic fibrosis. Anaesthesia *40*:448, 1985.

Laufer, P.O., et al.: Allergic bronchopulmonary aspergillosis and cystic fibrosis. J. Allergy Clin. Immunol. *73*:44, 1984.

Lester, L.A., et al.: Echocardiography in cystic fibrosis: a proposed scoring system. J. Pediatr. *97*:742, 1980.

Lester, L.A., et al.: Case report: aspiration and lung abscess in cystic fibrosis. Am. Rev. Respir. Dis. *127*:786, 1983.

Levitsky, S., Lapeu, A., and di Sant'Agnese, P.A.: Pulmonary resection for life-threatening hemoptysis in cystic fibrosis. JAMA *213*:125, 1970.

Levy, D.L., et al.: Effects of long-term nutritional rehabilitation on body composition and clinical status in malnourished children and adolescents with cystic fibrosis. J. Pediatr. *107*:225, 1985.

Lifschitz, M.K., et al.: Pneumothorax as a complication of cystic fibrosis. Am. J. Dis. Child. *116*:633, 1968.

Luck, S.R., et al.: Management of pneumothorax in children with chronic pulmonary disease. J. Thorac. Cardiovasc. Surg. *74*:834, 1977.

MacLusky, J., McLaughlin, F.J., and Levison, H.: Cystic fibrosis. I and II. Curr. Probl. Pediatr. *15*:1, 1985.

Mansell, A.L., et al.: Short-term pulmonary effects of total parenteral nutrition in children with cystic fibrosis. J. Pediatr. *104*:700, 1984.

Marmon, L., et al.: Pulmonary resection for complications of cystic fibrosis. J. Pediatr. Surg. *18*:811, 1983.

McLaughlin, F.J., Matthews, W.J., and Strieder, D.J.: Pneumothorax in cystic fibrosis: management and outcome. J. Pediatr. *100*:863, 1982.

Mearns, M.B., et al.: Pulmonary resection in cystic fibrosis—results in 23 cases, 1957–1970. Arch. Dis. Child. *47*:499, 1972.

Mitchell-Heggs, P.F., and Batten, J.C.: Pleurectomy for spontaneous pneumothorax in cystic fibrosis. Thorax *25*:165, 1970.

Moss, A.J.: The cardiovascular system in cystic fibrosis. Pediatrics *70*:728, 1982.

Olsen, M.M., et al.: Surgery in patients with cystic fibrosis. J. Pediatr. Surg. *22*:613, 1987.

Ostrer, H., and Hejtmancik, F.J.: Prenatal diagnosis and carrier detection of genetic diseases by analysis of deoxyribonucleic acid. J. Pediatr. *112*:679, 1988.

Penketh, A., et al.: Management of pneumothorax in adults with cystic fibrosis. Thorax *37*:850, 1982.

Penketh, A.R.L., et al.: Cystic fibrosis in adolescents and adults. Thorax *42*:526, 1987.

Porter, D.K., Von Every, M.J., and Mack, J.W.: Emergency lobectomy for massive hemoptysis in cystic fibrosis. J. Thorac. Cardiovasc. Surg. *86*:409, 1983.

Remy, J., et al.: Treatment of hemoptysis by embolization of bronchial arteries. Radiology *122*:33, 1977.

Rich, R.H., Warwick, W.J., and Leonard, A.S.: Open thoracotomy and pleural abrasion in the treatment of spontaneous pneumothorax in cystic fibrosis. J. Pediatr. Surg. *13*:237, 1978.

Robinson, D.A., and Branthwaite, M.A.: Pleural surgery in patients with cystic fibrosis. Anaesthesia. *39*:655, 1984.

Rubio, T.T.: Infection in patients with cystic fibrosis. Am. J. Med. *81*(Suppl. 1A):73, 1986.

Sahn, S.A., and Potts, E.D.: The effect of tetracycline on rabbit pleura. Am. Rev. Respir. Dis. *117*:493, 1978.

Schuster, S.R., and Fellows, K.E.: Management of major hemoptysis in patients with cystic fibrosis. J. Pediatr. Surg. *12*:889, 1977.

Schuster, S.R., et al.: Management of pneumothorax in cystic fibrosis. J. Pediatr. Surg. *18*:492, 1983.

Schuster, S., et al.: Pulmonary surgery for cystic fibrosis. J. Thorac. Cardiovasc. Surg. *48*:750, 1964.

Schwartz, E.E., and Holsclaw, D.S.: Pulmonary involvement in adults with cystic fibrosis. Am. J. Roentgenol. *122*:708, 1974.

Scully, R.E. (ed.): Case records of the Massachusetts General Hospital, Case 26-1977. N. Engl. J. Med. *296*:1519, 1977.

Shepherd, R., Cooksley, W.G.E., and Cooke, W.D.P.: Improved growth and clinical nutritional and respiratory changes in response to nutritional therapy in cystic fibrosis. J. Pediatr. *97*:351, 1980.

Shwachman, H., Kowalski, M., and Khaw, K.T.: Cystic fibrosis: a new outlook: 70 patients above 25 years of age. Medicine *56*:129, 1977.

Stern, R.C., et al.: Treatment and prognosis of massive hemoptysis in cystic fibrosis. Am. Rev. Respir. Dis. *117*:825, 1978a.

Stern, R.C., et al.: Treatment and prognosis of lobar and segmental atelectasis in cystic fibrosis. Am. Rev. Respir. Dis. *118*:821, 1978b.

Stowe, S.M., et al.: Open thoracotomy for pneumothorax in cystic fibrosis. Am. Rev. Respir. Dis. *111*:611, 1975.

Swersky, R.B., et al.: Endobronchial balloon tamponade of hemoptysis in patients with cystic fibrosis. Ann. Thorac. Surg. *27*:262, 1979.

Taussig, L.M., Belmonte, M.M., and Beaudry, P.H.: Staphylococcus aureus empyema in cystic fibrosis. J. Pediatr. *84*:724, 1974.

Tomashefski, J.F., Dahms, B., and Bruce, M.: Pleura in pneumothorax. Arch. Pathol. Lab. Med. *109*:910, 1985a.

Tomashefski, J.F., et al.: Pulmonary air cysts in cystic fibrosis: relation of pathologic features to radiographic findings and history of pneumothorax. Hum. Pathol. *16*:253, 1985b.

Thomassen, M.J., Demko, C.A., and Doershuk, C.F.: Cystic fibrosis: a review of pulmonary infections and interventions. Pediatr. Pulmon. *3*:334, 1987.

Trento, H., et al.: Massive hemoptysis in patients with cystic fibrosis: three case reports and a protocol for clinical management. Ann. Thorac. Surg. *39*:254, 1985.

Tribble, C.G., Selden, R.F., and Rodgers, B.M.: Talc poudrage in the treatment of spontaneous pneumothoraces in patients with cystic fibrosis. Ann. Surg. *204*:677, 1986.

Uflacker, R., et al.: Bronchial artery embolization in the management of hemoptysis: technical aspects and long-term results. Radiology *157*:637, 1985.

Vaisman, W., et al.: Energy expenditure of patients with cystic fibrosis. J. Pediatr. *111*:496, 1987.

Vasil, M.L.: *Pseudomonas aeruginosa*: Biology, mechanisms of virulence, epidemiology. J. Pediatr. *108*:800, 1985.

Wessel, H.U.: Lung function in cystic fibrosis. *In* Textbook of Cystic Fibrosis. Edited by J.D. Lloyd-Still. Boston, John Wright, PSG Inc., 1983, pp. 199–215.

READING REFERENCES

Doershuk, C.F., and Fink, R.J.: Pediatric Respiratory Therapy, 3rd ed., Chicago, Yearbook Medical Publishers, 1985.

Hodson, M.E., and Batten, J.C. (ed.): Cystic Fibrosis. London, Balliese, Tindall, 1983.

Lloyd-Still, J.D. (ed.): Textbook of Cystic Fibrosis. Boston, John Wright, PSG, Inc., 1983.

Taussig, L.M.: Cystic Fibrosis: New York, Thieme-Stratton, Inc., 1985.

CHAPTER 64

CONGENITAL VASCULAR LESIONS OF THE LUNG AND COMPRESSION OF THE TRACHEA AND ESOPHAGUS BY VASCULAR RINGS

James W. Kilman, Carl L. Backer, and Thomas W. Shields

The incidence of congenital vascular malformations of the lung is low despite the complex embryologic derivation of the pulmonary vasculature (see Chapter 1). Some of the anomalies can be associated with significant disability and still be amenable to appropriate surgical management. A classification of congenital abnormalities that affect the main branches of the pulmonary vessels and their tributaries was suggested by Ellis and associates (1964) and has been modified for completeness (Table 64–1). Although arbitrary, such a classification encourages more accurate diagnostic delineations of such defects, which may lead to eventual surgical repair in many.

Complex anomalies of the aorta and its branches also occur. Most of the clinically significant anomalies cause tracheal or esophageal obstruction in infants and young children, although some anomalies are asymptomatic throughout life. In an autopsy study, however, Liechty and associates (1957) described only 13 examples in 1000 adult specimens of variations of the aortic branching that could possibly have resulted in any tracheal or esophageal obstruction. Table 64–2 classifies the major clinically significant vascular anomalies of the great vessels in infants and children.

AGENESIS AND STENOSIS OF PULMONARY ARTERY

Agenesis and stenosis of pulmonary arteries are rare but provide unusual challenges in diagnosis and management. Most affected persons with these defects die at an early age from right ventricular failure and hypertension in the pulmonary artery of the unaffected side. A few patients are asymptomatic or are hampered by some dyspnea and recurrent pulmonary infections. The natural history of the anomaly is not well understood. Gregg (1941) reported that these anomalies are associated with maternal rubella.

In this abnormality, the affected lung has a small volume and decreased markings—the hyperlucent lung syndrome (Fig. 64–1). The thoracic cage is contracted, and ventilation is reduced. Ventilation–perfusion scans demonstrate vascular hypoperfusion, and decreased ventilation and obstructive bronchiolar disease can be demonstrated with bronchographic contrast material. Angiocardiography delineates the pulmonary artery anomaly. Stenosis of the pulmonary artery may occur at its origin (Fig. 64–2) or at isolated, multiple peripheral

Table 64–1. Classification of Congenital Vascular Lesions of the Lung

Abnormalities of the pulmonary circulation
  Pulmonary arteries
    Agenesis of a pulmonary artery
    Stenosis of a branch or branches of the pulmonary arteries
    Pulmonary arteriovenous fistula
  Pulmonary veins
    Abnormal pulmonary venous connection
    Varicosities of the pulmonary veins
  Lymphangiectasia

Modified with permission from Ellis, F.H., McGoon, D.C., and Kincaid, O.W.: Congenital vascular malformations of the lungs. Med. Clin. North Am. *48*:1069, 1964.

Table 64–2. Classification of Vascular Rings

Double aortic arch
Right aortic arch with left ligamentum
  With retroesophageal left subclavian artery
  With mirror image left innominate artery
Pulmonary artery sling
Left aortic arch
  Innominate artery compression
  Aberrant right subclavian
Miscellaneous

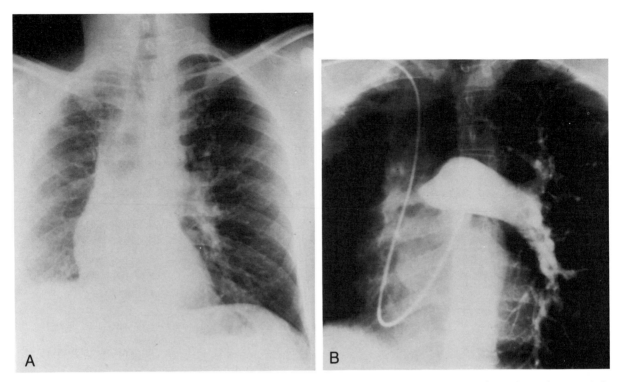

Fig. 64–1. Sawyer-James syndrome. *A,* PA chest roentgenogram demonstrating small right lung with decreased vascular markings. *B,* Pulmonary angiogram in a patient with agenesis of the right pulmonary artery and minimal vascular markings—hyperlucent lung syndrome.

sites. In agenesis of the pulmonary artery, an anomalous artery from the aorta (Fig. 64–3) usually supplies the involved lung, but dilated bronchial arteries may be the main source of the blood that maintains some viability of the affected lung.

Surgical treatment has been reported uncommonly, and although McGoon and Kincaid (1964) reported repair of multiple peripheral areas of stenosis, most have been at the origin of either main stem artery. The success of patch arterioplasty or graft replacement of absent or stenosed pulmonary arteries depends largely on the extent of the vascular anomaly and the degree of bronchial and parenchymal lung damage secondary to infection and fibrosis. Dilation by balloons has proved to be successful in certain cases of isolated, discrete stenosis of pulmonary arteries. Rocchini and associates (1984) reported that balloon dilation may be the procedure of choice for multiple stenotic lesions. In older patients with unilateral agenesis of the pulmonary artery, persistent respiratory infection is the most prominent complaint. Pneumonectomy is usually required, and care to identify and control any systemic artery to the lung is mandatory.

PULMONARY ARTERIOVENOUS FISTULAS

These congenital malformations result from errant capillary development, with incomplete formation or distintegration of the vascular septa that normally divide the primitive connections between the venous and arterial plexuses. Tobin (1966) verified that some pulmonary arteriovenous shunting exists in normal lungs. This shunting may be hemodynamically important in pathologic conditions associated with venous or arterial pulmonary hypertension, portal cirrhosis, and obstructive lung disease.

Classification

A review of the embryology of the pulmonary vascular system indicates that pulmonary arteriovenous abnormalities may occur as isolated or combined lesions at the arterial, capillary, or venous level. Anabtawi and colleagues (1965) presented an anatomic classification based on the size and position of arteriovenous communications (Table 64–3). The classification according to the blood supply has both hemodynamic and prognostic importance because the fistulas supplied by systemic arteries have the same hemodynamic consequences as arteriovenous fistulas of the general circulation have. Also, as Dines and associates (1974) noted, it is important to divide the entire group into those associated with Rendu-Osler-Weber disease—ROWD—also called hereditary hemorrhagic telangiectasis—HHT—and those not associated with it, because this stratification has important prognostic value. Patients with cutaneous telangiectasis—ROWD—more often have multiple pulmonary fistulas, a predictable progression of symptoms, and a higher rate of complications.

Pulmonary Arteriovenous Fistulas with Pulmonary Arterial Supply

Clinical Aspects

Congenital pulmonary arteriovenous fistulas occur more frequently in women and are transmitted as a dom-

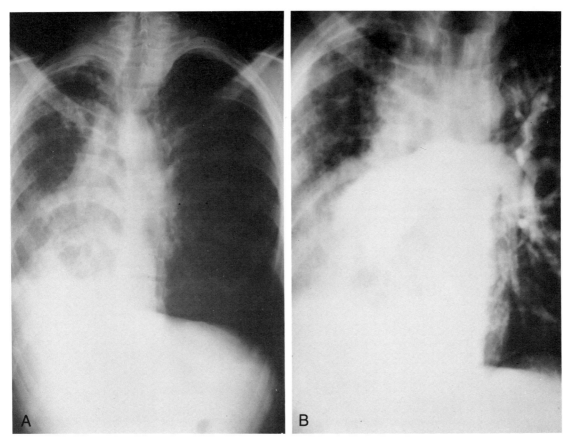

Fig. 64–2. *A*, PA chest roentgenogram of young adult man with severe pulmonary infection in the right lung with marked shift of the mediastinum and heart into the right hemithorax. *B*, Angiogram revealing agenesis of the right pulmonary artery.

inant gene with incomplete penetrance. Hodgson and Kaye (1963) reported a family that had hereditary hemorrhagic telangiectasis; 6.4% of those surveyed roentgenographically had pulmonary arteriovenous fistulas. Jeresaty and associates (1966) reported that symptoms began in childhood and consisted of dyspnea and easy fatigability in 25 to 50% of patients. Ellis and associates (1964) reported, however, that among 96 patients, only two had symptoms dating from childhood.

Exertional dyspnea, palpitations, and easy fatigability are the most frequent symptoms, usually appearing in the third or fourth decade of life, and are present in about 50% of patients. Hemoptysis is common when the fistula is associated with cutaneous telangiectasis—ROWD. A continuous bruit is present over the lesion in 75% of patients who have associated hereditary telangiectasis and in 38% of those who are without such an association. The typical bruit has a rough, humming, continuous sound that is accentuated in systole and with deep inspiration; the diastolic accentuation is more subtle. The audibility of the bruit can change with position. It may be associated with mitral valve prolapse in these patients.

The classic triad of cyanosis, polycythemia, and clubbing of the fingers or toes has been noted in about 20% of the patients. The presence of cyanosis indicates that at least 25 to 30% of the blood in the lesser circulation is being shunted from the right to the left side of the heart through the fistula.

Physiologic Findings

Po$_2$ and oxygen saturation are decreased. Intracardiac and intravascular pressure proximal to the fistula are normal; as a result, the cardiac output is usually normal, although it may be increased at times. The systemic blood pressure and the electrocardiographic findings are also normal. The heart is usually not enlarged. Blood volume studies reveal an increased red cell mass in most cases. The plasma volume remains normal.

Roentgenographic Features

In one half to two thirds of the patients, the fistulas are single. The remainder are multiple and may be bilateral in 8 to 10% of the patients. Roentgenograms of the chest show the fistulas as lobulated, fairly well defined densities connected to the hilar structures by broad linear shadows because of the dilated vascular connections (Fig. 64–4). Eighty percent of the lesions are subpleural or superficial. Usually, fistulas are seen more frequently in the lower than in the upper lobes. On fluoroscopy, they may be seen to pulsate or become smaller with the Valsalva maneuver. Also on fluoroscopy, because of the increased blood flow, there may be an increased amplitude of pulsation of the hilar vessels.

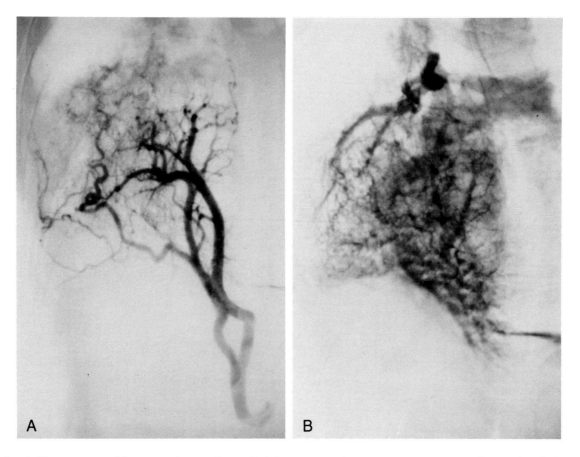

Fig. 64–3. *A*, This aortogram of the patient shown in Figure 64–2 demonstrates a large ectopic systemic artery that supplies the lower portion of the right lung and that arises from the subdiaphragmatic portion of the aorta. *B*, Delayed roentgenograms showing venous drainage through normal right pulmonary veins.

Table 64–3. Classification of Pulmonary Arteriovenous Malformations

I	Multiple small arteriovenous fistulas without aneurysm
II	Large single arteriovenous aneurysm—peripheral
IIIa	Large single arteriovenous aneurysm—central
IIIb	Large arteriovenous aneurysm with anomalous venous drainage
IIIc	Multiple small arteriovenous fistulas with anomalous venous drainage
IVa	Large single venous aneurysm with systemic artery communication
IVb	Large single venous aneurysm without fistula—undescribed
V	Anomalous venous drainage without fistula

Reproduced with permission from Anabtawi, I.N., Ellison, R.G., Ellison, L.T.: Pulmonary arteriovenous aneurysms and fistulas: anatomic variations, embryology, and classification. Ann. Thorac. Surg. 1:277, 1965.

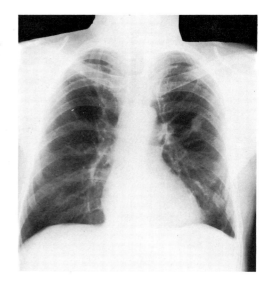

Fig. 64–4. Arteriovenous fistula in the left upper lobe with vascular connections to left hilus.

Computed tomography usually demonstrates the lesion sufficiently well to be diagnostic, but angiocardiography is the important diagnostic study to confirm the diagnosis and delineate the number of fistulas present (Fig. 64–5).

Additional Diagnostic Studies

Burke and Raffin (1986) suggested the use of noninvasive studies before the use of pulmonary angiography in patients suspected of having pulmonary arteriovenous fistulas. These studies include contrast echocardiography, described by Shub and associates (1976), and perfusion lung scintigraphy, reported by Lewis and colleagues (1978). A negative result excludes the presence of right-to-left shunt and thus excludes the presence of a fistula. A positive result confirms the suspected diagnosis without risk to the patient. In addition, perfusion lung scintigraphy provides a quantitative estimation of the magnitude of the shunt. Neither examination, however, supplants the use of contrast angiography in patients who are candidates for invasive therapy.

Complications

Stringer and associates (1955) noted 30 instances of serious complications or death among 140 patients with pulmonary arteriovenous fistulas. Dalton and co-workers (1967) recorded nine instances of intrapleural rupture. Massive hemoptysis is uncommon. White (1984) noted that paradoxic embolization and stroke as the result of a bland embolus to the brain may occur. Dines and associates (1974) observed a stroke to have occurred in 10% of all untreated patients followed for 4 to 10 years in whom a pulmonary AV fistula was seen on the roentgenogram or if there was hypoxemia on room air. Cerebral abscesses also have been reported, but none of 96 patients reported by Dines and colleagues (1983), however, had cerebral abscess or intrapleural rupture.

Treatment

Most patients with one or more pulmonary arteriovenous fistulas are candidates for resection or obliteration of the lesions. Only those few who have a small lesion—

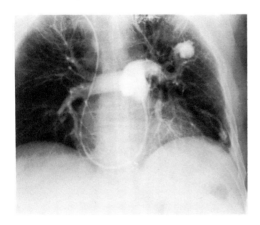

Fig. 64–5. Angiocardiogram delineating multiple arteriovenous fistulas: a large fistula in left upper lobe and an additional fistula in the left lower lobe.

10 to 15 mm in diameter—and who are asymptomatic with a minimal shunt may be observed. In this subset, however, the risk of paradoxic embolization is present as previously noted. In patients with Rendu-Osler-Weber disease, treatment is indicated in all patients, if at all possible, because the complication rate is highest in this group. Interventional therapy is likewise indicated in all symptomatic patients and even in those whose symptoms are minimal if the lesion can be identified on the standard chest roentgenogram or if hypoxemia is present when the patient breathes room air.

Single lesions are best managed by conservative surgical excision. Some multiple lesions may also be treated by excision, but most patients with multiple or bilateral lesions are best managed by roentgenographically guided embolization.

Surgical Therapy. Surgical excision of an isolated, single pulmonary arteriovenous fistula is successful, with minimal mortality and morbidity and little chance of recurrence of the lesion. Because most fistulas are located subpleurally, they can be removed with conservative local resections. As noted, multiple fistulas are occasionally suitable for resection. Patients with symptoms and one or more enlarging fistulas are candidates for operation. Dines and associates (1974) noted that patients with a single fistula and hereditary hemorrhagic telangiectasis—HHT—should be operated on because enlargement, symptoms, and complications are more frequent. Sperling and colleagues (1977) noted, however, that the combination of pulmonary hypertension and arteriovenous fistulas is a contraindication for surgical excision.

Embolic Obliteration. Selective roentgenographically guided embolization of multiple pulmonary arteriovenous fistulas unsuitable for surgical resection has proved to be a valuable therapeutic modality. The patients with multiple lesions are frequently severely disabled by the presence of the large right-to-left shunt, and occlusion of the shunts permits a return to a near-normal status.

Taylor and associates (1978) first reported therapeutic embolization of the fistula by pulmonary arterial catheterization and the use of small steel guide wires with 3 cm wool tails. Tadavarthy and colleagues (1975) had described the use of polyvinyl alcohol sponge—Ivalon—as an embolic agent, but its use has been infrequent in the management of PAVFs. The popular materials used at present are detachable silicone balloons devised by White and co-workers (1980) (Fig. 64–6) and stainless steel coils introduced by Gianturco and associates (1975).

The occluding element is placed precisely into the feeding pulmonary arterial branch beyond all of the artery's normal branches to the lung. Proper placement is guided by video monitoring or digital subtraction angiography, or both. White (1983) described his technique and pointed out that approximately 79% of the fistulas have a single feeding artery and a single draining vein, so occlusion is relatively easy to achieve; the remaining 21% have two or more feeding and draining branches, which makes the embolization process more difficult. Anderson and colleagues (1979) and Hatfield and Fried

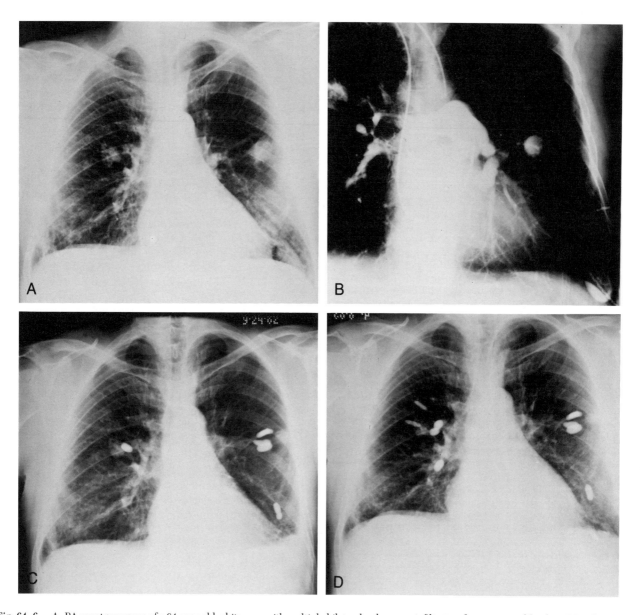

Fig. 64–6. *A*, PA roentgenogram of a 64-year-old white man with multiple bilateral pulmonary infiltrates, frequent nosebleeds, a PO$_2$ of 52 mmHg, and increasing shortness of breath. *B*, Pulmonary angiogram revealing multiple bilateral pulmonary arterial venous fistulas. *C*, PA roentgenogram in August 1982 after balloon embolization of a number of the fistulas by R.I. White, Jr. of Johns Hopkins University, with moderate symptomatic improvement. *D*, PA roentgenogram in March 1983 following balloon embolization of remaining AV fistulas, with complete relief of previous dyspnea and return of oxygen saturation and PO$_2$ levels to normal on room air. (Reproduced with permission of R.E. Otto.)

(1981) described the successful use of the Gianturco "mini" stainless-steel coil in patients with multiple fistulas. These coils (Fig. 64–7) cause clotting and obstruction of the fistula and can be seen on the postprocedure chest film (Fig. 64–8).

With proper technique and experience, the results are gratifying. With permanent occlusion of the fistulas by either of the occluding elements, the hypoxemia is corrected. Minimal pulmonary infarction may occur postocclusion, and chest pain may be troublesome early.

Wallenharyst and D'Souza (1988) reported a good result with the combined use of embolization of multiple bilateral small arteriovenous malformations and subsequent resection of a large subpleural AV fistula of the right lower lobe with maximal preservation of lung tissue by the resectional technique described by Bosher and associates (1959). In this approach the hilar vessels are temporarily controlled and the fistula resected with its feeding arteries and veins ligated with sacrifice of little or no lung tissue.

Systemic–Pulmonary Arteriovenous Fistulas

Pulmonary arteriovenous fistulas that have a systemic blood supply are rare. The bronchial arteries, internal mammary arteries, or aorta are the primary and immediate sources of the systemic arterial blood. Resection is indicated, although the extensive collateral circulation in the chest wall may provide formidable technical challenges. Involvement adjacent to the spinal column may preclude complete resection, but partial resection of the systemic arterial sources of blood, in particular, removes the threat of serious hemorrhagic and hemodynamic complications of high-output congestive failure (Fig. 64–9).

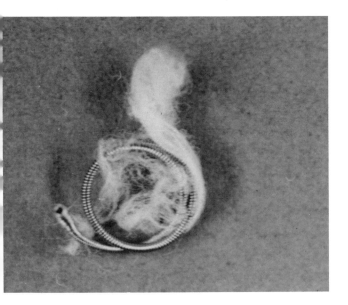

Fig. 64–7. Stainless-steel coil that can be inserted via cardiac catheter to occlude and thrombose a pulmonary arteriovenous fistula.

PULMONARY ARTERY ANEURYSMS

Aneurysmal dilation of the pulmonary artery secondary to associated congenital cardiovascular anomalies is not a rare entity, but true aneurysms of this vessel secondary to disintegration of its wall are indeed rare. Aneurysms consequent to long-standing hypertension or high pulmonary blood flow are most frequently associated with patent ductus arteriosus and by definition would be acquired and not congenital. This problem of etiology is not easily solved. Natelson and associates (1970) described aneurysms secondary to cystic medial necrosis of the pulmonary arteries that have caused striking clinicopathologic findings related to pulmonary hypertension, dissection, and rupture of the vessel. Ungaro and associates (1976) classified pulmonary artery aneurysms into specific causes—tuberculosis, syphilis, trauma—and nonspecific causes—mycotic, pulmonary hypertension, arteriosclerotic, those related to congenital defects in the vessel wall, and iatrogenic. Most so-called congenital aneurysms of the pulmonary artery, although acquired, are associated with some other congenital anomaly. Because the truly peripheral and often solitary aneurysms rupture in as many as 60% of patients, Ungaro and colleagues (1976) emphasized the necessity of definitive diagnosis and early treatment. Conservative pulmonary resection usually suffices.

Significant dilatation of both the right and the left pulmonary arteries may be present with isolated pulmonary valvular insufficiency or may be associated with the tetralogy of Fallot. This anomaly may result in the so-called Mickey Mouse heart, a sign named for its distinctive appearance on a plain chest film. This aneurysmal dilatation can cause airway problems with pressure on one or both main stem bronchi. Pierce and associates (1970) reported that an emphysematous lobe may be associated with pulmonary artery aneurysm of any etiology. Frequently, correction of the pulmonary valvular insufficiency by conduit replacement may remedy the problem, but resection of the enlarged vessels may be needed to cure the airway problems. Murphy and colleagues (1987) reported successful resection of a peripheral artery aneurysm using cardiopulmonary bypass.

ABNORMAL PULMONARY VENOUS CONNECTION

A complete discussion of anomalous pulmonary venous connections is beyond the scope of this text. Anomalous venous drainage of the right lung into the inferior vena cava—the scimitar syndrome, however, is often associated with bronchial anomalies, hypoplasia, and abnormal systemic arterial supply of the right lung. Although the abnormal left-to-right shunt may be the major cause of clinical problems in most patients with the syndrome, pulmonary symptoms—often of chronic severe pulmonary infection—may be the dominant clinical feature. Thus, consideration of the syndrome is important to the general thoracic surgeon.

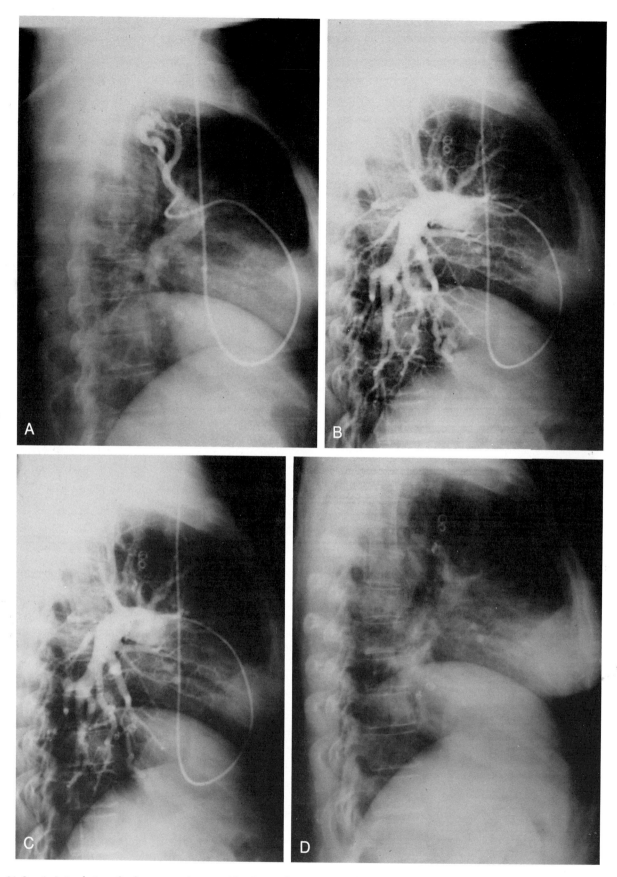

Fig. 64–8. *A*, Lateral view of pulmonary angiogram with selective demonstration of an upper lobe arteriovenous fistula in a patient with multiple fistulas and Rendu-Osler-Weber syndrome. *B*, The same patient with a nonselective pulmonary angiogram that demonstrates occlusion of the upper lobe fistula by the coil, which is visible on the film, and demonstration of a second fistula in the lower lobe. *C*, The same patient with both upper and lower lobe fistulas occluded by coils. *D*, The same patient's lateral chest film demonstrating multiple coils that have been used to occlude fistulas.

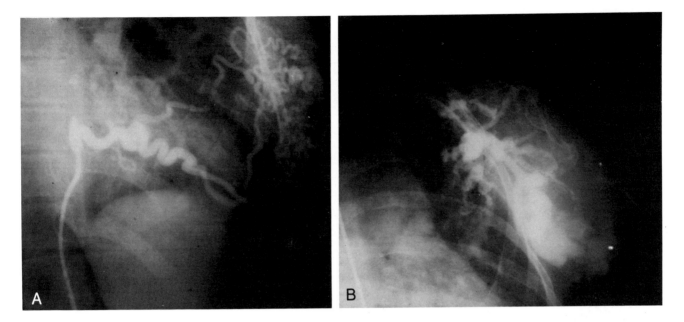

Fig. 64–9. *A*, Selective angiogram of an intercostal artery of a patient with a large systemic arteriovenous fistula of the chest wall. The fistula was draining into the lung. The patient had high-output congestive failure and was refractory to any occlusive therapy or surgical therapy of these multiple communications. *B*, Venous phase of the arteriovenous fistulas demonstrating drainage into the lung with rapid run-off into the pulmonary venous system.

Scimitar Syndrome

This syndrome consists of a constellation of abnormalities, the constant being total or partial anomalous pulmonary venous drainage of the right lung to the inferior vena cava. Neill and associates (1960) emphasized that the gently curved vertical shape of this vein on a chest roentgenogram resembles the curved Turkish sword or scimitar. Associated findings that may or may not be present are dextroposition of the heart, hypoplasia of the right lung and right pulmonary artery, malformation of the bronchial tree, and anomalous systemic arteries to the right lung from the abdominal aorta or its branches. Trell and colleagues (1971) reported that intracardiac defects are present in up to 40% of these patients.

Symptoms are related to the degree of left-to-right shunting, pulmonary hypertension, parenchymal lung disease, and associated intracardiac lesions. Kiely and co-workers (1967) documented in 70 cases that the more common symptoms were fatigue, dyspnea, decreased exercise tolerance, cough, recurrent respiratory tract infections, and failure to thrive. Chest roentgenograms show a small right lung, cardiac displacement to the right, and the shadow of the anomalous vein (Fig. 64–10). The electrocardiogram reveals right ventricular hypertrophy. Echocardiography is useful in identifying associated intracardiac lesions and the location of the anomalous vein penetrating the diaphragm. Cardiac catheterization and angiocardiography are diagnostic.

The decision for operative intervention must be individualized depending on the degree of symptoms and the findings at cardiac catheterization. For large left-to-right shunts, physiologic correction is preferred. Kirklin

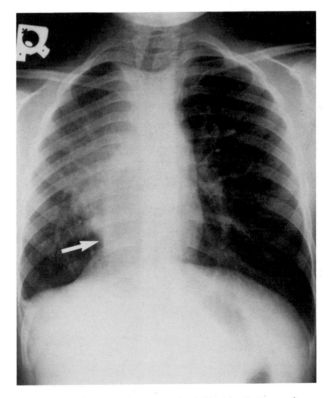

Fig. 64–10. Chest roentgenogram of a child with scimitar syndrome. Arrow points to the anomalous vein, which resembles a Turkish saber. Note the dextroposition of the heart and hypoplasia of the right lung.

and associates (1956) reported that either the anomalous vessel can be anastomosed directly to the left atrium or an intracardiac patch can be used to tunnel the flow from the anomalous vein to the left atrium through an atrial septal defect. Sanger and colleagues (1963) suggested that if inflammatory parenchymal changes are extensive, pulmonary resection or pneumonectomy should be considered. Resection eliminates the left-to-right shunt as well as the lung infection. In all instances, the systemic arterial supply to the lung is divided.

Results depend chiefly on the degree of preoperative pulmonary hypertension and associated cardiac lesions. Older patients with minimal symptoms have an excellent prognosis. Canter and associates (1986) noted that infants with cyanosis, failure to thrive, and severe pulmonary hypertension have a high mortality rate.

LYMPHANGIECTASIA

Primary pulmonary lymphangiectasia does occur or may be associated with generalized lymphangiectasia. Noonan and co-workers (1970) reported that this anomaly is associated with a syndrome that consists of pulmonary stenosis, atrial septal defect, and mental retardation. This anomaly has also been reported as a familial lesion by Scott-Emaukpor and associates (1981). The chest roentgenogram may show a pattern similar to hyaline membrane disease or may show cystic infiltrates. The patients may develop pleural effusions or chylothorax that require drainage. The only therapy is supportive, and the disease is usually progressive and fatal.

VASCULAR RINGS

Developmental malformations of the aortic arch may lead to the creation of a complete or nearly complete vascular ring encircling the trachea and the esophagus. Almost all clinically significant vascular rings become symptomatic in infants or young children and do so primarily because of tracheal compression with airway obstruction. Esophageal compression and obstruction are less important, although feeding difficulties may become apparent in the infant when solid foods are started. In most cases, the ring is an isolated defect, although it may be associated with intracardiac defects, the most common being tetralogy of Fallot. The various types of vascular rings are listed in Table 64–2 and are schematically represented in Figure 64–11.

Double Aortic Arch

Double aortic arch is the most common complete vascular ring that causes tracheoesophageal compression. Potts and associates (1948) noted that patients typically present in the first months of life with symptoms of stridor, respiratory distress, or a cough that sounds like a seal's bark.

Using the aortic arch model described by Edwards (1953), a double aortic arch results from persistence of the right fourth aortic arch. As a result, the ascending aorta divides into two arches that pass around the trachea

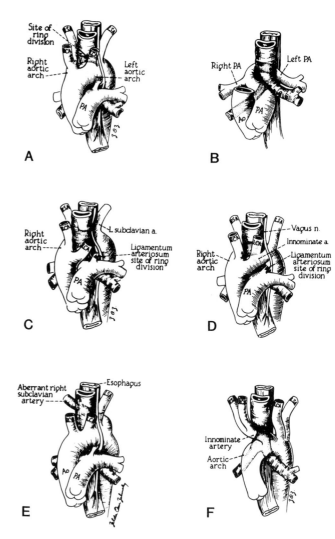

Fig. 64–11. Schematic illustration of the major vascular anomalies that cause tracheoesophageal compression. *A*, Double aortic arch, dominant left arch. *B*, Pulmonary artery sling. *C*, Right aortic arch with left ligamentum arteriosum and retroesophageal left subclavian artery. *D*, Right aortic arch with left ligamentum and mirror image left innominate. *E*, Left aortic arch with aberrant right subclavian artery. *F*, Anomalous innominate artery.

and esophagus and join posteriorly to form the descending aorta (Fig. 64–11A). Wychulis and associates (1971) showed that in two thirds of these infants, the right-sided—posterior—arch is dominant, and in one third, the left-sided—anterior—arch is dominant. The carotid and subclavian arteries originate symmetrically and separately from each arch. The tight, constricting ring thus formed compresses the trachea and esophagus.

The diagnosis can be suspected on examination of the chest roentgenogram because the location of the aortic arch in relation to the trachea is indeterminate. Ideally, the next study in these symptomatic infants is a barium esophagogram, which is generally diagnostic. The double aortic arch on an AP esophagogram appears as bilateral indentations of unequal size that are persistent in location. Computed tomography, magnetic resonance imaging, and angiography also demonstrate the double arch

(Fig. 64–12). These studies, however, may be misleading if a portion of the arch is atretic, which as Wychulis and associates (1971) noted can occur in 20 to 40% of patients.

All patients with double aortic arch and symptoms should be operated on; a narrowed trachea when further compromised by mucosal edema from even a mild upper respiratory infection can cause sudden respiratory arrest.

Severe symptoms usually are noted soon after birth, and release of the constricting vascular ring is indicated. Surgical approach is through a left thoracotomy except in cases of associated intracardiac lesions, in which simultaneous repair can be effected through a median sternotomy.

The ring is released by dividing the lesser of the two arches. This is done at a site selected to preserve brachiocephalic blood flow, usually where the lesser arch inserts into the descending aorta. The arch is divided between vascular clamps, and the stumps are oversewn with prolene sutures; simple ligation should not be done. The ligamentum arteriosum is also divided. Careful dissection is then performed around the trachea and esophagus to lyse any residual adhesive bands. Care must be taken not to injure the phrenic or recurrent nerves.

Results of surgical intervention are excellent, with almost no mortality. As Nikaidoh and associates (1972) reported, many children have residual noisy breathing for 6 months to 2 years, but this gradually resolves.

Right Aortic Arch

Right aortic arch with a left ligamentum arteriosum completing the vascular ring is almost as common as double aortic arch. The ring, however, is usually not as tight, and children typically present somewhat later in life, at 1 to 6 months of age. Symptoms are cough, respiratory distress, and stridor; in older children, dysphagia may be present.

Embryologically, right aortic arch results from persistence of the right fourth arch and deletion of the left fourth arch. Nikaidoh and associates (1972) showed that in two thirds of patients, the deletion occurs between the left carotid and subclavian arteries, and a retroesophageal left subclavian artery exists (Fig. 64–11C). In the other third, the left arch deletion occurs between the left subclavian artery and the descending aorta, and a mirror-image branching takes place with a left innominate artery (Fig. 64–11D). The left ligamentum between the descending aorta and left pulmonary artery completes the vascular ring.

The chest roentgenogram demonstrates an aortic arch to the right of the tracheal air column (Fig. 64–13). The single most effective diagnostic examination is the barium esophagogram. On AP projection there is a large right impression and a small left impression. The lateral projection shows a large posterior impression (Fig. 64–14).

The surgical approach is through a left thoracotomy, reserving median sternotomy for those patients with associated intracardiac lesions. The ring is released by dividing the ligamentum arteriosum. The origin of the retroesophageal subclavian artery may be dilated—Kommerele's diverticulum. This dilated area is a remnant of the left dorsal aortic root. As Wychulis and associates (1971) reported, this remnant may require resection to alleviate esophageal compression.

Pulmonary Artery Sling

This is an uncommon anomaly. In a review of the world literature, Koopot and associates (1975) identified 64 cases. Nearly all patients are symptomatic with respiratory distress, cyanosis, stridor, or apnea in the first month of life. Associated tracheobronchial anomalies are

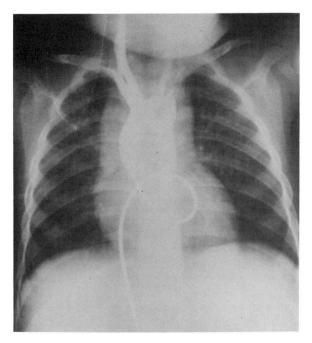

Fig. 64–12. Angiogram of a child with double aortic arch, both arches patent.

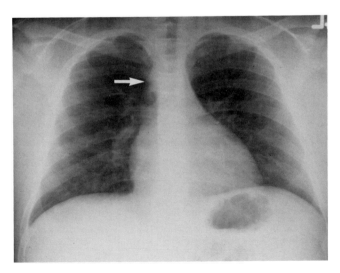

Fig. 64–13. This chest roentgenogram of a 16-year-old with right aortic arch and left ligamentum shows that the arch of the aorta (arrow) is to the right of the tracheal air column. The patient's esophagogram is shown in Fig. 64–14.

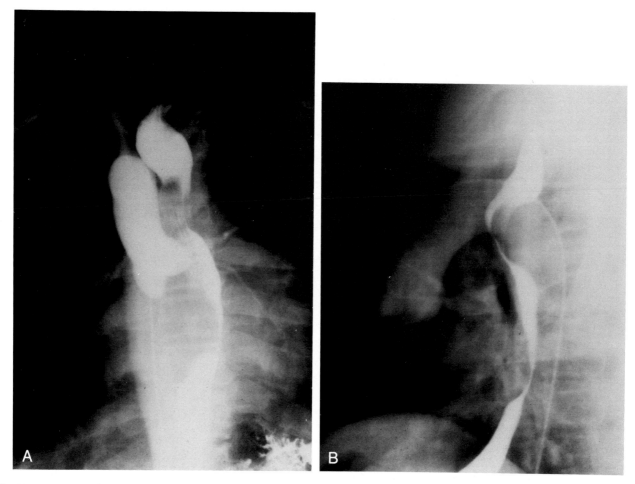

Fig. 64–14. *A,* AP and *B,* lateral views of an angiogram and esophagogram performed simultaneously in a patient with a right aortic arch and left ligamentum. The origin of the left subclavian artery is dilated, forming a Kommerele's diverticulum. The combination of the tight ligamentum and the diverticulum compress the esophagus.

common and aggravate the tracheal compression caused by the left pulmonary artery.

Sade and associates (1975) reported that pulmonary artery sling occurs when the developing left lung captures its arterial blood supply from derivatives of the right sixth aortic arch through capillaries caudad instead of cephalad to the lung bed. The left pulmonary artery originates from the right pulmonary artery and passes over the right main stem bronchus, behind the trachea, and anterior to the esophagus to reach the left lung. This results in a sling around the carina and right main stem bronchus (Fig. 64–11B).

A chest roentgenogram may show unilateral hyperaeration of the right lung field. A barium esophagogram shows anterior compression of the esophagus on the lateral views. Diagnosis requires angiography or computed tomography. Bronchoscopy should also be performed to rule out associated tracheal anomalies. As one of us (C.L.B.) and associates (1988) reported, up to one third of these patients have a complete vascular ring.

Surgical intervention should be undertaken as soon as the diagnosis is made because of the severity of respiratory difficulty. Left thoracotomy provides good expo-

sure. The pericardium is opened, and the left pulmonary artery is clamped and divided at its origin from the right pulmonary artery. It is then transposed anterior to the trachea and anastomosed to the main pulmonary artery. The first successful repair was reported by Potts (1954). Careful respiratory care is required postoperatively to keep the tracheobronchial tree free of secretions.

Innominate Artery Compression

Anterior compression of the trachea from anomalous origin of the innominate artery can cause stridor, respiratory distress, and apnea. The innominate artery appears to originate somewhat more posterior and leftward on the aortic arch than usual. Gross and Neuhauser (1948) first showed that as the innominate artery courses to the right, it can forcibly press on the trachea (Fig. 64–11F).

Enthusiasm for this diagnosis increased in the late 1970s when bronchoesophagologists switched from local to general anesthesia for bronchoscopy. As experience with these patients was gained, the selection criteria for surgery become more stringent. Radionuclide studies for gastroesophageal reflux, sleep studies, and neurologic evaluation—including CT and EEG—should all be performed to rule out other causes of apnea. Bronchoscopy should demonstrate at least a 50% obstruction of the tracheal lumen by the innominate artery compression. Anterior compression of the tracheal wall by the bronchoscope may compress the innominate artery and may temporarily obliterate the right radial pulse.

When indicated, suspension of the innominate artery is performed through a small right anterior thoracotomy incision. The thymus is mobilized and the adventitia of the innominate artery is suspended to the anterior chest wall, usually the periosteum of the sternum. Operative mortality is near zero. One of us (C.L.B.) and associates (1988) noted that when indicated results are excellent.

Miscellaneous Vascular Compression

Many vascular anomalies of the aortic arch system can cause tracheoesophageal compression, but not all require surgical intervention. A left aortic arch with aberrant right subclavian artery arising from the descending aorta may cause posterior indentation of the esophagus (Fig. 64–11E). Gross (1946) described this as the cause of dysphagia lusoria. As Beabout and associates (1964) showed, however, it is usually not a source of symptoms severe enough to cause surgical intervention unless there is aneurysmal dilatation of the subclavian origin.

In adults, however, when simple ligation of a symptomatic, compressive aberrant right subclavian artery is indicated, an approach, through a left thoracotomy, may result in vertebrobasilar or upper limb arterial insufficiency. If this occurs, a second procedure is necessary to anastomose the artery to the aorta or right common carotid artery. To negate the necessity of second procedure, Shumacker (1971), Pifarre (1971), Chaffin (1978), and Kalke (1987) and their colleagues suggested a one-stage procedure of division and anastomosis of the aberrant right subclavian artery through a single incision, preferably a median sternotomy. In the symptomatic patient, when an aneurysm of the aberrant vessel is present, however, Esposito and colleagues (1988) prefer a one-stage but two-incision approach because of the high incidence of complications with initial resection of the aneurysm. The major complications in their review of literature were those of upper limb ischemia and cerebral embolization and intraoperative hemorrhage. To obviate these, Esposito and colleagues (1988) suggested an initial approach through a right cervical incision to divide the right subclavian distal to the aneurysmal dilatation and anastomosis of the distal end to the right carotid artery to preserve blood flow to the distal distribution of the artery. The patient is then placed in a right lateral decubitus position and the aneurysm is excised through a left thoracotomy approach.

A cervical aortic arch may ascend into the neck and compress the trachea and esophagus. An anomalous left carotid artery compresses the trachea as it courses from right to left across the trachea. These anomalies are both well described by DeLaval (1983). Whitman and associates (1982) reported that a left aortic arch with right-sided ligamentum is another unusual cause of tracheoesophageal compression.

Prognosis

With proper and early identification of vascular rings in the infant or young child, surgical release of the tracheoesophageal compression may be accomplished with minimal morbidity and mortality. One of us (C.L.B.) and colleagues (1988) reported that satisfactory resolution of the signs and symptoms of the compression may be obtained in over 90% of the patients.

REFERENCES

Anabtawi, I.N., Ellison, R.G., and Ellison, L.T.: Pulmonary arteriovenous aneurysms and fistulas: anatomical variations, embryology, and classification. Ann. Thorac. Surg. *1*:277, 1965.

Anderson, J.H., et al.: "Mini" Gianturco stainless steel coils for transcatheter vascular occlusion. Radiology *132*:301, 1979.

Backer, C.L., et al.: Vascular anomalies causing tracheoesophageal compression: review of experience in children. Presentation at the Western Thoracic Surgical Association, Waikoloa, Hawaii, 1988.

Beabout, J.W., Stewart, J.R., and Kincaid, O.W.: Aberrant right subclavian artery: dispute of commonly accepted concepts. Am. J. Roentgenol. *92*:855, 1964.

Bosher, L.H., Jr., Blaki, D.A., and Byrd, B.R.: An analysis of the pathologic anatomy of pulmonary arteriovenous aneurysms with particular reference to the applicability of local excision. Surgery *45*:91, 1959.

Burke, C.M., and Raffin, T.A.: Pulmonary arteriovenous malformations, aneurysms, and reflections. Chest *89*:771, 1986.

Canter, C.E., et al.: Scimitar syndrome in childhood. Am. J. Cardiol. *58*:652, 1986.

Chaffin, J.S., Munnell, E.R., and Grantham, R.N.: Dysphagia lusoria: current surgical approach. J. Cardiovasc. Surg. *19*:311, 1978.

Dalton, M.L., Jr., et al.: Intrapleural rupture of pulmonary arteriovenous aneurysm: report of a case. Chest *52*:97, 1967.

DeLaval, M.: Vascular rings. *In* Surgery for Congenital Heart Defects. Edited by J. Stark and M. DeLaval. Orlando, FL, Grune & Stratton, 1983, p. 227.

Dines, D.E., et al.: Pulmonary arteriovenous fistulas. Mayo Clin. Proc. *49*:460, 1974.

Dines, D.E., et al.: Pulmonary arteriovenous fistulas. Mayo Clin. Proc. *58*:176, 1983.

Edwards, J.E.: Malformations of the aortic arch system manifested as "vascular rings." Lab. Invest. *2*:56, 1953.

Ellis, F.H., McGoon, D.C., and Kincaid, O.W.: Congenital vascular malformations of the lungs. Med. Clin. North Am. *48*:1069, 1964.

Esposito, R.A., et al.: Surgical treatment for aneurysm of aberrant subclavian artery based on a case report and review of the literature. J. Thorac. Cardiovasc. Surg. *95*:888, 1988.

Gianturco, C., Anderson, J.H., and Wallace, S.: Mechanical devices for arterial occlusion. Am. J. Roentgenol. *124*:428, 1975.

Gregg, N.M.: Congenital cataract following German measles in the mother. Trans. Ophthalmol. Soc. Australia *3*:35, 1941.

Gross, R.E.: Surgical treatment for dysphagia lusoria. Ann. Surg. *124*:532, 1946.

Gross, R.E., and Neuhauser, E.B.: Compression of the trachea by an anomalous innominate artery: case report. Am. J. Dis. Child. *75*:570, 1948.

Hatfield, D.R., and Fried, A.M.: Therapeutic embolization of diffuse pulmonary arteriovenous malformations. Am. J. Roentgenol. *137*:861, 1981.

Hodgson, C.H., and Kaye, R.L.: Pulmonary arteriovenous fistula and hereditary hemorrhagic telangiectasia: a review and report of 35 cases of fistula. Chest *43*:449, 1963.

Jeresaty, R.M., Knight, H.F., and Hart, W.E.: Pulmonary arteriovenous fistulas in children: report of two cases and review of literature. Am. J. Dis. Child. *111*:256, 1966.

Kalke, B.R., Magotra, R., and Doshi, S.M.: A new surgical approach to the management of symptomatic aberrant right subclavian artery. Ann. Thorac. Surg. *44*:86, 1987.

Kiely, B., et al.: Syndrome of anomalous venous drainage of the right lung to the inferior vena cava: a review of 67 reported cases and three new cases in children. Am. J. Cardiol. *20*:102, 1967.

Kirklin, J.W., Ellis, F.H., and Wood, E.H.: Treatment of anomalous venous connections in association with interatrial communications. Surgery *39*:389, 1956.

Koopot, R., Nikaidoh, H., and Idriss, F.S.: Surgical management of anomalous left pulmonary artery causing tracheobronchial obstruction: pulmonary artery sling. JTCVS *69*(2):239, 1975.

Lewis, A.B., Gates, G.F., and Stanley, P.: Echocardiography and perfusion scintigraphy in the diagnosis of pulmonary arteriovenous fistula. Chest *73*:675, 1978.

Liechty, J.D., Shields, T.W., and Anson, B.J.: Variations pertaining to the aortic arches and their branches: with comments on surgically important types. Q. Bull. Northwest. Univ. Med. School. *31*:136, 1957.

McGoon, D.C., and Kincaid, O.W.: Stenosis of branches of the pulmonary artery: surgical repair. Med. Clin. North Am. *48*:1083, 1964.

Murphy, J.P., et al.: Peripheral pulmonary artery aneurysm in a patient with limited respiratory reserve: controlled resection using cardiopulmonary bypass. Ann. Thorac. Surg. *43*:323, 1987.

Natelson, E.A., Watts, H.D., and Fred, H.L.: Cystic medionecrosis of the pulmonary arteries. Chest *57*:333, 1970.

Neill, C.A., et al.: The familial occurrence of hypoplastic right lung with systemic arterial supply and venous drainage: "Scimitar" syndrome. Bull. Johns Hopkins Hospital *107*:1, 1960.

Nikaidoh, H., Riker, W.L., and Idriss, F.S.: Surgical management of "vascular rings." Arch. Surg. *105*:327, 1972.

Noonan, J.A., et al.: Congenital pulmonary lymphangiectasis. Am. J. Dis. Child. *120*:314, 1970.

Pierce, W.S., et al.: Concomitant congenital heart disease and lobar emphysema in infants. Ann. Surg. *172*:951, 1970.

Pifarre, R., Niedballa, R.G., and Dieter, R.A., Jr.: Definitive surgical treatment of the aberrant retroesophageal right subclavian artery in the adult. J. Thorac. Cardiovasc. Surg. *61*:154, 1971.

Potts, W.J., Gibson, S., and Rothwell, R.: Double aortic arch: report of two cases. Arch. Surg. *57*:227, 1948.

Potts, W.J., Holinger, P.H., and Rosenblum, A.H.: Anomalous left pulmonary artery causing obstruction to right main bronchus: report of a case. JAMA *155*:1409, 1954.

Rocchini, A.P., et al.: Use of balloon angioplasty to treat peripheral pulmonary stenosis. Am. J. Cardiol. *54*:1069, 1984.

Sade, R.M., et al.: Pulmonary artery sling. JTCVS *69*(3):333, 1975.

Sanger, P.W., Taylor, F.H., and Robicsek, F.: The "scimitar syndrome," diagnosis and treatment. Arch. Surg. *86*:84, 1963.

Shumacker, H.B., Ischi, J.H., and Finnernan, J.C.: Unusual case of dysphagia due to anomalous right subclavian artery: A new approach for operative treatment. J. Thorac. Cardiovasc. Surg. *61*:304, 1971.

Scott-Emaukpor, A.B., et al.: Familial occurrence of congenital pulmonary lymphangiectasis. Am. J. Dis. Child. *135*:532, 1981.

Shub, C., et al.: Detecting intrapulmonary right-to-left shunt with contrast echocardiography: observations in a patient with diffuse pulmonary arteriovenous fistulas. Mayo Clin. Proc. *51*:81, 1976.

Sperling, D.C., et al.: Pulmonary arteriovenous fistulas with pulmonary hypertension. Chest *71*:753, 1977.

Stringer, C.J., et al.: Pulmonary arteriovenous fistula. Am. J. Surg. *89*:1054, 1955.

Tadavarthy, S.M., Moller, J.H., and Amplatz, K.: Polyvinyl-alcohol (Ivalon)—a new embolic material. Am. J. Roentgenol. *125*:609, 1975.

Taylor, B.G., et al.: Therapeutic embolization of the pulmonary artery in pulmonary arteriovenous fistula. Am. J. Med. *64*:360, 1978.

Tobin, C.E.: Arteriovenous shunts in the peripheral pulmonary circulation in the human lung. Thorax *21*:197, 1966.

Trell, E., et al.: The scimitar syndrome. Z. Kardiol. *60*:880, 1971.

Ungaro, R., et al.: Solitary peripheral pulmonary artery aneurysms: pathogenesis and surgical treatment. J. Thorac. Cardiovasc. Surg. *71*:566, 1976.

Wallenharyst, S.L., and D'Souza, V.: Combined radiologic and surgical management of arteriovenous malformations of the lung. Ann. Thorac. Surg. *45*:213, 1988.

White, R.I., Jr.: Angioarchitecture of pulmonary arteriovenous malformations: an important consideration before embolotherapy. Am. J. Roentgenol. *140*:681, 1983.

White, R.I., Jr.: Embolotherapy in vascular disease. Am. J. Roentgenol. *142*:27, 1984.

White, R.I., Jr., et al.: Detachable silicone balloons: results of experimental study and clinical investigations in hereditary hemorrhagic telangiectasia. Ann. Radiol. (Paris) *23*:338, 1980.

Whitman, G., Stephenson, L.W., and Weinberg, P.: Vascular ring: left cervical aortic arch, right descending aorta, and right ligamentum arteriosum. J. Thorac. Cardiovasc. Surg. *83*:311, 1982.

Wychulis, A.R., et al.: Congenital vascular ring: surgical considerations and results of operation. Mayo Clin. Proc. *46*:182, 1971.

READING REFERENCES

Hepburn, J., and Dauphinee, J.A.: Successful removal of hemangioma of the lung followed by the disappearance of polycythemia. Am. J. Med. Sci. *204*:681, 1942.

Kiphart, R.J., et al.: Systemic-pulmonary arteriovenous fistula of the chest wall and lung: a report of a case review of the literature. J. Thorac. Cardiovasc. Surg. *54*:113, 1967.

McCotter, R.E.: On the occurrence of pulmonary arteries arising from the thoracic aorta. Anat. Rec. *4*:291, 1910.

Smith, H.L., and Horton, B.T.: Arteriovenous fistula of the lung associated with polycythemia vera: report of a case in which the diagnosis was made clinically. Am. Heart J. *18*:589, 1939.

Wolfe, W.G., Anderson, R.W., and Sealy, W.C.: Hyperlucent lung. Ann. Thorac. Surg. *18*:172, 1974.

CHAPTER 65

BULLOUS AND BLEB DISEASES OF THE LUNG

Jean Deslauriers, Pierre Leblanc, and André McClish

Air space disorders are mostly medical problems, although patients may sometimes benefit from surgery in the management of specific complications such as pneumothorax or infection. The resection of compressive bullae or abnormal parenchyma to reduce symptoms is controversial and needs more clarification.

TERMINOLOGY

Pathologic

The National Heart Lung and Blood Institute as Snider and associates (1985) reported defines respiratory air space enlargement as an increase in air space as compared to the air space of normal lung. This definition applies to all varieties of air space enlargement distal to the terminal bronchiole, whether they are associated with fibrosis or not (Table 65–1). This enlargement can be simple and without evidence of destruction, as in postpneumonectomy hyperinflation (Fig. 65–1), or frankly pathological, as in emphysema or pulmonary fibrosis.

Emphysema

The American Thoracic Society (1962) defined emphysema as a condition of the lung characterized by abnormal and permanent enlargement of air spaces distal to the terminal bronchiole accompanied by destruction of their walls and without obvious fibrosis. Based on the

portion of acinus predominantly involved—an acinus being a unit of bronchopulmonary tissue distal to a terminal bronchiole, three pathologic subsets of emphysema have been described, and all three can be associated with bulla formation.

Centriacinar Emphysema. This develops in the proximal portion of the acinus. It is associated with inflam-

Table 65–1. Classification of Respiratory Air Space Enlargement

Simple air space enlargement
Congenital
Acquired
Emphysema
Centriacinar emphysema
Panacinar emphysema
Distal acinar emphysema (paraseptal)
Air space enlargement with fibrosis

National Heart, Lung, and Blood Institute (1985)

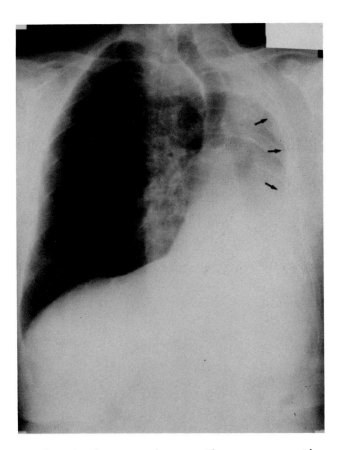

Fig. 65–1. Simple air space enlargement. Chest roentgenogram taken 4 years after left pneumonectomy for carcinoma. The right lung is hyperinflated with contralateral herniation (arrows).

matory destruction of respiratory bronchioles and is most common in the upper lung fields.

Panacinar Emphysema. In this form, all portions of the acinus are similarly destroyed, but the disease is predominant at the lung bases. The formation of a bulla is thought to result from intraparenchymal alveoli rupture.

Paraseptal Emphysema. This results from disruption of subpleural alveoli. Gaensler and associates (1983) noted that these tiny disruptions tend to coalesce into larger air spaces with eventual formation of giant subpleural bullae. These bullae are commonly located along the upper borders of the lung and are responsible for most spontaneous pneumothoraces.

In Gaensler and colleagues' review (1986) of 608 patients with abnormal air space disorders, 81% had emphysema and 19% had unrelated disorders, including air space enlargement proximal to the terminal bronchiole.

Air space enlargement associated with fibrosis is common but bears little clinical significance. It is seen with scarred tuberculosis—cicatricial emphysema—or with diffuse and chronic inflammatory diseases such as sarcoidosis, granulomatosis, or pneumoconiosis—honeycomb lung.

Clinical

Since the 1930s the terms blebs, cysts, and bullae have been given different meanings in the medical and surgical literature.

Pulmonary Bleb

Miller (1926) defined a pulmonary bleb (Fig. 65–2) as a well circumscribed intrapleural air space separated from the underlying parenchyma by a thin pleural covering. Blebs are small, peripheral, and nearly always located at the apex of the upper lobes. They also may

occur along the upper border of the superior segment of the lower lobes, as well as at the borders of any lobe. They are the result of subpleural alveolar rupture, which occurs when the elastic fibers in the alveoli have been stretched beyond the breaking point. Their outer wall is made of visceral pleura and the underlying lung is normal.

Air Cysts

Belcher and Siddons (1954) defined true pulmonary air cysts as congenital anepithelial air spaces unassociated with emphysema. Such cysts are rare, and most of them are attached to the lower lobes by a fibrous pedicle. When resected in the adult, they may be difficult to differentiate from acquired bullae.

Pulmonary Bullae

These were defined at the 1959 CIBA symposium as emphysematous spaces of more than 1 cm diameter in the inflated lung usually but not necessarily demarcated from surrounding lung by curved hairline shadows. It was recognized that bullous disease is secondary to emphysema and that bullae can be associated with any variety of emphysema. Witz and Roeslin (1980) proposed a clinical classification based on the presence or absence of obstructive lung disease in the nonbullous parenchyma.

Group I: Bullae Associated with "Almost" Normal Underlying Parenchyma. These bullae (Fig. 65–3) are well demarcated apical air spaces that almost invariably have a broad base of implantation within the parenchyma. Smaller bullae may also be visible over the remaining lung surface and, from a pathologic standpoint, they represent a variant of paraseptal emphysema. When they are large, the bullae compress adjacent lung but the patient remains relatively free of symptoms and the pul-

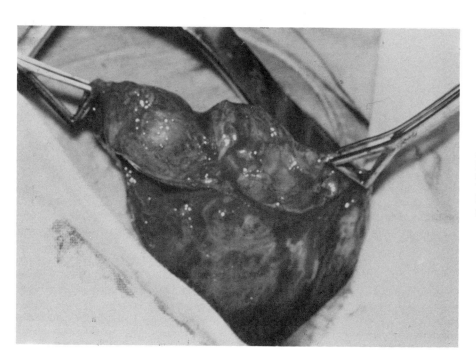

Fig. 65–2. Pulmonary blebs. Operative photograph showing well circumscribed subpleural blebs at the apex of the lung. This patient underwent transaxillary bullectomy for primary spontaneous pneumothorax.

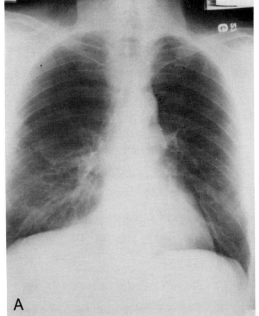

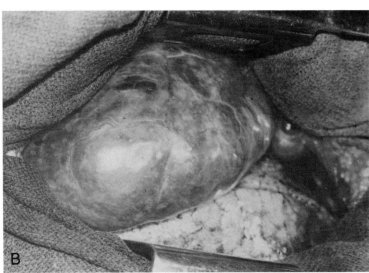

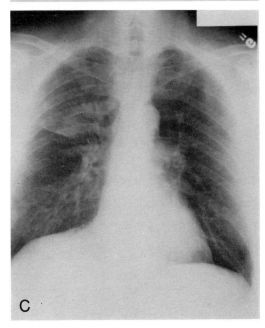

Fig. 65–3. Bulla associated with "almost" normal underlying parenchyma. A 52-year-old male was admitted for rapidly progressive dyspnea. *A,* His chest film shows decreased vascular markings in the right upper lobe area. Lung function was almost normal with an FEV_1 of 2.55 L—65% of predicted—and an FVC of 4.94 L—95% of predicted. *B,* The operative photograph shows a large bulla herniating through the thoracotomy wound with normal underlying parenchyma. *C,* After bullectomy the expanded lung fills the hemithorax.

monary function is close to normal. A giant bulla fills at least half of the hemithorax.

Group II: Bullae Associated with Diffuse Emphysema. This is essentially a local exaggeration of diffuse panacinar emphysema (Fig. 65–4). These bullae are usually multiple and can vary in extent and size. The symptoms depend on the size of the bullae, degree of compression, and severity of underlying emphysema.

Group III: Vanishing Lung. The vanishing lung has complete loss of parenchyma with virtually no signs of compression. It is often limited to a segment or lobe, but it can involve an entire lung. This abnormal air space has a broad base of implantation deep into the lung.

SURGERY FOR BULLOUS EMPHYSEMA

Chronic obstructive lung disease is a diffuse process with little if any surgical relevance. One possible exception to this rule is the individual with a nonfunctioning and compressive bulla for which resection may be followed by a lessening of dyspnea and to a lesser extent an improvement in pulmonary function. The potential for lung re-expansion and the compressive nature of the bulla are apparently key factors in predicting this clinical and physiologic improvement. Preoperative quantification of how much disability relates to the bulla and how much to the underlying emphysema is the single most

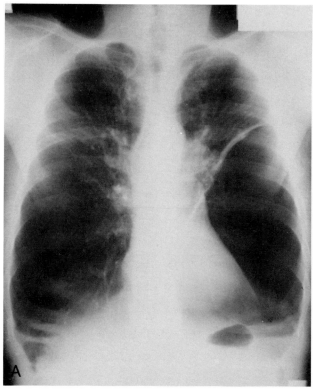

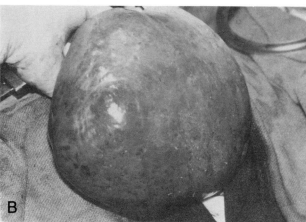

Fig. 65–4. Bulla associated with diffuse emphysema. This 47-year-old emphysematous man was admitted for worsening dyspnea. A, Chest roentgenogram shows bilateral basal bullae with flattening of the hemidiaphragms. Lung function was markedly impaired, with an FEV$_1$ of 0.3 L—8% of predicted—and a value for DL$_{CO}$ of 8.60 ml/min/mm Hg—49% of predicted. B, The operative photograph shows that the bulla is in fact a local exaggeration of diffuse panacinar emphysema.

important consideration when selecting patients for surgical intervention.

Rationale and Indications

The Nondyspneic Patient

In patients without ventilatory symptoms (Table 65–2), surgical intervention is mostly indicated for complications such as pneumothorax, infection, or hemoptysis that are clearly attributable to the bulla. Gaensler and colleagues (1986) noted that bullous emphysema predisposes to pneumothorax and that, in such circumstances, a pneumothorax can be troublesome for the following reasons: further reduction of function in already compromised patients; roentgenographic difficulties in diagnosing a pneumothorax when there are multiple bullae; and prolonged air leak that is often less responsive to tube drainage than when associated with primary spontaneous pneumothorax.

Infection of bullae is unusual, and most bullae containing a fluid level (Fig. 65–5) are only the site of an inflammatory reaction secondary to peribullous infection. Surgery is not indicated for this problem alone because significant shrinkage or gradual resolution may occur with clearance of the infection (Fig. 65–6).

Truly infected bullae (Fig. 65–7) should be managed conservatively, even though medical treatment is often unsuccessful because of the poor communications between the infected bulla and the bronchial tree. Surgical indications for resection are the same as for primary lung abscesses: failure of response to a 6-week course of adequate medical management; suspicion of occult bronchial carcinoma; and specific complications of the abscess, such as hemoptysis or free pleural space rupture. Dean and associates (1987) showed that percutaneous drainage of the abscess should be considered instead of resection for high risk patients.

Hemoptysis from an eroded artery is even more uncommon than infections. Berry and Oschner (1972) reported one of the few cases in which hemoptysis was

Table 65–2. Rationale and Indications for Surgery in Asymptomatic Patients with Apparently Normal Lung

Principal Indication for Surgery	Rationale
Pneumothorax (first episode or recurrence)	Further reduction of function in patients who may be compromised
	Radiologic difficulties of recognizing pneumothorax
	Prolonged air leak
True infection of bulla (pus within the bulla)	Failure of response of medical treatment
	Suspicion of occult carcinoma
	Specific complications: hemoptysis, pleural rupture
Massive hemoptysis	
Chest pain	Increased air trapping during hyperventilation
Preventive surgery (asymptomatic bulla)	Tendency of bulla to enlarge with time
	Possibility of permanent damage to compressed lung

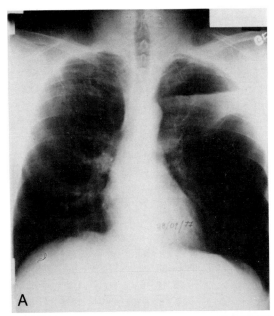

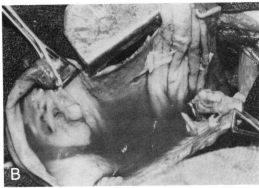

Fig. 65–5. Bulla containing an air-fluid level. *A,*This 35-year-old man with previous bullectomy on the right side has an asymptomatic loculation in the left upper lobe. *B,* At operation he was found to have a large bulla containing serous and noninfected fluid.

thought to be secondary to rupture of thin-walled pulmonary vessels passing through the alveolar wall and fibrous septae of a bulla. Because hemoptysis is seldom associated with bullous emphysema, another lesion in a different lung zone that could account for the bleeding should always be ruled out.

Gaensler (1983) and Witz (1980) and their associates described cases in which chest pain was the main symptom and sole indication for surgery. The pain was most often retrosternal and related to exercise, and in some cases it mimicked angina. This symptom was explained by overdistention of the bulla during hyperventilation with secondary mediastinal shift. All patients were improved following surgical removal of their bulla.

The Dyspneic Patient

Chronic and disabling dyspnea is the main indication for removing bullae associated with diffuse emphysema (Table 65–3). Hypothetically, surgical intervention could be beneficial to reduce airway resistance, reduce physiologic dead space, or remove a compressive bulla.

Reduction in Expiratory Airway Resistance. Ting and colleagues (1962) showed that bullae have little, if any, elastic recoil. At low volume, small variations in pressure bring important volumetric changes. At a critical level, however, compliance becomes extraordinarily low and the bulla cannot be stretched any more. When associated with emphysema, this low compliance decreases significantly the elastic recoil of the lungs and causes relaxation of the peribronchial tension. Ultimately it creates an "extrinsic airway obstruction" affecting the less diseased portions of parenchyma around the bulla.

Removal of bullae may improve the elastic recoil of the previously compressed lung tissue, thus reducing the tendency of airways to collapse on exhalation.

Reduction of Dead Space Ventilation. If a bulla is well ventilated and underperfused—high $\dot{V}/\dot{Q}$, the aim of surgery is to reduce this physiologic dead space and thereby decrease the work of breathing. Isotopic perfusion and ventilation studies have shown, however, that most bullae are neither perfused nor ventilated. The bulla was acting as a site of significant dead-space ventilation in only 1 of 14 patients studied by Pride and co-workers (1973).

Removal of a Compressive Bulla. Compression of relatively healthy lung near the bullae may impair overall gas exchange, with low $\dot{V}/\dot{Q}$ ratios in the compressed lung zone. Expansion of previously restricted lung should increase the VC and arterial oxygen saturation.

High intrathoracic pressures generated by the bullae may also result in major hemodynamic dysfunctions. Expiratory compression of the pulmonary arterial system and the systemic venous return significantly decreases cardiac output both at rest and during exercise. Lowering of intrathoracic pressures by removing the large bullae may correct some of these hemodynamic parameters and decrease the degree of dyspnea.

Bullous emphysema localized to the lower lobes may finally have a deleterious effect on the function of the diaphragm. Restoration of the normal diaphragmatic configuration can possibly improve its contractility.

Preventive Surgery

This is defined as the resection of asymptomatic bullae on the premise that most of them ultimately lead to serious and irreversible complications. Its role is unclear because of the limited number of studies describing the natural history of untreated and asymptomatic bullae. Boushy and associates (1968) observed that apical bullae tend to enlarge, but this enlargement was not seen in every case and it could not be predicted. They could not document any relationship between change in bulla size and deterioration of pulmonary function.

Most authors agree that preventive surgery is legitimate when the bulla occupies half or more of the hemithorax, compresses normal lung, or has enlarged over a period of years. Spear (1961) believed that any bulla occupying one third or more of the hemithorax would ultimately be associated with impaired drainage, infection, and permanent tissue damage to the adjacent compressed lung.

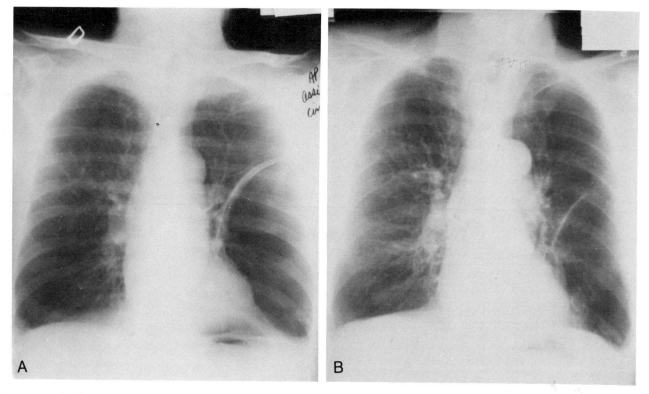

Fig. 65–6. Shrinkage of a bulla following peribullous infection. *A*, This 74-year-old man had a left basal bulla that shrank significantly. *B*, Following a 3-month episode of pulmonary infection.

Selection of Patients

Because of modern techniques for lung imaging and functional evaluation, guidelines have been proposed to help select individuals likely to benefit from surgery (Table 65–4). No single preoperative test, however, is considered to be an absolute predictor of improvement, and there are no absolute indications or contraindications to operation. Table 65–5 lists some ground rules for successful surgery.

Because the premise for successful surgery is the presence of a symptomatic, nonfunctioning, and compressive bulla, a complete evaluation should attempt to answer the following questions: Is there a localized or enlarging air space disorder, or both? Is the patient dyspneic, and if so, what is the pathogenesis of the dyspnea? Does the patient have associated chronic bronchitis, weight loss, or both? Is the area to be resected nonfunctional? Does the bulla compress adjacent lung, mediastinum, or diaphragm? What is the status of the compressed lung, and can this lung re-expand to become functional? What is the cardiac performance? Also, can the patient withstand an operation?

Delineation of Bullous Area

Bullae are recognized by increased radiolucencies—avascular areas—surrounded by arcuate hairline shadows—cyst wall. Their diagnosis, number, location, and volume can be estimated from standard PA and lateral roentgenograms of the chest, but films taken at maximum inspiration should be used to determine the true size of a given bulla. The observation that a bulla has enlarged is pertinent, especially if the enlargement is associated with concomitant deterioration in pulmonary reserve (Fig. 65–8).

Computed tomography is a sensitive diagnostic modality because it clearly shows the full extent of bullous disease, which is sometimes not discernible on simple PA and lateral views (Fig. 65–9). For this reason, CT should always be performed when evaluating patients with emphysema, whether they have obvious bullous disease or not. CT may also differentiate a pneumothorax from a large emphysematous bulla.

Dyspnea Index

Because the primary objective of operation is to relieve dyspnea, selection should be based on clinical considerations. Asymptomatic patients are not candidates for surgery unless they have a giant and compressive bulla—preventive surgery. As Pride and colleagues (1970) stated, the problem is to decide when surgery is justified in the absence of symptoms.

For patients with diffuse emphysema, the dyspnea must be disabling enough to limit work or everyday activities, or both despite adequate medical treatment. Incapacitating dyspnea associated with hypoxia and hypercapnia is not considered a contraindication to operation, but surgery for patients requiring mechanical ventilation is controversial.

Clinical evaluation must also rule out any other medical condition, such as heart failure, that may contribute to the intensity of dyspnea.

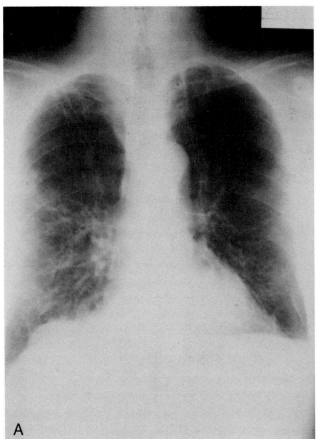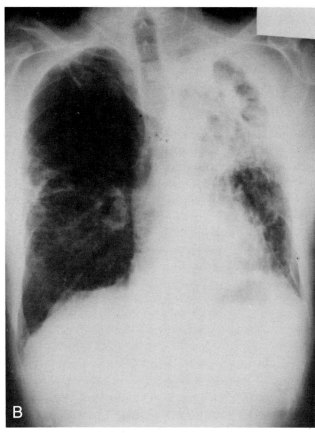

Fig. 65–7. True infection of the bulla. *A*, Initial chest roentgenogram of a 64-year-old man with bilateral apical bullae. *B*, This patient was readmitted 3 years later for high fever, chest pain and hemoptysis. His chest roentgenogram shows multiple loculations within the left bulla. At surgery, he had a pyogenic infection of the bulla.

Table 65–3. Rationale and Indications for Surgery in Dyspneic Patients with Diffuse Emphysema

Principal Indication	Rationale
Restoration of elastic recoil and reduction in airway resistance	Bullae increase the loss of elasticity of the emphysematous lung.
	Loss of elastic recoil causes an "extrinsic airway obstruction"
Removal of an area of dead-space ventilation	Reduction in volume of wasted ventilation
	Decrease in work of breathing
Expansion of previously collapsed lung	Increase in VC and FEV_1
	Improvement in gas exchange (higher $\dot{V}/\dot{Q}$ ratio and arterial Po_2)
Hemodynamic improvement	Increase in cardiac output
	Better exercise tolerance
Restoration of normal curve of diaphragm	Improvement in diaphragmatic function

Other Clinical Features

Gaensler and associates (1986) showed that virtually all patients with bullae have a history of smoking and that smoking cessation improves the chances for a good surgical result.

Patients with clinical signs of chronic bronchitis, bronchospasm, recurrent infections, or marked weight loss generally have a higher surgical risk and a lower chance of sustained good result. Some studies have shown, however, that improved postoperative pulmonary function often results in a return to normal eating habits and significant weight gain.

Function of the Bulla.

The distinction between communicating and noncommunicating bullae may be relevant to the understanding of the pathophysiology of a given bulla, but is relatively unimportant in making a surgical decision. Pulmonary areas that are to be resected, however, must be areas of poor perfusion.

Most bullae are nonventilated or poorly ventilated, so the change in size in inspiration and exhalation is small. The amount of trapped air in the bulla, however, as estimated by the difference between FRC calculated by the helium dilution method and by plethysmography, is

Table 65–4. Selection of Patients for Surgery

Area of Investigation	Diagnostic Technique	Most Suitable for Surgery	Least Suitable for Surgery
Anatomy of the Bulla			
Bullous area	PA and lateral chest films, CT	Large and localized apical bulla (>50%)	Multiple small bullae
		Unilateral disease	Bilateral disease
	Comparison with old films	Gradual enlargement	No enlargement
Clinical Appraisal			
Dyspnea index	Clinical evaluation	Rapidly progressive dyspnea	Slowly progressive dyspnea
			No dyspnea
Other clinical features		Nonsmokers	Smokers
		Pink puffers	Chronic bronchitis (blue bloaters)
		Minimal weight loss	Important weight loss
Function of the Bulla			
	Inspiratory/Expiratory films	Nonventilated bulla	Ventilated bulla
	Body plethysmography		
	Angiography	Nonperfused bulla	Perfused bulla
Compression Index			
	PA and lateral chest films	High index of compression (>3/6)	Low index of compression (<3/6)
	Pulmonary angiography		Vanishing lung syndrome
	CT		
State of Compressed Lung			
Overall function (extent of disease)	Chest film	Localized disease	Widespread emphysema
	Inspiratory/expiratory films		
	Pulmonary function studies	FEV_1 >40%	FEV_1 <35%
		Preserved $D_{L_{CO}}$ and Pa_{O_2} at rest	Reduced $D_{L_{CO}}$ and Pa_{O_2} at rest
		No hypoxemia during exercise	Hypoxemia during exercise
Regional function (potential for reexpansion)			
Perfusion	Angiography	Good capillary filling in compressed lung	Poor capillary filling
	Perfusion scans		
		Regional imbalance	No regional imbalance
Ventilation	Inspiratory/expiratory films	Good dynamic ventilation	Poor ventilation
	Ventilation scans		
Cardiac Performance			
	Chest film, ECG	Normal cardiac function	Right heart failure
	Heart catheterization		Cor pulmonale
			Pulmonary hypertension
Patient Medical Status			
		Younger age	Older age
			Severe intercurrent disease
		No respiratory failure	Frank respiratory failure
Choice of Operation			
		Bullectomy	Lobectomy, segmentectomy

Table 65–5. Ground Rules for Successful Surgery

Optimal preparation before surgery
Staged operations for bilateral disease
Stapling of the base of the bulla
Preservation of enough lung tissue for complete re-expansion
Proper tube drainage of the pleural space
Possibility of associated pleurectomy or pleural tent
External drainage as a surgical option

large. This difference reflects the true volume occupied by the bulla. After resection of such bullae, an increase in vital capacity and FEV_1 is expected.

Bullae that communicate freely have large volume variations between inspiratory and expiratory films, but small volume difference between plethysmographic and helium dilution measurements. Little change is expected in postoperative VC, but FEV_1 improves if the space taken by the bulla is replaced by normal lung parenchyma.

Compression Index

Once it is decided that an abnormal air space is present, the next step is to demonstrate that it is compressive. This is a key consideration, because re-expansion of com-

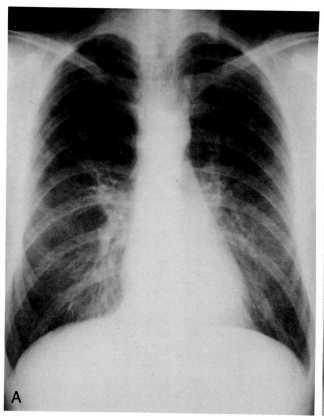

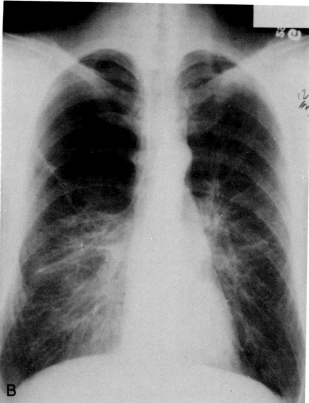

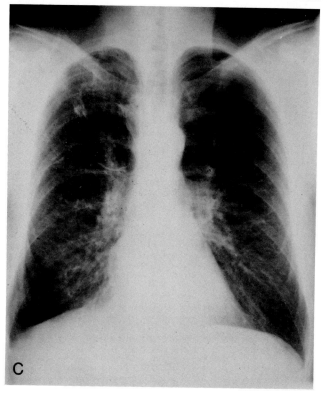

Fig. 65–8. Enlargement of a bulla. Serial roentgenograms demonstrating enlargement of an isolated right upper lobe bulla over an 8-year period. *A*, Only minimal overdistention. *B*, A well demarcated apical bulla. *C*, Following bullectomy, the underlying parenchyma re-expanded adequately.

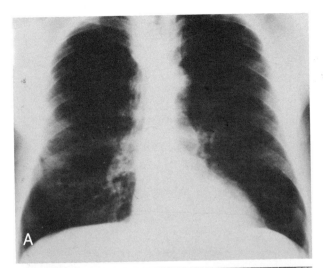

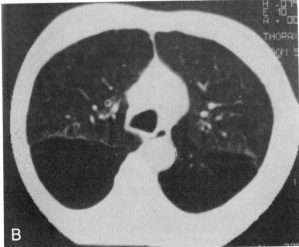

Fig. 65–9. Computed tomography scanning. This 53-year-old man was investigated for dyspnea. *A*, The standard PA chest film shows almost normal parenchyma. *B*, The CT scan demonstrates well demarcated bilateral basal bullae. Postoperatively, his FEV_1 rose from 1.1 L to 1.7 L and his VC from 2.9 L to 3.3 L. (Courtesy of Dr. Marcel Dahan).

pressed lung improves function and gas exchange, whereas overstretching of noncompressed parenchyma may ultimately lead to some functional loss. Laros and colleagues (1986) noted that in patients with vanishing lung syndrome, the destroyed lobe has a buffer function in preventing overexpansion of the remaining lung.

Brochard and associates (1986) described a simple but effective compression index based on initial roentgenologic data. Patients were rated 0 to 6, depending on the number of compression signs present: vascular crowding in the parenchyma adjacent to the hyperinflated lung; arcuate displacement of blood vessels in the periphery of the bulla; displacement of the hilum; mediastinal displacement during inspiration or exhalation or both; anterior mediastinal herniation of the lung; and displacement of lung fissures. They were able to correlate subjective results with the severity of compression.

Most of these signs can readily be seen on standard roentgenograms of the chest or CT scan, although pulmonary artery angiography is the most reliable and accurate technique of study. It is useful not only to document vascular crowding (Fig. 65–10) but also to assess capillary filling in the periphery of compressed parenchyma. Thinning or disruption of pulmonary capillaries (Fig. 65–11) suggests the presence of widespread emphysema and poor response to surgery.

State of Compressed Lung

Because diffuse emphysema is more likely to be associated with poor or at least short-lasting benefits, one major goal of preoperative workup is to assess its severity. By analysis of PA and lateral roentgenograms of the chest—including inspiratory and expiratory films, computed tomography, and simple pulmonary function studies, one can usually answer this question.

Pulmonary overdistention and attenuation of vascular shadows as seen on standard roentgenograms correlate poorly with the severity of disease. Computed tomography provides better information, but few data correlate image, function, and histopathology. Gaensler and associates (1986) showed that inspiration/expiration films—or fluoroscopic examination—may alleviate the need for additional and more elaborate studies. Large bullae showing no more trapping than the rest of the lung on expiration suggest that diffuse disease may cause the breathlessness.

Pride and associates (1973) showed that tests of overall function reflect the condition of the nonbullous lung and that they can be used to predict the possibility of generalized emphysema. Airflow limitation is probably the most significant functional abnormality seen in emphysema, and it can be estimated accurately by forced expiratory maneuvers. Several studies have stressed the importance of FEV_1 as a predictor of results following bullectomy. Fitzgerald and colleagues (1974) noted that patients with severe preoperative reductions in FEV_1 are less likely to to be improved following operation. Nakahara and co-workers (1983) also observed that symptomatic and functional improvement following bullectomy was less in patients whose FEV_1 was smaller than 35% of predicted. With large bullae, a low FEV_1 may indicate slow emptying of the bulla rather than diffuse emphysema, especially if the value of DL_{CO} is close to predicted value.

Patients with emphysema have a reduced capacity for oxygen or carbon monoxide transfer, or both. Abnormal CO diffusing capacity correlates well with the morphology of emphysema, but resting arterial PO_2 is often normal until the disease reaches its end stage. Arterial hypoxemia is best demonstrated during a graded exercise tolerance test—treadmill or stationary bicycle ergometer and the degree of desaturation correlates well with the values of DL_{CO} and the severity of emphysema. Hugh-Jones and Whinster (1978) noted that preserved DL_{CO}, together with minimal changes in blood gases during exercise, tend to be associated with sustained good results following bullectomy.

Although more difficult to predict, the potential for

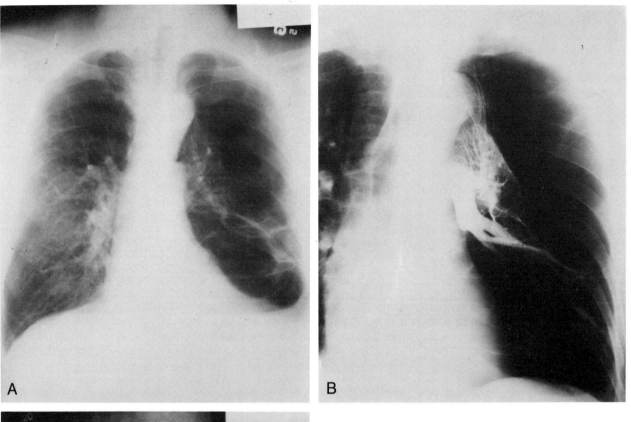

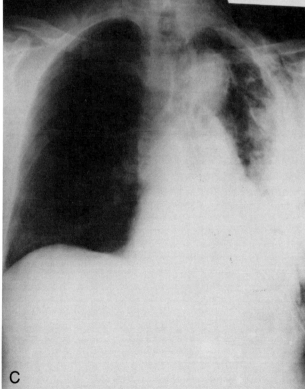

Fig. 65–10. Angiography. *A*, Chest roentgenogram of a 64-year-old man with previous left lower lobectomy and extensive bullous disease in the remaining upper lobe. *B*, The angiogram demonstrates a large bullous lesion with significant vascular compression. *C*, Postoperatively the lung expands adequately.

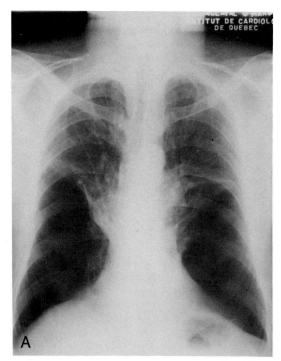

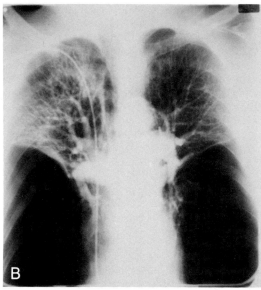

Fig. 65–11. Angiography. *A*, Chest roentgenogram and *B*, angiogram of a 57-year-old man with severe chronic obstructive lung disease and large basal bullae. This patient is not ideal for surgery because of a low index of compression. Peripheral capillaries in the left upper lung zone are significantly thinned.

re-expansion and function of the compressed lung can be assessed by angiography and by isotopic studies of regional lung function. Adequacy of perfusion—$\dot{Q}$—in the compressed lung is a prerequisite to functional recovery and is best demonstrated by dense capillary flow on angiography. Perfusion scans are less accurate, but they are easier to perform and they can be used for control during the follow-up period. Perfusion scans can also document regional imbalance—good perfusion on contralateral side and percentage of total perfusion—as they can delineate other areas of decreased perfusion not seen on roentgenograms of the chest.

Ventilation—$\dot{V}$—in the compressed lung is obviously more difficult to appreciate, but can be estimated from inspiration/exhalation roentgenograms of the chest and from ventilation scans. Dynamic ventilation per volume—$\dot{V}/V$ dynamic—calculated from ^{133}Xe washout half-time was reported by Nakahara and colleagues (1983) to be a good indicator of regional ventilatory efficiency as well as a good predictor of postoperative functional improvement (Fig. 65–12).

Selective pulmonary function studies—bronchospirometry, bronchoscopic regional function measurements, or bronchograms have not proved useful or practical in the selection for operation.

Cardiac Performance

Assessment of cardiac performance by heart catheterization may be indicated for patients with clinical signs of heart failure or cor pulmonale. With right heart failure, the surgical risk is higher, but Harris (1976) and others have shown excellent functional results. Pulmonary hypertension is common in bullous emphysema, but because it is often related to a restricted vascular bed in the compressed lung field, it does not contraindicate surgery.

Medical Status

Age alone is not an absolute contraindication for surgery, although emphysema is more severe and the expected operative morbidity is higher in older people. Woo-Ming and associates (1963) noted that the mean age at operation of patients who had a good result was 45.4 years, whereas the mean age of patients who experienced a fair or poor result was 54.5 years.

Operative Procedure

Choice of Operation

Since the 1930s, numerous surgical procedures have been proposed for the treatment of emphysema, but most have been abandoned because they were based on misconceptions about the pathophysiology of chronic obstructive lung disease.

There is now general agreement that the operative strategy should be to relieve compression while preserving all vascularized and potentially functioning lung tissue. This is best accomplished by limited resections, primarily local excision or plication of visible bullae, or both. Segmental resections are rarely indicated because

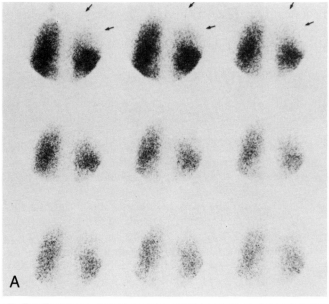

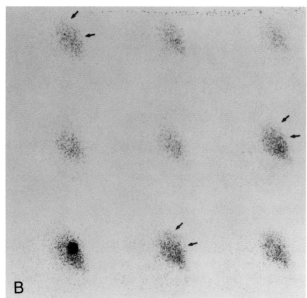

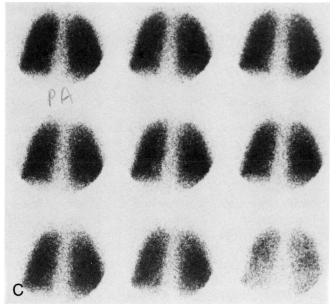

Fig. 65–12. Ventilation scan. *A*, PA view of a ventilation scan (¹³³Xe) showing poor ventilation in a right upper lobe bulla. *B*, The film taken during the washout shows trapping in the bulla but excellent ventilation and clearance of ¹³³Xe in all other lung zones. *C*, Postoperatively all lung zones return to normal. This patient is an ideal candidate for bullectomy.

bullous disease is seldom confined to an anatomic segment, and lobectomy—or pneumonectomy—should only be done when the entire lobe—or lung—is destroyed. Indeed, Gaensler and colleagues (1983) cautioned against performing lobectomy, because there is often funtional lung at the hilum even when the surgeon believes that the entire lobe is destroyed.

Before proceeding with operation, bronchoscopy should always be done to exclude a bronchial obstructive lesion.

Preoperative Preparation

Patients with chronic obstructive lung disease must have optimal preparation before bullectomy. Because the operative procedure is mostly elective, time must be spent preoperatively to teach methods for coughing, deep breathing, incentive spirometry, and chest physio-

therapy. Specific drug treatment must also be given to reverse airway obstruction and bronchospasm as well as to control any intercurrent pulmonary infection. In addition, every possible attempt should be made to discontinue smoking. If possible, corticosteroids should also be stopped, because they are almost invariably associated with poor healing and prolonged air leaks. Prophylaxis against deep vein thrombosis with subcutaneous low dose heparin—5000 IV twice daily— may be started the day of surgery.

Anesthesia

The technique of anesthesia must take into account the abnormal physiology of the emphysematous patient and the possibility of specific complications such as a tension pneumothorax occurring intraoperatively. In addition, the anesthetist must try to provide a quiet operative field during resection of the bulla.

Spontaneous Respiration. Because of increased peripheral airway resistance, it is best to maintain spontaneous respiration throughout most of the operation. The active expiration of emphysematous patients contributes significantly to the maintenance of satisfactory gas exchange, especially during anesthesia. All patients are intubated under topical anesthesia, and during the procedure, they are kept anesthetized by inhalation of a mixture of halothane and oxygen. Continuous administration of epidural narcotics perioperatively—the catheter is inserted before induction—has decreased the need for intravenous narcotics or anesthetic agents. When required, spontaneous respiration can be hand-assisted with low peak inspiratory pressures.

Once the operation is completed, assisted ventilation is discontinued as soon as the patient has regained full consciousness and his body temperature has returned to normal. Most patients are extubated in the recovery room unless they are unable to maintain adequate blood gases.

Intraoperative Complications. The possibility of tension pneumothorax or overdistention of the bulla precludes the use of nitrous oxide and restricts the indications for intermittent positive-pressure ventilation. What type of endotracheal tube should be used is controversial, but Benumof (1987) showed that a double-lumen tube is far safer than a single-lumen tube, especially if complications occur. Normandale and Feneck (1985) reported that high frequency ventilation with low tidal volume and airway pressure is a way to avoid pneumothorax or overdistention of the bulla.

We prefer initial intubation with a single-lumen tube that is replaced by a double-lumen tube once the patient is well anesthetized and hemodynamically stable. At the end of operation, the double-lumen tube is replaced by a single-lumen tube and the patient routinely bronchoscoped for aspiration of the blood and mucus.

The surgeon must be present in the operating room during induction because the pleural space may need quick decompression in the event of a pneumothorax. If intraoperative hypotension occurs, it is usually controlled by opening of the chest or the bulla, lightening of anesthesia, and replacement of blood volume.

Muscle Relaxants. At the time of bullectomy, muscle blocking agents—succinylcholine, 2% solution—can be administered to abolish diaphragmatic movements. Once the bullectomy is completed, the infusion is stopped and the patient is allowed to breathe spontaneously.

Technique

Most bullectomies are done through the standard posterolateral approach through the 5th or 6th interspace, although they could easily be performed through an anterolateral incision with presumably less interference with chest-wall mechanics and less incisional discomfort. Lima and associates (1981) reported four cases of severe bilateral bullous emphysema treated by bilateral resection through median sternotomy. Reduced disability and the ability to treat both lungs at once are possible benefits of surgery done through this approach. For most patients, however, we prefer bilateral staged operations where functional results of the first procedure can be evaluated before proceeding with contralateral thoracotomy (Table 65–5).

Pedunculated bullae are easily dealt with through suture-ligation of the pedicle and excision of the bulla. For patients with diffuse disease, the basic technique of plication is simple (Fig. 65–13). The development of surgical staplers has made the procedure even easier, and a modification of Naclerio's and Langer's method (1947), as reported by Nelems (1980), is now used.

The largest bulla is opened longitudinally and the cavity explored from within. Strands of fibrous septae are excised (Fig. 65–14) and long Allis forceps are applied from inside so that they grasp the pleura at the reflection of relatively normal parenchyma with the cyst cavity. The visceral pleura—cyst wall—is then folded back over the remaining raw surface of lung and the GIA stapler is applied along the base of the bulla. The stapler is applied as many times as necessary until the raw surfaces of the entire base of the cyst are closed off. This double layer of pleura acts as a buttress for the staples and reduces and may even prevent air leakage from the staple margin. Biological glues are useful to improve airtightness, but they limit pulmonary re-expansion somewhat when applied over lung surfaces.

The dilemma is to resect as much disease as possible while avoiding tissue reduction so extensive that it precludes lung re-expansion. In fact, the lung must be tailored to fit the hemithorax.

Some authors have stressed the importance of associating a pleurectomy or a pleural tent to the bullectomy. Eschapasse and Berthomieu (1980) advocated parietal pleurectomy, not only to prevent pneumothoraces but also to reinforce the periphery of the lung, in the hope of preventing further bulla formation. Pleural space reduction by tailoring the pleura—pleural tent, as Miscall and Duffy (1953) described, is useful when the lung is not large enough to fill the entire space. This tent is made out of parietal pleura mobilized from the apex and sutured to the lower border of the incision. Pneumoperitoneum is only occasionally indicated for patients with subpulmonic residual spaces. Because of the considerable air leak that follows bullectomy, two properly placed drainage tubes should be left in the pleural space.

External drainage of a bulla, reported by Head and Avery (1949), is a simple, useful, and expeditious technique that can be used as a temporary or sometimes permanent measure for patients considered to be at poor risk for thoracotomy. The procedure is done under local anesthesia and does not preclude later bullectomy. Because tension pneumothorax is a potentially serious complication of the technique, MacArthur and Fountain (1977) recommended that 2.5 cm of rib be removed over the center of the bulla and a purse-string suture be inserted between parietal pleura and cyst wall.

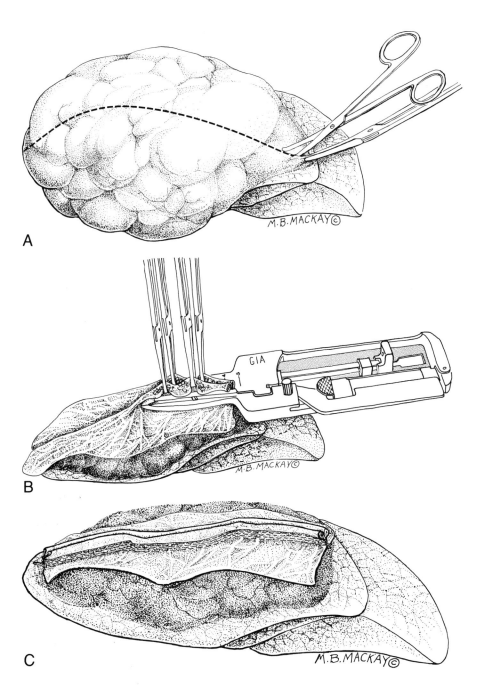

Fig. 65–13. Operative technique. *A*, Longitudinal opening of the bulla. *B*, Folding of visceral pleura over the raw surface of the lung and stapling of the entire base of the cyst. *C*, Completed bullectomy. (Courtesy of Dr. J.D. Cooper.)

A

B

C

Mortality

The reported mortality varies, but in general, age at operation, patient selection, surgical approach and technique, presence or absence of cor pulmonale, and severity of diffuse emphysema are excellent predictive variables.

Witz and Roeslin (1980) reported a mortality rate of 1.5% for 151 patients with relatively normal lung, but mortality was 11% in patients with diffuse emphysema. Most deaths resulted from respiratory failure, pleuro-

pulmonary infection, or contralateral pneumothorax. By contrast, only two deaths—2.3%—were clearly related to surgery in the series reported by Fitzgerald and associates (1974). This significant difference relates to patient selection, which was more standardized in Fitzgerald and associates' (1974) series—one institution—than in Witz and Roeslin's (1980) series—data collected from 27 institutions in five different European countries. In three series from the 1980s (Table 65–6), no operative fatalities occurred among 66 patients who underwent

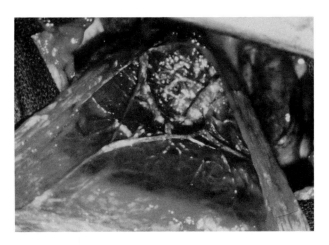

Fig. 65–14. Operative technique. Operative photograph showing trabeculations and fibrous septae that must be excised before stapling of the bulla.

bullectomy or lobectomy for bullous disease. The operative mortality for bullous emphysema should range between 1 and 5%.

Morbidity

Adequate postoperative care must include monitoring in an intensive care unit, prompt recognition and treatment of potential problems, early ambulation, drug treatment when needed, and above all, aggressive chest physiotherapy. This is possible only with appropriate pain control. New techniques such as epidural narcotic perfusion, cryoanalgesia, and patient-controlled intravenous analgesia have been significant developments in the prophylaxis of complications.

Most problems specific to bullectomy operations relate to delayed expansion of the remaining lung, prolonged air leaks or pleuropulmonary infections. All of these complications are troublesome, but eventually, most lungs re-expand and virtually every air leak stops.

Billig and associates (1968) noted that out of seven patients with persistent postoperative spaces, only one developed an empyema that required a second procedure.

Respiratory failure is uncommon if patients are well selected, and when a giant bulla is removed, the pulmonary function improves. Elective tracheotomy should be avoided, because most patients can maintain satisfactory gas exchange on spontaneous respiration. For de-

bilitated patients, nutritive support may be required before and after surgery.

Results

Assessing surgical results is difficult because nearly all reported series are small, and as Gaensler and colleagues (1986) pointed out, bulla size, preoperative evaluation, indications for surgery, type of surgery, and quality of follow-up vary among the various series. In addition, no randomized prospective clinical trial comparing standard medical therapy to surgery has ever been done. From our review of 45 clinical series written since 1960, it is obvious that only general concepts can be outlined.

One of the difficulties in reporting results is the choice of parameters considered representative of good results. Obviously, decreased dyspnea and improved exercise tolerance are the primary objectives of operative intervention. Such improvement may translate into a return to useful levels of activity or even a return to full-time employment. For some patients, an improvement in the severity of chronic bronchitis may also be noted, as well as better overall quality of life. As previously mentioned, a substantial weight gain can be expected after bullectomy.

Objective improvement is more difficult to quantitate and several authors have stressed the poor correlation between relief of dyspnea and documented improvement in pulmonary function. For most patients, pulmonary function studies improve only marginally, whereas considerable relief of dyspnea is noted. In general, the degree of improvement correlates reasonably well with increased air flow as measured by FEV_1, improved arterial oxygen saturations, and decreased trapped gas as measured by plethysmography.

Anatomic improvement is easier to demonstrate because the expanded lung nearly always fills the hemithorax and isotopic studies show an increased activity over previously radiolucent areas.

Early Results

With proper selection, approximately two thirds of patients experience significant postoperative relief of dyspnea whether they have widespread emphysema or not, and whether this improvement can be documented by pulmonary function studies or not. As Capel and Belcher (1957) observed, improvement is noted within 3 months of operation and is generally sustained for a period of 2 to 3 years postoperatively.

Table 65–6. Operative Mortality

Authors (year)	Years of Study	No. of Patients	No. of Operative Deaths	% Mortality
Witz (1980)	—	Group I : 151	2	1.5%
		Group II: 272	25	11.0%
Fitzgerald (1974)	1949–1972	84	2	2.3%
Laros (1986)	1958–1977	27	0	0.0%
O'Brien (1986)	1974–1981	20	0	0.0%
Connolly (1988)	1968–1988	19	0	0.0%

Table 67–7. Best Predictors of Good Postoperative Results

Early results
Bulla size and rate of enlargement
Degree of compression
State of underlying lung
Degree of regional asymmetry
Type of operation
Late results
Severity of emphysema

Determining the best predictors of early good results is more difficult (Table 65–7). Bulla size is an important variable in determining clinical and physiologic outcome. Capel and Belcher (1957) reported that patients with bigger cysts benefited more from operation. Gaensler and associates (1986) showed that when bullae had occupied less than one third of the lung, there was no postoperative improvement. With large bullae, however, postoperative increases of FEV_1 ranged from 50 to 200%. Patients likely to benefit from operation have well demarcated and enlarging apical bullae occupying at least 50% of the volume of the hemithorax. Cases of smaller bullae or multiple bullae disseminated throughout both lungs are less favorable.

Many regard the degree of compression as documented by chest roentgenograms or angiography as the most significant predictive variable. Gunstensen and McCormack (1973) noted that the worst results were in patients who did not have signs of compression. Brochard and colleagues (1986) showed that when the index of compression was equal to or greater than 3, all patients had significant postoperative clinical and functional improvement. No patients with an index lower than 2 improved.

Foreman and co-workers (1968) showed that perhaps the most useful information for selecting patients was given by the assessment of the compressed lung; it should be adequately perfused, as demonstrated by angiography, and have continued ability to wash out inhaled gas. Nakahara and associates (1983) observed that patients who did not benefit from bullectomy had disturbed ventilatory function in all lung regions, regardless of the location of the bulla. Patients with good results had relatively normal washout at the bases.

By comparing initial contribution of the involved lung with postoperative increase in FEV_1, Fitzgerald and colleagues (1974) noted a good correlation between regional imbalance and postoperative functional results. When the lung operated on contributed less than 10% of total function, FEV_1 always increased by more than 50% postoperatively. With a lung that initially contributed near-normal perfusion, there were small or no increases in postoperative FEV_1.

Plication of bullae results in larger increases in FEV_1 and better clinical results than lobectomy. Rogers and colleagues (1968) investigated the effect of surgical resection on airway conductance. They observed an increase in airway conductance in all patients who underwent bullectomy. These authors attributed this increase

to improved lung elastic recoil. In four of five patients who had lobectomy for carcinoma, there was a reduction both in the airway conductance and in the FRC with relatively little change in the conductance/volume ratio. Woo-Ming and associates (1963) noted that 12 of 28 patients who had a bullectomy had a good result, whereas only 2 of 15 patients who had lobectomy maintained a good result for any length of time.

Other factors that may be less predictive of early good results are a large amount of trapped air in the bulla as measured by plethysmography, a severe disability before surgery, and the absence of diffuse emphysema in the remaining lung.

Late Results

Although most series have shown good to excellent initial postoperative results, dyspnea gradually returns to preoperative levels after the fifth postoperative year. The severity of emphysema seems to be the main limiting factor for sustained good results. In Witz's series (1980), patients were divided into two groups. In group I patients—N = 151—with localized bullous disease and near-normal underlying lung, 73% were improved by surgery and most were able to return to work. In nearly all cases, this improvement persisted during the years of follow-up. In group II patients—N = 272—with more diffuse emphysema, only 50% were still improved after 5 years and 20% after 10 years. The degree of degradation paralleled the severity of emphysema.

In Fitzgerald and associates' (1974) series, 47 long-term survivors with a mean follow-up time of 9 years were divided into three groups. Group 1 patients—N = 16—with small and well demarcated bullae of the paraseptal emphysema type, all had sustained good results, and their long-term decline in function differed little from that of normal aging. In group II patients—N = 16—with larger but still localized bullae, initial good results were sustained for about 4 to 5 years, but then function declined, only to return to preoperative levels within 7 to 10 years. In 15 patients with diffuse emphysema—group III—the average decline in FEV_1 during the period of follow-up was 101 cc per year, and the functional improvement persisted for only one to two postoperative years. This annual decline is more than the expected 80 cc per year for patients with chronic obstructive lung disease and 28 cc per year for normal individuals.

Pearson and Ogilvie (1983) reviewed nine patients 5 to 10 years after surgery and all had gradual return to initial symptoms with an annual decline in FEV_1 of 82 cc/year. They found no new bullae on chest roentgenograms and no enlargement of pre-existing bullae.

This clinical information suggests that surgery for bullous disease associated with diffuse emphysema is worthwhile for short-term relief but that sustained improvement is highly unusual.

Conclusion

In bullous disease and generalized emphysema, it is sometimes more difficult to decide which individual should not have surgery. In general, asymptomatic patients, patients whose disease is not localized, and patients without roentgenologic evidence of compression should not have an operation. As Peters (1983) suggested, if bullous emphysema is only the end-stage manifestation of generalized degenerative changes in the lung, excision or stapling of the bullae has little benefit.

SURGERY FOR SPONTANEOUS PNEUMOTHORAX

Entry of air into the pleural space is always secondary to a disruption in the continuity of the pleural membrane—parietal, visceral or mediastinal. Although its occurrence is generally spontaneous or post-traumatic, a pneumothorax may be induced deliberately (Table 65–8).

Primary Spontaneous Pneumothorax

Pathogenesis

Primary spontaneous pneumothorax occurs predominantly in young healthy adults, predominantly in men—a ratio of 6:1. The overall incidence is estimated at 5 to 10 cases per 100,000 per year, but can be as high as 1 in 500 young men. Most primary pneumothoraces are caused by rupture of subpleural blebs in lungs that are otherwise normal—paraseptal emphysema. Air escape occurs when the distending pressure in the bleb exceeds the elastic strength of its wall and causes it to rupture intrapleurally.

The pathogenesis of apical blebs is unknown, although spontaneous pneumothoraces occur most often in tall and thin individuals. Withers and associates (1964) postulated that, in the tall and thin, the rapid growth rate of the lung relative to pulmonary vasculature causes ischemia and bleb formation at the apex, farther away from the main arterial supply of the pulmonary hilum. Perhaps higher transpulmonary pressures at the apex in tall individuals lead to greater alveoli-distending pressures. Spontaneous pneumothorax may also be associated with connective tissue disorders such as Marfan's syndrome.

Diagnosis

The predominant symptom of pneumothorax in young people is acute pleuritic chest pain, which often subsides over 24 hours. In most patients, the severity of symptoms is proportional to the magnitude of the pneumothorax,

but about 30% of patients have no pain or dyspnea. Contrary to traditional teaching, physical exertion is unrelated to the occurrence of pneumothorax.

Although the extent of collapse can best be quantified by measuring the diameters of the lung and hemithorax on a roentgenogram of the chest, most physicians estimate pneumothoraces without actual measurements. Jenkinson (1985) noted that this evaluation notoriously results in an underestimation of the pneumothorax. If the diagnosis is suspected but cannot be confirmed by a routine chest roentgenogram, a chest film taken during exhalation may accentuate the pneumothorax.

Management

Several questions should be answered before planning the management of a patient with pneumothorax: Is the pneumothorax large or small? Is the patient symptomatic or asymptomatic? Is it the first episode or a recurrence? Is it simple or complicated? Is the underlying lung normal or pathologic?

First Episode—Uncomplicated

Patients with less than 20% collapse, minimal symptoms, and no radiologic evidence of progression can be observed. Kircher and Swart (1954) showed by roentgenographic lung volume studies that the rate of air absorption from the pleural space is relatively constant at 1.25% per day—50 to 75 cc/day—when the fistula has sealed. Activities should be restricted, and 2 to 3 days of in-hospital observation may be needed to ensure that no complications develop.

The main argument for more aggressive management is the duration of therapy, which can be shortened by closed thoracostomy. Other indications for tube drainage are as follows: more than 20% collapse shown on the first roentgenogram, tension, disease of the contralateral lung, symptoms, or progression of the pneumothorax on successive roentgenograms.

Principles of Tube Drainage. The preferred site of insertion is the fourth or fifth interspace in the midaxillary line, although most textbooks still recommend the second space in the midclavicular line. It is not only more cosmetically acceptable—no obvious scar or danger of tube placement through breast tissue, but the technique of insertion is easier—no chest wall muscles to traverse—and safer—no danger of puncturing the internal mammary artery.

There are two accepted techniques for tube insertion: trocar method and blunt dissection. The trocar method is popular, but it is more likely to injure the lung or any other intrathoracic structure. Dissecting a tract with a Kelly hemostat clamp is safer and has replaced the trocar method in most institutions.

Although water-seal suction drainage has no documented advantage, most surgeons believe that a high negative intrapleural pressure promotes sealing of the leak against the parietal pleura and secondary pleural symphysis. One-way flutter valves—Heimlich valve—enable the pleural space to be evacuated without the encumbrance of a water-seal system. Mercier and as-

---

Table 65–8. Classification of Pneumothorax

Spontaneous Pneumothorax
  Primary (no identifiable pathology)
  Secondary (chronic obstructive lung disease or other pulmonary
    disorder)
  Catamenial
  Neonatal

Traumatic Pneumothorax
  Blunt or penetrating thoracic injuries
  Iatrogenic: mechanical ventilation, monitoring technique, postoperative

Diagnostic Pneumothorax

sociates (1976) showed that outpatient management with a flutter valve is safe, efficient, and economical.

The intercostal tube should stay in the pleural space for 24 hours after the air leak has stopped and the lung expanded. So and Yu (1982) suggested that leaving the tube for 3 to 4 days induces an inflammatory reaction and reduces the chances of recurrence. Mills and Baisch's (1965) observation supports the hypothesis that the recurrence rate is lower in patients whose oral temperature reached 101°F—38.3°C—who had a leukocytosis above 12,000/mm³, or who had roentgenologic evidence of pleural reaction over the apex.

First Episode—Complicated

Although most primary spontaneous pneumothoraces are uncomplicated, such problems as tension, hemorrhage, trapped lung, and persistent air leak may occur and force the surgeon to change the treatment plan.

Tension Pneumothorax. Tension pneumothorax requires immediate life-saving action. It occurs when a tear in the lung produces a one-way valve opened during inspiration—air flows into the pleural space—but closed during exhalation. As tension increases, the mediastinum shifts toward the contralateral side, causing interference with ventilation, venous return, and ultimately cardiac output.

Tension may develop at any time, and its onset is often sudden and dramatic. When the diagnosis is suspected, drainge by chest tube or large-bore needle should be done without roentgenographic confirmation of the pneumothorax. Once tension is relieved, further treatment is similar to that of patients with uncomplicated episodes.

Hemopneumothorax. Pleural effusion reportedly occurs in 15 to 20% of cases of pneumothorax, but frank hemothorax occurs in less than 5%. In general, the bleeding is arterial and secondary to a torn adhesion between visceral and parietal pleura. The bleeding point is nearly always on the chest wall side of the adhesion. The onset is often insidious and the diagnosis can be further delayed if a small chest catheter has been used to drain the space.

When lung expansion successfully tamponades the bleeding site, as is often the case, treatment can be conservative—tube drainage. In our experience, most of these individuals eventually need surgical intervention for control of the bleeding or space delocation. Grossman (1953) reported that blood in the pleural space may induce a chemical pleuritis that lowers the chances of a recurrence.

Persistent Air Leak. Although most air leaks have already sealed when the chest is drained or stop within the first 12 to 24 hours, 3 to 4% of patients have a persistent fistula after several days of drainage. When this problem occurs, the continuation of intercostal tube drainage for more than 10 days is inadvisable, and thoracotomy should be considered to close the fistula and obliterate the pleural space.

Failure to Expand and Chronicity. Despite proper tube placement and adequate suction, the lung may show only partial expansion on the postdrainage roentgeno-

grams. Among the factors responsible for delayed reexpansion, a large bronchopleural fistula or a trapped lung are the commonest. Management of these problems requires thoracotomy for direct closure of the fistula or decortication of the lung.

Special Problems. Spontaneous pneumothorax may be associated with a pneumomediastinum. Air is thought to leak into the mediastinum by dissection along the bronchi or the vascular sheaths of pulmonary vessels. This finding has no clinical consequence, although compression of the great vessels has been reported in children.

Bilateral simultaneous pneumothorax is rare, and has never been observed at our institution. In such a case, bilateral pleural drainage may be needed during the acute phase. Nonsimultaneous bilateral pneumothoraces are more common—5 to 10% of all cases, and parietal pleurectomy is recommmeded for any patient with an initial episode of pneumothorax on one side and a history of pneumothorax on the other.

Subcutaneous emphysema always indicates that drainage is inadequate. In some cases, the chest tube is malpositioned or obstructed, or one of the side holes is outside the pleural cavity. In other cases, the drainage system is not working properly or the amount of suction is inadequate for a large leak.

Treatment of pneumothorax in pregnant women should be conservative, with avoidance of thoracotomy. The obstetrician must be notified of the possibility of a pneumothorax—uni- or bilateral—occurring during delivery.

Thoracotomy may be indicated after the first episode in patients with an occupation in which a recurrence could be a hazard—airline personnel, divers, patients with demonstrable large bullae, or patients living in isolated areas.

Recurrence

Primary spontaneous pneumothorax tends to recur. The risk of recurrence after one episode is about 20%, but Gobbel and colleagues (1963) reported a 60 to 80% risk in patients who have suffered more than one previous episode. Most recurrences are ipsilateral—75%—and occur within 2 years of the first episode.

Risk factors include chronic obstructive lung disease, air leak for more than 48 hours during the first episode, and large air cysts seen on the roentgenogram (Table 65–9). The significance of the method of treatment used

Table 65–9. Risk Factors for Recurrence

Established
  More than one previous episode
  Chronic obstructive lung disease
  Air leak for more than 48 hours during first episode
  Large cysts seen on roentgenograms

Possible
  Nonoperative management of first episode (vs. tube drainage)
  Tube drainage for only 24 hours during first episode (vs. 3–4 days)
  Leukocytosis less than 12,000 and temperature less than 101°F
    (38.3°C) during the first episode

during the first episode and the duration of pleural space intubation is unknown.

To prevent recurrences, the pleural space should be obliterated and the diseased site resected. Pleural space obliteration is accomplished by chemical pleurodesis, mechanical abrasion, or parietal pleurectomy, and resection is by suture closure, wedge resection, or diathermy electrocoagulation.

Thorsrud (1965) noted that intrapleural instillation of chemical agents starts an inflammatory reaction of the pleural mesothelium with adhesion and fibrosis formation. The main inconveniences of these techniques are their toxicity—painful febrile reaction, pleural effusion, the nonuniformity of pleural adhesions—adhesions tend to form over the mediastinal or diaphragmatic surfaces, and the variability of results. Tetracycline—500 mg in 10 cc of isotonic sodium chloride—and talc are the only chemicals still used for pleurodesis, although Gaensler (1956) reported specific complications such as granulomas, fibrothorax, or induction of mesotheliomas related to the use of talc.

Scarification of the pleura is effective in preventing recurrences, especially when combined with bleb excision. The reported results have been consistently good, with minimal operative trauma and morbidity. This technique has the advantage of preserving an extrapleural plane should a future thoracotomy be needed.

Parietal pleurectomy creates an inflammatory surface that promotes fixation of the lung to the endothoracic fascia. Several authors have described pleurectomy as the most secure procedure to obtain permanent pleurodesis. Because the disease is nearly always limited to the lung apex, an apical pleurectomy, combined with bleb excision, is enough for definitive control of recurrences.

The operation one of us (J.D.) and associates (1980) prefer is performed through a transaxillary vertical approach with the patient in a 20° position on the operating table (Fig. 65–15). The arm is elevated and fixed to the anesthetic screen cross-bar. The surgical incision extends from the axilla along the external border of the pectoralis

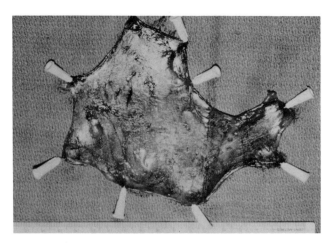

Fig. 65–16. Parietal pleurectomy. Strip of parietal pleura removed over the apex through the axillary incision.

major. No muscles are divided, and the chest cavity is entered through the third intercostal space. The apical blebs—or scarred apex—are excised with a stapling instrument, and the pleura stripped from the endothoracic fascia starting at the incision and over the apex (Fig. 65–16). Bleeding is meticulously controlled, and a large chest tube is left at the apex of the pleural space.

The procedure can be done in 30 to 45 minutes and produces significantly less morbidity than a standard thoracotomy, with an average hospital stay of five days after operation. Most patients return to work within 6 weeks of the procedure, and the long-term cosmetic appearance of the scar is satisfactory. When bilateral pleurectomy is advisable, it should be done in stages 10 to 30 days apart.

Secondary Spontaneous Pneumothorax

Pathogenesis

Secondary spontaneous pneumothorax occurs predominantly in people more than 45 years old with documented or roentgenographically apparent pulmonary disease. Most patients have chronic obstructive lung disease or bullous emphysema, but this may occur in other pulmonary pathologies (Table 65–10). Roentgenographically occult bronchial carcinoma must always be ruled out by bronchoscopy before planning therapy.

Catamenial pneumothoraces are nearly always right-sided. Maurer and associates (1958) postulated that air escapes from the fallopian tubes and reaches the pleural

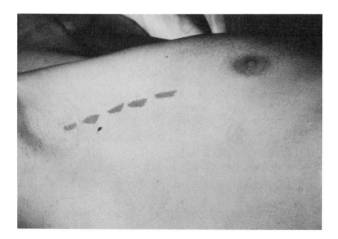

Fig. 65–15. Parietal pleurectomy. Transaxillary vertical approach to apical parietal pleurectomy.

Table 65–10. Pulmonary Disorders Frequently Associated with Secondary Pneumothorax

Chronic obstructive lung disease (bullous or diffuse emphysema)
Tuberculosis: active or inactive (scar or bulla formation)
Catamenial
Miscellaneous disorders
  Congenital: cystic fibrosis
  Endobronchial obstruction: neoplasm, foreign body
  Infection: pneumonia, lung abscess
  Diffuse disease: fibrosis, collagen, or interstitial disease
  Asthma

space through microscopic fenestrations in the diaphragm. In some cases, endometrial tissue has been found in the pleural space.

Diagnosis

The predominant symptom in emphysematous patients who develop a pneumothorax is an acute and often severe episode of shortness of breath, which can rapidly develop into frank respiratory failure. Because of compromised function, these patients often have only a minimal degree of lung collapse—5 to 10%—but severe hypoxia. Chest pain is almost never an important feature of the cliical presentation. In most cases, the diagnosis is readily made by a routine roentgenogram of the chest, but sometimes it is impossible to differentiate betweeen a pneumothorax and a large emphysematous bulla. As mentioned before, computed tomography of the chest may help in determining which of the two abnormalities is present.

Management

All patients with COPD and secondary pneumothorax should initially be treated by intercostal tube drainage for rapid re-expansion of functioning lung tissue. This simple therapeutic maneuver often dramatically improves the patient's clinical status.

In these patients air leaks generally last more than 10 days, but because of a significantly increased operative risk, tube drainage should be continued for longer than in primary pneumothoraces. Virtually all leaks stop if the pleural space is adequately drained, if the lung is fully expanded, and if the attending physician is patient. For individuals with moderate emphysema and acceptable operative risk, indications for thoracotomy are the same as in primary pneumothoraces.

If open thoracotomy is indicated and possible, a total parietal pleurectomy should be done without any attempt to excise hyperinflated lung parenchyma. For patients with prohibitive operative risk, pleural symphysis should be done by tetracycline—local anesthesia—or talc—general anesthesia—instillations.

Prognosis

Even though most patients with secondary spontaneous pneumothorax can be managed successfully, the morbidity may be prolonged, and death may even result from respiratory failure initiated by the occurrence of the pneumothorax, particularly in the older patient with extensive underlying pulmonary disease. Shields and Oilschlager (1966) reported a 16% mortality rate in an older age group of patients, most of whom also had other major disease processes. This mortality rate contrasts markedly with the zero mortality expected with the proper management of an uncomplicated primary spontaneous pneumothorax in the young.

SURGERY OF DIFFUSE EMPHYSEMA

Among the several but largely obsolete procedures that have been described to improve dyspnea in patients with diffuse emphysema, Brantigan and associates' (1959) approach was the most attractive, short of lung transplantation. The primary objective of the operation was to reduce lung volume through peripheral wedge resections, and in fact, the parenchyma was resected until the lung fit the pleural space on full exhalation. To reduce bronchial secretions and decrease the associated bronchospasm, total lung denervation was added to the procedure. The operation was intended to restore the physiologic mechanisms of circumferential pull on the smaller airways by improving the elastic recoil of the lung. In addition, Brantigan and colleagues hoped to increase diaphragmatic contractility by restoring its normal curvature. Postoperative follow-up studies showed little objective improvement, but patients were subjectively improved, with better exercise tolerance.

Knudson and Gaensler (1965) had reservations about this approach, arguing that it is difficult to believe that a disease characterized by extensive loss of parenchyma can be effectively treated by further resection of lung. Knudson and Gaensler (1965) further showed that mechanical distention of an already emphysematous lung may lead to accelerated deterioration.

Since then, little enthusiasm has been shown for the surgery for diffuse emphysema. In 1987, Sallerin and Dahan (personal communication) suggested that lung volume reduction may improve the dyspnea in nonbullous emphysema, by restoring impaired hemodynamic parameters. Georges and associates (1966) argued that positive expiratory pressure was not only responsible for bronchiolar obstruction and airflow limitation, but it also caused expiratory vascular obstruction with decreased right ventricular filling, increased pulmonary vascular resistance and ultimately fall in cardiac output. They also showed that these hemodynamic abnormalities worsened during exercise. Although Sallerin and Dahan (personal communication, 1987) did show some clinical and physiologic evidence of short-term improvement, pilot studies and controlled clinical trials are needed to quantitate possible benefits, improve the selection of patients, and eventually compare the results of surgical treatment to that of standard medical therapy.

REFERENCES

Bullous Emphysema

American Thoracic Society: Chronic bronchitis, asthma, and pulmonary emphysema: a statement by the committee on diagnostic standards for nontuberculous respiratory diseases. Am. Rev. Respir. Dis. 85:762, 1962.

Belcher, J.R., and Siddons, A.H.M.: Air-containing cysts of the lung. Thorax 9:38, 1954.

Benumof, J.L.: Sequential one-lung ventilation for bilateral bullectomy. Anaesthesiology 67:268, 1987.

Berry, B.E., and Oschner, A.: Massive hemoptysis associated with localized pulmonary bullae requiring emergency surgery. J. Thorac. Cardiovasc. Surg. 63:94:72.

Billig, D.M., Boushy, S.F., and Kohen, R.: Surgical treatment of bullous emphysema. Arch. Surg. 97:744, 1968.

Boushy, S.F., et al.: Bullous emphysema: clinical, roentgenologic, and physiologic study of 49 patients. Dis. Chest 54:17, 1968.

Brochard, L., et al.: Evaluation de l'efficacité du traitement chirurgical de l'emphysème pan-lobulaire. Rev. Mal. Respir. 4:187, 1986.

Capel, L.H., and Belcher, J.R.: Surgical treatment of large air cysts of the lung. Lancet 1:759, 1957.

Ciba Guest Symposium Report: Terminology, definitions and classification of chronic pulmonary emphysema and related conditions. Thorax 14:286, 1959.

Connolly, J.E., and Wilson, A.F.: Current status of surgery for bullous emphysema. J. Thorac. Cardiovasc. Surg. (in press.)

Dean, N.C., Stein, M.G., and Stulbarg, M.S.: Percutaneous drainage of an infected lung bulla in a patient receiving positive pressure ventilation. Chest 91:928, 1987.

Eschapasse, H., and Berthomieu, F.: La chirurgie de l'emphysème pulmonaire. Broncho-pneumologie 30:173, 1980.

Fitzgerald, M.X., Keelan, P.J., and Gaensler, E.A.: Surgery for bullous emphysema. Respiration 30:187, 1973.

Fitzgerald, M.X., et al.: Long-term results of surgery for bullous emphysema. J. Thorac. Cardiovasc. Surg. 68:566, 1974.

Foreman, S., et al.: Bullous disease of the lung: physiologic improvement after surgery. Ann. Intern. Med. 69:757, 1968.

Gaensler, et al.: Surgical management of emphysema. Clin. Chest. Med. 4:443, 1983.

Gaensler, E.A., Jederlinic, P.J., and Fitzgerald, M.X.: Patient work-up for bullectomy. J. Thorac. Imaging 1:75, 1986.

Gunstensen, J., and McCormack, R.J.M.: The surgical management of bullous emphysema. J. Thorac. Cardiovasc. Surg. 65:920, 1973.

Harris, J.: Severe bullous emphysema. Chest 70:658, 1976.

Head, J.R., and Avery, E.E.: Intra-cavitary suction (Monaldi) in the treatment of emphysematous bullae and blebs. J. Thorac. Surg. 18:761, 1949.

Hugh-Jones, P., and Whinster, W.: The etiology and management of disabling emphysema. Am. Rev. Respir. Dis. 117:343, 1978.

Laros, C.D., et al.: Bullectomy for giant bullae in emphysema. J. Thorac. Cardiovasc. Surg. 91:63, 1986.

Lima, O., et al.: Median sternotomy for bilateral resection of emphysematous bullae. J. Thorac. Cardiovasc. Surg. 82:892, 1981.

MacArthur, A.M., and Fountain, S.W.: Intracavitary suction and drainage in the treatment of emphysematous bullae. Thorax 32:668, 1977.

Miller, W.S.: A study of the human pleura pulmonalis: its relation to the blebs and bullae of emphysema. Am. J. Roentgenol. 15:399, 1926.

Miscall, L., and Duffy, R.W.: Surgical treatment of bullous emphysema. Dis. Chest 24:489, 1953.

Naclerio, E., and Langer, L.: Pulmonary cysts: special reference to surgical treatment of emphysematous blebs and bullae. Surgery 22:516, 1947.

Nakahara, H., et al.: Functional indications for bullectomy of giant bulla. Ann. Thorac. Surg. 35:480, 1983.

Nelems, J.M.B.: A technique for controlling bullous cysts of lungs: abstract of the postgraduate course in general thoracic surgery, University of Toronto, May, 1980.

Normandale, J.P., and Feneck, R.O.: Bullous cystic lung disease. Anaesthesia 40:1182, 1985.

O'Brien, C.J., Hughes, C.F., and Gianoutsos, P.: Surgical treatment of bullous emphysema. Aust. NZ J. Surg. 56:241, 1986.

Pearson, M.G., and Ogilvie, C.: Surgical treatment of emphysematous bullae: late outcome. Thorax 38:134, 1983.

Peters, R.M.: Indications for operative treatment of bullous emphysema (editorial). Ann. Thorac. Surg. 35:479, 1983.

Pride, N.B., et al.: Changes in lung function following the surgical treatment of bullous emphysema. Q. J. Med. 153:49, 1970.

Pride, N.B., Barter, C.E., and Hugh-Jones, P.: The ventilation of bullae and the effect of their removal on thoracic gas volume and tests of pulmonary function. Am. Rev. Respir. Dis. 107:83, 1973.

Rogers, R.M., Dubois, A.B., and Blakemore, W.S.: Effect of removal of bullae on airway conductance and conductance volume ratios. J. Clin. Invest. 47:2569, 1968.

Snider, G.L.: A perspective on emphysema. Clin. Chest. Med. 4:329, 1983.

Snider, G.L., et al.: The definition of emphysema. Am. Rev. Respir. Dis. 132:182, 1985.

Spear, H.G., et al.: The surgical management of large pulmonary blebs and bullae. Am. Rev. Respir. Dis. 87:186, 1961.

Ting, E.Y., Klopstock, R., and Lyons, H.A.: Mechanical properties of pulmonary cysts and bullae. Am. Rev. Respir. Dis. 87:538, 1963.

Witz, J.P., and Roeslin, N.: La chirurgie de l'emphysème bulleux chez l'adulte: ses résultats éloignés. Rev. Fr. Mal. Respir. 8:121, 1980.

Woo-Ming, M., Capel, L.H., and Belcher, J.R.: The results of surgical treatment of large air cysts of the lung. Br. J. Dis. Chest 57:79, 1963.

Spontaneous Pneumothorax

Deslauriers, J., et al.: Transaxillary pleurectomy for treatment of spontaneous pneumothorax. Ann. Thorac. Surg. 30:569, 1980.

Gaensler, E.A.: Parietal pleurectomy for recurrent spontaneous pneumothorax. Surg. Gynecol. Obstet. 102:293, 1956.

Gobbel, W.G., et al.: Spontaneous pneumothorax. J. Thorac. Cardiovasc. Surg. 46:331, 1963.

Grossman, L.A.: Recurrent bilateral spontaneous pneumothorax treated with artificial hemothorax. Ann. Intern. Med. 39:1303, 1953.

Jenkinson, S.G.: Pnemothorax. Clin. Chest Med. 6:153, 1985.

Kircher, L.T., and Swart, R.L.: Spontaneous pneumothorax and its treatment. J.A.M.A. 155:24, 1954.

Maurer, E.R., Schaal, J.A., and Mondez, F.L.: Chronic recurrent spontaneous pneumothorax due to endometriosis of the diaphragm. J.A.M.A. 168:2013, 1958.

Mercier, C., et al.: Outpatient management of intercostal tube drainage in spontaneous pneumothorax. Ann. Thorac. Surg. 22:163, 1976.

Mills, M., and Baisch, B.F.: Spontaneous pneumothorax: a series of 400 cases. Ann. Thorac. Surg. 1:286, 1965.

Shields, T.W., and Oilschlager, G.A.: Spontaneous pneumothorax in patients 40 years of age and older. Ann. Thorac. Surg. 2(3):377, 1966.

So, S., and Yu, D.: Catheter drainage of spontaneous pneumothorax: suction or no suction, early or late removal? Thorax 37:46, 1982.

Thorsrud, G.K.: Pleural reactions to irritants. Acta Chir. Scand. 355:1, 1965 (Suppl).

Withers, J.N., et al.: Spontaneous pneumothorax: suggested etiology and comparison of treatment methods. Am. J. Surg. 108:772, 1964.

Surgery for Diffuse Emphysema

Brantigan, O.C., Muellere, E., and Kress, M.B.: A surgical approach to pulmonary emphysema. Am. Rev. Respir. Dis. 80(supplement):194, 1959.

Georges, R., et al.: Données hémodynamiques sur l'emphysème diffus. J. Fr. Med. Chir. Thorac. 4:373, 1966.

Knudson, R. J., and Gaensler, E.A.: Surgery for emphysema. Ann. Thorac. Surg. 1:332, 1965.

SELECTED READINGS

Bullous Emphysema

Benfield, J.R., et al.: Current approach to the surgical management of emphysema. Arch Surg. 93:59, 1966.

Billig, D.M.: Surgery for bullous emphysema (editorial). Chest 70:572, 1976.

Boushy, S.F., Billig, D.M., and Lohen, R.: Changes in pulmonary function after bullectomy. Am. J. Med. 47:916, 1969.

Duffell, G.M.: The role of surgery in chronic obstructive pulmonary disease. Postgrad. Med. 54:197, 1973.

Knudson, R.J., and Gaensler, E.A.: Surgery for emphysema. Ann. Thorac. Surg. 1:332, 1965.

Laurenzi, G.A., Turino, G.M., and Fishman, A.J.P.: Bullous disease of the lung. Am. J. Med. 32:361, 1962.

Morgan, M.B.L., and Strickland, B.: Computed tomography in the assessment of bullous lung disease. Br. J. Dis. Chest 78:10, 1987.

Ogilvie, C., and Catterall, M.: Patterns of disturbed lung function in patients with emphysematous bullae. Thorax 14:216, 1959.

Wesley, J.R., Macleod, W.M., and Mullard, K.S.: Evaluation and surgery of bullous emphysema. J. Thorac. Cardiovasc. Surg. 63:945, 1972.

Spontaneous Pneumothorax

Clagett, O.T.: The management of spontaneous pneumothorax. J. Thorac. Cardiovasc. Surg. 55:761, 1965.

Clark, T.A., et al.: Spontaneous pneumothorax. Am. J. Surg. 124:725, 1972.

Deslauriers, J.: Spontaneous pneumothorax. Ann. R. Coll. Can. 21:9, 1980.

Weissberg, D.: Talc pleurodesis: a controversial issue. Poumon-Coeur 37:291, 1981.

Wied, U., et al.: Tetracycline versus silver nitrate pleurodesis in spontaneous pneumothorax. J. Thorac. Cardiovasc. Surg. 86:591, 1983.

Youmans, C.R., et al.: Surgical management of spontaneous pneumothorax by bleb ligation and pleural dry sponge abrasion. Am. J. Surg. 120:644, 1970.

CHAPTER 66

BACTERIAL DISEASES OF THE LUNG

R. Maurice Hood

Suppurative diseases of the lung, along with tuberculosis, formed the base for the development of thoracic surgery as a surgical specialty. Until the mid 1950s, they represented the bulk of the practice in this field. Antibiotics had an enormous impact on the incidence and management of these diseases. Since the 1940s, many changes in the incidence, the disease spectrum, and the clinical course of such disease have occurred. It seemed to many that surgical treatment of bronchiectasis and lung abscess had become obsolete and that the internist could easily cope with this disappearing group of diseases.

Unfortunately, suppurative disease did not disappear. Several factors combined to produce a new group of clinical problems and a small resurgence of lung abscess and empyema, including: (1) emergence of multiple antibiotic-resistant organisms, (2) an enormous increase in the number of immunosuppressed individuals, (3) the development of a drug-abuse culture, (4) continued immigration of people from the underdeveloped world who bring with them not only disease but the practices that result in disease, and (5) an increasingly aging population.

In the underdeveloped third world, suppurative bacterial pulmonary diseases still occur as frequently and severely as they did in the United Sates in the 1940s. Therefore, the basic surgical principles of management are essentially unchanged for surgeons working in these areas.

Also, postinfectious residua, such as fibrosing or sclerosing pneumonitis and organized nonresolving pneumonia, that pose diagnostic and surgical problems sometimes more difficult than surgeons faced earlier, have become more common in the United States.

BRONCHIECTASIS

Bronchiectasis is dilatation of bronchi. The pathogenesis of bronchiectasis has never been clearly understood. Previously, saccular bronchiectasis with its familiar symptomatology of large amounts of purulent sputum, recurring pulmonary infection, and hemoptysis was generally the complication of pertussis, a severe bacterial or viral pneumonitis, or an aspirated foreign body. Most of the cases seen today, however, are more insidious in presentation and many immune disorders and congenital abnormalities have a form of bronchiectasis as a complication or component of the underlying disease.

Any classification of bronchiectasis is probably inadequate, but classification may help to separate in the surgeon's thinking a varied group of patients (Table 66–1).

Saccular bronchiectasis follows a major pulmonary bacterial or viral infection or results from a foreign body or bronchial stricture and is the principal type with surgical implications. Cylindrical bronchiectasis consists of dilated bronchi that do not end blindly but communicate with lung parenchyma. In some patients this is only a mild degree of dilatation, but often is associated with immune disorders and other diseases.

Pseudobronchiectasis, first reported by Blades and Dugan (1944), is cylindrical dilatation of bronchi following acute pneumonic processes; it is associated with chronic cough and expectoration but is temporary and disappears after several weeks or months (Fig. 66–1). This process has no surgical implications.

Post-tuberculous bronchiectasis is a cylindrical dilatation of bronchi usually in the upper lobes in an area of healed or healing tuberculosis and is associated with

Table 66–1. Classification of Bronchiectasis

Postinfection saccular bronchiectasis
  Related to pertussis, bacterial and viral pneumonia, bronchial stricture, and retained foreign body
Cylindrial bronchiectasis
  Related to pulmonary infection
  Related to chronic aspiration (esophageal motility diseases—achalasia, tracheoesophageal fistula)
Pseudobronchiectasis
Post-tuberculous bronchiectasis
Genetic-related bronchiectasis

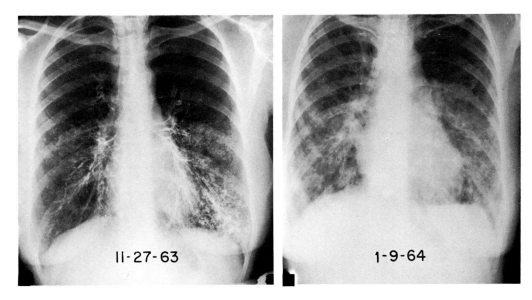

Fig. 66–1. A patient with Löffler's syndrome following bronchogram. She had fever, dyspnea, and sputum production for 3 weeks after the examination and then became asymptomatic. The roentgenograms showed little to no clearing in 1½ months.

extensive parenchymal fibrosis. Perhaps fibrosis and foreshortening of the bronchi accounts for some of the findings. These patients have no increase in sputum but seem to have an increased tendency to bleed. This finding was in the past a surgical indication, but is rarely seen today.

Several genetic syndromes are associated with some form of bronchiectasis (Table 66–2, Fig. 66–2). Whether the bronchiectasis is an acquired complication or a part of the genetic defect is not clear. A deficiency of bronchial cartilage may cause congenital bronchiectasis. Also, the uncommon widespread bilateral cystic bronchiectasis is congenital and is probably a form of sequestration. Kartagener's syndrome, with situs inversus, pansinusitis,

and bronchiectasis, is now thought to be a genetic disorder in which abnormal or nonfunctional respiratory mucosal cilia probably initiate the bronchial disease (Fig. 66–3). Wakefield and Waite (1980) reported abnormal and nonfunctioning cilia demonstrated by electron microscopy in a predominately Polynesian group of patients with bronchiectasis.

Despite this impressive array of genetic factors and syndromes, the fact that antibiotic therapy has radically changed the clinical course and incidence of the typical saccular bronchiectasis is also most irrefutable evidence that infection, bacterial, or viral, is the principal etiologic factor in the saccular form of the disease and that those with these genetic defects probably represent a subset

Table 66–2. Clinical Features of Familial Bronchiectasis

Disorder	Sinusitis	Otitis	Sperm	Situs Inversus	Skin Infections	Lobar Distribution	Genetics	Incidence
Cystic fibrosis	Yes	No	None	No	No	Upper, lower	AR	1/2,000
Immotile cilia syndrome	Yes	No	Immotile	Yes	No	Lower, middle	AR	1/20,000
Young syndrome	Yes	No	None	No	No	?	?	?
α_1-Anti-trypsin deficiency	No	No	Normal	No	No	?	AR	1/4,000
IgG deficiency	Yes	Yes	?	No	Yes	Lower, middle	AR, X, SP, AQ	Rare
IgA deficiency	Yes	No	?	No	No	Lower, middle	AR, SP, AQ	1/500 to 800
Williams-Campbell syndrome	No	No	?	No	No	Lower, middle	AR, SP, ?	Rare
Neutrophil deficiencies	Yes	Yes	?	No	Yes	?	AR, SP, X	Rare
Complement	?	?	?	No	?	?	?, AR	Very rare

AR, Autosomal recessive, X, X-linked recessive; SP, sporadic; AQ, acquired.

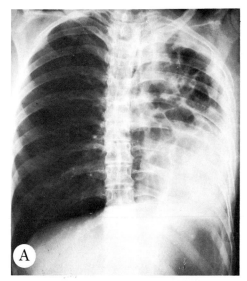

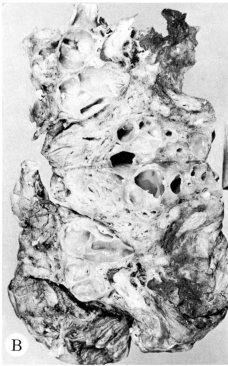

Fig. 66–2. Universal cystic bronchiectasis involving the entire left lung. *A*, Roentgenographic appearance. *B*, Gross specimen. Prior to pneumonectomy the patient was dyspneic, cyanotic, and produced large quantities of sputum. (Ferguson, T.B.: Congenital lesions of the lungs and emphysema. *In* Gibbon's Surgery of the Chest, 4th ed. Edited by D.C. Sabiston, Jr., and F.C. Spencer. Philadelphia, W.B. Saunders Co., 1982, Chapter 22.)

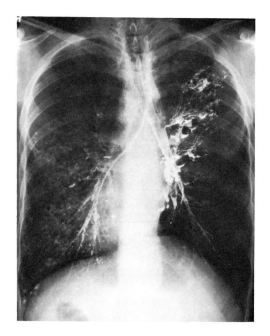

Fig. 66–3. Bronchogram in a patient with Kartagener's syndrome. Situs inversus of the thoracic and abdominal viscera is present. The patient had sinusitis and symptoms compatible with bronchiectasis. (Ferguson, T.B.: Congenital lesions of the lungs and emphysema. *In* Gibbon's Surgery of the Chest, 4th ed. Edited by D.C. Sabiston, Jr., and F.C. Spencer. Philadelphia, W.B. Saunders Co., 1982, Chapter 22.)

previously unrecognized because of the limited genetic knowledge and the previously high incidence of saccular bronchiectasis. The remainder of this discussion, however, will be confined to those with typical, saccular, postinfectious bronchiectasis.

One of the difficulties in discussing bronchiectasis today is that a new generation of surgeons and internists has never seen bronchiectasis of the preantibiotic era. Patients would produce from 100 cc to 500 cc of thick, unbelievably foul-smelling sputum per day. They were incapacitated by recurring infections, were socially ostracized because of their cough and odor, and had a life expectancy of less than 35 years.

Pathology

Gross

The uninvolved lung's volume is reduced even to the point of complete atelectasis; pleural adhesions are numerous, dense, and vascular. The cut lung shows grossly dilated subsegmental bronchi that are saccular, often as blind sacs surrounded by peribronchial consolidation (Fig. 66–4). The parenchyma is often airless, fibrosed, and sometimes showing pneumonitis and small abscesses. Lobar and peribronchial lymphadenopathy is extensive.

Microscopic

The involved bronchial walls show extensive destruction of musculature and cartilage with severe mucosal ulceration. Normal respiratory epithelium is replaced

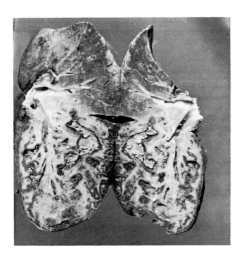

Fig. 66–4. Gross specimen of lung, removed because of bronchiectasis, showing extensive peribronchial infection and fibrosis.

with squamous metaplasia. There is peribronchial infiltration with inflammatory cells. Peribronchial microabscesses are common. Bronchial arteries are enlarged. The parenchyma shows a combination of fibrosis, acute and chronic pneumonitis, and occasionally abscess formation.

All of these changes vary in extent and severity. Like many other pulmonary diseases, bronchiectasis is segmental. Any number of segments bilaterally or unilaterally may be involved, but the disease primarily involves the basilar segments of the lower lobes, the middle lobe, and lingular segment of the left upper lobe. The right upper lobe, the remaining left upper lobe, and lower lobe superior segments are almost never involved. This anatomical fact is the basis of surgical resection as one form of therapy.

Clinical Findings

The child who shows retarded musculoskeletal development and inanition and occasionally cyanosis and who has a chronic cough producing large volumes of foul-smelling sputum poses no diagnostic problem. In the United States, however, a child or young adult who has an intermittently productive chronic cough and recurring pulmonary infections is more typical. In both groups, paranasal sinusitis is a constant or recurring problem. Hemoptysis is common and is usually minor, but with the severe form, exsanguinating hemoptysis can occur.

Physical Findings

These vary with severity but may include emaciation, pulmonary osteoarthropathy with marked clubbing and cyanosis, and dyspnea. Rales, wheezing, and ronchi may be audible over involved areas of the lung corresponding to the segmental distribution as described. In less advanced cases, fine rales over the involved segments may be the only finding.

Roentgenographic Findings

These may vary from normal roentgenograms of the chest in mild cases to atelectasis of involved areas in more

severe cases. Peribronchial infiltration produces visible bronchial shadows that adopt a curvilinear pattern characteristic of saccular disease (Fig. 66–5). The saccular lesions may also be visible. Pleural reaction and displaced fissures are common in advanced disease. Computed tomography can clearly show the dilated bronchi (Fig. 66–6), peribronchial infiltration, and parenchymal disease. These findings are diagnostic, making bronchography unnecessary unless it is needed for more accurate preoperative mapping (Fig. 66–7).

Bronchograms, if required, should be delayed until the patient's clinical condition is optimized by postural drainage and antibiotics. Attempting bronchography when copious volumes of sputum are being produced only results in nonfilling of multiple areas and necessitates a second procedure. I am fairly convinced that the procedure should be performed under a carefully administered topical anesthesia like that used for rigid bronchoscopy and that an intratracheal catheter, introduced through the nose, should be used. The radiologist-performed bronchogram is commonly frustrating because of the poor quality of films based on coughing and poor anesthesia. These films may be diagnostic but are largely useless for surgical mapping.

Oily Dionosil is used for bronchography. The quantity used for a bilateral study should not exceed 20 cc. Bronchography should not be done for at least 2 weeks following a clinical respiratory infection, and a surgical procedure should not be performed for at least 2 weeks after a bronchogram, which occasionally produces a pneumonitis. Although the contrast material disappears promptly, the oil base is only cleared over several weeks.

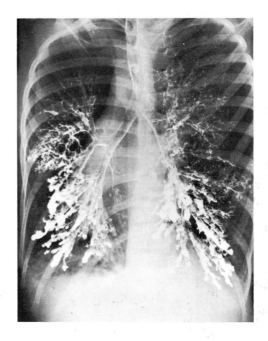

Fig. 66–5. A bilateral saccular bronchiectasis, characteristic of the preantibiotic era, involving the lower lobes, the lingula, and the right middle lobe. (Ferguson, T.B., and Burford, T.H.: The changing pattern of pulmonary suppuration: surgical implications. Dis. Chest 53:396, 1968.)

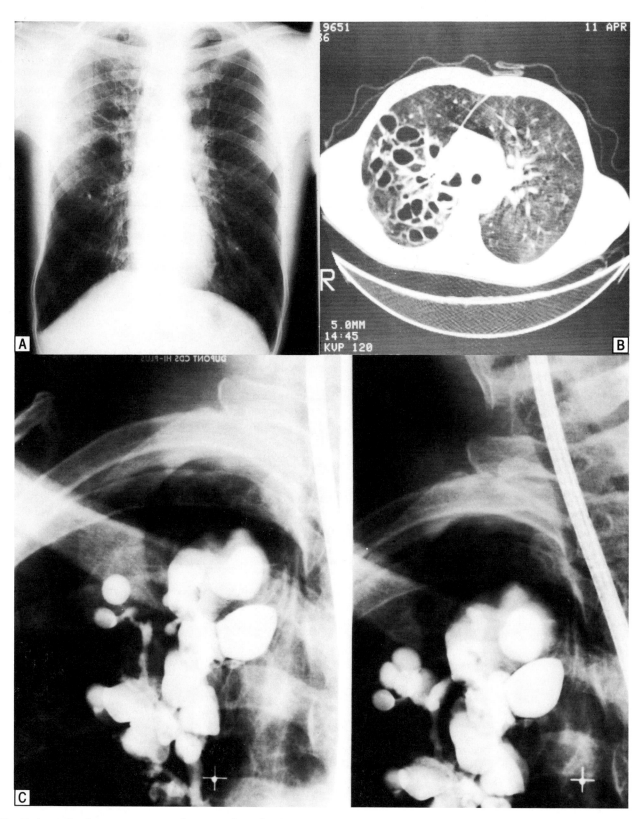

Fig. 66–6. *A,* PA chest roentgenogram of a patient admitted with a life-long history of pulmonary infection and hemoptysis demonstrating extensive cystic disease of the right lung. *B,* A CT film clearly illustrating the cystic nature of the bronchiectasis. *C,* A bronchogram confirms the diagnosis but adds no new information to that obtained from the CT examination.

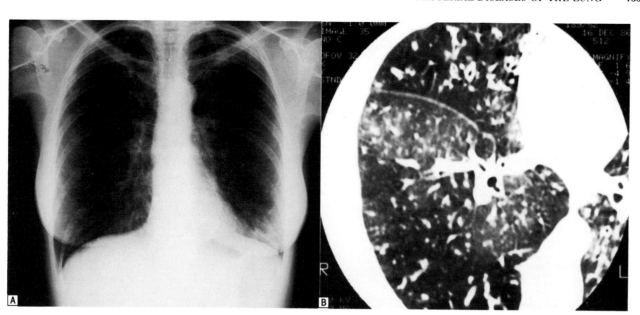

Fig. 66–7. *A,* A PA chest film made in a patient with frequent episodes of cough and minimal expectoration, suggesting the possibility of bronchiectasis. *B,* A CT examination shows dilated bronchi and peribronchial infiltration. Bronchography was not thought necessary for diagnosis or therapy.

Medical Management

For most patients seen today in the developed world, medical management is adequate (Fig. 66–8). Judicious use of systemic antibiotics based on current culture, mucolytic agents, nonirritant expectorants, postural drainage, humidification, and bronchial dilators are used. Some of these are best used by aerosol application. The patient should avoid the harsh winters of the northern and northeastern United States, if possible. An annual influenza vaccination is worthwhile.

The continuous use of antibiotics should be condemned because it results only in colonization of the patient with resistant organisms. Antibiotic use should be based on current culture and used in therapeutic amounts for brief periods.

Selection of Patients for Surgical Treatment

Surgical treatment is based on three premises: (1) the disease is segmental and nonchanging; (2) complete resection of all diseased areas based on good bronchograms is necessary if a good clinical result is to be obtained; and (3) complete resection of all disease prevents recurrence—this does not apply to those patients with immunologic or genetic abnormalities.

No patient should be considered for surgical treatment until a lengthy course of medical management, preferably under the direction of a pulmonary internist, has failed to relieve symptoms and prevent major illness. When structural damage to the lung is advanced, however, the disease is not reversible. In an underdeveloped area, where the disease is more likely to be advanced and medical facilities less than ideal, surgical management may be resorted to earlier and more often.

A high quality bronchogram supplemented by computed tomography, if available, is necessary to evaluate a patient for surgery. Breatnach (1985) and Moatoosamy (1985) and their associates demonstrated that computed tomography may be adequate for preoperative mapping without bronchography. Selection should include those patients who continue to have a cough productive of quantities of purulent sputum, those who have recurring major episodes of pneumonitis, and those with recurrent major hemoptysis.

Surgical patients must have localized disease that can be totally removed without removing an excess of functioning lung so that chronic respiratory insufficiency will not result. Ideally, the disease should be confined to one lobe, but bilateral, localized disease can also be resected successfully. Bronchoscopy should be performed by the surgeon primarily to discover anatomic abnormalities, bronchial stricture, and foreign bodies.

Before a final decision is reached and a recommendation for operation is made, the surgeon should determine with the patient the extent of symptoms and disability and whether these are sufficient to warrant one and occasionally two major operations. The surgeon should resist operating on a patient with minimal disability or performing an incomplete operation that resects "the worst" of the disease in the hope that the patient's condition will improve. A resection that intentionally does not remove all disease is meddlesome.

Pulmonary function studies are not often useful in selecting patients for operation. Serious preoperative pulmonary function disability usually places the patient outside surgical consideration.

In planning surgical resection, unless the disease is confined to a single lobe, segmental resection of one or a combination of segments may be planned. A common combination involves the lower lobe basilar segments

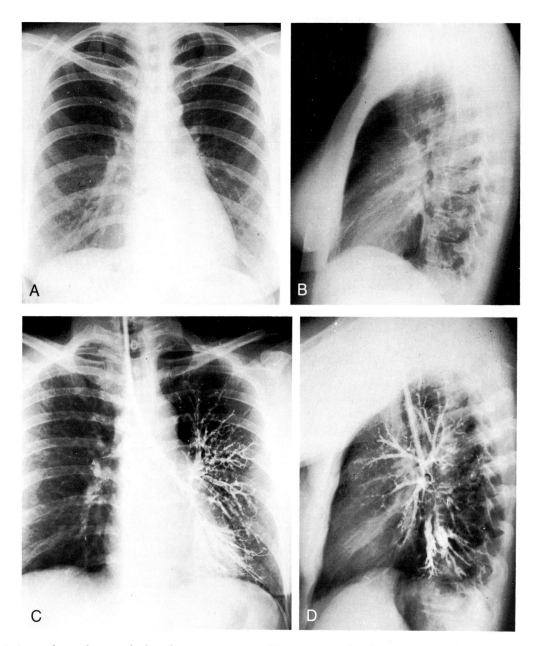

Fig. 66–8. *A,* A typical case of present-day bronchiectasis in a 43-year old woman who suffered recurrent lower respiratory tract infections every winter. The sputum became purulent with these episodes. *B,* The lesion in the retrocardiac portion of the left lower lobe is apparent on the lateral view only. *C* and *D,* The patient became symptom-free after a left lower lobectomy. (Ferguson, T.B., and Burford, T.H.: The changing pattern of pulmonary suppuration: surgical implications. Dis. Chest 53:396, 1968.)

and the middle lobe or lingular segment. Bilateral procedures might involve bilateral basilar segmentectomy and occasionally lingulectomy. The surgeon should leave the equivalent of at least two lobes intact, and the middle lobe should not be one of these.

Preoperative preparation involves maximizing the patient's medical condition, particularly by postural drainage several times daily. Cigarette smoking should be stopped at least 2 weeks preoperatively.

Results of Surgical Treatment

The surgery of bronchiectasis is in many ways a microcosm of the history of pulmonary surgery. Most of the techniques used today are products of the efforts of the surgeon to treat this disease. Brunn (1929), Churchill (1937, 1939), and Nissen (1931) were the earliest pioneers. Haight (1934), Blades and Kent (1940), and Lindskog and Hubbell (1955) made rapid progress in pulmonary resection for bronchiectasis.

Overholt and Langer (1947), in particular, developed segmental pulmonary resection for bronchiectasis to a fine art. Kergin (1950) and Borrie (1965), Sealy (1966), Ochsner (1949), Lindskog (1955) and Meade (1947) and their associates described the results obtained while bronchiectasis was still a common surgical disease. The results of pulmonary resection for bronchiectasis were excellent and the mortality less than 1%. The rejection of surgical therapy for bronchiectasis was not based on failure but on the striking change in the incidence of and the internist's improved ability to manage this entity.

Current reports of surgical treatment are few. Annest and associates (1982), Wilson and Decker (1982), Lewiston (1984), Vejlsted and associates (1982), and Sanderson and associates (1974) demonstrated that in properly selected patients, the results are good. The report of Wilson and Decker (1982) is representative. Of 96 patients who were operated upon, 75% were well or improved greatly, 21% improved, and 4% were unchanged. None died.

Certainly, surgical resection of localized bronchiectasis remains a valid and valuable option in managing this disease. Chronic disability in the patient for whom medical management fails is not a necessary result if the disease is resectable.

LUNG ABSCESS

Aspiration or putrid lung abscess, like saccular bronchiectasis untreated by antibiotics, is uncommon today. The classic abscess before the antibiotic era was a complication of oral surgical procedures such as dental surgery or tonsillectomy and was produced by aspirated material contaminated with the normal oral flora. Aspiration of food or vomitus because of illness or acute alcoholism caused many cases. An area of necrotizing pneumonia rapidly developed that usually drained into a bronchus and occasionally into the pleural space (Fig. 66–9). Before penicillin therapy, the mortality rate was over 30%. About 30 to 35% survived but with bronchiectasis or a pleurocutaneous fistula or both. The remaining third recovered and remained well.

This variety of lung abscess still occurs, but except in patients who do not seek medical care or who reside in developing nations, the course is modified by antibiotic therapy so rapidly that the cavity rarely develops, or if it does, resolution is prompt.

The incidence of lung abscess, at least in a major metropolitan area, increased markedly in the 1980s. The bacterial etiology has become varied, and organisms are producing lung abscesses that in the past were unknown as etiologic agents (Fig. 66–10, Table 66–3). The clinical course of some of the nosocomial infections is so rapid

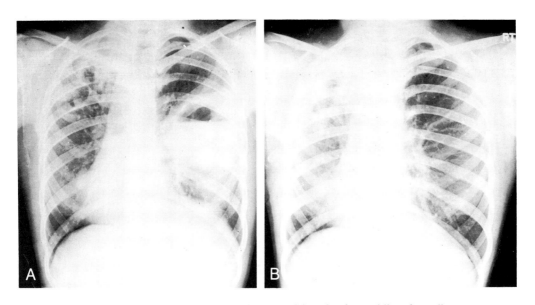

Fig. 66–9. *A,* Lung abscess of the preantibiotic era involving the left upper lobe. The abscess followed tonsillectomy. *B,* Same patient 3 weeks later showing spread to the right lung. (Ferguson, T.B., and Burford, T.H.: The changing pattern of pulmonary suppuration: surgical implications. Dis. Chest 53:396, 1968.)

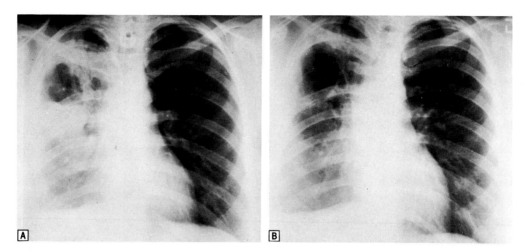

Fig. 66–10. Lung abscess in a patient with sclerosing mediastinitis *A*. The causative organism. *Herellea vaginicola,* is a pleomorphic gram-negative organism not ordinarily pathogenic for man. The diagnosis was made by transcutaneous aspiration of pus from the abscess cavity. On gentamicin therapy the patient made a complete clinical recovery with disappearance of the abscess in the right upper lung field (*B*).

and devastating that decisions about antibotic therapy and surgical measures must be made and acted upon quickly if a life is to be saved.

Aspiration Lung Abscess

This is the entity with which most physicians are familiar. The victim is usually an alcoholic, an elderly homeless person, or a malnourisshed individual, usually with a history of an episode of diminished consciousness or vomiting and aspiration.

Bacteriology

The organisms are derived from the mixed mouth flora, which includes staphylococci, nonhemolytic microaerophilic streptococci, fusiform bacilli, peptococcus, *Bacteroides melaninogenicus,* and *Bacteroides fragilis.* Many of these organisms are facultatively anaerobic. Some, but not all, are penicillin-sensitive. Eradicating the penicillin-sensitive organisms, however, terminates the infectious process in most patients. Edentulous patients rarely if ever develop a putrid abscess because they lack periodontal flora.

Pathology

Initially, contaminated material lodges in the distal bronchial system, where a rapidly spreading necrotizing pneumonitis develops. Within 24 to 48 hours, an extensive area of necrosis results in a multiloculated or uniloculated space that is filled with exudate, blood, and necrotic lung tissue. The abscess usually establishes communication with a bronchus and partially empties. The abscess contents have the characteristic odor of an anaerobic infection of the oral flora. The cavity is surrounded by a layer of pneumonitis of variable thickness with continuing necrosis. Unless the body's defenses modify the process, the necrosis may extend directly across fissures into an adjacent lobe or extend to the pleura and rupture into the pleural space. The infection may extend into the pleural space and produce an empyema without mechanical rupture of the abscess cavity. The infectious process extends by way of the lymphatics to hilar and mediastinal lymph nodes, which show marked hyperplasia and can necrose and become suppurative. Involvement of pulmonary veins causes he-

Table 66–3. Bacterial Classification of Lung Abscess

Primary (aspiration, putrid, anaerobic)
  Staphylococcus, fusiform bacilli, α nonhemolytic streptococcus/
  peptococci, *Bacteroides fragilis*
Specific infections
  Staphylococcus aureus, dermatitides
  Streptococcus—β hemolytic streptococcus
  Hemophilus influenzae
  Klebsiella
  Pseudomonas aeruginosa ⎫
  Proteus   ⎪
  Aerobacter   ⎬ usually nosocomial or in
  Escherichia coli   ⎪ immunosuppressed patients
  Candida albicans   ⎪
  Legionella pneumophila   ⎭

This list is not complete as numerous bacteria other than these may produce lung abscess, but this group is responsible for over 90% of the diseases seen.

matogenous extension of the process to the brain and other areas.

Clinical Picture

Several contributing factors promote the development of lung abscess (Table 66–4). One or more of these is almost invariably present, and their occurrence, associated with an acute fever, should arouse suspicion. The early clinical course is indistinguishable from that of any other acute pneumonic process and includes fever, cough, dyspnea, and often pleuritic chest pain. The cough is nonproductive early but as necrosis progresses and when a bronchial communication becomes established the foul-smelling contents of the abscess cavity are produced suddenly, usually with some degree of hemoptysis. The cough remains productive. The foul odor abates almost immediately with penicillin therapy. The fever and other symptoms usually improve somewhat with the initial bronchial drainage.

Occasionally the abscess ruptures into the pleural space, producing a pyopneumothorax that is often a tension pneumothorax. This event is catastrophic and the patient rapidly develops septic shock superimposed on acute respiratory distress and cyanosis. If untreated, the clinical course of this complication can be rapid, with increasing sepsis and death often within 24 hours.

Hemoptysis, although common, is usually minimal, but may become massive and life-threatening. Hemoptysis can usually be treated expectantly, but occasionally

Table 66–4. Contributing Factors to Origin of Lung Abscess

Dental caries and periodontal disease

Decreased state of consciousness
  Anesthesia
  Alcohol abuse
  Coma
  Convulsive disorders
  Drug abuse

Immunosuppression
  Steroid therapy
  Transplant
  Drug addiction
  Chemotherapy for malignancy
  Malnutrition
  Multiple trauma
  Debilitation
  Autoimmune syndrome

Neuromuscular and esophageal disease
  Esophageal obstruction
  Esophageal motility disorders, particularly achalasia
  Gastroesophageal reflux
  Inability to cough
  Absent cough and gag reflex

Bronchial obstruction
  Stricture
  Foreign body
  Neoplasm
  Bronchial compression

Generalized septicemia

necessitates bronchoscopic tamponade and urgent resection. Aggressive penicillin therapy is the best means of stopping the necrosis that results in hemorrhage.

Clinical complications of aspiration abscess include metastatic intracranial abscess, generalized septicemia, bronchogenic spread of infection to uninvolved areas of the lung, and, with rupture into the pleural space, empyema necessitans that may result in extensive spread of the anaerobic necrosing infection and air over the chest wall and even to remote areas. This in earlier times was referred to as "phlegmon" of the chest wall.

The clinical course is radically modified by antibiotic therapy, and the course described above is rarely seen and occurs in patients who present very late or have no access to medical care. The usual course is limited to the initial symptoms of fever, cough, and chest pain, which disappear within 3 to 5 days with no sequelae.

Roentgenographic Findings

The early finding is a localized but fairly extensive area of consolidation in a dependent segment. The most common sites are the lateral part of the posterior segment—axillary subsegment—of the right upper lobe (Fig. 66–11) and the superior segment of the right lower lobe. Uncommonly the middle lobe may be involved if the patient was prone at the time of aspiration. The apical-posterior segment of the left upper lobe and the superior segment of the left lower and lingular segments are less common sites of abscess (Fig. 66–12). The usual reason given for the right-sided predominance is the difference in the angle of the origin of the right main bronchus from the trachea.

As soon as a bronchial communication is established, an air-fluid level appears in the consolidated area. The wall is thick early but diminishes as the pneumonitis subsides because of both the patient's own defenses and the influence of antibiotic therapy.

The abscess in the untreated patient or the immunocompromised patient may enlarge rapidly. Pleural reaction becomes apparent if the process is near the surface of the lung or an interlobar fissure. Rapid growth predicts rupture into the pleural space if the process remains unchecked.

The CT examination is valuable in demonstrating cavitation within an area of consolidation, for evaluating the thickness and character of the abscess wall, and in determining the exact position of the process with regard to chest wall and interlobar fissures. The CT examination can also demonstrate bronchial occlusive disease proximal to the abscess. Standard roentgenograms sometimes do not help in distinguishing an empyema from an intrapulmonary or even interlobar fluid collection. Computed tomography is therefore vital to the study of lung abscess.

Differential Diagnosis

Several cavitary pulmonary diseases must be considered, including tuberculosis and mycoses. These produce cavitary lesions, but the clinical course of acute illness plus the air-fluid level in the cavity should make

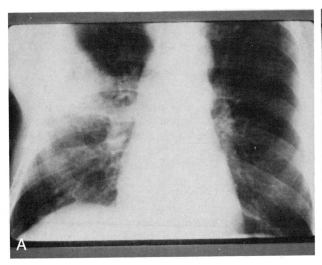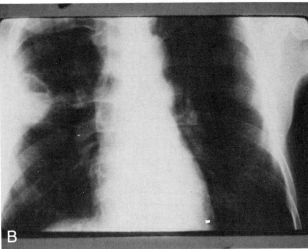

Fig. 66–11. *A,* A PA chest roentgenogram made the day of admission. The patient was a middle-aged male alcoholic. The abscess cavity with a large surrounding area of pneumonitis is seen in the lateral area of the posterior segment of the upper lobe, a typical position. *B,* A film made after six weeks of antibiotic therapy and general nutritional support demonstrating improvement but incomplete resolution. Lobectomy was performed.

the diagnosis apparent. Air-fluid levels are rare in these entities (Table 66–5).

Bacteriologic and serologic studies are also useful. Pulmonary cystic lesions such as intrapulmonary broncho- genic cysts and secondarily infected bullae can be con- fusing. The prior existence of these lesions as documented by old roentgenograms and the segmental location are not typical of lung abscess.

Squamous cell bronchial carcinoma produces cavitary lesions that are sometimes difficult to differentiate. The wall of the carcinomatous abscess is usually thicker and more irregular than that of the primary abscess. The absence of a clinical course of acute infection, the con- tinually enlarging cavity, and the failure to respond to antibiotic therapy help distinguish carcinoma (Fig. 66–14). Bronchoscopy and biopsy are diagnostic, al- though in far peripheral lesions thoracotomy may be re- quired to obtain a diagnosis.

Because an abscess distal to bronchial obstruction usu- ally occurs in an area of lobar pneumonitis and atelectasis but otherwise appears as a primary abscess, early bron- choscopy is indicated in all cases.

A localized empyema with bronchopleural fistula or a mediastinal bronchial or other mediastinal cyst with ero- sion into the lung, sometimes cannot be distinguished from lung abscess; this may have to be resolved at op- eration (Figs. 66–15, 66–16). Contrast material in com- puted tomography of the lung has been helpful.

Treatment

All available specimens for bacterial culture should be obtained and all pertinent roentgenographic studies completed before antibiotic therapy is begun.

Penicillin therapy requires from 3 to 20 million units in divided doses over 24 hours, with the higher levels used for patients who are more acutely ill.

Clindamycin has been recommended as the drug of choice; Lewison and associates (1983) reported a some- what faster clinical response, but Bartlett and Gorbach (1983) indicated that there is little difference and that if cost is to be considered then penicillin remains the drug of choice. Therapy must be continued from 4 to 12 weeks, depending on the clinical and roentgenographic re- sponse. Generally, the response is rapid and complete healing is effected in 10 to 16 weeks. The antibiotic ther- apy can be changed to oral therapy after the initial re- sponse, and Weiss and Cherniak's (1974) report suggests that the clinical response is as good with oral therapy as with parenteral therapy. Poor compliance with oral treat- ment out of the hospital makes this type of therapy im- practical for many patients of lower socio-economic lev- els.

Bronchoscopy with the goal of establishing and im- proving bronchial drainage should be an integral part of the management of lung abscess. If the abscess has not drained bronchially, the rigid bronchoscope is preferable to prevent dissemination of the abscess contents because of the small suction port of the fiber-optic bronchoscope. Bronchoscopy should be performed weekly until the acute clinical picture has subsided.

General supportive measures such as nutritional im- provement, cessation of drug and alcohol abuse, postural drainage, transfusion, and correction of serious dental disease are all adjuncts to medical therapy.

Indications for Surgical Treatment

There are few indications for surgical treatment of the putrid lung abscess, because most respond quickly to antibiotic therapy. The increased number of immuno- compromised patients, however, has increased the num- ber of patients requiring some operative procedure. Oc- casionally, a patient is admitted in a late stage of the disease with a gigantic abscess and in such poor general condition that a major surgical procedure is not possible.

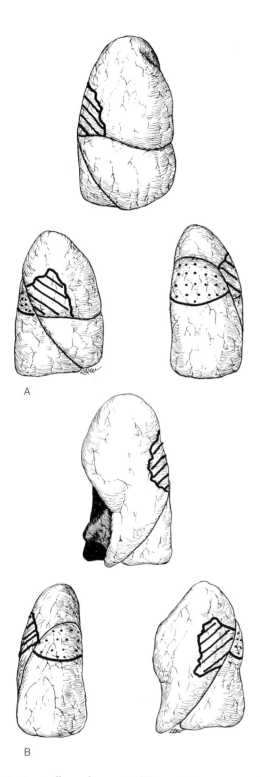

Fig. 66–12. Axillary subsegment of the posterior segment at the upper lobe and superior segment of the lower lobe. *A*, Right lung. *B*, left lung.

Table 66–5. Differential Diagnosis of Cavitary Lesions Other Than Bacterial Lung Abscess

Infectious
  Tuberculosis
  Mycosis
    Coccidiomycosis
    Histoplasmosis
  Infected pulmonary infarction

Parasitic
  Amoebic abscess
  Echinococcous cyst

Cavitary carcinoma

Cystic pulmonary disease
  Infected emphasematous bullus
  Infected bronchogenic cyst
  Pulmonary sequestration

Granulomatous disease
  Wegener's granuloma

The giant abscess—>6 cm—is unlikely to close under medical therapy and should be considered early for resection if the patient's condition permits. Some of these patients require catheter drainage using Monaldi's technique and occasionally rib resection with open drainage of the abscess (Fig. 66–17). Percutaneous catheter drainage under roentgenographic control has been increasingly recommended. The reports of Keller (1982) and Yellin (1985) and their associates are representative. Except in the extremely ill patient, a more adequate drainage of the cavity is indicated if drainage is indicated at all.

Lobectomy is the treatment of choice for the patient who does not respond adequately to medical management as reflected by a persistent or enlarging cavity and continued evidence of sepsis. Weekly chest roentgenograms should show progressive diminution of the abscess and disappearance of the surrounding pneumonitis. An

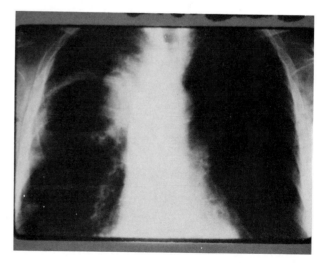

Fig. 66–13. A PA film in a 46-year old-male who presented 1 week earlier with a low grade fever and cough with minimal hemoptysis. This lesion proved to be a cavitary squamous cell carcinoma. A solid mass was never present.

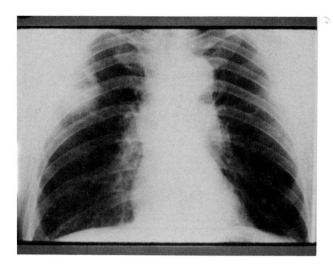

Fig. 66–14. *A,* PA chest roentgenogram in a 50-year-old alcoholic who presented in a state of malnutrition with cough and fever. Transbronchial biopsy revealed squamous cell carcinoma.

abscess that shows no change in 2 consecutive weeks should become a subject for surgical consideration if there is no further improvement.

Resection is also the procedure of choice for the patient with massive hemoptysis usually following intrabronchial tamponade. Once a massive hemorrhage has occurred, rebleed is highly likely and the initial mortality rate is higher than most physicians expect (Fig. 66–18). Gourin and Garzon (1974) found the mortality rate with early lobectomy was only 18%, compared with a 54% risk in patients with hemoptysis from all causes treated medically. Therefore, an early surgical decision should be

forthcoming when massive bleeding occurs—500 to 600 cc in 12 hours.

The catastrophic complication of rupture into the pleural space should be treated emergently by rib resection and drainage, and early resection should be considered if the patient's condition permits. Simple chest tube insertion is inadequate in this situation, and may only disseminate the anaerobic infection into the chest wall. Suction must be minimal or only water-seal drainage used because a large bronchopleural fistula is usually present.

Lobectomy for lung abscess can be technically difficult because of the vascular adhesions and marked hilar adenopathy. Blood loss is usually more than would be encountered in resection for other diseases.

Resection may be required when the diagnosis of carcinoma cannot be excluded and occasionally when no diagnosis is forthcoming and the cavitary disease is worsening. This situation is becoming less frequent, based on the information gained by computed tomography and by persistent efforts with the fiber-optic bronchoscope.

The results of surgical treatment are difficult to assess because the results depend heavily upon the characteristics of the patient population. The enormous increase in drug abuse, alcoholism, and AIDS, and the appearance of gram-negative bacteria as primary agents have increased the incidence of lung abscess and the associated mortality rate both for surgical and medically managed patients. Before 1980, mortality rates averaged between 5 and 10%. Hagan and Hardy (1983) found that the mortality rate in Jackson, Mississippi at that time was 28%, compared with 22% in the 1960s. Pohlsan and associates (1985) reviewed a series of 89 patients and found, in contrast to data from the preceding decade, that 23 required surgery and that 29% died apparently

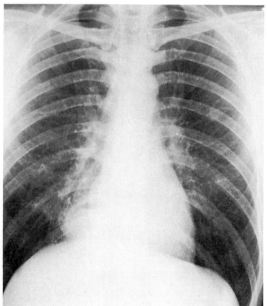
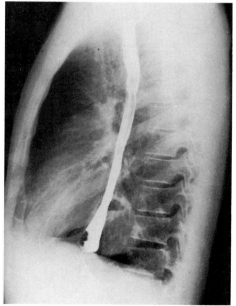

Fig. 66–15. Intralobar pulmonary sequestration. The patient had a long history suggestive of lung abscess. A large anomalous systemic artery arose from the abdominal aorta and penetrated the diaphragm to enter the right lower lobe. (Ferguson, T.B., and Burford, T.H.: The changing pattern of pulmonary suppuration: surgical implications. Dis. Chest 53:396, 1968.)

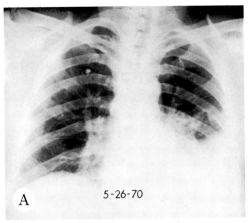

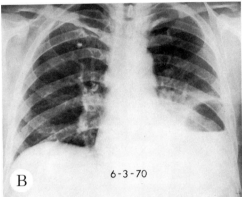

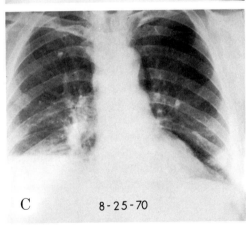

Fig. 66–16. Septic pulmonary embolus in the left lower lobe. Between the times roentgenograms A and B were taken, there was rapid destruction of lung tissue with large abscess formation and pyopneumothorax. Soon after the second roentgenogram, B, was obtained, closed chest drainage was instituted with subsequent complete recovery, as demonstrated in C.

from other causes but only 9% from the lung abscess. In a review of 41 deaths among 440 patients with lung abscess seen over a 10-year period at the Johns Hopkins hospital, alcoholism, seizure activity, and advanced age were important factors. Large abscesses were more likely to be fatal, and sudden rupture into the bronchus with aspiration of the abscess contents was a primary cause of death in several patients.

Lung Abscess—A Changing Disease

The change in bacterial etiology to such organisms as Staphylococcus. *Klebsiella pneumoniae, Escherichia coli,* proteus, enterobacter, and pseudomonas associated with the enormous increase in the population of immunosuppressed individuals has brought about an entirely new concept of lung abscess and its management. Several of these entities will be discussed separately.

Staphylococcal Lung Abscess in the Adult

In my experience, this is almost exclusively a complication of intravenous drug abuse. These patients present multiple injection-related infections that include local abscesses, suppurative thrombophlebitis, mycolic aneurysm of brachial and femoral arteries, pulmonary emboli, multiple lung abscesses (Fig. 66–19), empyema, and valvular endocarditis. It is frequently associated with AIDS and always with malnutrition and general debility (Fig. 66–20). Patients usually have a positive blood culture for staphylococci on admission. These patients have a high morbidity and mortality rate.

Gram-Negative Infections

Hospital-acquired gram-negative infections are usually pseudomonas, enterobacter, or proteus. The patients are often old, debilitated, surgical patients with major complications, or multiple trauma victims. As a rule, they are intensive care patients (Fig. 66–21). They have a beginning point of infection, such as aspiration, wound infection, or urosepsis. The infections are often fulminating, with life expectancy being only a few days. The organisms are resistant or have only a minimal sensitivity. Lung abscesses suddenly appear as an area of pneumonitis that rapidly excavates and enlarges (Fig. 66–22). Pleural involvement is almost 100%.

These patients often require abscess drainage and pleural drainage as an emergency. Unfortunately, the infection is systemic and often uncontrollable, and the pulmonary process represents only an incident in a fatal sequence.

Opportunistic Organisms

Candida albicans has become a major problem since 1985. In Pohlsan and associates' (1985) report, about one fourth of lung abscesses contained candida on culture. These have been particularly troublesome in cardiac surgical patients who develop sternal infections or who remain respirator-dependent for more than 5 to 6 days. A new entity in medicine is the occurrence of lung abscess from *Candida albicans* in an otherwise healthy patient. Schoenfell and associates (1983) reported such a patient.

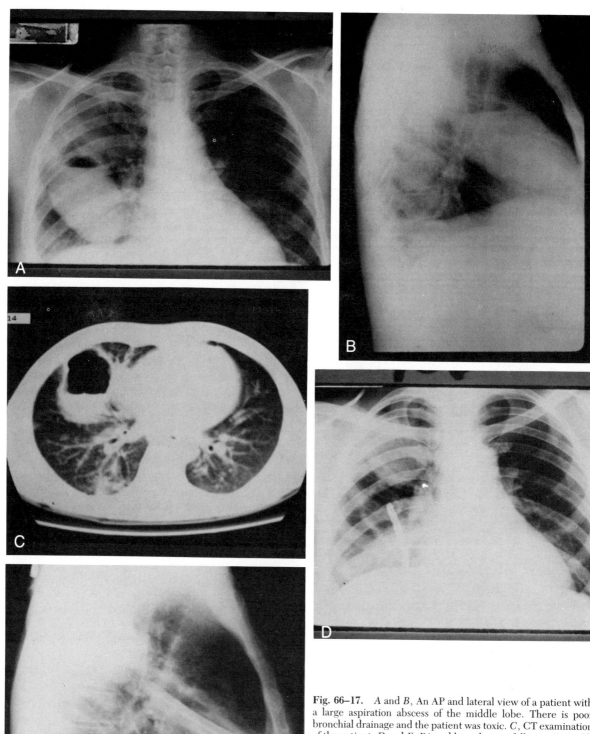

Fig. 66–17. *A* and *B*, An AP and lateral view of a patient with a large aspiration abscess of the middle lobe. There is poor bronchial drainage and the patient was toxic. *C*, CT examination of the patient. *D* and *E*, PA and lateral views following Monoldi drainage. The patient recovered. This patient was unresponsive to antibiotic therapy and shows the occasional need for surgical drainage. This patient was admitted in 1984.

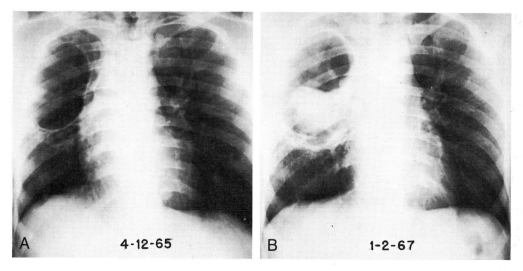

Fig. 66–18. *A*, This 24-year-old black man was asymptomatic in 1965. He returned in 1967 with massive pulmonary hemorrhage; an emergency pneumonectomy was necessary to save his life. *B*, A film taken just before the operation. The cavity is partially filled with fresh blood clot. Patient subsequently developed the typical renal lesions of Goodpasture's syndrome. (Ferguson, T.B., and Burford, T.H.: The changing pattern of pulmonary suppuration: surgical implications. Dis. Chest 53:396, 1968.)

Candida infections will probably continue to increase in incidence and severity (Fig. 66–23). Amphotericin B and surgical drainage remain the only avenues of treatment and at best have only limited success. A common denominator in the patients with gram-negative or candida infections has been progressive weight loss, often associated with anergy. These patients may be helped by parenteral or enteral hyperalimentation. Caloric intake may exceed 4000 calories before the negative nitrogen balance is reversed. Occasionally, anergy can also be reversed.

Legionella micdadei and *Legionella pneumophila* have been implicated in multiple lung abscess and have a high fatality rate.

Lung Abscess in Children

The incidence of lung abscess in children decreased markedly in the early antibiotic years. According to Ravitch and Fein (1961) *Staphylococcus aureus* replaced *Hemophilus influenzae* as the primary etiologic agent. Since then, occasional infections with *Hemophilus influenzae*, *Klebsiella pneumoniae*, and other organisms have reappeared. The typical aspiration abscess is always possible.

The differential diagnosis of suppurative pulmonary disease in children is more important and must include foreign body aspiration, chronic aspiration, cystic fibrosis, sequestration, various immune disorders, and bronchial compressive disease. Appropriate diagnostic procedures including bronchoscopy must be carried out.

Staphylococcal pneumonia and abscess is still the most common variety seen. Virtually unknown until the appearance of penicillin-resistant *Staphylococcus aureus* in the early 1960s, this entity developed into cyclic small epidemics. In one winter a large number of cases with a mortality rate between 10 to 15% would arise, then 3 to 4 years would elapse with only sporadic cases. This pattern ceased with the introduction of antibiotics effective against penicillin-resistant organisms.

Clinical Picture

Children, usually under age 2, present with acute symptoms of fever, prostration, and cough. The initial chest roentgenograms show usually bilateral multiple areas of pneumonic consolidation. Occasionally, the process is unilateral. Rapidly, thin-walled cavities, usually with an air-fluid level, appear and enlarge. These lesions are called pneumatoceles (Fig. 66–24) because of their thin walls and rapid growth. Pleural fluid is often visible within the first 24 hours and also rapidly accumulates. These abscesses tend to rupture into the pleural space and produce a tension pyopneumothorax that is life-threatening, particularly when the diagnosis is not anticipated and is made when respiratory distress suddenly appears. Chest tube insertion in these patients can be life-saving. Empyema often complicates the illness even without abscess rupture and usually requires drainage and debridement apart from the management of the abscess. Even with control of the infection, these cavities tend to persist but eventually close. They are probably not true abscess cavities. It is not usually necessary to resort to any surgical treatment if rupture or empyema does not occur.

Those patients with abscesses caused by *Hemophilus influenzae* are more likely to require drainage or resection. Lorenzo and associates (1985) described aspiration of the abscess percutaneously with a fluoroscopy-guided needle. Lacy and Koloske (1983) recommended open drainage of a large abscess cavity and Nonoyama and associates (1984) from Japan performed lobectomy in nine patients and drainage in one, all with satisfactory results. Organisms were staphylococcus, *Hemophilus influenzae*, and alpha hemolytic streptococcus. Four of ten

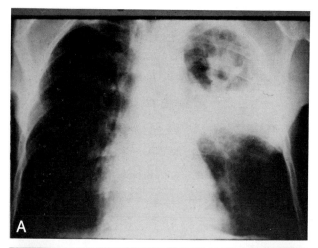

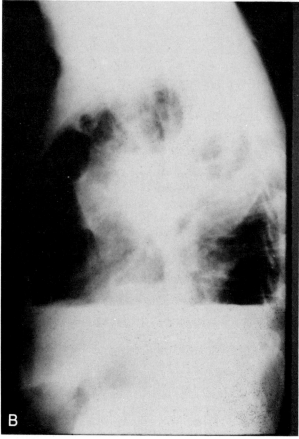

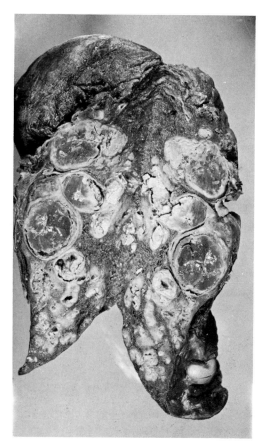

Fig. 66–20. Gross specimen of a lung showing multiple abscess cavities associated with hematogenous dissemination.

Fig. 66–19. *A* and *B*, PA and lateral views of an adult drug abuser made on the day of admission, demonstrating a large upper lobe abscess with a pyopneumothorax secondary to rupture. Emergency drainage was performed and subsequently a left upper lobectomy was performed. The organism was *Staphylococcus aureus* and was resistant to multiple antibiotics.

patients had negative cultures. Several required decortication.

I am reluctant to recommend needle aspiration of abscess cavities. If the pleura is not adherent, tension pyopneumothorax, which may be difficult to cope with in a roentgenographic suite, may result. Empyema that would not otherwise have occurred can also happen. Finally, I doubt that an abscess with a bronchial communication needs aspiration or that a one-time aspiration would be adequate drainage.

ORGANIZING PNEUMONITIS

Since the beginning of the antibiotic era, a well defined group of patients with pneumonitis has not followed a predictable course. Most patients show complete resolution under appropriate antibiotic therapy. Without therapy or with inappropriate therapy the process usually resolves completely, resolves with bronchiectasis as a sequela, or develops necrosis and abscess formation. Patients with organizing pneumonia, however, follow a separate course that produces confusion in diagnosis and management.

Clinical Course

Although the course varies considerably, it usually consists of an acute episode of cough, fever, chest pain,

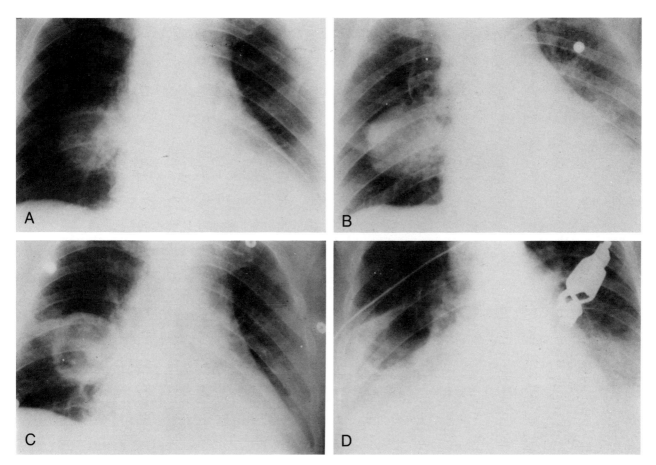

Fig. 66–21. *A*, Portable chest roentgenogram of an elderly general surgical patient 4 days after operation. Urosepsis was first noted, then cough and fever developed. This film postoperative 5 shows a large lower lobe abscess that as yet had no bronchial communication. Blood culture was positive for *Pseudomonas*. *B*, Twenty-four hours later the abscess had almost doubled in size. The patient was extremely ill. *C*, Forty-eight hours later the abscess had drained into the bronchus. Blood culture was still positive. *D*, Seventy-two hours later the abscess had ruptured into the pleural space. Patient now had septic shock. Pleural drainage was accomplished, but the patient died the same day.

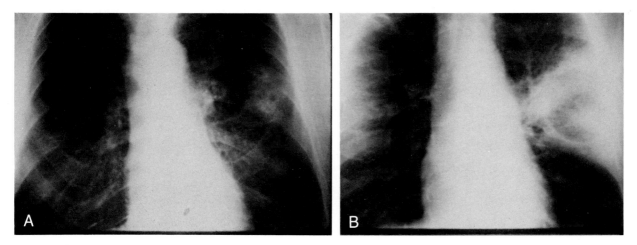

Fig. 66–22. *A*, PA chest roentgenogram in a postcolectomy patient who had developed fever and cough. This film demonstrates an area of pneumonitis with several small cavitary areas. *B*, Twenty-four hours later there is a giant lung abscess in the left upper lobe. Death occurred the same day after several hours of septic shock. Culture recovered *Pseudomonas*.

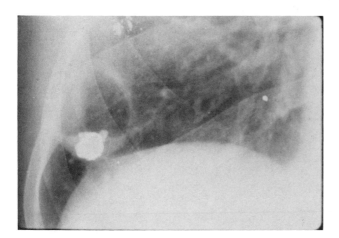

Fig. 66–23. A close-up photograph of the lower lobe area in a Vietnam War veteran who had been shot 17 years earlier. The bullet had been left in the lung. The patient presented with hemoptysis, cough, and fever. The film shows the foreign body lying in the center of an abscess cavity.

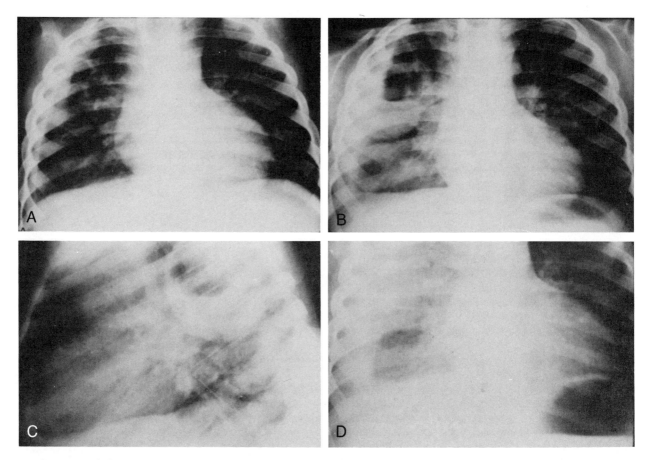

Fig. 66–24. *A*, Staphylococcal lung abscess in a 9-month-old child. Film on day of admission demonstrates pneumonitis, cluntialica, and pleural fluid of dispyema all present within 24 hours of onset of symptoms. *B*, PA chest roentgenogram 24 hours later showing marked progression of abscess, which is three times larger and has an air-fluid level. The empyema has also increased in volume. *C*, Lateral chest roentgenogram showing the posterior position of the abscess. *D*, Forty-eight hours after admission (day of operation) the empyema has increased. The abscess ruptured and produced a pyopneumothorax.

and expectoration of purulent material. With antibiotic therapy the patient improves clinically, although improvement may be slower than expected. The roentgenographic appearance shows the initial area of pneumonitis, but subsequent studies show incomplete or no resolution. Further resolution may occur slowly over several weeks in some patients. The involved area's volume then decreases progressively, possibly progressing to complete atelectasis. This process may be lobar or segmental.

The pathologic examination reveals the involved area to be airless and densely fibrotic, with bronchial distortion or bronchiectasis and pus exuding from the cut surface (Fig. 66–25). Microscopically, the lung structure is destroyed and replaced by fibrous tissue.

Whether this process results from delay of antibiotic therapy, inadequate dosage, improperly selected antibiotic, or other unidentified factors is unclear.

The clinical problem is the differential diagnosis and the appropriate management.

Differential Diagnosis

Obstructing carcinoma, bronchoalveolar carcinoma, tuberculosis, mycotic infection, foreign body aspiration, bronchial stricture from endobronchial disease, bronchial compression, pulmonary infarction, mucoid impaction, and lipoid pneumonia (Fig. 66–26) must be considered. Diseases that produce chronic aspiration, such as gastroesophageal reflux with or without diaphragmatic hernia, achalasia, pharyngoesophageal diverticulum, tracheoesophageal fistula—congenital or acquired—and vascular ring, must be excluded also.

Lipoid pneumonia, either exogenous from chronic ingestion of mineral oil or other agents, or endogenous

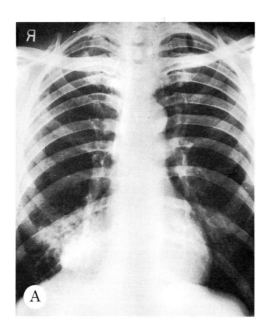

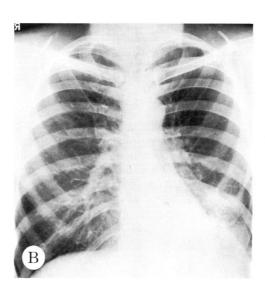

Fig. 66–26. Roentgenograms of the chest in two different patients. *A,* This patient had organizing pneumonia. *B,* This patient had epidermoid carcinoma. The roentgen-ray characteristics of the two are so similar that accurate roentgenographic differentiation is impossible.

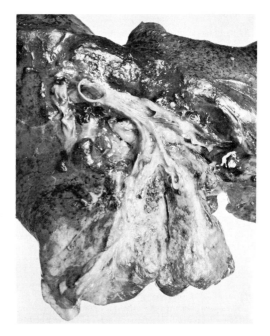

Fig. 66–25. Right lower lobe resected for organizing pneumonia showing extensive replacement of the parenchyma by scar tissue.

lipoid pneumonias that probably result from inflammatory or toxic injury to the lung (Fig. 66–27) must be ruled out. Lipoid pneumonia is poorly understood. Robbins and Sniffen (1949) called it cholesterol pneumonitis. Either form of lipoid pneumonia may not be distinguishable from carcinoma roentgenographically or grossly at operation.

Mucoid impaction produces a state that resembles organized pneumonia. Immunosuppression from AIDS, drug abuse, transplantation, and chemotherapy for malignant disease has produced various bacterial, mycotic, and parasitic infections that must be considered when response to therapy is atypical or incomplete.

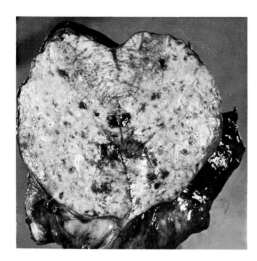

Fig. 66–27. Gross specimen of lobe removed in treatment for lipoid pneumonia.

This broad spectrum of diseases requires an extensive and time-consuming investigation by someone knowledgeable about pulmonary disease rather than just a continued course of multiple antibiotics.

Management

If the surgeon does not doubt the diagnosis, management may depend on the clinical course. Those patients with persistent continuous or repetitive episodes of cough, fever, expectoration, or hemoptysis should have the lesion resected. Those patients who are asymptomatic can under some circumstances be managed nonsurgically. This decision is difficult, because the etiology or pathologic nature of the process is rarely certain. Unfortunately, many internists follow the latter course.

The preferential decision once all pertinent diagnostic studies have been done is resection, preferably by lobectomy. If the process is completely resected and is not a part of some systemic disease process, the result should be curative. The results of major resection in the immunocompromised patient, however, are poor.

The most serious error is to advise a nonoperative approach when carcinoma cannot be excluded. Permitting a patient who is clinically chronically ill to remain ill when resection could produce a well patient also seems unwise.

REFERENCES

Bronchiectasis

Annest, L.S., Kratz, J.M., and Crawford, F.A.: Current results of treatment of bronchiectasis. J. Thorac. Cardiovasc. Surg. 83:546, 1982.

Borrie, J., and Lichter, I.: Surgical treatment of bronchiectasis: ten year survey. Br. Med. J. 22:637, 1965.

Blades, B., and Dugan, D.J.: Pseudobronchiectasis. J. Thorac. Surg. 13:40, 1944.

Blades, B., and Kent, E.M.: Individual ligation technique for lower lobe lobectomy. J. Thorac. Surg. 10:84, 1940.

Breatnach, E.S., Nath, P.H., and McElvin, R.B.: Pre-operative evaluation of bronchiectasis by computed tomography. J. Comput. Assist. Tomogr. 9:949, 1985.

Brunn, H.: Surgical principles underlying one-stage lobectomy. Arch. Surg. 18:490, 1929.

Churchill, E.D.: Lobectomy and pneumonectomy for bronchiectasis and cystic disease. J. Thorac. Surg. 6:286, 1937.

Churchill, E.D., and Belsey, R.: Segmental pneumonectomy in bronchiectasis: the lingular segment of the left upper lobe. Ann. Surg. 109:481, 1939.

Haight, C.: Total removal of the left lung for bronchiectasis. Surg. Gynecol. Obstet. 58:768, 1934.

Kergin, F.G.: The surgical treatment of bilateral bronchiectasis. J. Thorac. Surg. 19:257, 1950.

Lewiston, N.J.: Bronchiectasis in childhood. Pediatr. Clin. N. Am. 31:865, 1984.

Lindskog, G.E., and Hubbell, D.S.: An analysis of 215 cases of bronchiectasis. Surg. Gynecol. Obstet. 100:643, 1955.

Meade, R.H. Jr., Kay, E.B., and Hughes, F.A.: A report of 196 lobectomies performed at Kennedy General Hospital Chest Surgical Center from 1943 to 1946 with one death. J. Thorac. Surg. 16:1629, 1947.

Moatoosamy, I.M., et al.: Assessment of bronchiectasis by computed tomography. Thorax 40:920, 1985.

Nissen, R.: Extirpation eines ganzen Lungenflugels. Zentralbl. Chir. 58:3003, 1931.

Ochsner, A., DeBakey, M., and DeCamp, P.T.: Bronchiectasis, its curative treatment by pulmonary resection, an analysis of 96 cases. Surgery 25:518, 1949.

Overholt, R.H., and Langer, L.A.: A new technique for pulmonary segmental resection, its application in the treatment of bronchiectasis. Surg. Gynecol. Obstet. 84:257, 1947.

Sanderson, J.M., et al.: Bronchiectasis: results of surgical and conservative management: a review of 393 cases. Thorax 29:407, 1974.

Sealy, W.C., Bradham, R.R., and Young, W,.G., Jr.: Surgical treatment of multisegmental and localized bronchiectasis. Surg. Gynecol. Obstet. 123:80, 1966.

Vejlsted, H., Hjelms, E., and Jacobson, O.: Results of pulmonary resection of unilateral bronchiectasis. Scand. J. Thorac. Cardiovasc. Surg. 16:81, 1982.

Wakefield, S.J., and Waite, D.: Abnormal cilia in Polynesians with bronchiectasis. Am. Rev. Respir. Dis. 121:1003, 1980.

Wilson, J.F., and Decker, A.M.: The surgical management of childhood bronchiectasis: a review of 96 consecutive pulmonary resections in children with nontuberculous bronchiectasis. Ann. Surg. 195:354, 1982.

Pulmonary Abscess

Bartlett, J.G., and Gorbach, S.L.: Penicillin or clindamycin for primary lung abscess (editorial). Ann. Intern. Med. 98:546, 1983.

Gourin, A., and Garzon, A.A.: Operative treatment of massive hemoptysis. Ann. Thorac. Surg. 18:52, 1974.

Hagan, J.L., and Hardy, J.D.: Lung abscess revisited. Ann. Surg. 197:755, 1983.

Keller, F.S., et al.: Percutaneous interventional catheter therapy for lesions of the chest and lungs. Chest 81:407, 1982.

Lacey, S.R., and Koloske, A.M.: Pneumonostomy in the management of pediatric lung abscess. J. Pediatr. Surg. 18:625, 1983.

Lewison, M.E., et al.: Clindamycin compared with penicillin for the treatment of anaerobic lung abscess. Ann. Intern. Med. 98:466, 1983.

Lorenzo, R.L., et al.: Lung abscesses in children: Diagnostic and therapeutic needle aspiration. Radiology 157:779, 1985.

Nonayama, A., et al.: Surgical treatment of pulmonary abscess in children under ten years of age. Chest 85:356, 1984.

Pohlsan, E.C., et al.: Lung abscess: a changing pattern of disease. Am. J. Surg. 150:97, 1985.

Ravitch, N.M., and Fein, R.: The changing picture of pneumonia and empyema in infants and children. JAMA 175:1039, 1961.

Schachter, E.N., Kreisman, H., and Putman, C.: Diagnostic problems in suppurative lung disease. Arch. Intern. Med. 136:167, 1976.

Schoenfell, M.R., and Lapin, R.H.: Primary giant candida lung abscess response to miconazole. NY State J. Med. 83:1187, 1983.

Weiss, W., and Cherniack, N.S.: Acute nonspecific lung abscess: a controlled study comparing orally and parenterally administered penicillin G. Chest 66:348, 1974.

Yellin, A., Yellin, E.O., and Liberman, Y.: Percutaneous tube drainage: the treatment of choice for refractory lung abscess. Ann. Thorac. Surg. *39*:266, 1985.

Organizing Pneumonia

Robbins, L.L., and Sniffen, R.C.: Correlation between roentgenologic and pathologic findings in chronic pneumonitis of the cholesterol type. Radiology *53*:187, 1949.

READING REFERENCES

Abernathy, R.S.: Antibiotic therapy of lung abscess: effectiveness of penicillin. Dis. Chest. *53*:592, 1968.

Ackerman, L.V., Elliott, G.V., and Alanis, M.: Localized organizing pneumonia: its resemblance to carcinoma. Am. J. Roentgenol. *71*:988, 1954.

Adebonojo, S.A., et al.: Suppurative disease of the lung and pleura: a continuing challenge in developing countries. Ann. Thorac. Surg. *33*:40, 1982.

Afzelius, B.A.: A human syndrome caused by immotile cilia. Science *193*:317, 1976 (Abstract).

Alexander, J.C., Jr., and Wolfe, W.G.: Lung abscess and enpyema of the thorax. Surg. Clin. North Am. *60*:835, 1980.

Bartlett, J.G., and Finegold, S.M.: Anaerobic infections of the lung and pleural space. Am. Rev. Respir. Dis. *110*:56, 1974.

Bartlett, J.G., and Gorbach, S.L.: Treatment of aspiration pneumonia and primary lung abscess: Penicillin G vs. clindamycin. JAMA *234*:935, 1975.

Berg, R., Jr., and Burford, T.H.: Pulmonary paraffinoma (lipoid pneumonia). J. Thorac. Surg. *20*:418, 1950.

Brock, R.C.: Lung Abscess. Springfield, IL, Charles C Thomas, 1952.

Carden, D.L., and Gibb, K.A.: Pneumonia and lung abscess. Emerg. Med. Clin. North Am. *1*:345, 1983.

Chidi, C.C. and Mendelsohn, H.J.: Lung abscess: a study of the results of treatment based on 90 consecutive cases. J. Thorac. Cardiovasc. Surg. *68*:168, 1974.

Connors, J.P., Roper, C.L., and Ferguson, T.B.: Transbronchial catheterization of pulmonary abscesses. Ann. Thorac. Surg. *19*:254, 1975.

Davis, P.B., et al.: Familial bronchiectasis. J. Pediatr. *102*:177, 1983.

Dowling, J.N., et al.: Pneumonic and multiple lung abscesses caused by dual infection with *Legionella micdadei* and *Legionella pneumophila*. Am. Rev. Respir. Dis. *127*:121, 1983.

Ellis, D.A., et al.: Present outlook in bronchiectasis: Clinical and social study and review of factors influencing prognosis. Thorax *36*:659, 1981.

Ferguson, T.B., and Burford, T.H.: The changing pattern of pulmonary suppuration: surgical implications. Dis. Chest *53*:396, 1968.

George, S.A., Leonardi, H.K., and Overholt, R.H.: Bilateral pulmonary resection for bronchiectasis: a 40-year experience. Ann. Thorac. Surg. *28*:48, 1979.

Gluck, M.C., Levister, E.C., and Katz, S.: Pseudomonas abscess and empyema of the lung. Dis. Chest *54*:77, 1968.

Hollinger, W.M., and Gilman, M.J.: Primary lung abscess. J. Med. Assoc. Georgia *74*:78, 1985.

Jampolis, R.W., McDonald, J.R., and Clagett, O.T.: Mineral oil granuloma of the lungs: an evaluation of methods for identification of mineral oil in tissue. Surg. Gynecol. Obstet. *97*:105, 1953.

Kapila, R., et al.: Evaluation of clindamycin and other antibiotics in the treatment of anaerobic bacterial infections of the lung. J. Infect. Dis. *135*(Suppl.):S58, 1977.

Kurklu, E.U., Williams, M.A., and le Roux, B.T.: Bronchiectasis consequent upon foreign body retention. Thorax *28*:601, 1955.

Lawrence, G.H., and Rubin, S.L.: Management of giant lung abscess. Am. J. Surg. *136*:134, 1978.

Lindskog, G.E.: Bronchiectasis revisited. Yale Biol. Med. *56*:41, 1986.

Mengali, L.: Giant lung abscess treated by tube thoracostomy. J. Thorac. Cardiovasc. Surg. *90*:186, 1985.

Nemir, R.L.: Bronchiectasis. *In* Disorders of the Respiratory Tract in Children. Edited by E.L. Kendig and V. Chernik. Philadelphia, W.B. Saunders Co., 1983, pp. 446–469.

Ochsner, A.: Bronchiectasis: disappearing pulmonary lesion. NY State J. Med. *75*:1683, 1975.

Pappas, G., et al.: Pulmonary surgery in immunosuppressed patients. J. Thorac. Cardiovasc. Surg. *59*:882, 1970.

Ripe, E.: Bronchiectasis. I. A follow-up study after surgical treatment. Scand. J. Respir. Dis. *52*:96, 1971.

Schweppe, H.L., Knowles, J.H., and Kane, L.: Lung abscess: an analysis of the Massachusetts General Hospital cases from 1943 through 1956. N. Engl. J. Med. *265*:1039, 1961.

Stark, D.D., et al.: Differentiating lung abscess and empyema radiography and computed tomography. Am. J. Radiology *141*:163, 1983.

Stern, W.Z., and Subbaro, K.: Pulmonary complications of drug addiction. Semin. Roentgenol. *18*:183, 1983.

Takaro, T., et al.: Suppurative diseases of the lungs, pleurae, and pericardium. Curr. Probl. Surg. *14*:1, 1977.

Thoms, N.W., Puro, H.E., and Arbula, A.: The significance of hemoptysis in lung abscess. J. Thorac. Cardiovasc. Surg. *59*:617, 1970.

Wanner, A., et al.: Bedside bronchofiberscopy for atelectasis and lung abscess. JAMA *224*:1281, 1973.

CHAPTER 67

BRONCHIAL COMPRESSIVE DISEASES

R. Maurice Hood

Diseases that obstruct major airways have received little attention in thoracic surgical literature. Most surgeons are aware of the middle lobe syndrome, but its pathogenesis seems somewhat uncertain. Several diseases that produce bronchial or tracheal obstruction do so by extraluminal compression. Usually this subject deals with the so-called middle lobe syndrome or with atelectasis secondary to tuberculous lymphadenopathy. This chapter will endeavor to broaden the awareness of this group of diseases and put them into better perspective. Table 67–1 presents a classification of the various disease processes.

INFLAMMATORY LYMPHADENOPATHY

Primary Tuberculosis

Gross enlargement of hilar and mediastinal lymph nodes is a common finding and may be the principal feature of primary tuberculosis in some children. Why lymphadenopathy becomes so prominent in one patient but not in another is not understood. The comparatively small bronchial lumen in the child under 2 undoubtedly contributes to the frequency of atelectasis as a complication.

There may be a history of fever, but in underdeveloped areas the diagnosis of primary tuberculosis is rarely made. The child may present with wheezing or stridor or may be asymptomatic, and atelectasis of either upper lobe may be discovered on the roentgenogram (Fig. 67–1). Less commonly, obstructive emphysema of one or more lobes may result. With proper study, chest roentgenograms always reveal enlarged hilar and mediastinal nodes.

Diagnosis is made by chest roentogenogram, a positive tuberculin test, occasionally by positive sputum and by bronchoscopy. Bronchoscopy reveals that the bronchus is occluded from external pressure without endobronchial disease. Bronchoscopy is necessary to exclude foreign body and tuberculous bronchitis.

Treatment consists of antituberculous antibiotic ther-apy in the appropriate dosage for the age of the child. Surgical treatment is not usually required even though the atelectasis may persist for several weeks or months. A failure of medical therapy associated with evidence of parenchymal infection may be used as a surgical indication. Persistent obstructive emphysema with respiratory distress (Fig. 67–2) may require intervention. Rarely, nodes erode into the airway and discharge their caseous contents into the lumen.

Surgical resection of the obstructing nodes is usually all that is necessary to relieve the bronchial obstruction. Lobes that have developed fibrosis or bronchiectasis may require resection. Nakui and Nohl-Oser (1979) described seven cases requiring surgical treatment in England. Malatinszky and associates (1970) in Hungary reported a series of 173 patients with "tuberculous lymph node compression syndrome." All of their patients were over 20 years of age, with the average age being over 60. Treatment was not discussed.

Histoplasmosis

Histoplasmosis, because of its geographic distribution, is not a nationwide problem. For many years, calcified foci in the lung associated with calcified hilar nodes were assumed to be tuberculosis, and indeed they may be, but most of these patients have histoplasmosis (Fig. 67–3). The proliferative adenopathy of acute disease is not likely to be so extensive that it causes bronchial obstruction during the acute phase of the disease.

Bronchial compression by nodes involved with histoplasmosis usually occurs in adult life rather than childhood and by calcified, matted nodes that have obviously been present for many years. The middle lobe seems to be the lobe most commonly involved. Bronchial compression caused by histoplasmosis cannot be expected to resolve spontaneously or with therapy with amphotericin B, and if neoplasm, stricture (Fig. 67–4), and foreign body can be excluded, surgical resection of these nodes is indicated. Technically, this is not a simple procedure; adherence of these nodes to pulmonary vessels is dense and difficult to free surgically with safety.

Table 67–1. Classification of Bronchocompressive Diseases

Inflammatory lymphadenopathy
  Tuberculosis
  Histoplasmosis
  Sarcoidosis
  Nonspecific
Neoplastic lesions
  Benign
    Bronchogenic cyst
    Gastroenterogenous cysts
    Cystic hygroma
  Malignant
    Metastatic carcinoma producing enlargement of hilar nodes
    Primary malignancies
      Carcinoma of the lung
      Lymphomas
      Neurogenic tumors
      Miscellaneous
Sclerosing mediastinitis
Aberrant right upper lobe bronchus
Cardiovascular disease
  Enlarged vessels or chambers in normal position
    Enlarged left atrium
    Large left-to-right shunts with pulmonary and cardiac enlargement
    Tetralogy of Fallot—large aorta
    Pulmonary valve atresia—large pulmonary artery
    Pulmonary artery aneurysm
    Cardiomyopathy
  Abnormal vessels or abnormally positioned vessels
    Vascular ring—double arch, right arch, left ligamentum aberrant
      subclavian artery, left arch-right ligamentum aberrant innom-
      inate, anomalous left carotid
    Aberrant left pulmonary artery—pulmonary sling
    Pulmonary agenesis—abnormal position of aorta
    Patent ductus with pulmonary atresia
    Interrupted aortic arch with patent ductus arteriosus
    Corrected transposition of the great vessels
    Transposition of the great vessels—postoperative pulmonary
      artery dilatation
  Acquired aortic disease
    Aneurysm of the transverse arch
    Traumatic false aneurysm of the descending arch

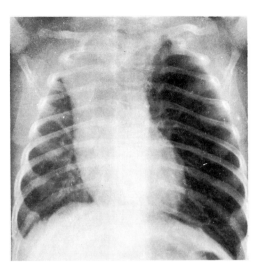

Fig. 67–1. This 2½-month-old infant has recurrent atelectasis in the right upper lobe. The child recovered on conservative therapy and eventually outgrew the problem. (Ferguson, T.B.: Congenital lesions of the lungs and emphysema. *In* Gibbon's Surgery of the Chest, 4th ed. Edited by D.C. Sabiston, Jr., and F.C. Spencer. Philadelphia, W.B. Saunders Co., 1982, Chapter 22.)

Other granulomatous diseases that involve lymph nodes could cause airway compression (Fig. 67–5) but are unusual. Because of the difficulty in identifying histoplasmosis, it is likely that most nonidentified diseases are caused by this organism rather than by tuberculosis.

Histoplasmosis is one of the etiologic agents in sclerosing mediastinitis and will be discussed separately.

Sarcoidosis

Sarcoidosis can also produce bronchial compression. Mendelson and associates described a patient with bilateral main bronchus compression producing severe respiratory obstruction. This responded to steroid therapy. Similar reports have been made by Munt (1973), Wescott and Noehren (1973), Stinson and Hargett (1981), and Sharma (1978). Because the adenopathy of sarcoidosis generally responds to steroid therapy, such nodes should rarely require resection.

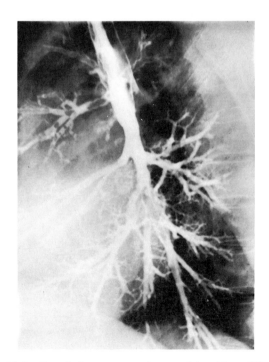

Fig. 67–2. Bronchial compressive disease of the right middle lobe showing angulation and narrowing of the lumen by a large calcified hilar lymph node. (Ferguson, T.B., and Burford, T.H.: The changing pattern of pulmonary suppuration: surgical implications. Dis. Chest 53:396, 1968.)

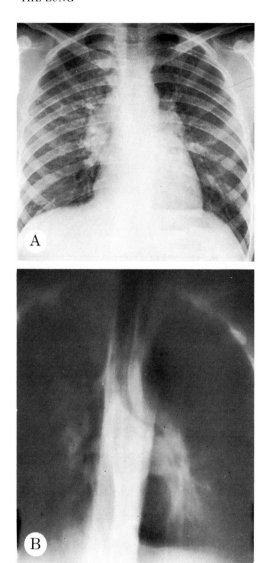

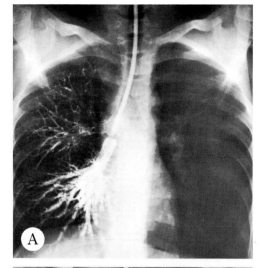

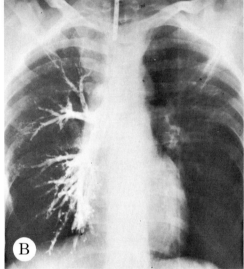

Fig. 67–3. *A,* Bilateral hilar adenopathy and parenchymal disease in an 11-year-old boy with proven disseminated histoplasmosis. *B,* Tomogram showing marked compromise of the right and left main stem bronchi by the inflammatory process.

Fig. 67–4. *A,* Stricture of the bronchus caused by inflammatory lymph node disease. Notice the pseudobronchiectasis of the right lower lobe. *B,* Postoperative bronchogram after resection of the stricture showing restoration of the lumen. The patient made a complete recovery.

Broncholithiasis

An isolated area of compressive bronchial disease is usually referred to as broncholithiasis. It is produced by a calcified hilar node eroding into a major bronchus. The most common symptom is recurrent hemoptysis that is often associated with obstructive pneumonitis or atelectasis. These patients frequently cough up calcified fragments of the eroding lymph node, hence the name broncholith. The etiologic agent is most often *Histoplasma capsulatum* and this is the primary complex of this disease. Tuberculous nodes can produce the same syndrome, and this disease is excluded by skin test and culture.

Because this situation is relatively rare, the more common bronchial occlusion by bronchogenic carcinoma with hemoptysis and obstruction must first be excluded. The mere presence of calcified hilar nodes is insufficient ev-

idence for benign bronchial obstruction, therefore repeated bronchoscopy and biopsy may be necessary. Biopsy of one of these eroding lymph nodes may result in brisk bleeding that may seem severe to the surgeon who has not experienced this entity.

Hemoptysis is a common symptom, and in at least half the instances the bronchoscopy fails to establish the diagnosis, but this should not deter the surgeon from using bronchoscopy for each patient with hemoptysis. The CT study clearly shows the relationship of the calcified node to the bronchial lumen. Attempts at biopsy must be cautious to avoid major bleeding.

This form of broncholithiasis should not be confused with the rare entity of true broncholithiasis. In this disease, for reasons not apparent, the patient periodically

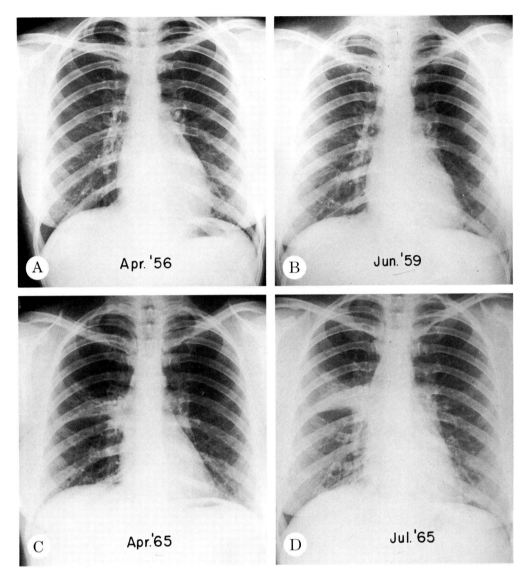

Fig. 67–5. Documentation of the development of bronchial compressive disease of right upper lobe over a 9-year period. Before 1963, the patient had a number of episodes of hemoptysis documented as originating from the right upper lobe. The offending calcified lymph node can clearly be seen in roentgenograms of April 1956 and June of 1959. After 1963 the patient began having recurrent episodes of right upper lobe pneumonitis. By July 1965, the patient was sufficiently symptomatic to require right upper lobectomy.

coughs up small calcified "casts" of terminal bronchi that look just like a cast of a bronchus. This process seems to be unrelated to pulmonary or other bronchial disease and is a benign process with no surgical implications.

MIDDLE LOBE SYNDROME

Graham and associates (1948) coined the term "middle lobe syndrome" in a report of two patients with atelectasis of the middle lobe produced by compression of the middle lobe bronchus by enlarged, nontuberculous lymph nodes (Fig. 67–6). These patients were symptomatic and had recurrent hemoptysis, cough, and pulmonary infection.

Since that time, many thoracic surgeons have referred to an atelectatic middle lobe as the middle lobe syndrome and carried out resection regardless of symptoms or a demonstrated pathologic basis.

It has been assumed that this entity is always caused by external bronchial compression by nodes whether demonstrated or not. Pulmonary internists have challenged this concept and often give their patients prolonged medical therapy without attempting anatomic or pathologic diagnosis.

Patients may present no symptoms or findings of illness other than the roentgenographic finding. Others may complain of cough, expectoration, hemoptysis, recurrent fever, and chest pain.

Roentgenographically, the principal finding is a contracted middle lobe that is usually airless. Hilar adeno-

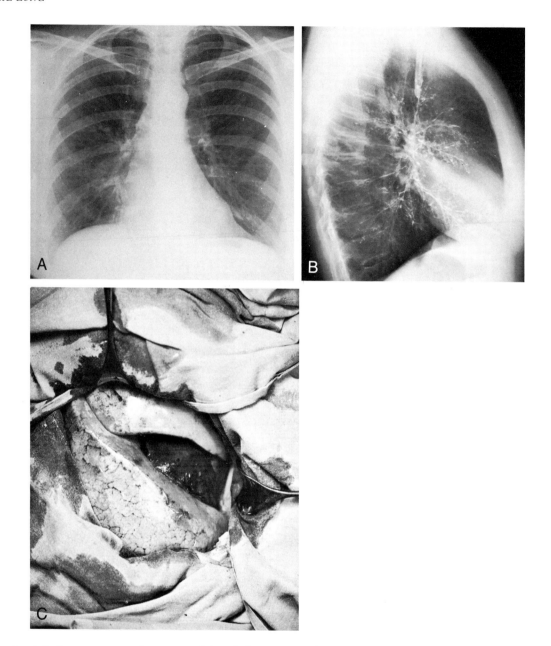

Fig. 67–6. A and B, Roentgenograms of a patient with bronchial compressive disease of the right middle lobe with complete atelectasis. Note obliteration of the right heart border by the inflammatory process. C, Appearance of the right middle lobe at the time of operation.

pathy, calcified or noncalcified, may or may not be present.

Pathology

The diagnosis cannot be assumed for there are several pathologic problems that may exist. Lindskog and Spear (1955) showed that several different etiologic situations were present. Paulson and Shaw (1949) noted, in contrast to other reports, that carcinoma of the middle lobe bronchus was a significant cause. Wagner and Johnston (1983), in their excellent collective review, found that in 22% of patients, middle lobe abscess was caused by carcinoma. Earlier reports suggested that carcinoma was rare in the middle lobe; this impression persists. Statistically, the standard concept of bronchial compression by lymph nodes producing atelectasis and chronic parenchymal disease is not common. Acute inflammatory disease of the middle lobe may result in atelectasis, bronchiectasis, pseudobronchiectasis, or even lung abscess. The lobe may not recover and may remain contracted or it may recover completely. Some patients have primary benign endobronchial disease that may include tuberculous bronchitis, foreign body, sarcoidosis, stricture of unknown etiology, and erosion of a calcified peribronchial node into the lumen of the bronchus. Other diseases could probably be included in this list.

Certainly the middle lobe bronchus is long, slender, and surrounded by lymph nodes (Fig. 67–7) and prob-

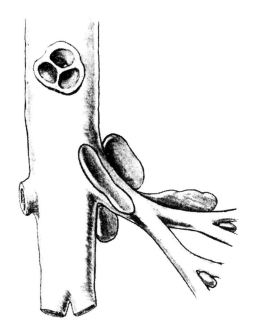

Fig. 67–7. Diagram of the middle lobe bronchus and the surrounding collar of lymph nodes. (Brock, R.C.: The Anatomy of the Bronchial Tree, 2nd ed. London, Oxford University Press, 1954, p. 122.)

ably has poorer drainage than other lobes (Fig. 67–8). At least for this and possibly for other reasons, it is more vulnerable than other areas of the lung.

The concept of the lack of collateral ventilation to the middle lobe as Culiner (1966) proposed is interesting, but fails to explain to my satisfaction the parenchymal disease usually present. However, his observation that the middle lobe bronchus is often nonobstructed in patients with the middle lobe syndrome is pertinent and agrees with my experience and many others'.

In some patients, inflammatory lymphadenopathy may have obstructed the bronchus and produced irreparable parenchymal disease then subsided, leaving an unobstructed bronchus (Fig. 67–9). Some patients may have primary parenchymal disease with no bronchial lesion at any time; they probably fit into the category of organizing or fibrosing pneumonitis.

Patients with immune disorders, chronic allergy, asthma, and septic fibrosis also may demonstrate middle lobe disease and atelectasis without bronchial compression.

Diagnosis should be based on complete studies of the middle lobe. Contraction of the middle lobe mandates bronchoscopy, CT scan, and bronchography to exclude neoplasm. Stricture, foreign body (Fig. 67–10), and active endobronchial disease must be identified. The extent of parenchymal disease and the presence and extent of bronchiectasis should be evaluated. Cytologic studies must be carried out.

Management

The treatment of middle lobe syndrome (Fig. 67–11) should be based on sound data. The concept of Graham and associates (1948) and of Paulson and Shaw (1949) that resection should be done in all cases probably is not tenable today. Certainly, after complete studies, those based on carcinoma and those in whom carcinoma cannot be excluded must be managed by resection.

Demonstrated bronchial stenosis or erosion of a calcified lymph node (Fig. 67–12) into the bronchus should also be treated by resection. Patients with bronchiectasis who are symptomatic are probably best treated by resection also.

Patients with only the finding of diminished volume of the middle lobe, in whom no obstruction of the bronchus can be identified, in whom carcinoma can be excluded, and who remain asymptomatic can be managed safely nonoperatively. However, the burden of responsibility for the missed diagnosis of carcinoma rests on the physician who opts for medical management.

In summary, the middle lobe syndrome as originally defined is uncommon and the term has been applied to a large group of pulmonary and bronchial diseases. Careful diagnostic studies are in order and management should be based on the results of these studies.

MEDIASTINAL TUMORS

Mediastinal cysts and neoplasms commonly cause respiratory obstruction in children but rarely do so in adults. A large bronchogenic or gastroenterogenous cyst may occlude either main bronchus or the trachea. The infant may present with varying degrees of respiratory distress and may require urgent surgical intervention to prevent death. Diagnosis is not usually possible except to identify a mass in children. Azizkhan and associates (1985) found that of 50 children with mediastinal tumors, 9 were found to have significant tracheobronchial compression. All nine presented with severe respiratory obstruction.

A small bronchogenic cyst or reduplication cyst in an infant or child—but rarely in an adult—can produce localized compression and obstruction of the trachea or either main bronchus. Balquet (1984a,b) described bronchial and trachea compression in 29 patients: 21 bronchogenic cysts and 8 esophageal duplication cysts. One patient developed saccular bronchiectasis from longstanding bronchial obstruction. Only one death occurred. Erosion with a fistula into the trachea or bronchus can occur and complicate the problem.

General anesthesia is safe for those without demonstrated compression but may be lethal in those with over a one-third decrease in luminal size of the airway. It is safest to establish the diagnosis by needle biopsy or lymph node biopsy with local anesthesia. Irradiation or chemotherapy, or both, is indicated based on the biopsy and occasionally should be given empirically when tissue diagnosis is not conclusive or obtainable. General anesthesia in those with tracheobronchial compression should be reserved for total resection and relief of airway compression. Azizkhan and associates (1985) proposed, in the patients with severe obstruction, cardiopulmonary bypass as a method of anesthesia and oxygenation for those with critical airway or impaired circulation.

Muscle relaxants should be avoided altogether. The protocol in the article is reproduced (Table 67–2) because

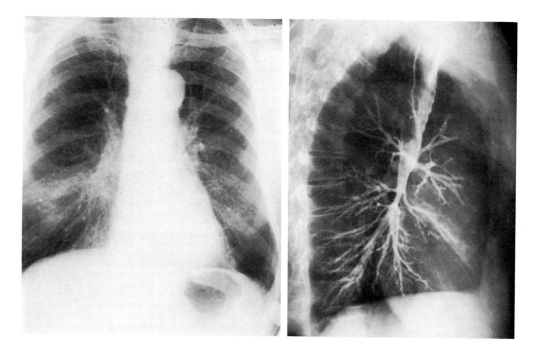

Fig. 67–8. Right middle lobe pneumonitis and atelectasis secondary to poor drainage. The right middle lobe bronchus is pushed downward by an adjacent node, but the bronchial lumen is not decreased in diameter. (Ferguson, T.B., and Burford, T.H.: The changing pattern of pulmonary suppuration: surgical implications. Dis. Chest 53:396, 1968.)

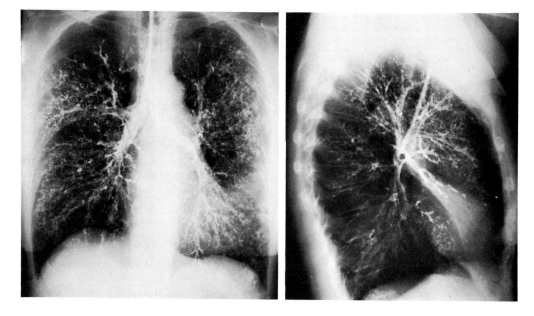

Fig. 67–9 Bronchial compressive disease of the lingular segment of the left upper lobe; a "middle lobe syndrome" on the left side. (Ferguson, T.B., and Burford, T.H.: The changing pattern of pulmonary suppuration: surgical implications. Dis. Chest 53:396, 1968.)

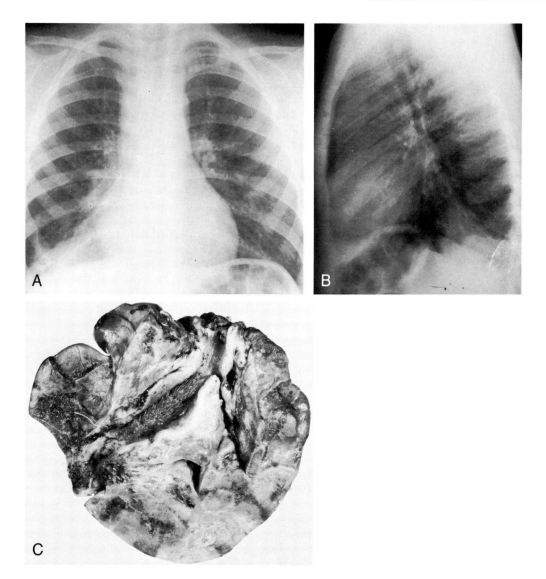

Fig. 67–10. *A* and *B*, Roentgenograms showing right lower lobe atelectasis in an asymptomatic 11-year-old boy. Bronchoscopy revealed complete occlusion of right lower lobe bronchus by granulation tissue. *C*, Resected right lower lobe showing timothy grass head in the bronchus. Notice that the spicules encourage progression of the foreign body into the distal part of the lung.

almost every thoracic surgeon has had the experience of having an irreversible cardiopulmonary arrest occur upon anesthesia induction in a small child with a mediastinal mass.

In adults, bronchial or tracheal obstruction may also occur from malignant neoplasm. Most often this is either a primary bronchial carcinoma with the primary tumor occluding a major bronchus by external pressure or metastatic lymph nodes producing compression. If the roentgenogram demonstrates what appears to be a primary tumor, the diagnosis is relatively simple, usually established by the CT scan.

Occasionally, however, the patient presents with bronchial or tracheal compression with respiratory distress and often associated with a superior vena caval syndrome with no evidence of pulmonary disease but only with mediastinal widening. These are usually undifferentiated carcinomas, often small cell tumors, but

the origin is not always apparent. Biopsy by needle or lymph node may not indicate the origin. I prefer, under these circumstances, to begin radiation therapy and chemotherapy simultaneously even if no microscopic diagnosis is available, because those with respiratory distress often die within 7 to 10 days. General anesthesia is also contraindicated in this group of patients, as is the use of relaxants.

SCLEROSING MEDIASTINITIS

This uncommon entity probably represents several separate diseases with similar gross pathologic behavior. Histoplasmosis can be and is responsible for some of these cases. Sclerosing Hodgkin's disease may produce an identical gross picture, and differentiating the two histologically may be difficult or impossible. Probably other etiologic agents exist, for in many cases no histo-

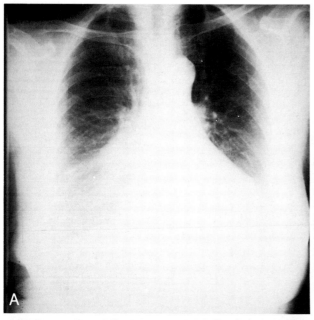

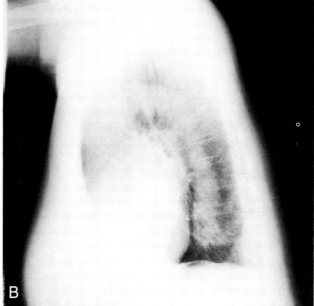

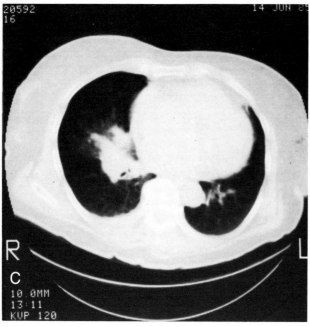

Fig. 67–11. *A* and *B*, PA and lateral chest films of a middle-aged woman with atelectasis of the middle lobe. The cause was not apparent. Bronchoscopy revealed external compression of the middle lobe bronchus, but no intraluminal lesion. *C*, CT examination shows a mass in the hilum compressing and occluding the bronchus. This was proven to be a small-cell carcinoma that was entirely extraluminal.

logic diagnosis other than fibrosis can be established. The trachea and main bronchi are affected and superior vena caval obstruction is usually present.

The standard chest roentgenogram is ordinarily interpreted as normal. The CT scan establishes the character of the disease but not its etiology.

Biopsy should be done with appropriate histologic and bacteriologic studies. Therapy, medical or surgical, seems to offer little.

ACQUIRED AORTIC DISEASE

Two separate entities can produce partial or complete occlusion of the left main bronchus. Traumatic false aneurysm of the descending aorta may become large enough to compress the left main bronchus in the subaortic area. Because this diagnosis is often missed in the immediate postinjury period, symptoms secondary to bronchial compression such as cough, wheezing, dyspnea, and hemoptysis may be the first symptoms of the aneurysm.

Chest roentgenograms are often read as a hilar or mediastinal mass (Fig. 67–13), and unless the history of injury is known, aortography may not be ordered. Some of these have been diagnosed at the time of exploratory operation. A CT study of this type of patient will establish the diagnosis.

An arteriosclerotic or luetic aneurysm of the aortic arch can also produce compression. Erosion or even destruction of the left main bronchus with obstructive emphy-

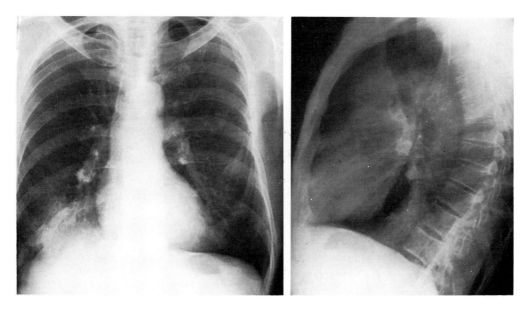

Fig. 67–12. Bronchial compressive disease in the right lower lobe. On both views the offending calcified lymph node is clearly seen. (Ferguson, T.B., and Burford, T.H.: The changing pattern of pulmonary suppuration: surgical implications. Dis. Chest 53:396, 1968.)

Table 67–2. Algorithm for Managing Children with Mediastinal Masses

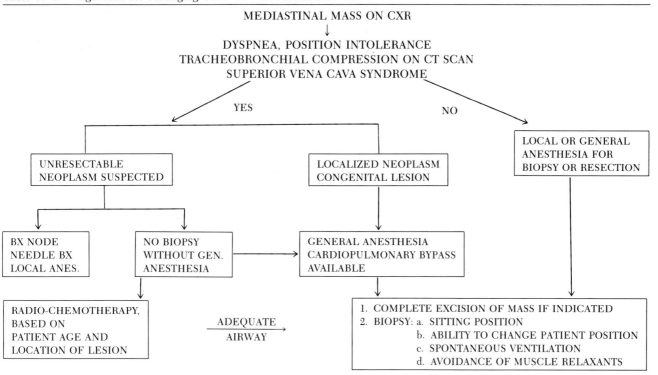

Azizkhan, R.G., et al.: Life-threatening airway obstruction as a complication to the management of mediastinal masses in children. J. Pediatr. Surg. 20:816, 1985.

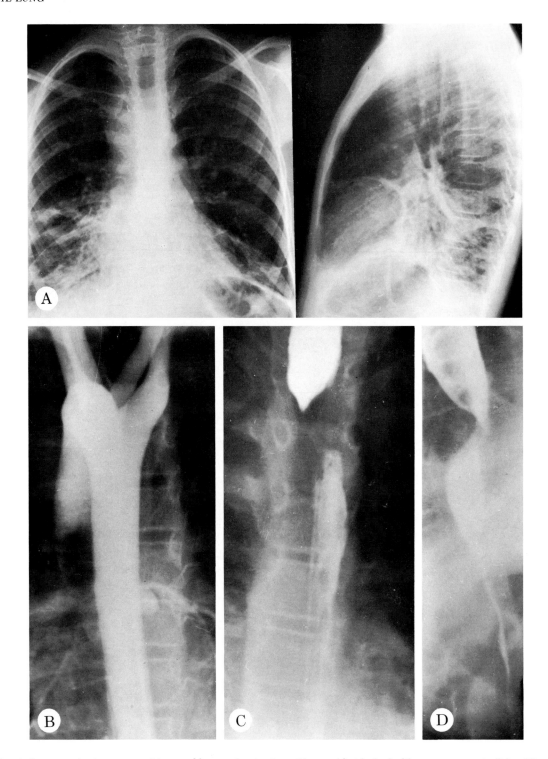

Fig. 67–13. *A*, Severe aspiration pneumonitis caused by vascular ring in an 11-year old girl who had been symptomatic all her life and exhibited growth failure. Extensive workup for mucoviscidosis, bronchiectasis, and collagen disease was performed before the true diagnosis was established. *B*, Posteroanterior arteriogram showing a right descending aortic arch and aberrant left subclavian artery. The first portion of this vessel is flattened where it crosses the esophagus. *C*, Posteroanterior esophagogram showing oblique indentation in the barium column at the level of the anomalous vessel. *D*, Lateral esophagogram showing posterior compression of the barium column caused by the aberrant artery. (Ferguson, T.B., and Burford, T.H.: The changing pattern of pulmonary suppuration: surgical implications. Dis. Chest 53:396, 1968.)

sema, pulmonary sepsis, or complete atelectasis is the clinical result. The pulmonary symptoms may be the first evidence of the aneurysm, and atelectasis may partially obscure the aneurysm. In one of my patients, the left main bronchus was totally eroded, and after the aneurysm was resected, with total arch replacement, pneumonectomy was required because of a 5-cm gap between the two ends of the eroded bronchus. Bronchial reanastomosis can be done in preference to pneumonectomy if the distal lung tissue appears to be normal.

The most serious error is to attempt bronchoscopy and biopsy without realizing that an aneurysm is present.

PRIMARY CARDIOVASCULAR DISEASE

Table 67–1 lists the cardiac and vascular abnormalities that can compress the trachea or main bronchi. These individual anomalies and results of disease are best studied as a part of the subject of congenital heart disease, which is outside the scope of this text. Some patients, however, present with symptoms and findings of airway compression without a history of cardiac or vascular disease.

An enlarged left atrium from either acquired mitral disease or congenital heart disease can compress and displace the left main bronchus. Any lesion that results in marked enlargement and increase in pressure of the pulmonary artery can compress the left main bronchus. These lesions include large left-to-right shunts, particularly associated with pulmonary hypertension. These may be large atrial or ventricular septal defects or a patent ductus arteriosus. Other less common lesions include patent ductus arteriosus with pulmonary valve atresia and interrupted aortic arch with patent ductus arteriosus. Corrected transposition of the great vessels and postoperative enlargement of the pulmonary artery following surgical correction of transposition can also occlude the left main bronchus.

The varieties of vascular ring involve primarily the distal trachea. The varieties noted include double aortic arch, a right descending aorta with a left ligamentum arteriosum, and a left descending arch with a left ligamentum arteriosum; an aberrant innominate artery arising to the left of its normal position and compressing the anterior wall of the trachea is rare. The aberrant right subclavian artery arising from the descending left aorta and coursing either between the trachea and esophagus or posterior to the esophagus can compress the trachea. Diagnosis of all of these lesions is not difficult once they are suspected, but too many children are treated for asthma or allergy before definitive studies are undertaken. (See Chapter 64.)

REFERENCES

Azizkhan, R.G., et al.: Life-threatening airway obstruction as a complication to the management of mediastinal masses in children. J Pediatr. Surg. 20:816, 1985.

Balquet, P.: Kystes bronchogéniques comprimant la trachée et les bronches souches. Chir. Pediatr. 25:270, 1984a.

Balquet, P.: Les duplications digestive comprimant la trachée et les bronches souches. Chir. Pediatr. 25:276, 1984b.

Berlinger, N.T., Long, C., and Foker, J.: Tracheobronchial compression in acyanotic congenital heart disease. Ann. Otol. Rhinol. Laryngol. 92:387, 1983.

Culliner, M.M.: The right middle lobe syndrome: a nonobstruction complex. Dis. Chest 50:509, 1966.

Graham, E.A., Burford, T.H., and Mayer, J.H.: Middle lobe syndrome. Postgrad. Med. 4:29, 1948.

Ichikawa, T., and Yokoyama, T.: A case report of bronchogenic cyst in an infant causing acute respiratory distress. Hiroshima J. Med. Sci. 34:39, 1985.

Lindskog, G.E., and Spear, H.C.: Middle lobe syndrome. N. Engl. J. Med. 253:489, 1955.

Malatinszky, I., et al.: Bronchopulmonary lesions associated with tuberculous lymph node compression—node compression syndrome. Tubercle 51:412, 1970.

Mendelson, D.S., Norton, K. Cohen, B.A., et al.: Case report: Bronchial compression: An unusual manifestation of sarcoidosis. J. Comput. Assist. Tomogr. 1:892, 1983.

Munt, D.W.: Middle lobe atelectasis in sarcoidosis. Am. Rev. Respir. Dis. 108:357, 1973.

Nakui, A.J., and Nohl-Oser, H.C.: Surgical treatment of bronchial obstruction in primary tuberculosis in children: report of seven cases. Thorax 34:464, 1979.

Paulson, D.L., and Shaw, R.R.: Chronic atelectasis and pneumonitis in the middle lobe. J. Thorac. Surg. 18:747, 1949.

Sharma, O.P.: Airway obstruction in sarcoidosis. Chest 73:6, 1978.

Stinson, J.M., and Hargett, D.: Prolonged lobar atelectasis in sarcoidosis. J. Natl. Med. Assn. 73:669, 1981.

Wagner, R.B., and Johnston, M.R.: Middle lobe syndrome. Ann. Thorac. Surg. 35:679, 1983.

Wescott, J.L., and Noehren, T.H.: Bronchial stenosis in chronic sarcoidosis. Chest 63:893, 1973.

READING REFERENCES

Albo, R.J., and Grimes, O.F.: The middle lobe syndrome: a clinical study. Dis. Chest 50:509, 1966.

Bradhan, R.R., Sealy, W.C., and Young, W.G., Jr.: Chronic middle lobe infection: factors responsible for its development. Ann. Thorac. Surg. 2:612, 1966.

Bertleson, S., et al.: Isolated middle lobe atelectasis: aetiology, pathogenesis, and treatment of the so-called middle lobe syndrome. Thorax 35:449, 1980.

Bray, R.J., and Fernandes, F.S.: Mediastinal tumor causing airway obstruction in anesthetized children. Anesthesiology 37:371, 1982.

Brock, R.C., Cann, R.J., and Dickinson, J.R.: Tuberculosis mediastinal lymphadenitis in childhood: secondary effects on the lungs. Guy's Hosp. Rep. 87:295, 1937.

Brock, R.C.: Post-tuberculous bronchostenosis and bronchiectasis of the middle lobe. Thorax 5:5, 1950.

Capitano, M.A., et al.: Obstruction of the airways by the aorta: an observation in infants with congenital heart disease. AJR 140:675, 1983.

Charrette, E.J.P., Winton, T.L., and Salerno, T.A.: Acute respiratory insufficiency from an aneurysm of the descending thoracic aorta. J. Thorac. Cardiovasc. Surg. 85:467, 1983.

Clarksan, P.M., Ritter, O.G., and Rahimtoola, S.H.: Aberrant left-pulmonary artery. Am. J. Dis. Child. 113:373, 1967.

Cochran, S.T., Gyepes, M.T., and Smith, L.E.: Obstruction of the airways by the heart and pulmonary vessels in infants. Pediatr. Radiol. 6:81, 1977.

Cohen, R., and Landing, B.H.: Tracheostenosis and bronchial abnormalities associated with pulmonary artery sling. Ann. Otol. 85:582, 1970.

Corno, A., et al.: Bronchial compression by diluted pulmonary artery. J. Thorac. Cardiovasc. Surg. 90:706, 1985.

Daig, D.T.: Atelectic bronchiectasis of the right middle lobe. Tubercle 27:173, 1946.

Dozier, R.R., et al.: Sclerosing mediastinitis involving major bronchi. Mayo Clin. Proc. 43:557, 1968.

Fearon, B., and Shorted, R.: Tracheobronchial compression by congenital cardiovascular anomalies in children: syndrome of apnea. Ann. Otol. 72:949, 1963.

Feigin, D.S., Eggleston, J.C., and Siegelman, S.S.: The multiple roentgen manifestations of sclerosing mediastinitis. Johns Hopkins Med. J. 144:1, 1979.

Gemliner, C.H., Mullins, C.E., and McMarmara, D.G.: Pulmonary artery sling. Am. J. Cardiol. 45:311, 1980.

Haller, J.A., Jr., et al.: Life-threatening respiratory distress from mediastinal masses in infants. Ann. Thorac. Surg. 19:364, 1975.

Harris, S.H., de Niord, R.N., and Teague, F.B., Jr.: Etiology and surgical management of middle lobe syndrome. Va. Med. Monthly 100:713, 1973.

Lenox, C.C., et al.: Pneumonectomy for intractable, left bronchial compression in transposition of the great arteries. J. Thorac. Cardovasc. Surg. 77:212, 1979.

Mandell, G.A., Lantrin, R., and Goodman, C.R.: Tracheobronchial compression in Hodgkin's lymphoma in children. AJR 139:1167, 1982.

McElvein, R.B., and Mayo, P.: Middle lobe disease. South. Med. J. 60:1029, 1967.

Miller, W.W., Park, C.D., and Waldhausen, J.A.: Bronchial compression from enlarged hypertensive right pulmonary artery with corrected transposition of great arteries, dextrocardia and ventricular septal defect. J. Thorac. Cardiovasc. Surg. 60:233, 1970.

Riokin, L.M., et al.: Massive atelectasis of the left lung in children with congenital heart disease. J. Thorac. Surg. 34:116, 1957.

Rudolph, A.M.: Pulmonary complications of congenital heart disease (Editorial). Pediatrics 43:757, 1969.

Sashegyi, B., and Malatinszky, I.: Bronchial pulmonary disease associated with tuberculous lymph nodes. Am. Rev. Resp. Dis. 97:880, 1968.

Simeak, C.: Middle lobe syndrome. Respiration 27:100, 1970.

Stanger, P., Lucas, R,.V., and Edwards, J.E.: Anatomic factors causing respiratory distress in acyanotic congenital cardiac disease. Special reference to bronchial obstruction. Pediatrics 43:760, 1969.

Todres, I.D., Reppert, S.M., and Walker, R.F.: Management of critical airway obstruction in a child with a mediastinal tumor. Anesthesiology 45:100, 1976.

Varkey, B., and Tristani, F.E.: Compression of pulmonary artery and branches by descending thoracic aortic aneurysm. Am. J. Cardiol. 34:610, 1974.

Verdant, A.: Chronic traumatic aneurysm of the descending thoracic aorta with compression of the tracheobronchial tree. Can. J. Surg. 27:278, 1984.

Yurdakul, Y., and Ayloc, A.: Surgical repair of tracheobroncheal compression by tuberculous lymph nodes. Br. J. Dis. Chest 73:305, 1979.

CHAPTER 68

PULMONARY TUBERCULOSIS AND OTHER MYCOBACTERIAL INFECTIONS OF THE LUNG

Thomas W. Shields

Symptomatic pulmonary disease caused by infections by *Myocbacterium tuberculosis,* or less often by other mycobacterial organisms, continues to be a significant health problem in the United States. Approximately 7% of the population is infected with the tubercle bacillus. Stead (1970) estimated the risk of developing clinical tuberculosis at 3.3% or one out of every 30 newly infected individuals. Sbarbaro (1975) projected that within 5 years, between 5 and 15% of those newly infected with *M. tuberculosis* will develop clinically significant disease and that 3 to 5% of those who do not will develop clinical disease sometime during their lifetime.

No age group, race, or sex is exempt from the disease; however, it is clinically manifested at present more often in the elderly, in minorities, and in many of the new immigrant groups. Although most of the clinical problems are effectively managed by antituberculous chemotherapy, surgical intervention is required on occasion to salvage some patients with the disease.

ETIOLOGY

Pulmonary tuberculosis is caused by the acid-fast organism, *Mycobacterium tuberculosis.* This bacillus produces invasive debilitating infection in man and is said to be so virulent that infection may be initiated by introduction of a single organism to an alveolar membrane of a susceptible person.

The bacilli responsible for the pulmonary infection are, most often, airborne, and the patient's history usually reveals a close contact with a person or persons having the disease. The disease is highly contagious, and outbreaks often are reported in closed populations of susceptible persons, such as the personnel of naval ships and crowded schools.

The initial infection of the lung most often results in the formation of a primary complex—the primary Ghon tubercle with secondary foci of tuberculosis in the hilar lymph nodes—and the development of hypersensitivity to the organism manifested by a cutaneous reaction to tuberculin or its derivatives. Occasionally, the primary infection in children results in progressive disease, such as the development of extensive pneumonia, granulomatous involvement of the hilar nodes, endobronchial disease, or miliary spread.

Most instances of clinical infection caused by the tubercle bacillus, however, are in persons already sensitized to the organism and, thus, represent a postprimary infection, frequently referred to, in the past, as reinfection tuberculosis. The postprimary infection may arise in any one of four ways: by direct progression of a primary lesion, by reactivation of a quiescent primary lesion, by hematogenous spread to the lungs, or by exogenous superinfection. Most instances of post-primary pulmonary tuberculosis are thought to arise either as progression of a primary lesion in the young or as reactivation of a dormant lesion–primary or postprimary—in the middle-aged or older person. Thus, most of the infections are considered to be of endogenous rather than of exogenous origin.

The structure and growth characteristics in culture of *M. tuberculosis* are discussed in Chapter 16.

With improved and more sophisticated methods of culture, other mycobacteria have been found to cause pulmonary disease in small percentage—3 to 5%—of patients thought to have infection caused by *M. tuberculosis.* In the past, most designated these organisms as atypical mycobacteria. They have been discussed and classified in Chapter 16. More than 50 species of the organisms have now been described, of which half, as reviewed by Wayne (1986), are recognized as pathogenic in varying degrees. The more important ones in man are *M. kansasii*—group I photochromogens—and *M. avium complex* or the Battey bacillus—group III nonchromogens and *M. fortuitum*—rapid growers. In patients with other underlying lung diseases such as chronic obstructive pulmonary disease, interstitial fibrosis, or pneumoconiosis, superimposed infections caused by *M. gor-*

donae, *M. simiae*, *M. szulgai*, *M. scrofulaceum*, *M. xenopi*, and *M. chelonei* have occasionally been reported.

Infections caused by *M. kansasii* tend to occur in a distinctly different group of patients than do those infections caused by *M. tuberculosis*. Lichtenstein and colleagues (1965), in summarizing their experience in Chicago, found that patients with infections caused by *M. kansasii* were more likely to be middle-aged men living in good economic surroundings, in contrast to patients with *M. tuberculosis*, who more commonly were living in overcrowded housing under poor economic conditions. In addition, *M. kansasii* does not appear to be contagious from human to human as is *M. tuberculosis;* only rare instances have been reported in which infection has occurred in more than one member of a family. Early experience showed that the highest incidence of *M. kansasii* infection was in midwestern cities; specifically Kansas City, Dallas, and Chicago. With increased awareness of the organism, isolates are being recognized now in many other parts of this country and the world.

Organisms from Runyon's group II scotochromogens are rarely associated with infection, although in one collected series, Kestle and associates (1967) reported 26 of 50 isolates of *M. scrofulaceum* associated with what was thought to be invasive infection. Gracey and Byrd (1970), however, found only one of 71 patients with sputum cultures containing these organisms to have pulmonary disease attributable to the organism. Infection from *M. scrofulaceum* does occur, however, in cervical lymph nodes, particularly in children. Ordinarily, the organism's virulence is considered to be low. A second scotochromogen, *M. gordonae* or the tap-water bacillus, which can be confused with *M. scrofulaceum*, is rarely associated with infection in human beings. Perhaps the most important aspect of the scotochromogenic mycobacteria, and particularly *M. scrofulaceum*, is the evidence from skin testing found by Smith (1967), as well as Klare and associates (1967), that inapparent infection has taken place with this organism in about half of the population of the United States by the time they are in their early twenties. Such evidence was gained by determining skin hypersensitivity by using a specific purified protein derivative—PPD—made from *M. scrofulaceum*—PPD-G—Gause strain. These studies showed that the organism is widely prevalent in the environment and is associated with inapparent infection in a much larger segment of the population than is *M. tuberculosis*. Recognition that there probably has been a previous subclinical infection with *M. scrofulaceum* may explain the increased isolation of this organism from patients who excrete viable organism but show little or no evidence of active infection.

Although as many as five mycobacterial species have been classified in the group III nonchromogens, only two are considered to be a significant cause of infection in man: *M. avium complex* and *M. xenopi*. The remaining organisms in group III are important only to the laboratory in the differentiation from *M. avium complex*—the Battey bacillus—and *M. xenopi*. Pulmonary infections with the Battey bacillus are similar to those caused by *M. kansasii* in that they are most common in an older age group and not as contagious as those caused by *M. tuberculosis*. Like infections from *M. kansasii*, infections from *M. avium complex* cluster geographically along the southern seaboard of the United States, where apparent prior contact with the organisms, as shown by skin testing, is about four times greater in children than is their contact with *M. tuberculosis*. *M. xenopi*, also formerly classified in Runyon's group III, was first isolated from the South African toad, *Xenopus laevis*. Pulmonary infection with *M. xenopi* has been described in England. Marks and Schwabacher (1965) reported that isolation of the organism from 50 patients was considered to be clinically significant in 20 and of doubtful significance in an additional six.

Infections with the rapidly growing mycobacteria in group IV are uncommon and, for the most part, are restricted to *M. fortuitum*. As with occasional infections from *M. scrofulaceum* and other weakly pathogenic strains of mycobacteria, *M. fortuitum* usually is seen as a complication of underlying and, most frequently, severe debilitating disease.

PATHOLOGY

Primary Pulmonary Tuberculosis

The primary infection is located most often in the peripheral portion of the mid-zone of the lung. The initial reaction to the invasion of *M. tuberculosis* bacilli is an exudative reaction in the involved, but still intact, alveolar spaces. With the development of hypersensitivity—usually within 6 weeks—caseous necrosis develops in the center of the lesion. At this point, healing is initiated in the lesion by the migation of fibroblasts. Progressive hyalinization and, eventually, calcification occur. Enlargement of the regional lymph nodes draining the primary infection also occurs. As noted, a few persons have progressive disease that, in reality, is a progression directly into postprimary pulmonary tuberculosis.

Postprimary Pulmonary Tuberculosis

This phase of the disease tends to be localized primarily in the apical and posterior segments of the upper lobes and the superior segments of the lower lobes, but other areas are not exempt. The process consists of foci of caseous necrosis with edema, hemorrhage, and mononuclear cell infiltration. These foci may coalesce, and the caseous areas may liquefy and empty into a bronchus. In addition to the caseous necrosis, tubercles continue to develop at the periphery of the necrotic lesions.

The tubercle is composed of a central mass of epithelioid cells in which Langhans's type of giant cells and varying degrees of caseation occur. The periphery is surrounded by lymphocytes, fibroblasts, and fibrous tissue (Fig. 68–1). With appropriate staining techniques, mycobacteria may be demonstrated within the lesion, usually at the junction of the epithelial cells and the caseous necrosis.

With progression of the disease, increased amounts of

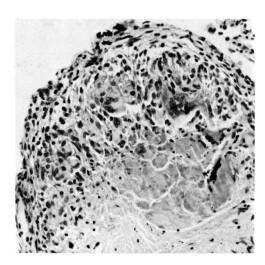

Fig. 68–1. Photomicrograph of tubercle in the lung.

lung tissue are destroyed and undergo caseation necrosis. Rupture of such large areas of necrosis into a bronchus results in the formation of the characteristic cavites seen in association with the disease. At the same time, attempts at healing take place and are represented by fibrosis and contracture of the involved areas. Depending on the resistance of the host, the virulence of the infecting organisms, and the adequacy of treatment, varying patterns of parenchymal destruction and associated healing may appear.

Early, the exudative, edematous phase is prominent; this stage may go on to complete healing with fibrosis, contracture, and, at times, calcification of the involved areas. In other patients, destruction of lung tissue exceeds the healing process, and caseation and subsequent cavitation are the major features. In some patients, the disease shows progression resembling an acute pneumonic process.

Initially, the cavities may be small and multiple and the walls irregular, thin, and pliable. These may fuse to form large or even giant cavities (Fig. 68–2). The walls

become thick and fibrous, and incomplete septa and trabeculations may appear within the cavities, representing surviving bronchovascular bundles. Because the blood supply of these trabeculae, as well as that of the wall of the cavity, is from the bronchial arterial system, erosion and rupture of these vessels may be the source of frequent hemoptysis. Multiple, bronchial communications are present, and with healing, the cavities become lined by a fibrous membrane. Extensive fibrosis and scarring occur in the adjacent parenchymal tissue (Fig. 68–3).

The tuberculous cavity may become secondarily infected by other bacteria, yeasts, or fungi, and these may contribute to the destructive process. Air-trapping may result from stenotic bronchi, now infrequently seen, and tension or giant cavities may develop. Smaller cavities may develop fibrous linings and come to resemble bronchiectatic sacs. Often, if this process does not occur, the cavity may become filled with inspissated caseous material. The lesion, thus, becomes a tuberculoma. The other cause of a tuberculoma—a large, conglomerate tubercle—is a parenchymal focus, either primary or postprimary. The tuberculoma resulting from the accumulation of caseous material in a cavity is associated most often with tuberculous bronchostenosis. This latter, as Lindskog and Liebow (1953) noted, results from one or several mechanisms: many small proliferative tuberculous lesions within the bronchial wall; extensive caseous necrosis within intramucosal tubercles; or necrosis of cartilage resulting from tuberculous chrondritis. These processes may occur in bronchi of any caliber, but with

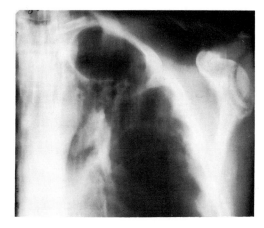

Fig. 68–2. AP laminogram of thin-walled, giant cavity in the left upper lobe. Several small cavities are seen below extending toward the hilus.

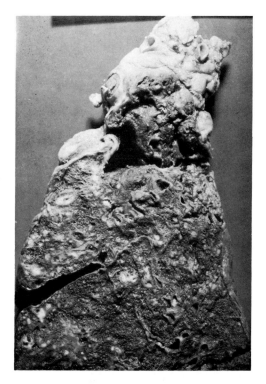

Fig. 68–3. Autopsy specimen of cut lung showing extensive apical pleural involvement, a large cavity in the apical area, plus numerous smaller cavities and fibrocaseous nodules throughout the lung tissue.

modern antituberculous chemotherapy, major bronchial involvement is rare.

Tuberculous bronchiectasis appears in upper lobes extensively involved by the disease process. This condition may result from healing and fibrosis of the tuberculous cavities, but also, the pathogenesis may resemble that of nontuberculous bronchiectasis (Chapter 66). True ectasia can be differentiated from fibrous-lined cavities by the multiple fistulous communications between the sacs in the latter.

Pleural involvement is frequent, and dense, fibrotic pleural adhesions are common. Pleural effusion also is common, and even so-called idiopathic pleural effusion may be the first clinical manifestation of the disease process.

Other Mycobacterial Infections

The pathologic changes observed in pulmonary disease produced by mycobacteria other than *M. tuberculosis* are essentially the same as those produced by *M. tuberculosis*, and no real differences are seen upon histologic examination of the tissue.

CLINICAL MANIFESTATIONS

Primary Infection

Most instances of primary infection caused by *M. tuberculosis* present no clinical manifestations and are discovered only at some later date by cutaneous tuberculin sensitivity or indirectly by the finding of a primary—Ghon—complex on a roentgenogram of the chest. Various factors influence the course of the initial infection and, of these, age, sex, heredity, and race, economic status, intercurrent disease, and psychologic factors are believed to be the most important.

Infants are thought to be the least resistant to continued activity of the organism, children from 5 years of age to puberty are apparently the most resistant, and a decrease in resistance extending into adult life appears to occur at puberty. Actually, however, the study of Myers and colleagues (1963) showed that, in many tuberculin reactors between birth and 5 years of age, only 8 to 9% developed clinical evidence of disease. Sixty percent of the patients with active disease recovered, whereas 40%—approximately 3% of the entire group—died because of tuberculosis. These data suggest that young children can resist the disease, although they do seem more prone to develop miliary tuberculosis and tuberculous meningitis than members of any other age group are.

Economic conditions, intercurrent disease, and social habits, as these affect the individuals, appear to be more important in the resistance to continued activity of the primary infection as well as to its progression into the postprimary state.

After the development of the primary complex and of tuberculin sensitivity, healing takes place in most persons without the development of any clinical manifestations. The disease in the small remainder progresses into one or more of the following clinical states: acute hematogenous dissemination with the development of miliary tuberculosis and tuberculous meningitis; extension to the pleura with development of pleurisy and pleural effusion; pulmonary parenchymal spread manifested as tuberculous pneumonia (Fig. 68–4); tracheobronchial tree compression by enlarged lymph nodes causing atelectasis; progression into the postprimary pulmonary disease evidenced by cavitation and extensive parenchymal involvement, or extrathoracic spread to other organ systems.

With pulmonary involvement, fever, cough, anorexia, weight loss, sweating, chest pain, lethargy, and dyspnea are common complaints. In the younger age group, erythema nodosum is a frequent finding and may be the initial presenting feature in as many as 12% of those with active disease.

Postprimary Infection

Many terms, such as adult progressive, reinfection, reactivation, and chronic pulmonary tuberculosis refer to postprimary tuberculosis. In many persons, tuberculosis is first discovered in a quiescent phase, an active phase of the postprimary infection having gone undetected. Such persons are asymptomatic and are classified as having inactive disease. Unfortunately, many patients who have active postprimary disease are also asymptomatic even in the presence of advanced disease.

About half of the new postprimary infections are found on routine roentgenographic screening of the chest. Of these, an estimated 10 to 30% occur in persons with active disease. The other patients are discovered by investigation of constitutional or respiratory symptoms, or both.

Generalized malaise, lassitude, easy fatigability, anorexia, and weight loss occur early in the course of active infection. Afternoon fever and night sweats are common. Any or all such symptoms are easily attributable to other, less serious diseases. In a susceptible person, such as the alcoholic, the drug addict, the immunosuppressed, the indigent, the diabetic, or one on corticosteriod medication, however, a high index of suspicion should be maintained in face of such general complaints.

Symptoms and signs referable to the lungs consists of cough, sputum production, hemoptysis, pleuritic chest pain, hoarseness, and shortness of breath.

Cough and sputum production are variable, but most patients with active disease have either one or both during the course of the disease. Hemoptysis is not an early symptom, but occurs in the presence of well established disease. Actually, it is not a common symptom. The expectoration is seldom profuse, although at times it may be massive and life-threatening. Generally, the hemoptysis is bright red, homogeneous, and self-limited. Persistent blood streaking of the sputum is unusual and should arouse the suspicion of bronchial carcinoma.

Chest pain is pleuritic and is affected by deep breathing and cough. It occurs infrequently in postprimary infection and, if the pain is persistent, the presence of

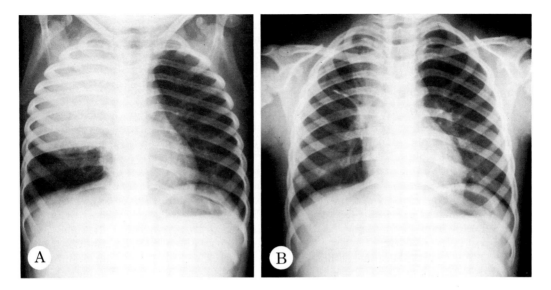

Fig. 68–4. *A,* PA roentgenogram of the chest of an infant with tuberculous pneumonia of the entire right upper lobe. *B,* After medical treatment, the patient at 3 years of age has a right upper lobe that is atelectatic and nonfunctioning.

carcinoma of the lung involving the pleura should be suspected.

Shortness of breath may result from pleural effusion, the extensive destruction of the lung parenchyma, or even from generalized toxemia with hyperventilation secondary to a high fever.

Other Mycobacteria-Infections

The clinical findings in patients with pulmonary infections caused by the other pathogenic mycobacteria resemble those present with disease caused by *M. tuberculosis.*

The patients, however, are more often middle-aged adults with average economic backgrounds. Pleural involvement is infrequent, and the chest roentgenogram often reveals that the disease is much more extensive than the symptoms suggest. Other mycobacterial infections, particularly those caused by *M. avium complex* are frequently seen in immunocompromised patients.

ROENTGENOGRAPHIC FEATURES

Primary Pulmonary Tuberculosis

The roentgenographic manifestations of primary infection with *M. tuberculosis,* as Fraser and Paré (1970) noted, may appear in the pulmonary parenchyma, in the hilar and mediastinal lymph nodes, in the tracheobronchial tree, and in the pleural space. The parenchymal involvement is most often in the midzone of the lung and resembles a pneumonic consolidation of variable size. The area is homogeneous in density, and the margins are ill defined, although an entire lobe may be involved with resultant sharply defined margins. Cavitation is uncommon in primary tuberculosis. Calcification may occur in the area of parenchymal involvement (Fig. 68–5).

Hilar or paratracheal lymph node enlargement appears

in almost all children with primary tuberculosis; it is less common in the adult. The enlargement may be bilateral or unilateral and hilar or paratracheal, or both.

Tracheobronchial involvement is common and, more often, results from compression by enlarged lymph nodes and, less commonly, from direct involvement of the structure by the disease process. Resultant partial or complete atelectasis of the lung distal to the obstruction occurs, although obstructive emphysema is occasionally present. Any lobe or segment may be involved, but because of the angle of the takeoff of the various segmental bronchi and the distribution of the lymph nodes about them, the anterior segment of the upper lobes and the medial segment of the middle lobe are more likely to be involved.

Pleural involvement with the development of an ef-

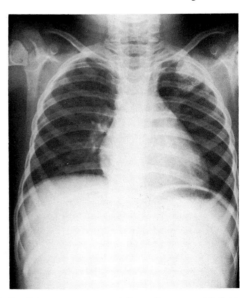

Fig. 68–5. PA roentgenogram of chest of 3½-year-old child with calcified residual of a primary infection in the left upper lobe.

fusion is more common in the young adult than in the child. The volume of the effusion is variable, and may be, but usually is not, associated with a demonstrable parenchymal lesion.

Postprimary Pulmonary Tuberculosis

Unlike primary tuberculosis, postprimary pulmonary tuberculosis is identified most often in the apical posterior segments of the upper lobes and less so in the superior segment of the lower lobes. An entire lobe or lung may, however, be involved in extensive disease. Rarely, the inflammatory processes may be isolated in the anterior segment of the upper lobes or in one of the basilar segments of the lung. If this situation occurs, particularly in the older patient, the possibility of carcinoma of the lung must be ruled out.

The roentgenographic features reflect the pathologic process present in the lung. Although the findings are often characteristic, definitive diagnosis of tuberculosis can be made only by the identification of the organism by culture or by microscopic examination of a specimen of the lung obtained at either operation or autopsy.

Many roentgenographic patterns can be identified in postprimary tuberculosis; Fraser and Paré (1970) listed local exudative lesions, local fibroproductive lesions, cavitation, bronchial spread and acute tuberculous pneumonia, miliary tuberculosis, bronchiectasis, bronchostenosis, and tuberculoma.

Local exudative lesions cause patchy or confluent alveolar consolidation. The lymphatic drainage markings radiating toward the hilus are accentuated.

Local fibroproductive lesions are defined more sharply, although their size and shape may vary. A decrease in lung volume evidences fibrosis and contracture, and the hilus and trachea are sometimes retracted toward the lesion (Fig. 68–6).

Cavitary lesions have moderately thick walls, but with healing, these tend to become thin; the inner surface linings are smooth, and air fluid levels are seen only infrequently (Fig. 68–7). The cavities may disappear following adequate therapy, but some persist as open "negative" cavities. Laminography may be necessary to verify the persistence of some cavities after therapy.

Active tuberculous infection in patients with a compromised immune system such as those with the acquired immune deficiency syndrome—AIDS—roentgenographically manifest a picture similar to that seen in children—primary pulmonary tuberculosis—rather than that normally seen in the adult with postprimary pulmonary tuberculosis, although in most if not all such patients, the infection is a postprimary reactivation. Pitchenik and Rubinson (1985) reviewed the roentgen findings in two groups of Haitian patients, one with and the other without AIDS. Table 68–1 summarizes their findings. Thus, in the immunocompromised adult host, atypical roentgenographic findings should alert the clinician to the possibility of tuberculosis.

Other Mycobacterial Infections

The roentgenographic manifestations of pulmonary disease caused by mycobacteria other than *M. tuberculosis* are generally those of moderate to far-advanced parenchymal involvement and may not be differentiated accurately from those of disease caused by *M. tuberculosis*. Some features, however, appear to be more characteristic of the infections caused by other mycobacteria. In infection with mycobacteria other than *M. tuberculosis*, cavitation with multiple, thin-walled cavities is more common than in infection with the tubercle bacillus; exudative lesions are uncommon, and hematogenous dissemination and pleural effusion are rare. Nonetheless, the two diseases rarely can be differentiated by the roentgenographic features alone. The observation that the patient with infection caused by mycobacteria other than *M. tuberculosis* is often less sick than the extensive roentgenographic findings suggest is important.

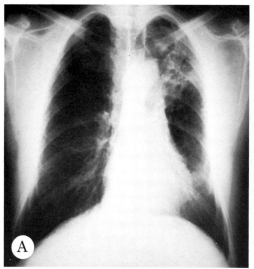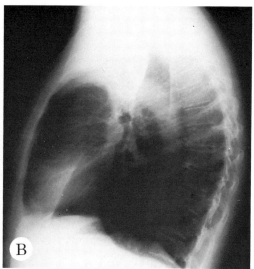

Fig. 68–6. PA *(A)* and lateral *(B)* chest roentgenograms of the chest showing fibrosis and contracture of the superior division—apical posterior and anterior segments—of the left upper lobe.

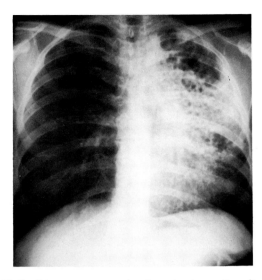

Fig. 68–7. PA roentgenogram showing extensive cavitary disease of the left lung.

DIAGNOSIS

The diagnosis of pulmonary tuberculosis may be suggested by the history and the clinical and roentgenographic manifestations, but depends soley on identification of the infecting organism or the histologic features and demonstration of the organism in a specimen of the lung.

Skin testing is important epidemiologically and the nonreaction to test doses of various strengths, except in certain circumstances, such as immunocompromise, miliary tuberculosis, or severe debilitation from the disease process, excludes the possibility of the disease.

The collection and treatment of material for culture of the organism is outlined in Chapter 16.

Bronchoscopy frequently is indicated, especially if the disease process is not responding well to therapy or if change in therapy is anticipated. The possibility of active endobronchial disease should be ruled out before surgical therapy, especially in those patients who continue to have the causative organisms in their sputum.

Special roentgenographic studies, such as laminography, and at times bronchography, as Langston and Tuttle (1966) recommended, should be performed in evaluating patients for possible surgical therapy. Computed tomography may help delineate the extent of associated parenchymal disease in patients with extensive pleural disease before any surgical decision is made.

Because many patients suspected of having tuberculosis are old, special care must be used to rule out the possibility of bronchial carcinoma. Although the risk of bronchial carcinoma in patients with pulmonary tuberculosis may be increased, the major problem is the coexistence of the two diseases. This problem is perplexing, particularly in the old patient with tuberculosis who has had stable roentgenographic findings and then manifests a change in the chest roentgenograms. Also, the old patient who initially presents with roentgenographic findings that suggest pulmonary tuberculosis and has a positive skin reaction to PPD causes concern if the smears and cultures of the sputum are negative for mycobacteria. A high index of suspicion must be maintained that these roentgenographic findings represent a bronchial carcinoma, and the patient must be evaluated and managed as if the disease process is carcinoma of the lung. Roentgenographic findings of unilateral prominence of one hilus; paratracheal node involvement; an atelectatic segment or lobe without mottling, linear streaking, or cavitation; homogeneous spread of the disease under adequate medical management; or a nodular density greater than 3 cm in diameter should suggest the possibility of carcinoma. If doubt remains, exploratory thoracotomy, when feasible, should be carried out after

Table 68–1. Results of Initial Pretreatment Chest Radiographs in Patients with Pulmonary Tuberculosis with and without Acquired Immune Deficiency Syndrome

Patients	Patients with AIDS 17		Patients without AIDS 30	
	No.	%	No.	%
Hilar and/or mediastinal adenopathy	10	59%	1	3%
Localized pulmonary infiltrates involving middle or lower lung field	5	29%	1	3%
Localized pulmonary infiltrates involving upper lobes	3	18%	29	97%
Diffuse interstitial miliary infiltrates*	1	6%	0	0%
Diffuse interstitial linear infiltrates†	2	12%	0	0%
Pulmonary cavities	0	0%	20	67%
No pulmonary infiltrates	6	35%	0	0%
Normal chest radiograph	2	12%	0	0%
Pleural effusion‡	2	12%	2	7%

*Two additional patients had miliary tuberculosis documented within 10 days of their initial chest radiography, which was technically good. The milary pulmonary lesions were seen on a follow-up chest radiograph in one of them and at autopsy in the other.

†Both patients with diffuse interstitial linear infiltrates has concurrent Pneumocystis carinii pneumonia.

‡Pleural effusions were small in the patients with AIDS.

Reproduced with permission from Pitchenik, A.E., and Rubinson, H.A.: The radiographic appearance of tuberculosis in patients with the acquired immune deficiency syndrome (AIDS). Am. Rev. Respir. Dis. *131*:393, 1985.

a short, intensive course of antituberculous chemotherapy.

TREATMENT

Medical Therapy

The primary treatment of pulmonary disease caused by *M. tuberculosis* is medical. Various combinations of the many antituberculous chemotherapeutic drugs are employed. When a single drug is used, no matter how specific, early development of bacterial resistance occurs. In contrast, when combinations of two or more agents are used, resistance is postponed or even prevented. In many clinics, these chemotherapeutic agents are divided into first-line and second-line drugs. The first-line drugs are isonicotinic acid hydrazide—INH, ethambutol—EMB, and rifampin. Streptomycin is used less frequently because its mode of administration by injection necessitates frequent patient visits. Pyrazinamide was not considered a first-line drug, but O'Brien and Snider (1985) noted that when it is added to the initial drug regimen, it can effectively reduce the length of treatment required. For this reason, this drug belongs in the first-line group. Second-line drugs include para-aminosalicylic acid—PAS, cycloserine, viomycin, ethionamide, capreomycin, and kanamycin. All of the aforementioned drugs carry some potential toxicity. Demonstration of individual patient toxicity or intolerance determines the drug regimen to be followed. Table 68–2 lists the dosage, toxicity, and tests for side effects of these drugs.

The principle of antituberculous chemotherapy is the action of the drugs on the metabolic processes of the tubercle bacillus. Table 68–2 lists the sites of action of the drugs, as well as whether they are bactericidal or bacteriostatic. For the drugs to have an effect, the organism must be actively metabolizing, although there is some indication that rifampin can kill even dormant organisms. Nonetheless, most organisms apparently do metabolize within a 2-year period because active treatment for 18 to 24 months reduces the relapse rate to less than 2%.

The American Thoracic Society (1983) suggested the following acceptable treatment regimens: (1) isoniazid and rifampin for 9 months with ethambutol or streptomycin for the initial 2 to 8 weeks—relapse less than 3%; (2) isoniazid and ethambutol for 18 months with the addition of streptomycin for the initial first to second month; and (3) isoniazid and streptomycin for 18 months. As noted, the addition of pyrazinamide to one of the aforementioned regimens during the initial 2 months of therapy may reduce treatment duration to 6 months without loss of treatment effectiveness.

Bacterial sensitivity studies are made routinely and may indicate the desirability of switching to other drugs. Some Asians and Hispanics as well as those persons with previous treatment or exposure to patients with drug-resistant organisms may have initial drug resistance. Certainly, if the initial regimen is clinically ineffective, addition or substitution of one of the second-line agents is indicated. Duration of treatment varies, depending upon individual patient response and the drug regimen selected.

Under adequate circumstances in cooperative patients, most pulmonary infections are controlled by such medical management. In patients who fail to adhere to the medical regimen or who have other serious associated disease, however, the failure rate, as Johnston and Wildrick (1974) noted, is 4 to 7%. Pitchenik and Rubinson (1985), as well as Dautzengberg and associates (1984), pointed out, however, that despite immunosuppression from AIDS or other causes, antituberculous drugs are apparently still effective.

The same chemotherapeutic agents are used, with some modifications, to treat infections caused by mycobacteria other than *M. tuberculosis*. Rifampin and isoniazid are the drugs most commonly employed, even though frequently the organisms, particularly *M. kansasii*, have been shown in vitro to be resistant to these drugs. Often these drugs are augmented by one or more of the second-line drugs. Therapy is given usually for 18 months. Response, as shown by conversion of the sputum and by the roentgenographic resolution of the parenchymal involvement, occurs slowly; often, conversion of the sputum is more pronounced than is roentgenographic evidence of resolution. In 20 to 30% of patients with infection caused by *M. kansasii*, the overall response is unsatisfactory. Therefore, more of the patients who have disease caused by this organism may become surgical candidates than of those who have infections caused by *M. tuberculosis*. Pulmonary disease caused by *M. avium complex*—the Battey bacillus—responds poorly. Medical therapy usually consists of four or more drugs. When the pathologic process is localized, most if not all of such patients with the disease are surgical candidates.

Pulmonary infections caused by *M. fortuitum* and *M. chelonei* are usually resistant to the standard antituberculosis agents. Young and Bailey (1988) advised medical therapy with cefoxitin and amikacin. Cefoxitin—200 mg/kg/day up to 12 g/day—and amikacin—15 mg/k/day—is given intravenously and continued for at least 12 weeks.

In patients with AIDS and disseminated *M. avium complex* infection, Masur and associates (1987) reported that clofazimine and ansamycin may be beneficial, although the experience with these drugs is limited.

Surgical Treatment

Present day surgical management of pulmonary tuberculosis and other atypical mycobacterial infections may be considered salvage therapy of past treatment failures. Resection of minor residual disease or open negative cavities is no longer indicated. Plombage thoracoplasty is obsolete and conventional thoracoplasty is rarely indicated except for some pleural complications that cannot be managed by decortication or transposition of muscle flaps.

Treatment failures can be classified into three categories: (1) failure of medical treatment—with modern management this should be no greater than 2 to 5% of

Table 68–2. Treatment of Mycobacterial Disease in Adults and Children

	Dosage		Most Common Side Effects	Tests for Side Effects	Remarks
	Daily Dose	Twice Weekly Dosage			
Commonly Used Agents					
Isoniazid	5 to 10 mg/kg up to 300 mg PO or IM	15 mg/kg PO or IM	Peripheral neuritis, hepatitis, hypersensitivity.	SGOT/SGPT (not as a routine).	Bactericidal to both extracellular and intracellular organisms. Pyridoxine 10 mg as prophylaxis for neuritis; 50 to 100 mg as treatment.
Rifampin	10 mg/kg up to 600 mg PO	10 mg/kg up to 600 mg PO	Hepatitis, febrile reaction, purpura (rare).	SGOT/SGPT (not as a routine).	Bactericidal to all populations of organisms. Orange urine and other body secretions. Discoloring of contact lens.
Streptomycin	15 to 20 mg/kg up to 1 g IM	25 to 30 mg/kg	8th nerve damage, nephrotoxicity.	Vestibular function, audiograms;* BUN and creatinine.	Bactericidal to extracellular organisms. Use with caution in older patients or those with renal disease.
Pyrazinamide	15 to 30 mg/kg up to 2 g PO	50 to 70 mg/kg	Hyperuricemia, hepatotoxicity.	Uric acid, SGOT/SGPT.	Bactericidal to intracellular organisms. Combination with an aminoglycoside is bactericidal.
Ethambutol	15 to 25 mg/kg	50 mg/kg PO	Optic neuritis (reversible with discontinuation of drug; very rare at 15 mg/kg), skin rash.	Red-green color discrimination and visual acuity.* Difficult to test in a child under 3 years.	Bacteriostatic to both intracellular and extracellular organisms, primarily used to inhibit development of resistant mutants. Use with caution with renal disease or when eye testing is not feasible.
Less Commonly Used Agents					
Capreomycin	15 to 30 mg/kg up to 1 g IM		8th nerve damage, nephrotoxicity.	Vestibular function, audiograms;* BUN and creatinine.	Bactericidal to extracellular organisms in cavities. Use with caution in older patients. Rarely used with renal disease.
Kanamycin	15 to 30 mg/kg up to 1 g IM		Auditory toxicity nephrotoxicity, vestibular toxicity (rare).	Vestibular function, audiograms;* BUN and creatinine.	Bactericidal to extracellular organisms. Use with caution in older patients. Rarely used with renal disease.
Ethionamide	15 to 30 mg/kg up to 1 g PO		GI disturbance, hepatotoxicity, hypersensitivity.	SGOT/SGPT	Bacteriostatic to both intracellular and extracellular organisms. Divided dose may help GI side effects; has a metallic taste. Avoid use during pregnancy.
Para-aminosalicylic acid (aminosalicylic acid)	150 mg/kg up to 12 g PO		GI disturbance, hypersensitivity, hepatotoxicity, sodium load.	SGOT/SGPT	Bacteriostatic to extracellular organisms only. GI side effects very frequent, making cooperation difficult.
Cycloserine	10 to 20 mg/kg up to 1 g PO		Psychosis, personality changes, convulsions, rash	Psychologic testing.	Bacteriostatic to both intracellular and extracellular organisms. Alcohol may aggravate psychiatric problems. Very difficult drug to use. Side effects may be blocked by pyridoxine, ataractic agents, or anticonvulsant drugs.

*Initial examination should be done at start of treatment.

Reproduced with permission of the American Thoracic Society: Treatment of tuberculosis and other mycobacterial disease. Am. Rev. Respir. Dis. *127*:790, 1983.

the patients; (2) surgically correctable complications of the disease; and (3) complications of previous operations for the disease.

Medical Treatment Failures

A few patients with *M. tuberculosis* continue to have parenchymal disease with persistently positive sputa despite adequate drug therapy. The organisms in most if not all such patients are drug-resistant. In such patients, surgical resection, preferably a lobectomy, rarely a pneumonectomy, may be the only way to attempt to eradicate the disease (Fig. 68–8). A lesser procedure such as a segmentectomy is contraindicated. Unfortunately, with resection under the aforementioned circumstances, the morbidity and potential mortality rates may be high, and theoretically, may be similar to those observed in the pre-antimicrobial chemotherapy era. Postoperative spread and the development of a bronchopleural fistula are the two major concerns. No large series of such patients have been reported, so the true risk remains unknown.

In patients with atypical mycobacterial organisms, most often *M. kansasii* or *M. avium complex* persistent, drug-resistant organisms in the sputum are common. Those with *M. kansasii* infection often remain well and resection is not indicated. In those patients with *M. avium complex* organisms whose disease is localized, however, resection, preferably a lobectomy when possible, appears to be beneficial. Moran and his associates (1983) carried out 40 resections in 37 patients with this type of infection and reported that 31 patients remained entirely free of their disease after the operative procedure.

Surgically Correctable Complications

These primarily consist of destroyed lung parenchyma with persistent pyogenic or superimposed mycotic infection, massive life-threatening hemoptysis, and pleural disease—empyema with or without underlying lung disease or a bronchopleural fistula. Infrequently a clinically significant bronchostenosis, an expanding blocked cavity, or tuberculous bronchiectasis involving the middle or lower lobes (Fig. 68-9) or entire lung may necessitate surgical intervention. The first two of the latter are rare and the last is really a variety of destroyed lung parenchyma.

In patients with destroyed lung parenchyma, persistent infection may be caused by either pyogenic or fungal organisms. Attempts should be made to control a pyogenic infection by appropriate antibiotics and postural drainage. When this therapy is unsuccessful or infection recurs often, the destroyed tissue should be resected. This need for resection occurs more often in patients with lower lung field disease or those with an entire destroyed lung. Odell and Henderson (1985) reported 169 pneumonectomies necessitated by a destroyed lung associated with secondary infection or hemoptysis.

Superimposed fungal disease is most commonly caused by *Aspergillus fumigatus*, but infections with *Monosporium apiospermum* organisms were reported by Jung and his colleagues (1977). Intracavitary mycetoma are

seen with either of these infections. Hemoptysis is a common complaint, and massive life-threatening hemorrhage may occur, particularly in those patients in whom the underlying disease process is pulmonary tuberculosis. Because of this possibility, resection is indicated in these patients, although a more conservative approach, as Faulkner (1978) and Jewkes (1983) and their associates suggested, may be appropriate in patients with minor episodes of hemoptysis and myectoma not associated with underlying tuberculosis.

Massive life-threatening hemoptysis in patients with tuberculosis may occur also in the absence of a fungal infection because of erosion into a bronchial artery or more rarely secondary to pulmonary arterial bleeding caused by rupture of a Rasmussen's aneurysm in cavitary tuberculosis.

The management of massive hemoptysis and the timing of surgical intervention pose difficult problems. Initially, the patient should be positioned to minimize as much as possible aspiration of the blood. Bronchoscopy is necessary to identify the site of bleeding and, should this fail, bronchial arteriography is indicated. Gourin and Garzon (1974) recommended prompt surgical resection for any individual who has bled more than 600 ml in 24 hours or less. With such a course of action, the mortality rate was 18%, as compared to a 75% rate in those treated conservatively after bleeding this amount in 16 hours. When active bleeding is present at the time of operation, these authors recommended single-lung anesthesia with balloon occlusion of the bronchus of the bleeding lung over the use of a double-lumen endotracheal tube for the conduct of anesthesia. Garzon and his associates (1982) repeated this recommendation. McCollum and his associates (1975), however, wrote that the use of the double-lumen tube is satisfactory. Gottlieb and Hillberg (1975) advocated endobronchial tamponade with a Fogarty balloon catheter to control the bleeding, either before surgical intervention or if such intervention is contraindicated.

With the development of the technique of bronchial artery embolization, the necessity of surgical intervention before control of the bleeding site has been markedly reduced. At present, the appropriate therapeutic plan is to identify the side and lobar origin of the bleeding by bronchoscopy; endobronchial tamponade is then established as necessary to prevent flooding of the remaining noninvolved lung. With the bleeding temporarily controlled, bronchial arteriography is done to identify the bleeding area and the appropriate vessel is then embolized with gel foam. Eckstein (1986) and Shetty (1986) and their co-workers reviewed the technique, results, and potential complications of this procedure. Control of the acute episode can be expected in over 75% of patients. In the series reported by Uflacker and associates (1983), bleeding was controlled by embolization alone in 26 of 33 patients; in the remaining 7, surgical resection was required following the embolization. In the presence of a mycetoma and residual pulmonary disease, however, rebleed rate was high—43%. This was accompanied by a high mortality rate if interval resection

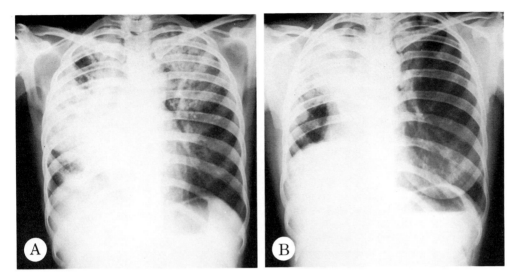

Fig. 68–8. *A*, PA roentgenogram of the chest showing extensive bilateral pulmonary tuberculosis. *B*, After prolonged antituberculous chemotherapy, the left lung is clear, but the right lung shows extensive parenchymal fibrosis and contraction. Sputum remained positive and pneumonectomy was required for control of the disease.

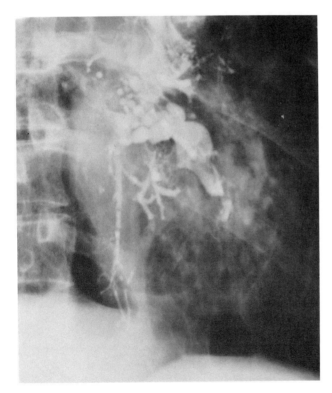

Fig. 68–9. Saccular tuberculous bronchiectasis of left lower lobe in adult patients with persistently positive sputa.

was not or could not be carried out. Thus, even though the bleeding is controlled by the initial embolization, elective resection of the involved area should be carried out when the patient's pulmonary function and the underlying disease are suitable for such a course of action. With this therapeutic approach, Uflacker and associates (1983) reported only an overall 7 to 9% mortality rate for the management of massive hemoptysis.

The management of pleural complications of pure or mixed tuberculous empyema with or without underlying lung disease has been discussed in Chapter 59. Decortication with or without pulmonary resection is usually indicated; on occasion, a pleuropneumonectomy may be necessary.

Complications of Previous Operations

These consist mainly of the migration of the plombage material subsequent to an earlier extraperiosteal plombage thoracoplasty or the occurrence and persistence of an empyema or bronchopleural fistula after a resectional procedure. The management of the migrating plomb is primarily the removal of the foreign material. The migration of the plomb—almost always a paraffin plomb—is a phenomenon of foreign body rejection. The migration is into the soft tissues external to the rib cage, and a lump forms beneath the muscles of the chest wall. When it occurs, it is most often localized posteriorly, although occasionally the axilla, subpectoral area, or even more rarely the supraclavicular region may be the site of the migration. This complication has developed as early as 5 or 6 months and as late as 10 or more years postoperatively. In a large series of wax plombage thoracoplasties, Fox and associates (1962) found that migration occurred in 25% of the patients. Simple removal is all that is indicated. Pyogenic infection of the residual space is rare. In contrast, Judd and colleagues (1954) noted that infection with fiberglass as a plombage material was high—26%. The management of postresectional complications of empyema or bronchopleural fistula is discussed in Chapters 32, 34, 35, and 59.

In patients with known or presumed tuberculosis, the question of the presence of malignant disease poses a problem, especially among patients with peripheral nodules; those who have a roentgenographic change in previously stable disease but whose sputum remains negative; and those with an undiagnosed pulmonary lesion but a positive tuberculin test. The management of these individuals requires appropriate diagnostic investigation, which may include thoracotomy.

In children, the indications for surgical intervention are few. A caseous pneumonic process may resolve much more slowly than in the adult; the decision concerning the advisability of operation frequently should be postponed for many months or years. In children, in addition to the indications as noted in adults, surgical treatment is required in the management of certain complications of progressive primary pulmonary tuberculosis. These complications are an uncontrolled, progressively enlarg-

ing primary parenchymal lesion with or without cavitation, persistent distal lobar or segmental atelectasis as the result of postprimary bronchostenosis, and clinically significant bronchiectasis (Fig. 68–10). Infrequently, bronchial obstruction may persist because of enlarged, involved peribronchial lymph nodes. With failure of response to medical therapy and persistence of symptoms, particularly respiratory distress, Nakvi and Nohl-Oser (1977) suggested excising or evacuating the caseous material to relieve the obstruction. Fortunately, these problems are encountered only infrequently. Although the overall incidence of surgical intervention, as Lees and associates (1967) reported, was approximately 5% in children with pulmonary tuberculosis under the age of 16 years, at present it is rare. Lowe and his associates (1980) reported that in a series of 140 children with pulmonary tuberculosis, surgical intervention was necessary in only 2 of these individuals for an incidence of only 1.4%.

Selection of the Surgical Procedure

In all patients with parenchymal disease that requires surgical intervention, resection is the procedure of

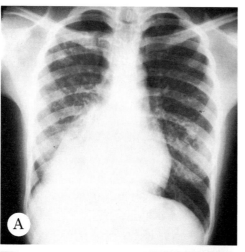

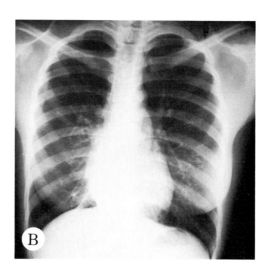

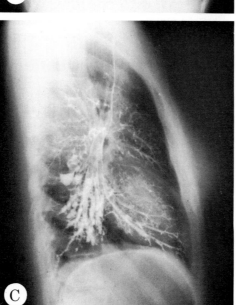

Fig. 68–10. *A,* PA roentgenogram of the chest of a 15-year-old girl with bilateral pulmonary tuberculosis and atelectasis of the right lower lobe. *B,* PA roentgenogram of chest, after 11 months of treatment, showing clearing of bilateral infiltrate but a completely atelectatic right lower lobe behind the border of the right side of the heart. *C,* Lateral view of the bronchogram showing extensive bronchiectatic changes throughout the entire right lower lobe.

choice. Conservation of pulmonary tissue to preserve as much pulmonary function as possible is indicated. Unfortunately, wedge resection or segmentectomy is rarely applicable for the control of the pulmonary disease that now requires resection. Lobectomy or pneumonectomy is most often necessary.

At times, particularly if the sputum contains drug-resistant strains of *M. tuberculosis*, or if it is thought that insufficient pulmonary tissue will remain after the resection to fill the normal-sized hemithorax, a preresection thoracoplasty may be performed.

Operative Techniques

The various types of pulmonary resections are discussed in Chapter 29 and do not differ in the surgical management of pulmonary tuberculosis. Extensive adhesions, however, that are frequently present between the parietal and visceral layers of the pleura over the areas of parenchymal involvement, render the mobilization of the lung difficult. Also, granulomatous involvement of the peribronchial nodes may cause these nodes to adhere markedly to the vascular and bronchial structures, which often makes the dissection of these structures tedious as well as hazardous. The management of associated tuberculous pleural disease is discussed in Chapter 59.

Postoperative Morbidity and Mortality

Complications are frequent after resections of the lung now required for the management of tuberculosis and the morbidity rates may range from 30 to 50%. Most of the complications are minor, such as asymptomatic persistent residual air spaces. Major complications, however, such as empyema, with or without a bronchopleural fistula; atelectasis as a consequence of retained secretions; postoperative intrapleural bleeding; and spread or reactivation of active tuberculous pulmonary disease may occur after surgical resection. The incidence of all complications is doubled when the preoperative sputum contains *M. tuberculosis*. If *M. kansasii* or *M. avium complex*—Battey bacillus—is present, however, the complication rate is similar to that in patients with *M. tuberculosis* infections and negative sputa. In children, the morbidity rates and complications are similar to those occurring in adults. In patients in whom the operations are done as an emergency life-saving maneuver, the mortality and morbidity rates are high.

Mortality varies with the selection of the patients and the extent of the surgical resections. The 60-day mortality rate after pneumonectomy varies from 8 to 12%—my associates and I (1970) reported a 10% rate. The rates after lobectomy have been 1.5% but may be as high as 20% in emergency operation for the control of massive bleeding.

Other Procedures

Thoracoplasty or cavernostomy rarely is performed in the treatment of pulmonary tuberculosis. A conventional thoracoplasty may be indicated to control a postresection empyema space but rarely, if ever, manage to parenchymal disease alone.

Cavernostomy is the external drainage of a tuberculous cavity. This procedure may be closed catheter drainage, as Monaldi (1939) proposed, or actual open marsupialization by direct and permanent opening of the chest wall over the cavity. Cautery, as Eloesser (1937) advocated, is used to induce cicatricial closure of the many bronchial communications in the exposed floor of such a cavity, and this technique may result in complete exteriorization of the cavity. The only current applications of cavernostomy are in a patient with a large cavity and persistent presence of tubercle bacilli in the sputum or massive bleeding that cannot be controlled otherwise, and insufficient pulmonary reserve to tolerate any major operative procedure, with resection or collapse. Although the procedure may permit temporary control of the bleeding, the outlook for any significant survival is almost nil.

Results of Surgical Therapy

Because surgical therapy is reserved almost exclusively for the failed group of patients or those with serious complications, the results of such intervention vary. When resistant primary tuberculous infection is controlled by a resection or a complication is corrected, the patient's prognosis is based on the functional status of the remaining lung tissue. As with any salvage procedure, the eventual results depend upon patient selection.

REFERENCES

American Thoracic Society: Treatment of tuberculosis and other mycobacterial disease. Am. Rev. Respir. Dis. *127*:790, 1983.

Dautzenberg, B., et al.: The management of thirty immunocompromised patients with tuberculosis. Am. Rev. Respir. Dis. *129*:494, 1984.

Eckstein, M.R., Waltman, A.C., and Athanasoulis, C.A.: The management of massive hemoptysis: control by angiographic methods. *In* Current Controversies in Thoracic Surgery. Edited by C.F. Kittle. Philadelphia, W.B. Saunders Co., 1986, pp. 255.

Eloesser, L.: Blocked cavities in pulmonary tuberculosis. J. Thorac. Surg. *7*:1, 1937.

Faulkner, S.L., et al.: Hemoptysis and pulmonary aspergilloma: operative versus nonoperative treatment. Ann. Thorac. Surg. *25*:389, 1978.

Fox, R.T., et al.: Extraperiosteal plombage thoracoplasty. J. Thorac. Cardiovasc. Surg. *44*:371, 1962.

Fraser, R.G., and Paré, J.A.P.: Diagnosis of Diseases of the Chest. Vol. II. Philadelphia, W.B. Saunders Co., 1970.

Garzon, A.A., Cerruti, M.M., and Golding, M.R.: Exsanguinating hemoptysis. J. Thorac. Cardiovasc. Surg. *84*:829, 1982.

Gottlieb, L.S., and Hillberg, R.: Endobronchial tamponade therapy for intractable hemoptysis. Chest *67*:482, 1975.

Gourin, A., and Garzon, A.A.: Operative treatment of massive hemoptysis. Ann. Thorac. Surg. *18*:52, 1974.

Gracey, D.R., and Byrd R.B.: Scotochromogens and pulmonary disease. Am. Rev. Respir. Dis. *101*:959, 1970.

Jewkes, J., et al.: Pulmonary aspergilloma: analysis of prognosis in relationship to hemoptysis and survey of treatment. Thorax *38*:572, 1983.

Johnston, R.F., and Wildrick, K.H.: "State of the art" review: the impact of chemotherapy on the care of patients with tuberculosis. Am. Rev. Respir. Dis. *109*:636, 1974.

Judd, A.R., Szypulski, J., and Kopernik, F.: The use of fiberglass in pulmonary tuberculosis. J. Thorac. Surg. 27:581, 1954.

Jung, J.Y., et al.: The role of surgery in the management of pulmonary monosporosis: a collective review. J. Thorac. Cardiovasc. Surg. 73:139, 1977.

Kestle, D.G., Abbott, V.D., and Kubica, G.P.: Differential identification of mycobacteria: subgroups of groups II and III (Runyon) with clinical significance. Am. Rev. Respir. Dis. 95:1941, 1967.

Klare, K.C., et al.: The prevalence of atypical mycobacterial tuberculin sensitivity in a selected population in New York City. Am. Rev. Respir. Dis. 95:103, 1967.

Langston, H.T., and Tuttle, W.M.: Pleuropulmonary tuberculosis. In Surgical Diseases of the Chest, 2nd ed. Edited by B. Blades. St. Louis, The C.V. Mosby Co., 1966, p. 185.

Lees, W.M., Fox, R.T., and Shields, T.W.: Pulmonary surgery for tuberculosis in children. Ann. Thorac. Surg. 4:327, 1967.

Lichtenstein, M.R., Takamura, Y., and Thompson, J.R.: Photochromogenic mycobacterial pulmonary infection in a group of hospitalized patients in Chicago. IL. Demographic studies. Am. Rev. Respir. Dis. 91:592, 1965.

Lindskog, G.E., and Liebow, A.A.: Chapter 9. In Thoracic Surgery and Related Pathology. New Haven, CT, Appleton-Century-Crofts, 1953, p. 191.

Lowe, J.E., et al.: Pulmonary tuberculosis in children. J. Thorac. Cardiovasc. Surg. 80:221, 1980.

Marks, J., and Schwabacher, H.: Infection due to Mycobacterium xenope. Br. Med. J. 1:32, 1965.

Masur, H., et al.: Effect of combined clofazime and ansamycin therapy on Mycobacterium avium-Mycobacterium intracellulare bacteremia in patients with AIDS. J. Infect. Dis. 155:127, 1987.

McCollum, W.B., et al.: Immediate operative treatment for massive hemoptysis. Chest 67:152, 1975.

Monaldi, V.: A propos du procede d'aspiration intracavitaire des cavernes pulmonaire selon Monaldi. Rev. Tuberc. 5:848, 1939.

Moran, J.F., et al.: Long-term results of pulmonary resection for atypical mycobacterial disease. Ann. Thorac. Surg. 35:597, 1983.

Myers, J.A., Bearman, J.E., and Dixon, H.: The natural history of tuberculosis in the human body. Am. Rev. Respir. Dis. 87:354, 1963.

Nakvi, A.J., and Nohl-Oser, H.C.: Surgical treatment of bronchial obstruction in primary tuberculosis in children: report of seven cases. Thorax 34:464, 1979.

O'Brien, R.J., and Snider, D.E.: Tuberculosis drugs—old and new. Am. Rev. Respir. Dis. 131:309, 1985.

Odell, J.A., and Henderson, B.J.: Pneumonectomy through an empyema. J. Thorac. Cardiovasc. Surg. 89:423, 1985.

Pitchenik, A.E., and Rubinson, H.A.: The radiographic appearance of tuberculosis in patients with the acquired immune deficiency syndrome (AIDS). Am. Rev. Respir. Dis. 131:393, 1985.

Sbarbaro, J.A.: Tuberculosis: the new challenge to the practicing clinician. Chest 68:436, 1975.

Shields, T.W., Fox, R.T., and Lees, W.M.: Changing role of surgery in the treatment of pulmonary tuberculosis. Arch. Surg. 100:363, 1970.

Shetty, P.C., and Magillijan, D.J.: The management of massive hemoptysis: treatment by bronchial artery embolization. In Current Controversies in Thoracic Surgery. Edited by C.F. Kittle. Philadelphia, W.B. Saunders Co., 1986, pp. 261.

Smith, D.T.: Diagnostic and prognostic significance of the quantitative tuberculin tests. Ann. Intern. Med. 67:919, 1967.

Stead, W.: Tuberculosis. In Harrison's Principles of Internal Medicine, ed. 6. Edited by M.M. Wintrobe, et al. New York, McGraw-Hill, 1970, p. 865.

Uflacker, R., et al.: Management of massive hemoptysis by bronchial artery embolization. Radiology 146:627, 1983.

Wayne, L.: The atypical mycobacteria: recognition and disease association. CRC Crit. Rev. Microbiol. 12:184, 1986.

Young, K., and Bailey, W.: Non-TB mycobacterial infections: a rapidly increasing danger. J. Resp. Dis. 9:20, 1988.

READING REFERENCES

Alexander, J.: The Collapse Therapy of Pulmonary Tuberculosis. Springfield, IL, Charles C Thomas, 1937.

Barrett, R.J., et al.: Pulmonary resection in the treatment of tuberculosis. J. Thorac. Surg. 36:803, 1958.

Chapman, J.S.: The Anonymous Mycobacteria in Human Disease. Springfield, IL, Charles C Thomas, 1960.

Fox, R.T., et al.: Extraperiosteal paraffin plombage thoracoplasty. J. Thorac. Cardiovasc. Surg. 44:371, 1962.

Fox, R.T., et al.: Bilateral extraperiosteal paraffin plombage for pulmonary tuberculosis. J. Thorac. Surg. 37:738, 1959.

Fox, R.T., et al.: Surgical considerations in "atypical" mycobacterial pulmonary disease. J. Thorac. Cardiovasc. Surg. 59:1, 1970.

Langston, H.T., Barker, W.L., and Pyle, M.M.: Surgery in pulmonary tuberculosis. Ann. Surg. 164:567, 1960.

Lees, W.M., Fox, R.T., and Shields, T.W.: Thoracic surgery for atypical mycobacterial pulmonary infection. Arch. Surg. 91:67, 1965.

Polk, J.W., Ponce, L., and Medina, M.: Surgical treatment in pulmonary infections due to atypical mycobacteria. Am. J. Surg. 113:739, 1967.

Shields, T.W., et al.: Persistent pleural air space following resection for pulmonary tuberculosis. J. Thorac. Cardiovasc. Surg. 38:523, 1959.

Steel, M.A., and Des Prez, R.M.: The role of pyrazinamide in tuberculosis chemotherapy. Chest 94:845, 1988.

CHAPTER 69

THORACIC ACTINOMYCETIC AND MYCOTIC INFECTIONS

Timothy Takaro

Actinomycetic infections, including actinomycosis and nocardiosis, have traditionally, albeit mistakenly, been classified and treated along with true fungal infections of the lungs in many textbooks for many years. "Actinomyces" literally means "ray fungus," for the radiating filaments in microcolonies, the formation of branching hyphae, and the production of spores. However, the actinomycetes are considered to be closer to bacteria than to fungi, and clearly respond to antibacterial rather than to antifungal agents. In the interests of common usage and expectation, however, they will be considered in this chapter.

THORACIC ACTINOMYCETIC INFECTIONS

Actinomycosis is a chronic infectious disease usually caused by *Actinomyces israelii*, rarely by *A. bovis*, and characterized by chronic suppuration, chronic sinus formation, and the discharge of purulent material containing yellow-brown "sulfur granules." These granules are actually microcolonies of the tangled hyphae of actinomycetes (Fig. 69–1). Because the organisms are anaerobic or microaerophilic, they require culturing under anaerobic conditions. They also require culturing of material from closed tissue spaces or from draining sinuses or abscesses; isolation from sputum or secretions from the mouth is not proof of infection, because the organism may reside normally in the oral cavity of man.

Clinical Features

There are three clinical syndromes: cervicofacial, thoracic, and abdominal. Thoracic actinomycosis usually results from bronchopulmonary infection following entry of organisms into the lungs through the oropharynx. Characteristically, the pleural and chest wall are involved, but as Eastridge and associates (1972) reported, this is usually preceded by some type of pulmonary infiltrate, or by dense hilar lymphadenopathy. The varieties of lung involvement are nonspecific, although Slade

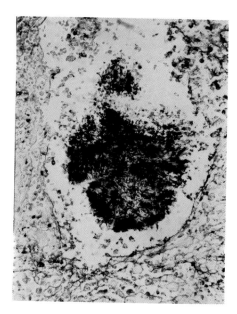

Fig. 69–1. Actinomycotic granule in a microabscess from a patient with actinomycosis. Note branching filaments in center of granule. Methenamine silver, × 200.

and colleagues (1973) emphasized that some of the presentations of actinomycosis may suggest bronchial carcinoma. The disease process may show extensions from one of the anatomic areas to the adjacent area: usually from the cervical or abdominal areas to the thoracic area (Fig. 69–2).

The roentgenographic manifestations of thoracic actinomycosis, as Balikian and associates (1978a) noted, although nonspecific, often involve the chest wall or pleurae, or both. Thus, pleural effusion or empyema, and rib erosion or periosteal involvement occur. Golden and associates (1985) emphasized the usefulness of body computed tomography in diagnosis. Rarely, as Datta and Raff (1974) reported, the pericardium may be involved.

The diagnosis of actinomycosis is difficult: first, be-

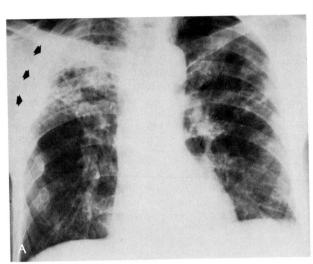
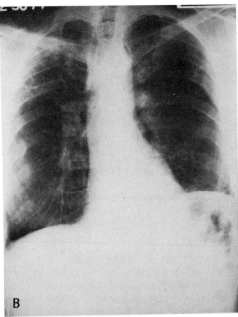

Fig. 69–2. Chronic thoracoabdominal actinomycosis. *A,* Fifty-year-old man with bilateral apical infiltrative disease was treated for presumptive diagnosis of pulmonary tuberculosis until left-sided pain, pleural fluid, and elevated diaphragm led to thoracotomy. A splenic actinomycetic abscess pointing through the diaphragm was removed; lung biopsy of extensive fibronodular disease also showed actinomycosis. Note pleural reaction, right upper lung (black arrows) and an elevated diaphragm left. The patient was treated with 20 million units of penicillin intravenously for 1 month, followed by 4 weeks of drug, 2.4 million units daily intramuscularly. *B,* Roentgenogram 2 years later. The disease process has cleared; except for elevated left diaphragm, chest roentgenogram is nearly normal. The disease did not recur over a 4-year follow-up period.

cause the disease is uncommon enough that it is not often suspected; second, because, being unsuspected, the anaerobic causative organism is often not given the appropriate cultural conditions; and third, because the roentgenographic resemblance to bronchial carcinoma often compels exploratory thoracotomy for diagnosis. Thus, in a series of 57 patients reported by Weese and Smith (1975), less than 10% were correctly diagnosed on admission.

Treatment

The drug of choice is penicillin. The dense fibrous tissue surrounding the colonies of organisms requires that high doses of antibiotics be used for long periods of time. McQuarrie and Hall (1968) recommended 20 million units of penicillin daily for 1 to 3 months. The tetracyclines, as Feingold and co-workers (1985) reported, are generally an adequate substitute when the patient is allergic to penicillin. The prognosis after effective treatment is good.

Exploratory thoracotomy on suspicion of carcinoma is the commonest indication for surgical intervention in patients with actinomycosis. Adequate and prolonged drug therapy is important following operation to prevent reactivation of disease or the development of empyema. If a preoperative diagnosis has been made, and excisional surgery is possible, for removal of a destroyed lobe, for example, it should be carried out under adequate drug coverage. Foley and associates (1971) reported that sometimes only drainage of an abscess or empyema may be possible, or necessary, but radical excision of sinus

tracts may also sometimes be feasible. Primary actinomycetic empyema is rare, as Harrison (1979) and Merdler (1983) and their associates noted, but may require decortication or pleural drainage as George and colleagues (1985) observed.

Nocardiosis is a chronic infectious disease usually caused by *Nocardia asteroides,* but occasionally also by *N. brasiliensis* and *N. madurae.* Some clinical features are similar to actinomycosis—chronic draining sinuses, "sulfur granules" in the exudate—but some differ, such as hematogenous dissemination from a pulmonary focus or central nervous system involvement, as both Frazier (1975) and Krick (1975) and their colleagues pointed out.

The organisms are aerobic, and occur not only in microcolonies, but also in coccobacillary or filamentous forms that are acid-fast and gram-positive. The former feature, as well as roentgenographic similarities, led in the past to confusion with the acid-fast bacilli of *Mycobacterium tuberculosis* (Fig. 69–3A).

Nocardia are widely distributed in soil, grains, and grasses, without a specific area of endemicity. It does not often occur as a saprophyte in man; thus, its presence in sputum, together with evidence of lung involvement, is presumptive evidence of disease.

The disease process varies widely, ranging from benign self-limited suppurative infections of the skin and subcutaneous tissues to pulmonary or generalized systemic infections. Balikian and associates (1978b) reported the roentgenographic features to be nonspecific pulmonary infiltrates resembling those of pulmonary tuberculosis, including solitary nodules and cavitation (Fig.

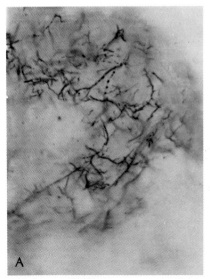

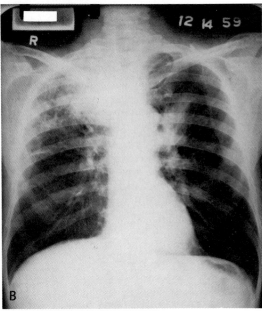

Fig. 69–3. Nocardiosis. *A*, Organisms of *Nocardia asteroides*. Gram's stain, × 1000. *B*, Roentgenogram of thorax showing bilateral pulmonary pneumonic infiltration. *Nocardia asteroides* was recovered from the sputum. The patient recovered after a course of sulfadiazine. (Takaro, T.: Thoracic actinomycetic and mycotic infections. *In* Practice of Surgery. Edited by H.S. Goldsmith. Hagerstown, MD, Harper & Row, 1978, Thoracic Surgery, Chap. 12.)

69–3*B*). Empyema caused by nocardia is also not rare. Central nervous system involvement—brain abscess or meningitis—which is ominous, may be the presenting picture, with minimal-appearing pulmonary disease.

The disease occurs primarily in immunosuppressed patients—85% of instances—including patients receiving organ transplants, being treated for malignancies, or those with AIDS. In the compromised host, cavitation or hematogenous dissemination, or both, may be accelerated. In the absence of a predisposing condition leading to the immunosuppressed state, nocardiosis may mimic bronchial carcinoma.

The diagnosis may be difficult to establish short of percutaneous lung aspiration, closed or open lung biopsy, or exploratory thoracotomy. The Gomori stain is useful, and aerobic culture media are necessary.

Treatment is primarily medical, sulfadiazine—4 to 8 g/day—or minocycline—100 mg BID being the mainstay. Prolonged treatment—at least 2 to 3 months, but sometimes longer—may be required. Surgical treatment may be required either to help make the diagnosis or, less frequently, to effect a cure. Drainage of empyemas and abscesses is indicated; with the use of specific drug coverage, this procedure has become safer.

THORACIC MYCOTIC INFECTIONS

Fungal infections of the lungs are not encountered commonly by most practicing thoracic surgeons. Exceptions are those surgeons practicing in the southwestern United States—the area endemic for coccidioidomycosis—and also those along the Mississippi Valley—the area of endemicity for histoplasmosis. Because mycotic lung infections mimic both bronchial carcinoma and pulmonary tuberculosis, however, they should frequently enter the differential diagnoses being considered by thoracic surgeons. Surgeons managing patients in organ transplantation programs also encounter fungal infections of the lungs more commonly than the average.

Two major considerations are worth noting: (1) the immunologically compromised patient i.e., the patient undergoing chemotherapy for malignancies, or steroidal therapy for a wide variety of conditions, and the patient with the acquired immune deficiency syndrome, is more likely to become infected by fungi, and (2) effective antifungal agents are now available against many of the fungal organisms. In most instances, the thoracic surgeon's role in fungal infections of the lungs is adjunctive: consultative and diagnostic. Both roles are important and require close collaboration with the pathologist and internist. Frequently, however, exploratory thoracotomy is necessary because of a strong suspicion of carcinoma especially, as Lillington (1982) and Godwin (1983) emphasized, in men over 40 years of age.

The laboratory diagnosis of fungal infection is discussed in detail in Chapter 16.

Histoplasmosis

This disease, probably the commonest of all fungal infections of lungs, is caused by the airborne spore *Histoplasma capsulatum*. Initially the disease was thought to be rare and almost always fatal. By 1945, however, the relationship between benign pulmonary calcifications and reactivity to skin testing with histoplasmin antigen was established, and widespread, almost universal subclinical infection with histoplasmosis in certain well-defined geographic areas of the United States was recognized. Some 30 million people are estimated to be infected, mostly along the Mississippi River and its tributaries (Fig. 69–4). Active disease, however, occurs uncommonly, only 1 in 2000 patients developing chronic

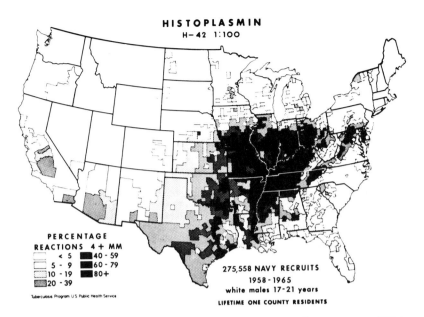

HISTOPLASMIN
H-42 1:100

PERCENTAGE
REACTIONS 4 + MM
< 5   40 - 59
5 - 9   60 - 79
10 - 19   80+
20 - 39

Tuberculosis Program U.S. Public Health Service

275,558 NAVY RECRUITS
1958 - 1965
white males 17 - 21 years
LIFETIME ONE COUNTY RESIDENTS

Fig. 69–4. Map of the United States showing areas of endemicity for histoplasmosis, based upon county of lifetime residence of naval recruits with positive histoplasmin skin test reactivity, shown as a percent of those treated. (Edwards, L.B., et al.: An atlas of sensitivity to tuberculin, PPD-B, and histoplasmin in the United States. Am. Rev. Respir. Dis. (Suppl)99:1, 1969.)

pulmonary disease, and dissemination occurring about 1 in 100,000 instances.

The organisms are found in soil, especially that contaminated by the droppings of fowl or bats. In tissue, yeast forms may appear packed in macrophages, or the stained capsules of dead organisms can be identified in the necrotic center of chronic granulomatous lesions (Fig. 69–5).

Goodwin and DesPrez (1978) classified the apparently bewildering variety of clinical presentations of histoplasmosis into three main pathogenetic categories: (1) benign—usually subclinical—infection of millions of otherwise normal people; (2) opportunistic infection; and (3) excessive host response characterized by excessive fibrosis (Table 69–1). The last two categories are of special diagnostic and therapeutic interest to the thoracic surgeon.

Pathogenesis and Symptomatology

Benign Infection of the Normal Host. In highly endemic areas, essentially the entire population becomes infected, without identifiable symptomatology, and often with conversion from a negative to a positive histoplasmin skin test as the only evidence of infection. Occasionally in infants and children, rarely in adults, cough, fever, and hilar lymphadenopathy mark the episode. Rarely the process progresses to the second or third categories. After an unusually heavy exposure to dust containing the spores of *H. capsulatum*, however, the clinical entity of acute histoplasmosis of either primary or reinfection types is recognized (Fig. 69–6). Roentgenographically, the primary type is characterized by scattered sparse to almost confluent small pneumonic or nodular infiltrates. The process is self-limiting, and may leave multiple nodular or calcific "buckshot" residues.

In fewer than 1% of the infections, dissemination or death occurs. The reinfection type produces a finer, more miliary granulomatous reaction. The roentgenographic characteristics occurring in an endemic area following exposure to dust contaminated with fowl or bat droppings, a positive skin test, and positive serologic findings—complement fixation—aid in confirming the diagnosis. An abbreviated course of amphotericin B is recommended for patients who remain ill more than 10 days to 2 weeks.

Opportunistic Infections. These infections occur on two bases: immunologic and structural. Goodwin and DesPrez (1978) conjectured that disseminated disease occurs as an opportunistic infection in a host with some immunologic deficiency. This deficiency is identifiable in patients on immunosuppressive medications or with lymphatic or hematopoietic malignancies. The pulmonary alveolar macrophage is probably parasitized by *H. capsulatum*, and provides not only nourishment and protection, but possibly transportation as well to all parts of the reticuloendothelial system. Disseminated histoplasmosis is a serious condition, for which full courses of amphotericin B are mandatory.

Chronic pulmonary histoplasmosis is postulated to occur as an opportunistic infection in an area of lung structurally damaged by centrilobular or bullous emphysema. Substantial roentgenologic evidence shows that chronic obstructive pulmonary disease sets the stage for chronic cavitary histoplasmosis. The organisms are found only in effusions in emphysematous spaces or in the necrotic lining of established cavities (Fig. 69–7).

According to this hypothesis, colonization of an emphysematous space, with spillover—bronchogenic spread—of antigen-laden effusion into adjacent areas of lung, accounts for the recognized interstitial pneumonitis and necrosis characteristic of this form of the disease.

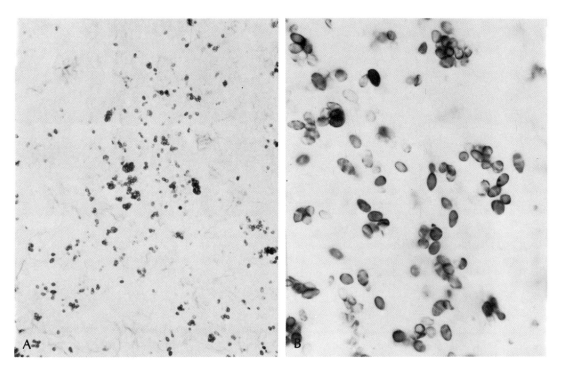

Fig. 69–5. *Histoplasma capsulatum* organisms. *A*, Nonviable capsules in necrotic area of a granuloma. Gomori's stain, × 780. *B*, Viable yeast forms in lymph node, × 1300.

Infection of cavity walls similarly is thought to be secondary to either colonization, or to dispersal of the same antigenic material from adjacent colonized spaces that causes, in other areas, pneumonitis and necrosis. Cavitary walls 2 mm or more thick suggest active disease that is likely to persist; thinner-walled cavities usually signify inactivity. Persistent thick-walled, 4mm or more, cavities appear to promote continuing necrosis and enlargement—the so-called marching cavities.

Symptomatology is nonspecific, resembling pulmonary tuberculosis as well as chronic obstructive lung disease. Cough, sputum, and hemoptysis are common, as are weight loss, low grade fever, and weakness. Symptoms of pulmonary insufficiency may be prominent.

Because the complement fixation test is of limited help

for various reasons, a positive diagnosis requires the demonstration of *H. capsulatum* in cultures of the sputum, which must be repeatedly and persistently tested for this fungus. The thicker-walled the cavity, the more readily are organisms identifiable by sputum cultures.

Treatment

Chronic cavitary histoplasmosis should be treated primarily by either amphotericin B or ketoconazole as Stamm and Dismukes (1983) outlined. A total dose of amphotericin B of about 2 g over a 10-week period is advocated. An effective alternative is 400 mg of ketoconazole per day for 6 to 12 months.

For disseminated disease, treatment with amphotericin B is urgently needed to prevent death. Stamm and Dismukes (1983) recommended at least 25 mg/kg body weight daily for a total dose of 2.5 g of amphotericin B. The pharmacologic effects of antimycotic agents and their toxicity and method of administration are outlined in detail by Bennett (1974) and Hermans (1977).

Goodwin and his colleagues (1976) found that treated patients fared better than untreated in every category of disease except the early lesion without persistent cavitation (Table 69–2).

Surgical excision is recommended for localized thick-walled cavities only if there has been no improvement after one or two courses of drug therapy, and if pulmonary function permits. Unfortunately, because chronic obstructive lung disease is almost the sine qua non of opportunistic infection of structurally damaged lung tissue by *H. capsulatum*, the risks and benefits of

Table 69–1. Classification of Histoplasmosis

Histoplasmosis in Normal Hosts—Acute Pulmonary Histoplasmosis
  Usual asymptomatic infection
  Occasional symptomatic infection
  Rare complications
    Pericarditis
    Mediastinal granuloma
    Mediastinal fibrosis
    Histoplasmomas
    Others
Opportunistic Infections
  Disseminated histoplasmosis (immune defect)
  Chronic pulmonary histoplasmosis (structural defect)

From Goodwin, R.A., et al.: Histoplasmosis in normal hosts. Medicine 60:232, 1981.

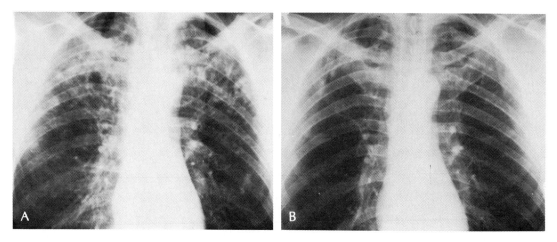

Fig. 69–6. Acute histoplasmosis. *A*, Thoracic roentgenogram of 48-year-old man who was asymptomatic when this routine film was made. Purified protein derivative (PPD) and histoplasmin skin tests were both positive. One sputum culture was reported to show *H. capsulatum*. Roentgenogram shows bilateral multiple soft infiltrates. No treatment was given. *B*, Thoracic roentgenogram 2 years later shows minimal residual fibrotic nodules. Patient remained well during the subsquent 5 years.

resection in many patients have to be carefully and individually assessed to determine what is in the patient's best interests.

Excessive Fibrosis: Healed Primary Lesion

The solitary pulmonary nodule, one of the commonest lesions seen by thoracic surgeons, in endemic areas is often a histoplasmoma. This benign lesion results from an excessive response to some antigenic stimulus to fibrogenesis in the necrotic center of the small—2 to 4 mm—primary focus containing *H. capsulatum*. Over a period of years, concentric layers of collagen are laid down, about 1 to 2 mm per year, resulting in a slowly enlarging and thus ominous-appearing nodular mass. Central or target calcification, however, or concentric laminar calcification that gives unequivocal evidence of the benign nature of the granulomatous reaction, can often be seen roentgenographically. This calcification is by far most commonly caused by histoplasmosis, but occurs also occasionally with tuberculosis and coccidioidomycosis (Fig. 69–8). Unfortunately, although over 50% of 1000 solitary pulmonary nodules in adults, mostly men, were benign granulomas, as Steele (1964) reported, 36% were malignant tumors. Therefore, unless the characteristic roentgenographic findings noted previously are identified by tomography, if not obvious on plain films

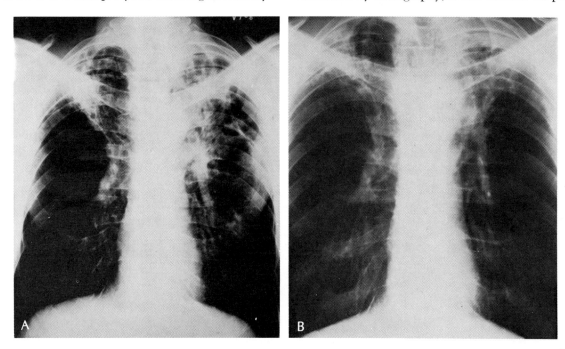

Fig. 69–7. Chronic cavitary histoplasmosis in a 53-year-old man. Initially, pulmonary tuberculosis was suspected; but ultimately sputum cultures and animal inoculation studies proved this to be chronic cavitary histoplasmosis. The patient received 2 g of amphotericin B over a 3-month period; ultimately, the lung lesions cleared. *A*, Thoracic roentgenogram prior to treatment. *B*, Appearance 6 months after completed treatment.

Table 69–2. Results of Treatment in 382 Lesions of Histoplasmosis in 228 Patients*

Types of Lesions	No. of Lesions	Conservative Treatment		Amphotericin Therapy		Surgical Resection	
		No. of Lesions	% Healed	No. of Lesions	% Healed	No. of Lesions	% Healed
Early, no persistent cavity	156	139	99+	6	100	11	100
Early, persistent cavity	44	25	16	11	55	8	100
Late, no persistent cavity	41	36	100	0		5	100
Late, thin-walled cavity	52	27	63	12	92	13	100
Late, thick-walled cavity	89	53	21	15	63	21	95*
Total Lesions	382	280		44		58	

*One surgical death.

Goodwin, R.A., et al.: Chronic pulmonary histoplasmosis. Medicine 55:413, 1976.

of the thorax, exploratory thoracotomy is often indicated as Godwin (1983) emphasized, especially in men over 40 (Fig. 69–9). On the other hand, if the diagnosis of a granuloma can be made by the characteristic roentgenographic findings, or by transbronchial brushing or percutaneous aspiration needle biopsy, or by evidence of an unchanging lesion for a period of several years, neither thoracotomy nor drug therapy may be needed. High resolution CT, which determines the density of the lesion, may also help. A high Hounsfeld unit number— >164—of the lesion—because of microcalcifications— denotes that the lesion is benign and that surgery is unnecessary.

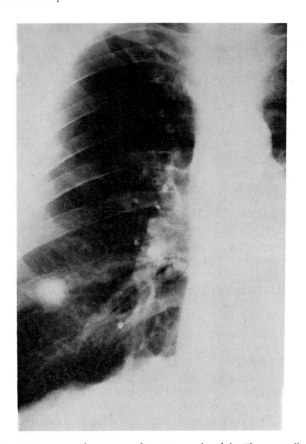

Fig. 69–8. *Histoplasma granuloma* in a male adult. This centrally calcified lesion remained unchanged for 10 years.

In hilar and mediastinal lymph nodes, this excessive encapsulating fibrogenetic response to the antigen of *H. capsulatum* may have serious consequences, depending on the region involved. In the right paratracheal region, superior vena caval syndrome or right bronchial stenosis may result; subcarinal lymph node involvement may produce stenosis of either or both main bronchi or the pulmonary veins; hilar lymph nodal involvement may cause either pulmonary arterial or bronchial stenosis. Mediastinal granulomas may be produced by the matting together of several large, caseous lymph nodes, presenting as mass lesions, in addition to giving rise to the aforementioned problems. Because of these serious complications, and the difficulties in managing them once they appear, excision of resectable asymptomatic mediastinal granulomas to forestall such difficult problems has been advocated by Ferguson and Burford (1965), as well as Dines (1979) and Zajtchuk (1973) and their associates and is probably appropriate.

Coccidioidomycosis

Coccidioidomycosis is a suppurative and granulomatous infectious disease that primarily attacks the lungs. Rarely, it occurs also in disseminated form.

Coccidioidomycosis bears several resemblances to histoplasmosis. This fungus occurs as a soil contaminant in sharply circumscribed geographic areas, resulting in subclinical infection in millions of persons, who are identifiable by a specific skin test, just as with histoplasmosis.

Drutz and Catanzaro (1978) made an exhaustive review of the disease.

Epidemiology

Fungal organisms occur in a well defined area of the southwestern part of the United States, including portions of California, Nevada, Arizona, New Mexico, and Texas (Fig. 69–10), as well as in Mexico and Central and South America. Infection results from the inhalation of spore-laden dust. About 10 million people in the United States have become infected, judging by skin tests. Agricultural and construction workers and others with similar outdoor pursuits are most likely to become infected. Archeologists are at special risk. Coccidioidomycosis is being diagnosed with increasing frequency in patients

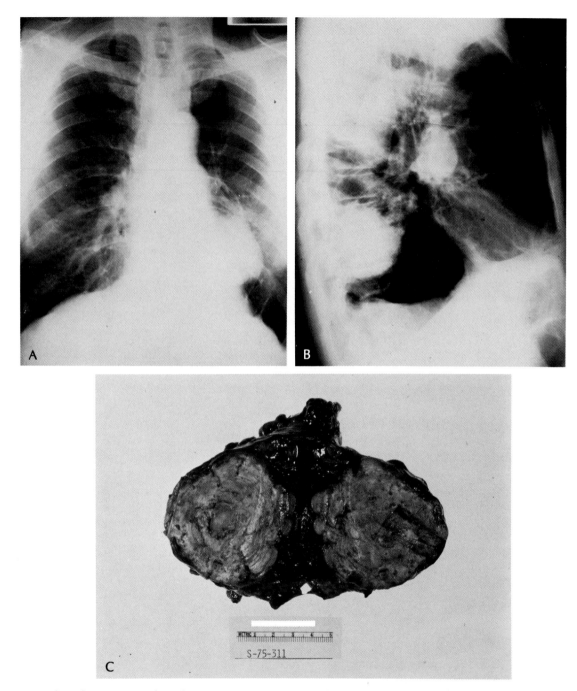

Fig. 69–9.   Giant histoplasmoma. *A*, and *B*, Thoracic roentgenograms, PA and lateral, of an asymptomatic 62-year-old man who was having a routine checkup. Diagnostic studies, including pulmonary angiography and thoracic aortography, did not disclose the nature of the lesion seen on the roentgenograms. *C*, Following exploratory thoracotomy on suspicion of bronchogenic carcinoma, a left lower lobectomy was performed. A large laminated fibrocollagenous granuloma with a necrotic center containing yeast cells morphologically consistent with *H. capsulatum* was found. This excessive degree of fibrogenesis is unusual.

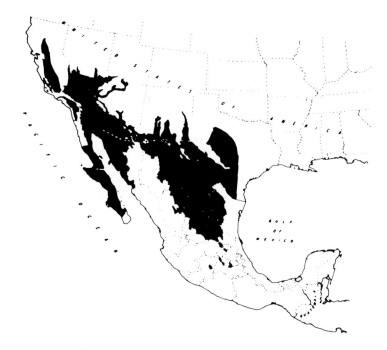

Fig. 69–10. Map showing area of endemicity of coccidioidomycosis in the United States and Mexico. (Ochoa, G.A.: Coccidioidomycosis in Mexico. *In* Coccidioidomycosis. Edited by L. Ajello. Tucson, University of Arizona Press, 1967.)

with acquired immune deficiency syndrome, according to Bronnimann and associates (1987).

Unlike most other fungus diseases, infection may also be acquired by inhalation of dust from fomites and from laboratory cultures of *Coccidioides immitis*. Therefore, such materials must be handled with special precautions.

Pathology

Pathologically, coccidioidomycosis resembles pulmonary tuberculosis. The primary complex is composed of a parenchymal pneumonitis and involvement of a regional lymph node or nodes, which may not be detected clinically. Reactivation of the primary complex may result in reinfection, with the development of caseous nodules, effusions, pneumonic areas, cavities, and calcified, fibrotic or ossified lung lesions (Fig. 69–11).

Extrapulmonary dissemination to lymph nodes, skin, spleen, liver, kidneys, bones, and meninges is more likely to occur in the primary than in the reinfection phase of the disease, and much more likely to afflict blacks, Filipinos, Native Americans, and Mexicans, by factors of five to ten times the incidence seen in whites.

The histologic characteristics of coccidioidomycosis lesions are those of granuloma formation with suppuration. With special stains, large—15 to 80μm—spherules, packed with tiny endospores when mature, or the endospores themselves can be seen (Fig. 69–12). Rarely, a mycetoma or "fungus ball" containing hyphae appears, as Bayer (1976), Thadepalli (1977), and Rohatgi (1984) and their associates reported.

Symptomatology

Most patients with primary infection have no symptoms. In about 25%, either mild or severe symptoms are

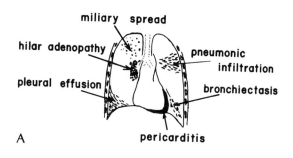

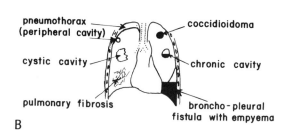

Fig. 69–11. Varieties of pulmonary manifestations of coccidioidomycosis. *A*, Acute stage; *B*, chronic stage. (Paulsen, G.A.: Pulmonary surgery in coccidioidal infections. *In* Coccidioidomycosis. Edited by L. Ajello, Tucson, University of Arizona Press, 1967.)

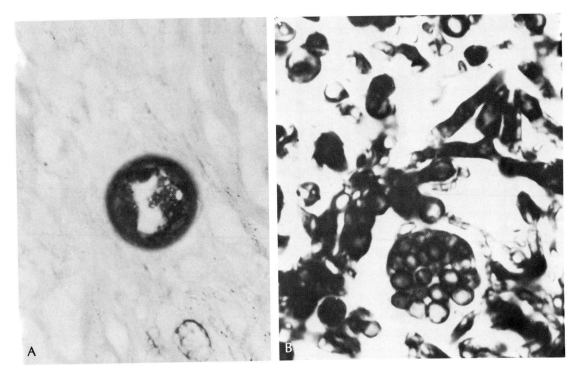

Fig. 69–12. *A*, Old spherule of *Coccidioides immitis* containing endospores, in an area of pulmonary fibrosis, × 1300. *B*, Organisms identified in a coccidioidal "fungus ball" in a cavitary lesion, showing both hyphae and spore forms, × 1300. This patient died of extensive cavitary coccidioidomycosis in spite of amphotericin B therapy 8 years after left pneumonectomy had been performed in an attempt to control his disease.

noted, which are nonspecific, and either referable to the respiratory tract or "flu-like," with malaise, headaches, and fever. Again, the condition is clustered among blacks and Filipinos. Symptoms may be pleuritic pain and cough productive of mucoid or, rarely, bloody sputum. Erythema multiforme, erythema nodosum, or less specific morbilliform rashes are observed occasionally, especially in women. Mild arthritic manifestations, which are called "desert rheumatism," also occur sometimes. The roentgenographic findings are nonspecific. In the acute stage, miliary lesions, pneumonic infiltrates, hilar adenopathy, or pleural and pericardial effusions may appear.

With chronic coccidioidomycosis, solitary nodules representing coccidioidal granulomas; chronic, usually, thin-walled cavities, sometimes with a fluid level; pneumothorax; fibrosis; or empyema may be manifestations of the disease.

Diagnosis

A positive culture of sputum, other body fluid or tissue is necessary for a definitive diagnosis. In acute coccidioidal pleural effusions, Lonky and associates (1976) noted that cultures of pleural biopsy specimens can be more rewarding than culturing the fluid. Recent conversion of the coccidioidin skin test to positive or positive serology, strongly suggests coccidiodomycosis. Although four serologic tests are available, early coccidioidal infection is usually detected only by the tube precipitin or the latex agglutination tests. Chick and co-workers (1973) noted that rising serial complement fixation tests mean

severe disease or even dissemination; a falling titer usually indicates regression or improvement.

Treatment

Many patients need no treatment at all. The most effective agent against coccidioidomycosis is amphotericin B, but because of the toxicity of this drug, indications for its use are limited: (1) the control of severe acute disease; (2) prevention of dissemination—especially in black patients, Filipinos, Native Americans, and Mexicans—the threat of which may be indicated by continuing elevation of the titer of the complement fixation test—1:64 or higher; (3) control of cavitary disease with sputum cultures positive for *C. immitis;* (4) arrest of dissemination of disease; (5) control of progressive chronic pulmonary lesions; (6) coverage during pulmonary resection or excision or drainage of abscesses, sinus tracts, lymph nodes, or necrotic bone; (7) preventive medical coverage in patients with active coccidioidomycosis, during corticosteroid therapy for whatever reason or during pregnancy. In the adult diabetic patient, Baker and associates (1978) also suggested using the drug in acute disease.

A suitable alternative agent, ketoconazole, as Stamm and Dismukes (1983) suggested, can be used for initial therapy for localized, non-life-threatening forms of coccidioidomycosis, including chronic pulmonary infections. Other triazoles are also coming into clinical trials, as Graybill (1986) reported.

The indications for resective surgery for coccidioidomycosis include localized granulomatous lesions and cav-

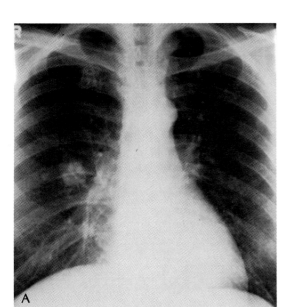

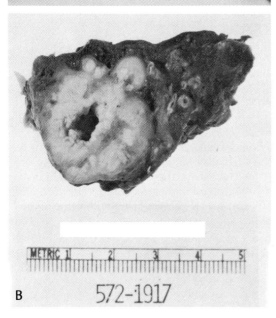

Fig. 69–13. Coccidioidal granuloma. *A*, Thoracic roentgenogram of 45-year-old asymptomatic male chronic smoker from Texas who was refused a job as a food handler because of this dense, irregularly shaped nodule in the superior segment of the right lower lobe. All diagnostic studies proved negative or normal. *B*, Chronic granuloma containing central cavitation found in resected segment. A small satellite nodule was also resected. Fungal stains showed typical spherules packed with endospores. (Takaro, T.: Lung infections and interstitial pneumonopathies. *In* Gibbon's Surgery of the Chest. Edited by D.C. Sabiston and F.C. Spencer. Philadelphia, W.B. Saunders Co., 1976.)

itary disease (Fig. 69–13). Although most undiagnosed solitary pulmonary nodules occurring in patients in the endemic area are coccidioidomas, Read (1972) and Cohen and associates (1972) found 26 to 35% to be malignant. Therefore, in the endemic area, the indications for resection of undiagnosed solitary pulmonary nodules must be individualized, as for histoplasmosis, because a known granuloma does not ordinarily necessitate resection.

Marks and colleagues (1967) reported that localized resections in over 700 patients were accompanied by a complication rate of approximately 10%, many of them air leaks or peripheral, small bronchopleural fistulae. For cavitary lesions, in most patients, resection is not indicated. When cavities persist more than 2 to 4 years, however, and are greater than 2 cm in diameter; when they are rapidly enlarging, thick-walled, or ruptured, or contain a fungus ball; when they are associated with severe or recurrent hemoptysis; when they occur in diabetic or pregnant patients; and when they coexist with pulmonary tuberculosis, surgical resection, preferably by lobectomy, is indicated as Nelson (1974) and Baker (1978) and Cunningham (1982) and their colleagues suggested. Some recommend drug coverage with amphotericin B, but it is not clear that the use of amphotericin B has resulted in significantly fewer complications of bronchopleural fistula, empyema, and recurrent cavitation.

North American Blastomycosis

This is a suppurative and granulomatous infectious disease caused by *Blastomyces dermatitidis*, a round, thick-walled single budding yeast cell, 5 to 20 μm in diameter.

Epidemiology

North American blastomycosis occurs mostly in the southeastern, south central, and midwestern states, especially in Arkansas, Kentucky, Mississippi, and Wisconsin, according to Klein and associates (1986) (Fig. 69–14). This disease is also an airborne infection of exogenous origin, the fungus having been identified in pigeon manure by Sarosi and Serstock (1976) and in soil by Klein and colleagues (1986). Thus, the incidence in some studies, as Busey and his associates (1964) noted, is highest among persons in close contact with the soil. Kitchen and his colleagues (1977), however, described an urban epidemic.

Pathology and Microbiology

North American blastomycosis characteristically induces a granulomatous and pyogenic reaction with microabscesses and giant cells and, occasionally, caseation, cavitation, and fibrosis. Primarily, the lungs, skin, bones, and genitourinary tract are affected. Skin lesions exhibit pseudoepitheliomatous squamous cell proliferation with microabscesses between areas of acanthotic epithelium. Special stains reveal the fungal organisms with the characteristic thick refractile walls (Fig. 69–15). Landis and Varkey (1976) as well as Laskey and Sarosi (1977) documented endogenous reinfection, as in pulmonary tuberculosis.

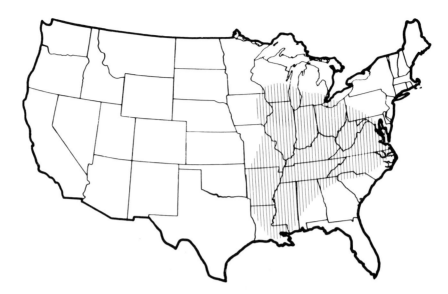

Fig. 69–14. Approximate area of endemicity in the United States for North American blastomycosis. (Adapted from Menges, R.W., et al.: Clinical and epidemiological studies on 79 canine blastomycosis cases in Arkansas. Am. J. Epidemiol. *81*:169, 1965.)

Symptomatology

The patient with blastomycosis is usually first seen because of symptoms referable to the skin or the lungs, or both.

The cutaneous manifestations begin as single and multiple papules or papulopustules that enlarge slowly, ulcerate, and exhibit elevated, cyanotic edges. Biopsies from such areas are more likely to yield the organisms than cultures of sputum are. The lesions may appear anywhere, on both exposed and unexposed portions of the skin, and are characterized by chronicity (Fig. 69–16). The patient may be unaware of the skin lesions. Healing may occur, leaving a soft noncontracting scar. The weight of clinical and pathologic evidence, as Rabinowitz and his associates (1976) pointed out, suggests that a primary pulmonary focus is present in practically all instances of both cutaneous and systemic North American blastomycosis.

After the cutaneous form, the next most common manifestations of blastomycosis are caused by pulmonary involvement. Cough—usually productive only of mucoid sputum, chest pain, and hemoptysis may occur; or mild fever, malaise, weight loss, weakness, and other nonspecific symptoms may be the only complaints. Physical signs are not characteristic or particularly helpful.

Thoracic Roentgenographic Findings

Cush and his colleagues (1976) noted that consolidation is characteristic in acute disease but also common in chronic blastomycosis. Fibronodular lesions, with or without cavitation, reminiscent of pulmonary tuberculosis are also common in chronic disease. Mass lesions, diffuse patterns, pleural involvement, and hilar lymphadenopathy also appear, but less commonly. Kinasewitz and colleagues (1984) recognized that major pleural disease indicates a poor prognosis. Many patients have been explored with the presumptive diagnosis of carcinoma of the lung.

Diagnosis

Most commonly, diagnosis is made by cultural demonstration of the organism in the sputum, in material from skin lesions, or from skeletal lesions: abscesses, sinuses, or biopsy material. Sutliff and Cruthirds (1973) advocated the examination of bronchial washings or sputum cytologic techniques for *B. dermatitidis*; Sanders and his associates (1977) confirmed the value of the latter. Several specimens may be required to demonstrate the organisms. Lung biopsy may be necessary to make the diagnosis, but unfortunately this procedure is occasionally followed by dissemination of the disease. The major differential diagnostic problem in endemic areas of blastomycosis is carcinoma of the lung, which Poe and associates (1972) emphasized. In patients with unrecognized pulmonary blastomycosis, unnecessarily radical operations may be performed with the mistaken diagnosis of tumor. A preoperative diagnosis is therefore important to avoid an unnecessary operation.

Because skin test and complement fixation test may be as often negative as positive, and because of the close antigenic similarity between coccidioidin, histoplasmin, and blastomycin, these serologic intracutaneous diagnostic tests are inadequate, and cannot be relied upon for a definitive diagnosis. Turner and Kaufman (1986) reported that serologic tests with improved diagnostic capabilities have been developed.

Treatment

Blastomycosis should be treated whenever the diagnosis can be made unequivocally by identifying the organism. Self-limited disease, however, was described by Sarosi and associates (1986). In any event, a presumptive diagnosis is not an adequate basis for therapy, because

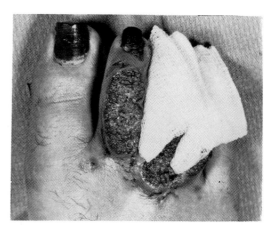

Fig. 69–16. Skin lesions of blastomycosis on dorsum of toes. Biopsy of characteristic raised edges showed multiple microabscesses containing *B. dermatitidis*. (Takaro, T.: Thoracic actinomycetic and mycotic infections. *In* Practice of Surgery. Edited by H.S. Goldsmith. Hagerstown, MD, Harper & Row, 1978, Thoracic Surgery, Chap. 12.)

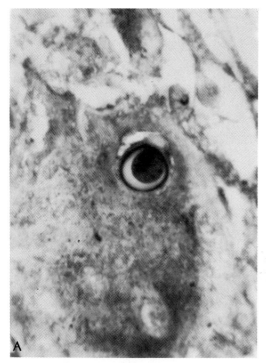

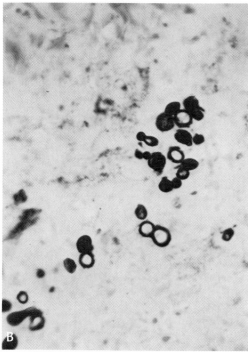

Fig. 69–15. Organisms of *B. dermatitidis* from resected lung tissue. *A*, Single thick-walled yeast form with refractile cell wall. *B*, Multiple yeast forms with single budding characteristic of this fungus. Periodic acid-Schiff stain, × 1100. (Takaro, T.: *In* Practice of Surgery. Edited by H.S. Goldsmith. Hagerstown, MD, Harper & Row, 1978, Thoracic Surgery, Chap. 12.)

the drugs used for treatment are toxic. Bradsher (1985) and McManus (1986) recommended ketoconazole as the treatment of choice because it is less toxic and easier to administer than amphotericin B. The National Institute of Allergy and Infectious Disease Mycoses Study Group (1985) recommended that the optimal dose is somewhere between 400 and 800 mg/day. For cavitary lesions or extensive disease or for systemic dissemination, amphotericin B is preferable (Fig. 69–17).

Resection is indicated when bronchial carcinoma is suspected after efforts have been made, especially in endemic areas, to rule out North American blastomycosis. Drug treatment with amphotericin B or ketoconazole should follow operation when the diagnosis is made only at the time of the thoracotomy. Resection of known blastomycotic cavitary lesions is indicated if they persist after adequate drug therapy with amphotericin B or ketoconazole, or both, because viable organisms are likely to persist in such lesions, even if they cannot be recovered in the sputum.

Pulmonary blastomycosis is still a serious disease, with a 5-year mortality rate of approximately 20%. Involvement of the genitourinary tract, the bones, and the nasal and oral mucosa is common.

Cryptococcosis

Definition

Cryptococcosis is a subacute or chronic infection caused by *Cryptococcus neoformans*—formerly known as *Torula histolytica*—which primarily attacks the bronchopulmonary tree but also has a special predilection for the central nervous system. This disease, like blastomycosis, histoplasmosis and coccidioidomycosis, was formerly thought to be a rare and invariably fatal infection, with meningitis the most prominent feature. Bronchopulmonary manifestations are apparently much more common than the dreaded meningeal form, however, and since the introduction of amphotericin B and 5-fluorocytosine even this form can be controlled. Duperval

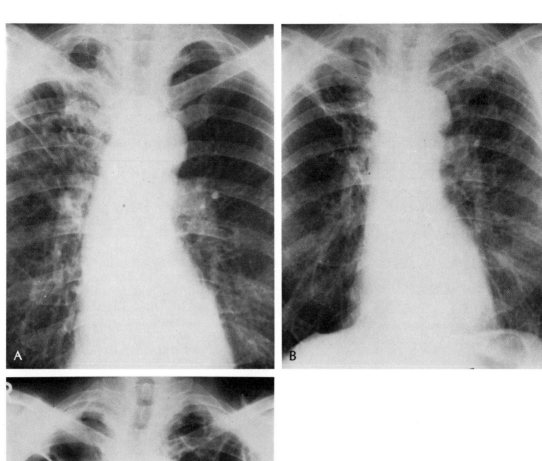

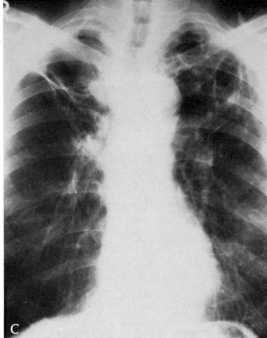

Fig. 69–17. Evolution of chronic pulmonary blastomycosis. *A*, Thoracic roentgenogram showing extensive right upper lung infiltrative lesion in a man with proven blastomycotic skin lesion of the nostril. Lesion was treated at first with potassium iodide. *B*, Four years later, bilateral cavitary disease is observed, but no organisms were seen in the sputum. *C*, Two-and-half years later, two thin-walled cavities in the left upper lobe, and an emphysematous bulla in the right upper lobe were noted. A number of sputum specimens showed *B. dermatitidis*. He was treated with 7 g of 2-hydroxystilbamidine. He has remained well.

and his colleagues (1977) noted that the number of immunocompromised patients with opportunistic infections with *C. neoformans* has increased; Gal and associates (1986) noted the infection in patients with acquired immune deficiency syndrome.

Epidemiology

Unlike histoplasmosis, coccidioidomycosis, and blastomycosis, cryptococcosis has no known geographic area of endemicity. Cryptococci may, however, be present in soil and dust contaminated by pigeon droppings; in this regard, it resembles histoplasmosis as well as North American blastomycosis.

Pathology

The organism *Cyptococcus neoformans* is a round, budding yeast form 5 to 20 μm in diameter—average 8 to 10 μm—with a sometimes wide gelatinous capsule that surrounds the organism and remains unstained. The usual special stains for fungi are all effective for demonstrating the organisms. The mucicarmine stain is specific. In fresh material the capsules can be demonstrated by mounting some of the specimen in a drop of diluted India ink (Fig. 69–18).

This infection is airborne, and the respiratory tract is the portal of entry. McDonnell and Hutchins (1985) described four basic morphologic patterns in the lungs: pulmonary granulomas; granulomatous pneumonias; diffuse alveolar and interstitial cryptococci accompanied by greater or lesser degrees of inflammatory response; and many alveolar and intravascular organisms in the lungs, where the primary route of infection was uncertain. The

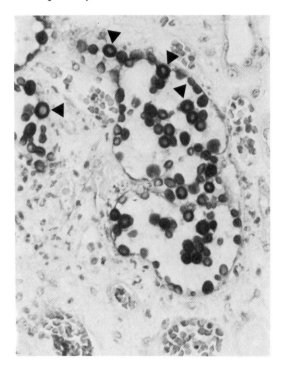

Fig. 69–18. Organisms of *Cryptococcus neoformans* showing thick capsules (arrows). Periodic acid-Schiff stain, × 780.

lesions are often solid, and the cut surface of the granuloma may be glairy or shiny, as in a mucoid carcinoma. Central necrosis and cavitation may occur but are uncommon, and calcification is rare. Duperval (1977) and Salyer (1974a) and their colleagues reported pleural effusions and empyemas, and dissemination to parts of the body other than the central nervous system has also been described.

Symptomatology

Pulmonary symptoms are nonspecific, insidious, or absent. Cough, bloody sputum, low-grade fever, weakness, and lethargy sometimes occur. Spontaneous remission may and probably does occur. Because cryptococcosis is often an opportunistic infection, the manifestations of the primary disease may overshadow those of cryptococcosis, and the diagnosis may become apparent only after abnormalities on thoracic roentgenograms call attention to the lungs, or symptoms referable to the central nervous system suggest meningitis.

Diagnosis

Cryptococcus may be isolated from sputum, bronchial washings, bronchial brushing, or percutaneous needle aspiration of the lungs, as well as from cerebrospinal fluid, where it should specifically be sought. Often the diagnosis is made from a resected lung specimen or at autopsy. No specific skin test for cryptococcosis is available, and serologic tests are not helpful.

The roentgenographic features of pulmonary cryptococcosis are not sufficiently characteristic to be of diagnostic help. Infiltrative, mass, nodular, and diffuse miliary lesions have all been described (Fig. 69–19). Pleural effusion is unusual, but is recognized more frequently than it once was, as Epstein (1972) and Littman (1968) and their associates as well as by the aforementioned authors noted.

Kerkering and colleagues (1981) pointed out that the diagnosis of cryptococcosis is often missed because it is not considered often enough in the differential diagnosis of abnormalities found on thoracic roentgenograms.

Treatment

Medical. The specific antifungal agents effective against *cryptococcus neoformans* are amphotericin B and 5-fluorocytosine—Ancobon. Although some difference of opinion exists, a reasonable policy, suggested by Hatcher (1971), Lewis (1972), and Smith (1976) and their colleagues, is that all patients with proven disease should receive antifungal therapy, because experience indicates that none who have received it have later developed meningitis. This view is more readily supportable because a less toxic regimen, described by Utz and Buechner (1971), uses orally administered 5-fluorocytosine together with low doses of amphotericin B—0.3 mg/kg. Kerkering and colleagues (1981) concluded that, because the natural history of untreated pulmonary disease in immunocomprised patients is extrathoracic dissemination, all such patients should receive antifungal treatment. On the other hand, otherwise normal patients with

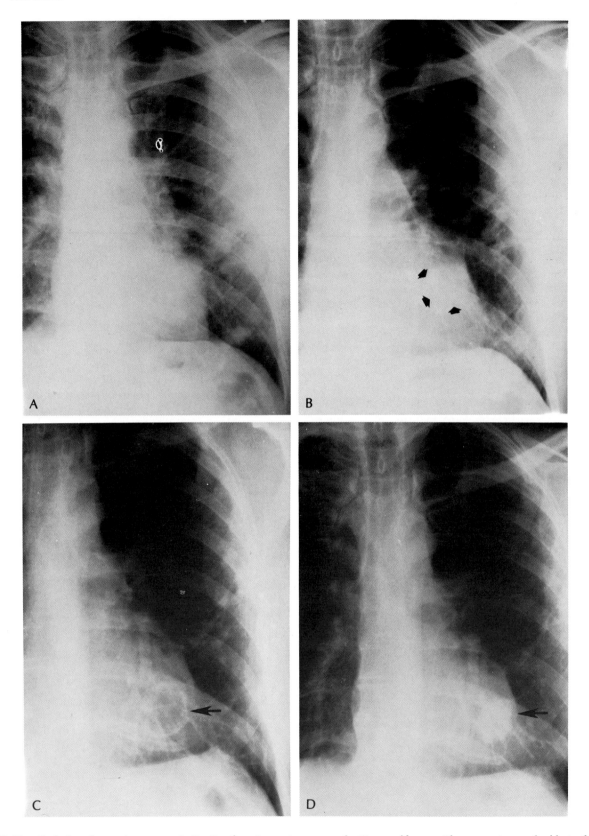

Fig. 69–19. Evolution of a cryptococcoma. *A,* Routine thoracic roentgenogram of a 54-year-old man with no symptoms referable to the chest showing scattered infiltrative lesions in the left lung. An open lung biopsy was carried out after an unrewarding diagnostic workup; biopsies showed multiple small granulomas containing numerous encapsulated yeast forms characteristic of cryptococci. Mouse virulence tests were confirmatory. Examination of spinal fluid showed no organisms. A course of treatment with amphotericin B was discontinued after 1.5 g had been administered, because of thrombosed veins. *B,* Four months later, a solitary nodule behind the cardiac shadow is seen (arrows): the infiltrative lesions have regressed. *C,* Eighteen months later, a thin-walled cavity is seen at the site of the solitary nodule (arrow). *D,* Forty months after the process was first noted, a dense, shrunken, irregular nodular lesion is noted (arrow). The patient remained without pulmonary symptoms.

pulmonary cryptococcosis in whom dissemination has been ruled out by appropriate studies generally do not require treatment.

Surgical. In the unusual event that the diagnosis of pulmonary cryptococcosis has been firmly established before operation, and pulmonary resection is being considered, Bennett (1974) as well as Utz and his associates (1975) recommended combined treatment with 5-fluorocytosine and amphotericin B. The combination may be additive, may permit a lower dose of amphotericin B to be used, may inhibit the emergence of resistance to 5-fluorocytosine, and may even obviate surgery. The spinal fluid should certainly be examined for evidence of the disease, as Sall and Bergeron (1971) noted, even if cryptococci are identified in sputum or by brush biopsy.

If, on the other hand, the diagnosis is made only after thoracotomy, on biopsied or resected lung tissue—the usual situation—opinions differ, as previously noted, regarding the need for antifungal therapy. One school of thought, represented by Geraci (1965), Hammerman (1973), and Kerkering (1981) and their colleagues, holds that active treatment may not be necessary if there is no evidence of central nervous system involvement and no organisms are found in cerebrospinal fluid.

Fortunately, even the dreaded meningeal form is no longer uniformly fatal. Recovery with drug treatment—sometimes requiring multiple courses—is now the rule rather than the exception.

Aspergillosis

Definition

In this condition the usually saprophytic *Aspergillus fumigatus*—or some other member of the species—has given rise to one of three distinctly different clinical syndromes; aspergillar bronchitis, aspergilloma—"fungus ball"—or invasive necrotizing aspergillous infection. Only the mycetoma is of special interest to surgeons. The first appears to be an allergic manifestation, and the last occurs as an opportunistic infection associated with hematogenous dissemination.

Pathogenesis

In the three clinical forms of aspergillosis, *A. fumigatus* is the fungus most commonly isolated, but *A. flavus*, *A. niger*, *A. nidulans*, and *A. clavatus* are other identified species. These filamentous fungi are found in soil and on decaying vegetation, and produce airborne spores especially abundantly at certain times of the year. Arnow and his associates (1978) pointed out that hospital air can become contaminated with aspergillus spores both from within—false ceilings—and without—ventilation systems—a serious consideration for immunosuppressed patients. In pathologic materials, usually only the coarse, fragmented, septate, branching hyphae appear either as short strands or as ball-like clusters, and can be identified only by isolation and culture (Fig. 69–20). Because aspergilli are saprophytic and ubiquitous, unless the material has been obtained under aseptic conditions, a diagnosis of aspergillosis cannot safely be made simply by culturing the fungi.

Most of the surgically resected lesions of aspergillosis are aspergillomas. A fungus ball is actually a matted sphere of hyphae, fibrin, and inflammatory cells, which appears grossly as a round or oval, friable, gray, red, brown, or yellow necrotic-looking mass. It is ordinarily found lying in an upper lobe cavity, the wall of which is often smooth and may be thick or thin with relatively little evidence of inflammatory reaction. The cavitary disease results from previous chronic lung disease such as tuberculosis, sarcoidosis, histoplasmosis, bronchiectasis, bronchogenic cyst, chronic lung abscess, or cavitating carcinoma. Rarely there is no obvious evidence of pre-existing pulmonary damage (Fig. 69–21).

Symptomatology

In certain cases, symptoms may be attributable to the mycetoma. Cough with bloody or blood-streaked sputum, however, frequently occurs, although histopathologic examination of the resected lesion may reveal no bleeding point. Sometimes hemopytsis is severe to exsanguinating.

Diagnosis

Finding aspergillus in the sputum alone does not justify the diagnosis of aspergillosis. If the clinical picture of aspergilloma is present and sputum cultures are positive for aspergillus, the diagnosis is probable.

Griepp (1975) reported that transtracheal aspirates or direct lung aspirates by thin-walled 18-gauge needles may provide a definitive diagnosis, and are especially useful in immunosuppressed patients.

Precipitating antibodies against *A. fumigatus* in the serum, skin sensitivity to aspergillus antigen, or characteristic roentgenographic shadows are confirmatory evidence. An aspergilloma can sometimes be identified roetgenographically as a mass shifting within a cavity or cyst on changes in position of the patient. Thus, in a roentgenogram of the thorax exposed in the upright position, a crescentic radiolucency above a rounded radiopaque lesion suggests aspergilloma (Fig. 69–22).

Treatment

Medical. Hammerman and his associates (1974) noted that medical treatment has been generally unsatisfactory. Isolated cures have been reported following treatment with iodides, nystatin, and hydroxystilbamidine, and with amphotericin B, which is the drug of choice. Eastridge (1976) suggested that amphotericin B's definite toxic effects have been overemphasized, and that treatment failures may sometimes be attributable to premature cessation of treatment, rather than lack of efficacy.

Surgical. This is controversial. According to Daly and colleagues (1986), management philosophy is more readily grasped when aspergillomas are classified as either simple—thin-walled localized cysts with little surrounding parenchymal disease—or complex—thick-walled cavities associated with gross evidence of parenchymal disease. Because the complication rate following surgery in the latter group is high, symptoms of hemoptysis or cough, or both, should be significant enough to warrant

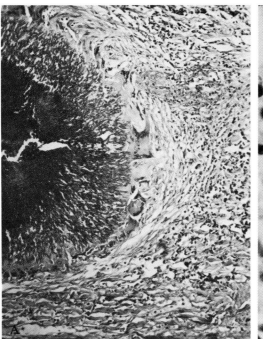
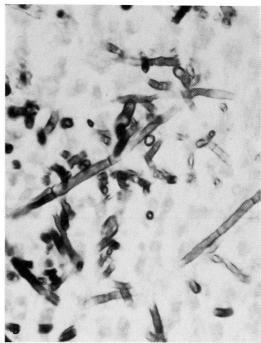

Fig. 69–20. Organisms of *Aspergillus fumigatus* in tissues. *A,* Small colony of aspergilli found in a resected carcinomatous lesion of the lung. Note mycelia radiating outward from darker center of the colony, × 250. (Takaro, T.: Lung infections and interstitial pneumonopathies. *In* Gibbon's Surgery of the Chest. Edited by D.C. Sabiston and F.C. Spencer. Philadelphia, W.B. Saunders Co., 1976.) *B,* Close-up of coarse, septate, fragmented mycelia of *A. fumigatus.* Round bodies are mycelia seen end-on. Gomori's stain. × 950. (Takaro, T.: Thoracic actinomycetic and mycotic infections *In* Practice of Surgery. Edited by H.S. Goldsmith. Hagerstown, MD, Harper & Row, 1978, Thoracic Surgery, Chap. 12.)

the risk of surgery. On the other hand, patients with simple aspergillomas with even minimal symptoms may be offered surgery because the risk is low and the likelihood of long-term cure is much improved as Eastridge (1972), Karas (1976), and Daly (1986) and their associates suggested.

Clearly, no unanimity of opinion exists in this regard—Varkey and Rose (1976) and Bower (1977) and Faulkner (1978) and their colleagues, as well as Pennington (1980), take differing views. Individualizing surgical management is clearly critical, as Battaglini (1985) and Butz (1985) and their colleagues emphasized. Allan and colleagues (1986) pointed out that additional surgical measures, short of pulmonary resection, in any event should be as conservative as possible. Eguchi and colleagues (1971) reported the use of cavernostomy; Daly and colleagues (1986) suggested the obliteration of the cavity by transposing muscle from the chest wall into the cavity; and Ramirez (1964) recommended endocavitary instillation of sodium iodide or amphotericin B. Remy and co-workers (1977) reported embolization of the bronchial arteries in a few patients with massive or repeated hemoptysis caused by aspergilloma, with early remission in four of six cases, but recurrence of bleeding in three of the four initially controlled.

Aspergillus empyema, or pleural aspergillosis, was reported by Herring and Pecora (1976) and others and has been treated by intrapleural amphotericin B, or nystatin, and by pleural drainage, pleurectomy, thoracoplasty, and repair of bronchopleural fistulae.

Candidiasis—Moniliasis

Definition

Candidiasis is usually an acute, subacute, or chronic superficial fungus infection caused by species of Candida—usually *C. albicans*—which commonly affects the skin or the oral, bronchial, or vaginal mucosa. Much less commonly, it can also be a deep or systemic infection, involving the lungs, bloodstream, endocardium, meninges, or almost any other organ. Other fungi of this genus that are occasionally pathogenic to man are *C. guiliermondii, C. stellatoidea, C. parakrusei,* and *C. tropicalis.*

Epidemiology

The organism occurs in the oropharynx of many normal individuals. It is a common hospital and laboratory contaminant, probably of universal distribution.

Pathogenesis

Candida organisms appear in fresh or potassium hydroxide preparations or on Gram's stain as small—2.5 to 4 μm—oval, thin-walled, budding cells with or without mycelial elements (Fig. 69–23). An acute or chronic granulomatous reaction may result. In systemic infections, both mycelial and yeast forms may appear in clusters surrounded by polymorphonuclear leukocytes, forming microabscesses. The fungi may also invade the tissues and blood vessel walls, with little evidence of inflammatory reaction in some instances. Thomas (1977) and Wray (1973) and their associates reported costal

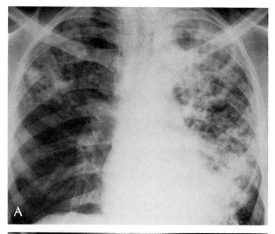

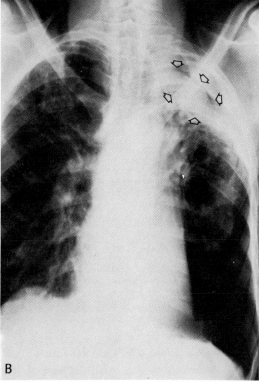

Fig. 69–21. Evolution of an aspergilloma. *A,* Thoracic roentgenogram in 1959 from a 30-year-old man with advanced cavitary pulmonary tuberculosis. He received multiple drug therapy for many months and sputum was last positive in 1962. *B,* Thoracic roentgenogram obtained in 1973 (14 years later) because of occasional mild hemoptysis, showing aspergilloma, or "fungus ball." Note radiolucent space between fungus ball and cavity wall (arrows). Severe chronic obstructive lung disease precluded resection, although the disease appeared to be localized. Chronic hemoptysis continued. There was little change in the patient's condition or in the appearance of the roentgenograms over a 2-year period. The patient ultimately died 16 years after the initial film, and 2 years after the discovery of the fungus ball, of "extensive pulmonary infection." Patients with this type of "complex" aspergilloma often do not do well following surgical therapy, but medical treatment also has little to offer.

chondritis as well as osteomyelitis of the sternum caused by candida.

Clinical Picture and Diagnosis

The importance of this opportunistic fungus infection lies in the slowly but steadily increasing incidence of disseminated disease noted during the past 25 years. This phenomenon is essentially iatrogenic, as Louria and colleagues (1962) noted; before the advent of broad-spectrum antibiotics, disseminated disease with invasion of internal organs, septicemia, and endocarditis were almost unheard of.

In the presence of intensive or prolonged antibiotic therapy, especially with multiple drugs, or of immunosuppressive therapy following organ transplantation, the normal bacterial flora of patients may be suppressed, allowing an overgrowth of the often-present saprophytic species of Candida. This type of suprainfection also occurs in patients with AIDS. Invasion then takes place through any portal of entry: the skin, the bloodstream—by way of needles or catheters used for intravenous therapy—the lungs, or the gastrointestinal tract. In the presence of altered host immunity or inhibited inflammatory response for any of various reasons, candida pneumonia, abscess—which Rubin and Alroy (1977) reported, or septicemia and generalized infection may result, often with a fatal outcome. Orringer and Sloan (1978) observed monilial esophagitis with stricture formation, and Spear and colleagues (1976) reported tracheal obstruction associated with candida fungus ball. Thus, although the presence of a species of Candida in the sputum of many healthy persons ordinarily is of no diagnostic or prognostic importance, the same cannot be said for the finding of Candida in bronchial or lung biopsies, in the bloodstream, or in deep tissue spaces. One cannot lightly dismiss such reports as reflecting laboratory contamination, especially not in immunosuppressed or otherwise compromised patients who have symptoms and signs of pneumonia, or of septicemia. Instead, one must assume that candida pneumonia or septicemia may be present, and Williams and his associates (1976) recommended that therapy with amphotericin B be given promptly if the patient is to have any chance of survival. On the other hand, Rosenbaum and co-workers (1974) suggested that some forms of candida pneumonia are self-limited and require no treatment.

As in the case of the other opportunistic fungi such as *Aspergillus fumigatus, Cryptococcus neoformans,* and Mucor, the circumstances that place a patient at risk are debility, senescence, prematurity, starvation, prolonged shock, multiple operations, multiple or mixed infections, bone marrow depression by lymphomas or antitumor drugs, radiation therapy, disseminated malignancies, immune deficiency, and antibiotic or steroid therapy.

Treatment

The combination of 5-fluorocytosine, and amphotericin B is the most promising regimen available. Of four patients with candida pneumonias reported by Howard and his associates (1978) who were treated with ampho-

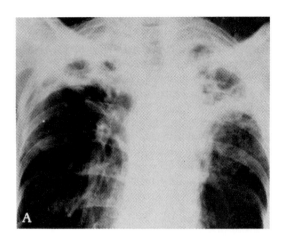
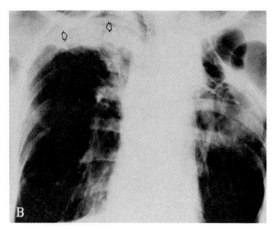
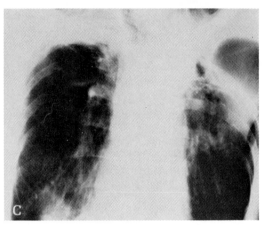

Fig. 69–22. Evolution of the bilateral cavitary disease with colonization by aspergilli; surgical treatment. *A*, Thoracic roentgenogram of a 55-year-old man with symptoms of gradually increasing weakness and weight loss. No positive findings on workup other than the destructive lung lesions. Pulmonary ventilatory function was only mildly impaired; segmental resection of the left upper lobe and four-rib thoracoplasty were carried out. Pathologic findings were nonspecific inflammatory disease with a cavity containing soft, brown masses, which proved to be colonies of *Aspergillus*. A chronic bronchocutaneous fistula developed and gradually closed after 3 months. *B*, Two years later, a distinct new "fungus ball" can be identified in the right upper cavity (arrows), with characteristic radiolucent area around the ball. There were few symptoms. *C*, Regression of the disease process in the right lung on roentgenogram 4 years later, without specific therapy.

tericin B—two of whom received 5-fluorocytosine also—all four made short-term recoveries, with two late deaths unrelated to the candida pneumonia. Early diagnosis and vigorous treatment give these patients a considerably more promising outlook than those with candida endocarditis. Dyess and associates (1985) reported that candida septicemia is associated with a mortality rate of 52%. On the other hand, Strinden and associates (1985) reported long-term survival in six of eight patients with septic thrombosis of the central veins caused by candida who had intensive therapy with amphotericin B.

Sporotrichosis

Sporotrichosis is a mycotic infection caused by *Sporotrichum schenckii*, a cigar-shaped, dimorphic organism that stains bright red with PAS stains. The disease is characterized by cutaneous and lymphatic involvement ordinarily, and pulmonary disease is relatively rare.

The causative organism is a saprophyte, under normal conditions, and is widely distributed in plants and soil. Thus, florists are especially susceptible. An epidemic involving miners exposed to infested mine timbers in South Africa was reported.

Pulmonary infection produces nonspecific symptoms resembling those of pulmonary tuberculosis: fever, hemoptysis, malaise, and weight loss. Similarly, roentgenographic findings mimic tuberculosis in the wide variety of presenting patterns, including hilar lymphadenopathy, pleural effusion, lobular consolidation, fibrosis, and multiple nodules. Michelson (1977) and Jay (1977) and Jung (1979) and their associates reported localized cavitary disease in over 50 patients. It is necessary not only to culture the organism, from sputum, bronchial washings, or lung tissue, but also to establish its pathogenicity for animals, because the organism is a saprophyte. The diagnostic value of serum agglutination tests for Sporotrichum is not established, but direct fluorescent antibody reliably identifies the organisms in specimens and tissue biopsies, according to Rohatgi (1980) (Fig. 69–24).

Optimal treatment for all patients with pulmonary sporotrichosis is not known with certainty. Although several patients have responded to potassium iodide treatment,

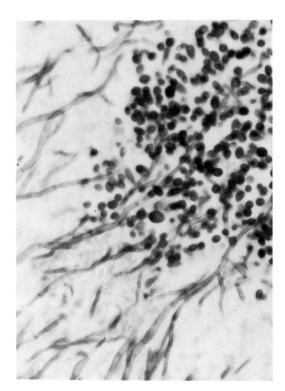

Fig. 69–23. Organisms of *Candida albicans*, showing both yeast and mycelial forms. Gomori's strain, × 1000. (Takaro, T.: Thoracic actinomycetic and mycotic infections *In* Practice of Surgery. Edited by H.S. Goldsmith. Hagerstown, MD, Harper & Row, 1978, Thoracic Surgery, Chap. 12.)

some have not. Similarly, a few successes with amphotericin B have been recorded, as well as a few failures. Pluss and Opal (1986) and Gerding (1986) concur that for pulmonary sporotrichosis with localized cavitary disease, early and complete surgical resection with concomitant chemotherapy with saturated solution of potassium iodide—SSKI—gives the best results. Amphotericin B is reserved for treatment failures using total doses up to 2 to 3 g. It is possible as Lopes-Berestein (1986) suggested, that the newly developing liposomal form of this drug will improve results.

Phycomycosis—Mucormycosis

This is a rare but potentially lethal fungus infection caused by genera belonging to the class Phycomycetes. These fungi are characterized structurally by broad—6 to 50 μm—nonseptate but branching hyphae (Fig. 69–25) that are difficult to culture. Among disease-causing organisms in this group are species of Absidia, Rhizopus, Mucor, Mortierella, and Basidiobolus.

These organisms are generally saprophytes, occurring as molds on manure and foods, and producing spores that can be inhaled. They are not ordinarily pathogenic to man. Under special conditions of immunosuppression or compromise, they can cause disease. In the lungs, the disease is characterized by blood vessel invasion, thrombosis, and infarction of invaded organs, with marked tissue destruction, cavitation, and abscess formation.

Phycomycosis is usually a rapidly fatal disease, occur-

ring especially in acidotic diabetics, in patients with lymphomas or leukemias, or in persons receiving intensive or prolonged antimetabolite, antibiotic, or steroid therapy. Extensive necrosis of areas around the face—paranasal sinuses, orbit, mucous membranes—and of the lung and the brain may occur in addition to cutaneous and subcutaneous infection. Murray (1975) reported massive fatal pulmonary hemorrhage. Gartenberg and associates (1978) reported two patients with necrotizing chest wall infections following aortocoronary bypass operation in which Elastoplast dressings were used; both died. Although amphotericin B is the only agent with some evidence of efficacy, of 18 survivors with pulmonary mucormycosis, 11 were managed by surgery alone, according to Bigby and colleagues (1986).

Early recognition, control of diabetes, and termination of antimetabolite, antibiotic, or steroid therapy are all important. Parfrey (1986) noted that, with increasing premortem diagnosis, allowing more vigorous management both surgically and medically, the prognosis of this grave infection is improving.

Pulmonary Monosporosis

This rare mycotic infection is caused by *Monosporium apiospermum*. This inhabitant of soil appears to act as a secondary invader of previously damaged lung tissue, such as a tuberculous cavity, a cyst, or a bronchial saccule. Sometimes—but not characteristically–a fungus ball is formed. Amphotericin B has not been effective. Jung and associates (1977) summarized the localized resections that were performed in ten patients, with two deaths. Conservative management is recommended for asymptomatic patients without cavitary disease or bronchiectasis. Resection is advocated for good-risk patients with localized cavitary disease, or to help make a definitive diagnosis when bronchial carcinoma is suspected.

Paracoccidioidomycosis—South American Blastomycosis

This chronic granulomatous infection involves the skin, mucous membranes, lymph nodes, and visceral organs, including the lungs; it is caused by *Paracoccidioides brasiliensis*, presumably a soil saprophyte.

It is endemic in South America and perhaps also in Central America, and was not recognized outside these areas before the 1970s, as Murray (1974) and Bouza (1977) and their colleagues noted. The organisms resemble *Blastomyces dermatitidis* in tissue (Fig. 69–26). Cavitary pulmonary disease occurs in about one third of the patients. The disease is fatal unless treated. The treatment of choice for chronic paracoccidioidomycosis, according to Stamm and Dismukes (1983), is ketoconazole. If therapy is continued for 1 year, the relapse rate is low—less than 10%. Surgical resection apparently has no place in this disease, other than lung biopsy, because bilateral disseminated and polymorphic lung lesions seem to be the rule.

ANTIMYCOTIC DRUGS

As stated earlier, not all patients with proven infections require treatment with antimycotic agents. Three stand-

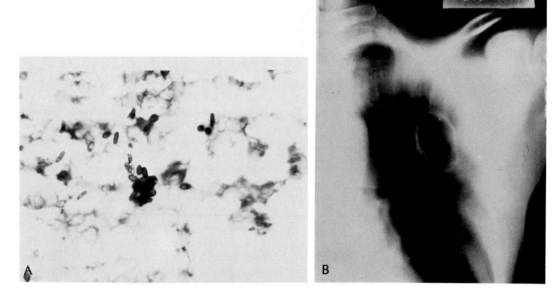

Fig. 69–24. Sporotrichosis. *A*, Cigar-shaped organisms of *Sporothrix schenckii* seen in resected lung specimen. PAS stain, × 1100. *B*, Thoracic roentgenogram showing cavitary lesion of pulmonary sporotrichosis. (Scott, S.M., et al.: Pulmonary sporotrichosis. N. Engl. J. Med. 265:453, 1961. Reprinted by permission from New England Journal of Medicine.)

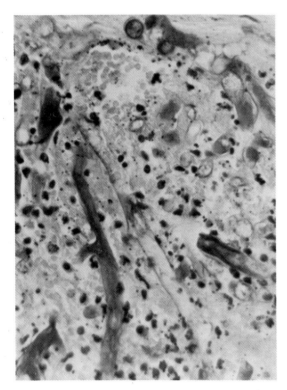

Fig. 69–25. Phycomycosis (mucormycosis). Broad, nonseptate hyphae of a phycomycete, probably *Mucor*, invading thrombosed pulmonary arterial wall. Hematoxylin & eosin stain, × 330. (Takaro, T.: Thoracic actinomycetic and mycotic infections. *In* Practice of Surgery. Edited by H.S. Goldsmith. Hagerstown, MD, Harper & Row, 1978, Thoracic Surgery, Chap. 12.)

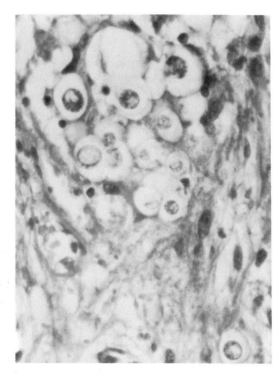

Fig. 69–26. Paracoccidioidomycosis (South American blastomycosis). Organisms of *Paracoccidioides brasiliensis,* in tissue. Note superficial resemblance to *Blastomyces dermatitidis.* (Takaro, T.: Thoracic actinomycetic and mycotic infections. *In* Practice of Surgery. Edited by H.S. Goldsmith. Hagerstown, MD, Harper & Row, 1978, Thoracic Surgery, Chap. 12.)

ard antifungal agents are available, and several others are under study.

Amphotericin B

As Table 69–3 shows, amphotericin B has the widest spectrum of effectiveness.

Amphotericin B is poorly absorbed from the gastrointestinal tract, and is effective only by the intravenous route. Because of its toxicity, it should be used only if the diagnosis is reasonably certain and spontaneous cure is unlikely. Suggested modes of administration include giving the patient a test dose of 1 mg of the drug in 250 ml of 5% glucose in water, over a 20- to 30-minute period, intravenously. On subsequent days, the dose is increased, advancing rapidly to a daily dose of about 0.5 mg to 0.6 mg/kg body weight, in 500 ml 5% dextrose in water over a 3- to 4-hour period. Fresh material should be made daily. Drug administration is begun only after obtaining baseline laboratory data—complete blood count, urinalysis, blood urea nitrogen, creatinine, serum potassium, and liver function studies. Hermans (1977) suggested that a flow sheet recording data to be obtained on a continuing basis is helpful. Certain toxic side effects—headache, nausea, vomiting, fever, hypotension, delirium—may be ameliorated or prevented by adding 25 to 50 mg of hydrocortisone sodium succinate to the infusion bottle, unless the patient is already receiving steroids. Blood pressure and pulse are monitored every half hour for the duration of the infusion; renal function is monitored twice weekly at first, until azotemia stabilizes—preferably at a level below 50 mg/dl with serum creatinine below 2 mg/dl. Then it can be checked once a week; and a double dose of drug can be given on alternate days, to diminish the patient's discomfort. A total dose of 3 g of amphotericin B is a common goal, but this regimen may be individualized in accordance with the severity of the patient's illness and the known prognosis without therapy of each fungal infection. Her-

mans (1977) recommended 2.5 g for histoplamosis; 1.5 g for blastomycosis and 2 g for nonmeningitic pulmonary coccidioidomycosis. According to Bennett (1974), as well as others, significant permanent reduction of renal function is unlikely in adults at total doses up to 4 g.

Flucytosine

5-Fluorocytosine

The range of effectiveness of this drug is narrower than that of amphotericin B, but it provides more effective treatment for pulmonary and meningeal cryptococcosis when used with amphotericin B, and it also allows lower doses of the latter to be used. This oral preparation is used in a dose of 150 mg/kg body weight, in divided doses, for several weeks to months. Besides mild side effects similar to those of amphotericin B, 5-fluorocytosine can cause leukopenia, anemia, and thrombocytopenia—and occasionally, pancytopenia. Rarely are these serious enough to require discontinuation of treatment. Harder and Hermans (1975), however, noted that when used in combination with amphotericin B, the renal damage caused by 5-fluorocytosine may lead to excessive blood levels of flucytosine.

Ketoconazole and Miconazole

Ketoconazole, an oral antifungal agent with relatively low toxicity, has proven its effectiveness. It is reportedly effective in patients with blastomycosis, histoplasmosis, and coccidioidomycosis, as reported in the Medical Letter (1986), and for nonmeningeal cryptococcosis as Dismukes and associates (1983) reported. Recommended dosage is 400 to 600 mg daily, and prolonged therapy—6 to 12 months or more—is required to treat the deep mycotic infections. Cauwenbergh (1986) suggested that ketoconazole may also be effective as a prophylactic against mycotic infections in immunocompromised patients.

Table 69–3. Currently Available Agents Against Actinomycetic and Fungal Infection

Infecting Organism	Drug of First Choice	Alternative Drugs
Actinomycosis	Penicillin	Broad-spectrum antibiotics
Nocardiosis	Sulfadiazine	Trimethroprim and sulfamethoxazole
Aspergillus species	Amphotericin B	No dependable alternative
Blastomyces dermatitidis	Amphotericin B or ketoconazole	
Candida species	Amphotericin B with or without flucytosine	Ketoconazole
Coccidioides immitis	Amphotericin B	Ketoconazole, miconazole
Cryptococcus neoformans	Amphotericin B with or without flucytosine	Ketoconazole
Histoplasma capsulatum	Amphotericin B	Ketoconazole
Mucor species	Amphotericin B	No dependable alternative
Paracoccidioides brasiliensis	Amphotericin B or ketoconazole	A sulfonamide, miconazole
Sporothrix schenckii	An iodide	Amphotericin B, ketoconazole

Adapted from Drugs for treatment of systemic fungal infections. Med. Lett. Drugs Ther. 28:41, 1986; Finegold, S.M., George, W.L., and Mulligan, M.E.: Anaerobic Infections. Part II. *In* Disease-A-Month. Edited by Nicholas J. Cotsonas, Jr. Chicago, Year Book Medical Publishers, Inc., 1985; and Wallace, R.J., Jr., et al.: Use of trimethoprim-sulfamethoxazole for treatment of infections due to Nocardia. Rev. Infect. Dis. 4:315, 1982.

Miconazole, given intravenously, may be useful for some patients with candidiasis, coccidioidomycosis, pseudallescheriasis, and paracoccidiodomycosis, as noted in the Medical Letter (1986). Itraconazole is under study for the treatment of paracoccidiodomycosis by Restrepo and colleagues (1987).

REFERENCES

Allan, A., Sethia, B., and Turner, M.A.: Recent experience of the treatment of aspergilloma with the surgical stapling device. Thorax 41:483, 1986.

Arnow, P.M., et al.: Pulmonary aspergillosis during hospital renovation. Am. Rev. Respir. Dis. 118:49, 1978.

Baker, E.J., Hawkins, J.A., and Waskow, E.A.: Surgery for coccidioidomycosis in 52 diabetic patients, with special reference to related immunologic factors. J. Thorac. Cardiovasc. Surg. 75:680, 1978.

Balikian, J.P., et al.: Pulmonary actinomycosis. Radiology 128:613, 1978a.

Balikian, J.P., Herman, P.G., and Kopit, S.: Pulmonary nocardiosis. Radiology 126:569, 1978b.

Battaglini, J.W., et al.: Surgical management of symptomatic pulmonary aspergilloma. Ann. Thorac. Surg. 39:512, 1985.

Bayer, A.S., et al.: Unusual syndromes of coccidioidomycosis. Diagnostic and therapeutic considerations: a report of 10 cases and review of the English literature. Medicine 55:131, 1976.

Bennett, J.E.: Chemotherapy of systemic mycoses. Parts I and II. N. Engl. J. Med. 290:30, 320, 1974.

Bigby, T.D., et al.: Clinical spectrum of pulmonary mucormycosis. Chest 89:435, 1986.

Bouza, E., et al.: Paracoccidioidomycosis (South American blastomycosis) in the United States. Chest 72:100, 1977.

Bower, G.C., et al.: Pulmonary aspergilloma: a report of 25 patients. Am. Rev. Respir. Dis. 115:90, 1977.

Bradsher, R.W., Rice, D.C., and Abernathy, R.S.: Ketoconazole therapy for endemic blastomycosis. Ann. Intern. Med. 103:872, 1985.

Bronnimann, D.A., et al.: Coccidioidomycosis in the acquired immunodeficiency syndrome. Ann. Intern. Med. 106:372, 1987.

Busey, J.F., et al.: Blastomycosis. I. A review of 198 collected cases in Veterans Administration Hospitals. Am. Rev. Respir. Dis. 89:659, 1964.

Butz, R.O., Zvetina, J.R., and Leininger, B.J.: Ten-year experience with mycetomas in patients with pulmonary tuberculosis. Chest 87:356, 1985.

Cauwenbergh, G.: Prophylaxis of mycotic infections in immunocompromised patients: a review of 27 reports and publications. Drugs Exp. Clin. Res. XII(5):419, 1986.

Chick, E., et al.: The use of skin tests and serologic tests in histoplasmosis, coccidioidomycosis, and blastomycosis, 1973. Am. Rev. Respir. Dis. 108:156, 1973.

Cohen, S.L., Gale, A.M., and Liston, H.E.: Report of a pilot study on noncalcified discrete pulmonary coin lesions in a coccidioidomycosis endemic area. Ariz. Med. 29:40, 1972.

Cunningham, R.T., and Einstein, H.: Coccidioidal pulmonary cavities with rupture. J. Thorac. Cardiovasc. Surg. 84:172, 1982.

Cush, R., Light, R.W., and George, R.B.: Clinical and roentgenographic manifestations of acute and chronic blastomycosis. Chest 69:345, 1976.

Daly, R.C., et al.: Pulmonary aspergilloma. Results of surgical treatment. J. Thorac. Cardiovasc. Surg. 92:981, 1986.

Datta, J.S., and Raff, M.J.: Actinomycotic pleuropericarditis. Am. Rev. Respir. Dis. 110:328, 1974.

Dines, D.E., et al.: Mediastinal granuloma and fibrosing mediastinitis. Chest 75:320, 1979.

Dismukes, W.E., et al.: Treatment of systemic mycoses with ketoconazole: emphasis on toxicity and clinical response in 52 patients. Ann. Intern. Med. 98:13, 1983.

Drutz, D.J., and Catanzaro, A.: Coccidioidomycosis. Parts I and II. Am. Rev. Respir. Dis. 117:559, 727, 1978.

Duperval, R., et al.: Cryptococcosis, with emphasis on the significance of isolation of *Cryptococcus neoformans* from the respiratory tract. Chest 72:13, 1977.

Dyess, D.L., Garrison, R.N., and Fry, D.E.: *Candida* sepsis. Arch. Surg. 120:345, 1985.

Eastridge, C.E.: Opportunistic infections due to aspergillosis. (Editorial) Ann. Thorac. Surg. 22:102, 1976.

Eastridge, C.E., et al.: Pulmonary aspergillosis. Ann. Thorac. Surg. 13:397, 1972.

Eguchi, S., et al.: Surgery in the treatment of pulmonary aspergillosis. Br. J. Dis. Chest 65:111, 1971.

Epstein, R., Cole, R., and Hung, K.K., Jr.: Pleural effusion secondary to pulmonary cryptococcosis. Chest 61:296, 1972.

Faulkner, S.L., et al.: Hemoptysis and pulmonary aspergilloma: operative versus nonoperative treatment. Ann. Thorac. Surg. 25:389, 1978.

Ferguson, T.B., and Burford, T.H.: Mediastinal granuloma—15-year experience. Ann. Thorac. Surg. 1:125, 1965.

Feingold, S.M., George, W.L., and Mulligan, M.E.: Anaerobic Infections. Part II. In Disease-a-Month. Edited by Nicholas J. Cotsonas, Jr. Chicago, IL, Year Book Medical Publishers, Inc., 1985.

Foley, T.F., Dines, D.E., and Dolan, C.T.: Pulmonary actinomycosis: report of 18 cases. Minn. Med. 54:593, 1971.

Frazier, A.R., Rosenow, E.C., III, and Roberts, G.D.: Nocardiosis: a review of 25 cases occurring during 24 months. Mayo Clin. Proc. 50:657, 1975.

Gal, A.A., et al.: The pathology of pulmonary cryptococcal infections in the acquired immunodeficiency syndrome. Arch. Pathol. Lab. Med. 110:502, 1986.

Gale, A.M., and Kleitsch, W.P.: Solitary pulmonary nodule due to phycomycosis (mucormycosis). Chest 62:752, 1972.

Gartenberg, G., et al.: Hospital-acquired mucormycosis (*Rhizopus rhizopodiformis*) of skin and subcutaneous tissue. N. Engl. J. Med. 299:1115, 1978.

George, R.B., Penn, R.L., and Kinasewitz, G.T.: Mycobacterial, fungal, actinomycotic, and nocardial infections of the pleura. Clin. Chest Med. 6:63, 1985.

Geraci, J.E., et al.: Focal pulmonary cryptococcosis: evaluation of necessity of amphotericin-B therapy. Proc. Staff Meet. Mayo Clin. 40:552, 1965.

Gerding, D.N.: Treatment of pulmonary sporotrichosis. Semin. Respir. Infect. 1:61, 1986.

Godwin, J.D.: The solitary pulmonary nodule. Radiol. Clin. North Am. 21:709, 1983.

Golden, N., et al.: Thoracic actinomycosis in childhood. Clin. Pediatr. 24:646, 1985.

Goodwin, R.A., Jr., and DesPrez, R.M.: Histoplasmosis. Am. Rev. Respir. Dis. 117:929, 1978.

Goodwin, R.A., Jr., et al.: Chronic pulmonary histoplasmosis. Medicine 55:413, 1976.

Graybill, J.R.: Azole antifungal drugs in treatment of coccidioidomycosis. Semin. Respir. Infect. 1:53, 1986.

Griepp, R.B.: In discussion of Henderson, R.D., et al.: Surgery in pulmonary aspergillosis. J. Thorac. Cardiovasc. Surg. 70:1088, 1975.

Hammerman, K.J., et al.: Pulmonary cryptococcosis: clinical forms and treatment. Am. Rev. Respir. Dis. 108:1116, 1973.

Hammerman, K.J., Sarosi, G.A., and Tosh, F.E.: Amphotericin-B in the treatment of saprophytic forms of pulmonary aspergillosis. Am. Rev. Respir. Dis. 109:57, 1974.

Harder, E.J., and Hermans, P.E.: Treatment of fungal infections with flucytosine. Arch. Intern. Med. 135:231, 1975.

Harrison, R.N., and Thomas, D.J.B.: Acute actinomycetic empyema. Thorax 12:406, 1979.

Hatcher, C.R., Jr., et al.: Primary pulmonary cryptococcosis. J. Thorac. Cardiovasc. Surg. 61:39, 1971.

Hauch, T.W.: Pulmonary mucormycosis: another cure. Chest 72:92, 1977.

Hermans, P.E.: Antifungal agents used for deep-seated mycotic infections. Mayo Clin. Proc. 52:687, 1977.

Herring, M., and Pecora, D.: Pleural aspergillosis: a case report. Am. Surg. 42:300, 1976.

Howard, R.J., Simmons, R.L., and Najarian, J.S.: Fungal infections in renal transplant recipients. Ann. Surg. 188:598, 1978.

Jay, S.J., Platt, M.R., and Reynolds, R.C.: Primary pulmonary sporotrichosis. Am. Rev. Respir. Dis. *115*:1051, 1977.

Jung, J.Y., et al.: The role of surgery in the management of pulmonary monosporosis: a collective review. J. Thorac. Cardiovasc. Surg. *73*:139, 1977.

Jung, J.Y., et al.: Role of surgery in the management of pulmonary sporotrichosis. J. Thorac. Cardiovasc. Surg. *77*:234, 1979.

Karas, A., et al.: Pulmonary aspergillosis: an analysis of 41 patients. Ann. Thorac. Surg. *22*:1, 1976.

Kerkering, T.M., Duma, R.J., and Shadomy, S.: The evolution of pulmonary cryptococcosis. Ann. Intern. Med. *94*:611, 1981.

Kinasewitz, G.T., Penn, R.L., and George, R.B.: The spectrum and significance of pleural disease in blastomycosis. Chest *86*:580, 1984.

Kitchen, M.S., Reiber, C.D., and Eastin, G.B.: An urban epidemic of North American blastomycosis. Am. Rev. Respir. Dis. *115*:1063, 1977.

Klein, B.S., et al.: Isolation of *Blastomyces dermatitidis* in soil associated with a large outbreak of blastomycosis in Wisconsin. N. Engl. J. Med. *314*:529, 1986.

Krick, J.A., Stinson, E.B., and Remington, J.S.: Nocardia infection in heart transplant patients. Ann. Intern. Med. *82*:18, 1975.

Landis, F.B., and Varkey, B.: Late relapse of pulmonary blastomycosis after adequate treatment with amphotericin-B: case report. Am. Rev. Respir. Dis. *113*:77, 1976.

Laskey, W., and Sarosi, G.A.: Endogenous reinfection in blastomycosis. Am. Rev. Respir. Dis. *115*:266, 1977.

Lewis, J.L., and Rabinovich, S.: The wide spectrum of cryptococcal infections. Am. J. Med. *53*:315, 1972.

Lillington, G.A.: Pulmonary nodules: solitary and multiple. Clin. Chest. Med. *3*:361, 1982.

Littman, M.L., and Walter, J.E.: Cryptococcosis: current status. Am. J. Med. *45*:922, 1968.

Lonky, S.A., et al.: Acute coccidioidal pleural effusion. Am. Rev. Respir. Dis. *114*:681, 1976.

Lopes-Berestein, G.: Liposomal amphotericin B in the treatment of fungal infections. Ann. Intern. Med. *105*:130, 1986.

Louria, D.B., Stiff, D.P., and Bennett, B.: Disseminated moniliasis in the adult. Medicine *41*:307, 1962.

Marks, T.S., Spence, W.F., and Baisch, B.F.: Limited resection for pulmonary coccidioidomycosis. *In* Coccidioidomycosis. Edited by L. Ajello. Tucson, University of Arizona Press, 1967, p. 73.

McDonnell, J.M., and Hutchins, G.M.: Pulmonary cryptococcosis. Hum. Pathol. *16*:121, 1985.

McManus, E.J., and Jones, J.M.: The use of ketoconazole in the treatment of blastomycosis. Am. Rev. Respir. Dis. *133*:141, 1986.

McQuarrie, D.G., and Hall, W.H.: Actinomycosis of the lung and chest wall. Surgery *64*:905, 1968.

Medical Letter: Drugs for treatment of systemic fungal infections. The Med. Lett. Drugs Ther. *28*:41, 1986.

Merdler, C., et al.: Primary actinomycetic empyema. South Med. J. *76*:411, 1983.

Michelson, E.: Primary pulmonary sporotrichosis. Ann. Thorac. Surg. *24*:83, 1977.

Murray, H.W.: Pulmonary mucormycosis with massive fatal hemoptysis. Chest *68*:65, 1975.

Murray, H.W., Littman, M.L., and Roberts, R.B.: Disseminated paracoccidioidomycosis (South American blastomycosis) in the United States. Am. J. Med. *56*:209, 1974.

Nelson, A.R.: The surgical treatment of pulmonary coccidioidomycosis. Curr. Probl. Surg. *11*:1, 1974.

National Institute of Allergy and Infectious Diseases Mycoses Study Group: Treatment of blastomycosis and histoplasmosis with ketoconazole. Ann. Intern. Med. *103*:861, 1985.

Orringer, M.B., and Sloan, H.: Monilial esophagitis. Ann. Thorac. Surg. *26*:364, 1978.

Parfrey, N.A.: Improved diagnosis and prognosis of mucormycosis. A clinicopathologic study of 33 cases. Medicine *65*:113, 1986.

Pennington, J.E.: Aspergillus lung disease. Med. Clin. North Am. *64*:475, 1980.

Pluss, J.L., and Opal, S.M.: Pulmonary sporotrichosis: review of treatment and outcome. Medicine *65*:143, 1986.

Poe, R.H., et al.: Pulmonary blastomycosis versus carcinoma—challenging differential. Am. J. Med. Sci. *263*:145, 1972.

Rabinowitz, J.G., Busch, J., and Buttram, W.R.: Pulmonary manifestations of blastomycosis: radiological support of a new concept. Radiology *120*(1):25, 1976.

Ramirez, R.J.: Pulmonary aspergilloma. N. Engl. J. Med. *271*:1281, 1964.

Read, C.T.: Coin lesion, pulmonary, in the Southwest (solitary pulmonary nodules). Ariz. Med. *29*:775, 1972.

Remy, J., et al.: Treatment of hemoptysis by embolization of bronchial arteries. Radiology *122*:33, 1977.

Restrepo, A., et al.: Itraconazole in the treatment of paracoccidioidomycosis: a preliminary report. Rev. Infect. Dis. *9*(Suppl. 1):S51, 1987.

Rohatgi, P.K.: Pulmonary sporotrichosis. South. Med. J. *73*:1611, 1980.

Rohatgi, P.K., and Schmitt, R.G.: Pulmonary coccidioidal mycetoma. Am. J. Med. Sci. *287*:27, 1984.

Rosenbaum, R.B., Barber, J.V., and Stevens, D.A.: *Candida albicans* pneumonia. Diagnosis by pulmonary aspiration, recovery without treatment. Am. Rev. Respir. Dis. *109*:373, 1974.

Rubin, A.H.E., and Alroy, G.G.: *Candida albicans* abscess of lung. Thorax *32*:373, 1977.

Sall, E.L., and Bergeron, R.B.: Pulmonary cryptococcosis—a case diagnostically confirmed by transbronchial brush biopsy. Chest *59*:454, 1971.

Salyer, W.R., and Salyer, D.C.: Pleural involvement in cryptococcosis. Chest *66*:139, 1974a.

Salyer, W.R., Salyer, D.C., and Baker, R.D.: Primary complex of cryptococcus and pulmonary lymph nodes. J. Infect. Dis. *130*:74, 1974b.

Sanders, J.S., et al.: Exfoliative cytology in the rapid diagnosis of pulmonary blastomycosis. Chest *72*:193, 1977.

Sarosi, G.A., and Serstock, D.S.: Isolation of *Blastomyces dermatitidis* from pigeon manure. Am. Rev. Respir. Dis. *114*(6):1179, 1976.

Sarosi, G.A., Davies, S.F., and Phillips, J.R.: Self-limited blastomycosis: a report of 39 cases. Semin. Respir. Infect. *1*:40, 1986.

Slade, P.R., Slesser, B.V., and Southgate, J.: Thoracic actinomycosis. Thorax *28*:73, 1973.

Smith, F.S., et al.: Pulmonary resection for localized lesions of cryptococcosis (torulosis): a review of eight cases. Thorax *31*:121, 1976.

Spear, R.K., Walker, P.D., and Lampton, L.M.: Tracheal obstruction associated with a fungus ball. Chest *70*:662, 1976.

Stamm, A.M., and Dismukes, W.E.: Current therapy of pulmonary and disseminated fungal diseases. Chest *83*:911, 1983.

Steele, J.D. (Ed.): Treatment of Mycotic and Parasitic Diseases of the Chest. Springfield, IL, Charles C Thomas, 1964.

Strinden, W.D., Helgerson, R.B., and Maki, D.G.: Candida septic thrombosis of the great central veins associated with central catheters. Ann. Surg. *202*:653, 1985.

Sutliff, W.D., and Cruthirds, T.P.: *Blastomyces dermatitidis* in cytologic preparations. Am. Rev. Respir. Dis. *108*:149, 1973.

Thadepalli, H., et al.: Pulmonary mycetoma due to *Coccidioides immitis*. Chest *71*:429, 1977.

Thomas, F.E., Jr., et al.: *Candida albicans* infection of sternum and costal cartilages: combined operative treatment and drug therapy with 5-fluorocytosine. Ann. Thorac. Surg. *23*:163, 1977.

Turner, S., and Kaufman, L.: Immunodiagnosis of blastomycosis. Sem. Respir. Infect. *1*:22, 1986.

Utz, J.P., and Buechner, H.A.: Mucormycosis (phycomycosis). *In* Management of Fungus Diseases of the Lungs. Edited by H.A. Buechner. Springfield, IL, Charles C Thomas, 1971.

Utz, J.P., et al.: Therapy of cryptococcosis with a combination of flucytosine and amphotericin-B. J. Infect. Dis. *132*:368, 1975.

Varkey, B., and Rose, H.D.: Pulmonary aspergilloma: a rational approach to treatment. Am. J. Med. *61*:626, 1976.

Wallace, R.J., Jr., et al.: Use of trimethoprim-sulfamethoxazole for treatment of infections due to Nocardia. Rev. Infect. Dis. *4*:315, 1982.

Weese, W.C., and Smith, I.M.: A study of 57 cases of actinomycosis over a 36-year period. Ann. Intern. Med. *135*:1562, 1975.

Williams, D.M., Krick, J.A., and Remington, J.S.: Pulmonary infection in the compromised host. Am. Rev. Respir. Dis. *114*:359, 593, 1976.

Wray, T.M., Bryant, R.E., and Killen, D.A.: Sternal osteomyelitis and costochondritis after median sternotomy. J. Thorac. Cardiovasc. Surg. *65*:227, 1973.

Zajtchuk, R., et al.: Mediastinal histoplasmosis: surgical considerations. J. Thorac. Cardiovasc. Surg. *66*:300, 1973.

READING REFERENCES

American Thoracic Society: Laboratory diagnosis of mycotic and specific fungal infections. Am. Rev. Respir. Dis. *132*:1373, 1985.

Beaman, B.L., et al.: Nocardial infections in the United States, 1972–1974. J. Infect. Dis. *134*:286, 1976.

Belcher, J.R., and Plummer, N.S.: Surgery in bronchopulmonary aspergillosis. Br. J. Dis. Chest *54*:335, 1960.

Cunningham, R.T., and Einstein, H.: Coccidioidal pulmonary cavities with rupture. J. Thorac. Cardiovasc. Surg. *84*:172, 1982.

Hermans, P.E.: Antifungal agents used for deep-seated mycotic infections. Mayo Clin. Proc. *58*:223, 1983.

Kerkering, T.M., Duma, R.J., and Shadomy, S.: The evolution of pulmonary cryptococcosis. Ann. Intern. Med. *94*:611, 1981.

Mills, S.A., Seigler, H.F., and Wolfe, W.G.: The incidence and management of pulmonary mycosis in renal allograft patients. Ann. Surg. *182*:617, 1975.

National Institute of Allergy and Infectious Disease Mycoses Study Group: Treatment of blastomycosis and histoplasmosis with ketoconazole. Ann. Intern. Med. *103*:861, 1985.

Restrepo, A., et al.: The gamut of paracoccidioidomycosis. Am. J. Med. *61*:33, 1976.

Scott, S.M., Peasley, E.D., and Crymes, T.P.: Pulmonary sporotrichosis: a report of two cases with cavitation. N. Engl. J. Med. *265*:453, 1961.

Soutter, D.I., and Todd, T.R.J.: Systemic candidiasis in a surgical intensive care unit. Can. J. Surg. *29*:197, 1986.

Steele, J.D. (Ed.): Treatment of Mycotic and Parasitic Diseases of the Chest. Springfield, IL, Charles C Thomas, 1964.

CHAPTER 70

PLEUROPULMONARY AMEBIASIS

Forrest C. Eggleston and Mohan Verghese

Pleuropulmonary amebiasis is almost invariably the result of perforation of an amebic liver abscess through the diaphragm. It accounts for 10% of all deaths from amebiasis. To understand its management, the nature of amebiasis and of the liver abscess it produces must be understood.

AMEBIASIS

Amebiasis is caused by the protozoan *Entamoeba histolytica*. The ameba's life cycle has three stages: trophozoite, precyst, and cyst (Fig. 70–1). Infection results from the ingestion of cysts, usually from contaminated food or water. Excystation occurs in the lower ileum. The resulting trophozoites are the active and growing stage of the parasite. Multiplication is by binary fission. The trophozoites can invade the mucosa of the bowel. Invasion is probably the result of physical means combined with production of the lytic substances from which the parasite derives its descriptive name. If the trophozoites do not invade the bowel, they become precysts and then cysts, finally being eliminated in the stool (Fig. 70–2).

According to the World Health Organization, the protozoan *Entamoeba histolytica* is present in the gastrointestinal tract of over 10% of the world's population. Fortunately, only about 10% of those harboring the parasite develop symptomatic infection. Although amebic infestation occurs throughout the world, clinical infection

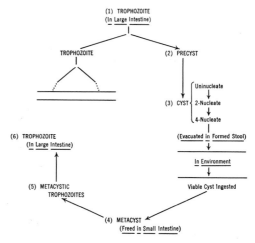

Fig. 70–2. Schematic representation of the life cycle of *E. histolytica*. (Modified from Faust, E.C., and Russell, P.F.: Clinical Parasitology, 7th ed. Philadelphia, Lea & Febiger, 1964.)

is far more frequent in tropical and subtropical climates, particularly in areas with inadequate sanitation, poor nutrition, poverty, and overcrowding. Stress, decreased resistance, and the administration of steroids can be important contributing factors.

Morphologic differences distinguish all species in the genus Entamoeba except for *E. histolytica* and *E. hartmanni*, which are identified primarily by size. *E. hartmanni* was formerly known as the "small race" of *E. histolytica*, and is now considered to be saprophytic. It is the "large race" of *E. histolytica* that produces disease in man. Several strains or species of ameba, morphologically indistinguishable but possibly differing in their pathogenic potential, make up the species complex known as *E. histolytica*. This may account for differences in clinical findings and therapeutic results in geographically separated centers.

Intestinal amebiasis may be acute or chronic. The acute form produces cramping abdominal pain, diarrhea, and tenesmus. The stool frequently contains blood. The chronic form may persist for a long time with alternating

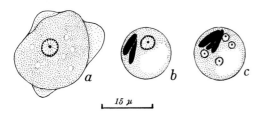

Fig. 70–1. *Entamoeba histolytica. a,* Trophozoite; *b,* immature cyst—precystic form; *c,* cystic or resistant form. (Modified from Faust, E.C., and Russell, P.E.: Clinical Parasitology, 7th ed. Philadelphia, Lea & Febiger, 1964.)

bouts of diarrhea and constipation. Many patient who develop liver abscesses, however, give no history of gastrointestinal symptoms.

AMEBIC LIVER ABSCESS

When amebae invade the colonic mucosa, particularly in the cecum, they may be carried to the liver through the portal venous system. There they lodge in the venules, producing thrombosis that is followed by an infarct, necrosis of liver tissue, and a localized abscess. This is not an abscess in the classic sense, but rather a collection of necrotic liver tissue with white blood cells and amebae in the center. The amebae in the periphery multiply, releasing lytic enzymes, resulting in additional necrosis and enlarging the abscess. No fibrous capsule or clear margin exists between the abscess and the surrounding tissue. Although the parasite does not normally stimulate the intense inflammatory response of other infective agents, it may do so under certain conditions, particularly if secondarily infected.

Because of the combination of the laminar flow of the portal venous system and the high incidence of cecal involvement, the right lobe of the liver is most commonly involved. In his review, Grigsby (1969) found that 85% of amebic liver abscesses were in the right lobe and 15% in the left lobe; both lobes were involved in 15 to 20% of cases. Our own figures are similar.

Although these abscesses may occur at any age, they are most frequent in the third to fifth decade of life. In adults, men are infected 7 to 9 times as often as women, whereas in children there is no sex difference.

Symptoms of an amebic liver abscess may be present for a few days to many months before patients seek help. In our and associates' (1978) experience the average duration was 33 days. Symptoms vary, and as a result, the diagnosis is not clear in one third of the cases.

Virtually all of the patients have pain, most commonly in the right hypochondrium—73%. Pain may also occur in the epigastrium, left hypochondrium, or right hemithorax. When associated with diaphragmatic irritation, it may be referred to the shoulder. The pain may be mild, moderate, or severe, and usually is constant. Many patients complain of a swelling in the upper abdomen. Anorexia, fever, and malaise are usual, and patients whose treatment has been delayed may have profound weight loss.

A history of diarrhea, although helpful in making a diagnosis, is given by less than half of all patients. Blood in the stool is noted in only about 25% of patients.

Examination of the abdomen shows a large, tender liver. Softening suggests imminent rupture of the amebic liver abscess. In addition, there is often tenderness on intercostal pressure. Pleural effusion is common. Jaundice is uncommon but when present is associated with a poor prognosis.

Proctosigmoidoscopy is useful only if punctate lesions are found in the mucosa or amebae are seen on examination of swab material.

Leukocytosis is the rule. Serologic tests, if positive, suggest current or previous invasive amebiasis. Except for the latex agglutination test, these procedures are time-consuming and many require considerable technical competence, which are definite disadvantages because many patients urgently need treatment.

The chest roentgenogram usually shows an elevated diaphragm, often accompanied by pleural effusion (Fig. 70–3). CT scanning (Fig. 70–4), ultrasonography (Fig. 70–5), and isotopic imaging all demonstrate both the presence and site of liver abscesses. When aspirated, the pus is usually reddish-brown or chocolate brown—the so-called anchovy sauce—although initially it may be yellowish or even white. Unless the amebic liver abscess was aspirated previously, it is bacteriologically sterile.

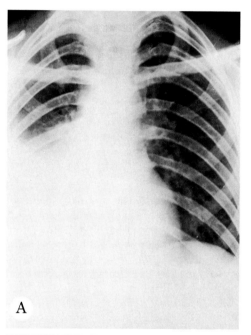

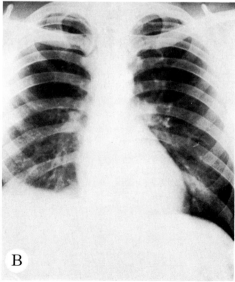

Fig. 70–3. Simple irritative pleuritis with effusion in the right hemithorax. *A,* Before treatment. *B,* After treatment.

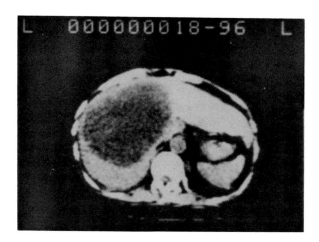

Fig. 70–4. CT scan showing a large abscess in the right lobe of the liver.

Amebae can be demonstrated in only about half of the abscesses.

Because of the lytic nature of the parasite and the lack of encapsulation of amebic liver abscesses, rupture occurs in from 10 to 30% of patients. The anatomic location of amebic liver abscesses makes upward or transdiaphragmatic rupture more frequent than downward or infradiaphragmatic rupture (Fig. 70– 6).

THORACIC AMEBIASIS

In amebiasis 70 to 97% of thoracic complications result from extension of an amebic liver abscess through the diaphragm. The type of complication depends upon whether the pleural space, the lung, or the pericardium is involved, either singly or in combination. We shall consider only pleural and pulmonary involvement.

Most patients have the clinical signs of an amebic liver abscess in addition to those related to the thoracic complication.

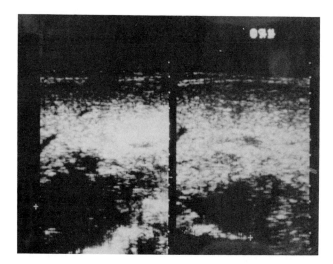

Fig. 70–5. Ultrasound. Parasagittal and subcostal sections showing a large liver abscess 6 cm below the skin.

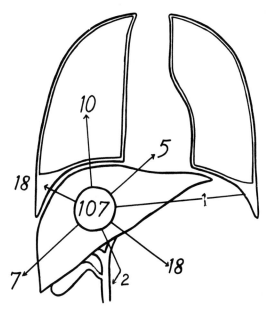

SITE OF 61 PERFORATIONS IN 52 PATIENTS

Fig. 70–6. Site of perforation in 107 consecutive patients operated on for amebic liver abscess. 34—65%—of perforations were into the thorax.

Pleural Involvement

An amebic liver abscess adjacent to the diaphragm produces irritation and a sympathetic pleural effusion. On the chest roentgenogram the diaphragm is elevated and fixed. The costophrenic angle is obliterated. Thoracentesis shows that the fluid is clear or serosanguineous and sterile on culture. Amebae are not present. This pleural effusion requires no specific therapy other than that for the causative liver abscess. Should it increase, however, it may presage the rupture of the abscess through the diaphragm and the development of frank empyema.

Amebic Empyema

Excluding sympathetic pleural effusion, amebic empyema is the most common of all the pleuropulmonary complications, occurring in 50 to 75% of patients with thoracic amebiasis. In 95%, the empyema is on the right side. Elevation of the diaphragm, friction rub, and effusion usually precede it. The onset can be either insidious or rapid and overwhelming (Fig. 70–7), depending on the size of the perforation and the volume of the abscess. It is accompanied by pain, dyspnea, and if massive, shock. Some patients complain of a "tearing" sensation. Roentgenograms of the chest show opacification of the ipsilateral lung field (Fig. 70–8).

On thoracentesis, purulent fluid is found, reddish-brown or bile-stained. Unless the lung is also involved, the fluid is sterile. Amebae are identified in less than 10% of cases.

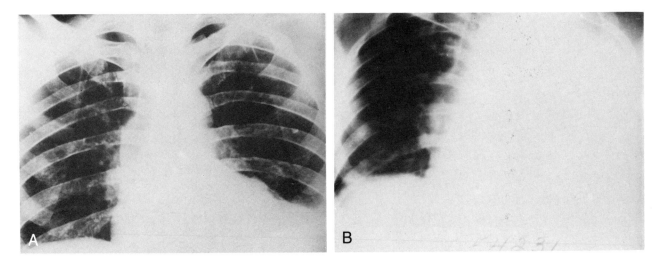

Fig. 70–7. *A*, This patient had an acute massive rupture of an amebic liver abscess into the left pleura. Roentgenogram taken before rupture. *B*, Same patient 12 hours later. This demonstrates the need for urgent treatment. (Reprinted from Eggleston, F.C.: Pitfalls in the surgical management of ALA. Trop. Doc. 9:178, 1979, with permission.)

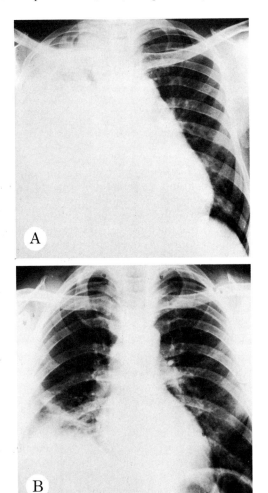

Fig. 70–8. Pure amebic empyema of the right hemithorax. *A*, Before treatment. *B*, After treatment.

Pleural thickening—often out of proportion to the duration of the empyema—follows rapidly, especially if there is secondary infection. Accordingly, treatment must be prompt and vigorous to avoid further complications. In addition to specific drug therapy, the pus must be removed rapidly. Although repeated aspirations—often combined with the instillation of streptokinase—have been recommended, we agree with Ibarra-Pérez (1981) that closed intercostal drainage with the largest cannula possible combined with strong suction offers the best chance for prompt and complete re-expansion of the lung. When carried out promptly, secondary surgical procedures other than an occasional rib resection are rarely required. Le Roux and his associates (1986) pointed out that subcostal drainage of the amebic liver abscess may be necessary when drainage persists or abscess becomes secondarily infected.

Should initial treatment be delayed or inadequate, re-expansion of the lung may be limited and decortication needed.

Mortality varies from 14 to 40%, depending upon the general condition of the patient and the delay in starting treatment.

Pulmonary Amebiasis

Two types of pulmonary amebiasis occur; the first results from rupture of an amebic liver abscess into the lung and the second is "metastatic," i.e., with no communication to the liver. The former is by far the more common.

When pleural symphysis precedes the transdiaphragmatic rupture of amebic liver abscess, the lung is directly involved, particularly the basal segments (Fig. 70–9), the middle lobe, or rarely the lingula. Following a few days of chest pain and nonproductive cough, the patient complains of expectoration of reddish brown or bile-stained material, sometimes in large quantities. Unless flooding of the tracheobronchial tree is overwhelming,

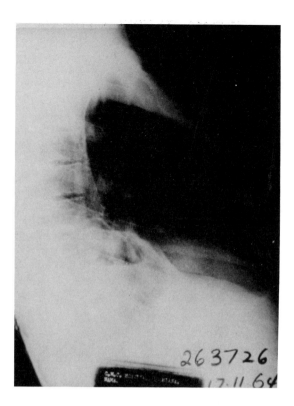

Fig. 70–9. Involvement of the right lower lobe basal segments by amebic abscess extending from the liver.

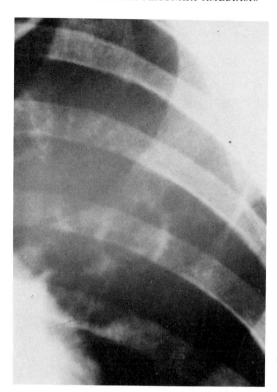

Fig. 70–10. Metastatic amebic lung abscess.

the prognosis is good and the patient's symptoms may be alleviated by drainage of the liver abscess.

Treatment consists of postural drainage, antibiotics to prevent secondary infection, and most importantly, specific antiamebic drug therapy. This complication carries the lowest mortality of any of the major complications of amebiasis.

Rarely, a persistent bronchobiliary fistula develops. Ragheb and his associates (1976) performed lung resection and closure of the fistulous tract. We prefer to drain the liver abscess transabdominally, as one of us (M.V.) and associates (1979) reported.

Occasionally, lung involvement is followed by bronchiectasis, usually mild—not severe enough to require resection. Indeed, we have never had to do one.

Metastatic pulmonary amebic lung abscesses are rare and result from hematogenous spread of amebae (Fig. 70–10). Symptoms resemble those of other lung abscesses, with fever, chest pain, cough, and hemoptysis. Occasionally they rupture into the pleura and produce a localized empyema (Fig. 70–11). Unless amebae can be demonstrated in the sputum or the pleural fluid, diagnosis is difficult and depends on finding evidence of amebiasis elsewhere.

Treatment is like that for any other lung abscess, with the addition of specific antiamebic drug therapy.

Pleural and Pulmonary Amebiasis

In about 25% of patients, both the pleura and lungs are involved. Treatment includes intercostal drainage

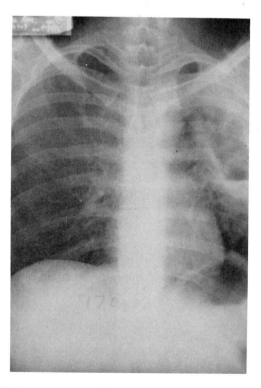

Fig. 70–11. Metastatic amebic lung abscess with rupture and localized empyema and bronchopleural fistula. Amebae seen on smear of empyema fluid.

Table 70–1. **Recommended Antiamebic Drug Schedule**

Drug	Route of Administration	Dose	Duration
Dehydroemetine	Intramuscular	1–1.5 mg/kg (maximum of 90 mg)	5–10 days
Metronidazole	Oral*	750 mg t.i.d. (children—35–50 mg/kg in 3 divided doses)	5–10 days
Chloroquine	Oral	600 mg b.i.d. followed by 300 mg b.i.d.	2 days 18 days

*Patients unable to tolerate metronidazole orally should be given it intravenously.

with strong suction, re-expansion of the lung, postural drainage, and appropriate antibiotics.

GENERAL CONSIDERATIONS

Rarely, an amebic liver abscess ruptures transdiaphragmatically following the institution of specific antiamebic therapy. Undoubtedly this rupture occurs in an already necrotic area of the diaphragm.

Patients with amebiasis, particularly those with pleuropulmonary complications, usually have been sick for a long time and are often economically disadvantaged and malnourished. Consequently, nutritional support is important.

ANTIAMEBIC CHEMOTHERAPY

Metronidazole is the drug of choice in the treatment of amebiasis. As Adams and MacLeod (1977) pointed out, many different acceptable drug regimens are available. Because relapse has been reported after the use of metronidazole alone and these patients become gravely ill, we prefer to use a combination of drugs (Table 70–1).

Dehydroemetine is cardiotoxic and the ECG must be monitored carefully. If there is any sign of toxicity, or the patient has known cardiac problems, we omit it. Chloroquine is generally well tolerated, and particularly effective in the liver. It is also relatively nontoxic. It should, however, be administered orally, which is not always possible in these seriously ill patients. Metronidazole produces little toxicity. Oral administration in high doses may be associated with nausea, anorexia, cramps, and diarrhea, which are less common with the intravenous route. Although metronidazole is carcinogenic in animals when given in large doses, it has not been proved carcinogenic in man. No evidence that drug resistance develops has yet been demonstrated.

Tinidazole—Fasigyn—is as effective as metronidazole, and can be better tolerated. Recommended dose for an amebic liver abscess is 800 mg three times daily for 5 days or 2 mg daily for 3 days. In children, 50 to 60 mg/kg is given up to a maximum of 2 g.

REFERENCES

Adams, E.B., and MacLeod, I.N.: Invasive amebiasis. II. Amebic liver abscess and its complications. Medicine 56:325, 1977.
Eggleston, F.C., et al.: The results of surgery in amebic liver abscess: experiences in 83 patients. Surgery 83:536, 1978.
Grigsby, W.P.: Surgical treatment of amebiasis. Surg. Gynecol. Obstet. 128:609, 1969.
Ibarra-Perez, C.: Thoracic complications of amebic abscess of the liver: report of 501 cases. Chest 79:672, 1981.
Le Roux, B.T., et al.: Pleuropulmonary amebiasis. In Diseases of the lung and pleural space. Part 1. Empyema thoracis and lung abscess. Curr. Probl. Surg. 23:73, 1986.
Ragheb, M.I., Ramadan, A.A.,and Khalil, M.A.H.: Intrathoracic presentation of amebic liver abscess. Ann. Thorac. Surg. 22:483, 1976.
Verghese, M., et al.: Management of thoracic amebiasis. J. Thorac. Cardiovasc. Surg. 78:757, 1979.

READING REFERENCES

Adams, E.B., and MacLeod, I.N.: Invasive amebiasis. I. Amebic dysentery and its complications. Medicine 56:315, 1977.
Beaver, P.C., Jung, R.C., and Cupp, E.W.: Clinical Parasitology. Philadelphia, Lea & Febiger, 9th ed., 1984.
Markell, E.K., Voge, M., and John, D.T.: Medical Parasitology. Philadelphia, W.B. Saunders, 1986.
Rodriguez, C.: Pulmonary and pleural amebiasis. In General Thoracic Surgery, 2nd ed. Edited by T.W. Shields. Philadelphia, Lea & Febiger, 1983.
Wolfe, M.S.: Amebiasis. In Hunter's Tropical Medicine, 6th ed. Edited by G.T. Strickland. Philadelphia, W.B. Saunders Co., 1976.

CHAPTER 71

HYDATID DISEASE OF THE LUNG

Homeros Aletras and Panagiotis N. Symbas

Hydatid disease, which is caused by the *Echinococcus granulosus* tapeworm and is known as echinococcosis or hydatidosis, has been acknowledged as a clinical entity since ancient times. Organs of sacrificed animals were described in the Talmud as "bladders full of water," and Hippocrates referred to hydatid disease in the aphorisms: "when the liver is filled with water and bursts into the epiploon, the belly is filled with water and the patient dies." Rudolphi (1808) first used the term "hydatid cyst" for the description of echinococcosis in man.

Echinococcosis is frequently encountered in the sheep-and cattle-raising regions of the world. This clinical entity has been most frequently observed in Australia, New Zealand, South Africa, South America, and the Mediterranean countries of Europe, Asia, and Africa. Although this disease, as Ginsberg and associates (1958) noted, has been rare in the United States and Canada, with the increase in mobility and migration of people, an increase in the frequency of this clinical entity can be expected in this part of the world. Therefore, the presence of hydatid disease should be considered in a patient who presents with a well-defined, spherical density of the lung, particularly a patient who has lived or traveled in an endemic area.

PATHOPHYSIOLOGY

The primary hosts for the infecting organism are the members of the Canidae family, usually dogs, wolves, and coyotes. Feline species are seldom naturally infected, but the parasite has been reported in the cat, wild cat, jaguar, and panther. The primary host contracts echinococcosis by ingesting mature and productive echinococcal cysts in the viscera of an intermediate host—sheep, goats, cattle, hogs, moose, reindeer, deer, elk, and other herbivorous animals. In the intestines of the primary host, the scolices of the hydatid cyst develop into a parasitic worm composed of a scolex, neck, and three proglottids—segments. The last proglottid, which is approximately half the length of the entire parasite, contains 400 to 800 ova. The proglottid matures and

breaks off from the scolex; the ova are released in the feces of the primary host, and are then ingested by intermediate hosts by ingesting contaminated grass, water, vegetables, and such. The larval stage, which cannot occur in the main host, begins in the intermediate host and leads to the development of pulmonary and hepatic hydatid cysts. These organs are then ingested by the primary hosts, and thus the cycle continues (Fig. 71–1).

Saidi (1976) emphasized that the ova are resistant to physical and chemical agents. In the gastrointestinal tract

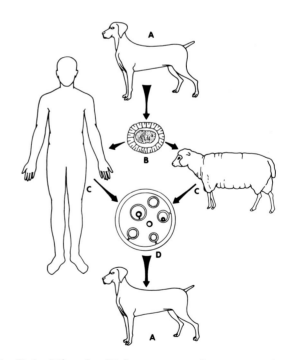

Fig. 71–1. Life cycle of *Echinococcus granulosus*. Primary host A ingests viscera of intermediate host C containing hydatid cyst → development of ova producing parasitic worm in intestine of primary host A → B ova shed with feces from primary host A contaminating vegetables, grass, etc. → ingestion of contaminated vegetable or grass by intermediate host C → development of hydatid cyst D in viscera of intermediate host C → ingestion of viscera of intermediate host C with hydatid cyst D by primary host A.

of the intermediate host, however, including man, the chitinous embryophore that surrounds the hexacanth embryo is lysed and the embryo is released. As Smyth (1968) described, the embryo, with the aid of its hooklets, attaches to and penetrates the mucosa of the duodenum and jejunum, enters the mesenteral venules, and proceeds to the portal vein. From the portal vein the embryo enters the liver, where it becomes embedded and, if it is not destroyed by phagocytosis, develops into a cyst. In most series of patients, such as that of Toole and associates (1960), the incidence of hepatic involvement in echinococcosis is 50 to 60%; Saidi (1976) reported an incidence of 70 to 80%. In the portal circulation, some of the embryos, whose diameters do not exceed 0.3 mm, may pass through the sinus capillaries of the liver and, by way of the hepatic veins and vena cava, proceed to the right side of the heart and the pulmonary capillaries, where they may become embedded. Here, as in the liver, the embryo that survives the phagocytosis hypertrophies, the hooklets disappear, and the embryo enters the larval stage.

The lungs are the second most common site of lodgement of the parasite, as Barrett (1947), Dew (1982), and others noted, with an incidence varying between 10% and 30%. The development of pulmonary echinococcosis presumes hepatic involvement, which is more difficult to diagnose than the pulmonary disease. In some reported cases in which pulmonary cyst(s) were removed, even though an intensive search was made for hepatic cyst(s), a positive diagnosis of hepatic involvement could not be made, even years later.

One alternative pathway of the parasites' entrance into the lung is via the lymphatic circulation: the embryo enters the lymphatics of the small intestine, proceeds to the thoracic duct, to the internal jugular vein, to the right side of the heart, and then to the lungs. Another possible route is a venal-venous anastomosis in the liver and the space of Retzius. Some researchers have supported the possibility of direct pulmonary exposure through the inhalation of air contaminated with echinococcus. As Chrysopathis (1966) pointed out, however, it is unsure whether the bronchial secretions can lyse the embryophore of the hexacanth to liberate the embryo. Other investigators, such as Barrett (1960), deny that an inhaled parasite could remain viable in the bronchial tree. Secondary pulmonary cysts may develop when ova enter the venous circulation because of rupture of extrapulmonary cysts. The site of the primary hydatid cysts producing secondary metastatic pulmonary echinococcus cysts in 31 patients was the heart in 64%, the liver in 26%, and the iliac bone in 10%. In such instances it is difficult to distinguish between primary and secondary cysts.

Peschiera (1974) pointed out that the most common areas of involvement of pulmonary echinococcosis are the right lung and both of the lower lobes. One of us (H.A.) (1968) and Barrett and Thomas (1952) noted that many cysts have a simultaneous development in either one or both lungs, with a reported incidence of 14 to 24%. Each cyst grows and matures independently of any developing coexisting cyst (Fig. 71–2).

Tsakayiannis and colleagues (1970) stated that it is unclear whether children are more likely to develop pulmonary than hepatic echinococcus cysts. Some evidence suggests that echinococcus cysts develop more rapidly in the lungs of children than of adults, which may explain the more common appearance of pulmonary echinococcal cysts in children. Sometimes the entire hemithorax of young children is occupied by parasitic cysts (Fig. 71–3). In these children, either the contamination must have occurred a few months after birth or the cysts grew rapidly.

Two types of hydatid cysts occur in humans, the unilocular and the alveolar. This discussion will be limited to the unilocular variety because these are the cysts of clinical importance in the lungs. A hydatid cyst is composed of the wall and the hydatid fluid. The wall of the cyst is composed of three zones, which are constantly present and independent of the shape the cyst finally assumes. Two of these zones, the laminated membrane and the germinal layer or germinative membrane, belong to the parasite, and one zone, the pericyst or adventitia, belongs to the host. The differentiation of these zones begins in the embryo and continues until the three discernible zones are developed.

The pericystic zone, also known as the adventitia or ectocyst, is rarely thicker than a few millimeters and is composed entirely of the host's cells. When the hexacanth embryo is embedded in the host's tissue, it causes a local reaction, and local migration of mononuclear leukocytes, lymphocytes, and eosinophils into the area. Polymorphonuclear leukocytes are not present, and their presence indicates that the parasite cannot implant at the particular site. The original cells are gradually replaced by fibroblasts so that this zone eventually is transformed into a thin and easily discernible capsule of fibrous matter, connective tissue, and compressed

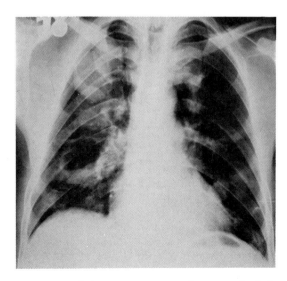

Fig. 71–2. Frontal chest roentgenogram showing multiple hydatid cysts of the lung.

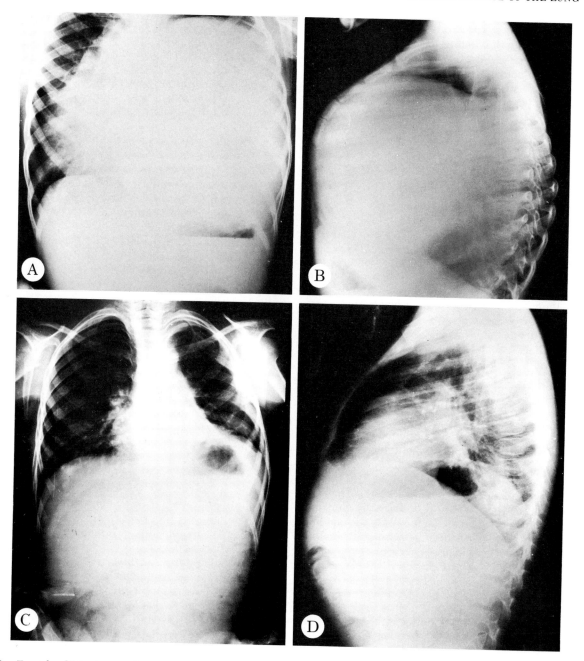

Fig. 71–3. Frontal and lateral pre- and postoperative chest roentgenograms of a 5-year-old boy with a giant left lower lobe hydatid cyst producing marked chest deformity.

parenchymal cells. Functionally, this layer provides mechanical protection and nutrition to the parasite. Therefore, whenever degenerative changes of the membrane develop, such as calcification, an amorphous degeneration or automatic absorption of the hydatid cysts occurs.

The laminated membrane is 1 to 3 mm thick and is surrounded by a pericystic layer. The membrane is white, gelatinous, rich in polysaccharides, and is characteristically laminated, which is often obvious to the naked eye. It is hyaline, elastic, with no host blood vessels entering into it and is easily discernible from the pericystic layer, which is vitally important to the surgeon. The laminated membrane, as described by Mor-

seth (1967), is composed of a plexus of fine fibers with a dispersed thick reticular substance, which, as Schwabe (1959) noted, is permeable to calcium, potassium, chlorides, water, and urea. Nutritional and other substances useful to the parasite traverse the membrane by diffusion, but active transport may also play a role. Agosin (1968) suggests that potassium and cyanide ions seem to affect the permeability of this membrane by causing a detachment of the germinal membrane from the rest of the cyst. Physiologic fluids of the host or even purulent fluids do not destroy this membrane, although the smallest break in the membrane may result in total rupture of the cyst and escape of its contents. The large cysts are especially vulnerable to rupture because of an increased pressure exerted by the fluid in the cyst.

The germinal layer, also known as the germinative membrane or endocyst, is the inner layer of the cystic wall. It is a thin, transparent membrane that is lined with small papillae, which are "brood capsules" at different stages of development. These capsules, which are formed by the proliferation of the cells of the germinal layer, develop buds of scolices. The scolices have suckers and hooks, and represent the mature parasite larvae. The germinative membrane is the living part of the parasite and produces the laminated membrane and reproduces the parasite. Some cysts cannot regenerate, but every undamaged cyst, regardless of size, must be considered capable of reproduction.

The daughter cysts, a rare finding in pulmonary echinococcosis, are produced from the germinal membrane, from the brood capsule, or from the scolices. Daughter cysts vary in size from a few millimeters to a few centimeters; their numbers range from a few to thousands and they contain viable scolices. Some of the daughter cysts may be degenerated, whereas others may contain their own daughter cysts.

The hydatid vesicle is filled with hydatid fluid, which is colorless and odorless and resembles crystal-clear water. The specific gravity of the fluid is 1.008 to 1.015; the pH is 6.7 to 7.2; and the concentration of sodium, potassium, chloride, and carbon dioxide is approximately that of the host's blood serum. The function of the hydatid fluid is similar to that of amniotic fluid, as it suspends the daughter cysts. A large production of hydatid fluid can disrupt the nutrition from the host to the interior of the cyst and cause the death of the parasite.

The parasitic cyst enlarges up to a certain limit, at which time either accidentally or because of symptoms produced by its presence, it becomes discernible and is removed. The rate of growth of any particular pulmonary cyst, which may be faster in children than in adults, varies; and their diameter can increase, as Sarsam (1971) and others noted, from a few millimeters up to approximately 5 cm a year. A cyst with a diameter of 10 cm contains approximately 400 ml of hydatid fluid, and any cyst that grows to a diameter of 6 to 7 cm must be removed. Usually the rate of growth of the echinococcus in the lungs is progressive and constant, but precipitous growth spurts can occur. The growth is rapid, much more so than in other organs, mainly because the pulmonary tissue is elastic and shows little resistance to the expansion in their size.

During the growth period of the cyst, it may rupture spontaneously or during coughing, sneezing, or any other cause of increased intra-abdominal pressure or after injury during diagnostic paracentesis. The rupture may occur within the boundaries of the pericystic layer, into the pleural space, or into a neighboring organ, bronchus or blood vessel. Rupture of the germinal membrane toward the interior of the cyst may result in the formation of daughter cysts; formation of daughter cysts after a rupture of the laminated membrane is rare. Rupture of the cyst toward the surrounding tissues may be followed by secondary echinococcosis, and the rupture into a blood vessel may lead to embolization of a portion of the cyst. Rupture of the cyst and evacuation of the cystic contents into a main bronchus may rarely result in spontaneous cure. Suppuration of the cyst can occur after rupture and secondary infection. In the course of their natural evolution, many cysts gradually cease growing and degenerate.

Although hydatid cysts of the liver commonly calcify, calcification of such a cyst in the lung is rare. The calcification, which resembles an eggshell, takes place in the adventitia of complicated cysts and does not always indicate that the hydatid is dead. The calcified lung cyst is almost always in communication with the bronchial tree and is probably infected.

Some investigators, including Bakir (1967), Saidi (1976), and Smyth (1968), have contended that the remaining pericystic cavity becomes obliterated after the cystic contents are evacuated through the bronchus or after excision of the cyst. Others, such as Kourias and Tobler (1957), Perez-Fontana (1948), and Peschiera (1964), have contended that the residual cavity persists, because of epithelialization of the adventitial sacs.

CLINICAL MANIFESTATIONS

Intact or simple hydatid cysts of the lung produce no characteristic symptoms. Their clinical manifestations depend on the site and size of the cyst. Small, peripherally located cysts are usually asymptomatic, whereas large cysts may manifest with symptoms of compression of adjacent organs. If the patient is symptomatic, he usually first complains of a nonproductive cough; and some patients, particularly those with centrally located cysts, may have blood-streaked sputum, although massive hemoptysis does not occur. Some patients complain of a dull aching pain or the sensation of pressure in the chest with no aggravating or relieving features. In children, who have a supple chest wall, a bulge in the ipsilateral chest may also be observed (Fig. 71–3).

Rupture of the hydatid cyst into an adjacent bronchus may be manifested by vigorous coughing and expectoration of a large amount of salty-tasting sputum, consisting of mucus, hydatid fluid, and occasionally fragments of the laminated membrane—generally described as "grapeskin" or frothy blood. In addition, the patient may develop a severe hypersensitivity reaction manifested by generalized rash, high fever, pulmonary congestion, and severe bronchospasm. Occasionally the intrabronchial rupture of the cyst manifests with sudden and severe dyspnea, which may lead to suffocation and death from complete tracheal obstruction by fragments from the hydatid membrane. Arce (1941) pointed out that the diagnosis of rupture of the hydatid cyst is unequivocally made when the hooklets of the parasite are found during the microscopic examination of the sputum. Fortunately, the intrabronchial evacuation of the hydatid cyst contents usually occurs without a catastrophic event. Rather, the patients may complain of repeated febrile episodes, chronic cough, and mucopurulent or dark bloody sputum.

When the hydatid cyst ruptures into the pleural space, the symptoms are usually insidious and moderate; they consist of dry cough, chest pain, moderate dyspnea, generalized malaise, and fever. These relatively mild clinical manifestations result from pre-existing pleural adhesions, which prevent the dissemination of the cyst contents into the whole pleural space. In some patients, particularly those without pre-existing pleural adhesions, the intrapleural rupture of the cyst produces an acute and dramatic clinical picture consisting of intense chest pain, persistent cough, severe dyspnea, and even cyanosis, shock, and suffocation. Frequently, symptoms of generalized urticaria, intense pruritus, severe anaphylactic shock, and even death can occur. The symptoms of the intrapleural rupture of the hydatid cyst are accompanied by the physical findings of localized or generalized hydropneumothorax.

DIAGNOSIS

The diagnosis of an intact echinococcus cyst is usually based on a suspicion resulting from an unexpected finding on a routine chest roentgenogram. Roentgenographically, the cyst appears as a smoothly outlined, dense, spherical opacity (Fig. 71–4). Sharma and Eggleston (1969) emphasized that the alteration from a spherical to an oval shape may only be observed during deep inhalation, the "Escudero-Nenerow" sign. The roentgenographic picture depends, for the most part, on the size and location of the cyst. The small cyst may appear as a small "vesicle" and is difficult to recognize until it grows large enough to present a clear image on the chest roentgenogram.

Centrally located cysts may compress the bronchovascular structures, presenting roentgenographically as

a depression or indentation at the site of pressure, the so-called notch sign. The cyst may also have a clear, crescent-shaped shadow on the top or on one side; this type is referred to as a "pneumocyst" by Dévé (1935), "perivesicular pneuma" by Arce (1941), "perivesicular meniscus" by Peschiera (1974), "moon sign" or "crescent sign" by Barrett and Thomas (1952), or "pulmonary meniscus sign" by Saidi (1976). This sign has been attributed to the air that enters the perivesicular space, becoming entrapped between the adventitia and the unruptured vesicle after vigorous coughing, straining, or direct trauma to the cyst, and it is the first roentgenographic sign of impending rupture of the cyst. A "double-dome arch" sign, as Arce (1941) noted, may appear when a small additional amount of air further enters the hydatid vesicle. The entrance of free air into the cyst and the perivesicular space, following the complete rupture of the laminated membrane, displaces the fluid, and this finding has been termed a "camalote" sign by Arce (1941) or a "waterlily" sign by Lagos Carcia and Segers (1924). This sign is produced by the floating membrane of the cyst (Fig. 71–5).

The three previously described diagnostic signs, however, are only roentgenographic rarities. Beggs (1985) reviewed the roentgenographic findings. Most present as a solid mass in the right lower lobe. They are multiple in 30% of patients and bilateral in 20%. Therefore every discrete radiologic lesion observed in any patients above the age of 3 years in an endemic area should be considered a hydatid cyst.

The roentgenographic pleural manifestations in the acute stage of rupture of the cyst vary from loculated hydropneumothorax to nonloculated partial, complete, or tension hydropneumothorax. The waterlily sign can also be observed in instances with rupture of the cyst into the pleura (Fig. 71–6).

Computed tomography, as Saksouk (1986) and Lewall (1986) and their associates reported, has greatly added to the diagnosis of hydatid disease of the lung, particu-

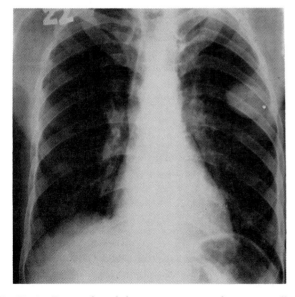

Fig. 71–4. Routine frontal chest roentgenogram showing a small peripheral hydatid cyst in the left upper lung field.

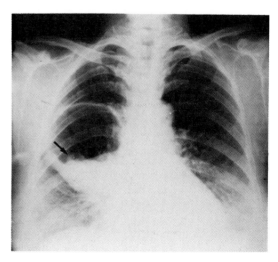

Fig. 71–5. Frontal chest roentgenogram of a ruptured echinococcal cyst in the right lower lung field with the cystic membrane floating on the hydatid fluid (arrow), a "water-lily sign."

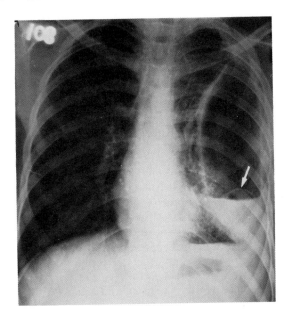

Fig. 71–6. Frontal chest roentgenogram showing a collapsed echinococcal membrane lying above the air-fluid level (arrow), a "water-lily sign," in a 15-year-old boy admitted with a pyothorax.

larly to the early discovery of coexistent small cysts in the lung and of pending or existing rupture of the cyst. Also, as Kalovidouris and colleagues (1984) noted, computed tomography appears to be valuable in the follow-up of patients who have had resection or evacuation of hydatid disease of the lung.

The diagnosis of echinococcal cyst may also be suspected because of eosinophilia which, as Faust and Russell (1964) and Aletras (1968) reported, occurred in 20 to 34% of the patients with echinococcosis. Because an increase of the eosinophils is also observed in many other pathologic states, this test has little diagnostic value. Tomography and bronchography add little information to the diagnosis and are rarely indicated. Pneumoperitoneum may be used to differentiate whether the cyst is in the liver or right lower lobe (Fig. 71–7).

Several clinical laboratory tests useful in the diagnosis of hydatid disease of the lung include the Casoni's intradermal test, the Weinberg complement fixation test, and the indirect hemagglutination test. The latex flocculation—particle fixation—test, the bentonite flocculation—BFT precipitin reaction—test, the immunodiffusion test, and the immunofluorescence test are, for the most part, used experimentally. The Casoni's intradermal test, first used by Casoni in 1911, is the most widely used and sensitive test. Imari (1962) reported this test to yield a positive reaction in 70 to 85% of the patients with uncomplicated cysts, and Sharma and Eggleston (1969) found a positive reaction in 92 to 100% of the patients with ruptured cyst. Other parasitic diseases caused by protozoa or metazoa, the sensitization of the host to animal proteins; and degenerative, allergic, or autoimmunologic diseases, however, can produce false-positive reactions.

The Weinberg complement fixation test, used first by

Ghedini (1906), is not specific. Its sensitivity rate was reported by Kagan (1968) and Kagan and co-workers (1966) to vary from 36 to 93%. Gräfe (1964) noted that it has a false-positive rate, especially in patients with neoplasms, of 28%.

The indirect hemagglutination test—IHA—first used by Garabedian and associates in 1957, is the clinical test of choice. Kagan and colleagues (1966, 1968) reported that its sensitivity ranges from 66 to 100%, whereas the false-positive results are few—1 to 2%.

TREATMENT

Medical treatment for hydatid disease of the lung was nonexistent until the 1980s; Benzimidazole compounds have shown encouraging results. Gil-Grande and associates (1983) reported the use of mebendazole with a 36 to 94% partial to complete response rate. Morris and colleagues (1985) used albendazole—10 mg/kg/day—with some remission in 15 of 22 patients. Response to this therapy is apparently related to the thickness of the cyst wall, which the drug must penetrate to reach the germinal layer. Young patients and patients with small cysts, in whom cyst walls are usually thin, have better response to this treatment. The failure rate of this therapy and the recurrence rate after the treatment is discontinued are apparently high and the side effects from the drugs considerable. As a result, until more data are available, this form of treatment at best may be considered in selected cases under close observation.

The surgical treatment has undergone considerable changes since the 1950s. Numerous surgical procedures based on the evacuation of the cyst through the chest wall in one or two stages have been used. These methods, although they may still be practiced by some, are not applicable when the cysts are near the hilum of the lung and are inadequate because secondary echinococcal cysts may develop in the surgical wound and a chronic bronchocutaneous fistula may be created.

The current treatment of the hydatid cyst of the lung is complete excision of the disease process with maximum preservation of the lung tissue. Peripherally located cysts of any size and small to medium-sized centrally located cysts should and can be excised without the sacrifice of lung parenchyma. Segmental resection is indicated principally in the treatment of large simple cysts that almost completely occupy the involved segment. It can also be used for complicated cysts of moderate size if the infection does not extend beyond the segmental plane.

Lobectomy should be performed when the size and number of cysts and the degree of infection exclude lesser procedures. The principal indications for lobectomy are: large cyst involving more than 50% of the lobe, cysts with severe pulmonary suppuration not responding to preoperative treatment, multiple unilobar cysts, and sequelae of hydatid disease, such as pulmonary fibrosis, bronchiectasis, or severe hemorrhage. Pneumonectomy is rarely indicated for the treatment of hydatid disease of the lung, and it should be used only when the whole

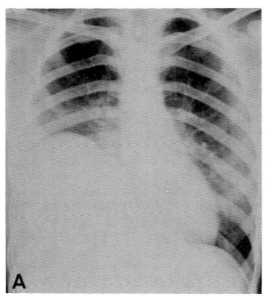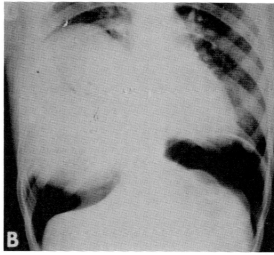

Fig. 71–7. *A*, Frontal chest roentgenogram showing radiodensity occupying the right lower lung field and the right upper quadrant. *B*, Pneumoperitoneum showing that the echinococcal cyst was involving the right lower lobe rather than the liver.

lung is involved in the disease process, leaving no salvageable pulmonary parenchyma.

The preoperative preparation of patients with hydatid disease of the lung is similar to the preparation of a patient undergoing thoracotomy for other comparable pulmonary lesions. Patients with small peripheral lesions require limited preparations, whereas patients with suppurative cysts should be treated with postural drainage, antibiotics, and other supportive measures until the suppurative process is as minimal as possible. Because echinococcal cysts not detected by the preoperative evaluation may exist in the liver or elsewhere, this possibility and the possibility for future surgical interventions should be brought to the patient's attention preoperatively, in addition to all the other information concerning the operative procedure.

Bilateral lung cysts should be resected in two stages (Fig. 71–8). In a patient with uncomplicated lung cysts, the lung with the larger cyst or with the greater number of cysts should be operated upon first. In a patient with a lung cyst greater than 4 to 5 cm in diameter of one lung and a ruptured cyst of the other lung, the intact cyst should first be removed to eliminate its future rupture. The lesions in the other lung are then resected 2 to 4 weeks after the first operation (Fig. 71–9).

Conventional general anesthesia is used for thoracotomy, and preparation should be made for the management of complications, such as blockage of the tracheobronchial tree by the cyst contents or anaphylactic reaction, which might occur during induction of anesthesia or during the operation from rupture of a hydatid cyst into the bronchus or pleural space.

A posterolateral thoracotomy, through the fifth, sixth, or seventh intercostal space or rarely through the bed of the fifth, sixth, or seventh rib, is performed, at the same time taking extreme care not to rupture the cyst. The

most superficial portion of an intact cyst, which is devoid of pulmonary parenchyma, is a round grayish-white area that is also devoid of blood vessels (Fig. 71–10*A*). The perimeter of this area is dark, ill defined, and blends into the normal lung tissue. This appearance, and particularly the elastic feel upon palpation of the mass, differentiate the hydatid cyst from a mitotic lesion. Needle aspiration, for establishing the diagnosis when evidence suggests that the mass lesion is a hydatid cyst, should be avoided because of the danger of spillage of the parasitic material and the subsequent inability to remove the cyst.

Several operative techniques are used to manage hydatid cyst of the lung, and their main objective is resec-

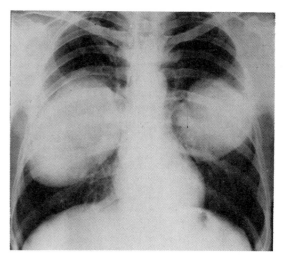

Fig. 71–8. Frontal chest roentgenogram showing two intact echinococcal cysts, one in each lung. Both were enucleated by separate thoracotomies at a 2-month interval.

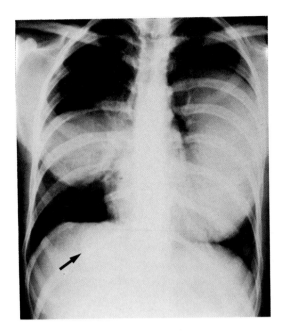

Fig. 71–9. Frontal chest roentgenogram showing three echinococcal cysts, one in each lung and one in the liver. Left hydatid cyst was removed first, and 6 weeks later the cyst from the right lung and liver were treated simultaneously.

tion of the intact or complicated cyst, while preserving as much lung as possible.

TREATMENT OF INTACT CYSTS

Resection by Enucleation Without Needle Aspiration

Excision of the intact hydatid cyst without needle aspiration is accomplished by careful separation of the laminated membrane from the pericystic zone. The separation of these two components of the parasitic cyst is feasible even though they are intimately adherent to one another. The enucleation of small cysts can usually be accomplished without difficulty. Large cysts, however, demand greater technical training and patience on the part of the surgeon because of the increased possibility of rupture during the separation of the pericystic zone from the laminated membrane. Because occasionally this complication is unavoidable, the surgical field must always be protected from the possibility of spillage of the parasitic material, with resultant contamination of the pleural space and surgical wound. Therefore, after the hydatid cyst is identified, the surgical wound and adjacent lung tissue are covered with packed gauzes steeped in normal saline solution so that only the area of the lung that contains the cyst is exposed. Because the gauze material filters *only* macroscopic-sized material, the hydatid fluid may still enter the pleural space and precipitate an allergic reaction. For this reason, before the dissection is begun, two well-functioning suction apparatuses must always be present. After the part of the lung containing the cyst is isolated, the tissue overlying the cyst is incised and the cyst is exposed. A cruciate or stellate incision is then made on the pericystic zone, and

with blunt dissection a small space is created between this zone and the laminated membrane. The separation of the two zones is continued with blunt dissection and direct visualization, which is facilitated by traction on Allis clamps applied on the edges of the pericystic zone (Fig. 71–10B). During the dissection, the endopulmonary pressure is lowered by the anesthesiologist to avoid the projection of the laminated membrane through the opening in the pericystic zone. After the two zones are completely separated, the anesthesiologist increases the endopulmonary pressure. With the current of air coming from the various bronchial openings, and the simultaneous even, steady, light pressure on the cyst from the surrounding lung, as a result of the increased endopulmonary pressure and the use of gravity, the cyst "pops" out into an ajacent kidney basin that contains a small amount of normal saline solution. Before and during the delivery of the cyst, the laminated membrane should never be grasped with an instrument; significant manual pressure on the pericystic zone should be avoided; and, in general, assistance in the "delivery" of the cyst must be careful to avoid its rupture. After the delivery of the cyst, the residual cavity, which is devoid of epithelium and always has some bronchial openings, must be appropriately managed (Fig. 71–10C).

The management of the residual cavity has historically passed through different stages. Posadas in 1899 advised only suturing of the bronchial openings. This practice, however, did not prevent air leak; thus fixation of the edges of the sutured pericystic zone to the thoracotomy incision was later added to this method. The same year Délbét advocated the folding of the pericystic zone by sutures, a method named "capitonnage." According to Crausaz (1967), pursestring sutures from the base of the pericystic cavity upward were used to obliterate the cavity. Allende and Langer in 1947 supplemented this method with suturing of the individual bronchial openings within the cavity. Closure of the bronchial openings at a more proximal point was introduced by Chrysospathis in 1966. To attain this closure, a probe was introduced through the bronchial opening and the surrounding pulmonary tissue was bluntly dissected along its length so that the bronchus could be closed more centrally.

Each of these methods, in the hands of their proponents, yielded good results. One of us (H.A.) favors, especially for a large pericystic cavity, closure of the bronchial openings; partial pericystectomy, that is, resection of the free portion of the pericystic zone; elimination of the residual cavity by capitonnage; and closure of its edges with continuous sutures. This method was introduced by Demirleau and Pernot in 1951. Saidi (1976) contended that the approximation and suturing of the residual cavity's edges are not necessary because the pulmonary parenchyma automatically obliterates the space and the surface of the lung at the site of the residual cavity will be covered by the pleura.

It is generally agreed, however, that the most important point in the management of the residual pericystic cavity is closure of patent bronchial openings. After the

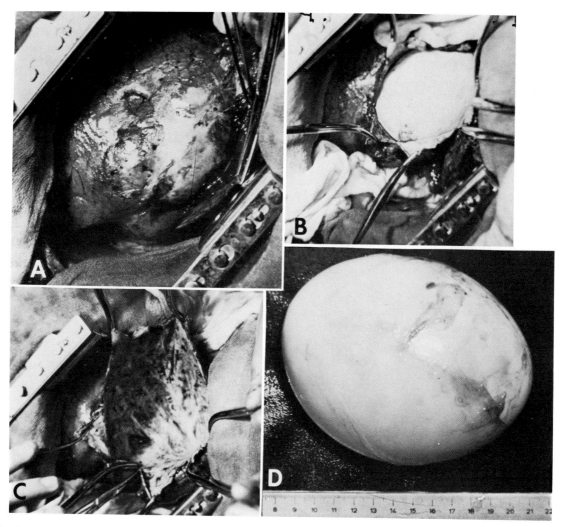

Fig. 71–10. Intraoperative photographs. *A*, The lung containing the hydatid cyst. Note the grayish white surface of the lung where the cyst is located. *B*, The hydatid cyst while being dissected. *C*, Residual pericystic cavity after the cyst has been removed. *D*, Hydatid cyst after it was excised.

grossly evident bronchial openings are closed, smaller opening can be easily detected by filling the residual cavity with normal saline solution. With the application of positive endopulmonary pressure, air escaping through any bronchial openings is visualized by the formation of bubbles. This maneuver must be repeated until sealing of all air leaks is achieved.

Removal of the Intact Cyst after Needle Aspiration

The danger of development of secondary hydatid cysts because of spillage of hydatid fluid as a result of violation of the integrity of the cyst by needle aspiration or rupture has led to the development of various chemical substances capable of rendering the hydatid fluid "sterile." These substances are generally used when the surgeon contemplates removing the intact cyst after needle aspiration. Formalin and formaldehyde solutions have mainly been used in the past as scolicidal agents during operation. The escape of these substances into the pericystic space causes irritation of the tissue, which results in impairment of healing and as Saidi (1976) noted, in

the formation of bronchial fistulas. Silver nitrate solution, 0.5%, has scolicidal properties and is used accordingly. Hypertonic saline solution, which is considered to have scolicidal properties, does not affect tissue healing; accordingly, one of us (H.A.) prefers this scolicidal agent.

Before the needle aspiration is begun, four Allis clamps and two suction machines, which are functioning well, should be available. The surgical wound and the lung, except for the segment containing the cyst, are covered with packed gauzes as was previously described. The lobe that contains the cyst is immobilized, the lung is maintained inflated, and a 20- or 21-gauge lumbar puncture needle, which is connected to a 20- or 50-ml glass syringe, is inserted into the prominent portion of the cyst, and is maintained immobile. The use of plastic syringes is not desirable because their relative nontransparency does not allow clear observation of the aspirated fluid. The hydatid fluid of the cyst should not be aspirated completely; a small residual amount must always be left in the cyst. The remaining fluid is then removed in one of two ways. First, after withdrawal of the aspirating needle, the wall of the parasitic cyst is incised and a suction tip connected to a suction apparatus is immediately introduced into the cyst and the remaining contents of the cyst are removed. The suction tip should be of the sump type with side holes to avoid the blocking of the suction channel by portions of membrane, or rarely by daughter cysts. While the preceding evacuation is carried out, a second suction apparatus is used to remove any hydatid fluid that may overflow from the cystic cavity, thus avoiding spillage of hydatid material. Second, after most of the hydatid cyst fluid is aspirated, instead of opening the pericystic and cystic wall, a trocar whose sidearm is connected to a suction apparatus is inserted in the cyst through the same orifice, immediately after the removal of the aspiration needle. The remaining hydatid contents are evacuated, the trocar is removed, the opening of the cyst is enlarged, and a second sump suction tip is introduced to withdraw the remaining contents of the cyst.

Throughout the entire period of evacuation of the parasitic contents of the cyst, the lungs must be kept expanded by maintaining constant positive pressure, because during the previously described maneuvers, rupture and detachment of the laminated membrane may occur and a small amount of hydatid fluid may escape into the pericystic space. With the maintenance of constant positive endobronchial pressure, none of the escaped parasitic fluid in the pericystic cavity can advance through the bronchial openings into the bronchial tree. Finally, the remainder of the laminated membrane is removed with sponge forceps, the residual cavity is cleaned, preferably with hypertonic saline solution, and the bronchial openings are closed in the manner described previously.

Pericystectomy

Pérez-Fontana (1951) described removal of the pericystic zone with the intact cyst. The technical difficulty with this method is the creation of an appropriate plane through the pulmonary tissue, near and around the parasitic cyst, with the resulting bleeding and air leak. This method can be easily applied in superficially located small cysts.

TREATMENT OF RUPTURED CYSTS

The management of ruptured cyst during the acute stages is mainly directed toward the prevention of major complications resulting from the evacuation of the cystic contents into the tracheobronchial tree or the pleural space. Preventive precautions include the maintenance of the airway free of secretions and cystic tissue by appropriate orotracheal suction or bronchoscopy, evacuation of the hydropneumothorax, and treatment of an anaphylactic reaction. After the acute period, the most conservative treatment should be used to save as much lung tissue as possible.

An infected cyst, with minimal damage to the adjacent lung parenchyma, is opened, its contents are evacuated, and the cavity is thoroughly irrigated. The bronchial openings with or without "capitonnage" of the residual cavity, are then closed and the pleural space is drained. When the cyst is infected and the lung parenchyma is irreversibly damaged, lobectomy is the operation of choice.

PROGNOSIS

In a series of 93 patients treated by one of us (H.A.), 80 underwent only excision of the cyst with individual closure of the bronchial openings and obliteration of the pericystic cavity; 12 patients underwent lobectomy and 1 a segmental resection. In a follow-up period of 2 to 16 years, no recurrences have been noted. Therefore, with appropriate treatment the prognosis is good.

REFERENCES

Agosin, M.: Biochemistry and Physiology of Echinococcus. World Health Organization Bulletin 39, 1968, p. 115.

Aletras, H.A.: Hydatid cyst of the lung. Scand. J. Thorac. Cardiovasc. Surg. 2:218, 1968.

Allende, J.M., and Langer, L.: Tratamiento de los quistes hidatidicos del pulmon. Boletin Y Trabajos. Academia Argentina di Chirugia 31:539, 1947.

Arce, J.: Hydatid cyst of the lung. Arch Surg. 43:789, 1941.

Bakir, F.: Serious complications of hydatid cyst of the lung. Am. Rev. Respir. Dis. 96:483, 1967.

Barrett, N.R.: Surgical treatment of the hydatid cyst of the lung. Thorax 2:21, 1947.

Barrett, N.R.: The anatomy and the pathology of multiple hydatid cysts in the thorax. Arris and Gale Lecture. Ann. Coll. Surg. Engl. 26:362, 1960.

Barrett, N.R., and Thomas, D.: Pulmonary hydatid disease. Br. J. Surg. 40:222, 1952.

Beggs, I.: The radiology of hydatid disease. Am. J. Radiol. 145:639, 1985.

Casoni, T.: La diagnosi biologica dell echinococcosi umana mediante l'intradermo-reazione. Folia Clinica Chimica et Microscopia Salsomaggiorie 4:5, 1911.

Chrysospathis, P.: Echinococcus cyst of the lung. Chest 49:278, 1966.

Crausaz, P.H.: Surgical treatment of the hydatid cyst of the lung and hydatid cyst of the liver with intrathoracic evolution. J. Thorac. Cardiovasc. Surg. 53:116, 1967.

Délbét, P.: Kystes hydatiques du foie traités par le capitonnage et la suture sans drainage. Bulletin et Memoires de la Société des chirurgiens de Paris 25, p. 30, 1899a.

Délbét, P.: Kystes hydatiques du foie traités par le capitonnage et la suture sans drainage. Semaine Médicale 19, 1899b.

Demirleau, J., and Pernot: Technique et indications therapeutiques de la kystectomie pour le traitement du kyste hydatique du poumon. J. Chir. 67:769, 1951.

Dévé, F.: Sur la stérilisation du sable hydatique par les solutions formolées et les solutions iodées. C.R. Soc. Biol. 119:352, 1935.

Dew, H.: Hydatid Disease: Its Pathology, Diagnosis, and Treatment. Sydney, Australasian Medical Publishing Company, 1928.

Faust, E.C., and Russell, P.F.: Craig and Faust's Clinical Parasitology. London, Kimpton, 1964, p. 678.

Garabedian, G.A., Matossian, R.M., and Djanian, A.Y.: An indirect hemagglutination test for hydatid disease. J. Immunol. 78:269, 1957.

Ghedini, G.: Ricerche sul siero di sangue di individuo affetto da cisti da echinococco e sul liquido in essa contenuto. Gazzetta degli Ospedali e della Cliniche 27:1616, 1906.

Gil-Grande, L.A., et al.: Treatment of liver hydatid disease with mebendazole: a prospective study of thirteen cases. Am. J. Gastroenterol. 78:584, 1983.

Ginsberg, M., Miller, J.M., and Surmonte, J.A.: Echinococcus cyst of the lung. Chest 34:496, 1958.

Gräfe, H.A.: Kritischer Beitrag zur Serodiagnostik der Echinokokkose des Menschen. Arch. Hyg. Bakteriol. *148*:367, 1964.

Imari, A.J.: Pulmonary hydatid disease in Iraq. Am. J. Trop. Med. Hyg. *11*:481, 1962.

Kagan, I.G.: A review of serological tests for the diagnosis of hydatid disease. World Health Organization Bulletin 39, 1968, p. 25.

Kagan, I.G., et al.: Evaluation of intradermal and serological tests for the diagnosis of hydatid disease. Am. J. Trop. Med. Hyg. *15*:172, 1966.

Kalovidouris, A., et al.: Postsurgical evaluation of hydatid disease with CT: diagnosis pitfalls. J. Comput. Assist. Tomogr. *8*:1114, 1984.

Kourias, B., and Tobler, A.L.: L'avenir eloigené des opérés pour kyste hydatique du poumon. Etude de 265 cas sur 305 opérés. Lyon Chir. *53*:209, 1957.

Lagos Carcia, C., and Segers, A.: Consideraciones sobre un caso de quiste hidatico pulmonar abierto in bronquios. Semin. Med. Bs. As. *31*:271, 1924.

Lewall, D.B., Bailey, T.M., and McCorkell, S.J.: Echinococcal matrix: computed tomographic, sonographic, and pathologic correlation. J. Ultrasound. Med. 5:33, 1986.

Morris, D.L., et al.: Albendazole: objective evidence of response in human hydatid disease. JAMA 253:2053, 1985.

Morseth, D.J.: Fine structure of the hydatid cyst and protoscolex of *Echinococcus granulosus*. J. Parasitol. 53:312, 1967.

Pérez-Fontana, V.: La patologia del guiste hidatico del pulmon. Arch. Int. Hidatid 8:47, 1948.

Pérez-Fontana, V.: Traitement chirurgical du kyste hydatique dus poumon. La méthode uruguayenne ou extirpation du perikyste. Arch. Int. Hidatid *12*:469, 1951.

Peschiera, C.A.: Hydatid cyst of the lung. *In* The Treatment of Mycotic and Parasitic Diseases of the Chest. Edited by J.D. Steele. Springfield, IL, 1964, p. 201.

Peschiera, C.A.: Hydatid cyst of the lung. *In* General Thoracic Surgery. Edited by T.W. Shields. Philadelphia, Lea & Febiger, 1972.

Posadas, A.: Traitement des kystes hydatiques. Rev. Chir. *19*:374, 1899.

Rudolphi, K.A.: Entozoorum Sive Verminum Intestinalium. Historia Naturalis, Vol. II, p. 247. Amsterdam, In Taberna, Libraria et Artinum, 1808. Cited by H. Dew, 1928.

Saidi, F.: Surgery of Hydatid Disease. Philadelphia, W.B. Saunders Co., 1976.

Saksouk, F.A., Fahl, M.H., and Rizk, G.H.: Computed tomography of pulmonary hydatid disease. J. Comput. Assist. Tomogr. *10*:226, 1986.

Sarsam, A.: Surgery of pulmonary hydatid cysts: review of 55 cases. J. Thorac. Cardiovasc. Surg. 62:663, 1971.

Schwabe, C.W.: Host-parasite relationship in echinococcosis: observations on the permeability of the hydatid cyst wall. Am. J. Trop. Med. Hyg. 8:20, 1959.

Sharma, S.K., and Eggleston, F.C.: Management of hydatid disease. Arch. Surg. 99:59, 1969.

Smyth, J.D.: In vitro studies and host-specificity in Echinococcus. World Health Organization Bulletin 39, 1968, p.5.

Toole, H., et al.: Considerations sur la thérapie actuelle des kystes hydatiques du poumon. Apprécition des procédés opératoires. Rev. Med. Moyen Orient *17*:358, 1960.

Tsakayiannis, E., Pappis, C., and Moussatos, P.: Late results of conservative surgical procedures in hydatid disease of the lung in children. Pediatr. Surg. 68:379, 1970.

CHAPTER 72

PULMONARY PARAGONIMIASIS AND ITS SURGICAL COMPLICATIONS

Ronald B. Dietrick

Several Paragonimus species infest man, *Paragonimus westermani* being the most common (Fig. 72–1). The disease is widespread, covering four continents. Not occurring naturally in the United States, paragonimiasis is found in much of East Asia, including Japan, Asian Russia, the Republic of Korea, the Republic of China, Tai-wan, and the Phillipines; in Southeast Asia, including Indonesia, Thailand, and the Indian subcontinent; in Africa, including Nigeria, the Cameroons, Gabon, and Zaire; in Honduras in Central America, and in Venezuela in South America.

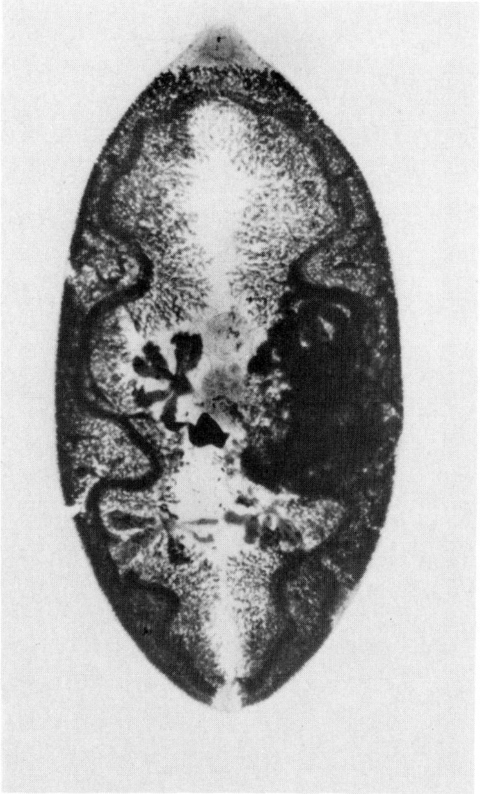

Etiology

Noble and Noble (1982) described the manner of infestation, which is the same everywhere. Eggs of *Paragonimus westermani* lying in moist soil or water hatch as miracidia and enter freshwater snails, from which they are subsequently released as cercariae. These enter freshwater crayfish, probably by ingestion, where they develop into metacercariae. When the flesh of raw crayfish is eaten by man, the metacercariae enter the gastrointestinal tract. Handling the raw flesh or its juice may result in the metacercariae being transferred from the hand into the mouth. Once in the small intestine, the metacercariae excyst, penetrate the intestine, and pass across the peritoneal cavity into the abdominal wall, where they reside in the muscles for about 7 days, only to re-enter the peritoneal cavity, migrate upward through the diaphragm, and wander in the pleural space. Here they penetrate the lungs, more on the right than on the left, to develop into mature worms. These become encysted, causing the basic pathologic lesion of the disease. They produce eggs, which enter a bronchus when the cysts rupture, to be coughed up and expectorated or swallowed, thus passing to the outer world in sputum or feces, completing the life cycle of the parasite.

PATHOLOGY

Gross Findings

Multiple cystic lesions form about the mature worms in the lung, as Yokogawa (1965) and Chung (1971) noted. Grossly, the cut surface of the lung shows slightly ele-

Fig. 72–1. *Paragonimus westermani.* Adult, ventral view. (Courtesy of M.D. Little.) (Reprinted with permission from Clinical Parasitology, 9th ed. Edited by P.C. Beaver, R.C. Jung, and E.W. Cupp. Philadelphia, Lea & Febiger, 1984.)

vated, oval, firm, resilient, nodular masses varying from yellowish-white to gray to reddish-brown. Serial section reveals these masses to be cystic, containing one parasite per cyst (Fig. 72–2), though on occasion more than one is found.

Microscopic Findings

Microscopically, early on, a layer of inflammatory cell infiltration, predominantly polymorphonuclear leukocytes, surrounds the parasites. The neutrophils are gradually replaced by eosinophils, and Charcot Leyden crystals sometimes appear in the necrotic center of the cyst. The eosinophils are gradually replaced by monocytes, lymphocytes, plasma cells, and young fibroblasts. The cyst wall then becomes more fibrotic and granulomata frequently appear near the cyst along with giant cells of the Langhans and foreign-body types. These often contain engulfed ova, but otherwise closely resemble the tubercle of pulmonary tuberculosis. In later stages, bronchial arteries form a new arteriolar network around the worm cyst, and these vessels may rupture and produce hemoptysis when a cyst communicates with a bronchus. Both acute and chronic pathologic changes may exist in the lung concomitantly.

CLINICAL FEATURES

Typically, patients infested by *Paragonimus westermani* tend to be older children or young adults, predominately males. A background of rural poverty is common, and many patients remember handling or eating raw or

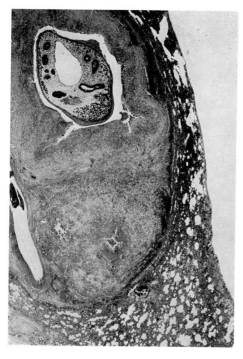

Fig. 72–2. *Paragonimus westermani.* Section of lung showing worm surrounded by infiltration and fibrous encapsulation. (Reprinted with permission from Human Helminthology, 1st ed. Edited by E.C. Faust. Philadelphia, Lea & Febiger, 1929.)

poorly cooked crayfish, if asked. They complain of cough productive of thick whitish sputum, very often blood-streaked, and some patients volunteer that their sputum smells "fishy." Many complain of pleuritic chest pain, fewer of dyspnea and lassitude. Strikingly, the patient often appears healthy, belying the severity of the reported symptoms. There is little fever or prostration, and patients remain active. Often the patient makes his own diagnosis in areas where the disease is endemic, coming to the physician for confirmation and treatment. Physical examination is not revealing, usually, though some patients have scattered fine rales and a few rhonchi throughout the chest. The clinical diagnosis depends more on the history than on the physical examination.

DIAGNOSIS

This is usually straightforward, provided the possibility is entertained. Many patients are diagnosed and treated for tuberculosis, which is often prevalent in areas where paragonimiasis is endemic, and indeed both diseases may afflict the same patient. A chest roentgenogram may show typical multiple, small, round, hazy infiltrations, often with tiny lucencies in the centers through both lungs. According to Chung (1971), on the chest roentgenogram the disease is indistinguishable from tuberculosis in about 40% of patients, and of these, many have been treated for tuberculosis.

Sputum examination helps reveal operculated paragonimus eggs in many cases, sometimes with Charcot Leyden crystals. Eggs may also appear in the feces, so fecal examination is often helpful, especially in children who swallow their sputum rather than spitting it out. The number of eggs shed depends on the severity of infestation, so lightly infested patients may have negative sputum and feces. When this is the case, an intradermal skin test is available, at least in Japan and South Korea. Positive reactions produce a wheal within 3 to 5 minutes, reaching a maximum in 15 minutes according to Yokogawa (1965), so the test may be performed in one visit. A minor difficulty is that the antigen may cross-react with antibodies to *Clonorchis sinensis*. In practice, skin tests are done for both diseases concurrently. Because the age groups, history, physical signs, and symptoms are so different in the two diseases, differentiation between the two is not difficult.

Further confirmation is available with a complement fixation test available from the Centers for Disease Control in Atlanta, Georgia. Although more time-consuming, it is more reliable, because the skin test may remain positive long after recovery, whereas the complement fixation test correlates with the presence of active disease, as Yokogawa and colleagues (1962) noted. Without the complement fixation test, a positive skin test is presumptive evidence of disease in the presence of typical symptoms and in the absence of tuberculosis.

Other laboratory tests have little value, except for frequent eosinophilia, but this is seen in many other parasitic infestations. Eosinophilia may be marked, and I saw one patient with an eosinophilia of over 70%.

CURRENT MEDICAL THERAPY

This is not difficult. Two drugs are effective. Bithionol has been used widely in East Asia for over 25 years, though it is still not generally available in the United States. It is effective in over 90% of patients treated with a course of 15 days. Side effects relating to the gastrointestinal tract are common but not usually severe, and may be decreased by treating on alternate days.

Praziquantel has been used with considerable success. Johnson and associates (1985) noted a positive response in seven of eight patients with treatment for only 2 days. He quoted several other series of patients, one of which contained 31 patients, with a cure rate of 87 to 100%. Side effects are said to be innocuous, and the shorter treatment time is an advantage. Overall, prognosis for cure is excellent no matter which of the two drugs is used.

COMPLICATIONS

There are three: pneumonthorax, pleural effusion, and pleural empyema. The first two occur early; the third is usually late. Only empyema is likely to require major intervention. A critical point in each is that failure to diagnose the underlying cause may lead to recurrent difficulty with a poor result.

Pneumothorax

Presumably this occurs when larvae traversing the pleural space penetrate the lung by breaching the pleura. Clinically, pneumothorax is uncommon and occurs early in the disease, about the time of pleuritic symptoms. Probably many small pneumothoraces occur, only to resolve without diagnosis, especially in underdeveloped areas where medical care is primitive. Pneumothorax should be treated with a superior—anterior—intercostal chest tube connected to underwater drainage on suction until air leakage ceases and the lung re-expands. Should fluid be present or develop, an inferior—posterior—tube should be added. The causative disease must be recognized and treated. Any fluid obtained should be examined for Paragonimus eggs.

Pleural Effusion

This complication occurs early also and more frequently than pneumothorax. Johnson and associates (1982) found effusion in five of nine patients reported. Early appearance is not surprising, because the larvae wander in the pleural space before entering the lung and cause an acute reaction. This too is related in time to symptoms of pleurisy. Again, it is likely that many cases of small pleural effusion go undiagnosed. Many patients with well established paragonimiasis have the haziness of old pleural reaction at the base of the thorax on the chest roentgenogram. When pleural effusion is diagnosed, it should be treated by drainage with an intercostal chest tube until drainage ceases and the pleural space seals off. The fluid should be examined for paragonimus eggs, and treatment for the disease given. The danger of not recognizing the underlying disease or failing to treat it is illustrated by Minh and colleagues (1981) who reported a patient with Paragonimus westermani infection who was tapped for recurrent pleural effusion repeatedly over a period of 24 months before the underlying disease was recognized and treated. Even after treatment, the patient was discharged with a loculated fluid collection in the chest, raising the possibility that there was actually an empyema.

Empyema

This complication often has an insidious onset, indolent nature, and long duration. I and associates (1981) reported 16 patients with such empyema, the shortest duration of symptoms being over 6.5 years. The likeliest explanation for the development of Paragonimus empyema is that it comes from a long-standing unresolved and heretofore undiagnosed pleural effusion. The time between the original symptoms of paragonimiasis and the diagnosis of empyema is so great that their relationship is not suspected. This probably explains why so few references are found in the literature to what must be a fairly frequent complication, particularly in endemic areas.

Slowly, over a period of years, an unresolved pleural effusion develops a pleural peel with encapsulation of the fluid, which becomes thick and pus-like. Unless secondary infection supervenes or the empyema has been drained with a chest tube, the pus is sterile. The symptoms are caused by restriction of the chest wall from the thick, tight peel, and loss of lung capacity from the size of the empyema. The patients are usually young men who complain of mild dyspnea with dull aching in the chest wall overlying the empyema.

If it has not already been done, these patients should *not* be treated with a chest tube (Fig. 72–3). Rather, a thoracentesis should be performed for bacteriologic studies. The pus obtained is usually moderately thick and yellow or brownish. When a chest tube has been inserted, bacterial contamination is common and a variety of organisms may be cultured.

Treatment is by decortication with re-expansion of the lung (Fig. 72–4). Both parietal and visceral pleural peel should be removed. The peel is often surprisingly thick, up to a centimeter, and amazingly easy to remove. On rare occasions, operculated Paragonimus eggs are found in the surgical specimen. Postoperatively, inferior and superior chest tubes are left in the pleural space until drainage ceases and the space has sealed off with the lung re-expanded. Results are uniformly good in patients who have not had a pre-operative chest tube, slightly less so in those who have.

In 16 patients I and associates (1981) reported, the results of decortication were good in 14—87.5%, satisfactory in 1— 6.3%, and poor in 1 who subsequently required a thoracoplasty for control of one of the four major complications that occurred in this group of patients.

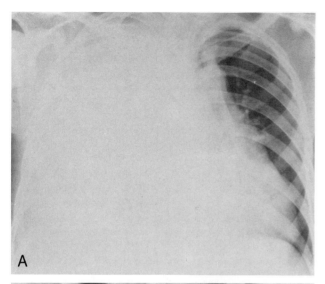

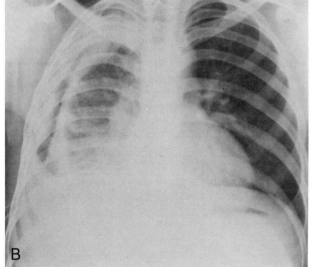

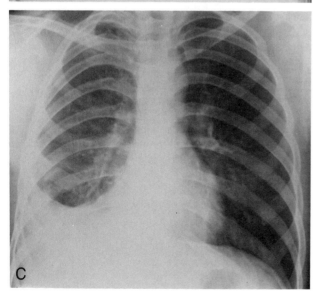

Fig. 72–3. *A,* Chest roentgenogram of an 18-year-old Korean male with *Paragonimus* empyema showing complete "white out" of right thorax and shift of heart to the left. *B,* Film taken after posterior tubing, on the medical service, showing residual space with incomplete expansion of the lung. Note the thick "peel" over the pleural surface of the lung. *C,* Decortication was delayed for almost two months after *B.* This roentgenogram, taken approximately three weeks after decortication, shows complete re-expansion of the lung, but some residual pleural thickening over the diaphragm, which remains elevated, slightly.

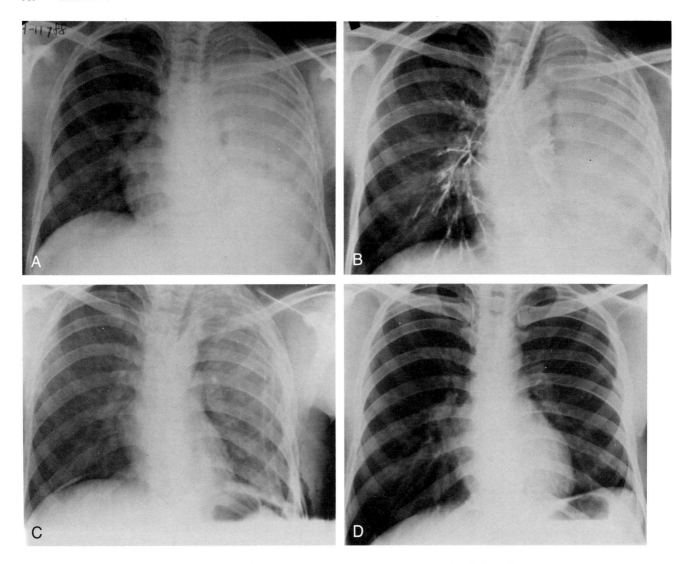

Fig. 72–4. *A*, Chest roentgenogram of a 19-year-old Korean male with *Paragonimus* empyema, taken before admission, showing massive empyema causing almost complete "white out" of the left thorax. *B*, Bronchogram 13 days later, revealing complete collapse of the left lung with "cut off" of all major bronchi. Note diminution of the left thorax with scoliosis. *C*, Roentgenogram taken 2 months later, shortly after left decortication. *D*, Chest roentgenogram 5 years after decortication showing excellent result. Note regeneration of sixth rib, slight elevation of left diaphragm laterally, and disappearance of scoliosis.

REFERENCES

Chung, C.H.: Human paragonimiasis, (pulmonary distomiasis, endemic hemoptysis). *In* Pathology of Protozoal and Helminthic Diseases, Edited by R.A. Marcial-Rojas. Baltimore, Williams & Wilkins Co., 1971, p. 531.

Dietrick, R.B., and Sade, R.M., and Pak, J.S.: Results of decortication in chronic empyema with special reference to paragonimiasis. J. Thorac. Cardiovasc. Surg. *82*:58, 1981.

Johnson, J.R., et al.: Paragonimiasis in the United States. Chest *82*:168, 1982.

Johnson, R.J., et al.: Paragonimiasis: diagnosis and the use of praziquantel in treatment. Rev. Infect. Dis. *7*:200, 1985.

Minh, V., et al.: Pleural paragonimiasis in a Southeast Asian refugee. Am. Rev. Respir. Dis. *124*:186, 1981.

Noble, R.R., and Noble, G.A.: Parasitology, The Biology of Animal Parasites, 5th ed. Philadelphia, Lea & Febiger, 1982, p. 179.

Yokogawa, M., Tsuji, M., and Okura, T.: Studies on the complement fixation test for paragonimiasis as the method of criterion of cure. Jpn. J. Parasitol. *11*:117, 1962.

Yokogawa, M.: Paragonimus and paragonimiasis. Adv. Parasitol. *3*:99, 1965.

CHAPTER 73

DIFFUSE LUNG DISEASE

Harold Stern, Ronald B. Ponn, and Allan L. Toole

Thoracic surgeons are often asked to help solve the diagnostic problem posed by patients with diffuse lung diseases. Although these diseases are not cured or palliated by operation, the knowledgeable surgeon should play a meaningful role in determining the timing, method, and wisdom of invasive diagnostic efforts in these often seriously ill patients. Cooperation among medical specialists is the key to optimal patient care as well as clinical-pathologic studies that advance our understanding of these diseases. Beryllium disease, discussed by Hardy (1961); farmer's lung, noted by Emanuel and associates (1964) and Hapke and colleagues (1968); and desquamative interstitial pneumonia, defined by Liebow (1965) and Gaensler (1969) and their co-workers are excellent examples of such studies. Epler and colleagues' (1985) elucidation of the syndromes of bronchiolitis obliterans organizing pneumonia resulted from the collaboration of pulmonologist, radiologist, pathologist, and thoracic surgeon.

Since Hamman and Rich (1935) described rapidly progressive pulmonary fibrosis, the number of disorders classified as diffuse diseases* has grown greatly. Despite wide variation in etiology, acuity, and outcome, these diseases are grouped together because of clinical, roentgenographic, and histologic similarities.

CLINICAL FEATURES AND PATHOPHYSIOLOGY

Patients most often present with shortness of breath. The dyspnea associated with many infections as well as with acute hypersensitivity reactions often arises abruptly and progresses rapidly. In other instances, e.g., pneumoconioses, shortness of breath develops insidiously many years after exposure to an offending agent. A nonproductive cough is common in both acute and chronic illnesses. Pleuritic chest pain, wheezing, and hemoptysis may occur. Anginal chest pain can result from chronic cor pulmonale. Fever and other nonspecific con-

*Also known as diffuse interstitial lung disease, diffuse infiltrative lung disease, miliary lung disease, and diffuse alveolar damage.

stitutional symptoms may be present in cases of diffuse lung disease caused by infection, certain systemic illnesses, or lymphoma. Other extrapulmonary manifestations may be more specific and suggest a diagnosis. Examples include uveitis and erythema nodosum in sarcoidosis, skin rashes and arthralgias in the collagen vascular diseases, diabetes insipidus in esoinophilic granuloma, and otitis in Wegener's granulomatosis. Occasionally, the first symptoms may result from spontaneous pneumothorax. Pneumothorax in patients with advanced disease can be life-threatening. Light (1983) pointed out that the still compliant, less involved areas of lung collapse more than the diseased portions. The result is often profound respiratory compromise with roentgenographically small pneumothoraces (Fig. 73–1).

Evaluation of patients with diffuse lung disease must include a careful occupational, travel, and environmental history, however remote. A history of contact with animals, travel to areas where certain fungi or parasites are endemic, exposure to organic dusts, mold, asbestos or plastics, a lifestyle associated with acquired immune deficiency syndrome, use of certain medications, and prior radiation therapy can help establish a diagnosis. History alone provided an etiologic diagnosis in one fifth of the patients reported by Gaensler and associates (1964).

The pathophysiology underlying the symptoms of diffuse lung disease involves lung volumes, flows, and ventilation-perfusion abnormalities. Fulmer (1982) described the variable pulmonary function derangements in these disorders. In early cases of slowly progressive disease, lung volumes may be normal; but with advancing fibrosis, vital capacity and total lung capacity decline. In contrast, the acute alveolitis of hypersensitivity pneumonitis causes early reduction in lung volumes. In other cases, small airway obstruction by bronchiolitis or peribronchial fibrosis may produce an obstructive pattern or at least modulate any change in volumes. Carrington and associates (1977) showed that in lymphangioleiomyomatosis—LAM—such airway narrowing characteristically produces emphysematous changes and increased lung volumes. The granulomas of sarcoidosis and Wegener's

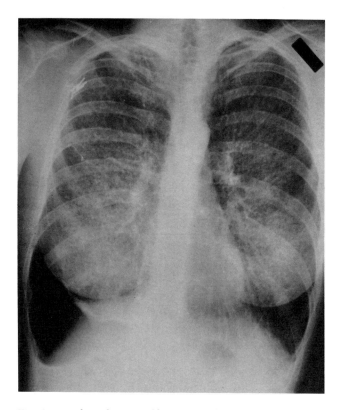

Fig. 73–1. Thirty-five-year-old woman with lymphangioleiomyomatosis presented with severe dyspnea. Chest film showed a right basal pneumothorax under tension (depressed hemidiaphragm). Tube thoracostomy caused immediate relief.

granulomatosis can occur in larger bronchi and cause airflow obstruction. In all these situations, the classic restrictive picture may be replaced by a combined restrictive and obstructive pattern.

Diffusion impairment is evident even in early diffuse lung disease. The major cause of hypoxemia, however, is not decreased oxygen diffusion, but ventilation-perfusion mismatch with resultant right-to-left shunt and widened alveolar-arterial oxygen gradient. With early involvement, arterial oxygen tension at rest may be maintained by hyperventilation, with hypoxemia provoked only by exertion. With progressive fibrosis, resting hypoxemia occurs. Because ventilatory capacity generally remains intact, hypercapnia occurs only in the end stage.

PATHOGENESIS AND PATHOLOGY

Although the airways, the alveolar spaces, and the pulmonary vasculature are involved to some degree in many diffuse lung diseases, the principal site of ultimate damage is the connective tissue of the pulmonary interstitium (Fig. 73–2). The normal interstitium contains collagen, elastin, fibroblasts, lymphocytes, histiocytes, and occasional leukocytes and is bounded by the alveolar epithelium and the capillary endothelium (Fig. 73–3). Weibel (1968) showed that the total tissue barrier between air and blood may be 0.2 μm or less.

An acute alveolitis is the usual finding in early diffuse

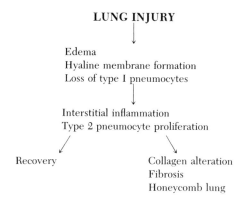

LUNG INJURY

Edema
Hyaline membrane formation
Loss of type I pneumocytes

Interstitial inflammation
Type 2 pneumocyte proliferation

Recovery   Collagen alteration
                  Fibrosis
                  Honeycomb lung

Fig. 73–2. Pathogenesis of the lung injury.

lung disease, with inflammatory and immune cells appearing in the interstitium in variable ratios. Often, these inflammatory cells spill over into the alveolar lumina. Eosinophils and macrophages predominate in the eosinophilic pneumonias, lymphocytes in sarcoidosis, special histiocytes in histiocytosis X, and macrophages, lymphocytes, and plasma cells in idiopathic pulmonary fibrosis. The degree of cellularity correlates with disease activity and may have important clinical applications (Fig. 73–4). In some cases, monocyte activation and granuloma formation occur. Early, alveolar and interstitial edema, hyaline membrane formation, and replacement of type I and type II pneumocytes also occur. This nonspecific response has also been called diffuse alveolar damage—DAD. Alveolitis can result from a wide variety of lung injuries mediated by different mechanisms. For example, Schatz and associates (1979) showed that T-lymphocytes are involved in the granuloma formation of sarcoidosis. Reynolds (1982) described the role of immune complexes and cell-mediated immune reactions in hypersensitivity pneumonitis. Leukocyte chemotactic factors have been identified in some diffuse lung diseases.

If not reversed, the alveolitis results in permanent collagen alteration and eventual interstitial fibrosis. The

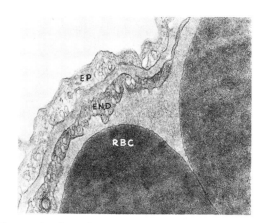

Fig. 73–3. Alveolar wall. Type 1 alveolar epithelial cell—EP—separated from the endothelium—END—by a basement membrane. RBC = red blood cell. Magnification: approximately ×24,000. (Courtesy Klaus Bensch, M.D.)

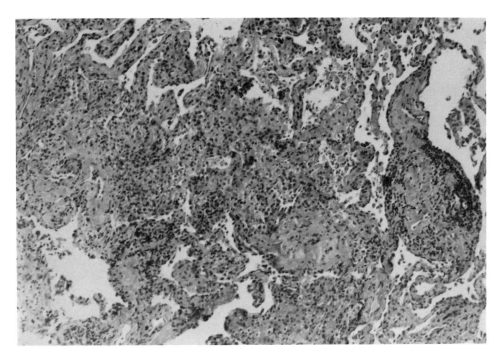

Fig. 73–4. Open biopsy specimen from a middle-aged man with dyspnea and bilateral infiltrates. There is marked interstitial thickening and infiltration with inflammatory cells as well as some fibrosis. There was a good clinical response to steroids. (Courtesy of Darryl Carter, M.D.)

final histologic pattern is marked fibrosis, decreased cellularity, distention of distal airways, replacement of alveoli by scar, and cyst formation, and end-stage "honeycomb" lung. At this point, pathologic evaluation is nonspecific and rarely provides a diagnosis or aids in treatment. In early stages of disease, in contrast, the presence of granulomas, the degree of cellularity and the types of inflammatory cells, the presence of bronchiolitis obliterans with organizing pneumonia, or the demonstration of vasculitis may allow for a more specific diagnosis and successful treatment.

ROENTGENOGRAPHIC FEATURES

Diffuse lung diseases classically appear in chest roentgenograms as widespread infiltrative densities. The picture is usually nonspecific and rarely can be relied on alone either to establish a diagnosis or to assess physiologic severity. Nevertheless, considerable information can be gained by comparing serial chest films, by noting certain patterns or zones of involvement, and by examining extrapulmonary structures.

Felson (1967) and Fraser and Paré (1977) described the roentgenographic patterns in diffuse lung disease. Involvement of the alveolar spaces produces an acinar pattern, consisting of scattered small, nodular densities with poorly defined margins. Filling of alveoli with inflammatory cells, hyaline membranes, or edema fluid can result in an air bronchogram. Among the processes associated with an acinar pattern are desquamative interstitial pneumonia, pulmonary alveolar proteinosis, bronchioloalveolar carcinoma, lymphoma, and some cases of sarcoidosis—"alveolar" sarcoidosis.

Involvement of the interstitium causes several patterns. A granular or ground-glass appearance consists of a diffuse haziness caused by generalized mild thickening of the interstitium and is common in the early stages of many diffuse lung diseases such as asbestosis, eosinophilic pneumonia, berylliosis, and hemosiderosis. A predominantly nodular pattern often appears in silicosis, miliary tuberculosis, and talcosis. The reticular pattern is formed by a network of linear densities caused by significant thickening of the interstitium. This mesh-like appearance is described as fine, medium, or coarse, and correlates with the disease stage as documented for idiopathic pulmonary fibrosis and rheumatoid lung. A combination of linear and nodular densities produces a reticulonodular pattern, as in lymphangitic carcinoma, lymphoma, and sarcoidosis. The presence of air cysts surrounded by thick walls, with gross deformation of the pulmonary parenchyma, is termed "honeycombing." It appears late in many diffuse lung diseases but is characteristic of lymphoangioleiomyomatosis, histiocytosis X, idiopathic pulmonary fibrosis, and end-stage sarcoidosis.

Some diffuse lung diseases predominate in certain areas of the lung. Eosinophilic granuloma, silicosis, histiocytosis X, and sarcoidosis involve the upper zones. A basal distribution is characteristic of rheumatoid lung, asbestosis, and idiopathic pulmonary fibrosis. Bergin and Müller (1987) used CT scanning to delineate axial—central, middle, and peripheral compartments of the pulmonary parenchyma and described a predilection of certain diseases for each of these zones.

Abnormal extraparenchymal findings may also aid diagnosis. Examples include pleural plaques in asbestosis, hilar adenopathy in lymphoma and sarcoidosis, pneu-

Table 73–1. Granulomatous Disease

Infection
   Tuberculosis
   Atypical mycobacteria
   Fungi
   Schistosoma
   Filaria
Unknown Cause
   Sarcoidosis
   Wegener's granulomatosis
   Lymphomatoid granulomatosis
   Allergic granuloma
   Eosinophilic granuloma
   Histiocytosis X
Inhalation
   Organic dust pneumoconioses
     (hypersensitivity pneumonitis)
   Inorganic dusts—silica, beryllium

mothorax in eosinophilic granuloma, histiocytosis X, and lymphangioleiomyomatosis—LAM— and pleural effusion seen commonly with collagen-vascular disorders and LAM but rarely in sarcoidosis or silicosis.

Roentgenography is most helpful when constellations of findings are considered and correlated with the patient's clinical course and presentation. Epler and associates (1978) found, however, that the chest film was normal in 10% of 458 symptomatic patients with biopsy-documented diffuse lung disease.

CLASSIFICATION

Diffuse lung diseases may be classified in two distinct ways, etiologically and pathologically. Neither scheme is completely satisfactory because of overlapping. For example, ample evidence suggests that berylliosis in the chronic form is a hypersensitivity disease with granuloma formation. Acute toxic berylliosis, however, has also been described. Therefore, a purely etiologic classification would require two listings, one under hypersensitivity diseases and the other under acute inhalation damage. From the pathologic point of view, berylliosis would have to be classified both under granulomatous disease and under acute alveolar damage.

In Tables 73–1 and 73–2, we have divided the diseases into granulomatous and nongranulomatous categories with subclassification by etiology or associated disease. In this text, some nongranulomatous processes are grouped according to histology. Neither the tables nor the discussions are meant to be all-inclusive.

Granuloma

Granulomatous diseases may all have a common background of hypersensitivity. This sensitivity may be to micro-organisms, be it to bacteria, fungi, or as yet unknown agents. Granulomas may tend to form when tissues have prolonged contact with the offending antigen. Both cell-mediated allergic responses and humoral antibodies may cause granulomas. The granulomas of tuberculosis may resemble those of sarcoidosis and ber-

ylliosis. Common characteristics include the presence of asteroid bodies and Schaumann bodies within giant cells. Distinct granulomas occur in farmer's lung disease, which as Pepys and associates (1963) reported, is a hypersensitivity to the thermophilic actinomycete *Micropolyspora taeni*. Other sarcoid-like reactions are seen in patients with maple bark disease and pigeon breeder's lung. As Carrington and Liebow (1966) discussed, Wegener's granulomatosis may be confined to the lung or may be a part of a systemic process. Granulomas may occur in the alveolar walls themselves or near arterioles or in larger vessels or bronchi (Figs. 73–5 through 73–7).

Nongranulomatous Pulmonary Disease

Nongranulomatous diffuse lung disease may be caused by infection, inhalation, drug sensitivities, irradiation, systemic diseases, neoplasm, or unknown cause.

Interstitial Pneumonias

Liebow (1968) described the histologic features of the interstitial pneumonias. In usual interstitial pneumonia—UIP—there is a spectrum of changes, from normal lung to interstitial inflammation to severe fibrosis. Chronic inflammatory cells appear in the interstitium but a few cells appear in the alveoli. In desquamative interstitial pneumonia—DIP—the histology is more homogeneous. The air spaces are filled with alveolar macrophages. Interstitial eosinophils and plasma cells are more common than in UIP. There is alveolitis and thickening of the interstitium, but less fibrosis than in UIP. In lymphocytic interstitial pneumonia—LIP—many mature lymphocytes, some plasma cells, and a few immunoblasts accumulate. Bronchiolitis associated with interstitial inflammation is termed bronchiolitis interstitial pneumonia—BIP. In BIP there is edematous granulation tissue within distal bronchioles and alveolar ducts, extending into the alveoli with varying amounts of interstitial inflammation. In giant cell interstitial pneumonia—GIP—bizarre multinucleate giant cells appear in the alveoli.

Carrington and associates (1978) noted that UIP and DIP represent two distinct clinicopathologic syndromes, with DIP being more amenable to treatment with steroids. Scadding and Hinson (1967), Patchefsky and associates (1973), and Tubbs and colleagues (1977), on the other hand, consider DIP to be the early cellular phase and UIP the later, fibrotic phase of the same process. In fact, progression from DIP to UIP has been documented.

Interstitial pneumonias occur in patients with no known exposure or underlying illness as well as in association with specific diseases and injuries (Figs. 73–8 through 73–11). Fishman (1978) pointed out that they may represent a nonspecific inflammatory response to injuries of varying type, duration, and severity. In addition, patients with interstitial pneumonias of unknown cause may have a clinical course and response to treatment different from those of patients with associated diseases. The current tendency is to separate those pneumonias with known causes from the idiopathic. This has led to some confusion regarding terminology. Table 73–3 attempts to summarize the situation.

Table 73–2. Nongranulomatous Disease

Unknown Cause
  Idiopathic pulmonary fibrosis
  Lymphocytic infiltrative disorders
  Pulmonary alveolar proteinosis
  Amyloidosis
  Glycogen storage disease
  Hemosiderosis
  Goodpasture's syndrome
  Pulmonary alveolar microlithiasis
  Ankylosing spondylitis

Collagen Vascular
  Dermatomyositis
  Lupus
  Rheumatoid arthritis
  Scleroderma
  Sjögren's

Neoplasm
  Leukemia
  Lymphoma
  Pseudolymphoma ?
  Lymphangioleiomyomatosis ?
  Hematogenous metastases
  Lymphangitis carcinoma
  Mycosis fungoides
  Kaposi's sarcoma
  Bronchoalveolar carcinoma
  Pulmonary adenomatosis

Inhalation
  Inorganic dust—asbestos, beryllium,
    cadmium, iron, tungsten titanium,
    etc.
  Organic dust—farmer's lung, bagas-
    sosis, bird fancier's lung, etc.
  Fumes and gases—acid, chlorine, ox-
    ygen toxicity, etc.

Infection
  Bacteria, viruses, mycoplasma, pro-
    tozoa, rickettsia

Drugs
  Chemotherapeutic —bleomycin,
    methotrexate, cyclophosphamide,
    etc.
  Cardiovascular—amiodarone, pro-
    cainamide, hydralazine, etc.
  Antibiotics—nitrofurantoin, PAS,
    sulfonamides
  Miscellaneous—diphenylhydantoin,
    methysergide

Physical Injury
  Radiation
  Aspiration
  Blast injury
  Deceleration injury
  Thermal injury

Most clinicians prefer the term idiopathic pulmonary fibrosis—IPF—for the syndrome of slowly progressive pulmonary inflammation and fibrosis of unknown etiology. In Britain, the designation cryptogenic fibrosing alveolitis is preferred. The prognosis is poor for patients with advanced fibrosis at the time of biopsy. Dreisen and associates (1978), however, found a correlation among circulating immune complex levels, immunofluorescent studies of biopsy specimens, degree of cellularity, and response to treatment in patients with IPF. Whether DIP is a distinct process or a type of early IPF remains unresolved.

Similarly, bronchiolitis obliterans with interstitial in-

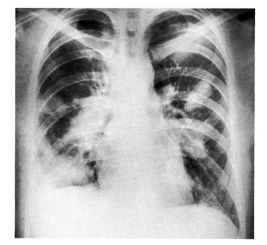

Fig. 73–5. Wegener's granuloma in a 28-year-old male who complained of dyspnea. Biopsy of one of the right lower lobe masses revealed Wegener's granuloma. The patient died in 4 months of progressive pulmonary involvement despite therapy with steroids and immunosuppressive agents.

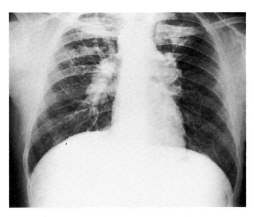

Fig. 73–6. Sarcoidosis in a 21-year-old man with typical linear, mediastinal, and diffuse parenchymal involvement.

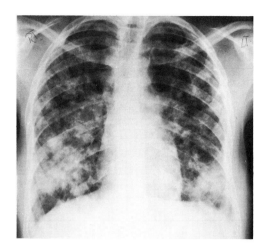

Fig. 73–7. Advanced sarcoidosis in a 24-year-old man. Numerous discrete and confluent densities are present, with minimal node involvement.

flammation can be postinfectious or related to connective tissue diseases, drugs, and inhalation injury. In addition, bronchiolitis with or without organizing pneumonia has been reported following marrow transplantation by Ralph and associates (1984) and after heart-lung transplantation by Burke and co-workers (1984). Epler and associates (1985) reviewed the clinical characteristics of patients with IPF whose biopsies showed bronchiolitis obliterans organizing pneumonia—BOOP. They showed that patients with idiopathic BOOP have a high rate of favorable response to prolonged steroid treatment and should, therefore, be regarded as a distinct clinical group.

Lymphocytic interstitial pneumonia—LIP—occurs in association with immunologic diseases such as Sjögren's syndrome, systemic lupus erythematosus, myasthenia gravis, and chronic active hepatitis. Dysproteinemia is present in most cases of LIP even when not associated with a defined syndrome. Reports by Oleske and asso-

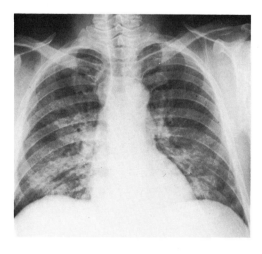

Fig. 73–8. Leukemia and UIP in a 57-year-old man who had a 3 week history of extreme dyspnea when first seen. Acute myelogenous leukemia. pH 7.51, P_{CO_2} 30 mm, P_{O_2} 47 mm. Lung biopsy revealed leukemic infiltration and organizing interstitial pneumonia.

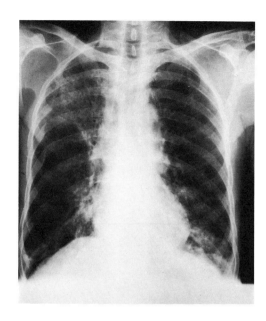

Fig. 73–9. Progressive dyspnea in a 57-year-old man with chronic myelogenous leukemia treated with busulfan. Biopsy revealed changes consistent with UIP. No leukemic infiltrates or organisms were seen.

ciates (1983) of LIP in children of mothers at risk for acquired immune deficiency syndrome and by Morris and colleagues (1987) of LIP in adults with AIDS or AIDS-related complex further support an immunologic etiology. Most cases are treated with steroids. The relationship of LIP to lymphoma is debated (see Chapter 77). Progression to malignant lymphoma is common. Some investigators believe that LIP is a low-grade malignant lymphoma from the outset. Lymphomatoid granulomatosis may also be a malignant lymphoma. Finally, most "pseudolymphomas" of the lung may, in fact, be small lymphocytic lymphomas. Kennedy (1985) and Herbert (1985) and their colleagues discussed this complex area.

Too few cases of giant cell interstitial pneumonia have been reported to determine if GIP represents a true clinicopathologic entity. Measles pneumonia can produce a similar picture.

Primary Alveolar Diseases

Several diseases appear to involve primarily the alveolar lumina. Pulmonary alveolar proteinosis—PAP—is an example of such a process in which proteinaceous material stuffs the alveoli. This proteinaceous material is periodic-acid-Schiff-stain—PAS—positive. Rosen and associates (1958) noted a close resemblance between PAP and *Pneumocystic carinii* pneumonia. PAP may also be associated with fungal disease, notably nocardiosis. Electron microscopy has shown that the predominant cell within the alveoli is the type II alveolar cell.

Idiopathic pulmonary hemosiderosis and the pulmonary phase of Goodpasture's syndrome also may be classified within this category, and are characterized by intra-alveolar hemorrhage and masses of hemosiderin-laden phagocytes.

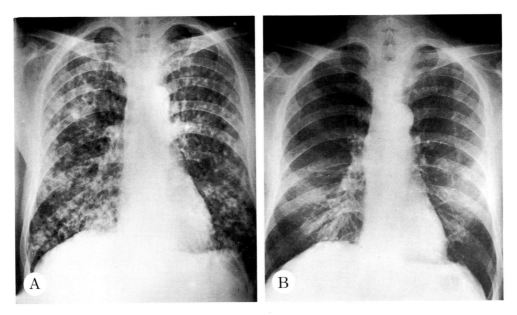

Fig. 73–10. *A,* Noxious fume inhalation in a 60-year-old man with high fever, dyspnea, and cough. Nitric acid fume exposure. Histologic examination showed active alveolitis. *B,* Follow-up roentgenogram of the chest made 1 year later.

Primary Vascular Lesions

Heart disease is probably the commonest cause of pulmonary arteriolar disease. Collagen diseases, especially progressive systemic sclerosis, can affect the pulmonary arterioles. Pulmonary hypertension may be a late effect of occlusions of the multiple pulmonary arterioles by the granulomatous response to *Schistosoma mansoni* ova. Chronic hypoxia, whether caused by lung disease, heart disease, or high altitude, may cause marked medial muscular hypertrophy.

Pulmonary Allergic Responses

Gell and Coombs (1968) classified four main mechanisms of allergic reactions: type I—anaphylactic; type II—cytotoxic; type III—complex mediated; and type IV—delayed hypersensitivity. Types I, II, and III result from antigen-antibody reactions, whereas type IV is a T-cell mediated immune response.

Type I pulmonary hypersensitivity consists of bronchospasm, either alone or as part of generalized anaphylaxis, and is mediated by IgE immunoglobulins or reagins—skin sensitizing antibodies. When the inhaled

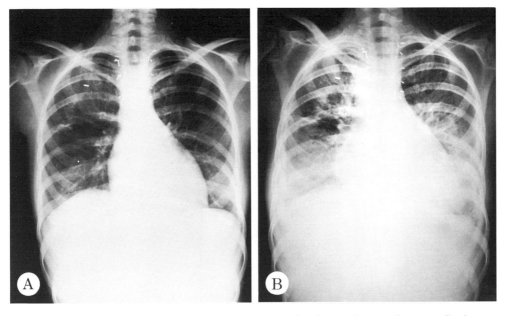

Fig. 73–11. *A,* Diffuse systemic sclerosis in a 23-year-old woman with previous dorsal sympathectomy for Raynaud's phenomenon secondary to scleroderma. *B,* Roentgenogram made 4 months later, shortly before death, shows marked progression of the interstitial process. This patient had pulmonary insufficiency.

Table 73–3.   The Interstitial Pneumonias

Histology	Clinical Syndrome	Known Associations
Usual interstitial pneumonia (UIP)	Idiopathic pulmonary fibrosis (IPF)—advanced	Collagen vascular disease Infection (viral, mycoplasma) Drugs Inhalation injury Radiation
Desquamative interstitial pneumonia (DIP)	DIP ? early IPF ?	Same
Bronchiolitis interstitial pneumonia (BIP)	Bronchiolitis obliterans organizing pneumonia (BOOP)	Same plus Marrow transplantation Heart-lung transplantation
Lymphocytic interstitial pneumonia (LIP)	LIP—unclassified	Sjögren's Lupus Myasthenia Phenytoin AIDS
Giant-cell interstitial pneumonia (GIP)	GIP ?	Measles pneumonia

antigen encounters the antibody on the mast cell surface, potent pharmacologic agents, such as histamine, serotonin, kinins, and eosinophil chemotactic substances, are released. Type II sensitivity consists of the binding of IgM and IgG antibodies to cellular and tissue antigens. Complement may or may not be involved in the process. Drugs may combine with erythrocytes, platelets, or leukocytes, with subsequent production of antibodies to the drug-cell complex. The antigen-antibody reaction allows the destruction of the cells—hemolytic anemia, thrombocytopenia, or leukopenia. Goodpasture's syndrome may be a result of destruction of the alveolar basement membrane by antibodies. Immunofluorescent studies establish this diagnosis by demonstrating deposits of immunoglobulins along the basement membranes. Type III reactions are mediated by IgM and IgG antibodies or precipitins that combine with antigen. These complexes may be deposited on vessel walls, may cause release of vasoactive amines from platelets, or may result in the release of lysosomal enzymes from neutrophils. Edema formation, vasculitis, and neutrophilic infiltration result. Examples of type III response are serum sickness and extrinsic alveolitis caused by organic dust inhalation. Type IV reactions are caused by release of lymphokines from T-lymphocytes, resulting in inflammation—tuberculin test. No circulating antibodies are demonstrable. Granulomatous reactions are type IV responses.

Inhalation of pituitary snuff may result in an acute asthmatic—type I—response or, less commonly, produce an alveolitis that is a manifestation of type III hypersensitivity. The lesions of polyarteritis also suggest a type III response. Byssinosis is a type I response caused by the inhalation of cotton dust. Spores of *Cryptostroma corticale* appear in the giant cells of maple bark lung. *Schistosoma* ova appear in the pulmonary granulomas of schistosomiasis. Precipitating antibodies against moldy hay appear in the sera of most patients with farmer's lung. Many of the entities mentioned in this chapter apparently may be caused by hypersensitivity responses

of one or more types. Only the allergen needs to be discovered (Fig. 73–12).

Pulmonary Eosinophilias

Liebow and Carrington (1969a) discussed eosinophilic responses within the lung extensively. Various agents can cause eosinophilic infiltration. Among the eosinophilic pneumonias are Löffler's syndrome, consisting of wandering pulmonary infiltrations that are self-limited and of short duration, prolonged pulmonary eosinophilia, tropical eosinophilia caused by various parasitic infestations, eosinophilic pneumonias induced by chemical agents, especially nitrofurantoin, penicillin, and para-

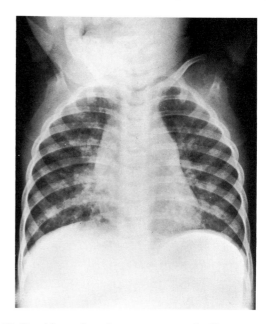

Fig. 73–12.   Allergic lung disease in a 3-month-old infant who had had respiratory distress since 7 weeks of age. Diagnosis was made by finding precipitins to milk. Resolution took place when milk was removed from the diet.

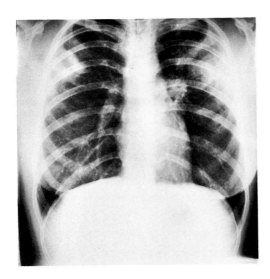

Fig. 73–13. Eosinophilic pneumonia in a 21-year-old woman who had a 1-month history of fever and migratory infiltrates bilaterally. Marked eosinophilia was present. The patient responded rapidly to steroid therapy.

aminosalicylic acid. Liebow and Carrington (1969a) and Carrington and associates (1969) described prolonged eosinophilic pneumonia (Figs. 73–13, 73–14, and 73–15).

Disseminated Neoplasm

Bronchioloalveolar carcinoma can emerge as diffuse pulmonary disease, although this possibility is far less common in our experience than the localized form associated with scars, as Raeburn and Spencer (1953) noted. This is probably a result of earlier recognition of the pulmonary cancer, because diffuse involvement may

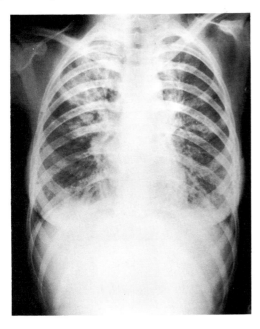

Fig. 73–14. Eosinophilic pneumonia in a 14-year-old girl with a 1-month history of cough, wheezing, and chest pain. Changing pulmonary infiltrates. WBC 50,000, 80% eosinophils. Good response to steroids.

occur in patients whose original lesion was localized. Spread is along the alveolar walls, and the neoplasm may actually be airborne from one portion of the lung to another, resulting in bilateral diffuse disease in extreme instances. Lobar consolidation may also occur (Fig. 73–16A and B).

Carcinoma of the lung may metastasize by lymphangitic spread, often on the same side as the primary lesion, which may remain small and difficult to identify. Hematogenous and lymphangitic spread are common manifestations of metastatic cancer from primary sites, which may be obvious from the outset or escape detection until an autopsy is performed. In most patients, the primary invasion of the lungs is by multiple tumor emboli to small pulmonary arteries and subsequent invasion of periarterial lymphatics. Pulmonary hypertension may result from hematogenous disseminated disease (Fig. 73–17).

Hodgkin's disease may metastasize as multiple miliary nodules. Leukemic infiltrations of different natures can occur during the course of various types of blood dyscrasias, and restrictive lung disease may occur in these patients. Interstitial pneumonitis— without tumor-cell infiltration—may occur in patients with leukemia; UIP may be associated with busulfan therapy.

Radiation Pneumonitis

Radiation therapy may result in diffuse infiltration of the lung noted roentgenographically. In addition, radiation bronchiolitis as well as pleuritis may occur, depending on the dosage and individual susceptibility. End-stage fibrosis, contraction, and atelectasis of an entire lobe, but rarely of a lung, may occur.

A review of the original port films or diagrams is often helpful because radiation changes can be sharply delineated. These changes can be seen after therapy for bronchial carcinoma as well as radical radiation therapy for mediastinal lymphomas and carcinoma of the breast. Thus, differential diagnosis becomes difficult in the patient with Hodgkin's disease who has had radiation therapy to the mediastinum and supraclavicular areas, has had chemotherapy and steroids, and develops bilateral upper lobe infiltrations.

Opportunistic Infections of the Lung

Altered host resistance to infection may result from congenital or acquired states, steroid therapy, or cancerocidal and immunosuppressive agents. Normally nonpathogenic organisms are given the opportunity to cause clinical infection. Opportunistic pulmonary infections have become more common and complex in this era of transplantation, advanced cancer treatment, aggressive support of patients with multiple organ failure, and continuing spread of the acquired immune deficiency syndrome. Bacteria, protozoans, fungi, and viruses may all cause infection in these patients (Table 73–4 and Figs. 73–18 through 73–22).

Bacterial pneumonia caused by gram-negative organisms, staphylococcus, or pneumococcus, is common in immunocompromised patients. Other less common bacterial infections may occur as well. *Nocardia asteroides*

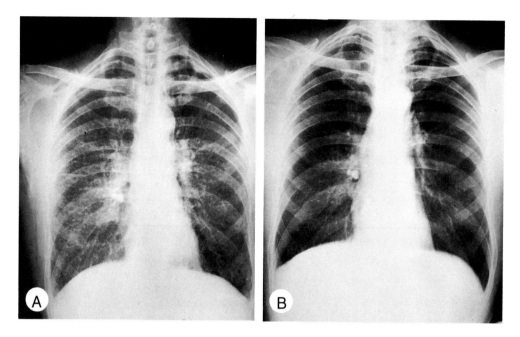

Fig. 73–15. *A*, Nitrofurantoin lung in a 60-year-old man treated with nitrofurantoin for 13 days. The patient was first seen with dyspnea, fever, WBC 17,000, 16% eosinophils. *B*, Five days after cessation of nitrofurantoin administration the infiltrates began to clear. Roentgenogram, made 2 years after the one shown in *A*, demonstrates clear lung fields.

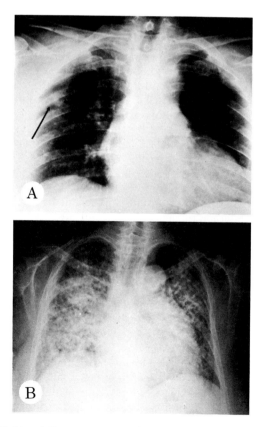

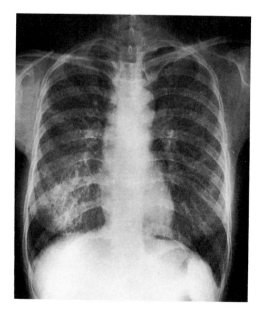

Fig. 73–16. *A*, Roentgenogram made in 1963 of a 68-year-old woman with a 1.5-cm lesion in the right upper lung field. No diagnosis was made at this time and no therapy was given. *B*, Roentgenogram made in 1965. The diagnosis of diffuse bronchioalveolar cell carcinoma was made following lung biopsy.

Fig. 73–17. Metastatic carcinoma and granuloma in a 50-year-old woman with a history of thyroidectomy and radical neck dissection for carcinoma. Biopsy revealed nodules of papillary adenocarcinoma (thyroid) and noncaseating granulomas.

Table 73–4. Pulmonary Infiltrates in the Immunocompromised Host

Bacteria	Protozoa
Gram-negative and positive	Pneumocystis
Nocardia	Toxoplasma
Legionella	Viruses
Tuberculosis	Cytomegalovirus
Atypical mycobacteria	Herpes
	Varicella—zoster
Fungi	Noninfectious
Aspergillus	Radiation pneumonitis
Candida	Chemotherapy lung
Histoplasma	Transplantation bronchiolitis
Cryptococcus	Idiopathic pulmonary fibrosis—
Blastomyces	interstitial pneumonia
Coccidioides	Neoplasm—lymphoma, leukemia,
Sporotrichum	Kaposi's sarcoma

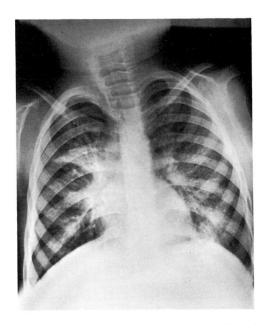

Fig. 73–19. Opportunistic infection in a 5-year-old child with agammaglobulinemia who suffered repeated gram-positive and gram-negative infections.

may cause lung and brain abscesses in addition to diffuse infiltrates. Legionella usually appear as a nosocomial epidemic among compromised patients. Cordes and associates (1980) described the association of legionella pneumonia with hyponatremia, confusion, hematuria, and bradycardia. Chastre and co-workers (1987) showed that pulmonary fibrosis can progress even after successful treament of acute legionella pneumonia. Interestingly, patients with AIDS seem not to be at increased risk for community-acquired Legionnaires' disease, according to Polsky and associates (1986). Atypical mycobacterial infection, especially with *M. avium*, is common in AIDS. Also, Handwerger and associates (1987) found infection with *M. tuberculosis* in 15% of hospitalized AIDS patients.

Pneumocystis carinii pneumonia—PCP—has become the epitome of opportunistic infection. PCP has long been recognized in renal transplant patients and in patients with leukemia and lymphoma. It is the most common diffuse lung infection in AIDS and is responsible for considerable morbidity and mortality. PCP can pursue a rapid course with early respiratory failure or present as a more indolent infection. The mortality rate for PCP in AIDS patients is 30%. Recurrences are common. Shelhamer and associates (1984) showed persistence of the protozoan in transbronchial biopsy specimens even after prolonged treatment and clinical improvement. Toxoplasmosis is a protozoal disease that involves the lung in its disseminated form, but more often is confined to the central nervous system.

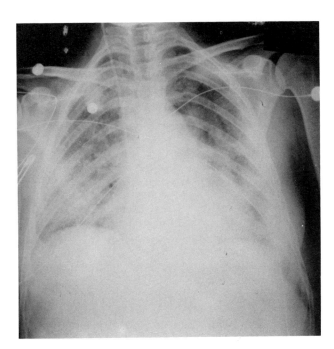

Fig. 73–18. Thirty-year-old intravenous drug abuser with AIDS presented with sepsis and respiratory distress. *Pneumocystis carinii* pneumonia documented by bronchoalveolar lavage.

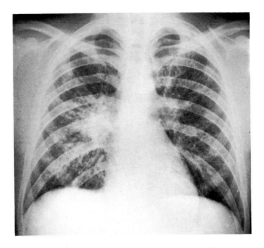

Fig. 73–20. Opportunistic infection in a 32-year-old man with a 2½-year history of progressive sarcoiodosis. The patient died of cryptococcosis of lung, brain, and meninges.

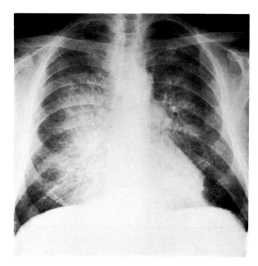

Fig. 73–21. Opportunistic infection in a 71-year-old man with monocytic leukemia who was treated with 6-mercaptopurine and prednisone and multiple broad-spectrum antibiotics for gram-negative infection. Sputum culture showed *Cryptococcus, Aspergillus,* and *Candida.*

Fungal infections of the lung are discussed in Chapter 69. Among the fungi, Candida and Aspergillus are the most commonly encountered opportunistic pathogens. The lung may be involved alone or as part of a disseminated infection. Pulmonary infection may result in abscess formation as well as diffuse infiltrates. Demonstration of the organism in tissues samples is necessary for a definitive diagnosis. These two organisms cause problems in impaired hosts so commonly that prophylactic antifungal treatment is often used in neutropenic leukemic patients. Cryptococcal pneumonia and meningitis occur in patients with impaired cellular immunity, especially Hodgkin's disease. Zunger and colleagues (1986) demonstrated a significant incidence in AIDS patients as well. Disseminated histoplasmosis is increasingly common in AIDS patients living in endemic areas.

Cytomegalovirus—CMV—is the most frequent cause of viral pneumonia in immunocompromised patients and often coexists with PCP. Superinfection with bacterial pathogens is also common. Herpes simplex and varicella zoster pneumonia occur less often, the latter usually associated with a typical rash. Viral serology and examination of skin lesions are helpful. Intranuclear inclusions appear in sputum samples but are nonspecific. Tissue biopsy is often needed.

Pulmonary infiltrates in immunocompromised patients may, of course, be from causes other than infection. Fever, dyspnea, and infiltrates may be caused by radiation pneumonitis or lymphangitic tumor spread. Many chemotherapeutic agents produce pneumonitis, usually without fever. Patients with immunologic and collagen vascular diseases can develop interstitial pneumonias and pulmonary fibrosis that mimic infection. Transplant recipients may develop bronchiolitis. Garay and colleagues (1987) showed that the clinical presentation of pulmonary Kaposi's sarcoma in AIDS may be indistinguishable from opportunistic infection. Ramaswamy and associates (1985) documented that AIDS patients can present with febrile syndromes and alveolitis/pulmonary fibrosis in the absence of concurrent lung infection.

The principles Lurie and Duma (1970) stressed regarding opportunistic infection remain applicable. Because of an altered host response, one should not be misled by aberrant or "atypical" clinical or pathologic findings. For the same reasons, serologic tests may be confusing. Because many infections develop in the wake of previous infections, residual tissue reactions or damage may complicate pathologic interpretation. Prior or concomitant antibiotics may have killed the primary pathogen so that it can no longer be cultured and identified. Subsequent overgrowth by saprophytic organisms may occur and add to interpretive difficulty. Because opportunistic infections are often mixed, all isolates must be carefully evaluated before final conclusions are drawn.

DIAGNOSIS

When essential noninvasive methods fail to produce a diagnosis, an invasive surgical procedure may be required. Examination of sputum for fungi, tubercle bacilli, cells, and fat may be unrewarding. Skin tests rarely help except to show anergy.

Bronchoscopy with vigorous bronchoalveolar lavage—BAL—is becoming more useful because of refined laboratory techniques, as Stover (1984) and Daniele (1985) and their associates noted. In addition to a search for infectious agents, cell types and their immune properties can be evaluated. *Pneumocystis carinii* is seen with the Grocott stain. Helper and suppressor T-cell analysis may aid the diagnosis of sarcoidosis. Immunofluorescent examination using monoclonal antibodies is being inves-

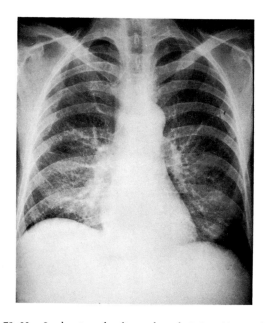

Fig. 73–22. Leukemia and miliary tuberculosis in a 63-year-old patient with chronic leukemia who developed diffuse bilateral infiltration. Needle aspiration of the lung revealed *Mycobacterium tuberculosis.* Prompt response to chemotherapy was obtained.

tigated intensively and may extend the value of BAL. As much as 500 cc of lavage fluid may be used to irrigate a segmental bronchus. We feel that this is excessive and recommend a maximum of 200 cc. The contents of millions of alveoli may be sampled by this method. Critically ill patients may need ventilatory support. Complications of BAL are few, although severely hypoxic patients may not tolerate the procedure.

Transbronchial lung biopsy—TBLB—is best performed with fluoroscopic control. This assures that the biopsy forceps is in a peripheral location and away from main vessels. However, with this technique only 25 to 50 alveoli are sampled with each bite. According to Carter (1987), this method has been helpful mainly in the diagnosis of granulomas, neoplasms, and PCP, as well as some other infectious processes. The small sample size does not lend itself to a definitive diagnosis or staging of the interstitial pneumonias. The same limitations may hold true for pneumoconioses, hypersensitivity reactions, vasculitides and the like. Complications of TBLB include hemorrhage and pneumothorax. Coagulopathy is a contraindication to its use.

Transthoracic fine-needle aspiration may diagnose confluent infiltrates, especially in a search for pathogens such as fungi, Pneumocystis and Legionella. It is of no value in the interstitial pneumonias. Cutting or large-needle biopsy improves the diagnostic yield but the complication rate is excessive. Lung biopsy with the aid of the thoracoscope may be valuable. Thoracoscopy is becoming popular once again and has been helpful in our hands when there is evidence of pleural involvement by the process. A diagnostic thoracotomy may be carried out at the same sitting if frozen sections obtained with the thoracoscopic biopsy forceps are negative. Boutin and associates (1982) had impressive results and recommended this as a definitive initial diagnositic procedure in diffuse lung disease.

Prescalene lymph node biopsy has been the mainstay in our diagnosis of sarcoidosis. If the disease is clinically and roentgenographically suspect, even in the absence of palpable nodes, we perform a right prescalene lymph node biopsy under local anesthesia in an outpatient facility. The yield has been almost 100%. Of course, cultures of nodal tissues for fungus and tuberculosis are taken. Palpable supraclavicular nodes should be biopsied in all cases if the diagnosis has not been obtained by simpler means.

Mediastinoscopy should be undertaken only if the expected yield is high, as evidenced by enlarged mediastinal nodes on plain films or on CT scanning. Some prefer mediastinoscopy over scalene node biopsy for the confirmation of suspected sarcoidosis. Anterior mediastinotomy or the Chamberlain procedure has the advantage that a simultaneous lung biopsy can be obtained by entering the pleural cavity. Both procedures require general anesthesia. Complications include hemorrhage and recurrent nerve or phrenic nerve injury.

Open lung biopsy provides the highest diagnostic yield. Its advantages include large specimen size, choice of affected areas by direct vision, and accurate hemosta-

sis. Small, muscle-sparing incisions can be made in the axilla or anteriorly with low morbidity. In chronic processes, Gaensler and Carrington (1980) showed a mortality of only 0.3%. Despite wide variation in the reported mortality in acutely ill patients requiring open lung biopsy, significant morbidity in this group of patients is the rule. Specimens should include active disease with "normal" adjacent lung and avoid "burned-out" areas. Thus, the activity of the alveolitis or other processes can be assessed accurately. Any appropriate area of lung may be chosen. We have not avoided the middle lobe or the lingula as often suggested. Wetstein (1986) showed concordance between biopsies from the lingula and other sites in acute cases. Proper handling of the specimens is crucial. If possible, the pathologist should be informed of the contemplated procedure and the specimen divided under sterile conditions on a side table in the operating room and submitted to the various laboratories. If one suspects lipoid pneumonia, a portion of the specimen should be saved for frozen section analysis because the usual fixation methods dissolve lipid. In an acutely ill patient, frozen section and immediate examination in the appropriate bacteriologic setting should be carried out. Frozen section should be performed even in elective biopsies to assure that an area with appropriate pathology has been biopsied.

The patient's clinical course should determine the tempo of the evaluation. In chronic cases that remain undiagnosed after a careful clinical examination, biopsy is indicated. Biopsy is not indicated in cases of obvious end-stage honeycomb lung or when a change in therapy is unlikely, except for legal reasons. Transbronchial biopsy is generally performed first and may be sufficient in sarcoidosis, granulomatous diseases, neoplasm, and some infections, but is generally inadequate in cases of less specific histology such as idiopathic pulmonary fibrosis and the pneumoconioses. Serial bronchoalveolar lavage may help in following activity and response to treatment, but its role in initial diagnosis has not been established. Open lung biopsy should be performed if bronchoscopic studies are nonspecific.

The difficulty of clinical decision-making is compounded in acute cases, especially those involving suspected infections in immunocompromised patients. Despite the high yield of combined TBLB and BAL in this setting, up to 10% of cases remain undiagnosed. Coagulopathy, mechanical ventilation, and hypoxemia may preclude TBLB and BAL. In other cases, clinical deterioration occurs despite appropriate treatment for a documented infection. Open lung biopsy should be considered in such patients, although there is controversy regarding its benefit. Pass and associates (1986) reported that open lung biopsy led to therapeutic changes in many of their AIDS patients. Fitzgerald and colleagues (1987) found that open lung biopsy was useful when bronchoscopy was contraindicated or nondiagnostic but not when deterioration occurred during treatment for proven infection. Potter and associates (1985) showed no significant differences in mortality comparing open lung biopsy and empiric antibiotics in cancer patients. Rossiter and co-workers (1979) likewise found no difference in mortality rates comparing patients with and without a specific diagnosis after OLB. On the other hand, although the finding of a noninfectious process such as Kaposi's sarcoma or lymphoma may not alter outcome, it may permit more reasonable decisions by physicians, patient and family. If LIP becomes more common in AIDS victims, open lung biopsy will be indicated more often because the response to steroids may be excellent.

TREATMENT

A complete discussion of therapy for the diffuse lung diseases is beyond the scope of this chapter. Certain general rules apply. If an etiologic agent such as a drug, fume, or dust is identified, it should be removed. Infections are treated with specific antimicrobials, including antiviral agents if indicated. Steroids may be helpful in patients with active alveolitis from any cause as well as those with collagen vascular disease, lymphocytic infiltrations, progressive sarcoidosis, histiocytosis X, and eosinophilic pneumonia. Chemotherapy is indicated for neoplastic infiltrates if palliation is likely. Antimetabolites may have a role in treating Wegener's granulomatosis and some vasculitides. In extensive fibrosis, supportive care is all that can be offered.

REFERENCES

Bergin, C.J., and Müller, N.L.: CT of interstitial lung disease: a diagnostic approach. Am. J. Radiol. 148:9, 1987.

Boutin, C., et al.: Thoracoscopic lung biopsy. Experimental and clinical preliminary study. Chest 82:44, 1982.

Burke, C.M., et al.: Post-transplant obliterative bronchiolitis and other late sequelae in human heart-lung transplantation. Chest 86:824, 1984.

Carrington, C.B., et al.: Chronic eosinophilic pneumonia. N. Engl. J. Med. 280:786, 1969.

Carrington, C.B., and Liebow, A.A.: Limited forms of angiitis and granulomatosis of the Wegener's type. Am. J. Med. 41:497, 1966.

Carrington, C.B., et al.: Lymphangioleiomyomatosis: physiologic-pathologic-radiographic correlation. Am. Rev. Respir. Dis. 116:977, 1977.

Carrington, C.B., et al.: Natural history and treated course of usual and desquamative interstitial pneumonia. N. Engl. J. Med. 298:801, 1978.

Carter, Darryl. M.D.: Personal communication.

Chastre, J., et al.: Pulmonary fibrosis following pneumonia due to acute Legionnaires' disease. Chest 91:57, 1987.

Cordes, L.G., et al.: Legionellosis. Med. Clin. North Am. 64:529, 1980.

Daniele, R.P., et al.: Bronchoalveolar lavage: role in pathogenesis, diagnosis, and management of interstitial lung disease. Ann. Intern. Med. 102:93, 1985.

Dreisen, R.B., et al.: Circulating immune complexes in the idiopathic interstitial pneumonias. N. Engl. J. Med. 298:353, 1978.

Emanuel, D.A., et al.: Farmer's lung: clinical, pathologic, and immunologic study of 24 patients. Am. J. Med. 37:392, 1964.

Epler, G.R., et al.: Normal chest roentgenograms in chronic diffuse infiltrative lung disease. N. Engl. J. Med. 298:934, 1978.

Epler, G.R., et al.: Bronchiolitis obliterans organizing pneumonia. N. Engl. J. Med. 312:152, 1985.

Felson, B.: The roentgen diagnosis of disseminated pulmonary alveolar diseases. Semin. Roentgenol. 2:3, 1967.

Fishman, A.P.: UIP, DIP, and all that (Editorial). N. Engl. J. Med. 298:843, 1978.

Fitzgerald, W., et al.: The role of open lung biopsy in patients with the acquired immunodeficiency syndrome. Chest 91:659, 1987.

Fraser, R.B., and Paré, J.A.P.: Diagnosis of Diseases of the Chest. Philadelphia, W.B. Saunders Co., 1977.

Fulmer, J.D.: Interstitial lung diseases. Clin. Chest. Med. 3:457, 1982.

Gaensler, E.A., and Carrington, C.B.: Open biopsy for chronic diffuse infiltrative lung disease: clinical, roentgenographic, and physiologic correlations in 502 patients. Ann. Thorac. Surg. 30:411, 1980.

Gaensler, E.A., Goff, A.M., and Prowse, C.M.: Desquamative interstitial pneumonia. N. Engl. J. Med. 274:113, 1966.

Gaensler, E.A., Moister, V.B., and Hamm, J.: Open-lung biopsy in diffuse pulmonary disease. N. Engl. J. Med. 270:1319, 1964.

Garay, S.M., et al.: Pulmonary manifestations of Kaposi's sarcoma. Chest 91:39, 1987.

Gell, P.G.H., and Coombs, R.R.A.: Clinical Aspects of Immunology. Oxford, Blackwell Scientific Publications, 1968.

Hamman, L., and Rich, A.R: Fulminating diffuse interstitial fibrosis of the lungs. Trans. Am. Clin. Climatol. Assoc. 51:154, 1935.

Handwerger, S., et al.: Tuberculosis and acquired immune deficiency syndrome at a New York hospital: 1978–1985. Chest 91:176, 1987.

Hapke, E.J., Seal, R.M.E., and Thomas, G.O.: Farmer's lung: clinical, radiographic, functional, and serologic correlation of acute and chronic stages. Thorax 23:451, 1968.

Hardy, H.L.: Beryllium disease: a continuing diagnostic problem. Am. J. Med. Sci. 242:150, 1961.

Herbert, A., et al.: Lymphocytic interstitial pneumonia identified as lymphoma of mucosa associated lymphoid tissue. J. Pathol. 146:129, 1985.

Kennedy, J.L., et al.: Pulmonary lymphomas and other pulmonary lymphoid lesions: a clinicopathologic and immunologic study of 64 patients. Cancer 56:539, 1985.

Liebow, A.A.: New concepts and entities in pulmonary diseases. In The Lung. Edited by A.A. Liebow and D.E. Smith. Baltimore, Williams & Wilkins, 1968.

Liebow, A.A., and Carrington, C.B.: The eosinophilic pneumonias. Medicine 48:251, 1969a.

Liebow, A.A., and Carrington, C.B.: The interstitial pneumonias. In Frontiers of Pulmonary Radiology. Edited by M. Simon, E.J. Potchen, and J. LeMay. New York, Grune & Stratton, 1969b.

Liebow, A.A., Steer, A., and Billingsley, J.G.: Desquamative interstitial pneumonia. Am. J. Med. 39:369, 1965.

Light, R.W.: Pleural Diseases. Philadelphia, Lea & Febiger, 1983.

Lurie, H.I., and Duma, R.J.: Opportunistic infections of the lungs. Hum. Pathol. 1:233, 1970.

Morris, J.M., et al.: Lymphocytic interstitial pneumonia in patients at risk for the acquired immune deficiency syndrome. Chest 91:63, 1987.

Oleske, J., et al.: Immune deficiency syndrome in children. JAMA 249:2345, 1985.

Pass, H.I., et al.: Indications for and diagnostic efficacy of open-lung biopsy in the patient with acquired immunodeficiency syndrome (AIDS). Ann. Thorac. Surg. 41:307, 1986.

Patchefsky, A.S., et al.: Desquamative interstitial pneumonia: relationship to interstitial fibrosis. Thorax 28:680, 1973.

Pepys, J., et al.: Farmer's lung: thermophilic actinomycetes as a source of "farmer's lung hay" antigen. Lancet 2:607, 1963.

Polsky, B., et al.: Bacterial pneumonia in patients with the acquired immunodeficiency syndrome. Ann. Intern. Med. 104:38, 1986.

Potter, D., et al.: Prospective randomized study of open lung biopsy versus empirical antibiotic therapy for acute pneumonitis in nonneutropenic cancer patients. Ann. Thorac. Surg. 40:422, 1985.

Raeburn, C., and Spencer, H.: Study on origin and development of lung cancer. Thorax 8:1, 1953.

Ralph, D.D., et al.: Rapidly progressive airflow obstruction in marrow transplant recipients. Am. Rev. Respir. Dis. 129:641, 1984.

Ramaswamy, G., Jagadha, V., and Tchertkoff, V.: Diffuse alveolar damage and interstitial fibrosis in acquired immune deficiency syndrome patients without concurrent pulmonary infection. Arch. Pathol. Lab. Med. 109:408, 1985.

Reynolds, H.Y.: Hypersensitivity pneumonitis. Clin. Chest Med. 3:503, 1982.

Rosen, S.H., Castleman, B., and Liebow, A.A.: Pulmonary alveolar proteinosis. N. Engl. J. Med. 258:1123, 1958.

Rossiter, S.J., et al.: Open lung biopsy in the immunosuppressed patient. J. Thorac. Cardiovasc. Surg. *77*:338, 1979.

Scadding, J.G., and Hinson, K.F.W.: Diffuse fibrosing alveolitis (diffuse interstitial fibrosis of the lungs). Thorax *22*:291, 1967.

Schatz, M., Patterson, R., and Fink, J.: Immunologic lung disease. N. Engl. J. Med. *300*:1310, 1979.

Shelhamer, J.H., et al.: Persistence of *Pneumocystis carinii* in lung tissue of AIDS patients treated for Pneumocystis pneumonia. Am. Rev. Respir. Dis. *130*:1161, 1984.

Stover, D.E., et al.: Bronchoalveolar lavage in the diagnosis of diffuse pulmonary infiltrates in the immunosuppressed host. Ann. Intern. Med. *101*:1, 1984.

Tubbs, R.R., et al.: Desquamative interstitial pneumonitis. Chest *72*:159, 1977.

Weibel, E.R.: Airways and respiratory surface. *In* The Lung. Edited by A.A. Liebow and D.E. Smith. Baltimore, Williams & Wilkins, 1968.

Wetstein, L.: Sensitivity and specificity of lingular segmental biopsies of the lung. Chest *90*:383, 1986.

Zunger, A., et al.: Cryptococcal disease in patients with acquired immune deficiency syndrome: diagnostic features and outcome. Ann. Intern. Med. *104*:234, 1986.

CHAPTER 74

LUNG TRANSPLANTATION

G. Alexander Patterson and Joel D. Cooper

Active surgical interest in organ transplantation developed in the 1950s, following Medawar's (1944) establishment of the immunologic basis of allograft rejection. Metras (1950) in France and Hardin and Kittle (1954) in the U.S. demonstrated the feasibility of canine lung transplantation. Hardy and associates (1963) reported the first human lung transplant. The patient survived for 18 days, demonstrating not only the technical feasibility of the operation in humans but also the capability of the transplanted lung to function. This short-lived success stimulated worldwide interest in transplantation.

During the 1970s and 1980s, organ transplantation developed rapidly with the repeated demonstration of long-term clinical success with transplantation of kidney, heart, and liver. Success with lung transplantation, however, lagged far behind. In the twenty years following Hardy's (1963) initial attempt, approximately 40 lung or lobe transplants were performed worldwide without restoration of any patient to normal health for a significant period of time. Only one recipient was actually discharged from the hospital, a 23-year-old patient of Derom and co-workers' (1971) who underwent right-lung transplantation for advanced silicosis. The patient was discharged from hospital 8 months following transplantation but died a short while later with chronic rejection, sepsis, and bronchial stenosis. Most recipients succumbed within 2 weeks of transplantation, usually from primary respiratory failure, sepsis, or rejection. Of the first 38 transplants performed, only 9 patients survived more than 2 weeks and 6 of these died in the first month from bronchial anastomotic disruption. This was also the outcome of our initial attempt at lung transplantation reported by Nelems and associates (1980), when in 1978, a young ventilator-dependent victim of inhalation burns died of bronchial anastomotic disruption 3 weeks after right-lung transplantation.

After this experience, we began a laboratory program to evaluate factors affecting bronchial anastomotic healing following lung transplantation. The initial experiments involved canine lung autotransplantation. In these experiments, animals were randomized to a treatment group receiving standard immunosuppression consisting of azathioprine and prednisone or to a control group receiving no immunosuppression. The treated animals demonstrated significant bronchial complications similar to those following clinical lung transplantation. Lima and our associates (1981) reported that these included ischemia, necrosis, and disruption of the bronchial anastomosis.

It was subsequently shown that this adverse effect on bronchial healing was caused entirely by the prednisone and that azathioprine did not prejudice satisfactory healing of bronchial anastomoses. Goldberg and colleagues (1983) reported further studies that demonstrated that cyclosporine did not have any negative impact on bronchial anastomotic healing.

Another major factor in adverse bronchial anastomotic healing is ischemia of the donor bronchus. The bronchial artery circulation is not reconstituted at the time of lung transplantation, leaving the donor bronchus completely devoid of native arterial circulation. We postulated that a pedicled flap of abdominal omentum wrapped around the anastomosis would not only buttress the suture line in case of partial disruption, but also would aid in the development of a collateral circulation to the donor bronchus and improve healing. In a series of canine experiments, Morgan (1983) and Dubois (1984) and their colleagues in our laboratory demonstrated that this bronchial omentopexy did in fact improve bronchial healing and promoted rapid restoration of bronchial circulation through collateral vessels from the omentum.

CLINICAL LUNG TRANSPLANTATION

Following this laboratory success, we embarked on a limited program of clinical lung transplantation. The Toronto Lung Transplant Group's (1985) initial attempt was in a victim of paraquat poisoning with hepatic, renal, and respiratory failure requiring mechanical ventilation as well as membrane oxygenator support. A right lung transplant initially functioned well but after several days sustained damage from high levels of residual circulating paraquat. A subsequent left lung transplantation was performed with restoration of satisfactory pulmonary gas exchange, but the patient died 10 weeks following initial lung transplantation, having never recovered renal function.

Selection of Recipients

On reviewing the world experience with lung transplantation, we concluded that poor recipient selection significantly contributed to the unfavorable outcome, as with our paraquat victim. We decided to employ at least initially strict criteria for recipient selection in the hopes of improving the outcome (see Table 74–1). Patients with bilateral pulmonary sepsis seemed ill suited for unilateral lung transplantation because the remaining infected lung would not only contaminate the transplanted lung but would serve as a focus for systemic infection following institution of immunosuppression. In emphysema, unilateral lung transplantation might result in hyperexpansion of the contralateral native lung, with mediastinal shift and crowding of the transplanted lung. We have, to date, excluded ventilator-dependent patients from consideration, as such individuals usually have airway sepsis, multisystem failure, and in general insufficient stamina to permit rapid recovery and cessation of ventilatory assistance early in the postoperative period.

We therefore concluded that patients with end-stage fibrotic lung disease represented ideal candidates for single lung transplantation. The restrictive airway disease and increased vascular resistance in the native lung would lead to preferential ventilation and perfusion of the transplanted lung, thereby avoiding a ventilation-perfusion imbalance or any significant degree of wasted ventilation.

Unfortunately, patients with end-stage pulmonary fibrosis are at one time or other frequently treated with high dose prednisone in an attempt to retard the progression of the disease. Because of the negative impact of corticosteroids on bronchial anastomotic healing, we require all transplant recipients to be weaned from prednisone entirely for at least 1 month before transplantation. In most of these end-stage patients, little if any active inflammation remains and cessation of corticosteroid therapy can usually be accomplished without adverse effect.

We have attempted to identify recipients who are

Table 74–1. Criteria for Lung Transplantation, Toronto Lung Transplant Program

Measurable deterioration in pulmonary function

Expected survival of less than 18 months

Absence of
    Other organ failure
    Psychosocial derangement
    History of malignancy
    Steroid medication

Capable of participation in preoperative pulmonary rehabilitation program

Age: less than 60 years

likely to die of their pulmonary disease within a period of 12 to 18 months without a transplant. Such patients are oxygen-dependent and demonstrate a marked fall in oxygen saturation with exercise. They usually have had an increasing requirement for oxygen administration during the preceding 12 months. In addition, all of these patients have had progressive, measurable deterioration in pulmonary function. These patients have some degree of pulmonary hypertension, but this is usually moderate so cor pulmonale is not present. Right ventricular function is evaluated noninvasively using echocardiography and gated nuclear angiography to compute the first-pass right ventricular ejection fraction.

Patients with end-stage pulmonary fibrosis generally have excellent respiratory muscle strength because of the chronic workload of ventilating low compliance, fibrotic lungs. Suitable transplant candidates must be judged capable of participating in a graded preoperative exercise rehabilitation program. Marked improvement in exercise tolerance is usually achieved during this period of preoperative rehabilitation. Prospective recipients with significant psychosocial problems are excluded because of the considerable stress that the preoperative assessment, long waiting, and postoperative recovery impose. Furthermore, the need for strict patient compliance and co-operation is essential to ensure a satisfactory long-term result. Table 74–1 outlines the general criteria for recipient selection.

Donor Selection

The lack of suitable donors is currently the major obstacle to more widespread application of lung transplantation. Only a fraction of organ donors have lungs that remain suitable for lung transplantation. We require that the donor chest roentgenogram be entirely clear and that the arterial oxygen tension exceed 300 mm Hg when 100% oxygen is administered, with 5 cm positive end-expiratory pressure. We also require that bronchoscopy reveal no purulent secretions. Donor and recipient must be matched for ABO compatibility, but prospective histocompatibility matching has not been used.

Lung Preservation

To minimize ischemic injury to the lung, we initially used only donors whose families would permit transfer of the donor to our hospital so that removal of the lung and its subsequent transplantation were carried out in adjacent operating rooms. With increasing experience, we have abandoned this policy, and at present, most donor lungs are excised elsewhere and transported to our hospital for implantation.

After excision from the heparinized donor, the lung graft is immersed in Eurocollins solution at 4°C. Using this simple technique we have satisfactory results with ischemic periods up to 4 hours. To date, we have not used the technique reported by Hakim and associates (1987) of flushing with cold electrolyte solution that is routinely used for heart-lung transplants at other centers. We also have no experience with use of vasodilator agents given to improve the efficacy of pulmonary artery flush which Hakim (1987), Jurmann (1986) and Hachida (1986) and their colleagues reported. We expect that flush techniques that are superior to simple immersion and that will extend the period of safe ischemia up to 12 hours or longer will be developed. Handa and associates (1987) reported limited success with such a technique in animals.

Size Matching

For purposes of size matching, the vertical and transverse roentgenologic dimensions of the chest are used. The transverse diameter is measured at the level of the apex of the diaphragm and the vertical measurement on each side from the apex of the chest to the diaphragm. As donor lateral films are usually not available, one must rely on portable anteroposterior films in most situations, and exact comparison with the intended recipient is often difficult. Body weight, height, and chest circumference are also used in an attempt to assess the suitability of the match. Originally we selected a donor lung of approximately the same size as the recipient chest. With experience, however, we realized that an oversized donor lung was not only satisfactory but actually desirable. With pulmonary fibrosis, the recipient's chest is contracted because of the nature of the disease process. Insertion of a larger lung allows restoration of a more normal chest configuration and provides better lung function. The combination of the recipient chest with a larger donor lung is facilitated if the left side is used for transplantation, as the left diaphragm descends more readily than the right and the mediastinum shifts easily towards the right (Fig. 74–1).

Operative Procedure

Choice of Side

We have performed lung transplantation on either side, but in general prefer the left for several technical reasons: (1) It is generally easier to clamp the left atrium proximal to the pulmonary veins and obtain a large atrial cuff on the left side. On the right side, the pulmonary veins enter the left atrium near the interatrial groove. (2) For this same reason, separate extraction of the donor heart for cardiac transplantation is easier if the donor's left lung is to be used for lung transplant, because on the left, larger atrial cuffs can be preserved on the heart and lung grafts. (3) The recipient bronchus is longer on the left, making the bronchial anastomosis somewhat easier. (4) For the aforementioned reasons, an oversized donor lung may be more easily accommodated on the left than on the right.

If the recipient has had a major thoracotomy on the left side, we favor a right-lung transplant.

Donor Preparation

At the present time, as Todd and we (1988) reported, most donor lungs are extracted in conjunction with separate cardiac extraction. To facilitate such coordination and to minimize the delay of the cardiac team, the heart is removed initially, leaving behind a small cuff of left atrium attached to the donor lung. Immediately following inflow occlusion and cardioplegic arrest, the cardiac extraction is performed in situ. The superior and inferior venae cavae and the ascending aorta are divided, as is the common pulmonary artery just proximal to its bifurcation. This leaves the base of the heart attached only by the left atrium. Careful incision of the left atrium is then carried out to leave an adequate left atrial cuff on both the heart and the lung side of the division. Separate excision of the heart requires only a few minutes more than ordinarily required for routine cardiac extraction. Following the cardiac removal, the trachea is divided at its midpoint with the distal end stapled. The two lungs are extracted en bloc and immersed in a bag containing 4°C Eurocollins solution. This bag is then placed on ice for transportation. Just before implantation, the donor lung is trimmed from the specimen, dividing the donor bronchus two rings proximal to the upper lobe takeoff and the ipsilateral pulmonary artery at its origin. We leave large flaps of pericardium attached to the hilum of the donor lung as one route for systemic revascularization of the bronchial circulation.

Anesthesia

Before induction of anesthesia, a Swan-Ganz thermal-dilution catheter is inserted into the recipient and positioned into the pulmonary artery of the lung opposite the one to be transplanted. This position is verified by chest roentgenogram. An arterial line permits continuous blood pressure monitoring and frequent arterial blood gas analysis. Pulse oximetry and continuous end tidal CO_2 monitoring are also employed. Endotracheal intubation is achieved using a technique that allows for unilateral lung ventilation. For patients undergoing a left lung transplant, a left bronchial blocker—Fogarty No. 14 Fr. venous occlusion catheter*—is inserted temporarily into the distal trachea, after which a standard single-lumen endotracheal tube is inserted. A flexible bronchoscope is then inserted through the endotracheal tube, and under direct vision, the tip of the bronchial blocker is positioned into the proximal left main bronchus, about 2 cm distal to the carina. The balloon is inflated with 5 to 7 cc of air to verify complete occlusion of the left main bronchus, after which the balloon is deflated and the bronchoscope removed. For patients undergoing right lung transplant, a left double-lumen endotracheal tube is inserted and the appropriate position verified by clinical assessment and fiber-optic bronchoscopy.

Technique

After anesthetic induction and intubation, the patient is maintained in a supine position. The abdomen and groin on the side of the proposed transplant are prepped and draped. A small upper midline incision is made and the greater omentum is withdrawn through the wound. It is usually necessary to dissect the omentum from the transverse colon to provide adequate mobilization. Additional omental length can be obtained if necessary by

---

*Model #62-080-8, American Hospital Supply

dividing the right or left vascular arcade. A tunnel is made immediately behind the xyphisternum by blunt dissection. This tunnel is enlarged to several finger breadths and the leading edge of the omentum is placed into the tunnel before abdominal wound closure. This portion of the procedure generally requires 15 to 20 minutes.

During this time, the anesthetist performs a thorough assessment of hemodynamics and gas exchange while ventilating both lungs. The lung to be transplanted is then collapsed by inflation of the bronchial blocker and hemodynamic and gas exchange measurements repeated after approximately 15 minutes. At this point, a preliminary decision is made about whether the patient can likely be managed without cardiopulmonary bypass during replacement of the lung. If bypass is thought likely to be required, the femoral vessels on the side of the proposed thoracotomy are exposed and prepared at this time. Otherwise, no groin dissection is performed, but the groin area is always draped in the field when preparing for the thoracotomy, should the need for intraoperative extracorporeal support arise.

When the abdomen has been closed, the patient is suitably positioned for a posterolateral thoracotomy. The chest, abdomen, and ipsilateral groin are prepped and draped in the field. A thoracotomy is made through the bed of the resected fifth rib and any adhesions between the lung and chest wall, diaphragm, or mediastinum are divided using electrocautery, rather than blunt or sharp dissection, as much as possible. The pulmonary veins are isolated outside the pericardium and the proximal pulmonary artery is encircled within the pericardium. On the left side, this dissection is facilitated by division of the ligamentum arteriosum. On the right, division of the azygous vein and elevation of the vena cava assures adequate exposure of the right main pulmonary artery.

During this mobilization, the lung is collapsed, if tolerated, to facilitate dissection. Intolerance of single-lung ventilation is an indication that extracorporeal bypass may be required. A vascular clamp is then temporarily placed on the proximal pulmonary artery and the artery is completely occluded. If this maneuver produces hemodynamic instability or deterioration of gas exchange, the clamp is removed and the femoral vessels prepared for cardiopulmonary bypass. The main bronchus is encircled just above the upper lobe takeoff, with special care not to dissect tissue from around the recipient bronchus proximal to the point of proposed division.

If the previous temporary occlusion of the pulmonary artery was well tolerated, the pulmonary artery is again clamped proximally in preparation for lung extraction. If the previous trial occlusion was not well tolerated, partial venoarterial bypass is instituted before the pulmonary artery is reclamped. The first branch to the upper lobe is isolated and divided between ligatures. The pulmonary artery is subsequently divided just distal to this point, providing additional length for the anastomosis as well as a somewhat smaller caliber lumen to reduce the usual discrepancy between a large recipient pulmonary artery and a normal donor pulmonary artery.

The two pulmonary veins are then ligated outside the pericardium and the veins are divided peripheral to these ligatures. The pulmonary artery is divided transversely just beyond the ligated first branch, and the bronchus is divided transversely immediately proximal to the upper lobe bronchus. After removal of the recipient lung, the pericardium is opened circumferentially around the stumps of the pulmonary veins and a large atrial clamp is placed as centrally as possible on the left atrium without impinging on the contralateral pulmonary veins. On the right side, it may be necessary to dissect into the interatrial groove to mobilize enough left atrium to allow satisfactory proximal placement of the atrial clamp. After hemodynamic stability has been ensured, the previously placed ligatures on the pulmonary veins are removed and the cleft of atrium between the pulmonary veins is divided to create a large left atrial cuff. This cuff is then fashioned to match the size of the donor atrial cuff.

Lung Implantation

When hemostasis has been achieved, the previously prepared deflated donor lung is positioned posteriorly in the chest. The atrial anastomosis is performed first. The posterior wall of the atrial anastomosis is performed from the front using a continuous 3-0 polypropylene suture. The front wall of the atrial anastomosis is similarly performed without need to reposition the lung. The donor and recipient pulmonary arteries are then trimmed as necessary, and proper orientation is accomplished. The previously ligated first branch of the recipient pulmonary artery is of assistance in ensuring proper orientation. The posterior wall of the pulmonary artery anastomosis is then performed with continuous 5-0 polypropylene suture. The anterior wall is constructed but left untied to allow subsequent back bleeding through the anastomosis.

The bronchial anastomosis is performed with interrupted 4-0 Vicryl sutures with knots placed on the exterior of the bronchus as much as possible. Following completion of the bronchial anastomosis, the left atrial clamp is released, permitting back bleeding through the untied pulmonary artery suture line. This back bleeding should occur within several minutes and is sometimes aided by gentle inflation of the lung. With appropriate back bleeding accomplished, or after several minutes if no back bleeding is apparent, the pulmonary artery clamp is released to flush the pulmonary artery. The suture line is then secured and the clamp is removed from the pulmonary artery.

The mediastinal pleura is then opened just above the diaphragm anteriorly and the omentum withdrawn from its retrosternal position. The omentum is brought inferior and then posterior to the hilum of the lung. The apex is passed anterior to the bronchial anastomosis between the bronchus and the pulmonary artery, wrapped around the bronchus, and secured to itself. This creates a broad blanket of omentum completely encircling the anastomosis and separating it from the atrium and pulmonary artery suture lines. The omentum is secured in this position with several interrupted sutures (Fig. 74–1).

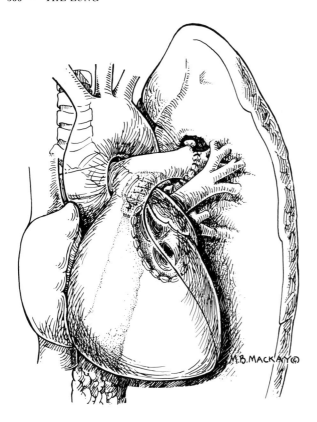

Fig. 74–1. A completed left lung transplantation. After completion of the left atrial anastomosis, a left main pulmonary artery anastomosis is constructed immediately distal to the first branch of the recipient left main pulmonary artery. The bronchial anastomosis is then completed and circumferentially wrapped with omentum.

The free edge of the donor pericardium is then loosely attached to the omentum as a route for collateral circulation from the omentum, through the donor pericardium to the bronchial circulation at the hilum of the lung. Two chest tubes are placed and the chest is closed in a standard fashion. The bronchial anastomosis is checked bronchoscopically and any secretions aspirated. The average blood requirement for this procedure has been one unit. We and our associates (1987) reported this technique of single-lung transplantation. The completed implantation is shown in Fig. 74–1.

Use of Extracorporeal Bypass

If contralateral ventilation or temporary clamping of the proximal pulmonary artery before excision of the diseased lung indicates the need for extracorporeal support, partial venoarterial bypass is instituted through the femoral vessels. This is begun after the lung has been completely mobilized and continues until circulation is restored to the transplanted lung. Extracorporeal bypass has been required in four of fifteen single-lung transplants performed in our center.

Results

The Toronto Lung Transplant Group (1986, 1988) reported fifteen patients with end-stage pulmonary fibrosis who have undergone single-lung transplantation in our center. Two patients underwent right lung transplant and 13 underwent left lung transplant. There have been four postoperative deaths, two related to poor donor selection, one caused by viral pneumonia, and one caused by an accidental venous air embolism on the tenth postoperative day. Of the eleven survivors, two subsequently died, one from chronic rejection at 6 months, and one from B cell lymphoma at eight months. Seven patients have survived more than 1 year, the patient with the longest survival was alive and well more than 4 years following transplantation (Figs. 74–2, 74–3).

Bronchial Healing

No patient has died from complications of bronchial anastomotic healing. Of the 11 long-term survivors, 9 had normal bronchial healing. Two patients developed partial necrosis of the donor bronchus just distal to the anastomosis. Both patients required repeated pulse doses of steroids in the early postoperative period because of rejection. Neither individual developed a bronchovascular or bronchopleural fistula, presumably because of the protection afforded by the encircling omental wrap (Fig. 74–4). Both individuals required repeated bronchial dilatation and were ultimately treated by endoscopic insertion of a short silicone rubber stent into the left main bronchus. This has remained in place for 1 year in one case, and 3 years in the other, without further difficulty.

DOUBLE-LUNG TRANSPLANTATION

Patient Selection

Patients with chronic bilateral pulmonary sepsis such as cystic fibrosis or bronchiectasis, or patients with emphysema, are not suitable candidates for single-lung transplantation, for reasons previously noted. We were impressed by the early results Reitz and colleagues (1982) obtained with combined heart-lung transplantation at Stanford for patients with pulmonary hypertension and cor pulmonale. A few patients with bilateral septic disease and emphysema have also undergone combined heart-lung transplant at several centers, including our own.

Significant problems, however, are associated with combined heart-lung transplantation, including a severe lack of suitable donor grafts for this procedure. With the proliferation of successful cardiac transplant programs around the world, most available donor hearts are employed for isolated cardiac transplantation. This is not surprising, given the excellent results of cardiac transplantation compared with those generally observed with heart-lung recipients, as Dawkins (1985) and Griffith (1987) and their colleagues reported. This markedly limits the number of donors for those patients awaiting combined heart-lung transplantation. A definite advantage of isolated lung transplantation, whether single or double, is the feasibility of employing heart and lung grafts of the same donor for use in two recipients.

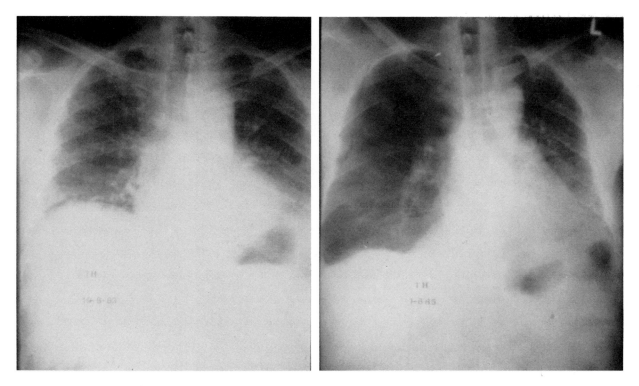

Fig. 74–2. Preoperative (*A*) and 21-months postoperative (*B*) chest films from a patient who underwent right lung transplantation. Note that, by mediastinal shift and depression of the ipsilateral diaphragm, a much larger donor lung can be implanted in such patients with restrictive lung disease.

It was initially thought that pulmonary rejection could be monitored by simple transvenous endomyocardial biopsy. Griffith and associates (1985) recognized that pulmonary and cardiac rejection can occur asynchronously. Combined heart-lung transplantation, therefore, does not offer any advantage over isolated lung transplantation with respect to postoperative rejection monitoring.

We also recognized that combined heart-lung transplantation was not ideal for recipients with adequate or recoverable right ventricular function. The recipient must give up his own heart unnecessarily. The recipient must accept transplantation of two major organ systems,

each of which is associated with its own problems, including rejection of one independent of the other. Dawkins and co-workers (1985) reported development of advanced coronary sclerosis after several years in recipients of heart and heart-lung transplants. The donor heart would be best used in an individual requiring heart transplantation without prejudicing the use of the lungs for the recipient with pulmonary disease.

The concept of simultaneous en bloc bilateral pulmonary transplantation is not new and was demonstrated in dogs by Vanderhoeft and associates (1972). Dark and we and associates (1986) developed a model of en bloc

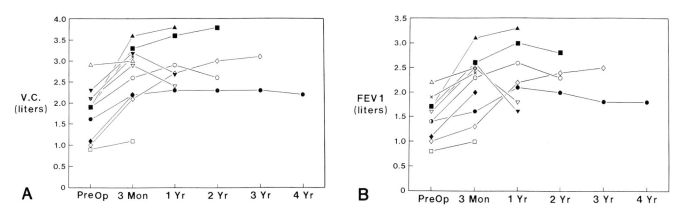

Fig. 74–3. Vital capacity (*A*) and 1-second forced expired volume (*B*) in nine patients after single lung transplantation. Marked increases in volumes and flow rates were observed in all patients.

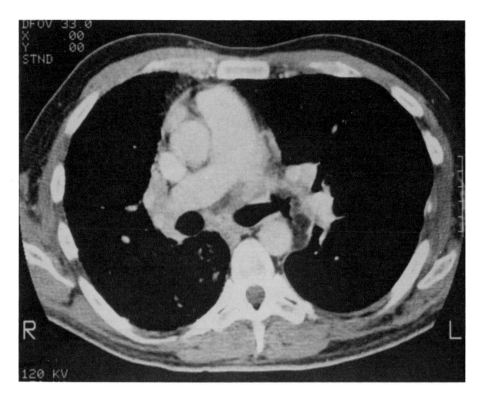

Fig. 74–4. Computerized tomogram of a patient with bronchial anastomotic disruption after single lung transplantation. The extrabronchial mediastinal cavity is contained by the omentum, which is readily apparent in this figure. This disruption granulated over a course of 1 month, and the patient was left with a residual fibrous stricture that has been managed by transbronchoscopic insertion of a Silastic stent.

double-lung transplantation that preserves the recipient heart, and we (1988a,b) obtained experimental and clinical success with this procedure.

Technique of Double-Lung Transplantation

Donor Procedure

The donor extraction was outlined in the previous section. When cardiac extraction is performed in anticipation of preparation of a double-lung graft, great care must be taken to preserve an adequate atrial cuff around the pulmonary veins, particularly on the right side. The donor graft consists of both lungs attached by the trachea and main bronchi, the pulmonary artery and both its branches, and an atrial cuff containing the orifices of all four pulmonary veins (Fig. 74–5).

Recipient Procedure

Monitoring lines are inserted as for a single-lung transplantation. The patient is then anesthetized and a single-lumen endotracheal tube inserted. A median sternotomy is performed with extension of the incision into the epigastrium. Through the inferior end of this incision, the omentum is mobilized in a length adequate to reach up into the posterior mediastinum. A small transverse incision is made in the diaphragm several centimeters anterior to the esophageal hiatus for better passage of the omentum into the posterior mediastinum.

The superior and inferior venae cavae, the ascending aorta, the main pulmonary artery, and the trachea are encircled before institution of cardiopulmonary bypass. The patient is then heparinized and cardiopulmonary

bypass instituted using double venous and ascending aortic cannulation. The temperature is maintained above 30°C to prevent fibrillation of the heart.

All four pulmonary veins are stapled inside the pericardium. Both pulmonary arteries are stapled, the right inside the pericardium between the vena cava and aorta and the left outside the pericardium and the hilum of the lung so as to minimize the likelihood of injury to the recurrent laryngeal nerve.

At this point, both lungs are excised, dividing the pulmonary ligaments and hilar structures using electrocautery. The excision is carried out lateral to the previously placed vascular staple lines. The main bronchus on each side is isolated and divided between two staple lines, so as to prevent contamination of the field.

Through the right pleural space, the right main bronchus is then grasped firmly and retracted inferiorly and to the right. The bronchus is then carefully dissected from the mediastinal structures using electrocautery. This dissection is carried down the left main bronchus to completely free up that structure as well. The dissection is continued so as to completely mobilize both main bronchi and the distalmost portion of the trachea. Care is taken not to extend the dissection proximally more than one ring above the carina, so as not to devascularize the recipient trachea.

At this point, the heart is lifted gently upwards and to the right to expose the left atrium. The pulmonary veins on both sides are separated from the pericardium from within the pericardium. The small defects thereby created in the pericardium are enlarged to create a pleural pericardial window through which the donor lungs

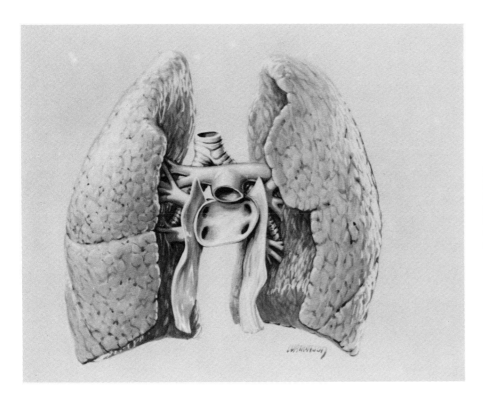

Fig. 74–5. A double lung graft with both lungs attached by a cuff of left atrium containing all pulmonary vein orifices, main pulmonary artery, and short segment of supracarinal trachea. Note the large pericardial flaps, which are left attached to the donor specimen.

will be passed into the respective pleural spaces. On the left this incision in the pericardium runs from the diaphragm to the pulmonary artery behind the phrenic nerve. On the right the window runs behind the venae cavae and right atrium from the diaphragm to a point superior to the right pulmonary artery.

The omentum is now brought up through the opening previously created in the diaphragm, behind the heart and up to the level of the recipient's distal trachea.

The donor specimen is then introduced into the field. A long clamp is inserted from the superior mediastinum between the aorta and vena cava down behind the heart but in front of the omentum. The trachea is then drawn up posterior to the heart to lie in the visceral—central—portion of the mediastinum. The lungs are placed in the respective pleural cavities through the previously created pleural pericardial windows. The donor and recipient trachea are each divided 1 to 2 rings above their respective carinae. An end-to-end tracheal anastomosis is constructed immediately proximal to the donor carina using a running suture on the posterior wall and interrupted Vicryl sutures on the anterior wall. The omentum is wrapped completely around the tracheal anastomosis and secured in that position. Bronchoscopic assessment of the tracheal anastomosis is then made. The lungs are gently inflated.

The aorta is then cross-clamped and 1 L of cold cardioplegia administered via the aortic root to arrest the heart. The heart is then lifted upward and to the right to expose the back of the left atrium. The left inferior pulmonary vein stump is amputated and this atriotomy elongated inferolaterally towards the right inferior pulmonary vein and supralaterally toward the atrial appendage. Care is taken in making this incision to stay well away from the coronary sinus. The donor atrial cuff is then sewn to this atriotomy using a running suture of 3-0 polypropylene (Fig. 74–6). The donor and recipient main pulmonary arteries are then aligned and cut to suitable size and length. An end-to-end anastomosis is made. The suture line is left open so that adequate air removal from the right side of the heart can be achieved through this anastomosis (Fig. 74–7).

During the pulmonary artery anastomosis, the patient is rewarmed. The air is removed from the heart through the right atrial ventricular vent and the pulmonary artery anastomosis, as well as through the left atrial appendage, the apex of the left ventricle, and the cardioplegia catheter. Once circulation has been re-established, the donor pericardial flaps are brought inside the recipient pericardium and secured in that position to re-create a cradle for the heart. Atrial and ventricular pacing wires are inserted and both pleural spaces and the mediastinum drained by separate tubes. The sternum is closed in the usual manner. We and co-workers (1988b) described the technical details of this procedure.

Results

We have performed 11 double-lung transplants in patients ranging from 17 to 43 years of age. Five patients had emphysema, 4 because of α-1 antitrypsin deficiency. One patient had bronchiolitis obliterans. Another patient had end-stage eosinophilic granuloma. Two patients had chronic bronchiectasis, and one patient had cystic fibrosis. One patient had primary pulmonary hypertension. All patients were judged by nuclear angiography and echocardiography to have adequate or recoverable right

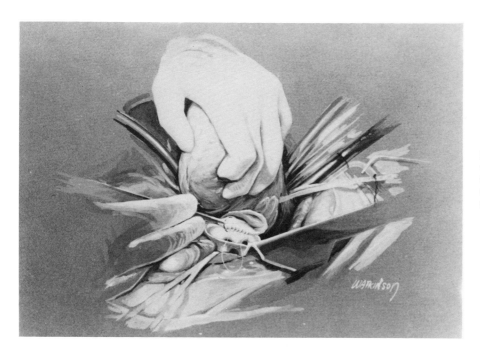

Fig. 74–6. Retraction of the heart upward and to the right provides excellent exposure for creation of the recipient atriotomy and performance of the left atrial anastomosis.

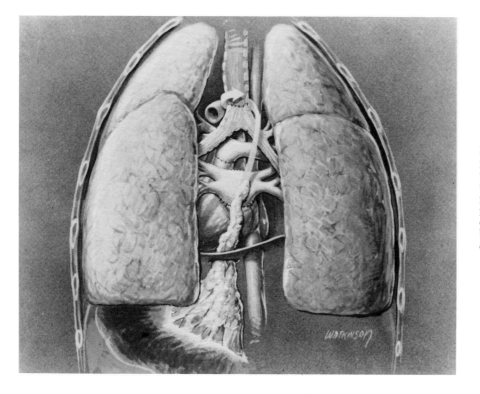

Fig. 74–7. A posterior view of the completed left lung implantation showing the tracheal left atrial and main pulmonary artery anastomosis. The omentum is depicted drawn through a defect in the diaphragm immediately anterior to the esophageal hiatus. The omentum is passed behind the heart and wrapped circumferentially around the tracheal anastomosis.

heart function. The one operative death resulted from tracheal and main bronchial necrosis. The other seven patients survived and returned to normal levels of activity without oxygen supplementation (Figs. 74–8, 74–9).

Two postoperative hemorrhages required reexploration, but airway complications have been the most significant long-term problem in the management of these patients. It was apparent from the outset that airway complications might occur. The additional length of ischemic donor airway in a double-lung graft increased the possibility of airway necrosis. Ladowski and colleagues (1984) reported, however, that a collateral circulation permits retrograde flow from the pulmonary artery to bronchial artery circulation. We anticipated that this collateral flow alone would not provide adequate circulation to the donor trachea and proximal main bronchi. For this reason, we employed a tracheal anastomotic omentopexy as we have done in single-lung transplantation, to establish antegrade bronchial flow through collateral circulation at the suture line. This supplements the retrograde bronchial artery flow originating from the pulmonary circulation. Nonetheless, one patient developed a fatal airway necrosis. One other patient developed a late left main bronchial and tracheal anastomotic stricture that persisted despite repeated dilatations. Another patient developed a local area of necrosis involving the membranous trachea and a short segment of the right

lateral wall (Fig. 74–10). This patient developed local stricture, which also has required repeated bronchoscopic dilatation. Silastic endobronchial stents placed in both of these patients allowed them a perfectly normal level of activity without symptoms.

Two of these patients with airway necrosis had significant systemic hypotension during the immediate postoperative period, which may have decreased perfusion pressure within the pulmonary circulation as well as reducing retrograde circulation from pulmonary artery to bronchial artery circulation.

IMMUNOSUPPRESSION

All patients receive a single dose of cyclosporine A— 5 mg/kg, and intravenous azathioprine—1.5 mg/kg—immediately before transplantation. The early postoperative immunosuppression consists of oral cyclosporine, 10 mg/kg/day in divided doses. Doses are adjusted to achieve plasma cyclosporine trough levels of 150 to 200 ng/ml. Azathioprine 1.5 mg/kg/day, and Minnesota antilymphocyte globulin—MAG—10 to 15 mg/kg/day are given intravenously. As adequate levels of cyclosporine are observed with oral administration, the MAG is discontinued. When bronchoscopic assessment reveals satisfactory bronchial anastomotic healing—usually within 2 to 3 weeks, prednisone 0.5 mg/kg/day is begun. This

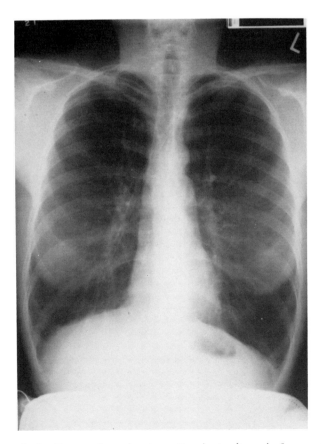 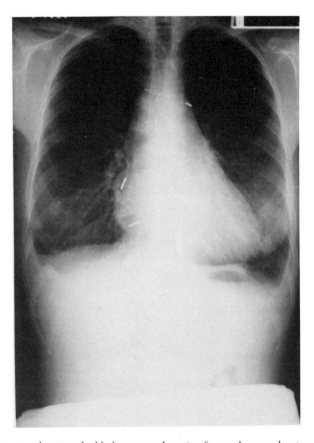

Fig. 74–8. Preoperative and postoperative chest radiographs from a patient undergoing double lung transplantation for emphysema due to α-1 antitrypsin deficiency. The diaphragm and intercostal spaces return to a normal configuration within days after double lung transplant.

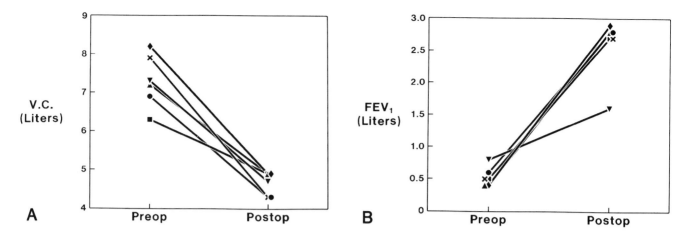

Fig. 74–9. Vital capacity (A) and 1-second forced expired volume (B) in six patients undergoing double lung transplantation for obstructive lung disease. Note the marked decrease in vital capacity and increase in flow rate in all patients.

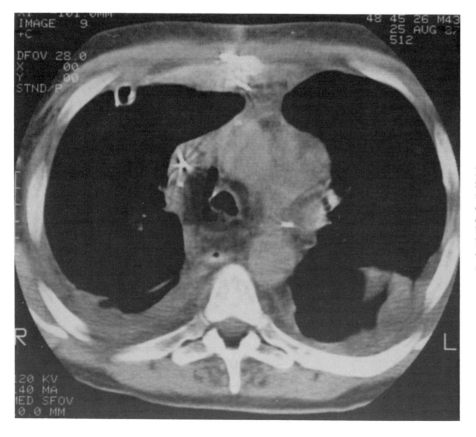

Fig. 74–10. Computerized tomogram from a patient following the double lung transplantation. Note the mediastinal air cavity to the right of the trachea: the trachea and cavity are completely surrounded by omentum. The tracheal defect healed by granulation, leaving a chronic stricture, which has been treated by transbroncho-scopic placement of a Silastic stent.

dosage is then gradually reduced over the ensuing several months with most patients receiving approximately 15 mg of prednisone on alternate days. Double-lung transplant recipients have remained on higher doses of prednisone in an attempt to prevent the development of bronchiolitis obliterans, a complication that, as Burke and associates (1987) reported, appears to be a manifestation of chronic rejection. Though this complication has frequently been reported by Burke and colleagues (1984) and others in heart-lung recipients, we have not experienced this complication in any of our single- or double-lung recipients to date.

REJECTION

Rejection remains a major problem of clinical lung transplantation. The diagnosis is imprecise and is made on clinical grounds. Typically, the patient experiences a low grade pyrexia, leukocytosis, an increased alveolar arterial oxygen gradient, a perihilar flare on the chest roentgenogram and a general feeling of malaise accompanied by modest dyspnea. This constellation of clinical findings cannot accurately differentiate rejection from pulmonary infection, or, on occasion, from pulmonary edema. We have found quantitative perfusion scanning valuable in the diagnosis of rejection following single-lung transplantation. Graph perfusion progressively increases during the first month postoperatively. During rejection episodes, perfusion to the transplanted lung decreases significantly relative to baseline values. Rejection cannot be accurately determined by quantitative perfusion scanning following double-lung or heart-lung transplantation, because both lungs are equally affected by rejection.

The most reliable diagnostic test for rejection is the patient's clinical response to an intravenous bolus of methylprednisolone. In general, acute rejection episodes are markedly reversed within hours of this treatment. With a clinical diagnosis of rejection so confirmed, patients receive two more successive daily intravenous bolus doses of methylprednisolone 5 to 10 mg/kg.

PROBLEMS IN CLINICAL LUNG TRANSPLANTATION

Rejection

A more reliable way to obtain a clinical diagnosis of rejection must be found so the patient can be treated specifically for rejection episodes rather than being treated for rejection, infection, and fluid overload, all at the same time. Higenbottam and colleagues (1987) reported that the Papworth group has had encouraging results using systematic multiple transbronchial biopsy for heart-lung recipients. Griffith (1987) and Paradis (1988) and their associates noted that bronchoalveolar lavage has been used to advantage by the Pittsburgh group. We do not have extensive experience with this modality during the early postoperative period in pa-

tients with a suspected rejection episode. More sensitive and specific noninvasive modalities are required.

Donor Availability

The supply of donor lungs is severely limited. If all suitable local donors were made available, the supply would be significantly augmented, but this goal is difficult to achieve. Therefore, improved methods of preservation that would permit long-distance procurement are essential. Adequate preservation for periods of up to 5 to 6 hours is not difficult and has been achieved with relatively simple techniques, but truly reliable procurement times of 12 to 24 hours are not feasible at present. Hakim (1987), Jurmann (1986) and Hachida (1986) and colleagues, as well as others, have described many interesting techniques and pharmacologic agents to enhance preservation, but no safe, consistent means of preserving lungs for more than 4 to 6 hours has yet been demonstrated.

Airway Anastomotic Healing

This remains a major clinical problem. It appears to be a more frequent and troublesome problem following double-lung transplantation, but we have experienced some difficulty even in single-lung transplantation, as Griffith and associates (1987) have following heart-lung transplantation. Several potential solutions could be considered. The most obvious ones are to augment the bronchial artery circulation directly or to decrease the length of ischemic donor airway. The former solution could be achieved by direct reconnection of the bronchial circulation at the time of transplantation. This would prove technically difficult, although likely not impossible.

Alternatively, the donor airway could be shortened. This would be feasible in double-lung transplantation by performing two bronchial anastomoses rather than a single tracheal anastomosis. This would be technically feasible, but would expose the patient to the risk of two airway anastomoses rather than a single tracheal anastomosis. As we have experienced some complication with bronchial anastomosis following single-lung transplantation, this risk is not negligable.

SUMMARY

Selected patients with terminal lung disease have been managed effectively by lung transplantation. Strict selection criteria for donors and recipients, attention to technical detail, and avoidance of perioperative corticosteroids increase the likelihood of success following pulmonary transplantation. The underlying pulmonary diseases determines the appropriate procedure. At present, we recommend unilateral lung transplantation for patients with end-stage pulmonary fibrosis, double-lung transplantation for patients with obstructive lung disease or bilateral pulmonary sepsis, and combined heart-lung transplantation for patients with the combination of irreversible cardiac and pulmonary disease. Clinical and experimental evidence suggests that the adverse effects of pulmonary hypertension on the right ventricle may be reversible in many cases following restoration of normal pulmonary vascular resistance. For patients with primary pulmonary hypertension, therefore, the application of single- or double-lung transplantation seems promising. Further clinical experience with all three forms of transplantation will be required before a final evaluation of the role, benefits, and long-term results of each is made. Apparently, however, transplantation for end-stage lung disease can produce a degree of success already achieved with other forms of organ transplantation.

REFERENCES

Burke, C.M., et al.: Post-transplant obliterative bronchiolitis and other late lung sequelae in human heart-lung transplant. Chest 86:824, 1984.

Burke, C.M.: Lung immunogenicity rejection and obliterative bronchiolitis. Chest 92:547, 1987.

Cooper, J.D.: Technique of successful lung transplantation in humans. J. Thorac. Cardiovasc. Surg. 93:173, 1987.

Dark, J.H.: Experimental en-bloc double-lung transplantation. Ann. Thorac. Surg. 42:394, 1986.

Dawkins, K.D., et al.: Long-term results, hemodynamics, and complications after combined heart-lung transplantation. Circulation 71:919, 1985.

Derom, F., et al.: Ten-month survival after lung homotransplantation in man. J. Thorac. Cardiovasc. Surg. 61:835, 1971.

Dubois, P., Choiniere, L., and Cooper, J.D.: Bronchial omentopexy in canine lung allotransplantation. Ann. Thorac. Surg. 38:211, 1984.

Goldberg, M., et al.: A comparison between cyclosporin A and methylprednisolone plus azathioprine on bronchial healing following canine lung allotransplantation. J. Thorac. Cardiovasc. Surg. 85:821, 1983.

Griffith, B.P., et al.: Asynchronous rejection of heart and lungs following cardiopulmonary transplantation. Ann. Thorac. Surg. 40:488, 1985.

Griffith, B.P., et al.: Heart-lung transplantation: lessons learned and future hopes. Ann. Thorac. Surg. 43:6, 1987.

Hachida, M., et al.: Efficacy of verapamil in prolonging ischemic time for lung preservation. Surg. Forum 37:331, 1986.

Hakim, M., et al.: Distant procurement and preservation of heart-lung homografts. Transplantation Proceedings 19:3535, 1987.

Handa, M., et al.: 48-hour simple hypothermic preservation of the canine lung transplant: study of buffer action of the modified extracellular perfusate. ISHOKU. Jap. J. Transpl. 21:288, 1987.

Hardin, C.A., and Kittle, C.F.: Experience with transplantation of the lung. Science 119:97, 1954.

Hardy, J.D.: Lung homotransplantation in man. JAMA 186:1065, 1963.

Higenbottam, T., et al.: The diagnosis of lung rejection and opportunistic infection by transbronchial lung biopsy. Transplant. Proc. 19:3777, 1987.

Jurmann, M.J., et al.: Prostacycline as an additive to single crystalloid flush: improved pulmonary preservation in heart-lung transplantation. J. Heart. Trans. 5:384, 1986.

Ladowski, J.S., Hardesty, R.L., and Griffith, B.P.: The pulmonary artery blood supply to the supracarinal trachea. Heart Trans. 4:40, 1984.

Lima, O., et al.: Effects of methylprednisolone and azathioprine on bronchial healing following lung autotransplantation. J. Thorac. Cardiovasc. Surg. 82:211, 1981.

Medawar, P.B.: The behaviour and fate of skin autografts and skin homografts in rabbits. J. Anat. 78:176, 1944.

Metras, H.: Note preliminaire sur la graffe totale du poumon chez le chien. Fr. Acad. Sci. 1176, 1950.

Morgan, W.E., et al.: Improved bronchial healing in canine left lung reimplantation using omental pedicle wrap. J. Thorac. Cardiovasc. Surg. 85:139, 1983.

Nelems, J.M., et al.: Human lung transplantation. Chest 78:569, 1980.

Paradis, I.L., et al.: Immunologic risk factors for human chronic lung rejection. Am. Rev. Respir. Dis. 137(4S):46, 1988.

Patterson, G.A., et al.: Experimental and clinical double-lung transplantation. J. Thorac. Cardiovasc. Surg. 95:70, 1988a.

Patterson, G.A., et al.: Technique of successful clinical double-lung transplantation. Ann. Thorac. Surg. 45:626, 1988b.

Reitz, D.A., et al.: Heart-lung transplantation: successful therapy for patients with pulmonary vascular disease. N. Engl. J. Med. 306:557, 1982.

Todd, T.R., et al.: Separate extraction of cardiac and pulmonary grafts from a single organ donor. Ann. Thorac. Surg. (in press).

Toronto Lung Transplant Group: Sequential bilateral lung transplantation for paraquat poisoning. J. Thorac. Cardiovasc. Surg. 89:734, 1985.

Toronto Lung Transplant Group: Unilateral lung transplantation for pulmonary fibrosis. N. Engl. J. Med. 314:1140, 1986.

Toronto Lung Transplant Group: Experience with single-lung transplantation for pulmonary fibrosis. JAMA 259:2258, 1988.

Vanderhoeft, P., et al.: Bloc allotransplantation of both lungs with pulmonary trunk and left atrium in dogs. Thorax 27:415, 1972.

CHAPTER 75

BRONCHIAL ADENOMA

Robert J. Ginsberg, H. Shennib, and Donald L. Paulson

The term "adenoma," originally used by Mueller in 1882, is a misnomer. These tumors are an interesting group of low grade malignant neoplasms arising from the epithelium, ducts, and glands of the tracheobronchial tree. These lesions account for approximately 0.5 to 1% of all bronchial tumors and no more than 1 or 2% of all bronchial tumors undergoing surgical resection. Included in this group are: carcinoid tumor, adenoid cystic carcinoma, mucoepidermoid tumor, bronchial mucous gland adenoma, and rarely a mixed tumor of salivary gland type.

CLINICAL FEATURES

The carcinoid tumor is by far the most frequent and accounts for 85 to 90% of all bronchial "adenomas" seen; most of the rest are adenoid cystic carcinomas—cylindroma. In our (D.L.P. and R.J.G.) (1971) series reported in the first edition of this book, of 71 patients with these tumors, 61 had carcinoid tumors, 9 had adenoid cystic carcinomas, and 1 had a mucoepidermoid tumor. The patients' ages ranged from 14 to 71 years with a mean age of 48 years. Although in our series the tumors occurred in women almost twice as often as in men, in the literature the sex ratio is about equal.

SIGNS AND SYMPTOMS

The symptoms and physical findings associated with bronchial adenoma depend on the location of the tumor—central or peripheral. The peripheral tumors are most often asymptomatic, presenting as solitary pulmonary nodules on roentgenographic studies of the chest (Fig. 75–1). The proximally located tumors grow partially or wholly within a bronchus. Partial or complete endobronchial obstruction and its sequelae, as well as the vascularity of the tumor, account for the symptoms. Cough, hemoptysis, and recurrent infection constitute the classic triad of symptoms (Table 75–1).

Because of the small size and slow growth of these tumors, symptoms may persist for many years before the

Table 75–1. Signs and Symptoms of Bronchial Adenoma in 71 Patients

	No. of Patients	%
Cough	33	47
Recurrent infection	32	45
Hemoptysis	27	39
Pain	14	19
Wheeze	12	17
Asymptomatic	15	21

underlying cause is discovered. A history of wheezing or recurrent infection dating back many years is common (Fig. 75–2). One of our patients had recurrent hemoptysis for 40 years before diagnosis and treatment of a bronchial adenoma. These tumors frequently masquerade clinically as bronchial asthma, chronic bronchitis, or bronchiectasis, particularly if the tumor produces incomplete obstruction and is located in the trachea or proximal portions of the bronchial tree.

Incomplete obstruction leads to cough, wheezing, or recurrent distal infection with its sequelae. On occasion, a unilateral hyperlucent segment, lobe, or lung is identified on the chest roentgenogram because of a ball-valve mechanism. Complete obstruction may result in obstructive pneumonitis with pain, fever, and dyspnea. Bronchiectasis or chronic lung abscesses are found in patients with long-standing undiagnosed tumors, eventually resulting in total destruction of lung tissue distal to the obstruction (Fig. 75–3).

Stridor can be the presenting symptom in tracheal or main stem bronchial tumors. Adenoid cystic carcinomas (Fig. 75–4). often present this way because these tumors are most frequently found in the lower trachea or main stem bronchi. Occasionally, this high airway obstruction becomes life-threatening.

Recurrent hemoptysis, another frequent symptom, results from ulceration of the mucosa overlying the tumor or simply from chronic inflammation distally. This is most commonly seen in carcinoid tumors and, in women, has

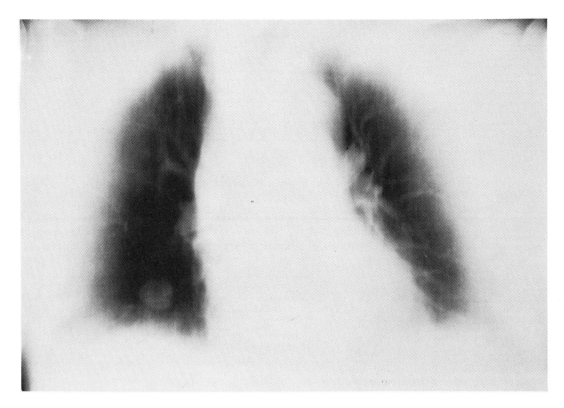

Fig. 75–1. Tomogram of an asymptomatic peripheral carcinoid adenoma.

been noted to be accentuated during times of menstrual flow.

The carcinoid syndrome occurs infrequently and exclusively in patients with large primary tumors or extensive hepatic metastases.

DIAGNOSIS

No single investigative modality is sufficient to diagnose the presence of a bronchial adenoma in all patients, but by various radiographic techniques and bronchoscopy, most tumors can be located and correctly identified. Fine-needle aspiration biopsy of peripheral lesions can be accurate, but histologic examination of tumor tissue is the only completely reliable means of diagnosis.

Roentgenographic Studies

Standard roentgenograms of the chest may reveal a tumor mass or changes in pulmonary parenchyma caused by tracheobronchial obstruction. In approximately one fourth of our patients—19 of 71—a routine roentgenogram of the chest showed no abnormality (Fig. 75–5A). Tomograms may detect an otherwise undetectable central lesion and may delineate an endobronchial component of the tumor not readily apparent on routine studies. Computed tomography can further delineate the endobronchial and parenchymal component of the tumor (Fig. 75–5B), although this is an unessential examination in the investigation of most patients. In the past, bronchography was used frequently to outline the endobronchial obstruction and to demonstrate irreversible bronchiectasis in the bronchial tree distally. With current, more sophisticated techniques such as computed tomography, this examination is now rarely indicated.

None of these radiologic techniques accurately differentiates these tumors from other benign and malignant neoplasms, although one may suspect their nature by the roentgenographic appearance.

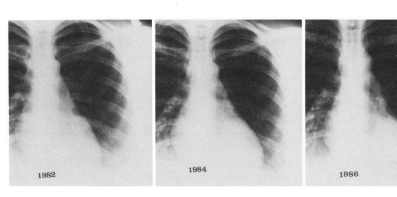

Fig. 75–2. Serial roentgenograms of a retrocardiac bronchial adenoma demonstrating slow growth over a 4-year period.

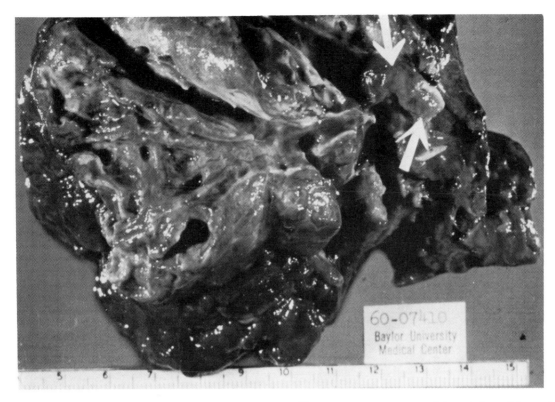

Fig. 75–3. Gross specimen of a typical polypoid bronchial carcinoid resected by superior segmentectomy of the right lower lobe, wedge resection of the bronchus intermedius, and bronchoplasty. Note the bronchiectasis and abscesses distally.

Bronchoscopy

Except in the presence of a peripheral nodule, bronchoscopy should be successful in identifying all tumors situated within and proximal to the segmental orifices. Approximately 75% of all carcinoid tumors and virtually all adenoid cystic carcinomas are visible endoscopically.

Accurate identification of the tumors requires bronchial biopsy. Wilkins (1963) and Donahue (1968) and their associates, among others, have written about massive bleeding following biopsies of carcinoid tumors. Indeed, these vascular tumors do tend to bleed, but almost all severe postbronchoscopic hemorrhages result from attempts at partial or complete removal of the tumor by this means. Care must be taken in performing such biopsies. These tumors present submucosally and do require deeper biopsies than other malignant bronchial neoplasms require. We and Rozenman and associates (1987) continue to perform bronchoscopic biopsies of these tumors, using a dilute epinephrine solution for vasoconstriction before and after biopsy. Some authors recommend general anesthesia and rigid bronchoscopy for airway control, in case uncontrollable hemorrhage occurs during fiber-optic bronchoscopic examination. Adenoid cystic and mucoepidermoid tumors are not highly vascular and do not tend to bleed.

Transbronchoscopic fine-needle aspiration biopsy of the submucosal tumor for cytologic examination may help in diagnosing carcinoid tumors when biopsy is unwarranted or unhelpful.

Frozen-section examination of the biopsy material may be misleading. Because of their similarity to small cell carcinoma, carcinoid tumors have occasionally been misdiagnosed by this technique, but examination of permanent hematoxylin and eosin preparations usually leads to an accurate diagnosis, although unfortunately mistaken diagnoses—especially atypical carcinoids versus small cell carcinoma—have been made by this method as well.

Nodal Staging

Preoperative nodal staging by mediastinoscopy has little value in typical carcinoid tumors or adenoid cystic carcinomas unless mediastinal involvement is suspected, but it may be useful, especially when atypical carcinoid tumors or high grade mucoepidermoid carcinomas are present.

Biochemical Studies

Unless the carcinoid syndrome is suspected, screening patients with suspected bronchial carcinoids for serotonin and its breakdown products—5-hydroxyindoleacetic acid—in blood or urine has limited value.

CARCINOID TUMORS

Pathology

Carcinoid tumors constitute 80 to 90% of all bronchial adenomas. Experimental evidence has suggested that

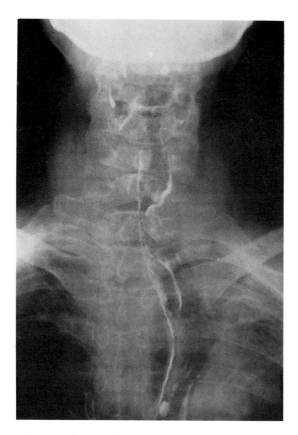

Fig. 75–4. Tracheogram demonstrating the high airway obstruction of an adenoid cystic carcinoma of the upper trachea.

these tumors arise from stem cells of the bronchial epithelium rather than from APUD—amine precursor uptake of amino acid decarboxylase—cells that migrated from the neural crest. Gould and associates' (1983) review of the histogenesis and differentiation of bronchial carcinoids and their proposed relationship with other pulmonary tumors with neuroendocrine features is excellent.

Typical Carcinoid

Most of these tumors are situated centrally; 20% are located in the main stem bronchi, approximately 60% in the lobar and segmental bronchi, and another 20% are located peripherally (Table 75–2). Carcinoid tumors infrequently involve the carina or trachea and, rarely, multiple or multicentric tumors are discovered in one patient.

Bronchoscopically they appear as highly vascularized pink to purplish soft tumors, covered by intact epithelium (Fig. 75–6). Large areas of ulceration are rare. A few tumors are polypoid with a definite stalk, but most are sessile. Because the bulk of the tumor is usually extraluminal, they have been called iceberg tumors. They penetrate the bronchial wall and may extend into the pulmonary parenchyma and peribronchial lymph nodes.

Microscopically, the tumor consists of uniform round to polygonal cells with small oval nuclei and finely gran-

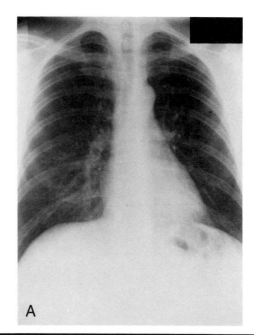

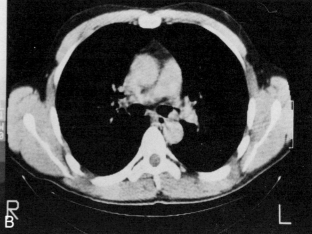

Fig. 75–5. *A,* A chest roentgenogram called "normal." There is an endobronchial carcinoid in the distal left main stem bronchus. *B,* An endobronchial carcinoid of the left main stem bronchus demonstrated by computed tomography. Note the minimal involvement of the bronchial wall.

Table 75–2. Location of Tumor in 61 Carcinoid Tumors

	Right	Left
Main bronchus	4	5
Upper lobe bronchi	4	2
Bronchus intermedius	12	—
Middle lobe bronchus	2	—
Lower lobe bronchi	11	8
Peripheral	9	4
Total	42	19

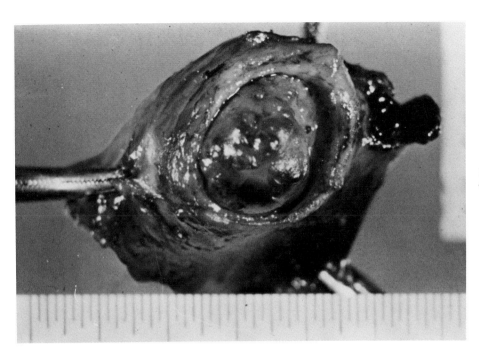

Fig. 75–6. "Bronchoscopic" view of a carcinoid adenoma.

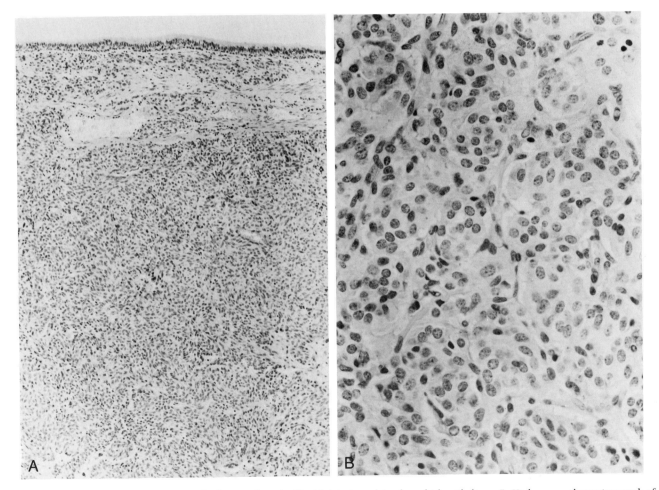

Fig. 75–7. *A*, Low power photomicrograph of a typical carcinoid with intact overlying bronchial epithelium. *B*, High power photomicrograph of a typical carcinoid tumor comprised of nests of regular polygonal cells separated by a network of capillary vessels reflecting the vascularity of the tumor.

ular chromatin. The cytoplasm is abundant and eosinophilic. Mitosis is infrequent. The cells may be spindle-shaped, particularly in peripherally located tumors. The cells are arranged in small clusters or interlacing cords, or both, separated by highly vascular connective tissue (Fig. 75–7). The stroma may show osseous metaplasia, which may be secondary to necrosis within the tumor or necrosis of compressed bronchial cartilage with secondary ossification (Fig. 75–8). This may be reflected by calcification seen by computed tomography. The overlying bronchial epithelium may undergo squamous metaplasia, but frank ulceration or invasion by tumor is rare. As Bertelsen and colleagues (1985) noted, only 10 to 15% of "typical" carcinoid tumors present with lymph node metastases.

Ultrastructurally, Bensch and associates (1965) described that these tumors consist of closely packed cells with small but well formed desmosomes and numerous neurosecretory granules. The size, shape, and density of the neurosecretory granules (Fig. 75–9) are heterogeneous.

Atypical Carcinoids

This group of carcinoid tumors, which displays both malignant histologic features and aggressive behavior, was described by Englebreth-Holm (1944–1945) and Von Albertini (1951) but most accurately by Arrigoni and associates (1972). Warren and colleagues (1985) referred to these tumors as "well differentiated neuroendocrine car-

cinomas." In contrast to typical carcinoids, more than 50% of these tumors are located peripherally, and 50 to 70% of cases present with lymph node or distant metastases. In some instances it is difficult to differentiate an atypical carcinoid from a small cell anaplastic carcinoma.

Histologically, while retaining a "carcinoid-like" pattern, they display unmistakable pleomorphism with mitotic activity, nuclear abnormalities, peripheral palisading, and necrosis (Fig. 75–10). In any series, about 10% of carcinoids are "atypical."

Oncocytic Carcinoid

This is a subtype of the typical carcinoid tumor. They are composed of a variable admixture of large eosinophilic oncocytes and cells characteristic of the typical carcinoid.

Tumorlets and Multiple Peripheral Carcinoids

Whitwell (1955) coined the term pulmonary tumorlet to describe isolated foci of atypical hyperplastic bronchial epithelium. Tumorlets were initially regarded as forms of early invasive or in situ small cell carcinoma. They are usually an incidental finding at autopsy or in lungs resected for infection or tumor. Miller and co-workers (1978) described them particularly in patients with restrictive pulmonary disease.

Immunohistochemical staining has demonstrated differences in secretory products between tumorlets and typical carcinoids. Because of the similarity in staining

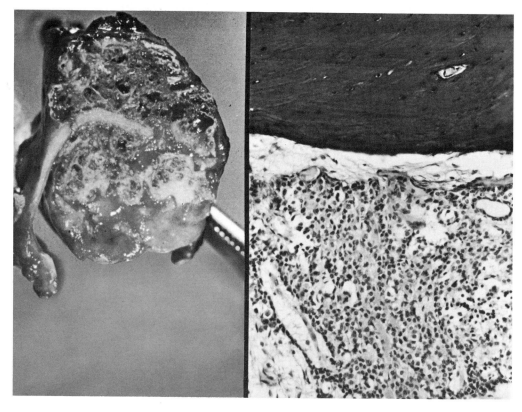

Fig. 75–8. Gross and microscopic appearance of a carcinoid adenoma with osseous metaplasia. Note the large, extrabronchial component of this tumor.

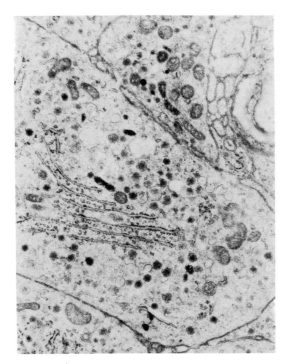

Fig. 75–9. High power electron photomicrograph (×2300) of a carcinoid adenoma reviewing secretion granules, typical of neurosecretory cells. (Reproduced with permission from Toker, C.: Observations on the ultrastructure of a bronchial adenoma (carcinoid-type). Cancer 19:1943, 1966.)

patterns between tumorlets and normal bronchial epithelium, Cutz and associates (1982) suggested that tumorlets are hyperplastic proliferations rather than neoplasms, although D'Agati and Perzin (1985) described one case with peribronchial lymph node metastases.

Carcinoid Syndrome

The carcinoid syndrome is a well defined clinical entity consisting of well described cutaneous, cardiovascular, gastrointestinal, and respiratory manifestations. It was first described in and most commonly occurs with metastatic carcinoid tumors of the gastrointestinal tract, but this syndrome occasionally occurs in association with bronchial carcinoids.

The syndrome occurs in bronchial tumors only when the primary tumor is large or when liver metastases have occurred, often many years after removal of the primary tumor. An interesting phenomenon is the left-sided cardiac valvular abnormalities found in the carcinoid syndrome associated with large primary tumors of the lung, unlike the right-sided valvular lesions found with hepatic metastases.

Carcinoid syndrome is rare in pulmonary tumors, perhaps because bronchial carcinoids reportedly contain less serotonin per gram of tissue than do intestinal carcinoids. Possibly, this reduced level can be attributed to the lung's high content of monoamine oxidase, which can detoxify the serotonin.

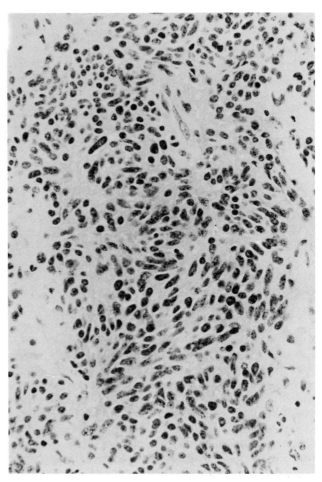

Fig. 75–10. A high power photomicrograph of an atypical carcinoid tumor consisting of ribbons of polygonal cells that show greater pleomorphism and mitotic activity than those seen in a typical carcinoid tumor.

Other Endocrinopathies

Like small cell carcinoma, bronchial carcinoids have also been associated with various other endocrine disorders, including Cushing's syndrome—increased ACTH production; excessive pigmentation—MSH; inappropriate ADH secretion; and hypoglycemia. In addition, the multiple endocrine syndrome—MEA—has been reported in association with these tumors.

Treatment

Unless distant metastatic disease is evident, the principles of treatment of carcinoid tumors include complete removal of the primary lesion with preservation of as much normal lung tissue as possible. Because most of these tumors are only locally invasive, the most conservative resection that allows complete removal of the tumor is indicated wherever possible.

Endoscopic Resection

Endoscopic removal of carcinoid tumors was a frequent mode of treatment before the advent of modern techniques in surgery, anesthesia, and postoperative care, permitting removal of pulmonary tissue with low morbidity and mortality. Because most of these tumors are largely extraluminal, and frequently only a small portion of the tumor is visible and accessible to bronchoscopy, incomplete removal with recurrence was common. The highly vascular connective tissue within the tumor made this mode of therapy fraught with dangers, including exsanguinating hemorrhage. Personne and colleagues (1986) reported the advent of the Nd-YAG laser has reduced the risk of hemorrhage in endoscopic removal of these tumors by photocoagulation. It is not recommended, however, that carcinoids be primarily treated by this technique because local recurrence is inevitable except for the rare occasion when a polypoid tumor, easily accessible, is on a narrow, uninvolved stalk.

Occasionally, when thoracotomy is contraindicated for other reasons, transbronchoscopic removal of the tumor may be warranted to alleviate bronchial obstruction and perhaps to provide long-term asymptomatic management.

Surgical Resectional Therapy

Keeping in mind the locally invasive nature of this tumor, complete removal with preservation of as much normal lung as possible is the goal of treatment. Destroyed, functionless lung tissue distal to the lesion should also be removed. The types of procedures performed in our original series are listed in (Table 75–3).

Surgical staging is a necessary adjunct to any thoracotomy. Biopsies of the lymph nodes located in the bronchopulmonary segment, lobar areas, and hilum should be performed. Frozen-section analysis is required. In those patients who have local metastases, a more extensive cancer operation with lymph node dissection is required, and mediastinal nodes should be sampled and removed if necessary.

Bronchotomy. Bronchotomy and simple wedge excision of the bronchial wall are used on occasion. Polypoid tumors accessible by bronchotomy can thus be removed with the attached bronchial wall. Unfortunately, this simple bronchotomy approach is rarely applicable.

Sleeve Resection. Main stem bronchial tumors or tumors located in the bronchus intermedius occasionally, as Frist and associates (1987) described, can be removed by sleeve resection of the bronchus, preserving all pul-

monary tissue. This is preferable to pneumonectomy or bilobectomy. On occasion, carinal resection is required.

Wedge Resection. This may be appropriate for the occasional small peripheral typical carcinoid tumor.

Segmental Resection. This is the procedure of choice for many tumors arising distal to the origin of the tertiary bronchi. Tumors originating in the orifice of the superior segment of the lower lobes can be treated by segmental resection combined with sleeve resection of the lower lobe bronchus, preserving all basal segments.

Lobectomy. Lobectomy with or without a bronchoplastic procedure is the most common operation because most of these tumors occur in or near the origins of the lobar bronchi. A concomitant sleeve resection of the main stem bronchus is required if the orifice of the lobar bronchus or the adjacent main stem bronchus is involved by tumor. Addition of the bronchoplastic procedure permits preservation of distal normal lung tissue that otherwise would have to be sacrificed and is preferable to pneumonectomy.

Pneumonectomy. This rarely should be used in the treatment of this tumor. Since one of us (D.L.P.) and Shaw (1955) introduced bronchoplastic procedures, few patients have required pneumonectomy. Only in the rare instance of destruction of all lobes by a proximal tumor should pneumonectomy ever be considered.

The margin of the bronchial resection must be examined by frozen section at the time of operation. If microscopic tumor is found at the margin of resection, a more proximal resection is required. Although some surgeons, such as Smith (1969) and McCaughan and colleagues (1985), advocate a complete mediastinal node dissection in all patients because of the possibility of occult microscopic involvement, we prefer nodal staging by frozen section at the time of surgery rather than the more extensive node dissection, unless atypia or nodal involvement is identified at frozen-section analysis.

Radiation Therapy

Bronchial carcinoids are radiation resistant; this modality should never be considered as the primary treatment when surgical resection can be performed. Baldwin and Grimes (1967) and others, however, have reported a few inoperable patients who had a good response to irradiation. Postoperative irradiation has been recommended in atypical carcinoids with lymph node metastases when complete surgical resection has not been accomplished or mediastinal lymph nodes are involved. The benefit of this treatment has not been documented.

Chemotherapy

Combination chemotherapy similar to that used in small cell carcinoma has been effective in managing metastatic carcinoid tumors, although the response rate to this chemotherapy is not as high as that seen in small cell carcinoma. Some authors advocate adjuvant chemotherapy for atypical carcinoids that have demonstrated mediastinal nodal spread at the time of surgery. This is usually recommended in combination with mediastinal radiation therapy.

Table 75–3. Treatment of Carcinoid Adenoma

Types of Procedure	No. of Patients
Pneumonectomy	6
Lobectomy	23
with bronchoplasty	5
Bilobectomy	10
with bronchoplasty	1
Segmentectomy	9
with bronchoplasty	1
Bronchoplasty (no lung removed)	3
Thoracotomy (unresectable)	2
Refused surgery	1
Total	61

The Carcinoid Syndrome

Total removal of large primary tumors associated with the carcinoid syndrome ablates the symptoms of the syndrome. Once hepatic metastases have occurred, the management of the syndrome can become more difficult.

Prognosis

Carcinoid tumors grow slowly, and the natural history is prolonged. We have seen one patient with symptoms of 40 years' duration without treatment and a second patient, who refused surgical treatment, alive and well 20 years later.

Five-year survival rates after resection depend on the aggressiveness of the tumor. Almost all typical carcinoid tumors without lymph node metastases are cured by adequate surgical treatment. One should expect a 90% or greater 5-year survival in this group of patients as Hurt and Bates (1984) and Wilkins (1984), Brandt (1984), Okike (1976), and McCaughan (1985) and their colleagues reported.

Once lymph node metastases have occurred with typical carcinoids, less than 70% of patients survive 5 years disease-free as McCaughan (1985) and Okike (1976) and their associates reported.

Atypical carcinoids, with their frequent incidence of lymph node and distant metastases, have a much lower 5-year survival rate, no greater than 50%. In this latter group of tumors, the role of postoperative adjuvant chemotherapy and irradiation has not been adequately assessed. More aggressive management might result in increased survival.

ADENOID CYSTIC CARCINOMA

This malignant tumor, also called cylindroma, adenocystic basal cell carcinoma, adenomyoepithelioma, and pseudoadenomatous basal cell carcinoma, is a slowly growing malignant lesion similar in most respects to adenoid cystic carcinoma of the major and minor salivary glands. These tumors are much less common than carcinoid tumors, constituting about 10% of all bronchial "adenomas," are much more aggressive, and have a poorer prognosis. As with carcinoid tumors, there is an equal sex incidence and similar age range, the commonest incidence occurring in the fifth decade of life.

Pathology

Unlike carcinoid tumors, adenoid cystic carcinomas occur most frequently in the lower trachea at the level of the carina and the orifices of the main bronchi. Approximately two thirds are located in this area and another one third within the origins of the major bronchi. Rarely are they situated peripherally. Most of the peripheral tumors identified later prove to be metastatic from another primary site.

Although distant metastases tend to occur late in the course of the disease, approximately one third of patients have evidence of metastases at the time of first treatment, commonly along perineural lymphatics, to regional lymph nodes, or distally to liver, bone, and kidneys. Bronchoscopically, the tumor appears as a convex broad-based mass with intact pink epithelium overlying it (Fig. 75–11).

Microscopically, these tumors are identical to those in the salivary glands. The most characteristic pattern is the reticular type, in which strands, columns, and clumps of cells are embedded in a connective tissue stroma. The strands of cells interconnect to enclose cystic spaces (Fig. 75–12). Less common variants include the spindle-cell type, which is composed of parallel arrays of fusiform cells, and the solid type, in which solid masses of cells form either continuous sheets or discrete rounded clumps. The tumor tends to be infiltrative and involve nerves, accounting for the frequent finding of submucosal and perineural spread far beyond the obvious gross tumor (Fig. 75–13). Balazs (1986) described the ultrastructure of these tumors well.

Treatment

Because adenoid cystic carcinomas are of low grade malignancy but are locally invasive, often permeating lymphatics, the aims of curative therapy include a generous en bloc excision of the tumor. Preservation of as much normal lung tissue as possible is another goal of treatment.

If complete excision is impossible, therapy should be aimed at local control of the tumor to relieve airway obstruction.

Endoscopic Excision

Bronchoscopic removal cannot be considered curative therapy but can be used effectively in relieving airway obstruction before definitive surgery or as palliation when surgery is contraindicated because of the extent of the disease.

Laser photocoagulation—Nd-YAG—has proved to be extremely effective to locally ablate the obstructing tumor and has replaced mechanical debridement as the bronchoscopic procedure of choice. Long-term palliation in inoperable cases can be achieved by repeated endoscopic removal of tumor. Frequently, as Personne and associates (1986) described, this is used conjointly with radiation therapy.

Surgical Therapy

A tumor arising in lobar or main stem bronchi can be dealt with by lobectomy, sleeve resection, or a combination of both. Because of the high incidence of perineural lymphatic invasion, submucosal extension, and lymph node metastases, wide local excision, including peribronchial tissue and a hilar node dissection, should be performed. Frozen-section examination of the margins of resection is mandatory.

Lesions occurring in the trachea and carina are challenging surgical problems. Modern techniques of mobilization and reconstruction of the trachea allow up to 8 cm of tracheal length to be excised with end-to-end anastomoses.

Perelman and Koroleva (1987) proposed the following

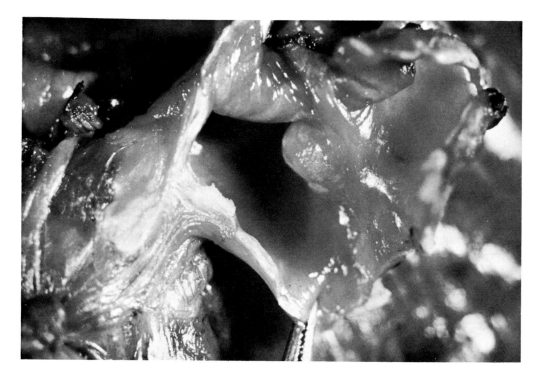

Fig. 75–11. Intraoperative view of the interior of the carina (trachea to left) showing an adenoid cystic carcinoma of the carina after preoperative radiotherapy. The pre- and postoperative tracheograms are shown in Fig. 75–14. (Courtesy of F.G. Pearson).

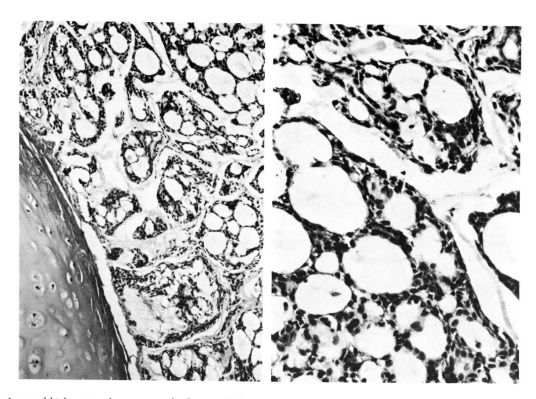

Fig. 75–12. Low and high power photomicrograph of a typical adenoid cystic carcinoma with pseudoacinar pattern.

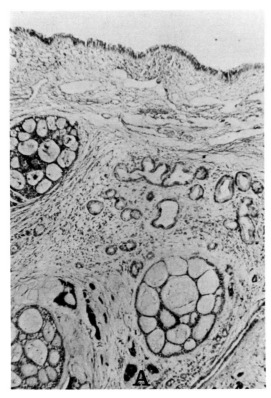
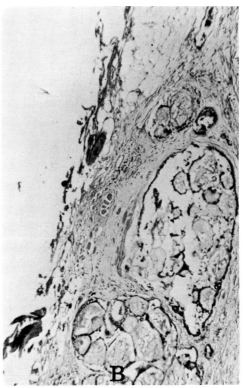

Fig. 75–13. Photomicrographs demonstrating submucosal *(A)* and perineural lymphatic *(B)* microscopic spread of an adenoid cystic carcinoma well beyond a grossly identifiable tumor. Note the overlying intact epithelum in *A*.

principles in the management of these tumors: (1) Routine perioperative biopsies are performed at different levels around the tumor, including submucosa, to determine proximal and distal spread. Preoperative endoscopic biopsy proximal and distal to the tumor can help guide the surgeon as to the extent of resection. (2) If the tumor is believed to be circumscribed, sleeve resection should be performed with frozen-section guidance. (3) If extensive submucosal involvement is detected at preoperative endoscopy or intraoperatively before tracheal resection, serious consideration should be given to abandoning the attempt at resection, considering the limits of mobilization that can be accomplished in the trachea.

Although tracheal prostheses can be used to extend the length of tracheal resection, these prostheses are fraught with complications and should be avoided wherever possible, as Pearson and colleagues (1984) noted.

Carinal tumors can be dealt with successfully using two-lung anesthesia through a sternotomy or a high right thoracotomy approach (Fig. 75–14). Cardiopulmonary bypass is rarely necessary. These lesions should be managed by only the most experienced thoracic surgeons. Although the process is malignant, the risks of resection must be weighed against the life expectancy of the patient if palliative endoscopic treatment and irradiation are used. This latter treatment can be effective for long-term control.

A single pulmonary metastasis with a localized endotracheal or endobronchial tumor does not necessarily contraindicate a surgical approach. The solitary metastasis can be removed as part of the surgical procedure.

Radiation Therapy

Although adenoid cystic carcinomas are fairly radiation resistant, those occurring in the airway have been treated successfully and appear to be more sensitive than those occurring in other salivary gland sites. Perelman and Koroleva (1987) found that these tumors are more sensitive than squamous cell carcinomas of the trachea.

Radiation therapy should be considered in all inoperable patients as part of the palliative approach. Rostom and Morgan (1978) reported that radiation doses in the curative range—greater than 5500 rads—are required and the response is usually slow. Munsch and associates (1987) suggested that before irradiation, if airway obstruction is a problem, laser or cryoablation of the tumor or an indwelling T-tube stent is warranted. Ryan and associates (1986) reported that the combination of intraluminal brachytherapy and external beam irradiation allows higher doses of radiation therapy to the tumor.

Although surgical therapy remains the treatment of choice, a radiation therapy approach can lead to long-term survival and occasionally cure.

If residual tumor remains after resection, postoperative irradiation is indicated. As Pearson and associates (1984) and Grillo (1983) noted, the question of whether preoperative or postoperative irradiation, or both, as a combined modality approach is valuable has not been answered. Because of the high incidence of perineural

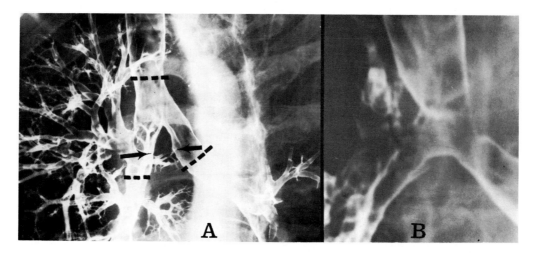

Fig. 75–14. *A,* Preoperative tracheogram of an adenoid cystic carcinoma of the carina after preoperative radiotherapy. The arrows indicate the lower extent of tumor involvement, and the broken lines indicate extent of resection. *B,* Postoperative tracheogram showing the appearance after resection of the carina and right upper lobe. For reconstruction, the bronchus intermedius and left main bronchus were anastomosed to the resected lower end of the trachea (Courtesy of F.G. Pearson).

lymphatic invasion, it would appear to be advantageous to sterilize the lymphatics before surgical excision. Because of the high doses required, however, preoperative irradiation may lead to significant postoperative complications.

Chemotherapy

The role of chemotherapy in this disease is undefined and at present of little known value.

Prognosis

Adenoid cystic carcinoma is inherently a more malignant tumor than the carcinoid tumor. Because of its tendency to permeate lymphatics, metastasize to regional lymph nodes, and infiltrate surrounding structures such as pleura and pericardium, this tumor is prone to recur locally unless adequately excised. Its natural history, however, is prolonged, and long-term survival, measured in decades, with persistent disease is common. Before modern tracheal surgical techniques were developed, only 30% of patients could be expected to survive without recurrent disease. Grillo (1983), however, reported that 12 of 16 patients were disease-free after 5 years. Similarly, Pearson (1984) reported that 50% of patients were disease-free 2 to 18 years after tracheal resection. Perelman and Koroleva (1987) reported a 65% 5-year and 56% 10-year survival rate in resected patients.

Owing to its low biologic activity, even after incomplete surgical excision, long survival periods can occur even with persisting or recurrent disease. For this reason, aggressive treatment of these tumors, palliative or curative, is warranted.

MUCOEPIDERMOID CARCINOMA

These carcinomas are rare bronchial tumors, accounting for less than 1% of the bronchial "adenomas" encountered. As with the other types, they are seen most commonly in persons in the fifth decade of life, but have been reported in patients as young as 10 and as old as 75 years of age. Sex incidence is approximately equal.

Pathology

Reichle and Rosemond (1966) reported that mucoepidermoid carcinomas are found in the same location as carcinoid tumors. As with other mucoepidermoid tumors, those arising in the bronchial tree may be either of high or low grade malignancy, most of them being of the latter variety. Endoscopically, the tumor appears either as a polypoid submucosal mass located in the main stem or peripheral bronchi or as an infiltrative mass (Fig. 75–15).

Microscopically, the tumors resemble those found in the salivary glands. They are composed of three characteristic cell types—mucous, squamous, and intermediate cells. The three types are seen in varying proportions in different tumors. The low grade tumors have a high proportion of mucous cells, whereas the high grade tumors have a high proportion of squamous cells (Fig. 75–16). The tumor may have a predominantly solid growth pattern or mixed solid and cystic pattern.

The low grade variety can infiltrate the bronchial wall but does not invade vessels or metastasize to lymph nodes. The high grade variety metastasizes to regional lymph nodes and distantly like other bronchial carcinomas.

Treatment

The principles of treatment outlined for carcinoid tumors apply to the mucoepidermoid variety, low grade type. These procedures should include complete removal of tumor with preservation of as much normal lung tissue as possible. Segmentectomy, lobectomy, or rarely pneumonectomy with or without sleeve resection, may be required. Preoperative bronchial biopsies and intra-

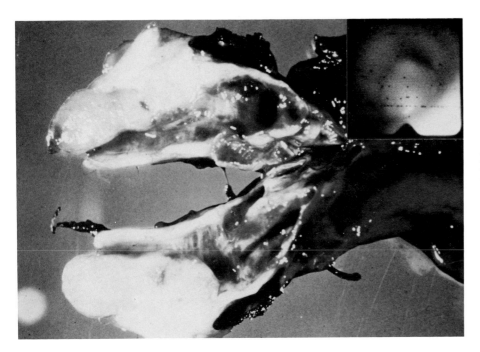

Fig. 75–15. A low grade mucoepidermoid tumor almost completely obstructing the bronchus intermedius. The inset shows the bronchoscopic appearance (upper right).

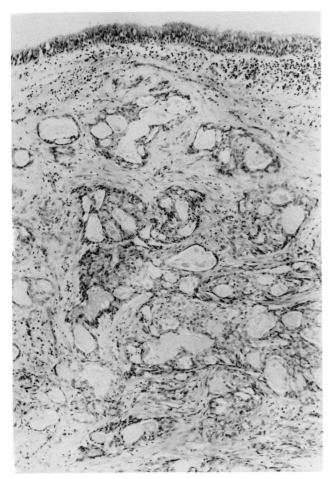

Fig. 75–16. A low grade mucoepidermoid tumor comprised of mucinous cysts and mixed with solid collections of squamoid cells. The overlying bronchial epithelium is intact.

operative surgical staging of lymph nodes should be performed to identify the more malignant variety.

The high grade malignant mucoepidermoid carcinoma should be investigated and managed with the same philosophy as that used for other carcinomas, the treatment depending upon the local and regional extent of disease.

Prognosis

The low grade malignant mucoepidermoid tumor can be completely cured by adequate surgical removal. Although few high grade mucoepidermoid carcinomas have been reported, the results of surgical therapy seem to be similar to those seen for bronchial carcinoma, according to the local and distant spread of the disease at the time of treatment.

MUCOUS GLAND ADENOMA

Mucous gland adenomas, also known as bronchial cyst adenomas, or papillary cystadenomas, are rare, with only a few examples reported in the English literature by Weinberger (1955), Gilman (1956), Weiss (1961), Kroe (1967), and Emory (1973) and their associates. These are the only true "adenomas" of the bronchus, being benign with no invasive or metastatic tendencies. Of the tumors reported, more occurred on the right side than on the left and the sex incidence was equal.

Pathology

With rare exceptions, these tumors have been located in major bronchi. Endoscopically they appear as firm pink masses with intact overlying epithelium (Fig. 75–17).

Histologically they are composed of numerous small mucus-filled cysts lined by well differentiated epithelium similar to mucous glands (Fig. 75–18).

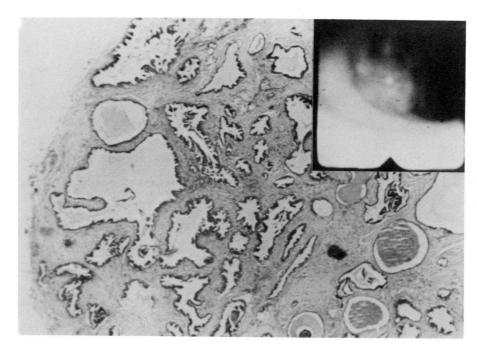

Fig. 75–17. A low powered photomicrograph of a mucous gland adenoma. The inset shows the endoscopic appearance (upper right).

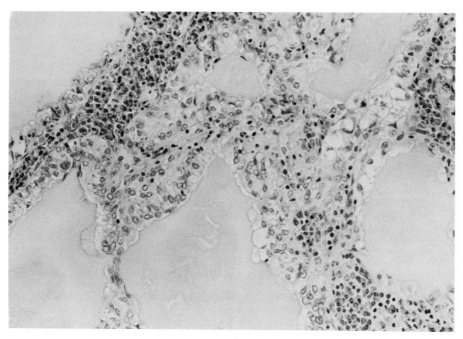

Fig. 75–18. A high powered view of a mucous gland adenoma consisting of cysts of various diameters lined by columnar mucous cells. A chronic inflammatory reaction separates the tubules.

Treatment

Even though mucous gland adenomas rarely have a stalk, these benign tumors can be completely removed endoscopically by curettage, cryotherapy, or laser ablation. Follow-up endoscopy at intervals is mandatory to ensure completeness of removal. Thoracotomy and surgical resection is only indicated when distal lung has been destroyed or endoscopic removal is contraindicated or incomplete.

Prognosis

Complete removal of these tumors endoscopically or surgically results in permanent cure.

MIXED TUMORS, SALIVARY GLAND TYPE

Payne and colleagues (1965) reported two bronchial tumors histologically similar to mixed salivary gland tumors. Both of these examples showed infiltrative tendencies; one patient required a second procedure for removal of local recurrences. Survival in both patients was over 10 years. Wide surgical excision can be curative.

REFERENCES

Arrigoni, M.G., Woolner, L.B., and Bernatz, T.E.: Atypical carcinoid tumours of the lung. J. Thorac. Cardiovasc. Surg. *64*:413, 1972.
Baldwin, J.N., and Grimes, O.F.: Bronchial adenomas. Surg. Gynecol. Obstet. *124*:813, 1967.

Balazs, M.: Adenoid cystic (cylindromatous) carcinoma of the trachea: an ultrastructural study. Histopathology 10:425, 1986.

Bensch, K.G., Gordon, G.B., and Miller, L.R.: Electron microscopic and biochemical studies on the bronchial carcinoid tumour. Cancer 18:592, 1965.

Bertelsen, S., et al.: Bronchial carcinoid tumours: a clinical pathologic study of 82 cases. Scand. J. Thorac. Cardiovasc. Surg. 19:105, 1985.

Brandt, B., et al.: Bronchial carcinoid tumours. Ann. Thorac. Surg. 38:63, 1984.

Cutz, E., et al.: Immunoperoxidase staining for serotonin, bombesin, calcitonin, and leu–enkephalin in pulmonary tumorlets, bronchial carcinoids, and oat cell carcinomas. Laboratory Investigation 46:16A, 1982.

D'Agati, V., and Perzin, K.A.: Carcinoid tumorlets of the lung with metastases to a peribronchial lymph node: report of a case and review of the literature. Cancer 55:2472, 1985.

Donahue, J.K., Weichert, R.R., and Ochsner, J.L.: Bronchial adenoma. Ann. Surg. 167:873, 1968.

Emory, W.B., Mitchel, W.T., and Hatch, H.B.: Mucus gland adenoma of the bronchus. Am. Rev. Respir. Dis. 108:1407, 1973.

Englebreth-Holm, J.: Benign bronchial adenomas. Acta Chir. Scand. 90:383, 1944–1945.

Frist, W.H., et al.: Bronchial sleeve resection with and without pulmonary resection. J. Thorac. Cardiovasc. Surg. 93:350, 1987.

Gilman, R.A., Klassen, K.P., and Scarpelli, D.G.: Mucus gland adenoma of the bronchus. Am. J. Clin. Pathol. 26:151, 1956.

Gould, V.E., et al.: Neuroendocrine components of the bronchopulmonary tract: hyperplasias, dysplasias, and neoplasms. Lab. Invest. 48:519, 1983.

Grillo, H.C.: Tracheal tumours: diagnosis and management. In Thoracic Oncology. Edited by N.C. Troy and H.C. Grillo. New York, Raven Press, 1983.

Hurt, R., and Bates, M.: Carcinoid tumours of the bronchus: a 33-year experience. Thorax 39:617, 1984.

Kroe, D.J., and Pitcoc, J.A.: Benign mucus gland adenoma of the bronchus. Arch. Pathol. 84:539, 1967.

McCaughan, B.C., Martini, N., and Bains, M.J.: Bronchial carcinoids: review of 124 cases. J. Thorac. Cardiovasc. Surg. 89:8, 1985.

Miller, M., Mark, G., and Kanarek, D.: Multiple peripheral pulmonary carcinoid and tumorlets of carcinoid type with restrictive and obstructive lung disease. Am. J. Med. 65:373, 1978.

Mueller, H.: Zur Entstehungsgeschichte: der Bronchialweiterungen. Inaug. Diss. Halle Vol. 15, 1882.

Munsch, C., Westaby, S., and Sturridge, M.: Urgent treatment for a nonresectable, asphyxiating tracheal cylindroma. Ann. Thorac. Surg. 43:663, 1987.

Okike, N., Bernatz, P., and Woolner, L.B.: Carcinoid tumours of the lung. Ann. Thorac. Surg. 22:270, 1976.

Paulson, D.L., and Shaw, R.R.: Preservation of lung tissue by bronchoplastic procedures. Am. J. Surg. 89:347, 1955.

Paulson, D.L., and Ginsberg, R.J.: Bronchial adenoma. In General Thoracic Surgery. Edited by T.W. Shields. Philadelphia, Lea & Febiger, 1972.

Payne, W.S., Schier, J., and Woolner, L.B.: Mixed tumours of the bronchus (salivary gland type). J. Thorac. Cardiovasc. Surg. 49:663, 1965.

Pearson, F.G., Todd, T.R.J., and Cooper, J.D.: Experience with primary neoplasms of the trachea and carina. J. Thorac. Cardiovasc. Surg. 88:511, 1984.

Perelman, M.I., and Koroleva, N.S.: Primary tumours of the trachea. In International Trends in General Thoracic Surgery, Vol. 2. Edited by N.C. Delarue, and H. Eschapasse. Philadelphia, W.B. Saunders Co., 1987.

Personne, C., et al.: Indications and technique for endoscopic laser resection in bronchology. J. Thorac. Cardiovasc. Surg. 91:710, 1986.

Reichle, F.A., and Rosemond, G.P.: Mucoepidermoid tumours of the bronchus. J. Thorac. Cardiovasc. Surg. 51:443, 1966.

Rostom, A.Y., and Morgan, R.L.: Results of treating primary tumours of the trachea by irradiation. Thorax 33:387, 1978.

Rozenman, J., et al.: Bronchial adenoma. Chest 92:145, 1987.

Ryan, K.L., Lowy, J., and Harrell, J.H.: Management of adenoid cystic carcinoma. Chest 89:503s, 1986.

Smith, R.A.: Bronchial carcinoid tumours. Thorax 24:98, 1969.

Turnbull, A.D., et al.: Mucoepidermoid tumours of bronchial glands. Cancer 28:539, 1971.

Von Albertini, A.: Patholisch-anatomisches Kurzreferat zum Thema Lungenkrebs. Schweiz. Med. Wochensch. 81:659, 1951.

Warren, W.H., et al.: Neuroendocrine neoplasms of the bronchopulmonary tract. J. Thorac. Cardiovasc. Surg. 89:819, 1985.

Weinberger, M.A., Katz, S., and Davis, E.W.: Peripheral bronchial adenoma of mucus gland type. J. Thorac. Surg. 29:626, 1955.

Weiss, L., and Ingram, M.: Adenomatoid bronchial tumours: a consideration of the carcinoid tumours and salivary tumours of the bronchial tree. Cancer 14:161, 1961.

Whitwell, F.: Tumourlets of the lung. J. Pathol. Bacteriol. 70:529, 1955.

Wilkins, E.W., et al.: A continuing clinical survey of adenomas of the tracheum bronchus in a general hospital. J. Thorac. Cardiovasc. Surg. 46:279, 1963.

Wilkins, E.W., et al.: Changing times and surgical management of bronchopulmonary carcinoid tumor. Ann. Thorac. Surg. 38:339, 1984.

CHAPTER 76

CARCINOMA OF THE LUNG

Thomas W. Shields

Since the second decade of the twentieth century, the incidence of carcinoma of the lung has risen alarmingly in all economically developed countries of the world. It now stands as one of the commoner causes of death from cancer and is, in fact, the most common cause of death in all men with cancer. The highest recorded mortality rate for this disease is in the United Kingdom. The death rates per 100,000 population in Finland, Austria, several other western European countries, and the Union of South Africa also exceed the rate in the United States.

Formerly, the greater increase in incidence of the disease was in men, but at present a more rapid increase is seen in women. Although carcinoma of the lung is still more common in men, the ratio of distribution in men and women is less than 3:1, whereas it was 8:1 only a decade ago. The marked rise in the frequency of the disease in both sexes has been associated with the introduction of certain environmental factors prevalent in the twentieth century: cigarette smoking, urban air pollution, and specific industrial exposure (Table 76–1).

ETIOLOGY

The nature of the interaction of these environmental factors with the cells of the respiratory tract and the subsequent development of carcinoma, is not fully understood. Particle size, the distribution and retention of particles within the respiratory tract, the response of the respiratory mucosa to irritation, and the eventual penetration and intracellular location of the carcinogen are important. Auerbach and his associates (1961) and Auerbach and Stout (1964) recorded changes in the bronchial epithelium of chronic smokers, including the loss of cilia, an increase in the number of cell rows, and the presence of atypical cells in the thickened epithelium. As Kotin (1968) noted, these findings suggest "a progression of changes from initial goblet cell hyperplasia to metaplasia, metaplasia with atypism, and ultimately carcinoma in situ and invasive cancer."

These studies support the observation of a probable causative relationship between cigarette smoking and the development of bronchial carcinoma. A vast amount of epidemiological evidence accumulated by Doll and Hill (1952), Dorn (1959), Wynder (1961), Boucot and associates (1964, 1966), and others supports this observation. Initially it was believed that this correlation applied only to squamous and undifferentiated small cell carcinomas, but it is now recognized that this correlation applies to adenocarcinoma as well. The former tumors are rare in nonsmokers. Overall, lung carcinoma is four to ten times more common in cigarette smokers than in nonsmokers. Statistically, the risk increases with the number of cigarettes smoked per day as well as the number of years the person has been smoking. Cessation of smoking for a long period of time appears to lower the risk. Various factors in the smoke have been suggested as causative agents, but none as yet has been proved to be the essential one.

In contrast, various agents found in industrial exposure have been related to the development of bronchial carcinoma, most notably asbestos, radioactive material—^{210}Po being one of the more important of these—arsenic, chromates, and nickel. Less certainly, coal tar and petroleum products have been implicated. These products also are present in varying quantities in the atmosphere, particularly in urban areas.

The role of atmospheric pollution in the development of lung carcinoma is much more difficult to elucidate. Various carcinogenic agents, such as 3,4-benzopyene, 1,12-benzoperylene, arsenous oxide, radioactive substances, nickel, and chromium compounds, as well as incombustible aliphatic hydrocarbons, also are present in the atmosphere. The unknown nature of action of these various substances, the combined effect of cigarette smoking, and the presence of chronic bronchitis in many persons make the problem of the pathogenesis of lung carcinoma difficult to solve.

HISTOGENESIS

Most investigators believe that all varieties of lung cancer arise from endodermal cells. Under varying in-

Table 76–1. Epidemiologic Factors in the Development of Lung Cancer

General Environment

Cigarette Smoke
Polluted Urban Air

Occupational Environment

Occupation	Agents
Radioactive ore mining and smelting	Radioactivity, alpha, beta, gamma
Coke oven operators	Hydrocarbons
Gas works operators	Hydrocarbons
Chromium ore refining	Chromates
Nickel ore refining	
Asbestos mining and use	
Welders, steam fitters Short order cooks Crane operators Foundry workers	Exposure to high temperature fumes

Adapted from Kotin, P.: Carcinogenesis of the lung. *In* The Lung. Edited by A.A. Liebow and D.E. Smith. Baltimore, Williams & Wilkins, 1968, p. 206; and The International Academy of Pathology.

fluences—chemical initiators and chemical promoters—the mucus-goblet cells of the bronchial epithelium may "dedifferentiate" and then differentiate into one of the varieties of lung cancer. Yesner (1977, 1986) suggested a Y diagram with small cell carcinoma at the bottom, large cell carcinoma at the fork and epidermoid and adenocarcinomas at the arms. All these cell types secrete big ACTH, as Gewirtz and Yallow (1974) demonstrated, although in varying amounts as Bondy (1981) noted (Table 76–2). There is a varying degree of heterogenicity in most carcinomas of the lung, especially in large and in far-advanced lesions. This heterogenicity has been observed in many patients with recurrent or residual disease of an originally pure small cell tumor after treatment with chemotherapy, as Ginsberg (1983), Valdivieso (1982), and Prager (1984) and associates and others have noted.

The smaller, earlier lesions tend to be more homogeneous. The biologic factors that direct carcinogenesis to establish dominately one cell line remain unknown. Clonal selection and the presence of oncogenes, such as C *myc* and *ras*, and chromosomal deletions seen in lung cancer cells may help elucidate the histogenesis of the varying types of lung cancers.

PATHOLOGY

Gross Characteristics

Bronchial carcinoma occurs more frequently in the right lung than in the left, in a ratio of approximately

**Table 76–2. "Big" ACTH as a Marker in Lung Cancer*:
ACTH[+] >100 pg/ml**

Cell Type	No. Pts. Examined	% Positive
Small Cell	27	63
Squamous	86	92
Adenocarcinoma	40	80
Large Cell	11	64

[+]ACTH, "big" ACTH and pro-ACTH
*Modified from Bondy, P.K., Yale J. Biol. Med. *54*:181, 1981.

6:4. The upper lobes are involved more often than the lower lobes, and the middle lobe is involved the least frequently of all. In the upper lobes, the tumor is most likely to be located in the anterior segment, although the other segments are not spared as the site of origin.

The tumor's anatomic site of origin may be classified as: (a) the central zone: the main stem, the lobar bronchi, and the primary segmental bronchi of the lower lobe; (b) the segmental or intermediate zone: the third, fourth, and possibly the fifth order segmental bronchi; and (c) the peripheral zone: the remainder of the distal bronchi and bronchioles. In the roentgenographic localization of lung tumors, zones (a) and (b) may be considered the central area and zone (c) the peripheral area.

According to Meyer and Liebow (1965), approximately 50 to 60% of carcinomas of the lung originate in the peripheral area. Of those carcinomas that arise in the central and segmental zones—the central area—20 to 40% arise in the former and 60 to 80% in the latter.

Grossly, the tumors in the central and segmental zones appear as a firm, irregular mass of varying size. Intraluminal growth of the mass may occlude partially or completely the bronchial lumen, although obstruction also may be caused by circumferential narrowing of the lumen. Extrabronchial spread may extend for a variable distance into the adjacent lung parenchyma. The tumor is generally homogeneous, with a whitish-gray cut surface. The endobronchial surface is almost always ulcerated. Atelectasis or secondary inflammatory change, including secondary bronchiectasis, pneumonitis, or lung abscess distal to the site of the tumor, is frequently present.

The peripherally located tumors are firm, irregular, and may or may not appear to be demarcated from the surrounding lung tissue. The cut surface is homogeneous. The smaller lesions are usually solid, although the larger ones may reveal central necrosis with cavitation. Umbilication or puckering of the overlying adjacent visceral pleura is often present. The blood supply of both the centrally and the peripherally located bronchial carcinomas is from the bronchial arteries.

Microscopic Characteristics

Many histologic classifications of lung tumors have been suggested. One derived from the classification adopted in 1981 by the Expert Committee on Lung Cancer formed by the World Health Organization, however, is appropriate. Table 76–3 shows a modified classification.

At present it is common to divide all these tumors into two subgroups: the non-small cell cancers—epidermoid carcinoma, adenocarcinoma, and undifferentiated large cell carcinoma—and the small cell cancers.

Non-Small Cell Tumors

Epidermoid Carcinoma

The well differentiated epidermoid tumors have polygonal or prickle-type cells, stratification, and intercellular bridge formation. Individual cells keratinize or tend to form epithelial pearls or both; the nuclei may be uniform, pelomorphic, or giant. The moderately differentiated tumors have polygonal or prickle-type cells, stratification, intercellular bridge formation, and some keratinization. The poorly differentiated tumors are composed predominantly of anaplastic cells, with little but still distinct evidence of intercellular bridge formation or individual cell keratinization or both. A tumor without these latter markers should not be placed in this category (Fig. 76–1).

These squamous cell tumors constitute approximately 35% of all lung carcinomas. They may occur in either the central or peripheral areas, although two thirds are found in the central area. Squamous cell tumors grow relatively slowly and tend to metastasize late. The centrally located lesions tend to extend peribronchially so that frequently the lumen is constricted by extrinsic pressure but has a grossly normal-appearing mucosal pattern. The peripherally located squamous cell tumors tend to undergo central necrosis with resultant cavitation.

Table 76–3. Histologic Classification of Bronchial Carcinoma

Squamous Cell—Epidermoid—Carcinoma
  Spindle cell (squamous) variant
Adenocarcinoma
  Acinar adenocarcinoma
  Papillary adenocarcinoma
  Bronchioloalveolar carcinoma
  Solid carcinoma with mucus formation
Large Cell Undifferentiated Carcinoma
  Giant cell variant
  Clear cell variant
Undifferentiated Small Cell Carcinoma
  Oat cell—typical small cell—carcinoma
  Intermediate—polygonal, fusiform—cell type
  Combined—mixed—cell type
Adenosquamous carcinoma

Adenocarcinoma

The well differentiated tumors are composed of cuboidal to columnar epithelial cells with fairly uniform round nuclei, have adequate to abundant pink or vacuolated cytoplasm, and are arranged in distinct acinar or glandular patterns and supported by a fibrous stroma. The cells may show papillary intraluminal growth or contain mucicarmine-positive vacuoles or secretions. The moderately differentiated tumors are composed of nests, cords, or isolated cells, occasionally arranged in an acinar or glandular pattern (Fig. 76–2). The cytoplasm is supported by a fibrous or desmoplastic stroma, and the cells may contain mucicarmine-positive vacuoles or secretions. The poorly differentiated tumors are composed predominantly of anaplastic cells of variable size and shape, with minimal but distinct evidence of acinar formation. Mucicarmine-positive vacuoles may be present. Tumors without distinct acinar formation should not be placed in this category.

Adenocarcinomas account for approximately 25 to 50% of all carcinomas of the lung. Vincent and associates (1977) reported an increasing incidence of adenocarcinoma; they found more adenocarcinomas than epidermoid tumors. This observation has been confirmed by numerous investigators, including Yesner and Carter (1982), who reported in an all male population of veterans in a two-decade period a 7% increase in adenocarcinomas of the lung and an associated drop of 4% in squamous cell tumors and a 3% drop in small cell carcinomas. Amemiya and Oho (1982) noted a similar preponderance of adenocarcinoma in the Japanese.

The usual glandular variety of adenocarcinoma arises in the peripheral area of the lung, although one fourth or even more in my own recent experience may occur in the central area. Many of the tumors arise in conjunction with lung scars—the so-called scar carcinoma—and areas of chronic interstitial fibrosis. Such tumors may represent the response to chronic irritation. Clinically, these scar carcinomas behave as typical adenocarcinomas. The growth rate of the adenocarcinoma is intermediate between that of the epidermoid and the undifferentiated small cell types. These tumors tend to spread by way of the vascular system early in the course of the disease, but lymphatic spread may occur late. They also may become large without undergoing central necrosis.

Bronchioloalveolar/papillary cell carcinoma is a highly differentiated adenocarcinoma that spreads along the alveolar walls (Fig. 76–3). Microscopically, the alveolar spaces are lined by cuboidal or nonciliated columnar epithelium in layers or in papillary formation. The alveolar spaces may be filled, or even distended, with this proliferating epithelium. Occasionally, single cells or clusters containing large multinucleated giant cells may appear lying free. The nuclei are hypochromatic, and mitosis is not common. The cytoplasm is acidophilic and abundant. Distant spread as well as nodal metastases is infrequent. These tumors constitute 1.5 to 7% of all bronchial carcinomas, with an average incidence of 2.5%. Grossly, it may occur in one of three forms: solitary

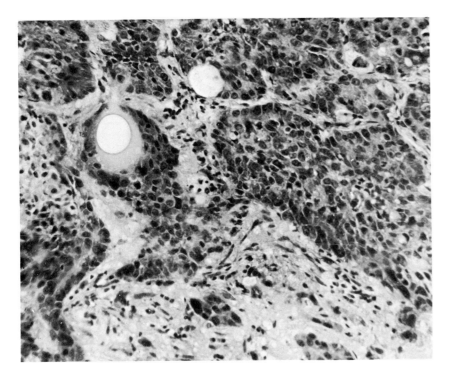

Fig. 76–1. Photomicrograph of squamous cell carcinoma of the lung.

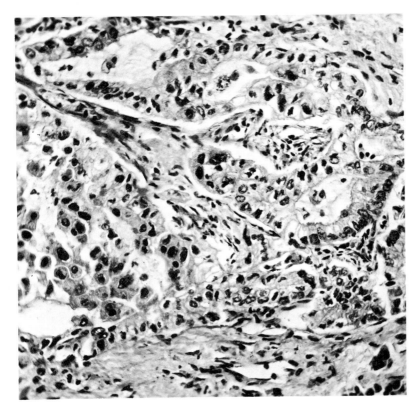

Fig. 76–2. Photomicrograph of adenocarcinoma of the lung.

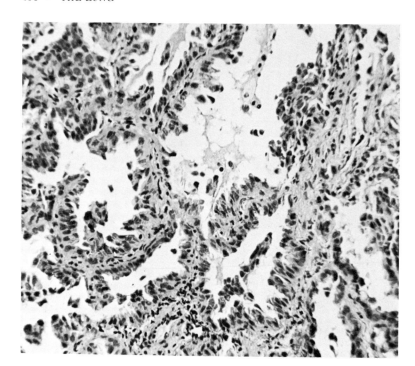

Fig. 76–3. Photomicrograph of bronchioloalveolar cell carcinoma.

nodule, multinodular, and diffuse or pneumonic type. The first is the most common and comprises two thirds of the tumors of this subclassification. The remainder, the multinodular and diffuse forms, usually do not represent a surgical problem (Chapter 73). The more common peripherally located solitary lesions of this cell type, however, are usually asymptomatic. Generally, the solitary type of this highly differentiated tumor has a much better prognosis than do the other types of adenocarcinomas arising in the lung.

Undifferentiated Large Cell Carcinoma

These heterogeneous tumors, which cannot be classified readily either as squamous cell carcinomas or as adenocarcinomas, are considered anaplastic tumors that show no apparent evidence of differentiation. Tumors composed of stratifying cells without evidence of intercellular bridge formation or keratin production are included in this group. Individual cells have enlarged, irregular vesicular or hyperchromatic nuclei that may have prominent nucleoli. The cell may have abundant cytoplasm (Fig. 76–4).

Because of the lack of uniformity in the criteria for the histologic diagnosis of these lesions, their actual incidence is unknown but probably is between the 4.5% recorded by Shinton (1963) and the 15% recorded by Yesner and associates (1965). These tumors may occur in either the central or the peripheral zone, although the latter site is probably somewhat more common. They spread earlier and have a relatively poorer prognosis than more differentiated non-small cell types have.

The so-called giant cell tumor is a variety of the undifferentiated large cell tumors. A varying combination of cell types may occur in this lesion: pleomorphic, anaplastic-multinuclear cells, and spindle cells. The clinical course of these lesions is rapidly fatal. Fortunately, this variety is uncommon and constitutes less than 1% of all lung tumors.

Mixed Cell Types

The most common of the mixed cell types of non-small cell tumors is the adenosquamous variety. This type makes up approximately 1% of all lung tumors, and its diagnosis is based on light microscopy. These tend to be peripheral lesions, and their biologic behavior apparently depends upon the predominant cell type.

Small Cell Tumors

Undifferentiated small cell tumors are subdivided morphologically into three cell types: the oat cell, the intermediate, and the combined or mixed cell types. The oat cell—typical small cell—and intermediate cell types, although different histologically, have similar biologic behavior. The combined—mixed cell—and the small cell-large cell variant types, however, do behave somewhat differently, especially in response to therapy.

Typical Small Cell Tumors

These are characterized by clusters, nests, or sheets of small, round, oval, or spindle-shaped cells with small, dark, round nuclei, with delicate chromatin and without prominent nucleoli. Cytoplasm is scanty and the cells are supported by a vascular fibrous stroma (Fig. 76–5).

Intermediate Cell Tumors

These are composed of clusters or sheets of small cells with more fusiform or polygonal nuclei. Cystoplasm is more distinct but still scanty and the nuclear chromatin is clumped.

Combined Cell Types

Mixed tumors may be composed of any combination of the various non-small cell types—large, epidermoid,

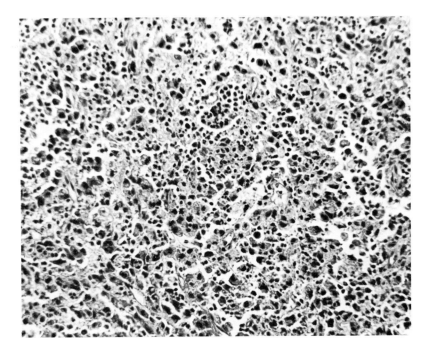

Fig. 76–4. Photomicrograph of undifferentiated large cell carcinoma of the lung.

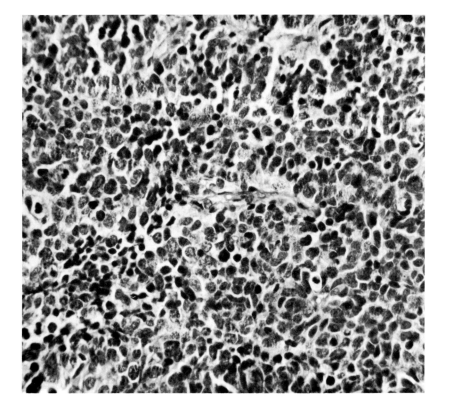

Fig. 76–5. Photomicrograph of undifferentiated small cell carcinoma of the lung.

or adenocarcinoma—with the small cell type cell. Intermediate small cell elements mixed with large cell elements is apparently the most common combination.

Gross Features

Various types of small cell tumors constitute approximately 15 to 35% of all bronchial carcinomas. Approximately four fifths of these arise in the central area, and the remainder arise in the peripheral area of the lung. Tumors arising in either region involve the hilar and mediastinal lymph nodes early. Central necrosis within the tumor or changes in the distal parenchyma of the lung occur less frequently than in squamous cell tumors.

Biologic Behavior

The small cell tumors have been studied extensively in cell cultures, and such cultures can be established in 75% of small cell tumors. The cultures can be separated into two cell lines: the classic cell line and the variant lines. The former is characterized by tight spherical aggregates and has a doubling time of 50 hours and low colony-forming efficiency, whereas the latter grows in much looser aggregates of floating cell lines and has a faster doubling time and a greater colony-forming efficiency. The classic line corresponds to the pure small cell carcinoma, expresses the usual production of the various biologic substances, and contains many dense granules. The variant lines have few granules, produce fewer biologically active substances, and less of them and resemble the combined cell types clinically.

Regardless of the cell line, however, these tumors are highly malignant and spread early by way of both the lymphatic and the vascular systems. Many believe that most if not all small cell tumors have spread systemically by the time of initial diagnosis.

Electron Microscopic Features

Study of the ultrastructure of the various types of bronchial carcinomas by electron microscopy may help to resolve some of the difficulties in their classification. Generally, as Nagaishi and associates (1965) observed, tumor cells have degenerated and bizarre mitochondria and have more free ribosomes, fewer profiles of granular endoplasmic reticulum, and more lipid granules than do normal cells. The Golgi apparatus is usually poorly developed.

Razzuk and associates (1970) reported certain ultrastructural features for the various cell types of bronchial carcinoma. Squamous cell carcinoma was made up of polygonal cells showing distinct cell membranes and numerous desmosomes between adjacent cells. Tonofilaments, keratohyalin granules, and some keratin pearls were dominant features. Adenocarcinoma was composed of cuboidal- to columnar-shaped cells. Aggregates of chromatin were dispersed inside the nuclei. Microvilli, acinar formation, desmosomes, and terminal bars were identified. Well developed Golgi apparatuses with secretory vacuoles were frequently present. Secretory granules, resembling those of goblet cells, were present in most examples of alveolar cell tumors. Undifferen-

tiated large cell carcinoma showed marked variation in cell shape. Cell membranes were often indistinct. Large nuclei with abundant cytoplasm and numerous organelles were present. Occasionally, tonofilaments were identified, but no distinctive features were present to permit categoric determination of cell type. Warren and associates (1985) suggested that dense-core granules and predominately neuroendocrine differentiation appear in 40% of the so-called large cell tumors. Undifferentiated small cell carcinoma revealed marked cellular pleomorphism, but the shape of the cell was usually round to ovoid in transection. Some cells adjacent to the basement membrane possessed "pseudopod-like" processes extending between adjacent cells. Cell membranes were often indistinct. The nuclei were large, often with eccentric nucleoli, and were surrounded by a narrow zone of cytoplasm. Although Razzuk and associates (1970) identified no neurosecretory cytoplasmic granules, Bensch and co-workers (1968) found these granules in the undifferentiated small cell tumors, which many authors, including Warren and associates (1985), have confirmed. These neurosecretory granules and the observed production of many biologically active substances by the small cell have led many to include these tumors in the APUD system and to classify these tumors as neuroendocrine tumors of the lung. This proposes a cell origin for these tumors different from that of the non-small cell carcinomas. As noted previously under histogenesis, however, this is not a universally held concept.

METASTASIS OF BRONCHIAL CARCINOMA

Carcinoma of the lung has three modes of spread. Its dissemination occurs by direct extension and by lymphatic and hematogenous metastases.

Direct Extension

The lesion may extend directly into the adjacent pulmonary parenchyma, across the fissure, along the bronchus of origin, and also into adjacent structures in the thorax. Many tumors situated in the central area extend directly along the bronchus.

Cotton (1959) studied this bronchial extension and noted five important factors in this type of spread; first, direct extension continuous with the tumor in the bronchial wall and the adjacent parabronchial tissues; second, direct extension into bronchi other than the bronchus of origin, particularly by tumors arising close to a segmental or a major lobar bronchial orifice; third, invasion of the submucosal lymphatics in the bronchial wall; fourth, extension of the tumor proximally along the lumen of the bronchus by papillary or polypoid process without further attachment to the bronchial wall; and fifth, the presence of epithelial metaplasia, particularly if the epithelial change shows atypical proliferative features. He found that spread into the bronchial wall beyond the palpable mass occurred in only 12% of patients with lung cancer, and the maximum distance of the spread was three quarters of an inch—1.9 cm. This extent of spread essentially agrees with Griess and colleagues' (1945) results; they found that the proximal extension of tumor in the bronchial wall could be removed satisfactorily if the line of resection included 1.5 cm of grossly normal bronchus. Polypoid extension of the tumor into the lumen of the bronchus without bronchial wall involvement was observed as far as 2.5 to 3.2 cm. Submucosal lymphatic spread was noted in only 6% of the tumors and these specimens had extensive lymph node involvement. Cotton (1959) found epithelial metaplasia beyond the tumor in 31 of 100 specimens, but is was extensive in only 8 specimens. In these, it extended as far as 5 cm. All these factors are important considerations in the surgical treatment of carcinoma of the lung.

More important, however, is that direct extension occurs into adjacent structures within the thorax. The sites commonly involved are the pleura, pulmonary vessels, chest wall, the superior sulcus area and its adjacent neurogenic and bony structures, the diaphragm, the pericardium, and the heart and great vessels. Although direct extension from the tumor may involve the superior vena cava, the contiguous nerves—the recurrent laryngeal and phrenic nerves, and the esophagus, these structures more frequently are invaded by secondary extension from metastatic disease within the mediastinal lymph nodes.

Lymphatic Metastasis

This spread is common in patients with carcinoma of the lung. Ochsner and DeBakey (1942) reported regional node metastases in 72.2% of 3047 lung cancer patients studied. Cell type, as noted, affects the rate of incidence; it occurs in undifferentiated small cell carcinoma, undifferentiated large cell carcinoma, adenocarcinoma, and squamous cell carcinoma, in the order of decreasing frequency.

In an extensive study of the lymphatic spread of the disease, Nohl (1956), Greschuchna and Maassen (1973) and Hata and associates (1981) showed that the lymphatic pathways from the individual lobes to the mediastinum are constant (Chapter 5). The important area in each lung is the lymphatic sump of Borrie (1952). The interlobar nodes that make up the sump are located in the region between the upper lobe bronchus and the superior segmental and middle lobe bronchi on the right and the upper lobe bronchus and superior segmental bronchus on the left. All three lobes on the right drain into the sump region. The drainage of the upper lobe can be to the nodes on the lateral aspect of the bronchus intermedius, but most commonly is to the nodes on the superior surface of the upper lobe bronchus and the just proximal portion of the right main stem bronchus and the anterior trunk of the pulmonary artery; then to those beneath the azygos vein—the azygos nodes, also called the superior tracheobronchial nodes—which are continuous proximally with nodes of the lower paratracheal area. The middle and right lower lobes drain not only to the lateral nodes in the sump but also to the nodes on the medial surface of the bronchus intermedius, which are contiguous with the inferior tracheobronchial—subcarinal—nodes. Drainage also may occur to the pulmo-

nary ligament and paraesophageal nodes. The drainage of the left upper lobe is to the left sump, which drains to the nodes in the aortic window, the paratracheal area, the anterior mediastinum, and the subcarinal area. The left lower lobe drains to the sump area and to the subcarinal nodes. As with right lower lobe tumors, nodes in the pulmonary ligament and paraesophageal nodes may be involved frequently with left lower lobe tumors. Transgression of the fissure or massive lymphatic involvement, however, may change these specific patterns.

The spread of tumor from the pulmonary nodes to the tracheobronchial and other mediastinal nodes is usually ipsilateral. Contralateral spread, however, does occur. From the right such contralateral spread is unusual; Nohl-Oser (1972) (see Chapter 5) reported this spread in only 4% of patients with right upper lobe tumors and 5% of those with right lower lobe tumors. On the left, however, patients with upper lobe lesions had a 9.3% incidence of contralateral spread, and those with lower lobe tumors had a 28% incidence. Greschuchna and Maassen (1973) reported a higher incidence of bilateral or contralateral spread—a total of 21% in 540 patients with nodal metastases from bronchial carcinoma routinely investigated by mediastinoscopy. In an update of his continuing experience, Maassen (1985) noted that 30% percent of his patients had stage III disease and that the incidence of positive mediastinal nodes was 71% in this group. The high incidence of advanced disease obviously influenced the high rate of contralateral spread originally reported. Certainly in early disease—clinical stage I—the overall incidence of contralateral spread in my own experience, as determined by CT scanning and mediastinal exporation when indicated, is much less. Nevertheless, Hata's (1981) lymphoscintigraphy findings suggest that contralateral lymph flow does indeed occur.

Although lymphatic metastases usually progress from lobar to hilar and thence to the various mediastinal node stations, skip metastasis directly to mediastinal nodes without involvement of either lobar or hilar nodes may occur. Martini (1983b, 1987) and Libshitz (1986) and their associates reported that in patients with complete resections who were found to have mediastinal node involvement, lobar or hilar nodal disease was absent in 27 to 29%. Lymph nodes in the cervical region and those in the para-aortic region below the diaphragm also are often involved. Axillary lymph nodes are involved only rarely. Inguinal lymph nodes are involved infrequently and, when such involvement is noted, it is usually caused by hematogenous spread.

Hematogenous Spread

Blood-borne metastases are common in patients with bronchial carcinoma. Direct invasion of the smaller branches of the pulmonary veins occurs in many of the patients with these tumors. At times, a major vein may be filled with tumors, which may extend even as far as the left atrium. Invasion of the pulmonary artery also occurs.

Detectable blood vessel invasion on histologic examination of the tumor is thought to portend an unfavorable prognosis; although in reviewing data from the Veterans Administration Surgical Oncology Group's lung studies, I (1983) did not find that parenchymal blood vessel invasion had prognostic significance. Interestingly, however, parenchymal lymphatic vessel invasion even in the absence of lymph node metastases suggests a poor prognosis. Likewise, the finding of tumor cells in the circulation has not been well correlated with the prognosis. The fate of these circulating cells is undetermined in the individual patient, but these cells are certainly responsible for the development of metastatic deposits in distant organs at one time or another in the host-tumor relationship.

The organs and structures most commonly involved are the brain, liver, lungs, skeletal system, adrenal glands, kidneys, and pancreas (Table 76–4). Skeletal metastases are usually osteolytic; they occur most commonly in the ribs, spine, femur, humerus, and pelvis. Metastatic deposits distal to the knee or elbow are rare. Although, as Clain (1965) noted, the incidence of bony metastasis from carcinoma of the lung is less than that from four other primary sites—prostate gland, breast, kidney, and thyroid gland—the lung is second only to the breast as the most common primary site of metastases to bone.

Metastatic deposits may occur in the skin and subcutaneous tissue, myocardium, thyroid gland, small intestine, spleen, and ovary. Although deposits in these locations are uncommon, the lung is the most common primary site responsible for secondary metastases in the heart, and after carcinoma of the breast and melanoma, the lung is the next most common primary site for metastases to the skin and subcutaneous tissue. This variety of metastasis occurs in 1 to 4% of all patients with bronchial carcinoma.

CLINICAL MANIFESTATIONS

The average patient with carcinoma of the lung is a man in the sixth or seventh decade of life who is a heavy cigarette smoker and who resides in an urban area. All age groups are affected, but the disease is rare in persons under 30 years of age.

Five percent of the patients are asymptomatic, and in this group the tumor is discovered only on routine roentgenographic examination of the chest. In much fewer, the tumor may be roentgenographically occult, with only a positive sputum cytology suggesting the presence of a tumor. Most patients, however, have one or more symptoms related to the presence of the tumor. The symptoms may be designated as bronchopulmonary, extrapulmonary intrathoracic, extrathoracic metastatic, extrathoracic nonmetastatic, and nonspecific. On the average, symptoms have been present for 3 to 6 months by the time the patient seeks medical advice.

Bronchopulmonary Symptoms

Symptoms arising from involvement of the lung are caused by irritation, ulceration, or obstruction—or a combination of these—of a bronchus, and to septic complication within the lung parenchyma distal to the tumor.

In a review of 4000 patients with carcinoma of the lung, Le Roux (1968a) reported that 75% had cough as one of the major symptoms, and this symptom was severe in 40% of the patients. Hemoptysis, generally episodic blood-streaking of the sputum, was present in 57% of the patients and was the first symptom in 4%. Chest pain, frequently a dull ache, and dyspnea were also common complaints. Febrile respiratory symptoms were present in 22% of these patients, but unfortunately, they often are misinterpreted by the physician. Frequently, they are promptly, if only temporarily, ameliorated by antibiotic therapy, and further delay occurs before the proper diagnosis is made. Wheezing and stridor also occur but are uncommon.

Extrapulmonary Intrathoracic Symptoms

Other symptoms of chest disease result from growth of the tumor beyond the confines of the lung. These symptoms are caused by involvement of the pleura, chest wall, mediastinal structures, and contiguous nerves. Approximately 15% of the patients complain of such symptoms with or without associated bronchopulmonary symptoms. Hoarseness from paralysis of a vocal cord resulting from involvement of the left recurrent laryngeal nerve or rarely of the right recurrent laryngeal nerve, and the superior vena caval syndrome (Chapter 89) each occur in approximately 5% of patients with carcinoma of the lung. Severe pain in the chest wall caused by direct involvement of the chest wall by tumor and pain down the arm caused by involvement of the branches of the brachial plexus from tumors located in the superior sulcus occur less frequently. A Horner's syndrome is frequently present in the latter situation. Dysphagia from partial obstruction of the esophagus by tumor in the paraesophageal lymph nodes occurs in approximately 1% of the patients, as does massive pleural effusion from metastatic involvement of the pleura. The latter results

Table 76–4. Incidence of Organ Involvement by Metastatic Disease from Carcinoma of the Lung

	Liver (%)	Lung (%)	Skeleton (%)	Adrenals (%)	Kidneys (%)	Brain (%)	Pancreas (%)
Ochsner and De Bakey (1941–1942)							
3047 autopsies	33.3	23.3	21.3	20.3	17.5	16.5	7.3
Galluzzi and Payne (1955)							
741 autopsies	39.0	—	15.0	33.0	15.0	—	—
Spencer (1968)							
1000 autopsies	38.5	—	15.5	26.4	14.3	18.4	—

in severe dyspnea and is occasionally the presenting complaint. Varying amounts of pleural effusion may occur in as many as 10% of the patients. Paralysis of either leaf of the diaphragm caused by involvement of the ipsilateral phrenic nerve is rarely symptomatic.

Nonspecific Symptoms

Many patients experience weight loss, weakness, anorexia, lassitude, and malaise, with or without other symptoms. In 10 to 15% of the patients, these symptoms instigate the initial visit to the physician. Their causes are obscure, but when they are severe, metastatic intra-abdominal spread of the tumor—to liver, adrenal glands, pancreas, or para-aortic nodes—should be suspected.

Extrathoracic Metastatic Symptoms

Symptoms resulting from metastatic spread of the tumor outside of the thorax account for a few of the presenting or major complaints of patients with carcinoma of the lung. In 3 to 6%, neurologic symptoms caused by intracranial metastases may be present. Most often, these symptoms are hemiplegia, epilepsy, personality changes, confusion, speech defects, or at times only headache. Bone pain and pathologic fracture from metastatic involvement occur in 1 to 2% of the patients. Rarely, jaundice, ascites, or an abdominal mass is the major complaint. Masses in the neck, muscle, or subcutaneous tissue are rare.

Extrathoracic Nonmetastatic Symptoms

Approximately 2% of patients with bronchial carcinoma seek medical advice because of systemic symptoms and signs not related to spread of the tumor (Table 76–5). None of these manifestations is specific, and each may occur in association with other malignant lesions. These paraneoplastic syndromes occur in more patients with carcinoma of the lung than is generally appreciated.

Metabolic Manifestations

Most of these manifestations result from the secretion of endocrine or endocrine-like substances by the tumor. At times, these syndromes may be produced by tumors that are still resectable, but unfortunately most are found in association with small cell carcinomas.

Cushing's Syndrome. Most of the patients with this syndrome associated with nonadrenocortical, nonpituitary tumors have bronchial carcinoma, which occurs most often in patients with small cell carcinoma. These patients differ from those with classic Cushing's syndrome. The sex ratio is reversed, the patients tend to be older, hypokalemic alkalosis is more prominent and the patients have fewer physical stigmas of typical Cushing's syndrome and a more rapid, fulminating clinical course. Significant amounts of adrenocorticotropic hormone—ACTH—have been demonstrated in the tumor tissue and blood of many of these patients. By physiologic, physiochemical, and immunochemical tests, the ectopic ACTH is indistinguishable from the normal hormone, although the tumors have physiologic autonomy because dexamethasone fails to suppress the levels of end prod-

Table 76–5. Classification of Extrapulmonary Manifestations of Carcinoma of the Lung

Metabolic
 Cushing's syndrome
 Excessive antidiuretic hormone
 Hypercalcemia
 Ectopic gonadotropin
Neuromuscular
 Carcinomatous myopathy
 Peripheral neuropathies
 Subacute cerebellar degeneration
 Encephalomyelopathy
Skeletal
 Clubbing
 Pulmonary hypertrophic osteoarthropathy
Dermatologic
 Acanthosis nigricans
 Scleroderma
 Other dermatoses
Vascular
 Migratory thrombophlebitis
 Nonbacterial verrucal endocarditis
 Arterial thrombosis
Hematologic
 Anemia
 Fibrinolytic purpura
 Nonspecific leukocytosis
 Polycythemia

ucts of ACTH in the urine. Excessive quantities of hydroxycorticosteroids—17-OHCS—are readily demonstrable in the urine; the normal levels are usually less than 12 mg per day. Blocking the synthesis of steroids with the appropriate drugs has not been valuable except for short-term relief of symptoms of hyperadrenocorticism. At times, aldactone may relieve the hypokalemic alkalosis. Although the incidence of response is unknown, the signs and symptoms of the syndrome may be ameliorated by appropriate chemotherapy when the tumor is of the undifferentiated small cell type.

Excessive Antidiuretic Hormone Production. This occurs most often in patients with small cell tumors. One third of the patients with this type of tumor have some degree of hyponatremia. Bondy and Gilby (1982) reported it to be more common in women than in men—54% versus 25%. In 12 such patients, Bartter and Schwartz (1967) reported the positive immunoassay of an arginine-vasopressin-like material. The symptoms are water intoxication with anorexia, nausea, and vomiting, accompanied by increasingly severe neurologic complications. Hypotonicity of the plasma, hyponatremia, persistent renal sodium loss, relative hypertonicity of the urine, or absence of clinical evidence of fluid depletion, and normal renal and adrenal function may be the presenting situation. Treatment consists of fluid restriction in the mild cases. Hypertonic saline solution when used should be infused carefully. Demeclocyline, which produces a reversible pharmacologic nephrogenic diabetes insipidus, has been suggested as a good therapeutic alternative. An appropriate chemotherapeutic regimen also is indicated.

Hypercalcemia. This is a frequent complication of malignant disease, and although it often represents bony metastases, it may be caused by excessive secretion of a polypeptide, similar to parathyroid hormone, by the tumor. An accompanying hypophosphatemia frequently occurs. Most of the tumors associated with hypercalcemia are of the squamous cell type. Clinically, the patient may have somnolence and mental changes as well as anorexia, nausea, vomiting, and weight loss. Frequently, the tumors are resectable, and this has resulted in a reversal of the abnormal calcium levels in the blood. Recurrence of the tumor has led to a return of the hypercalcemia. At recurrence, as well as preoperatively, the hypercalcemia can be controlled by neutral phosphate or saline infusions, combined with furosemide-induced diuresis. Plicamycin—a single dose at 25 mg per kg body weight—is the most effective treatment.

Ectopic Gonadotropin Production. This occurs rarely in association with carcinoma of the lung. Gonadotropin production has been documented in some male patients with tender gynecomastia, often associated with hypertrophic pulmonary osteoarthropathy. In one patient reported by Faiman and his associates (1967), radioimmunoassay of blood samples taken at operation showed increased gonadotropin activity after passage through the lung containing the tumor. Gonadotropic activity of the tumor tissue also was established. These tumors resemble undifferentiated large cell carcinoma histologically. Adenocarcinomas also produce human chorionic gonadotropin in tissue culture.

Other Hormone Levels. Elevated levels of calcitonin have been documented by numerous investigators, including Gilby (1976) and Hansen (1980) and associates. Its production occurs mostly in small cell tumors. Increased levels of growth hormone occur in patients with lung cancer of all types.

The production of prolactin, serotonin, gastrin, insulin, or somatostatin by lung cancer has not been supported by convincing evidence in the literature.

Neuromuscular Manifestations

The carcinomatous neuromyopathies are the most frequent extrathoracic, nonmetastatic manifestions of carcinoma of the lung. If they are specifically looked for, one or more types of neuromyopathy can be found in approximately 15% of these patients. In the combined series of patients with such manifestations reported by Morton and his colleagues (1966), 56% had small cell carcinoma, 22% squamous cell carcinoma, 16% anaplastic tumor, and 5% adenocarcinoma. Half of the patients had no other symptoms of the lung tumor, and in one third, the neuromyopathy preceded, by 1 year or more, the symptoms or the dignosis of the carcinoma.

Carcinomatous Myopathies. These are the more common syndromes. The two types seen are the myasthenic-like syndrome and polymyositis. The former—the Eaton-Lambert syndrome—is probably a defect of neuromuscular conduction and is characterized by weakness and marked fatigability of the proximally located muscles of the extremities, particularly those of the pelvic girdle and thighs. Polymyositis resembles the myasthenic syndrome, except that muscular wasting is more prominent, and a primary degeneration of the muscle fibers occurs.

Peripheral Neuropathy. This may be purely sensory, with pain and paresthesias followed by complete sensory loss in the extremities. Often, however, this is found in association with motor neuropathy, as evidenced by muscular weakness and wasting. Neuropathologic findings consist of loss of neurons in the dorsal root ganglia and selective degeneration of the posterior roots and columns of the spinal cord. The anterior roots are relatively unaffected.

Subacute Cerebellar Degeneration. This results in a rapidly progressive loss of cerebellar function. Ataxic gait, lack of coordination, vertigo, nystagmus, and dysarthria are the characteristic features. Diffuse degeneration and depletion of Purkinje cells, as well as other degenerative changes, occur in the cerebellum.

Encephalomyelopathy. This is manifested by a wide range of psychiatric disorders, such as dementia, deterioration of memory, and mood disorders. If the brain stem is involved, the symptoms depend on the distribution of the lesions. Pyramidal tract signs and pseudobulbar palsy may occur.

The cause and pathogenesis of these neuropathies are unclear. The current hypothesis is that they arise as autoimmune or altered immune responses to substances produced by the tumor cells.

The recognition and differentiation of these neuromyopathies from metastatic lesions are important, because resection of the lung tumor may be possible. Remission of the symptoms may occur after successful removal of the tumor.

Skeletal Manifestations

The most frequent peripheral sign of bronchial carcinoma is clubbing of the fingers, which at times is associated with generalized hypertrophic pulmonary osteoarthropathy. The periosteal proliferation and new-bone formation (Fig. 76–6) at the ends of the long bones may occur before other symptoms of the lung lesion arise.

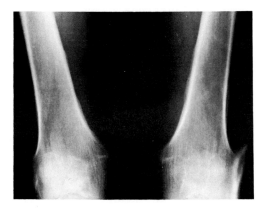

Fig. 76–6. Roentgenogram of the lower end of both femurs showing marked periosteal changes in a patient with bronchial carcinoma and hypertrophic pulmonary osteoarthropathy.

The clinical features and theories of pathogenesis of these skeletal signs are discussed in Chapter 60.

The incidence of hypertrophic pulmonary osteoarthropathy in patients with carcinoma of the lung has been reported to be from 2 to 12%. Yacoub (1965) noted an incidence of 4%. Interestingly, hypertrophic pulmonary osteoarthropathy was not found in patients with small cell tumors, but its incidence in patients with the other three major cell types was equally distributed.

Dermatologic Manifestations

The development of acanthosis nigricans in the adult may be associated with bronchial adenocarcinoma. Scleroderma, dermatomyositis, erythema gyratum, acquired ichthyosis, and nonspecific dermatoses also may occur in patients with bronchial carcinoma.

Vascular Manifestations

Thrombophlebitis, recurrent or migratory, was the first indication of the presence of bronchial tumor in 0.3% of the patients reported by Le Roux (1968a). Nonbacterial veruccal—marantic—endocarditis, characterized by deposition of sterile fibrin plaques on the heart valves and resultant arterial embolization, may occur. The mechanism by which either of these complications takes place is unknown.

Hematologic Manifestations

These signs are nonspecific. Normocytic, normochromic anemia, fibrinolytic purpura, erythrocytosis, and nonspecific leukocytosis have been reported in patients with bronchial carcinoma.

ROENTGENOGRAPHIC FEATURES

The roentgenographic findings caused by carcinoma of the lung may result from the tumor itself; changes in the pulmonary parenchyma distal to a bronchus obstructed by the tumor—atelectasis, infection, or both; and spread of the tumor to extrapulmonary intrathoracic sites—hilar and mediastinal lymph nodes, pleura, chest wall, and other mediastinal structures. Thus, the findings vary with the location, the cell type, and the length of time that the tumor has been present.

Garland (1966) estimated that when a lung tumor is first detectable on a chest roentgenogram, it has completed three fourths of its natural history. Rigler (1957) observed that the roentgenographic abnormality frequently antedates the first symptoms or signs of the disease by seven or more months. These early features are, unfortunately, subtle, and often are appreciated only in retrospect.

Early Roentgenographic Features

The early signs visible in the roentgenograms of the chest, as Rigler (1966) noted, are produced directly by the tumor itself. These signs may be listed as: a density within the lung parenchyma, that is, a homogeneous density—a rounded nodule with sharp borders or with irregular and poorly defined borders—or a linear-shaped lesion, nonhomogeneous in density; cavitation within a solid tumor; a segmental, indistinct, poorly defined dense area; a nodular streaked, local infiltration along the course of a blood vessel; segmental consolidation; a roughly triangular lesion arising in the apex and extending toward the hilus; a mediastinal mass—an uncommon early sign; an enlargement of one hilus; segmental or lobar obstructive emphysema—a rare finding in carcinoma of the lung; and segmental atelectasis.

The relative incidences of these various early changes are difficult, if not impossible, to discern, because most patients have more advanced disease when first seen. In all patients with bronchial carcinoma, however, the roentgenogram of the chest is abnormal in 97 to 98%, and the abnormality is most suggestive of tumor in over four fifths of all these patients.

Usual Roentgenographic Manifestations

Byrd and his associates (1969) classified these manifestations as hilar, pulmonary parenchymal, and intra-

Table 76–6.   Classification of Radiographic Abnormalities Associated with Bronchial Carcinoma

Region Involved	Type of Involvement
Hilus	Hilar prominence: slight enlargement of structures in hilar area without discrete mass Hilar mass: discrete mass limited to hilar area Perihilar mass: discrete mass limited to perihilar area with center within 4 cm of hilus
Pulmonary parenchyma	Small mass: single mass 4 cm or less in diameter within substance of lung, not necessarily with well-defined border Large mass: single mass greater than 4 cm in diameter within substance of lung, not necessarily with well-defined border Apical mass: single mass of any size limited to apex of lung Multiple masses: two or more masses of any diameter within substance of lung Hypertranslucency: increased radiolucency of lung lobe or segment Evidence of bronchial obstruction: collapse, consolidation, or pneumonitis in lung, lobe, or segment
Intrathoracic extrapulmonary structures	Mediastinal mass or widening: local or diffuse enlargement of normal mediastinal shadow Chest wall: erosion or interruption in normal contours of chest-wall structures or vertebrae Pleural effusion Elevation of hemidiaphragm

Byrd, R.B., et al.: Radiographic abnormalities in carcinoma of the lung as related to histological cell type. Thorax *24*:573, 1969.

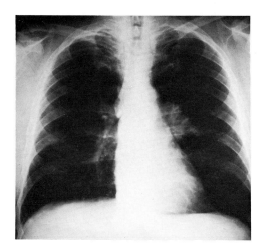

Fig. 76–7. PA roentgenogram of the chest showing a left hilar mass. Mediastinotomy revealed metastatic squamous cell carcinoma in the subaortic lymph nodes.

thoracic extrapulmonary (Table 76–6 and Figs. 76–7 through 76–14). In their review of the chest roentgenograms of 600 patients with carcinoma of the lung, a hilar abnormality either alone or associated with other abnormalities was present in 41% of the patients. Obstructive pneumonitis, collapse, or consolidation was also present in 41%. A large parenchymal mass was present in 21.7% and a small mass in 20.3%; multiple masses were present in only 1.1%. An apical mass was found in 2.6% of the patients, and in no patient was hypertranslucency seen. The various extrapulmonary intrathoracic manifestations were present in 11%, mediastinal widening and pleural effusion being the more common of these. Amemiya and Oho (1982) (Table 76–7) and Swett and associates (1982) noted that a peripheral nodular mass is now the most common roentgenographic presentation of bronchial carcinoma.

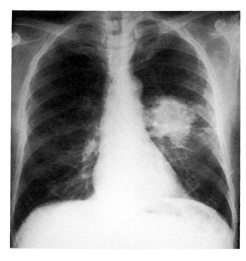

Fig. 76–8. PA roentgenogram of the chest showing a large perihilar mass located in the left upper lobe. Undifferentiated cell carcinoma on biopsy. Pulmonary function precluded resection.

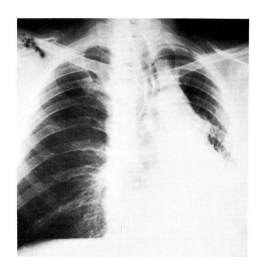

Fig. 76–9. PA roentgenogram of the chest showing atelectasis of the left lower lobe. Squamous cell carcinoma present in the left main stem bronchus.

Influence of Cell Type

Certain roentgenographic patterns are characteristic of the various cell types. From Byrd and his associates' (1969) study, several generalities can be made.

Squamous cell carcinoma most often presents the picture of obstructive pneumonitis, collapse, or consolidation. A hilar abnormality also is often present. Approximately one third of the squamous cell tumors appear as a peripheral mass, two thirds of which are usually larger than 4 cm. Cavitation is more common in these peripheral squamous cell carcinomas than in other lung carcinomas and occurs in one fifth of the patients with these tumors. Cavitation, in these instances, results from necrosis within the tumor mass, but cavitation and abscess formation also may occur distal to a bronchus obstructed by tumor. When both types of cavities are combined, they constitute approximately 50% of all lung abscesses seen in patients over 50 years of age. Also, in 3 to 4% of squamous cell tumors, the roentgenogram of the chest may show no abnormality, the tumor being located in a main stem bronchus and producing no changes in the parenchyma distal to it.

Adenocarcinomas are most often peripheral masses, and two thirds of these are larger than 4 cm. Cavitation is rare, and either a hilar abnormality or an obstructive parenchymal lesion is noted only infrequently.

Large cell undifferentiated carcinomas are most likely to be peripheral lesions—approximately 60%—and two thirds of these also are larger than 4 cm. Cavitation occurs in only about 6% of these peripheral lesions. A hilar abnormality and parenchymal changes are each present in association with about one third of these tumors. Ten percent of the patients with this type of tumor have mediastinal widening.

Small cell undifferentiated tumors appear primarily as hilar abnormalities—78%. They are associated with mediastinal widening in 13% of the patients. A parenchymal obstructive lesion occurs in slightly less than 40% and a

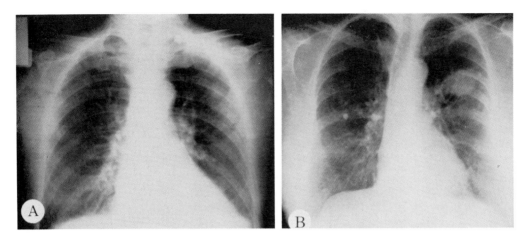

Fig. 76–10. Roentgenograms of two peripheral pulmonary masses. *A*, PA roentgenogram of the chest showing a small peripheral mass located in second anterior interspace on the left. A diagnosis of squamous cell carcinoma was made on microscopic examination of the resected lobe. *B*, PA roentgenogram of the chest showing a large peripheral mass in the left upper lobe. The tumor was found to be an adenocarcinoma on microscopic examination of the resected lobe.

peripheral mass in 29% of the subjects, three fourths being smaller than 4 cm.

Chest Roentgenography as a Screening Procedure

Because roentgenograms of the chest of almost all patients with carcinoma of the lung show an abnormality and the abnormality frequently antedates any symptoms, frequent chest roentgenograms have been suggested for high-risk populations to detect the disease earlier.

Such projects to date, however, have not yielded encouraging results. Gilbertsen (1964) reported a detection rate of 1 carcinoma in 5378 survey roentgenographic examinations, and Virtama (1962) found a detection rate of 0.41 per thousand, although in persons over 60 the rate was 9.89. Boucot (1961) and Weiss (1966, 1971) and their associates found a minimal yield and little or no gain in survivorship of patients who developed lung tumor while

under observation in the Philadelphia Project. Brett (1968) likewise found that early detection in a similar prospective study did not significantly reduce the mortality from lung carcinoma.

The National Cancer Institute has sponsored three randomized controlled trials of screening for early lung cancer by periodic sputum cytologic examinations and chest roentgenograms. The techniques were somewhat different in the three trials, which were reported by Melamed and associates (1984), Tockman (1986), and Sanderson (1986). As a prototype, however, the Mayo Lung Study, reported by Fontana and Sanderson (1986), is described briefly. Men over 45 years of age without known cancer of the lung who smoked one or more packs of cigarettes daily were initially screened by sputum studies and roentgenograms of the chest. Those found to have a lung cancer—a prevalence case— were treated

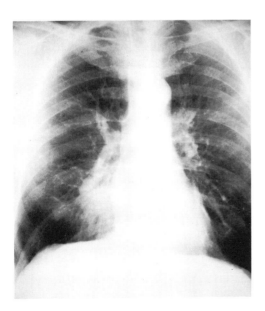
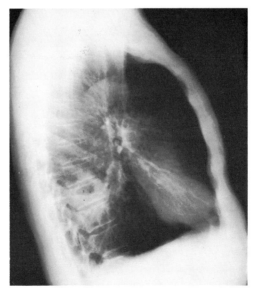

Fig. 76–11. PA and lateral roentgenograms of the chest revealing a carcinomatous—squamous cell—abscess in the right lower lobe.

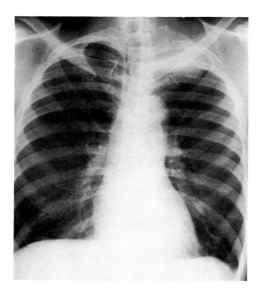

Fig. 76–12. PA roentgenogram of the chest showing the typical appearance of carcinoma of the lung located in the left superior sulcus. Rib erosion was evident in both the first and second ribs.

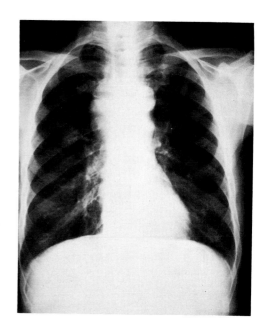

Fig. 76–14. PA roentgenogram of the chest showing a peripheral mass at the anterior end of the right third rib and a large superior mediastinal mass. Node biopsy revealed undifferentiated large cell carcinoma.

as indicated. The other patients without tumor were randomized into two groups, one group to undergo repeat screening examinations every four months. In the other group, the control group; at least yearly screening was recommended. Any tumor subsequently found in either group was an incidence case. The initial screening identified a prevalence rate of 8.3/1000. Of these cases, 65% were detected by roentgenography alone, 19% by cytology alone and 16% by both modalities. Only half of the roentgenographically identified tumors could be resected for cure, whereas almost all of the ones identified by cytology were resected. The poorest group—only 3 of 15 patients could be resected—was that in which both studies were positive. There was a 30% 5-year post-treatment survivorship. The incidence in the group screened every four months was 5.5 incidence cases/1000 person-years of surveillance. Only 44% of the "incidence" cancers were picked up by the screening tests; 20% of these were detected by cytology alone and the other 80% by roentgenographic abnormalities. The other 56% of new cancers were discovered because of symptoms or a non-

Table 76–7. Roentgenographic Findings in 200 Patients with Lung Cancer

Tumor in the Periphery of the Lung	39.5%
Hilar Tumor	19.5%
Atelectasis	13.5%
Pleural Effusion	7.0%
Hilar Invasion	5.0%
Normal	4.0%
Infiltrative Shadow in the Periphery	3.0%
Other	8.5%

Adapted with permission from Amemiya, R., Oho, K.: X-ray diagnosis of lung cancer. In Hayata, Y., (ed): Lung Cancer Diagnosis, New York, Igaku-Shoin, 1982.

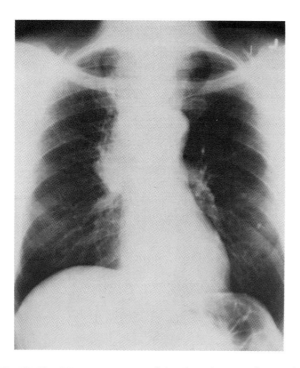

Fig. 76–13. PA roentgenogram of the chest showing a large right hilar mass and a widened superior mediastinum. Biopsy revealed epidermoid carcinoma.

study chest roentgenogram obtained for other reasons. In the control group the incidence was 4.3 cases/1000 person-years. The patients with cytologically detected lesions did well—80% 5-year survival with noncancer deaths excluded. The survival in the asymptomatic patients with radiologically discovered tumors was only approximately 40%. Those patients with symptomatic tumors did poorly—only a 10% long-term survival. Unfortunately, despite the better lung cancer detection, resectability rates and survival rates in the screened group as compared to the control group, there was no overall difference between the two groups in either total mortality or mortality as a result of lung cancer. No survival differences were detected in either of the other two studies as well. Thus routine screening, especially cytologic screening, remains inappropriate for the general population and some even question the use of routine roentgenograms of the chest as a screening modality.

Special Roentgenographic Studies

In addition to the routine roentgenograms of the chest taken with the patient in the posteroanterior and lateral positions, other roentgenograms of the chest can be obtained with the patient in the right or left anterior oblique, the lordotic, or other special positions to delineate further any suspected lesion. Other roentgenographic studies—laminography, 55° oblique tomography, bronchography, contrast study of the esophagus, angiography, azygography, and pneumomediastinography, as well as radioisotopic scanning of the lungs—can be obtained to aid further in the diagnosis and determination of appropriate therapy in patients with bronchial carcinoma.

Computed Tomography and Magnetic Resonance Imaging

Computed tomography in patients suspected of having lung cancer has become almost routine. Like any other noninvasive examination, however, it cannot distinguish inflammatory tissue from cancer tissue. It is excellent for demonstrating vertebral body invasion but not invasion of the ribs or other adjacent structures—pericardium, aorta, or chest wall. With contrast infusion it may suggest invasion or encirclement of vital structures in the mediastinum. Unsuspected pleural fluid also may be found. Its greatest use however, is in determining roentgenologically nondemonstrable mediastinal lymph node enlargement. Lymph nodes smaller than 1 cm may be considered normal in most instances. Metastatic disease, however, may be present in 4 to 6% of such normal-sized nodes, but in almost all instances such nodes can be resected completely. Lymph nodes from 1 to 2 cm in size are considered indeterminate and a high percentage contain tumor, but in 15 to 20% the enlargement is caused by inflammation. Thus, all enlarged nodes should be further evaluated by one of the various biopsy techniques.

The enlarged lymph nodes identified on the CT scan can be designated and mapped by the schema suggested by the American Thoracic Society (1983) (Fig. 76–15)

(Table 76–8). The identification of enlarged nodes and their anatomical location may permit a more appropriate use of either mediastinoscopy or mediastinotomy for mediastinal exploration. Lymph nodes over 2 to 3 cm can generally be seen on standard films. When this is the case, a CT scan need not be done and biopsy only is indicated.

High resolution CT can also be used to determine the calcium content of peripheral solitary masses. This is discussed in the following section on the asymptomatic solitary pulmonary nodule.

The role of magnetic resonance imaging in evaluating the patient with lung cancer has yet to be determined. MRI appears to be no better in determining lymph node involvement but may in time be more valuable in demonstrating local invasion of adjacent structures. Also, it can be used effectively when contrast material is contraindicated. Likewise, it can produce views in the coronal and sagittal planes, which at times may be helpful (see Chapter 14).

Asymptomatic Solitary Pulmonary Nodule

A circumscribed, solitary, peripheral lung mass—the pulmonary coin lesion—in the symptomless patient, as noted, frequently represents a relatively early primary carcinoma of the lung. Often, however, it is an inflammatory mass, a vascular lesion, a benign tumor, or even a solitary metastasis in the lung (Table 76–9).

Several criteria have been suggested for designating a roentgenographic shadow as a coin lesion. It should be spherical or ovoid, relatively well demarcated, and small, and it should be surrounded by air-containing lung, although it may be located just beneath the visceral pleura of the lung. The actual margins of the lesion may vary from ill defined to sharply demarcated, and the size may vary from less than 1 cm to over 6 cm. I believe, however, that no lesion larger than 3 cm should be included in the category. Rarely is a solitary lesion smaller than 1 cm recognized on the standard roentgenogram, the limit of visibility being 0.7 to 0.8 cm. Calcification may be present and, occasionally, small satellite lesions may also appear.

In determining clinically whether the lesion is benign or malignant, certain roentgenographic features, size, contour, calcification, and growth, are helpful, but in no one patient, with few exceptions, can these features be considered absolutely diagnostic.

Siegelman and associates (1980) suggested using computed tomography to evaluate the density of the lesion to determine its benignancy or malignancy. Benign lesions have high densities because of microcalcification and thus have high Hounsfield numbers—HU—and malignant ones have lower densities because they lack microcalcifications. Although this group succeeded in determining the nature of most solitary peripheral nodules—a CT number greater than 164 HU indicated benignancy and a lower one probable malignancy—other groups such as Swett and associates (1982) have had difficulty in reproducing their results. To overcome this problem, a special lung nodule simulator has been de-

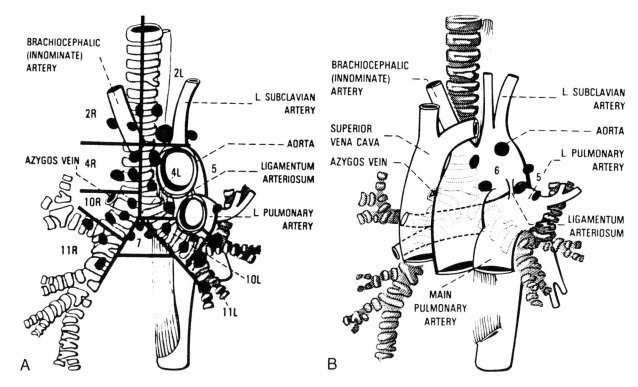

Fig. 76–15. *A*, ATS map of regional pulmonary nodes. *B*, Separation of nodal stations 5 and 6 requires anterior thoracostomy. (Reproduced with permission of the American Thoracic Society: Clinical staging of primary lung cancer. Am. Rev. Respir. Dis. *127*:659, 1983.)

veloped so that a standard reference can be applied to any scanner. Thus, measurements should be accurately reproduced and can be compared to the nodules of reference.

In addition to tumor density determinations, the use of high resolution CT—HRCT—with scans 1.0 to 1.5 mm thick through the nodule, as Aberle (1987) pointed out, permits precise definition of the interface of the nodule with the adjacent parenchyma, as well as determination of the calcium content. As noted, HRCT nodule densitometry is predicated on both qualitative and quantitative observations, which may indicate the benignancy of a lesion. The calcification should represent over 10% of the nodule and the pattern of calcification should be symmetric, such as central, diffuse, laminated, or popcorn in distribution. Aberle (1987) noted that coin lesions larger than 2 to 3 cm or those with spiculated margins may be malignant. The percentage of benign and malignant lesions in any given series of coin lesions varies with the patient selection and the definition of such a lesion. In the general population, 5% of such lesions discovered by a routine roentgenographic survey are carcinomas. In series in which resections have been performed, however, 50% of such masses in patients over 50 years of age are carcinomas. Further, this percentage increases with the advancing age of the patient group.

Steele (1963), in reviewing a series of 887 resected, solitary pulmonary nodules in males, found that 316 were malignant, 65 were benign tumors, 474 were granulomas, and the remaining 32 were miscellaneous lesions. Of the malignant lesions, approximately 8% were met-

astatic, but in only 3 of these 26 patients was there no history of treatment of a previous malignant tumor; 2 of these patients had carcinoma of the kidney and 1 had an undetected primary carcinoma of the lung. Thus, only 1% of all of the patients with malignant lesions and less than 0.4% of all the patients with coin lesions had metastatic disease in the lungs from either an unknown or an asymptomatic tumor elsewhere in the body. Consequently, any extensive evaluation of the patient with a coin lesion for a possible occult primary tumor has little potential reward. I believe that extensive evaluation is not indicated unless the patient has symptoms relating to a specific organ system or the routine laboratory studies reveal an abnormality, such as hematuria, that suggests the possibility of an occult tumor. Nystrom and associates (1979) documented the futility of routine roentgenographic evaluation of asymptomatic organ systems.

In evaluating a coin lesion, a standard history, a physical examination, and laboratory and roentgenographic studies should be obtained. Bronchoscopy is optional in the diagnostic evaluation. Skin tests should be performed for *Mycobacterium tuberculosis* and the fungi. Sputum smears for detecting acid-fast organisms and cytologic studies should be made, and laminographic study of the lesion carried out. When the issue of the presence of calcification remains unresolved, CT and HRCT may be done.

Any previous roentgenograms of the chest should be reviewed when available. Nathan and his associates (1962) noted that in patients over 40, solitary peripheral

Table 76–8.   Proposed Definitions of Regional Nodal Stations for Prethoracotomy Staging

X	Supraclavicular nodes.
2R	Right upper paratracheal (suprainnominate) nodes: nodes to the right of the midline of the trachea between the intersection of the caudal margin of the innominate artery with the trachea, and the apex of the lung. (Includes highest R mediastinal node.) (Radiologists may use the same caudal margin as in 2L.)
2L	Left upper paratracheal (supra-aortic) nodes: nodes to the left of the midline of the trachea between the top of the aortic arch and the apex of the lung. (Includes highest L mediastinal node.)
4R	Right lower paratracheal nodes: nodes to the right of the midline of the trachea between the cephalic border of the azygos vein and the intersection of the caudal margin of the brachiocephalic artery with the right side of the trachea. (Includes some pretracheal and paracaval nodes.) (Radiologists may use the same cephalic margin as in 4L.)
4L	Left lower paratracheal nodes: nodes to the left of the midline of the trachea between the top of the aortic arch and the level of the carina, medial to the ligamentum arteriosum. (Includes some pretracheal nodes.)
5	Aortopulmonary nodes: subaortic and para-aortic nodes, lateral to the ligamentum arteriosum or the aorta or left pulmonary artery, proximal to the first branch of the LPA.
6	Anterior mediastinal nodes: nodes anterior to the ascending aorta or the innominate artery. (Includes some pretracheal and preaortic nodes.)
7	Subcarinal nodes: nodes rising caudal to the carina of the trachea but not associated with the lower lobe bronchi or arteries within the lung.
8	Paraesophageal nodes: nodes dorsal to the posterior wall of the trachea and to the right or left of the midline of the esophagus. (Includes retrotracheal, but not subcarinal nodes.)
9	Right or left pulmonary ligament nodes: nodes within the right or left pulmonary ligament.
10R	Right tracheobronchial nodes: nodes to the right of the midline of the trachea from the level of the cephalic border of the azygos vein to the origin of the right upper lobe bronchus.
10L	Left peribronchial nodes: nodes to the left of the midline of the trachea between the carina and the left upper lobe bronchus, medial to the ligamentum arteriosum.
11	Intrapulmonary nodes: nodes removed in the right or left lung specimen plus those distal to the main stem bronchi or secondary carina. (Includes interlobar, lobar, and segmental nodes.)*

*Post-thoracotomy staging: nodes could be divided into stations 11, 12, 13 according to the AJC classification.

With permission of American Thoracic Society: Clinical staging of primary lung cancer. Am. Rev. Respir. Dis. *127*:659, 1983.

lesions with a doubling time of less than 37 days are almost always benign, as are those lesions with a doubling time of more than 465 days. Most malignant lesions have a doubling time between 37 and 280 days. Meyer (1973) noted a relationship between the doubling time and prognosis. Those patients with doubling times of less than 80 days had the least favorable prognosis and those with doubling times over 150 days the most favorable.

If the lesion has been unchanged for years or if any one of three specific types of calcification—laminar layers, large central core, or popcorn distribution of the calcium—appears, the lesion can be considered benign and may be observed periodically roentgenographically.

When acid-fast organisms are present in the sputum the patient should receive appropriate antituberculous chemotherapy and the lesion should be re-evaluated within 2 to 3 months. When none of these features is present, particularly if the patient is over 34 years of age, the lesion should be removed for diagnosis as well as treatment. I question the routine use of percutaneous transthoracic needle biopsy, although when the lesion is likely a hamartoma, a needle biopsy is indicated (see Chapter 77).

Cummings and his colleagues (1986a, b) evaluated the decision process in the management of the solitary peripheral nodule extensively. The size of the lesion, the age of the patient, and the smoking history are the important factors that should be considered. The larger the lesion, the older the patient, and the more the patient smokes cigarettes, the more likely it is that the lesion is malignant.

DIAGNOSTIC PROCEDURES

In addition to various roentgenographic studies used to diagnose carcinoma of the lung, several surgical and laboratory procedures are employed, more or less routinely, to evaluate patients with suspected tumors of the lung.

Cytologic Studies

Cytologic examination of sputum has been highly rewarding in patients suspected of having carcinoma of the lung. With appropriate cytologic study of several sputum specimens, tumor cells are found in 45% to as many as 90% of the patients. Oswald and his associates (1971) reported that in patients with primary lung cancer, the study of one or more sputum samples yielded a 59% positive result, three samples a 69%, and four samples an 85% positive result. They found a false-positive incidence of only 0.7%, although in most laboratories the reported incidence is approximately 2 to 3%.

Cell type as determined by cytologic study agrees with the final histologic diagnosis in approximately 85% of patients. Lange and Høeg (1972) found that the comparison of cytologic and histologic diagnosis in a group of lung carcinomas showed that well differentiated epidermoid carcinomas, undifferentiated small cell carcinomas, and adenocarcinoma could be effectively typed by cytology. Kato (1982) found the accuracy of cytologic diagnosis and definitive diagnosis to be 90 to 100% in small cell carcinoma, 92 to 96% in squamous cell carcinoma and 87 to 97% in adenocarcinoma. The undifferentiated carcinomas, the poorly differentiated epidermoid carcinomas, and combined carcinomas were more difficult to type correctly.

Cytologic studies are most often positive in patients with large tumors that involve the main bronchi. Peripheral lesions frequently do not communicate with a bronchus, and the results in patients with such lesions are less rewarding.

To improve the yield in patients with more peripherally placed lesions, bronchial brushing has been carried

Table 76–9.   Causes of Coin Lesion

Neoplasms	Inflammatory lesions	Malformations
Primary carcinoma	Tuberculoma and tuberculous lesions	Arterio-venous malformation
Solitary metastases	Histoplasmosis	Vascular endothelioma
Primary sarcoma	Coccidioidomycosis	Sequestrated segment
Bronchial adenoma	Cryptococcus	Traumatic lesions
Reticuloses	Nonspecific granuloma	Haematoma
Mixed tumor	Chronic lung abscess	Hernias
Fibroma	Lipoid pneumonia	Cysts
Myxoma	Massive fibrosis	Bronchogenic
Neurogenic tumors	Rheumatoid granuloma	Pericardial
Lipoma	Gumma	Dermoid
Hibernoma	Parasitic lesions	Teratoma
Mesothelioma	Hydatid cysts	Infarct
Leiomyoma	Ascaris lumbricoides	
Plasmocytoma	Mycetoma	
Thymoma		
Endometriosis		

Bateson, E.M.: Analysis of 155 solitary lung lesions illustrating the differential diagnosis of mixed tumors of the lung. Clin. Radiol. *16*:60, 1965.

out via a bronchial catheter under fluoroscopic, image-intensifier guidance systems and during fiber-optic bronchoscopic examination. Fennesy (1968), Hattori and Matsuda (1971), and Faber and associates (1973), as well as others, reported excellent results with these techniques.

Cytologic Screening

Because of the high diagnostic yield in known bronchial carcinoma, cytologic study of the sputum had been suggested as a screening procedure. As noted in the aforementioned section on screening procedures (p. 905), this technique cannot be recommended for the general population. Although cytologic screening is the least successful method of prospective screening even in heavy smokers, when a positive cytologic smear is the only evidence of cancer—roentgenographic occult disease—resection once the disease is located is highly effective. In such patients, every effort to locate the disease, including repeated fiber-optic bronchoscopy with or without differential mucosal staining techniques, is indicated. Resection without identification of a lesion is not recommended. Of course, disease in the oral pharynx and esophagus must be ruled out in the patient's evaluation.

Tumor Markers

Various substances, including the aforementioned hormone-like substances, are produced in excess in some patients with carcinoma of the lung. The value of these hormonal substances, particularly "big" ACTH—the biologically inactive precursor form—described by Ayvazian (1975) and Gewirtz (1974) and their colleagues, as well as the oncofetal carcinoembryonic antigen—CEA—and the products associated with increased cell turnover, β_2-microglobulin and polyamines, in diagnosis of patients with bronchial carcinoma and in predicting prognosis after surgical treatment has been studied. Unfortunately, despite the observation that these levels may be elevated in patients with bronchial carcinoma, the levels are not diagnostic because these substances may be elevated by other nonspecific causes. Elevated levels of these substances are frequently found in smokers, particularly patients with chronic lung disease. Yalow and her associates (1979) reported that the measurement of pre- and postoperative immunoreactive "big" ACTH had no value in predicting either remission or long-term survival. On the other hand, Concannon (1978) and Vincent (1979) and their colleagues suggested that CEA levels may have prognostic value in the postoperative period. The nonspecific origins of β_2-microglobulin and the polyamines, as Hallgren (1980) and Durie (1977) and their associates noted, render them poor tumor markers in the patient with bronchial carcinoma.

Tumor biomarkers are more common in small cell carcinoma (Table 76–10), and a few may be helpful in following therapeutic responses. Also, these may help differentiate the "classic" oat cell and intermediate cell types from the variant form, which usually produces less of these substances. The variant form responds poorly to chemotherapy, as numerous investigators have noted.

Roentgenographic Studies

Although no roentgenographic technique can establish a histologic diagnosis, appropriate studies can demonstrate involvement that may preclude resection. Involvement of the main stem pulmonary artery, demonstrated by angiocardiography, or fixation and distortion of the esophagus, revealed by a barium swallow, are examples.

Pulmonary Angiography

Although this study is used infrequently in evaluating resectablity of centrally located tumors, Sanders and associates (1962) reported several findings indicating nonresectablity with this angiographic procedure. The most important were: involvement of the ipsilateral pulmonary artery within 1.5 cm of its origin on the left and involvement just proximal to the takeoff of the truncus anterior branch on the right, involvement of the pulmonary veins

Table 76–10. Candidates for Tumor Biomarkers in Lung Cancer

Substance	Frequency of occurrence in (cell type)	
	Small cell	Non-small cell
Polypeptide hormones		
ACTH[a]	+ +	+
ADH (Arginine vasopressin)[a,b] neuro-physins	+ +	±
Calcitonin[b]	+ + +	+
Bombesin[c] (gastrin-releasing peptides)	+ + +	+
Human placental lactogen		
Human chorionic gonadotropin	+	+
Parathyroid hormone	–	+
Growth hormone		
Enzymes		
Dopa decarboxylase[c]	+ +	–
Neuron-specific enolase[b]	+ +	–
Histaminase[c]	+ +	–
Creatine kinase[c]	+ +	–
Biogenic amines[c]		
Serotonin	+	–
5-Hydroxytryptophan	+	–
Histamine	+	–
Tumor-associated antigens		
Carcinoembryonic antigen[b]	+ +	+ +
Cell surface proteins[c]		
Morphologic markers[c]		
Electron-dense granules[b]	+ +	±
Specific chromosome abnormality	+	–

[a]Clinical syndrome associated with elevated marker level
[b]Clinically useful for monitoring therapy
[c]Primarily identified in tumor tissue
Reproduced with permission of Krauss, S.: Peptide hormones as tumor markers in lung cancer patients. *In* Peptide Hormones in Lung Cancer. Edited by K. Havemann, G. Sorenson, and C. Group. Recent Results Cancer Res. *99*:177, 1985.

as they enter the pericardium, and involvement of either innominate vein or the superior vena cava.

Azygography

This study, now only infrequently done, may reveal mediastinal lymph node involvement as well as involvement of the vena cava by the tumor. Gray and colleagues (1968), in the preoperative evaluation of 40 patients with bronchial carcinoma, found that 90% of those with gross abnormality demonstrated by azygography had nonresectable carcinoma. The examination was considered abnormal when a blockage or frank interruption of the radiopaque material appeared in the venous pattern or when reflux of the contrast medium away from the heart, either to the vertebral plexus or into the inferior vena cava, occurred.

Benfield and his associates (1969) combined azygography with intravenous pulmonary angiography in selecting patients with carcinoma of the lung for thoracotomy. Of the 34 patients deemed to have an unresectable tumor according to the study, 22 underwent an explor-

atory thoracotomy, and none of these had a resectable lesion. Unfortunately, resection was possible in only 19 of 35 patients who were judged to have resectable lesions. Thus, if the study yields positive results, it provides a helpful evaluation, but if negative, it has little value.

Pneumomediastinography

This examination was also suggested as a diagnostic procedure. Bariety and his associates (1965) insufflated filtered air into the mediastinal space and made tomograms and routine roentgenographic views of the chest to evaluate 250 patients with primary bronchial carcinoma. Pneumomediastinography in these patients did not establish a definitive diagnosis but helped delineate adhesions, infiltration of tumor, and hilar adenopathy. Little additional information, however, was gained by this special examination.

Laminography

In my experience, laminography, except to demonstrate the presence or absence of a central core or laminar calcification in peripheral solitary lesions has been of little or no value in helping to determine the nature of a parenchymal infiltrate, particularly that located in the hilar or perihilar area. Laminograms of the hilus taken in the 55° oblique position, however, help determine the presence or absence of lobar or hilar adenopathy but are not particularly suitable for evaluating the mediastinum.

Bronchography

This procedure is beneficial for a few patients to differentiate a benign parenchymal inflammatory process from an obstructive process caused by tumor in a peripheral bronchus beyond the field of bronchoscopic vision. Ikeda (1968), Eno (1976), and Osada (1982) reported that the Japanese have used this procedure extensively, but it is not frequently used in Europe or America.

Computed Tomography and Magnetic Resonance Imaging

The value of computed tomography and magnetic resonance imaging of the lungs and mediastinum in patients with carcinoma of the lung has been discussed in the section on Roentgenographic Features, page 901.

Radionuclide Studies

Ernst (1969), Maxfield (1971), and DeLaude (1974) and their associates found that radionuclide scanning of the lung is satisfactory for identifying the primary tumor. DeMeester and colleagues (1976, 1979) found that ^{67}Ga scanning may help identify metastatic deposits in the mediastinal lymph nodes. When the primary lung tumor concentrates ^{67}Ga and the mediastinum does not, mediastinal exploration is usually unrewarding. When the primary tumor picks up ^{67}Ga and overshadows the mediastinum or when the mediastinum concentrates ^{67}Ga, mediastinal exploration is indicated. DeMeester and associates (1976) recommended the use of specialized whole-body scans after the administration of ^{67}Ga to identify its concentration in distant metastatic sites. Brereton and colleagues (1978), however, were of the opinion that this technique is inferior to multiorgan system scans.

The routine use of multiple organ system scanning to detect occult metastatic sites is contraindicated. Ramsdell and associates (1977) and others have shown that when no signs nor symptoms of the specific organ system involvement are present, such investigations are unrewarding. CT scan or MRI of the brain in patients with adenocarcinoma has been suggested because of the high incidence of failure in this site that Mountain (1980), Immerman (1981), Martini (1983a), Feld (1984) and associates and the Ludwig Lung Cancer Study Group (1987) reported. Whether or not this would be useful, let alone cost-effective, remains to be evaluated. Hooper and associates (1984) wrote that in asymptomatic patients with any non-small cell tumor, CT of the brain is not indicated because of the low yield. MRI may, however, improve the yield in this situation.

Surgical Diagnostic Procedures

Bronchoscopy

The tracheobronchial tree in all patients suspected of having a tumor of the lung should be examined with either the rigid or flexible fiber-optic bronchoscope. An exception may be made in patients with a small, peripheral lesion with no evidence of hilar or mediastinal lymphadenopathy. Direct visualization of the tumor or positive biopsy findings, or both, are obtained in 25 to 50% of the patients. A higher positive diagnostic yield may be secured if many patients with far-advanced disease are included in any given series. Also, cell type influences the rate of positive findings. Small cell tumors are identified proportionately more often than squamous cell or large cell undifferentiated tumors are, and adenocarcinomas are identified least frequently of all.

In addition to actual assessment of the tumor, other valuable information can be obtained at bronchoscopy. The length of normal bronchus proximal to the tumor and the status of the carina can be determined. During bronchoscopy with the rigid scope, the mobility and rigidity of either main stem bronchus, as well as the bronchus intermedius on the right, can be evaluated.

Lymph Node Biopsy

Excision of lymph nodes in the supraclavicular fossa or in the mediastinum is indicated in many patients with bronchial carcinoma. Any palpable cervical lymph nodes should be excised for histologic study; most of these are involved by tumor. Biopsy of nonpalpable lymph nodes in the scalene area is no longer indicated in patients with suspected or known carcinoma of the lung. Ginsberg (personal communication), however, does recommend its use in all patients with superior sulcus tumors that are potentially resectable, as well as in patients with known large adenocarcinomas in the upper lobes. The former recommendation may be valid, but I don't believe the latter is.

Mediastinal exploration in many institutions is the standard preoperative method of evaluating the status of the mediastinal lymph nodes in most patients with potentially resectable carcinoma of the lung. This may be done by mediastinoscopy, as Carlens (1959) described, or by an extended cervical mediastinoscopy for left upper lobe lesions as Ginsberg and associates (1987) described, or through an anterior mediastinotomy, introduced by McNeill and Chamberlain (1966).

Pearson (1968) and associates (1982), Sarin and Nohl-Oser (1969), Paulson and Urschel (1971), Maassen (1985), and Coughlin (1985) and Cooper (1986) and their associates recommended mediastinoscopy as a routine procedure in all potentially operable patients. Approximately 27 to 34% of these patients have metastases to the mediastinal lymph nodes, but the examination is unrewarding in approximately 70% of the patients submitted to the procedure. Moreover, 10 to 20% of the patients with positive nodes may have resectable lesions. Martini and associates (1983b, 1985b) believe that such exploration is not indicated in any potential surgical candidate unless the mediastinum is grossly abnormal. With this approach, Martini and Flehinger (1987) reported that a complete resection could be carried out in 53% of the patients found to have unsuspected N2 disease. With either approach, a significant number of patients have an unnecessary invasive procedure.

I believe in a selective approach as reported by Backer and our group (1987). In patients with peripheral lesions and normal hilar and mediastinal shadows on standard roentgenograms of the chest, mediastinal exploration is not indicated in patients with non-small cell tumors. Involved mediastinal nodes are found in only approximately 5% of such patients. In patients in whom the hilus is enlarged, the mediastinal shadow is suggestively abnormal, or either structure is obscured by overlying tumor or parenchymal disease, a CT scan is done. When the scan is negative—nodes smaller than 1 cm, except for multiple small nodes 0.5 cm in size with known adenocarcinoma—no preoperative mediastinal exploration is done. Tumor involvement of the mediastinal nodes smaller than 1 cm is found in less than 5% at operation. When the nodes are 1 cm or larger, preoperative exploration is done and tumor involvement is present in 80 to 85% of such patients. This result contrasts markedly with the 27 to 34% positive yield in routine explorations. When the roentgenogram of the chest reveals a grossly abnormal mediastinal shadow, biopsy only is done to confirm the presence of tumor.

Needle Biopsy

Lauby and his associates (1965) suggested percutaneous, transthoracic needle biopsy as a routine for indeterminate, solitary peripheral lesions. Sagel (1978) and Mark (1978) and their associates found this procedure to be more accurate than flexible fiber-optic bronchoscopy in the diagnosis of peripheral tumors; it is even more accurate with CT-guided, fine-needle aspiration biopsy. In patients who have resectable lesions, however, other than establishing the diagnosis preoperatively, the procedure per se has little to do with the ultimate management of the patients. Needle biopsy is important in those patients who refuse operation, who are unsuitable for resection, or who have a nonresectable lesion in whom other diagnostic techniques have been unsuccessful.

Needle biopsy of the pleura in the presence of pleural effusion is positive for tumor in 60 to 75% of patients with proved bronchial carcinoma. In these patients, this procedure has a higher incidence of positive yield than bronchoscopy, scalene node biopsy, or even cytologic study has.

Transbronchoscopic needle biopsy has become popular in some institutions. It may be useful in the patient with an abnormal carina or enlarged paratracheal lymph nodes demonstrated by CT scan. Shure (1984) and Brynitz (1985) and associates and Wang (1986) described the techniques and results of this procedure.

Biopsy of Suspected Metastatic Deposits

This procedure is indicated when the physical findings or radionuclide or CT scan are positive. Patients with an apparently resectable tumor of the lung who have a positive liver scan should undergo either a needle or an open biopsy of the liver before a decision for definitive therapy is made. When mediastinal CT is done, routine scanning of the upper abdomen should be done as well. Occasionally, an occult lesion in the liver—3 to 6.5% in asymptomatic patients with normal liver functions—or enlargement of an adrenal gland is identified. Enlargement of the adrenal gland of less than 2 cm usually results from a benign tumor, but over 3 cm usually results from a malignant tumor (Fig. 76–16). In either situation, biopsy confirmation must be obtained. In patients with minimal local disease—T1N0—adrenal enlargement usually results from primary adrenal disease, although on rare occasions the adrenal is involved by metastases. The possibility of metastatic disease is increased when the mediastinal lymph nodes are involved—N2 disease. Pagani (1984) found unsuspected adrenal metastasis in

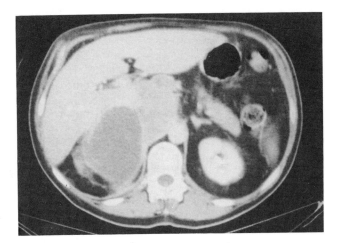

Fig. 76–16. CT scan of upper abdomen revealing a large adrenal mass. Percutaneous needle biopsy revealed the mass to be an occult metastatic large cell carcinoma from a simultaneous primary in the lung.

7.8% of patients thought to have only local chest disease; the extent of the local disease, however, was unrecorded.

Thoracotomy

Despite the many techniques available, many patients with bronchial carcinoma—approximately 20 to 25%—are operated on without a histologic diagnosis. Thus, exploratory thoracotomy becomes one of the most efficient means of diagnosis, particularly in those patients who have a resectable tumor. Thoracotomy, however, should not be used for diagnosis if the lesion does not appear to be resectable. One should avoid this procedure especially in elderly patients or in those with insufficient pulmonary reserve. In these patients, the surgical diagnostic techniques that have been described, as well as the various aforementioned roentgenographic and other studies, are invaluable.

STAGING

Once the diagnosis has been established and the extent of the disease determined, the patient's disease can be classified and staged by various morphologic, clinical, and functional classifications. The two most useful are Karnofsky and Burchenal's (1949) functional classification (Table 76–11) and the revised International Clinical Staging System, reported by Mountain (1986a) (Table 76–12), of the original staging schema of the American Joint Committee for Cancer Staging and End Results Reporting—AJC—(1973). In this classification, T designates the primary tumor, N the regional lymph nodes, and M distant metastasis. The staging can be determined after standard diagnostic evaluation—clinical classification; after surgical evaluation–post-thoracotomy classification; or after surgical resection—postsurgical treatment or pathologic classification.

With assignment of the TNM categories, the tumor can be staged as an occult carcinoma or as an invasive carcinoma: stage I, II, IIIa, IIIb, or IV (Table 76–13). The stage grouping is primarily applicable to patients with tumors of a cell type other than undifferentiated small cell; tentative clinical classification of even patients with this tumor, however, is helpful in their management.

As to the AJC's initial inclusion of T1N1 disease in stage I, the revised stage grouping answers many of the questions I and my associates (1977, 1980) and others raised. Also, it better differentiates surgical stage III—now stage IIIa—disease from locoregional, nonsurgical lesions—now stage IIIb disease. Unfortunately, a problem with the staging grouping of N2 disease persists. Only 10 to 20% of patients with N2 disease have tumor involvement that can be completely resected. Most patients with N2 disease—those with grossly enlarged nodes on standard roentgenograms of the chest and positive biopsy, as well as most of those patients with positive nodes determined by prethoracotomy mediastinal exploration—are at present nonsurgical candidates. Therefore, most patients with N2 disease really belong in stage IIIb. The system recognizes that cervical lymph

Table 76–11. Karnofsky Scale of Performance Status

Condition	Percentage	Comments
A: Able to carry on normal activity and to work. No special care is needed.	100	Normal, no complaints, no evidence of disease
	90	Able to carry on normal activity, minor signs or symptoms of disease
	80	Normal activity with effort, some signs or symptoms of disease
B: Unable to work. Able to live at home, care for most personal needs. A varying degree of assistance is needed.	70	Cares for self. Unable to carry on normal activity or to do active work
	60	Requires occasional assistance, but is able to care for most of his needs
	50	Requires considerable assistance and frequent medical care
C: Unable to care for self. Requires equivalent of institutional or hospital care. Disease may be progressing rapidly.	40	Disabled, requires special care and assistance
	30	Severely disabled, hospitalization indicated although death not imminent
	20	Hospitalization necessary, very sick, active supportive treatment necessary
	10	Moribund, fatal processes progressing rapidly
	0	Dead

node involvement should be considered an extension of locoregional disease rather than distant metastases, and it separates extrathoracic metastatic disease as stage IV disease.

TREATMENT

When the diagnosis is established, slightly less than one fourth of the patients with carcinoma of the lung have stage I or II disease, one fourth have stage IIIa or IIIb disease, and half have disseminated stage IV disease. The therapeutic modalities available are surgical resection, radiation therapy, chemotherapy, immunotherapy, and supportive care.

Patients with non-small cell tumors who have stage I or II disease and many patients with stage IIIa disease are surgical candidates. The rare patient with either a peripheral T1N0M0 or T2N0M0 undifferentiated small cell tumor may also be a surgical candidate, as I and my colleagues (1982a) and others, including Meyer (1982), Shepherd (1983), Merkle (1985), and Ohta (1986) and their associates and Maassen (1985) have noted.

Contraindication to Definitive Resection

Based on the Stage of Tumor

For most patients who have extrapulmonary intrathoracic manifestations and all those with extrathoracic metastatic manifestations, with rare exceptions, surgical therapy is not indicated.

Most patients with extrapulmonary intrathoracic manifestations have stage IIIb disease because of a T4 lesion or extracapsular N2 disease or N3 disease. None of these patients, as a rule, are candidates for resection, although at times direct phrenic nerve involvement may be re-

sected along with the adjacent pericardium. I have found this to be rare, and I believe that documented phrenic nerve involvement is a contraindication to exploration. Pleural effusion is infrequently not caused by the tumor, and resection may be possible. As Decker and associates (1978) noted, however, in a group of 73 patients with cytologically negative pleural fluid, resection was only possible in 5.5%.

Many patients with inoperable disease present with an enlarged mediastinal shadow because of metastatic mediastinal node disease—N2 or N3 disease—even in the absence of local symptomatology or signs. Martini and associates (1985b, 1987) stated that complete resection is rarely possible in such patients. Biopsy proof of such disease contraindicates surgery.

Considerable controversy about whether resection should be carried out for N2 disease discovered before thoracotomy—a positive preoperative mediastinal exploration—persists. The extensive writings of Pearson and his group—Pearson (1982); Cooper (1986); Martini (1979) and associates (1980, 1983b, 1985b, 1987); the European investigators—Bergh and Schersten (1965), Bergh and Larsson (1971), and Maassen (1985); and Japanese authors—Naruke (1976, 1978), Shimizu (1982), and Watanabe (1982)—attest to this problem. I (1986) believe that preoperatively discovered N2 disease, except under special circumstances—disease confined to within the capsule, low superior mediastinal location, only one or two stations and nodes involved, and lack of fixation—is a contraindication to resection, as is, of course, any N3 disease—contralateral lymph node involvement. Even with a fairly aggressive approach, only 10 to 20% of the patients with positive nodes—N2 disease—discovered by mediastinal exploration are surgical candidates.

Luke and associates (1986) of Toronto explored 20% of

Table 76–12. Definitions of T, N, and M Categories for Carcinoma of the Lung

Category	Description
T: Primary Tumors	
TX	Tumor proven by the presence of malignant cells in bronchopulmonary secretions but not visualized roentgenographically or bronchoscopically, or any tumor that cannot be assessed, as in a retreatment staging.
T0	No evidence of primary tumor.
TIS	Carcinoma in situ
T1	A tumor that is 3.0 cm or less in greatest dimension, surrounded by lung or visceral pleura, and without evidence of invasion proximal to a lobar bronchus at bronchoscopy.
T2	A tumor more than 3.0 cm in greatest dimension, or a tumor of any size that either invades the visceral pleura or has associated atelectasis or obstructive pneumonitis extending to the hilar region. At bronchoscopy, the proximal extent of demonstrable tumor must be within a lobar bronchus or at least 2.0 cm distal to the carina. Any associated atelectasis or obstructive pneumonitis must involve less than an entire lung.
T3	A tumor of any size with direct extension into the chest wall (including superior sulcus tumors), diaphragm, or the mediastinal pleura or pericardium without involving the heart, great vessels, trachea, esophagus, or vertebral body, or a tumor in the main bronchus within 2 cm of the carina without involving the carina.
T4	A tumor of any size with invasion of the mediastinum or involving heart, great vessels, trachea, esophagus or vertebral body or carina or presence of malignant pleural effusion.
N: Nodal Involvement	
N0	No demonstrable metastasis to regional lymph nodes.
N1	Metastasis to lymph nodes in the peribronchial or the ipsilateral hilar region, or both, including direct extension.
N2	Metastasis to ipsilateral mediastinal lymph nodes and subcarinal lymph nodes.
N3	Metastasis to contralateral mediastinal lymph nodes, contralateral hilar lymph nodes, ipsilateral or contralateral scalene or supraclavicular lymph nodes.
M: Distant Metastasis	
M0	No (known) distant metastasis
M1	Distant metastasis present

Table 76–13. Stage Grouping of TNM Subsets

	Stage Grouping		
Occult Carcinoma	TX	N0	M0
Stage 0	TIS	Carcinoma in situ	
Stage I	T1	N0	M0
	T2	N0	M0
Stage II	T1	N1	M0
	T2	N1	M0
Stage IIIa	T3	N0	M0
	T3	N1	M0
	T1–3	N2	M0
Stage IIIb	Any T	N3	M0
	T4	Any N	M0
Stage IV	Any T	Any N	M1

their patients with positive prethoracotomy N2 disease. The disease was completely resected in 56% of the patients explored, representing 12% of the total number with preoperatively identified N2 involvement. Coughlin and associates (1985) explored 10.6% of their patients with positive prethoracotomy N2 disease. Resection was done in 80% of these patients which represented only 8.2% of this entire group.

With or without adjuvant therapy, long-term survival in this select group, as Pearson (1982) and Coughlin (1985) and their colleagues reported, is approximately 18 to 20%. When the number of surviving patients is related to the entire group with mediastinoscopically positive lymph nodes, however, salvage is only around 1%.

Extrathoracic metastatic disease, either blood-borne distant metastases or lymphatic involvement outside the ipsilateral hemithorax, must be considered in almost all instances to be an absolute contraindication to any definitive surgical procedure. On rare occasions, a patient presents with a solitary brain metastasis at the time of identification of an otherwise resectable lung carcinoma. When the metastasis is indeed solitary, as determined by MRI and other studies as indicated, the cerebral lesion should be excised, followed by whole-brain irradiation. This, as Mandell and associates (1986) noted, gives the best chance for local control. Resection of the primary lung tumor may then be considered if all other sites are free of metastases—a CT scan of the mediastinum and upper abdomen and a bone scan should be negative. The primary disease should preferably be T1 but certainly no greater than T2, and the regional nodes should be negative. Resection then can be done, and an occasional long-term survivor may be obtained. Sundaresan and associates (1983, 1985) and Martini (1986b) reported that 37.5% of such patients have survived at least 24 months. Magilligan and associates (1986) concurred with this aggressive approach.

Infrequently, a solitary adrenal metastasis is identified. Preoperatively, this finding rules out resection of the primary. On the rare occasions, such a metastasis is identified in a previously resected patient. Attempts to remove the "solitary" adrenal metastasis should be discouraged; complete removal of all tumor is not possible because a regional en bloc resection is impossible in this location.

Based on the Tumor Location or Cell Type

Tumors involving the main stem carina or encroaching upon the tracheal wall, thus precluding an adequate length of proximal bronchus for safe closure of the stump, are considered nonresectable. Rarely, under ideal circumstances, a small, highly differentiated tumor can be removed by a tracheal-sleeve pneumonectomy with a bronchoplastic procedure to repair the tracheal wall or opposite main stem bronchus. Jensik (1972a, 1982), Deslauriers (1985), and Dartevelle (1988) and their associates and Faber (1987) reported experience in managing such lesions with tracheal-sleeve pneumonectomy.

Patients with undifferentiated small cell tumors, except those with stage I and possibly stage II lesions, are not surgical candidates even though the tumor may be thought to be confined to the ipsilateral hemithorax. All such patients are best managed by chemotherapy or chemotherapy plus irradiation. Adjuvant surgical resection after chemotherapy, as Meyer (1986) and his colleagues (1979, 1982) suggested, is under investigation by many groups, including the North American Lung Cancer Study Group, but not enough data have been obtained to define its role. The reports of Prager and associates (1984) and Meyer (1984, 1985), however, have not been too encouraging, especially in patients with N2 disease.

Based on the Patient's Medical Condition

Most contraindications for resection not related to the tumor are related either to the lungs or the heart. Rarely does advanced age alone or other systemic disease states preclude surgical resection. At times, the determination of what constitutes insufficient pulmonary reserve for tolerance of the required pulmonary resection, at best, is difficult to make. The patient's ventilatory studies and blood gas determination must be evaluated not only in terms of what is normally expected for that patient, but also in light of the extent of the disease process and known associated physiologic derangements, as judged by the roentgenographic findings, as well as by the nature of the planned resection.

No single set of values can determine at what level impaired function makes resection too hazardous. Ali (1976) noted, however, that the reduction of the FEV_1 to 1 L or less—40% of predicted normal—contraindicates a major resection, as does an MVV of less than 45 to 50% of predicted normal. Bronchoradiospirometry, as Kristersson and associates (1972) suggested, may predict postoperative FEV_1. As Olsen and colleagues (1974a, b) noted, and Ali (1980a, b, 1986), Cooper (1980), and Wernly (1980) and their associates concurred, when the predicted value of FEV_1 is 800 ml or greater, the patient should be able to tolerate a pneumonectomy. Of course, marked impairment of the ventilatory function from whatever cause, pulmonary emphysema severe enough to lead to hypercarbia, hypoxia at rest or after mild exercise, and marked pulmonary hypertension contraindicate surgical intervention. Arterial blood gases indicate the level of risk. A PO_2 of 60 to 80 torr and a PCO_2 of 35 to 45 torr indicate low risk in pulmonary resection. A PO_2 of less than 50 torr indicates a high risk, and a PCO_2 of greater than 45 torr indicates an even higher risk; the latter finding generally is considered by most to contraindicate any pulmonary resection.

Interest in the value of exercise tolerance as a measure of the patient's ability to tolerate a pulmonary resection has been renewed. The clinical stair climbing test provides a subjective estimation of the patient's cardiopulmonary reserve. The standard exercise tolerance test, however, as Reichel (1972) suggested, supplies more objective data. Bechard and Wetstein (1987) correlated postoperative morbidity and mortality of lung resection, the extent of which was based on the preoperative FEV_1, with preoperative exercise O_2 consumption— $M\dot{V}O_2$. In

a group of 50 patients selected on the results of the FEV_1 values, the mortality was 4% and the morbidity was 12%. When these results were stratified on the bases of the $M\dot{V}O_2$, there was a 29% mortality and 43% morbidity in the 7 patients with an $M\dot{V}O_2$ of less than 10 ml/kg/min. In the 28 patients with an $M\dot{V}O_2$ greater than 10 mL/kg/min but less than 20 ml/kg/min there were no deaths, but the morbidity rate was 10.7%. In the 15 patients with an $M\dot{V}O_2$ of greater than 20 ml/kg/min, no morbidity nor mortality was noted. Although these data should be confirmed, they do suggest that exercise testing should be valuable in evaluating the ability of a patient to successfully undergo a pulmonary resection.

Cardiac catheterization with balloon occlusion of the pulmonary artery on the side of the proposed operation, as Sloan and his associates (1955) suggested, can be used in patients with borderline function as an additional procedure to aid in assessing the functional reserve. Because of the development of radiospirometric methods, however, this study is rarely indicated.

Cardiac contraindications include recent myocardial infarct, uncontrolled heart failure or an uncontrollable arrhythmia. Steen and associates (1978) confirmed the findings of Tarhan and colleagues (1972) from the same institution of a 27% reinfarction rate in patients operated upon within 3 months of the initial infarction, an 11% incidence when the infarction had occurred 3 to 6 months previously, and a 4% to 5% reinfarction rate when the interval was greater than 6 months. With reinfarction, the mortality rate was 69%. In Tarhan and associates' (1972) series the mortality rate approached 80% when the reinfarction occurred within the first 48 hours of the operation. Thus, if at all possible, resection should be deferred until after the third month following an infarction.

To evaluate the patient's status, the history and electrocardiogram—ECG—are sufficient when both are normal. When the ECG is abnormal, an arrhythmia is present, or there is a history of angina, a previous myocardial infarct, or controlled failure, a stress test should be performed. When this is normal, other studies need not be done. If the stress test is not completed or is equivocal, ^{201}Tl scan to evaluate myocardial perfusion should be done. When either the stress test or ^{201}Tl scan is abnormal, a coronary angiogram should be obtained. When a patient is a candidate for myocardial revascularization or other cardiac procedures and has a resectable lung cancer, both procedures should be done at the same time if possible through a median sternotomy. In general, the pulmonary lesion should be completely resectable by a lobectomy or even a more limited procedure—a wedge or local resection. Piehler and colleagues (1985) reported a successful pneumonectomy, but this procedure's role, if any exists, is limited in this situation. The pulmonary resection should be done without systemic anticoagulation present, usually after its reversal following completion of the cardiac procedure. A staged procedure may be necessary but is best avoided when possible.

Kirsh and associates (1976b) noted age per se is not a contraindication, although pneumonectomy should be avoided whenever possible in most patients over 70. Lobectomy and lesser resections are reasonably tolerated, and the long-term survival, as the aforementioned authors and Bates (1970) and Harviel and his associates (1978) reported, is comparable to that seen in younger patients. Patients under 40 do poorly as a group, as Pemberton and colleagues (1983) noted, but this results from late diagnosis rather than poor response to appropriate therapy.

When no contraindications are present and the patient accepts the recommendation for surgical therapy, the ultimate resectability of the tumor is determined at thoracotomy.

Thoracotomy Findings

Despite the use of the various diagnostic techniques in the preoperative evaluation of patients with bronchial carcinoma to exclude those who have nonresectable lesions, some patients are found at thoracotomy to have nonresectable tumors. This finding may be caused by previously undetected seeding of the parietal pleura by the tumor or direct involvement of adjacent structures, such as the esophagus, vena cava, and vertebral bodies. Extensive metastatic involvement of mediastinal lymph nodes, with extracapsular growth and fixation to adjacent structures, that prevents complete excision of the tumor and its spread also contraindicates resection.

N2 disease per se, however, does not preclude a definitive, potentially complete resection. When involved mediastinal lymph nodes are discovered initially at thoracotomy, in contrast to involved mediastinal nodes identified preoperatively, the patient's prognosis appears to be less unfavorable. Such nodes, even though enlarged, frequently have the metastatic growth confined within the capsule and are not fixed to adjacent structures. These nodes may have been missed during a mediastinal exploration—a false negative node—or may be in a patient in whom the disease was believed to be clinically stage I or II only and no preoperative mediastinal exploration was done or the nodes were smaller than 1 cm on CT examination. In patients who are considered clinically to have only stage I or II disease, Martini and associates (1985b, 1987) recorded a 29% 5-year actuarial survival, and in the false-negative mediastinal node group, Pearson (1982) and Patterson (1987) and associates noted similar actuarial survivals. Although opinions differ somewhat, most believe that among patients with N2 disease, resection is more favorable in those with only one node and station involved, the node being located in the lower portion of the superior mediastinum—low paratracheal or superior tracheobronchial stations, although subcarinal location of the node does not rule out resection; in whom the primary tumor is a T1 or even a T2 lesion rather than a T3 lesion, and in whom complete resection of all tumor is possible.

Tumor involvement of the hilar structures, which even with extended techniques precludes safe management and control of either the vascular structures or the bronchial stump, contraindicates resection. In some patients, when it has been determined preoperatively that the patient could tolerate only a lobectomy, the extent of the tumor in the lung necessitates a pneumonectomy, and thus resection must be abandonded.

The percentage of patients in whom one or more of these local contraindications are found varies with the preoperative selection of the patients and the aggressiveness of the individual surgeon in the operative management of carcinoma of the lung. In many series, this figure is between 20 and 25%, although Abbey Smith (1957), by aggressive surgical policy, reduced it to 3%, and both Pearson (1968) and Sarin and Nohl-Oser (1969), with routine mediastinoscopy reduced the nonresectability rate at thoracotomy to approximately 5%.

This percentage must be kept as low as possible, because appreciable morbidity occurs after exploratory thoracotomy for a nonresectable bronchial carcinoma. The mortality rates are likewise high; many groups have reported an 8 to 10% rate within the first 30 postoperative days.

In the patients in whom the tumor is judged resectable, the appropriate operative procedure is carried out. If a tissue diagnosis of the tumor has not been obtained before exploration, biopsy of the lesion and frozen-section examination of the specimen to confirm the diagnosis of carcinoma are indicated if the contemplated procedure is more extensive than a lobectomy. A pneumonectomy or any other extended operative procedure should not be done only on the suspicion of cancer.

Definitive Surgical Resection

Lobectomy

At present, a lobectomy is done more often than is a pneumonectomy. In the CCNU and hydroxyurea lung trial of the Veterans Administration Surgical Oncology Group I and my associates (1982b) reported, a lobectomy was done in 66.5% of the patients, a pneumonectomy in 25.7%, a bilobectomy in 6.7%, and a segmental resection in 1%. In the Lung Cancer Study Group trials reported by Ginsberg and associates (1983), the percentages were 67.9 for lobectomy, 25.6 for pneumonectomy and 6.4 for lesser resections.

A standard lobectomy, in which the resection encompasses the entire disease process, is an excellent procedure in the management of localized non-small cell carcinomas. The standard procedure should be accomplished with lymph node sampling of the lymphatic drainage areas described by Nohl-Oser (Chapter 5) or with a standard or radical lymph node dissection as Martini (1976) and associates (1983b, 1987) and Naruke and colleagues (1976, 1988) described. The Lung Cancer Study Group and others suggested that sampling of each possibly involved ipsilateral lymph node station as well as the subcarinal area is adequate in evaluating the disease at thoracotomy. In either case, mediastinal lymph node dissection or extensive sampling only, the precise anatomic location of the various lymph nodes removed should be recorded, using one of the lymph node maps developed by the American Joint Committee (1973) (Fig. 76–17), Naruke and colleagues (1976), Martini and as-

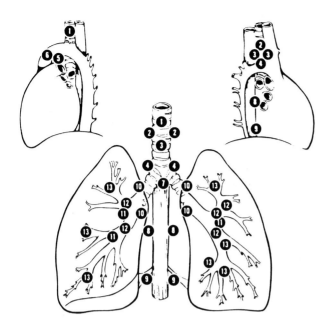

N2 Nodes

- • Superior Mediastinal Nodes
  1. Highest Mediastinal
  2. Upper Paratracheal
  3. Pre- and Retrotracheal
  4. Lower Paratracheal
     (including Azygos Nodes)

- • Aortic Nodes
  5. Subaortic (aortic window)
  6. Para-aortic (ascending aorta or phrenic)

- • Inferior Mediastinal Nodes
  7. Subcarinal
  8. Paraesophageal (below carina)
  9. Pulmonary Ligament

N1 Nodes

10. Hilar
11. Interlobar
12. Lobar
13. Segmental

Fig. 76–17. AJC classification of regional lymph nodes. (Reproduced with permission of the American Thoracic Society: Clinical staging of primary lung cancer. Am. Rev. Respir. Dis. *127*:659, 1983.)

sociates (1983), or the American Thoracic Society (1983). Region 4 on the right side in the AJC map (Fig. 76–17) includes the azygos nodes, which are placed in section 10R in the ATS map (Fig. 76–15). This area of confusion has yet to be resolved, but it would appear appropriate to consider any node cephalad to the inferior border of the azygos vein a superior tracheobronchial node and thus a superior mediastinal lymph node.

The advantages of a lobectomy are that it permits conservation of lung parenchyma and that it is better tolerated in the long term than is a pneumonectomy. The 30-day postoperative mortality is approximately 3%, half of that recorded for pneumonectomy. In patients over 70 years of age, the mortality may be increased but remains much less than that for pneumonectomy in this population group.

The morbidity experienced after a lobectomy, however, may be significant. Cardiac arrhythmias occur in 15 to 20% of patients over 60 years of age. Respiratory complications are common, and for patients in the poor-

risk groups, vigorous postoperative ventilatory care is necessary. The immediate physiologic derangement may be severe, and the initial functional loss is out of proportion to the anatomic tissue loss. Over time, function gradually increases so that the final loss is less than half of the initial loss. The final functional status is appropriate for the amount of pulmonary tissue remaining.

In the presence of metastatic involvement of the lobar and hilar nodes, a lobectomy may be less satisfactory, as I (1961) and Iascone and associates (1986) noted. When the primary lesion is in the right upper lobe and to a lesser extent, in the left upper lobe, however, lymph node dissection may be as adequate with a lobectomy as with a pneumonectomy. This is not true when the primary tumor is in one of the other three lobes and the nodal involvement is in the area of the lymphatic sump (Chapter 5).

Sleeve lobectomy and bilobectomy are modifications of the standard lobectomy. A bilobectomy can be carried out on the right lung. A right upper and middle lobectomy can be done when a tumor in the anterior segment has spread across a complete or incomplete minor fissure into the middle lobe or vice versa. A middle and right lower bilobectomy has been suggested as a routine procedure when the tumor is in either of these lobes, because theorectically this assures a more complete excision of the lymphatic drainage area of these two lobes. In the absence of any gross evidence of lymph node spread, however, I do not do this procedure routinely. Keller and colleagues (1988) reported 166 bilobectomies in patients with lung carcinoma. The indications were tumor extending across a fissure in 45%, absent fissure in 21%, endobronchial location of the tumor in 14%, extrinsic tumor or nodal invasion of the bronchus intermedius in 10%, vascular invasion in 5%, and miscellaneous indications in 5%. The postoperative morbidity rate was somewhat greater than that after lobectomy, and the mortality rate was 4.2%—slightly higher than that reported after a lobectomy but less than that observed after a pneumonectomy.

A sleeve lobectomy consists of resection of the lobe plus a segment of the adjacent main stem bronchus, with bronchoplastic repair of the bronchus by an end-to-end anastomosis to preserve the distal normal pulmonary parenchyma (Chapter 30). The advantage of a sleeve lobectomy is that it preserves uninvolved lung tissue that would be sacrificed by pneumonectomy. This procedure is most often applicable when the tumor is in the right upper lobe orifice and at times when the tumor is in the left upper lobe orifice. A bronchoplastic procedure is rarely appropriate when any of the other lobar orifices are involved by a non-small cell carcinoma. Faber (1984) and Deslauriers (1986) and their co-workers, among others, have published excellent series of this procedure. Gross lymph node involvement generally contraindicates sleeve lobectomy, although Naef (1974) stated strongly that sleeve lobectomy may be indicated as a palliative procedure in some patients. Involvement of the pulmonary artery also usually contraindicates resection. Bennett and Abbey Smith (1979) and Toomes and Vogt-

Moykopf (1985), however, reported long-term survival of patients who underwent a simultaneous angioplastic procedure along with the bronchial sleeve resection. The postoperative complications associated with the procedure are those normally seen after a lobectomy plus those attendant to the bronchial anastomosis. These may include bronchial disruption, bronchovascular fistula, and angulation or kinking of the bronchial repair. Suture granulation occasionally occurs, and unfortunately the local recurrence rate is high. The latter, however, should not deter surgeons from using the procedure, as satisfactory long-term survival rates have been reported. More importantly, the survival rates in patients in whom the procedure is done electively, as Weisel and associates (1979) noted, are not statistically different from those in patients with comparable stages of disease who undergo pneumonectomy.

Pneumonectomy

A standard pneumonectomy is required when a lobectomy or one of its modifications is not sufficient to remove the local disease or its metastases to the lobar or hilar lymph nodes. Unfortunately, it sacrifices more lung tissue than does lobectomy and is accompanied by higher rates of postoperative morbidity and mortality, particularly in patients over 70 years of age. In properly selected patients, the mortality rate is approximately 6%; in those over 70 years of age, it may be as high as 15 to 30%, although with a judicious selection of patients for the operation, it can be kept as low as 6%. The late development of pulmonary hypertension and subsequent ventilatory disability, however, are additional disadvantages of the procedure, particularly in older patients.

A pneumonectomy can be modified to include an extensive en bloc dissection of the mediastinal lymph nodes or the intrapericardial ligation of the pulmonary vessels. The modifications, alone or combined, have the same disadvantages as standard pneumonectomy. A third modification is a supra-aortic pneumonectomy on the left when the lesion is high in the left main stem bronchus. A fourth modification is a pneumonectomy with a tracheal-sleeve resection (Chapter 31). This extensive procedure carries a high mortality, although Dartevelle and colleagues (1988) reported one of only 10%.

Lesser Procedures

In an effort to preserve a more functional lung in older patients and in those with major pulmonary function defects, segmentectomy has been advocated. Current data suggest that in patients with small, peripheral lesions and without lymph node involvement—T1N0M0— a segmentectomy may be an adequate operation for lung carcinoma. Any segment can be resected, but the segments most commonly removed are those of the upper lobes. The advantage of a segmentectomy is that the least amount of pulmonary tissue is excised, with all the subsequent benefits to the patient. The mortality rate is low, 2 to 5%, although morbidity may be caused by prolonged air leak from the raw segmental surfaces.

In the patient in whom a possible prolonged air leak after segmentectomy would be detrimental to survival, such as an older patient with minimal pulmonary reserve, a wedge resection or even a local cautery excision may be considered as a compromise procedure. No true controlled studies have been done to determine whether a wedge resection is as satisfactory as a segmentectomy or lobectomy under similar circumstances.

All of the aforementioned procedures can be extended to include en bloc removal of any structures into which the primary tumor has extended, as long as the structure is not vital to the life and well-being of the patient. Portions of the lateral chest wall, the diaphragm, the pericardium, the left atrium, a lateral segment of the superior vena cava, and the apex of the chest cage— superior sulcus lesion—can be removed. The morbidity and mortality rates for such procedures are usually greater than for the standard procedure, but when they are properly indicated, the long-term results justify their use.

Because of the advantages and disadvantages of the various procedures, the selection of the operative procedure for a given patient is not blind adherence to any one operation as the only procedure of choice, but should be determined by the physiologic status of the patient and the topographic extent of the tumor at operation.

After deciding which procedure would be best tolerated by the patient, the operation then may be selected either as the definitive procedure of choice or as a compromise procedure, as determined by the topographic extent of the tumor at operation.

Topographically, tumors can be categorized into five groups: group I, solitary peripheral tumor without lymph node involvement or transgression of a fissure; group II, solitary peripheral tumor with gross lobar or hilar lymph node involvement or transgression of a fissure; group III, tumor in a lobar or main stem bronchus without lymph node involvement; group IV, tumor in a lobar or main stem bronchus with gross lobar or hilar but resectable lymph node involvement; and group V, tumor with direct extension to contiguous structures beyond the visceral pleura.

Choice of Operative Procedure

In group I tumors, lobectomy is the definitive procedure in all patients; when the tumor is in the right lower or middle lobe, bilobectomy has been recommended to ensure a more complete removal of the lymphatic drainage. This is not always necessary when the tumor is a T1N0M0 lesion. A segmentectomy, particularly in the upper lobes or superior segment of the lower lobes, can be used in selected patients when the tumor is confined to the segment. The upper division of the left upper lobe or either basilar segmental groups can be considered to be segments. In group II lesions, a standard pneumonectomy is the definitive procedure, although when the tumor is in the upper lobe—particularly on the right—a lobectomy with nodal dissection may be considered a definitive procedure. When disease extends across the fissure, a bilobectomy on the right may be considered. Elsewhere, a lobectomy with node dissection, or wedge resection of the disease extending across the fissure, or both, can be used as a compromise procedure in the elderly, poor-risk patient, or one with markedly reduced pulmonary or cardiac reserves. For those with group III tumors, a pneumonectomy or, when feasible, a lobectomy with a sleeve resection of the bronchus may be considered as the definitive procedure. With group IV tumors, a standard or extended pneumonectomy, depending on the need for intrapericardial ligation of the hilar vessels, may be used as the procedure of choice; a lobectomy with a sleeve resection as Naef (1971, 1973) suggested and reported by Deslauriers and associates (1986) may be considered in the poor-risk patient. Massive nodal involvement, however, contraindicates a bronchoplastic procedure in any patient. In group V tumors, the extent of parenchymal resection is governed similarly to resection in the other four groups, and is performed to enable an en bloc resection of the locally involved extrapulmonary structure.

The techniques of the standard operative procedures and the major variations have been discussed in Chapters 29 to 33. Most surgeons prefer a standard, posterolateral thoracotomy in most patients with carcinoma. Urschel and Razzuk (1986) recommended resection through a median sternotomy. The approach is unsatisfactory, however, for a left lower lobectomy, a left pneumonectomy, or excision of the chest wall or a superior sulcus tumor. If a bronchoplastic procedure is contemplated, some recommend the prone position with a posterior thoracotomy. As noted, mediastinal, subcarinal, and paraesophageal lymph nodes should be removed and appropriately labeled; usually, no true en bloc removal of these lymph nodes and of the surrounding tissues can be performed. Martini and Flehinger (1987), however, advised that an en bloc dissection of the mediastinal nodes should be carried out in all patients undergoing a pulmonary resection for cure. They stated that three mediastinal lymph node compartments are amenable to en bloc resection: the superior or paratracheal compartment on the right, the aorticopulmonary window on the left, and the subcarinal and inferior-posterior compartments on either side. Enlarged nodes anterior to the vena cava on the right are simply excised, as are enlarged nodes in the supra-aortic compartment on the left. Nodes in the superior mediastinum on the left are also simply excised because access to this area is limited by the great vessels, and an en bloc removal is not readily possible. Intrapericardial ligation of the vessels, as a rule, is done only to facilitate the safe ligation of these structures if adequate length cannot be obtained otherwise. In all patients in whom a pneumonectomy or an extended or bronchoplastic procedure is contemplated, dissection and isolation of the vascular structures are carried out to determine the feasibility of the operation before an irrevocable step, such as ligation and divison of the vessels, is undertaken.

In extended resections, resultant defects are repaired as indicated. Defects in the diaphragm may be closed by simple suture or by advancing the diaphragm up the chest wall; occasionally one or more lower ribs may be resected to accomplish this closure. Pericardial defects may be left widely open on the left—small defects should be closed—and all defects regardless of size always should be closed on the right to prevent herniation of the heart in the postoperative period. If large, the defect may be closed with the pericardial fat pad, a free pleural graft, or a prosthetic material.

Standard vascular techniques can be employed to excise involved portions of the atrium, pulmonary artery, and the vena cava. Rarely, if ever, is complete transection and replacement of the vena cava indicated in the treatment of a bronchial carcinoma.

Some manage involvement of the parietal pleura without extension into the chest wall by developing an extrapleural plane and stripping away the lung and parietal pleura from the chest wall. When no tumor is seen at the margin on frozen section, nothing futher is done; if tumor extends to the margin, chest wall resection is then carried out. Unfortunately, the few available data, which were reported by Trastek and associates (1984), can be interpreted to suggest that excision of the parietal pleura alone even when the tumor extension is confined to this structure is less satisfactory than an en bloc resection of the adjacent chest wall. I believe that when a tumor is fixed to the parietal pleura, no attempt should be made to strip it away, but that an en bloc resection of the parietal pleura and the adjacent chest wall should be done initially. The only exception to this is the attempt, as a compromise procedure to strip the parietal pleura off the vertebral column when a tumor is fixed in this area, because no further resection is indicated in this situation.

In patients with direct invasion of the chest wall, extension of the tumor to the vertebral bodies, transverse processes, or sternum, as well as pleural seeding or extension to structures outside the chest wall, generally obviates curative resection. Also, many believe that only infrequently should a chest wall excision be done when a pneumonectomy is required to treat the pulmonary extent or nodal spread of the disease. The presence of involved lymph nodes, as Piehler (1982), Patterson (1982), and McCaughan (1985) and associates noted, has a serious deleterious effect on survival. When an en bloc excision is performed, the extent of the chest wall excision should include one rib and the intercostal space above, as well as below, the gross involvement and several inches beyond the tumor both anteriorly and posteriorly. Reconstruction of the chest wall is important to prevent paradoxic motion of the decostalized area, for even after pneumonectomy, this motion produces severe postoperative difficulties. Various techniques can be used to achieve this reconstruction. In defects of the upper posterior chest wall, the mediastinal pleura, if intact, can be freed and attached to the lower margin of the defect to create a dome-like support, but most often, support by the adjacent muscles of the chest wall and scapula suffices. In anterior or lateral defects, a prosthesis, such as fascia lata, Marlex mesh with or without the addition of methyl methacrylate or a Gore-tex soft tissue patch, is required. In resections of the lower chest wall, the diaphragm can be brought to the upper margin to close off the defect.

When the tumor involves the apex of the chest and adjacent structures—the lower portion of the bronchial plexus, the so-called superior sulcus lesion—and no vertebral body invasion or Horner's syndrome is present, an en bloc resection may be carried out as described in Chapter 33. Preoperative irradiation is used initially, and it is recommended that radiation therapy in the range of 3000 to 3500 rads be given in a period of 2 weeks. This dose is thought to limit growth, to block adjacent lymphatics, and to destroy nests of malignant cells in the perineural sheaths. One month after completion of this therapy, if there is no evidence of distant spread, resection is undertaken. When lymph nodes are positive or when extensive vertebral bony involvement is present, resection is contraindicated. In such instances, further irradiation is indicated.

The results of combined therapy have been satisfactory. Not only has an acceptable 5-year salvage rate been obtained, but also most patients note relief of the severe pain, even though they eventually may die of the disease. The addition of postoperative irradiation may increase the long-term salvage rate, even when the resection has been incomplete.

Palliative Surgical Resection

Palliative resection of a carcinoma of the lung, as I noted (1974), should be defined strictly as a procedure that leaves gross or microscopically identifiable tumor behind at its completion. Such resections have been of little or no benefit. Abbey Smith (1971, 1981), however, has written that incomplete resection can be carried out

with some hope of success, particularly when the only disease remaining is left on the arterial wall.

Most distressing symptoms resulting from pain, bleeding, or infection can be controlled reasonably well by the judicious use of radiation therapy, chemotherapy, antibiotics, and narcotics; even bronchial artery embolization can be used to control massive hemoptysis. The addition of a noncurative resection, with attendant morbidity and mortality, as well as the subsequent reduction of the ventilatory reserves of the patient, is not justified. Hara and his colleagues (1984), in a review of a large series of patients with stage III disease, showed that palliative resection confers no survival benefit over thoracotomy alone or even to only nonsurgical palliative measures (Fig. 76–18). Burt and associates (1987) at Memorial Hospital reported a 22% 5-year actuarial survival in 33 patients with direct mediastinal extension who underwent an incomplete resection supplemented with brachytherapy—intraoperative ^{125}I implantation or placement of catheters for postoperative ^{192}Ir afterloading. There were no long-term survivors with incomplete resection only. Thus I believe incomplete resections alone have little or no indication in patients with lung carcinoma regardless of the patient's age or general condition. At times, unfortunately, gross tumor or more commonly microscopic tumor at the bronchial margin of the resection is not identified until the bronchus has been divided or until histologic examination of the stump has been carried out. As a rule, as with other incomplete resections, this portends a poor prognosis for the patient. A small subset of such patients with squamous cell carcinoma present only in the submucosa or mucosal layers of the bronchus, however, may unexplainably survive without recurrence of the disease process.

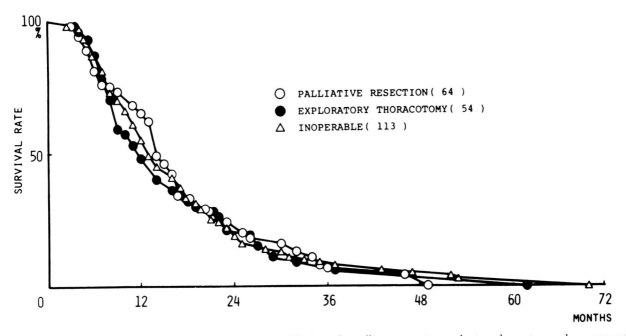

Fig. 76–18. Survival curves of patients with stage III carcinoma of the lung after palliative resection, exploratory thoracotomy only, or no surgical therapy. (Reproduced with permission of Hara, N., et al.: J. Surg. Oncol. 25:153, 1984.)

I (1974) suggested that tumors present at the cut margin of the bronchial stump be divided into three categories. The first is macroscopic gross disease at the margin proved by histologic examination. The second is a grossly normal margin but with microscopically proved peribronchial tumor, and the third is a grossly normal margin but with microscopic submucosal or mucosal tumor. The prognosis of the first type is poor, and radiation therapy is indicated to control local disease. The prognosis of the second variety is somewhat better, and the possibility of a more proximal resection to get above the level of the tumor should be considered. In those with mucosal or submucosal tumor involvement only, approximately one quarter of the patients may survive without further therapy (Table 76–14). Jeffery (1972) and Soorae and Stevenson (1979) recorded similar long-term survival. Additional therapy, however, may be elected after further evaluation of the bronchial stump by endoscopic biopsy and evaluation of the general condition of the patient. Another variety of tumor involvement of a grossly normal-appearing stump is the presence of tumor in the lymphatics of the bronchial wall. In this circumstance, a more proximal resection usually reveals the same lymphatic involvement; and as a consequence further resection is contraindicated. Radiation therapy may be used as a palliative measure; but as Soorae and Stevenson (1979) noted, the prognosis is poor in this subset.

Results of Surgical Treatment

The overall 5-year salvage rates after surgical resection vary from as low as 7.5% to as high as 45%, the average figures usually being between 20% and 35%. The prognosis after resection is primarily dependent on the post-surgical—pathologic—TNM classification of the tumor (Table 76–15). Williams and his associates (1981) reported that patients with T1N0M0 lesions had an 80% probability, those with T2N0M0 a 62% probability, and those with T1N1M0 lesions had a 52% probability of surviving 5 years tumor-free. In a similar study that I and my colleagues (1980) reported, the actuarial survival at 5 years was 54% in patients with T1N0M0 lesions and 40% in patients with T2N0M0 lesions. When lymph nodes were involved—T1N1M0 or T2N1M0—the 3-year survival was respectively 37% and 40%. Martini and associates (1983a) reported a 56% and a 48% 5-year survival for patients with T1N1M0 and T2N1M0 disease, respectively. With T3N0-1M0 disease it is 35%.

A major factor affecting the postsurgical results is the absence or presence of lymph node metastases and their location. Study of the data from the Veterans Administration Surgical Oncology Group (VASOG), presented by me and my associates (1975), revealed that in 2349 patients, the 5-year survivals in those without lymph node involvement was 33.7%; with lobar nodes involved, 20.1%; with hilar nodes involved, 17.4%; and with mediastinal nodes involved, only 8.9%. The 10-year survivals were 20.4%, 10.6%, 9.8%, and 4.7% respectively. In more selected series of patients with N2 disease reported by Martini (1985b), Martini and Flehinger (1987), Pearson (1982) and Patterson (1987) and associates, approximately a 29% 5-year actuarial survival has been observed.

Tumor size is also an important prognostic factor. In patients with peripheral lesions, Higgins and associates (1975), Soorae and Abbey Smith (1977), Freise and associates (1978), and Treasure and Belcher (1981) documented that patients with smaller lesions—T1—do better than those with larger ones—T2. Moreover, the larger the T2 lesion, the poorer the prognosis.

Deslauriers and associates (1988) addressed the effect of a satellite tumor nodule or nodules on the prognosis of a resected lung tumor. These investigators identified 84 lung tumors associated with satellite tumor nodules; only 15.5% of the nodules had been identified by initial roentgenograms of the chest. This represented 7.6% of the resected specimens in their series of 1105 lung tumors. The 5-year survival rate was 21.6% for those with a satellite tumor nodule compared to 44% for those patients in whom no satellite tumor nodules were found. Interestingly, the adverse effect on 5-year survival was

Table 76–14. Survival of Patients with Residual Tumor at Bronchial Margin

	Gross Tumor	Microscopic Peribronchial	Microscopic Bronchial Submucosal	Total
No.	12	24	31	67
Postoperative deaths	5	3	5	13
Bronchopleural fistula	2	3	2	7
_____ Survival _____				
1 to 3 months	1	7	2	10
4 to 6 months	2	2	4	8
7 to 12 months	3	7	2	12
Over 12 months	1	5	18	24
	1>2 yrs.	2>2 yrs.	6>2 yrs.	
		1>3 yrs.	3>3 yrs.	
		1>4 yrs.	1>4 yrs.	
		1>5 yrs.	2>5 yrs.	
			6<5 yrs.	

Reproduced with permission from Shields, T.W.: The fate of patients after incomplete resection of bronchial carcinoma. Surg. Gynecol. Obstet. 139:569, 1974.

Table 76–15. Survival Relative to TNM Classification

TNM Subset	Clinical No.	Clinical % Surviving	Surgical No.	Surgical % Surviving
T1N0M0	591	61.9	429	68.5
T2N0M0	1,012	35.8	436	59.0
T1N1M0	19	33.6	67	54.1
T2N1M0	176	22.7	250	40.0
T3N0M0	221	7.6	57	44.2
T3N1M0	71	7.7	29	17.6
Any N2M0	497	4.9	168	28.8
Any M1	1,166	1.7	—	—
Total	3,753		1,436	

Reproduced with permission from Mountain, C.E.: A new international staging system for lung cancer. Chest 89:225S, 1986.

more pronounced in stage I tumors, 32% versus 54.4%, than in either stage II and III patients, although poor survival rates of 12.5% and 5.6% were reported respectively in these two stage groups. They suggested that when a satellite tumor nodule is present, the tumor should probably be included in the T3 category and the patient staged as having IIIa disease.

Cell type, other than undifferentiated small cell carcinoma, generally is reported to have little significance in those patients resected for potential cure in whom the lymph nodes are found to be uninvolved. The aforementioned Veterans Administration Study and the data presented by Paulson and Reisch (1976) and Stott and associates (1976) documented this finding. Feld (1984) and Read (1988) and their colleagues, however, reported that patients with squamous cell tumors have a better prognosis than do those with adenocarcinoma or large cell undifferentiated tumors, even in the absence of lymph node metastases. In reviewing some of the unpublished data from the VASOG lung trial, I found this to be true in the T2N0 group but not in the T1N0 patients (Fig. 76–19). Read and associates (1988), however, found that squamous cell lesions have a more favorable prognosis even in the T1N0 group. When lymph nodes are involved, patients with epidermoid carcinoma do better than patients with the other cell types (Fig. 76–20).

The tumor's location, as well as the sex and age of the patient, also affects the prognosis. Tumors in the peripheral zone generally have a better prognosis than those in the central zone. Tumors in the upper lobes have a better prognosis than do those arising in the lower lobes.

Williams and associates (1981) and Mountain (1986b) noted the better prognosis of women versus men with stage I disease. The difference was significantly better at 5 years, and in Mountain's series it was primarily in patients with adenocarcinoma. Patients over the age of 70 have a poorer prognosis than those patients 69 or younger.

When a lobectomy is the procedure of choice, not only is the immediate mortality rate less than after a pneumonectomy, but the 5-year survival rates are better and are frequently in the range of 40% to as high as 68%

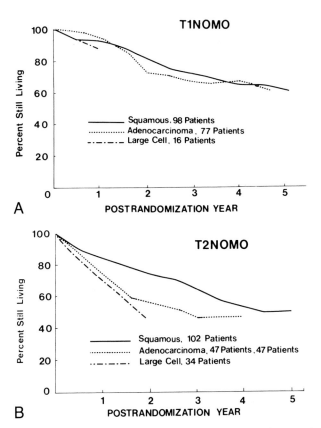

Fig. 76–19. *A,* Survival curves of patients with T1N0M0 disease relative to cell type. *B,* Survival curves of patients with T2N0M0 disease relative to cell type. (Reproduced with permission of Shields, T.W.: Surg. Clin. N. Am. *61*:1279, 1981.)

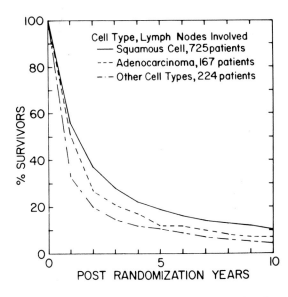

Fig. 76–20. Survival curves for patients with the three histologic cell types with metastatic lymph node involvement. (Shields, T.W., et al.: Relationship of cell type and lymph node metastasis to survival after resection of bronchial carcinoma. Ann. Thorac. Surg. *20*:506, 1975.)

Table 76–16. Five-Year Survival After Pneumonectomy and Lobectomy for Treatment of Bronchial Carcinoma

	Lobectomy (%)	Pneumonectomy (%)
Le Roux (1968b)	40	20
Thomeret et al. (1970)	37	20
Dillon and Postlethwait (1971)	31	26
Inberg et al. (1972)	31.9	23.5
Weiss (1974)	29.5	16.5
Ashor et al. (1975)	41	26
DeBesse et al. (1976)	31.4	31
Vincent et al. (1976)	20.1	15.3
Kirsh et al. (1976a)	38	30
Paulson and Reisch (1976)	34.5	15.5
Freise et al. (1978)	32.8	22.9
Williams et al. (1981)	68	45

(Table 76–16). Martini (1986a) reported a long-term survival of 83% for patient with T1N0M0 lesion and one of 65% for T2N0M0 lesions. All but 5% of these patients—six with T2N0M0 disease—had undergone a lobectomy.

With sleeve resection and a bronchoplastic procedure in selected patients, Rees and Paneth (1970) obtained a 35% 5-year survival rate. Paulson (1970), Jensik (1972b), Weisel (1979), and Toomes (1985) and their associates reported 39%, 30%, 36%, and 34%, respectively. Deslauriers and colleagues (1986) reported an actuarial 5-year survival of 67% in patients with N0 disease, and one of 63% in those with N1 disease. In Toomes and Vogt-Moykopf's (1985) series, the addition of an angioplastic procedure reduced survival to only 14% at 5 years. In patients who require a pneumonectomy, the mortality rate is higher and the 5-year survival rates are only approximately 20 to 45% (Table 76–16).

With lesser procedures, the long-term survival rates depend somewhat upon whether or not the operations were done as compromise procedures because of the patient's age or poor physiologic status or as an elective procedure in an otherwise healthy patient. Bennett and Abbey Smith (1979) and Jensik (1986) reported 5-year survivals of over 55% in large series of segmentectomies, and Errett and colleagues (1985) reported a 6-year survival of 69% after a wedge resection in selected patients with peripheral T1N0M0 lesions.

In regard to extended resections, Grillo and his coworkers (1966) reported only a 16% survival rate after chest wall resections. Piehler (1982) and Patterson (1982) and their associates, however, reported overall survival rates of over 32%. In the younger patient and those without lymph node involvement, the actuarial 5-year survival may be even greater than 80%. Survival figures for other types of extended resections are difficult to obtain. Trastek and associates (1984), however, reported an actuarial 5-year survival for en bloc resection of adjacent thoracic parieties, other than chest wall resection, of 38% for patients with T3N0 disease. The rate was 29% for those with T3N1 or T3N2 disease. Burt and colleagues (1987) reported a 9% 5-year survival in 49 patients who underwent a complete resection of direct mediastinal extension of the tumor. Most of these patients had N2

disease as well as the T3 disease. The best results were observed in the subsets of those patients whose resected disease involved a pulmonary vein, the phrenic nerve, the esophagus, or the pericardium.

Resection of superior sulcus lesions results in approximately a 35% 5-year survival. Paulson (1985) reported a survival of 44% when no lymph nodes were involved; in this group of patients, 33% survived 10 years and 30% survived 15 years. With the addition of postoperative irradiation, Shahian and associates (1987) achieved a 56% 5-year survival in these patients with superior sulcus tumors, even when the resection was incomplete.

Survival after resection of N2 disease has been discussed previously (pp. 913 and 920). The results of resection when N2 disease is present can be summarized briefly. Patients with clinically—standard roentgenographic examination—detectable N2 disease have a low resectability rate and the few patients who do undergo complete excision have a less than 10% 5-year survival—which represents only a 1% survival of all patients in this group, according to the studies of Martini and associates (1983b, 1985b, 1987). Approximately 10 to 20% of those patients whose positive N2 disease is discovered on preoperative mediastinal exploration subsequently can have the disease resected, usually after radiation therapy. Coughlin (1985) and Pearson (1982) and their associates reported 5-year survival rates of 19% to as high as 41% in selected subsets of such patients, but when the survival data in these aforementioned series are extrapolated to include the entire number of patients initially comprising the study groups, the 5-year survival is reduced to approximately 1%. Also Gibbons (1972) and Fosburg and associates (1979) reported no survivors following resection in the presence of preoperatively proved N2 metastases. In those patients in whom the involvement of the mediastinal nodes is unknown until the time of thoracotomy and a complete resection has been carried out, Pearson (1982), Patterson (1987), Martini (1987) and Naruke (1988) and their associates and Neptune (1988) reported 5-year survival rates varying from 19% to as high as 42%, the average rate being approximately 30%. Five-year survival, according to the report of Martini and Flehinger (1987), is influenced by the T status, the number of nodal stations involved, and the number of involved nodes. The histologic subtype, the location of the nodal station involved, the size of the involved node, and the presence or absence of N1 disease—27% of their patients had skip metastases to the N2 nodes without N1 involvement—had little influence on the rate of long-term survival.

Patterns of Failure in Surgically Treated Patients

Most treatment failures occur within the first 3 years after resection. Most of the deaths occur during the first 12 to 24 months. The percentage then falls gradually until the end of the third year. Few patients succumb during the fourth year and a slightly greater number than this during the fifth year. I and Robinette (1973) found that only infrequently thereafter does a patient die of the original disease. Belcher and Rehahn (1979) as well as

Abbey Smith (1971), however, reported a continued high recurrence rate even after the fifth and tenth years.

In autopsy studies by Rasmussen (1964) and Spijut and Mateo (1965) of patients who had undergone surgical resection and who died before the sixth postoperative year, the percentage of patients without evidence of tumor was 15 to 17%. In the Veterans Administration Surgical Oncology Group studies of men after resection of a lung carcinoma reported by me and Robinette (1973), 22.3% of the patients dying within the first 5 years postoperatively had no known evidence of recurrence or metastatic cancer. In other studies, comprised of different population groups, reported by Belcher and Rehahn (1979) and the Ludwig Lung Cancer Study Group (1987), this number has varied from 10 to 15% to as high as 23 and 25%. The explanation of the differences may be the number of women, the socioeconomic factors, and the age distribution within the reported groups. When this figure is subtracted from those who died within the 5-year period, the number of "true" treatment failures can be determined.

From this subset, another category of persons can be identified, that is: those who have gross, but occult, metastatic disease at the time of operation. Although such patients represent in the true sense treatment failures, they are in reality failures of selection. This subset represents from 10 to 30% of patients operated upon for carcinoma of the lung as determined by autopsy studies of patients dying within the first 30 postoperative days. In 1964, Rasmussen found the incidence of occult gross disease to be 14%. The incidence of such occult macrometastases tends to vary, as would be expected, with the cell type and the extent of the disease within the chest. Rocmans and colleagues (personal communication) reported that patients with N0 disease had an incidence of less than 10%, whereas those with N1 or N2 disease had an incidence of over 30%. Matthews and associates (1977) found the incidence of distant metastases in patients with T1 non-small cell tumors to be 11%. The incidence was greater in those with adenocarcinoma—27%—than in those with squamous cell carcinoma—9%. In the patients who had T2 lesions, the incidence of distant macrometastases was 15%. In those with squamous cell carcinoma or adenocarcinoma, incidences were 12.6% and 40%, respectively. In each group the patients with lymph node metastases or with adenocarcinoma had more occult macrometastases than the other patients who had neither of these features.

When the number of patients with occult macrometastases is subtracted from the known treatment failures, a reasonable estimate of the number of patients who harbor micrometastases can be made in each subset of the treatment groups. The importance of this information is that micrometastases may be more likely to be susceptible to either adjuvant local or systemic therapy, or both. It is reasonable, therefore, to attempt to define the initial site of failure from the growth of undetectable micrometastases in each postsurgical stage subgroup so that more appropriate adjuvant therapy can be used.

Previous autopsy studies of cancer deaths after an initial successful resection revealed a high incidence of local recurrence as well as a high incidence of distant metastases, but the initial sites of recurrence were unrecorded. The data from recent studies have attempted to answer this question, but the data have not always been in total agreement. It is evident, however, that initial distant metastasis is much more common than local recurrence, in contrast to the earlier autopsy findings. In our own study with Immerman and colleagues (1981), however, we found locoregional recurrence to be common in patients who had metastases in regional lymph nodes in the resected specimen. In patients with treatment failure in the T1N0 category, either locoregional recurrence—including supraclavicular lymph node metastases—or distant metastasis occurred in 28%; in the T2N0 category, recurrent disease occurred in 50%; and in the T1N1 plus T2N1 group—stage II disease—64% of the patients had recurrent disease. In Pairolero and associates' (1984) study, the recurrence rates were 28.8% in patients with T1N0 lesions, 40.5% with T2N0 lesions, and 66.7% with T1N1 lesions. The Ludwig Lung Cancer Study Group (1987) observed rates of 49% in T1N0, 55.6% in T2N0 and 67% in stage II disease. The sites of first failure were distant metastases to the brain, bone, liver, or contralateral lung in most of the patients in the series reported by Mountain (1980), Martini (1983a), Feld (1984), and Pairolero (1984) and their associates. In each, the brain was the most common site. In contrast to these series, the Ludwig Lung Cancer Study Group (1987) reported the highest initial failure rate in patients with stage I disease to be in the ipsilateral hemithorax—locoregional failure—as did Iascone and associates (1986). The reasons for this are unexplained.

Similar studies have not been reported in patients with stage IIIa disease. Martini and associates (1983b), however, who used postoperative local irradiation, noted distant metastases to be common in patients with N2 disease: over 85% in the patients with recurrent disease. Iascone and colleagues (1986) also noted a high incidence of distant failure in the presence of N2 disease. Local recurrence, however, is common when adjuvant local radiation therapy has not been given to patients with N2 disease.

Adjuvant Therapy

As noted, 28% to over 75% of patients with lung carcinoma, depending upon the stage of the disease at the time of resection, die from recurrent carcinoma. Obviously, some form of ajuvant therapy is indicated in many of these patients. Unfortunately, with rare exceptions, irradiation, chemotherapy, or immunotherapy has not been successful to date.

Radiation Therapy

Initial studies using preoperative irradiation reported by Bromley and Szur (1955) and Bloedorn and Cowley (1960) suggested the efficacy of such an approach. Prospective, randomized studies reported by Warram (1975) and by me (1972), however, revealed no benefit relative to long-term survival with the routine use of preoperative irradiation. In fact, in the Veterans Administration study (Fig. 76–21), those patients who were resected after preoperative irradiation did less well than those who underwent resection only. Because of these studies, the routine use of preoperative irradiation is contraindicated.

The use of adjuvant preoperative radiation therapy in patients selected to undergo resection of a superior sulcus lesion has been noted. The use of preoperative irradiation, however, in patients with direct chest wall involvement in other locations has been questioned. Patterson and his colleagues (1982) approve of this therapy and suggest that their satisfactory 5-year survival rate of 56% results from its use. Piehler and his colleagues (1982), however, reported a similar survival rate in such patients without the use of this adjuvant modality. A controlled prospective study is obviously necessary.

Prospective studies of postoperative irradiation have been carried out only infrequently; Van Houtte and colleagues (1980) and the Lung Cancer Study Group's study reported by Weisenburger (1984) and Holmes and associates (1985) are two such series. Previously, numerous nonrandomized series reported by Kirsh (1971, 1976a, b, 1982), Green (1975), and Martini (1980, 1983b) and their associates have suggested that such therapy is beneficial when resected mediastinal lymph nodes have been found to contain tumor. Kirsh and his associates (1971) found such therapy especially beneficial in those patients with epidermoid carcinoma; although Martini and associates (1980, 1983b) noted similar favorable results in patients with adenocarcinoma.

In the aforementioned randomized study by the Lung Cancer Study Group, however, survival was not improved in patients with stage II and III squamous cell carcinoma of the lung who received postoperative irradiation as compared to those who did not. A marked reduction in the incidence of local recurrence, however, was seen in the patients receiving radiation therapy. Van Houtte and colleagues (1980) also noted fewer local recurrences in their patients who received postoperative irradiation, but likewise no survival benefit.

Chemotherapy

Numerous prospective randomized trials of postoperative adjuvant chemotherapy have been carried out.

Unfortunately, none of the studies reported by Slack (1970), and by Stott (1976), me (1974, 1977, 1982b), and Hara (1985) and colleagues have reported any benefit with its use.

Isolated reports of benefit in selected randomized patients, however, have been recorded. Newman and co-workers (1983) reported improved survival with a regimen of cyclophosphamide (C), doxorubicin (A), methotrexate (M), and procarbazine (P)—CAMP—in patients with T1N1M0 and T2N1M0 resected non-small cell carcinoma. Holmes and associates (1985) reported prolonged disease-free survival in patients with resected stage II and III adenocarcinoma or large cell carcinoma who received a regimen of cyclophosphamide (C), doxorubicin (A), and cisplatin (P)—CAP—as opposed to those who received intrapleural bacille Calmette-Guérin vaccine—BCG—and levamisole. Nonetheless, despite the isolated favorable reports, it is the consensus of most investigators attending the Non-Small Cell Lung Cancer Workshop (1987) that routine adjuvant chemotherapy is not indicated. Moreover, in our study (1982b), adjuvant chemotherapy may have harmed those patients with the more favorable lesions—T1N0M0 and T2N0M0. Nonetheless, continued prospective trials with new agents and different combinations are indicated in patients in whom more extensive disease has been resected, as the Lung Cancer Study Group's trial suggested.

Neoadjuvant Therapy

There has been recent interest in the use of preoperative chemotherapy with or without radiation therapy in marginally resectable or nonresectable stage IIIa disease, particularly in those with known N2 involvement, in an attempt to convert the local disease into a resectable lesion. The more commonly used regimens have used cisplatin and fluorouracil infusion with 30 to 40 Gy of irradiation, as Taylor and associates (1987) reported. In their series of 64 patients, 61% underwent resection after completion of the neoadjuvant therapy and in 23%—9 patients or 14% of the initial number of patients—the tumor had been sterilized. Martini and colleagues (1988) reported similar results of preoperative chemotherapy alone in patients with N2 disease. The regimens used

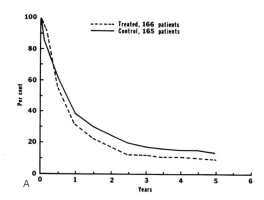
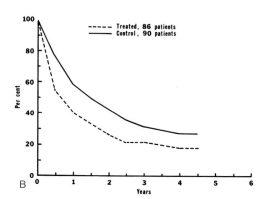

Fig. 76–21. *A,* Percentage of survivors of all patients admitted to the lung preoperative radiation therapy study from the date of randomization. *B,* Percentage of survivors after surgical resection based on the date of operation. (Redrawn from Shields, T.W., et al.: Preoperative x-ray therapy as an adjuvant in the treatment of bronchogenic carcinoma. J. Thorac. Cardiovasc. Surg. 59:49, 1970.)

consisted of cisplatin with vindesine or vinblastine with or without mitocyin C. In 41 patients, 71% had a major roentgenographic response, 27 patients were explored, and complete resections were carried out in 21 patients—51% of the total group. Eight patients had total sterilization of their tumor—19% of the initial group. How these results will translate into long-term survival remains to be seen.

Immunotherapy

Both active and passive immunotherapeutic techniques have been under investigation as adjuvant measures. Tumor-specific antigens are the most promising of the former. Intrapleural instillation of bacille Calmette Guérin vaccine—BCG, the use of *Corynebacterium parvum*, or the oral administration of levamisole have been the passive agents that have undergone extensive trials.

McKneally and his associates (1976, 1979, 1981) reported improved survival in patients with stage I tumors who received intrapleural instillation of BCG vaccine postoperatively than in those patients who did not. The trial reported by Mountain and Gail (1981), however, failed to show any benefit from its use. Millar and his associates (1982) noted similar negative results. Moreover, Bakker and his associates (1981, 1982) noted possible harmful effects from its use.

Randomized trials with the use of *C. parvum* and BCG vaccine reported by the Ludwig Lung Cancer Study Group (1985, 1987) showed that the use of *C. parvum* was detrimental with respect to survival and the use of BCG was associated with a decrease in the disease-free interval.

Amery (1976) reported that levamisole, an immunoreconstituter, given orally favorably influenced survival, especially in patients with larger epidermoid tumors. Anthony and his colleagues (1979), however, did not observe any benefit from its use and reported a higher mortality in the patients receiving the drug than in the control group. At present, adjuvant immunotherapy has no apparent place in the lung cancer patient with completely resected local disease.

Prospects for Adjuvant Therapy

The prospects of adjuvant therapy are discouraging. Patients with stage T1N0 disease probably are not candidates for either local or systemic adjuvant therapy. Patients with T2N0 disease should benefit from systemic therapy if an effective chemotherapeutic regimen could be identified. Patients with stage II—T1N1 and T2N1—disease also would be candidates for effective systemic therapy. Patients with stage IIIa—T3N0 or N1—disease likewise need systemic therapy as do those with stage IIIa—any TN2—disease; in this latter category, however, local therapy—irradiation—would also seem to be helpful, at least in controlling the local disease.

Second Primary Lung Tumor

A second primary lung tumor in patients surviving a resection for a bronchial carcinoma is being recognized more frequently, particularly in patients whose resected tumor was initially occult—cytologically positive but roentgenographically negative. Martini and colleagues (1985) reported an incidence of new primaries of 38%. Generally, the incidence is much lower in the standard population group operated upon; LeGal and Bauer (1961) noted new primaries in 6.4% of patients surviving 30 months or more. In the VASOG studies, I and my colleagues (1973, 1978) reported an incidence of approximately 10% in patients surviving 5 years or longer. Pairolero and colleagues (1984) reported a high incidence of second primary lung tumor in their patients with stage I disease; the incidence was 25.6%, which is much higher than that reported elsewhere.

Jensik (1986) reported that 20% of his population group has had sequential resections for second primary lung lesions. Martini and associates (1985a) noted an incidence of only 11% in his stage I patients. The new lesion usually arises in the opposite lung (Fig. 76–22), although after lobectomy the second tumor may occur in the same lung. In this situation, such a new lesion must be differentiated from a recurrence of the initial lesion. Most double primary tumors occur nonsynchronously, although bilateral and multiple unilateral synchronous tumors have been reported. When a new lesion arises in the same or opposite lung, its nature must be ascertained so that appropriate therapy can be used.

To be considered second primary lung tumors, each lesion must be distinct and the possibility that one is a metastasis of the other must be excluded. The latter possibility may be difficult to resolve. By considering such factors as the time interval, the site of the second lesion, the histologic patterns of each tumor, and the lack of evidence of recurrent local—especially nodal metastasis—or distant metastatic disease, a reasonable clinical assumption can be made.

Once the new tumor is assumed to be a new primary lesion, definitive surgical therapy, if possible, should be undertaken. Jensik (1986) reported a cumulative survival after resection of the second primary lung tumor of 33% at 5 years, 20% at 10 years, and 13% at 15 years. The type of treatment used is governed by the extent of the previous resection, the physiologic reserves of the patient, and the topographic extent of the tumor. Although standard operations for carcinoma should be carried out, when feasible, local excision of the second tumor may be justified in many situations. One such patient of mine, who underwent a pneumonectomy and subsequent wedge resection of a new tumor in the remaining lung, survived over 10 years. Kittle and colleagues (1985) reported 15 limited resections—14 for a second primary—after a previous pneumonectomy with only one postoperative death. Long-term survival of over 30 months was observed in six patients. When definitive resection is contraindicated, appropriate radiation therapy should be employed.

The possibility that a second cancer may occur elsewhere, as well as the possibility that a second primary lesion may arise in the lung, requires a change in the postoperative evaluation of the patient who has undergone successful resection of a bronchial carcinoma. In

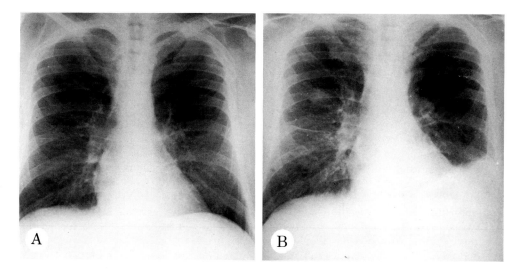

Fig. 76–22. *A*, PA roentgenogram of the chest showing a peripheral mass in left first intercostal space. Lobectomy was performed. The lesion was found to be a squamous cell carcinoma on microscopic examination. *B*, PA roentgenogram of the chest of same patient shown in *A* 6 years later, revealing an ill-defined mass off the anterior end of the third rib on the right. Lobectomy was performed; this second lesion was a bronchioloalveolar cell carcinoma. The patient is living and well 10 years after the second resection.

the past, one or two yearly visits after the third year were considered adequate. Clinical and roentgenographic examination at least four times a year throughout the remaining life span of the patient is more appropriate. Cytologic examination and bronchoscopy are not indicated unless findings indicate the necessity of either procedure.

Radiation Therapy

Radiation therapy of bronchial carcinoma is discussed in detail in Chapters 92 and 93. Several statements, however, may be made here concerning this modality.

Radiation therapy continues to be a major therapeutic modality in the management of carcinoma of the lung. It is used in selected patients as a curative therapeutic agent but finds its greatest application as a palliative measure in patients with disseminated disease.

Radical irradiation for cure is indicated in those patients with resectable lesions—stage I, II, or IIIa disease—who either refuse or who are unable to undergo the indicated operative procedure. In patients with stage I or II disease, Smart (1966) reported a 22.5% 5-year survival and Hilaris and Martini (1979), using brachytherapy, reported a long-term survival rate of 33%. Most patients who are candidates for definitive radiation therapy for attempted cure, however, have nonresectable stage IIIa or IIIb disease. In such patients, Guttman (1971) reported a 7%, Johnson (1977) a 6%, and Hilaris and Martini (1979) a 7% 5-year survival.

Radiation therapy may be used also as an adjuvant measure preoperatively in patients with superior sulcus tumors. In patients with other involvement of the chest wall, data to support its use are lacking. Postoperatively, radiation therapy as an adjuvant may be indicated in those patients in whom examination of the resected specimen reveals metastatic tumor in the mediastinal lymph nodes to reduce the incidence of local recurrence.

Whether or not the morbidity entailed is justified only to control local recurrence remains unanswered.

Irradiation, however, finds its greatest use as a palliative measure in patients with nonresectable lesions who have specific complaints such as pain in the chest wall, hemoptysis, the superior vena caval syndrome, and supraclavicular metastases, and in selected patients with bronchial obstruction. Relief of metastatic bone pain or of symptoms caused by cranial metastases is also a major indication for its use.

Its routine use, either in all patients with nonresectable disease caused by intrathoracic or distant spread or as a preoperative or postoperative measure in patients who have undergone a resection, cannot be defended by the present data provided by the literature. Like surgical therapy, the use of radiation therapy must be selected and tailored. Whether irradiation should be accomplished by external radiation only or, on occasion, from an internal source—brachytherapy—by the interstitial implantation of radioactive seeds, as Hilaris and his colleagues (1975, 1983) recommended, is not resolved.

Chemotherapy

Chemotherapy is discussed in detail in Chapters 96 and 97. Patients with undifferentiated small cell carcinoma are the major candidates for this modality. All such patients, including those with small cell tumors classified as T1N0 or T2N0 lesions who may have undergone initial resection, should be treated by one of the effective multiple-drug regimens currently in use. Prophylactic brain irradiation, as Tulloh (1977) and Jackson (1977) and their associates reported, is suggested for patients who are complete responders because it almost completely prevents the occurrence of cerebral metastases even though it does not prolong survival time. The role and timing of irradiation of the primary site and mediastinum are undetermined but are under active investigation.

Approximately 80 to 85% of the patients with small-cell carcinoma respond to chemotherapy, and in half of these the response is complete; remission of disease may last as long as 2 years. Patients with localized disease—stage I, II, and localized stage IIIa or IIIb disease—as Livingston (1978), Mandelbaum (1978), and Greco (1978) and their associates noted, are more likely to experience a complete response than are those with disseminated—now termed stage IV—disease. A poor performance status also adversely affects the degree and duration of response.

Patients with non-small cell tumors do not respond to chemotherapy as favorably as the aforementioned patients. Multiple drug regimens continue to be investigated for each of the non-small cell types. Generally, only patients with symptomatic disseminated disease should receive chemotherapy, and preferably their performance status should be 50 or above as measured on the Karnofsky scale (Table 76–11).

Immunotherapy

The interest in immunotherapy began with the observation of a possible salutatory effect on survival of the occurrence of a postoperative empyema after a resection of a lung carcinoma. Le Roux (1965), Takita (1970), and Ruckdeschel and associates (1972) reported survival rates of approximately 35% in a few such patients. Cady and Cliffton (1967), as well as Lawton and Keehn (1972), however, noted no such increase in survival. Pastroino and his colleagues (1982) likewise reported no such benefit. Those patients with postoperative empyema had a 5-year survival of 24% compared to 35% in those who did not develop this complication. Nonetheless, great interest in passive immunotherapy was stimulated, but numerous prospective trials of adjuvant immunotherapy, as noted in the section on Adjuvant Therapy, have not supported its use. Studies with active immunization continue, but what the role of immunotherapy will be is yet unknown.

Endobronchial Management of Lung Cancer

Although for years recurrent tumor obstructing the lower trachea or main stem bronchi has been coagulated endoscopically to prevent death from strangulation, the development of laser technics has made this endoscopic approach much more satisfactory.

Both the carbon dioxide and the neodymium-YAG lasers have been used to remove obstructing cancer tissue. Experimentally, phototherapy with hematoporphyrin derivative has also been evaluated.

Laser Therapy

This is better suited than phototherapy with hematoporphyria derivative for this task. The YAG laser is more appropriate than the CO_2 laser because it can be used through the flexible fiberscope, its light wavelength is not absorbed appreciably by either water or blood, and its energy can penetrate several millimeters. The CO_2 laser requires rigid-tube endoscopy, its depth of penetration is less than a millimeter, and to be effective it requires an absolutely dry field.

The YAG laser produces a thermal necrosis that debulks the tumor, and it controls any superficial bleeding. The technique is not without danger. Bleeding from perforation of a large vessel may occur, as may late hemorrhage from tumor necrosis. Cortese (1986) suggested the following as indications for YAG laser therapy: (1) the airway obstruction has been unresponsive to other reasonable therapy; (2) the lesion protrudes into the bronchial lumen without obvious extension beyond the cartilage; (3) the axial length of the endobronchial component of the tumor is less than 4 cm; (4) the bronchoscopist can see the bronchial lumen; and (5) functioning lung tissue exists beyond the obstruction. Wolf and Sabiston (1986) reported satisfactory palliation of severe obstruction or hemoptysis in 79% of 43 patients with advanced malignant tumors involving the trachea or main stem bronchi by the use of the YAG laser.

Bronchoscopic Phototherapy with Hematoporphyrin Derivative— HpD-PT

This also can be used to manage advanced, previously treated tumor causing significant airway obstruction. To date, HpD-PT has not been as successful as either the carbon dioxide or the neodymium-YAG lasers; but clinical trials are being carried out to define its usefulness and to improve its technique.

HpD-PT has been used more successfully in managing roentgenographically occult superficial squamous cell carcinoma than in removing obstruction. The tumor must be an in situ carcinoma or an invasive carcinoma limited to microinvasion of less than the full thickness of the bronchial wall. Hayata (1982) and Cortese (1984) and associates described the use of HpD-PT to eradicate such superficial lesions. Edell and Cortese (1987) reported the use of the modality for the treatment of 38 bronchial carcinomas in 36 patients. A complete response was observed in 13 patients—14 tumors. Of the 14 tumors, 3 recurred and required alternative therapy, as did the 26 carcinomas that did not respond completely with the initial HpD-PT therapy. All tumors that responded were radiographically occult, were less than 3 cm² in surface area, and appeared superficial at bronchoscopy. Two of the three patients with local recurrence after initial complete response died of carcinoma. Of the patients who had only partial responses, most died of carcinoma or because of hemoptysis. This form of therapy is indicated in only a highly select group of patients and in no way replaces the standard forms of therapy.

PROGNOSIS

The prognosis for patients with carcinoma of the lung continues to be poor. The overall survival rate remains less than 10%, the usual reported 5-year survival rates being 6 to 8%. Individual survival is determined by the cell type of the tumor, the site, the local spread as well as the presence or absence of distant spread at the time of discovery, the therapy, the age and sex of the patient, and the immunologic interplay of the host-tumor relationship. Although no definitive prognosis can be assigned to any one patient, broad generalizations can be made, although marked individual variations occur. In fact, a few proved bronchial carcinomas have undergone spontaneous regression with long-term survival after no or totally inadequate therapy. Unfortunately, however, most patients with bronchial carcinoma die of their disease.

The cell type of the tumor is critical. Because of the biologic nature of the various cell types, the clinical stage in which each most frequently is discovered, and the applicability of definitive therapy, the 5-year survival rates for bronchioloalveolar cell carcinoma are 30 to 35%; for sqamous cell carcinoma 8 to 16%; for adenocarcinoma 5 to 10%; and for undifferentiated small cell carcinoma, less than 3%.

The extent of the local disease and the presence or absence of lymphatic or blood-borne metastases, or both, are important in determining the prognosis of the patient.

Those patients who are first seen with extrathoracic metastatic disease or extrapulmonary intrathoracic disease that contraindicates exploration have the poorest prognosis as a group. They usually receive either no or only palliative therapy. Most die within 6 months, and fewer than 20% survive the first year. Two to five percent may survive the second year, and rarely a patient may live longer, but no survivors are expected by the fifth year. All patients, with rare exceptions, who have metastatic tumor in the brain, liver, or lung are dead within 6 months and most are dead within 3 months. Those with osseous metastases have slightly longer survival periods, but almost all are dead within 1 year, and half die within the first 6 months. The patients with extrathoracic lymph node metastases, such as in cervical nodes, do poorly, and the average survival time is approximately 3 months. Most of these patients are dead within 6 months. Of patients with lymph node involvement manifested by intrathoracic findings of a superior vena caval syndrome, two thirds die within 6 months, and almost all within 1 year. Rarely, a patient may survive 3 or 5 years after radiation therapy. In those patients with recurrent laryngeal nerve paralysis, the prognosis is somewhat better, because this paralysis is usually associated with a squamous cell carcinoma. Approximately two thirds of the patients survive 6 months; one fourth, 1 year; and one tenth, 2 years. An occasional patient survives 3 to 5 years. Only 20% of the patients whose tumor has spread to the pleura, and in whom a malignant pleural effusion is present, survive as long as 6 months, and only a few live more than 1 year.

Patients with extrathoracic, nonmetastatic, manifestations generally have a poor prognosis, particularly those with endocrine manifestations. Almost all those manifestations, except hypercalcemia and ectopic gonadotropin secretion, are associated with small cell tumors. Le Roux (1968a) reported that patients with a pulmonary hypertrophic osteoarthropathy, despite the high resectability rate for the tumor, likewise do not do well.

Of these patients, all those who do not undergo resection die within a year. Of the patients whose tumor is resected, 88% die within 3 years and only a few survive 5 years.

Patients with bronchial carcinoma who undergo an exploratory thoracotomy but are found to have nonresectable disease because of local spread of the tumor usually receive postoperative radiation therapy. Thus, the true natural course of the disease in this situation is difficult to determine because the effect of the radiation therapy must be considered. Generally, 15% of the patients die within the first 3 months and about half within the first 6 months. Approximately 30% live longer than a year. Only 3 to 5% survive for 2 years, and these patients usually die before the end of the third year, although rarely a patient survives for 5 or more years.

The prognosis of the patients who undergo an incomplete resection of their tumor is poor. I (1974) reported the results of such resections that had been done in the VASOG studies. Seventy-five percent of these patients were dead within one year. Although 8.5% survived three years, no patient with incomplete excision of mediastinal disease or lymph nodes survived that length of time. With the use of postoperative brachytherapy after incomplete resection, however, Burt and associates (1987) reported an improved survival in selected patients in this subset.

The prognosis of patients in the various stage groups I, II, and IIIa after complete resections has been discussed previously. These surviving patients are those who make up almost all of the overall 6 to 8% survivors of the entire patient group with carcinoma of the lung.

REFERENCES

Abbey Smith, R.: The results of raising the resectability rate in operation for lung carcinoma. Thorax 12:79, 1957.

Abbey Smith, R.: Cure of lung cancer from incomplete surgical resection. Br. Med. J. 2:563, 1971.

Abbey Smith, R.: The importance of mediastinal lymph node invasion by pulmonary carcinoma in selection of patients for resection. Ann. Thorac. Surg. 25:5, 1978.

Abbey Smith, R.: Evaluation of the long-term results of surgery for bronchial carcinoma. J. Thorac. Cardiovasc. Surg. 82:325, 1981.

Aberle, D.: Application of computed tomographic and magnetic resonance imaging in chest diseases. Presented at American College of Surgeons 73rd Annual Clinical Congress, San Francisco, October 12, 1987.

Ali, M.K.: Preoperative pulmonary function evaluation of the lung cancer patient. In Cancer Patients Care at M.D. Anderson Hospital and Tumor Institute. Edited by R.L. Clark and C.D. Rowe. Chicago, Year Book Medical Publishers, 1976, pp. 224–231.

Ali, M.K., et al.: Predicting loss of pulmonary function after pulmonary resection for bronchogenic carcinoma. Chest 77:337, 1980a.

Ali, M.K., et al.: Physiologic evaluation of the patient with lung cancer. In Lung Cancer: Current Status and Prospects for the Future. Edited by C.F. Mountain, and D.T. Carr. Austin, University of Texas Press, 1980b, p. 99.

Ali, M.K., et al.: Physiological evaluation of the patient with lung cancer: annual clinical conference on cancer, In Lung Cancer: Current Status and Prospects for the Future. Vol. 28. Edited by C.F. Mountain, and D.T. Carr. Austin, The University of Texas System Cancer Center, 1986, pp. 99—104.

Amemiya, R., and Oho, K.: X-ray diagnosis of lung cancer. In Lung Cancer Diagnosis. Edited by Y. Hayata. Igaku-Shoin, Tokyo, New York, 1982, p. 4.

American Joint Committee for Cancer Staging and End Results Reporting: Clinical staging system for carcinoma of the lung. Chicago, 1973.

American Thoracic Society: Clinical staging of primary lung cancer. Am. Rev. Respir. Dis. 127:659, 1983.

Amery, W.: Levamisole in resectable human bronchogenic carcinoma. Cancer Immunol. Immunother. 1:159, 1976.

Anthony, H.M., et al.: Levamisole and surgery in bronchial carcinoma patients: increase in deaths from cardiorespiratory failure. Thorax 34:4, 1979.

Ashor, G.L., et al.: Long-term survival in bronchogenic carcinoma. J. Thorac. Cardiovasc. Surg. 70:581, 1975.

Auerbach, O., and Stout, A.P.: Histopathological aspects of occult cancer of the lung. Ann. NY Acad. Sci. 114:803, 1964.

Auerbach, O., et al.: Changes in bronchial epithelium in relation to cigarette smoking and in relation to lung cancer. N. Engl. J. Med. 265:253, 1961.

Ayvazian, L.F., et al.: Ectopic production of big ACTH in carcinoma of the lung: its clinical usefulness as a biologic marker. Ann. Rev. Respir. Dis. 111:279, 1975.

Backer, C.L., et al.: Selective preoperative evaluation for possible N2 disease in carcinoma of the lung. J. Thorac. Cardiovasc. Surg. 93:337, 1987.

Bakker, W., et al.: Postoperative intrapleural BCG in lung cancer: lack of efficacy and possible enhancement of tumour growth. Thorax 36:870, 1981.

Bakker, W., et al.: Complications of postoperative intrapleural BCG in lung cancer. Ann. Thorac. Surg. 33:267, 1982.

Bariety, M., et al.: Twelve years' experience with gas mediastinography. Dis. Chest. 48:449, 1965.

Bartter, F.C., and Schwartz, W.B.: The syndrome of inappropriate secretion of antidiuretic hormone. Am. J. Med. 42:790, 1967.

Bates, M.: Results of surgery for bronchial carcinoma in patients aged 70 and over. Thorax 25:77, 1970.

Bateson, E.M.: An analysis of 155 solitary lung lesions illustrating differential diagnosis of mixed tumours of the lung. Clin. Radiol. 16:51, 1965.

Bechard, D., and Wetstein, L.: Assessment of exercise oxygen consumption as preoperative criterion for lung resection. Ann. Thorac. Surg. 44:344, 1987.

Belcher, J.R., and Rehahn, M.: Late deaths after resection for bronchial carcinoma. Br. J. Dis. Chest. 73:18, 1979.

Benfield, J.R., et al.: Azygograms and pulmonary arteriograms in bronchogenic carcinoma. Arch. Surg. 99:406, 1969.

Bennett, W.F., and Abbey Smith, R.: Segmental resection for bronchogenic carcinoma: a surgical alternative for the compromised patient. Ann. Thorac. Surg. 27:169, 1979.

Bensch, K.G., et al.: Oat-cell carcinoma of the lung. Cancer 22:1163, 1968.

Bergh, N.P., and Larsson, S.: The significance of various types of mediastinal lymph-node metastases in lung cancer. In Mediastinoscopy: Proceedings of an International Symposium. Edited by O. Jepsen, and H.R. Sorenson. Odense, Odense University Press, 1971.

Bergh, N.P., and Schersten, T.: Bronchogenic carcinoma: a follow-up study of a surgically treated series with special reference to the prognostic significance of lymph node metastases. Acta Chir. Scand. (Suppl.) 347:1, 1965.

Bloedorn, F.G., and Cowley, R.A.: Irradiation and surgery in the treatment of bronchogenic carcinoma. Surg. Gynecol. Obstet. 111:141, 1960.

Bondy, P.K., and Gilby, E.D.: Endocrine function in small cell undifferentiated carcinoma of the lung. Cancer 50:2147, 1982.

Borrie, J.: Pulmonary carcinoma of the bronchus. Ann. R. Coll. Surg. Engl. 10:165, 1952.

Boucot, K.R., Cooper, D.A., and Weiss, W.: The Philadelphia Pulmonary Neoplasm Research Project. Ann. Intern. Med. 54:363, 1961.

Boucot, K.R., et al.: The natural history of lung cancer. Am. Rev. Respir. Dis. 89:519, 1964.

Boucot, K.R., et al.: Cigarettes, cough, and cancer of the lung. JAMA 196:985, 1966.

Brereton, H.D., et al.: Gallium scans for staging small cell lung cancer. JAMA 249:666, 1978.

Brett, C.Z.: The value of lung cancer detection by six-monthly chest radiographs. Thorax 23:414, 1968.

Bromley, L.I., and Szur, L.: Combined radiotherapy and resection for carcinoma of the bronchus. Lancet 2:937, 1955.

Brynitz, S., and Struve-Christensen, E.: Transcarinal mediastinal needle biopsy as a supplement to bronchoscopic evaluation of neoplastic lung diseases. Endoscopy 17:18, 1985.

Burt, M.E., et al.: Results of surgical treatment of stage III lung cancer invading the mediastinum. Surg. Clin. North Am. 67(5):987, 1987.

Byrd, R.B., et al.: Radiographic abnormalities in carcinoma of the lung as related to histological cell type. Thorax 124:573, 1969.

Cady, B., and Cliffton, E.E.: Empyema and survival following surgery for bronchogenic carcinoma. J. Thorac. Surg. 53:102, 1967.

Carlens, E.: Mediastinoscopy. Dis. Chest 36:343, 1959.

Clain, A.: Secondary malignant disease of bone. Br. J. Cancer 19:15, 1965.

Concannon, J.P., et al.: Prognosis value of carcinoembryonic antigen (CEA) plasma levels in patients with bronchogenic carcinoma. Cancer 42:1477, 1978.

Cooper, J.D., and Ginsberg, R.J.: The use of mediastinoscopy in lung cancer: preoperative evaluation. In Current Controversies in Thoracic Surgery. Edited by C.F. Kittle. Philadelphia, W.B. Saunders Co., 1986, p. 162.

Cooper, W.R., Guerrant, J.L., and Teates, C.D.:Prediction of postoperative respiratory function in patients undergoing lung resection. Va. Med. 107:264, 1980.

Cortese, D.A.: Endobronchial management of lung cancer. Chest 89:234S, 1986.

Cortese, D.A., and Kinsey, J.H.: Hematoporphyrin derivative phototherapy in the treatment of bronchogenic carcinoma. Chest 86:8, 1984.

Cotton, R.E.: The bronchial spread of lung cancer. Br. J. Dis. Chest. 53:142, 1959.

Coughlin, M., Deslauriers, J., and Beaulieu, M.: Role of mediastinoscopy in pre-treatment staging of patients with primary lung cancer. Ann. Thorac. Surg. 40:556, 1985.

Cummings, S.R., Lillington, G.A., and Richard, R.J.: Managing solitary pulmonary nodules: the choice of strategy is a "close call." Am. Rev. Respir. Dis. 134:435, 1986a.

Cummings, S.R., Lillington, G.A., and Richard, R.J.: Estimating the probability of malignancy in solitary pulmonary nodules: a Bayesian approach. Am. Rev. Respir. Dis. 134:449, 1986b.

Dartevelle, P.G., et al.: Tracheal-sleeve pneumonectomy for bronchogenic carcinoma: report of 50 cases. Ann. Thorac. Surg. 46:68, 1988.

DeBesse, B., et al.: La survie du carcinome epidermoide bronchique opère. Ann. Chir. Thorac. Cardiovasc. 15:25, 1976.

Decker, D.A., et al.: The significance of cytologically negative pleural effusion in bronchogenic carcinoma. Chest 74:640, 1978.

DeLaude, F.H., et al.: 67Ga-citrate imaging in untreated primary lung cancer: preliminary report of cooperative group. J. Nucl. Med. 15:408, 1974.

DeMeester, T.R., et al.: Gallium-67 scanning for carcinoma of the lung. J. Thorac. Cardiovasc. Surg. 72:699, 1976.

DeMeester, T.R., et al.: The role of gallium-67 scanning in the clinical staging and preoperative evaluation of patients with carcinoma of the lung. Ann. Thorac. Surg. 28:451, 1979.

Deslauriers, J.: Technical considerations in stage III disease: involvement of the main carina. In International Trends in General Thoracic Surgery, Vol. 1, Lung Cancer. Edited by N.C. Delarue and H. Eschapasse. Philadelphia, W.B. Saunders Co., 1985, p. 139.

Deslauriers, J., et al.: Long-term clinical and functional results of sleeve lobectomy for primary lung cancer. J. Thorac. Cardiovasc. Surg. 92:871, 1986.

Deslauriers, J., et al.: Carcinoma of the lung: evaluation of satellite nodules as a factor influencing prognosis after resection. J. Thorac. Cardiovasc. Surg. (in press).

Dillon, M.L. and Postlethwait, R.W.: Carcinoma of the lung. Ann. Thorac. Surg. 11:193, 1971.

Doll, R., and Hill, A.B.: A study of the etiology of carcinoma of the lung. Br. Med. J. 2:1271, 1952.

Dorn, H.F.: Tobacco consumption and mortality from cancer and other diseases. Public Health Rep. 74:581, 1959.

Durie, B.G.M., Salmon, S.E., and Russell, D.H.: Polyamines as markers of response and disease activity in cancer chemotherapy. Cancer Rev. 37:214, 1977.

Edell, E.S., and Cortese, D.A.: Bronchoscopic phototherapy with hematoporphyrin derivative for treament of localized bronchogenic carcinoma: a 5-year experience. Mayo Clin. Proc. 62:8, 1987.

Eno, K.: Bronchographic studies of lung cancer: correlation with histologic types. Jpn. J. Lung Cancer 16:43, 1976 (in Japanese).

Ernst, H., Kruger, J., and Vassal, K.: Lung scanning as a screening method for cancer of the lung. Cancer 23:508, 1969.

Errett, L.E., et al.: Wedge resection as an alternative procedure for peripheral bronchogenic carcinoma in poor risk patients. J. Thorac. Cardiovasc. Surg. 90:656, 1985.

Faber, L.P.: Results of surgical treatment of stage III lung carcinoma with carinal proximity: the role of sleeve lobectomy versus pneumonectomy and the role of sleeve pneumonectomy. Surg. Clin. N. Am. 67:1001, 1987.

Faber, L.P., et al.: Flexible fiberoptic bronchoscopy. Ann. Thorac. Surg. 16:163, 1973.

Faber, L.P., Jensik, R.J., and Kittle, C.F.: Results of sleeve lobectomy for bronchogenic carcinoma in 101 patients. Ann. Thorac. Surg. 37:279, 1984.

Faiman, C., et al.: Gonadotropin secretion from a bronchogenic carcinoma. N. Engl. J. Med. 227:1395, 1967.

Feld, R., et al.: Site of recurrence in resected stage I non-small cell lung cancer: a guide for future studies. J. Clin. Oncol. 2:1352, 1984.

Fennesy, J.J.: Bronchial brushing and transbronchial forceps biopsy in the diagnosis of pulmonary lesions. Dis. Chest 53:377, 1968.

Fontana, R.S., and Sanderson, D.R.: Screening for lung cancer: a progress report. In Lung Cancer: Current Status and Prospects for the Future. Edited by C.F. Mountain and D.T. Carr. Austin, University of Texas Press, 1986, p. 51.

Fosburg, R.G., Hopkins, G.B., and Kan, M.K.: Evaluation of mediastinum by gallium-67 scintigraphy in lung cancer. J. Thorac. Cardiovasc. Surg. 77:76, 1979.

Freise, G., Gabler, A., and Leibig, S.: Bronchial carcinoma and long-term survival. Retrospective study of 433 patients who underwent resection. Thorax 33:228, 1978.

Galluzzi, S., and Payne, P.M.: Bronchial carcinoma. Br. J. Cancer 9:511, 1955.

Garland, L.H.: The rate of growth and natural duration of primary bronchial cancer. Am. J. Roentgenol. 96:604, 1966.

Gewirtz, G., and Yalow, R.S.: Ectopic ACTH production in carcinoma of the lung. J. Clin. Invest. 53:1022, 1974.

Gibbons, J.P.R.: The value of mediastinoscopy in assessing operability of carcinoma of the lung. Br. J. Dis. Chest. 66:162, 1972.

Gilbertsen, V.A.: X-ray examination of the chest. JAMA 188:1082, 1964.

Gilby, E.D., Reis, L.H., and Bondy, P.K.: Ectopic hormones as markers of response to therapy in cancer. In Proceedings of the Sixth International Symposium on the Biological Characteristics of Human Tumors. Excerpta Medica International Congress Series No. 375, New York, Elsevier-North Holland Publishing Company, 1976.

Ginsberg, R.J., et al.: Chemotherapy followed by adjuvant surgery in the treatment of limited small cell carcinoma (SCLC). In Proc. 13th International Congress Chemotherapy, Edited by K.H. Spitzy and K. Karrer. Vienna, 1983.

Ginsberg, R.J., et al.: Extended cervical mediastinoscopy—a single staging procedure for bronchogenic carcinoma of the left upper lobe. J. Thorac. Cardiovasc. Surg. 94:673, 1987.

Gray, F.W., Schorr, R.T., and Heilbrom, H.: Interosseous azygography. J. Thorac. Cardiovasc. Surg. 55:389, 1968.

Greco, F.A., et al.: Treatment of oat cell carcinoma of the lung: complete remission, acceptable complications, and improved survival. Br. Med. J. 2:10, 1978.

Green, N., et al.: Post-resection irradiation for primary lung cancer. Radiology 116:405, 1975.

Greschuchna, D., and Maassen, W.: Die lymphogenen Absiedlungswege des Bronchialkarzinoms. Stuttgart, Thieme Verlag, 1973.

Griess, D.F., McDonald, J.R, and Clagett, O.T.: The proximal extension of carcinoma of the lung in the bronchial wall. J. Thorac. Surg. 14:362, 1945.

Grillo, H.C., Greenberg, J.J., and Wilkins, E.W.: Resection of bronchogenic carcinoma involving thoracic wall. J. Thorac. Cardiovasc. Surg. 51:417, 1966.

Guttman, R.J.: Radical supervoltage therapy in inoperable carcinoma of the lung. In Carcinoma of the Bronchus. Edited by T.J. Deeley. New York, Appleton-Century-Crofts, 1971.

Hallgren, R., Nou, E., and Lundquist, G.: Serum β_2 microglobulin in patients with bronchial carcinoma and controls. Cancer 45:780, 1980.

Hansen, M., et al.: Hormonal polypetides and amine metabolites in small cell carcinoma of the lung, with special references to stage and subtypes. Cancer 45:1432, 1980.

Hara, N., et al.: Assessment of the role of surgery for stage III bronchogenic carcinoma. J. Surg. Oncol. 25:153, 1984.

Hara, N., et al.: Surgical adjuvant chemotherapy for lung cancer. In Recent Advances in Chemotherapy: Proceedings of the 14th International Congress on Chemotherapy. Edited by J. Ishigami. Tokyo, University of Tokyo Press, 1985, p. 155.

Harviel, J.D., McNamara, J.J., and Straehley, C.J.: Surgical treatment of lung cancer in patients over the age of 70 years. J. Thorac. Cardiovasc. Surg. 75:802, 1978.

Hata, E., Troidl, H., and Hasegawa, T.: In vivo Unterschungen der Lymphdrainage des Bronchialsystem beim menschen mit der Lymphoszintigraphie—eine neue diagnostische Technik. In Behandlung des Bronchialkarzinoms: Resignation oder neue Ansatze: Symposium Kiel. New York, G. Thieme Verlag, 1981.

Hattori, S., and Matsuda, M.: TV brushing method for early diagnosis of small peripheral lung cancer. In Carcinoma of the Bronchus. Edited by T.J. Deeley. New York, Appleton-Century-Crofts, 1971, p. 53.

Hayata, Y., et al.: Hematoporphyrin derivative and laser photoradiation in the treatment of lung cancer. Chest 81:269, 1982.

Higgins, G.A., Shields, T.W., and Keehn, R.J.: The solitary pulmonary nodule. Ten-year follow-up of Veterans Administration-Armed Forces Cooperative Study. Arch. Surg. 110:570, 1975.

Hilaris, B.S., and Martini, N.: Interstitial brachytherapy in cancer of the lung: a 20-year experience. Int. J. Radiat. Oncol. Biol. Phys. 5:1951, 1979.

Hilaris, B.S., et al.: Interstitial irradiation for unresectable carcinoma of the lung. Ann. Thorac. Surg. 20:491, 1975.

Hilaris, B.S., et al.: Value of perioperative brachytherapy in the management of non-oat cell carcinoma of the lung. Int. J. Radiat. Oncol. Biol. Phys. 9:161, 1983.

Holmes, E.C., et al.: A randomized comparison of the effects of adjuvant therapy on resected stages II and III non-small cell carcinoma of the lung. Ann. Surg. 202:335, 1985.

Hooper, R.G., et al.: Computed tomographic scanning of the brain in initial staging of bronchogenic carcinoma. Chest 85:774, 1984.

Iascone, C., et al.: Local recurrence of resectable non-oat cell carcinoma of the lung. Cancer 57:471, 1986.

Ikeda, S.: Bronchography of lung cancer. In Atlas of Lung Cancer. Edited by S. Ishikawa. Tokyo, Nakayama Shoten, 1968, p. 186 (in Japanese).

Immerman, S.C., et al.: Site of recurrence in patients with stage I and II carcinoma of the lung resected for cure. Ann. Thorac. Surg. 32:23, 1981.

Inberg, M.V., et al.: Facilities for surgery and survival prospects in lung carcinoma. Scand. J. Thorac. Cardiovasc. Surg. 6:297, 1972.

Jackson, D., et al.: The value of prophylactic cranial irradiation in small cell carcinoma of the lung: a randomized study. Proc. A.A.C.R.-A.S.C.O. 18:319, 1977.

Jeffery, R.M.: Survival in bronchial carcinoma: tumor remaining in the bronchial stump following resection. Ann. R. Coll. Surg. (Engl.) 51:55, 1972.

Jensik, R.J.: The extent of resection for localized lung cancer: segmental resection. In Current Controversies in Thoracic Surgery. Edited by C.F. Kittle. Philadelphia, W.B. Saunders Co., 1986, p. 175.

Jensik, R.J., et al.: Tracheal-sleeve pneumonectomy for advanced carcinoma of the lung. Surg. Gynecol. Obstet. 134:231, 1972a.

Jensik, R.J., et al.: Sleeve lobectomy for carcinoma. A ten-year experience. J. Thorac. Cardiovasc. Surg. 64:400, 1972b.

Jensik, R.J., et al.: Survival following resection for second primary bronchogenic carcinoma. J. Thorac. Cardiovasc. Surg. 82:658, 1981.

Jensik, R.J., et al.: Survival in patients undergoing tracheal-sleeve pneumonectomy for bronchogenic carcinoma. J. Thorac. Cardiovasc. Surg. 84:489, 1982.

Johnson, R.R.J.: Radiotherapy—primary and/or adjuvant modality. In Perspectives in Lung Cancer: Frederick E. Jones Memorial Symposium in Thoracic Surgery. Columbus, Ohio, 1976. New York, S. Karger, 1977, p. 74.

Karnofsky, D.A., and Burchenal, J.H.: The clinical evaluation of chemotherapeutic agents in cancer. In Evaluation of Chemotherapeutic Agents. Edited by C.M. McLeod. New York, Columbia University Press, 1949.

Kato, H.: Sputum cytology diagnosis. In Lung Cancer Diagnosis. Edited by Y. Hayata. Tokyo, Igaku-Shoin, 1982, p. 85.

Keller, S.M., Kaiser, L.R., and Martini, N.: Bilobectomy for bronchogenic carcinoma. Ann. Thorac. Surg. 45:62, 1988.

Kirsh, M.M., and Sloan, H.: Mediastinal metastases in bronchogenic carcinoma: Influence of postoperative irradiation, cell type, and location. Ann. Thorac. Surg. 33:459, 1982.

Kirsh, M.M., et al.: Treatment of bronchogenic carcinoma with mediastinal metastases. Ann. Thorac. Surg. 12:11, 1971.

Kirsh, M.M., et al.: Carcinoma of the lung: results of treatment over ten years. Ann. Thorac. Surg. 21:371, 1976a.

Kirsh, M.M., et al.: Major pulmonary resections for bronchogenic carcinoma in the elderly. Ann. Thorac. Surg. 22:369, 1976b.

Kittle, C.F., et al.: Pulmonary resection in patients after pneumonectomy. Ann. Thorac. Surg. 40:294, 1985.

Kotin, P.: Carcinogenesis of the lung. In The Lung. Edited by A.A. Liebow and D.E. Smith. Baltimore, Williams & Wilkins, 1968. p. 203.

Kristersson, S., Lindell, S.E., and Svanberg, L.: Prediction of pulmonary function loss due to pneumonectomy using ^{133}Xe-Radiospirometry. Chest 62:694, 1972.

Lange, E., and Høeg, K.: Cytologic typing of lung cancer. Acta Cytol. 16:327, 1972.

Lauby, V.W., et al.: Value and risk of biopsy of pulmonary lesions by needle aspiration. J. Thorac. Cardiovasc. Surg. 49:159, 1965.

Lawton, R.L., and Keehn, R.J.: Bronchogenic cancer, sepsis and survival. J. Surg. Oncol. 5:466, 1972.

LeGal, Y., and Bauer, W.C.: Secondary primary bronchogenic carcinoma. J. Thorac. Surg. 41:114, 1961.

Le Roux, B.T.: Empyema thoracis. Br. J. Surg. 52:89, 1965.

Le Roux, B.T.: Bronchial Carcinoma. London, E. and S. Livingstone, Ltd., 1968a.

Le Roux, B.T.: Bronchial carcinoma. Thorax 23:136, 1968b.

Libshitz, H.I., et al.: Patterns of mediastinal metastases in bronchogenic carcinoma. Chest 90:229, 1986.

Livingston, R.B.: Small-cell carcinoma of the lung: combined chemotherapy and radiation. Ann. Intern. Med. 88:194, 1978.

Ludwig Lung Cancer Study Group: Adverse effect of intrapleural Corynebacterium parvum as adjuvant therapy in resected stage I and II non-small cell carcinoma of the lung. J. Thorac. Cardiovasc. Surg. 89:842, 1985.

Ludwig Lung Cancer Study Group: Patterns of failure in patients with resected stage I and II non-small cell carcinoma of the lung. Ann. Surg. 205:67, 1987.

Ludwig Lung Cancer Study Group: Immunostimulation with intrapleural BCG as adjuvant therapy in resected non-small cell lung cancer. Cancer (in press).

Luke, W.P., et al.: Prospective evaluation of mediastinoscopy for assessment of carcinoma of the lung. J. Thorac. Cardiovasc. Surg. 91:53, 1986.

Maassen, W.: Accuracy of mediastinoscopy. In International Trends in General Thoracic Surgery, Vol. 1, Lung Cancer. Edited by N.C. Delaure and H. Eschapasse. Philadelphia, W.B. Saunders Co., 1985, p. 42.

Maassen, W., Greschuchna, D., and Martinez, I.: The role of surgery in the treatment of small cell carcinoma of the lung. Recent Results Cancer Res. 97:107, 1985.

Magilligan, D.J., Jr., et al.: Surgical approach to lung cancer with solitary cerebral metastasis: twenty-five years' experience. Ann. Thorac. Surg. 42:360, 1986.

Mandelbaum, I., et al.: Combined therapy for small cell undifferentiated carcinoma of the lung. J. Thorac. Cardiovasc. Surg. 76:292, 1978.

Mandell, I., et al.: The treatment of single brain metastasis from non-oat cell lung carcinoma. Cancer 58:641, 1986.

Mark, J.B.D., Marlin, S.I., and Castellino, R.A.: The role of bronchoscopy and needle aspiration in the diagnosis of peripheral lung masses. J. Thorac. Cardiovasc. Surg. 76:266, 1978.

Martini, N.: Improved methods of recording data in lung cancer. Clin. Bull. Memorial Sloan-Kettering Cancer Center 6:93, 1976.

Martini, N.: Identification and prognosis implications of mediastinal lymph node metastases in carcinoma of the lung. In Lung Cancer: Progress in Therapeutic Research. Edited by F. Muggia and J. Rozencweig. New York, Raven Press, 1979.

Martini, N.: The extent of resection for localized lung cancer: lobectomy. In Current Controversies in Thoracic Surgery. Edited by C.F. Kittle. Philadelphia, W.B. Saunders Co., 1986a, p. 171

Martini, N.: Rationale for surgical treatment of brain metastasis in non-small cell lung cancer. Ann. Thorac. Surg. 42:357, 1986b.

Martini, N., et al.: Prospective study of 445 lung carcinomas with mediastinal lymph node metastases. J. Thorac. Cardiovasc. Surg. 89:390, 1980.

Martini, N., and Flehinger, B.J.: The role of surgery in N2 lung cancer. Surg. Clin. North Am. 67(5):1037, 1987.

Martini, N., et al.: Prognostic significance of N1 disease in carcinoma of the lung. J. Thorac. Cardiovasc. Surg. 86:646, 1983a.

Martini, N., et al.: Results in resection in non-oat cell carcinoma of the lung with mediastinal lymph node metastases. Ann. Surg. 198:386, 1983b.

Martini, N., Ghosen, P., and Melamed, M.R.: Local recurrence and new primary carcinoma after resection. In International Trends in General Thoracic Surgery, Vol. 1, Lung Cancer. Edited by N.C. Delarine and H. Eschapasse. Philadelphia, W.B. Saunders Co., 1985a, p. 164.

Martini, N., et al.: Management of stage III disease: alternate approaches to the management of mediastinal adenopathy. In International Trends in General Thoracic Surgery, Vol. 1, Lung Cancer. Edited by N.C. Delarue and H. Eschapasse. Philadelphia, W.B. Saunders Co., 1985b, p. 108.

Martini, N., et al.: The effects of preoperative chemotherapy on the resectability of non-small cell lung carcinoma with mediastinal node metastases (N2MO). Ann. Thorac. Surg. 45:370, 1988.

Matthews, M.J.: Morphologic classification of bronchogenic carcinoma. Cancer Chemother. Rep. 3:229, 1973.

Matthews, M.J., Pickren, J., and Kanhowa, S.: Who has occult metastases? Residual tumor in patients undergoing surgical resections for lung cancer. In Perspectives in Lung Cancer. Edited by D.S. Yuhn. Frederick E. Jones Memorial Symposium in Thoracic Surgery. Basel Karger, 1977, p. 9.

Maxfield, W.S., Hatch, H.B., Jr., and Nelson, J.R.: Forecast of prognosis after radiotherapy. In Carcinoma of the Bronchus. Edited by T.J. Deeley. New York, Appleton-Century-Crofts, 1971.

McCaughan, B.C., et al.: Chest wall invasion in carcinoma of the lung. J. Thorac. Cardiovasc. Surg. 89:836, 1985.

McKneally, M.F., et al.: Regional immunotherapy with intrapleural BCG for lung cancer. J. Thorac. Cardiovasc. Surg. 72:333, 1976.

McKneally, M.F., et al.: Regional immunotherapy of lung cancer using intrapleural BCG: summary of a four-year randomized study. In Lung Cancer: Progress in Therapeutic Research. Edited by F.M. Muggia and M. Rozencweig. New York, Raven Press, 1979, p. 471.

McKneally, M.F., et al.: Four-year follow-up on the Albany experience with intrapleural BCG in lung cancer. J. Thorac. Cardiovasc. Surg. 81:485, 1981.

McNeill, T.M., and Chamberlain, I.M.: Diagnostic anterior mediastinotomy. Ann. Thorac. Surg. 2:532, 1966.

Melamed, M.R., et al.: Screening for early lung cancer: results of the Memorial Sloan-Kettering study in New York. Chest 86:44, 1984.

Merkle, N.M., et al.: Problems of oat cell carcinoma: surgical resection. In International Trends in General Thoracic Surgery. Edited by

N.C. Delarue and H. Eschapasse. Philadelphia, W.B. Saunders Co., 1985, p. 190.

Meyer, E.C., and Liebow, A.A.: Relationship of interstitial pneumonia honeycombing and atypical epithelial proliferation to carcinoma of the lung. Cancer 18:322, 1965.

Meyer, J.A.: Growth rate versus prognosis in resected primary bronchogenic carcinomas. Cancer 31:1468, 1973.

Meyer, J.A.: Surgical resection as an adjunct to chemotherapy for small cell carcinoma of the lung. In Bronchial Carcinoma. Edited by M. Bates. Berlin, Springer-Verlag, 1984, p. 177.

Meyer, J.A.: Effect of histologically verified TNM stage on disease control in treated small cell carcinoma of the lung. Cancer 55:1747, 1985.

Meyer, J.A.: Five-year survival in treated stage I and II small cell carcinoma of the lung. Ann. Thorac. Surg. 42(6):668, 1986.

Meyer, J., et al.: Selective surgical resection in small cell carcinoma of the lung. J. Thorac. Cardiovasc. Surg. 77:243, 1979.

Meyer, J.A., et al.: Phase II trial of extended indications for resection in small cell carcinoma of the lung. J. Thorac. Cardiovasc. Surg. 83:12, 1982.

Millar, J.W., et al.: Five-year results of a controlled study of BCG immunotherapy after surgical resection in bronchogenic carcinoma. Thorax 37:57, 1982.

Morton, D.L., Itabashi, H.H., and Grimes, O.F.: Nonmetastatic neurological complications of bronchogenic carcinoma. J. Thorac. Cardiovasc. Surg. 51:14, 1966.

Mountain, C.F.: The biologic operability of stage III non-small cell lung cancer. Ann. Thorac. Surg. 40:60, 1985.

Mountain, C.F.: A new international staging system for lung cancer. Chest 89:225S, 1986a.

Mountain, C.F.: Selecting patients for surgical treatment of lung cancer. In Lung Cancer: Current Status and Prospects for the Future. Edited by C.F. Mountain and D.T. Carr. Austin, University of Texas Press, 1986b, p. 161.

Mountain, C.F., and Gail, M.H.: Surgical adjuvant intrapleural BCG treatment for stage I non-small cell lung cancer: preliminary report of the National Cancer Institute Lung Cancer Study Group. J. Thorac. Cardiovasc. Surg. 82:649, 1981.

Mountain, C.F., et al.: Present status of postoperative adjuvant therapy for lung cancer. Cancer Bull. 32:108, 1980.

Naef, A-P.: Chirurgie tracheobronchique et fonction respiratoire. Rev. Therap. 28:738, 1971.

Naef, A-P.: Tracheobronchial reconstruction. Ann. Thorac. Surg. 15:301, 1973.

Naef, A-P., and deGruneck, J.S.: Right pneumonectomy or sleeve lobectomy in the treatment of bronchogenic carcinoma. Ann. Thorac. Surg. 17:168, 1974.

Nagaishi, C., et al.: Electron microscopic observations of the human lung cancer. Exp. Med. Surg. 23:177, 1965.

Naruke, T., Suemasu, K., and Ishikawa, S.: Surgical treatment for lung cancer with metastasis to mediastinal lymph nodes. J. Thorac. Cardiovasc. Surg. 71:279, 1976.

Naruke, T., Suemasu, K., and Ishikawa, S.: Lymph node mapping and curability at various levels of metastasis in resected lung cancer. J. Thorac. Cardiovasc. Surg. 76:832, 1978.

Naruke, T., et al.: The importance of surgery to non-small cell carcinoma of the lung with mediastinal lymph node metastasis. Ann. Thorac. Surg. (in press).

Nathan, M.H., Collins, V.P., and Adams, R.A.: Differentiation of benign and malignant pulmonary nodules by growth rate. Radiology 79:221, 1962.

Neptune, W.B.: Primary lung cancer surgery in stage II and stage III. Arch. Surg. 123:583, 1988.

Newman, S.B., et al.: The treatment of modified stage II (T1N1M0, T2N1M0) non-small cell bronchogenic carcinoma. J. Thorac. Cardiovasc. Surg. 86:180, 1983.

Nohl, H.C.: An investigation into the lymphatic and vascular spread of carcinoma of the bronchus. Thorax 11:172, 1956.

Nohl-Oser, H.C.: Lymphatics of the lung. In General Thoracic Surgery. 3rd ed. Edited by T.W. Shields. Philadelphia, Lea & Febiger, 1988.

Non-small Cell Lung Cancer Workshop. Key Biscayne, Florida, November 6–10, 1987.

Nystrom, J.S., et al.: Identifying the primary site in metastatic cancer of unknown origins. JAMA 241:381, 1979.

Ochsner, A., and DeBakey, M.: Significance of metastasis in primary carcinoma of the lungs. J. Thorac. Surg. 11:357, 1942.

Ohta, M., et al.: The role of surgical management of small cell carcinoma of the lung. Jpn. J. Clin. Oncol. 16:289, 1986.

Olsen, G.N., Block, J., and Tobias, J.A.: Prediction of postpneumonectomy function using quantitative macroaggregate lung scanning. Chest 66:13, 1974a.

Olsen, G.N., et al.: Pulmonary function evaluation of the lung resection candidate: a prospective study. Am. Rev. Respir. Dis. 111:379, 1974b.

Osada, H.: Bronchography. In Lung Cancer Diagnosis. Edited by Y. Hayata. Tokyo, Igaku-Shoin, 1982, p. 68.

Oswald, N.C., et al.: The diagnosis of primary lung cancer with special reference to sputum cytology. Thorax 26:623, 1971.

Pagani, J.J.: Non-small cell lung carcinoma adrenal metastases: computed tomography and percutaneous needle biopsy in their diagnosis. Cancer 53:1058, 1984.

Pairolero, P.C., et al.: Postsurgical stage I bronchogenic carcinoma: morbid implications of recurrent disease. Ann. Thorac. Surg. 38:331, 1984.

Pastroino, U., et al.: Empyema following lung cancer resection: risk factors and prognostic value on survival. Ann. Thorac. Surg. 33:320, 1982.

Patterson, G.A., et al.: Combined pulmonary and chest wall resection for carcinoma of the lung: benefits of adjuvant radiotherapy. Ann. Thorac. Surg. 34:692, 1982.

Patterson, G.A., et al.: Significance of metastatic disease in subaortic lymph nodes. Ann. Thorac. Surg. 43:155, 1987.

Paulson, D.L.: Technical considerations in stage III disease: the superior sulcus lesion. In International Trends in Thoracic Surgery. Vol. 1, Lung Cancer. Edited by N.C. Delarue and H. Eschapasse. Philadelphia, W.B. Saunders Co., 1985, p. 121.

Paulson, D.L., and Reisch, J.S.: Long-term survival after resection for bronchogenic carcinoma. Ann. Surg. 184:324, 1976.

Paulson, D.L., and Urschel, H.C., Jr.: Selectivity in the surgical treatment of bronchogenic carcinoma. J. Thorac. Cardiovasc. Surg. 62:554, 1971.

Paulson, D.L., et al.: Bronchoplastic procedures for bronchogenic carcinoma. J. Thorac. Cardiovasc. Surg. 59:38, 1970.

Pearson, F.G.: An evaluation of mediastinoscopy in the management of presumably operable bronchial carcinoma. J. Thorac. Cardiovasc. Surg. 55:617, 1968.

Pearson, F.G., et al.: Significance of positive superior mediastinal nodes identified at mediastinoscopy in patients with resectable cancer of the lung. J. Thorac. Cardiovasc. Surg. 83:1, 1982.

Pemberton, J.H., et al.: Bronchogenic carcinoma in patients younger than 40 years. Ann. Thorac. Surg. 36:509, 1983.

Piehler, J.M., et al.: Bronchogenic carcinoma with chest wall invasion: factors affecting survival following en bloc resection. Ann. Thorac. Surg. 34:684, 1982.

Piehler, J.M., et al.: Concomitant cardiac and pulmonary operations. J. Thorac. Cardiovasc. Surg. 90:662, 1985.

Prager, R.L., et al.: The feasibility of adjuvant surgery in limited state small cell carcinoma: a prospective evaluation. Ann. Thorac. Surg. 38:622, 1984.

Ramsdell, J.W., et al.: Multiorgan scans for staging lung cancer. J. Thorac. Cardiovasc. Surg. 73:653, 1977.

Rasmussen, P.S.: Metastasis in lung cancer: a study based on a series of pulmonary resections. Dan. Med. Bull. 2:60, 1964.

Razzuk, M.A., et al.: Observations of ultrastructural morphology of bronchogenic carcinoma. J. Thorac. Cardiovasc. Surg. 59:581, 1970.

Read, R.C., et al.: Diameter, cell type, and survival in stage I primary non-small-cell lung cancer. Arch. Surg. 123:446, 1988.

Rees, G.M., and Paneth, M.: Lobectomy with sleeve resection in the treatment of bronchial tumours. Thorax 25:160, 1970.

Reichel, J.: Assessment of operative risk of pneumonectomy. Chest 62:570, 1972.

Rigler, L.G.: A roentgen study of the evolution of carcinoma of the lung. J. Thorac. Cardiovasc. Surg. 34:283, 1957.

Rigler, L.G.: The earliest roentgenographic signs of carcinoma of the lung. JAMA 195:655, 1966.

Ruckdeschel, J.C., et al.: Postoperative empyema improves survival in lung cancer. N. Engl. J. Med. 287:1013, 1972.

Sagel, S.S., et al.: Percutaneous transthoracic aspiration needle biopsy. Ann. Thorac. Surg. 26:399, 1978.

Sanders, D.E., Delarue, N.C., and Lau, G.: Angiography as a means of determining resectability of primary lung cancer. AJR 87:884, 1962.

Sanderson, D.R.: Lung cancer screening: the Mayo Clinic study. Chest 89:324S, 1986.

Sarin, C.L., and Nohl-Oser, H.C.: Mediastinoscopy. Thorax 24:585, 1969.

Shahian, D.M., Neptune, W.B., and Ellis, F.H.: Pancoast tumors: improved survival with preoperative and postoperative radiotherapy. Ann. Thorac. Surg. 43:32, 1987.

Shepherd, F.A., et al.: Reduction in local recurrence and improved survival in surgically treated patients with small cell lung cancer. J. Thorac. Cardiovasc. Surg. 86:498, 1983.

Shields, T.W.: Lobectomy in the treatment of bronchogenic carcinoma. Surg. Gynecol. Obstet. 112:1, 1961.

Shields, T.W.: Preoperative radiation therapy in the treatment of carcinoma. Cancer 30:1388, 1972.

Shields, T.W.: The fate of patients after incomplete resection of bronchial carcinoma. Surg. Gynecol. Obstet. 139:569, 1974.

Shields, T.W.: Prognostic significance of parenchymal lymphatic vessel and blood vessel invasion in carcinoma of the lung. Surg. Gynecol. Obstet. 157:185, 1983.

Shields, T.W.: The use of mediastinoscopy in lung cancer: the dilemma of mediastinal lymph nodes. In Current Controversies in Thoracic Surgery. Edited by C.F. Kittle. Philadelphia, W.B. Saunders Co., 1986, p. 145.

Shields, T.W., and Keehn, R.J.: Postresection stage grouping in carcinoma of the lung. Surg. Gynecol. Obstet. 145:725, 1977.

Shields, T.W., and Robinette, C.D.: Long-term survivors after resection of bronchial carcinoma. Surg. Gynecol. Obstet. 136:759, 1973.

Shields, T.W., et al.: Preoperative x-ray therapy as an adjuvant in the treatment of bronchogenic carcinoma. J. Thorac. Cardiovasc. Surg. 59:49, 1970.

Shields, T.W., Robinette, C.D., and Keehn, R.J.: Bronchial carcinoma treated by adjuvant cancer chemotherapy. Arch. Surg. 109:329, 1974.

Shields, T.W., et al.: Relationship of cell type and lymph node metastasis to survival after resection of bronchial carcinoma. Ann. Thorac. Surg. 20:501, 1975.

Shields, T.W., et al.: Adjuvant cancer chemotherapy after resection of carcinoma of the lung. Cancer 40:2057, 1977.

Shields, T.W., et al.: Long term survivors after resection of lung carcinoma. J. Thorac. Cardiovasc. Surg. 76:439, 1978.

Shields, T.W., et al.: Pathological stage grouping of patients with resected carcinoma of the lung. J. Thorac. Cardiovasc. Surg. 80:400, 1980.

Shields, T.W., et al.: Surgical resection in the management of small cell carcinoma of the lung. J. Thorac. Cardiovasc. Surg. 84:481, 1982a.

Shields, T.W., et al.: Prolonged intermittent adjuvant chemotherapy with CCNU and hydroxyurea after resection of carcinoma of the lung. Cancer 50:1713, 1982b.

Shields, T.W., et al.: Pathologic stage grouping of patients with resected carcinoma of the lung. J. Thorac. Cardiovasc. Surg. 80:400, 1980.

Shimizu, N., et al.: The surgical treatment of N2 lung cancer. Presented at the III World Conference on Lung Cancer. The Secretariat of the III World Conference on Lung Cancer. National Cancer Center, Tsukiji, Tokyo, Japan, 1982, p. 114 (abstract).

Shinton, N.K.: The histologic classification of lower respiratory tract tumors. Br. J. Cancer 17:1, 1963.

Shure, D., and Fedullo, P.F.: The role of transcarinal needle aspiration in staging of bronchogenic carcinoma. Chest 86:693, 1984.

Siegelman, S.S., et al.: A CT of the solitary pulmonary nodule. AJR 135:1, 1980.

Slack, N.H.: Bronchogenic carcinoma. Nitrogen mustard as a surgical adjuvant and factors influencing survival. University Surgical Adjuvant Lung Project. Cancer 25:987, 1970.

Sloan, H., et al.: Temporary unilateral occlusion of the pulmonary artery in the preoperative evaluation of thoracic patients. J. Thorac. Surg. 39:591, 1955.

Smart, J.: Can lung cancer be cured by irradiation alone? JAMA 195:1034, 1966.

Soorae, A.S., and Abbey Smith, R.: Tumour size as a prognostic factor after resection of lung carcinoma. Thorax 32:19, 1977.

Soorae, A.S., and Stevenson, J.M.: Survival with residual tumor on the bronchial margin after resection for bronchogenic carcinoma. J. Thorac. Cardiovasc. Surg. 78:175, 1979.

Spencer, H.: Pathology of the Lung. 2nd ed. London, Pergamon Press, 1968, p. 860.

Spijut, H.J., and Mateo, L.E.: Recurrent and metastatic carcinoma in surgically treated carcinoma of the lung. Cancer 18:1462, 1965.

Steele, J.D.: The solitary pulmonary nodule. J. Thorac. Cardiovasc. Surg. 46:21, 1963.

Steen, P.A., Tinker, J.H., and Tarhan, S.: Myocardial reinfarction after anesthesia and surgery. JAMA 239:2566, 1978.

Stott, H., et al.: Five-year follow-up of cytotoxic chemotherapy as an adjuvant to surgery in carcinoma of the bronchus. Br. J. Cancer 34:167, 1976.

Sundaresan, N.M., and Galicich, J.H.: The surgical treatment of single brain metastases from non-small cell lung cancer. Cancer 55:1382, 1985.

Sundaresan, N.M., Galicich, J.H., and Beattie, E.J.: Surgical treatment of brain metastases from lung cancer. J. Neurosurg. 58:661, 1983.

Swett, H.A., Nagel, J.S., and Sostman, H.D.: Imaging methods in primary lung carcinoma. Clin. Chest Med. 3:331, 1982.

Takita, H.: Effect of postoperative empyema on survival of patients with bronchogenic carcinoma. J. Thorac. Cardiovasc. Surg. 59:642, 1970.

Tarhan, S., et al.: Myocardial infarction after general anesthesia. JAMA 220:1451, 1972.

Taylor, S.G., et al.: Simultaneous cisplatin fluorouracil infusion and radiation followed by surgical resection in regionally localized stage III, non-small cell lung cancer. Ann. Thorac. Surg. 43:87, 1987.

Thomeret, G., Dubost, C., and Grenier, G.: Etude statistique des resultats a distance de 299 exereses pour cancer du poumon. Ann. Chir. Thorac. Cardiovasc. 9:489, 1970.

Tockman, M.S.: Survival and mortality from lung cancer in a screened population: the Johns Hopkins study. Chest 89:324S, 1986.

Toomes, H., Vogt-Moykopf, I.: Conservative resection for lung cancer. In International Trends in General Thoracic Surgery, Vol. 1, Lung Cancer. Edited by N.C. Delarue and H. Eschapasse. Philadelphia, W.B. Saunders Co., 1985, p. 88.

Trastek, V.F., et al.: En bloc (non-chest wall) resection for bronchogenic carcinoma with parietal fixation: factors affecting survival. J. Thorac. Cardiovasc. Surg. 87:352, 1984.

Treasure, T., and Belcher, J.R.: Prognosis of peripheral lung tumours related to size of the primary. Thorax 36:5, 1981.

Tulloh, M., Maurer, L., and Forcier, R.: A randomized trial of prophylactic whole brain irradiation in small cell carcinoma of lung. Proc. A.A.C.R.-A.S.C.O. 18:268, 1977.

Urschel, H.C., Jr. and Razzuk, M.A.: Median sternotomy as a standard approach for pulmonary resection. Ann. Thorac. Surg. 41:130, 1986.

Valdivieso, M., et al.: Increasing importance of adjuvant surgery in the therapy of patients with small cell lung cancer. Proc. Am. Soc. Clin. Oncol. 1:c-576, 1982.

Van Houtte, P., et al.: Postoperative radiation therapy in lung cancer: a controlled trial after resection of curative design. Int. J. Radiat. Oncol. Biol. Phys. 6:983, 1980.

Vincent, R.G., et al.: Surgical therapy of lung cancer. J. Thorac. Cardiovasc. Surg. 71:581, 1976.

Vincent, R.G., et al.: The changing histopathology of lung cancer: a review of 1682 cases. Cancer 39:1647, 1977.

Vincent, R.G., et al.: Carcinoembryonic antigen as a monitor of successful surgical resection of 130 patients with carcinoma of the lung. In Lung Cancer: Progress in Therapeutic Research. Edited by F. Muggia and M. Rozencweig. New York, Raven Press, 1979, p. 191.

Virtama, P.: Mass miniature radiography of the Finnish State Railways. Ann. Med. Intern. Fenniae *51*,Suppl.:37, 1962.

Wang, K.P.: Needle biopsy for the diagnosis of intrathoracic lesions: transbronchial needle biopsy. *In* Current Controversies in Thoracic Surgery. Edited by C.F. Kittle. Philadelphia, W.B. Saunders Co., 1986, p. 92.

Warram, J.: Preoperative irradiation of cancer of the lung: final report of a therapeutic trial. Cancer *36*:914, 1975.

Warren, W.H., et al.: Neuroendocrine neoplasms of the bronchopulmonary tract: a classification of the spectrum of carcinoid to small cell carcinoma and intervening variants. J. Thorac. Cardiovasc. Surg. *89*:819, 1985.

Watanabe, Y., et al.: Results of treatment for lung cancer with N2 disease. Presented at the III World Conference on Lung Cancer. The Secretariat of the III World Conference on Lung Cancer. National Cancer Center, Tsukiji, Tokyo, Japan, 1982, p. 114 (abstract).

Weisel, R.D., et al.: Sleeve lobectomy for carcinoma of the lung. J. Thorac. Cardiovasc. Surg. *78*:839, 1979.

Weisenburger, T., Hill, M.L., and Pearson, F.: Recurrence patterns in resected stage II/III epidermoid lung cancer: preliminary report. Proc. Am. Soc. Clin. Oncol. *3*:232, 1984.

Weiss, W.: Operative mortality and five-year survival rates in men with bronchogenic carcinoma. Chest *66*:483, 1974.

Weiss, W., Boucot, R., and Cooper, D.A.: Growth rate in the detection and prognosis of bronchogenic carcinoma. JAMA *198*:1246, 1966.

Weiss, W., Boucot, R., and Cooper, D.A.: The Philadelphia Pulmonary Neoplasm Research Project. Surgical factors in bronchogenic carcinoma. JAMA *216*:2119, 1971.

Wernly, J.A., et al.: Clinical value of quantitative ventilation-perfusion lung scans in the surgical management of bronchogenic carcinoma. J. Thorac. Cardiovasc. Surg. *80*:535, 1980.

Williams, D.E., et al.: Survival of patients surgically treated for stage I lung cancer. J. Thorac. Cardiovasc. Surg. *82*:70, 1981.

Wolfe, W.G., and Sabiston, D.C., Jr.: Management of benign and malignant lesions of the trachea and bronchi with the neodymium-yttrium-aluminum-garnet laser. J. Thorac. Cardiovasc. Surg. *91*:40, 1986.

World Health Organization: Histologic Typing of Lung Tumors, 2nd ed., Geneva, 1981.

Wynder, E.L.: An appraisal of the smoking-lung-cancer issue. N. Engl. J. Med. *264*:1235, 1961.

Yacoub, M.H.: Relation between the histology of bronchial carcinoma and hypertrophic pulmonary osteoarthropathy. Thorax *20*:537, 1965.

Yalow, R.S., et al.: Plasma and tumor ACTH in carcinoma of the lung. Cancer *44*:1789, 1979.

Yesner, R.: A unified concept of lung cancer. *In* Proceedings of the Veterans Administration Third Diagnostic Electron Microscopy Conference. Washington, D.C. Veterans Administration, 1977, p. 29.

Yesner, R.: Heterogenicity of small cell carcinoma of the lung. *In* Lung Cancer: Current Status and Prospects for the Future. Edited by C.F. Mountain and D.T. Carr. Austin, University of Texas Press, 1986, p. 3.

Yesner, R., and Carter, D.: Pathology of carcinoma of the lung: changing patterns. Clin. Chest Med. *3*:257, 1982.

Yesner, R., Gerstl, B., and Auerbach, O.: Application of the World Health Organization classification of lung carcinoma to biopsy material. Ann. Thorac. Surg. *1*:33, 1965.

READING REFERENCES

Carney, D.N.: Recent advances in the biology of small cell lung cancer. Chest *89*:253S, 1986.

Hankins, J.R., et al.: Surgical management of lung cancer with solitary cerebral metastasis. Ann. Thorac. Surg. *46*:24, 1988.

Hansen, M., and Pedersen, A.G.: Tumor markers in patients with lung cancer. Chest *89*:219S, 1986.

CHAPTER 77

BENIGN AND LESS COMMON MALIGNANT TUMORS OF THE LUNG

Thomas W. Shields and Philip G. Robinson

Benign and malignant tumors of the lung other than bronchial carcinomas, bronchial carcinoids, and adenoid cystic carcinomas are infrequently encountered. Martini and Beattie (1983) reported that less than 1% of the lung tumors resected at their institution are benign. The less common malignant lesions are identified even less frequently in most clinical practices.

BENIGN TUMORS OF THE LUNG

Benign tumors may be derived from all cell types present in the lung and may be parenchymal or endobronchial in location. Table 77–1 lists the various lesions.

Hamartoma

The most common benign tumor is the hamartoma; Arrigoni and associates (1970) reported that they comprise 77% of all benign tumors of the lungs. Bateson

Table 77–1. Benign Tumors of the Lung

Solitary
  Hamartoma
  Fibrous polyps and papillomas
  Granular cell myoblastoma—granular cell tumor
  Leiomyoma
  Fibroma
  Lipoma
  Neurilemoma
  Neurofibroma
  Inflammatory pseudotumor—plasma cell granuloma
  Sclerosing hemangioma
  Benign clear-cell tumor—sugar tumor
  Chemodectoma—paraganglioma
  Glomus tumor
  Benign teratoma
  Pulmonary hyalinizing granuloma
  Pulmonary meningioma
Multiple
  Benign metastasizing leiomyoma
  Lymphangioleiomyomatosis

(1973) described this lesion as a benign true neoplasm of fibrous connective tissue of the bronchi encased by a passively included lining of respiratory epithelium. Most often hamartomas contain cartilage (Fig. 77–1), and the tumor is frequently referred to as a "chondroma" or as a "chondromyxoid hamartoma."

Ninety percent of these lesions present as a solitary peripheral mass (Fig. 77–2A, B), but rarely there are multiple lesions. Eight to ten percent occur as endobronchial lesions. These tumors are most common in the middle-aged adult, although no age group is exempt. Arrigoni and associates (1970) reported that pulmonary hamartomas are observed twice as often in men as in women. Slow growth of the lesion may be observed (Fig. 77–2C, D), but the "doubling-time" almost always is well above the "doubling-time" of a malignant lesion (See Chapter 76).

Most patients with peripherally located lesions are asymptomatic. Only those few patients who have an endobronchial lesion have symptoms, including cough, hemoptysis, and frequently repeated or persistent pulmonary infection.

Roentgenographically, the peripheral lesion, most often located in the lower lung fields, appears as a smooth and well circumscribed mass; at times the margins appear lobulated or, more specifically, bosselated (Fig. 77–3). The usual size is 1 to 2 cm, but larger lesions are occasionally observed. Calcifications have been reported to be present in 10 to 30% of these lesions. On CT examination, however, Ledor and associates (1981) found identifiable calcification in less than 5% of these tumors. The calcification occurs most often in a "popcorn" distribution. This can be seen on a standard tomogram, but high resolution CT scans may demonstrate it more readily (Fig. 77–4). Siegelman and colleagues (1984) reported that fatty tissue was identified in 50% of the hamartomas evaluated by CT. Thus, even though it is a benign lesion, the CT number—Hounsfield unit—is most often low and therefore of no diagnostic significance.

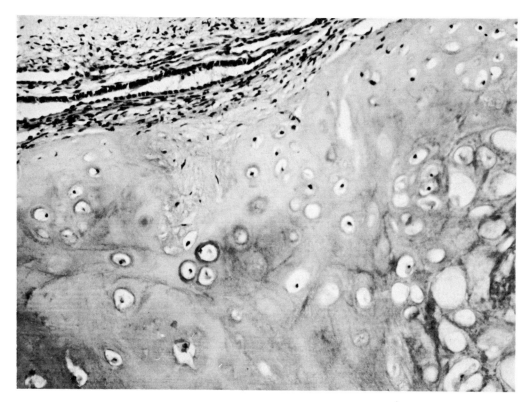

Fig. 77–1. Photomicrograph of a hamartoma. Note the predominance of cartilage cells (×110).

The endobronchial lesions per se are undetectable roentgenographically except that distal parenchymal lung changes—atelectasis, obstructive pneumonia, or abscess formation—may suggest an obstructing, endobronchial lesion.

Bronchoscopy and biopsy are indicated in any patient with pulmonary symptoms: cough, hemoptysis, repeated pulmonary infection, or atelectasis. Endoscopy is not an essential diagnostic step in patients with a peripheral lesion.

Hamper and colleagues (1985) reported that percutaneous, transthoracic needle aspiration biopsy yields diagnostic information in 85% of hamartomas. Care must be taken in aspirating these peripheral lesions because of their firm consistency; the aforementioned authors reported a 50% incidence of postaspiration pneumothorax, which is twice the incidence after biopsy of other peripheral nodules. The histologic examination of the aspiration has higher diagnostic yield than cytologic examination of the aspirated specimen has. One may suspect that the lesion is a hamartoma when fibromyxomatous tissue, which stains metachromatically with Giemsa or Wright stain, and fragments of low columnar epithelium are present. When fragments of cartilage are present cytologically, the aspiration is diagnostic of a hamartoma. Cartilage is more often demonstrated by standard histologic examination of the aspirated material. Therefore, if the diagnosis of a hamartoma is suspected from the standard roentgenographic and CT studies, a needle aspiration biopsy is indicated, particularly in a patient who is a poor candidate for a major operation.

When the diagnosis is known in a patient with a peripherally located hamartoma, Nili and associates (1979) reported that the patient may be observed without surgical intervention. If a prethoracotomy diagnosis has not been made, thoracotomy and excision are indicated. The least possible amount of normal pulmonary tissue should be excised. At times when a suspected hamartoma is palpated within the lung, the mass is readily moved and may be advanced to just beneath the visceral pleural surface. Incision of the pleura and enucleation of the mass can then be readily carried out. When there is any fixation of the mass within the parenchyma of the lung, a standard resection—wedge, segmentectomy, or even at times a lobectomy—as necessary must be done. A pneumonectomy should be avoided if at all possible.

When the hamartoma is endobronchial, a lobectomy or segmentectomy, as one of us (T.W.S.) and Lynn reported (1958), is most often required to remove the tumor as well as the chronically infected pulmonary parenchyma distal to the lesion.

Recurrence after excision of a hamartoma is unknown. A second, separate primary hamartoma rarely occurs later.

Other Benign Tumors

Benign tumors of epithelial, mesenchymal, or lymphoid origin are rare. These tumors may either be endobronchial or peripheral. The symptomatology depends upon whether a bronchus is irritated or a bronchial lumen is occluded partially or completely by an endobronchial

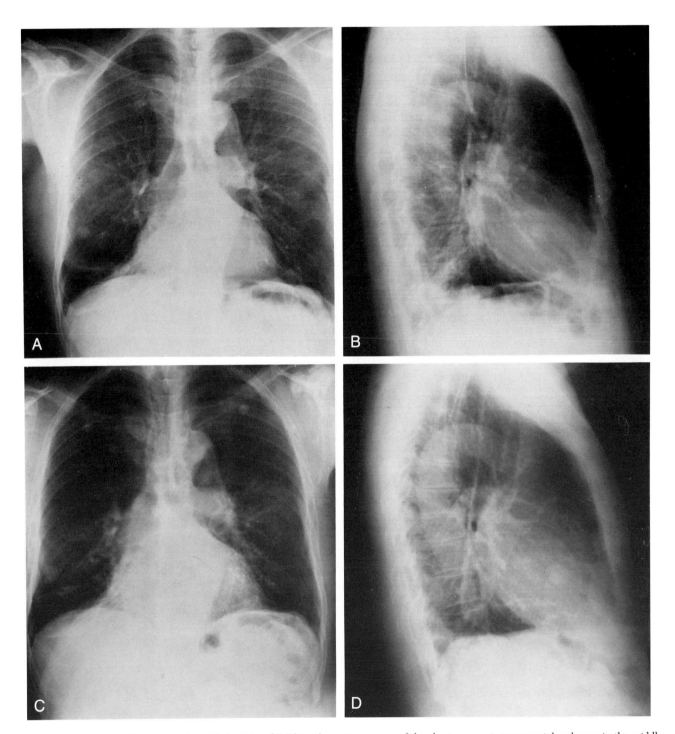

Fig. 77–2. Hamartoma demonstrated on (A) the PA and (B) lateral roentgenograms of the chest, presenting as a peripheral mass in the middle lobe. (C) PA and (D) lateral roentgenograms of the chest of the peripheral hamartoma showing slow growth of the mass over a 4-year period.

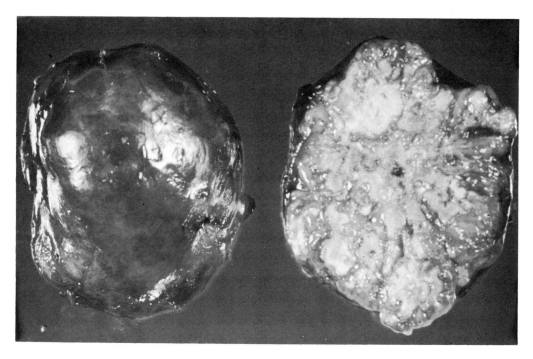

Fig. 77–3. Gross specimen of a resected hamartoma showing typical bosselated appearance.

lesion. The peripherally located tumors are almost always asymptomatic.

Fibrous polyps and papillomas originate from the mucosa and are confined to the bronchial lumen. These lesions may be removed endoscopically, or occasionally a bronchotomy or sleeve resection may be necessary. When irreversible parenchymal damage distal to the lesion is present, surgical resection of the destroyed lung tissue is required.

Granular cell myoblastomas are found in the larger bronchi; Oparah and Subramanian (1976) reviewed the features of these lesions. These tumors are now believed to originate from Schwann cells and are frequently referred to simply as granular cell tumors. Most are sessile or polypoid growths with smooth surfaces arising in the wall of a large bronchus, although they may occur as a peripheral nodule. Distal obstruction is frequently present in association with the endobronchial lesions. These rare tumors are seen in middle-aged adults. Resection of the tumor and any associated damaged lung tissue is indicated.

Leiomyomas account for about 2% of the benign tumors of the lung. They may occur in the trachea, bronchus, or pulmonary parenchyma (Table 77–2). As Hurt (1984), Arrigoni and associates (1970), and White and colleagues (1985) noted, the distribution is approximately equal between a tracheobronchial or parenchymal location. The tumor is most often discovered in young and middle-aged adults and is more common in women than in men. Surgical resection is the treatment of choice. In selected patients with endobronchial lesions without distal destroyed lung tissue, laser resection of the tumor may be possible. Archambeaud-Mouveroux and associates (1988) reported successful management of a benign bronchial leiomyoma by endoscopic use of a neodymium-yttrium aluminum garnet laser.

Fibromas as well as benign neurogenic tumors—neurilemoma or neurofibroma—occur, but nothing distinctive is evident in these tumors.

Lipomas arise most often from the wall of the tracheobronchial tree—80%. The lesion is more common in men than in women. Local resection by bronchotomy or sleeve resection should be done whenever possible if the parenchyma distal to the lesion is normal.

Inflammatory pseudotumor is a benign lung tumor that may be postinflammatory and that has various names, depending on the predominant cellular element. Other names include plasma cell granuloma, fibroma, fibrous histiocytoma, fibroxanthoma, xanthoma, and mast cell granuloma. Berardi and associates (1983) reviewed this subject and found that these tumors could occur in patients from 1 to 73 years with an average age of 29.5 years. There was no predilection for either sex. Most—74%—of the patients were asymptomatic. Roentgenographically, a well-defined solitary nodule appears in the lung. Surgical resection is diagnostic and curative. Prognosis is excellent. Spencer (1984), Bahadori and Liebow

Table 77–2. Reported Cases of Leiomyoma of the Lower Respiratory Tract

Site	No. of Cases	%
Trachea	12	16
Bronchus	22	33
Parenchyma	34	51
Total	68	

Reproduced with permission from White, S.H., et al.: Leiomyomas of the lower respiratory tract. Thorax 40:306, 1985.

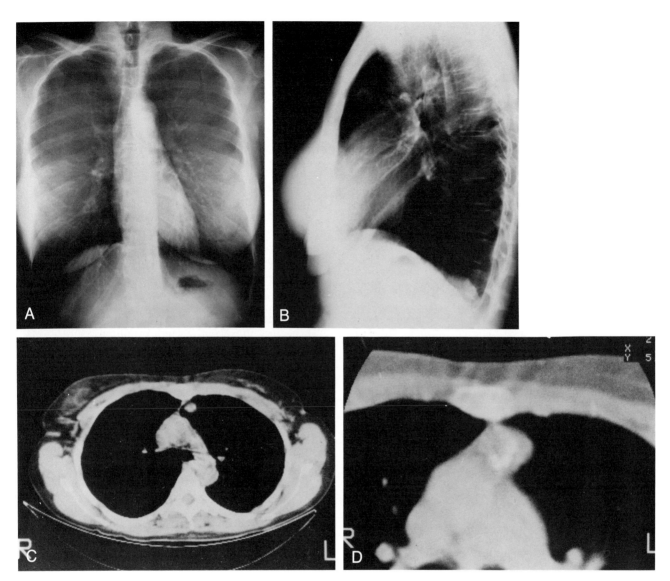

Fig. 77-4. *A*, PA roentgenogram of calcified lesion overlying aortic knob on the left. *B*, Lateral roentgenogram shows the lesion to be in the anterior segment of the left lung. *C*, CT exam showing calcification within the mass. *D*, Enhanced CT revealing popcorn-like calcifications in the mass, typical of a hamartoma.

(1973), and Warter and colleagues (1987) reviewed this subject.

Sclerosing hemangioma originally described by Liebow and Hubbell (1956), is a benign lung tumor of undetermined histogenesis. Katzenstein and associates (1982) described 51 cases Liebow saw after his 1956 description. She noted that the patients ranged in age from 15 to 69 years, with an average age of 42 years. Eighty-four percent of the patients were women. Most—78%— of the patients were asymptomatic. Those who were symptomatic complained of hemoptysis or vague chest pain, or both. On roentgenographic study it appears as a solitary nodule that is found more often in one of the lower lobes. Surgical excision of the tumor is curative.

Benign clear cell tumor or sugar tumor of the lung is a benign lung tumor of unknown histogenesis. Andrion and colleagues (1985), however, suggested from their light microscopic, histochemical, and ultrastructural study of the tumor that it is derived from either epithelial nonciliated bronchiolar—Clara cells—epithelium or epithelial serous cells. The tumor was first reported by Liebow and Castleman (1963), who later published a series of 12 cases (1971). Seventy-five percent of the lesions occurred in patients between 45 and 59 years of age. The tumors were equally distributed between men and women. All of the patients were asymptomatic. Roentgenographically, the lesions were solitary and peripheral and ranged in size from 1.5 to 3 cm. Excision is curative. The pathologic differential diagnosis is important in these tumors, because they could represent a metastatic renal cell carcinoma or a primary clear cell carcinoma of the lung. These sugar tumors are so rare that the surgeon must rule out renal cell carcinoma before accepting the lesion as a true benign clear cell tumor.

Singh and colleagues (1977) reviewed the primary pulmonary paraganglioma or chemodectoma. Few cases were reported, and the tumors were not absolutely distinguished from carcinoid tumors. This distinction remains a problem.

A glomus tumor—glomangioma—is a tumor derived from the cells of a special arteriovenous shunt, the Sucquet-Hoyer canal. These tumors are rare and should be differentiated from hemangiopericytomas, carcinoids, and paragangliomas.

Teratomas are rare lung tumors. Many of the older cases may represent anterior mediastinal tumors that extended into the lung. Most occur in the anterior segment of the left upper lobe, and resection is curative.

Pulmonary hyalinizing granuloma is a tumor of dense hyalinized connective tissue that occurs in the lung as a result of inflammatory or postinflammatory changes. Engleman and associates (1977) first described the lesion. Yousem and Hochholzer (1987a) summarized 24 cases. The tumor occurs in patients between 24 and 77 years of age with an average age of 42.3 years. The lesions are equally distributed between men and women. Patients may be asymptomatic or complain of cough, shortness of breath, chest pain, or weight loss. The lesions are nodular and vary from a few millimeters to 15 cm in greatest dimension. Many of the patients have multiple lesions, with most being bilateral.

Pulmonary meningioma is a rare benign tumor of the lung. Chumas and Lorelle (1982) and Kemnitz (1982), Fu-lin (1983), and Unger (1984) and their associates reported examples of this rare pulmonary tumor. It represents more of a problem to the clinician who sees a nodule on the chest roentgenogram than to the patient. The histogenesis of this tumor in the lung may be from a chemodectoma or from the pleural surface of the lung. Wende (1983) and Miller (1985) and their colleagues reported cases of metastatic meningioma from the cranium, and the patient should be examined to exclude this source.

Rare multiple benign peripheral lesions such as the benign metastasizing leiomyoma may also be seen. The exact nature of the lesion remains undetermined. These tumors occur in young women and are frequently associated with a leiomyoma of the uterus. Growth of the lesion may or may not occur, and regression can occur after oophorectomy. Winkler and colleagues (1987) suggested resection of the pulmonary lesions when feasible. Another smooth muscle lesion that occurs in the lung is lymphangioleiomyomatosis—LAM—which Corrin and associates (1975) and Carrington and associates (1977) described. The disease is rare and is seen in women during their reproductive years. The smooth muscle in the lung proliferates, resulting in a secondary obstruction of airways, veins, and lymphatics. These changes can produce emphysema, pneumothoraxes, pulmonary hemorrhages with hemoptysis, and a chylothorax. If the disease is left untreated, it slowly progresses and results in respiratory insufficiency and death. Adamson and associates (1985) as well as Banner and colleagues (1981) suggested that hormonal manipulation may be valuable in treating these patients, so it would be appropriate for the surgeon to take some of the fresh lung tissue at the time of biopsy and send it for estrogen- and progesterone-receptor assays.

MALIGNANT TUMORS

Most of these lesions are sarcomas, but they also include the pulmonary blastoma, the carcinosarcoma, the primary pulmonary lymphomas, and the rare primary malignant melanoma and malignant teratoma (Table 77–3). Nascimento and colleagues (1982) reported that over 50% of the malignant lesions are initially asymptomatic. Most are peripheral. Resection, when feasible, is the treatment of choice, and adjuvant chemotherapy, when applicable, should be used. Radiation therapy has only a minor role in management except for patients with lymphoma. In most instances the prognosis is poor.

Soft-Tissue Sarcomas

Primitive mesenchymal cells are present in every organ of the human body. They proliferate and normally mature into fat, fibrous tissue, muscle, cartilage, or bone. Tumors of mesenchymal origin may arise from the stromal elements of the bronchial or vascular wall or from the interstices of lung parenchyma. They usually expand toward the lung parenchyma, but occasionally they expand intraluminally. Only rarely do they invade and break through the bronchial epithelium. As a result, these tumors do not exfoliate cells, and diagnosis by cytologic examination of expectorations or of tracheobronchial washings is uncommon. They usually appear as well-circumscribed and encapsulated masses in lung parenchyma (Fig. 77–5). When peripherally located, they may invade the adjacent pleura and chest wall. They metastasize by way of the bloodstream and rarely by lymphatic invasion. They generally spread by local invasion, and as Watson and Anlyan (1954) noted, metastases to distant organs are usually late manifestations of the disease process. Only rarely do these tumors cavitate. Microscopically, these tumors present a wide range of cellular differentiation. They occur at almost any age with equal frequency in either sex. Fadhli and colleagues (1965) reported the age range to be 4 to 83 years. They occur with equal frequency in either lung. As Martini and associates (1971) reported, they vary in diameter from 1 to 15 cm or more, with an average diameter of 6 to 7 cm. Many are asymptomatic and are only detected on a routine roentgenogram of the chest. When the pa-

Table 77–3. Less Common Malignant Tumors of the Lung

Soft-tissue sarcomas
  Parenchymal and bronchial sarcomas
  Sarcomas of large vessel origin
  Sarcomas of small vessel origin
Carcinosarcoma
Pulmonary blastoma—embryoma
Lymphoma
Malignant melanoma
Malignant teratoma

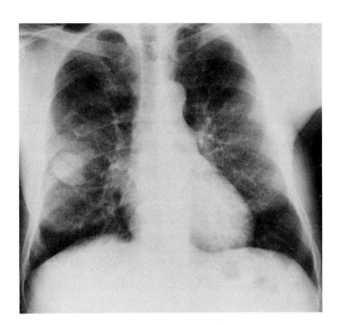

Fig. 77–5. PA chest roentgenogram revealing recurrent fibrosarcoma of the right lung following previous wedge resection of a "fibromatous" tumor from the middle lobe.

tient is symptomatic, chest pain, cough, dyspnea, and hemoptysis are the most common presenting symptoms. Fever, fatigue, anorexia, and weight loss usually are late manifestations. On roentgenograms of the chest, the tumor usually appears as a sharply demarcated mass density within the lung substance at the hilus or in the lung periphery. The lesions are usually solitary and confined to one lung. Peripheral tumors invading the chest wall may be associated with varying degrees of pleural effusion. Tumors obstructing a bronchus (Fig. 77–6)— approximately 15%—may result in distal parenchymal changes.

Dail (1988) categorized the soft-tissue sarcomas arising within the lung into three groups: (1) parenchymal and bronchial-endobronchial sarcomas, (2) sarcomas of large vessel origin, and (3) sarcomas of small vessel origin.

Parenchymal and Bronchial-Endobronchial Sarcomas

Fibrosarcoma, leiomyosarcoma, rhabdomyosarcoma, neurogenic sarcoma, chondrosarcoma, osteosarcoma, malignant mesenchymoma, liposarcoma, and malignant fibrous histiocytoma all come under this category. The occurrence of any of these sarcomas as primaries in the lung is rare. Table 77–4 lists the distribution of some of these lesions in adults and children in the series reported by Nascimento (1982), Hartman (1983), and McCormack (1988) and their associates.

Fibrosarcomas and leiomyosarcomas occur both endobronchially and peripherally in the lung. Guccion and Rosen (1972) reported 16 endobronchial fibrosarcomas and 8 endobronchial leiomyosarcomas. Most of the patients in these two groups tended to be children or young adults. All of the patients were symptomatic with cough or hemoptysis. These endobronchial lesions were confined to the bronchus and did not invade into the adjacent

pulmonary parenchyma. These patients tend to do well following surgical removal of the lesion. An explanation for this better prognosis is that endobronchial lesions are symptomatic and are detected clinically at an earlier stage. Intraparenchymal leiomyosarcomas and fibrosarcomas have a worse prognosis than endobronchial ones.

The peripheral lesions are solid, although Goldthorn and associates (1986) reported cavitation in a fibrosarcoma in a child.

Some investigators believe that the larger—thus slow-growing—tumors have a better prognosis than the smaller, peripheral lesions. Nascimento and colleagues (1982), however, reported that only those patients with small tumors—2 to 3 cm—survived over 5 years. Shaw and associates (1961) reported that leiomyosarcomas have a relatively good prognosis, and Yellin and associates (1984) reported a 45% 5-year survival rate after resection of leiomyosarcomas. Martini and colleagues (1971) reported that with the exception of this latter variety of tumor, all patients with pulmonary soft-tissue sarcomas succumb to their disease within 3 years. Guccion and Rosen (1972) found that the mitotic rate, size of the tumor, and involvement of adjacent structures—chest wall, diaphragm, and mediastinum—were all prognostic indicators.

Pulmonary rhabdomyosarcomas are rare. Most of the reported tumors replaced one or more pulmonary lobes and tended to invade local structures, especially the pulmonary veins and bronchi. Luck and colleagues (1986) summarized a few cases in children in whom the tumor was associated with a congenital adenomatoid malformation—as the pulmonary blastoma is on occasion. Lee (1981) and Avignia (1984) and their colleagues reviewed pulmonary rhabdomyosarcoma.

Liposarcoma, neurogenic sarcoma, chondrosarcoma, osteosarcoma, malignant mesenchymoma, and malignant fibrous histiocytoma, which Yousem and Hochholzer (1987b) reviewed, are rare. The prognosis of all these variants of spindle cell sarcoma, with the exception of the leiomyosarcomas and the endobronchial fibrosarcomas is poor. Survival beyond a year is rare.

Sarcomas of Large Vessel Origin

A pulmonary trunk sarcoma is a primary sarcoma arising within the pulmonary artery or, as Mandelstramm (1923) described, from the pulmonary valve of the heart. In Wackers (1969), Bleisch (1980), and Baker (1985) and their associates' reviews, fibrosarcoma, fibromyxosarcoma, and leiomyosarcoma make up the majority of the cell types of these intravascular tumors. They may spread distally within the vascular tree or extend outside the vessel to invade the lung tissue. The patients present with chest pain, dyspnea, and a new onset of a systolic heart murmur; one third may also have cough, hemoptysis, and palpitations. A late manifestation is right-sided heart decompensation. Moffat and colleagues (1972) reported the roentgenographic features. The lesion presents most often as a lobulated parahilar mass. Angiography may reveal multiple defects within the pulmonary artery. CT and MRI scans may help determine the extent

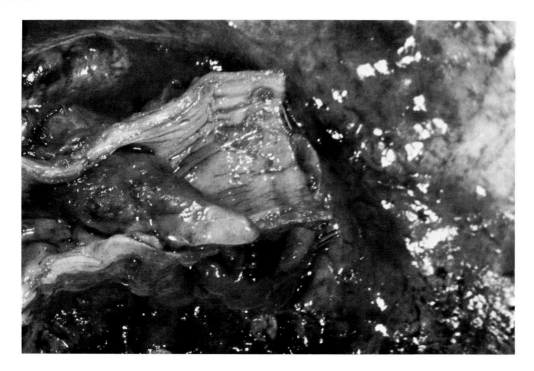

Fig. 77–6. Malignant endobronchial sarcoma.

of the disease. Pulmonary hypertension with proximal dilatation of the vessels is a constant feature. Treatment is by resection, but this is rarely possible; the prognosis for survival is poor.

Sarcomas of Small Vessel Origin

Angiosarcoma, epithelioid hemangioendothelioma, hemangiopericytoma, and hemangioendothelioma are malignant or potentially malignant vascular tumors that occur in the lung. Kaposi's sarcoma, which is a vascular neoplasm, will not be discussed here because it has not been described as having a primary pulmonary origin. According to Enzinger and Weiss (1983), the term hemangioendothelioma should only be used to designate a group of vascular tumors that cannot be accurately classified histologically as to their ultimate biologic behavior. Angiosarcomas are rare in the lungs. Yousem (1986) believes they are most likely to be metastases from an angiosarcoma of the right ventricle, pulmonary arterial

trunk, or extrathoracic site. Spragg and associates (1983) reviewed the literature and presented ten possible cases of angiosarcoma arising in the lung, but some doubts about whether these cases are all true pulmonary angiosarcomas exist. An angiosarcoma can be associated with a hemothorax or hypertrophic pulmonary osteoarthropathy, or both. The prognosis is poor.

An epithelioid hemangioendothelioma was first described by Dail and Liebow in 1975, and Dail and colleagues (1983) reviewed an additional 19 cases. They initially called this tumor an intravascular bronchioloalveolar tumor—IVBAT, but they now prefer the term "sclerosing endothelial tumor"—SET. Weiss and Enzinger (1982) published 41 cases of an identical tumor occurring in soft tissue and proposed the name epithelioid hemangioendothelioma, which has become widely accepted. Weiss and colleagues (1986) published a combined review of lesions in soft tissue, lung, liver, and bone. Wenisch and Lulay (1980) reported that in the

Table 77–4. Distribution of Soft-Tissue Sarcomas

Cell Type	Nascimento, et al. (1982) (Adults)	McCormack and Martini (1988) (All Age Groups)	Hartman and Shochat (1983) (Children)
Pulmonary blastoma	0	1	14
Fibrosarcoma	9	2	—
Leiomyosarcoma	4	16	9
Rhabdomyosarcoma		5	6
Hemangiopericytoma	3	1	3
Osteosarcoma	2	—	—
Myxosarcoma	—	—	1
Spindle cell sarcoma	—	13	—
Angiosarcoma	—	2	—
Malignant fibrous histiocytoma	—	3	—

lung these tumors occur in patients from 4 to 70 years of age, with one third of the patients being under the age of 30. The tumor occurs four times more commonly in women than it does in men. Most of the patients are asymptomatic or complain of a nonproductive cough. Chest roentgenograms reveal many small—1 cm in diameter—nodular densities in both lung fields. The average survival after diagnosis is 4.6 years, but Miettinen and associates (1987) reported a patient who survived for 24 years with repeated surgical excisions. Death from pulmonary insufficiency is the usual course of this disease.

Hemangiopericytomas of the lung are unusual. These sarcomas are derived from the ubiquitous capillary pericytic cell and are commonly located in the soft tissues of the thigh and retroperitoneum. Yousem and Hochholzer (1987c) found that pulmonary hemangiopericytomas occurred with equal frequency in men and women; average age of patient was 46.1 years. About one third of the patients were asymptomatic. The symptomatic patients complained of chest pain, hemoptysis, dyspnea, and cough. One patient had pulmonary osteoarthropathy. Roentgenograms of the chest usually show a lobulated, well circumscribed, homogenous soft tissue density, but other findings may be present (Fig. 77–7). The treatment is surgical excision. Prognosis is variable; indicators of malignant behavior are chest symptoms, size of the tumor—>8 cm, pleural and bronchial wall invasion, tumor giant cells, greater than three mitoses per ten high power fields, and tumor necrosis. Shinn and Ho (1979) noted that tumors 5 cm or larger had metastasis 33% of the time, and 10 cm or larger had metastasis 66% of the time. Davis and co-workers (1972) demonstrated that most recurrences took place within 2 years of diagnosis. Enzinger and Smith (1976) and Feldman and Seaman (1964) reported that chemotherapy and radiation therapy do not consistently help the patient.

Carcinosarcoma

Cabarcos and associates (1985) reviewed the literature on carcinosarcomas. The consensus is that they are malignant neoplasms that contain both epithelial and mesenchymal components. The epithelial component is usually squamous cell carcinoma, and the mesenchymal component is usually fibrosarcoma. Carcinosarcomas comprise 0.3% of all pulmonary neoplasms and are most often found in a proximal bronchus. They occur more often in men than in women—5:1. Approximately 87% develop in patients over the age of 50 years. These tumors frequently have a slow rate of growth. The major portion of the growth can be endobronchial, with little propensity to infiltrate the bronchial wall, but extensive invasion into the surrounding lung does occur. Metastases to the regional lymph nodes and to distant organs is common. Bronchial biopsy may be followed by excessive hemorrhage but is nonetheless indicated for the preoperative evaluation of the lesion. Surgical resection, when possible, is the indicated treatment. In most series, 75% to 80% of the patients die within the first year after resection.

Pulmonary Blastoma—Embryoma

Barnard (1952) first reported this lung lesion and called it an embryoma. Spencer (1961) reviewed Barnard's case, added three cases of his own, and renamed the tumor pulmonary blastoma. A pulmonary blastoma is a malignant tumor of the lung whose histogenesis is uncertain. Spencer (1961) thought that the pulmonary blastoma arose from pluripotential embryonic cells of the mesoderm. This lesion is differentiated from the carcinosarcoma by the fact that it forms gland-like structures that are lined by epithelial cells with a clear cytoplasm and that these glands are set in a primitive-looking stroma. The lesion is always peripherally located. Francis and

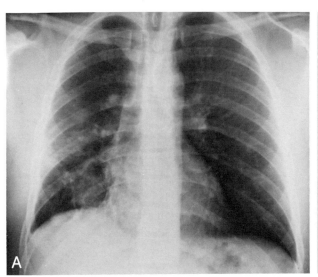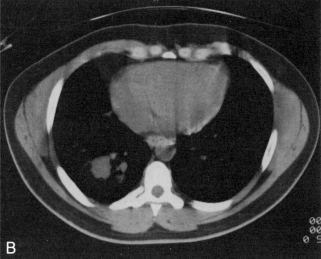

Fig. 77–7. *A*, PA roentgenogram of the chest revealing a 5-cm mass in the right lower lobe. Suggestion of additional masses evident on the levels of the second and third anterior interspaces. *B*, CT scan revealing mass in right lower lobe with multiple satellite lesions. Histologic examination of resected specimen revealed a poorly differentiated hemangiopericytoma.

Jacobsen (1983) reviewed 72 cases and added 11 of their own. A pulmonary blastoma may occur at any age. A biphasic age distribution is seen; the first peak of incidence is in the first decade of life and the second peak in the seventh decade. Three fourths are discovered in the adult. The average age is just under 40. Men are affected three times as often as women, although in infants the sex ratio is equal. Most tumors are large—over 10 cm. Metastases to the lymph nodes and brain occur. Treatment is surgical excision. Most patients die of the tumor within one year, but approximately 16% of patients survive 5 years or longer; survival as long as 10 to over 20 years has been reported.

Primary Pulmonary Lymphoma

Lymphomas of the lung can be divided into Hodgkin's lymphoma and non-Hodgkin's lymphoma. Primary lymphomas of the lung are rare. L'hoste and colleagues (1984) reported that only 0.34% of all lymphomas originate in the lung. Furthermore, primary pulmonary lymphomas represent only 0.5% of all lung tumors. Secondary involvement of the lung by lymphoma is common. Risdall and associates (1979) found lung involvement at autopsy in 39 of 79 patients with non-Hodgkin's lymphoma. Most of those lymphomas that involved the lung were of the large cell—histiocytic—type. In Hodgkin's disease, Kern and associates (1961) reported secondary lung involvement to be as high as 40%, although Fisher and colleagues (1962) believed that it was somewhat less. The prognosis of primary lymphoma of the lung is much better than that of secondary involvement of the lung (Fig. 77–8).

Non-Hodgkin's Lymphoma

The multiple classification schemes for non-Hodgkin's lymphoma have confused clinicians and pathologists alike. These schemes are those of Jackson and Parker (1947), Rappaport (1966), Lukes and Collins (1975), the Kiel classification reported by Lennert (1978) and the Working Formulation of the Non-Hodgkin's Lymphoma

Pathologic Classification Project (1982). The older terms of Jackson and Parker (1947), such as lymphosarcoma and reticulum cell sarcoma, should not be used because so many different lesions were included under these two headings. Costa and Martin's (1985) classification of pulmonary lymphoid disorders is both practical and useful (Table 77–5). Table 77–6 shows the clinical stage grouping of primary pulmonary lymphomas.

The rare primary pulmonary lymphomas may occur in any of the deposits of lymphoid elements normally present in the lung, such as in the peribronchial tissue, in the interstices of the lung parenchyma, or in the intrapulmonary and subpleural lymph nodes. The intrapulmonary and subpleural lymph nodes are normally present, particularly in persons over 25 years of age. Trapnell (1964) demonstrated by pulmonary lymphangiography that 18% of normal persons had intrapulmonary nodes within the lung parenchyma.

It is difficult for the pathologist to separate benign lymphoid lesions, lymphocytic interstitial pneumonia—LIP—and pseudolymphoma—PSL—of the lung from primary pulmonary lymphocytic lymphomas (Table 77–7). Kradin and Mark (1983) applied the term nodular lymphoid hyperplasia to pseudolymphoma—PSL—and diffuse lymphoid hyperplasia to lymphocytic interstitial pneumonia—LIP. These may both be better terms for these two lesions. Until they become more widely used, they unfortunately serve to confuse clinicians.

Saltzstein (1963) addressed the problem of separating benign lymphoid lesions from the malignant ones by proposing three criteria for pulmonary lymphomas. His criteria were "immature" lymphocytes, absence of germinal centers, and involvement of hilar lymph nodes. Despite Saltzstein's criteria for differentiating benign from malignant lymphoid lesions, there are reports of LIP and PSL progressing to lymphoma. Turner and associates (1984) tried to clarify the situation with regard to pulmonary lymphoid lesions by proposing that a pattern of lymphangitic spread and a monomorphic cell population could be used to separate the malignant lesions

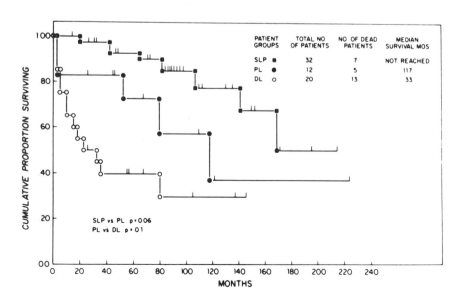

PATIENT GROUPS	TOTAL NO OF PATIENTS	NO OF DEAD PATIENTS	MEDIAN SURVIVAL MOS
SLP ■	32	7	NOT REACHED
PL ●	12	5	117
DL ○	20	13	33

SLP vs PL p=006
PL vs DL p=01

Fig. 77–8. Survival curves of patients with primary and secondary lymphoma of the lung. SLP: Survival curve of patients with small lymphocytic proliferation including those with small cell lymphocytic lymphoma as well as pseudolymphoma or lymphocytic interstitial pneumonia. PL: Survival curve of patients with presumed primary lymphoma of the lung, limited to one or both lungs, exclusive of primary Hodgkin's disease. DL: Survival curve of patients with disseminated lymphoma of extrapulmonary origin involving the lungs. (Reproduced with permission of Kennedy, J.L., et al.: Pulmonary lymphomas and other pulmonary lymphoid lesions: a clinicopathologic and immunologic study of 64 patients. Cancer 56:539, 1985.)

Table 77–5. Pulmonary Lymphoreticular Disorders

Rappaport Classification	Working Formulation
Benign Primary Pulmonary Lymphoproliferative Lesions	
Pseudolymphoma—PSL[1]	
Lymphocytic interstitial pneumonia—LIP[2]	
Primary Non-Hodgkin's Lymphoma of the Lung	
Low-grade	
Well-differentiated lymphocytic—WDL	Small lymphocytic
Nodular, poorly differentiated lymphocytic—PDL	Follicular, predominantly small cleaved cells
Intermediate-grade	
Nodular histiocytic	Follicular, predominantly large cells
Diffuse, poorly differentiated lymphocytic	Diffuse, small cleaved cells
Diffuse, mixed lymphocytic and histiocytic	Diffuse, mixed small and large cells
High-grade	
Diffuse histiocyte	Large cell, immunoblastic
Lymphoblastic	Lymphoblastic, convoluted cells
Angiocentric Immunoproliferative Lesions—AIL	
Lymphocytic vasculitis	
Lymphomatoid granulomatosis—LYG	
Angiocentric large cell lymphoma	
Plasma Cell Disorders	
Waldenstrom's macroglobulinemia	
Plasmacytoma	
Multiple myeloma	
Hodgkin's Disease	

[1]Pseudolymphoma is also known as nodular lymphoid hyperplasia.
[2]Lymphocytic interstitial pneumonia is also known as diffuse lymphoid hyperplasia.
Modified with permission from Costa, J., and Martin, S.: Pulmonary lymphoreticular disorders. *In* Surgical Pathology of the Lymph Nodes and Related Organs. Edited by E.S. Jaffe. Philadelphia, W.B. Saunders Co., 1985, p. 282.

Table 77–6. Clinical Staging Grouping of Pulmonary Non-Hodgkin's Lymphoma*

Stage	Extent of Disease
IE	Lung only involved
II1E	Lung and hilar nodes involved
II2E	Lung and mediastinal nodes involved
II2EW	Lung and adjacent chest wall or diaphragm involved
III and IV	Disseminated disease

*Modified Ann Arbor Classification.
Reproduced with permission from L'hoste, R.J., et al.: Primary pulmonary lymphomas. Cancer 54:1397, 1984.

from the benign ones. With regard to Saltzstein's criteria, they pointed out that germinal centers could be seen with lymphomas and that hilar lymph nodes are not always involved when a lymphoma is present. Hence, the lack of hilar lymph node involvement should not be used to support the diagnosis of a benign lymphoid process. In conclusion, there probably are truly benign lymphoid lesions of the lung—LIP and PSL, but unfortunately the current histologic criteria do not always allow for a clear distinction of LIP and PSL from lymphocytic lymphoma. Therefore, LIP and PSL must be viewed as potentially premalignant lesions.

Lymphocytic Interstitial Pneumonia—LIP

Carrington and Liebow (1966) first described lymphocytic interstitial pneumonia, and Liebow and Carrington (1973) further defined it as being widespread pulmonary infiltrates composed of lymphocytes, plasma cells, and histiocytes. In some cases, germinal centers are present and the term "diffuse lymphoid hyperplasia" has also been applied to this condition. Colby and Carrington (1983) and Turner and colleagues (1984) believed that some of the cases reported in the past actually represented diffuse, well differentiated lymphocytic lymphomas presenting in the lung. Most patients with LIP are adult women, usually in their fifth through seventh decades. These patients have nonspecific symptoms, such as dry cough, dyspnea, weight loss, and occasionally fever. Typical roentgenologic features are diffuse bilateral lower lobe reticular infiltrates. Small—1 cm—or large— 1 to 3 cm—nodules or patchy consolidations may be present on the chest roentgenogram. Patients with LIP can have diseases with immunologic abnormalities such as Sjögren's syndrome—one third of cases—collagen vascular diseases, autoimmune diseases, and immunodeficiency diseases, including the acquired immune deficiency syndrome—AIDS. The course of LIP varies. Patients have been treated with corticosteroids and immunosuppressive drugs, but the response is difficult to judge because of the occurrence of spontaneous remissions.

Pseudolymphoma—PSL

As noted, Saltzstein (1963) attempted to establish histologic criteria to separate malignant lymphocytic pulmonary infiltrates from benign ones. He termed the be-

Table 77–7. Differentiation of Lymphoma, Lymphocytic Interstitial Pneumonia, and Pseudolymphoma

	Lymphoma (Small Lymphocytes)	Lymphocytic Interstitial Pneumonia	Pseudolymphoma
Clinical			
Pulmonary symptoms	+	+ + +	+
Systemic symptoms	+ +	+	+
Adenopathy (when present)	+ + + +	0	0
Histologic			
Pleomorphic infiltrate	0	+ +	+ + +
Germinal centers	+	+ +	+ +
Node involvement	+ + + +	0	0
Cartilage destruction	+ + +	0	±
Pleural invasion	+ + +	0	±
Immunologic Stain			
Monoclonal cells	+	0	0
Polyclonal cells	0	+	+
Roentgenographic			
Solitary lesion	+ +	0	+ +
Multiple lesions	+ + +	0	+
Adenopathy	+ + + +	0	+
Effusion	+ + +	0	+
Diffuse lesion	+	+ + +	0

From Seminar in Pulmonary and Mediastinal Diagnosis. Given by the Armed Forces Institute of Pathology in October, 1986. Reproduced with permission of Michael N. Koss, M.D., Associate Professor of Pathology, University of Southern California Medical Center, Los Angeles, California.

nign lymphocytic proliferations pseudolymphomas—PSL—or as they were later called, nodular lymphoid hyperplasias of the lung. Koss (1983), Herbert (1984), and Weiss (1985) and their colleagues, as well as others, have reinterpreted many of the lesions that were called PSL as well differentiated lymphocytic lymphomas. True PSL are reactive lymphoid proliferations that manifest themselves in the lung as one or several masses or as localized infiltrates. Koss and associates (1983) reviewed 23 pseudolymphomas and found that the lesions were usually discovered in asymptomatic patients on routine roentgenograms of the chest. The patients ranged in age from the third to the eighth decade with a mean age of 51 years. Many of the symptomatic patients had fever. Resection of a true pseudolymphoma is both diagnostic and curative. The lesion has a low rate of recurrence at the original surgical site. The prognosis is excellent providing that the pathologist has made the correct diagnosis. Table 77–7 shows the differentiating clinical, pathologic, and roentgenographic features of LIP, PSL, and small cell lymphocytic lymphoma.

Small Cell Lymphocytic Lymphoma

When the lung is involved with non-Hodgkin's lymphoma, 50 to 60% of the cases in various series are proliferations of small lymphocytes or lymphocytes with plasmacytoid features. Patients with pulmonary lymphocytic lymphomas—small cell—range in age from the second to the ninth decade of life, with a peak at the sixth decade. There is an equal distribution between men and women. One third of the patients are asymptomatic, and their lesions are found on routine chest roentgenograms. Symptomatic patients complain of cough, dyspnea, chest pain, and hemoptysis. Treatment may be limited to surgical removal of the mass or additional radiation therapy,

chemotherapy, or both, if other factors suggest the need. The prognosis of small cell lymphocytic lymphomas of the lung is excellent. Koss and associates (1983) reported a 5-year survival of 70% and L'hoste and co-workers (1984) a survival of 83%. Kennedy and colleagues (1985) reported a 9.75-year median survival for a group of 12 patients, and Turner and associates (1984) reported a median 4-year survival for a group of 33 patients of whom only one died of lymphoma. The survival data for large cell—histiocytic—lymphomas of the lung is less clear because there are fewer reported cases.

Large Cell—Histiocytic—Lymphoma

The large cell—histiocytic—lymphoma is more common in women than in men. The lesions tend to occur in the fifth and sixth decades of life. Hilar lymph nodes are always involved. The lesions tend to occur in the upper lobes, although an entire lung may be involved. Chest wall and pleural involvement can occur. Cavitation may occur with the mixed—large and small—cell types. When feasible, surgical resection should be attempted. When the hilar nodes are positive, postoperative radiation therapy is indicated. In patients with widespread disease, chemotherapy is the treatment of choice. These are more aggressive tumors than the small cell lymphocytic lymphomas, and the prognosis is correspondingly poorer (Fig. 77–8). L'hoste and colleagues (1984) reported late recurrence in 53% of their patients. The recurrences can occur within months or many years after the initial treatment. In general, these patients do not survive as long as patients with small cell lymphocytic lymphomas. The prognosis of patients with primary non-Hodgkin's lymphoma of the lung, despite frequent recurrences, is better than that of patients with initial systemic disease.

Lymphomatoid Granulomatosis—LYG

This is an atypical lymphoreticular infiltrate that involves the vessels of the lung and other organs—skin and brain. Lymphomatoid granulomatosis was first described in 1972 by Liebow and colleagues. The lesion had certain histologic features of lymphoma and Wegener's granulomatosis, hence the name lymphomatoid granulomatosis. Since the original description, the knowledge of extranodal lymphomas has grown considerably. Weis and associates (1986) examined the subject of peripheral T-cell lymphomas and concluded from their cases and the existing literature that LYG is an example of a peripheral T-cell lymphoma. Lymphomatoid granulomatosis usually affects middle-aged adults, with a slight predominance in men. Patients present with cough, shortness of breath, and chest pain as well as fever, malaise, and weight loss. The roentgenographic findings are multiple bilateral nodular densities. In a study of 15 patients, Fauci and colleagues (1982) found that cyclophosphamide and prednisone could be beneficial to these patients. Katzenstein and co-workers (1979), however, reported that two thirds of the patients died despite treatment with corticosteroids or chemotherapy or both; the median survival was 14 months. Koss and colleagues (1986) reported that 38% of the patients with LYG died within a year of diagnosis. In summary, this disease should be viewed as a peripheral T-cell lymphoma that primarily involves the lung and has a poor prognosis.

Plasma Cell Disorders

Waldenstrom's macroglobulinemia, plasmacytoma, and multiple myeloma may in rare instances originate in the lung. Noach (1956) first reported Waldenstrom's macroglobulinemia to involve the lung. Systemic manifestations such as lymphadenopathy, splenomegaly, and weight loss may be present.

Plasmacytomas may occur in the lung, but they are rare. They may be forerunners of disseminated disease. Treatment is excision when possible, but in most instances chemotherapy is the modality of choice.

Multiple myeloma may involve the lung as a solitary mass or as part of a systemic disease.

Primary Pulmonary Hodgkin's Disease

Primary Hodgkin's disease of the lung is rare. Kern and colleagues (1961) reviewed 18 cases of primary pulmonary Hodgkin's disease, and Yousem and associates (1986) reviewed an additional 15 cases. In the latter series the patients ranged from 19 to 82 years—mean 45 years. Women were affected twice as often as men; the affected women tended to be older than the men. Patients complained of cough, fever, and weight loss and all but two were symptomatic. Roentgenographically, most showed a nodular pattern that could be solitary or multiple. Seven patients has unilateral disease and eight, bilateral disease. Patients received various chemotherapeutic agents. Six patients died of their disease between 3 to 49 months after diagnosis; in contrast, seven of the patients survived from 10 to 82 months after diagnosis.

Patients who were older than 60 years and who had bilateral lesions on chest roentgenograms had a worse prognosis.

Summary

In view of the pathologist's difficulty in interpreting lymphoid lesions of the lung, the surgeon should take some extra steps if he suspects a lymphoid lesion. The hilar lymph nodes should be sampled both for diagnosis and staging, and some of the tumor should be frozen for immunologic marker studies. Most lymphoid markers are destroyed in paraffin-embedded tissue. Marker studies on pseudolymphomas and lymphoid interstitial pneumonia demonstrate polyclonal staining for heavy chains—IgG, IgA, IgM—and light chains—kappa, lambda—of immunoglobulins; B-cell lymphomas show monoclonal staining. Also, some of the fresh unfixed tissue should be sent for flow cytometry studies, which produce information about the cell cycle, the DNA content of the cells, and immunologic markers. The phase of the cell cycle reveals whether the cells are rapidly proliferating. The DNA content differentiates diploid cell populations from aneuploid stem cell populations. Flow cytometry can give a percentage distribution of immunologic markers, whereas frozen sections only give an architectural distribution of the markers. These two ways of performing immunologic markers complement each other. In conclusion, new scientific techniques are offering more ways for the surgeon and the oncologist to evaluate lymphoid lesions of the lung. The crucial step is to consider the possibility of a lymphoid lesion and then collect the appropriate fresh, frozen, and formalin-fixed tissue.

Malignant Melanoma of the Bronchus

Almost all malignant melanomas of the lung are metastatic lesions. Only Salm's (1963) case report excluded an alternative primary site for the tumor by postmortem examination. Other cases of primary melanoma of the bronchus have been reported, but complete proof of the absence of a remote site of origin is lacking. Melanomas discovered in the bronchus behave like a primary carcinoma of the lung, resulting in bronchial obstruction. If a melanoma is encountered and no history or evidence of a simultaneous or previous primary can be elicited, resection if possible should be carried out.

Malignant Teratomas

Intrapulmonary teratomas are uncommon; half of these may be malignant. Day and Taylor (1975) reviewed the available literature and noted that for some unexplained reason most malignant teratomas occurred in the left upper lobe. In the past, some malignant lesions have been confused with the pulmonary blastomas. The prognosis of the malignant teratoma is poor.

REFERENCES

Adamson, D., et al.: Successful treatment of pulmonary LAM with oophorectomy and progestrone. Am. Rev. Respir. Dis. *132*:916, 1985.

Andrion, A., et al.: Benign clear cell ('sugar') tumor of the lung: a light microscopic, histochemical, and ultrastructural study with a review of the literature. Cancer 56:2657, 1985.

Archambeaud-Mouveroux, F., et al.: Bronchial leiomyoma: report of a case successfully treated by endoscopic neodymium-yttrium aluminum garnet laser. J. Thorac. Cardiovasc. Surg. 95:356, 1988.

Arrigoni, M.G., et al.: Benign tumors of the lung: a ten-year surgical experience. J. Thorac. Cardiovasc. Surg. 60:589, 1970.

Avignina, A., et al.: Pulmonary rhabdomyosarcoma with isolated small bowel metastases: a report of a case with immunohistological and ultrastructural studies. Cancer 53:1948, 1984.

Bahadori, H., and Liebow, A.A.: Plasma cell granulomas of the lung. Cancer 31:191, 1973.

Baker, P.B., and Goodwin, R.A.: Pulmonary artery sarcoma: a review and report of a case. Arch. Pathol. Lab. Med. 109:35, 1985.

Banner, A.S., et al.: Efficacy of oophorectomy in lymphangioleiomyomatosis and benign metastasizing leiomyoma. N. Engl. J. Med. 305:204, 1981.

Barnard, W.G.: Embryoma of lung. Thorax 7:299, 1952.

Bateson, E.M.: So-called hamartoma of the lung: a true neoplasm of fibrous connective tissue of the bronchi. Cancer 31:1458, 1973.

Berardi, R.S., et al.: Inflammatory pseudotumors of the lung. Surg. Gynecol. Obstet. 156:89, 1983.

Bleisch, V.R., and Kraus, F.T.: Polypoid sarcoma of the pulmonary trunk: analysis of the literature and report of a case with leptomeric organelles and ultrastructural features of rhabdomyosarcoma. Cancer 46:314, 1980.

Cabarcos, A., Gomez Dorronsoro, M., and Lobo Beristain, J.L.: Pulmonary carcinosarcoma: a case study and review of the literature. Br. J. Dis. Chest 79:83, 1985.

Carrington, C.B., and Liebow, A.A.: Lymphocytic interstitial pneumonia (Abstract). Am. J. Pathol. 48:36a, 1966.

Carrington, C.B., et al.: Lymphangioleiomyomatosis: Physiologic-Pathologic-Radiologic Correlations. Am. Rev. Respir. Dis. 116:977, 1977.

Chumas, J.C., and Lorelle, C.A.: Pulmonary meningioma: a light- and electron-microscopic study. Am. J. Surg. Pathol. 6:795, 1982.

Colby, T.V., and Carrington, C.B.: Lymphoreticular tumors and infiltrates of the lung. Pathol. Annu. 18:27, 1983.

Corrin, B., Liebow, A.A., and Friedman, P.J.: Pulmonary lymphangiomyomatosis: a review. Am. J. Pathol. 79:348, 1975.

Costa, J., and Martin, S.: Pulmonary lymphoreticular disorders. In Surgical Pathology of the Lymph Nodes and Related Organs. Edited by E. Jaffee. Philadelphia, W.B. Saunders Co., 1985, p. 289.

Dail, D.H.: Uncommon tumors. In Pulmonary Pathology. Edited by D.H. Dail and S.P. Hammar. New York, Springer-Verlag, 1988, p. 847.

Dail, D., and Liebow, A.A.: Intravascular bronchioalveolar tumor (Abstract). Am. J. Pathol. 78:6, 1975.

Dail, D.H., et al.: Intravascular, bronchiolar, and alveolar tumor of the lung (IVBAT): an analysis of twenty cases of a peculiar sclerosing endothelial tumor. Cancer 51:452, 1983.

Davis, Z., et al.: Primary pulmonary hemangiopericytoma. J. Thorac. Cardiovasc. Surg. 64:882, 1972.

Day, D.W., and Taylor, S.A.: An intrapulmonary teratoma associated with thymic tissue. Thorax 30:582, 1975.

Engleman, P., et al.: Pulmonary hyalinizing granuloma. Am. Rev. Respir. Dis. 115:997, 1977.

Enzinger, F.M., and Smith, B.H.: Hemangiopericytoma. Hum. Pathol. 7:61, 1976.

Enzinger, F.M., and Weiss, S.W.: Soft Tissue Tumors. St. Louis, C.V. Mosby Co., 1983, p. 409.

Fadhli, H.A., Harrison, A.W., and Shaddock, S.H.: Primary pulmonary leiomyosarcoma. Dis. Chest 48:431, 1965.

Fauci, A.S., et al.: Lymphomatoid granulomatosis: prospective clinical and therapeutic experience over 10 years. N. Engl. J. Med. 306:68, 1982.

Feldman, F., and Seaman, W.B.: Primary thoracic hemangiopericytoma. Radiology 82:998, 1964.

Fisher, A.M.H., Kendall, B., and Van Leuven, B.D.: Hodgkin's disease: a radiologic survey. Clin. Radiol. 13:115, 1962.

Francis, D., and Jacobsen, M.: Pulmonary blastoma. Curr. Top. Pathol. 73:265, 1983.

Fu-lin, Z., et al.: Lung ectopic meningioma: a case report. Chinese Med. J. 96(4):309, 1983.

Goldthorn, J.F., et al.: Cavitating primary pulmonary fibrosarcoma in a child. J. Thorac. Cardiovasc. Surg. 91:932, 1986.

Guccion, J.G., and Rosen, S.H.: Bronchopulmonary leiomyosarcoma and fibrosarcoma: a study of 32 cases and review of the literature. Cancer 30:836, 1972.

Hamper, U.M., et al.: Pulmonary hamartoma: diagnosis by transthoracic needle aspiration biopsy. Radiology 155:15, 1985.

Hartman, G.E., and Shockat, S.J.: Primary pulmonary neoplasms of childhood: a review. Ann. Thorac. Surg. 36:108, 1983.

Herbert, A., Wright, D.H., and Isaacson, P.G.: Primary malignant lymphoma of the lung: histopathologic and immunologic evaluation of nine cases. Hum. Pathol. 15:415, 1984.

Hurt, R.: Benign tumors of the bronchus and trachea: 1951–1981. Ann. R. Coll. Surg. Engl. 66:22, 1984.

Jackson, H., and Parker, F.: Hodgkin's Disease and Allied Disorders. New York, Oxford University Press, 1947.

Katzenstein, A.L., Carrington, C., and Liebow, A.A.: Lymphomatoid granulomatosis: a clinicopathologic study of 152 cases. Cancer 43:360, 1979.

Katzenstein, A.L., Gmelich, J.T., and Carrington, C.B.: Sclerosing hemangioma of the lung: a clinicopathologic study of 51 cases. Am. J. Surg. Pathol. 4:343, 1982.

Kemnitz, P., Spormann, H., and Heinrich, P.: Meningioma of lung: first report with light and electron microscopic findings. Ultrastruct. Pathol. 3:359, 1982.

Kennedy, J.L., et al.: Pulmonary lymphomas and other pulmonary lymphoid lesions: a clinicopathologic and immunologic study of 64 patients. Cancer 56:539, 1985.

Kern, W.H., Crepeau, A.G., and Jones, J.C.: Primary Hodgkin's disease of the lung: report of 4 cases and review of the literature. Cancer 14:1151, 1961.

Koss, M.N., et al.: Primary non-Hodgkin's lymphoma and pseudolymphoma of the lung: a study of 161 patients. Hum. Pathol. 14:1024, 1983.

Koss, M., et al.: Lymphomatoid granulomatosis: a clinicopathologic study of 42 patients. Pathol. (Sydney) 18:283, 1986.

Kradin, R.L., and Mark, E.J.: Benign lymphoid disorders of the lung, with a theory regarding their development. Hum. Pathol. 14:857, 1983.

Ledor, K., et al.: CT diagnosis of pulmonary hamartomas. CT 5:343, 1981.

Lee, S.H., Reganchary, S.S., and Paramesk, J.: Primary pulmonary rhabdomyosarcoma: a case report and review of the literature. Hum. Pathol. 12:92, 1981.

Lennert, K.: Malignant Lymphomas Other Than Hodgkin's Disease. New York, Springer-Verlag, 1978.

L'hoste, R.J., et al.: Primary pulmonary lymphomas. Cancer 54:1397, 1984.

Liebow, A.A., and Carrington, C.B.: Diffuse pulmonary lymphoreticular infiltration associated with dysproteinemia. Med. Clin. North Am. 57:809, 1973.

Liebow, A.A., and Castleman, B.: Benign "clear cell" tumors of the lung. (Abstract) Am. J. Pathol. 43:13a, 1963.

Liebow, A.A., and Castleman, B.: Benign clear cell ("sugar") tumors of the lung. Yale J. Biol. Med. 43:213, 1971.

Liebow, A.A., and Hubbell, D.S.: Sclerosing hemangioma (histiocytoma xanthoma) of the lung. Cancer 9:53, 1956.

Liebow, A., Carrington, C., and Friedman, P.: Lymphomatoid granulomatosis. Hum. Pathol. 3:457, 1972.

Luck, S.R., Reynolds, M., and Raffensperger, J.G.: Congenital bronchopulmonary malformations. Curr. Probl. Surg. 23:251, 1986.

Lukes, R.J., and Collins, R.D.: New approaches to the classification of lymphomata. Br. J. Cancer 2(Suppl.):1, 1975.

Mandelstramm, M.: Über primary Neubildung des Herzens. Virch. Arch. Pathol. Anat. 245:43, 1923.

Martini, N., and Beattie, E.J., Jr.: Less Common Tumors of the Lung. In General Thoracic Surgery, 2nd ed. Edited by T.W. Shields. Philadelphia, Lea & Febiger, 1983, p. 780.

Martini, N., Hajdu, S.I., and Beattie, E.J., Jr.: Primary sarcoma of lung. J. Thorac. Cardiovasc. Surg. 61:33, 1971.

McCormack, P.M., and Martini, N.: Primary Sarcomas and Lymphomas of Lung. *In* International Trends in General Thoracic Surgery, Vol. 5. Edited by N. Martini and I. Vogt-Moykopf. St. Louis, C.V. Mosby Co., 1988 (in press).

Miettinen, M., et al.: Intravascular bronchioloalveolar tumor. Cancer *60*:2471, 1987.

Miller, D.C., et al.: Benign metastatizing meningioma. J. Neurosurg. *62*:763, 1985.

Moffat, R.E., Chang, C.H.J., and Slaven, J.E.: Roentgen considerations in primary pulmonary artery sarcoma. Radiology *104*:283, 1972.

Nascimento, A.G., Unni, K.K., and Bernatz, P.E.: Sarcomas of the lung. Mayo Clin. Proc. 57:355, 1982.

Nili, M., et al.: Multiple pulmonary hamartomas: a case report and review of the literature. Scand. J. Thorac. Cardiovasc. Surg. *13*:157, 1979.

Noach, A.S.: (Pulmonary involvement in Waldenstrom's macroglobulinemia.) Ned. Tijdschr. Geneeskd. *100*:3881, 1956.

The Non-Hodgkin's Lymphoma Pathologic Classification Project: National Cancer Institute-sponsored study of classification on non-Hodgkin's lymphoma. Cancer *49*:2112, 1982.

Oparah, S.S., and Subramanian, V.A.: Granular cell myoblastoma of the bronchus: report of 2 cases and review of the literature. Ann. Thorac. Cardiovasc. Surg. *22*:199, 1976.

Rappaport, H.: Tumors of the hematopoietic system. Atlas of Tumor Pathology, Fascicle 8. Washington, D.C., Armed Forces Institute of Pathology, 1966.

Risdall, R., Hoppe, T.R., and Warnke, R.: Non-Hodgkin's lymphoma: a study of the evolution of the disease based upon 92 autopsied cases. Cancer *44*:529, 1979.

Salm, R.: A primary malignant melanoma of the bronchus. J. Pathol. Bacteriol. 85:121, 1963.

Saltzstein, S.L.: Pulmonary malignant lymphomas and pseudolymphomas. Classification, therapy and prognosis. Cancer *16*:928, 1963.

Shaw, R.R., et al.: Primary pulmonary leiomyosarcomas. J. Thorac. Cardiovasc. Surg. *41*:430, 1961.

Shields, T.W., and Lynn, T.E.: Endobronchial hamartoma: a case report. Arch. Surg. 76:358, 1958.

Shinn, M.S., and Ho, K.J.: Primary hemangiopericytoma of lung: radiography and pathology. AJR *133*:1077, 1979.

Siegelman, S.S., et al.: CT of pulmonary hamartoma. Presented at the American Roentgen Ray Society, 84th Annual Meeting, Las Vegas, Nevada, April 1984.

Singh, G., Lee, R.E., and Brooks, D.H.: Primary pulmonary paraganglioma: report of a case and review of the literature. Cancer *40*:2286, 1977.

Spencer, H.: Pulmonary blastoma. J. Pathol. *82*:161, 1961.

Spencer, H.: The pulmonary plasma cell/histiocytoma complex. Histopathology 8:903, 1984.

Spragg, R.G., et al.: Angiosarcoma of the lung with fatal pulmonary hemorrhage. Am. J. Med. *74*:1072, 1983.

Trapnell, D.H.: Recognition and incidence of intrapulmonary lymph nodes. Thorax *19*:44, 1964.

Turner, R.R., Colby, T.V., and Doggett, R.S.: Well-differentiated lymphocytic lymphoma: a study of 47 cases with primary manifestation of the lung. Cancer *54*:2088, 1984.

Unger, P.D., Gella, S.A., and Anderson, P.J.: Pulmonary lesions in a patient with neurofibromatosis. Arch. Pathol. Lab. Med. *108*:654, 1984.

Wackers, F.J., van der Schoot, J.B., and Hamper, J.R.: Sarcoma of the pulmonary trunk associated with hemorrhagic tendency: a case report and review of the literature. Cancer 23:339, 1969.

Warter, A., Satge, D., and Roeslin, N.: Angioinvasive plasma cell granuloma of the lung. Cancer 59:435, 1987.

Watson, W.L, and Anlyan, A.J.: Primary leiomyosarcoma: a clinical evaluation of six cases. Cancer 7:250, 1954.

Weis, J.W., et al.: Peripheral T-cell lymphomas: Histologic, immunologic, and clinical characterization. Mayo Clin. Proc. *61*:411, 1986.

Weiss, L.M., Yousem, S.A., and Warnke, R.A.: Non-Hodgkin's lymphomas of the lung. Am. J. Surg. Pathol. 9:480, 1985.

Weiss, S.W., and Enzinger, F.M.: Epithelioid hemangioendothelioma:

a vascular tumor often mistaken for a carcinoma. Cancer *50*:970, 1982.

Weiss, S.W., et al.: Epithelioid hemangioendothelioma and related lesions. Semin. Diagn. Pathol. 3:259, 1986.

Wende, S., et al.: Lung metastasis of a meningioma. Neuroradiology *24*:287, 1983.

Wenisch, H.J.C., and Lulay, M.: Lymphogenous spread of an intravascular bronchioloalveolar tumour: case report and review of the literature. Virchows Arch. [A] *387*:117, 1980.

White, S.H., et al.: Leiomyomas of the lower respiratory tract. Thorax *40*:306, 1985.

Winkler, T.R., Burr, L.H., and Robinson, C.L.N.: Benign metastasizing leiomyoma. Ann. Thorac. Surg. 43:100, 1987.

Yellin, A., Rosenman, Y., and Lieberman, Y.: Review of smooth muscle tumours of the lower respiratory tract. Br. J. Dis. Chest 78:337, 1984.

Yousem, S.A.: Angiosarcoma presenting in the lung. Arch. Pathol. Lab. Med. *110*:112, 1986.

Yousem, S.A., and Hochholzer, L.: Pulmonary hyalinizing granuloma. Am. J. Clin. Pathol. 87:1, 1987a.

Yousem, S.A., and Hochholzer, L.: Malignant fibrous histiocytoma of the lung. Cancer 60:2532, 1987b.

Yousem, S.A., and Hochholzer, L.: Primary pulmonary hemangiopericytoma. Cancer 59:549, 1987c.

Yousem, S.A., et al.: Primary pulmonary Hodgkin's disease: a clinicopathologic study of 15 cases. Cancer 57:1217, 1986.

READING REFERENCES

General

Carter, D., and Eggleston, J.C.: Tumors of the lower respiratory tract, Series 2. Washington, D.C.: Armed Forces Institute of Pathology 1980, p. 221.

Churg, A.: Tumors of the Lung. *In* Pathology of the Lung. Edited by W. Thurlbeck. New York, Thieme Medical Publishers, Inc., 1988, p. 311.

Dail, D.H., and Hammar, S.P.: Pulmonary Pathology. New York, Springer-Verlag, 1987.

Dunnill, M.S.: Rare Pulmonary Tumors. *In* Pulmonary Pathology, 2nd ed. Edited by M.S. Dunnill. New York, Churchill Livingstone, Inc., 1987, p. 413.

Madewell, J.E., and Feigan, D.S.: Benign tumors of the lung. Semin. Roentgenol. *12*:175, 1977.

Spencer, H.: Rare Pulmonary Tumors. *In* Pathology of the Lung, 4th ed. Edited by H. Spencer. New York, Pergamon Press, 1985, p. 933.

Connective Tissue Tumors, Benign

Orlowski, T.M., Stasiak, K., and Kolodziej, J.: Leiomyoma of the lung. J. Thorac. Cardiovasc. Surg. 76:257, 1978.

Schraufnagel, D.E., Morin, J.E., and Wang, N.S.: Endobronchial lipoma. Chest 75:97, 1979.

Epithelial Tumor

Spencer, H., Dail, D.H., and Arneaud, J.: Noninvasive bronchial epithelial papillary tumors. Cancer 45:1486, 1986.

Fibrous Histiocytoma, Benign and Malignant

Bedrossian, C.W.M., et al.: Pulmonary malignant fibrous histiocytoma: light and electron microscopic studies of one case. Chest 75:186, 1979.

Silverman, J.F., and Coalson, J.J.: Primary malignant myxoid fibrous histiocytoma of the lung: light and ultrastructural examination with review of the literature. Arch. Pathol. Lab. Med. *108*:49, 1984.

Viguera, J.L., et al.: Fibrous histiocytoma of the lung. Thorax 31:475, 1976.

Granular Cell Myoblastoma (Granular Cell Tumor)

O'Connell, D.J., MacMahon, H., and DeMeester, T.R.: Multicentric tracheobronchial and oesophageal granular cell myoblastoma. Thorax 33:596, 1978.

Valenstein, S.L., and Thurer, R.J.: Granular cell myoblastoma of the bronchus: case report and literature review. J. Thorac. Cardiovasc. Surg. 76:465, 1978.

Hamartoma

Becker, R.M., ViLorio, J., and Chiu, C.: Multiple pulmonary leiomyomatous hamartomas in women. J. Thorac. Cardiovasc. Surg. 71:631, 1976.

Bennett, L.L., Lesar, M.S., and Tellis, C.J.: Multiple calcified chondrohamartomas of the lung: CT appearance. J. Comput. Assist. Tomogr. 9:180, 1985.

Koutras, P., Urschel, H.C., Jr., and Paulson, D.L.: Hamartoma of the lung. J. Thorac. Cardiovasc. Surg. 61:768, 1971.

Minasian, H.: Uncommon pulmonary hamartomas. Thorax 32:360, 1977.

Petheram, I.S., and Heard, B.E.: Unique massive pulmonary hamartoma: case report with review of hamartoma treated at Brompton Hospital in 27 years. Chest 75:95, 1979.

Ramzy, I.: Pulmonary hamartomas: cytologic appearances of fine-needle aspiration biopsy. Acta Cytol. 20:15, 1976.

Shah, J.P., et al.: Hamartomas of the lung. Surg. Gynecol. Obstet. 136:406, 1973.

Spencer, H.: Hamartomas, Blastoma and Teratoma of the Lung. In Pathology of the Lung, 4th ed. Edited by H. Spencer. New York, Pergamon Press, 1985, p. 1061.

Tomashefski, J.F., Jr.: Benign endobronchial mesenchymal tumors: Their relationship to parenchymal pulmonary hamartomas. Am. J. Surg. Pathol. 6:531, 1982.

Lymphangioleiomyomatosis—LAM

Graham, M.L., et al.: Pulmonary lymphangiomyomatosis: with particular reference to steroid-receptor assay studies and pathologic correlation. Mayo Clin. Proc. 59:3, 1984.

Luna, C.M., et al.: Pulmonary LAM associated with tuberous sclerosis: treatment with tamoxifen and tetracycline pleurodesis. Chest 88:473, 1985.

Lymphomas

Freeman, C., Berg, J.W., and Cutler, S.J.: Occurrence and prognosis of extranodal lymphoma. Cancer 29:252, 1972.

Gibbs, A.R., and Seal, R.M.E.: Primary lymphoproliferative conditions of lung. Thorax 33:140, 1978.

Greenberg, S.D., and Jenkins, D.E.: Xanthomatous inflammatory pseudotumors of the lung. South. Med. J. 68:754, 1975.

Greenberg, S.D., et al.: Pulmonary lymphoma versus pseudolymphoma: a perplexing problem. South. Med. J. 65:775, 1972.

Hurt, R.L., and Kennedy, W.P.U.: Primary lymphosarcoma of the lung. Thorax 29:258, 1974.

Rubin, M.: Primary lymphoma of lung. J. Thorac. Cardiovasc. Surg. 56:293, 1968.

Neural Tumors

Davidson, K.G., Walbaum, P.R., and McCormack, R.J.M.: Intrathoracic neural tumors. Thorax 33:359, 1978.

Reed, J.C., Hallet, K.K., and Feigin, D.S.: Neural tumors of the thorax: subject review from the AFIP. Diagn. Radiol. 126:9, 1978.

Pseudotumors

Graham, M.L., et al.: Pulmonary lymphangiomyomatosis: with particular reference to steroid-receptor assay studies and pathologic correlation. Mayo Clin. Proc. 59:3, 1984.

Spoto, G., Jr., Rossi, N.P., and Allsbrook, W.C.: Tracheobronchial plasma cell granuloma. J. Thorac. Cardiovasc. Surg. 73:804, 1977.

Pulmonary Blastoma

Ashworth, T.G.: Pulmonary blastomas: a true congenital neoplasm. Histopathol. 7:585, 1983.

Gibbons, J.R.P., McKeown, F., and Field, T.W.: Pulmonary blastoma with hilar lymph node metastases: survival for 24 years. Cancer 47:152, 1981.

Spencer, H.: Hamartomas, Blastoma and Teratoma of the Lung. In Pathology of the Lung, 4th ed. Edited by H. Spencer. New York, Pergamon Press, 1985, p. 1061.

Pulmonary Sarcoma

Cameron, E.W.J.: Primary sarcoma of the lung. Thorax 30:516, 1975.

Ramanathan, T.: Primary leiomyosarcoma of the lung. Thorax 29:482, 1974.

Sawamura, K., et al.: Primary liposarcoma of the lung: report of a case. J. Surg. Oncol. 19:243, 1982.

Wick, M.R., et al.: Primary pulmonary leiomyosarcomas: a light and electron microscopic study. Arch. Pathol. Lab. Med. 106:510, 1982.

Teratomas, Benign and Malignant

Ali, M.Y., and Wong, P.K.: Intrapulmonary teratoma. Thorax 19:228, 1964.

Gantam, H.P.: Intrapulmonary malignant teratoma. Am. Rev. Respir. Dis. 200:863, 1969.

Holt, S., Peverall, P.B, and Boddy, J.E.: A teratoma of the lung containing thymic tissue. J. Pathol. 126:85, 1978.

Spencer, H.: Hamartomas, Blastoma and Teratoma of the Lung. In Pathology of the Lung, 4th ed. Edited by H. Spencer. New York, Pergamon Press, 1985, p. 1061.

CHAPTER 78

SECONDARY TUMORS IN THE LUNG

Patricia McCormack and Nael Martini

Metastatic tumor from cancer elsewhere in the body often occurs in the lungs. Autopsy studies by Turner and Jaffe (1940) and Willis (1952) demonstrated that pulmonary metastases were present at death in up to 30% of patients who died of malignant disease. Fallon and Roper (1967) reported that 12% of patients who died with pulmonary metastases had resectable lesions. Minor (1950) concluded from clinical and autopsy data that 1.2% of all patients with malignant disease have solitary pulmonary metastasis at some time during the course of their disease. Marcove (1975), in a study of 184 patients, noted that in primary sarcomas, the lungs fill with metastases before other sites are involved. In carcinomas, however, in less than 50% of patients with metastases is the lung the only organ involved. This difference is essential in treatment planning. In half of the patients, the pulmonary lesions are the only metastatic spread. The lesions are usually multiple and bilateral, although in approximately 10% of cases, the secondary tumor is solitary.

PATHOLOGY

The metastatic pathway may be by direct infiltration, by lymphatic-borne metastases, and most importantly by blood-borne metastases. True intrabronchial spread—airborne metastasis—if it occurs at all, is rare.

Most metastatic tumors reach the lungs by way of the pulmonary arteries, although a few may travel by way of the bronchial arteries. Most are spherical masses and solid lesions (Fig. 78–1), although cavitation may occur. Chaudhuri (1970) wrote that cavitation is best explained by thromboses and consequent ischemia. The origin of the blood supply of these secondary tumors is not as definitely established as it is for primary tumors of the lung. Cudkowicz and Armstrong (1953) could not demonstrate an increase in the bronchial artery pattern to these secondary growths.

Rarely, a lymphatic-borne tumor embolus may lodge in the submucosal lymphatics of a major bronchus and, with growth, may closely simulate a primary tumor of the bronchus. The reported incidence of this isolated involvement is about 2%, although Shepherd (1982) reported that 28% of 90 patients with pulmonary metastases evaluated for surgical resection had endobronchial involvement. Renal and colorectal carcinomas cause isolated endobronchial involvement more often than other primary tumors reportedly do, but carcinoma in other sites, such as the breast, pancreas, adrenal glands, and uterine cervix, as well as melanoma, has been implicated.

Diffuse permeation of the pulmonary lymphatics occurs more often and results in typical clinical and roentgenographic findings of lymphangitic carcinomatosis (Fig. 78–2). The common primary lesions that spread in this manner are tumors arising in the stomach, breast, lung, prostate, and pancreas, and occasionally the ovary, as Spencer (1968) noted.

Whether metastatic lesions in the lung may act as a secondary source of blood-borne tumor emboli to other sites remains undetermined, but lymphatic invasion and involvement of bronchial and hilar lymph nodes are not unusual. The mode of spread to these structures is not known, perhaps the secondary lung lesion is the major source, although the possibility of blood-borne metastases to the lymph node from the original tumor cannot be ruled out. Metastatic disease may also involve the pleura, diaphragm, and chest wall and the adjacent structures in the mediastinum.

SYMPTOMS

In the absence of involvement of the pleura, major bronchi, or other contiguous structures, the secondary tumors of the lung, even when extensive, usually remain asymptomatic. Most are discovered on a routine roentgenogram of the chest or at autopsy. Hemoptysis, cough, fever, pain, and dyspnea predominate when symptoms are present at all. Rarely, hypertrophic pulmonary osteoarthropathy has been reported. Because pulmonary metastases usually have few symptoms, the benefits of treatment must be measured in terms of prolonged survival.

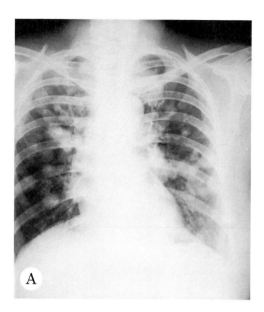

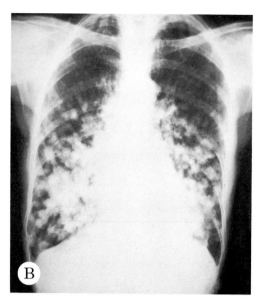

Fig. 78–1. PA roentgenograms of the chest showing: *A*, bilateral metastases to lungs from a primary carcinoma of breast; *B*, bilateral metastases to lungs from a primary thyroid carcinoma.

DIAGNOSIS

The nature of the pulmonary lesions is usually readily suspected by clinical and roentgenographic findings. Chang (1979) compared acuity and accuracy of the chest roentgenogram, plain tomograms, and the CT scan in detecting pulmonary lesions. The chest roentgenogram detects a 9 mm nodule, 90% of which are malignant; the standard chest tomogram can detect a 7 mm nodule, only 60% of which are malignant; and the CT scan of the chest can detect a 3 mm nodule, only 45% of which are malignant. Most of the lesions are nodular, but may appear as infiltrative, lymphangitic, miliary, or even massive, consolidative lesions. A tissue diagnosis, however, is necessary to establish the pathology of the lesion. Bronchoscopy, cytologic examination of the sputum, percu-

taneous needle biopsy, and direct open lung biopsy have been used with varying degrees of success.

Adkins and his associates (1968) reported 50 patients presenting with a solitary lung nodule following treatment of a malignancy elsewhere in the body. In 9 patients the intrathoracic mass was benign, usually a granuloma; a new primary lung carcinoma was found in 9 patients and a metastatic lesion in the other 32.

In patients with known primary cancer outside the lung, multiple pulmonary lesions are almost always metastatic, but a solitary pulmonary lesion in patients with known cancer elsewhere raises one of three possibilities: a new and separate cancer of the lung (Fig. 78–3), a

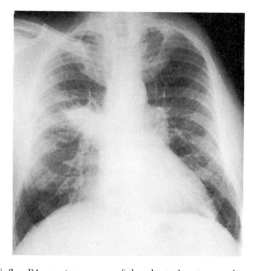

Fig. 78–3. PA roentgenogram of the chest showing a solitary right hilar mass—squamous cell carcinoma—in a patient who had undergone a left forequarter amputation 1 year previously for the treatment of a rhabdomyosarcoma in the left scapular region. The patient survived over 10 years after right pneumonectomy.

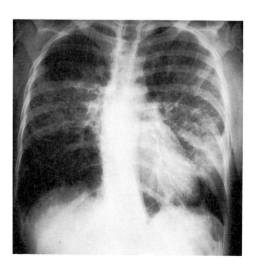

Fig. 78–2. PA roentgenogram of the chest showing lymphangitic carcinomatosis from breast carcinoma.

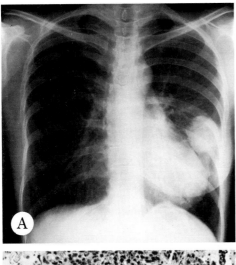

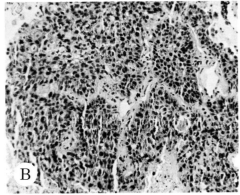

Fig. 78–4. *A,* PA roentgenogram of the chest showing solitary metastasis in the left lung from a primary breast carcinoma. *B,* Photomicrograph of metastatic carcinoma of the breast in the lung.

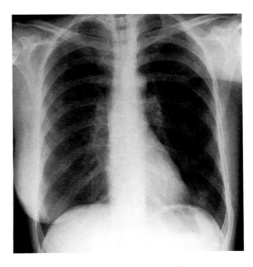

Fig. 78–5. PA roentgenogram of the chest showing a solitary lesion located at the anterior end of the left sixth rib. The patient previously had a breast carcinoma. The lung lesion proved to be a benign granuloma.

are not operative candidates or who will not accept surgery.

TREATMENT

Surgical resection is the procedure of choice for most patients with a solitary metastasis in the lung. Although this group constitutes 10% or less of all patients with pulmonary metastasis, the results of resection are satisfactory. Based on these results, as well as the development of some effective chemotherapeutic regimens, a more aggressive policy of resection for multiple and even bilateral metastatic lesions has evolved. Many reports, such as those of Martini (1971), McCormack (1978), Cliffton (1967), Han (1981) and Mountain (1984) and their associates, validated such an approach. The role of resection, however, is changing, and criteria for the proper selection of the best treatment modality for each patient must be carefully applied. In selecting patients for operative intervention, several guidelines should be followed. First, the primary tumor must be controlled or controllable. Second, the lungs must contain the only evidence of metastatic disease. Third, no other treatment modality must offer comparable results. Fourth, the patient must be at low operative risk. The surgical guideline to follow is removal of all tumor while conserving functioning lung tissue.

The extent of the metastatic disease work-up depends on the tumor type. In sarcomas, the lungs are the predominant organ of metastasis; therefore, brain, bone, and liver scans need be done only when abnormal laboratory results or the patient's symptoms dictate the need for more specific tests. The paucity of positive scans in the absence of objective evidence of disease contraindicates their routine use.

In carcinomas, metastases are not necessarily confined to lung. A meticulous search for other organ involvement, particularly the liver and bone, becomes man-

metastasis from the known primary cancer (Fig. 78–4), or a benign unrelated lesion (Fig. 78–5). Tissue diagnosis becomes necessary. In general, a solitary pulmonary lesion is more likely to be a metastasis if the primary lesion is a sarcoma or a melanoma. In our experience it is more likely to be a new lesion if the known primary tumor is in the head and neck or breast. Casey and associates (1984), however, reported that in 3% of 1416 patients with breast cancer, either a synchronous—25%—or a metachronous—75%—solitary pulmonary nodule was identified, and only 52% of these lesions were new lung carcinomas. Five percent were benign lesions, and 43% proved to be metastases from the primary breast carcinoma. In patients with known gastrointestinal or genitourinary tumors, a solitary lung lesion has an equal chance of being a metastasis or a new lung lesion.

Todd (1981) reviewed 2114 aspiration needle biopsies. Of 974 cancers, 112 were secondary lesions. The exact tissue of origin was determined in 46% of these metastases.

If the patient is at low operative risk, a thoracotomy should be performed instead of a needle biopsy. If the latter is positive, surgery is needed; if negative, thoracotomy is necessary to establish the nature of the lesion. Therefore, needle biopsy is reserved for patients who

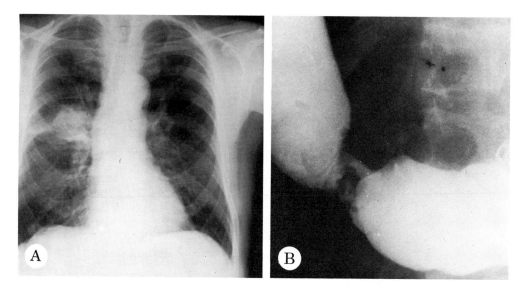

Fig. 78–6. *A*, PA roentgenogram of the chest showing right parahilar squamous cell carcinoma. *B*, Spot film of barium study of the colon revealing a simultaneously occurring adenocarcinoma of the sigmoid colon.

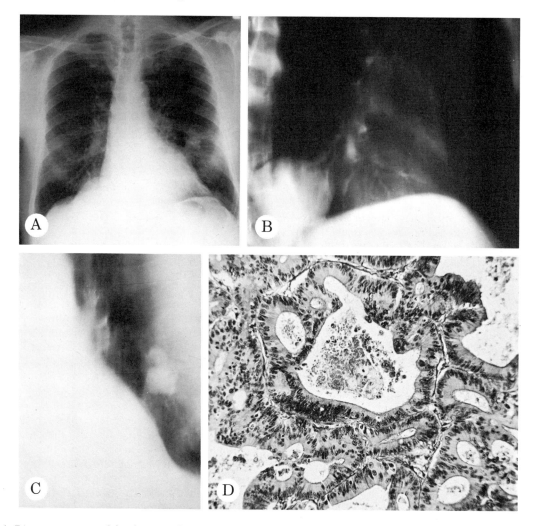

Fig. 78–7. *A*, PA roentgenogram of the chest revealing a solitary mass in the posteroinferior portion of the right lung and a second solitary mass in the left lung located in the fourth left anterior intercostal space. Both masses proved to be metastatic adenocarcinoma from the colon. *B*, Lateral laminogram demonstrating the right lung mass. *C*, AP laminogram showing the left lung mass. *D*, Photomicrograph of metastatic lesion in one resected specimen. The patient survived 5 years following resections of the metastatic lesions.

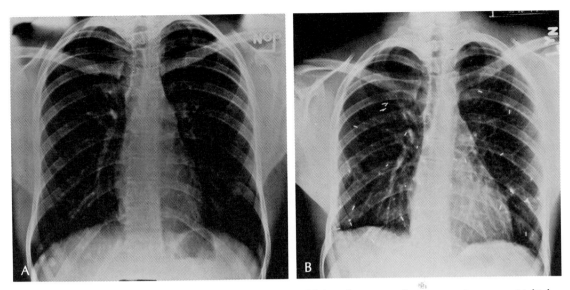

Fig. 78–8. *A*, Preoperative roentgenogram of chest in a 21-year-old male with bilateral metastases from osteogenic sarcoma. Multiple small tumor nodules are seen. *B*, Postoperative roentgenogram after bilateral thoracotomy; 19 metastases were excised from the right lung and 15 from the left lung. Clips have been placed to identify the site of excisions.

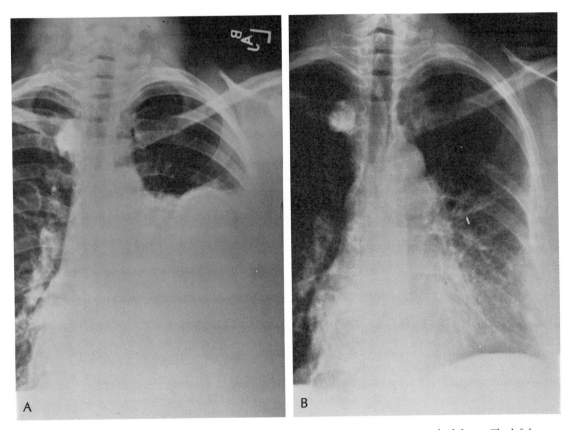

Fig. 78–9. *A*, PA roentgenogram of chest in a 43-year-old woman with metastatic osteogenic sarcoma to both lungs. The left lung mass opacifies nearly two thirds of the left pleural cavity. *B*, Chest roentgenogram after left thoracotomy and resection of large pedunculated solitary tumor derived from the lingula of the left upper lobe.

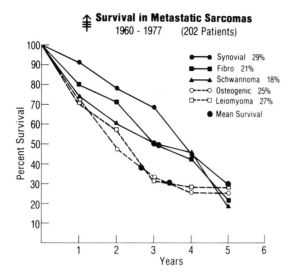

Fig. 78–10. Survival in metastatic sarcomas. 1960–1977, 202 patients. (McCormack, P.M., and Martini, N.: The changing role of surgery in pulmonary metastases. Ann. Thorac. Surg. 28:139, 1979.)

datory, but the efficacy of routine nuclide scans in this regard has not been resolved.

Tumor doubling time of less than 40 days has been advocated as a contraindication to resection, but when the lungs contain the only metastatic tumor, and this tumor can be resected, waiting for any length of time to ascertain doubling time may be counterproductive, as is demonstrated in many patients with metastatic sarcoma of the lung.

If the lung lesion and another distant primary lesion are discovered synchronously, one must determine whether the two lesions are related (Fig. 78–6). When they are not related, one must decide which of the two lesions is more threatening to the life of the patient, and if surgical intervention is decided upon, in what sequence the two operations would be better tolerated. The simultaneous occurrence of solitary bilateral lesions (Fig. 78–7) or multiple lesions in the same lung poses a difficult therapeutic decision, and individualization must be the rule.

One of us (N.M.) and associates (1971) carried out multiple, sequential resections in selected patients with osteogenic sarcoma. Also, Cliffton (1967), Kilman (1969), and Han (1981) and their associates reported encouraging results in children with multiple and bilateral metastatic disease in the lungs treated with a combination of surgical resection and irradiation or chemotherapy, or both.

The following course of action is recommended when a metastatic pulmonary lesion or lesions develops after adequate treatment of the primary tumor. If the primary tumor is known to be senstive to chemotherapy, as in lymphomas or myeloid tumors, the appropriate chemotherapeutic regimen is given. Similarly, if the primary tumor is sensitive to radiation therapy and if the port of treatment to the metastases can be kept small, this modality is used. If little or no response is noted after treatment by radiation therapy or chemotherapy, surgical re-

section is indicated. Unfortunately, however, no effective nonsurgical treatment is available for most sarcomas and carcinomas. Surgical treatment of metastases in this group of patients becomes an important modality.

Neither size nor number of metastases necessarily precludes excision, provided lung tissue can be conserved (Figs. 78–8 and 78–9). The type of surgical resection varies with the size, number, and location of the tumor. When the resection is performed for multiple metastases, conservation of lung tissue is crucial. Wedge resection is the procedure of choice when multiple lesions are present. Bilateral metastases may be removed through a median sternotomy approach or by staged posterolateral thoracotomies. Each approach has advantages. Complete resection of tumor must be the goal. Selection of a proper incision depends on which approach ensures this outcome at the least cost to the patient. Multiple thoracotomies may be needed to control recurrent disease, and the initial criteria should be reapplied each time resection is considered. One of us (N.M.) and associates (1971) reported a 27% long-term survival rate. Mountain and associates (1984) reported their 20-year experience of a 33% long-term survival rate for single and multiple metastases.

In surgical resection of a solitary lesion, lobectomy is recommended when the known primary is a carcinoma. Diagnosis by frozen section is often unsatisfactory in differentiating primary from metastatic disease. Permanent pathologic diagnosis is needed to confirm that the new lesion is not a second primary carcinoma of the lung. In this group of patients, mediastinal exploration and lymph node dissection are also recommended, because regional node metastases occur often. If the solitary pulmonary lesion is a sarcoma, a wedge resection or segmentectomy is sufficient, unless the lesion is central and precludes excision without performing a lobectomy. A lobectomy is indicated when a lesser resection will not completely remove the metastatic lesion. Only in select instances is a pneumonectomy justified for a solitary metastasis that cannot be removed with a lesser resection.

The role of external radiation therapy in metastatic disease to the lung has been limited to the rare instance in which the treatment could be applied through a limited portal. Techniques using radioactive iodine implantable seeds at the time of thoracotomy in nonresectable lesions has been useful in controlling the metastasis, with prolonged survival in some patients, as we (P.M. and associates, 1978) reported. In all series, major operative morbidity has been low and the mortality rates reported are from 0 to 3%.

Advances in chemotherapy have altered the role of surgical resection in several tumor types. Only 8% of patients with seminomatous testicular carcinoma require surgical resection of lung metastases because of the effective combination chemotherapy with vinblastine, actinomycin D, and bleomycin. Resection in these patients is reserved until after chemotherapy and is used to establish the diagnosis of a solitary metastasis or to remove lesions that grow despite chemotherapy and those that shrink but do not disappear. Operation in these instances

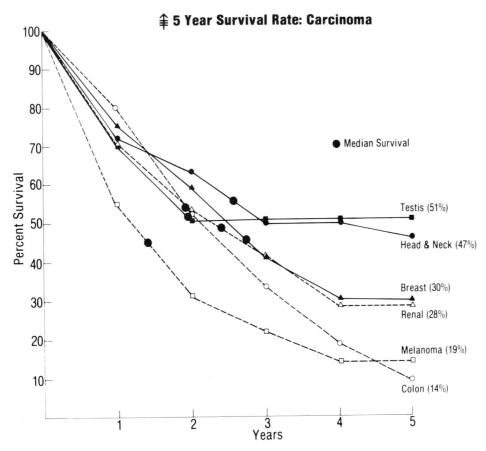

Fig. 78–11. Survival in metastatic carcinoma. 1960–1977, 246 patients. (McCormack, P.M., and Martini, N.: The changing role of surgery in pulmonary metastases. Ann. Thorac. Surg. *28:*139, 1979.)

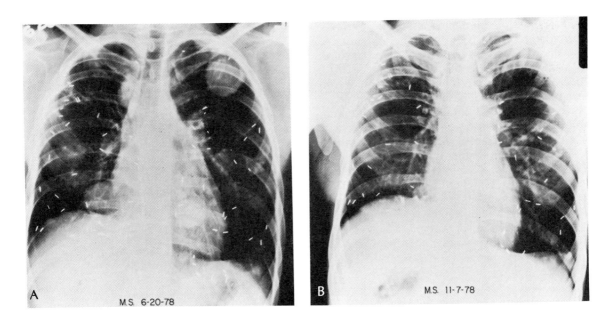

Fig. 78–12. Twenty-three-year-old male who had hip disarticulation in December, 1973, for osteogenic sarcoma of the distal femur. Bilateral lung metastases were first evident in June, 1974. Since then he has had 4 thoracotomies and intensive chemotherapy with high dose methotrexate and doxorubicin HCl (Adriamycin) with response. *A*, Chest film of June, 1978, demonstrates further recurrence of metastases despite this treatment. *B*, Chest film of November, 1978, shows resolution of these lesions after treatment with high dose cisplatin. Metal clips identify sites of resected metastases. He is now alive and well 5 years after initial treatment of his metastases.

is carefully timed to permit further chemotherapy induction if the resected lesion contains viable tumor cells. Many authors have reported finding mature teratomas or benign fibromas in these resected metastases.

Chemotherapy is the treatment of choice for pulmonary metastatic lesions of choriocarcinoma, with remission rates exceeding 85% for isolated pulmonary nodules. As Sink and associates (1981) reported, however, thoracotomy is indicated when such lesions fail to respond to multiple courses of combination chemotherapy and no other areas of gross disease are demonstrable. Excellent results can be expected following total resection of these lesions.

A special treatment plan is used for those patients with osteogenic sarcoma who present with pulmonary metastases. Patients with diffuse bilateral pulmonary metastases are first treated with intensive chemotherapy. Any residual pulmonary disease not responding to the medical treatment is then surgically removed. Patients presenting with one solitary metastasis or a few of similar size are candidates for an initial thoracotomy followed by adjuvant, but intensive, chemotherapy. The pathologic specimen in these resected metastases frequently shows "mature bone," indicating the chemotherapeutic response. The effectiveness of the chemotherapy on a specific tumor can be assessed by a pathologic study of the resected lesion, and treatment plans may be altered accordingly.

In metastatic colon carcinoma Kemeny and associates (1978) reported a 50% response rate following use of a combination of methyl lomustine—MeCCNU, vincristine sulfate—Oncovin, 5-fluorouracil, and streptozotocin for patients with colon metastases to lung alone. This report was of a 2-year follow-up only, and further evaluation will be necessary before the role of resection can be assessed for multiple metastatic lesions in the lung from colon carcinoma. Resection of a solitary metastatic lesion from the colon, however, remains the procedure of choice. Although, as Schulten and associates (1976) reported, a solitary metastasis is observed in only 2% of patients who have undergone resection of colorectal carcinoma, the results in this group of patients are satisfactory.

Metastatic mammary carcinoma has always merited special attention. We have found that the lungs are seldom the sole site of metastatic disease in these patients, and a meticulous search for other metastases is merited. The response of these patients to chemotherapy or hormonal manipulation is well documented. Surgical intervention is reserved for those rare instances in which the tumor becomes refractory to other treatment modalities.*

---

*Editor's Footnote. A solitary pulmonary lesion, in contrast to multiple lesions, in a breast cancer patient without evidence of any other systemic involvement, however, requires resection since as Casey and associates (1984), as well as the authors, have noted that it represents either a new lung primary or, infrequently, a benign lesion in half or even more of such instances.

Patients with a previous malignant melanoma present a more troublesome problem. Resection of even a solitary pulmonary metastasis yields poor prolongation of survival. Pogrebniak and associates (1988)

RESULTS

Pulmonary metastases are usually asymptomatic. The benefits of treatment, therefore, must be measured by length of survival. Five-year survival rates from surgical treatment of pulmonary metastases reportedly range from 15 to 44%, varying with tumor types and site of origin of the primary tumor (Figs. 78–10 and 78–11). The overall figure for 5-year survival with surgical treatment in solitary metastases is approximately 25%, and for multiple metastases 15%. No universal agreement exists about the effect of cell type on prognosis. The relationship of prognosis to the time interval before discovery of the metastatic lesions is also debated.

PROGNOSIS

The prognosis of patients with multiple pulmonary metastases is poor. Our overall survival results lead us to conclude that one third of the patients die within 1 year of surgical treatment of the metastases. Because of effective chemotherapy, we believe that the prognosis can be improved by combining surgery and chemotherapy (Fig. 78–12). Therefore, a diligent watch for pulmonary metastases in all cancer patients and a positive approach when they are found will continue to improve the survival statistics.

The prognosis of patients with solitary pulmonary metastases is favorable. The 5-year survival for such patients when treated by surgical resection approximates the overall 5-year survival results of primary lung cancer adequately treated by resection. None of the long-term survival rates, however, including those reported by Patterson (1982) and Wright (1982) and their associates, approach those after resection of stage I bronchial carcinoma.

REFERENCES

Adkins, P.C., et al.: Thoracotomy on the patient with previous malignancy: metastasis or new primary? J. Thorac. Cardiovasc. Surg. 56:351, 1968.

Cahan, W.G., Castro, E.B., and Hajdu, S.I.: The significance of a solitary lung shadow in patients with colon carcinoma. Cancer 33:414, 1974.

Casey, J.J., et al.: The solitary pulmonary nodule in the patient with breast cancer. Surgery 96(4):801, 1984.

Chang A.E., et al.: Evaluation of computed tomography in the detection of pulmonary metastases. Cancer 43:913, 1979.

Chaudhuri, M.R.: Cavitary pulmonary metastases. Thorax 25:375, 1970.

Cliffton, E.E., and Pool, J.L.: Treatment of lung metastases in children with combined therapy. J. Thorac. Cardiovasc. Surg. 54:403, 1967.

Cudkowicz, L., and Armstrong, J.B.: The blood supply of malignant pulmonary neoplasms. Thorax 8:152, 1953.

---

recorded only a 13-month median survival in 33 patients after resection of the metastatic pulmonary disease. These authors, however, continue to recommend resection, since in their series of 49 patients, 16 of their patients—33%—had benign disease. These patients experienced a mean survival of 169 months, significantly greater than that of patients with metastatic tumor. One can question that the observed survival was influenced by the resection, but certainly a better prognosis can be assigned to the patient when benign disease is found.

Fallon, R.H., and Roper, C.L.: Operative treatment of metastatic pulmonary cancer. Ann. Surg. *166*:263, 1967

Han, M., et al.: Aggressive thoracotomy for pulmonary metastatic osteogenic sarcoma in children and young adolescents. J. Pediatr. Surg. *16*:928, 1981.

Kemeny, N., Yagoda, A., and Golbey, R.: Methyl CCNU (MeCCNU), 5-fluorouracil (5-FU), vincristine, and streptozotocin, (MOF-Strep) for metastatic colorectal carcinoma. A.S.C.O. Abstracts, Orlando, FL, Grune & Stratton, 1978.

Kilman, J.W., et al.: Surgical resection for pulmonary metastases in children. Arch. Surg. *99*:158, 1969.

Marcove, R.C., Martini, N., and Rosen, G.: Treatment of pulmonary metastases in osteogenic sarcoma. Clin. Orthop. *111*:65, 1975.

Martini, N., et al.: Multiple pulmonary resections in the treatment of osteogenic sarcoma. Ann. Thorac. Surg. *12*:271, 1971.

McCormack, P.M., et al.: Pulmonary resection in metastatic carcinoma. Chest *73*:163, 1978.

Minor, G.R.: A clinical and radiologic study of metastatic pulmonary neoplasms. J. Thorac. Surg. *20*:34, 1950.

Mountain, C.F., McMurtrey, M.J., and Hermes, K.E.: Surgery for pulmonary metastasis: a 20-year experience. Ann. Thorac. Surg. *38*:323, 1984.

Patterson, G.A., et al.: Surgical management of pulmonary metastases. Can. J. Surg. *25*:102, 1982.

Pogrebniak, H.W., et al.: Resection of pulmonary metastases from malignant melanoma: Results of a 16-year experience. Ann. Thorac. Surg. *46*:20, 1988.

Schulten, M., Heiskell, C.A., and Shields, T.W.: The incidence of solitary pulmonary metastasis from carcinoma of the large bowel. Surg. Gynecol. Obstet. *143*:727, 1976.

Shepherd, M.: Endobronchial metastatic disease. Thorax 37:362, 1982.

Sink, J.D., Hammond, C.B., and Young, W.G., Jr.: Pulmonary resection in the management of metastases from gestational choriocarcinoma. J. Thorac. Cardiovasc. Surg. *81*:830, 1981.

Spencer, H.: Pathology of the Lung, 2nd ed. London, Pergamon Press, 1968.

Todd, T.R., et al.: Aspiration needle biopsy of thoracic lesions. Ann. Thorac. Surg. *32*:154, 1981.

Turner, J.W., and Jaffe, H.L.: Metastatic neoplasms: clinical and roentgenographical study of involvement of skeleton and lungs. Am. J. Roentgenol. *43*:479, 1940.

Willis, R.A.: The spread of tumours in the human body. London, Butterworth and Co., Ltd., 1952.

Wright, J.O., III, Brandt, B., III, and Ehrenhaft, J.L.: Results of pulmonary resection for metastatic lesions. J. Thorac. Cardiovasc. Surg. *83*:94, 1982.

The Esophagus

CHAPTER 79

CONGENITAL ANOMALIES OF THE ESOPHAGUS

Darroch W.O. Moores, Lewis W. Britton, III, and Martin F. McKneally

Understanding the development of congenital anomalies of the esophagus is facilitated by reviewing the early embryogenesis of the esophagus and trachea from the primitive foregut. The discussion of the topic by Gray and Skandalakis (1972) is excellent. We have followed their lucid presentation closely, and quoted from it liberally in the following summary, with permission of the authors.

The cranial end of the esophagus and trachea becomes demarcated with the appearance of a median ventral diverticulum of the foregut 22 to 23 days after fertilization. The tracheal diverticulum becomes a groove in the floor of the esophagus, and elongation of both structures begins. Rosenthal (1931) described that ridges of cells appear on the lateral walls, and the eventual fusion of these ridges divides the foregut into tracheal and esophageal channels. Incomplete fusion results in the various forms of tracheoesophageal fistulae (Fig. 79–1). The lung buds develop at the distal end of the tracheal primordium, reducing the amount of tissue at the level of the tracheal bifurcation so that the diameter of the esophageal channel becomes smaller than it was at an earlier stage. It is here that most esophageal atresias and stenoses develop.

During the seventh and eighth weeks, the esophageal epithelium proliferates until the lumen is nearly filled with cells and irregular vacuoles within the cellular mass, forming communicating channels. By the tenth week, the vacuoles coalesce, and a single lumen is restored. Division of the foregut into the trachea and esophagus results from the development of separate organ-forming fields, on opposite sides of the foregut. The anterior portion of the endoderm differentiates directly into tracheal mucosa and the posterior portion into esophageal mucosa.

Should the balance between the organ-forming fields be upset, the division of endoderm becomes inequitable or incomplete. If imbalance occurs, the tracheal field usually dominates the esophageal field. Complete or segmental esophageal atresia results when a disproportionate amount of endoderm becomes organized into the trachea, leaving too little from which to form an esophagus.

ESOPHAGEAL ATRESIA AND TRACHEOESOPHAGEAL FISTULA

Esophageal atresia with or without tracheoesophageal fistula is the most common serious congenital anomaly of the esophagus. Sulamaa and associates (1952) and Myers (1974) estimated its incidence at 1 in 3000 to 4500 births. Esophageal atresia may occur as an isolated anomaly, but more commonly is associated with esophago-respiratory fistula. The fistula usually arises from the distal trachea but may arise from a main stem bronchus. Kluth (1976) compiled an atlas of all reported variations of this anomaly. A reasonable approximation of the incidence of tracheoesophageal anomalies cited here are from a large collective series reported by Holder and colleagues (1964). Esophageal atresia with distal tracheoesophageal fistula is the most common variant—86.5% (Fig. 79–2A). Esophageal atresia without tracheoesophageal fistula—7.7% (Fig. 79–2B), tracheoesophageal fistula without esophageal atresia—4.2% (Fig. 79–2C), esophageal atresia with proximal tracheoesophageal fistula—0.8% (Fig. 79–2D), and esophageal atresia with both proximal and distal tracheoesophageal fistulae—0.7% (Fig. 79–2E) are less common variants. Approximately 50% of these infants had other associated congenital anomalies. These anomalies ranged from minor lesions to lesions incompatible with life. Associated anomalies are the major cause of death in children with esophageal atresia. The defects that pose the greatest threats to life are congenital heart disease and intestinal atresia.

Clinical Presentation

Infants with esophageal atresia and distal tracheo-esophageal fistula present at birth with excessive drooling. Feeding produces choking, coughing, and cyanosis because of aspiration. Aspiration of gastric contents into the lungs through the fistula may cause atelectasis and

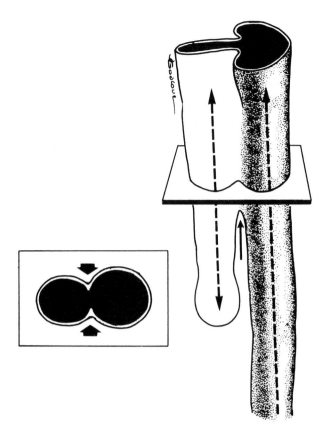

Fig. 79–1. Division of the primitive foregut, with stippled area showing the future esophageal portion. Arrows indicate the local morphogenic movements. (Reproduced with permission from Gray, S.W., and Skandalakis, J.E.: Embryology for Surgeons. Philadelphia, W.B. Saunders Co., 1972, p. 64.)

pneumonia. These complications can be prevented by maintaining a high degree of suspicion, early diagnosis, and prompt treatment.

Diagnosis

When esophageal atresia is suspected, a radio-opaque gastric tube should be passed, and the diagnosis confirmed by roentgenograms of the chest. If the tube passes into the stomach, no esophageal atresia exists, but the child may still have isolated tracheoesophageal fistula without atresia of the esophagus. In children with esophageal atresia, the proximal pouch usually ends blindly at the level of the first or second thoracic vertebra. The orogastric tube passes approximately 10 mm; because it may curl in the proximal pouch, roentgenographic evaluation is mandatory. Approximately 1 cc of dilute barium can be instilled through the orogastric tube to outline the proximal pouch if the diagnosis of esophageal atresia is in doubt (Fig. 79–3A). If a barium study is performed, the barium must be retrieved through the tube to avoid pulmonary aspiration of the barium. If barium appears in the trachea, it must be determined whether the barium was aspirated from above or entered through an associated proximal tracheoesophageal fistula or laryngeal cleft. We prefer to inject air instead of barium through the catheter into the proximal pouch. Air is safe

and outlines the pouch clearly, as seen in Fig. 79–3B. The disadvantage of air, compared to barium, is the possibility of missing an associated proximal tracheoesophageal fistula. We accept this risk, because the associated proximal tracheoesophageal fistula is infrequent, and when present is usually small and open only intermittently. Ensuring that a proximal tracheoesophageal fistula does not exist may therefore require a large volume of barium and considerable time. A policy of routinely searching for proximal fistulae during surgical dissection of the proximal pouch provides better protection against missing these variants.

The roentgenogram should be evaluated carefully for additional information. The status of the lungs, heart size, intestinal gas pattern, and associated vertebral anomalies should be determined. Esophageal atresia with a gasless abdominal pattern on the roentgenogram indicates esophageal atresia without tracheoesophageal fistula. If gas is seen in the intestine, tracheoesophageal fistula is present. Right-sided aortic arch occurs in 5% of children with esophageal atresia and must be specifically looked for on the child's roentgenogram. If the side of the aortic arch is difficult to determine on the existing film, high kV airway films, as Berdon and associates (1979) described, should be obtained to clarify this question (Fig. 79–4). As Harrison and co-workers (1977) reported, the presence of a right-sided aortic arch has major significance, as it necessitates repair through the left chest.

ESOPHAGEAL ATRESIA WITH DISTAL FISTULA

Initial Management

Once a diagnosis is made, the infant must be protected from aspiration. The proximal pouch is decompressed with a sump catheter. Replogle (1963) designed a sump catheter especially for this purpose (Fig. 79–5), which is effective and currently commercially available. The child is placed in the prone position or with the head elevated at 45° to minimize aspiration. Antibiotics are started and a rapid but complete evaluation of the child's status is carried out. Respiratory status is evaluated and associated congenital anomalies sought. The abdominal gas pattern should be assessed to rule out associated gut atresia. Rectal examination is performed to look for imperforate anus. Cardiac evaluation by echocardiography is indicated if clinical signs suggest the possibility of congenital heart disease. Following initial measures to prevent aspiration and full assessment, therapy is dictated by the child's status and associated anomalies.

Waterston and associates (1962) published a classification of infants with esophageal atresia with or without tracheoesophageal fistula depending upon the birth weight, associated anomalies, and the presence or absence of pneumonia (Table 79–1). The classification has been used extensively since it was first described and serves as an excellent framework by which to classify these infants and decide management. Healthy, full-term

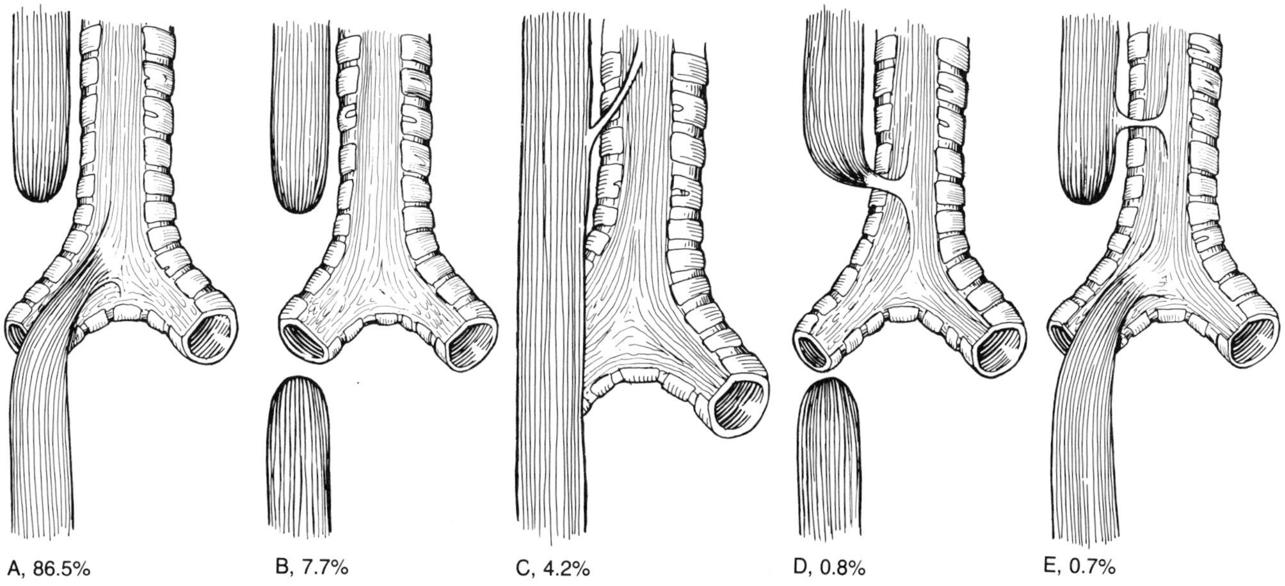

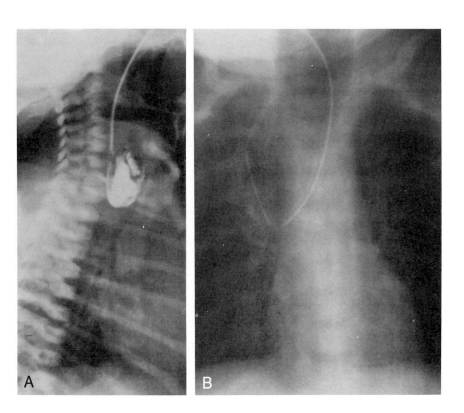

Fig. 79–2. *A*, Esophageal atresia with distal tracheoesophageal fistula. *B*, Esophageal atresia without tracheoesophageal fistula. *C*, Tracheoesophageal fistula without esophageal atresia. *D*, Esophageal atresia with proximal tracheoesophageal fistula. *E*, Esophageal atresia with both proximal and distal tracheoesophageal fistulae.

A, 86.5% B, 7.7% C, 4.2% D, 0.8% E, 0.7%

Fig. 79–3. *A*, Esophagogram of infant with esophageal atresia; barium outlines the proximal pouch. *B*, Roentgenogram of infant with esophageal atresia. Air distends and outlines the proximal pouch.

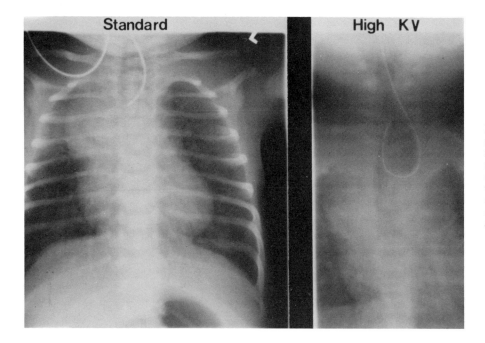

Fig. 79–4. Standard and high KV roentgenogram of infant with esophageal atresia. The high KV roentgenogram shows deviation of the trachea to the right, indicating a left aortic arch. (Reproduced with permission from McKneally, M.F., et al.: Surgical treatment of congenital esophageal atresia. Ann. Thorac. Surg. 38:606, 1984.)

Table 79–1. Waterston Risk Classification—Esophageal Atresia and Tracheoesophageal Fistula*

	Birth Weight	Associated Major Anomalies
Group A	>2500 g	none
Group B	1800–2500 g	none
Group C	<1800 g	present

*The presence of significant pneumonia moves the patient into the next greater risk group.

Reproduced with permission from Holder, T.M.: Esophageal atresia and tracheoesophageal fistula. *In* Pediatric Esophageal Surgery. Edited by K.W. Ashcraft and T.M. Holder. Orlando, FL, Grune and Stratton, 1986.

babies of normal birth weight with no other major anomalies and without pneumonia—Waterston A—are candidates for immediate repair. Children with pneumonia—Waterston B—as their only complicating factor are usually managed by delayed primary repair. Initially, proximal sump decompression, gastrostomy under local anesthesia—to prevent further gastric aspiration, appropriate antibiotics, and supportive measures are begun. Once the pneumonia has cleared, primary repair is carried out.

Infants with respiratory distress syndrome or severe pneumonia may require mechanical ventilatory support. Because poor pulmonary compliance requiring high pressure ventilation causes massive air leak across the fistual into the gut, mechanical ventilation may become impossible. Thoracotomy with division of the fistula is carried out following gastrostomy. No attempt at primary anastomosis is made at this time. The distal segment is tied at its origin from the trachea and divided flush with the trachea. The proximal tracheal end is closed with interrupted fine absorbable sutures. We prefer 5-0 Vicryl

suture for this closure. The distal segment is tacked to the spine to prevent retraction. Once the lungs have matured and the child has stabilized, gastrointestinal continuity is established by delayed primary esophageal repair.

Low birth weight infants with other severe congenital abnormalities—Waterston group C—are the most difficult to manage. The treatment must be individualized,

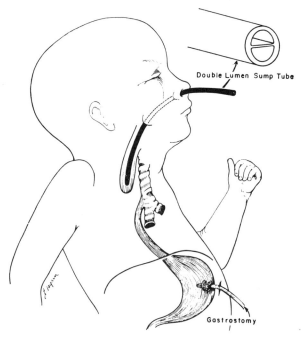

Fig. 79–5. Replogle double-lumen sump catheter designed to decompress the proximal pouch in infants with esophageal atresia. (Reproduced with permission from Replogle, R.L.: Esophageal atresia: plastic sump catheter for drainage of the proximal pouch. Surgery 54:296, 1963.)

and the most serious and life-threatening congenital anomaly dealt with first. Congenital cyanotic heart disease may require early surgical intervention in the neonatal period. Associated gut atresia must be assessed and either repaired at the time of gastrostomy or staged with the esophageal repair. Infants with gut anomalies preventing enteral nutrition should have a central line placed for intravenous alimentation. Severe associated anomalies requiring immediate treatment can be managed by proximal pouch decompression and gastrostomy. The cardiac anatomy should be defined early to allow shunting or ductus ligation at the time of thoracotomy for fistula division.

Operative Approach

The proximal esophageal pouch, which usually ends at the level of T1 to T2, becomes dilated and thickened from continual fetal swallowing against obstruction. If present, the distal fistula usually arises just above the carina on the membranous portion of the trachea, but may arise from any point on the trachea or from a main stem bronchus. The distal esophageal segment has much thinner walls and smaller diameter than the proximal pouch. Its blood supply is segmental, arising from the aorta. The length of the gap between the proximal and distal pouches varies, depending on the length of the proximal pouch and the site of origin of the distal segment from the airway. There may be no appreciable gap between the ends or there may be muscular continuity of the esophageal wall despite luminal discontinuity (Fig. 79–6). Commonly, the gap is about 1 to 2 cm, but it may be substantially longer.

Successful repair of esophageal atresia with tracheoesophageal fistula is gratifying. Reconstruction may be fairly straightforward or technically difficult because of a

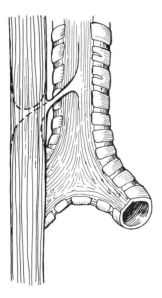

Fig. 79–6. Esophageal atresia with distal tracheoesophageal fistula. Muscular continuity of the proximal and distal esophageal pouches obscures the pathology. The proximal mucosal pouch ends blindly within the muscular wall. The tracheoesophageal fistula arises from the distal pouch.

long distance between the proximal and distal segments. Expert pediatric anesthesia is essential to facilitate the operative management of these infants.

We prefer to perform gastrostomy during the initial operative management of esophageal atresia with tracheoesophageal fistula. It provides immediate decompression, allows alimentation by drip feeding from the first postoperative day, and is associated with little morbidity. The gastrostomy can be performed under local anesthesia before intubation or under general anesthesia. Some authors manage patients routinely without gastrostomy, as Bishop (1985) and Yeh (1986) and their colleagues described.

The thoracotomy is performed on the side opposite the aortic arch. The approach may be transpleural or extrapleural. The extrapleural approach is slightly more tedious, but adds a measure of protection in the event of anastomotic leak. Leakage is confined by the pleura, does not produce empyema, and heals rapidly. Anastomotic leak with intrapleural repair is more dangerous, leads to empyema, and may cause prolonged drainage and sepsis.

A fourth interspace thoracotomy is carried down to the level of the pleura, which is then reflected medially using a moist sponge. The vagus nerve runs along the mediastinum onto the distal esophageal segment and serves as a good landmark. The tracheoesophageal fistula is identified and may be immediately occluded by pressure with a Kitner cotton dissector. It is divided nearly flush with the trachea and the tracheal side closed with interrupted fine absorbable suture. We prefer 5-0 Vicryl. Excessive mobilization of the distal esophageal segment is avoided to prevent devascularization, as the blood supply of the distal segment is segmental. Identification of the proximal pouch is facilitated by downward pressure on the nasogastric tube by the anesthesiologist and a traction suture is placed in its distal tip. The proximal pouch is mobilized, with a careful search on the tracheal side for another tracheoesophageal fistula. Dudgeon and associates (1972) reported that the proximal fistula is more common than previously thought, and may arise high. The proximal pouch should be mobilized as far up into the neck as possible (Fig. 79–7). If a proximal fistula is found, it is divided and closed.

Following mobilization of the proximal pouch, the esophageal ends are brought together for anastomosis. The two esophageal ends usually differ in size and thickness. The proximal pouch is large and thick; the distal esophagus is thin and is narrow at its tracheal insertion. This tissue should not be dilated, but excised back several millimeters to a point where healthy esophageal mucosa is encountered. The distal segment is incised longitudinally for a short distance to decrease luminal discrepancy between the two segments. The tip of the proximal pouch is excised.

Following mobilization of the proximal pouch and preparation of the distal pouch, a large gap between the two esophageal ends may remain. Livaditis and colleagues (1972) and de Lorimier and Harrison (1980) described that single or multiple myotomies (Fig. 79–8)

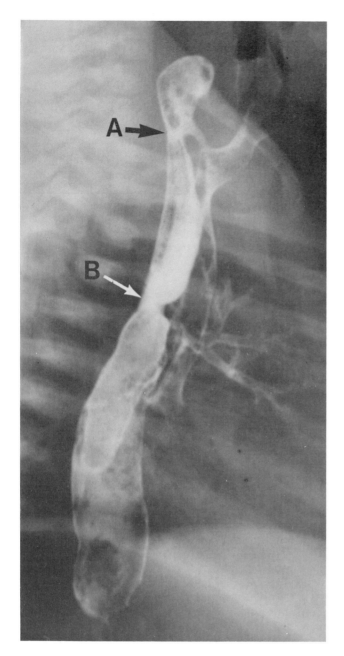

Fig. 79–7. This esophagogram illustrates a high proximal fistula (A) which was missed at previous repair of esophageal atresia with distal tracheoesophageal fistula (B).

down to submucosa can be carried out on the proximal pouch to increase the length of the proximal pouch and reduce tension on the anastomosis. Each myotomy lengthens the proximal pouch by approximately 8 to 10 mm. We have found Kimura and co-workers' (1987) technique of spiral myotomy (Fig. 79–9) to be an excellent means of increasing length. Distention of the proximal pouch with a Foley catheter passed through the mouth into the pouch by the anesthesiologist aids in the myotomy.

The anastomosis is carried out in a single-layer or two-layer technique. The original technique Haight (1957)

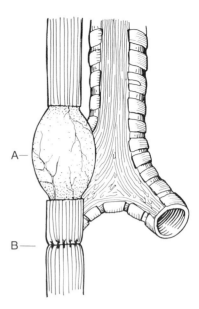

Fig. 79–8. Esophageal myotomy (A) performed to increase the length of the proximal pouch to relieve tension on esophageal anastomosis (B).

described is a two-layer telescoping anastomosis (Fig. 79–10). In the Haight technique, the mucosa of the proximal pouch is anastomosed to the full thickness of the distal segment. The muscularis of the proximal pouch is then brought down over the first suture line and secured by a second row of sutures. We prefer a single layer of fine interrupted sutures, full thickness on both the upper and lower segments. Manning and associates (1986) reported that this single-layer technique is faster and easier than the Haight technique. There is a slightly higher risk of anastomotic leak, but a lower incidence of stricture formation than with the two-layer anastomosis. We use

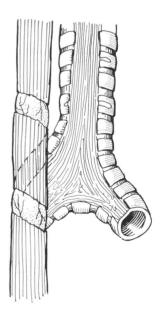

Fig. 79–9. Spiral myotomy is an excellent technique for increasing the length of the proximal pouch to avoid excessive anastomotic tension.

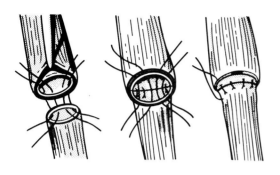
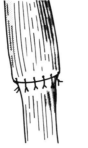
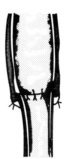

Fig. 79-10. Haight anastomosis. The mucosa of the proximal pouch is anastomosed to the full thickness of the distal segment. The muscularis of the proximal pouch is then brought down over the suture line and secured by a second row of sutures. (Adapted from Beal, J.M., Holman, C.W., and Haight, C.: Congenital atresia of the esophagus with tracheoesophageal fistula. *In* John L. Madden's Atlas of Technics in Surgery, 2nd edition, Vol. 2. East Norwalk, CT, Appleton-Century-Crofts, 1964.)

absorbable oiled 5-0 Vicryl sutures for this anastomosis, as we believe nonabsorbable sutures may play a role in the recurrence of tracheoesophageal fistula following initial repair. Kafrouni (1970) and Manning (1986) and their colleagues reported that the incidence of recurrence following initial repair is between 5% and 11%. Following completion of the anastomosis, a nasogastric tube is passed across the anastomosis and distally into the stomach. Surrounding tissue or pleura is interposed between the two suture lines to decrease the chance of refistulization. A chest drain is placed near the anastomosis and left until the integrity of the anastomosis is proven by the postoperative barium swallow.

Postoperative Care

Postoperatively the endotracheal tube is usually removed when the child returns to the neonatal intensive care unit. Intravenous fluids are maintained and antibiotics are continued. Gastrostomy feeding is started on the first or second postoperative day and is increased as tolerated. Unless complications arise, we perform a barium swallow at 7 days postoperatively to assess the anastomosis and the motility of the esophagus and to detect gastroesophageal reflux (Fig. 79-11). If the barium swallow shows no leakage, oral feeding is begun and advanced. Elevation of the head of the bed is continued in babies with roentgenographically demonstrated reflux, which occurs in approximately half of those tested. The gastrostomy feeding is decreased proportionately and discontinued when full oral intake has been achieved.

The gastrostomy tube may be removed before discharge or left in place until the first postoperative visit. If anastomotic narrowing is a concern, the tube may be left in place while reassessment, endoscopy, and dilation are performed.

ESOPHAGEAL ATRESIA WITHOUT TRACHEOESOPHAGEAL FISTULA

Isolated esophageal atresia causes polyhydraminos because the fetus cannot swallow and absorb the amniotic fluid. The clinical presentation at birth resembles atresia associated with tracheoesophageal fistula, with excessive drooling and coughing, choking, and cyanosis after feeding. The abdomen, however, is usually scaphoid and the roentgenogram reveals no gas in the abdomen. These infants are at risk for aspiration of saliva or feedings. They cannot aspirate gastric acid, as no fistula exists. The surgeon must be alert to the possibility of a proximal tracheoesophageal fistula in these infants. The proximal fistula usually arises 1 to 2 cm from the tip of the proximal pouch but may arise much higher, just below the cricopharyngeus (Fig. 79-7).

In esophageal atresia without tracheoesophageal fistula, the distal pouch is thin-walled and small, and frequently extends only a short distance—1 to 2 cm—above the diaphragm. The long gap between the two ends of the esophagus makes primary anastomosis difficult. Howard and Myers (1965), Lafer and Boley (1966), Hendren and Hale (1975), and de Lorimier and Harrison (1980) described techniques for stretching the proximal and distal pouches. Pouch stretching can be carried out by conventional bougienage or by electromagnetic bougienage, which Hendren and Hale described in 1975. The dilatation is carried out over a period of time, up to 2 months. This delay allows for growth in the child, which may well be the most significant factor in elongation of the pouches. During the period of pouch dilatation, the

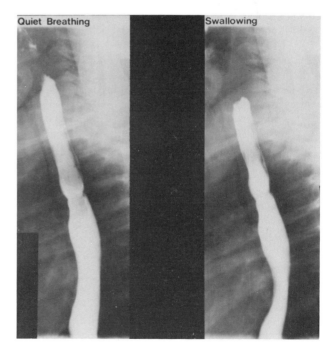

Fig. 79-11. Esophagogram performed at 7 days following repair of esophageal atresia and distal tracheoesophageal fistula. Failure of barium clearance with swallowing indicates poor esophageal motility.

proximal pouch is kept decompressed and the baby is fed through a gastrostomy.

Operative Approach

At the time of thoracotomy for repair, the proximal and distal pouches are extensively mobilized, and myotomy is performed on the distal as well as the proximal pouches. To maximize mobilization, Holder (1986) suggested a second cervical incision to allow better access for cervical esophageal mobilization and proximal pouch myotomy. With the combination of pouch dilatation and multiple myotomies, the esophageal ends can usually be brought together. These anastomoses are often performed under considerable tension, and therefore the risk of anastomotic leak and stricture is increased.

In children in whom the esophageal ends cannot be brought together, the proximal pouch is brought out as an end cervical esophagostomy and the distal segment resected and oversewn. The children are maintained on gastrostomy feeding until colon interposition is carried out to establish gastrointestinal continuity. Although immediate replacement of the esophagus has been advocated, we prefer a staged approach, interposing the colon after a period of growth. The patient should be allowed to taste food when gastrostomy feedings are given to preserve an interest in eating by mouth. The techniques of esophageal replacement with the colon are discussed in Chapter 40 and with various gastric tubes in Chapter 39.

TRACHEOESOPHAGEAL FISTULA WITHOUT ESOPHAGEAL ATRESIA

Haight (1957), and Waterston (1962) and Kappelman (1969) and their associates reported tracheoesophageal fistula without esophageal atresia in 1.8 to 4% of children with congenital tracheoesophageal fistula. These children are more likely to have normal birth weight. The fistula is usually high, occurring at or above the second thoracic vertebra. Holder and colleagues (1964) reported a 27% incidence of associated congenital anomalies, much lower than the 50% incidence found in infants with both tracheoesophageal fistula and esophageal atresia.

This type of tracheoesophageal fistula has been called the H-type TEF, but the tracheal end of this anomaly is always higher than the esophageal end, more closely resembling the letter N than the letter H (Fig. 79–2C). This offset keeps the fistula closed most of the time. As a result, patients with isolated tracheoesophageal fistula are usually discovered at an older age than patients with esophageal atresia. The symptoms are present from birth but tend to be more subtle. Holman and associates (1986) reported that the diagnosis may not be made for several months or even many years. These authors discovered an isolated congenital tracheoesophageal fistula in a 52-year-old adult. Typically, however, the infant has paroxysms of severe choking and coughing brought on by feeding. Recurrent pneumonia is common. Liquids tend to cause more trouble than solids. Abdominal distension and excessive flatus is caused by passage of air across the fistula into the gut.

Demonstration of an isolated tracheoesophageal fistula may be difficult; if it is suspected, the child should undergo a barium swallow with cinefluoroscopy in the prone position by an expert pediatric radiologist. These fistulae tend to open intermittently. The cinefluoroscope is positioned to image the fistula in the lateral position. If barium swallow does not reveal the fistula, esophagoscopy is carried out under general anesthesia and positive pressure ventilation. Careful examination of the proximal esophagus under saline irrigation may reveal air passing through the fistula into the esophagus. The membranous trachea should be inspected carefully using the rigid ventilating bronchoscope. Once the fistula is found, Holder (1986) recommends passing a catheter through it at the time of bronchoscopy. The catheter is brought back out through the mouth and left in position to aid in identifying the fistula at the time of surgical exploration.

Operative Approach

Blank and colleagues (1967) found, in a review of patients with isolated tracheoesophageal fistulas, that the fistula arises at or above the level of T2 in 70% of cases. The operative approach is through a right transverse cervical incision. The fistula is found by retracting the esophagus laterally. A large suction catheter in the esophagus facilitates this dissection. Care must be taken to avoid damage to the recurrent laryngeal nerve. The fistula is divided and oversewn with absorbable sutures, then the strap muscles are interposed to reduce the risk of recurrence. Isolated tracheoesophageal fistulae occurring below T2 are best approached transthoracically on the side opposite the aortic arch.

RESULTS OF TREATMENT

Manning and associates (1986) reported 50 years of experience with the management of esophageal atresia and tracheoesophageal fistula from the University of Michigan. This series of 426 children with this anomaly includes Haight's (1957) first recorded successful repair. The incidence of new cases and the number of associated anomalies remained constant over this period. The long-term survival improved from 36% before 1950 to 84% during the 1970s and 1980s. In the last nine year of their review, they reported no postoperative deaths in the Waterston group A or group B infants. In Waterston group C infants the postoperative mortality rate was 18.2% over the same time period, and almost all of these deaths resulted from associated anomalies. Louhimo and Lindahl (1983) reported similar excellent results in 500 consecutively treated infants with esophageal atresia with or without tracheoesophageal fistula from 1947 to 1978 at the University of Helsinki in Finland.

We have treated 103 infants at the Albany Medical Center with esophageal atresia. Since 1970 the survival has improved to 85% overall survival with no deaths in the Waterston group A or group B children. There have

Table 79–2.   Esophageal Atresia and Tracheoesophageal Fistula Results of Treatment Related to Waterston Risk Groups Albany Medical Center Hospital

	Group A	Group B	Group C
1951–1987 Total: 103 patients treated			
Total	57	18	28
No. of survivors	54	11	6
% survivors	94	61	21
Overall survival 1951–1987: 71/103 (69%)			
1970–1987 Total: 49 patients treated			
Total	31	6	12
No. of survivors	31	6	5
% survivors	100	100	42
Overall survival 1970–1987: 42/29 (85%)			

*There have been no deaths since 1982 in any patients with esophageal atresia with or without tracheoesophageal fistula.

been no deaths in any Waterston group in the past 5 years (Table 79–2).

ESOPHAGEAL MOTILITY AFTER SUCCESSFUL REPAIR

Haight (1957) noted abnormal esophageal motility by fluoroscopy in the lower segment of the esophagus following primary repair of esophageal atresia. Nakazato and associates (1986), by microdissection and point-count morphometric studies, demonstrated abnormal Auerbach plexes in the distal esophagus and to a lesser extent in the proximal esophagus in patients with esophageal atresia and tracheoesophageal fistula.

Kirkpatrick (1961) and Desjardins (1964) and their colleagues reported cinefluoroscopic evidence of disordered motor activity of the esophagus in infants with tracheoesophageal fistula. Typically, no coordinated esophageal stripping wave occurs. This disordered activity can be present throughout the entire esophagus or, more commonly, confined to the distal segment below the anastomosis. Manometric studies in children and young adults following repair of esophageal atresia and tracheoesophageal fistula have yielded conflicting results. Lind and co-workers (1966) reported failure of relaxation of the lower esophageal sphincter with swallowing, and motor activity indistinguishable from achalasia. Studies by Burgess (1968) and Orringer (1977) and their associates failed to substantiate these findings. They found normal function of the lower esophageal sphincter in response to swallowing, and an aperistaltic segment extending both proximally and distally to the anastomosis. Burgess and colleagues (1968) found normal resting lower esophageal sphincter tone in all patients. Orringer and associates (1977), on the other hand, demonstrated lack of a distal high pressure zone in five—23%—of 22 patients studied. In every patient with a demonstrable lower esophageal high pressure zone, they found normal relaxation with swallowing. Disordered motor activity was found in 21—95%—of 22 children and young adults with esophageal atresia. Fifty-nine percent were found to

have moderate to severe gastroesophageal reflux demonstrated by pH reflux testing. Roentgenographic evidence of gastroesophageal reflux was documented in only 2 of the 22 patients. This surprisingly low incidence of roentgenographically proven reflux is probably related to the fact that barium studies carried out as part of a routine follow-up program did not focus specifically on the question of reflux. Since 1974, 29 patients treated at Albany Medical Center for esophageal atresia and tracheoesophageal fistula have been carefully studied roentgenographically in the early postoperative period for the presence or absence of gastroesophageal reflux. Reflux was noted in 48%. These results indicate that postoperative gastroesophageal reflux can often be detected by careful roentgenographic studies carried out during the first few weeks of life. Severe gastroesophageal reflux in conjunction with impaired acid clearance in these children exposes the esophageal mucosa to the damaging effects of gastric acid for prolonged periods.

Strictures (Fig. 79–12A) were found by follow-up esophagograms in 24 of 103 patients operated upon at Albany Medical Center Hospital. Fifteen—62%—of these strictures required dilatation (Fig. 79–12B) and five—20%—required surgical revision of the anastomosis. Of the 24 strictures, five had anastomotic leak, and tension was considered excessive in three. In the last six

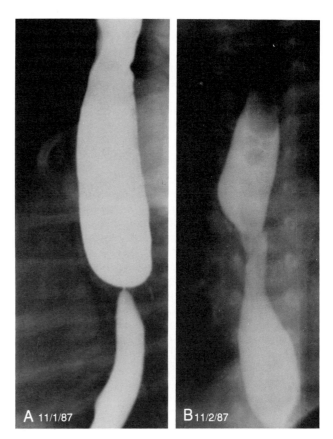

Fig. 79–12. A, Esophagogram at 6 weeks following repair of esophageal atresia with distal tracheoesophageal fistula. A tight stricture is seen at the anastomosis. B, Esophagogram taken 24 hours following dilatation.

cases of anastomotic stricture, four had significant reflux demonstrated by esophagogram. Of 24 patients with reflux, strictures developed in nine—37%. Although tension, leakage, and tissue handling are potentially culpable in the formation of strictures, acid reflux is clearly a contributing factor in the development of esophageal strictures. Pieretti (1974) and Randolph (1974, 1983) and their colleagues, as well as Fonkalsrud (1979), have urged that antireflux procedures be performed to interrupt the pattern of recurrence of anastomotic strictures associated with primary reconstruction in esophageal atresia. The early prophylactic application of fundoplication for the prevention of anastomotic strictures and pulmonary complications of reflux might be appropriate if the subset of patients at high risk for development of these complications could be identified accurately. Unfortunately, the initial roentgenographic findings at birth do not provide guidelines for incorporating fundoplication into the treatment plan at the time of initial gastrostomy. It seems rational to attempt to identify those infants with significant gastroesophageal reflux early in the postoperative period and to treat the reflux aggressively to prevent anastomotic and pulmonary complications.

CONGENITAL ESOPHAGEAL STENOSIS

Although the most common cause of esophageal narrowing or stricture in children is secondary to reflux esophagitis, congenital esophageal stenosis does occur, and three types have been described: (1) esophageal web; (2) intraluminal rests of cartilaginous tracheobronchial tissue; and (3) segmental hypertrophy of the muscularis and submucosa of the esophageal wall. Infants presenting with symptoms suggestive of esophageal stenosis should undergo barium swallow and esophagoscopy; pH monitoring should be carried out to evaluate the role of gastroesophageal reflux in the stenosis.

Esophageal Web

Esophageal webs most commonly occur in the middle third of the esophagus. They are similar to other mucosal diaphragms seen throughout the gastrointestinal tract. Symptoms and presentation of esophageal web depend upon whether the web is complete or incomplete. Complete webs cause signs at birth similar to esophageal atresia: excessive salivation and coughing and choking spells associated with attempts to feed. Incomplete webs present later with regurgitation and dysphagia when solid foods are introduced. On barium swallow the esophageal web presents a sharp shelf at the point of obstruction. Esophageal dilatation is the best method of treating esophageal webs. Repeated dilatation may be necessary to achieve long-term relief. Huchzermeyer and associates (1979) reported the use of cautery ablation accompanied by esophageal dilatation for the treatment of such esophageal webs. Experience with laser vaporization is too preliminary to assess, but seem rational.

Esophageal Stenosis

Esophageal stenosis secondary to tracheobronchial remnants becomes symptomatic when solid foods are started in the first year of life but may be recognized considerably later. Scherer and Grosfeld (1986) reviewed the reported series of esophageal stenosis secondary to tracheobronchial remnants. The condition affected both sexes equally. Predominant symptoms were dysphagia, vomiting or regurgitation of undigested food, failure to thrive, and recurrent aspiration pneumonia. Nishina and colleagues (1981) reviewed 81 cases of esophageal stenosis secondary to tracheobronchial remnants in Japan; 17.3% of patients had associated anomalies. Esophageal atresia was the most frequent, followed by anorectal anomalies. Cardiovascular anomalies were uncommon. The tracheobronchial remnant has the appearance of an esophageal stricture with proximal esophageal dilatation. Esophageal stenosis secondary to cartilaginous tracheobronchial remnant generally requires local esophageal resection and primary anastomosis.

Segmental Hypertrophy

Segmental hypertrophy of the esophagus contains only mucosal or submucosal elements. The cause of this anomaly is unknown but is thought to be related to a remnant of a perforated esophageal web.

CONGENITAL LARYNGOTRACHEOESOPHAGEAL CLEFT

Laryngotracheoesophageal clefts are rare congenital malformations that result from the failure of fusion of the two lateral primordia of the cricoid cartilage and the rostral advancement of the tracheoesophageal septum. Roth (1983) and Hof (1987) and their associates reported a 50% incidence of other associated congenital anomalies. The most common of these anomalies is esophageal atresia with tracheoesophageal fistula.

Laryngotracheoesophageal cleft was first described by Richter in 1792. Pettersson (1955) performed the first successful repair of this defect, and he (1969) classified laryngotracheal clefts into three types, depending upon the severity of the lesion (Fig. 79–13). Type I—the cleft extends from the arytenoid notch down to the lower part of the cricoid cartilage; i.e., only the cricoid cartilage is split. Type II—the cleft extends farther down and involves several tracheal cartilages. Type III—the cleft extends throughout the entire trachea to the carina. This defect has also been called persistent esophagotrachea by Zachary and Emery (1961) and Griscom (1966). Roth and colleagues (1983) reported a collective review of 82 cases from the world literature. Table 79–3 summarizes the presenting symptoms. Aspiration and cyanosis after feeding was found in more than 50% of the cases reviewed. According to Roth and colleagues (1983), the combination of a low soundless cry, stridor, and increased production of saliva should lead to the diagnosis of laryngeal cleft. Pneumonia is commonly seen on the chest roentgenogram. An orogastric tube may appear shifted forward on the lateral roentgenogram. Similarly, an oral endotracheal tube appears shifted posteriorly through the cleft into the esophagus.

Barium swallow with cinefluoroscopy reveals massive

I   II   III

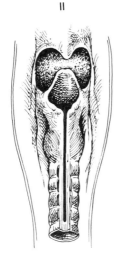

UVULA
TONGUE
EPIGLOTTIS
EPIGLOTTIC
FOLDS
CRICOID
LAMINA
CLEFT
TRACHEA
PARS
MEMBRANACEA

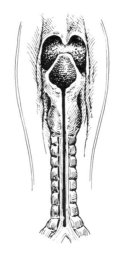

Fig. 79–13. Congenital laryngotracheo-esophageal clefts.

Table 79–3. Incidence of Leading Symptoms of Laryngotracheoesophageal Cleft in Newborn and Young Infants

Symptoms	Incidence
Aspiration and cyanosis after feeding	53%
Postpartum asphyxia	33%
Increased production of mucus	23%
Recurrent pneumonia	16%
Voiceless crying	16%
Stridor	10%
Impaired swallowing	5%

Reproduced with permission from Roth, B., et al.: Laryngo-tracheo-oesophageal cleft: clinical features, diagnosis, and therapy. Eur. J. Pediatr. 140:41, 1983.

aspiration of contrast material into the tracheobronchial tree. If laryngeal cleft is suspected, a contrast agent suitable for bronchography such as Lipiodol should be used. Differentiation between a high tracheoesophageal fistula or pharyngeal incoordination leading to aspiration may be difficult, as Delahunty and Cherry (1969) noted.

Endoscopy is the most important diagnostic measure. The cleft may not be seen during inspiration because of overlying mucosa. The probe Berkovits and associates (1974) described is useful for diagnosing and measuring the length of the esophageal cleft (Fig. 79–14). The most common operative technique for repair consists of exposure of the cleft through a lateral pharyngoesopha-

gotomy and repair with two flaps. The cumulative mortality rate among the series reported by Roth in 1983 was 39 of 85—46%. Twenty-four patients died before diagnosis was made. Ninety-two percent of the 14 patients with type III defects died, as did 41% of the 31 patients with type II defect, and 43% of the patients with type I defect. Forty-eight patients underwent repair of the defect. Thirteen—27%—of these patients died.

Hof and colleagues (1987) reported a series of 17 patients with laryngotracheoesophageal cleft. Only one patient in this series—6%—died. This one death occurred in a patient with a type III defect. Hof found gastroesophageal reflux in four cases following repair of the laryngotracheoesophageal cleft. In three of these cases the gastroesophageal reflux was believed to be responsible for breakdown of the surgical repair. The fourth patient had recurrent aspiration that disappeared after fundoplication. Hof and his colleagues concluded that all patients with laryngotracheoesophageal cleft should be evaluated preoperatively for gastroesophageal reflux and treated by fundoplication and gastrostomy before laryngotracheal surgery if gastroesophageal reflux is found.

SUMMARY

Surgical treatment of esophageal anomalies has become safe and effective in most cases. The advances in neonatal intensive care, improvements in suture material and magnification, and the innovative contributions of

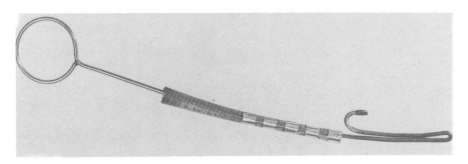

Fig. 79–14. Probe used to measure laryngotracheoesophageal clefts. (Reproduced with permission from Berkovits, R.N.P., Bax, N.M.A., and van der Schans, E.J.: Surgical treatment of congenital laryngotracheo-oesophageal cleft. Prog. Pediatr. Surg. 21:36, 1987.)

the many surgeons have brought the results of treatment to a gratifyingly high level of reliability. It does not restore a normal esophagus, but provides a reasonably functional conduit. The problem of reflux must be treated vigilantly in the preoperative period and should be carefully assessed and appropriately treated after repair as well.

REFERENCES

Berdon, W.E., et al.: Plain film detection of right aortic arch in infants with esophageal atresia and tracheoesophageal fistula. J. Pediatr. Surg. 14:436, 1979.

Berkovits, R.N.P., et al.: Congenital laryngotracheoesophageal cleft. Arch. Otolaryngol. 100:442, 1974.

Berkovits, R.N.P, Bax, N.M.A., and van der Schans, E.J.: Surgical treatment of congenital laryngotracheo-oesophageal cleft. Prog. Pediatr. Surg. 21:36, 1987.

Bishop, P.J., et al.: Transpleural repair of esophageal atresia without a primary gastrostomy: 240 patients treated between 1951 and 1983. J. Pediatr. Surg. 20:823, 1985.

Blank, R.H., Connar, R.G., and Carlton, L.M., Jr.: Problems encountered in the management of congenital esophageal anomalies. South. Med. J. 60:1180, 1967.

Burgess, J.N., Carlson, H.C., and Ellis, F.H., Jr.: Esophageal function after successful repair of esophageal atresia and tracheoesophageal fistula: a manometric and cinefluorographic study. J. Thorac. Cardiovasc. Surg. 56:667, 1968.

Delahunty, J.E., and Cherry, J.: Congenital laryngeal cleft. Ann. Otol. Rhinol. Laryngol. 78:96, 1969.

de Lorimier, A.A., and Harrison, M.R.: Long gap esophageal atresia: primary anastomosis after esophageal elongation by bougienage and esophagomyotomy. J. Thorac. Cardiovasc. Surg. 79:138, 1980.

Desjardins, J.G., Stephens, C.A., and Moes, C.A.F.: Results of surgical treatment of congenital tracheoesophageal fistula, with a note on cinefluorographic findings. Ann. Surg. 160:141, 1964.

Dudgeon, D.L., Morrison, C.W., and Woolley, M.M.: Congenital proximal tracheoesophageal fistula. J. Pediatr. Surg. 7:614, 1972.

Fonkalsrud, E.W.: Gastroesophageal fundoplication for reflux following repair of esophageal atresia: experience with nine patients. Arch. Surg. 114:48, 1979.

Gray, S.W., and Skandalakis, J.E.: Embryology for Surgeons: The Embryological Basis for the Treatment of Congenital Defects. Philadelphia, W.B. Saunders Co., 1972.

Griscom, N.T.: Persistant esophagotrachea: the most severe degree of laryngotracheo-esophageal cleft. Am. J. Roentgenol. Radium Ther. Nucl. Med. 97:211, 1966.

Haight, C.: Some observations on esophageal atresias and tracheoesophageal fistulas of congenital origin. J. Thorac. Surg. 34:141, 1957.

Harrison, M.R., et al.: The significance of right aortic arch in repair of esophageal atresia and tracheoesophageal fistula. J. Pediatr. Surg. 12:861, 1977.

Hendren, W.H., and Hale, J.R.: Electromagnetic bougienage to lengthen esophageal segments in congenital esophageal atresia. N. Engl. J. Med. 293:428, 1975.

Hof, E., et al.: Deleterious consequences of gastroesophageal reflux in cleft larynx surgery. J. Pediatr. Surg. 22:197, 1987.

Holder, T.M.: Esophageal atresia and tracheoesophageal fistula. In Ashcraft, K.W., and Holder, T.M. (Eds.): Pediatric Esophageal Surgery. Orlando, FL, Grune & Stratton, Inc., 1986, p. 29.

Holder, T.M., et al.: Esophageal atresia and tracheoesophageal fistula: a survey of its members by the surgical section of the American Academy of Pediatrics. Pediatrics 34:542, 1964.

Holman, W.L., et al.: Surgical treatment of H-type tracheoesophageal fistula diagnosed in an adult. Ann. Thorac. Surg. 41:453, 1986.

Howard, R., and Myers, N.A.: Esophageal atresia: a technique for elongating the upper pouch. Surgery 58:725, 1965.

Huchzermeyer, H., Burdelski, M., and Hruby, M.: Endoscopic therapy of a congenital esophageal stricture. Endoscopy 4:259, 1979.

Kafrouni, G., Baick, C.H., and Woolley, M.M.: Recurrent tracheoesophageal fistula: a diagnostic problem. Surgery 68:889, 1970.

Kappelman, M.M., et al.: H-type tracheoesophageal fistula: diagnostic and operative management. Am. J. Dis. Child. 118:568, 1969.

Kimura, K., et al.: A new approach for the salvage of unsuccessful esophageal atresia repair: a spiral myotomy and delayed definitive operation. J. Pediatr. Surg. 22:981, 1987.

Kirkpatrick, J.A., Cresson, S.L., and Pilling, G.P., IV: The motor activity of the esophagus in association with esophageal atresia and tracheoesophageal fistula. Am. J. Roentgenol. Radium Ther. Nucl. Med. 86:884, 1961.

Kluth, D.: Atlas of esophageal atresia. J. Pediatr. Surg. 11:901, 1976.

Lafer, D.J., and Boley, S.J.: Primary repair in esophageal atresia with elongation of the lower segment. J. Pediatr. Surg. 1:585, 1966.

Lind, J.F., Blanchard, R.J., and Guyda, H.: Esophageal motility in tracheoesophageal fistula and esophageal atresia. Surg. Gynecol. Obstet. 123:557, 1966.

Livaditis, A., Radberg, L., and Odensjo, G.: Esophageal end-to-end anastomosis: reduction of anastomotic tension by circular myotomy. Scand. J. Thorac. Cardiovasc. Surg. 6:206, 1972.

Louhimo, I., and Lindahl, H.: Esophageal atresia: primary results of 500 consecutively treated patients. J. Pediatr. Surg. 18:217, 1983.

Manning, P.B., et al.: Fifty years' experience with esophageal atresia and tracheoesophageal fistula beginning with Cameron Haight's first operation in 1935. Ann. Surg. 204:446, 1986.

Myers, N.A.: Oesophageal atresia: the epitome of modern surgery. Ann. R. Coll. Surg. Engl. 54:277, 1974.

Nakazato, Y., Landing, B.H., and Wells, T.R.: Abnormal Auerbach plexus in the esophagus and stomach of patients with esophageal atresia and tracheoesophageal fistula. J. Pediatr. Surg. 21:831, 1986.

Nishina, T., Tsuchida, Y., and Saito, S.: Congenital esophageal stenosis due to tracheobronchial remnants and its associated anomalies. J. Pediatr. Surg. 16:190, 1981.

Orringer, M.B., Kirsh, M.M., and Sloan, H.: Long-term esophageal function following repair of esophageal atresia. Ann. Surg. 186:436, 1977.

Pettersson, G.: Inhibited separation of larynx and the upper part of trachea from oesophagus in a newborn: report of a case successfully operated upon. Acta Chir. Scand. 110:250, 1955.

Pettersson, G.: Laryngo-tracheo-oesophageal cleft. Z. Kinderchir. 7:43, 1969.

Pieretti, R., Shandling, B., and Stephens, C.A.: Resistant esophageal stenosis associated with reflux after repair of esophageal atresia: a therapeutic approach. J. Pediatr. Surg. 9:355, 1974.

Randolph, J.: Experience with the Nissen fundoplication for correction of gastroesophageal reflux in infants. Ann. Surg. 198:579, 1983.

Randolph, J.G., Lily, J.R., and Anderson, K.D.: Surgical treatment of gastroesophageal reflux in infants. Ann. Surg. 180:479, 1974.

Replogle, R.L.: Esophageal atresia: plastic sump catheter for drainage of the proximal pouch. Surgery 54:296, 1963.

Richter, C.F.: Dissertatio medico de infanticido in artis obstetriciae. (Thesis). Leipzig, 1792.

Rosenthal, A.H.: Congenital atresia of the esophagus with tracheoesophageal fistula: report of eight cases. Arch. Pathol. 12:756, 1931.

Roth, B., et al.: Laryngo-tracheo-oesophageal cleft: clinical features, diagnosis and therapy. Eur. J. Pediatr. 140:41, 1983.

Scherer, L.R., and Grosfeld, J.L.: Congenital esophageal stenosis, esophageal duplication, neurenteric cyst and esophageal diverticulum. In Pediatric Esophageal Surgery. Edited by K.W. Ashcraft and T.M. Holder. Orlando, FL, Grune & Stratton, Inc., 1986, p. 53.

Sulamaa, M., Gripenberg, L., and Ahvenainen, E.K.: Prognosis and treatment of congenital atresia of the esophagus. Acta Chir. Scand. 102:141, 1952.

Waterston, D.J., Carter, R.E.B., and Aberdeen, E.: Oesophageal atresia: tracheo-oesophageal fistula: a study of survival in 218 infants. Lancet 1:819, 1962.

Yeh, M.-L., et al.: Treatment of esophageal atresia with distal tracheoesophageal fistula: are gastrostomy and prophylactic esophageal dilatation necessary? Int. Surg. 71:169, 1986.

Zachary, R.B., and Emery, J.L.: Failure of separation of larynx and trachea from the esophagus: persistent esophagotrachea. Surgery 49:525, 1961.

READING REFERENCES

Holder, T.M., and Ashcraft, K.W.: Esophageal atresia and tracheo-esophageal fistula. Curr. Probl. Surg. *6*:1, 1966.

Ladd, W.E.: The surgical treatment of esophageal atresia and tracheoesophageal fistula. N. Engl. J. Med. *230*:625, 1944.

Lanman, T.H.: Congenital atresia of the esophagus: a study of thirty-two cases. Arch. Surg. *41*:1060, 1940.

Leven, N.L.: Congenital atresia of the esophagus with tracheoesophageal fistula: report of successful extrapleural ligation of fistulous communication and cervical esophagostomy. J. Thorac. Surg. *10*:648, 1941.

CHAPTER 80

MOTOR DISTURBANCES OF DEGLUTITION

Earle W. Wilkins, Jr.

Advancements toward understanding the physiology of motor dysfunction of the esophagus, including its upper and lower sphincters, are less than 100 years old. Standard modalities for study of the esophagus have been roentgenographic observation by the barium esophagogram, esophagoscopy by open rigid and fiber-optic techniques, and esophageal manometry. Manometric observation has been uniquely effective in the diagnosis of motor disorders of the esophagus.

The barium swallow carried out with cinefluorography provides a unique opportunity for the clinician to observe and study esophageal peristalsis and, in particular, the function of the lower esophageal sphincter. Computed tomography—assessing a thickened muscle wall—and radionuclide scintigraphy—measuring liquid or solid food bolus transit time—and a gamma camera detecting tagged technetium sulfur colloid activity are also used to evaluate the esophagus. It has been suggested that scintigraphy could be used as a screening test for esophageal motility disorders; Mughal and associates (1986), however, disagree.

Provocative testing of esophageal dysmotility has proved effective in the differential diagnosis of esophageal pain from that of coronary artery disease. Richter and associates (1985) indicated that edrophonium is the safest and most effective agent. It does not produce coronary artery spasm or provoke chest pain in normal subjects. Esophageal balloon inflation and upright solid food ingestion as Mellow (1982) suggested are other provocative testing methods.

Maas and associates (1985) developed an ambulatory manometry system that permits 24-hour testing—monitoring—of esophageal motility on an outpatient basis. Coupled with electrocardiographic recording, this should enhance the understanding and documentation of the cause of chest pain in patients with motor dysfunction of the esophagus.

THE UPPER ESOPHAGEAL SPHINCTER

As Henderson (1976) noted, the upper—proximal—sphincter of the esophagus functions as a part of a triad of anatomic structures: the pharynx, the cricopharynx, and the adjacent upper portion of the esophagus. Jones and associates (1986) emphasized pharyngoesophageal relationships in roentgenologic diagnosis when simultaneous disorders represent related phenomena.

The sphincter itself is the cricopharynx, or cricopharyngeus muscle, which maintains constant closure of the entrance into the esophagus except for the specific relaxation that accompanies normal deglutition. It is composed of striated muscle and, as with most sphincters, has a double innervation derived from sympathetic and parasympathetic sources. The sympathetic supply comes from fine branches of the ganglia of the cervical sympathetic chain; the parasympathetic, from the vagus, including the recurrent laryngeal nerve, the glossopharyngeal nerve, and bulbar roots of the spinal accessory nerve. The complexity of innervation is a most important factor in comprehending dysfunction of the upper sphincter, particularly in central nervous system disease or following orolaryngeal or thyroid operation.

Henderson's classification, which differentiates primary from secondary and idiopathic disorders, is useful in discussing motor disturbances of the upper esophageal sphincter. Table 80–1 presents a modification of his classification. Many of these entities have no surgical therapy and are included in a surgical text primarily for general comprehension and differential diagnosis.

Primary Myogenic or Neurogenic Disorders

Myasthenia Gravis

This serious neurologic disease is characterized by failure of myoneural impulse transmission. Particularly in its bulbar form, the skeletal muscles of the pharynx, cricopharyngeus, and upper quarter of the esophagus are affected, causing an unusual form of dysphagia accompanied frequently by coughing, choking, and regurgitation of food through the nose. This sequence is not caused by obstruction of the cricopharyngeus or failure in its relaxation; rather, it results from weakness of the muscles of the soft palate and resulting inability to close

Table 80–1. Motor Disorders of the Upper Esophageal Sphincter

Primary (Myogenic and/or Neurogenic)
Myasthenia gravis
Muscular dystrophy
Cerebrovascular disease
Bulbar poliomyelitis
Secondary
Gastroesophageal reflux
Caustic burns
Post orolaryngeal surgery
Idiopathic
Cricopharyngeal bar or achalasia
Pharyngoesophageal diverticulum
Globus hystericus

off the nasopharynx. Nasal regurgitation, in general, connotes neuromuscular impairment and only infrequently results from obstruction. In myasthenia gravis the pharyngeal swallowing symptoms may be mild in the morning but become progressively more disabling as the day progresses.

Medical treatment is based on cholinergic—anticholinesterase—medication, including neostigmine bromide—Prostigmin—and pyridostigmine bromide—Mestinon. Edrophonium chloride—Tensilon—can be used as a diagnostic test and is useful as a prompt measure for differentiating myasthenia gravis from other myoneurogenic disorders causing dysphagia. Manometric study has not been extensively investigated in this disease; the tracing in Fig. 80–1 identifies the weakness in skeletal muscles of deglutition, whereas the smooth muscle of the distal two thirds of the esophagus shows normal propulsile conduction.

Surgical removal of the thymus has proved moderately successful in the management of myasthenia gravis (Chapter 91). When the patient with the bulbar form of the disease responds, as I (1981) noted, the patient's difficulty in swallowing may be greatly ameliorated.

Muscular Dystrophy

Fischer and his associates (1965) reported on esophageal motility in neuromuscular disorders including myotonia, a manifestation of muscular dystrophy that involves degeneration of the striated muscle and is of unknown cause. Motor activity in the skeletal portion of the pharynx and esophagus is impaired and, as in myasthenia gravis, results in difficulty in swallowing and in nasal regurgitation. Unlike those in myasthenia gravis, these symptoms are constant, without relation to fatigue or response to medication.

Oculopharyngeal muscular dystrophy produces dysphagia, according to Victor and his colleagues (1962). A familial disease of late life characterized by dysphagia and progressive ptosis of the eyelids, it is rare and thus far poorly understood. Henderson (1976) reported manometric testing of three patients with the condition, including one subjected to cricopharyngeal myotomy. Improvement in the patient who underwent myotomy is difficult to explain in the presence of a manometrically

normal cricopharynx and proximal esophagus. There is no proved rationale for surgical intervention in any form of muscular dystrophy associated with dysphagia.

Cerebrovascular Disease

Some older patients who have experienced cerebrovascular accident from hemorrhage, thrombosis, or embolism are troubled by difficulty in swallowing, including choking and aspiration. In this situation the difficulty seems to stem from either weakness or paralysis, or both, of pharyngeal muscle and from incoordination of the swallowing complex so that cricopharyngeal relaxation is out of sequence; that is, it does not occur at the appropriate time in pharyngeal contraction. Whether one can have the latter phenomenon from a small central nervous system vascular lesion without a concomitant major symptomatic stroke is not completely understood.

Nonvascular central nervous system lesions are said also to produce pharyngoesophageal motor dysfunction, as in parkinsonism, amyotrophic lateral sclerosis, and the congenital Riley-Day syndrome. The incidence of dysphagia in these various diseases is obscure because no manometric evaluations have been reported.

Bulbar Poliomyelitis

This illness is almost never encountered today, yet its propensity to produce difficulty in swallowing must be recorded. The cause of the dysphagia is apparently paralysis of pharyngeal muscles with an intact and normal cricopharyngeus muscle. This imbalance results in physiologic obstruction by the upper esophageal sphincter. Any possibility of improvement by cricopharyngeal myotomy would seem to be counter-balanced by the pharyngeal paralysis and the resulting coughing, choking, and nasal regurgitation so common in lack of neurologic control in swallowing.

Secondary Motor Disorders

Gastroesophageal Reflux

Much has been written, for example by Smiley (1972) and by Henderson and his associates (1976), about the apparent relationship between gastroesophageal reflux and motor disturbances of the upper esophageal sphincter. It has never been demonstrated whether, in the presence of reflux, the discomfort of dysphagia in the neck is caused by obstruction at the level of the distal esophagus—and referred to or felt in the neck—or to secondary spasm of the upper sphincter. Henderson (1976) described an indirect method of measurement, the response time in the act of swallowing a 1-cm marshmallow from the exact moment of swallowing to the exact moment of obstruction. "If obstruction occurs within one second of swallowing, the block is the pharyngoesophageal level, whereas if obstruction is recognized in 4 to 8 seconds, it is in the distal esophagus."

When gastroesophageal reflux is documented by roentgenographic study, such as the water siphon test, or by either esophageal pH recording or esophagoscopic observation, reflux to the level of the upper esophageal

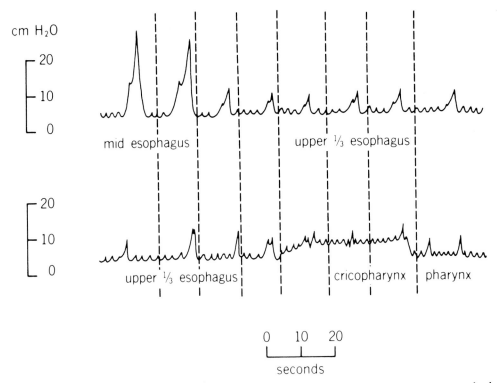

Fig. 80–1. Myasthenia gravis. Esophageal manometric tracings of motor activity in pharynx, cricopharynx, upper third and mid-esophagus illustrating the weak contractions of the first three (skeletal muscle) in contrast with the latter (smooth muscle). (Henderson, R.D.: Motor Disorders of the Esophagus. Baltimore, MD, Williams & Wilkins, 1976.)

sphincter may produce secondary sphincteric spasm. Failure of this apparent protective mechanism, as in more elderly patients in the horizontal position of sleep, can result in coughing and choking from laryngeal irritation or frank tracheal aspiration. Actual manometric assessment of the upper sphincter has been carried out more extensively by British investigators such as Hunt and co-workers (1970), but interpretations are not uniform. Henderson (1976), in a major analytical study, concluded that a pharyngeal-cricopharyngeal incoordination in some patients with cervical dysphagia is like that described by Ellis and colleagues (1969) in patients with pharyngoesophageal diverticulum.

Clearly, both esophageal sphincters should be evaluated in patients with reflux, but conclusions should be drawn with care and these patients individually assessed. Cricopharyngeal myotomy, for instance, to relieve true secondary cervical dysphagia can enhance the possibility of aspiration if the underlying gastroesophageal reflux is untreated.

Caustic Burns

The swallowing of solid caustic agents, particularly flakes or pellets of sodium hydroxide—caustic soda or lye—produces maximal burns of the mouth, pharynx, and upper esophageal sphincter, in contrast to liquid drain cleaners, which cause extensive burning throughout the esophagus and stomach. The damage is almost instantaneous, and little can be done at the initial treatment except to ensure the removal of gross remaining substance from the oral pharynx. The ultimate dysphagia occurring at the upper esophageal sphincter level is secondary to cicatricial scarring at both mucosal and muscle levels rather than the result of any neuromotor imbalance. Surgical management is exceedingly complex and difficult, often requiring extensive plastic surgical reconstruction.

Post Orolaryngeal Surgical Procedures

The complexity of innervation of the cricopharynx suggests that anatomic disturbances in innervation, particularly in extensive resectional procedures for malignant disease, as in radical laryngectomy with neck dissection, can be expected to produce motor disturbance of the upper esophageal sphincter. This motor disturbance is more likely to be symptomatic if relative obstruction or perhaps incoordination—pharyngoesophageal dyskinesia—is produced. Duranceau and associates (1976) described marked derangements in both the upper esophageal sphincter and the body of the esophagus, but not in the lower esophageal sphincter, in 10 patients after laryngectomy. Myotomy of the pharyngoesophageal junction as a possible avenue of therapy needs documentary study.

Gibbons and associates (1985) noted the possibility of a second carcinoma distal to the neopharynx following total laryngectomy: 4 cases in 35 studied with esophagogram for dysphagia.

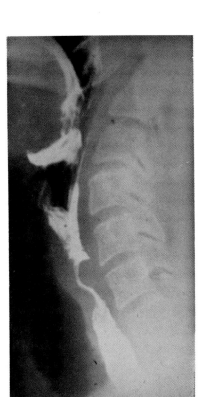

Fig. 80–2. Cricopharyngeal bar. An unusually prominent intrusion upon the barium esophagogram silhouette at the level of the upper esophageal sphincter. It was accompanied by cervical dysphagia and was relieved by sphincteric myotomy.

Idiopathic Motor Disorders

Cricopharyngeal Bar or Achalasia

Cricopharyngeal bar is a roentgenologic term describing a prominent indentation of the pharyngoesophageal column of barium seen, according to Seaman (1966), in 5% of normal patients studied for the presence of this abnormality. The bar apparently correlates with the upper esophageal sphincter (Fig. 80–2). In the absence of diverticulum, some patients presenting with cervical dysphagia may show a prominence of the cricopharynx. Manometry has shown high cricopharyngeal pressures.

Sutherland (1962) discussed obstruction at this level in terms of cricopharyngeal achalasia, defined in its basic Greek derivation as failure in relaxation, not in analogy to esophageal achalasia with loss of ganglionic innervation. He described manometric sphincteric hypertension, recognizable muscle hypertrophy at operation, and effective relief by cricopharyngeal myotomy. The term may be misleading; the role of this operative procedure requires continuing investigation.

As Jones (1986) reported, in the absence of neurologic disease, cricopharyngeal prominence may be the clue to esophageal disease.

Pharyngoesophageal Diverticulum

Diverticula at this level may be related to obstruction at the cricopharynx or to pharyngosphincteric incoordination. The subject is discussed in Chapter 81.

Globus Hystericus

Once the common explanation for cervical dysphagia, this psychiatric manifestation of swallowing difficulty must, if it exists at all, be relegated to the bottom of the differential diagnosis spectrum until appropriate study has excluded organic disease. The symptom, dysphagia, at any level can never be assumed psychiatric in origin.*

BODY OF THE ESOPHAGUS

Centimeter for centimeter, much greater attention has been focused on the extremities of the esophagus—containing its two sphincters—than on the body. Nonetheless, motor disturbances of the body of the esophagus play an important role in disruption of the normal process of deglutition. Transport of food and drink from mouth to stomach is generally included in the term swallowing, and the symptom of dysphagia is applied to difficulties incurred at any level of the esophagus.

An intact neuromuscular anatomy is necessary for the orderly propagation of the esophageal peristalsis. This motor activity consists of primary, secondary, and tertiary or segmental contractions. The first are progressive, conducted peristaltic contractions initiated by swallowing. Secondary contractions are progressive waves that occur without initiation by a swallow. Segmental contractions are nonperistaltic and invariably signify disordered motility. Disturbances in motility may result from primary neurogenic or myogenic abnormalities, from the efforts of abnormalities originating outside the esophagus—secondary—or from a variety of diseases in which the cause of the esophageal disorder remains unexplained (Table 80–2).

Primary Neurogenic or Myogenic Disorders

Achalasia

The definition by Ellis (1969) remains most descriptive and pertinent. "Esophageal achalasia is . . . a disease of unknown etiology characterized by absence of peristalsis

Table 80–2. Motor Disorders of the Body of the Esophagus

Primary (Neurogenic and/or Myogenic)
Achalasia
Diffuse esophageal spasm
Supersqueeze ("nutcracker") esophagus
Progressive systemic sclerosis
Secondary
Secondary disordered motor activity
Midesophageal and epiphrenic diverticulum
Metastatic carcinomatous neuropathy
Uncertain Relationship to Systemic Disease
Multiple sclerosis
Diabetic neuropathy
Sjögren's syndrome
Intramural pseudodiverticulosis

*E.M. Thorton: The Freudian Fallacy: An Alternative View of Freudian Theory, Doubleday, 1984, suggests that "globus hystericus" is not hysterical but a manifestation of a form of epilepsy.

in the body of the esophagus and failure of the inferior sphincter to relax in response to swallowing." The term itself, translated from the Greek "failure to relax," is here used to include cardiospasm, megaesophagus, idiopathic esophageal dilatation, aperistalis of the esophagus, and aganglionic or amyenteric achalasia.

The cause is not known. Chagas' disease—parasitic infestation with *Trypanosoma cruzi*—largely a South American disease, produces similar dysfunction of the esophagus but often involves other organs as well. The characteristic pathology of idiopathic achalasia described by Cassella and associates (1965) lies in deficiency of, or changes in, the ganglia of Auerbach's plexus, often more prominent in the body of the esophagus itself. Friesen and colleagues (1983) found by electron microscopy marked loss of small nerve fibers and a paucity of granules in the remaining fibers with secondary nonspecific smooth muscle changes—filament disarray and fiber mottling, among other changes—in the esophagus in achalasia.

Some progress has been made in the experimental production of such pathologic changes. Motility derangement and dilatation of the esophagus have been created by stereotactic bilateral destructive lesions in the nucleus ambiguus in the medulla of the dog or in the dorsal motor nuclei of the vagus nerves in the cat.

Jones and associates (1983) found a statistically significant increase of serum antibody titres against measles virus in 18 patients with achalasia compared with age-matched controls—several viral and bacterial agents were assessed.

The symptoms produced by achalasia are variable and may be nonspecific. The initiation of swallowing is normal but dysphagia is appreciated by failure of emptying of the esophagus. The degree of dysphagia may be inversely related to the degree of esophageal dilatation; the larger the esophagus, the less the sense of dysphagia. Esophageal emptying is by gravity and patients are sometimes aware of the sudden gush of food into the stomach. Regurgitation of partially digested food is common. Nocturnal regurgitation may produce cough, choking, or aspiration, the last more often in the elderly. Malodorous breath is common. Weight loss is frequent. Because of difficulties in eating, some victims isolate themselves during meals. This pattern has produced the impression that achalasia is psychogenic, but no evidence supports this theory.

A variant of typical achalasia exists in patients who have unusually marked dysphagia combined with spastic pain, apparently associated with residual disordered peristalsis that is ineffective in overcoming the unrelaxed lower esophageal sphincter. Sanderson and his colleagues (1967) termed this condition "vigorous achalasia" although it is probably the same phenomenon Sweet (1956) described as type II achalasia.

The severity of achalasia, as measured in the degree of megaesophagus, is usefully recorded in three stages, as Henderson and associates (1972) suggested: stage I—minimal—esophageal diameter < 4 cm; stage II—moderate—esophageal diameter 4 to 6 cm; and stage III—severe—esophageal diameter > 6 cm. Most patients with vigorous achalasia have stage I disease; thus, the dilatation is minimal but the symptoms may be major. This staging process is provided by measurement of the maximal diameter of the esophagus on standard roentgenograms of the chest during the barium esophagogram. More important roentgenologically, however, is the dynamic appearance of peristaltic activity. Peristalsis is usually absent, although forceful erratic contractions are common in vigorous achalasia.

Although the diagnosis of achalasia is usually suggested by the esophagogram, endoscopy and manometry are important components of the investigational workup. Achalasia may be roentgenologically confused with distal esophageal stricture or carcinoma of the cardia of the stomach, unfortunately misleadingly labeled "pseudoachalasia" by Kahrilas and associates (1987). These conditions can usually be differentiated by a combination of direct visualization, with the fiber-optic or rigid esophagoscope, and the passage of the larger Maloney mercury dilators. These dilators usually pass through the narrowed lower segment in achalasia, but not in tight stricture or carcinoma. The manometric tracing of achalasia is characteristic (Fig. 80–3). Manometry is therefore the ultimate diagnostic test. Besides failure of full relaxation of the lower esophageal sphincter, peristaltic response in the smooth muscle portion of the body of the esophagus is absent during both wet and dry swallows. The pressure in the lower sphincter is usually, but not always, elevated. Katz and associates (1986) reported that 7 of 23 achalasia patients had esophageal aperistalsis but complete lower esophageal sphincter relaxation. In vigorous achalasia, nonpropagated motor waves occur in

Table 80–3. Manometric Criteria for Esophageal Motility Disorders

Achalasia
  Absence of peristalsis in esophageal body*
  Incomplete lower sphincter relaxation*
  Elevated lower sphincter pressure (varying with laboratory)†
  Increased intraesophageal baseline pressure relative to gastric†
Diffuse Esophageal Spasm
  Simultaneous, nonperistaltic contractions occurring after more than 10% of wet swallows*
  Periods of normal peristalsis*
  Sometimes spontaneous and/or repetitive contractions†
  Contractions may have increased amplitude or duration†
  Lower sphincter pressure may be elevated in one third of patients†
Nutcracker Esophagus
  Mean peristaltic amplitude in distal esophagus greater than 180 mm Hg*
  Normal peristaltic sequence preserved*
  Contractions may be prolonged†
Hypertensive Lower Esophageal Sphincter
  Lower sphincter pressure greater than 2 standard deviations above normal mean with normal relaxation*
  Normal peristalsis†

*Required for diagnosis
†Often associated but not required for diagnosis
Modified with permission from Katz, P.O., and Castell, D.O.: Review: esophageal motility disorders. Am. J. Med. Sci. 290(2):61, 1985.

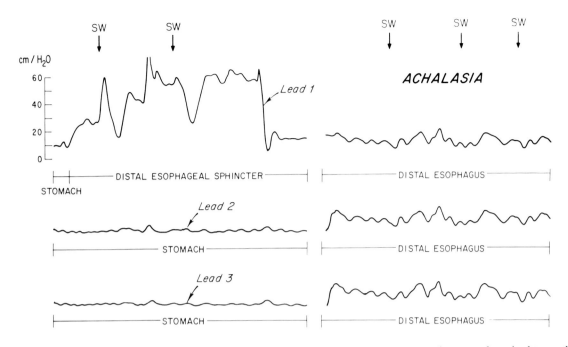

Fig. 80–3. Achalasia. The manometric tracings of classic achalasia of the esophagus. (Left) A hypertensive lower esophageal sphincter illustrating failure of complete relaxation in the proximal lead; (Right) superimposable tracings in all three leads in the lower body of the esophagus with complete absence of conducted peristalsis.

the body of the esophagus and have unusually high amplitude.

Treatment of esophageal achalasia remains controversial. In 1965 Kramer pointed out that no controlled prospective study has compared the accepted therapeutic techniques of esophageal myotomy with pneumatic or hydrostatic dilatation. Csendes and co-workers (1981) attempted a prospective randomized comparative study, but only 18 patients were dilated and 20 patients operated upon, finding permanent improvement in all surgical patients and 50% of the patients who were dilated.

Myotomy, to be successful, must be single, contrasted with the original double Heller (1913) technique, complete through the muscularis mucosae, and undermining laterally to permit outward bulging of mucosa and to minimize subsequent fibrotic closure (Fig. 80–4). The procedure can be performed transabdominally, particularly in children, or transthoracically. The latter is preferred if residual doubt exists about the accuracy of the diagnosis. The myotomy need extend only a few millimeters onto the surface of the stomach. As Ellis and Olsen (1969) noted, an antireflux procedure is necessary if hiatal incompetency is present or if the hiatal anatomy is compromised by extensive operative dissection. Some experienced general thoracic surgeons now combine myotomy extended onto the gastric wall with an antireflux procedure. Duranceau and collaborators (1982) reported using a 2-cm total fundoplication. Murray and his group (1984) applied a complementary fundoplication in selected patients in whom circumstances suggested high risk of reflux esophagitis. Nelems and associates (1980), noting that incomplete myotomy and reflux esophagitis constituted the principal failures of the modified Heller operation, advised adding the Belsey fundoplication—

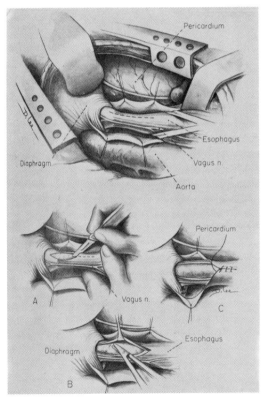

Fig. 80–4. Modified Heller esophagomyotomy. (Top) Intended line of muscle incision and minimal disturbance of crural attachments. *A,* Sharp scalpel myotomy. *B,* Lateral undermining of muscle layers. *C,* Optional closure of mediastinal pleura. (Ellis, F.H., et al.: Ann. Surg. *16*:64, 1967.)

they also commented that gastroplasty is contraindicated in patients with achalasia. The problem in adding an antireflux procedure is to avoid a too obstructive repair for the patient who has no esophageal peristalsis. I prefer to limit the myotomy on the cardia, as Ellis and associates (1984) suggested, adding a modified Belsey antireflux technique. Okike and his colleagues (1979) reported the results of myotomy. Of 458 modified Heller esophagomyotomy procedures, 90% showed good or excellent results; only one hospital death occurred and only 6% showed poor results. Ellis and associates (1984) studied 115 myotomy patients before and after operation and found 91% improved by the operation without antireflux procedure. Ellis (1960) noted that 19% of patients with achalasia developed carcinoma, but Pierce and his associates (1970) found the incidence to be only 2.7%. A good result from myotomy apparently does not minimize the possibility of subsequent development of carcinoma. Follow-up, therefore, must be vigilant.

The technique of effective dilatation of the lower esophageal sphincter begins with cleansing of the esophagus; emptying of retained food is best accomplished by lavage with a large orally swallowed tube of the Ewald type. Using topical anesthesia, the pneumatic bougie is passed under fluoroscopic control and dilated only when properly positioned astride the esophagogastric junction. Proper dilatation produces sharp, localized, severe pain. Pain persisting long after dilatation or blood on the dilator must cause concern and be followed with prompt Gastrografin esophagography.

Among the many advocates of primary pneumatic balloon dilatation of the lower esophageal sphincter in achalasia patients are: Jacobs and colleagues (1983), who reported highly successful results in 30 patients solely with pneumatic dilatation under fluoroscopic control; Witzel (1981), who used an inflatable polyurethane balloon assembly attached to a small fiber-optic gastroscope in 39 patients without complication; and Fellows and associates (1983), who assessed 50 patients undergoing pneumatic dilatation, 29 of whom required one procedure, 21 requiring repeated dilatations as many as four or more times. Esophagomyotomy was necessary in five—10%—of Fellows' patients, primarily those under age 45.

Slater and Sicular (1982) described the management of five patients incurring perforation from forced dilatation in a 9-year experience. Operation with a two-layer closure of the laceration was converted into successful Heller esophagomyotomy on the contralateral aspect of the distal esophagus. In my experience, early recognition of perforation by routine postdilatation Gastrografin swallow is essential for this approach; closure of the laceration is also enhanced by pleural or intercostal muscle buttress.

The modified Heller esophagomyotomy is preferred in children and in patients with vigorous achalasia. Buick and Spitz (1985) advocated that the modified Heller myotomy be combined with a short, loose Nissen fundoplication in children. Azizkhan and colleagues (1980) recommended myotomy in all children under 9 and

dilatation as initial procedure thereafter. The combination of low morbidity and improving results from myotomy has resulted in increasing application of surgery in preference to bag dilatation.

Diffuse Esophageal Spasm—DES

The term primary disordered motor activity, popularized by Henderson (1976), is replaced by diffuse esophageal spasm, as Creamer and his co-workers (1958) suggested. Other terms have included pseudodiverticulosis and curling, corkscrew, or spindled esophagus, all of which roentgenologically demonstrate segmental spasm. In DES the smooth muscle portion of the esophagus has lost its normal peristaltic motor coordination and has spontaneous activity, repetitive waves, prolonged contractions, and high amplitude contractions. The lower esophageal sphincter is usually normal, both in tone and in its ability to relax in response to swallowing. The cause of DES is not known. The principal entity to be differentiated is achalasia. In DES, the Auerbach ganglion cells are normal.

The prime symptom is severe spastic pain, which occurs somewhat inconstantly upon swallowing either liquid or solid food; it apparently corresponds to peristaltic segmental contractions. In addition, dysphagia, regurgitation, and progressive weight loss are common. Henderson (1976) described the major roentgenographic features on the barium swallow as "marked motor spasm in the lower two thirds of the organ and an increase in esophageal wall thickness to 5 mm or more." Nevertheless, the diagnosis is seldom made by a barium examination alone. The esophagoscopic findings are nondiagnostic. Esophageal manometry is, however, specific. The lower sphincter is usually normal—although in one third of the patients it may be elevated—as are the upper skeletal muscle portion and the cricopharyngeus muscle. The abnormality, confined to the lower two thirds or smooth muscle portion of the esophagus, consists of spastic motor waves of prolonged duration and unusually high amplitude, brought on by swallowing but lacking coordinated propulsive propagation. The amplitude is frequently in excess of 100 cm H_2O (Fig. 80–5). Richter and Castell (1984) regard "simultaneous contractions after wet swallows" the diagnostic finding on manometry in symptomatic patients.

Various medicinal agents are advocated for the relief of the symptoms of primary esophageal motor disorders, including calcium channel blockers, metoclopramide, hydralazine, bethanecol, and isosorbide. The calcium channel blockers—nifedipine, verapamil, diltiazem—seem to effectively decrease the amplitude of esophageal peristaltic contractions and lower the sphincter pressure. Hongo and colleagues' (1984) studies have been thorough in this regard, especially in correlation with plasma nifedipine levels; but Thomas and colleagues (1986) reported the side effects may be unacceptable in young workers, precluding prolonged use.

Pneumatic dilatation is not indicated, physiologically, because the lower sphincter is not the site of the abnormality. The treatment of choice is a long esophago-

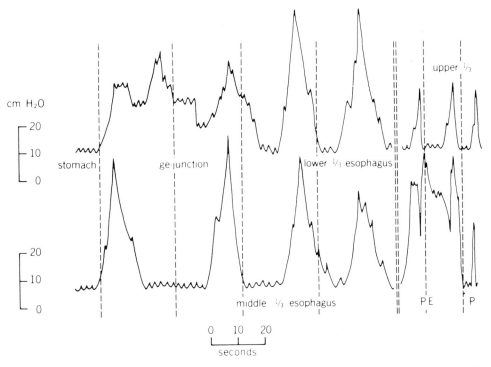

Fig. 80–5. Diffuse esophageal spasm (DES). The manometric tracing illustrating a normal lower esophageal sphincter and spastic motor waves of long duration and high amplitude, lacking coordinated propagation. (Henderson, R.D.: Motor Disorders of the Esophagus. Baltimore, MD, Williams & Wilkins, 1976.)

myotomy, the length of the segment of abnormal motility on the esophageal manometric tracing. Smooth muscle thickening is common. The myotomy is carried distally through the esophagogastric junction. Proximally, it is better to carry the myotomy to the apex of the intrathoracic esophagus than to be uncertain of the adequacy of its length. An antireflux procedure is included if roentgenologic evidence suggests hiatal hernia or demonstrable reflux appears on the standard acid reflux test. Henderson and associates (1987) reported a 5-year review of 34 patients surgically treated with myotomy from the apex of the chest through the high pressure zone and total fundoplication antireflux repair; "30 patients eat normally without dysphagia or spontaneous pain."

Supersqueeze—Nutcracker—Esophagus

Gelfand and Botoman (1987) used the term supersqueeze esophagus for a condition of high amplitude and prolonged peristaltic swallowing waves seen in patients with noncardiac chest pain. They prefer this term to "nutcracker" esophagus, which implies a peristalsis. Dysphagia is an inconsistent symptom; when present, it does direct attention to the esophagus. Its absence creates a problem in differential diagnosis for which manometry is the decisive test.

Katz and associates (1986) reported a review of 910 patients evaluated for noncardiac chest pain in 3 years—1983 to 1985—in Castell's laboratory; 255 had abnormal manometric tracings. The "nutcracker", as they called it, esophagus was found in 48% of patients with abnormal tracings. Provocative testing with edrophonium was

more useful in reproducing pain than in other motility disorders. This response is like that in patients with vigorous achalasia and diffuse esophageal spasm in demonstrating supersensitivity of a parasympathetically denervated organ to cholinergic agents—Cannon's law (1939). Unanswered is whether esophageal contraction abnormalities represent a diffuse gastrointestinal neuromuscular derangement, as Clouse and Eckert (1986) discussed.

Treatment programs are thus far inconclusive. Both Traube's group (1984) and Richter and associates (1984) suggested a specific effect of calcium channel blockers—nifedipine and diltiazem—in reducing the high amplitude contractions. Mellow (1982) reported the apparent value of long-term oral hydralazine in decreasing amplitude and duration of chest pain in patients with primary, painful esophageal motility disorders. Long-acting nitrates, in particular isosorbide, have been in general use for all esophageal motor disorders but produce troublesome side effects, such as headache and flushing.

No one has yet proved any role for esophagomyotomy in this condition. It therefore is advisable for the gastroenterologist to juggle the available drugs seeking maximal response in the individual patient. Gelfand and Botoman (1987) in fact suggest that symptoms may moderate with time.

Progressive Systemic Sclerosis

Involvement of the esophagus may occur in various collagen disorders, most frequently in progressive systemic sclerosis or scleroderma. Pathologic changes include smooth muscle atrophy, in the lower two thirds; deposition of collagen in connective tissue; and subintimal arteriolar fibrosis. Although the lesion seems largely myogenic, Auerbach's plexus may be damaged.

The essential abnormalities noted at roentgenologic examination are esophageal atony, often missed unless the patient is examined recumbent, and the associated presence of hiatal hernia, and gastroesophageal reflux. Stricture may be present. The flexible fiberscope makes endoscopic evaluation safe and effective. The typical manometric pattern (Fig. 80–6) reveals low amplitude peristaltic contractions, and disordered motor activity in the lower two thirds of the esophagus plus a reduction in tone in the lower esophageal sphincter.

No specific treatment exists for scleroderma of the esophagus. Standard medical methods are used to prevent and treat esophagitis and stricture: dietary control, antacids, postural elevation for sleep, and Maloney mercury bougienage. If surgical resection becomes inevitable, replacement with jejunum or colon may create a special problem because either organ may be, or become, involved in the disease process. Esophageal lengthening with a modified antireflux procedure, such as gastroplasty with a short fundoplication, appears to be the operation of choice at this time. The various techniques are discussed in Chapter 83.

DeMerieux and colleagues (1983) reported that esophageal abnormalities in polymyositis and dermatomyositis resemble those in scleroderma. Dysmotility is a basic feature of systemic sclerosis patients with the CREST syndrome—calcinosis, Raynaud's phenomenon, esophageal dysmotility, sclerodactyly, and telangiectasia.

Secondary Motor Disorders

Secondary Disordered Motor Activity

Henderson (1976) defined this entity as "the response of the esophagus to injury, such as infection—candidiasis, ingestion of a foreign body or a chemical irritant—lye, acid . . . or the most common injury due to reflux of gastric contents into the esophagus." In general, the greater the severity of the inflammatory process, the greater the disruption of the normal motor function. Once inflammation involves the muscular layers of the esophagus and particularly when fibrosis ensues, the maximum interference with orderly peristalsis ensues. Full-thickness circumferential fibrosis may be accompained by complete loss of peristalsis.

Chapter 82 presents a detailed consideration of gastroesophageal reflux.

Two types of motor changes may, singly or together, accompany reflux. The first set of changes includes those that occur when the lower esophageal sphincter is in the thorax: respiratory negativity on the motility tracing, a double respiratory reversal, or lowered activity or tone of the sphincter. The second type of motor changes occurs in the body of the esophagus and may include low amplitude primary peristaltic contractions, simultaneous contractions sometimes with high spikes, or spontaneous contractions, not initiated by swallowing. The basic factor in differential diagnosis from primary motility disorders such as achalasia is the presence of an underlying pattern of conducted peristaltic movement.

Midesophageal and Epiphrenic Diverticula

Diverticula in these locations are usually the result, and not the cause, of esophageal motility disorders; a

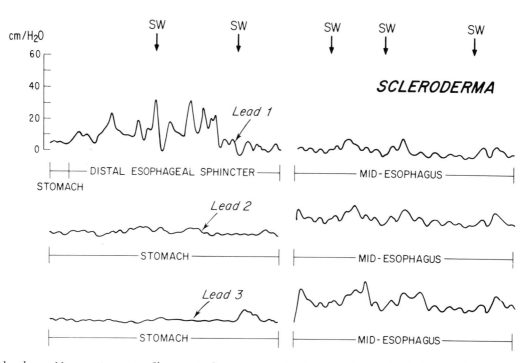

Fig. 80–6. Scleroderma. Manometric tracings of hypotensive lower esophageal sphincter and low-amplitude disordered peristalsis involving lower two thirds of esophagus.

few paracarinal diverticula may indeed be traction diverticula. The pulsion diverticula are mentioned here to draw attention to the need for esophageal manometric study in all such patients. Rivkin and associates (1984) described 34 patients studied both roentgenologically and manometrically; all demonstrated a motility disorder. When symptoms are sufficient to warrant operation, excision of the diverticulum must be accompanied by correction of the underlying pathophysiologic abnormality: antireflux repair or esophagomyotomy, or both. There is no nonsurgical therapy.

Metastatic Carcinomatous Neuropathy

Simeone and his associates (1976) reported a unique case of esophageal aperistalsis secondary to metastatic invasion of the myenteric plexus. The patient, with a proved bronchial carcinoma, had severe nonobstructive dysphagia. A cine-esophagogram revealed a totally atonic esophagus. Postmortem examination showed no gross changes involving the esophagus, in particular no evidence of esophagitis. Microscopic sections, however, clearly demonstrated carcinomatous invasion of the ganglia of Auerbach's plexus and the terminal branching of the vagus nerves. From this evidence Simeone and associates (1976) drew the inference that motor disorders of the esophagus can result from secondary carcinomatous involvement of the myenteric plexus.

Motor Disorders with Uncertain Relation to Systemic Disease

Multiple Sclerosis

Daly and his colleagues (1962) reported that esophageal function is occasionally altered in multiple sclerosis. The mechanism of dysfunction is not clear, but it apparently involves both interference with motor peristaltic activity and failure of distal esophageal sphincter relaxation.

Diabetic Neuropathy

While studying both esophageal function and peripheral neuropathy, Hollis and colleagues (1977) evaluated 50 unselected patients with diabetes mellitus, in contrast with 14 age-matched healthy subject controls. Twenty-eight patients—56%—demonstrated an abnormal esophageal motility: frequent spontaneous contractions and reduced primary peristaltic activity. Peristaltic amplitude, however, was unaffected in comparison with controls and also unchanged when the diabetes mellitus patients were grouped into those with or without peripheral neuropathy. Velocity of esophageal peristalsis was reduced in the diabetic peripheral neuropathy patient in comparison with controls or non-neuropathic diabetic patients. Resting lower esophageal sphincteric pressures were similar in all groups. The significance of these determinations in the clinical management of diabetic patients and the etiologic relationship of the abnormalities require further clarification.

Stewart and his associates (1976) studied 31 patients with diabetes mellitus, 23 of whom had either gastro-intestinal or genitourinary symptoms related to autonomic neuropathy. They found reduced lower esophageal sphincteric pressure, diminished amplitude of esophageal peristalsis, and delayed esophageal emptying in a 15° Trendelenburg position. They observed no esophageal motor hypersensitivity to cholinergic drugs.

Sjögren's Syndrome

Ramirez-Mata and associates (1976) evaluated esophageal manometric tracings in 10 unselected patients with primary Sjögren's syndrome, patients without clinical evidence of other connective tissue disorder. They concluded that the uniform pattern of esophageal dysfunction in these patients differs from the motility disorders in other distinct connective tissue entities and may therefore be a distinct entity in itself. This conclusion warrants additional investigation and confirmation. The specific motor changes consist of absent or decreased contractility in the upper third of the esophagus—the skeletal muscular segment. In 4 of the 10 patients, this pattern extended to lower levels in the body of the esophagus. The authors believed these changes could not be explained simply by oropharyngeal dryness or mucosal atrophy.

Intramural Pseudodiverticulosis

Beauchamp and colleagues (1974) suggested this term for multiple, tiny protrusions from the esophageal wall accompanying variable periods of dysphagia, usually in older patients, with an area of narrowing or stricture. They suggested the likely origin as a diffuse inflammatory process in the esophagus but regarded stricture formation and *Candida albicans* superinfection as secondary manifestations. Trier and Bjorkman (1984) reported that intramural pseudodiverticulosis is common in patients with candidiasis; symptoms include odynophagia, dysphagia, and bleeding. Treatment includes oral nystatin—Mycostatin—in candidiasis.

THE LOWER ESOPHAGEAL SPHINCTER

The lower esophageal sphincter—LES—or gastroesophageal high pressure zone, lies in the terminal 4 cm of the esophagus. Unlike the upper sphincter, it cannot be defined either anatomically or surgically. Botha (1962) described a zone of muscle thickening, arising from the inner circular muscle layer, seen by stripping away the esophageal mucosa. Its effectiveness as a barrier against gastric reflux into the esophagus stems, at least in part, from its normal location in the intra-abdominal segment of esophagus. There is also an element of neurologic control of the high pressure zone—HPZ—in which increase in intragastric pressure results in augmentation of lower esophageal sphincter tone. But the principal component of sphincter control may well be hormonal. Gastrin release from the gastric antrum results in increased tone of the lower sphincter; both secretin and cholecystokinin produce decreased tone in the gastroesophageal junction. Aggestrup and colleagues (1983) suggested that a reduced number of vasoactive intestinal polypeptide fibers contributes to incomplete LES relaxation, at least

Table 80–4. Motor Disorders of the Lower Esophageal Sphincter

Hypertensive Sphincter
Achalasia
Giant muscular hypertrophy
Postvagotomy dysphagia
Schatzki's ring
Hypotensive Sphincter
Hiatal hernia and gastroesophageal reflux
Chalasia

in patients with achalasia. Diliwari and associates (1975) showed the effects of the prostaglandins on sphincter tone: $F_2\alpha$ caused increased pressure in the lower esophageal sphincter, and E_2 reduced the intrinsic tone.

Table 80–4 presents abnormalities of the lower esophageal sphincter. These abnormalities fall into two distinct groups, those with a hypertensive sphincter and those with a hypotensive sphincter. Some of the abnormalities have already been discussed under Body of the Esophagus; the hypotensive sphincter associated with gastroesophageal reflux is discussed in greater detail in Chapter 82.

Hypertensive Sphincter

Achalasia

One of the essentials in the diagnosis of achalasia is failure of relaxation of the lower sphincter. In the normal sphincter, relaxation must be complete and responsive to the arrival of an orderly peristaltic wave from above. In achalasia, little or no relaxation may occur, or as much as 70% relaxation may exist. In addition, pressures generated within the lower esophageal sphincter may be as high as 40 cm H_2O. Pressures of 20 cm H_2O or less are still consistent with the diagnosis of achalasia if relaxation does not occur in the normal fashion. Henderson (1976) reported one additional abnormality, the early contraction of the sphincteric zone in patients with achalasia, beginning at 2 to 3 seconds after deglutition, rather than the usual 5 to 10 seconds.

Giant Muscular Hypertrophy

This uncommon condition results in marked thickening in the circular muscle of the esophagus including the area of the high pressure zone and the distal body of the esophagus. The number of patients studied manometrically is insufficient to be certain of the exact nature of the motor disorder, but clinically a hypertensive lower sphincter is at least partially responsible for the severe dysphagia produced. A modified Heller esophagomyotomy, to be effective in relief of that dysphagia, must be lengthy, usually to the level of the aortic arch. In this respect, the condition resembles DES. In one unusual case, Wall and associates (1967) reported smooth muscle hypertrophy extending onto the proximal stomach.

Postvagotomy Dysphagia

Uncommonly, patients experience dysphagia following bilateral truncal vagotomy. Andersen and his asso-

ciates (1966) reported 10 such patients in a series of 1300 patients who underwent vagotomy. A few of these patients proved to have periesophageal fibrosis, apparently secondary to surgical dissection of the vagal fibers. Most, however, demonstrated a motility disorder characterized by failure of relaxation of the lower esophageal sphincter and some simultaneous contractions within the distal esophagus—as with achalasia. The dysphagia may be transient. Maloney mercury bougienage is the primary effective management. Rarely, an esophagomyotomy may be necessary.

Schatzki's Ring

This entity is generally defined as a sharply outlined narrowing of the distal esophagus precisely at the squamocolumnar juncture at the proximal edge of a small sliding hiatal hernia (Fig. 80–7). It is caused by submucosal fibrosis that results in adherence of the undersurfaces of the two types of mucosa, producing a circumferential ring. If sufficiently tight, it causes dysphagia. Manometric evidence is insufficient to label it a condition of hypertensive sphincter; yet the clinical significance is similar. Further, the ring lies at or near the lower end of the normal gastroesophageal high pressure zone. Its management seems best accomplished by Maloney mercury bougienage, rather than more extensive procedures such as mucosal excision of the ring. Ottinger and I (1980) noted that hiatal hernia repair in such patients seems to be fraught with an usually high incidence of recurrent symptoms.

Hypotensive Sphincter

Hiatal Hernia and Gastroesophageal Reflux

Certainly the most common esophageal motor disorder is the hypotensive sphincter, which seems largely responsible for the phenomenon of pathophysiologic gastroesophageal reflux, with or without a sliding hiatal hernia. The clinical significance of this abnormality is thoroughly discussed in Chapter 82.

Chalasia

Berenberg and Neuhauser (1950) introduced this term, referring to the phenomenon of hypotensive lower esophageal sphincter in infants. In the embryologic development of the esophagus, the area of the lower esophagus apparently lies well within the thorax and descends before birth to its normal position. The clinical syndrome of free reflux of an ingested meal, however, may persist beyond the neonatal period and indicates hypotension in the lower sphincter. This condition, in the absence of hiatal herniation of the stomach, is properly referred to as chalasia. Care must be taken to keep infants with chalasia in the upright position following feeding.

Fortunately, the powerful upper esophageal sphincter usually protects against regurgitation into the pharynx and the potential serious complication of tracheal aspiration. Nonetheless, surgical antireflux procedures may be necessary in the infant or young child to prevent the threatening complications of esophagitis and aspiration.

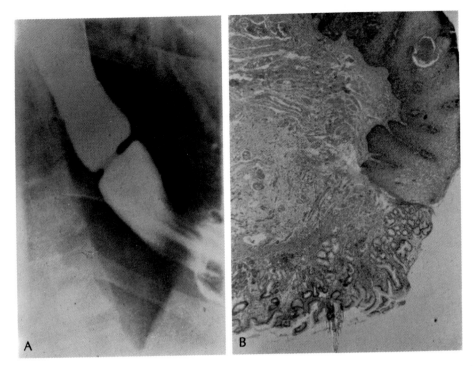

Fig. 80–7. Schatzki ring. *A*, The barium esophagogram with the symmetric constriction at the esophagogastric junction above a sliding hiatal hernia. *B*, A biopsy photomicrograph illustrating the squamocolumnar mucosal junction at the ring.

Such a procedure is best accomplished by the transabdominal approach utilizing a Nissen fundoplication.

REFERENCES

Aggestrup, S., et al.: Lack of vasoactive intestinal polypeptide nerves in esophageal achalasia. Gastroenterol. *84*:924, 1983.

Anderson, H.A., Schlegel, J.F., and Olsen, A.M.: Postvagotomy dysphagia. Gastrointest. Endosc. *12*:13, 1966.

Azizkhan, R.G., Tapper, D., and Eraklis, A.: Achalasia in childhood: a 20-year experience. J. Pediatr. Surg. *15*:452, 1980.

Beauchamp, J.M., et al.: Esophageal intramural pseudodiverticulosis. Radiology *113*:273, 1974.

Berenberg, W., and Neuhauser, E.B.D.: Cardioesophageal relaxation (chalasia) as a cause of vomiting in infants. Pediatrics 5:414, 1950.

Botha, G.S.M.: The Gastro-Oesophageal Junction. London, J & A Churchill Ltd., 1962.

Buick, R.G., and Spitz, L.: Achalasia in children. Brit. J. Surg. 72:341, 1985.

Cannon, W.B.: A law of denervation. Am. J. Med. Sci. *198*:737, 1939.

Cassella, R.R., Ellis, F.H., Jr., and Brown, A.L., Jr.: Fine structure changes in achalasia of the esophagus. I. Vagus nerves. Am. J. Pathol. *46*:279, 1965.

Clouse, R.E., and Eckert, T.C.: Gastrointestinal symptoms of patients with esophageal contraction abnormalities. Dig. Dis. Sci., *31*:236, 1986.

Creamer, B., Donoghue, E., and Code, C.F.: Pattern of esophageal motility in diffuse spasm. Gastroenterology 34:782, 1958.

Csendes, A., et al.: A prospective randomized study comparing forceful dilatation and esophagomyotomy in patients with achalasia of the esophagus. Gastroenterol. *80*:789, 1981.

Daly, D.D., Code, C.F., and Anderson, H.A.: Disturbances of swallowing and esophageal motility in patients with multiple sclerosis. Neurology *12*:250, 1962.

DeMerieux, P., et al.: Esophageal abnormalities and dysphagia in polymyositis and dermatomyositis. Arthritis Rheumat. *26*:961, 1983.

Diliwari, J.B., et al.: Response of the human cardia sphincter to circulating prostaglandins F2 alpha and E2 and to anti-inflammatory drugs. Gut *16*:137, 1975.

Duranceau, A., et al.: Alteration in esophageal motility after laryngectomy. Am. J. Surg. *131*:30, 1976.

Duranceau, A., LaFontaine, E.R., and Vallieres, B.: Effects of total fundoplication on function of the esophagus after myotomy for achalasia. Am. J. Surg. *143*:22, 1982.

Ellis, F.G.: The causes of death in achalasia of the cardia. Ann. R. Coll. Surg. Engl. *53*:663, 1960.

Ellis, F.H., Jr., and Olsen, A.M.: Achalasia of the Esophagus. Major Problems in Clin. Surg. Vol. 9. Philadelphia, W.B. Saunders Co., 1969.

Ellis, F.H., Jr., et al.: Cricopharyngeal myotomy for pharyngoesophageal diverticulum. Ann. Surg. *170*:340, 1969.

Ellis, F.H., Jr., Crozier, R.E., and Watkins, E., Jr.: Operation for esophageal achalasia: results of esophagomyotomy without an antireflux operation. J. Thorac. Cardiovasc. Surg. *88*:344, 1984.

Fellows, I.W., Ogilvie, A.L., and Atkinson, M.: Pneumatic dilatation in achalasia. Gut *24*:1020, 1983.

Fischer, R.A., et al.: Esophageal motility in neuromuscular disorders. Ann. Intern. Med. *63*:229, 1965.

Friesen, D.L., Henderson, R.D., and Hanna, W.: Ultrastructure of the esophageal muscle in achalasia and diffuse esophageal spasm. Am. J. Clin. Pathol. *79*:319, 1983.

Gelfand, M.D., and Botoman, V.A.: Esophageal motility disorders: a clinical overview. Am. J. Gastroenterol. *82*:181, 1987.

Gibbons, R.G., et al.: Esophageal lesions after total laryngectomy. Am. J. Roentgenol. *144*:1197, 1985.

Heller, E.: Extramukose Cardioplastik beim chronischen Cardiospasmus mit Dilatation des Oesphagus. Mitt. Grenzgeb. Med. Chir. 27:141, 1913.

Henderson, R.D.: Motor disorders of the esophagus. Baltimore, Williams & Wilkins, 1976.

Henderson, R.D.: The Esophagus: Reflux and Primary Motor Disorders. Baltimore, Williams & Wilkins, 1980.

Henderson, R.D., et al.: Diagnosis of achalasia. Can. J. Surg. *15*:190, 1972.

Henderson, R.D., Woolf, C., and Marryatt, G.: Pharyngoesophageal dysphagia and gastroesophageal reflux. Laryngoscope 86:1531, 1976.

Henderson, R.D., Ryder, D., and Marryall, G.: Extended esophageal myotomy and short total fundoplication hernia repair in diffuse esophageal spasm: five-year review in 34 patients. Ann. Thorac. Surg. 43:25, 1987.

Hollis, J.B., Castell, D.O., and Braddom, R.L.: Esophageal function in diabetes mellitus and its relation to peripheral neuropathy. Gastroenterology 73:1098, 1977.

Hongo, M., et al.: Effects of nifedipine on esophageal motor function in humans: correlation with plasma nifedipine concentration. Gastroenterol. 86:8, 1984.

Hunt, P.S., Connell, A.M., and Smiley, T.B.: The cricopharyngeal sphincter in gastric reflux. Gut 11:303, 1970.

Jacobs, J.B., Cohen, N.L., and Mattel, S.: Pneumatic dilatation as the primary treatment for achalasia. Ann. Otol. Rhinol. Laryngol. 92:353, 1983.

Jones, B., et al.: Pharyngoesophageal interrelationships: observations and working concepts. Gastrointest. Radiol. 11:123, 1986.

Jones, D.B., et al.: Preliminary report of an association between measles virus and achalasia. J. Clin. Pathol. 36:655, 1983.

Kahrilas, P.J., et al.: Comparison of pseudoachalasia and achalasia. Am. J. Med. 82:439, 1987.

Katz, P.O., et al.: Apparent complete lower esophageal sphincter relaxation in achalasia. Gastroenterol. 90:978, 1986.

Kramer, F.: Progress in gastroenterology: esophagus. Gastroenterology 49:439, 1965.

Maas, L.C., et al.: 24-hour ambulatory manometry in diagnosis of esophageal motor disorders causing chest pain. South. Med. J. 78:810, 1985.

Mellow, M.H.: Effect of isosorbide and hydralazine in painful primary esophageal motor disorders. Gastroenterol. 83:364, 1982.

Mughal, M.M., Marples, M., and Bancewicz, J.: Scintigraphic assessment of oesophageal motility: what does it show and how reliable is it? Gut 27:946, 1986.

Murray, G.F., et al.: Selective application of fundoplication in achalasia. Ann. Thorac. Surg. 37:185, 1984.

Nelems, J.M., Cooper, J.D., and Pearson, F.G.: Treatment of achalasia: esophagomyotomy with antireflux procedure. Can. J. Surg. 23:588, 1980.

Netscher, D., Larson, G.M., and Polk, H.C., Jr.: Radionuclide esophageal transit: a screening test for esophageal disorders. Arch. Surg. 121:843, 1986.

Okike, N., et al.: Esophagomyotomy for achalasia of the esophagus. Ann. Thorac. Surg. 32:119, 1979.

Ottinger, L.W., and Wilkins, E.W., Jr.: Late results in patients with Schatzki rings undergoing destruction of ring and hiatus herniorrhaphy. Am. J. Surg. 139:591, 1980.

Pierce, W.S., MacVaugh, H., III, and Johnson, J.: Carcinoma of the esophagus arising in patients with achalasia of the cardia. J. Thorac. Cardiovasc. Surg. 59:335, 1970.

Ramirez-Mata, M., Pena Ancira, F.F., and Alarcon-Segovia, D.: Abnormal esophageal motility in primary Sjögren's syndrome. J. Rheumatol. 3:63, 1976.

Richter, J.E., and Castell, D.O.: Diffuse esophageal spasm: a reappraisal. Ann. Intern. Med. 100:242, 1984.

Richter, J.E., et al.: Edrophonium: a useful provocative test for esophageal chest pain. Ann. Intern. Med. 103:14, 1985.

Rivkin, L., Bremner, C.G., and Bremner, C.H.: Pathophysiology of mid-oesophageal and epiphrenic diverticula of the oesophagus. S. Afr. Med. J. 66:127, 1984.

Sanderson, D.R., et al.: Syndrome of vigorous achalasia: clinical and physiologic observations. Dis. Chest. 52:508, 1967.

Seaman, W.B.: Cineroentgenographic observations of the cricopharyngeus. Am. J. Roentgenol. Radium. Ther. Nucl. Med. 96:922, 1966.

Simeone, J., Burrell, M., and Toffler, R.: Esophageal aperistalsis secondary to metastatic invasion of the myenteric plexus. Am. J. Roentgenol. 127:862, 1976.

Slater, G., and Sicular, A.A.: Esophageal perforations after forceful dilatation in achalasia. Ann. Surg. 195:186, 1982.

Smiley, T.B.: Pressure studies in the upper esophagus in relation to hiatus hernia. Paper 15. Surgery of the Oesophagus: the Coventry Conference. Edited by R.A. Smith and R.E. Smith. London, Butterworth, 1972.

Stewart, I.M., et al.: Oesophageal motor changes in diabetes mellitus. Thorax 31:278, 1976.

Sutherland, H.D.: Cricopharyngeal achalasia. J. Thorac. Cardiovasc. Surg. 43:114, 1962.

Sweet, R.H.: Surgical treatment of achalasia of the esophagus. N. Engl. J. Med. 254:87, 1956.

Thomas, E., et al.: Nifedipine therapy for diffuse esophageal spasm. South. Med. J. 79:847, 1986.

Traube, M., et al.: Effects of nifedipine in achalasia and in patients with high-amplitude peristaltic esophageal contractions. JAMA 252:1733, 1984.

Trier, J.S., and Bjorkman, D.J.: Esophageal, gastric, and intestinal candidiasis. Am. J. Med. 77:39, 1984.

Victor, M., Hayes, R., and Adams, R.D.: Oculopharyngeal muscular dystrophy, a familial disease of late life characterized by dysphagia and progressive ptosis of the eyelids. N. Engl. J. Med. 267:1267, 1962.

Wall, M.H., et al.: Giant esophagus; an unusual case of massive idiopathic hypertrophy and dilatation of the esophagus and proximal stomach. Ann. Thorac. Surg. 4:60, 1967.

Wilkins, E.W., Jr.: Thymectomy. In Modern Technique in Cardiac-Thoracic Surgery. Mt. Kisco, NY, Futura Publishing, 1981.

Witzel, L.: Treatment of achalasia with a pneumatic dilator attached to a gastroscope. Endoscop. 13:176, 1981.

READING REFERENCES

Cannon, W.B.: The acid closure of the cardia. Am. J. Physiol. 23:105, 1908.

Kronecker, H., and Meltzer, S.: Der Schluckmechanismus, seine Erregung und seine Hemmung. Arch. Anat. Physiol. Suppl. 1883, p. 328.

Schatzki, R.: The lower esophageal ring: long-term follow-up of symptomatic and asymptomatic rings. Am. J. Roentgenol. 90:805, 1963.

CHAPTER 81

ESOPHAGEAL DIVERTICULA

Victor F. Trastek and W. Spencer Payne

Esophageal diverticula are acquired conditions of the esophagus that occur almost exclusively in adults. Congenital esophageal diverticula are rare and probably are best classified as a variant of esophageal or alimentary duplication.

By definition, an esophageal diverticulum is a completely epithelial-lined blind pouch or pocket leading from the main lumen of the esophagus. Three specific types are commonly recognized: pharyngoesophageal—Zenker's pulsion diverticulum; epiphrenic or supradiaphragmatic—pulsion diverticulum; and parabronchial—traction diverticulum. Pulsion diverticula probably result from transmural pressure gradients that develop from within the esophagus to produce a herniation of mucosa through a weak point in the investing musculature. Traction diverticula result from the cicatricial contracture outside the esophagus, usually from inflammation in neighboring tracheobronchial lymph nodes affected by specific granulomatous diseases, especially histoplasmosis or tuberculous infections. Because these diverticula result from an external pulling force, they are called traction diverticula. Typically, they present as a broad-mouthed, conical deformity composed of all layers of the esophageal wall.

Although all three major types of esophageal diverticula can produce significant symptoms and disability, the pulsion diverticula at the upper or lower ends of the esophagus are the most frequently symptomatic. Symptoms and complications are mainly related to esophageal obstruction, esophageal retention, regurgitation, and secondary respiratory aspiration. Traction or midesophageal diverticula rarely produce difficulties, though bleeding, fistula formation, and esophageal obstruction have been reported. With a full understanding, esophageal diverticula offer a particularly rewarding opportunity for both precise diagnosis and effective treatment.

PHARYNGOESOPHAGEAL DIVERTICULUM

The pharyngoesophageal diverticulum is the most common of the symptomatic esophageal diverticula.

Characteristically, it presents as a posterior protrusion of pharyngeal mucosa between the oblique fibers of the inferior constrictor muscles of the pharynx, just cephalad to the transverse fibers of the cricopharyngeus muscle. Although this diverticulum was first described in 1769 by the English surgeon Ludlow, the name of the German surgeon Zenker became eponymically associated with the condition as a consequence of his lucid review in 1874.

Pathophysiology

The cause of pharyngoesophageal diverticulum is not known. Because it is usually seen in patients more than 50 years of age, and rarely in those less than 30 years old (Fig. 81–1), it is considered an acquired condition. However, Negus (1950) concluded that the constant site of origin just above the cricopharyngeus muscle suggests the possibility of an anatomic weak point in muscular layers, as well as some distal obstructive role of the cricopharyngeus muscle. Although considerable speculation regarding the nature of this obstruction has developed since the report of Zenker and von Ziemssen (1874), most of the disorders described have been based more

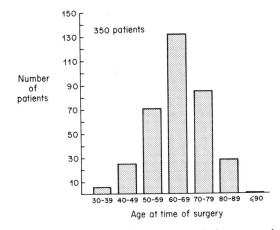

Fig. 81–1. Age distribution of 350 patients with pharyngoesophageal diverticulum treated at the Mayo Clinic (1964 through 1971).

on theory than on fact. Smiley and associates (1970) and Hunt and associates (1970) suggested that gastroesophageal reflux results in a reflex increase of the resting tone of the cricopharyngeus muscle.

A retrospective review of Mayo Clinic material (Table 81–1) revealed a high incidence—33%—of associated esophageal conditions, but it did not confirm the universal incidence of hiatal hernia, as Smiley and associates (1970) suggested. In an unpublished prospective study of 75 patients, we saw a nearly 97% incidence of anatomic hiatal hernia. Reflux symptoms, however, were rare, and only 1 of the 75 required antireflux surgery at the time of diverticulectomy. Furthermore, Winans (1972) was unable to confirm the contention of Smiley and associates that reflux causes elevation of cricopharyngeal pressure, and he suggested that the orientation of the catheter orifice during pressure recording of the cricopharyngeus affects the magnitude of pressure recorded. Finally, manometric studies conducted at the Mayo Clinic by Ellis and associates (1969) failed to confirm the presence of either achalasia or hypertension of the cricopharyngeus in patients with this diverticulum. Nevertheless, those studies did define an abnormal temporal relationship between pharyngeal contraction and sphincteric relaxation and contraction with swallowing. In patients with diverticula, upper esophageal sphincteric contraction occurred before completion of pharyngeal contraction. Thus, premature contraction of the upper sphincter was implicated as characteristic of pharyngoesophageal diverticulum. Although these studies provide a definite pattern of the events occurring in patients with diverticula, they fail to define the cause of the observed incoordination. The fact that premature sphincteric contraction was noted in small, early diverticula, as well as in large, established ones, strongly implicates cricopharyngeal incoordination as their cause. Although most of the patients with diverticula are of an age in which cerebrovascular disease may be present, associated overt neurologic deficits are rare in these patients.

Thus, the act of swallowing in the presence of cricopharyngeal incoordination, combined with the usual pressure phenomena during deglutition, is now believed to generate sufficient transmural pressure to allow mucosal herniation through an anatomically weak point in the posterior pharynx above the cricopharyngeus muscle. Because of the recurrent nature of pressures involved and the constant distention of the sac with ingested material, the established diverticulum enlarges rapidly and descends dependently. The neck of the diverticulum hangs over the cricopharyngeus, and the sac becomes interposed between the esophagus and the vertebrae. Indeed, the advanced diverticulum may come to lie in the same vertical axis as the pharynx, permitting selective filling of the sac, which may compress and angulate the adjacent esophagus anteriorly. These anatomic changes obstruct swallowing. Moreover because the mouth of the diverticulum is above the cricopharyngeus, spontaneous emptying of the diverticulum is unimpeded and often associated with laryngotracheal aspiration, as well as regurgitation into the mouth.

Symptoms and Diagnosis

Although the pharyngoesophageal diverticulum may be asymptomatic or may not be suspected until after complications develop, most are symptomatic from the onset. Characteristically, the symptoms are progressive and consist of high cervical esophageal dysphagia, foul breath, noisy deglutition, and spontaneous regurgitation with or without coughing, choking, or strangling episodes. The regurgitated food is characteristically fresh and undigested and is not bitter, sour, or contaminated by gastroduodenal secretions. If the condition is neglected, weight loss, hoarseness, asthma, respiratory insufficiency, pulmonary sepsis, or a soft, palpable cervical mass may occur. Although the chief complications of pharyngoesophageal diverticulum are nutritional and respiratory, Wychulis and associates (1969) recorded that the diverticulum may occasionally be the site of a primary malignancy. Futhermore, diverticular perforation may occur with any esophageal intubation or instrumentation or with the accidental ingestion of a foreign body.

Diagnosis is confirmed by roentgenographic examination (Fig. 81–2). Usually, this diagnostic study is the only one required. Studies of esophageal motility and esophagoscopy are rarely indicated, and then only to assess some unusual associated clinical or roentgenographic feature. Complete esophageal obstruction caused by impacted food bolus or foreign body, suspected diverticular neoplasm, and distal esophageal abnormalities are chief indications for endoscopy. When required, esophagoscopy in patients with a diverticulum should probably use a previously swallowed thread as a guide.

Treatment

The treatment of a pharyngoesophageal diverticulum is surgical. All patients with such diverticula should be considered candidates for treatment, irrespective of the size of the diverticulum. Treatment is best done on an elective prophylactic basis while the pouch is small or of moderate size and before complications have occurred. When nutritional or respiratory complications are present, or when neoplasm is suspected, surgical interven-

Table 81–1. Associated Esophageal Conditions in 110 of 331 Patients Who Underwent Pharyngoesophageal Diverticulectomy at the Mayo Clinic, 1958 Through 1971

Associated Condition	No. of Patients
Esophageal hiatal hernia	77
Other esophageal diverticula	26
Achalasia of esophagus	5
Diffuse spasm of esophagus	1
Primary cancer of diverticulum	1
Total	110

Welsh, G.F., and Payne, W.S.: The present status of one-stage pharyngo-esophageal diverticulectomy. Surg. Clin. North Am. 53:953, 1973.

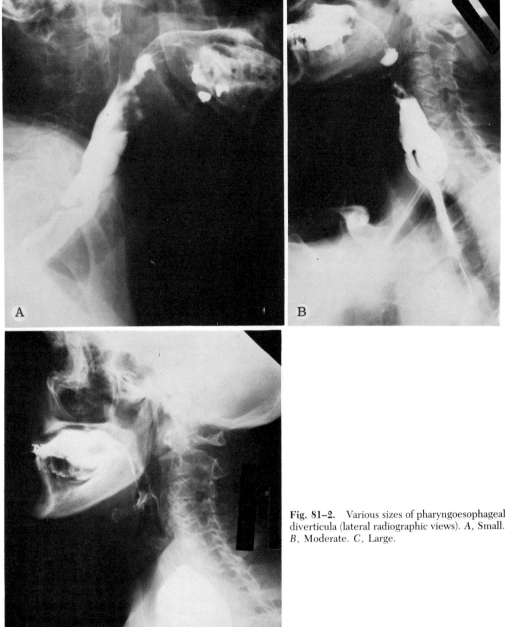

Fig. 81–2. Various sizes of pharyngoesophageal diverticula (lateral radiographic views). *A*, Small. *B*, Moderate. *C*, Large.

tion becomes urgent. Diverticular perforation is a surgical emergency.

Evolution of Current Surgical Management

Just before 1900, various innovative procedures were carried out for the treatment of this diverticulum, not all of which were successful. These procedures included one-stage extirpation, invagination, and diverticulopexy. Because of the high morbidity and mortality associated with these early efforts, a two-stage diverticulectomy was developed by Goldmann in 1909, and subsequently popularized by C.H. Mayo—cited by Terracol and Sweet (1958)—and by Lahey and Warren (1954) in this country. To prevent subsequent spread of infection, the first stage of this operation was designed to seal the fascial planes of the neck. At the second-stage operation, diverticulectomy could be performed without risk of sepsis, though a temporary fistula frequently occurred. Largely through the pioneering efforts of Harrington (1939), Sweet (1947), Shallow and Clerf (1948), and Clagett—Clagett and Payne (1960), Payne and Clagett (1965)—a safe, highly successful one-stage diverticulectomy was evolved and continues to be the preferred method.

Other approaches have been used successfully. Dohlman and Mattsson (1959) employed a peroral endoscopic diathermic division of the septum or common wall between the diverticulum and the esophagus. This technique was popularized in the United States by Holinger and Schild (1969) and by van Overbeek (1977) in the Netherlands. Sutherland (1962) employed cricopharyngeal myotomy alone; Cross and his associates (1961) used it as an adjunct to extirpation, and Belsey (1966) as an adjunct to diverticulopexy. Because of our experience, reported by Ellis and associates (1969), with cricopharyngeal myotomy, we now recommend this procedure alone for small diverticula and reserve the one-stage diverticulectomy for larger sacs, as Welsh and one of us (W.S.P.) (1973) noted. Since the 1970s we have added myotomy to diverticulectomy in hopes of further improving the highly satisfactory results of diverticulectomy alone.

Preoperative Preparation

Most patients undergoing surgical treatment require little or no preoperative preparation. Rarely are nutritional deficiencies severe enough to require preoperative parenteral hyperalimentation or gastrostomy. Prompt repair of the diverticulum provides the best means of correcting most deficiences. Suppurative lung diseases, too, often require definitive resolution of the diverticular problem before they can be effectively managed. Occasionally, esophageal bougienage temporarily ameliorates esophageal obstructive symptoms and temporarily palliates nutritional and respiratory complications, but the patient is usually best served by prompt surgical treatment of the diverticulum.

Surgical Techniques

Two techniques are currently employed at our institution: cricopharyngeal myotomy alone for the small sacs (Fig. 81–3) and one-stage pharyngoesophageal diverticulectomy with cricopharyngeal myotomy for the larger ones (Fig. 81–4).

Either regional cervical blocks or general anesthesia can be used satisfactorily, but currently almost all patients receive general anesthesia with a cuffed endotracheal tube. This technique controls not only the inspired gas concentrations and ventilation but also the airway, and prevents intraoperative respiratory aspiration. Various incisions can be used to obtain surgical exposure, whether myotomy or diverticulectomy is planned. Right-handed surgeons find the left cervical approach (Figs. 81–3 and 81–4) easiest for exposing most diverticula, unless an uncommon right-sided origin of the diverticulum is noted before operation. We have used both horizontal and oblique lower cervical incisions with equal ease and cosmetic result. Usually, we employ an oblique incision along the anterior border of the sternocleidomastoid, extending from the level of the hyoid bone to a point 1 cm above the clavicle. After the incision has been deepened, surgical exposure of the retropharyngeal space and the diverticulum is obtained by retracting the sternocleidomastoid muscle and carotid sheath laterally and the thyroid gland and larynx medially. The diverticulum can be recognized promptly as arising from the posterior wall of the pharynx at a point just above the level where the omohyoid muscle crosses the incision (Fig. 81–4).

The apex of the diverticulum is grasped with an Allis forceps and is elevated into the wound. Dissection of the diverticulum is carried down to its neck or site of origin. Dissection of the neck of the diverticulum must be performed carefully so as not to injure the mucosa. Whether myotomy or diverticulectomy is to be performed, the surgeon must thoroughly dissect out the diverticulum, identifying the margins of the pharyngeal muscular defect through which the mucosal sac protrudes.

Cricopharyngeal Myotomy

After the diverticulum is freed to its neck, a scalpel is used to make a vertical incision in the transverse fibers of the cricopharyngeal muscle (Fig. 81–3b). Beginning immediately below the neck of the diverticulum, this incision is carried down to the mucosa and extended distally onto the esophagus. The total length of the extramucosal myotomy is about 3 cm. As with other esophagomyotomies, divided muscle must be dissected from approximately half of the circumference of the mucosal tube to assure complete muscle division and allow the mucosa to protrude freely through the myotomy (Fig. 81–3b). When the dissection is properly and appropriately performed, one sees the narrow-necked mucosal diverticulum transformed into a broad-based, diffuse mucosal bulge. The cervical incision is closed around two small Penrose drains brought from the retropharyngeal space to the outside through the lower end of the incision. Oral intake can be resumed during the immediate postoperative period; drains are removed and hospital convalescence is completed in 48 to 72 hours.

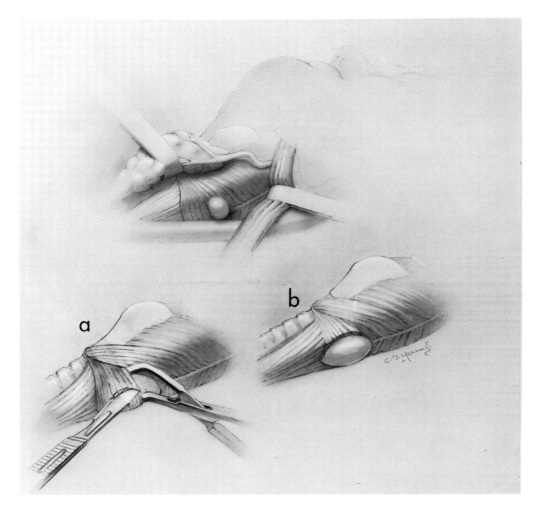

Fig. 81–3. Technique of cricopharyngeal myotomy. Myotomy alone is employed for the treatment of small pharyngoesophageal diverticula. Surgical exposure of the retropharyngeal space is gained through an oblique left cervical incision oriented along the anterior border of the sternomastoid muscle (not shown). Retraction of the sternomastoid and carotid sheath laterally and the thyroid, pharynx, and larynx medially provides necessary exposure of the diverticulum, which is located at a cervical level where the omohyoid crosses the surgical field. (Note that the omohyoid in the upper center of drawing has been retracted cephalad to show the diverticulum.) After connective tissue is dissected from the mucosal sac to identify the defect in the posterior pharyngeal wall (*a*), a right-angle forceps is used to develop a dissection plane inferiorly between the muscularis and the mucosa. A posterior midline extramucosal myotomy is effected with a scalpel from the neck of the small sac inferiorly for a distance of 3 cm. With retraction of the ends of the cut muscle (*b*), an almond-shaped diffuse bulge of mucosa through the myotomy is seen. A small Penrose drain is brought from the region of the myotomy and retropharyngeal space through the lower end of the cervical wound to the outside, and the platysma and skin are closed in layers around the drain.

Pharyngoesophageal Diverticulectomy With Myotomy

Surgical exposure through a cervical incision is the same as for myotomy. After the diverticulum is freed to its neck, the surrounding ring of muscular tissue is clearly defined. With the diverticulum held cephalad, a dissection plane is developed between the muscularis and the mucosa just below the neck of the diverticulum (Fig. 81–4*a*). A vertical 3-cm long myotomy is made. The neck of the mucosal sac is amputated and closed, simply by applying a curved clamp to the neck of the sac at right angles to the long axis of the esophagus (Fig. 81–4*c*). Care is taken to avoid drawing too much of the esophageal mucosa into the clamp by placing a catheter in the esophageal lumen before applying the curved clamp. By the cut-and-sew technique, the sac is amputated and the

mucosal defect closed. Alternatively, as Hoehn and one of us (W. S. P.) (1969) suggested, one of the commercially available stapling devices can be used. Since the 1970s we use the TA stapling devices for transecting and closing the diverticular neck. Stapling improves the speed and accuracy of closure (Fig. 81–5). The mucosal closure, be it suture or staple line, is covered with a row of vertical sutures placed in the pharyngoesophageal musculature (Fig. 81–4*e* and *f*). Soft Penrose drains are brought from the area of repair to the outside through the incision, which is closed around them. A small suction wound catheter placed in the retropharyngeal space is equally effective. Diet is resumed the morning after operation. If drainage is minimal, the surgical drains are removed 48 to 72 hours after operation, and the patient is ready

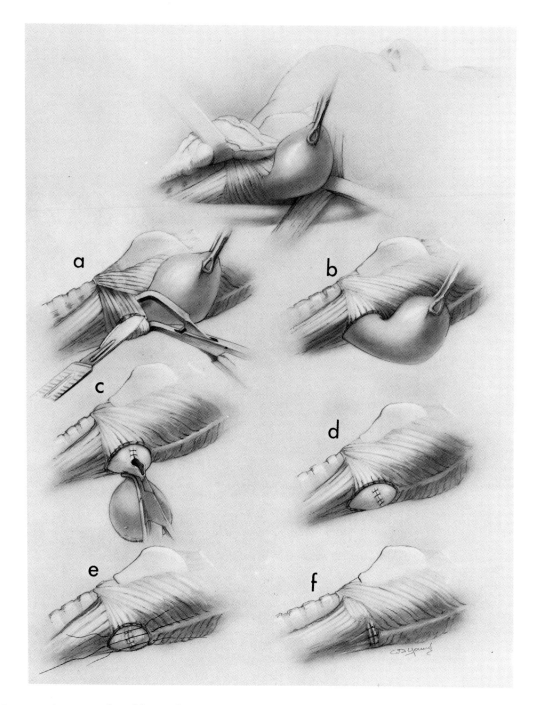

Fig. 81–4.   One-stage pharyngoesophageal diverticulectomy with myotomy. This procedure is employed in the management of medium- and large-sized diverticula. *Top*, Medium-sized diverticulum exposed through left cervical incision, as for myotomy alone. Note that the omohyoid has been retracted cephalad and the diverticulum has been dissected out to its neck and its apex held cephalad. A right-angle forceps (*a*) is used to develop a dissection plane between the muscularis and the mucosa just below the neck of the sac in preparation for extramucosal myotomy with the scalpel. After a 3-cm vertical myotomy is completed (*b*), the neck of the mucosal sac appears to have widened. With a No. 28-F catheter in the esophagus (*c*), a curved clamp is placed across the neck of the diverticulum at right angles to the long axis of the esophagus at the point of planned amputation. With a cut-and-sew technique, the sac is amputated stepwise and closed using fine vascular silk (5-0) placed so that tied knots are within the esophageal lumen. Alternatively, a stapling device can be used. Diverticulectomy and closure are completed (*d*). Vertical absorbable sutures are placed in the edges of the muscular defect after myotomy and diverticulectomy (*e*). This completed transverse closure (*f*) provides a muscular layer closure over the mucosal suture line, which further minimizes leakage without restitution of the cricopharyngeus. Drainage and closure are effected, as with myotomy alone.

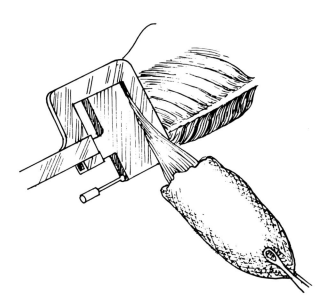

Fig. 81–5. As an alternative to the cut-and-sew techique (Fig. 81–4c) of diverticulectomy, since 1969 we have routinely used the TA stapling device to transect and close the neck of the diverticulum. Depending on the size of the diverticulum, a TA-15, TA-30, or TA-55 stapling device has been selected. Most require TA-30 with 4.8-mm staples. Note that the stapling device is oriented at right angles to the long axis of the esophagus and that an indwelling 28F esophageal catheter is used to prevent stenosis and minimize the length of any luminal narrowing. The use of a stapling device greatly enhances the speed and accuracy of diverticular neck amputation and closure. Myotomy and burying of the staple line are effected as illustrated in Figure 81–4. (Reproduced with permission from Payne, W.S., and Reynolds, R.R.: Surgical treatment of pharyngoesophageal diverticulum [Zenker's diverticulum]. Surg. Rounds 5:18, 1982. Copyright ©1982 by Romaine Pierson Publishers, Inc., Port Washington, New York.)

to leave the hospital on the fourth or fifth postoperative day.

Results

As Clagett and one of us (W.S.P.) (1960) reported, the results of the one-stage pharyngoesophageal diverticulectomy have been most gratifying. From 1944 through 1971, 809 patients were treated at the Mayo Clinic by this means, and the operative mortality was 1.4%. The chief complications were recurrent nerve palsy—2.8%—and esophagocutaneous fistula—2.5%. Generally, both of these complications are only temporary problems that clear spontaneously in a matter of days or weeks. In a 5- to 14-year follow-up of 164 surgical patients, Welsh and one of us (W.S.P.) (1973) found that 93% either were asymptomatic or had such rare and mild symptoms that they could be classified as having an excellent–82%—or a good—11%—result. Only 11—7%—of the 164 had poor results, with or without anatomic recurrence, and required additional treatment. During the past 15 years, we have incorporated cricopharyngeal myotomy with equally satisfactory results. One of our (W.S.P.) and Reynolds' (1982) late follow-up results show little change in the incidence of late diverticular recurrence, which has been minimal in either event. Any roentgenographic recurrence is less likely to be symptomatic if the initial diverticulectomy was accompanied by myotomy. We

continue to use myotomy both for this reason and for theoretical considerations.

A word of caution on reoperation for recurrent pharyngoesophageal diverticulum: a review of Huang and associates (1984a) of this aspect of diverticular surgery clearly indicated an increased risk of early postoperative morbidity. Indeed, when our results of reoperation were analyzed separately from those for primary operations, almost all the morbidity recorded in the total experience was confined to patients undergoing second or third procedures. Fortunately, long-term results were essentially at the same satisfactory level in both groups.

Cricopharyngeal myotomy alone is required relatively uncommonly in our experience and has been restricted to treatment of the smaller diverticula. In 24 operations reviewed, no deaths or complications occurred and hospital stay has been shortened from the usual 5 days with diverticulectomy to 3 days with myotomy.

Cancer arising in Zenker's diverticulum is rare, but apparently more common than in the general population. It appears to occur in chronically neglected or retained diverticula. Huang and associates (1984b) reported that in two patients with cancer totally confined to the sac, simple diverticulectomy provided long-term survival. More aggressive management would seem indicated if there is extension beyond the sac.

EPIPHRENIC OR PULSION DIVERTICULUM OF THE THORACIC ESOPHAGUS

Pulsion diverticula of the thoracic esophagus occur less frequently than those in the pharyngoesophageal region. During the 1950s through the 1980s at the Mayo Clinic, the relative incidence of these two types of diverticula remained approximately 1 to 5. The ages of our patients with thoracic diverticula have ranged from 25 to 80 years at the time of diagnosis, with a ratio of 2 to 1 for men to women. Pulsion diverticula of the thoracic esophagus have been encountered at almost every esophageal level, but because of their predilection for the lower 10 cm of the thoracic esophagus, they are generally referred to as epiphrenic or, less frequently, supradiaphragmatic diverticula. Most of the diverticula develop as a mucosal protrusion or herniation between the muscular fibers on the right side of the thoracic esophagus, and when large, they may protrude into the right pleural space. Although this type of diverticulum was first described by Deguise in 1804, little progress was made in basic understanding and management of the condition until modern techniques for clinical investigation and thoracic surgical intervention became available.

Etiology, Development, and Pathophysiology

Most, if not all, of these diverticula result from functional or mechanical esophageal obstruction. This characteristic was probably first appreciated by Vinson in 1934 and subsequently emphasized by Harrington (1939), Goodman and Parnes (1952), Cross (1961), Effler and associates (1959), Habein and their co-workers (1956a, b), and by Allen and Clagett (1965).

The inference is that these diverticula develop as a mucosal protrusion through some weak point in the esophageal musculature, such as occurs in the evolution of pharyngoesophageal diverticulum. The forces involved, however, are more definable, although the site of protrusion varies. Significantly, most of these diverticula develop in the portion of the esophagus invested with smooth muscle. The pathogenesis of the symptoms of epiphrenic diverticulum is less clear. Many patients are asymptomatic at the time of diagnosis. In others, although symptoms seem to be compatible with a diverticulum, they are difficult to differentiate from identical symptoms caused by almost ubiquitous associated esophageal conditions.

Debas and associates (1980) completed a review of 65 patients with epiphrenic diverticulum in whom roentgenographic, endoscopic, and manometric studies were performed. Fifty patients—77%—had manometric evidence of abnormal motility: 21 with diffuse spasm, 13 with achalasia, 6 with hypercontracting lower esophageal sphincter, and 10 with nonspecific motor disturbance. Of the 15 patients—23%—with normal esophageal motility, 13 had a hiatal hernia, and 5 of these had a high-grade organic distal esophageal stricture. Only 8 of the 65 patients studied had no definable organic or functional abnormality associated with the esophageal diverticulum. Although this information confirms the wisdom of performing esophagomyotomy concomitantly with diverticulectomy in most patients, it also indicates the possibility of individualization of therapy when complete studies can be performed before operation. Furthermore, this review suggests that organic obstruction to the distal portion of the esophagus, as well as functional obstruction, must be identified to plan effective treatment.

Symptoms and Diagnosis

Most patients with epiphrenic diverticula either have been asymptomatic or have had such mild symptoms at diagnosis that extensive investigation and therapy are not warranted. In others, symptoms seem to be compatible with a diverticulum, but at times symptoms have been difficult to differentiate from associated mechanical and functional conditions. Dysphagia, esophageal retention, and regurgitation are frequent and characteristic of diverticula, but symptoms of associated diaphragmatic hernia, esophagitis, stricture, diffuse spasm, or achalasia may be dominant and identical. Secondary symptoms of respiratory aspiration are seen, but less frequently than in patients with pharyngoesophageal diverticulum. Primary carcinoma has been occasionally noted with epiphrenic diverticula, as Allen and Clagett (1965) reported, as have rare benign neoplasms, particularly leiomyoma and lipoma.

Roentgenographic examination of the esophagus is the most reliable means of determining the presence of a pulsion diverticulum of the thoracic esophagus (Fig. 81–6). Endoscopic examination and studies of esophageal motility are essential in evaluating patients and defining the nature and severity of associated conditions. Esoph-

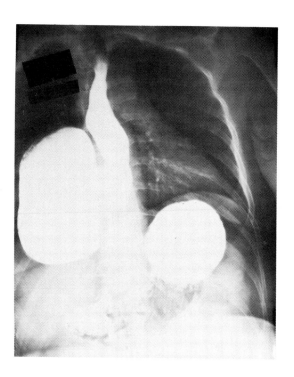

Fig. 81–6. Esophagus with huge epiphrenic diverticulum occupying approximately half of the right thorax. Note associated sliding esophageal hiatal hernia.

agoscopy also may be required not only for diagnosing the condition but also for removing retained debris from the sac before operation in patients with severe retention and regurgitation.

Treatment, Techniques, and Results

Treatment is surgical and is indicated chiefly in patients with symptoms, particularly when the symptoms are progressive or incapacitating. Simple medical measures often provide good temporary control in mildly symptomatic patients. Diverticulectomy should be considered when an operation is planned for the management of associated esophageal conditions, even when symptoms cannot be definitely attributed to the diverticulum. Surgical treatment also should be considered for any diverticulum that is progressively enlarging and for any that is already large, irrespective of symptoms.

Clairmont performed the first extirpation of an epiphrenic diverticulum in 1927, using an extrapleural approach. A transpleural approach was first reported by Barrett in 1933. The technique currently employed at the Mayo Clinic is a transthoracic diverticulectomy, usually with a long extramucosal esophagomyotomy (Fig. 81–7). The frequently associated sliding esophageal hiatal hernia is repaired at operation. One of the nonobstructive antireflux procedures is advised. Any associated esophageal obstructive condition must be corrected at or before operation, not only to prevent suture-line leak and diverticular recurrence but also to relieve the symptoms from the associated condition. No operative mortality has occurred, and long-term results in 18 patients treated in this manner have been good. In our total experience with 55 patients who underwent surgical

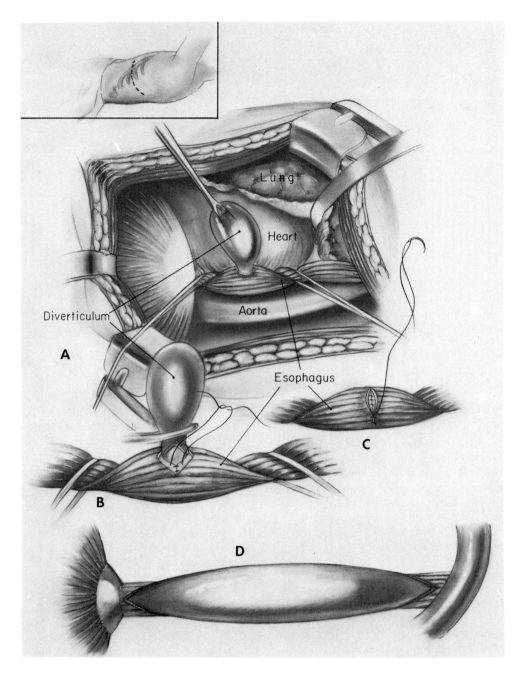

Fig. 81–7. Surgical management of pulsion diverticulum of the lower portion of the esophagus. *Inset*, Placement of left posterolateral thoracotomy incision. *A*, Exposure of diverticulum obtained when the chest is entered through the bed of the left eighth rib. Note that the esophagus has been delivered from its mediastinal bed, tapes have been passed around the esophagus, and the esophagus has been rotated to bring the diverticulum into view. The neck of the mucosal diverticulum has been dissected, identifying the defect in the esophageal muscular wall. *B*, Cut-and-sew technique of diverticulectomy. Note that amputation and closure are effected in a transverse axis. Mucosal sutures are tied with knots within the esophageal lumen. *C*, Closure of esophageal musculature over mucosal suture line. *D*, Site of diverticular incision has been rotated back to the right and is not visible. A long esophagomyotomy, extending from esophagogastric junction to aortic arch, has been performed. The musculature of the esophagus has been freed from approximately 50% of circumference of the esophageal mucosal tube to allow mucosa to bulge through the muscular incision. Frequently associated sliding esophageal hiatal hernia is shown; when present, it should be repaired at operation. (Payne, W.S.: Diverticula of the esophagus. *In* The Esophagus. Edited by W.S. Payne and A.M. Olsen. Philadelphia, Lea & Febiger, 1974, p. 207.)

treatment for epiphrenic diverticulum, 2 deaths have occurred. One death happened with induction of anesthesia, which resulted in regurgitation and massive respiratory aspiration before the operation was performed. The other death occurred after operation, as a consequence of suture-line leak and empyema. Four patients in the series had late recurrent epiphrenic diverticula. Although the failure to use esophagomyotomy in conjunction with diverticulectomy may be associated with recurrence or suture-line complication and postoperative death, these sequelae are not inevitable results of its omission. One may infer from the data, however, only that every effort should be made to correct associated esophageal conditions to minimize postoperative complications and symptoms. We have found that early radiographic examination of the esophagus using absorbable contrast medium—Gastrografin—before starting an oral diet is particularly valuable in the postoperative management of these patients. This examination permits a final assessment of the suture line at the diverticulectomy site and evaluation of an unobstructed esophagogastric lumen. When leak or obstruction is encountered, parenteral hyperalimentation is continued for 3 weeks before restudy and resumption of oral diet. Patients are generally asymptomatic after operation if associated esophageal conditions have been adequately dealt with at operation.

TRACTION, MIDESOPHAGEAL, OR PARABRONCHIAL DIVERTICULUM

The incidence of these diverticula appears to parallel that of specific granulomatous disease, especially tuberculosis or histoplasmosis. Esophageal involvement by mediastinal granuloma is uncommon but may present as esophageal compression, stricture, diverticulum, or sinus tract or tracheoesophageal fistula, as Dukes (1976) and MacCarty (1979) and their associates pointed out. Traction diverticula, however, are usually of only passing clinical interest. Because of the configuration and size of these diverticula (Fig. 81–8), symptoms are rare. Occasionally, dysphagia or odynophagia occurs, presumably caused by compression, stricture, or inflammation in the diverticulum. Local esophagitis may occur, suggesting that the discharging caseous material may irritate the esophageal mucosa. Fistulization to the tracheobronchial tree occasionally results from inflammatory necrosis of the originating granuloma. Similar but rarer communications have been found between the esophagus and the great vessels, as Powell (1957) and Cheitlin and associates (1961) noted, but most hemorrhagic manifestations are probably caused by friable granulation tissue or erosion of small bronchial or esophageal vessels by calcific debris, as Schick and Yesner (1953) and Jonasson and Gunn (1965) pointed out.

When the condition is symptomatic, surgical treatment is indicated. After the process is defined by roentgenographic studies and by esophagoscopy, surgical intervention usually can be undertaken without fear of complication by specific organisms, because inciting bac-

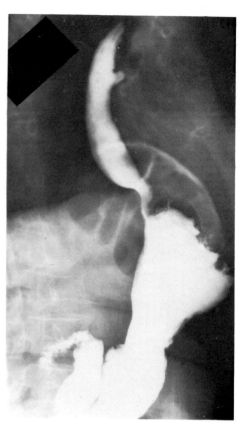

Fig. 81–8. Esophagus with traction diverticulum in middle third of thoracic portion in relation to subcarinal lymph nodes. Patient was asymptomatic. (Payne, W.S.: Diverticula of the esophagus. *In* The Esophagus. Edited by W.S. Payne and A.M. Olsen. Philadelphia, Lea & Febiger, 1974, p. 207.)

teria generally have been eliminated. Local excision of the diverticulum and adjacent inflammatory mass, with layer closure of the esophagus over an indwelling 40 to 50 Fr catheter, is usually all that is required for the symptomatic uncomplicated traction diverticulum. Fistulas with the respiratory tract or blood vessels require similar excisions and closure of the airway or vessel as well (Fig. 81–9). Recurrence of fistula is minimized by the interposition of viable pleural pedicle, connective tissue, or muscle. As with any esophageal suture line, care should be taken to eliminate any distal esophageal obstruction.

Among the causes for acquired, nonmalignant esophagorespiratory fistulas seen at the Mayo Clinic, Wychulis and associates (1966) found that infection by tuberculosis or fungi was second only to trauma in frequency. Others, including Davis and co-workers (1956) and Hutchin and Lindskog (1964), have commented on the occurrence of this occult but common cause for acquired tracheoesophageal fistula. The chance that such a fistula would develop in a patient with a traction diverticulum of the esophagus probably is remote, yet such a possibility should be considered in a patient with chronic suppurative lung disease or in one with symptoms of cough after swallowing. In evaluating such patients, roentgen-

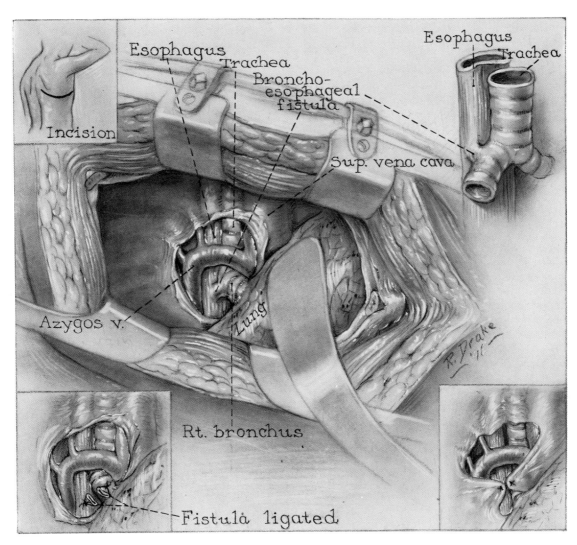

Fig. 81–9. Technique for closing acquired esophagobronchial fistula as a complication of a traction diverticulum of the esophagus. *Upper left inset*, Right posterolateral thoracotomy incision. *Center*, Surgical exposure. Lung has been retracted anteriorly. Note the relationship of the esophagus, right main bronchus, and fistula to neighboring sutures. *Upper right and lower left insets*, Fistula before division and after division and ligation. *Lower right inset*, Method of interposing pedicles of mediastinal pleura between esophageal and bronchial closures. (Reproduced with permission from Payne, W.S., and Clagett, O.T.: Pharyngeal and esophageal diverticula. *In* Current Problems in Surgery. Edited by M.M. Ravitch, et al. Copyright ©1965 by Year Book Medical Publishers, Inc., Chicago.)

ographic examination of the esophagus should be performed. Cinefluoroscopy during the ingestion of contrast medium usually defines the site and size of a communication and aids in screening many other patients suspected of having a fistula. Many of the latter patients are actually aspirating ingested material through the larynx because of some other mechanism than fistula. Leisurely study of a cine filmstrip provides a more precise diagnosis. Endoscopic examination of both the esophagus and the tracheobronchial tree is indicated, and the orifices of the fistula usually can be identified. The introduction of methylene blue or other dye into the esophagus during bronchoscopy may facilitate this identification. Appropriate biopsy material should be obtained for histopathologic and microbiologic study, although viable organisms are rarely identified. If symptoms suggest chronic pulmonary suppuration, bronchography or CT scan of the lungs is indicated to delineate the extent of bronchiectasis that might require surgical management at the time of fistula repair.

In addition to division of the fistula and repair of the esophagus and airway, attention must be paid to correction of distal esophageal obstruction, whether it is organic or is one of the specific esophageal motility disturbances. A particularly useful maneuver under such circumstances is the passage of a 40 to 50 Fr esophageal dilator using a previously swallowed thread as a guide. Its easy passage to the stomach assures the absence of an organically obstructed esophagus. Although traction diverticula are rarely complicated by specific esophageal motility disturbances, esophageal manometry is the most reliable means of defining these conditions.

Esophagovascular fistulas such as those reported by Schick and Yesner (1953), Powell (1957) and Jonasson and Gunn (1965) are rare complications of traction diverticula. Impressive hemorrhage may occur without communication with a major vessel; this may provide additional time for orderly study and treatment. All too often, initial bleeding is sudden, massive, and fatal when major vessels are involved. In addition to standard endoscopic and roentgenographic studies, selective arteriography during active bleeding can help define the site of hemorrhage.

AN OVERVIEW OF THORACIC-ESOPHAGEAL DIVERTICULA

Most esophageal diverticula are readily classifiable as either pulsion or traction type. One should be cautious in ascribing any thoracic esophageal diverticulum to either traction or pulsion on the basis of anatomic location alone. We have seen typical epiphrenic pulsion diverticula complete with associated motility disturbances located at the level of carinal lymph nodes which at operation had no relationship to these nodes, nor were nodes affected by any disease process. In contrast, we have seen mediastinal and pulmonary granulomas produce symptomatic traction diverticula in the lower 10 cm of the esophagus—a location suggestive of a pulsion diverticulum. Also, typical pulsion diverticula have been encountered with significant peridiverticulitis or ancient granulomas in which a traction element could not be ruled out.

Although such lesions may pose some classification problems for the purist, they do emphasize the need for complete esophageal evaluation before operation to define possible etiologic and complicating associated functional and organic pathologic changes of the esophagus that must be considered along with the diverticulum. The concept of a pulsion-traction diverticulum is appealing in some circumstances but probably represents nothing more than the progression of a pre-existing traction diverticulum as a pulsion diverticulum in a patient who subsequently develops functional or organic esophageal obstruction and in whom the mucosal sac merely develops at the vulnerable predetermined site.

Furthermore, it is probably inappropriate to rely too rigidly on a purist's view that pulsion diverticula are only mucosal protrusions without a muscular coat, because pulsion diverticula may have a thin layer of attenuated muscle and connective tissue adherent to the external surface of the mucosal sac. Only when well organized, thick layers of completely investing musculature are present should one seriously consider the diverticulum to be congenital, and then it is probably best classified as a duplication of the foregut. In many of these congenital malformations, the mucosal lining proves to be glandular and not squamous epithelium. An epithelialized sinus tract or an intramural esophageal abscess should be not be confused with a diverticulum. Diffuse intramural microdiverticulosis of the esophagus, as Andrén and Theander (1956) reported, is seen occasionally in association with esophageal moniliasis but also may occur without specific cause, as Castillo and associates (1977) emphasized. The microdiverticula are believed to be dilated esophageal submucosal glands. Approximately half of the patients develop esophageal strictures that respond to bougienage. The clinical course is generally benign.

REFERENCES

Allen, T.H., and Clagett, O.T.: Changing concepts in the surgical treatment of pulsion diverticula of the lower esophagus. J. Thorac. Cardiovasc. Surg. 50:455, 1965.

Andrén, L., and Theander, G.: Roentgenographic appearances of esophageal moniliasis. Acta Radiol. 46:571, 1956.

Barrett, N.R.: Diverticula of the thoracic oesophagus: report of a case in which the diverticulum was successfully resected. Lancet 1:1009, 1933.

Belsey, R.: Functional disease of the esophagus. J. Thorac. Cardiovasc. Surg. 52:164, 1966.

Castillo, S., et al.: Diffuse intramural esophageal pseudodiverticulosis: new cases and review. Gastroenterology 72:541, 1977.

Cheitlin, M.D., Kamin, E.J., and Wilkes, D.J.: Midesophageal diverticulum: report of a case with fistulous connection with the superior vena cava. Arch. Intern. Med. 107:252, 1961.

Clagett, O.T., and Payne, W.S.: Surgical treatment of pulsion diverticula of the hypopharynx: one-stage resection in 478 cases. Dis. Chest. 37:257, 1960.

Clairmont: Cited by Moynihan, B.: Diverticula of the alimentary canal. Lancet 1:1061, 1927.

Cross, F.S., Johnson, G.F., and Gerein, A.N.: Esophageal diverticula: associated neuromuscular changes in the esophagus. Arch. Surg. 83:525, 1961.

Davis, F.W., Katz, S., and Peabody, J.W., Jr.: Broncholithiasis, a neglected cause of broncoesophageal fistula. JAMA 160:555, 1956.

Debas, H.T., et al.: Pathophysiology of lower esophageal diverticulum and its implications for treatment: Surg. Gynecol. Obstet. 151:593, 1980.

Deguise, F.: Dissertation sur l'anévrisme, suivie de propositions médicales sur divers objets, et des aphorismes d'Hippocrate sur le spasme. Thesis, Paris, 1804.

Dohlman, G., and Mattsson, O.: The role of the cricopharyngeal muscle in cases of hypopharyngeal diverticula: a cineroentgenographic study. Am. J. Roentgenol. 81:561, 1959.

Dukes, R.J., et al.: Esophageal involvement with mediastinal granuloma. JAMA 236:2313, 1976.

Effler, D.B., Barr, D., and Groves, L.K.: Epiphrenic diverticulum of the esophagus: surgical treatment. Arch Surg. 79:459, 1959.

Ellis, F.H., Jr., et al.: Cricopharyngeal myotomy for pharyngo-esophageal diverticulum. Ann. Surg. 170:340, 1969.

Goldmann, E.E.: Die zweizeitige Operation von Pulsiondivertikeln der Speiseröhre: nebst Bemerkungen über den Oesophagusmund. Beitr. Klin. Chir. 61:741, 1909.

Goodman, H.I., and Parnes, I.H.: Epiphrenic diverticula of the esophagus. J. Thorac. Cardiovasc. Surg. 23:145, 1952.

Habein, H.C., Jr., et al.: Surgical treatment of lower esophageal pulsion diverticula. Arch. Surg. 72:1018, 1956a.

Habein, H.C., Jr., Moersch, H.J., and Kirklin, J.W.: Diverticula of the lower part of the part of the esophagus: a clinical study of one hundred forty-nine nonsurgical cases. Arch. Intern. Med. 97:768, 1956b.

Harrington, S.W.: Pulsion diverticula of hypopharynx: a review of forty-one cases in which operation was performed and a report of two cases. Surg. Gynecol. Obstet. 69:364, 1939.

Hoehn, J.G., and Payne, W.S.: Resection of pharyngoesophageal diverticulum using stapling device. Mayo Clin. Proc. 44:738, 1969.

Holinger, P.H., and Schild, J.A.: The Zenker's (hypopharyngeal) diverticulum. Ann. Otol. Rhinol. Laryngol. 78:679, 1969.

Huang, B., Payne, W.S., and Cameron, A.J.: Surgical management for recurrent pharyngoesophageal (Zenker's) diverticulum. Ann. Thorac. Surg. 37:189, 1984a.

Huang, B., Unni, K.K., and Payne, W.S.: Long-term survival following diverticulectomy for cancer in pharyngoesophageal (Zenker's) diverticulum. Ann. Thorac. Surg. 38:207, 1984b.

Hunt, P.S., Connell, A.M., and Smiley, T.B.: The cricopharyngeal sphincter in gastric reflux. Gut 11:303, 1970.

Hutchin, P., and Lindskog, G.E.: Acquired esophagobronchial fistula of infectious origin. J. Thorac. Cardiovasc. Surg. 48:1, 1964.

Jonasson, O.M., and Gunn, L.C.: Midesophageal diverticulum with hemorrhage: report of a case. Arch. Surg. 90:713, 1965.

Lahey, F.H., and Warren, K.W.: Esophageal diverticula. Surg. Gynecol. Obstet. 98:1, 1954.

Ludlow, A.: A case of obstructed deglutition, from a preternatural dilation of, and bag formed in the pharynx. Med. Observations Inquiries, Soc. Phys. (London) 3:85, 1769.

MacCarty, R.L., et al.: Radiographic findings in patients with esophageal involvement by mediastinal granuloma. Gastrointest. Radiol. 4:11, 1979.

Negus, V.E.: Pharyngeal diverticula: observations on their evolution and treatment. Br. J. Surg. 38:129, 1950.

Payne, W.S., and Clagett, O.T.: Pharyngeal and esophageal diverticula. Curr. Probl. Surg. April 1965, pp.1–31.

Payne, W.S., and Reynolds, R.R.: Surgical treatment of pharyngoesophageal diverticulum (Zenker's diverticulum). Surg. Rounds 5:18, 1982.

Powell, M.E.A.: A case of aortic-oesophageal fistula. Br. J. Surg. 45:55, 1957.

Schick, A., and Yesner, R.: Traction diverticulum of esophagus with exsanguination: report of a case. Ann. Intern. Med. 39:345, 1953.

Shallow, T.A., and Clerf, L.H.: One stage pharyngeal diverticulectomy: improved technique and analysis of 186 cases. Surg. Gynecol. Obstet. 86:317, 1948.

Smiley, T.B., Caves, P.K., and Porter, D.C.: Relationship between posterior pharyngeal pouch and hiatus hernia. Thorax 25:725, 1970.

Sutherland, H.D.: Cricopharyngeal achalasia. J. Thorac. Cardiovasc. Surg. 43:114, 1962.

Sweet, R.H.: Pulsion diverticulum of the pharyngoesophageal junction: technic of the one-stage operation; a preliminary report. Ann. Surg. 125:41, 1947.

Terracol, J., and Sweet, R.H.: Diseases of the Esophagus. Philadelphia, W.B. Saunders Co., 1958, p. 264.

van Overbeek, J.J.M.: The Hypopharyngeal Diverticulum: Endoscopic Treatment and Manometry. Assen, Netherlands, Van Gorcum, 1977.

Vinson, P.P.: Diverticula of the thoracic portion of the esophagus: report of forty-two cases. Arch. Otolaryngol. 19:508, 1934.

Welsh, G.F., and Payne, W.S.: The present status of one-stage pharyngo-esophageal diverticulectomy. Surg. Clin. North Am. 53:953, 1973.

Winans, C.S.: The pharyngoesophageal closure mechanism: a manometric study. Gastroenterology 63:768, 1972.

Wychulis, A.R., Ellis, F.H., Jr., and Anderson, H.A.: Acquired nonmalignant esophagotracheobronchial fistula: report of 36 cases. JAMA 196:117, 1966.

Wychulis, A.R., Gunnlaugsson, G.H., and Clagett, O.T.: Carcinoma occurring in pharyngo-esophageal diverticulum: report of three cases. Surgery 66:976, 1969.

Zenker, F.A., and von Ziemssen, H.: Krankheiten des Oesophagus. In Handbuch der speziellen Pathologie und Therapie, Vol. 7, Part 1. Suppl. Edited by H. von Ziemssen. Leipzig, F.C.W. Vogel, 1874.

CHAPTER 82

ESOPHAGEAL HIATAL HERNIA AND GASTROESOPHAGEAL REFLUX

David B. Skinner

Hiatal hernia and gastroesophageal reflux are among the most common conditions diagnosed in human beings residing in North America and Europe. These two diagnoses are rarely made in other parts of the world. Hiatal hernia was not diagnosed in living human beings until after the development of radiographic visualization of the esophagus at the beginning of this century. Until midcentury, hiatal hernia was thought to be an anatomic curiosity of significance similar to that of other hernias through the abdominal wall. Surgical treatment stressed anatomic repair. Gastroesophageal reflux was not recognized as the cause of the common complaints of heartburn and the complications of esophagitis, stricture, bleeding, and pulmonary aspiration until Allison's classic description of the complications of reflux gained wide notice (1951). Current knowledge of these two conditions has been based entirely upon observations and experimental studies carried out within the past 30 years.

Hiatal hernia is noted on barium swallow examination in many adults regardless of their symptoms. At least 10% of the adult population of the United States is thought to have a known hiatal hernia. Radiologists report that they demonstrate this finding in more than half of the patients undergoing barium swallow examination if vigorous maneuvers are employed. The commonly seen type I, axial, or sliding hiatal hernia by itself causes no specific symptoms or complications and should be considered an irrelevant anatomic variation frequently seen in adult patients and not requiring further investigation or treatment.

Gastroesophageal reflux is a normal event following ingestion of a meal or during induced belching or burping. Pathologic degrees of reflux may occur and cause the symptoms of heartburn and regurgitation and the complications related to esophagitis or aspiration. Although hiatal hernia and reflux are both common problems and are frequently associated, each may occur independently from the other. They should be regarded as separate entities. Among the large population of in-

dividuals harboring a hiatal hernia, only an estimated 5% have persistent symptomatic reflux.

ANATOMIC CONSIDERATIONS

To understand the abnormalities involved in either hiatal hernia or gastroesophageal reflux, a review of the normal anatomy is necessary. The esophagus passes from the thorax into the abdomen through the esophageal hiatus of the diaphragm. The hiatus is usually composed of muscle fibers arising from the right crus of the diaphragm, although fibers from both crura contribute to the hiatal opening in some individuals. The esophagus then continues for 2 to 3 cm within the abdomen before entering the stomach.

The intra-abdominal portion of the esophagus is held beneath the diaphragm by the insertion of the phrenoesophageal membrane into the submucosal tissue of the esophagus 3 to 4 cm above the junction of esophageal muscle with the gastric pouch. The phrenoesophageal fascial membrane is an extension of the endoabdominal fascia lining the inner surface of the transversus abdominus muscle and the diaphragm. As this fascia leaves the margins of the hiatus, it is joined by a thin contribution from the endothoracic fascia lining the superior surface of the diaphragm. The collagen fibers of this fused endoabdominal and endothoracic fascia, the phrenoesophageal membrane, penetrate through the muscle layer of the distal esophagus and insert into the connective tissue in the esophageal submucosa. Normally the membrane is short so the muscle of the diaphragm is close to the muscle of the esophageal wall.

No definite anatomic sphincter muscle is present in the distal esophagus of primates. Other species such as the dog, bat, and opossum have a well developed anatomically distinct sphincter at the gastroesophageal junction. Such a sphincter muscle is not identifiable in primates. The sphincter-like action of the human distal esophagus, which normally prevents gastroesophageal reflux, follows Laplace's law. Force necessary to distend a tube is inversely proportional to the radius of the tube. When a tube of small diameter such as the esophagus abruptly enters a pouch of large diameter such as the stomach, Laplace's law predicts that it will require more force to distend the distal esophagus than the stomach, and that the esophagus will remain closed while the stomach dilates. The normally closed distal esophagus is opened during the act of swallowing or vomiting. When the longitudinal muscle layer of the esophagus contracts, the esophagus shortens. Shortening of the esophagus pulls against the insertion of the phrenoesophageal membrane, which tethers the distal esophagus. Because the membrane fibers enter the esophagus at an angle, this shortening effect tends to pull open the distal esophagus. This opening is recorded as relaxation of the distal esophagus during swallowing when manometry is performed, and permits normal physiologic reflux, belching, or vomiting. This theory of distal esophageal function appears to account for the sphincter-like actions observed.

HERNIAS OF THE ESOPHAGEAL HIATUS

Anatomic Varieties

Herniations of abdominal viscera through the esophageal hiatus may be classified into several types (Fig. 82–1). In the common type I, axial, or sliding hiatal hernia, the phrenoesophageal membrane is somewhat stretched but is intact circumferentially. This thinning or stretching of the membrane permits a small pouch of gastric cardia to protrude upward through the esophageal hiatus. Because the membrane is intact, the distal several centimeters of esophagus below the membrane still are within the abdominal pressure compartment and the hernia remains intra-abdominal. In most individuals with this weakening of the membrane, the normal intra-abdominal location of the distal esophagus is maintained so that no abnormal gastroesophageal reflux occurs. This type of hernia in the absence of abnormal reflux has *no* medical significance.

The uncommon type II, rolling, or paraesophageal hernia is caused by a specific defect in the phrenoesophageal membrane. This defect usually occurs at the anterolateral reflection of the peritoneum from the greater abdominal sac off the anterior wall of the intra-abdominal esophagus. This defect permits a protrusion of peritoneum to herniate upward alongside the esophagus. The stomach, being the most immediately adjacent organ to the peritoneum at this point, enters the hernial sac. Because the thoracic side of the defect is subject to less than atmospheric pressure while abdominal pressure is positive, this type of hernia tends to enlarge progressively. Eventually, most or all of the stomach may herniate upward into the chest. At the extreme, this hernia appears during radiographic studies as an upside-down stomach with the cardiac and pylorus being adjacent to each other. The entire gastric fundus, body, and antrum are herniated into the thoracic cavity. Frequently this condition is associated with some type of gastric volvulus,

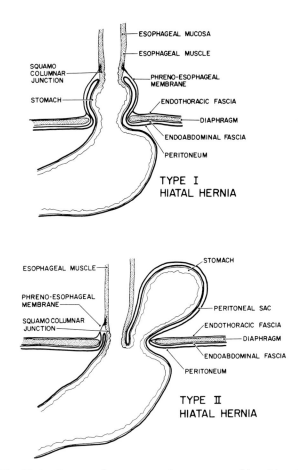

Fig. 82–1. Diagram demonstrating the two types of hiatal hernia. The type I hiatal hernia is not a true hernia in that the endoabdominal fascial lining of the abdomen remains intact. In the type II hernia, a defect in the fascia allows a peritoneal sac to pass through the opening in the hiatus and enter the pleural cavity.

which introduces the serious risk of gastric obstruction, infarction, or strangulation; bleeding; or acute intrathoracic dilatation. This rare type of hiatal hernia may be lethal, and should be repaired surgically when it is diagnosed, even if the patient is asymptomatic.

Combinations or variants of the type I and type II hiatal hernia are seen, and may be labeled type III or type IV hernia. A type III hiatal hernia has elements of both the type I and type II hernia, and the patient is exposed to the risks and associated complications of both types of hernia. As the type II hernia enlarges, frequently the phrenoesophageal membrane is stretched so that a type I component is often seen in conjunction with the type II hiatal hernia. In this case the gastric fundus is herniated into the thorax at a level cephalad to the cardia.

When abdominal organs other than the stomach enter the hernial sac, a new complicating element is introduced. Accordingly, this type of hernia is labeled a type IV hernia. Usually these hernias are large and contain stomach and adjacent organs such as colon or spleen. Infarction of these other organs may determine the clinical course of the patient.

GASTROESOPHAGEAL REFLUX

As noted, gastroesophageal reflux is a normal phenomenon and in most people the refluxed material is quickly cleared from the lower esophagus and produces no symptoms or injury to the esophageal mucosa. In a few individuals, however, the reflux occurs more frequently than normal and clearing of the acid-peptic juice is delayed. The resulting esophageal irriation produces heartburn, and damage to the esophageal muscosa may occur. In as many as 80% of such patients the aforementioned type I esophageal hiatal hernia may be demonstrated, but in the remaining 20% such a finding is absent.

Pathophysiology of Reflux

The precise abnormality causing gastroesophageal reflux remains controversial and uncertain. Some evidence suggests that patients suffering from gastroesophageal reflux have a lower-than-normal insertion of the phrenoesophageal membrane, and have lost most or all of the intra-abdominal esophagus. In this situation it is believed that reflux occurs because the entire esophagus is subjected to less than atmospheric thoracic pressure, which tends to enlarge the lumen and permit reflux to occur. Another possible mechanism explaining gastroesophageal reflux would be increased tension on the phrenoesophageal membrane so that the distal esophagus is frequently pulled open. This mechanism may account for the frequency of reflux symptoms in overweight patients or the frequency of reflux noted during straining or abnormal postures. Abnormal reflux may persist early in life, indicating that it is a congenital condition in some patients. On the other hand, it is more common for reflux symptoms to develop later in life, suggesting that in most patients it is an acquired condition. Both theories of the cause of reflux, abnormally low insertion of the membrane or undue tension on the membrane, can be used to explain acquired reflux. For example, in an obese patient the angle of entry of the phrenoesophageal membrane into the distal esophagus may be filled in with fatty tissue and effectively lower the extension of the abdominal cavity onto the distal esophagus and reduce the intra-abdominal portion. Patients who are heavy smokers or drinkers of alcohol frequently have a nonspecific esophagitis. Inflammation associated with this condition may lead to adherence between the phrenoesophageal membrane and the distal esophagus and in effect reduce the intra-abdominal segment. The precise anatomic cause of abnormal reflux in all patients is not certain. The evidence and theories described, however, all involve some abnormality of the phrenoesophageal membrane.

Various other theories have been proposed to explain the normal competency of the cardia and abnormal gastroesophageal reflux. These theories concern some specialized hormonal receptors and muscle function of the distal esophagus, abnormalities of muscle sensitivity to neurohumoral stimuli, and abnormal balance between hormones that tighten or relax foregut muscle. To date, none of these theories is substantiated, and none appear as likely or as well supported as the theories involving the insertion of the phrenoesophageal membrane and length of intra-adominal esophagus.

Once abnormal gastroesophageal reflux develops, several patterns of reflux may be noted. DeMeester and colleagues' (1976) studies of normal volunteers showed that brief periods of reflux occur normally after an ingested meal. Following a larger meal, the number of episodes of reflux may increase. The esophagus usually clears regurgitated material by swallows and peristaltic action. The exposure of the esophageal muscosa to the regurgitated gastric contents is normally brief, and not sufficient for irritation of the muscosa to occur or for the patient to be aware of symptoms.

As pathologic reflux develops, an increase in the number of postprandial bouts of reflux and a prolongation of the time of contact of regurgitated material with esophageal muscosa are noted. At this stage the patient may be aware of the symptoms of heartburn and regurgitation.

Two distinct patterns of abnormal reflux are observed. In some patients the cardia and distal esophagus remain competent to reflux while the patient is lying flat, but permit frequent regurgitation when the patient is upright. Such patients have an increased amount of reflux during normal daytime activities and may be highly symptomatic at this time. When they are reclining at night, however, the cardia may function competently and no nocturnal reflux may be observed. Because swallowing and esophageal peristalsis are defense mechanisms against prolonged contact of noxious gastric contents with the esophageal mucosa, these patients may be protected against developing esophagitis by frequent swallowing during the day.

In another pattern of reflux, the regurgitation of gastric contents occurs mainly when the patient is reclining. Such patients may have normal physiologic postprandial reflux while upright during the day, but may regurgitate at night. If reflux occurs while the patient is asleep, no symptoms may be noted and the voluntary act of swallowing may not occur. This situation permits prolonged contact of gastric contents with the mucosa and penetration through the mucosa to stimulate an inflammatory response. In such patients, inflammation and esophagitis may develop without the patient being aware of significant symptoms during the day. In most patients requiring surgical treatment for symptoms and complications of reflux, both upright and supine reflux of gastric contents occurs. Such patients have both daytime symptoms and prolonged low pH in the esophagus during the night with an associated higher risk of esophagitis. Little and associates (1980) described prolonged or delayed gastric emptying as the factor predisposing to nocturnal or supine reflux. Pure upright daytime refluxers have rapid gastric emptying and do not retain a volume of secretion in the stomach at night.

When regurgitated gastric contents remain in prolonged contact with the esophageal muscosa, penetration through the squamous epithelium may occur and stimulate an inflammatory response. Chronic irritation of the esophageal mucosa from various causes such as reflux, smoking, ingestion of spicy foods, and ingestion of alcohol or hot beverages may all cause a nonspecific alteration in the esophageal epithelium. To the esophagoscopist, this mucosa appears more red than normal. A biopsy shows hyperplasia of the basal layers of the esophageal epithelium and proximity of the rete pegs to the surface, often with neovascularization in the epithelium. This neovascularization accounts for the red appearance of the lower esophagus. At this stage no inflammatory reaction and no ulceration exist, so this condition is not a true form of esophagitis, and is a nonspecific finding. Such grade I esophagitis proved only by microscopic changes on biopsy is not specifically caused by reflux and is not an indication for antireflux therapy.

More prolonged contact of regurgitated material with the mucosa may lead to breakdown of the mucosa and frank ulceration. This condition is classifed as grade II esophagitis and is readily visible through the esophagoscope. Biopsies show definite inflammatory changes in the submucosa and breakdown and ulceration of the mucosa. With continued and prolonged reflux causing ulcerative esophagitis, the healing process involves the laying down of granulation tissue and collagen. This action in turn leads to a stiffening and thickening of the esophageal wall. At this stage a grade III esophagitis is diagnosed. If the abnormal reflux is permitted to continue further, the esophageal lumen may become narrowed both by shortening of the collagen fibers laid down during repair and by the edema of the esophageal wall and spasm of esophageal muscle. Roentgenographic studies demonstrate a stricture of the distal esophagus, and difficulty may be encountered in passing the esophagoscope through the narrowed area. Reflux-induced strictures of the esophagus are classified as grade IV esophagitis and represent an advanced stage of the complications from gastroesophageal reflux.

In some patients subject to chronic reflux, the repair process of the ulcerated mucosa apparently involves the regeneration and advancement of columnar epithelium proximally into the esophagus. The squamocolumnar junction in such patients may advance cephalad up the esophagus. When more than 3 cm of this glandular epithelium is found in the esophagus, a diagnosis of Barrett's esophagus or esophagus lined with columnar epithelium is made. This condition is thought most often to be a complication of chronic reflux. It is usually associated with ulceration at the junction of the squamous and columnar epithelium if reflux persists. The development of adenocarcinoma of the esophagus in this epithelium is repeatedly reported (see Chapter 84).

Other complications caused by abnormal gastroesophageal reflux are laryngeal and pulmonary changes. If the regurgitated substances frequently pass through the cricopharyngeal sphincter into the hypopharynx, they may be aspirated into the larynx and trachea. Inflammatory vocal cord polyps may occur. More severe aspiration causes repeated bouts of pneumonia, severe and recurrent bronchitis, lung abscess, or bronchiectasis in rare cases when foreign substances lodge in the lung. Asthma attacks may be triggered in susceptible individuals.

CLINICAL PROBLEMS

The surgeon must be careful in evaluating patients suspected of having a clinically significant hiatal hernia or gastroesophageal reflux, or both. Numerous upper abdominal pathologic conditions as well as cardiac problems may mimic the findings presented by these patients. The appropriate cause must be determined and objective pathology demonstrated before instituting surgical therapy for the repair of what in reality is an asymptomatic hiatal hernia.

Signs and Symptoms

Hiatal Hernia

The common type I or sliding hiatal hernia causes no specific symptoms by itself. When symptoms do occur, they result from the association of gastroesophageal reflux with this condition.

Specific symptoms may occur from a type II or type III hiatal hernia related to the gastric pouch within the hernia sac. Patients may complain of dysphagia from compression of the distal esophagus by the adjacent gastric hernia. Postprandial fullness, early satiety, and postprandial vomiting may be noted. Ulcerations in the herniated pouch may cause chronic anemia or frank gastrointestinal bleeding. Preforations of the gastric pouch occur, causing the symptoms of acute mediastinitis or empyema. A dramatic and life-threatening illness may be caused by this type of hernia when gastric volvulus, obstruction, and infarction develop. Acute dilatation of the intrathoracic stomach may cause respiratory distress and compromise. If mediastinal shift is caused by the overdistended stomach, vascular embarrassment may occur as well.

In a type IV hiatal hernia, symptoms may be related to the presence of other organs within the hernial sac. Most commonly this organ is the colon, and the patient may note a change in bowel habits or colonic obstruction.

Reflux

The clinical symptoms of gastroesophageal reflux may be typical or atypical and vary widely. The symptom Allison (1951) described, thought to be classic for gastroesophageal reflux, is epigastric or substernal burning pain, often described by the patient as heartburn. When heartburn is elicited by stooping, straining, or lying flat, and relieved by standing upright, the postural aggravation of the symptom highly suggests reflux. When heartburn is accompanied by regurgitation of sour or bitter-tasting material into the mouth, again related to posture, the diagnosis may be made with some certainty clinically. Symptoms caused by complications of reflux include dysphagia from stricture of the esophagus or spasm of esophageal muscle. More severe chest pain may be caused by spasm of esophageal muscle triggered by abnormal reflux. In some patients, the chest pain caused by reflux mimics the pain of angina pectoris, and may even be relieved by nitrites, which relax esophageal muscle. Patients with esophagitis may complain of painful swallowing or odynophagia. This symptom is frequently elicited by the ingestion of hot or extremely cold liquids or spicy or highly seasoned foods. Patients with esophagitis frequently have bleeding from the distal esophagus and may present with a chronic anemia and guaiac-positive stools. Rarely, massive hematemesis and upper gastrointestinal bleeding is demonstrated to come from a diffuse hemorrhagic esophagitis caused by reflux. In patients with abnormal columnar epithelium in the lower esophagus, a gastric ulcer may develop in this epithelium and may penetrate deeply through the esophageal wall, causing massive hemorrhage as well as pain. Pulmonary symptoms caused by aspiration of refluxed gastric contents include cough while lying flat at night and in association with regurgitation, postprandial cough associated with symptomatic reflux, and symptoms associated with more severe respiratory illness such as pneumonia or lung abscess.

Other atypical symptoms caused by gastroesophageal reflux may mimic various other diseases, including biliary tract disease, duodenal or gastric ulcer disorders, or pancreatitis. An unusual symptom complex associated with abnormal reflux is a feeling of a foreign object in the throat, difficulty in initiating swallowing, and a feeling of choking. This symptom complex may be diagnosed as "globus hystericus," and is thought to be caused by irritation of the upper esophagus caused by high regurgitation from the stomach. In a few patients this is the only symptom, and it is frequently misdiagnosed.

Diagnosis

Hiatal Hernia

The diagnosis of hiatal hernia is made by roentgenographic studies. On occasion, the diagnosis may be made by seeing an air-fluid level in the posterior mediastinum behind the heart. This finding is particularly true for a type II hiatal hernia. More frequently, the diagnosis is made by a barium swallow examination. The recording of the examination in a cineradiographic study facilitates later study of esophageal function. Radiologists report that they are able to demonstrate a type I hiatal hernia in many patients while applying compression to the abdomen. Because this diagnosis has no significance, the efforts employed by the radiologist to demonstrate the hiatal hernia are of little consequence to the clinical management of the patient. Complications of a type II or type III hiatal hernia may be demonstrated if the radiologist finds evidence of gastric ulceration, volvulus, or retention of barium in the hiatal hernia pouch.

Reflux

Roentgenography is less successful in making a diagnosis of abnormal gastroesophageal reflux. Spontaneous reflux is difficult to demonstrate. Among a large group of patients eventually proved to have abnormal reflux, roentgenographic studies, including cineroentgenography, demonstrate spontaneous reflux in only approximately 40%. Complications of reflux may be observed. The diagnosis of stricture is usually first made by barium swallow. Deep or multiple ulcers of the distal esophagus

are demonstrated by roentgenographic examination. Cineroentgenography may demonstrate secondary muscle spasm and motor disorders, which may accompany gastroesophageal reflux, or may be part of another esophageal disorder. Some radiologists advocate the so-called "water sipping" test to increase the diagnosis of reflux. During this test the patient is asked to swallow water while the radiologist compresses the abdomen and barium-filled stomach. Reflux of barium into the esophagus under these circumstances is a normal finding, however, and does not indicate pathologic reflux. The pulmonary complications of reflux are frequently documented by roentgenography.

Because roentgenography is frequently unsuccessful in demonstrating reflux spontaneously, esophageal function tests are used to improve diagnostic accuracy. Esophageal manometry—as described in Chapter 17—may demonstrate evidence of a large hiatal hernia. Manometry frequently shows reduced amplitude of the distal esophageal high pressure zone in patients with pathologic reflux. Studies demonstrate a considerable overlap in distal esophageal pressures between normal individuals and those who have reflux. For this reason, manometry alone is not a satisfactory diagnostic technique for gastroesophageal reflux. Several conditions that may cause symptoms mimicking reflux are diagnosed by manometry. These conditions include achalasia, in which regurgitation is frequent; scleroderma, which is often associated with reflux; and diffuse esophageal spasm. Manometry is essential to exclude these conditions. In achalasia the distal esophageal high pressure zone fails to relax with swallowing, and none of the esophageal contractions are progressive and peristaltic. In scleroderma, esophageal contraction is completely absent and the distal esophageal high pressure zone is reduced or eliminated. In diffuse esophageal spasm, the distal esophageal high pressure zone is frequently normal, but multiple synchronous high amplitude contractions occur in the body of the esophagus with some interspersed normal peristaltic contractions.

The use of the intraluminal esophageal pH probe has proved the most effective technique for demonstrating abnormal reflux. A standardized test for esophageal reflux, as described by Kantrowitz and associates (1969), has been employed at several institutions. In this test, a load of 0.1 N HCl is placed in the stomach, and a pH electrode is positioned 5 cm above the high pressure zone. The patient is asked to perform a series of respiratory actions, including coughing, deep breathing, a Valsalva maneuver, and a Müller maneuver, in each of several body positions. Normal subjects reflux no more than twice during the performance of these maneuvers, whereas patients with abnormal reflux have frequent drops of pH in the distal esophagus or maintain a low pH throughout the course of the study. Because this test involves strenuous maneuvers, a small incidence of false positive examinations occurs, and because the test is short, it may not accurately reflect the true occurrence of reflux under normal conditions. Because of the small but persistent incidence of false positive and false negative examinations with a standardized pH acid reflux test, 24-hour pH monitoring is useful in patients in whom the diagnosis is in doubt. In this test, the pH electrode is left in place 5 cm above the high pressure zone over a 24-hour period while the patient eats a neutral pH diet and spends approximately half the time in the supine position and half the time in the upright position. Johnson and DeMeester (1974) provided a quantitative score for reflux to aid in interpretation of this test. To date, this method is the most sensitive and accurate method for assessing normalcy of the gastroesophageal junction.

In patients in whom symptoms suggest the possibility of gastroesophageal reflux, and reflux is demonstrated spontaneously on barium swallow examinations or by esophageal pH studies, esophagoscopy is indicated to document the degree of esophagitis complicating reflux. Esophagitis is a tissue diagnosis and requires direct observation of the distal esophagus to ascertain whether ulcerations, fibrosis, or stricture are present. The flexible fiber-optic esophagoscope is generally satisfactory for this examination. Only in patients with a stricture is rigid tube endoscopy still occasionally necessary to facilitate bougienage during the examination and the deeper biopsies of the wall of the esophagus necessary to exclude carcinoma.

From an analysis of symptoms, roentgenographic findings, esophageal function tests, and endoscopy, it becomes clear whether a patient is suffering from abnormal gastroesophageal reflux and its complications. Based on this information, decisions about therapy are made.

Indications for Treatment

No treatment is indicated for patients with a type I hiatal hernia who complain of vague or nonspecific symptoms and do not have abnormal gastroesophageal reflux. The presence of a hiatal hernia itself is not an indication for medical or surgical treatment. All patients demonstrating a type II, type III, or type IV hiatal hernia should undergo surgical repair regardless of severity of symptoms if the patient is otherwise a satisfactory candidate for a major surgical procedure. Operation is indicated because of the grave risk of serious complications from these rare types of hernias.

Indications for medical or surgical treatment for gastroesophageal reflux depend on the findings obtained during the diagnostic evaluation. Patients with symptomatic reflux not previously treated, those shown by objective testing to have reflux, and those who have mild grade I or no esophagitis are treated medically. Patients with documented reflux who demonstrate ulcerative grade II esophagitis persisting on medical treatment are candidates for operation to correct the reflux before the esophagitis progresses to fibrosis and stricture or bleeding. Those with more advanced esophagitis such as fibrosis and stricture are nearly always surgical candidates if their general condition permits major operation.

Patients with clearly documented evidence of recurring aspiration as a cause of pulmonary disease are surgical candidates even in the absence of severe esophagitis. Great care must be taken in making this diagnosis,

because cough may precede and cause reflux, and chronic cough and reflux are frequent conditions that may co-exist but be unrelated. In analyzing the symptoms and reflux pattern in patients with known abnormal gastroesophageal reflux, less than 10% have well documented episodes of aspiration caused by reflux.

In the absence of ulcerative or advanced esophagitis, documented aspiration, or severe bleeding from esophagitis, medical therapy is employed. If patients do not respond to medical therapy for reflux that has been clearly demonstrated to be the cause of symptoms, surgical treatment may be employed to relieve symptoms. In such instances, care must be taken to document that reflux is the cause of the symptoms and is clearly abnormal. A prolonged course of medical treatment is usually advisable, generally 6 months or more, by a physician knowledgeable and interested in the medical treatment of this condition before a surgical procedure is considered for symptomatic relief.

Treatment

The medical treatment for gastroesophageal reflux stresses alteration of the conditions that may predispose to reflux. These changes include dietary, postural, and pharmacologic measures. Patients are instructed to remain upright after meals, and to sleep with the head of the bed elevated on 6-inch blocks. Antacids are prescribed 1 hour following meals and at bedtime. Patients are advised to take smaller meals to avoid gastric distention, and to avoid irritants to the esophageal muscosa such as spicy foods, alcohol, and smoking. Obese patients must lose weight and undertake a physical conditioning program. Postural maneuvers that aggravate reflux should be avoided whenever possible. On occasion, this may interfere seriously with a patient's work, and may thus be a factor in the eventual decision to undertake surgical correction. In highly symptomatic cases, a 6-week trial of cimetidine or ranitidine is employed to determine whether further symptomatic improvement can be achieved. If gastric emptying is prolonged, metoclopramide may be helpful. Cholinergics such as bethanecol or urecholine are rarely successful in controlling reflux and may introduce troublesome secondary symptoms.

When the indications for surgical management are present, the operation performed should be an antireflux repair. There is no indication for a simple hiatal hernia repair. Even in patients with type II, III, and IV hiatal hernia, the degree of dissection necessary to reduce the hernia will almost surely set the stage for subsequent gastroesophageal reflux unless an antireflux repair is performed. As a practical matter, an antireflux procedure is the only operation widely used today for gastroesophageal reflux, hiatal hernia, or both. Patients with advanced esophagitis causing stricture may require a more extensive procedure. This operation is discussed in Chapter 83.

An antireflux procedure should restore those factors that normally are important in controlling reflux. This means the creation of a narrow-diameter intra-abdominal

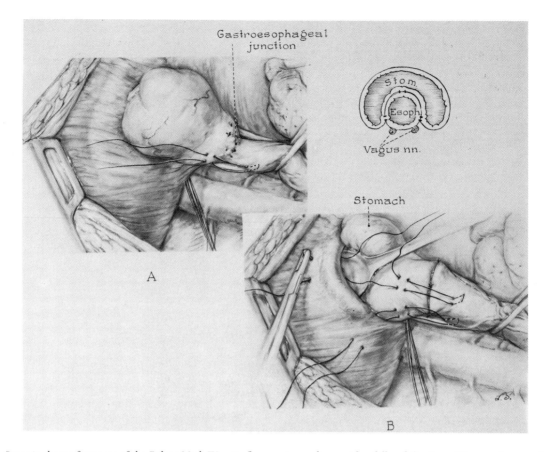

Fig. 82–2. Steps in the performance of the Belsey Mark IV antireflux repair are shown. After full mobilization of the esophagus and insertion of sutures in the crura posteriorly, a first row of plicating sutures is passed between the stomach and esophagus. When these have been tied, a second row of sutures is passed through the diaphragm, stomach, and esophagus and mattressed back in a reverse direction. As shown on the inset, three such sutures are placed approximately 270° around the circumferences of the esophagus anteriorly. When all the sutures are tied, a 4-cm segment of esophagus is restored to the abdominal location. (Belsey, R.H.R., and Skinner, D.B.: Surgical treatment: thoracic approach. *In* Gastroesophageal Reflux and Hiatal Hernia. Edited by D.B. Skinner, et al. Boston, Little, Brown & Co., 1972, p. 138.)

distal esophagus. When patients are adequately prepared with preoperative medical therapy to reduce inflammation, edema, and spasm, it is almost always possible to restore an intra-abdominal segment of distal esophagus. In patients with severe esophagitis, recurrence after previous operation, or marked obesity, a thoracic approach is preferred so that the esophagus can be mobilized all the way to the arch of the aorta to facilitate creation of the intra-abdominal segment of esophagus. In patients with less severe esophagitis or undergoing operation for the first time, an abdominal exposure of the distal esophagus is generally adequate to accomplish a satisfactory anti-reflux repair. The abdominal approach is particularly indicated in patients having other intra-abdominal disease requiring surgical correction. Vagotomy and gastric drainage procedures have no place in the treatment of gastroesophageal reflux. These gastric acid-reducing maneuvers are used only for specific indications such as active and symptomatic duodenal ulcer disease.

Several types of anti-reflux operations are described, all of which employ the basic principle of restoring an intra-abdominal segment of esophagus and maintaining the distal esophagus at a narrow diameter as it enters

the gastric pouch. Antireflux repairs receiving the greatest attention in recent years are those developed by Belsey and reported by me and Belsey (1967), Nissen (1961), and Hill (1967). Each re-establishes the intra-abdominal esophagus and employs a partial plication of gastric wall around the esophagus to prevent its overdistention.

The Belsey operation, entitled the Mark IV repair by its developer, is performed through a thoracic incision (Fig. 82–2). The term Mark IV indicates that previous types of repairs employed failed to correct reflux. Through a left sixth interspace thoracotomy the lower half of the esophagus from the aortic arch down to the diaphragm is fully mobilized, and all of the attachments of the cardia are divided. Excess phrenoesophageal membrane and fibrofatty tissue around the cardia are removed to facilitate adherence of the gastric fundus to the distal esophagus. The vagus nerves are carefully preserved. The repair is accomplished by two layers of sutures imbricating the gastric fundus around two thirds of the circumference of the lower esophagus for a distance of 4 cm upward from the gastroesophageal junction. The first row of three mattress sutures is placed between the stomach and esophagus, and the second row of three sutures passes through the nearby edge of the tendinous

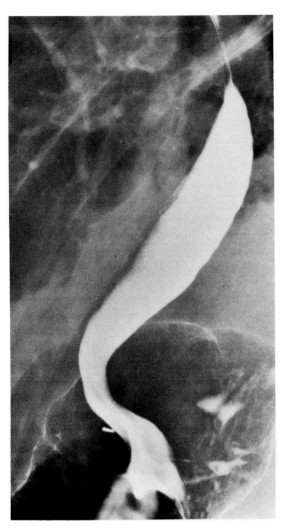

Fig. 82–3. A postoperative barium swallow following the Mark IV antireflux repair shows the characteristic appearance of plication of stomach onto the esophagus and the 4-cm segment of intra-abdominal esophagus. The clip marks the esophagogastric junction.

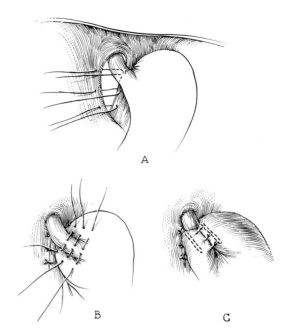

Fig. 82–4. Steps in the performance of the Nissen fundoplication operation performed through an abdominal incision. Sutures are placed in the crura posteriorly to narrow the hiatus. After full mobilization of the fundus, the stomach is passed behind the esophagus and a series of sutures is placed through the stomach and esophagus. When these are tied, approximately a 4-cm segment of esophagus should be restored within the abdomen. (Zuidema, G.D.: Surgical treatment: abdominal approach. *In* Gastroesophageal Reflux and Hiatal Hernia. Edited by D.B. Skinner, et al. Boston, Little, Brown & Co., 1972, p. 154.)

portion of diaphragm as well as gastric fundus and esophagus. Sutures are placed in the esophageal crura posteriorly to narrow the hiatus, which helps to maintain the bulky repair within the abdomen. Following completion of this repair, the surgeon leaves a chest tube in place. The patient begins swallowing liquids as soon as bowel sounds return. A barium swallow performed before discharge should demonstrate a 3- to 4-cm segment of intra-abdominal esophagus with adjacent gastric fundus (Fig. 82–3). Long-term results from this operation are reported from the innovator's clinic by Orringer and his associates (1972). Results are based on patient interview at intervals, and repeat barium swallow and endoscopic examination in patients complaining of any symptoms. Among more than 250 patients followed more than 10 years, the known success rate of the operation is 85%. Fifteen percent of patients have evidence of symptoms, recurrent hiatal hernia, or recurrent gastroesophageal reflux, or are lost to follow-up. Recurrences are demonstrated to occur as long as 10 years after the operation, so long-term follow-up is essential in the evaluation of an operation of this type used for the treatment of a benign disease.

The fundoplication operation described by Nissen can be employed through an abdominal or a thoracic approach. The thoracic approach is selected for obese patients, those with extensive esophagitis, or those having a recurrence following previous operation. When performed through the thorax, the mobilization of the esophagus is identical to that employed for the Belsey Mark IV operation. After mobilization of the esophagus through either the thoracic or abdominal approach, several short gastric arteries between stomach and spleen are ligated and divided to facilitate mobilization of the stomach. The posterior wall of the gastric fundus is brought behind the esophagus around to the medial side. A series of sutures is placed through the anterior fundus of the stomach, the wall of the esophagus, and the posterior fundus brought behind the esophagus (Fig. 82–4). In this way the gastric fundus is used to encompass the entire circumference of distal esophagus. A 3- to 4-cm length of wrap is measured. The wrap must be performed over a large bougie or performed in such a way that it will easily admit the operator's finger through the completed fundoplication. As with the Mark IV operation, the diaphragmatic crura are approximated posteriorly to prevent the bulky reconstruction from passing into the chest. Some surgeons advocate leaving the fundoplica-

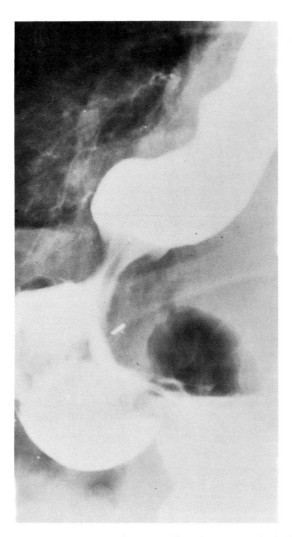

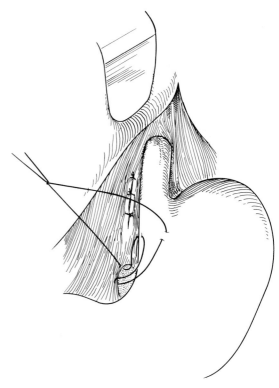

Fig. 82–6. A schematic representation of one of the sutures used for the Hill posterior gastropexy and calibration of the cardia. The crura have already been closed with sutures. The arcuate ligament has been dissected, and sutures are placed on the posterior and anterior aspect of the gastroesophageal junction to cause a partial plication of stomach around the intra-abdominal esophagus and to hold the 4 cm of abdominal esophagus to the arcuate ligament.

Fig. 82–5. A postoperative barium swallow after a Nissen fundoplication shows the pseudotumor effect of the repair and the intra-abdominal segment of esophagus. The repair must not be too tight. The clip marks the esophagogastric junction.

tion in the lower thorax. This practice has several disadvantages, including progressive enlargement of the iatrogenic hiatal hernia, retention of gastric secretions and food within the intrathoracic pouch, leading to ulceration or perforation in some cases, and hemorrhage from the gastric pouch. For these reasons, most surgeons do not advocate intrathoracic placement of the fundoplication except under difficult circumstances when the repair simply cannot be delivered into the abdomen. Because the more circumferential wrap may make later passage of a nasogastric tube difficult, a tube is left within the stomach until bowel action has completely returned. A postoperative barium swallow should demonstrate the pseudotumor effect of the fundoplication and a 4-cm segment of distal swallowing tube passing through the wrap into the stomach (Fig. 82–5). No air-fluid level should be present in the lower esophagus. Good results have been reported in approximately 85 to 90% of patients in several series, with follow-ups of variable duration up to the 10-year experience reported for the Belsey Mark IV

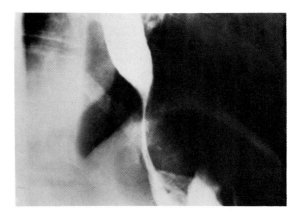

Fig. 82–7. Postoperative barium swallow following a Hill repair shows a satisfactory segment of intra-abdominal esophagus anchored posteriorly with the plication of stomach on the esophagus. (Zuidema, G.D.: Surgical treatment: abdominal approach. *In* Gastroesophageal Reflux and Hiatal Hernia. Edited by D.B. Skinner, et al. Boston, Little, Brown & Co., 1972, p. 157.)

operation. The full fundoplication has proved to be an effective valve in preventing reflux, as this repair is mechanically competent even in the absence of the infradiaphragmatic position. For this reason, however, the incidence of inability to vomit, gaseous retention in the stomach, and postoperative dysphagia, as Woodward and his associates (1971) reported, is somewhat higher for the Nissen fundoplication than for the other types of repairs. On rare occasions the symptoms of the "gas bloat" syndrome may be sufficient to require taking down of this repair and converting it to some other type of antireflux operation.

Posterior gastropexy with calibration of the cardia described by Hill (1976) is performed through an abdominal incision. After full mobilization of the cardia and lower esophagus through the hiatus, the repair is started. The arcuate ligament which overlies the aorta above the celiac axis is dissected free. Sutures are placed from the posterior aspect of the gastroesophageal junction through this ligament. Additional sutures are placed from the anterior aspect of the cardia through the ligament to cause a partial or 180° imbrication of stomach around the medial aspect of the intra-abdominal esophagus. Hill advocates placing these sutures using intraluminal manometry to judge the degree of compression of the esophagus achieved (Fig. 82–6). Hill reports a target of 50 mm Hg of pressure in the distal esophagus. Several of these sutures are placed in the anterior and posterior aspects of the cardia until the desired pressure effects are achieved. The crura are approximated to maintain the intra-abdominal location of the distal esophagus now anchored to the arcuate ligament. Postoperative barium swallow examination should show a 4-cm segment of intra-abdominal esophagus of small diameter adjacent to the large gastric fundic pouch (Fig. 82–7). Results reported with this repair include a low incidence of recurrent hernia through the hiatus, and a variable success rate in controlling reflux depending on the specific technique described by the operating surgeon. At least 90% of patients in Hill's own experience are said to be free of symptoms and reflux documented by pH reflux testing during a follow-up of variable time duration.

Each of these repairs has proved to be remarkably effective in the early postoperative period, both in eliminating hiatal hernia and in controlling reflux. A decision about the most effective repair over the long term awaits the completion of several ongoing long-range prospective studies comparing the different repairs as performed by the same team of surgeons in several institutions. At present, it is not possible to say which is the best repair. A surgeon should master the techniques for one or more of these repairs, and use them for carefully selected patients. In this way, relief of the symptoms and compli-

cations of gastroesophageal reflux, and the elimination of hiatal hernia can be achieved for over a decade in at least 85% of such patients.

REFERENCES

Allison, P.R.: Reflux esophagitis, sliding hiatal hernia, and the anatomy of repair. Surg. Gynecol. Obstet. 92:149, 1951.
DeMeester, T.R., et al.: Patterns of gastroesophageal reflux in health and disease. Ann. Surg. 184:459, 1976.
Hill, L.D.: An effective operation for hiatal hernia: an eight-year appraisal. Ann. Surg. 166:681, 1967.
Hill, L.D.: Transabdominal hiatal herniorrhaphy with median arcuate ligament repair. Surgical Techniques Illustrated 1:59, 1976.
Johnson, L.F., and DeMeester, T.R.: Twenty-four hour pH monitoring of the distal esophagus: a quantitative measure of gastroesophageal reflux. Am. J. Gastroenterol. 62:325, 1974.
Kantrowitz, P.A., et al.: Measurement of gastroesophageal reflux. Gastroenterology 56:666, 1969.
Little, A.G., et al.: Pathogenesis of esophagitis in patients with gastroesophageal reflux. Surgery 88:101, 1980.
Nissen, R.: Gastropexy and "fundoplication" in surgical treatment of hiatal hernia. Am. J. Dig. Dis. 6:954, 1961.
Orringer, M.B., Skinner, D.B., and Belsey, R.H.R.: Long-term results of the Mark IV operation for hiatal hernia and analyses of recurrences and their treatment. J. Thorac. Cardiovasc. Surg. 63:25, 1972.
Skinner, D.B., and Belsey, R.H.R.: Surgical management of esophageal reflux and hiatus hernia. J. Thorac. Cardiovasc. Surg. 53:33, 1967.
Skinner, D.B., et al. (Eds.): Gastroesophageal Reflux and Hiatal Hernia. Boston, Little, Brown & Co., 1972.
Woodward, E.R., Thomas, H.F., and McAlhany, J.C.: Comparison of crural repair and Nissen fundoplication in the treatment of esophageal hiatus hernia and peptic esophagitis. Ann. Surg. 173:783, 1971.

READING REFERENCES

Boesby, S., et al.: Failures after surgical treatment of patients with hiatus hernia and reflux symptoms: a pathophysiological study. Scand. J. Gastroenterol. 17:219, 1982.
Bombeck, C.T., Dillard, D.H., and Nyhus, L.M.: Muscular anatomy of the gastroesophageal junction and role of phrenoesophageal ligament. Autopsy study of sphincter mechanism. Ann. Surg. 164:643, 1966.
Booth, D.J., Kemmerer, W.T., and Skinner, D.B.: Acid clearing from the distal esophagus. Arch. Surg. 96:731, 1968.
Ellis, F.H., Jr., and Crozier, R.E.: Reflux controlled by fundoplication: A clinical and manometric assessment of the Nissen operation. Ann. Thorac. Surg. 38:387, 1984.
Gregorie, H.B., Jr., Cathcart, R.S., III, and Gregorie, R.J.: Surgical treatment of intractable esophagitis. Ann. Surg. 199:580, 1984.
Henderson, R.D.: Dysphagia complicating hiatal hernia repair. J. Thorac. Cardiovasc. Surg. 88:922, 1984.
Jonsell, G., and DeMeester, P.: Comparison of diagnostic methods for selection of patients for antireflux operations. Surgery 95:2, 1984.
McCallum, R.W., et al.: Effects of metoclopramide and bethanechol on delayed gastric emptying present in gastroesophageal reflux patients. Gastroenterology 84:1573, 1983.
O'Sullivan, G.C., et al.: Interaction of lower esophageal sphincter pressure and length of sphincter in the abdomen as determinants of gastroesophageal competence. Am. J. Surg. 143:40, 1982.
Piehler, J.M., et al.: The uncut Collis-Nissen procedure for esophageal hiatal hernia and its complications. Probl. Gen. Surg. 1:1, 1984.

CHAPTER 83

BENIGN STRICTURES OF THE ESOPHAGUS

Robert D. Henderson

Benign strictures of the esophagus account for approximately 8% of esophageal disease requiring surgical management. In adult practice, 7% are reflux-related peptic strictures of the gastroesophageal junction. All other strictures of the esophagus are rare. The classification of these strictures is seen in Table 83–1.

CONGENITAL STRICTURES

These strictures are rare, but Spitz (1973) found them in the lower esophagus. They may be related or unrelated to congenital atresias and tracheobronchial fistulae. They are already present at birth and become symptomatic when solid food is introduced to the infant's diet. Because of their rarity, a pattern of treatment has not been established, but a fully patent esophagus can be obtained by either dilatation or surgery.

Table 83–1. Classification of Benign Strictures of the Esophagus

CONGENITAL
   Tracheobronchial remnants
ACQUIRED
   Reflux Related
      Lower esophageal peptic stricture
      Allison-Johnston stricture and Barrett's esophagus
      Schatzki's ring
      Midesophageal stricture
      Cricopharyngeal web
      Scleroderma and peptic stricture
      Pre-existing strictures—effects of reflux
   Traumatic Strictures
      Caustic ingestion
      Foreign body ingestion
      Late results of spontaneous or traumatic perforation
      Previous surgical resections
   Infection
      Monilia esophagitis
   Rare Diseases
      Behçet's disease
      Pemphigus

ACQUIRED STRICTURES

Strictures may be complications of various disease processes; the most common is caused by uncontrolled reflux of gastric juice into the lower esophagus. Strictures also recur in association with collagen disease, after caustic burns, after trauma, and with other serious disease processes.

Reflux-Related Strictures

Lower esophageal peptic strictures are by far the commonest reflux-related strictures. Although some of the etiologic factors are clearly understood, many are not. Etiologic aspects can be considered under the following headings: reflux control mechanisms, the quality of the refluxed bolus; esophageal motor activity, and resistance factors in the esophageal mucosa.

Reflux Control Mechanisms

Various factors have been considered important in reflux control, including the intra-abdominal segment of esophagus, the high pressure zone—HPZ—tone, the angle of entry of esophagus and stomach, the mucosal rosette, the diaphragm and its esophageal attachments, neurologic control of the esophagus, gastric neurogenic reflux mechanisms to the HPZ, and hormonal control mediated through gastrin and secretin (Fig. 83–1).

The most important factors in reflux control have been shown by Botha (1962), Pope (1967), and me (1976) and many others to be the HPZ tone and the intra-abdominal segment of esophagus; neurologic and hormonal reflexes, however, may play an added minor role in modifying the tone of HPZ in response to a meal. Whereas gastrin was considered important in reflux control, Snape and Cohen (1976) showed that in physiological concentrations this hormone is of minor importance.

In the normal subject, reflux can occur intermittently, but when the control mechanisms break down, the frequency and volume of the refluxed bolus increase.

Quality of the Refluxed Bolus

I (1978a) and my associates (1972) showed that the quality of the refluxed bolus is important in determining

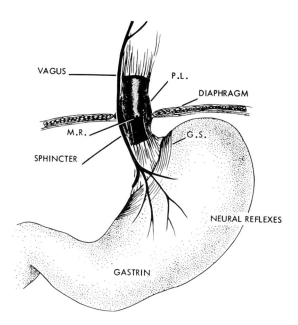

Fig. 83–1. Many factors are involved in the maintenance of reflux control. The esophagus is maintained in correct anatomic position by the diaphragm and phrenoesophageal ligament together with the vascular fixation of the stomach. The mucosal rosette is variable and most likely not significant. The sphincter (high pressure zone), the intra-abdominal segment of esophagus, and the gastric sling fibers are probably the most important factors in reflux control. Neurogenic and hormonal reflux mechanisms are involved in negation of sphincteric tone. M.R. = mucosal rosette; P.L. = phrenoesophageal ligament; G.S. = gastric sling fibers.

its effect on the esophagus. In most patients the refluxed bolus consists of gastric acid and food, but particularly in those with previous gastric surgery, bile may become a significant added constituent. With continued reflux, the esophageal mucosa becomes sensitive and even in the absence of ulceration, heartburn may develop.

Heartburn may occur in patients with neutralized gastric acid, indicating that acid is not the sole factor. Bile acids are the active constituent in bile reflux and these acids may produce esophageal injury on their own, or their action may be augmented by bile salts precipitating out of the bile acids.

Esophageal Motor Activity

Motor activity of the esophagus is important in preventing damage from the refluxed bolus. In patients with a healthy esophagus, motor activity rapidly empties the esophagus and avoids injurious contact of the refluxed bolus and mucosa. When motor activity is damaged, Booth and colleagues (1968) showed, esophageal clearance is prolonged and the potential for added injury is increased.

Resistance Factors in the Esophageal Mucosa

Mucosal resistance factors are poorly understood. Most likely they are important and may well be suppressed in patients who have other systemic disease. Esophageal symptoms often worsen following operation for other diseases, and in some patients requiring prolonged gastric drainage, NG-tube stricture may develop.

When the esophagus is irritated, mucous secretions from racemose glands are copious and augmented by increased salivation. Aylwin (1953) suggested that the neutralizing effects of these secretions may be an important protective mechanism. In diseased states, particularly those associated with shock or dehydration, this defense mechanism may be inactivated.

Evidence from several sources indicates the importance of the intra-abdominal segment of esophagus and the tone of the HPZ (Fig. 83–2). When this mechanism breaks down with loss of the segment or decrease of HPZ tone, reflux is likely to occur. Reflux has been shown to damage the tone of the HPZ and to increase esophageal disordered motor activity—DMA. Increased DMA prolongs esophageal emptying time and exposes the esophagus to further damage. Decreased HPZ tone, induced by reflux, further predisposes to reflux. These self-perpetuating processes continue with progressive esophageal injury unless interrupted by effective therapy.

Effects of Reflux

In most patients with reflux the esophageal mucosa can cope well with the acid or bile irritation. In only a few does mucosal ulceration appear. Once ulceration occurs, the inflammatory process spreads through the esophageal wall, and Donnelly (1973) and I (1976) and our associates showed that the wall becomes thickened by scar and inflammation. Stricture is the end product of ulceration and results from granulation and scar contracture. In most patients, stricture occurs only after years of symptomatic reflux, but in a few patients, the process develops rapidly.

Peptic Stricture

Symptomatology

The basic symptoms of reflux are present in most patients with peptic stricture (Table 83–2). Dysphagia is a common symptom of gastroesophageal reflux, occurring in 81% of this group of 193 patients requiring surgery

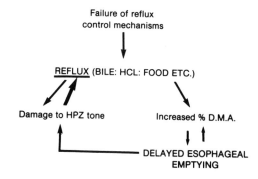

Fig. 83–2. When reflux control breaks down, gastric content refluxes into the esophagus. This material includes acid, bile, and food. The refluxed bolus is poorly cleared from the esophagus because of secondary disordered motor activity (DMA). Delayed emptying increases both esophageal and sphincteric damage and further promotes reflux.

Table 83–2. Symptoms of Gastroesophageal Reflux in 193 Patients*

Symptom	%
Heartburn	99.5
Reflux	87
Aspiration	31.5
Nausea and vomiting	79
Total dysphagia	81
Mechanical	8
Motor	73
—Gastroesophageal	67.5
—Pharyngoesophageal	50
—Pharyngoesophageal and aspiration	23

*The two most diagnostic symptoms of reflux are recognizable reflux to the throat and dysphagia. In this group, 94.2% of patients had one or both of these symptoms.

for reflux. In many patients the symptom is mild and intermittent, but it can be severe whether or not a stricture is present. Of this group, 8% had a peptic stricture.

Differentiation of mechanical—stricture induced—dysphagia from a motor—spastic—esophageal dysphagia is not always possible by history alone. Typically in motor dysphagia, the food sticking is variable and occurs mostly with solids but may also be induced by liquids. In almost all such patients occasional meals are swallowed without dysphagia. By contrast, a mechanical obstruction tends to be bolus-size specific, and the food particle, if too large, obstructs at the stricture site.

Two other factors affect the descent of the food bolus (Fig. 83–3). In patients with poor esophageal motor power, no driving force is available to pass the bolus through the stricture, so even a mild degree of narrowing produces a profound dysphagia. This problem is typical of the patient with scleroderma and an adynamic esophagus. The other important factor is stricture length, because with a long stricture, the food bolus is more likely to impact in the middle of the strictured segment. Because of stricture length, the peristaltic force of contracture does not affect the impacted food bolus.

Investigation

A peptic stricture is a sign of advanced reflux disease and should be carefully evaluated before proceeding to treatment. When the facilities are available, the following studies should be conducted: roentgenographic studies, manometry with pH studies and acid perfusion, and esophagoscopy with biopsy and brushing.

The roentgenologic appearance is usually typical (Fig. 83–4). Berridge and co-workers (1966) showed that peptic stricture occurs at the squamocolumnar junction and has clearly delineated margins, allowing fairly accurate separation from a malignancy. Palmer (1968) and Payne (1970) showed that the same disease of scar contracture that produces a stricture also produces esophageal shortening and a roentgenologically irreducible hiatal hernia. Roentgenologic reflux is usually demonstrable, but with a tight stricture, the narrowing may reduce or prevent symptomatic and roentgenologic reflux.

Manometrically, because of the advanced nature of reflux damage, the HPZ tone is low and DMA is severe in the body of the esophagus. I (1977), Ellis (1976), and

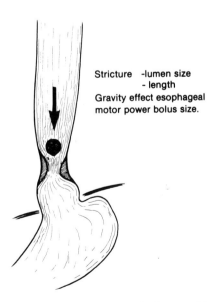

Fig. 83–3. When a stricture is present, the descent of the food bolus is affected by stricture lumen, food consistency, and the effects of esophageal motor power.

Stricture -lumen size
- length
Gravity effect esophageal motor power bolus size.

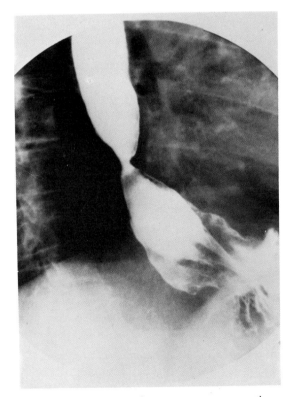

Fig. 83–4. In this patient a tight stricture is present at the squamocolumnar junction in association with a shortened esophagus and fixed hiatal hernia. Radiologically the lumen smoothly narrows and shows no evidence of deep ulceration, as might be seen with an esophageal carcinoma.

DeMeester and his associates (1974) found that these motor changes, although often severe, are reversible by effective reflux control.

Manometry is important in excluding other disease. The two most important differential diagnoses in patients with a peptic stricture are malignancy and scleroderma. Whereas Kelly (1968) stated that malignancy gives a variable motor response in the esophagus, it is unlikely to show the advanced motor damage of reflux. Scleroderma and related collagen disorders may be complicated by a peptic stricture, although Creamer (1956) showed that it can be recognized by the typical manometric changes. Recognition of scleroderma is important because it may alter the therapeutic approach.

Endoscopic evaluation is mandatory in the investigation and management of a peptic stricture. Malignancy must be excluded by direct brushing and by biopsy. Unless kept constantly in mind, early malignancies will be missed (Fig. 83–5). Ulcerative esophagitis predisposes to malignancy.

Medical Management

The principles of medical management are well established: dietary control, bed elevation, antacids, and the use—when necessary—of medications such as cimetidine and metoclopramide.

Reflux occurs mostly after eating and is aggravated by slow gastric emptying. Fried and fatty foods should be avoided, and high bulk or acidic foods may produce irritation. Depending on the severity of the stricture, the particle size of swallowed food may have to be reduced. Total esophageal occlusion is rare with benign disease, but in the occasional severe peptic stricture, only liquids can be tolerated.

Bed elevation protects the esophagus from gravity-induced reflux and is an important part of medical management. Also, to avoid night reflux, the patient should be instructed not to eat before going to bed.

Antacids are still the mainstay of therapy and should be used with each meal and at night. Fordtran and his colleagues (1973) showed that liquid antacids give the most immediate relief, although tablets can be carried for convenience.

Cimetidine was the first H_2-blocking medication to be introduced. These drugs suppress the production of gastric acid and pepsin. The rare but important side effects include hepatic and renal injury, possible hematopoietic suppression, gynecomastia, impotence, diarrhea, neurologic symptoms and a possible effect on spermatogenesis.

Ranitidine is a more recently introduced H_2 blocker that is active in lower dose levels and is less likely to afect liver or brain.

Famotidine is yet another H_2-blocking medication, active in even smaller doses. Its incidence of side effects may be even lower, but long-term studies are not yet available.

All of these medications are effective in duodenal ulcer disease and somewhat less effective with gastric ulcers caused by mixed etiologic factors.

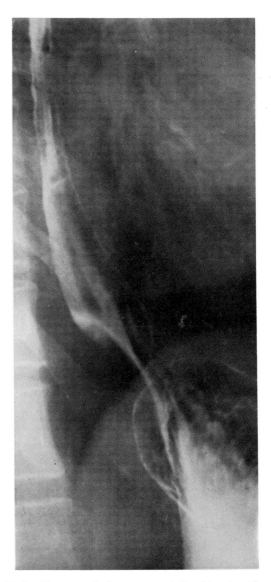

Fig. 83–5. This patient had a symptomatic hiatal hernia with severe dysphagia. Although radiologically there is no evidence of carcinoma, at endoscopy a mucosal squamous carcinoma was recognized and a biopsy was performed. Without endoscopy the malignancy would not have been noted and would have presented as an obstruction at a later date.

Reflux symptoms are often improved, but many patients have partial or no relief, and Behar and associates (1978) showed that ulceration is rarely healed by H_2-blocking medications.

Occasionally in bile gastritis, cholestyramine is used to eliminate bile salts. This medication is seldom effective in giving symptomatic relief, even when bile is a significant constituent of the refluxed bolus.

Justin-Besancon and his colleagues (1964) and Johnston (1971) showed that metoclopramide increases HPZ tone, increases gastric motor activity, and relaxes the pyloric sphincter. In some patients, significant symptomatic improvement results. Neurologic side effects of this medication are its main disadvantage. Domperidone, a more recently introduced cholinergic medication, has a similar mode of action and appears to be equally effective, but its side effects, although similar, are rarely as severe.

Esophageal Dilatation

The six possible methods of esophageal dilatation include: direct vision dilatation, indirect mercury-weighted dilatation, guided dilatation, retrograde dilatation, balloon dilatation, and intra-operative dilatation.

Direct vision dilatation requires rigid esophagoscopy with visualization of the stricture. Gum elastic bougies can be guided through the stricture to disrupt the stricture margin. This used to be the most common form of dilatation but now should rarely be used because of major limitations. The rigid endoscope does carry a significant added risk. As the bougie is being passed, the tip is poorly controlled and may become trapped in a wall irregularity so that the force of dilatation may be directed against the wall, risking perforation. The bougie size is limited by the esophagoscope size and the ability of the operator to see the stricture with the bougie in place. Although it is possible to dilate up to No. 50 Fr with a dilating endoscope, most instruments limit safe dilatation to No. 28 to 36 Fr bougie size (Fig. 83–6).

Indirect mercury-weighted dilatation is the simplest and safest method. This is safest under local anesthesia, in which the patient's recognition of pain controls the force used. I have used Maloney bougies with a gargle of viscous local anesthetic in several thousand indirect dilatations without a perforation.

This method is effective in most patients, but ineffective with tight strictures. The smaller the stricture lumen, the narrower the bougie has to be. With a bougie of less than No. 40 Fr dilatation force is reduced and generally ineffective.

Guided dilatation is the most effective method for managing the tight stricture. Under local or general anesthesia a guide wire can be passed through the fiberoptic flexible endoscope and guided under roentgenologic control into the stomach. The endoscope is removed, and graded bougies are then passed over the guide wire and into the stomach.

Several types of bougie are available. The Enid-Peustow is a metal olive-tipped bougie with a flexible metal handle. The olive must be changed each time before passage to give graded dilatation. Celestin bougies are two solid bougies, each of which is shaped to allow 3 grades of dilatation with one passage. Savary bougies are made of Silastic and are taper-tipped. These bougies are flexible and, because of their gradual taper, are, I believe, the safest method of guided dilatation (Fig. 83–7).

The system of retrograde dilatation is mostly of historic interest. A thread is passed into the stomach and brought out through a gastrostomy. Tucker bougies can be attached and pulled back and forth through the stricture. The newer methods of bougienage are simpler, avoid a gastrostomy, and have largely replaced Tucker bougies.

Balloon dilatation is also possible using flexible endoscopy. Fine balloons are placed across the stricture and dilated as the balloon is distended. I have no personal experience with this method.

Intraoperative dilatation is useful rarely in strictures that have not responded to the standard methods. Hegar dilators can be passed retrograde through a gastrostomy while the esophagus is held and can be inspected under direct vision. The risk of perforation is high as these strictures are of the most severe type. Occasionally I have used Maloneys per os with the surgeon passing the bougie and keeping one hand sterile in the chest to gradually ease the bougie through the stricture.

In general I prefer indirect Maloney bougienage and guided Savary bougienage. Using this approach, almost all strictures are safely dilatable and can usually be maintained at No. 60 Fr lumen size.

Surgical Management

Various surgical approaches are possible in the management of a peptic stricture (Table 83–3). Each of these will be outlined briefly, with a more detailed description

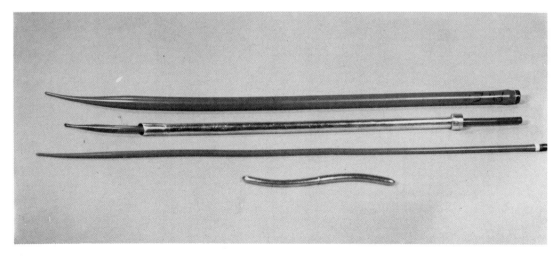

Fig. 83–6. The upper bougie is a No. 60 Fr Maloney bougie. It is compared with a No. 26 Fr gum elastic filling the lumen of an esophagoscope, a No. 26 Maloney, and a No. 20 Hegar dilator.

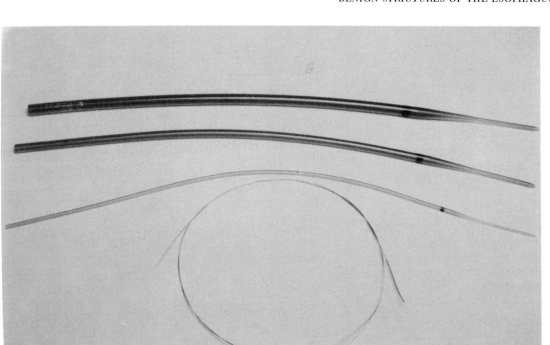

Fig. 83–7. Savary bougies are passed over a guide wire. Tapered Silastic tips allow safe stricture dilatation.

of the procedure that I consider most effective and reliable.

Undilatable Strictures. These are rare, but if intraoperative dilatation using the Hegar dilators is not possible or if the esophagus tears badly during intraoperative dilatation with Hegar bougies, then resection and interposition can be used. Although the techniques of surgical resection are described elsewhere, their relative value in benign esophageal replacement should be considered.

Whenever possible, the esophagus should be preserved, but if resection is necessary, the most commonly used replacement is the left colon. This approach has the advantage of well established reliability and is adaptable to replacement of distal esophagus as well as total esophageal replacement.

Small bowel interposition, as described by Merendino (1958), has been used successfully, although reported experienced is scant.

Bowel interposition has the advantage of preserving stomach below the diaphragm and is less likely to result in nutritional problems than esophagogastric anastomosis

Table 83–3. Classification of Operative Repairs

Undilatable Strictures (rare)
   Esophageal resection and replacement by colon, small bowel, or
      stomach
Dilatable Strictures
   Standard hernia repair using methods of Belsey, Hill, or Nissen
Dilatable Stricture—plastic procedure
   Thal-Nissen
   Intrathoracic Nissen
   Partial fundoplication gastroplasty
   Total fundoplication gastroplasty

is. Stomach as a replacement organ does have some advantages in older patients whose blood supply to the colon or small bowel may be less reliable. Pearson (1969) and I (1971) and our colleagues showed that under these circumstances an end-to-end esophagogastric anastomosis with 4-cm invagination effectively controls reflux and usually gives a good clinical result.

Most patients with bowel or stomach replacement of distal esophagus return to normal and comfortable eating. Reflux is effectively controlled by the intra-abdominal segment of colon or small bowel, or by the invagination technique of esophagogastric anastomosis. If these patients do develop gastric or esophageal problems, little more can be done, and for this reason these procedures should be carefully restricted.

Standard Hiatal Hernia Repair. Belsey (1977), Skinner and Belsey (1967), Hill (1977) and associates (1970), or Nissen's (1977) methods carry a higher recurrence rate in the presence of stricture and esophageal shortening than in the management of the uncomplicated hiatal hernia. Standard hernia repairs must be constructed under tension with a resultant higher incidence of breakdown and recurrence. Because of these difficulties, most surgeons have abandoned standard repair as a method of managing peptic stricture, although both the Hill repair and the Nissen have been described as being valuable in the presence of stricture.

Plastic Repair. The Thal (1968) operation was described as a method of handling esophageal shortening and stricture. Thal split the esophagus longitudinally, opening the strictured lumen and using stomach as a patch. Although this operative approach immediately relieves dysphagia, it carries definite problems. Reflux is inadequately controlled so that restricturing may occur. The intrathoracic stomach, produced by the Thal procedure, may become ulcerated because of poor emptying or may, because of hiatal weakness, allow a paraesophageal hernia. These problems carry with them a delayed threat to life.

Woodward and associates (1970) modified the Thal procedure to produce a Thal-Nissen intrathoracic fundoplication. Although this method effectively controls reflux, it does not avoid the difficulties of ulceration in the intrathoracic stomach or the potential to develop a paraesophageal hernia (Fig. 83–8).

The intrathoracic Nissen effectively controls reflux and can be used in conjunction with stricture dilatation to give good immediate results; again, the problems of an intrathoracic stomach are significant and this approach should be avoided.

Gastroplasty. This operative approach was originally developed by Collis (1961). The procedure lengthens the esophagus by cutting a tube from the lesser curvature of stomach. This gastroplasty tube is then retained below the diaphragm and used for reflux control. Esophageal strictures can be dilated intraoperatively and, with good reflux control, remain fully patent or require only occasional early dilatation.

Collis developed the gastroplasty tube and used his own hernia repair for reflux control. The results were not completely satisfactory because of a high incidence of continued moderate to severe reflux.

Pearson (1977) and associates (1973, 1978) modified Collis' operative approach, using a modified Belsey fundoplication for reflux control. Although his results are better than those of Collis, he reported a high incidence of reflux. I (1978b) have been unable to reproduce Pearson's results, using a similar operative approach (Fig. 83–9).

Because of failure to achieve reflux control with the Belsey or partial fundoplication gastroplasty—PFG—I (1977) developed the total fundoplication gastroplasty—

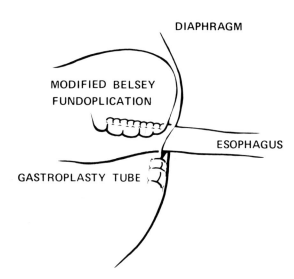

Fig. 83–9. In the Belsey or partial fundoplication gastroplasty, the gastroplasty tube is cut in the same manner as for a total fundoplication gastroplasty (Fig. 83–10). The method of fundoplication varies with each author's report; however, basically a 270° wrap is completed around the gastroplasty tube, incorporating if possible the distal 2 cm of esophagus. This wrapped gastroplasty tube is then reduced below the diaphragm and fixed in this position by crural closure.

TFG—as a method of reflux control. This operative approach will be described in more detail.

Total Fundoplication Gastroplasty. The choice of incision for TFG can vary with the preoperative pathology. I (1985b) reported the use of a transabdominal incision for primary hernia repairs in patients with normal esophageal length and reserved the thoracoabdominal or thoracic incisions for revision surgery and for patients with reflux-induced esophageal scar shortening.

The distal esophagus and gastric fundus are mobilized. Posterior crurae are repaired with No. 1 silk sutures. The gastroplasty tube is fashioned over a No. 60 Fr Maloney bougie. At this stage the new fundus is passed posterior to the gastroplasty tube and distal esophagus and the fundic tip brought medially. The first step in suture fixation is to approximate stomach to the gastroplasty tube and distal 1 cm of esophagus with 5 mattress 2-0 silk sutures (Fig. 83–10). This creates stability and an intra-abdominal length of 6.5 cm. Completion fundoplication is accomplished by approximately the tip of the fundus to the fundic body over a tailored distance of 1.5 cm using 3 mattress 2-0 silk sutures (Fig. 83–11).

The fundoplication creates a flap-valve mechanism, preventing reflux, but with the reduced length of fundoplication, the degree of competence is controlled and these patients do not have dysphagia or eructation.

I have reported this technique (1985a) in 351 patients, with 5 to 8.5 years of follow-up. In this study, 93.1% of patients became asymptomatic, 4% improved, and 2.9% had significant residual or recurrent symptoms.

This operative technique is safe and effective and is my approach to the management of dilatable esophageal strictures secondary to reflux.

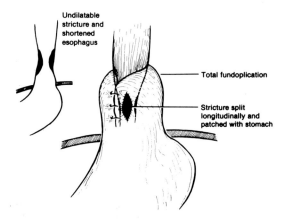

Fig. 83–8. The Thal-Nissen procedure has been advocated for the management of a tight stricture. The stricture is opened longitudinally and patched with a free graft of skin and then stomach. Reflux control is maintained by an intrathoracic fundoplication.

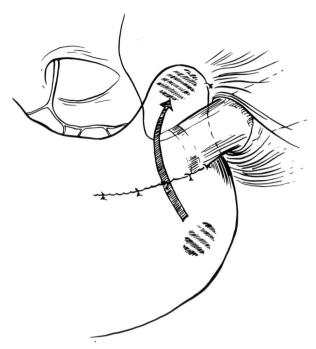

Fig. 83–10. The gastroplasty tube is 5 cm long and No. 60 Fr in diameter. In preparation for fundoplication, gastric fundus is mobilized laterally to the distal 1.5 cm of esophagus and the gastroplasty tube suture line using 5-000 silk mattress sutures. This suture line creates 6.5 cm of intra-abdominal esophagus.

OTHER STRICTURES RELATED TO REFLUX

Most reflux strictures are at the squamocolumnar junction, but other strictures do occur and variations of the typical peptic stricture also occur.

Schatzki's Ring

Although a Schatzki's ring, as Goyal and his colleagues (1971) noted, occurs exactly at the squamocolumnar junction, it is quite different in its significance from the mere tight peptic stricture (Fig. 83–12). With a Schatzki's ring, only minor inflammatory changes occur, and the ring is a thin, submucosal, fibrous band. The presence or absence of a ring has little to do with the severity of reflux

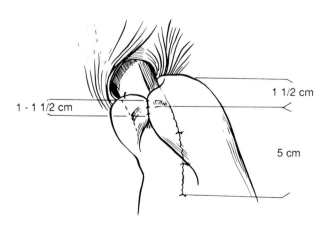

Fig. 83–11. Complete fundoplication is over a distance of 1 to 1.5 cm using 3-00 silk mattress sutures. The fundoplication is tailored to lie on the medial aspect of the esophagus.

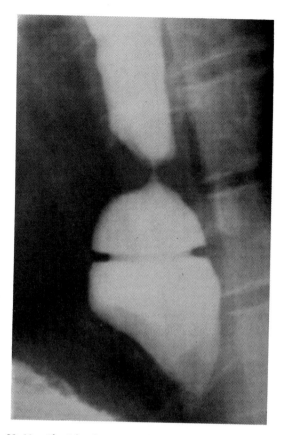

Fig. 83–12. The Schatzki ring is at the squamocolumnar junction and is narrow and symmetrical in outline. Almost always it is associated with a recognizable hiatal hernia.

symptoms. The only symptom definitely associated is dysphagia, and this symptom tends to be minor and bolus-size related.

The stricture itself is not an indication for surgical management. If dysphagia is present, a single dilatation with a No. 60 Fr Maloney bougie is usually effective. Operative intervention for reflux control is carried out only when clinically indicated because of intractable symptoms.

Midesophageal Stricture

These strictures are uncommon. They may be associated with ectopic gastric mucosa but may also occur in the squamous-lined esophagus. When present and related to reflux, they can be treated like a standard peptic stricture except that great care is necessary at endoscopy to brush and biopsy this stricture, because malignancy must be excluded.

Allison-Johnston Stricture and Barrett's Esophagus

The origin of a gastric-lined esophagus is controversial. In its early embryonic state, the esophagus is lined by columnar epithelium, but with development, this columnar lining is replaced by squamous lining. Islands of ectopic columnar mucosa may persist in the adult esophagus. With reflux, ulceration of the squamocolumnar junction denudes the lower esophagus. When re-epithelialization takes place, the mucosa may be of a gastric type. Progressive replacement may result in extensive gastric lining in the lower esophagus. In a few patients, Barrett (1957) found gastric lining progressing to the level of the aortic arch and just above. Whether this type of clearly delineated esophageal replacement is secondary to reflux or is congenital has not been decided. Almost all patients with extensive gastric lining in the esophagus have a hiatal hernia and reflux (Fig. 83–13).

An Allison-Johnston stricture commonly develops at the new squamocolumnar junction. Although this stricture resembles the Schatzki's ring at the HPZ, it may progress and cause major mechanical obstruction.

Patients with a Barrett's esophagus have increased risk of carcinoma—adenocarcinoma, high esophageal stricture, and reflux symptomatology, which is often severe. Naef and colleagues (1975) showed that malignancy must be excluded, both by roentgenologic methods and by endoscopic biopsy. If no malignancy is present, management can be based on symptom severity.

The strictures can be dilated. Some patients' reflux symptoms are not severe, but in my experience, most are severe and unresponsive to conservative management. The presence of gastric mucosa in the thoracic esophagus should not deter the surgeon from operative reflux control. Once reflux has been stopped, the Allison-Johnston stricture resolves with appropriate dilatation and the patient returns to normal eating without heartburn symptoms.

Most of these patients have a thick-walled, shortened

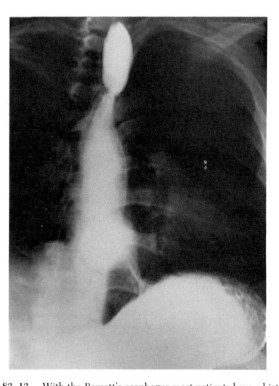

Fig. 83–13. With the Barrett's esophagus most patients have a hiatal hernia with reflux. The body of the eosphagus is replaced by gastric mucosa and frequently a stricture forms at the squamocolumnar junction.

esophagus; for such patients, esophageal lengthening and total fundoplication gastroplasty is the operative procedure of choice.

Cricopharyngeal Web

Web-like strictures at the cricopharyngeal junction have been reported to be related to hypochromic anemia and malignancy. This association is rare. Most such strictures are associated with active reflux, and the stricture itself is inflammatory. When the patient refluxes at night, the gastric reflux bolus lodges below the first competent sphincter—the cricopharyngeus—and I and my co-workers (1976) showed that it produces a local inflammation and muscle incoordination.

Strictures at this level are rare, but may be present with major symptoms of cricopharyngeal dysphagia and aspiration of the swallowed food bolus. Occasionally with solid particles, aspiration and tracheal obstruction may lead to asphyxia and death.

Roentgenographic examinations help establish a diagnosis, but without a careful search for this stricture, it can easily be missed. Endoscopy and biopsy are mandatory, and at the same time the stricture can be dilated to No. 60 Fr.

Once the stricture has been dilated, the major dysphagia symptoms and the risk of aspiration are under good control. Further management depends on the severity and responsiveness of reflux symptoms to standard medical management.

SCLERODERMA AND RELATED COLLAGEN DISEASES

Patients with scleroderma and related collagen diseases may lose esophageal motor power in the lower two thirds of the eosphagus. Most commonly this loss occurs in scleroderma—Stevens and associates (1964) found an 86% incidence of adynamic esophagus—and is commonly associated with Reynaud's phenomenon.

With an adynamic esophagus, HPZ tone is markedly reduced and esophageal motor activity has low amplitude.

Patients with an adynamic esophagus may be totally asymptomatic, and swallowing may occur by gravity alone. When reflux occurs, esophageal wall inflammation and stricture develop early and may be severe. The general symptoms resemble those of patients with normal esophageal motor function. When a stricture develops, food obstruction is disproportionately severe because of the loss of peristaltic motor power.

For effective relief of dysphagia, the esophagus must be dilated to No. 60 Fr. Even a mild peptic stricture produces severe dysphagia.

When surgical intervention is contemplated, my and Pearson's (1973) experience indicates that esophageal lengthening by gastroplasty is necessary, the addition of a shortened and modified total fundoplication wrap is essential for good reflux control.

I prefer a TFG with completion of fundoplication only 5 mm long—one stitch. Although this procedure allows reflux control, it avoids the difficulty of excess competence and dysphagia that may occur with a 3-cm fundoplication.

TRAUMATIC ESOPHAGEAL STRICTURES

When the esophagus was previously damaged by caustic ingestion, reflux aggravates a pre-existing stricture.

The esophageal shortening process caused by scar maturation may result in the development of a hiatal hernia and reflux. When caustic strictures reactivate, reflux should always be evaluated as a possible causative factor.

Caustic Burns of the Esophagus

The cause of and pathologic conditions associated with acute caustic burns are described in Chapter 45. Only the late sequelae will be considered.

Borrie (1945) showed that management in late-stage disease consists of dilatation and diet modification to avoid major food obstruction. Once the inflammatory response has completely resolved, the patient is left with a single or multiple fibrous stricture of varying length and tightness. Dilatation therapy follows the principles already outlined. When initially seen, these patients should undergo endoscopic studies and be dilated under direct vision. A successful dilatation allows a lumen size of No. 34 Fr. Indirect bougienage may then successfully increase lumen size to No. 60 Fr. The stricture's density, however, may be a limiting factor; particularly with long strictures, effective dilatation may not be possible.

Once maximum possible dilatation has been achieved, these patients can usually be followed with dietary care to avoid hard solid food, and further endoscopy or dilatation is carried out only when necessary or if a food bolus obstructs.

Some such patients do not have a satisfactory esophageal lumen and require esophageal resection and interposition. Occasionally, endoscopy and dilatation result in esophageal perforation, necessitating esophageal reconstruction.

Late Complications of Trauma

As previously described, esophageal shortening may result in symptomatic reflux. The first indication of reflux may be reactivation of a previously quiescent stricture.

Carcinoma may also develop as a late complication of caustic stricture. These malignant growths usually present as increasing dysphagia and may be recognized earlier if attention is paid to biopsy and brushing of strictures at the time of endoscopy.

Foreign Body Ingestion

The cricopharynx is the narrowest part of the gastrointestinal tract, and most swallowed objects, once through the cricopharynx, pass into the stomach. Although exceptions exist, most objects sticking in the esophagus do so because of a sharp edge that impinges on mucosa.

Boyd (1951) showed that foreign bodies in the esophagus are badly tolerated and produce recognizable symptoms of pain and dysphagia. If left in the esophagus, they may disimpact and pass to stomach. Many produce perforation of pleura or aorta, or because of ulcercation, may produce a stricture.

Treatment initially is endoscopic removal of the foreign body. If this procedure fails, the foreign body must be removed by thoracotomy. Complications of an impacted foreign body may require emergency operation.

Sequelae of Spontaneous, Traumatic, or Postoperative Esophageal Fistulae

Esophageal fistulae are a rare cause of stricture, and even major fistulous tracts usually close spontaneously without stenosis. Strictures, should they develop, almost always can be managed effectively by bougienage once healing is complete.

Previous Surgical Resections of Esophagus

Various types of stricture can develop at the site of a previous operation. Most resective esophageal procedures entail anastomosis of the esophagus to another organ—stomach, small bowel, or colon. The most common exception is end-to-end esophageal anastomosis in children with esophageal atresia.

Esophagogastric anastomoses may initially cause stricture from suture reaction and operative trauma; delayed strictures may, however, result from gastroesophageal reflux.

Dilatation of an end-to-end suture line stricture must

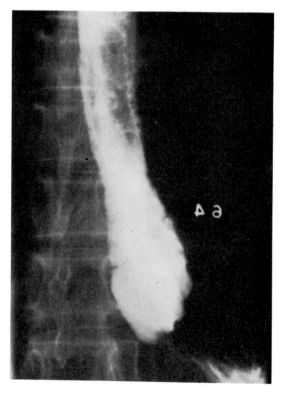

Fig. 83–14. In patients with monilia esophagitis a superficial, severe, ulcerative esophagitis is present. The mucosal ulceration can be recognized radiologically.

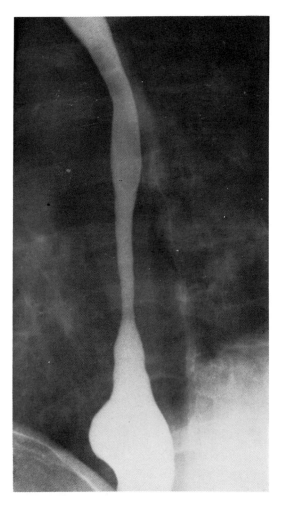

Fig. 83–15. In Behçet's disease, esophageal ulceration may be present in the absence of reflux. In the patient illustrated, a 10-cm diffuse narrowing has required repeated dilatation to allow for adequate swallowing.

be performed cautiously. The esophageal wall is not as thickened and fibrosed as in esophagitis and may rupture with even minor dilating pressure.

Monilia Esophagitis and Stricture

Jensen and colleagues (1964) showed that moniliasis develops secondary to antibiotic or steroid therapy; it can also occur in debilitated and immunosuppressed patients. Most often a painful red mouth with characteristic multiple small monilial plaques indicates the presence of the disease. The esophagus itself develops a fulminating infection that is usually recognizable endoscopically because of its severity.

The ulcerative process affects the mucosa, rarely extending through the esophageal wall.

Painful dysphagia is the most common symptom, again usually present in a debilitated patient.

Roentgenology studies by Sheft and Shrago (1970) showed a characteristic extensively ulcerated esophagus (Fig. 83–14). Orringer and Sloan (1978) showed that this ulceration can progress to stricture formation.

When the problem is recognized, oral nystatin—mycostatin—is the treatment of choice and usually gives satisfactory results. Unrecognized disease can progress to severe stricture formation and occasionally to fistulization with the tracheobronchial tree.

When a stricture develops, it can usually be successfully treated by dilatation. Based on past experience, dilatation should be carried out carefully because the esophageal wall is not as thickened and scarred as with a peptic esophagitis and perforation can occur more readily.

RARE CAUSES OF ESOPHAGEAL STRICTURE

Behçet's Disease

This rare autoimmune disease can occasionally be associated with diffuse esophageal ulceration and secondary stricture formation (Fig. 83–15).

Berlin (1960) and Arma and associates (1971) showed that diagnosis of this process depends upon its coexistent systemic manifestations. Roentgenologically, a stricture may be demonstrable in the absence of reflux. Manometric changes are nonspecific.

Because of its rarity, no established modalities of therapy are available. In my experience with one such patient, intermittent bougienage allowed an adequate diet.

Pemphigus

Minkin (1973) and Raque (1970) and their co-workers found that pemphigus occasionally involves the esophagus and causes secondary stricture formation and hemorrhage. This disorder should be considered whenever the typical skin manifestations of pemphigus are associated with symptomatic dysphagia.

Management includes treatment of the systemic disorder with the possible addition of esophageal dilatation.

REFERENCES

Aylwin, J.A.: Physiological basis of reflux oesophagitis in sliding hiatal diaphragmatic hernia. Thorax 8:38, 1953.
Arma, S., et al.: Dysphagia in Behçet syndrome. Thorax 26:155, 1971.
Barrett, N.R.: The lower esophagus lined by columnar epithelium. Surgery 41:881, 1957.
Behar, J., et al.: Cimetidine in the treatment of symptomatic gastroesophageal reflux. Gastroenterology 73:441, 1978.
Belsey, R.: Mark IV repair of hiatal hernia by the trans-thoracic approach. World J. Surg. 1:475, 1977.
Berlin, C.: Behçet's disease as a multiple symptom complex; report of ten cases. A.M.A. Arch. Dermatol. 82:73, 1960.
Berridge, F.R., Friedland, G.W., and Tagart, R.E.B.: Radiological landmarks at the oesophago-gastric junction. Thorax 21:499, 1966.
Borrie, J.: Management of corrosive burns of the esophagus. Aust. N.Z. J. Surg. 25:62, 1955.
Booth, D.J., Kemmerer, W.T., and Skinner, D.B.: Acid clearing from the distal esophagus. Arch. Surg. 96:731, 1968.
Botha, G.S.M.: The Gastro-Oesophageal Junction. Boston, Little, Brown and Co., 1962.
Boyd, G.: Esophageal foreign bodies. Can. Med. Assoc. J. 64:102, 1951.
Collis, J.L.: Gastroplasty. Thorax 16:197, 1961.
Creamer, B., Andersen, H.A., and Code, C.F.: Esophageal motility

in patients with scleroderma and related diseases. Gastroenterologia (Basel) 86:763, 1956.

DeMeester, T.R., Johnson, L.F., and Kent, A.H.: Evaluation of current operations for prevention of gastroesophageal reflux. Ann. Surg. 180:511, 1974.

Donnelly, R.J., Everall, P.B., and Watson, D.A.: Hiatus hernia with and without esophageal stricture: experience with the Belsey Mark IV repair. Ann. Thorax. Surg. 16:301, 1973.

Ellis, F.H.: The effects of fundoplication on the lower esophageal sphincter. Surg. Gynecol. Obstet. 143:1, 1976.

Fordtran, J.S., Morawski, S.G., and Richardson, C.T.: In vivo and in vitro evaluation of liquid antacids. N. Engl. J. Med. 288:923, 1973.

Goyal, R.K., Bauer, J.L., and Spiro, H.M.: The nature and location of lower esophageal ring. N. Engl. J. Med. 284:1175, 1971.

Henderson, R.D.: Motor Disorders of the Esophagus. Baltimore, Williams & Wilkins, 1976.

Henderson, R.D.: Reflux control following gastroplasty. Ann. Thorac. Surg. 24:206, 1977.

Henderson, R.D.: Gastroesophageal reflux following gastric operation. Ann. Thorac. Surg. 26:563, 1978a.

Henderson, R.D.: The gastroplasty tube as a method of reflux control. Can. J. Surg. 21:264, 1978b.

Henderson, R.D., and Marryatt, G.V.: Total fundoplication gastroplasty (Nissen gastroplasty): five-year review. Ann. Thorac. Surg. 39:74, 1985a.

Henderson, R.D., and Marryatt, G.V.: Transabdominal total fundoplication gastroplasty to control reflux: a preliminary report. Can. J. Surg. 28:127, 1985b.

Henderson, R.D., and Pearson, F.G.: Preoperative assessment of esophageal pathology. J. Thorac. Cardiovasc. Surg. 72:512, 1976.

Henderson, R.D., and Pearson, F.G.: Surgical management of esophageal scleroderma. J. Thorac. Cardiovasc. Surg. 66:868, 1973.

Henderson, R.D., Lind, J.F., and Feaver, B.: Invagination for control of reflux after esophagogastric anastomosis. Can. J. Surg. 14:195, 1971.

Henderson, R.D., et al.: The role of bile and acid in the production of esophagitis and the motor defect of esophagitis. Ann. Thorac. Surg. 14:465, 1972.

Henderson, R.D., Woolf, C., and Marryatt, G.: Pharyngoesophageal dysphagia and gastroesophageal reflux. Laryngoscope 86:1531, 1976.

Hill, L.D.: Progress in the surgical management of hiatal hernia. World J. Surg. 1:425, 1977.

Hill, L.D., Gelfand, M., and Bauermeister, D.: Simplified management of reflux esophagitis with stricture. Ann. Surg. 172:638, 1970.

Jensen, K.B., et al.: Esophageal moniliasis in malignant neoplastic disease. Acta Med. Scand. 175:455, 1964.

Johnston, A.G.: Controlled trial of metoclopramide in the treatment of flatulent dyspepsia. Br. Med. J. 2:25, 1971.

Justin-Besancon, J., Laville, C., and Thominet, M.: Le metoclopramide et ses homologues: introduction à leur étude biologique. C.R. Acad. Sci. (Paris) 258:4384, 1964.

Kelly, M.L., Jr.: Intraluminal manometry in the evolution of malignant disease of the esophagus. Cancer 21:1011, 1968.

Merendino, K.A., and Thomas, G.I.: The jejunal interposition operation for substitution of the esophagogastric sphincter: present status. Surgery 4:1112, 1958.

Minkin, W., Seliger, G., and Auerbach, R.: Esophageal stenosis in benign mucous membrane pemphigoid. Ann. Otol. 82:384, 1973.

Naef, A.P., Savary, M., and Ozyello, L.: Columnar lined lower esophagus: an acquired lesion with malignant predisposition. Report on 140 cases of Barrett's esophagus with 12 adenocarcinomas. J. Thorac. Cardiovasc. Surg. 70:826, 1975.

Nissen, R., Rosetti, J., and Siewert, R.: 20 years in the management of reflux disease using fundoplication. Chirurgie 48:634, 1977.

Orringer, M.B., and Sloan, H.: Monilia esophagitis: an increasingly frequent cause of esophageal stenosis. Ann. Thorac. Surg. 26:364, 1978.

Palmer, E.D.: The hiatus hernia-esophagitis-esophageal stricture complex: twenty year prospective study. Am. J. Med. 44:566, 1968.

Payne, W.S.: Surgical treatment of reflux esophagitis and stricture associated with permanent incompetence of the cardia. Mayo Clin. Proc. 45:553, 1970.

Pearson, F.G.: Surgical management of acquired short esophagus with dilatable peptic stricture. World J. Surg. 1:463, 1977.

Pearson, F.G., and Henderson, R.D.: Experimental and clinical studies of gastroplasty in the management of acquired short esophagus. Surg. Gynecol. Obstet. 136:737, 1973.

Pearson, F.G., Henderson, R.D., and Parrish, R.M.: An operative technique for control of reflux following esophagogastrostomy. J. Thorac. Cardiovasc. Surg. 58:668, 1969.

Pearson, F.G., Cooper, J.D., and Nelems, J.M.: Gastroplasty and fundoplication in the management of complex reflux problems. J. Thorac. Cardiovasc. Surg. 76:664, 1978.

Pope, C.E., II: A dynamic test of sphincter strength; its application to the lower esophageal sphincter. Gastroenterology 52:779, 1967.

Raque, C.J., Stein, K.M., and Samitz, M.H.: Pemphigus vulgaris involving the esophagus. Arch. Dermatol. 102:371, 1970.

Sheft, D.J., and Shrago, G.: Esophageal moniliasis. The spectrum of the disease. J.A.M.A. 213:1859, 1970.

Skinner, D.B., and Belsey, R.H.R.: Surgical management of esophageal reflux and hiatal hernia: long term results with 1030. J. Thorac. Cardiovasc. Surg. 53:33, 1967.

Snape, W.J., and Cohen, S.: Hormonal control of esophageal function. Arch. Intern. Med. 136:538, 1976.

Spitz, L.: Congenital esophageal stenosis distal to associated atresia. J. Pediatr. Surg. 8:973, 1973.

Stevens, M.B., et al.: Aperistalsis of the esophagus in patients with connective-tissue disorders and Raynaud's phenomenon. N. Engl. J. Med. 270:1218, 1964.

Thal, A.P.: A unified approach to surgical problems of the esophagogastric junction. Ann. Surg. 168:542, 1968.

Woodward, E.R., Rayl, J.E., and Clarke, J.M.: Esophageal hiatus hernia. Curr. Probl. Surg. 1:62, 1970.

CHAPTER 84

BARRETT'S ESOPHAGUS

David M. Shahian and F. Henry Ellis, Jr.

Barrett's esophagus is the presence of a columnar epithelial lining of the distal esophagus. Although identification of the condition is attributed to Barrett (1950), who believed it to represent intrathoracic stomach, the first report was actually by Tileston in 1906. Subsequent work by Allison and Johnstone (1953) and Bosher and Taylor (1951) correctly localized the columnar epithelium to the esophagus, a fact Barrett (1957) later acknowledged. Barrett's esophagus is defined as a significant length, usually greater than 3 cm, of columnar-lined tubular esophagus.

INCIDENCE

The prevalence of Barrett's esophagus is difficult to determine because many patients with this condition are asymptomatic. The percentage of patients found to have Barrett's esophagus within a given study group varies proportionately with the severity of reflux symptoms. Naef and colleagues (1975) found Barrett's esophagus in 2% of all patients having upper gastrointestinal endoscopy. It was present in 4% of patients in Burbige and Radigan's (1978) series, in 0.6% of patients in Dees and colleagues' (1978) endoscopy series, and in 2%, as Herlihy and associates (1984) reported. Naef and associates (1975) found Barrett's esophagus in 11%, Borrie and Goldwater (1976) in 4.5%, Starnes and colleagues (1984) in 9.1%, Herlihy and associates (1984) in 14%, and Sarr and co-workers (1985) in 8% of patients who underwent endoscopy because of symptomatic reflux esophagitis. Winters and associates (1987) detected Barrett's esophagus at endoscopy in 12.4% of patients with chronic reflux symptoms and in 36% of patients with esophagitis. Spechler and associates (1983) found Barrett's esophagus in 44% of patients with reflux strictures, an advanced complication of reflux esophagitis.

PATHOGENESIS

Barrett's esophagus was originally thought to be congenital. Johns (1952) demonstrated that fetal ciliated columnar epithelium is present within the esophagus up to the 17th week of gestation and is then replaced in both orad and aborad directions by squamous epithelium. Persistence of this fetal columnar epithelium could result in Barrett's esophagus.

A preponderance of evidence, however, now supports the view that Barrett's esophagus is usually an acquired condition secondary to chronic gastroesophageal reflux. It is almost always seen in association with reflux, and sequential endoscopic studies by Naef and colleagues (1975), Borrie and Goldwater (1976), Mossberg (1966), Goldman and Beckman (1960), and Endo and associates (1974) documented progressive cephalad columnar epithelialization in the presence of continuing reflux. Chronic reflux causes destruction of the normal squamous epithelium and repopulation by columnar epithelium. The source of the latter could be esophageal submucosal glands or congenital columnar epithelial rests within the esophagus, but the most likely explanation is orad migration of cells from the gastric cardia or esophagogastric junction. Bremner and associates (1970) demonstrated experimentally that the combination of mucosal denudation, hiatus hernia, destruction of the lower esophageal sphincter—LES—and gastric hypersecretion can repopulate the lower esophagus with columnar epithelium, and they further showed that the submucous glands were not the source of these new cells. The clinical observation that Barrett's esophagus develops only in patients with the most severe reflux was predictable from Bremner and associates' studies, because only experimental animals with histamine-stimulated hyperacidity as well as reflux had consistent repopulation by columnar epithelium.

This experimental evidence linking Barrett's esophagus to chronic reflux has been corroborated by numerous clinical studies. Burbige and Radigan (1978) and Herlihy and associates (1984) demonstrated low LES pressures and low amplitude contractions in the esophageal body in patients with Barrett's esophagus. They also observed qualitative motor abnormalities, including repetitive contractions, tertiary contractions, and aperistalsis.

Iascone and associates (1983) performed detailed functional studies. Their data from patients with Barrett's esophagus, patients with reflux esophagitis without Barrett's esophagus, and normal control subjects appear to confirm the experimental observation that the potential for the development of Barrett's epithelium increases proportionately with the severity of reflux and acid exposure. Compared with both normal controls and patients with reflux but no Barrett's epithelium, patients with Barrett's esophagus had lower LES pressures, longer esophageal exposure to a pH of less than 4 in both the upright and supine positions, and greater frequency and duration of reflux episodes. These data suggest that the esophagus of those patients with reflux who ultimately develop Barrett's esophagus has more acid exposure.

Several specific clinical settings in which Barrett's esophagus has been observed tend to confirm this pathogenetic scheme. Diminished LES pressure and impaired esophageal peristalsis apparently provide an ideal milieu for the development of Barrett's metaplasia. Barrett's esophagus has been documented in scleroderma by Agha and Dabich (1985) and McKinley and Sherlock (1984) and in postmyotomy achalasia by Feczko and associates (1983). Both conditions are associated with diminished LES pressure and aperistalsis of the esophageal body. Gastric hypersecretion in Zollinger-Ellison syndrome has also resulted in Barrett's esophagus, as Symonds and Ramsey (1980) and Karl and co-workers (1983) described, despite the potentially ameliorating effect of gastrin in increasing LES pressure. Meyer and colleagues (1979) noted Barrett's esophagus after total gastrectomy, and Spechler and associates (1981) noted it following lye ingestion. This suggests that any chronic or severe injury to esophageal squamous mucosa can lead to repopulation by columnar epithelium, although by far the commonest cause remains acid peptic injury.

Although most cases of Barrett's esophagus are acquired secondary to reflux, evidence supports a congenital origin in some patients. Naef and Savary (1972) and Borrie and Goldwater (1976) observed a bimodal age distribution, which led to the hypothesis that childhood cases may be congenital and adult cases a result of reflux. Postlethwait and Musser's (1974) finding of total columnar-lined esophagus on autopsy in a neonate supports this explanation. Nonetheless, Rothstein and Dahms' (1985) and Hassall and associates' (1985) careful analysis of childhood cases demonstrates that most of these young patients have gastroesophageal reflux. In children, reflux may be less clinically apparent because its manifestation is less often heartburn than vomiting or pulmonary symptoms.

The familial occurrence of Barrett's esophagus also has been cited in support of a genetic or inherited cause. Barrett's esophagus has been observed in two brothers by Borrie and Goldwater (1976), in sexagenarian identical twins by Gelfand (1983), in a father and two sons by Everhart and associates (1983), in a father and three sons by Crabb and associates (1985), and in two sisters who presented with Barrett's esophagus at the same age by Prior and Whorwell (1986). In all of these cases, however, it is more likely that the inherited tendency is not for Barrett's esophagus itself but for the development of gastroesophageal reflux.

PATHOLOGY AND CELLULAR FUNCTION

Barrett's esophagus is not simple re-epithelialization of injured esophageal lining by cephalad migration of gastric mucosa. Barrett's epithelium consists of a heterogeneous collection of cell types and patterns, some resembling gastric body and cardiac mucosa and others resembling gastric mucosa that has undergone intestinal metaplasia. Paull and associates (1976) carefully studied Barrett's epithelium using suction biopsy samples obtained under manometric control and have identified three types of mucosa.

The first, a gastric fundic type, resembles the mucosa of the body and fundus of the stomach. It may contain chief and parietal cells and has a gastric foveolar pattern. Goblet cells do not appear.

The second type, junctional epithelium, resembles gastric cardia epithelium. It, too, has a foveolar pattern and cardiac mucous glands, but chief and parietal cells are not present.

The third epithelial type, specialized columnar epithelium, is unlike any other in the gastrointestinal tract. In addition to being the commonest type observed in Barrett's esophagus in adults, it is also the kind most often implicated in the development of dysplasia and adenocarcinoma. It has a villous structure with glycoprotein secretion, mucous glands, and intestinal-like goblet cells. Occasional neuroendocrine and Paneth cells also appear but no parietal or chief cells. Trier (1970) observed that specialized columnar epithelium, unlike normal intestinal columnar mucosa, does not absorb micellar lipids. Specialized columnar epithelium resembles that in type IIB incomplete intestinal metaplasia of the stomach, a process Jass (1980) considered premalignant. This epithelium has some structural and functional resemblance both to gastric and intestinal mucosa. Unlike complete intestinal metaplasia, it has mucous-secreting rather than absorbing cells, in association with intestinal-like goblet cells.

Paull and associates (1976) also found distinct zonation among the three types of mucosa described. Specialized columnar epithelium was always most proximal, the gastric fundic type was most distal, and the junctional epithelium was situated between the two others.

Thompson and associates (1983) performed complete sectioning of eight surgically resected esophagi that contained Barrett's epithelium and adenocarcinoma. Unlike Paull and associates (1976), they found neither the three distinct epithelial types nor a consistent pattern of zonation. When examined in toto rather than by random suction biopsies, Barrett's epithelium appears to be a complex mosaic of cell types, including surface goblet and mucous, absorptive, mucous neck, mucous gland, neuroendocrine, Paneth, chief, and parietal cells. Varying degrees of differentiation toward gastric or intestinal mucosa were observed, interspersed with areas of inflammatory atrophy. The surface architecture was heterogeneous, varying from flat foveolar to villous. Ozzello and associates (1977) and Keen and associates (1984) reported similar histologic findings without obvious zonation. Zwas and associates (1986) confirmed the ultrastructural heterogeneity of Barrett's epithelium by scanning electron microscopy; their studies demonstrated a wide range of microvillar lengths, widths, cell types, and patterns in specialized columnar epithelium.

Barrett's epithelium is capable of a wide range of functional activity, including the secretion of acid and pepsin, gastrointestinal hormones, and mucins. This is consistent with the hypothesis that it derives from metaplastic transformation either of gastric cardiac epithelium or of a pluripotential stem cell. Mangla and associates (1976, 1980) and Hershfield and colleagues (1965) demonstrated pepsinogen and gastrin secretion by Barrett's epithelium, and Ustach and associates (1969) documented acid secretion. Barrett's epithelium itself secretes little acid, particularly in comparison to the amount refluxed. Acid and pepsin secretion occurs only from the gastric fundiclike epithelium, not from specialized or junctional types.

Buchan and associates' (1985) immunocytochemical analysis confirmed the presence of enterochromaffin—serotonin-containing—endocrine cells, gastrin, and somatostatin in fundic and junctional epithelium, but not in specialized columnar epithelium. Banner and colleagues (1983) studied hormonal function in Barrett's adenocarcinoma and contiguous Barrett's epithelium. They also documented the presence of a wide spectrum of gastrointestinal tract hormones, including somatostatin, gastrin, serotonin, substance P, and bombesin.

Lee (1984) investigated mucin secretion by mucous and goblet cells in Barrett's epithelium. Whereas normal gastric surface mucous cells produce neutral mucins, the mucin secreted in Barrett's esophagus is a heterogeneous mix of neutral and acidic mucins, including sialomucins and sulfomucins. Although sulfomucin production does not occur in normal gastric cardiac mucosa and is characteristic of premalignant type IIB intestinal metaplasia, Peuchmaur and co-workers (1984) found it in 53% of patients with benign Barrett's esophagus. Zwas and associates (1986) confirmed this heterogeneity of mucin by demonstrating both colonic-like—acid, sulfated—and small intestinal-like—acid, nonsulfated—types. The presence of acid, sulfated mucins in 43% of patients in Zwas and colleagues' study and in 53% in Peuchmaur and associates' suggest that this finding is common in benign Barrett's epithelium and may not be a useful screening tool for dysplasia or adenocarcinoma.

CLINICAL PRESENTATION

An unknown but probably substantial proportion of patients with Barrett's esophagus are asymptomatic, despite objective data by Iascone and colleagues (1983) that they have significant reflux. This has led to the teleologic argument that Barrett's epithelium, which replaces injured squamous mucosa, is less sensitive to acid peptic injury. Most symptomatic patients with Barrett's esophagus are white men between the ages of 55 and 60, often with a history of alcohol or tobacco use. They commonly present with heartburn or regurgitation secondary to reflux. They may also experience dysphagia or weight loss because of esophageal stricture.

COMPLICATIONS

Stricture and Ulceration

A middle or upper esophageal stricture occurring at the inferior border of the squamous epithelium suggests Barrett's esophagus. Agha (1986), Shapir and colleagues (1985), Chen and co-workers (1985), and Lackey and associates (1984), however, demonstrated that strictures in Barrett's esophagus occur with equal or even greater frequency in the distal third. This may be secondary to healing of a Barrett's ulcer or from an earlier stricture at the squamocolumnar junction with subsequent ascension of Barrett's epithelium. Ulceration is another presentation of Barrett's esophagus and may also be of two different types. A high, shallow ulcer in the squamous epithelium may occur, and this is typical of ulcers associated with reflux esophagitis. The classic Barrett's ulcer occurs within the columnar epithelium and is deep and sharply circumscribed like a gastric ulcer. It may cause hemorrhage, or it may perforate into the mediastinum or pleural space. Occult bleeding from Barrett's epithelium may also result in chronic anemia.

Dysplasia

Adenocarcinoma is the most ominous complication of Barrett's esophagus, and it is now recognized that dysplastic changes precede carcinoma in situ and invasive malignancy. A similar progression of neoplastic changes has been observed in carcinoma of the cervix and colon and in cutaneous melanoma. Studies of cell proliferation in Barrett's epithelium by Herbst and associates (1978) and Pellish and colleagues (1980) suggest that Barrett's epithelium, particularly the specialized columnar type that has been linked clinically to dysplasia and carcinoma, has some neoplastic growth characteristics. Presumably, by identifying dysplasia in patients with Barrett's epithelium, those at high risk for adenocarcinoma may be identified and closely observed and may possibly even undergo prophylactic resection.

The histologic characteristics of dysplasia include decreased cellular specialization and loss of mucin production, increased nuclear cytoplasmic ratio, increase in the number of mitotic figures, loss of orientation, cellular crowding, and nuclear stratification (Fig. 84–1). Changes secondary to inflammation must be excluded. Numerous grading schemes have been proposed, but Riddell and associates' (1983) is the most commonly used.

Dysplastic changes are uncommon in Barrett's epithelium in the absence of adenocarcinoma. Schmidt and associates (1985) reported low grade dysplasia in 2 of 38 patients with benign Barrett's esophagus, and Skinner and colleagues (1983) found dysplasia in 2 of 23 patients

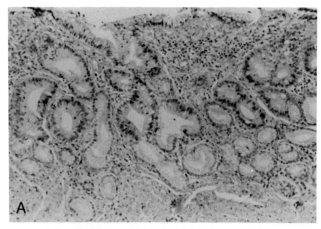

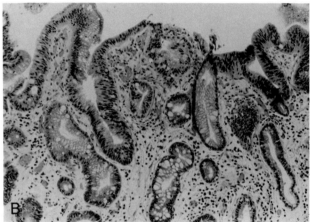

Fig. 84–1. Photomicrographs of esophageal mucosa in two patients with Barrett's esophagus. *A*, Mild dysplasia. *B*, Marked dysplasia.

without cancer. Harle and associates (1985) reported that 10% of patients with benign Barrett's epithelium had dysplasia. Herlihy and associates (1984) reported a 15% prevalence of low grade dysplasia, and Peuchmaur and colleagues (1984) found no dysplasia among 17 patients with benign Barrett's epithelium. Of 107 patients with Barrett's esophagus who were free of adenocarcinoma, Spechler and associates (1984) found only four with low grade dysplasia and none with high grade dysplasia. Spechler and Goyal (1986) estimated the overall prevalence of dysplasia in apparently cancer-free patients with Barrett's epithelium to be 5 to 10%.

In contrast to the overall infrequency of dysplasia in benign Barrett's epithelium, it occurs in many patients with associated adenocarcinoma. These dysplastic changes occur most commonly in specialized columnar epithelium, which is also the type most closely associated with the development of carcinoma. Thompson and colleagues (1983) sectioned eight tumors and found associated multifocal dysplasia in all of them, carcinoma in situ in seven, invasive carcinoma in six, and metastases in three. Haggitt and colleagues (1978) noted multifocal dysplasia associated with carcinoma in 10 of their 12 patients, and Harle and associates (1985) reported dysplasia in 68% of patients with Barrett's carcinoma.

Schmidt and colleagues (1985) found dysplasia in 18 of 23 patients with Barrett's adenocarcinoma, which included 7 patients with continuous transition from high grade dysplasia to carcinoma. In two of these patients, esophagectomy was carried out prophylactically for high grade dysplasia, and carcinoma was found in sectioning of the specimen. Kalish and colleagues (1984) found dysplasia adjacent to Barrett's adenocarcinoma in 21 of their 23 cases. Smith and associates (1984) found dysplasia adjacent to Barrett's adenocarcinoma in 100% of their cases and high grade dysplasia in 89%. Lee (1985) emphasized the significance of high grade dysplasia. In his study, of four patients who underwent prophylactic esophagectomy because of high grade dysplasia, three were found to have invasive carcinoma in the permanent sections.

Barrett's adenoma, described by Stillman and Selwyn (1975) and McDonald and associates (1977), is a unique, macroscopic manifestation of dysplasia in columnar-lined esophagus. Of six patients with esophageal adenoma recently reviewed by Lee (1986), five had adjacent dysplastic epithelium. Lee suggests that adenoma in Barrett's esophagus is a polypoid or nodular form of dysplasia, a macroscopic form within an otherwise flat field of dysplastic mucosa. It may have premalignant potential similar to that of microscopic dysplasia.

Given the significant association between high grade dysplasia and adenocarcinoma, even when carcinoma is not found on random endoscopic biopsies, such patients may be considered to be at substantially higher risk to have occult carcinoma or to develop carcinoma subsequently. Prophylactic esophagectomy is recommended in the otherwise good risk patient. Low grade dysplasia warrants close follow-up and endoscopic biopsy every 3 to 6 months. Because smoking and alcohol consumption may be additive risk factors for the development of carcinoma, they should be discontinued by all patients with Barrett's esophagus.

Adenocarcinoma

Since the initial reports of Carrie (1950) and Morson and Belcher (1952), approximately 200 cases of adenocarcinoma associated with Barrett's esophagus have been described (Fig. 84–2). Although this suggests that Barrett's epithelium is a premalignant state, the risk of carcinoma developing in a patient with Barrett's epithelium has yet to be characterized accurately. Several factors have contributed to the lack of consistent data. First, it is often difficult to distinguish adenocarcinomas arising in Barrett's esophagus from ascending carcinomas of the gastric cardia and from those arising de nova from esophageal submucosal glands or congenital rests. Kalish and associates (1984) compared carcinoma of the gastric cardia with Barrett's adenocarcinoma and found them morphologically similar, although there is a greater incidence of dysplasia and specialized columnar epithelium associated with Barrett's adenocarcinoma. Because carcinomas of the cardia are often excluded in reviews of Barrett's adenocarcinoma and because Barrett's epithelium may be obscured by tumor overgrowth, the actual prev-

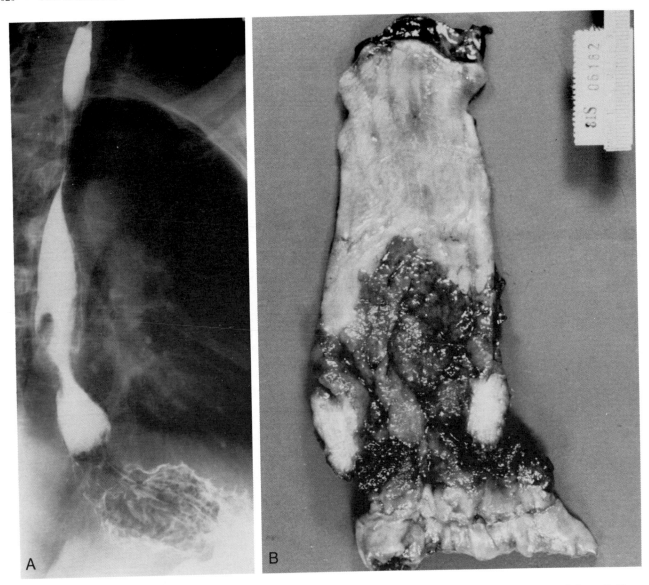

Fig. 84–2. Carcinoma developing in Barrett's mucosa. *A,* Esophageal roentgenogram. *B,* Macroscopic specimen. (From Shahian, D.M., and Ellis, F.H., Jr.: Tumors of the esophagus. *In* Thoracic and Cardiovascular Surgery, 4th ed. Edited by W. Glenn, et al. East Norwalk, CT, Appleton-Century-Crofts, 1983.)

alence of carcinomas in this location that arise from Barrett's epithelium may be underestimated.

Primary esophageal adenocarcinoma is uncommon, probably representing only 5 to 10% of all esophageal carcinomas. Haggitt and associates (1978) and Levine and colleagues (1984) found that 86 to 100% of these primary esophageal adenocarcinomas may actually arise from Barrett's epithelium. Thus, Barrett's adenocarcinoma, adenocarcinoma of the esophagogastric junction, and primary esophageal adenocarcinoma may all have a similar pathogenetic mechanism related to Barrett's epithelium.

Many studies of Barrett's adenocarcinoma are also flawed by their misuse of the statistical terms "incidence" and "prevalence." Prevalence is the percentage of malignant cases found at a given time within a population of patients with Barrett's esophagus, whereas incidence refers to the subsequent risk of cancer developing in

initially cancer-free patients. The malignant potential of Barrett's epithelium may be exaggerated by the use of prevalence data describing the frequency of adenocarcinoma in patients undergoing endoscopy or surgical resection. This population is skewed toward patients who are most symptomatic and ignores the potentially large population of patients with Barrett's esophagus who have not sustained a complication and who do not seek medical help. There is a broad range of reported prevalence data for adenocarcinoma discovered coincidentally with Barrett's epithelium (Table 84–1).

Only four groups have specifically investigated the subsequent risk of adenocarcinoma in patients with Barrett's esophagus who are initially cancer-free. Cameron and associates (1985) found one occurrence in 441 patient-years of follow-up. This incidence was 30 times greater than that in the general population of Minnesota

Table 84–1. Prevalence of Adenocarcinoma in Barrett's Esophagus

Authors	Year	Prevalence (%)
Naef et al.	1975	9
Borrie and Goldwater	1976	0
Radigan et al.	1977	26
Skinner et al.	1983	46
Levine et al.	1984	37
Spechler et al.	1984	7
Sprung et al.	1984a	22
Starnes et al.	1984	37
Cameron et al.	1985	15
Harle et al.	1985	25
Sarr et al.	1985	15
Saubier et al.	1985	13
Achkar et al.	1986	14

but not a statistically significant detriment to survival—age- and sex-corrected. Spechler and associates (1984) reported one case in 175 patient-years of follow-up, a 42.5-fold greater risk than in the general population, and Achkar and associates (1986) reported one occurrence in 160 patient-years of follow-up. At the Lahey Clinic, Sprung and associates (1984a) reviewed 41 patients followed up a total of 162 patient-years. Adenocarcinoma developed in two patients after 3.5 and 4.3 years of surveillance for an incidence of one patient per 81 patient-years of follow-up. Thus, a patient with Barrett's esophagus may be reassured that, although the risk of cancer developing is increased, it is still small.

Barrett's adenocarcinoma usually develops in white men with an average age of 60 years. They commonly have a 7- to 10-year history of reflux symptoms and often use alcohol and tobacco. Their presenting symptoms resemble those of squamous carcinoma of the esophagus, usually dysphagia and weight loss. Skinner and associates (1983), Harle and co-workers (1985), and Sanfey and colleagues (1985) found diminished symptoms of reflux in patients with Barrett's adenocarcinoma, suggesting relative insensitivity to acid.

At the time of diagnosis, adenocarcinoma associated with Barrett's esophagus is similar in macroscopic characteristics to other esophageal cancers, and in two thirds of the cases is stage III because of full-thickness penetration of the esophageal wall and lymph node involvement. Witt and associates (1983) and Meuwissen and colleagues (1983) noted multifocal carcinoma, again emphasizing that the entire Barrett's epithelium is at risk. Adenocarcinoma is not the only histologic type associated with Barrett's epithelium. Haggitt and Dean (1985) and Resano and colleagues (1985) identified squamous and adenosquamous tumors and postulated that these result from islands of residual squamous epithelium within Barrett's esophagus. Smith and associates (1984) found three patients with two separate adenocarcinomas, another patient with adenocarcinoid tumor, another with adenosquamous tumor, and another with adenocarcinoma and a separate distinct focus of squamous carcinoma.

Increased frequencies of other aerodigestive carcino-

mas have been associated with Barrett's adenocarcinoma. Spechler and associates (1984) noted that carcinomas of the head, neck, and lung are more common in these patients, which may be explained by common genetic or environmental factors. Songtag and associates (1985) observed benign and malignant neoplasms of the colon in 45% of patients with Barrett's esophagus. They suggest that routine investigation of the bowel in such patients may prove a more useful surveillance tool than follow-up studies of the esophagus itself.

DIAGNOSIS

Halpert and associates (1984), Robbins and co-workers (1978), and Agha (1986) reviewed the roentgenographic findings of Barrett's esophagus. These are nonspecific and include hiatus hernia, reflux, and mucosal thickening and irregularity secondary to esophagitis. The classic high strictures (Fig. 84–3) or deep Barrett's ulcers are the most specific findings suggestive of Barrett's epithelium. Although Levine and colleagues (1983) have as-

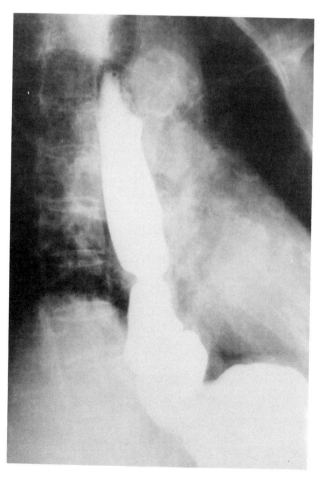

Fig. 84–3. Esophageal roentgenogram in a patient with Barrett's esophagus. Note small sliding esophageal hiatus hernia with an esophageal stricture several inches proximal to the esophagogastric junction. (From Ellis, F.H., Jr.: The esophagus. *In* The Practice of Surgery. Edited by H.S. Goldsmith. Philadelphia, J.B. Lippincott Co., 1983.)

sociated a fine reticular pattern of the mucosa on barium studies with Barrett's esophagus, reports by Vincent and associates (1984), Shapir and co-workers (1985), and Chen and associates (1985) indicated that this is both an insensitive and nonspecific marker of significant esophageal disease.

Endoscopy remains the definitive technique by which to establish a diagnosis of Barrett's esophagus. Desbaillets and Mangla (1976) reviewed the specific characteristics. Barrett's epithelium appears as a slightly irregular, pink-red epithelium, often with edema, erosions, ulcerations, and residual islands of squamous epithelium. This contrasts with the smooth, pink-white squamous mucosa typically seen in the normal esophagus (Fig. 84–4). Herlihy and associates (1984) noted circumferential and island types of columnar epithelium, the latter presumably representing an earlier stage of the disease. Ransom and associates (1982) described limited and extended varieties of Barrett's epithelium, depending on whether it is located less than 30 cm from the incisors. The diagnosis may be equivocal in some patients, particularly when the Barrett's epithelium is of limited extent. Skinner and associates (1983) required at least 3 cm of columnar epithelial-lined tubular esophagus proximal to the normal esophagogastric junction. Spechler and associates (1984) required either the demonstration of specialized columnar epithelium on esophageal biopsy at any level or the presence of gastric fundic or junctional epithelium cephalad to the LES. Burbige and Radigan (1978) suggested the use of Lugol's solution, which stains only squamous epithelium black, to aid in endoscopic diagnosis. Bozymski and colleagues (1982) advocated the use of manometrically guided suction biopsies to assure that specimens are taken from above the LES.

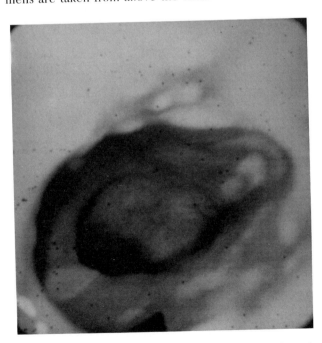

Fig. 84–4. Endoscopic appearance in a patient with Barrett's esophagus. White mucosa is squamous epithelium with erosion. Gray mucosa is Barrett's epithelium with islands of squamous epithelium.

Pertechnetate radionuclide scanning to identify Barrett's epithelium, described by Mangla and Brown (1976), is insensitive. A major shortcoming is its inability to detect the clinically most important specialized columnar epithelium. Herlihy and associates (1984) noted that the electrical potential difference is high across Barrett's epithelium and is low in typical reflux. This has not been used extensively, but it may have application as a screening device.

TREATMENT AND RESULTS

Continued reflux results in cephalad progression of Barrett's epithelium and may be associated with an increasing risk of dysplastic changes and carcinoma. Most investigators believe that, once identified, Barrett's esophagus should be treated. Iascone and associates (1983) observed that symptoms do not correlate well with objective measurements of reflux, and the latter should be the end point of therapy. Medical treatment may be used initially, including such common methods as elevating the head of the bed, weight loss, avoidance of smoking, avoidance of food before bedtime, and dietary modifications. Antacids should be employed as well as cimetidine—Tagamet—or ranitidine—Zantac—to further decrease acid production. Metoclopromide—Reglan—has been employed to increase LES pressure and enhance gastric emptying, and bethanechol—Urecholine—increases esophageal clearance. Follow-up studies by Castell (1985), Kothari and co-workers (1980), Humphries (1982), Wesdorp and associates (1981), and Delpre and colleagues (1984) document that esophagitis in Barrett's epithelium may be treated medically with reasonable success. Patel and associates (1982) also documented regression of Barrett's epithelium and resolution of dysplastic changes in three patients after aggressive medical treatment. Other reports, however, suggest a less favorable response. Starnes and associates (1984) documented progression of Barrett's epithelium to adenocarcinoma in one patient undergoing medical therapy. Overall, 75% of their patients treated surgically had relief of symptoms, compared with 15% in the medical program. Skinner and associates (1983) observed a progression to high grade dysplasia in one patient treated medically for 3 years.

These results led some to advocate a surgical antireflux procedure for all patients with Barrett's esophagus and objective evidence of reflux. Skinner and associates (1983) documented that in patients with benign Barrett's epithelium, antireflux surgery increases LES pressure and renders most patients asymptomatic. Whether or not effective antireflux operation can cause regression of Barrett's epithelium remains controversial. Naef and associates (1975) and Starnes and co-workers (1984) observed no regression of columnar epithelium after antireflux surgery, whereas Radigan and associates (1977) and Ransom and colleagues (1982) did document such regression. Harle and co-workers (1985) reported regression in only one of 13 patients after antireflux operation, but objective testing to document elimination of reflux was not performed. Brand and associates (1980) reported a 40% regression of columnar to squamous epithelium after antireflux operation, although the adequacy of their biopsy methods and sampling techniques has been questioned. Skinner and associates (1983) emphasized that spurious regression of metaplastic epithelium may occur. Repositioning of the esophagogastric junction after an antireflux procedure may give the appearance that the squamocolumnar junction is more distal. Furthermore, these investigators observed squamous epithelial regeneration overlying areas of Barrett's epithelium. This might obscure the columnar epithelium endoscopically, but would not reduce its malignant potential.

The ability of antireflux surgery to reverse or stabilize dysplastic changes is also controversial. Skinner and associates (1983) observed regression of low grade dysplasia in one patient after successful antireflux operation. Skinner (1985) reported no dysplasia and no carcinoma in patients who had objective documentation of reflux control. Abstracts by Pinotti and associates (1986) and Gasparri and co-workers (1986) also reported regression or stabilization of Barrett's epithelium and no incidence of adenocarcinoma after successful antireflux operation.

In contrast to these favorable results, adenocarcinoma occurring after antireflux operation has been described by Starnes and colleagues (1984), Haggitt and associates (1978), Naef and co-workers (1975), Hamilton and colleagues (1984), and Sanfey and associates (1985). Objective evidence of reflux control has not been adequately documented in some of these patients. Sprung and associates (1984b) at our institution followed up 15 patients who had previously undergone antireflux operation for Barrett's esophagus. In four of the 15—27%—partial regression of Barrett's epithelium was demonstrated. In two other patients adenocarcinoma and dysplasia developed at 3.6 years and 3.5 years, respectively. Survival after esophagectomy for Barrett's adenocarcinoma is comparable to that for other esophageal carcinomas as Witt and associates (1983), Skinner and colleagues (1983), and Sanfey and co-workers (1985) reported.

In summary, the goal of treatment of Barrett's esophagus is the elimination of reflux and esophagitis, as documented by objective testing. Although it may be possible to accomplish this medically, surgical antireflux procedures probably offer more consistent results and should be employed if medical treatment fails. Subsequent to treatment, endoscopy should be performed to assess reflux control, resolution of esophagitis, and regression or progression of metaplasia and dysplasia. Identification of low grade dysplasia warrants close endoscopic surveillance at 3- to 6-month intervals. High grade dysplasia is often associated with occult adenocarcinoma and should be considered an indication for operation in otherwise good risk patients. Barrett's adenocarcinoma is treated by standard esophageal resection. All Barrett's epithelium must be removed in addition to the tumor, and some groups advocate total thoracic esophagectomy.

REFERENCES

Achkar, E., et al.: The clinical features and biological behavior of adenocarcinoma of the esophagus complicating Barrett's esophagus. Abstracts of the 3rd World Congress of the International Society for Diseases of the Esophagus and the 3rd International Conference on Diseases of the Esophagus, Munich, West Germany, Sept. 14–19, 1986, p. 94.

Agha, F.P.: Radiologic diagnosis of Barrett's esophagus: critical analysis of 65 cases. Gastrointest. Radiol. 11:123, 1986.

Agha, F.P., and Dabich, L.: Barrett's esophagus complicating scleroderma. Gastrointest. Radiol. 10:325, 1985.

Allison, P.R., and Johnstone, A.S.: The oesophagus lined with gastric mucous membrane. Thorax 8:87, 1953.

Banner, B.F., et al.: Carcinoma with multidirectional differentiation arising in Barrett's esophagus. Ultrastruct. Pathol. 4:205, 1983.

Barrett, N.R.: Chronic peptic ulcer of oesophagus and 'oesophagitis.' Br. J. Surg. 38:175, 1950.

Barrett, N.R.: The lower esophagus lined by columnar epithelium. Surgery 41:881, 1957.

Borrie, J., and Goldwater, L.: Columnar cell-lined esophagus: assessment of etiology and treatment: a 22-year experience. J. Thorac. Cardiovasc. Surg. 71:825, 1976.

Bosher, L.H., Jr., and Taylor, F.H.: Heterotopic gastric mucosa in the esophagus with ulceration and stricture formation. J. Thorac. Surg. 21:306, 1951.

Bozymski, E.M., Herlihy, K.J., and Orlando, R.C.: Barrett's esophagus. Ann. Intern. Med. 97:103, 1982.

Brand, D.L., et al.: Regression of columnar esophageal (Barrett's) epithelium after anti-reflux surgery. N. Engl. J. Med. 302:844, 1980.

Bremner, C.G., Lynch, V.P., and Ellis, F.H., Jr.: Barrett's esophagus: congenital or acquired? An experimental study of esophageal mucosal regeneration in the dog. Surgery 68:209, 1970.

Buchan, A.M.J., Grant, S., and Freeman, H.J.: Regulatory peptides in Barrett's oesophagus. J. Pathol. 146:227, 1985.

Burbige, E.J., and Radigan, J.: Characteristics of the columnar-cell lined esophagus, abstract. Gastroenterology 74:1015, 1978.

Cameron, A.J., Ott, B.J., and Payne, W.S.: The incidence of adenocarcinoma in columnar-lined (Barrett's) esophagus. N. Engl. J. Med. 313:857, 1985.

Carrie, A.: Adenocarcinoma of the upper end of the oesophagus arising from ectopic gastric epithelium. Br. J. Surg. 37:474, 1950.

Castell, D.O.: Medical management of the patient with Barrett's esophagus. In Barrett's Esophagus: Pathophysiology, Diagnosis and Management. Edited by S.J. Spechler and R.K. Goyal. New York, Elsevier, 1985, pp. 199–209.

Chen, Y.M., et al.: Barrett esophagus as an extension of severe esophagitis: analysis of radiologic signs in 29 cases. AJR 145:275, 1985.

Crabb, D.W., et al.: Familial gastroesophageal reflux and development of Barrett's esophagus. Ann. Intern. Med. 103:52, 1985.

Dees, J., van Blankenstein, M., and Frenkel, M.: Adenocarcinoma in Barrett's esophagus: a report of 13 cases, abstract. Gastroenterology 74:1119, 1978.

Delpre, G., et al.: Prolonged cimetidine therapy in ulcerated Barrett's columnar-lined esophagus. Am. J. Gastroenterol. 79:8, 1984.

Desbaillets, L.G, and Mangla, J.C.: Endoscopic diagnosis of Barrett's esophagus. Endoscopy 8:65, 1976.

Endo, M., et al.: A case of Barrett's epithelialization followed up for five years. Endoscopy 6:48, 1974.

Everhart, C.W., Jr., Holtzapple, P.G., and Humphries, T.J.: Barrett's esophagus: inherited epithelium or inherited reflux? J. Clin. Gastroenterol. 5:357, 1983.

Feczko, P.J., et al.: Barrett's metaplasia and dysplasia in postmyotomy achalasia patients. Am. J. Gastroenterol. 78:265, 1983.

Gasparri, G., et al.: Barrett's esophagus: is there a real regression after antireflux surgery? Abstracts of the 3rd World Congress of the International Society for Diseases of the Esophagus and the 3rd International Conference on Diseases of the Esophagus, Munich, West Germany, Sept. 14–19, 1986, p. 92.

Gelfand, M.D.: Barrett esophagus in sexagenarian identical twins. J. Clin. Gastroenterol. 5:251, 1983.

Goldman, M.C., and Beckman, R.C.: Barrett syndrome: case report with discussion about concepts of pathogenesis. Gastroenterology 39:104, 1960.

Haggitt, R.C., and Dean, P.J.: Adenocarcinoma in Barrett's epithelium. In Barrett's Esophagus: Pathophysiology, Diagnosis, and

Management. Edited by S.J. Spechler and R.K. Goyal. New York, Elsevier, 1985, pp. 153–166.

Haggitt, R.C., et al.: Adenocarcinoma complicating columnar epithelial-lined (Barrett's) esophagus. Am. J. Clin. Pathol. 70:1, 1978.

Halpert, R.D., Feczko, P.J., and Chason, D.P.: Barrett's esophagus: radiological and clinical considerations. J. Can. Assoc. Radiol. 35:120, 1984.

Hamilton, S.R., et al.: Adenocarcinoma in Barrett's esophagus after elimination of gastroesophageal reflux. Gastroenterology 86:356, 1984.

Harle, I.A., et al.: Management of adenocarcinoma in a columnar-lined esophagus. Ann. Thorac. Surg. 40:330, 1985.

Hassall, E., Weinstein, W.M., and Ament, M.E.: Barrett's esophagus in childhood. Gastroenterology 89:1331, 1985.

Herbst, J.J., et al.: Cell proliferation in esophageal columnar epithelium (Barrett's esophagus). Gastroenterology 75:683, 1978.

Herlihy, K.J., et al.: Barrett's esophagus: clinical, endoscopic, histologic, manometric, and electrical potential difference characteristics. Gastroenterology 86:436, 1984.

Hershfield, N.B., et al.: Secretory function of Barrett's epithelium. Gut 6:535, 1965.

Humphries, T.J.: Long-term treatment and endoscopic follow-up of patients with Barrett's esophagus. Gastrointest. Endosc. 28:134, 1982.

Iascone, C., et al.: Barrett's esophagus: functional assessment, proposed pathogenesis, and surgical therapy. Arch. Surg. 118:543, 1983.

Jass, J.R.: Role of intestinal metaplasia in the histogenesis of gastric carcinoma. J. Clin. Pathol. 33:801, 1980.

Johns, B.A.E.: Developmental changes in the oesophageal epithelium in man. J. Anat. 86:431, 1952.

Kalish, R.J., et al.: Clinical epidemiologic, and morphologic comparison between adenocarcinomas arising in Barrett's esophageal mucosa and in the gastric cardia. Gastroenterology 86:461, 1984.

Karl, T.R., Pindyck, F., and Sicular, A.: Zollinger-Ellison syndrome with esophagitis and Barrett mucosa. Am. J. Gastroenterol. 78:611, 1983.

Keen, S.J., Dodd, G.D., Jr., and Smith, J.L., Jr.: Adenocarcinoma arising in Barrett esophagus: pathologic and radiologic features. Mt. Sinai J. Med. (N.Y.) 51:442, 1984.

Kothari, T., Mangla, J.C., and Kalra, J.: Barrett's ulcer and treatment with cimetidine. Arch. Intern. Med. 140:475, 1980.

Lackey, C., Rankin, R.A., and Welsh, J.D.: Stricture location in Barrett's esophagus. Gastrointest. Endosc. 30:331, 1984.

Lee, R.G.: Mucins in Barrett's esophagus: a histochemical study. Am. J. Clin. Pathol. 81:500, 1984.

Lee, R.G.: Dysplasia in Barrett's esophagus: a clinicopathological study of six patients. Am. J. Surg. Pathol. 9:845, 1985.

Lee, R.G.: Adenomas arising in Barrett's esophagus. Am. J. Clin. Pathol. 85:629, 1986.

Levine, M.S., et al.: Barrett esophagus: reticular pattern of the mucosa. Radiology 147:663, 1983.

Levine, M.S., et al.: Adenocarcinoma of the esophagus: relationship to Barrett mucosa. Radiology 150:305, 1984.

Mangla, J.C., and Brown, M.: Diagnosis of Barrett's esophagus by pertechnetate radionuclide. Am. J. Dig. Dis. 21:324, 1976.

Mangla, J.C., et al.: Pepsin secretion, pepsinogen, and gastrin in "Barrett's esophagus": clinical and morphological characteristics. Gastroenterology 70:669, 1976.

Mangla, J.C., Camp, R., and Dalton, D.: Agar gel electrophoretic patterns of pepsinogen zymograms in Barrett's esophagus. Biochem. Med. 24:39, 1980.

McDonald, G.B., Brand, D.L., and Thorning, D.R.: Multiple adenomatous neoplasms arising in a columnar-lined (Barrett's) esophagus. Gastroenterology 72:1317, 1977.

McKinley, M., and Sherlock, P.: Barrett esophagus with adenocarcinoma in scleroderma. Am. J. Gastroenterol. 79:438, 1984.

Meuwissen, S.G.M., et al.: Quadruple cancer in a columnar-lined (Barrett) esophagus. J. Clin. Gastroenterol. 5:71, 1983.

Meyer, W., Vollmar, F., and Bär, W.: Barrett esophagus following total gastrectomy: a contribution to its pathogenesis. Endoscopy 11:121, 1979.

Morson, B.C., and Belcher, J.R.: Adenocarcinoma of the oesophagus and ectopic gastric mucosa. Br. J. Cancer 6:127, 1952.

Mossberg, S.M.: The columnar-lined esophagus (Barrett syndrome)—an acquired condition? Gastroenterology 50:671, 1966.

Naef, A.P., and Savary, M.: Conservative operations for peptic esophagitis with stenosis in columnar-lined lower esophagus. Ann. Thorac. Surg. 13:543, 1972.

Naef, A.P., Savary, M., and Ozzello, L.: Columnar-lined lower esophagus: an acquired lesion with malignant predisposition. Report on 140 cases of Barrett's esophagus with 12 adenocarcinomas. J. Thorac. Cardiovasc. Surg. 70:826, 1975.

Ozzello, L., Savary, M., and Roethlisberger, B.: Columnar mucosa of the distal esophagus in patients with gastroesophageal reflux. Pathol. Annu. 12:41, 1977.

Patel, G.K., et al.: Resolution of severe dysplastic (CA in situ) changes with regression of columnar epithelium in Barrett's esophagus on medical treatment, abstract. Gastroenterology 82:1147, 1982.

Paull, et al.: The histologic spectrum of Barrett's esophagus. N. Engl. J. Med. 295:476, 1976.

Pellish, L.J., Hermos, J.A., and Eastwood, G.L.: Cell proliferation in three types of Barrett's epithelium. Gut 21:26, 1980.

Peuchmaur, M., Potet, F., and Goldfain, D.: Mucin histochemistry of the columnar epithelium of the oesophagus (Barrett's oesophagus): a prospective biopsy study. J. Clin. Pathol. 37:607, 1984.

Pinotti, H.W., et al: Barrett esophagus (late results of conservative management). Abstracts of the 3rd World Congress of the International Society for Diseases of the Esophagus and the 3rd International Conference on Diseases of the Esophagus, Munich, West Germany, Sept. 14–19, 1986, p. 92.

Postlethwait, R.W., and Musser, A.W.: Changes in the esophagus in 1,000 autopsy specimens. J. Thorac. Cardiovasc. Surg. 68:953, 1974.

Prior, A., and Whorwell, P.J.: Familial Barrett's oesophagus. Hepatogastroenterology 33:86, 1986.

Radigan, L.R., et al.: Barrett's esophagus. Arch. Surg. 112:486, 1977.

Ransom, J.M., et al.: Extended and limited types of Barrett's esophagus in the adult. Ann. Thorac. Surg. 33:19, 1982.

Resano, C.H., et al.: Double early epidermoid carcinoma of the esophagus in columnar epithelium. Endoscopy 17:73, 1985.

Riddell, R.H., et al.: Dysplasia in inflammatory bowel disease: standardized classification with provisional clinical applications. Hum. Pathol. 14:931, 1983.

Robbins, A.H., et al.: Revised radiologic concepts of the Barrett esophagus. Gastrointest. Radiol. 3:377, 1978.

Rothstein, F.C., and Dahms, B.B.: Barrett's esophagus in children. In Barrett's Esophagus: Pathophysiology, Diagnosis, and Management. Edited by S.J. Spechler and R.K. Goyal. New York, Elsevier, 1985, pp. 129–141.

Sanfey, H., et al.: Carcinoma arising in Barrett's esophagus. Surg. Gynecol. Obstet. 161:570, 1985.

Sarr, M.G., et al.: Barrett's esophagus: its prevalence and association with adenocarcinoma in patients with symptoms of gastroesophageal reflux. Am. J. Surg. 149:187, 1985.

Saubier, E.C., et al.: Adenocarcinoma in columnar-lined Barrett's esophagus: analysis of 13 esophagectomies. Am. J. Surg. 150:365, 1985.

Schmidt, H.G., et al.: Dysplasia in Barrett's esophagus. J. Cancer Res. Clin. Oncol. 110:145, 1985.

Shapir, J., DuBrow, R., and Frank, P.: Barrett oesophagus: analysis of 19 cases. Br. J. Radiol. 58:491, 1985.

Skinner, D.B: The columnar-lined esophagus and adenocarcinoma. Ann. Thorac. Surg. 40:321, 1985.

Skinner, D.B., et al.: Barrett's esophagus: comparison of benign and malignant cases. Ann. Surg. 198:554, 1983.

Smith, R.R., et al.: The spectrum of carcinoma arising in Barrett's esophagus: a clinicopathologic study of 26 patients. Am. J. Surg. Pathol. 8:563, 1984.

Sontag, S.J., et al.: Barrett's oesophagus and colonic tumours. Lancet 1:946, 1985.

Spechler, S.J., and Goyal, R.K.: Barrett's esophagus. N. Engl. J. Med. 315:362, 1986.

Spechler, S.J., et al.: Barrett's epithelium complicating lye ingestion with sparing of the distal esophagus. Gastroenterology *81*:580, 1981.

Spechler, S.J., et al.: The prevalence of Barrett's esophagus in patients with chronic peptic esophageal strictures. Dig. Dis. Sci. *28*:769, 1983.

Spechler, S.J., et al.: Adenocarcinoma and Barrett's esophagus: an overrated risk? Gastroenterology *87*:927, 1984.

Sprung, D.J., Ellis, F.H., Jr., and Gibb, S.P.: Incidence of adenocarcinoma in Barrett's esophagus, abstract. Am. J. Gastroenterol. *79*:817, 1984a.

Sprung, D.J., Ellis, F.H., Jr., and Gibb, S.P.: Regression of Barrett's epithelium after antireflux surgery, abstract. Am. J. Gastroenterol. *79*:817, 1984b.

Starnes, V.A., et al.: Barrett's esophagus: a surgical entity. Arch. Surg. *119*:563, 1984.

Stillman, A.E., and Selwyn, J.L.: Primary adenocarcinoma of the esophagus arising in a columnar-lined esophagus. Am. J. Dig. Dis. *20*:577, 1975.

Symonds, D.A., and Ramsey, H.E.: Adenocarcinoma arising in Barrett's esophagus with Zollinger-Ellison syndrome. Am. J. Clin. Pathol. *73*:823, 1980.

Thompson, J.J., Zinsser, K.R., and Enterline, H.T.: Barrett's meta-plasia and adenocarcinoma of the esophagus and gastroesophageal junction. Hum. Pathol. *14*:42, 1983.

Tileston, W.: Peptic ulcer of the oesophagus. Am. J. Med. Sci. *132*:240, 1906.

Trier, J.S.: Morphology of the epithelium of the distal esophagus in patients with midesophageal peptic strictures. Gastroenterology *58*:444, 1970.

Ustach, T.J., Tobon, F., and Schuster, M.M.: Demonstration of acid secretion from esophageal mucosa in Barrett's ulcer. Gastrointest. Endosc. *16*:98, 1969.

Vincent, M.E., et al.: The reticular pattern as a radiographic sign of the Barrett esophagus: an assessment. Radiology *153*:333, 1984.

Wesdorp, I.C.E., et al.: Effect of long-term treatment with cimetidine and antacids in Barrett's esophagus. Gut *22*:724, 1981.

Winters, C., Jr., et al.: Barrett's esophagus: a prevalent, occult complication of gastroesophageal reflux disease. Gastroenterology *92*:118, 1987.

Witt, T.R., et al.: Adenocarcinoma in Barrett's esophagus. J. Thorac. Cardiovasc. Surg. *85*:337, 1983.

Zwas, F., et al.: Scanning electron microscopy of Barrett's epithelium and its correlation with light microscopy and mucin stains. Gastroenterology *90*:1932, 1986.

CHAPTER 85

BENIGN TUMORS, CYSTS, AND DUPLICATIONS OF THE ESOPHAGUS

Thomas W. Shields

BENIGN TUMORS

Benign tumors of the esophagus are rare. Moersch and Harrington (1944) found only 15 instances in 11,000 patients complaining of dysphagia. Plachta (1962) found 90 benign tumors in 19,982 consecutive autopsies over a 50-year period, an incidence of less than 0.5%.

Benign esophageal tumors can be classified according to their location within the structure—intraluminal, submucosal, or intramural—or according to their histologic type (Table 85–1). The most common of these tumors is the leiomyoma, which is almost always intramural. The esophageal polyp is the second most common lesion and is intraluminal. Hemangiomas and granular cell myoblastomas are less common and are most often submucosal.

Clinical Features

The signs and symptoms of the benign esophageal tumors depend primarily on the location of the tumor. Those located intraluminally obstruct the lumen to a varying extent. Dysphagia, vomiting, and weight loss are the more common features. Bernatz and associates (1958) noted that many patients have aspiration pneumonitis, cough, substernal distress, and gastrointestinal bleeding. The tumor itself is sometimes regurgitated into or even out of the patient's mouth. Rarely, the regurgitated tumor obstructs the airway and kills the patient.

Submucosal lesions may produce obstruction with consequent dysphagia, but many are asymptomatic and are found only incidentally or at autopsy. Hemorrhage may occur in patients with a hemangioma and may be fatal.

Intramural tumors are frequently asymptomatic. When symptoms are present, dysphagia and vague chest pain are the more common complaints. Pyrosis is likewise relatively common, but is considered mainly as a symptom of coexistent esophageal pathology. Weight loss is an inconsistent finding and bleeding is a rarity.

Diagnosis

The diagnostic evaluation of patients with symptoms referable to the esophagus consists of appropriate roentgenographic studies and endoscopy. Occasionally a large intramural esophageal lesion may be recognized on the standard chest roentgenograms as a mediastinal lesion in the visceral compartment (Fig. 85–1) or as widening of the mediastinal shadow as a result of dilatation of the

Table 85–1. Histologic Classification of Benign Tumors of the Esophagus

Epithelial
Papilloma
Polyps
Adenoma
Cysts
Nonepithelial
Myoma
Leiomyoma
Fibromyoma
Lipomyoma
Fibroma
Vascular
Hemangioma
Lymphangioma
Mesenchymal and others
Reticuloendothelial
Lipoma
Myxofibroma
Giant cell
Neurofibroma
Osteochondroma
Heterotopic
Gastric mucosa
Melanoblastic
Sebaceous gland
Granular cell myoblastoma
Pancreatic gland
Thyroid nodule

Adapted from Nemir, P., Jr., et al.: Curr. Probl. Surg. *13*:1, 1976.

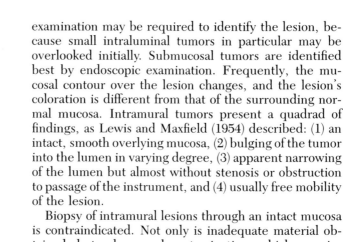

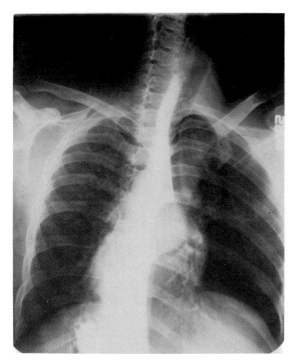

Fig. 85–1. Oblique roentgenogram of chest of barium esophagogram showing an extrinsic rounded mass indenting the esophageal lumen. Enucleation revealed the mass to be a leiomyoma.

esophagus. Calcification may be identified in a leiomyoma. Most often, however, the esophageal lesion is only identified by evaluation of the esophagus by a barium swallow.

Intraluminal tumors may be outlined by the barium column. Movement of the mass may be noted and the normal peristaltic wave may be interrupted just above the tumor and at the level of attachment of the pedicle. At times, the intraluminal tumor may be mistaken for an ingested foreign body. Submucosal tumors are identified rarely by this roentgenographic study. Intramural tumors, however, present a characteristic smooth, crescent type of defect in the contour of the esophageal lumen, as Schatzki and Hawes (1950) described (Fig. 85–2). Characteristically, the lesion meets the normal esophageal wall at a sharp angle. The mucosal folds over the tumor are obliterated but appear on the opposite normal wall.

Other specialized roentgenographic studies such as angiography and pneumomediastinography, reported respectively by Ben-Menachem and associates (1977) and Perasalo and Laustela (1955), are indicated only infrequently. Only in the most difficult situations diagnostically, such as when an aneurysm or a vascular malformation cannot be ruled out, may such an examination be justified. Computed tomography with contrast infusion or magnetic resonance imaging should usually obviate these studies.

Esophagoscopy is indicated in all these patients. An intraluminal tumor, its pedicle, and its attachments may be visualized by appropriate maneuvers. More than one

examination may be required to identify the lesion, because small intraluminal tumors in particular may be overlooked initially. Submucosal tumors are identified best by endoscopic examination. Frequently, the mucosal contour over the lesion changes, and the lesion's coloration is different from that of the surrounding normal mucosa. Intramural tumors present a quadrad of findings, as Lewis and Maxfield (1954) described: (1) an intact, smooth overlying mucosa, (2) bulging of the tumor into the lumen in varying degree, (3) apparent narrowing of the lumen but almost without stenosis or obstruction to passage of the instrument, and (4) usually free mobility of the lesion.

Biopsy of intramural lesions through an intact mucosa is contraindicated. Not only is inadequate material obtained, but submucosal contamination, which may interfere with subsequent treatment, results. Biopsy of intraluminal and submucosal tumors, however, may be accomplished generally without difficulty.

Differential diagnosis of benign tumors of the esophagus includes carcinoma of the esophagus, enterogenous cysts and esophageal duplications, vascular rings and aneurysms, tumors and cysts involving the visceral compartment of the mediastinum, and other intrinsic esophageal diseases.

Leiomyoma

The true incidence of this smooth muscle tumor in the esophagus is probably greater than recorded in the literature. I found 11 such tumors in 700 autopsies (1959), whereas Daniel and Williams (1950) found none in 4000 autopsies. The incidence found undoubtedly reflects the vigor with which these tumors were sought. Clinically, however, these lesions constitute only 5 to 10% of all gastrointestinal leiomyomas. Seremetis and associates (1976) collected 838 documented examples of this tumor located in the esophagus.

Most clinically evident leiomyomas of the esophagus occur in the middle and lower thirds of the thoracic portion of the structure, and only a few occur in the upper third. The incidence is reported to be approximately 40%, 50%, and 10%, respectively. Only rarely are they identified in the cervical portion of the esophagus. According to Seremetis and associates (1976), less than 3% of the lesions are multiple. Diffuse leiomyomatosis of the esophagus was described by Linder and Vogt-Moykopf (1970) and reviewed by Kabuto and colleagues (1980). The latter believe that only patients with numerous confluent myomatous nodules should be included in this category. Ninety-nine percent of clinically evident leiomyomas are intramural, and only the remaining few are intraluminal polypoid tumors.

Leiomyomas are found more commonly in men than in women, a ratio of 2 to 1. None have been reported in infants or young children under the age of 12, but any other age group may be affected.

Intramural tumors are sharply demarcated, round or ovoid, generally smooth, but at times lobulated. The size varies. Infrequently, the growth may be circumferential or even assume the configuration of a horseshoe. In such

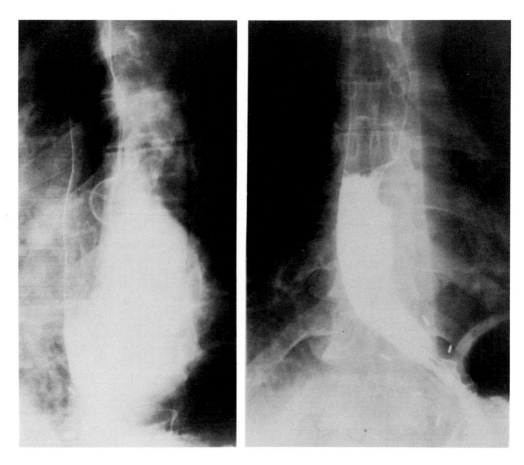

Fig. 85–2. Roentgenogram of chest with barium esophagogram revealing typical smooth filling defect of a small intraluminal leiomyoma.

instances, the lumen may be partially or completely obstructed.

Grossly, the lesion is firm, is usually nodular on cut section, and has a sharp line of demarcation from the surrounding esophagus. Microscopically, the smooth muscle cells are arranged in strands and whorls. The tumor cells sometimes tend to palisade. Hydropic, fatty, and hyaline degenerative changes, as well as calcification, may occur within the lesion.

Polyp of the Esophagus

This rare lesion tends to occur more commonly in older men, although women and persons of other age groups are not exempt. The lesion almost always arises in the cervical esophagus at the level of the cricoid cartilage. Polyps have been found infrequently in the middle and lower thirds of the thoracic portion of the esophagus. Most often the polyp is single.

Grossly, the lesion is located intraluminally; it is long and cylindrical and may have a long pedicle. Occasionally, the mass may be large enough to produce marked dilatation of the esophagus. Microscopically, the polyps are composed of a heterogeneous group of connective tissue elements covered by mucosa, which at times may be secondarily ulcerated. The fibrous element may vary

from a loose myxoid to a dense collagenous tissue. Fatty tissue may comprise a greater or lesser amount of tumor. As Bernatz and associates (1958) suggested, the term "fibrolipoma" describes these polyps accurately. Other histologic varieties of polyps have been reported rarely. Hamartoma, lymphangioma, eosinophilic granuloma, and pure lipoma have been identified in the esophagus.

Lipoma

This benign lesion of the esophagus is uncommon. Most have been recorded as intraluminal polyps. Kinnear (1955) and Ochsner and Ochsner (1957) recorded submucous lipomas, and Tolis and I (1967) reported one located intramurally.

Hemangioma

Generally appearing as submucosal lesions of varying size, they only rarely become polypoid in form. The lesion may appear as a dark, purplish-red nodule in the submucosa. Microscopically, it may be a simple capillary hemangioma, mixed, or more often a cavernous hemangioma.

Hemangiomas constitute approximately 2 to 3% of all benign tumors of the esophagus, and more than half are not discovered until a postmortem examination. The symptomatic lesions present with dysphagia and other symptoms of a large intraluminal polyp or with signs and symptoms of gastrointestinal hemorrhage. Hanel and associates (1981) reviewed the 23 case reports in the literature, added one case report of their own, and outlined the investigation and management of these lesions, which in essence does not differ from that of other benign lesions of the esophagus. Interestingly, endoscopic biopsy of the lesion has not been hazardous.

Neurofibroma and Neurinoma

These lesions are similar to leiomyomas, except for their histologic appearance. This tumor is more common in patients with generalized neurofibromatosis.

Granular Cell Myoblastoma

This lesion, which most commonly is found in the skin, tongue, or breast, has been identified in the esophagus by Paskin (1972) and Farrell (1973) and their associates. Howe and Postlethwait (1981) reviewed 27 case reports from the literature and added 2 of their own. In an esophageal location it is readily confused with a benign stricture, but responds poorly to dilatation. It appears as a whitish, firm area beneath the mucosa. Grossly, the lesion is generally a nodule beneath the mucosa distinct from the muscularis. Microscopically, the tumor is composed of large polyhedral cells with faintly staining cytoplasm and small regular nuclei. The current opinion is that the cells are neural—Schwann cells–in origin. Malignant change has been reported in other sites, but no such instance has been recorded in those located in the esophagus. Despite the low malignant potential, however, invasion does occur, and Howe and Postlethwait (1981) recommended removing even the asymptomatic ones.

Papilloma

This unusual lesion is defined as a growth primarily of mucosal origin. It appears as a sessile, lobulated lesion of varying size. The lesions is covered with squamous epithelium and has a fibrovascular core.

Other Tumors

A true adenoma has been described on several occasions. Postlethwait and Detmer (1975) reported an aberrant thyroid nodule in the esophageal wall.

Treatment

The generally accepted treatment of benign intraluminal, submucosal, and intramural tumors of the esophagus has been surgical removal of the lesion. One exception had been the original management of hemangiomas; radiation therapy was employed in several patients. Even these lesions, however, are now being excised surgically.

The tumor's location and the extent of involvement of the normal esophagus dictate the surgical approach. Intraluminal tumors occasionally can be removed endoscopically when the stalk is accessible and the tumor is small enough to be controlled safely by this approach.

When the size of the lesion or its stalk precludes this approach, cervical exploration or thoracotomy, depending on the location of the origin of the stalk, is indicated. Once the esophagus is free from the surrounding tissues, a longitudinal incision is made through the wall of the esophagus into the lumen on the side opposite the origin of the stalk. The incision should be large enough to permit delivery of the tumor out of the esophagus and to permit isolation and safe division and ligature of the stalk at its site of origin. After the tumor has been removed, the incision in the esophagus is closed in layers with a continuous fine absorbable suture to approximate the mucosa and with interrupted nonabsorbable sutures to close the muscular layer. Esophageal resection rarely is necessary.

Intramural and submucosal tumors are managed most often by the appropriate thoracotomy, incision of the mediastinal pleura, and mobilization of that portion of the esophagus containing the tumor. Schorlemmer and co-workers (1983) recommended a cervical approach for esophageal leiomyoma in the upper third of the thoracic esophagus to avoid the morbidity of a standard thoracotomy. An extension of this approach would be a limited median sternotomy for exposure of the upper thoracic esophagus, as Orringer (1984) suggested. The normal or thinned-out portion of the musculature overlying the tumor is incised longitudinally, and enucleation of the mass by both blunt and sharp dissection is carried out (Fig. 85–3). Generally, enucleation can be accomplished without injury to the esophageal mucosa. When an opening does occur, however, repair of the rent with a continuous fine absorbable suture may be carried out. The incision in the esophageal wall is closed with interrupted fine nonabsorbable sutures. Drainage of the pleural space and closure of the thoracotomy then is carried out

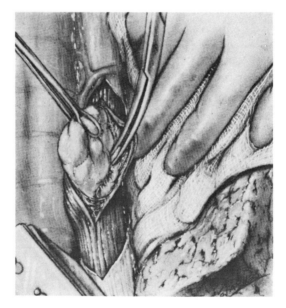

Fig. 85–3. Enucleation of a leiomyoma of the esophagus. (Postlethwait, R.W. (Ed): Surgery of the Esophagus. New York, Appleton-Century-Crofts, 1979, p. 325.)

in a standard manner. Only rarely is excision of the esophagus necessary for the removal of benign tumors, and it should be avoided because of the increase in mortality when this procedure is necessary. The mortality rate after enucleation was less than 2% and at present is probably near zero, whereas the mortality rate can be 10% or greater when resection is carried out.

Despite the low or even zero mortality rate after enucleation, the removal of small, asymptomatic, intramural lesions in adults is questionable. When after thorough diagnostic evaluation the lesion is judged without question a benign tumor or cyst, recommendation for excision of the tumor may be withheld without undue jeopardy to the patient. If symptoms do develop or if growth of the lesion is noted on periodic follow-up evaluation, surgical removal then may be carried out.

Prognosis

The prognosis of patients after identification and removal of benign tumors of the eosphagus is excellent. Malignant degeneration has not been recorded in most of the histologic varieties, and even in the few instances in which it has been reported, the question of whether the lesion was malignant from its inception remains.

CYSTS

Esophageal cysts are uncommon, although in the Mayo Clinic data reported by Andersen and Pluth (1974), esophageal cysts were second only to the leiomyomas as the most common benign "tumor" of this organ.

Esophageal cysts probably originate from displaced cells of the embryonic foregut and may be considered a variant of an enterogenous cyst. The cyst may be incorporated in the wall of the esophagus, may be connected to it by a fistulous tract, or may be only contiguous to it. Because during its development the mucosa of the esophagus is composed initially of pseudostratified columnar epithelium and later by squamous epithelium, an esophageal—enterogenous—cyst may be lined by any of the aforementioned epithelia.

Grossly, the cyst generally is a rounded structure found in an intramural location with splaying out of the longitudinal muscle fibers of the esophagus over it. Usually the cyst can be separated from the esophageal mucosa without difficulty. When the cyst is opened, its contents may be either a clear mucoid or brownish serous material. Microscopic examination of the cyst may reveal a flattened-out epithelial lining or one of typical sqamous, ciliated columnar, or pseudostratified columnar epithelium. At times the lining may resemble gastric mucosa, although this is more common in the larger duplication cysts than in the simple esophageal cysts.

Symptoms

Simple cysts may be symptomatic in the infant or child because of the size of the lesion, with its resultant compression of adjacent respiratory structures or obstruction of the esophageal lumen. In adults, most are asymptomatic, although respiratory distress, dysphagia, and pain have been reported. Sudden onset of severe pain may represent bleeding into the cyst. This condition is rare in the adult and is seen more often in infants and children. Infection of the cyst's contents has occurred, but likewise is unusual in the adult.

Diagnosis

As with benign tumors, the diagnosis is suggested most often by roentgenographic and endoscopic studies. The smaller intramural cysts present the aforementioned typical features described for benign intramural tumors of the esophagus (Fig. 85–4). Biopsy of a suspected cyst is contraindicated.

Treatment

The treatment of either a large or a symptomatic cyst is surgical excision, which may be accomplished by enucleation without injury to the mucosa in most instances. Rarely, esophageal resection is required. Small, asymptomatic cysts in the adult probably do not need to be removed.

DUPLICATIONS

Duplication of the esophagus is a less common lesion than the simple cyst. It should, however, be considered a foregut cyst. Of all duplications of the gastrointestinal tract, 20% occur in the thorax. The duplication is lined with any of the cell types that line simple cysts, and the wall contains all layers of the normal esophagus. The second lumen may or may not communicate with the esophagus or the hypopharynx. In some instances, the duplication is associated with vertebral abnormalities and malformations of the spinal cord. This combination is referred to as the split notochord syndrome. In this situation the "duplication" or cyst may in reality be a neurenteric cyst (see Chapter 90).

Symptoms

The symptoms of duplication of the esophagus depend on its size and on the presence of infection, either of which may cause pain or malfunction of the esophagus. In infants with duplication of the esophagus—neurenteric cyst—Waterston (1972) noted that the duplication was frequently lined by gastric mucosa. When either a vertebral or a spinal anomaly was present, this gastric mucosal lining was almost always present. With this lining, peptic ulceration and erosion into the tracheobronchial tree may occur, with resultant hemoptysis. When a connection to the gastrointestinal tract is present, melena may be a presenting sign. In Pokorny and Goldstein's (1984) review, the enteric thoracoabdominal duplications connected to the gastrointestinal tract in over two thirds of the children. The major symptoms were respiratory in neonates and pain and melena in the older child.

Diagnosis

The duplication may be recognized initially as a mass in the visceral compartment of the mediastinum that may

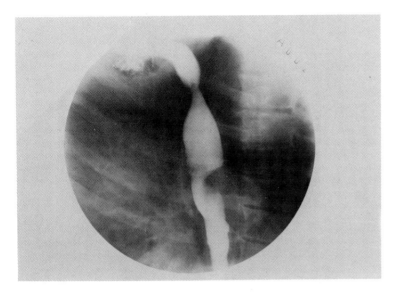

Fig. 85–4. Roentgenogram of chest during barium swallow reveals a filling defect from a duplication cyst.

extend into one or the other paravertebral spaces. Vertebral anomalies may be sought with standard roentgenographic or computed tomographic examination of the thoracic spine. Contrast evaluation of the lumen of the esophagus and esophagoscopy reveals varying degrees of displacement or indentation of the esophageal lumen.

Treatment

Some duplications may be excised without difficulty. When only a common mucosal wall is present between the esophagus and the duplication, the partition may be divided, as Ansell and Edwards (1958) suggested. In infants, adherence of the duplication to surrounding structures, as well as its vascularity, frequently make complete removal hazardous. Waterston (1972) suggested in such situations that only a small incision be made into the lesion—permitting removal of the mucosal lining but leaving the wall intact. Haller and colleagues (1975) also reported partial excision with complete removal of the lining.

Prognosis

The prognosis of patients with duplication of the esophagus, even infants with associated vertebral or spinal cord anomalies, is satisfactory with appropriate surgical intervention. Most of the deaths, as Postlethwait (1979) noted, occurred in those patients receiving only supportive therapy.

REFERENCES

Anderson, H.A., and Pluth, J.R.: Benign tumors, cysts, and duplications of the esophagus. *In* The Esophagus. Edited by W.S. Payne and A.M. Olsen. Philadelphia, Lea & Febiger, 1974, p. 225.

Ansell, G., and Edwards, F.R.: Double oesophagus. J. Faculty Radiologists 9:154, 1958.

Ben-Menachem, Y., et al.: Angiographic characteristics of esophageal leiomyoma. Am. J. Roentgenol. 128:479, 1977.

Bernatz, P.E., et al.: Benign, pedunculated, intraluminal tumors of the esophagus. J. Thorac. Surg. 35:503, 1958.

Daniel, R.A., Jr., and Williams, R.B., Jr.: Leiomyoma of the esophagus. J. Thorac. Surg. 19:800, 1950.

Farrell, K.H., et al.: Granular cell myoblastoma of the esophagus—incidence and surgical treatment. Ann. Otol. Rhinol. Laryngol. 82:784, 1973.

Haller, J.A., Jr., et al.: Life-threatening respiratory distress from mediastinal masses in infants. Ann. Thorac. Surg. 19:364, 1975.

Hanel, K., Tolley, N.A., and Hunt, D.R.: Hemangioma of the esophagus: an unusual cause of upper gastrointestinal bleeding. Dig. Dis. Sci. 26:257, 1981.

Howe, W.R., and Postlethwait, R.W.: Granular cell myoblastoma of the esophagus. Surgery. 89:701, 1981.

Kabuto, T., et al.: Diffuse leiomyomatosis of the esophagus. Dig. Dis. Sci. 25:388, 1980.

Kinnear, J.S.: Lipoma of the oesophagus: report of a case. Br. J. Surg. 42:439, 1955.

Lewis, B., and Maxfield, R.G.: Leiomyoma of the esophagus. Case report and review of the literature. Int. Abstr. Surg. 99:105, 1954.

Linder, F., and Vogt-Moykopf, I.: Diffuse leiomyomatose des oesophagus. Langenbecks Arch. Chir. 328:42, 1970.

Moersch, H.J., and Harringon, S.W.: Benign tumors of the esophagus. Ann. Otol. Rhinol. Laryngol. 53:800, 1944.

Ochsner, S., and Ochsner, A.: Lipoma of the esophagus. Surgery 42:787, 1957.

Orringer, M.B.: Partial median sternotomy: anterior approach to the upper thoracic esophagus. J. Thorac. Cardiovasc. Surg. 87:124, 1984.

Paskin, D.L., Hull, J.D., and Cookson, P.J.: Granular cell myoblastoma: a comprehensive review of 15-years' experience. Ann. Surg. 175:501, 1972.

Perasalo, O., and Laustela, E.: Benign muscle wall tumors of the esophagus. Report of two cases. Ann. Chir. Gynaecol. 44:145, 1955.

Plachta, A.: Benign tumors of the esophagus. Review of literature and report of 99 cases. Am. J. Gastroenterol. 38:639, 1962.

Pokorny, W.J., and Goldstein, I.R.: Enteric thoracoabdominal duplications in children. J. Thorac. Cardiovasc. Surg. 87:821, 1984.

Postlethwait, R.W.: Surgery of the Esophagus. New York, Appleton-Century-Crofts, 1979.

Postlethwait, R.W., and Detmer, D.E.: Ectopic thyroid nodule in oesophagus. Ann. Thorac. Surg. 19:98, 1975.

Schatzki, R., and Hawes, L.E.: Tumors of the esophagus below the mucosa and the roentgenological differential diagnosis. Rev. Gastroenterol. 17:991, 1950.

Schorlemmer, G.R., Battaglini, J.W., and Murray, G.F.: Cervical approach to esophageal leiomyomas. Ann. Thorac. Surg. 35:469, 1983.

Seremetis, M.G., et al.: Leiomyomata of the esophagus: an analysis of 838 cases. Cancer 38:2166, 1976.

Shields, T.W.: Leiomyoma of the esophagus. Q. Bull. Northwest. Univ. Med. School 33(1):29, 1959.

Tolis, G.A., and Shields, T.W.: Intramural lipoma of the esophagus. Ann. Thorac. Surg. 3:60, 1967.

Waterston, D.: Oesophageal disease in infancy and childhood, excluding oesophagotracheal fistula. *In* Surgery of the Oesophagus, The Coventry Conference. Edited by R.A. Smith and R.E. Smith. New York, Appleton-Century-Crofts, 1972, p. 81.

CHAPTER 86

SQUAMOUS CELL CARCINOMA OF THE ESOPHAGUS

Thomas W. Shields

Squamous cell carcinoma of the esophagus is uncommon except in isolated endemic areas, but is generally devastating to the patient. Usually, by the time the disease becomes clinically evident, it is incurable. The physician's role is then relegated to attempting to palliate the symptoms in the best possible manner with the least morbidity and mortality. Of course, in a few patients with early disease and in even fewer with more advanced disease, cure may be obtained by appropriate therapy, which most believe is surgical resection with immediate restoration of gastrointestinal continuity with or without preoperative or postoperative adjuvant therapy.

INCIDENCE

In North America, squamous cell carcinoma of the esophagus represents 1.5 to 2% of all cancers and approximately 7% of all gastrointestinal neoplasms. It is three times more common in black men than in white men. Interestingly, a high incidence—13.6 per 100,000 individuals—is seen in French men, as Lambert and his colleagues (1978) noted. The highest reported incidence is from China, where Armstrong (1980) reported a rate of 32 per 100,000. Lower, but still high, rates are seen in Iran, Singapore, Puerto Rico, Chile, and Japan (Fig. 86–1).

In certain small geographic areas throughout the world, the incidence has almost reached epidemic proportions. In China near the southern slopes of the Tai-hang mountain range, cancer of the esophagus is the most common cause of death in the men and women, an incidence of over 130 per 100,000 persons. In the Caspian littoral area of Iran, the incidence is 93 per 100,000 men and 110 per 100,000 women. In the Transkei district in South Africa, 47% of all tumors in men and 36% in women are esophageal in origin.

ETIOLOGY

No specific etiologic agent is known, but poverty and malnutrition are noted in most areas. Nutritional defi-

ciencies are common in all population groups with a high incidence of the disease. Most diets in these areas are deficient in protein, certain trace elements, and multiple vitamins. In each area, other predisposing factors usually are present.

Heredity

Tylosis, an inherited autosomal dominant trait, is associated with a 35% risk of esophageal cancer. This is the only known hereditary condition, other than the possible hereditary association in a few high incidence Chinese families reported by Yang (1980).

Dietary Factors

Alcohol and tobacco, especially in combination, may be implicated in many areas. This is true in North America and France. The ingestion of hot, spicy foods and hot beverages also has been implicated in other geographic areas. The marked concentration of nitrosamines and their precursors in food and water in areas of China with high incidences of esophageal carcinoma has also been noted, as have ingestion of bracken fern in Japan, *Fusarium moniliforme*-contaminated cereal in Transkei, and wheat flour contaminated with fine silica in areas in Iran where the disease is common.

Several conditions of the esophagus that produce chronic irritation or metaplastic strictures are thought to predispose to the development of esophageal carcinoma. Persons with lye burns, Plummer-Vinson syndrome, or achalasia are reported to have a significantly increased incidence of the disease. Patients with peptic reflux esophagitis and resultant columnar-lined esophagus also have an increased incidence, but the cell type is an adenocarcinoma rather than a squamous cell carcinoma.

Sex

In North America and Europe, the disease is more common in men, but in areas of high prevalence, men and women may be equally affected. In some areas, such

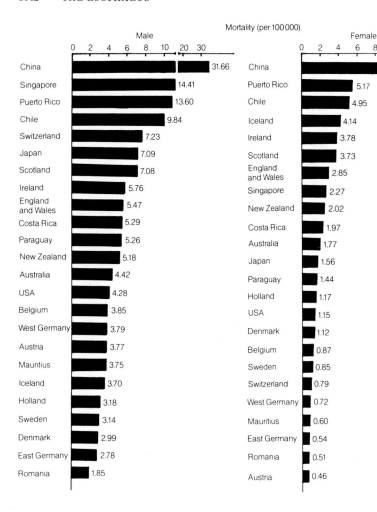

Fig. 86–1. Age-adjusted mortality for esophageal cancer in selected countries. (Reproduced with permission of Huang, G.J., and Wu, Y.K. (Eds): Carcinoma of the Esophagus and Gastric Cardia. Berlin, Springer-Verlag, 1984, p. 4.)

as the Province of Mazardaran in Iran, the incidence seen in women exceeds that seen in men. These observations, as well the aforementioned data, strongly suggest that extrinsic factors are the most likely cause of the disease.

Summary

The disease is prevalent in widely separated geographic areas. These areas, urban or rural, are economically poor, and dietary deficiencies are common. Ingestion of potential chemical carcinogens or their precursors have been documented in many of the affected populations. Epithelial irritation with hyperplasia and dysplasia is common in these endemic areas. Lastly, the risk of developing the disease appears to increase with age, further suggesting the major influence of environmental agents.

PATHOLOGY

Squamous cell carcinoma is rare before the age of 30, and the incidence increases with age. In most single and collected series such as that of Postlethwait (1986), the highest incidence is in the sixth and seventh decades of life.

Location

Squamous cell carcinoma of the thoracic and abdominal portions of the esophagus are most commonly located in the middle third of the thoracic esophagus; this region of the esophagus, as noted in Chapters 6 and 7, is from the level of the tracheal carina to the level of the inferior pulmonary veins. In the collected series Postlethwait (1986) reported, this location represented the site of approximately 50% of the squamous cell lesions. Thirty to forty percent of lesions arise in the lower third, including the abdominal portion of the organ. Only 10 to 20% occur in the upper third—from the thoracic inlet to the level of the tracheal carina. Most of the aforementioned percentages are based on surgical material. Liu (1976), in a series of 3663 patients in whom the diagnosis was based on balloon cytology, esophagoscopy, and roentgenographic contrast studies, reported the tumor to be located in the upper third of the esophagus in 11.7%, the middle third in 63.4%, and the lower third in 24.9%. These figures may represent more accurately the true distribution of the squamous cell tumors.

Macroscopic Features

The early stages of the disease are encountered infrequently in North America or Europe. Such lesions are more commonly seen in certain locations in China and other endemic areas, where routine screening is frequently practiced. The early lesions may be occult, erosive (Fig. 86–2), plaque-like, or papillary (Fig. 86–3). These early lesions are generally small, but may involve the entire circumference of the mucosa. The plaque-like lesion is the most common type seen, the next is the erosive type, and the papillary type is encountered only rarely. These lesions generally invade only the mucosa and submucosa, but the papillary type may invade the muscular wall of the esophagus.

Mannell (1982) described the lesions in the more advanced stages of the disease as fungating, ulcerative, or infiltrative tumors. The fungating lesions project into the lumen and appear as a filling defect. These lesions may also present as a flat plaque or as multiple polypoidal excrescences. The ulcerative tumor appears as an ulcerative lesion with regular or irregular everted edges with a deep base and associated infiltration of the esophageal wall with stenosis of the lumen (Fig. 86–4). The infiltrative tumor is characterized by extensive intramural spread. A marked desmoplastic response is usually present, producing a tight stricture of esophagus (Fig. 86–5). Occasionally, the tumor spread is superficial only, resulting in the so-called superficial spreading type. Other descriptive terms for the various gross forms have been

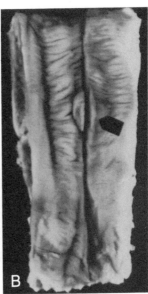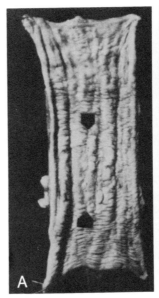

Fig. 86–3. Early esophageal carcinoma. *A*, Plaque-like type. *B*, Papillary type. (Reproduced with permission from Huang, G.J., and Wu, Y.K.: Carcinoma of the Esophagus and Gastric Cardia. Berlin, Springer-Verlag, 1984, p. 82.)

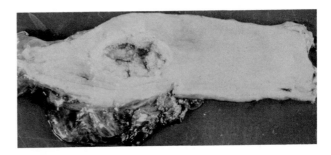

Fig. 86–4. Late esophageal carcinoma, fungating type.

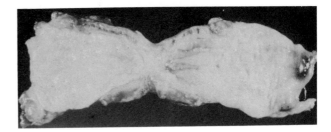

Fig. 86–5. Late esophageal carcinoma.

used by other investigators; Akiyama and his colleagues (1981) divided the various types into protuberant, ulcerative, superficial, exophytic, and miscellaneous types, and Liu and Zhou (1984) divided them into medullary, fungating, ulcerative, scirrhous, and intraluminal types. The various descriptions of the different types overlap. Actually, it is not the gross descriptions per se, but the extent of the growth in or through the wall of the esophagus and the presence or absence of lymph node metastases, that are important.

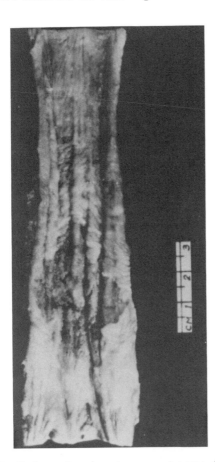

Fig. 86–2. Early esophageal carcinoma, erosive type. (Reproduced with permission of Huang, G.J., and Wu, Y.K.: Carcinoma of the Esophagus and Gastric Cardia. Berlin, Springer-Verlag, 1984, p. 4.)

Microscopic Features

Early-stage squamous cell tumors can be divided into intraepithelial, intramucosal, and submucosal carcinomas. The first is the typical carcinoma in situ with the basement membrane intact. In the second, the tumor cells penetrate the basement membrane and infiltrate the lamina propria or part of the muscularis mucosae. In the third variety, the cells have penetrated through the muscularis mucosae into the submucosa, but have not reached the muscular layer (Fig. 86–6). No lymph node metastases should be seen with any of these aforementioned early lesions. In the more advanced stages of squamous cell carcinoma, a greater or lesser distance of the muscular layers of the esophagus are invaded, or as is often the case, the tumor cells may extend through the wall into the adventitia. The degree of differentiation varies from well differentiated to poorly differentiated. Sixty percent of the tumors are moderately differentiated. Lymph node metastases are frequently present with these more advanced histologic forms.

Ultrastructure

The cancer cells' sizes, shapes, and arrangements differ from normal cells'. The tumor cells have markedly enlarged nuclei, these usually contain one or more nucleoli. The nuclear/cytoplasmic ratio is reversed. The cytoplasm may contain more mitochondria, with irregular sizes and shapes, and more free ribosomes and tonofilaments.

Metastasis

Sqamous cell carcinoma of the esophagus may spread by direct extension and by lymphatic or hematogenous metastases. In the advanced pathologic stages of the disease, in contrast to the early pathologic stages, direct extension through the wall of the esophagus is common, as are lymphatic metastases. Akiyama and associates (1981) found the latter in approximately 60% of their patients who underwent resection of the esophagus. Mandard and associates (1981) reported it in 75% in autopsy series. Hematogenous spread is also common in autopsy specimens. Liu (1980) found an incidence of 63%, and Mandard and associates (1981) reported it to be 50%. At the time of diagnosis, however, the incidence of distant metastases is generally believed to be only 25 to 30%.

Intraesophageal Spread

The tumor's microscopic spread is much greater than its macroscopic extent. Because the esophagus shrinks markedly once it is excised, even more so when it is fixed in formalin, the true extent of cephalad and caudad spread of the tumor cells is difficult to determine. Miller

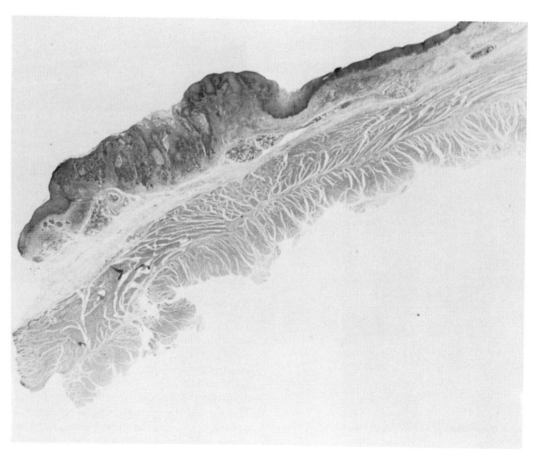

Fig. 86–6. Photomicrograph of early esophageal carcinoma with tumor spread confined to the submucosa of the wall of the esophagus.

(1962), however, allowing for shrinkage of the fixed specimen to one third of its in situ length, found that proximal—cephalad—spread was 3 cm in 64% of the specimens, 6 cm in 22%, 9 cm in 11%, and as great as 10.5 cm in 3% of the specimens. Wong (1987a) noted the marked correlation between the length of the resected esophageal segment above the tumor and the incidence of recurrence at the site of the proximal anastomosis (Table 86–1). His observations support the necessity of resecting a sufficiently long segment of the esophagus, as Miller (1962) suggested. Microscopic spread distal—caudal—to the gross tumor, for some unexplained reason, extends for a shorter distance than does proximal spread; Burgess and associates (1951) found this to be approximately only 4 cm beyond the tumor. Submucosal lymphatic spread occurs often. This may result in tumor emboli producing "skip" or satellite nodules, as Watanabe and associates (1979) described; these have serious prognostic import.

Direct Extension

After penetration of the adventitial layers covering the esophagus, the tumor may invade adjacent structures or organs. In the upper third, the tissues of the mediastinum, the great vessels, the trachea, and the anterior longitudinal ligament of the vertebral column may be involved. The recurrent nerves may also be involved, as well as the thoracic duct. The pleura and lung may also be invaded. In the middle third, the left main stem bronchus, the aorta, the thoracic duct, pericardium, pleura, lung, and the anterior longitudinal ligament may be invaded. In the lower third, in addition to some of the aforementioned structures, the diaphragm, stomach and even at times the liver may be involved by direct extension of the tumor. Roberts (1980) noted that at postmortem examination of untreated patients, the tumor spread in one third of the specimens is restricted to only the periesophageal tissues.

Lymphatic Spread

The direction of lymph flow in the extensive lymphatic network of the esophagus is primarily longitudinal rather than transverse or segmental (Chapter 7). This concept is supported both experimentally and clinically. The direction of the flow may be either cephalad or caudad. Experimentally, as well as clinically, the flow from the

upper third tends to be cephalad and from the lower two thirds caudad. Tanabe and associates (1986), in a clinical investigation with lymphoscintigraphy using ^{99m}Tc rhenium colloid, found that flow from the upper third was primarily ascending to the upper mediastinum and neck. From the middle third it was both ascending to the upper mediastinum and neck and descending into the abdomen. From the lower third the main flow was descending to the abdomen. These flow patterns generally are observed clinically, although flow in either direction from any site in the esophagus may be observed.

In a series of autopsy studies, Postlethwait (1986) recorded that the supraclavicular nodes were involved in 6.9%. In two small surgical series, Sannohe (1981) and Ide (1974) and their associates recorded that the supraclavicular nodes were involved in approximately 19%. Anderson and Lad (1982), in an autopsy series, reported a 15% incidence, which is probably a more representative figure than those of the aforementioned autopsy or surgical series. In contrast, spread below the diaphragm is more common. Akiyama and associates (1981) reported an incidence of nodal metastases in the superior gastric area in 31.8% of patients with tumors located in the upper third, 32.8% in patients with tumors of the middle third, and 61.5% in those with tumors of the lower third. These figures are similar to those reported by Ide and associates (1974). Although caudad spread is more common than cephalad spread, the flow is not exclusively in any one direction. Supraclavicular and superior mediastinal lymph nodes may be involved when the tumor is in the lower third, and abdominal nodes may be involved when the tumor is in the upper third.

The incidence of lymphatic metastasis in surgical specimens ranges from 40 to 60%. The overall incidence is undoubtedly higher. The incidence is related to the depth of invasion of the primary tumor in the wall and its extent beyond the wall. Lu and associates (1987) reported significant differences in the rates relative to these features in their surgical population (Table 86–2).

The various lymph nodal stations were discussed in Chapter 7. The first nodal group may be termed either the epiesophageal or paraesophageal nodes—station 1—and are adjacent to or contained within the adventitial sheath of the esophagus. The second nodal stations con-

Table 86–1. Proximal Resection Margin and Anastomotic Recurrence

Length of Margin (cm)	No. of Patients	Percent
0–2	1/4	25
2–4	2/11	18
4–6	2/13	15
6–8	2/26	8
8–10	1/15	7
>10	0/26	0

Reprinted with permission from Wong, J.: Esophageal resection for cancer: the rationale of current practice. Am. J. Surg. *153*:18, 1987a.

Table 86–2. Degree of Invasion and Lymph Node Status of 504 Resected Specimens of Esophageal Cancer

Degree of Invasion	No. of Resected Specimens	Lymph Node Metastasis	%
Submucosa	1	0	0
Muscularis	175	52	29.7*
Full thickness	273	118	42.2*
Adjacent tissue	55	38	69.1*
Total	504	208	41.3

*Proportion is significantly different at a $p < .05$. Reproduced with permission of Lu, Y. K., et al.: Cancer of esophagus and esophagogastric junction: analysis of results of 1025 resections after 5 to 20 years. Ann. Thorac. Surg. *43*:176, 1987.

sist of the periesophageal, the celiac, and the perigastric lymph node groups within the mediastinum and upper abdomen. These second station nodes, as well as those of the first station, constitute the regional nodes of the esophagus. The third nodal stations consist of the supraclavicular, lateral thoracic, or more distal subdiaphragmatic regions—the distal node groups. Figure 86–7 illustrates the incidence of involvement of these various stations.

The American Joint Committee (1983) suggested that in staging the involvement of the lymph nodes all intrathoracic groups—station 1 and station 2 above the diaphragm—be considered N1 disease and all extrathoracic stations—stations 2 and 3 beneath the diaphragm or station 3 in the neck—be considered M1 disease, that is, distant metastases. In a newer TNM classification suggested by the Japanese Committee for Registration of Esophageal Carcinoma (1985), N1 disease is considered either intrathoracic and perigastric or celiac lymph node involvement or both—stations 1 and 2. More distal abdominal or cervical node involvement—station 3—is considered metastasis, distant lymph nodes—M, LYN. The involvement of these various lymph nodes groups has therapeutic and prognostic importance.

Distant Metastases

Visceral metastases may be present in 25 to 30% of the patients at the time of diagnosis and are late manifestations of the disease. In Mandard and associates' (1980) autopsy report, 40% of the patients with well differentiated squamous cell carcinoma of the esophagus had visceral metastases, and 87% of those with undifferentiated squamous cell carcinoma had such spread. The total rate was 50% of all patients with squamous cell carcinoma of the esophagus. In the order of decreasing frequency, the lung, liver, pleura, bone, kidney, and adrenal gland were involved. Liu (1980) and Yamashita (1979) reported similar but not identical results. The nervous system was involved in only 2.7% of the specimens, excluding the undifferentiated tumors. Anderson

and Lad (1982) reported only a 1% incidence of metastases to the brain.

CLINICAL MANIFESTATIONS

Symptoms of early carcinoma of the esophagus are recognized infrequently, and then usually only in retrospect, in patients discovered to have early tumors on cytologic screening in high incidence areas such as in China. Huang and Wu (1984a) described that retrosternal discomfort or pain and sensation of friction, burning, or slow passage of food during swallowing are present in approximately 90% of such patients. These symptoms usually are intermittent and may be present for years. Our group identified several patients with early carcinoma who presented only with odynophagia. Most patients, however, ignore such symptoms and only become alarmed when swallowing becomes progressively difficult.

The major symptom of late carcinoma is progressive dysphagia that results from obstructing intraluminal tumor or stenosis by circumferential growth of the tumor to involve at least two thirds or more of the esophageal wall, as Edwards (1974) pointed out. The dysphagia may be intermittent initially, but soon becomes persistent first to solid foods, then to soft foods, and eventually even to liquids. Pain on swallowing is less common, although vague, ill defined pain is reported frequently. Significant melena or hematemesis is observed only infrequently. Anemia may be present to varying degrees. Significant weight loss is almost always present. Symptoms of regurgitation, vomiting, and periodic aspiration with cough are common.

With progression of the tumor through the wall of the esophagus and invasion of adjacent structures, symptoms that indicate incurability develop, including persistent back pain caused by involvement of the paravertebral fascia, hoarseness caused by involvement of the recurrent nerve, hiccoughs from involvement of the phrenic nerves or diaphragm, and difficulty in breathing caused by tracheal obstruction. Symptoms of a tracheoesophageal fistula, acute mediastinitis, or lethal massive hematemesis may occur if the tumor erodes into the tracheobronchial tree, the mediastinum, or a great vessel.

On physical examination, cachexia is often evident. Supraclavicular nodes may be palpable. Occasionally, osteoarthropathy as well as clubbing of the fingers or toes is seen. The liver may be palpable, but symptoms and signs of hematogenous visceral metastasis, even though it is present in approximately 25% of the patients when first seen, are unusual.

Laboratory examinations may reveal the presence of anemia, hypoproteinemia, hypercalcemia, and abnormal liver function tests. Hypercalcemia is more common than previously appreciated. Stephens (1973), Benrey (1974), and Chandrasekhara (1975) and their associates reported it in approximately 15% of the patients with squamous cell carcinoma of the esophagus.

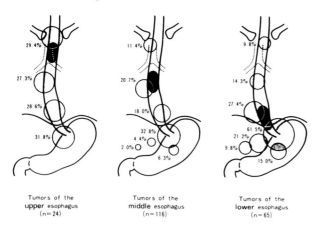

Tumors of the
upper esophagus
(n=24)

Tumors of the
middle esophagus
(n=116)

Tumors of the
lower esophagus
(n=65)

Fig. 86–7. Incidence and sites of lymph node metastases from squamous cell carcinoma in the upper, middle, and lower thirds of esophagus. (Reproduced with permission of Akiyama, H., et al.: Principles of surgical treatment for carcinoma of the esophagus: analysis of lymph node involvement. Ann. Surg. *194*:438, 1981.)

CYTOLOGIC SCREENING

Diagnostic cytology and biopsy of visible endoscopic lesions are additive, with approximately a 10% increase in the number of positive diagnoses obtained by cytologic smear. The greatest value of cytologic studies, however, is in screening of asymptomatic persons in high incidence areas. The Chinese obtain smears of the esophageal mucosa with an abrasive balloon catheter. The cells are classified as normal, mild hyperplasia, marked dysplasia, near-carcinoma, and early carcinoma. The latter two categories are considered early tumors—carcinoma in situ or early invasive carcinoma. Huang (1984a) reported successfully detecting such early cancer in populations with a high incidence of the disease by this technique in 1% of the persons with no symptoms. Shu and associates (1981) noted that approximately 15% of patients with marked dysplasia discovered during such examinations develop true carcinoma within 1 to 12 years, whereas only 1% with mild hyperplasia do so. These investigators found no cancers in a control group with normal cytology that was followed for 5 years.

ROENTGENOGRAPHIC FEATURES

Standard PA and Lateral Roentgenograms

Standard chest roentgenograms reveal an abnormal finding in 47.5% of the patients with esophageal cancer, according to Lindell and his associates (1979). The more important abnormalities seen are an abnormal azygo-esophageal line, a widened mediastinum, a posterior tracheal indentation or mass, and a widened retrotracheal stripe. In addition to these findings, hilar or superior mediastinal adenopathy may be suspected, and evidence of pulmonary metastases may be present. Compression, displacement or irregularity of the tracheal air column may appear, as well as secondary pulmonary infiltrates caused by aspiration and secondary infection. Pleural fluid—metastatic effusion or an empyema—is rarely seen at presentation.

Contrast Studies

The barium swallow is an essential diagnostic study for patients with the late lesions that are seen in most patients; the swallow almost always suggests an esophageal malignancy (Fig. 86–8). The fungating lesions present with a variable filling defect, and the junction between normal esophagus and tumor is usually abrupt and clear. Greater or lesser obstruction to the barium meal may be present. The ulcerative lesions usually present as a large, punched-out ulcer. The edges of the ulcer are elevated. Obstruction of the barium column is mild. The infiltrative tumors result in fusiform or annular stenosis. The infiltrative lesion is usually short and the wall may appear smooth. Obstruction of the barium meal is usually marked.

Except in the aforementioned infiltrative lesions, esophageal tumor length varies and is frequently over 5 cm. The length of the lesion, however, does not correlate with the degree of tumor penetration into or through the wall of the esophagus. Nonetheless, Mannel (1982), as well as others, believe that tumors longer than 10 cm are usually incurable. A more reliable sign of incurability or nonresectability—the result of growth beyond the esophageal wall—is an abnormality in the esophageal axis seen on barium swallow. Normally, as Klinkhamer (1969) described, the esophagus has a major curve at the aortic arch and at the left main stem bronchus; in the remainder of its length above and below these structures the esophagus is smooth and straight. With infiltration of the local mediastinal tissues by tumor growing beyond the wall, this straight axis is disrupted, and the barium column may become tortuous, angulated, or deviated from its normal course (Fig. 86–9). Some benign conditions may also cause axis abnormalities, but these usually can be readily differentiated from tumor. Akiyama and associates (1972) found that 74% of the esophagus tumors that had penetrated the wall were associated with axis abnormalities and that only 10% of those still confined within the wall had demonstrable axis changes. Thus, as Mannel (1982) noted, an axis abnormality is a fairly sensitive criterion for tumor growth beyond the esophagus proper, although it is not absolute. The demonstration of a tracheoesophageal fistula or a sinus tract into the mediastinum, pleural space, or pulmonary parenchyma on barium swallow, however, is almost always caused by penetration of the tumor beyond the confines of the esophageal wall (Fig. 86–10).

In contrast to these late roentgenographic findings, the demonstration of roentgenographic changes on barium swallow in early esophageal cancer is difficult. Wang and Su (1984) described four varieties: erosive—thickened, interrupted and tortuous mucosal folds; plaque-like—small filling defects in interrupted mucosal folds; papillary—small, defined filling defects protruding into the esophageal lumen; flat—no defect but a rigid and less distensible area of the esophageal wall. Most of these are noticed only in patients in whom there is a high index of suspicion of the disease in an area of high incidence or whose cytologic smear is positive.

Computed Tomography

Computed tomography—CT—of the chest and upper abdomen has become routine in the evaluation of patients with squamous cell carcinoma of the thoracic portion of the esophagus. Moss and associates (1981) classified the CT findings into four stages: stage I, intraluminal mass without esophageal wall thickening; stage II, esophageal wall thickening; stage III, contiguous spread of the tumor into adjacent structures—trachea, bronchi, aorta, or pericardium; and stage IV, evidence of distant metastases. The first two are self-explanatory, for normally the esophagus is a thin-walled structure with or without contained air. Contiguous spread is identified by the absence or obliteration of the normal fat planes between the esophagus and adjacent mediastinal structures (Figs. 86–11, 12). Unfortunately, these planes are frequently absent in the undernourished, emaciated person, and consequently the CT examination has less value in many patients with long-

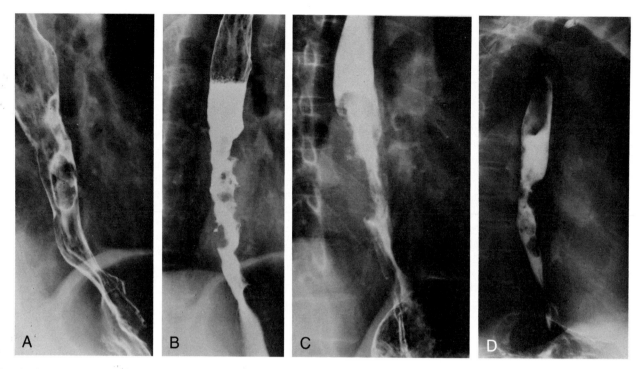

Fig. 86–8. Roentgenograms of barium swallows demonstrating typical "late" squamous cell carcinomas of the esophagus. *A,* Polypoid lesion. *B,* Multiple polypoid tumor. *C,* Long, ulcerative tumor. *D,* Stenotic, infiltrative tumor.

standing carcinoma of the esophagus. When the nutritional status is adequate and the fat plane is obliterated, however, Thompson and associates (1983) found that the tumor extends to the adjacent structure in at least 90% of the patients. Only 21% of the patients whose fat planes were preserved had tumor extension beyond the esophageal wall; an accuracy of 88%. Another sign of direct invasion, as Halvorsen and Thompson (1984) noted, is a mass that indents or displaces the tracheobronchial tree.

Computed tomography is also believed to be valuable in identifying lymph nodes in the mediastinum and below the diaphragm. Lymph nodes 1 to 1.5 cm or larger may be involved with tumor, but such enlargement may be caused by inflammation. The examination is best for identifying enlarged superior mediastinal and subcarinal lymph nodes (station 2 nodes), but I have found it un-

reliable for identifying paraesophageal nodes (station 1 nodes). Thompson and associates (1983) concur. Controversy surrounds its value in demonstrating enlarged nodes below the diaphragm. Thompson and associates (1983) found that 69% of the patients with positive subdiaphragmatic lymph node involvement were identified by computed tomography, but 31% were not. Likewise, when lymph node involvement was thought to be absent, the examination was falsely negative in 23%. Therefore, it is an insensitive diagnostic technique. This has been my experience as well, and Lea and associates' (1984) data confirm the insensitivity of the examination in evaluating lymph node involvement.

Examination of the upper abdomen may, however, reveal unsuspected liver or adrenal metastases, so the examination is still worthwhile. As in patients with lung

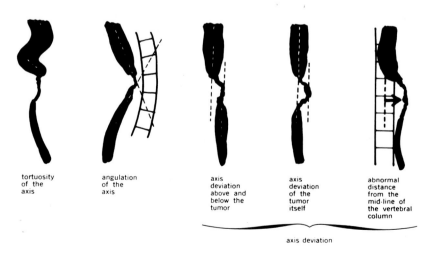

tortuosity of the axis

angulation of the axis

axis deviation above and below the tumor

axis deviation of the tumor itself

abnormal distance from the mid-line of the vertebral column

axis deviation

Fig. 86–9. Schematic representation of axis deviation of the esophagus caused by extramural extension of esophageal carcinoma usually associated with nonresectability for potential cure. (Reproduced with permission from Akiyama, H., et al.: The esophageal axis and its relationship to the resectability of carcinoma of the esophagus. Ann. Surg. *176*:30, 1972.)

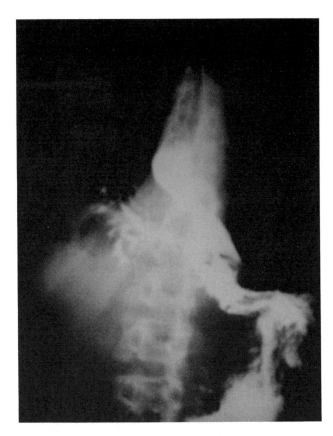

Fig. 86–10. Roentgenogram of contrast study demonstrating a malignant esophageal mediastinal-pulmonary sinus tract associated with a perforated carcinoma of the esophagus.

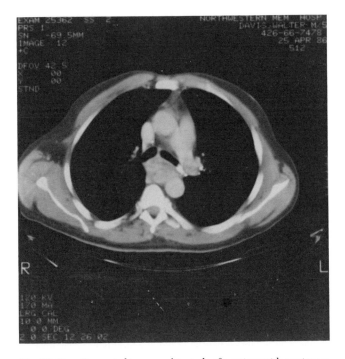

Fig. 86–11. Computed tomographic study of a patient with carcinoma of the esophagus confined to the esophageal wall with preservation of normal mediastinal fat planes.

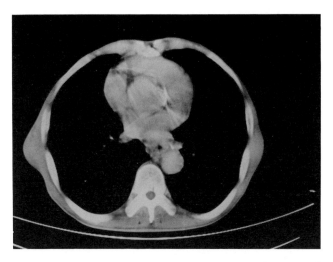

Fig. 86–12. Computed tomographic study of patient with extramural spread of a squamous cell carcinoma with obliteration of normal fat planes between the lesion and the aorta and anterior longitudinal spinal ligament.

cancer, however, histologic proof of such metastatic disease must be obtained if the suspected spread of the disease will affect the therapeutic decision.

Magnetic Resonance Imaging

Lehr and colleagues (1988) reported the use of MRI in prethoracotomy staging of carcinoma of the esophagus. They found it to have low sensitivity and specificity in determining involvement of adjacent structures or the presence of lymph node metastases. In their study, CT was equally of little value.

Radionuclide Studies

Radionuclide scans have found little use in the evaluation of patients with esophageal carcinoma. Kondo and associates (1982) evaluated 68 patients with ^{67}Ga scans and concluded that the scans are of little use for routine staging, but that they might have some use in planning radiation therapy in nonsurgical candidates.

ENDOSCOPY

Endoscopic evaluation of the esophagus is essential in all patients suspected to have a carcinoma of the esophagus. The location of the lesion, the presence of satellite nodules, the degree of obstruction, and the longitudinal and circumferential extent of the lesion should be determined in all patients. Bronchoscopy should also be done in all patients with upper or middle third lesions to identify any extension to the tracheobronchial tree. Even those patients with lower third lesions should undergo bronchoscopy to evaluate the tracheal carina for the possible involvement of the subcarinal lymph nodes, although computed tomography may be better for this determination.

Esophagoscopy

The technique of rigid and flexible fiber-optic esophagoscopy is covered in Chapter 18. The endoscopic features of late carcinoma are recognized readily, although at times the associated stenosis by submucosal infiltration of the tumor prevents actual identification of the tumor. Biopsy and cytologic smears should be done in all cases. The biopsy specimen should be taken from the edge of the lesion and not from the necrotic center. As a rule, three or more biopsy specimens should be taken. These should not be deep, because perforation of the esophageal wall should be avoided. A positive tissue diagnosis should be obtained in over 90% of tumors.

In patients with early carcinoma identified in high risk groups by cytologic screening, the endoscopic changes are subtle and may be difficult to recognize. There may be mucosal erosion, focal congestion, and roughness of the mucosa. A small nodule, a minute ulcer, or even a small tumor mass may be observed.

When no lesion can be identified, mucosal staining with toluidine blue or Lugol's solution or both has been used. Zhang (1984) reported that with toluidine blue, which stains the tumor cells but not the normal mucosa, positive staining was observed in 57 of 62 patients with positive balloon cytology, 14—26.9%—of whom were initially negative under direct vision. Wang (1981) reported similar results. Lugol's solution, on the other hand, stains the normal mucosa but not the tumor cells. Mandard (1980) and Volkov (1981) and their colleagues, as well as others, have reported its use. The role of hematoporphyrin derivative fluorescence for localization of early lesions of the esophagus, as Doiron and associates (1979) suggested for identification of early lung cancer, has not been fully investigated but is under study.

Bronchoscopy

Bronchoscopy is indicated in the evaluation of the patients with tumors in the upper two thirds of the esophagus to rule out fixation, invasion, or fistulization into the tracheobronchial tree. As Giuli and Sancho-Garnier (1986) noted, however, frank invasion found at thoracotomy may be interpreted as normal in 7% or just as compression in 20% of the patients on routine bronchoscopy.

Endoscopic Ultrasonography

Takemoto and associates (1986a, b) investigated the depth of carcinomatous invasion in and through the esophageal wall with endoscopic ultrasonography. Five layers of the esophageal wall can be identified, and Takemoto and colleagues (1986b) correctly identified the depth of invasion of the tumor in 75% of the patients studied. In addition, Ogino (1984) and Kumegawa (1985) and their associates identified enlarged regional esophageal lymph nodes by this technique. Whether or not such studies will affect the preoperative staging and therapy of squamous cell cancer remains to be seen.

STAGING

Accurate staging of squamous cell carcinoma is important for therapeutic as well as for prognostic considerations. Preoperative staging should rule out resection for patients whose disease is so extensive that effective or even reasonable palliation, let alone potential cure, by surgical excision or bypass is so remote that aggressive surgical therapy is contraindicated. It should also identify those patients in whom either therapeutic irradiation or surgical excision should be considered palliative at best, as well as to single out those few patients in whom a potential cure is possible.

In the pretherapeutic assessment, all of the aforementioned diagnostic studies, as well as biopsy of suspected metastatic sites and the obtaining of organ scans as necessary, are important. As in carcinoma of the lungs, routine organ scans are not indicated. CT scans or radionuclide scans should be done only if warranted by clinical or laboratory findings. Biopsy of suspicious metastatic sites is always indicated, particularly when cervical lymph nodes are enlarged. Biopsy of mediastinal nodes should be guided by the findings on CT examination. Laparotomy for biopsy of infradiaphragmatic nodes generally should be done only as part of a planned operative procedure and not as a preoperative measure.

The American Joint Committee for Cancer Staging and End-Results Reporting (1983) suggested a TNM system for clinical staging of esophageal cancer, but unfortunately, lesions of the cervical portion of the esophagus are included, so the system is somewhat cumbersome. Table 86–3 presents a reasonable modification. Even so, the designation of involvement of cervical and all subdiaphragmatic lymph nodes as M1 disease is probably inappropriate. Akiyama and co-workers (1984) as well as the Japanese Committee for Registration of Esophageal Carcinoma (1985) noted long-term survival in patients with positive infradiaphragmatic lymph nodes in specific

Table 86–3.   Clinical Staging of Intrathoracic Esophageal Carcinoma

Category	Stage	Extent of Lesion
Primary Tumor		
T1	I	Lesion ≤5 cm long that produces no obstruction, not involving the whole circumference and not extending beyond the esophagus.
T2	II	Lesion >5 cm long, involving total circumference and not extending beyond the esophagus, or a tumor of any size that produces obstruction.
T3	III	Direct extraesophageal spread
Lymph Nodes		
N0	I	No nodes involved
N1	II	Local nodes positive
NY		Nodes not assessable
Metastases		
M0	I	No distant metastases
M1	III	Distant nodes* or visceral metastases

*Cervical or celiac lymph nodes

Reproduced with permission of the American Joint Committee for Cancer Staging and End Results Reporting. *In* Manual for Staging Cancer, 2nd ed. Edited by O.H. Beahrs and M.H. Myers. Philadelphia, J.B. Lippincott Co., 1983, p. 61.

locations (Chapter 7). They suggested that the para-esophageal lymph nodes should be designated N1 disease and also that the other regional mediastinal lymph nodes and certain subdiaphragmatic lymph nodes—the paracardiac nodes, the left gastric nodes, and celiac axis nodes—should be considered N1 disease. The other, more distant, subdiaphragmatic nodes, as well as the cervical lymph nodes, could be considered distant metastases, or better yet M, LYN disease.

The American Joint Committee for Cancer Staging and End-Results Reporting (1983) postsurgical classification takes into account the depth of invasion of the tumor into or through the esophageal wall, and the Japanese Committee (1985) published data that suggest that this feature is as important prognostically as lymph node involvement. Tables 86–4 and 86–5 present the Japanese Committee's suggested system.

Regardless of which system or combination of systems

Table 86–4. Postsurgical Staging of Intrathoracic Esophageal Carcinoma: Proposed New Japanese Classification

Category	Extent of Lesion
Primary Tumor	
T1	Tumor invades into but not beyond the submucosa
T2	Tumors extends into but not beyond the muscularis propria
T3	Tumor invades into the adventitia
T4	Tumor invades contiguous structures
Lymph Nodes	
N0	No node involvement
N1	Regional nodes involved*
Metastases	
M0	No distant metastases
M1 LYN	Distant lymph nodes involved†
M1	Visceral metastases

*Mediastinal or proximal intra-abdominal nodes (station no. 2—Chapter 7)

†Supraclavicular or distant intra-abdominal nodes (station no. 3—Chapter 7)

Adapted with permission from the Japanese Committee for Registration of Esophageal Carcinoma: A proposal for a new TNM classification of esophageal carcinoma. Jpn. J. Clin. Oncol. *14*:625, 1985.

Table 86–5. Postsurgical Stage Grouping of Intrathoracic Esophageal Carcinoma

	T	N	M
Stage I	T1	N0	M0
Stage IIa	T2	N0	M0
	T3	N0	M0
Stage IIb	T1	N1	M0
	T2	N1	M0
Stage III	T3	N1	M0
	T4	N0	M0
	T4	N	M0
Stage IV	any T	any N	M1

Adapted with permission from the Japanese Committee for Registration of Esophageal Carcinoma: A proposal for a new TNM classification of esophageal carcinoma. Jpn. J. Clin. Oncol. *14*:625, 1985.

is used, the TNM designations are most important in staging the postoperative patient relative to his or her potential prognosis. In the preoperative patient, the T status and N status cannot be determined accurately with any confidence. In the inoperable patient, however, clinical staging is important in arriving at an alternative therapeutic choice.

SELECTION OF THERAPY

Most patients with squamous cell carcinoma of the thoracic portions of the esophagus have late tumors. Many have distant metastases when the diagnosis is established. Many of those who only have regional disease are not candidates for curative surgery but may be markedly benefitted by surgical excision and replacement of the esophagus. Others may obtain relief with a surgical bypass, irradiation, chemotherapy, and other therapeutic maneuvers—intubation, photocoagulation, or endoscopic dilatation. A few patients with localized disease and those with early tumors may indeed have curable tumors.

Thus, the selection of the appropriate therapeutic approach may be difficult. Many factors enter into the final decision, and it remains unknown which is the best treatment regimen for the disease. Palliation rather than cure, except in the early cases, may be the ultimate, realistic therapeutic goal. It is difficult, however, to appraise palliation, and the morbidity and mortality of any approach must be considered in the final therapeutic decision.

SURGICAL THERAPY

Unless the patient has proven distant metastases or evidence of regional spread beyond the field of reasonable surgical excision, such as a malignant tracheobronchial fistula, most believe that surgical resection is the procedure of choice. The resectability rate varies markedly in the many reported series. Akiyama and associates (1981) reported a resectability rate of 54.5% and Wu and Huang (1984) a rate of 83.4%. In a collected series of over 22,514 patients, Postlethwait (1986) reported 48.2% of cases to be operable. Resection was performed in 63.9% of the operable group, but this represented only 30.8% of the entire group. In many of the reported series, other than those from Asia, the higher the resectability rate, the higher the mortality rate.

Most tumor resections are primarily intended to palliate dysphagia, because spread beyond the muscular esophageal wall or lymph node metastases, or both, are usually present, which reduces the chance for cure to a minimal level. Of course, those few patients with early tumors confined to the esophagus and without lymph node metastases may be expected to have a significant survival rate.

Selection of the Surgical Procedure

There is no unanimity of opinion about which is the better operation for the removal of the esophagus. Each surgeon or surgical group has a procedure or procedures of choice for removing tumors in various locations of the thoracic esophagus. The technical aspects of the various surgical options are discussed in Chapter 38. As with the esophagectomy itself, opinions also vary about the extent as well as the necessity of regional lymph node dissection.

Akiyama and associates (1981) employed a modified Lewis technique with a total thoracic esophagectomy and subsequent esophagogastric anastomosis in the neck. An extensive lymph node dissection is done in both the thorax and in the abdomen, including resection of the lesser curve of the stomach in almost all instances. Wong (1981) reported using multiple approaches for tumors at different levels. For those lesions in the middle third he also uses the modified Lewis technique, but now most often constructs the anastomosis high in the apex of the chest (1987b). Huang and Wu (1984b) use many approaches, similar to those described by Wong (1981), depending upon the location of the lesion. The surgeons at the Mayo Clinic, as Payne and colleagues (1986) reported, and at the Lahey Clinic as Ellis and associates (1983) noted, use a similar approach for middle-third lesions and a left-sided approach for lower-third lesions, as do most other surgeons in North America. Orringer (1984b), with Sloan (1978) and with Orringer (1983), reported using almost exclusively a nonthoracic transhiatal esophagectomy, as did Steiger (1981), Szentpetery (1979), and Stewart (1985) and their associates. Skinner (1983) continues to advocate a radical esophagectomy, as described in Chapter 38, as the preferred procedure. Resection of the proximal stomach, tail of the pancreas, and spleen as Scanlon and associates (1956) once advocated, is rarely, if ever, indicated for squamous cell carcinoma of the esophagus.

I prefer, as do Ginsberg and Pearson (1983), a total thoracic esophagectomy with restoration of esophagogastric continuity by an anastomosis in the neck. More of the esophagus is resected, and the morbidity and mortality from an anastomotic leak is less. Either a modified Lewis technique or a nonthoracotomy, transhiatal esophagectomy is done, depending on the location of the lesion, its response to adjuvant therapy—chemotherapy at our institution—and the presence of lymph node metastasis within the abdomen. In all cases, with the rare exception of early lesions located in the upper third, the abdominal phase of the procedure, to assess the presence and extent of intra-abdominal spread, should be the initial step to determine whether or not the lesion should be excised. What constitutes contraindication to resection in this regard again varies. Some surgeons consider liver metastasis or fixed celiac lymph nodes absolute contraindications, whereas others, such as Wong (personal communication, 1986), do not. The decision is philosophical and depends upon many factors in any given situation.

Restoration of esophagogastric continuity is routinely done at the time of esophagectomy. Delayed restoration is rarely practiced. The stomach is the organ of choice (Chapter 39), but at times the colon (Chapter 40), as Isolauri and associates (1987) advocated, may be used as the conduit. Only infrequently is the jejunum used. The pros and cons of these various substitutes are discussed in the aforementioned chapters. The route of replacement, posterior mediastinal, retrosternal, or infrequently subcutaneous, is again the choice of the surgeon. The posterior mediastinal position is the shortest route, although the organ does lie in the resected tumor bed and also may limit somewhat the dose of postoperative irradiation.

Morbidity and Mortality

The morbidity of esophagectomy is significant, and is relative to patient selection and the operation performed. The major complications have been discussed in Chapter 38. Respiratory complications, which seem to be exaggerated in patients who have received preoperative irradiation—although this is not substantiated by data in the literature—are most frequent.

The mortality rates vary, as do the morbidity rates. Akiyama (1980) reported a mortality of only 0.8% and Huang (1984b) and Endo and associates (1982) reported rates of 4%. In North America, rates of 10 to 12%, as Skinner (1983) and Orringer and Orringer (1983) reported, are common, although Ellis and associates (1983) reported a rate of 1.3%, similar to Akiyama's. In Europe, the mortality rates are frequently in the range of 14 to 19%, as Giuli and Sancho-Garnier (1986) reported, and Launois and his associates (1983) reported 17.8%, although both groups' more recent mortality rates were only approximately 2.6%. These rates, of course, reflect patient selection—age, cardiovascular risk, respiratory risk, the inclusion of all hospital deaths, as well as other factors, as Wong (1981) noted. Ideally, in North America and Europe with the population at risk, a mortality rate of 5% should be acceptable.

Surgical Results

Long-term survival after resection of late squamous cell carcinoma of the esophagus is poor. Five-year survival rates of less than 5 to greater than 30% have been recorded. In contrast, results of surgical excision of early tumors are good. Huang and colleagues (1981a, b) reported a 5-year survival rate of 86%.

The extent of the lesion through the various layers of the esophageal wall or beyond it, and the presence or absence of metastatic disease in regional or distant lymph nodes, appear to be the more important factors in survival. The site of the tumor within the esophagus is also somewhat relevant. Wu and Huang (1984) reported a 5-year survival rate of 31.3% for lesions originating in the lower third, and one of only 14.3% for those arising in the middle or upper thirds. When there was no gross disease beyond the esophageal wall it was 28.9%, and only 20.2% when such disease was evident. When regional nodes were negative, the rate was 32.1%, and when positive, the rate was 13.6%. Akiyama and associates (1981) reported a 53.8% 5-year survival when the lymph nodes were uninvolved, and a 15.3% survival when metastatic disease was present. These authors noted that subdiaphragmatic nodal involvement did not preclude long-term survival.

Lu and associates (1987) reported a resectability rate of 81.2% and a 5-year survival rate of 28.2% in patients with complete resections. Late survival rates of all resected patients were 20%, 12%, and 7.4% at 10, 15, and 20 years, respectively. The best results were observed in patients with lower-third lesions confined to the wall and without lymph node metastases; a 5-year survival of 64.2%. This is similar to the long-term survival rate of 60.8% recorded by the Japanese Committee for Registration of Esophageal Carcinoma (1985) for patients with disease classified as T1N0M0 (Table 86–8). Tables 86–6, 86–7, and 86–8 show the other survival rates based on the new Japanese TNM classification. Data in these tables clearly permit the observation of the effects of the local extent and the metastatic spread of the disease on the patients' prognoses. Only 35% of the patients operated upon have reasonably localized disease without lymph node metastases.

Surgical Resection Plus Adjuvant Therapy

Because of the low resectability rates and generally poor survival rates, except in the patients with early disease, many surgeons have advocated adjuvant therapy. This primarily has been preoperative radiation ther-

Table 86–6. 5-Year Survival for Carcinoma of the Thoracic Esophagus by Depth of Invasion: New Japanese Staging System

T Status*	Total No. of Cases	Relative 5-Year Survival Rate
T1	233	48.54%
T2	673	29.53%
T3	1814	22.07%
T4	527	7.98%
Total	3211	23.16%

*T1—epithelium to the submucosa
T2—invasion of muscular layers
T3—tumor invading the adventitia
T4—tumor invading contiguous structure
Adapted with permission from the Japanese Committee for Registration of Esophageal Carcinoma: A proposal for a new TNM classification of esophageal carcinoma. Jpn. J. Clin. Oncol. *14*:625, 1985.

Table 86–7. 5-Year Survival for Carcinoma of Thoracic Esophagus by Nodal Involvement: New Japanese Staging System

N Status*	Total No. of Cases	Relative 5-Year Survival Rate
N0	1263	39.54
N1	1210	17.04
M1 LYN	738	4.98
Total	3211	23.16

*N0—no involvement
N1—paraesophageal, mediastinal, or proximal intra-abdominal nodes involved (regional nodes)
M1 LYN—metastases to lymph nodes in supraclavicular area and more distant lymph nodes in abdomen (distant nodes)
Adapted with permission from the Japanese Committee for Registration of Esophageal Carcinoma: A proposal for a new TNM classification of esophageal carcinoma. Jpn. J. Clin. Oncol. *14*:625, 1985.

Table 86–8. 5-Year Survival for Carcinoma of the Thoracic Esophagus by New Japanese TNM Classification

Stage	Total No. of Cases	Relative 5-Year Survival Rate (%)
T1N0	149	60.78
T1N1	54	30.84
T2N0	338	41.55
T2N1	189	23.11
T3N0	642	38.85
T3N1	716	17.44
T4N0	121	15.92
T4N1	213	8.64
M1 LYN	687	5.33
M1	102	1.58

Reproduced with permission from the Japanese Committee for Registration of Esophageal Carcinoma: A proposal for a new TNM classification of esophageal carcinoma. Jpn. J. Clin. Oncol. *14*:625, 1985.

apy, but various preoperative chemotherapeutic regimens with or without irradiation are now under investigation.

Preoperative Radiation Therapy

Many advocate preoperative radiation for potential candidates for surgical resection. Akiyama (1981), Huang (1981c), Van Andel (1979), Parker (1976) and their associates strongly support its use. Reportedly, the tumor frequently becomes smaller and softer and presents with less infiltration, so the tissue planes are more readily developed. Huang and associates (1981c) reported that in 408 patients with borderline resectability, 82% could be resected after preoperative irradiation and the 5-year survival rate was 31.6%. Others also have reported improved long-term survival rates; unfortunately, these are difficult to substantiate from the presented data. In the few reported prospective, controlled trials, the addition of preoperative irradiation has not been shown to be beneficial. Launois and colleagues (1981) reported one of these trials in great detail, and both the long-term survival rates and average survival times were greater in the surgery alone group: 11.5% versus 9.5% and 8.2 months versus 4.5 months. Wong (1981), in a preliminary report, found no significant differences in the 5-year survival between surgery alone and surgery plus preoperative radiation therapy in patients with middle-third lesions (Fig. 86–13).

Postoperative Irradiation

Routine postoperative radiation therapy after a potential curative resection has evoked little enthusiasm. In Wong's (1981) preliminary report its use conferred no survival benefit (Fig. 86–13). Most surgeons, however, do recommend its use postoperatively when gross or microscopic tumor has been left in the thorax or abdomen at the time of resection. Gu (1984) suggested that when postoperative radiation therapy is used, the dose should be large enough to be curative and the course of irradiation should be begun within 2 weeks after the operation.

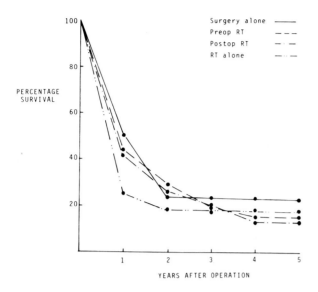

PERCENTAGE SURVIVAL

Surgery alone ———
Preop RT − − −
Postop RT − · −
RT alone − · · −

YEARS AFTER OPERATION

Fig. 86–13. Pulmonary results of a controlled trial for middle-third squamous cell tumors of the esophagus using four modalities of treatment. There is no significant difference in 5-year survival between the modalities. (Used with permission from Wong, J.: Management of carcinoma of the oesophagus: art or science? J. R. Coll. Surg. Edinb. 26:138, 1981.)

Chemotherapy

Even though various drugs such as bleomycin, mitomycin C, doxorubicin, 5-fluorouracil, methotrexate, cisplatin, and vindesine have shown varying degrees of antitumor activity against squamous cell carcinoma of the esophagus—as Kelsen (1984) summarized—none are used as single agents in an adjuvant setting. As a rule, two or more drugs are given in combination preoperatively with or without supplemental irradiation. At present, most of the chemotherapeutic regimens used are cisplatin-based. Many preliminary studies—the reports

of Kelsen (1981), Bains (1982), Steiger (1981), Leichman (1984a, b), Shields (1984), Miller (1985), Parker (1985), Popp (1986), Wolfe (1987) and Hilgenberg (1988) and their associates—have been encouraging, but as yet there is no clear evidence that the multimodality approach is superior to either surgery or irradiation alone.

In one major approach summarized by Leichman and colleagues (1984a) (Fig. 86–14), two courses of a combination of cisplatin and 5-fluorouracil plus a concurrent course of radiation therapy was given to 138 patients. Sixty-eight percent of the patients were then subjected to esophagectomy, and of these 22% had no tumor in the resected specimens. Only a few in the latter group had developed recurrent disease at the time of the report. Some have suggested, therefore, that resection may be unnecessary when no disease is evident on the preoperative restaging after completion of the chemotherapeutic-irradiation course. Campbell and his associates (1985), however, found endoscopy and biopsy to be unreliable for detecting all persistent tumor and suggested that resection should be done even when persistent tumor cannot be identified. Austin and his colleagues (1986) agree that surgical resection should remain a necessary phase in the overall treatment plan.

Our own group—Shields and co-workers (1984), as well as DenBesten (personal communication, 1985) and Hilgenberg and associates (1988)—deleted the radiation therapy preoperatively in our trial. Three courses of cisplatin and 5-fluorouracil are given preoperatively and irradiation is given postoperatively only when the resection has been judged incomplete. The tumor response to the preoperative chemotherapy was approximately 45 to 50%. Acceptable but significant toxicity—stomatitis and leukopenia—was noted, but no chemotherapeutic deaths occurred. Most responses were partial, but even in the few "complete" responders, tumor was present in the resected specimen. Median survival has been in-

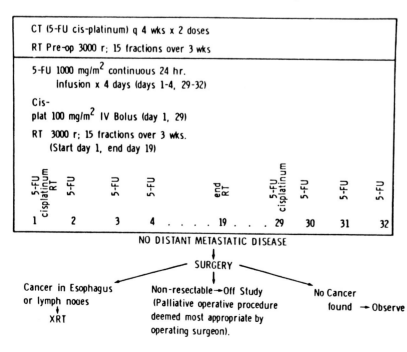

CT (5-FU cis-platinum) q 4 wks x 2 doses
RT Pre-op 3000 r; 15 fractions over 3 wks

5-FU 1000 mg/m² continuous 24 hr.
    Infusion x 4 days (days 1-4, 29-32)
Cis-
plat 100 mg/m² IV Bolus (day 1, 29)
RT 3000 r; 15 fractions over 3 wks.
    (Start day 1, end day 19)

5-FU cisplatinum RT | 5-FU | 5-FU | 5-FU | end RT | 5-FU cisplatinum | 5-FU | 5-FU | 5-FU
1   2   3   4 . . . . 19 . . . 29   30   31   32

NO DISTANT METASTATIC DISEASE
↓
SURGERY
↓
Cancer in Esophagus or lymph nodes ←— Non-resectable→Off Study (Palliative operative procedure deemed most appropriate by operating surgeon). —→ No Cancer found → Observe
↓
XRT

Fig. 86–14. Scheme of the second Wayne State University pilot study of multimodality treatment of squamous cell carcinoma of the esophagus. (Reproduced with permission of Leichman, L., et al.: Combined preoperative chemotherapy and indication therapy for cancer of the esophagus: the Wayne State University, Southwest Oncology Group and Radiation Therapy Oncology Group experience. Semin. Oncol. 11:178, 1984.)

creased over the historic controls, but it is too soon to judge the effect on long-term survival. We believe, as do Campbell and associates (1985) and others, that resection remains important in these patients.

What the final role and the exact combination of agents in the multimodality therapy for squamous cell carcinoma of the esophagus will be remains to be seen. Continued trials are necessary, and eventually, randomized trials should be done. Unfortunately, the imprecision of present-day clinical staging remains a major drawback to such trials.

Fate of the Surgically Resected Patient

Because long-term survival is uncommon even in the patient resected for cure, the prognosis of the surgical patient group as a whole must be understood. In Isono and colleagues' (1985) study most patients who died after an initial successful resection died of recurrent disease. Most of these patients had received preoperative irradiation to the local area and postoperative irradiation to the neck and upper thorax. In 147 patients in this setting, the recurrence involved the lymph nodes in 42.2%, visceral organs—lung, liver, bone, brain, etc.—in 40.1%, the remnant of the esophagus in 7.5%, the local site in 6.8%, and the peritoneum in 3.4%. The number of patients without disease was not noted, but in studies quoted by these authors (Tables 86–9, 86–10) of autopsy cases in Japan of patients who had initially undergone successful resection, lymph node recurrence was observed in all but 22.2% and visceral metastases in all but 5.2%. Most recurrences occurred within 2 years of the operative procedure. Discovery of lymph node involvement was most common within the first year and was identified only rarely after 3 years. Survival after recurrence averaged slightly less than 4 months. Visceral metastases also were discovered more commonly in the first postoperative year, and survival after identification of recurrence was again approximately 4 months. The finding of local recurrence was similar to the aforementioned groups. Recurrence in the esophagus was much later as

a rule, but survival was not different once the recurrence was identified.

The patients who survive 5 years or more after resection, as Hzuka and colleagues (1985) noted, tend to have the following prognostic factors present at the time of the operation: small tumor—less than 5 cm long; no invasion of the adventitia; no lymph node involvement; and age under 60. Women had a higher 5-year survival than men. Of their 102 5-year survivors—a long-term survival rate of 20.7%—32 patients died by the time of their report. Recurrence was noted in only three of these patients, but eight—one fourth—developed a secondary primary in a different organ system; a situation similar to that of long-term survivors after resection of a lung cancer. Unfortunately, their follow-up data were incomplete in half of the patients, but they assumed most died of other diseases of the elderly.

Palliative Surgical Procedures

In many patients, surgical excision is only palliative, even when the operation is done for cure. In a large series of autopsies of patients who died within 30 days of the operation, as Isono and associates (1985) recorded, persistent tumor was identified in the various lymph node groups in 31.9% and in distant organs in 27.7% (Tables 86–9 and 86–10). In addition to these patients, there are many in whom gross tumor is left behind knowingly, and many in whom no resection can be accomplished. For these patients, surgical bypass procedures, endoscopic dilatation, esophageal intubation, and photodynamic therapy are available to attempt to palliate the patient's inability to swallow and at times to ameliorate the symptoms caused by a malignant tracheoesophageal fistula, which occurs in 10 to 15% of all patients with squamous cell carcinoma of the esophagus. This is the commonest cause of an acquired tracheoesophageal fistula in the adult. The life expectancy is approximately 4 months after its occurrence.

Surgical Bypass for Palliation

Most authors believe that esophagectomy, even when tumor is left behind, affords the best palliation with the

Table 86–9. Rate of Recurrence in Lymph Nodes in Autopsied Cases After Resection of Esophageal Cancer

Location of Lymph Node	Persistent Positive Lymph Nodes in Patients Dying in Postoperative Period (549 Cases)	Autopsy Incidence of Lymph Node Metastases (Late Deaths) (883 Cases)
Cervical	7.5%	29.8%
Paratracheal	9.1%	27.2%
Mediastinal	3.1%	14.3%
Bifurcation	3.8%	11.3%
Pulmonary hilar	5.5%	23.7%
Paraesophageal	2.4%	3.2%
Para-aortal	3.6%	16.4%
Paracardial	3.5%	9.7%
Retroperitoneal	4.2%	17.4%
Parapancreatic	2.6%	13.6%
No Involvement	68.1%	22.2%

Adapted with permission from Isono, K.: Recurrence of intrathoracic esophageal cancer. Jpn. J. Clin. Oncol. *15*:49, 1985. (From the Annual of the Pathological Autopsy Cases in Japan, 1970–1980.)

Table 86–10. Metastasis to Organs in Autopsied Cases of Esophageal Cancer after Surgery

Sites of Metastases	Direct Operative Deaths Within 30 Days (549 Cases)	Cases of Recurrence Late Deaths (883 Cases)
Lung	8.2%	56.9%
Liver	6.6	42.8
Bone	2.4	23.7
Accessory Kidney	1.6	15.2
Kidney	0.9	13.4
Pancreas	2.2	12.1
Stomach	1.5	8.8
Esophagus	1.3	4.3
None present	72.3	5.2

Adapted with permission from Isono, K.: Recurrence of intrathoracic esophageal cancer. Jpn. J. Clin. Oncol. *15*:49, 1985. (From the Annual of the Pathological Autopsy Cases in Japan, 1970–1980.)

least morbidity and mortality. Keagy and associates (1984) and Orringer (1983b) presented convincing data in this regard. At times, however, this is impossible to accomplish, particularly in the presence of an impending or an existing malignant tracheobronchial-esophageal fistula. In this and other similar circumstances, gastric bypass through a substernal route with exclusion of the esophagus has been advocated. Huang (1984c) reported the mortality to be as low as 4.7%. Wong (1981) performs a modified Kirschner (1920) operation, which was reintroduced by Ong (1973), in which the distal esophagus is defunctionalized by a long Roux-en-Y loop of jejunum. Unfortunately, the mortality and morbidity rates were not reported. In both the United States and South Africa, however, gastric bypass is accompanied by a mortality of 21 to 25%, as Orringer (1983a, 1984a) with Sloan (1975) and Conlan and associates (1983) recorded. Thus, the decision to carry out a bypass as a palliative maneuver is difficult and has to be made on an individual basis. Symbas (1984) reported a lesser mortality rate in a few patients in whom the esophagus was stapled off above and below the fistula along with the bypass procedure. Duranceau and Jamieson (1984) recommended that in the management of patients with malignant tracheoesophageal fistula, either peroral intubation to seal off the fistula or, preferably, initial surgical exclusion of the esophagus be done. In the latter situation, esophagogastric continuity can subsequently be restored when the

patient's general condition improves enough to warrant a major bypass procedure.

Esophageal Intubation

These procedures vary and are described in Chapter 87. The morbidity and mortality rates vary with the patient selection and the skill of the operator. Early death may occur in an average of 10 to 12.5% as a complication of the placement or migration of the prosthesis, but may even be as high as 25 to 65% in the presence of a tracheobronchial-esophageal fistula, as Boyce (1984) and Duranceau and Jamieson (1984) recorded in their reviews.

Photodynamic Therapy and Endoscopic Laser Therapy

Fleischer and Kessler (1983) reported that endoscopic removal of the obstructing tissue by YAG laser temporarily alleviated dysphagia in a few patients. McCaughan and associates (1985) reported photodynamic therapy after intravenous injection of a hematoporphyrin derivative in 16 patients, with reasonable palliation of the obstructive symptoms. The eventual role of these two approaches for the relief of dysphagia in the inoperable patient is not yet established.

RADIATION THERAPY

Irradiation, both for potential cure and for palliation, is used throughout the world as the major therapeutic modality in those patients unsuitable for resection. In many institutions it remains the therapy of choice in lesions of the upper third of the thoracic portion of the esophagus. The subject is presented in full in Chapter 94. Radiation therapy, however, only results in approximately a 20% 2-year survival and less than a 10% 5-year survival in most series (Table 86–11). The major problem in most patients is the failure to control the local disease for any prolonged period. Initial palliation occurs in most, however, and is well worth the effort in the nonsurgical patients.

Because many patients with squamous cell carcinoma of the esophagus in China are treated by irradiation, many long-term survivors have been observed. Yang and associates (1983) analyzed 1136 5-year survivors. The important prognostic factors were a lesion less than 5 cm long, a lesion located in the upper-third segment, and

Table 86–11. 5-Year Survival Rates with Radiation Therapy Alone in Patients with Esophageal Carcinoma

Author	No. of Patients	Rad Dose	5-Year Survival in %
Frazier et al. (1970)	79	3000–6000/3–6	1.5
X'ian Mc (1974)*	2310	?	9.3
Pearson (1977)	212	5000/4 weeks	14.0
Earlam & Cuhna-Melo (1980)†	8489	Various	6.0
Yin et al. (1980)	3798	?	8.4
Linxian (1981)*	1081	?	16.4
Newaishy et al. (1982)	4421	5000–5500/4 weeks	9.0

*Chinese data quoted by Gu, X.Z.: Radiation therapy for carcinoma of the esophagus. *In* Carcinoma of the Esophagus and Gastric Cardia. Edited by G.J. Huang and Y.K. Wu. Berlin, Springer-Verlag, 1984.
†Collected Series 1954–1979

one that was sensitive to irradiation. Most long-term survivors received a dose of between 50 and 80 Gy. Of these long-term survivors, 404 patients subsequently died. Late local recurrence and hematogenous spread or lymph node metastases were found in 50% of the patients at the time of death. Even this late in the illness, loss of local control was a major factor in mortality.

The addition of chemotherapy to the radiation therapy program, as well as the use of radiosensitizers, is under investigation. Whether or not these will add additional long-term survivors remains to be seen.

CHEMOTHERAPY

Chemotherapy is not a primary treatment modality. Its use is restricted basically to the adjuvant mode. Alone, the various drug regimens have little to offer, but investigation for the development of better drug regimens for use in extensive disease must be continued.

PROGNOSIS

Except for the very early cases, the prognosis of the patient with squamous cell carcinoma of the esophagus remains poor. Approximately only 10% or fewer of the patients survive for a prolonged period regardless of the various treatment regimens available. High quality palliation is the major goal, along with minimal initial morbidity or mortality. This requires the proper selection of the various treatment modalities for each patient. Continued efforts to identify patients with early lesions must continue. In this group, the success of surgical resection is highly satisfactory. In endemic areas, the use of balloon cytology has been rewarding. To identify and evaluate the high risk groups in America and Western Europe remains the problem.

REFERENCES

Akiyama, H.: Surgery for carcinoma of the esophagus. Curr. Probl. Surg. 17:53, 1980.
Akiyama, H., Kogure, T., and Itai, Y.: The esophageal axis and its relationship to the resectability of carcinoma of the esophagus. Ann. Surg. 176:30, 1972.
Akiyama, H., et al.: Principles of surgical treatment for carcinoma of the esophagus: analysis of lymph node involvement. Ann. Surg. 194:438, 1981.
Akiyama, H., et al.: Development of surgery for carcinoma of the esophagus. Am. J. Surg. 147:9, 1984.
American Joint Committee For Cancer Staging and End-Results Reporting: Cancer of esophagus. In Manual for Staging of Cancer, 2nd ed. Edited by O.H. Beahr and M.H. Myers. Philadelphia, J.B. Lippincott Co., 1983, p. 61.
Anderson, L.L., and Lad, T.E.: Autopsy findings in squamous cell carcinoma of the esophagus. Cancer 50:1587, 1982.
Armstrong, B.: The epidemiology of cancer in the People's Republic of China. Int. J. Epidemiol. 9:305, 1980.
Austin, J.C., Postier, R.G., and Elkins, R.C.: Treatment of esophageal cancer: the continued need for surgical resection. Am. J. Surg. 152:592, 1986.
Bains, M., et al.: Treatment of esophageal carcinoma by combined preoperative chemotherapy. Ann. Thorac. Surg. 34:521, 1982.
Benrey, J., Graham, D.Y., and Goyal, R.K.: Hypercalcemia and carcinoma of the esophagus (Letter). Ann. Intern. Med. 80:415, 1974.

Boyce, H.W., Jr.: Palliation of advanced esophageal cancer. Semin. Oncol. 11:186, 1984.
Burgess, H.M., et al.: Carcinoma of the esophagus: clinicopathologic study. Surg. Clin. North. Am. 31:965, 1951.
Campbell, W.R., et al.: Therapeutic alternatives in patients with esophageal cancer. Am. J. Surg. 150:665, 1985.
Chandrasekhara, R., Pilz, C.G., and Levitan, R.: Hypercalcemia associated with esophageal carcinoma in the absence of bone metastasis. Am. J. Dig. Dis. 20:173, 1975.
Conlan, A.A., et al.: Retrosternal gastric bypass for inoperable esophageal cancer: a report of 71 patients. Ann. Thorac. Surg. 36:396, 1983.
Doiron, D.R., et al.: Fluorescence bronchoscopy for detection of lung cancer. Chest 76:27, 1979.
Duranceau, A., and Jamieson, G.G.: Malignant tracheoesophageal fistula. Ann. Thorac. Surg. 37:346, 1984.
Edwards, D.A.W.: Carcinoma of the oesophagus and fundus. Postgrad. Med. J. 50:223, 1974.
Elam, R., and Cunha-Melo, R.J.: Oesophageal squamous cell carcinoma. II. A critical review of radiotherapy. Br. J. Surg. 67:457, 1980.
Ellis, F.H., Jr., Gibb, S.P., and Watkins, E., Jr.: Esophagogastrectomy: a safe, widely applicable, and expeditious form of palliation for patients with carcinoma of the esophagus and cardia. Ann. Surg. 198:531, 1983.
Endo, M., et al.: Surgical treatment of thoracic esophageal cancer, including clinical evaluation of early esophageal cancer. In Cancer of the Esophagus, Vol. II. Edited by C.J. Pfeiffer. Boca Raton, FL, CRE Press, Inc., 1982.
Fleischer, D., and Kessler, F.: Endoscopic Nd:YAG laser therapy for carcinoma of the esophagus: a new form of palliative treatment. Gastroenterology 85:600, 1983.
Frazier, A.G., Lefitt, S.H., and Degiorgi, L.S.: Effectiveness of irradiation therapy in the treatment of carcinoma of the esophagus. Am. J. Roentgenol. 108:830, 1970.
Ginsberg, R.J., and Pearson, F.G.: Squamous cell carcinoma of the esophagus. In General Thoracic Surgery, 2nd ed. Edited by T.W. Shields. Lea & Febiger, Philadelphia, 1983.
Giuli, R., and Sancho-Garnier, H.: Diagnostic, therapeutic, and prognostic features of cancer of the esophagus: results of the international study conducted by the OESO group (790 patients). Surgery 90:614, 1986.
Gu, X.Z.: Radiotherapy for carcinoma of the esophagus. In Carcinoma of the Esophagus and Gastric Cardia. Edited by G.J. Huang and Y.K. Wu. Berlin, Springer-Verlag, 1984.
Halvorsen, R.S., and Thompson, W.M.: Computed tomographic evaluation of esophageal carcinoma. Semin. Oncol. 11:113, 1984.
Hilgenberg, A.D., et al.: Preoperative chemotherapy, surgical resection, and selective postoperative therapy for squamous cell carcinoma of the esophagus. Ann. Thorac. Surg. 45:357, 1988.
Huang, G.J.: What is the value of abrasive cytology? In Cancer of the Esophagus. 1984: One Hundred and Thirty-five Questions. Edited by R. Giuli. Paris, S.A. Maloine, Editeur, 1984a, p. 320.
Huang, G.J.: Results of treatment of carcinoma of the esophagus. In Cancer of the Esophagus 1984: One Hundrend and Thirty-five Questions. Edited by R. Giuli. Paris. S.A. Maloine, Editeur, 1984b, p. 58.
Huang, G.J.: Palliative treatment. In Carcinoma of the Esophagus and Gastric Cardia. Edited by G.J. Huang and Y.K. Wu. Berlin, Springer-Verlag, 1984c.
Huang, G.J., and Wu, Y.K.: Clinical diagnosis. In Carcinoma of the Esophagus and Gastric Cardia. Edited by G.J. Huang and Y.K. Wu. Berlin, Springer-Verlag, 1984a.
Huang, G.J., and Wu, Y.K.: Operative technique for carcinoma of the esophagus. In Carcinoma of the Esophagus and Gastric Cardia. Edited by G.J. Huang and Y.K. Wu. Berlin, Springer-Verlag, 1984b.
Huang, G.J., et al.: Diagnosis and surgical treatment of early esophageal carcinoma (English abstract). Chin. Med. J. 94:229, 1981a.
Huang, K.C. (G.J.), et al.: Diagnosis and surgical treatment of early esophageal carcinoma. In Medical and Surgical Problems of the Esophagus, Vol. 43. Edited by S. Stipa, R.H.J. Belsey, and A.

Moraldi. Serona Symposia, New York, Academic Press, Inc., 1981b.

Huang, G.J., et al.: Combined preoperative irradiation and surgery in esophageal carcinoma: report of 408 cases. Clin. Med. J. 94:73, 1981c.

Hzuka, T., Kato, H., and Watanabe, H.: One hundred and two 5-year survivors of esophageal carcinoma after resective surgery. Jpn. J. Clin. Oncol. 15:369, 1985.

Ide, H., et al.: Lymph node metastases of thoracic esophageal cancer. Shujutsu 18:1355, 1974.

Isolauri, J., Markkula, H., and Autio, V.: Colon interposition in the treatment of carcinoma of the esophagus and gastric cardia. Ann. Thorac. Surg. 43:420, 1987.

Isono, K., et al.: Recurrence of intrathoracic esophageal cancer. Jpn. J. Clin. Oncol. 25:49, 1985.

Japanese Committee for Registration of Esophageal Carcinoma: A proposal for a new TNM classification of esophageal carcinoma. Jpn. J. Clin. Oncol. 14:625, 1985.

Keagy, B.A., et al.: Esophagogastrectomy as palliative treatment for esophageal carcinoma: results obtained in the setting of a thoracic surgery residency program. Ann. Thorac. Surg. 38:611, 1984.

Kelsen, D.P.: Chemotherapy of esophageal cancer. Semin. Oncol. 11:159, 1984.

Kelsen, D.P., et al.: Combined modality therapy of esophageal carcinoma. Cancer 48:31, 1981.

Kirschner, M.B.: Ein neues Verfahren der Oesophagoplastik. Langenbeck's Arch. Klin. Chir. 114:606, 1920.

Klinkhamer, A.C.: Esophagogastrotomy in anomalies of the aortic arch system. Amsterdam, Excerpta Medica Foundation, 1969.

Kondo, M., et al.: Ga-67 scans in patients with intrathoracic esophageal carcinoma planned for surgery. Cancer 49:1031, 1982.

Kumegawa, H., et al.: Study of endoscopic ultrasonography for esophageal carcinoma. Jpn. J. Med. Ultrasonic 12:207, 1985.

Lambert, R., Audigier, J.C., and Tuyns, A.J.: Epidemiology of oesophageal cancer in France. In Carcinoma of the Oesophagus. Edited by W. Silber. Capetown, South Africa, A.A. Balkema, 1978, pp. 23–28.

Launois, B., et al.: Preoperative radiotherapy for carcinoma of the esophagus. Surg. Gynecol. Obstet. 153:690, 1981.

Launois, B., et al.: Results of the surgical treatment of carcinoma of the esophagus. Surg. Gynecol. Obstet. 156:753, 1983.

Lea, J.W., Prager, R.L., and Bender, H.W.: The questionable role of computed tomography in preoperative staging of esophageal cancer. Ann. Thorac. Surg. 38:s479, 1984.

Lehr, L., Rupp, N., and Siewert, J.R.: Assessment of resectability of esophageal cancer by computed tomography and magnetic resonance imaging. Surgery 103:344, 1988.

Leichman, L., et al.: Combined preoperative chemotherapy and indication therapy for cancer of the esophagus: the Wayne State University, Southwest Oncology Group and Radiation Therapy Oncology Group experience. Semin. Oncol. 11:178, 1984a.

Leichman, L., et al.: Preoperative chemotherapy and radiation therapy for patients with cancer of the esophagus: a potentially curative approach. J. Clin. Oncol. 2:75, 1984b.

Li, K.H., Kao, J.C., and Wu, Y.K.: A survey of the prevalence of carcinoma of the esophagus in North China. In Selected papers on cancer research. Edited by the Chinese Academy of Medical Sciences. Shanghai Scientific and Technical Publishers, 1962, pp. 215. Quoted by Liu, F.R., and Zhou, C.N. In Carcinoma of the Esophagus and Gastric Cardia. Edited by G.J. Huang and Y.K. Wu. New York, Springer-Verlag, 1984.

Lindell, M.M., Jr., Hill, C.A., and Libshitz, H.I.: Esophageal cancer: radiographic chest findings and their prognostic significance. AJR 133:461, 1979.

Liu, F.S.: Autoptic analysis of 41 cases of esophageal cancer (in Chinese with English abstract). Natl. Med. J. China 60:218, 1980.

Liu, F.S.: Pathology of esophageal cancer (in Chinese). Cancer Res. Prev. Treat. 3:1976. (Quoted by Liu, F.S., and Zhou, C.N. In Carcinoma of the Esophagus and Gastric Cardia. Edited by G.J. Huang and Y.K. Wu. Berlin, Springer-Verlag, 1984, p. 79.

Liu, F.S., and Zhou, C.N.: Pathology of carcinoma of the esophagus. In Carcinoma of the Esophagus and Gastric Cardia. Edited by G. Huang and Y.K. Wu. Berlin, Springer-Verlag, 1984.

Lu, Y.K., Li, Y.M., and Gu, Y.Z.: Cancer of esophagus and esophagogastric junction: analysis of results of 1025 resections after 5 to 20 years. Ann. Thorac. Surg. 43:176, 1987.

Mandard, A.M., et al.: In situ carcinoma of the esophagus: macroscopic study with particular reference to the Lugol test. Endoscopy 12:51, 1980.

Mandard, A.M., et al.: Autopsy findings in 111 cases of esophageal cancer. Cancer 48:329, 1981.

Mannell, A.: Carcinoma of the esophagus. Curr. Probl. Surg. 19:555, 1982.

McCaughan, J.S., Jr., Williams, T.E., and Bethel, B.H.: Palliation of esophageal malignancy with photodynamic therapy. Ann. Thorac. Surg. 40:113, 1985.

Miller, C.: Carcinoma of the thoracic esophagus and cardia. Br. J. Surg. 49:507, 1962.

Miller, J.J., McIntyre, B., and Hatcher, C.R., Jr.: Combined treatment approach in the surgical management of carcinoma of the esophagus: a preliminary report. Ann. Thorac. Surg. 40:289, 1985.

Moss, A.A., et al.: Esophageal carcinoma: preoperative staging by computed tomography. Am. J. Roentgenol. 136:1051, 1981.

Newaishy, G.A., et al.: Results of radical radiotherapy of squamous cell carcinoma of the oesophagus. Clin. Radiol. 33:347, 1982.

Ogino, Y., et al.: Diagnosis of esophageal cancer by means of endoscopic ultrasonography. Stomach Intestine 19:1291, 1984.

Ong, G.B.: The Kirschner operation: a forgotten procedure. Br. J. Surg. 60:221, 1973.

Orringer, M.B.: Esophageal carcinoma: what price palliation? (Editorial.) Ann. Thorac. Surg. 36:377, 1983a.

Orringer, M.B.: Palliative procedures for esophageal cancer. Surg. Clin. North Am. 63:941, 1983b.

Orringer, M.B.: Substernal gastric bypass of the excluded esophagus: results of an ill-advised operation. Surgery 96:467, 1984a.

Orringer, M.B.: Transhiatal esophagectomy without thoracotomy for carcinoma of the thoracic esophagus. Ann. Surg. 200:282, 1984b.

Orringer, M.B., and Orringer, J.S.: Esophagectomy without thoracotomy: a dangerous operation? J. Thorac. Cardiovasc. Surg. 85:72, 1983.

Orringer, M.B., and Sloan, H.: Substernal gastric bypass of the excluded thoracic esophagus for palliation of esophageal carcinoma. J. Thorac. Surg. 70:836, 1975.

Orringer, M.B., and Sloan, H.: Esophagectomy without thoracotomy. J. Thorac. Cardiovasc. Surg. 76:643, 1978.

Parker, E.F., and Gregorie, H.B.: Carcinoma of the esophagus: long-term results. JAMA 235:1018, 1976.

Parker, E.F., et al.: Chemoradiation therapy and resection for carcinoma of the esophagus: short term results. Ann. Thorac. Surg. 40:121, 1985.

Payne, W.S., et al.: Current techniques for the surgical management of malignant lesions of the thoracic esophagus and cardia. Mayo Clin. Proc. 61:564, 1986.

Pearson, J.F.: The present status and future potential of radiotherapy in the management of esophageal cancer. Cancer 39:882, 1977.

Popp, M.B., et al.: Improved survival in squamous esophageal cancer. Arch. Surg. 121:1330, 1986.

Postlethwait, R.W.: Surgery of the Esophagus, 2nd ed. East Norwalk, CT, Appleton-Century-Crofts, 1986.

Roberts, J.G.: Cancer of the oesophagus: How should tumor biology affect treatment? Br. J. Surg. 67:791, 1980.

Sannohe, Y., Hiratsuka, R., and Doki, K.: Lymph node metastases in cancer of the thoracic esophagus. Am. J. Surg. 141:216, 1981.

Scanlon, E.F., et al.: The treatment of carcinoma of the esophagus. Q. Bull. Northwest Univ. Med. Sch. 30:144, 1956.

Shields, T.W., et al.: Multimodality approach to the treatment of carcinoma of the esophagus. Arch. Surg. 119:558, 1984.

Shu, Y.J., Yuan, X.Q., and Jin, S.P.: Further investigations of the relationship between dysplasia and cancer of the esophagus. Chin. Med. J. 1:39, 1981.

Skinner, D.B.: En bloc resection for neoplasms of the esophagus and cardia. J. Thorac. Cardiovasc. Surg. 85:59, 1983.

Steiger, Z., and Wilson, R.F.: Comparison of the results of esophagectomy with and without a thoracotomy. Surg. Gynecol. Obstet. 153:653, 1981.

Steiger, Z., et al.: Eradication and palliation of squamous cell carcinoma of the esophagus with chemotherapy, radiotherapy, and surgical therapy. J. Thorac. Cardiovasc. Surg. *82*:713, 1981.

Stephens, R.L., Hansen, H.H., and Muggia, F.M.: Hypercalcemia in epidermoid tumors of the head and neck and esophagus. Cancer *31*:1487, 1973.

Stewart, J.R., et al.: Transhiatal (blunt) esophagectomy for malignant and benign esophageal disease: clinical experience and technique. Ann. Thorac. Surg. *40*:343, 1985.

Symbas, P.W., et al.: Tracheoesophageal fistula from carcinoma of the esophagus. Ann. Thorac. Surg. *38*:382, 1984.

Szenpetery, S., Wolfgang, T., and Lower, R.R.: Pull-through esophagectomy without thoracotomy for esophageal carcinoma. Ann. Thorac. Surg. *27*:399, 1979.

Takemoto, T., et al.: Endoscopic ultrasonography. Clin. Gastroenterol. *15*:305, 1986a.

Takemoto, T., Ito, T., and Okita, K.: Endoscopic ultrasonography in the diagnosis of esophageal carcinoma, with particular regard to staging it for operability. Endoscopy *18*(Suppl. 3):22, 1986b.

Tanabe, G., et al.: Clinical evaluation of the esophageal lymph flow system based on RI uptake of dissected regional lymph nodes following lymphoscintigraphy. Nippon Geka Gakkai Zasshi *87*:315, 1986.

Thompson, W.M., et al.: Computed tomography for staging esophageal and gastroesophageal cancer: a re-evaluation. Am. J. Radiol. *141*:951, 1983.

Van Andel, J.F., et al.: Carcinoma of the esophagus: results of treatment. Ann. Surg. *190*:684, 1979.

Volkov, B.P., et al.: Chromoesophagogastroduodenoscopy. Vestn. Khir. *127*:27, 1981.

Wang, G.Q.: Endoscopic diagnosis of early oesophageal carcinoma. J. R. Soc. Med. *74*:502, 1981.

Wang, Z.Y., and Su, J.H.: Radiologic diagnosis. *In* Carcinoma of the Esophagus and Gastric Cardia. Edited by G.J. Huang and Y.K. Wu. Berlin, Springer-Verlag, 1984.

Watanabe, H., Iizuka, N., and Hirata, K.: Examination of esophageal cancer with intramural skip or separate satellite nodules. Geka Shinryo *21*:1096, 1979.

Wolfe, W.G., et al.: Early results with combined modality therapy for carcinoma of the esophagus. Ann. Surg. *205*:563, 1987.

Wong, J.: Management of carcinoma of oesophagus: art or science. J. R. Coll. Surg. Edinb. *26*:138, 1981.

Wong, J.: Esophageal resection for cancer: the rationale of current practice. Am. J. Surg. *153*:18, 1987.

Wong, J.: Stapled esophagogastric anastomosis in the apex of the right chest after subtotal esophagectomy for carcinoma. Surg. Gynecol. Obstet. *164*:569, 1987b.

Wu, Y.K., and Huang, G.J.: Surgical treatment. *In* Carcinoma of the Esophagus and Gastric Cardia. Edited by G.J. Huang and Y.K. Wu. Berlin, Springer-Verlag, 1984.

Yamashita, N.: A statistical analysis concerning the routes of dissemination of cancer of the esophagus based on the autopsy records. J. Jpn. Soc. Cancer Ther. *14*:1146, 1979.

Yang, C.S.: Research on esophageal cancer in China: a review. Cancer Res. *40*:2633, 1980.

Yang, A-Y, et al.: Long-term survival of radiotherapy for esophageal cancer: analysis of 1136 patients surviving for more than 5 years. Int. J. Radiol. Oncol. Biol. Physiol. *9*:1769, 1983.

Zhang, D.W.: Fiberesophagoscopic diagnosis. *In* Carcinoma of the Esophagus and Gastric Cardia. Edited by G.J. Huang and Y.K. Wu. Berlin, Springer-Verlag, 1984.

CHAPTER 87

SURGICAL PALLIATION OF INOPERABLE CARCINOMA OF THE ESOPHAGUS

Robert J. Ginsberg and Paul F. Waters

Carcinoma of the esophagus, be it squamous cell carcinoma or adenocarcinoma, continues to be lethal, with minimal hope of total cure. At diagnosis, fewer than 5% of patients have localized disease without regional node involvement. Another 50% of patients have locoregional disease. The rest present with distant metastases. It is unlikely that more than 10% of patients presenting with carcinoma of the esophagus will be cured of their tumor. For the rest, the most one can hope for is palliation of symptoms. The aim of palliation in the group with advanced disease is to improve the quality of the limited life remaining for the patient.

DYSPHAGIA

The most frequent symptom requiring surgical palliation is dysphagia. Obstructing tumors of the esophagus vary in the amount of dysphagia produced, but the progressive interference with the ability to eat is surely one of the most distressing symptoms one can have. When the patient aspirates or can only swallow liquids because of complete obstruction, intervention, often surgical, is required. The ability to swallow saliva and to eat as normally as possible is the goal of palliative treatment.

ASPIRATION

Pulmonary symptoms resulting from aspiration of saliva, caused by complete dysphagia, or of food, because of esophagorespiratory fistulae, is life-threatening and can be ameliorated surgically.

PAIN

Thoracic pain caused by invasion of an unresectable tumor cannot be relieved surgically, other than by neurosurgical ablative techniques. These patients are best treated nonsurgically.

SURGICAL CONSIDERATIONS

Regardless of the palliative technique employed, the morbidity and mortality of any procedure are significant, because of the advanced stage of the disease and the poor nutritional status of most patients. The more major the surgical intervention, the more likely postoperative complications are. The selection of the appropriate palliative technique should be modulated by several factors, including: the experience of the surgeon, the expected survival time of the patient, and the general condition of the patient at the time of intervention. One must always remember that nonsurgical methods of palliation are available. Radiation therapy can effectively shrink a tumor and alleviate pain and dysphagia. Combination chemotherapy has been used effectively for the same purpose. Chapters 86 and 94 discuss these modalities. Neither of these nonsurgical treatments has been effective in managing a tracheoesophageal fistula, and in fact they may aggravate the condition.

We will deal exclusively with those surgical procedures aimed at improving the ability to swallow without dysphagia or aspiration, including palliative resection, esophageal bypass, esophageal dilatation, esophageal intubation, laser ablation, and gastrostomy or jejunostomy.

PALLIATIVE ESOPHAGEAL RESECTION

The philosophy regarding palliative esophageal resection depends on the criteria used to define unresectable disease. These vary from surgeon to surgeon and from institution to institution.

Whenever a carcinoma of the esophagus can be completely resected without the expectation of leaving residual disease, a "curative" resection should be considered for the patient. All patients with local disease or disease limited to regional—N1—lymph nodes are likely to be considered for this form of curative therapy. In many instances, unfortunately, at the time of surgery, only an incomplete "palliative" resection can be performed.

Those patients with lymph node involvement beyond the regional area—M1 LYN—or metastatic disease—M1—cannot be considered curable by surgical resection. We believe that only in exceptional circumstances should surgical resection be performed as a palliative maneuver in these patients. A successful surgical resection without postoperative complications provides good swallowing function quickly, but palliative resections are prone to excessive postoperative complications and mortality. In noncurative resections, the median survival time is less than 6 months, the combined mortality and morbidity rate exceeds 30%, and virtually no patient survives 5 years. In these patients, we believe that irradiation offers as much hope for palliation as surgical resection, without the attendant postoperative problems, especially in tumors above the carina. Stoller and Brumwell (1984) demonstrated equal palliation by surgery or radiation therapy. Obstructing circumferential tumors below the carina are at times best treated by a palliative, incomplete resection, despite the inability to cure. In this location, the stricture produced by irradiation can result in significant dysphagia and poor quality of life. Adenocarcinomas respond less quickly to radiation therapy and the symptoms during the remaining few months of life may not be palliated by this modality. Giuli and Gignoux (1980), however, reported that an incomplete resection results in recurrent local disease in approximately 40% of the patients with early recurrent dysphagia. This must be considered before a palliative resection for patients whose tumor cannot be completely resected is recommended.

ESOPHAGEAL BYPASS

In a small group of patients with esophageal carcinoma, resection is not technically possible but nutritional and respiratory status and life-expectancy are such that esophageal bypass can be considered as the prime mode of therapy to ameliorate the dysphagia. Included in this group are those in whom radiation therapy may be contraindicated—impending or actual tracheoesophageal fistula or obstructing lesions at the lower end of the esophagus—or where irradiation or chemotherapy, or both, have failed.

The morbidity and mortality of such bypass procedures, however, are excessive (Table 87–1). In Orringer (1984) and Conlan and associates' (1983) series, the op-

erative mortality rates exceeded 20%, complication rates exceeded 50%, and median survival was less than 6 months. Orringer (1984) has abandoned this approach.

The simplest method of bypass uses the presternal or retrosternal route, with the anastomosis in the neck performed by laparotomy and neck incision. The left or right intrathoracic approach, however, can be used, with the anastomosis created in the chest, above the obstruction, or in the neck.

Gastric Tubes

Bypass using whole stomach—our own preference (Fig. 87–1)—or reversed—(Fig. 87–2) as Heimlich (1972) advocated—or nonreversed greater curvature gastric tubes—(Fig. 87–3) as Postlethwaite (1979) suggested—provides satisfactory swallowing. When using the entire stomach, the esophagus may be totally excluded and closed proximally and distally or, as recommended by Ong (1973), drained distally by a Roux-en-Y or simple jejunal loop (Fig. 87–4).

Advocates of greater curvature gastric tubes—reversed or nonreversed—claim that the simplicity and rapidity of fashioning these tubes far outweighs the slightly higher "leak" rate at the cervical esophageal anastomosis.

Fundal Bypass

A modified Popovsky procedure mobilizing the fundus of the stomach to bypass localized esophagogastric tumors (Fig. 87–5) has been successful in highly selected cases. This technique was well described by Popovsky in 1980.

Colon Segments

Although any portion of the colon may be used, we prefer an isoperistaltic left colon transplant, with a vascular pedicle based on the left colic artery, placed in the retrosternal position (Fig. 87–6). We use this approach when gastric transposition cannot be considered.

Jejunal Loops

The jejunum has a much more tenuous blood supply than the colon or stomach and is the least preferred bypass tube from neck to abdomen, but intrathoracic bypass using a Roux-en-Y jejunal loop, as Kirschner (1920) described and Ong (1973) used, is feasible, especially in esophagogastric tumors in which the stomach must also be bypassed (Fig. 87–7).

When recommending any of these bypass procedures,

Table 87–1. **Results of Large Series of Bypass Procedures Performed for Unresectable Carcinoma of the Esophagus**

Author	No. of Patients	Route	Organ	Mortality (%)	Anastomotic Leaks (%)	Median Survival
Hugier et al. (1970)	63	Presternal	Gastric tube	24	—	—
Wang et al. (1981)	142	Retrosternal	Stomach	41.5	47.2	5
Conlan (1982)	71	Retrosternal	Stomach	21	24	5
Orringer 1984)	37	Retrosternal	Stomach	24	20	6

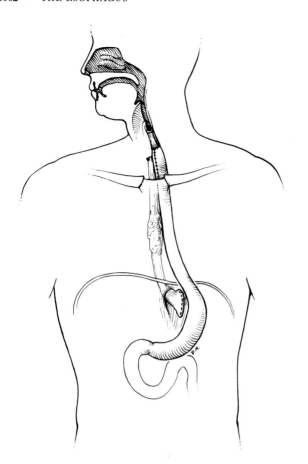

Fig. 87–1. Whole stomach bypass using the retrosternal route. Note that the esophagus has been excluded proximally and distally.

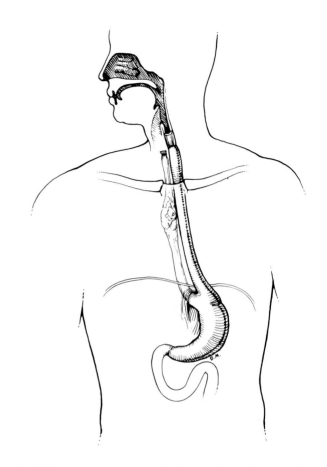

Fig. 87–2. A reversed gastric tube bypass. The esophagus has been excluded proximally but is drained adequately distally through the gastroesophageal junction.

one must remember that the patient has a limited life span and that any procedure should be aimed at a rapid recovery and discharge from the hospital with successful palliation of dysphagia.

Unfortunately, all of these bypass procedures have high morbidity and in-hospital mortality rates. One must be selective in recommending esophageal bypass for a patient with advanced, inoperable esophageal carcinoma.

Extracorporeal Tubes

Akiyama and Hatano (1968) and Skinner and De-Meester (1976) advocated permanent extracorporeal bypass using plastic tubes inserted into a preformed cervical esophagostomy and abdominal gastrostomy. This approach, however, has not been accepted as a usual means of palliation. The patient's disfigurement and distress seem to us to far outweigh the possible benefits of this type of palliative procedure.

ESOPHAGEAL DILATATION

Simple repeated esophageal dilatation rarely provides satisfactory swallowing ability for any significant duration. Usually the patient's symptoms are relieved for a few days or weeks at the most.

Dilatation, however, is usually necessary before per-oral intubation or laser ablation. We prefer using either Maloney bougies (Fig. 87–8) if a guide-wire is not required, or Savary bougies after the stricture has been successfully negotiated by a guide-wire under fluoroscopic control (Fig. 87–10). In most cases this can be performed satisfactorily with local anesthesia.

Many of these patients have already received radiation therapy, and care must be taken to dilate the stricture gradually, because the risk of perforation by splitting the postirradiated carcinomatous stricture is significant. Often the procedure must be repeated, gradually increasing the bougie size over a few sessions to obtain a satisfactory lumen.

ESOPHAGEAL INTUBATION

Various prostheses have been developed to intubate the esophagus, thereby relieving severe dysphagia or aspiration from tracheoesophageal fistulae. None of these prostheses allows perfectly normal swallowing. In most instances, little more than a minced or pureed diet can be tolerated. In most series, median survival after tube insertion is only about 3 months, with few if any patients surviving beyond 1 year.

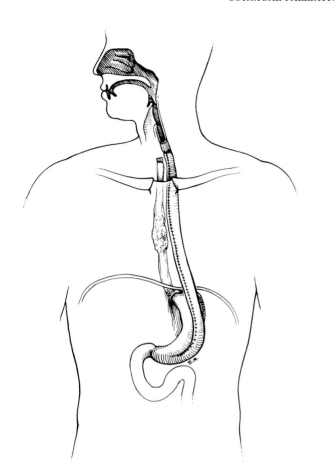

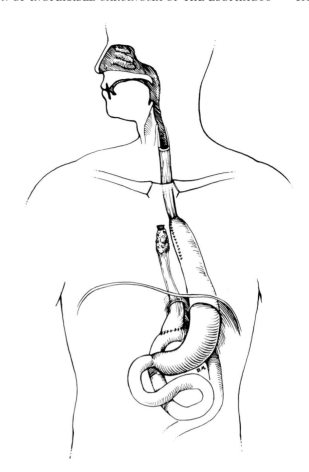

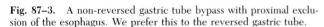

Fig. 87–3. A non-reversed gastric tube bypass with proximal exclusion of the esophagus. We prefer this to the reversed gastric tube.

Fig. 87–4. An intrathoracic gastric bypass excluding the esophagus proximally but draining the distal esophagus into a loop of jejunum.

The ideal tube should be easy to place, should remain in position without migrating proximally or distally, should remain patent on a reasonable diet, and should not erode into surrounding mediastinal structures. As yet, no tube is ideal.

Although there are many designs, most tubes can be categorized by the technique of insertion—"push" per os or "pull" by way of laparotomy and gastrotomy.

Peroral Intubation—"Push" Method

This is, by far, the most common technique currently employed. With flexible endoscopy, it can be applied successfully to tumors throughout the thoracic esophagus. The method usually does not require general anesthesia but does require preinsertion dilatation. We generally prefer the armored rubber tubes—Celestin or Atkinson—or silastic tubes—Savary (Fig. 87–11). Proctor-Livingston tubes have been used with success in South Africa.

Technique

Before insertion is attempted, a full-length barium esophagogram is obtained and flexible endoscopy is performed to assess the site and length of the stricture. If necessary, following endoscopy a guide-wire is passed through the tumor under fluoroscopic control. Careful

dilatation over the guide-wire using Savary bougies is carried out until an appropriate size—usually 14 mm—is reached. Care must be taken not to dilate the stricture larger than the tube itself lest the tube be inserted too far distally. Local—preferred—or general anesthesia can be used.

Once the tumor is dilated, the prosthesis is pushed into place using an introducing system tube designed for this purpose (Fig. 87–12). Fluoroscopic control is valuable. Either the guide-wire or the endoscope is used as a guide (Fig. 87–13).

To avoid reflux, after intubation of tumors in the thoracic esophagus it is desirable for the tube not to traverse the gastroesophageal junction. At least 4 cm of tube distal to the tumor, however, is necessary. Once the tube has been seated, endoscopy confirms adequate placement of the tube.

Following the procedure and before beginning oral feeding, a roentgenogram of the chest and contrast esophagogram—with Gastrografin—are performed to rule out perforation and ensure the correct position of the prosthesis. The patient is instructed to eat carefully, using liberal amounts of liquid, especially carbonated beverages, to "flush" the tube. The patient is also advised not to lie completely supine after meals or while sleeping

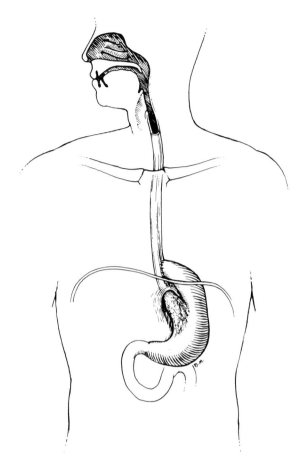

Fig. 87–5. A simple fundal bypass for a small gastroesophageal obstructing carcinoma.

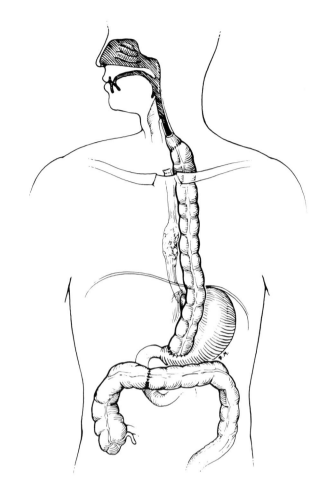

Fig. 87–6. A retrosternal colon bypass with exclusion of the proximal esophagus. We prefer an isoperistaltic left colon based on the ascending branch of the left colic artery.

to avoid reflux and aspiration—a significant late complication.

If placed accurately and atraumatically, these endoesophageal prostheses afford excellent palliation of dysphagia and can occlude an esophagorespiratory fistula.

Obstructing lesions in the cervical esophagus are difficult to treat by intubation. On occasion, we have successfully introduced a Montgomery salivary tube (Fig. 87–14), seating the flange above the cricopharyngeus muscle. If the flange must be seated below the upper esophageal sphincter, there is a significant risk of erosion into the trachea. This tube is designed for cervical strictures following laryngopharyngectomy, when the airway has been isolated by a tracheostomy.

Rigid endoscopy under anesthesia can be used for the occasional difficult case (Figs. 87–15, 87–16).

Morbidity

Complications of the procedure occur in about 20% of cases and include perforation, erosion of the tube into contiguous structures with fatal hemorrhage or a pleural fistula, upward migration and regurgitation of the tube, and dislodgement and passage of the tube beyond the lesion into the stomach. Occasionally, further tumor growth proximally can occlude the tube. For this latter problem, we have successfully inserted a second tube

above the first one on a few occasions when the original tube could not be replaced. Table 87–2 lists results of the peroral technique.

Intubation via Laparotomy—"Pull" Method

Although previously the most common approach, this technique is now usually reserved for those cases where the peroral technique cannot be used.

Technique

A left subcostal, paramedian, or midline laparotomy incision is appropriate. A high gastrotomy is performed. The anesthetist passes the introducer of the tube system orally if it was not already placed before the procedure. If this fails, retrograde dilatation by a bougie or retrograde insertion of a nasogastric tube to the mouth enables the surgeon to pull the introducer—attached by the anesthetist—through the obstruction. We prefer the Celestin or Fell tube, which is designed for this technique and permits gradual dilatation of the lumen (Fig. 87–17).

Using the introducer as a lead, the surgeon pulls the tube down the esophagus as the anesthetist facilitates the passage of the tube through the pharynx. The tube

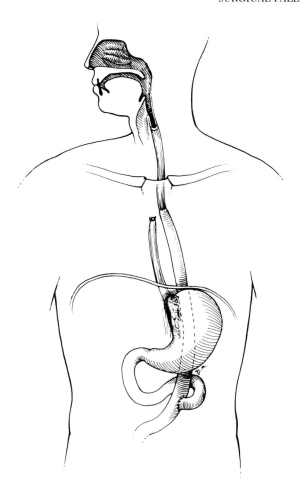

Fig. 87–7. An interthoracic Roux-en-Y esophageal jejunal bypass with exclusion of the proximal esophagus.

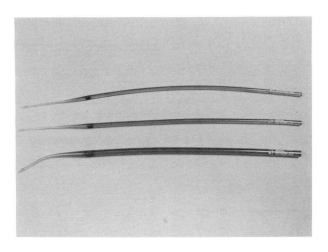

Fig. 87–9. Savary bougies for utilization with guide-wires.

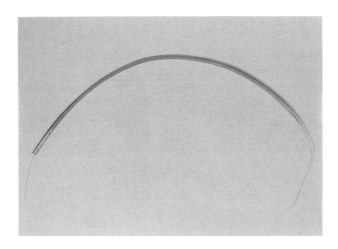

Fig. 87–10. An example of a Savary bougie with the guide-wire in place.

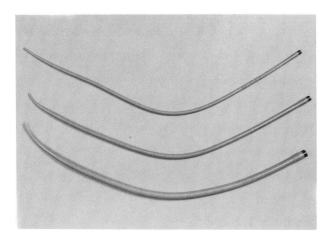

Fig. 87–8. Maloney bougies which we utilize for esophageal dilatation when guide-wires are not required.

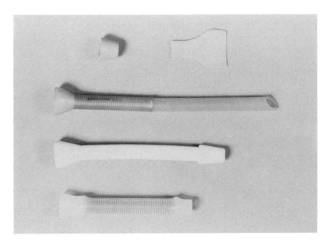

Fig. 87–11. Three examples of endoprostheses designed for "push" technique. Note the distal flange in an attempt to prevent proximal slippage and the rubber dam in an attempt to prevent reflux.

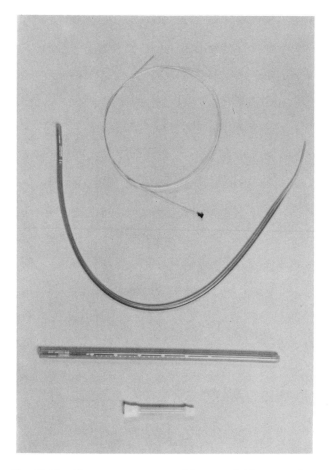

Fig. 87–12. The equipment required for peroral dilatation and intubation of a malignant obstruction.

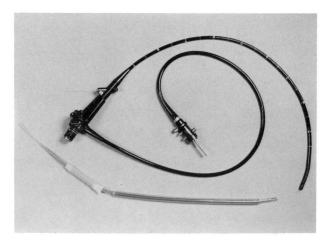

Fig. 87–13. The equipment assembled for intubation of a malignant obstruction. See text.

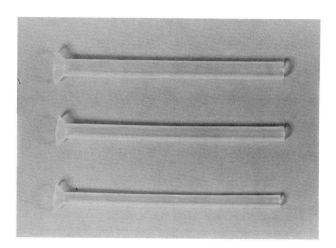

Fig. 87–14. Examples of Montgomery salivary tubes for use in proximal esophageal obstruction. The proximal flange should be placed above cricopharyngeus and is designed for use if a tracheostomy has been performed.

is then "seated" securely in place by traction (Fig. 87–18). Excess tube is removed distally using a guillotine shear. Ideally, the tube tip should lie above the gastroesophageal junction to avoid gastric reflux. With distal tumors, however, this placement is impossible, because the distal end must reside in the stomach; in these cases, many authors advocate suturing the tube to the anterior wall of the stomach to prevent proximal displacement. Because of high postoperative rate of wound infection, any technique to avoid this should be used, such as perioperative antibiotics and delayed skin closure. Flexible per-oral endoscopy before closing the gastrostomy incision is advisable to confirm the tube's placement. Table 87–3 presents the results of this technique.

Results of Esophageal Intubation

Most authors currently favor the peroral "push" method over the pull method. Kratz and colleagues (1988) demonstrated a lower complication rate—13% versus 58%, lower mortality rate—6% versus 40%, and longer median survival—3 versus 2 months—when using the peroral route.

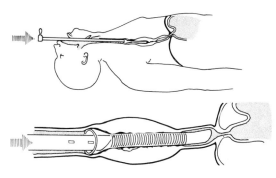

Push-through

Fig. 87–15. "Push" method utilizing rigid endoscopic techniques. Note that the end of the tube is above the gastroesophageal junction to avoid reflux. This is preferred whenever possible.

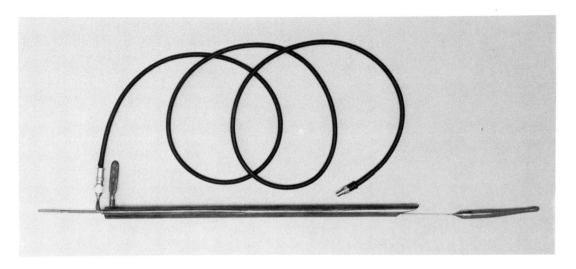

Fig. 87–16. A Negus esophagoscope with proximal lighting. This larger endoscope will allow forceful dilatation with gum-tipped bougies to a No. 38 size.

Table 87–2. Results of Recent Series of Intubations of the Esophagus Using the Peroral—Push—Technique

Author	No. of Patients	Tube	1-Month Mortality (%)	Median Survival (months)
Ogilvie (1982)	118	Celestin	11	4
Den Hartog Jager (1979)	200	Tygon	2	3
Proctor (1980)	2000	Proctor-Livingston	16.5 (2 weeks)	3
Anghorn (1981)	1045	Proctor-Livingston	16	6
Chavy et al. (1986)	77	Celestin	5	3.2

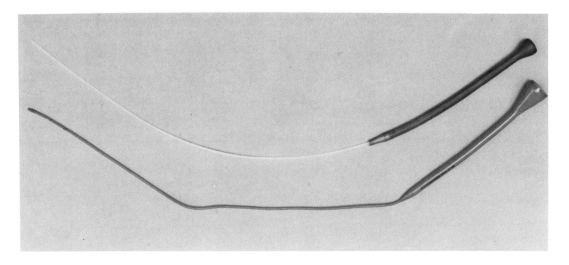

Fig. 87–17. A Celestin (top) and Porge tube (bottom) used for "pull" method of intubation.

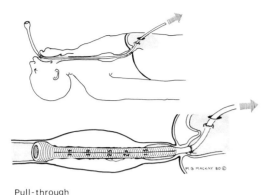

Pull-through

Fig. 87–18. "Pull" method. The tube eventually is cut off above the gastroesophageal junction whenever possible.

GASTROSTOMY AND JEJUNOSTOMY

Percutaneous or operative gastrostomy or jejunostomy can be used to maintain the nutrition of a patient but fails to deal with the problem of dysphagia. We seldom employ this technique. On rare occasions, however, this approach may be useful as an adjunct to other palliative techniques and can be especially important if the patient is receiving radiation therapy or chemotherapy, or both, for palliation.

LASER PROCEDURES

Restoration of swallowing ability by endoscopic removal of tumor by either photocoagulation therapy—CO_2 or Nd-YAG lasers—or photodynamic treatment—hematoporphyrin sensitization and argon pumped dye laser excitation—has been used with encouraging success. With either modality, exophytic fungating tumors are more amenable to palliation than tumor extrinsically compressing the esophagus.

Photocoagulation Therapy

Both the CO_2 and Nd-YAG lasers destroy tumor. The latter laser is preferable because it can be delivered by fiber-optic endoscopy. Patients need not be anesthetized for the procedure. After the 3 or 4 sessions required to produce an adequate lumen, repeated treatments at monthly or more frequent intervals may be required to maintain the lumen.

The advantages of this technique are the absence of mortality or major morbidity, although perforation oc-

curs in 4 to 5% of cases (Table 87–4). In expert hands, up to 90% of obstructing lesions can be opened up, allowing the patient to swallow liquids or semisolid foods. Because this procedure can be done on an ambulatory basis, it may prove to be valuable as a palliative procedure in the preterminal patient. Failure with this therapy still allows treatment with an endoprosthesis.

Photodynamic Therapy

The use of hematoporphyrin derivatives to sensitize malignant tumors to 630 ± 2 nm light—red—argon pumped dye laser—is effective in those tumors that are accessible to the argon laser beam. Skin, bladder, rectal, and pulmonary tumors have all been treated in this fashion. Obstructing esophageal tumors have been opened up by presensitizing the patients with hematoporphyrin derivatives and then using the laser endoscopically to destroy the tumor. It is believed that the mechanism of action is the production of intracellular singlet oxygen radicals, which destroy the tumor cells.

McCaughan (1985) and Thomas (1987) and their colleagues have reported that this technique has been successful in re-establishing a swallowing function. Usually two treatments are applied 3 and 6 days after the injection of hematoporphyrin. Within 1 to 3 weeks, the patient's ability to swallow improves. The treatment can be repeated if dysphagia recurs. Unfortunately, the patient must avoid direct sunlight for 1 month—a distinct disadvantage for someone with a limited life expectancy.

This type of therapy is in its infancy, and the exact application for palliation of esophageal tumors is unknown. Possibly, this type of treatment can be used in combination with irradiation or chemotherapy to improve its effect.

TRACHEOESOPHAGEAL FISTULA

The only modalities that can deal with this problem are exclusion, bypass, and intubation. None of these treatments is very successful. Once cachexia or pneumonia has complicated the problem, it is unlikely that any therapy will palliate symptoms or prolong survival. Only a few "early," healthy, nonseptic patients benefit from palliative treatment of this morbid complication.

CONCLUSIONS

The palliation of obstructing or fistulizing carcinomas of the esophagus is not always easy. Regardless of the

Table 87–3. Results of Recent Series of Intubations of the Esophagus Using the Transabdominal—Pull—Technique

Author	No. of Patients	Tube	1-Month Mortality (%)	Median Survival (months)
Wang et al. (1984)	334	Mousseau-Barbin (modified)	8.1	5
Kairaluoma et al. (1977)	108	Celestin	16.0	5
Saunders (1979)	105	Celestin	34.0	3
Diamanties (1983)	228	Celestin	31.0	2.2

Table 87–4.   Early Results with the Use of Nd-YAG Laser Therapy for Palliation of Obstructing Esophageal Cancer

Author	No. of Patients	No. of Initial Treatments (median)	Mortality	Average Duration of Palliation (months)
Fleischer (1984)	40	3.0	0	3–6
Riemann et al. (1985)	18	3.5	0	N/S
Rontal et al. (1986)	32	3.2	0	2–10
Wetstein et al. (1987)	40	3.3	0	

treatment, the perioperative morbidity and mortality are high. One cannot expect the median survival of these patients to be greater than 3 to 6 months, with the occasional patient's symptoms being palliated for up to a year. Despite the multitude of surgical techniques available, no one technique suits every patient. The surgeon must be cautious in choosing that technique which affords the patient adequate palliation with minimal morbidity and a short in-hospital stay.

REFERENCES

Akiyama, H., and Hatano, S.: Esophageal cancer: palliative treatment. Jap. J. Thorac. Surg. *21*:391, 1968.

Anghorn, H.B,.: Intubation in the treatment of carcinoma of the esophagus. World J. Surg. 5:535, 1981.

Chavy, A.L., et al.: Esophageal prosthesis for neoplastic stenosis: a prognostic study of 77 cases. Cancer 57:1426, 1986.

Conlan, A.A., et al.: Retrosternal gastric bypass for inoperable esophageal cancer: a report of 71 patients. Ann. Thorac. Surg. 36:396, 1983.

Den Hartog Jager, F.C, Bartelsman, J.F., and Tytgat, G.N.: Palliative treatment of obstructing esophagogastric malignancy by endoscopic positioning of plastic prosthesis. Gastroenterology 77:1008, 1979.

Giuli, R., and Gignoux, M.: Treatment of carcinoma of the esophagus: retrospective study of 2400 patients. Ann. Surg. 192:44, 1980.

Heimlich, H.J.: Esophagoplasty with reverse gastric tube. Am. J. Surg. 123:80, 1972.

Hugier, M., et al.: Results of 117 esophageal replacements. SGO *124*, 1058, 1970.

Kirschner, M.B.: Arch. Klin. Chir. *114*:606, 1920.

Kairaluoma, M.I., et al.: Celestin tube palliation of unresectable esophageal carcinoma. J. Thorac. Cardiovasc. Surg. 73:783, 1977.

Kratz, J.M., et al: A comparison of endoesophageal devices: improved results with Atkinson tube. J. Thorac. Cardiovasc. Surg. (in press).

McCaughan, J.S., et al.: Palliation of esophageal malignancy with photodynamic therapy. Ann. Thorac. Surg. *40*:113, 1985.

Ogilvie, A.L., et al.: Palliative intubation of esophagogastric neoplasms at fiberoptic endoscopy. Gut 23:1060, 1974.

Ong, G.B.: The Kirschner operation—a forgotten procedure. Br. J. Surg. *60*:221, 1973.

Orringer, M.B.: Substernal gastric bypass of the excluded esophagus—results of an ill-advised operation. Surgery 96:467, 1984.

Popovsky, J.: Esophagogastrostomy in continuity for carcinoma of the esophagus. Its use for unresectable tumors of the lower third of the esophagus and cardia. Arch. Surg. *115*:637, 1980.

Postlethwaite, R.W.: Technique for isoperistaltic gastric tube for esophageal by-pass. Ann. Surg. *189*:673, 1979.

Procter, D.S.: Esophageal intubation for carcinoma of the esophagus. World J. Surg. *4*:451, 1980.

Riemann, J.F., Rucks, C.E., and Demling, L.: Combined therapy of malignant stenoses of the upper gastrointestinal tract by means of laser beam and bouginage. Endoscopy *171*:43, 1985.

Rontall, E., et al.: Laser palliation for esophageal carcinoma. Laryngoscope 96:846, 1986.

Saunders, N.R.: Celestin tube in the palliation of the esophagus and cardia. Br. J. Surg. 66:419, 1979.

Skinner, D.B., and DeMeester, T.R.: Permanent extracorporal esophagogastric tube for esophageal replacement. Ann. Thorac. Surg. 22:107, 1976.

Stoller, J.L., and Brumwell, M.L.: Palliation after operation and after radiotherapy for cancer of the esophagus. Can. J. Surg. 27:491, 1984.

Thomas, R.J., et al.: High-dose photoradiation of esophageal cancer. Ann. Surg. *206*:193, 1987.

Wang, P.Y., et al.: A spiral-grooved endoesophageal tube for management of malignant esophageal obstruction. Ann. Thorac. Surg. 39:503, 1985.

Wetstein, L., et al.: A prospective evaluation of endoscopic Nd-YAG laser therapy in squamous cell carcinoma of the esophagus. Chest 92:62S, 1987 (abst).

CHAPTER 88

LESS COMMON MALIGNANT TUMORS OF THE ESOPHAGUS

Gordon F. Murray and G. Edward Rozar, Jr.

The less common malignant tumors of the esophagus share all too common clinical behavior and pathologic features with typical epidermoid esophageal carcinoma. The poor outcome for patients with squamous cell carcinoma persists despite advances in diagnostic and surgical techniques. Unfortunately, survival rates for patients with primary adenocarcinoma and other rare epithelial malignant lesions of the esophagus are equally discouraging. Neither the cell type nor the degree of histologic differentiation is significant in the prognosis, which is uniformly poor regardless of the treatment received. The uncommon polypoid carcinomas and sarcomas of the esophagus have a somewhat better prognosis when amenable to resection, but spread beyond the esophagus is rapidly fatal. Thus, cancer of this mediastinal organ, however unusual, is often lethal.

Table 88–1 lists malignant tumors of the esophagus other than typical epidermoid carcinoma. The unusual glandular carcinomas include the simple adenocarcinoma, cylindroma, and adenoacanthoma. Less common epitheliomatous lesions of the esophagus are the verrucous carcinoma, polypoid carcinoma, oat cell carcinoma, and melanoma. Of the few remaining primary esophageal malignant tumors, the true sarcomas are most notable. Rarely, the esophagus may be involved by metastatic tumor.

ADENOCARCINOMA

Invasion of the lower esophagus by gastric cancer is common and must be carefully excluded to determine the true incidence of primary adenocarcinoma of the esophagus. Malignant lesions involving the esophagogastric junction are almost invariably of gastric origin and may extend as high as the carina and aortic arch. Only rarely is esophageal adenocarcinoma explained by primary neoplastic change within the squamous-lined esophagus. Turnbull and Goodner (1968) found primary adenocarcinoma in the anatomic esophagus in 45 of 1859

Table 88–1. Less Common Malignant Tumors of the Esophagus

PRIMARY TUMORS
  Malignant Epithelial Tumors
    Adenocarcinoma
      Type "ordinaire"
      Adenoid cystic carcinoma (cylindroma)
      Mucoepidermoid carcinoma
      Adenocanthoma
      Choriocarcinoma
    Variants of Squamous Cell Carcinoma
      Verrucous carcinoma
      Polypoid carcinoma
        Carcinosarcoma
        Pseudosarcoma
    Small cell carcinoma
    Melanoma
  Malignant Mesenchymal Tumors
    Leiomyosarcoma
    Rhabdomyosarcoma
    Fibrosarcoma
    Chondrosarcoma
    Osteosarcoma
    Liposarcoma
    Kaposi's sarcoma
  Lymphoma
METASTATIC TUMORS TO THE ESOPHAGUS

patients with esophageal cancer at the Memorial Sloan-Kettering Cancer Center. Similar carefully documented studies have established that primary adenocarcinoma accounts for approximately 3% of all esophageal carcinomas. The sex, race, and age of patients with adenocarcinoma follow closely the pattern in patients with epidermoid carcinoma. The signs and symptoms, roentgenologic presentation, and endoscopic findings also do not distinguish these tumors from the squamous cell lesions. Diagnosis must be established by biopsy or cytologic examination.

A review of the glandular epithelial structures that may

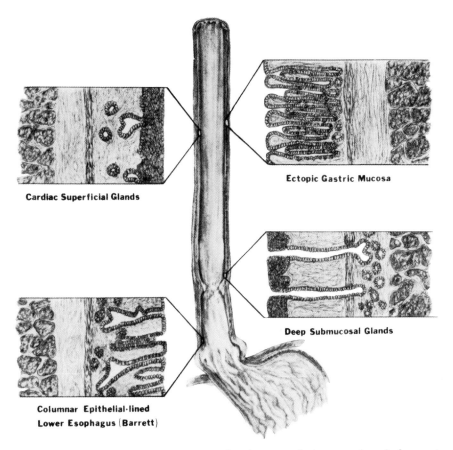

Fig. 88–1. Sources of columnar epithelium in the esophagus recognized in the origin of primary esophageal adenocarcinoma.

occur within the esophagus is essential to an understanding of the development of esophageal adenocarcinoma. Four sources of columnar epithelium in the esophagus have been recognized (Fig. 88–1). Superficial and deep submucosal glands constitute a part of the normal anatomy of the esophagus. Heterotopic islands of aberrant gastric mucosa occur in many organs of the body, including the esophagus. Only since the 1950s has the acquired nature of the columnar epithelial-lined lower esophagus been appreciated. The glandular epithelium in all of these conditions is premalignant.

The superficial esophageal glands arise in tall columnar epithelium that Johns (1952) noted in the embryo. Localization of the superficial glands in the adult to the upper and lower ends of the esophagus corresponds to the embryonal foci of the columnar epithelium. These mucus-secreting glands occupy an area in the lamina propria and are indistinguishable from the cardiac glands of the stomach. Although Hewlett (1900) suggested that these glands might give rise to adenocarcinoma, documented instances are difficult to find; nevertheless, Goldman (1952), Scicchitano (1962), and Raphael (1966) and their colleagues described malignant lesions that probably arose from the superficial glands of the esophagus. Goldfarb's (1967) well illustrated case report removes all doubt that adenocarcinoma may arise in the cardiac submucosal glands of the esophagus. The histo-logic structure of these lesions is adenocarcinoma "type ordinaire" as commonly seen in the stomach.

The deep esophageal submucosal glands develop mainly during the postnatal period and are found throughout the length of the esophagus. Columnar cells line the ducts that pierce the muscularis mucosa to reach the squamous epithelium. Although the deep glands are mucus-secreting, serous cells may be found, giving an appearance identical with minor salivary glands. Esophageal adenoid cystic carcinoma or cylindroma (Fig. 88–2), is incontrovertible evidence of primary esophageal glandular carcinoma, a tumor well known in the major salivary glands and oropharyngeal region, but with no counterpart in the stomach. Azzopardi and Menzies (1962) reported four examples of cylindroma in the esophagus histologically identical to that seen in the salivary glands. Rarely, true mucoepidermoid tumors that resemble lesions of the major salivary glands microscopically appear in the esophagus. The tumors show distinct epidermoid features with evidence of intracellular mucus secretion. Doubtless, these tumors also arise in the deep submucosal glands of the esophagus. Because of their submucosal origin, these tumors often present as intramural masses.

Islands of gastric mucosa sometimes replace portions of the squamous lining of the esophagus (Fig. 88–3). These areas of heterotopic epithelium usually consist of cardiac glands, but they may contain parietal cells. The

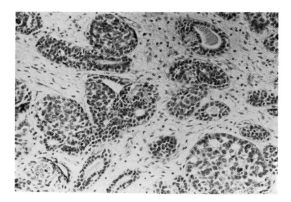

Fig. 88–2. Adenoid cystic carcinoma of the esophagus. (Sobin, L.H.: Histologic Typing of Gastric and Oesophageal Tumours. Geneva, World Health Organization, 1977.)

frequency of such patches varies, but Rector and Connerly (1941) found patches in 7.8% of 1000 consecutive pediatric autopsies. The heterotopic tissue was found most often in the upper third of the esophagus. Postlethwait and Musser (1974) found 1 neonatal esophagus completely lined by columnar epithelium among 200 specimens studied. Carrie (1950) reported apparently the first example of adenocarcinoma arising from a patch of ectopic gastric epithelium; the concept is now established by many reports. The gastric origin of the tumor is evident, because in situ malignant changes can be found in remnants of the heterotopic epithelium and the tumor is morphologically identical to gastric carcinoma. A variant of adenocarcinoma shows a concomitant squamous metaplastic element and is designated adenocanthoma. The lesion is principally a well differentiated adenocarcinoma with groups of squamous cells surrounded by glandular tumor. Distinct from these tumors is the squamous cell carcinoma with pseudoglandular degeneration characterized by its lack of mucus secretion, and the rare composite adenosquamous malignancy with aggressive glandular and epidermoid elements. McKechnie and Fechner's (1971) report suggested that metaplasia of esophageal adenocarcinoma forms hormonally active choriocarcinoma. This tumor is rare, and it may be a

giant cell variant of adenocarcinoma that is attempting trophoblastic differentiation.

The columnar epithelial-lined lower esophagus, or Barrett's esophagus, is usually a reparative response to gastroesophageal reflux. The relationship of this finding and the occurrence of adenocarcinoma in the columnar-lined esophagus is discussed in Chapter 84.

Treatment

Surgical resection is the treatment of choice for adenocarcinoma of the esophagus. Extensive infiltration of the wall and lymphatics is common, so frozen section examination of the proximal margin is advisable. Palliative radiation therapy may result in a gratifying clinical response in a few patients for up to 1 year. Only surgical excision permits survival of 5 years or more. Whether effective antireflux operation prevents cancer in the columnar epithelium-lined esophagus remains unproved.

Berenson and associates (1978) emphasized that the finding of carcinoma in situ in patients with Barrett's esophagus should lead to a consideration of resection of the affected portion of the mucosa. Most patients with adenocarcinoma in the columnar-lined lower esophagus have undergone resection and esophagogastrostomy. As examination of resected specimens has shown scattered changes of diffuse atypia or carcinoma in situ, Poleynard and his colleagues (1977) recommended complete extirpation of all columnar epithelium when curative resection is contemplated. In a series by Witt and associates (1985) of 19 patients with adenocarcinoma arising from Barrett's esophagus, 7 had multicentric disease.

Prognosis

The prognosis of adenocarcinoma of the esophagus is uniformly poor, regardless of site of origin or treatment received. Turnbull and Goodner (1968) reported only one 5-year survivor among 45 patients with adenocarcinoma—2.2%. Of 20 patients with adenocarcinoma reported by Hankins and associates (1974), only 2 survived more than 1 year, and the average survival period was 5.6 months. As in the simple adenocarcinoma, the mucoepidermoid tumors of the esophagus show a high degree of malignancy. They are extensively invasive, and metastases are generally present. Ming (1973) emphasized that the relatively benign course of adenocystic carcinomas in other areas is not applicable to the esophageal lesions. The latter generally demonstrate extensive intramural spread, and distant metastases are frequent. Allard and associates (1981) reported a case in a 75-year-old man, and they suggested that this tumor, like squamous cell carcinoma, should be treated by radical excision. Symptomatic malignancy in patients with Barrett's esophagus is not expected to behave differently from other types of adenocarcinoma, but early detection and excision may improve the prognosis of patients with primary esophageal adenocarcinoma arising in a columnar-lined lower esophagus. Esophagoscopy with directed biopsy and cytology is the best screening procedure.

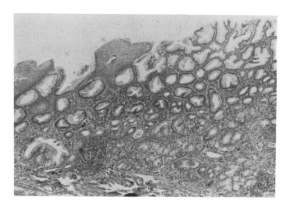

Fig. 88–3. Gastric heterotopia, upper esophagus. (Sobin, L.H.: Histologic Typing of Gastric and Oesophageal Tumours. Geneva, World Health Organization, 1977.)

UNUSUAL VARIANTS OF SQUAMOUS CELL CARCINOMA

Verrucous Carcinoma

A distinct morphologic variant of the squamous cell carcinoma of the esophagus is the verrucous carcinoma. This tumor is a papillary or warty, cauliflower epidermoid growth that is well differentiated histologically and shows marked acanthosis and hyperkeratosis (Fig. 88–4). Verrucous squamous carcinoma is most frequently found in the oral cavity; it has also been found on the larynx, glans penis, and vulva. Verrucous carcinoma of the esophagus is rare. Minielly and colleagues (1967) found only five instances among all esophageal carcinoma cases seen at the Mayo Clinic since 1906. Chronic retention of esophageal contents may have contributed to the development of these verrucous lesions. Two of the patients had a history of long-standing achalasia, and in two patients a diagnosis of esophageal diverticulum had been made several years before the discovery of esophageal carcinoma. The two surgical specimens showed a moderate degree of associated leukoplakia. Leukoplakia, commonly associated with verrucous squamous carcinoma in other sites such as the oral cavity or the penis, is rarely encountered in the esophagus except with achalasia or esophageal diverticulum.

The natural history of verrucous squamous carcinoma in the esophagus, as in other sites, is that of a slowly growing but gradually invasive neoplasm. Meyerowitz and Shea's (1971) report of a patient with a verrucous carcinoma at the lower end of the esophagus for almost 7 years before diagnosis and surgical resection illustrates the indolent growth of verrucous carcinoma. The slowly progressing infiltrative tumor characteristically becomes large but does not metastasize. No distant metastasis of verrucous carcinoma has been reported. Lymph nodes adjacent to the tumor may be involved by direct extension. Diagnosis may be difficult because the growth is well differentiated, and the biopsy specimen should be deep enough to demonstrate invasion. Early recognition of the lesion requires clinical suspicion of this growth,

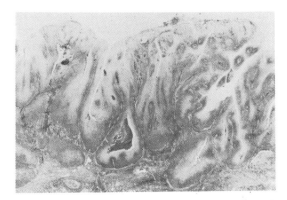

Fig. 88–4. Verrucous squamous cell carcinoma of the esophagus with typical blunt contours of deep margin. (Sobin, L. H.: Histologic Typing of Gastric and Oesophageal Tumours. Geneva, World Health Organization, 1977.)

particularly in the presence of achalasia or esophageal diverticulum.

Verrucous carcinoma of the esophagus, as in other sites, ideally should be treated by en bloc surgical resection. Radiation therapy alone is not an advisable form of therapy. Goethals and associates (1963) stated that irradiation may cause a tumor to regress, but the treatment may also make the low grade lesion anaplastic and aggressive. Irradiation rarely effects a cure. Since verrucous carcinoma of the esophagus follows the usual growth pattern of this tumor elsewhere in the body, the outlook for these patients should be more favorable than it is for patients with the usual type of epidermoid carcinoma. Unfortunately, most patients in whom verrucous carcinoma of the esophagus has been documented died as a result of their tumor. Minielly and colleagues (1967) explained the poor prognosis of the esophageal lesion by the close proximity of vital mediastinal structures, the technical hazards of esophageal resection, and the frequent delay in diagnosis. Thus, early recognition and reduction in operative mortality by improved surgical techniques may result in a better prognosis for future patients.

Polypoid Carcinoma

Polypoid carcinoma with spindle-cell sarcomatous features is a rare variant of squamous carcinoma seen most commonly in the mouth, fauces, and upper respiratory tract, and less often in the esophagus. When these tumors are present in the esophagus, they are usually in the middle third. Many tumors apparently develop in response to radiation therapy for either benign conditions or typical squamous carcinoma, but this association is not reported for esophageal lesions. The exophytic esophageal tumors have been termed either carcinosarcoma or pseudosarcoma, based on the degree of intermingling and metastatic potentiality of carcinomatous and sarcomatous elements. Hence, carcinosarcoma is characterized histologically by the presence of intimate mingling of the carcinomatous and sarcomatous elements in the primary tumor; and metastatic potential is assigned to either the epithelial or sarcomatous component, or both. By contrast, in pseudosarcoma the carcinomatous element, in situ or invasive, is confined to the surface epithelium adjacent to the base of the polyp (Fig. 88–5). Only the carcinomatous component of the polypoid pseudosarcoma has been considered to have metastatic potential, but Martin and Kahn (1977) and Osamura and associates (1978) described polypoid esophageal malignancies with all of the morphologic features of a pseudosarcoma and definite evidence of metastasis of the spindle cell element (Fig. 88–6). Matsusaka and associates (1976b) failed to demonstrate any significant differences in the clinicopathologic features of carcinosarcoma and pseudosarcoma. Thus, no important distinction can be made between the two tumors, and Osamura (1978) proposed the unifying term polypoid carcinoma.

The idea that the sarcomatous elements of polypoid carcinoma arise from transformation of squamous cells was proposed at the turn of the century, and this view-

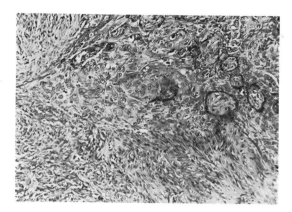

Fig. 88–5. Focus of squamous carcinoma in upper half of photomicrograph adjacent to sarcoma in lower half in section from base of polyp. Hematoxylin-eosin stain, ×125. (Martin, M.R., and Kahn, L.B.: So-called pseudosarcoma of the esophagus. Arch. Pathol. Lab. Med. *101*:607, 1977. Copyright 1977, American Medical Association.)

point represents the current consensus. Electron microscopic studies supporting the squamous origin of the sarcomatous-like cells resolved the controversy. Shields and colleagues (1972) reported the first electron microscopic studies of a polypoid carcinoma of the esophagus (Fig. 88–7). Many cells exhibited desmosomal attachment with neighboring cells with well developed junctional complexes including tonofilaments (Fig. 88–8). A few cells had many typical branching tonofibrils (Fig. 88–9). Tonofibrils appear only in epithelial cells, predominately squamous, and are thought to be related to the process of keratinization. Well developed tonofilament-associated desmosomes are also common in epithelial tumors, especially in those of squamous cell origin. Thus, Shields and associates (1972) concluded that the spindle-shaped cells in the polypoid tumor were of squamous cell origin. Battifora (1976) described further ultrastructural evidence of the squamous origin of the spindle cell element of polypoid esophageal carcinoma. The latter findings suggest that the sarcomatous component of the tumor originates from mesenchymal met-

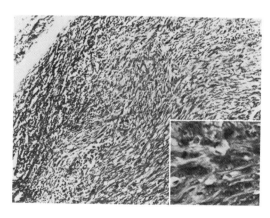

Fig. 88–6. Metastatic sarcoma in lymph node. Inset shows detail of spindle cells and several mitoses, including abnormal forms. Hematoxylin-eosin stain, ×125; inset ×320. (Martin, M.R., and Kahn, L.B.: So-called pseudosarcoma of the esophagus. Arch. Pathol. Lab. Med. *101*:607, 1977. Copyright 1977, American Medical Association.)

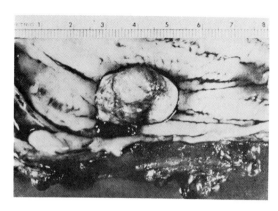

Fig. 88–7. Polypoid pseudosarcoma of the oesophagus. (Shields, T.W., et al.: Pseuodosarcoma of the oesophagus. Thorax 27:474, 1972.)

aplasia of squamous cells and that collagen is produced by these metaplastic cells.

Wide surgical resection of polypoid carcinoma of the esophagus is the treatment of choice and most effectively palliates the patient's obstructive symptoms—dysphagia and pulmonary aspiration. The extent of surgical resection and subsequent reconstruction of gastrointestinal continuity depends on the level of the lesion rather than the estimated degree of malignancy. Local excision has invariably resulted in recurrence of the tumor. Radiation therapy has met with only limited success, and long-term survival is unusual.

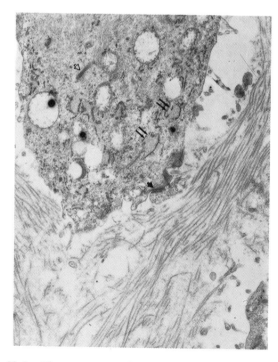

Fig. 88–8. Electron micrograph of pseudosarcoma of the esophagus showing portion of a spindle cell and a small segment from another cell. At point of contact a well-developed desmosome is present (solid arrow). The cytoplasm is rich in tonofilaments that in places form bundles (hollow arrow). Several distended cisternae of rough endoplasmic reticulum are visible (double arrows). Collagen fibers abound in the vicinity of the cell, ×22,000.

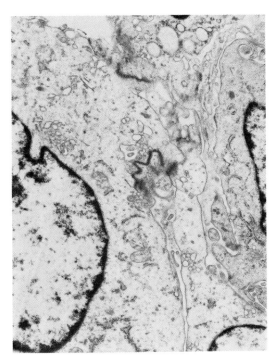

Fig. 88–9. Electron micrograph of pseudosarcoma of the esophagus showing the contact site of four tumor cells. Well-developed desmosomes are prominent and numerous, ×22,000.

Although a clear correlation between gross appearance and biologic behavior is not established, the polypoid carcinoma carries a better prognosis than typical squamous cell carcinoma of the esophagus because it rarely penetrates deeply into the esophageal wall. Diagnosis may be more prompt, because the polypoid pattern of growth results in early obstructive symptoms. Tumors up to 15 cm wide have been reported. At the time of evaluation, extraesophageal disease is usually absent; local invasion or metastases occur late, if at all. Early reported deaths were most often caused by complications of reconstructive surgery. Reports of long-term survival with wide surgical excision support the conclusion that polypoid carcinoma is often potentially curable.

SMALL CELL CARCINOMA

The existence of a small cell anaplastic carcinoma of the esophagus with a striking morphologic and biologic resemblance to oat cell carcinoma of the lung is gaining recognition. Bensch and associates (1968) showed that oat cell carcinoma of the lung and bronchial carcinoid tumors are endocrine polypeptide-producing tumors—apudomas—derived from cells that resemble argentaffin—Kulchitsky—cells in the intestinal tract. The cells, which possess long cytoplasmic processes, contain characteristic cytoplasmic granules referred to as neurosecretory-type granules. The intracellular neurosecretory-type granules display argentaffinic or, more commonly, argyrophilic properties, depending on the ability of the granules to reduce silver compounds. Small cell tumors with microscopic appearance similar to pulmonary oat

cell carcinoma and bronchial carcinoid may occur whenever argyrophilic cells are present. On the basis of the embryologic derivation of the esophagus from the foregut, argyrophilic neurosecretory cells can be expected in the esophagus. Brenner and associates (1969) discussed the probability of the presence of these cells in a report describing a carcinoid tumor in the distal esophagus. Demonstration of argyrophilic cells in the basal epithelium of the normal human esophagus was accomplished by Tateishi and co-workers (1974). Subsequently, Matsusaka and associates (1976a) found intracytoplasmic argyrophilic granules in three autopsy specimens of esophageal anaplastic carcinoma with an oat cell pattern. Tateishi and colleagues (1976) used electron microscopy and assay for ACTH content to study six patients with esophageal malignancies resembling pulmonary oat cell carcinoma; the three tumors studied contained neurosecretory-type granules, and ACTH activity in the tumor tissues was detected by bioassay or radioimmunoassay in three of the four tumors tested. They concluded that the oat cell carcinoma of the esophagus represents a distinct histopathologic entity clearly distinguishable from other types of esophageal carcinoma. These tumors are histologically identical to oat cell carcinoma of the lung, but clinically evident ectopic production of ACTH has not been a presenting feature. The tumor is composed of uniform small cells with hyperchromatic nuclei and little cytoplasm. The undifferentiated cells are arranged in solid sheets, or ribbon and streaming patterns (Fig. 88–10). Cook and colleagues (1976) emphasized that squamous cell carcinoma is often found adjacent to the esophageal oat cell lesion. The precise histogenetic relationship of the two tumor components is not clear, but derivation from the same cell of origin with divergent differentiation is possible. Sato and associates (1986) reported a case of a well differentiated squamous cell carcinoma and a non-oat cell small cell carcinoma without squamous differentiation. This non-oat cell tumor is thought to be a variant of squamous cell carcinoma.

Oat cell carcinoma and carcinoid tumor of the esophagus appear to behave like their pathologic counterparts in the lung. The carcinoid tumor is normally a locally

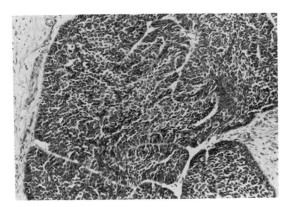

Fig. 88–10. Undifferentiated carcinoma, esophagus. A distinct form referred to as oat cell carcinoma is described in the text. (Sobin, L.H.: Histologic Typing of Gastric and Oesophageal Tumours. Geneva, World Health Organization, 1977.)

spreading but relatively benign neoplasm. The esophageal oat cell carcinoma is the anaplastic highly malignant form of the argyrophilic cell tumor. These tumors are usually fungating, polypoid lesions that ulcerate and are located in the middle or lower third of the esophagus. Most tumors have been identified at postmortem examination, which usually reveals extensive metastases. All six of the carefully studied patients described previously underwent surgical resection. Of the six patients, four died with widespread tumor recurrences within 9 months of operation; and one of the two surviving patients was alive with tumor recurrence at 14 months postoperatively. Oat cell carcinoma of the esophagus should be recognized as a separate entity, because its natural history and response to therapy may differ from ordinary esophageal carcinoma's. Progress in the treatment of oat cell carcinoma of the lung suggests that adjunctive combination chemotherapy and radiation therapy should be considered in the management of this unusual esophageal malignancy.

MELANOMA

Primary melanoma occurs most commonly in the skin. The second most common site is the eye. Rarely, malignant melanoma has arisen from the esophagus (Fig. 88–11). The prerequisite for primary esophageal melanoma, that is, the natural occurrence of melanoblasts in the esophageal mucosa, has been established. De La Pava and colleagues (1963) reported that, in 4 of 100 esophagi studied, typical melanoblasts with melanin granules and dendrites were found in the basal layer of the esophageal epithelium. These authors speculated that the melanoblasts, present in the upper third of the esophagus in 2 specimens and in the middle third in 2 specimens, migrated to the esophagus from the neural crest. Piccone and associates (1970) recorded the fourth example of a primary malignant melanoma of the esophagus associated with esophageal melanosis and the first with melanosis of the entire esophagus. The absence of melanosis in most melanomas of the esophagus indicates that the tumor more commonly originates in some other

way: an origin from some of the few normally occurring melanoblasts, from metaplasia of normal esophageal basal epithelial cells, or from ectopic melanoblast-containing epithelium included within the esophagus during development.

The presence of junctional changes in the overlying or adjacent epithelium is considered unequivocal evidence of a primary cutaneous malignant melanoma. Allen and Spitz (1953) broadened the concept of junctional change as an essential criterion of primacy to include visceral melanoma. Optimally, the diagnosis of primary esophageal melanoma should be based on the following criteria: (1) the tumor should have the characteristic histology of a melanoma and contain melanin; (2) the tumor should arise from an area of junctional change in squamous epithelium; (3) the adjacent epithelium should demonstrate junctional change with the presence of melanin-containing cells; and (4) careful evaluation must exclude skin, ocular, or anal mucosal primary melanomatous malignancy. In the esophagus, a rapidly growing tumor may ulcerate the adjacent epithelium, and direct origin from junctional epithelium is difficult to establish clearly. On the other hand, metastatic malignant melanoma of the esophagus has been reported only rarely. This infrequent reporting is curious, because melanoma in the stomach or small bowel is almost always a secondary deposit.

Nearly all primary esophageal melanomas present a shaggy, polypoid appearance roentgenographically, unlike metastatic lesions, which usually involve the muscularis and appears extrinsic and smooth in contour. Remarkably, the primary tumor usually grows to considerable size within the esophageal lumen before obstructive symptoms appear. Odynophagia is a prominent symptom, probably related to the frequent finding of ulcerated mucosa. The characteristic finding at endoscopy is a lobulated tumor situated on a wide pedicle in the mid- or lower esophagus. Gross pigmentation has been present in varying degrees, and the tumor may be black, brown, or gray. Most tumors are ulcerated and friable and bleed easily. Usually a single melanoma is present, but satellite lesions may be seen. The nature of the tumor should be determined by direct biopsy.

Because these tumors exhibit wide lateral growth, radical surgical excision with restoration of swallowing would appear to offer the best palliation of symptoms and the only hope of cure. Radiation therapy has been ineffective, and a role for chemotherapy has not been defined. The esophageal lesion is no less fatal than malignant melanoma found elsewhere in the body. The prognosis is grave because widespread disease usually develops rapidly, followed by a fulminating, deteriorating clinical course. Spread to the regional lymph nodes is most frequent, and the lungs, liver, and pancreas are often sites of distant metastases. Most patients die of their disease within 2½ years of its discovery and treatment, and nearly half die within 6 months. Chalkiadakis and associates (1985) reported a 4.2% 5-year survival.

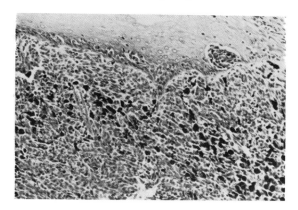

Fig. 88–11. Malignant melanoma of the esophagus. The primary tumor is heavily pigmented. (Sobin, L.H.: Histologic Typing of Gastric and Oesophageal Tumours. Geneva, World Health Organization, 1977.)

MALIGNANT MESENCHYMAL TUMORS

Sarcomatous lesions of the esophagus are rare. Leiomyosarcoma is the most frequent sarcoma, and leiomyoma is the commonest benign esophageal tumor. Rhabdomyosarcoma is far less common. The distinguishing pathologic feature of these muscle tumors is their frequently pedunculated gross configuration. In this regard they may resemble benign esophageal polyps and tumors, and the surgeon must be alert to the malignant potential of the polypoid esophageal lesion. The polypoid sarcoma tends to remain superficial within the esophageal wall, and nodal or distant metastasis is uncommon. Thus, esophageal sarcoma, unlike esophageal carcinoma, has a favorable prognosis following successful surgical resection.

Leiomyosarcoma

Leiomyosarcoma, with a ratio of two men to one woman, is more common, however, in women than squamous cell carcinoma; the latter tumor is predominant in men, with a ratio of approximately five to one. The age incidence of the two malignancies is much the same. The simultaneous occurrence of leiomyosarcoma and squamous cell carcinoma in the esophagus as separate tumors has received attention but is rare. Leiomyosarcomas are equally distributed throughout the esophagus, despite the relative paucity of smooth muscle in the proximal third. Although infiltration into adjacent structures may occur, the tumor is usually a bulky, polypoid intraluminal mass that may reach great size before producing obstructive symptoms (Fig. 88–12A).

The histologic distinction between well differentiated leiomyosarcoma and leiomyoma may be difficult; clinical behavior is the only true indication of the malignant nature of the lesion. Light microscopic findings of interlacing spindle-shaped pleomorphic cells with numerous mitotic figures is characteristic of leiomyosarcoma (Fig. 88–12B). In general, tumors with frequent mitotic figures and cellular anaplasia are more aggressive and

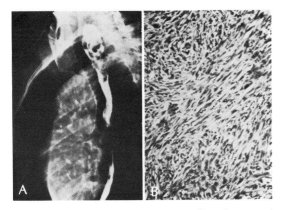

Fig. 88–12. Leiomyosarcoma. *A*, Barium swallow shows a polypoid mass in the upper thoracic and cervical esophagus. *B*, Photomicrograph of the polyp demonstrates large spindle-shaped cells with numerous mitoses. Hematoxylin-eosin stain, × 150. (DeMeester, T.R., and Skinner, D.B.: Polypoid sarcomas of the esophagus. Ann. Thorac. Surg. *20*:405, 1975.)

have a higher incidence of lymph node and distant organ metastasis. Gaede and associates (1978) emphasized that ultrastructural demonstration of the absence or scarcity of organelles in smooth muscle tumors may help determine malignant potential. Abnormal nucleoli visible with the electron microscope are apparently further evidence of malignancy.

Extragastric leiomyoblastoma primary in the esophagus has been reported (Fig. 88–13). Leiomyoblastoma, unlike leiomyosarcoma, has cells with eccentrically placed nuclei and large vascular spaces in the cytoplasm, giving the cells an epithelioid appearance resembling that of a signet-ring cell (Fig. 88–13C). Unlike adenocarcinoma, the cytoplasmic vacuoles do not react to periodic acid-Schiff, mucicarmine, and fat stains. Similar to leiomyosarcoma, the clinical behavior of these tumors appears to parallel the microscopic presence of nuclear pleomorphism and mitotic activity.

Surgical resection is the treatment of choice and is responsible for most of the recorded 5-year survivals. Postlethwait (1986) tabulated 52 reported patients who had resection and noted that 17 patients were alive, 5 for more than 5 years. One patient was alive 12 years after resection. The value of palliative radiotherapy in producing regression of bulky tumors and marked, often prolonged, symptomatic improvement is noteworthy. Combined surgery and irradiation might improve the somewhat favorable prognosis of leiomyosarcoma.

Rhabdomyosarcoma

Rhabdomyosarcoma of the esophagus is a curiosity. Postlethwait (1986) recorded 14 examples. Ming (1973) suggested that this tumor may well be a poorly differentiated leiomyosarcoma, particularly if it occurs in the distal esophagus where striated muscle cells are normally absent. Rhabdomyosarcoma has also been reported as a component of polypoid carcinoma. Microscopic diagnosis of rhabdomyosarcoma appears to be difficult and is based on the presence of cells shaped like a tennis racket, with one long protoplasmatic projection. Some authors regard identification of transverse cross striation as an essential diagnostic criterion. Unlike rhabdomyosarcoma in other sites, lymph node metastases are encountered.

Treatment of rhabdomyosarcoma does not differ from that of other esophageal sarcomas, and surgery is preferred, but no long-term survivors have been reported with esophageal resection. Radiation therapy is not effective; among the soft tissue sarcomas, rhabdomyosarcoma is the least radiosensitive.

Fibrosarcoma

Although fibrosarcoma was often cited in the early literature as the most common esophageal sarcoma, Stout and Lattes (1957) knew of no undoubtedly accurate report of primary fibrosarcoma arising in the esophagus. Very few examples have been recorded since then, and it is likely that many earlier reports were examples of leiomyosarcoma. Goodner and associates (1963) reported one fibrosarcoma among 1456 esophageal malignancies from 1926 through 1961. It is of interest that two reported

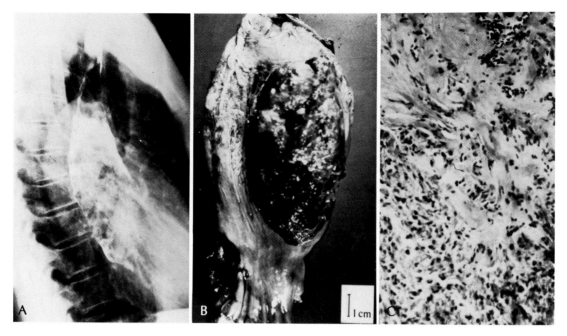

Fig. 88–13. Leiomyoblastoma. *A,* Barium swallow reveals a large polypoid mass within the middle third of the esophagus. *B,* Surgical specimen shows a 9-cm polypoid tumor within the esophagus with necrosis and hemorrhagic changes on its surface. *C,* Photomicrograph of the pedicle portion of the polyp demonstrates cells containing eccentric nuclei with cytoplasmic vacuolization. Hematoxylin-eosin stain, × 150. (DeMeester, T.R., and Skinner, D.B.: Polypoid sarcomas of the esophagus. Ann. Thorac. Surg. 20:405, 1975.)

patients received thyroid irradiation 29 and 30 years prior to the recognition of cervical esophageal fibrosarcoma. Long-term survival has been achieved with polypoid fibrosarcoma by wide surgical excision.

Chondrosarcoma

Yaghmai and Ghahremani (1976) reported a varicoid chondrosarcoma of the lower esophagus. Malignant degeneration of a cartilaginous tracheobronchial remnant was implicated in the pathogenesis of the tumor. Cartilaginous nodules and rings—tracheobronchial choristoma—cause segmental stenosis of the esophagus in children. Cell aggregates of chondrosarcoma are occasionally found within esophageal polypoid carcinoma, and metaplasia of mesenchymal cells is the prevalent consideration in that instance.

Other Sarcomas

Mansour and associates (1983) described a case of a liposarcoma of the cervical esophagus. The presenting symptoms were respiratory, and the tumor was excised locally because the pedicle was not involved. McIntyre and associates (1982) reported osteosarcoma, which is rare in the esophagus, as a polypoid mass in the lower esophagus of a 70-year-old man. This tumor penetrated the muscle layers, and it was treated by esophagogastrectomy. Umerah (1980) reported the case history of a 23-year-old black man with Kaposi's sarcoma of the foot with polypoid defects in the lower half of the esophagus. An autopsy confirmed esophageal involvement with Kaposi's sarcoma. Several authors have described esophageal Kaposi's sarcoma in patients with AIDS. Pass and associates (1984) reported that 2 of 15 patients with AIDS

had this lesion; one had cytomegalovirus esophagitis plus Kaposi's sarcoma of the esophagus, and the other had isolated Kaposi's sarcoma of the esophagus. Unsuspected tumors were found in three patients on postmortem exam in this series. The authors suggested that esophageal Kaposi's sarcoma should be suspected if the patient has cutaneous evidence of the sarcoma and concomitant dysphagia.

LYMPHOMA

Involvement of the gastrointestinal tract, including the esophagus, by lymphoma and Hodgkin's disease is frequently found at autopsy. In most instances, widespread and extensive disease is noted. Less often, gastrointestinal involvement is clinically evident. The stomach, small bowel, and colon are affected, in decreasing order of frequency. Lymphomas localized to the hollow viscus and its regional lymph nodes may be the only manifestations of disease, and these should be referred to as primary gastrointestinal lymphomas.

Primary malignant lymphoma of the esophagus is rare. Nevertheless, lymphocytic—lymphosarcoma, histiocytic—reticulum cell sarcoma, and Hodgkin's—nodular sclerosing—lymphomas have each been recorded as primary in the esophagus. Most patients are asymptomatic, but esophageal obstruction and perforation have been described. Lymphomatous infiltration of the distal esophageal myenteric plexus may simulate achalasia; Davis and associates (1975) reported dramatic clinical and manometric reversal with chemotherapy alone. Radiation therapy or chemotherapy or both should be considered for most patients with esophageal lymphoma.

Marked regression of the tumor is generally reported, with long-term symptom-free survival.

Extramedullary plasmacytomas of primary gastrointestinal origin are rare. Ahmed and colleagues (1976) documented in a 67-year-old man the first primary extramedullary esophageal plasmacytoma. The diagnosis of solitary primary plasmacytoma of the esophagus requires: (1) absence of Bence Jones proteinuria, (2) normal serum electrophoresis, (3) normal bone marrow biopsy, and (4) absence of distant metastases on liver scan and bone survey. Surgical excision is the treatment of choice for the obstructive lesion, with adjuvant radiation therapy if the nodes are involved.

METASTATIC TUMORS TO THE ESOPHAGUS

Metastatic tumors to the esophagus usually result from direct extension from contiguous organs such as the stomach, lung, pharynx, larynx, and thyroid, but it can occur by way of the mediastinal lymph nodes or by blood-borne metastasis. Metastatic lesions to the esophagus originating from the prostate, pancreas, testes, eye, tongue, tibia, liver, uterus, breast, skin, and lung and the wrist synovium have been described. Among the rare examples of metastasis from a distant tumor, breast carcinoma is by the far the most common. The mechanism of lymphatic spread of carcinoma of the breast to the esophagus is uncertain, but the internal mammary chain may be involved in breast cancer, and progression to the periesophageal lymphatics by an intercostal pathway is possible.

About half of the patients with metastatic involvement of the esophagus present with dysphagia. The esophagogram usually demonstrates a smooth concentric stricture or indentation of the esophageal lumen with intact mucosa (Fig. 88–14). Esophagoscopy demonstrates a smooth concentric or nodular narrowing without mucosal abnormality. Biopsies usually show only normal epithelium, and the risk of perforation is inordinately high. Polk and coauthors (1967) believe the diagnosis of metastatic breast carcinoma may be accepted without histologic confirmation when the characteristic barium-swallow and endoscopic findings are noted in a postmastectomy patient with dysphagia.

Bougienage is contraindicated for metastatic malignant lesions of the esophagus. Catastrophic perforation of diffusely infiltrated, friable esophageal wall is often reported. Radiation therapy, with or without chemotherapy or hormone therapy, is the treatment of choice and has produced significant improvement in some patients. In selected patients, surgical resection with restoration of alimentary continuity may be an acceptable alternative.

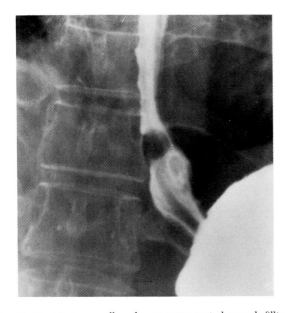

Fig. 88–14. Barium swallow demonstrates typical smooth filling of metastatic breast carcinoma in the distal esophagus.

REFERENCES

Ahmed, N., et al.: Primary extramedullary esophageal plasmacytoma: first case report. Cancer *38*:943, 1976.
Allard, M., et al.: Primary adenoid cystic carcinoma of the esophagus. Can. J. Surg. *24*:405, 1981.
Allen, A.C., and Spitz, S.: Melanoma: a clinicopathologic study. Cancer *6*:1, 1953.
Azzopardi, J.G., and Menzies, T.: Primary oesophageal adenocarcinoma: configuration of its existence by the finding of mucous gland tumors. Br. J. Surg. *49*:497, 1962.
Battifora, H.: Spindle cell carcinoma: ultrastructural evidence of squamous origin and collagen production by the tumor cells. Cancer *37*:2275, 1976.
Bensch, K.G., et al.: Oat-cell carcinoma of the lung: its origin and relationship to bronchial carcinoid. Cancer *22*:1163, 1968.
Berenson, M.M., et al.: Malignant transformation of esophageal columnar epithelium. Cancer *41*:554, 1978.
Brenner, S., Heimlich, H., and Widman, M.: Carcinoid of esophagus. N.Y. State J. Med. *69*:1337, 1969.
Carrie, A.: Adenocarcinoma of the upper end of the oesophagus arising from ectopic gastric epithelium. Br. J. Surg. *37*:474, 1950.
Cook, M.G., Eusebi, V., and Betts, C.M.: Oat-cell carcinoma of the oesophagus: a recently recognized entity. J. Clin. Pathol. *29*:1068, 1976.
Davis, J.A., et al.: Reversible achalasia due to reticulum-cell sarcoma. N. Engl. J. Med. *293*:130, 1975.
De La Pava, S., et al.: Melanosis of the esophagus. Cancer *16*:48, 1963.
DeMeester, T.R., and Levin, B.: Cancer of the Esophagus. Orlando, FL, Grune & Stratton, Inc., 1985.
Gaede, J.T., et al.: Leiomyosarcoma of the esophagus: report of two cases, one with associated squamous cell carcinoma. J. Thorac. Cardiovasc. Surg. *75*:740, 1978.
Goethals, P.L., Harrison, E.G., Jr., and Devine, K.D.: Verrucous squamous carcinoma of the oral cavity. Am. J. Surg. *106*:845, 1963.
Goldfarb, T.G.: Esophageal gland adenocarcinoma of the mid-esophagus. Am. J. Clin. Pathol. *48*:281, 1967.
Goldman, J.L., Marshak, R.H., and Friedman, A.I.: Primary adenocarcinoma of the esophagus simulating a benign lesion. J.A.M.A. *149*:144, 1952.
Goodner, J.T., Miller, T.R., and Watson, W.L.: Sarcoma of the esophagus. Am. J. Roentgenol. Radium Ther. Nucl. Med. *89*:132, 1963.
Hankins, J.R., et al.: Adenocarcinoma involving the esophagus. J. Thorac. Cardiovasc. Surg. *68*:148, 1974.
Hewlett, A.W.: The superficial glands of the esophagus. J. Exp. Med. *5*:319, 1900.
Johns, B.A.E.: Developmental changes in the oesophageal epithelium in man. J. Anat. *86*:29, 1952.
Mansour, K.A., et al.: Pedunculated liposarcoma of the esophagus: a first case report. J. Thorac. Cardiovasc. Surg. *86*:447, 1983.

Martin, M.R., and Kahn, L.B.: So-called pseudosarcoma of the esophagus. Arch. Pathol. Lab. Med. *101*:604, 1977.

Matsusaka, T., Watanabe, H., and Enjoji, M.: Anaplastic carcinoma of the esophagus: report of three cases and their histogenetic consideration. Cancer *37*:1352, 1976a.

Matsusaka, T., Watanabe, H., and Enjoji, M.: Pseudosarcoma and carcinosarcoma of the esophagus. Cancer *37*:1546, 1976b.

McIntyre, M., Webb, J.N., and Browning, G.C.: Osteosarcoma of the Esophagus. Hum. Pathol. *13*:680, 1982.

McKechnie, J.C., and Fechner, R.E.: Choriocarcinoma and adenocarcinoma of the esophagus with gonadotropin secretion. Cancer *27*:694, 1971.

Meyerowitz, B.R., and Shea, L.T.: The natural history of squamous verrucose carcinoma of the esophagus. J. Thorac. Cardiovasc. Surg. *61*:646, 1971.

Ming, S.: Tumors of the esophagus and stomach. Fascicle 7. Washington, D.C., Armed Forces Institute of Pathology, 1973.

Minielly, J.A., et al.: Verrucous squamous cell carcinoma of the esophagus. Cancer *20*:2078, 1967.

Osamura, R.Y., et al.: Polypoid carcinoma of the esophagus: a unifying term for "carcinosarcoma" and "pseudosarcoma." Am. J. Surg. Pathol. *2*:201, 1978.

Pass, H.I., et al.: Thoracic manifestations of the acquired immune deficiency syndrome. J. Thorac. Cardiovasc. Surg. *88*:654, 1984.

Piccone, V.A., et al.: Primary malignant melanoma of the esophagus associated with melanosis of the entire esophagus: first case report. J. Thorac. Cardiovasc. Surg. *59*:864, 1970.

Poleynard, G.D., et al.: Adenocarcinoma in the columnar-lined (Barret) esophagus. Arch. Surg. *112*:997, 1977.

Polk, H.C., Jr., Camp, F.A., and Walker, A.W.: Dysphagia and esophageal stenosis: manifestation of metastatic mammary cancer. Cancer *20*:2002, 1967.

Postlethwait, R.W.: Surgery of the Esophagus. 2nd ed. New York, Appleton-Century-Crofts, 1986.

Postlethwait, R.W., and Musser, A.W.: Changes in the esophagus in 1,000 autopsy specimens. J. Thorac. Cardiovasc. Surg. *68*:953, 1974.

Raphael, H.A., Ellis, F.H., Jr., and Dockerty, M.B.: Primary adenocarcinoma of the esophagus. Ann. Surg. *162*:785, 1966.

Rector, L.E., and Connerly, M.L.: Aberrant mucosa in the esophagus in infants and in children. Arch. Pathol. *31*:285, 1941.

Sato, T., et al.: Small cell carcinoma (non-oat cell type) of the esophagus concomitant with invasive squamous cell carcinoma and carcinoma in situ. Cancer *57*:328, 1986.

Scicchitano, L.P., and Camishion, R.C.: Primary adenocarcinoma of the esophagus. Am. J. Surg. *104*:531, 1962.

Shalkiadakis, G., et al.: Primary malignant melanoma of the esophagus. Ann. Thorac. Surg. *39*:472, 1985.

Shields, T.W., Eilert, J.B., and Battifora, H.: Pseudosarcoma of the oesophagus. Thorax *27*:472, 1972.

Stout, A.P., and Lattes, R.: Atlas of tumor pathology: tumors of the esophagus. Section 5, Fascicle 20. Washington, D.C., Armed Forces Institute of Pathology, 1957.

Tateishi, R., et al.: Argyrophil cells and melanocytes in esophageal mucosa. Arch. Pathol. *98*:87, 1974.

Tateishi, R., et al.: Argyrophil cell carcinoma (apudoma) of the esophagus: a histopathologic entity. Virchows Arch. Pathol. Anat. Histol. *371*:283, 1976.

Turnbull, A.D.M., and Goodner, J.T.: Primary adenocarcinoma of the esophagus. Cancer *22*:915, 1968.

Umerah, B.C.: Kaposi's sarcoma of the esophagus. Br. J. Radiol. *53*:807, 1980.

Witt, T.R., et al.: Adenocarcinoma in Barrett's esophagus. J. Thorac. Cardiovasc. Surg. *85*:337, 1983.

Yaghmai, I., and Ghahremani, G.G.: Chondrosarcoma of the esophagus. Am. J. Roentgenol. *126*:1175, 1976.

READING REFERENCES

Adenocarcinoma

Cameron, J.L., et al.: Carcinoma arising in Barrett's esophagus. Surg. Gynecol. Obstet. *161*:570, 1985.

Dawson, J.L.: Adenocarcinoma of the middle oesophagus arising in an oesophagus lined by gastric (parietal) epithelium. Br. J. Surg. *51*:940, 1940.

Faintuch, J., Shepard, K.V., and Levin, B.: Adenocarcinoma and other unusual variants of esophageal cancer. Semin. Oncol. *11*:196, 1984.

Lortat-Jacob, J.L., et al.: Primary esophageal adenocarcinoma: report of 16 cases. Surgery *64*:535, 1968.

McCorkle, R.G., and Blades, B.: Adenocarcinoma of the esophagus arising in aberrant gastric mucosa. Am. J. Surg. *21*:781, 1955.

Sjogren, R.W., Jr., and Johnson, L.F.: Barrett's esophagus: a review. Am. J. Med. *74*:313, 1983.

Variants of Squamous Cell Carcinoma

Agha, F.P., and Keren, D.F.: Spindle-cell squamous carcinoma of the esophagus: a tumor with biphasic morphology. AJR *145*:541, 1985.

Enrile, F.T., et al.: Pseudosarcoma of the esophagus (polypoid carcinoma of esophagus with pseudosarcomatous features). Cancer *31*:1197, 1973.

Olmsted, W.W., Lichtenstein, J.E., and Hyams, V.J.: Polypoid epithelial malignancies of the esophagus. AJR *140*:921, 1983.

Odes, H.S., et al.: Varicoid carcinoma of the esophagus. Am. J. Gastroenterol. *73*:141, 1980.

Parkinson, A.T., Haidak, G.L., and McInerney, R.P.: Verrucous squamous cell carcinoma of the esophagus following lye stricture. Chest *57*:489, 1970.

Postlethwait, R.W., Wechsler, A.S., and Shelburne, J.D.: Pseudosarcoma of the esophagus. Ann. Thorac. Surg. *19*:198, 1975.

Razzuk, M.A., et al.: Pseudosarcoma of the esophagus: a case report. J. Thorac. Cardiovasc. Surg. *61*:650, 1971.

Talbert, J.L., and Cantrell, J.R.: Clinical and pathologic characteristics of carcinosarcoma of the esophagus. J. Thorac. Cardiovasc. Surg. *45*:1, 1963.

Oat Cell Carcinoma

Azzopardi, J.G., and Pollock, D.J.: Argentaffin and argyrophil cells in gastric carcinoma. J. Pathol. Bacteriol. *86*:443, 1963.

Ho, K.J., et al.: Small cell carcinoma of the esophagus: evidence for a unified histogenesis. Hum. Pathol. *15*:460, 1984.

Horai, T., et al.: A cytologic study on small cell carcinoma of the esophagus. Cancer *41*:1890, 1978.

Ibrahim, N.B., Briggs, J.C., and Corbishley, C.M.: Extrapulmonary oat-cell carcinoma. Cancer *54*:1645, 1984.

Imura, H., et al.: Studies on ectopic ACTH-producing tumors. II. Clinical and biochemical features of 30 cases. Cancer *35*:1430, 1975.

Karnad, A., and Poskitt, T.R.: Small cell carcinoma of the esophagus: case report and review of the literature. J. Tenn. Med. Assoc. *77*:451, 1984.

Melanoma

DasGupta, T.K., Brasfield, R.D., and Paglia, M.A.: Primary melanomas in unusual sites. Surg. Gynecol. Obstet. *128*:841, 1969.

Frable, W.J., Kay, S., and Schatzki, P.: Primary malignant melanoma of the esophagus: an electron microscopic study. Am. J. Clin. Pathol. *58*:659, 1972.

Montgomery, A.C.V.: Primary malignant melanoma of the oesophagus. Clin. Oncol. *2*:239, 1976.

Saibil, E., and Palayew, M.J.: Primary malignant melanoma of the esophagus. Am. J. Gastroenterol. *61*:63, 1974.

Takubo, K.P.: Primary malignant melanoma of the esophagus. Hum. Pathol. *14*:727, 1983.

Wood, C.B., and Wood, R.A.B.: Metastatic malignant melanoma of the esophagus. Am. J. Dig. Dis. *20*:786, 1975.

Sarcomas

Almeida, J.M.: Leiomyosarcoma of the esophagus. Chest *81*:761, 1982.

Athanasoulis, C.A., and Aral, I.M.: Leiomyosarcoma of the esophagus. Gastroenterology *54*:271, 1968.

Borrie, J.: Sarcoma of esophagus: surgical treatment. J. Thorac. Surg. *37*:413, 1959.

DeMeester, T.R., and Skinner, D.B.: Polypoid sarcomas of the esophagus: a rare but potentially curable neoplasm. Ann. Thorac. Surg. *20*:405, 1975.

Turnbull, A.D., et al.: Primary malignant tumors of the esophagus other than typical epidermoid carcinoma. Ann. Thorac. Surg. *15*:463, 1973.

Wobbes, T., et al.: Rhabdomyosarcoma of the esophagus. Arch. Chir. Neerl. *27*:69, 1975.

Lymphoma

Agha, F.P., and Schnitzer, B.: Esophageal involvement in lymphoma. Am. J. Gastroenterol. *80*:412, 1985.

Allen, A.W., et al.: Primary malignant lymphoma of the gastro-intestinal tract. Ann. Surg. *140*:428, 1954.

Carnovale, R.L., et al.: Radiologic manifestations of esophageal lymphoma. Am. J. Roentgenol. *128*:751, 1977.

Deodhar, L.P., and Purandare, S.M.: Lymphomas of the gastrointestinal tract. J. Postgrad. Med. *18*:95, 1972.

Freeman, C., Berg, J.W., and Cutler, S.J.: Occurrence and prognoses of extranodal lymphomas. Cancer *29*:252, 1972.

Kirsch, H.L., et al.: Esophageal perforation: an unusual presentation of esophageal lymphoma. Dig. Dis. Sci. *28*:371, 1983.

Nissan, S., Bar-Moar, J.A., and Levy, E.: Lymphosarcoma of the esophagus: a case report. Cancer *34*:1321, 1974.

Stein, H.A., Murray, D., and Warner, H.A.: Primary Hodgkin's disease of the esophagus. Dig. Dis. Sci. *26*:457, 1981.

Weyand, C.M., Goronzy, J.J., and Huchzermeyer, H.: Presentation of an unrecognized lymphoma as esophageal tumor. Endoscopy *18*:61, 1986.

Worgan, D., and Baldock, C.R.: Lymphosarcoma of the oesophagus. J. Laryngol. Otolaryngol. *90*:207, 1976.

Metastatic Tumors

Atkins, J.P.: Metastatic carcinoma to the esophagus: endoscopic considerations with special reference to carcinoma of the breast. Ann. Otolaryngol. Rhinol. Laryngol. *75*:356, 1966.

Biller, H.F., et al.: Breast carcinoma metastasizing to the cervical esophagus. Laryngoscope *92*:999, 1982.

Gore, R.M., and Sparberg, M.: Metastatic carcinoma of the prostate to the esophagus. Am. J. Gastroenterol. *77*:358, 1982.

Laforet, E.G., and Kondi, E.S.: Postmastectomy dysphagia. Am. J. Surg. *121*:368, 1971.

Orringer, M.B., and Skinner, D.B.: Unusual presentations of primary and secondary esophageal malignancies. Ann. Thorac. Surg. *11*:305, 1971.

Vansant, J.H., and Davis, R.K.: Esophageal obstruction secondary to mediastinal metastasis from breast carcinoma. Chest *60*:93, 1971.

Zarian, L.P., Berliner, L., and Redmond, P.: Metastatic endometrial carcinoma to the esophagus. Am. J. Gastroenterol. *78*:9, 1983.

The Mediastinum

CHAPTER 89

INFECTIONS OF THE MEDIASTINUM AND THE SUPERIOR VENA CAVAL SYNDROME

Robert W. Jamplis and P. Michael McFadden

Mediastinitis is a serious inflammatory condition of the mediastinal structures that may result in various acute or chronic disorders. Knowledge of the anatomy and the fascial planes is essential to the understanding of the relationship between mediastinitis and infections of the neck and abdomen (Fig. 89–1). The pretracheal space is bounded by the treachea posteriorly and the pretracheal fascia anteriorly and contains the thyroid gland. The prevertebral—retrovisceral—space is bounded posteriorly by the prevertebral fascia and anteriorly by the buccopharyngeal fascia. The carotid sheaths form the lateral boundaries. The compartment extends from the base of the skull to the upper retroperitoneal space. These fascial planes connect the neck to the anterior and visceral mediastinum and to the retroperitoneal space within the abdomen. Infections in the neck may travel inferiorly because of the effects of gravity and negative intrathoracic pressure. The visceral mediastinum is involved more commonly by way of the prevertebral space. Rarely, the anterior mediastinum is involved by way of the pretracheal space. Infections may spread inferiorly from the mediastinum to the retroperitoneal area, and less frequently they may travel superiorly from the abdomen to the mediastinum. Mediastinal infections almost never spread superiorly to involve the fascial compartments of the neck.

ACUTE MEDIASTINITIS

This occurs secondary to perforation of adjacent organs, by direct extension of infection from those organs, or by fascial spread of infections from the neck or abdomen. If the pathophysiologic factors go unrecognized and treatment is delayed, serious illness and even death may ensue.

Etiology

The most common cause of acute mediastinitis is postoperative infection following the median sternotomy incision in cardiac surgery. The mediastinitis that follows is serious and often fatal, because of extension to the cardiotomy incision, particularly when an intracardiac prosthesis is present. The incidence of this condition varies between 1 and 6% of all cardiac operations. The usual organisms are pseudomonas and staphylococci, which often display different antibiotic sensitivities. Predisposing factors apparently include instability of the sternum because of faulty closure or contributory factors such as diabetes, chronic obstructive pulmonary disease, steroid use, tracheostomy, prolonged perfusion time, postoperative hemorrhage requiring re-exploration of the sternotomy wound, and a low cardiac output following surgery. Nevertheless, most coronary artery bypass grafts remain patent despite mediastinal infection.

Another common cause of acute mediastinitis is esophageal injury secondary to instrumentation during either endoscopy, bougienage, or placement of a nasogastric tube. Perforation of the cervical esophagus occurs occasionally in patients with arthritic spurs of the cervical vertebrae that puncture the posterior wall of the esophagus at the time of endoscopy or when an endotracheal tube is present. This perforation often occurs just below the cricopharyngeus muscle. Since achalasia and most strictures of the esophagus are located at or near the cardioesophageal junction, it stands to reason that the distal thoracic esophagus is most frequently injured during bougienage and therapeutic, pneumatic or hydrostatic, dilatations.

Noninstrumental esophageal perforation secondary to postemetic rupture—Boerhaave's syndrome; spontaneous perforation of an esophageal carcinoma; or leakage from an intrathoracic anastomotic suture line frequently results in a virulent, necrotizing, and often fatal mediastinitis.

Likewise, whereas penetrating wounds of the esophagus, trachea, or major bronchi can be rapidly fatal, small ones can produce a smoldering infection. Occasionally, the erosion by a foreign body of the tracheobronchial

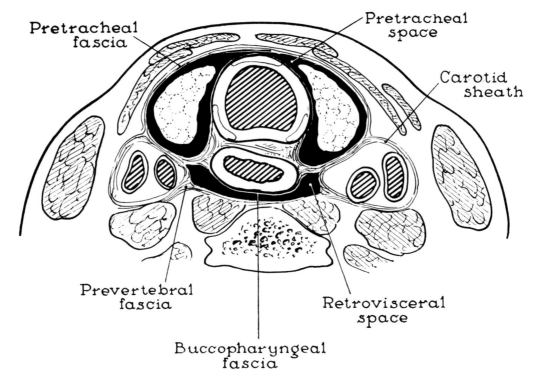

Fig. 89–1. Cross section of the neck at the seventh cervical vertebra. The retrovisceral and pretracheal spaces extend directly into the mediastinum. (Seybold, W.D., Johnson, M.A., III, and Leary, W.V.: Perforation of esophagus: analysis of 50 cases and account of experimental studies. Surg. Clin. North Am. *30*:1155, 1950.)

tree or esophagus leads to a mediastinal infection. In both of these conditions, a localized abscess often results.

In the preantibiotic era, dental infections, periotonsillar abscesses, Ludwig's angina, and postanginal sepsis often resulted in neck infections that spread to the mediastinum by way of the fascial planes. It is rare now, but still may occur when treatment is delayed or the organism is particularly virulent.

Finally, osteomyelitis of the vertebrae and ribs, lung abscesses, empyema, metastatic infections, and subphrenic and retroperitoneal abscesses cause acute mediastinitis only rarely.

Clinical Manifestations and Diagnosis

Diagnosis of acute mediastinitis following cardiac operation through a median sternotomy incision is sometimes difficult. One must have a high index of suspicion, as the infection can be indolent and frank pus may not be seen. A thin, clear watery discharge in the presence of mild sternal instability often heralds sternal wound infection and mediastinitis. In the obvious instance, one finds fever, leukocytosis, and a painful swelling over the sternum. Purulent drainage bubbling up from a wound dehiscence confirms the diagnosis.

Esophageal perforation following instrumentation may go unnoticed at first if the perforation is small, or it may result in severe immediate prostration with larger perforations. The clinical manifestations depend upon the size of the perforation, the virulence of the organism, the host resistance, and the length of time before the condition is recognized. Should neck pain and tender-

ness along with dysphagia and malaise occur soon after esophagoscopy, the diagnosis is almost certain. These symptoms, accompanied by crepitation in the supraclavicular area, fever, chills, and leukocytosis, are diagnostic of perforation. Prompt treatment can prevent spread of the infection inferiorly and prevent the development of acute mediastinitis.

Should a perforation of the middle or lower esophagus occur following one of the aforementioned causes and result in leakage of esophageal contents into the mediastinum a rapid onset of symptoms, such as severe substernal chest and epigastric pain, nausea, retching, fever, chills, and leukocytosis, is common. Shock often transpires. Cervical crepitus is not usually present, but epigastric tenderness and abdominal guarding, as well as dullness and decreased breath sounds at the lung bases, are commonly found on physical examination. Infrequently, the process is indolent, and a localized abscess may develop. The diagnosis and management of perforations of the esophagus are dealt with in Chapter 45.

The occasional instance of postanginal sepsis may also lead to acute mediastinitis. In this condition, the history of a unilateral painful swelling a week or more following a dental or pharyngeal infection is most important. The swelling in the neck may be accompanied by dysphagia, hoarseness, chills, and fever. Pain is particularly intense when the head is turned away from the involved side. If the condition is left untreated, it commonly spreads inferiorly by way of the retrovisceral space to involve the mediastinum and often the pericardial and pleural cavities as well. Jugular vein thrombophlebitis and carotid artery arteritis are frequent complications of this syndrome.

Roentgenography can be considerably helpful in establishing a diagnosis of acute mediastinitis. Early in the disease, the roentgenograms may be negative. As it progresses, a posteroanterior film of the chest shows a widening of the mediastinal shadow and the lateral view might reveal an increased opacity of the substernal space. Involvement of the mediastinal soft tissues is often associated with gas within the tissues and air-fluid levels indicating abscess cavities. Pleural and pericardial effusions frequently develop concomitantly with the mediastinal infection. These findings, however, often occur as a late manifestation of the disease.

Roentgenograms of the neck may reveal a loss of the normal cervical lordosis as well as the presence of air or an increase in the soft tissue space between the vertebrae and the esophagus. An esophagogram with a water-soluble contrast medium can delineate the exact site of the perforation. This technique is best in lower esophageal perforations. Fluoroscopy, tomography, angiography, ultrasound studies, and computed tomography can be helpful if the diagnosis remains in doubt. Coaxial white cell scanning and magnetic resonance imaging techniques show considerable promise in early detection of mediastinal infections.

Occasionally, the substernal pain associated with mediastinitis may be confused with a myocardial infarction or pulmonary embolism. These conditions, however, are easily ruled in or out by the history, electrocardiogram, serum myocardial enzymes, arterial blood gases, lung scan, and pulmonary arteriography.

Treatment

If untreated, acute mediastinitis can rapidly lead to a fulminating illness and death. Therefore, early recognition and immediate vigorous treatment is imperative for optimal results. Most importantly the surgeon must have a high index of suspicion if signs and symptoms of infection should appear following a median sternotomy incision or after esophagoscopy or esophageal dilatation. The same holds true for penetrating wounds and foreign bodies of the neck, thorax, and upper abdomen, as well as in persistent pharyngitis or following esophageal and pulmonary operations.

In severely ill patients, the primary treatment may have to be directed toward alleviating septic shock and establishing an adequate airway. Appropriate antibiotic therapy is also indicated from the outset. The sine qua non in treatment, however, is incision and drainage while the disease is still localized and before septicemia ensues.

Once a sternotomy wound becomes infected, the wound must be reopened widely for adequate drainage and debridement. Extreme caution must be taken not to disturb the coronary artery grafts, which may be present beneath the sternum from the original operation. If pus or fluid is encountered, a Gram stain of the material should be obtained and cultures and drug sensitivities sent for aerobic and anaerobic pathogens as well as for fungi and acid-fast bacilli. Appropriate intravenous antibiotics should be started and the wound widely debrided. Foreign bodies, such as Teflon buttresses along a suture line, and devitalized and infected tissue should be removed. Following debridement, a decision about whether to use closed or open drainage is best made on the basis of the extent and duration of the infection. If the infection is not extensive and it has been recognized early, a closed method might be considered. This is accomplished by placing two large catheters in the mediastinum and closing the sternum over them with wires. The fascia can be approximated with absorbable sutures. The subcutaneous tissues and skin are left open and managed with local wound care in anticipation of a delayed wound closure or healing by secondary intention. Antibiotic solutions of 1-g neomycin sulfate and 50,000 U of bacitracin in a liter of 0.5 normal saline solution can be instilled through the ingress catheter at the rate of 50 to 100 ml/hour and aspirated from the egress catheter by continuous suction. This method usually requires 1 to 2 weeks of irrigation to successfully manage the infection. If, however, the infection is severe or diagnosis has been significantly delayed, the open method can and should be used (Fig. 89–2). The entire wound is merely left open, with the heart and other organs exposed. It is packed with 0.5% povidone-iodine-soaked sponges that are changed every 4 to 6 hours. It may take weeks for the wound to granulate, and therefore nutritional support with enteral or parenteral hyperalimentation is usually indicated. A tracheostomy and positive-pressure ventilation are often necessary because of chest instability and poor ventilatory mechanics. With the use of myocutaneous flaps, large granulating areas can be filled in and covered, with excellent cosmetic results. Usually, the pectoralis major muscles are used, with or without rib grafts and Marlex mesh (see Chapter 48).

Early and limited neck infections resulting from esophageal perforations following endoscopy, foreign bodies, or small penetrating wounds, or subsequent to dental or oropharyngeal infections, can successfully be treated

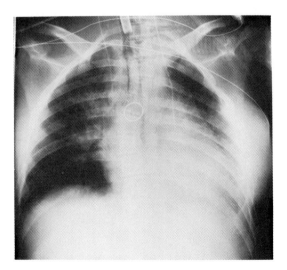

Fig. 89–2. Acute mediastinitis secondary to open heart surgery. Note air in the mediastinum.

with antibiotics alone. If this is not immediately effective, however, drainage must be carried out. The safest plan is to treat the condition with antibiotics and drainage from the outset. Drainage is easily accomplished by a cervical mediastinotomy. An incision is made along the anterior border of the sternocleidomastoid muscle starting at the sternal notch on the involved side. The muscle, along with the carotid sheath, is retracted laterally while the thyroid gland and trachea are retracted medially. Care must be taken to avoid injuring the recurrent laryngeal nerve. This incision exposes the esophagus and the retrovisceral space (Fig. 89–3). If this procedure is performed early, pus will probably not be encountered and adequate drainage with Penrose drains is all that is required. No attempt to find and close the rent in the esophagus is necessary unless it is large. If large and early, an accurate two-layer closure of the esophageal perforation along with adequate drainage may suffice. Cervical fistulae, however, usually close rapidly with adequate drainage aided by hyperalimentation.

Should infection in the prevertebral space reach the visceral compartment of the mediastinum, or should mediastinitis develop after an esophageal dilatation and perforation of the middle or lower esophagus, surgical drainage must be undertaken. This drainage in the past was almost exclusively done through a posterior mediastinotomy. The posterior angles of three or four ribs were resected through a vertical paraspinal incision and drainage effected. The prevertebral space can be entered via this approach without violating the pleura.* The most common and direct approach, however, is drainage of mediastinal infection transpleurally by tube thoracostomy with or without thoracotomy and mediastinotomy.

Treatment of mediastinal infections from adjacent organs, such as lung, pleural cavity, vertebrae, chest wall, and diaphragm, is directed toward the primary lesion.

---

*Editor's Footnote: Although infrequently indicated, a posterior mediastinotomy is a satisfactory approach for the drainage of a contained chronic mediastinal abscess or the removal of an impacted esophageal foreign body that cannot be extracted by an endoscopic approach. The technique is seen in Figure 89–4. A right-sided posterior mediastinotomy, however, is recommended rather than the left-sided approach shown, except in the most inferior portion of the thorax, since this affords better access to the esophagus and avoids the descending thoracic aorta.

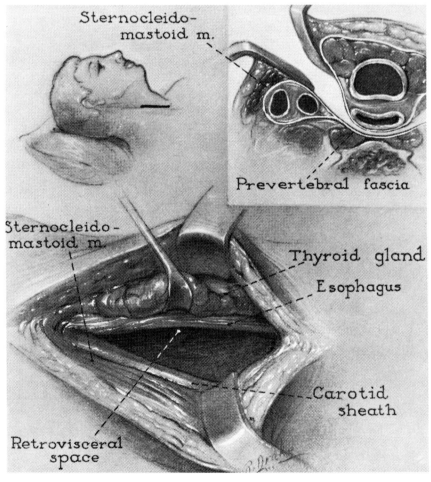

Fig. 89–3. Exposure of the esophagus and the retrovisceral space by the transcervical approach. The mediastinum as far as the aortic arch can be drained from the supraclavicular incision. (Seybold, W.D., Johnson, M.A., III, and Leary, W.V.: Perforation of esophagus: analysis of 50 cases and account of experimental studies. Surg. Clin. North Am. 30:1155, 1950.)

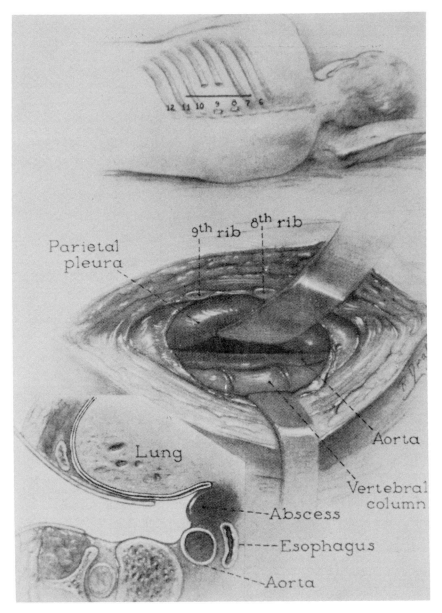

Fig. 89–4. Posterior mediastinotomy to unroof a chronic mediastinal abscess. Note the proximity of the pleura to the collection of purulent material (lower left). (Reproduced with permission from Seybold, W.D., Johnson, M.A., III, and Leary, W.V.: Surg. Clin. N. Amer. *30*:1155, 1950.)

CHRONIC MEDIASTINITIS

This is less common than acute mediastinitis. The acute form usually either resolves completely or causes death. Only rarely does it develop into a chronic inflammation.

Etiology

Although a chronic localized abscess occasionally results from inadequate treatment of acute suppurative mediastinitis, the most common cause of chronic infection in the mediastinum is granulomatous disease. In the past this condition was usually attributed to tuberculosis. Currently, fungi and, in particular, *Histoplasma capsulatum* (Fig. 89–5*A* and *B*) and *Coccidioides immitis*, are

most commonly the offending organisms. These organisms usually involve the lung parenchyma at first, but inevitably, spread to the mediastinum occurs through the pulmonary lymphatic drainage, resulting in chronic mediastinal node enlargement.

Chronic fibrous mediastinitis deserves special mention. This lesion is an exuberant growth of chronic inflammatory and dense fibrous tissue within the mediastinum. It usually occurs in adults between the ages of 20 and 45. It formerly was called nonspecific or idiopathic. Current opinion is that it is probably the end-stage granulomatous process of *Histoplasma capsulatum* in affected mediastinal lymph nodes.

The mechanism of transition from a mediastinal granuloma to the desmoplastic entity known as chronic fi-

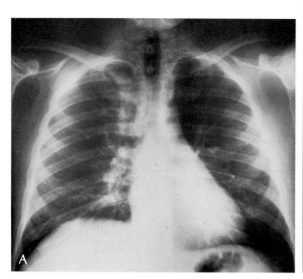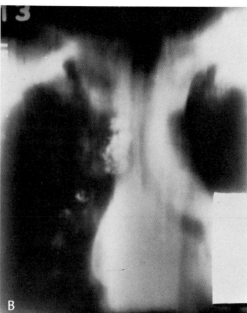

Fig. 89–5. *A*, Right paratracheal mediastinal tumor proved to be a histoplasmoma at exploration. *B*, Tomogram of same histoplasma granuloma. Note extensive calcification in the tumor and in the hilum.

brous mediastinitis is speculative at best, but evidence for this transition mounts as the presence of histoplasmosis in these lesions is seen more frequently. Although lymph nodes infected with tuberculous and coccidioidal organisms both heal with calcification, this is particularly true in histoplasmosis. Only in histoplasmosis is this extravagant collagenous process recognized with any regularity. Likewise, because of the fascial planes connecting the neck, chest, and abdomen, evidence suggests that the same etiologic factors may be responsible for retroperitoneal fibrosis, chronic fibrous mediastinitis, and Riedel's struma of the thyroid gland.

Clinical Manifestations and Diagnosis

Diagnosing chronic mediastinitis is usually more difficult than diagnosing the acute form. If a localized abscess forms as a sequela to an unrecognized or poorly treated acute mediastinitis, the diagnosis can be made by the history, the symptoms, the appearance and localization on roentgenogram, ultrasound, white cell scan, computed tomography, and magnetic resonance imaging. Percutaneous needle aspiration of the abscess and endoscopy can often help obtain specimens for smear and culture.

The usual granulomatous form of the disease may be preceded by many symptoms or may be asymptomatic before detection of mediastinal widening or masses on chest roentgenography. Chronic changes usually appear in the mid and superior portions of the mediastinum. Flu-like symptoms of malaise, fever, and cough, indicating an early systemic infection with the granulomatous organisms may be difficult to elicit, but one must not wait for the appearance of late signs and symptoms such as weakness, weight loss, anorexia, anemia, and pain

before making a diagnosis. Calcified lymph nodes, although not always harboring viable organisms, can lead to specific symptoms. Irritation of the bronchus by these structures can cause a dry, persistent, hacking cough. If erosion occurs through the bronchial wall, the patient may cough up "stones" or broncholiths. Should calcific nodes compress a bronchus, distal chronic obstructive pneumonitis may result, as occurs in "middle lobe syndrome." Sequelae include abscess formation and ultimately empyema if the condition is allowed to continue untreated. Because most instances are caused by fungal infection, it is important to know the geographic area in which the patient resides or has traveled. The results of skin tests and serum antibodies are also helpful. The definitive diagnosis, however, rests with the identification of the organism in the sputum, in the needle biopsy aspirate, or within the histologic specimen itself, which can be obtained by scalene or deep jugular lymph node biopsy, mediastinoscopy, mediastinotomy, or if necessary, by an exploratory thoracotomy. Other mediastinal tumors and cysts, aneurysms, collapsed or cystic lobes of the lung, and digestive tract lesions must be considered in the differential diagnosis.

The cicatrization in chronic fibrous mediastinitis can involve the major airways, the large vessels, and the esophagus, and thereby lead to various significant symptoms. On the other hand, the patient may be completely asymptomatic. If the trachea, bronchi, and esophagus are extensively involved, a dry cough, chest pain, dyspnea, dysphagia and interscapular pain are often present. More common and more disturbing, however, are the symptoms stemming from compression of the superior vena cava, pulmonary veins, and other thin-walled, low pressure blood and lymph vessels. Roentgenograms of the chest may appear normal, but more commonly a widening of the mediastinal shadow and marked calcification of the subcarinal, hilar, and paratracheal lymph nodes is apparent. Compression and narrowing of the superior vena cava, the large pulmonary arteries and veins, and the tracheobronchial tree and circumferential narrowing of the esophagus may be observed. Angiography, tomography, esophagograms, bronchography, computed tomography, and magnetic resonance imaging can be considerably helpful in making the diagnosis. Should any or all of these symptoms and signs arise in a young adult, an exhaustive attempt to establish a diagnosis of histoplasmosis should be made.

Treatment

If a chronic mediastinal pyogenic abscess is encountered, it must be incised and drained. The type of thoracotomy incision chosen should provide for the most direct and dependent drainage. Adjuvant antibiotics should be administered.

If acid-fast bacilli are found in the mediastinal granulomatous process, antituberculous drug therapy should be initiated. If either coccidioidomycosis or histoplasmosis is proved, no therapy is probably in order unless the symptoms are severe. The appropriate drug to use when antifungal therapy is indicated is discussed in detail in Chapter 69.

An operative procedure should not be contemplated as a form of therapy except in broncholithiasis and "middle lobe syndrome." In these conditions, lobectomy is often necessary. An attempt to remove a granulomatous lymph node adherent to the superior vena cava can be dangerous, as massive hemorrhage, which may be difficult to control, may ensue. Also, these nodes rarely lead to serious complications.

Only symptomatic treatment is available for chronic fibrous mediastinitis. Fortunately, the process occurs gradually and usually allows for the development of collateral vessels, which usually prevent the distressing symptoms of superior vena caval obstruction. Operation for chronic fibrosing mediastinitis is indicated only for diagnostic purposes.

SUPERIOR VENA CAVAL SYNDROME

The superior vena cava is locked in a tight compartment in the mediastinum immediately adjacent and anterior to the trachea and right main bronchus. It is surrounded by lymph nodes draining the entire right chest and lower portion of the left chest. Any extrinsic pressure, encasement, or actual invasion of the superior vena cava causing an obstruction of venous return from the head and upper extremities leads to unmistakable signs and symptoms. These characteristics, which were first described by William Hunter in 1757, are called the superior vena caval syndrome.

Etiology

Malignant disease accounts for well over 90% of all superior vena caval obstructions, with three quarters of

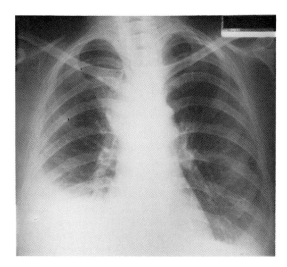

Fig. 89–6. Right upper lobe undifferentiated large cell bronchial carcinoma presenting with superior vena caval obstruction.

these caused by bronchial carcinoma of the right upper lobe (Fig. 89–6). These central lesions often result in distal obstructive pneumonitis, usually with involvement of the right hilar and mediastinal lymph nodes. Lymphomas, and to a lesser extent metastatic carcinomas, malignant thymomas, and malignant germ cell tumors are at fault about 20% of the time.

Less than 5% of cases of superior vena caval syndrome are caused by benign disease, usually a large substernal goiter, chronic fibrous mediastinitis (Fig. 89–7), or a thrombus within the vessel itself. Although aneurysms of the ascending aorta and innominate artery were among the leading causes of this syndrome in the 1950s and 1960s, they are now rare.

Iatrogenic causes, such as thrombosis subsequent to placement of a transvenous endocardial pacemaker electrode, a central venous line, or a Swan-Ganz catheter have been implicated. Although intravenous thrombosis occurs more frequently than previously appreciated, su-

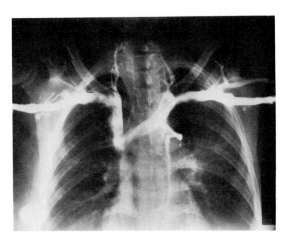

Fig. 89–7. Complete obstruction of the superior vena cava and azygos veins with the filling of inferior vena cava via the hemiazygos vein. Biopsy revealed an indeterminate granulomatous process in the mediastinum.

perior vena caval obstruction and superior vena caval syndrome are rare. A recognized complication of the Mustard operation used for the correction of transposition of the great vessels is obstruction of the superior vena cava by the intracardiac baffle created during the operation.

Clinical Manifestations and Diagnosis

Superior vena caval syndrome is directly related to obstruction of the venous drainage of the head, neck, and upper extremities, with a concomitant increase in venous pressure. The signs and symptoms can be dramatic. The eyes are often affected first. The patient may complain of tearing, swelling of the eyelids, and proptosis. Headache, dizziness, tinnitus, and a "bursting" sensation in the head upon bending forward follow in short succession. The face may become red, edematous, and cyanotic. Swelling of the neck, arms, and upper chest occurs, and the veins of the neck and upper extremities become distended (Fig. 89–8). Dilated venous channels may appear over the upper anterior chest wall. These symptoms are greatly exaggerated when the azygos vein is also obstructed.

The venous hypertension is likely to produce cerebral vascular thrombosis and hemorrhage, with dire consequences. Should the thin-walled pulmonary veins also be obstructed, pulmonary hypertension can develop.

Because most superior vena caval obstructions are caused by carcinoma of the lung, it follows that involvement of structures contiguous with the superior vena cava, such as the trachea and right main stem bronchus, may lead to airway obstruction and respiratory distress. The respiratory distress varies from a mild, irritative cough to severe pain and incapacitating dyspnea.

The phrenic, vagus, and sympathetic nerves traverse the superior mediastinum, and their involvement can lead to paralysis of the right diaphragm, hoarseness, or Horne's syndrome, respectively.

The posteroanterior and lateral roentgenograms of the chest usually reveal the cause of the superior vena caval obstruction. A right hilar mass with right upper lobe obstructive pneumonitis—volume loss—suggests bronchial carcinoma. A smooth right superior mediastinal mass with tracheal deviation usually indicates a substernal thyroid and this at times, may be substantiated by radioiodine scanning. Malignant lymphoma or metastatic disease presents with prominent mediastinal lymphadenopathy, which is best delineated by computed tomog-

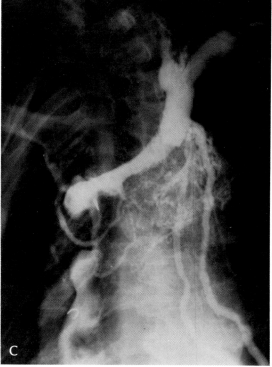

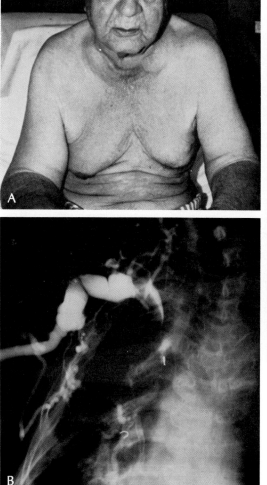

Fig. 89–8. *A,* Appearance of 65-year-old man with superior vena caval obstruction caused by malignancy. Note the swelling of the neck, arms, and upper chest as well as the puffiness of the face. Dilated veins over the chest and cyanosis of the face and arms were present. *B,* Venogram showing complete obstruction of the superior vena cava with filling of collateral channels. *C,* Later phase of venogram showing filling of the inferior vena cava via the hemiazygos veins—intercostal and lateral thoracic branches and internal mammary veins.

raphy. An aortic or innominate artery aneurysm suspected on the roentgenogram is often confirmed by fluoroscopic examination. Arteriography remains the standard method for diagnosis of vascular lesions, but MRI may be just as valuable.

The roentgenogram of the chest is usually not helpful in instances of thrombosis or chronic fibrous mediastinitis except to reveal the common hilar mediastinal calcifications found in the latter. A normal roentgenogram in a patient with superior vena caval obstruction in the absence of previous instrumentation or operative procedure is almost pathognomonic of chronic fibrous mediastinitis (Fig. 89–9).

Retinoscopy reveals edema and venous engorgement, as one would expect. Venography by a catheter in the superior vena cava introduced through the neck or arm, although somewhat risky, can be useful in locating the exact site of the obstruction and can help verify the diagnosis in chronic fibrous mediastinitis. The role of radionuclide scanning in superior vena caval syndrome is discussed in Chapter 15.

Diagnostic procedures to determine the cause and define the site of obstruction can be hazardous. Complications such as massive hemorrhage, acute respiratory obstruction, and propagation of thrombus from the operative site are common. Therefore, although surgical procedures should be performed for tissue diagnosis, they should be well planned and accomplished judiciously.

The easiest and least risky procedure to obtain a definitive diagnosis is sputum cytology, especially if carcinoma is suspected. Sputum may be induced, if necessary, by heated aerosol inhalation. A supraclavicular fat pad biopsy of the scalene and deep cervical lymph nodes is also relatively safe, as it is performed under direct vision. Mediastinoscopy and mediastinotomy, in experienced hands, are safe procedures and have the best chance to succeed in obtaining diagnostic tissue. Per-

cutaneous needle aspiration biopsy, however, is contraindicated because of the likelihood of severe hemorrhage. One must remember that in this condition the increased venous pressure often simulates arterial pressure. Percutaneous transvenous biopsy of a lesion protruding into the lumen of the superior vena cava can be used to obtain tissue using an endomyocardial bioptome under fluoroscopic control. With this procedure a thrombus may form at the remaining tumor site, which may cause further obstruction of the vena cava. Bronchoscopy in a patient with respiratory distress can be risky, as it may increase the mucosal edema already present and lead to further respiratory insufficiency. Finally, if tissue absolutely must be obtained for a therapeutic decision and other attempts have failed, exploratory thoracotomy may be elected. Good exposure can be obtained, and hemorrhage, should it occur, can be managed readily.

Treatment

When the manifestations of superior vena caval obstruction are severe and rapidly progressive, one should proceed immediately with emergent radiation therapy, especially if the index of suspicion is high for a radiation-sensitive process. Under these circumstances, irradiation should be initiated even in the absence of a definitive tissue diagnosis. The patient is usually given steroids, and rapid, high-dose, supravoltage irradiation is instituted, using 400 rads in the midplane daily for 4 days. This treatment is both safe and effective, particularly in poorly differentiated tumors, such as small cell undifferentiated carcinoma and lymphoma. In these conditions, tumor size decreases faster than the edema from the irradiation can develop, but the reverse may happen in well-differentiated tumors. In these situations, edema may lead to serious respiratory distress. Further diagnostic steps can more readily and safely be undertaken after symptoms have been controlled with irradiation.

Because malignancies cause 95% of cases of superior vena caval syndrome, and because essentially all of the malignancies are inoperable, further radiation therapy is probably indicated. This therapy is accomplished by using the conventional low-dose fractionation—200 rads daily. The best long-term results are seen with the lymphomas. Of all patients with superior vena caval syndrome with malignancies, 10 to 20% survive more than 2 years.

Medical measures such as salt restriction, diuretics, and steroids to reduce edema should be initiated. Chemotherapy in small cell undifferentiated carcinoma and certain lymphomas is indicated as adjunctive therapy along with irradiation. In those instances of idiopathic and septic thrombophlebitis or iatrogenic thrombosis of the superior vena cava, anticoagulants, antibiotics, and occasionally fibrinolytic agents should be prescribed.

Operation should be considered only in superior vena cava obstruction secondary to a substernal goiter or vascular aneurysm. The goiter should be removed through a cervical incision if possible because its blood supply stems from the neck, but preparation should be made for sternotomy in case uncontrollable hemorrhage oc-

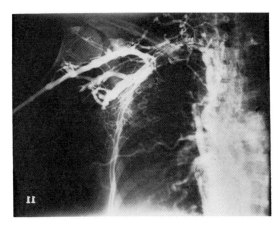

Fig. 89–9. Occlusion of the right subclavian vein, innominate vein, and superior vena cava caused by chronic fibrous mediastinitis in a young woman with a normal chest roentgenogram. Note the extensive collateral vessels via the large azygos and hemiazygos veins draining downward to the inferior vena cava. Other dilated channels include intercostal vessels, internal mammary veins, and lateral thoracic branches.

curs. Resection of an aneurysm in this instance would probably require cardiopulmonary bypass.

Operative intervention in superior vena caval syndrome secondary to chronic fibrous mediastinitis is not only contraindicated but can be meddlesome. This disease is usually self-limited because its slow, insidious progress permits the development of extensive venous collaterals, which are often interrupted by operative intervention. Elaborate collateral pathways are present in superior vena caval obstruction via the internal mammary, azygos, lateral thoracic, and vertebral veins whereby the venous blood from the head, neck, and arms eventually returns to the right heart by way of the inferior vena cava. Only when irradiation and other forms of therapy fail, which is seldom, and the obstruction becomes unbearable, should bypass surgery be contemplated. In the past, autogenous and synthetic grafts to bypass the obstruction have been unsuccessful, usually because of thrombosis. Some limited success has been realized by anastomosis between the azygos vein, if uninvolved in the obstruction, and the inferior vena cava. Also, a reversed in situ saphenous vein graft mobilized and anastomosed to the dilated jugular neck vein through a subcutaneous tunnel has been tried. The contralateral saphenous vein can be used, if necessary, to obtain more length. Thrombectomy in acute superior vena caval obstruction has also been described. The best results seem to follow the use of a spiral saphenous vein graft bypassing the obstruction from the left jugular-subclavian vein to the right atrium. Nevertheless, optimism about the success of these procedures should be guarded.*

REFERENCES

Anderson, R.P., and Li, W.: Segmental replacement of superior vena cava with spiral vein graft. Ann. Thorac. Surg. 36:85, 1983.

Dartevelle, P., et al.: Replacement of the superior vena cava with polytetrafluoroethylene grafts combined with resection of mediastinal—pulmonary malignant tumors: Report of thirteen cases. J. Thorac. Cardiovasc. Surg. 94:361, 1987.

Doty, D.B.: Bypass of superior vena cava: Six years' experience with spiral vein graft for obstruction of superior vena cava due to benign and malignant disease. J. Thorac. Cardiovasc. Surg. 83:326, 1982.

Masuda, H., et al.: Total replacement of superior vena cava because

*Editor's Footnote: The editor concurs that there are only a few indications for the replacement of the superior vena cava. It is rarely, if ever, indicated in patients with benign obstruction of the vessel. Its replacement is also not indicated in patients in whom the vessel is involved by direct extension or by metastatic lymph node involvement from a bronchial carcinoma. The vessel's replacement, however, is indicated when it is directly involved by an invasive thymoma or other locally malignant anterior mediastinal tumor. This is especially true when there are no signs of superior vena caval obstruction present clinically. Once clinical obstruction is present, replacement of the cava is less successful. Patency is dependent upon adequate flow through the graft. As noted by the authors, the best results in this country have been obtained by the interposition of a spiral saphenous vein graft. Doty (1982), Anderson and Li (1984), and others described this technique and the results of its use. In Europe, Dartevelle and associates (1987) and, in Japan, Nakahara (1988) and Masuda (1988) and their colleagues reported the successful use of expanded or ringed polytetrafluoroethylene—PTFE—grafts in patients with malignant involvement of the vessel. The grafts were especially successful when the tumor was a malignant thymoma.

of invasive thymoma: Seven years' survival. J. Thorac. Cardiovasc. Surg. 95:1083, 1988.

Nakahara, K., et al.: Thymoma: Results with complete resection and adjuvant postoperative irradiation in 141 consecutive patients. J. Thorac. Cardiovasc. Surg. 95:1041, 1988.

READING REFERENCES

Acute and Chronic Mediastinitis

Barois, A., et al.: Treatment of mediastinitis in children after cardiac surgery. Intensive Care Med. 4:35, 1978.

Bryant, L.R., Spencer, F.C., and Trinkle, J.K.: Treatment of median sternotomy infection by mediastinal irrigation with an antibiotic solution. Ann. Surg. 169:914, 1969.

Case Records of the Massachusetts General Hospital: Case 15—1978. N. Engl. J. Med. 298:894, 1978.

Cheanvechai, C., Travisano, F., and Effler, D.B.: Treatment of infected sternal wounds. Cleve. Clin. Q. 39:43, 1972.

Culliford, A.T., et al.: Sternal and costochondral infections following open heart surgery: a review of 2,596 cases. J. Thorac. Cardiovasc. Surg. 72:714, 1976.

Dye, T.C., et al.: Sclerosing mediastinitis with occlusion of pulmonary veins: manifestations and management. J. Thorac. Cardiovasc. Surg. 74:137, 1977.

Engelman, R.M., Saxena, A., and Levitsky, S.: Delayed mediastinal infection after ventricular aneurysm resection. Ann. Thorac. Surg. 25:470, 1978.

Enquist, R.W., Blanck, R.R., and Butler, R.H.: Nontraumatic mediastinitis. J.A.M.A. 236:1048, 1976.

Hewlett, T.H., Steer, A., and Thomas, D.E.: Progressive fibrosing mediastinitis. Ann. Thorac. Surg. 2:345, 1966.

Jimenez-Martinez, M., et al.: Anterior mediastinitis as a complication of median sternotomy incisions: diagnostic and surgical considerations. Surgery 67:929, 1970.

Kay, H.R., et al.: Use of computed tomography to assess mediastinal complications after median sternotomy. Ann. Thorac. Surg. 36:706, 1983.

Kittredge, R.D., and Nash, A.D.: The many facets of sclerosing fibrosis. Am. J. Roentgenol. Radium Ther. Nucl. Med. 122:288, 1974.

Lee, A.B., Jr., Schimert, G., and Shatkin, S.: Total excision of the sternum and thoracic pedicle transposition of the greater omentum; useful strategems in managing severe mediastinal infection following open heart surgery. Surgery 80:433, 1976.

Lillington, G.A., and Jamplis, R.W.: A Diagnostic Approach to Chest Diseases. Baltimore, Williams & Wilkins, 1977.

MacManus, W., and Okies, J.E.: Mediastinal wound infection and aortocoronary graft patency. Am. J. Surg. 132:558, 1976.

Martini, N., et al.: Comparative merits of conventional, computed tomographic, and magnetic resonance imaging in assessing mediastinal involvement in surgically confirmed lung carcinoma. J. Thorac. Cardiovasc. Surg. 90:639, 1985.

Miller, D.R., Murphy, K., and Cesario, T.: *Pseudomonas* infection of the sternum and costal cartilages: report of three cases. J. Thorac. Cardiovasc. Surg. 76:723, 1978.

Moncada, R., et al.: Mediastinitis from odontogenic and deep cervical infection: anatomic pathways of propagation. Chest 73:497, 1978.

Neuhof, H.: Acute infections of the mediastinum with special reference to mediastinum suppuration. J. Thorac. Cardiovasc. Surg. 6:184, 1936.

Payne, W.S., and Larson, R.H.: Acute mediastinitis. Surg. Clin. North Am. 49:999, 1969.

Poon, P.Y., et al.: Magnetic resonance imaging of the mediastinum. J. Can. Assoc. Radiol. 37:173, 1986.

Rholl, K.S., Levitt, R.G., Glazer, H.S.: Magnetic resonance imaging of fibrosing mediastinitis. Am. J. Radiol. 145:255, 1985.

Rice, D.H., Batsakis, J.G., and Coulthard, S.W.: Sclerosing cervicitis—homologue of sclerosing retroperitonitis and mediastinitis. Arch. Surg. 110:120, 1975.

Schowengerdt, C.G., Suyemoto, R., and Main, F.B.: Granulomatous and fibrous mediastinitis: a review and analysis of 180 cases. J. Thorac. Cardiovasc. Surg. 57:365, 1969.

Serry, C., et al.: Sternal wound complications. J. Thorac. Cardiovasc. Surg. 80:861, 1980.

Starr, M.G., Gott, V.L., and Townsend, T.R.: Mediastinal infection after cardiac surgery. Ann. Thorac. Surg. 38:414, 1984.

Sutherland, R.D., et al.: Postoperative chest wound infections in patients requiring coronary bypass: a controlled study evaluating prophylactic antibiotics. J. Thorac. Cardiovasc. Surg. *73*:944, 1977.

Thurer, R.J., et al.: The management of mediastinal infection following cardiac surgery: an experience utilizing continuous irrigation with povidone-iodine. J. Thorac. Cardiovasc. Surg. *68*:962, 1974.

Weinreb, J.C., Mootz, A., and Cohen, J.M.: MRI evaluation of mediastinal and thoracic inlet venous obstruction. Am. J. Radiol. *146*:677, 1985.

Weinstein, R.A., et al.: Sternal osteomyelitis and mediastinitis after open heart operation: pathogenesis and prevention. Ann. Thorac. Surg. *21*:442, 1976.

Wieder, S., and Rabinowitz, J.G.: Fibrous mediastinitis: a late manifestation of mediastinal histoplasmosis. Radiology *125*:305, 1977.

Superior Vena Caval Syndrome

Armstrong, P., Hayes, D.R., and Richardson, P.J.: Transvenous biopsy of carcinoma of bronchus causing superior vena caval obstruction. Br. Med. J. *1*:662, 1975.

Bonchek, L.I., Geiss, D.M., and Farley, G.: Emergency thrombectomy for acute thrombosis of superior vena cava. J. Thorac. Cardiovasc. Surg. *77*:922, 1979.

Chetty, K.G., and Glauser, R.L.: Suspected superior vena cava syndrome: the role of the Swan-Ganz catheter. Chest *72*:673, 1977.

Cooley, D.A., and Hallman, G.L.: Superior vena caval syndrome trated by azygos vein-inferior vena cava anastomosis: report of a successful case. J. Thorac. Cardiovasc. Surg. *47*:325, 1964.

Cumming, G.R., and Ferguson, C.C.: Obstruction of superior vena cava after the Mustard procedure for transposition of the great arteries. J. Thorac. Cardiovasc. Surg. *70*:242, 1975.

Davenport, D., et al.: Response of superior vena cava syndrome to radiation therapy. Cancer *38*:1577, 1976.

Fiore, A.C., et al.: Prosthetic replacement for the thoracic vena cava. J. Thorac. Cardiovasc. Surg. *84*:560, 1982.

Gladstone, D.J., et al.: Relief of superior vena caval syndrome with autologous femoral vein used as a bypass graft. J. Thorac. Cardiovasc. Surg. *89*:750, 1985.

Hunter, W.: History of aneurysm of the aorta with some remarks on aneurysm in general. M. Obser. Inq. (London) *1*:323, 1757.

Kumar, P.P.: Value of radiotherapy in superior vena caval syndrome. J. Natl. Med. Assoc. *70*:111, 1978.

Lesavoy, M.A., Norberg, H.P., and Kaplan, E.L.: Substernal goiter with superior vena caval obstruction. Surgery *77*:325, 1975.

Lewis, R.J., Sisler, G.E., and MacKenzie, J.W.: Mediastinoscopy in advanced superior vena cava obstruction. Ann. Thorac. Surg. *32*:458, 1981.

Lochridge, S.K., Knibbe, W.P., and Doty, D.B.: Obstruction of the superior vena cava. Surgery *85*:14, 1979.

Lokich, J.B., and Goodman, R.: Superior vena cava syndrome: clinical management. J.A.M.A. *231*:58, 1975.

Mahajan, V., et al.: Benign superior vena cava syndrome. Chest *68*:32, 1975.

Miller, D.B.: Palliative surgery for benign superior vena caval syndrome. Am. J. Surg. *129*:361, 1975.

Perez, C.A., Presant, C.A., and Van Amburg, A.L., III: Management of superior vena cava syndrome. Semin. Oncol. *5*:123, 1978.

Skinner, D.B., Salzman, E.W., and Scannell, J.G.: Challenge of superior vena caval obstruction. J. Thorac. Cardiovasc. Surg. *49*:824, 1965.

Taylor, G.A., et al.: Bypassing the obstructed superior vena cava with a subcutaneous long saphenous vein graft. J. Thorac. Cardiovasc. Surg. *68*:237, 1974.

Williams, D.R., and Demos, N.J.: Thrombosis of superior vena cava caused by pacemaker wire and managed with streptokinase. J. Thorac. Cardiovasc. Surg. *68*:134, 1974.

Wilson, E.S.: Systemic to pulmonary venous communication in the superior vena caval syndrome. Am. J. Roentgenol. *127*:247, 1976.

Yakirevich, V., et al.: Fibrotic stenosis of the superior vena cava with widespread thrombotic occlusion of the major tributaries: an unusual complication of transvenous cardiac pacing. J. Thorac. Cardiovasc. Surg. *85*:632, 1983.

CHAPTER 90

PRIMARY TUMORS AND CYSTS
OF THE MEDIASTINUM

Thomas W. Shields

Various tumors and cysts occur in the mediastinum. They occur in all age groups, although they are apparently more common in young and middle-aged adults. Most of these masses are discovered on routine roentgenographic examination of the chest in an asymptomatic patient, but these lesions may produce specific or nonspecific symptoms and signs. Generally, benign lesions—the majority of mediastinal tumors and cysts—are asymptomatic, but malignant lesions may also be asymptomatic. Most malignant tumors, however, produce clinical findings, as do some of the benign tumors. The precise nature of a lesion in the mediastinum, as elsewhere, cannot be determined without histologic examination of the tissue. Nonetheless, a reasonable, tentative, preoperative diagnosis for each lesion frequently can be made by considering its location in the mediastinum, the age of the patient, the presence or absence of local or constitutional symptoms and signs, and the association of a specific systemic disease state.

MEDIASTINAL COMPARTMENTS

Although the anteroposterior limits of the mediastinum are the undersurface of the sternum anteriorly and the anterior surface of the vertebral bodies posteriorly, the paravertebral—costovertebral—regions bilaterally have usually been included as a portion of the mediastinum in any discussion of mediastinal masses.

Many anteroposterior divisions of the space have been suggested, but I find it satisfactory to divide the mediastinum into three regions: the anterior compartment, the visceral compartment, and the paravertebral sulci. All compartments extend from the thoracic inlet to the diaphragm. The lateral limits bilaterally are the mediastinal surfaces of the parietal pleurae.

The anterior space is bounded anteriorly by the undersurface of the sternum and posteriorly by an imaginary line formed by the anterior surfaces of the great vessels and the pericardium. The visceral compartment, also known as the middle mediastinum or central space, extends posteriorly from the posterior limit of the anterior compartment to the anterior longitudinal spinal ligament. The paravertebral sulci—costovertebral regions—are potential spaces along each side of the vertebral bodies and adjacent ribs (Fig. 90–1). The term "posterior mediastinum" is best not used, because in the literature, both a portion of the central space—the area posterior to the trachea and heart—and the paravertebral areas have been interchangeably referred to by the term. Each of the tumors and cysts arising in the mediastinum has, as a rule, a predilection for one of the three regions, although migration or enlargement into an adjacent space is common (Table 90–1).

The major lesions occurring in the anterior mediastinum are thymomas, lymphomas, and germ cell tumors—teratomas. Less common masses are of vascular or mesenchymal origin. Rarely, true aberrant thyroid tissue is found. Displaced parathyroid tissue also is found in this compartment.

In the visceral compartment, enterogenous cysts—bronchogenic, esophageal, and gastric cysts—and primary as well as secondary tumors of the lymph nodes constitute the majority of lesions. Pleuropericardial cysts and cystic lymphangiomas, which most often occur in the anterior cardiophrenic angle, arise posterior to the anterior surface of the heart and thus are properly assigned to this compartment. Miscellaneous lesions of lymph nodes, thoracic duct cysts, and other rare cysts also occur in the visceral compartment.

Most lesions arising in the paravertebral sulci are tumors of neurogenic origin. Neurenteric cysts and, rarely, vascular lesions are also found in this locality.

Fibromas, lipomas, and their malignant components are rare but may occur in any of the three compartments. In addition, many lesions arising outside the mediastinum may project into the various compartments and masquerade as primary mediastinal masses on a roentgenogram of the chest.

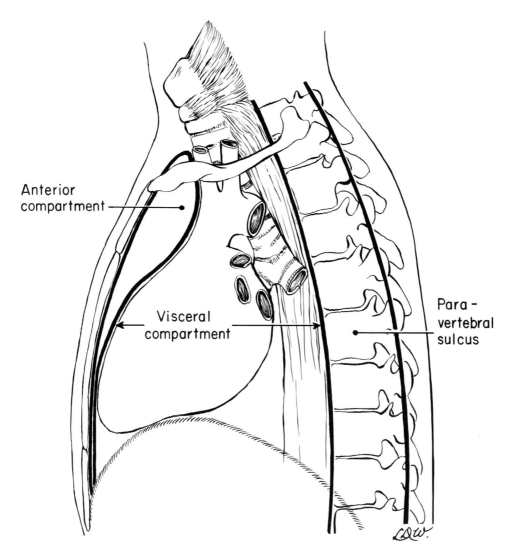

Fig. 90–1. Schematic illustration of mediastinal compartments as seen from the left.

Table 90–1. **Common Location of Tumors and Cysts in the Mediastinum**

Anterior Mediastinum	Middle Mediastinum	Paravertebral Sulci
Thymoma	Enterogenous cyst	Neurilemoma
Lymphoma	Lymphoma	Neurofibroma
Germ cell tumor	Mesothelial cyst—pleuropericardial	Ganglioneuroma
Lymphangioma	Mediastinal granuloma	Neuroblastoma
Hemangioma	Lymphoid hamartoma	Fibrosarcoma
Parathyroid adenoma	Thoracic duct cyst	Lymphoma
Thymic cyst		Gastroenteric cyst
Lipoma		Paraganglioma
Fibroma		Pheochromocytoma
Aberrant thyroid		Askin tumor

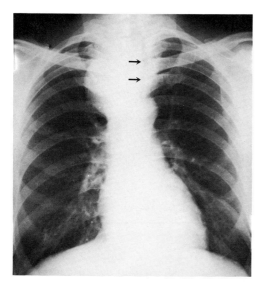

Fig. 90–2. PA roentgenogram of chest showing large substernal thyroid with deviation of the trachea to the left.

LESIONS MASQUERADING AS MEDIASTINAL TUMORS

Lesions masquerading as mediastinal tumors may arise from structures in the cervical region, thoracic skeleton, spinal canal, heart and great vessels, esophagus, lungs, and structures below the diaphragm.

The most frequent lesion from the cervical region is a substernal extension of a thyroid goiter. This lesion usually is located anteriorly in the superior portion of the mediastinum but may be found in a retrotracheal position. Almost always a mass can be palpated in the neck, and tracheal deviation is apparent. Dyspnea frequently is present and, rarely, a superior vena caval syndrome may occur if the mass fills the thoracic inlet. On roentgenographic study of the chest, tracheal deviation is readily seen and calcifications are often apparent within the mass (Fig. 90–2); a CT scan may show the mass, with displacement of the trachea and great vessels (Fig. 90–3). Radioactive ^{131}I scans occasionally yield positive indication of the presence of the goiter, but more often do not,

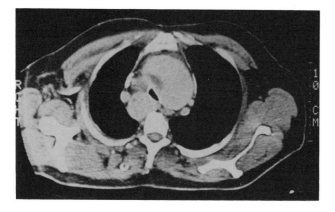

Fig. 90–3. CT of substernal thyroid with marked compression but not obstruction of the great vessels. Distortion and deviation of trachea are evident.

because many, if not most, of these goiters are nonfunctioning. The blood supply of this thyroid tissue is from the vessels in the neck, and thus a cervical approach is indicated for its excision. On rare occasions, a second incision in the anterior thorax or an upper median sternotomy may be necesary to facilitate removal of the goiter. The use of a thoracic approach alone is contraindicated, not only because the blood supply arises from the neck but also because injury to either or both recurrent laryngeal nerves may occur when the mass is removed solely by way of this route.

Cystic hygromas arising in the neck also frequently extend into the thorax. In fact, most lymphangiomas in the mediastinum represent a portion or an extension of a cervical lesion. When excision is indicated, a combined cervical and thoracic approach, as Mills and Grosfeld (1973) described, is necessary.

Lesions of the thoracic skeleton that project into the mediastinum are usually bony tumors. Tumors of the sternum are rarely confusing, but posteriorly, chondromas and chondrosarcomas of the heads of the ribs or vertebral bodies may look like mediastinal tumors. Ewing's sarcoma of a rib rarely masquerades as a primary mediastinal tumor. Infrequently, a tuberculous paravertebral abscess resembles a mediastinal mass on roentgenographic examination, but the associated bony and intervertebral disc destruction, as well as the clinical course of the patient, should lead to the appropriate diagnosis.

Infrequently, a lesion that presents in a paravertebral sulcus is an anterior meningocele from the spinal canal. It is usually asymptomatic and is readily confused with a primary neurogenic tumor. Almost all of the patients are young to middle-aged adults, and the ratio of men to women is about equal. Eighty percent of these meningoceles are associated with peripheral neurofibromatosis or skeletal abnormalities, or both. The skeletal deformities are kyphoscoliosis, enlarged intervertebral foramina, erosion of adjacent ribs or vertebral bodies, and developmental abnormalities, such as fused vertebrae or hemivertebrae. The diagnosis is confirmed by myelography, pneumomyelography being the preferred method. If the diagnosis is established by preoperative study, no treatment is necessary unless symptoms result from the lesion's size or erosion of adjacent bone. If excision is undertaken, YaDeau and associates (1965) advised that the neck of the sac be dissected to the intervertebral foramen, isolated, transfixed, and divided. The sac is then excised. In the past, infection of the pleura or meninges was the major complication, occasionally resulting in death. With the use of antibiotics, however, neither of these infections should occur with any frequency. Rarely, a thoracic vertebral chordoma may present primarily as a mediastinal tumor. Three to fifteen percent of all chordomas arise in the thoracic spine and, of these, a third, as Levowitz and associates (1966) reported, present as a paravertebral mass. The tumor arises from embryonic remnants of the primitive notochord within the axial skeleton. It is a slowly growing malignant tumor that destroys the adjacent vertebrae; bony changes have been noted in almost all patients with this tumor. Symptoms most often are related to the involvement of the spinal cord and adjacent neurogenic structures.

Ectopic extramedullary hematopoietic tissue also can masquerade as a paravertebral mass. The lesion may appear unilateral on routine roentgenograms of the chest, but laminograms or CT examination frequently reveal the mass to be bilateral (Fig. 90–4). Catinella and associates (1985) reported extramedullary hematopoiesis in the anterior mediastinal compartment, but this is an unusual location for this tissue. Development of the ectopic mass of hematopoietic tissue is noted in patients with spherocytosis, thalassemia, or other severe, long-term, hemolytic disease processes. Needle biopsy may be performed if the diagnosis is in doubt. No specific therapy of the hematopoietic mass is indicated.

Mediastinal masses of vascular origin must be differentiated from true mediastinal tumors. These masses may be either arterial or venous in origin and, as Kelley and colleagues (1978) noted, may arise from either the systemic or pulmonary systems (Table 90–2). The normal vascular anatomy and the various congenital anomalies and disease states of these structures must be kept in mind when a mediastinal mass is encountered roentgenographically. Angiography is usually the most helpful diagnostic study, but radionuclide flow studies and computed tomography may also be helpful. Magnetic resonance imaging should be valuable in evaluating suspected vascular abnormality, because of the imaging characteristics of blood-filled structures (see Chapter 14).

A few lesions of the esophagus, such as achalasia, epiphrenic diverticulum, esophageal duplications, a large leiomyoma, and large extramural spread or a contained perforation of an esophageal carcinoma may appear as mediastinal tumors on initial roentgenographic studies of the chest. In esophageal carcinoma, a CT scan may suggest the diagnosis because of pockets of air in the mass (Fig. 90–5). Barium studies of the esophagus, endoscopy, and manometric studies may help establish the appropriate diagnosis. Surgical treatment should be carried out as indicated.

Tumors of the lung, both benign and malignant, may be confused with mediastinal tumors. Occasionally, an extralobar sequestration may be initially thought to be a mediastinal tumor. Appropriate studies, including aortography, establish the diagnosis, although on occasion, thoracotomy is necessary.

Lesions originating below the diaphragm may simulate a primary mediastinal tumor or cyst. Hernias through the esophageal hiatus posteriorly or the foramen of Morgagni anteriorly often are confusing. These subjects are discussed in Chapters 54, 55, and 82. Infrequently a pancreatic pseudocyst may present as a mass in the visceral compartment behind the heart. Johnston and his colleagues (1986) reviewed this subject and presented an example of this unusual complication of pancreatic disease. The clinical presentation should alert one to the possibility that the retrocardiac mass is a pseudocyst. Confirmation is best obtained by CT of the chest and abdomen, which demonstrates the extension of the cyst from the abdomen into the chest. Treatment is by internal drainage through a laparotomy approach.

RELATIONSHIP OF AGE TO TYPE OF MEDIASTINAL LESION

The incidence and types of the many primary mediastinal tumors and cysts vary with the age of the patient group under consideration. In infants and children, the collected series reveal the lesions—in the order of decreasing frequency—to be neurogenic tumors, enterogenous cysts, germ cell tumors, lymphomas, angiomas and lymphangiomas, thymic tumors, and pericardial cysts (Table 90–3). Comparable series in adults are less

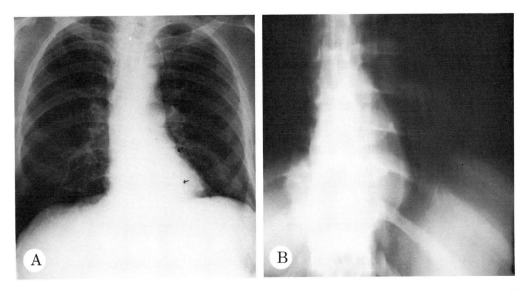

Fig. 90–4. *A*, PA roentgenogram of chest showing an ill-defined mass behind the heart on the left. *B*, Laminogram showing bilateral nature of the ectopic, hematopoietic tissue. (Drake, C.T., et al.: Ectopic hematopoietic tissue masquerading as a mediastinal tumor. Ann. Thorac. Surg. *1*:743, 1965.)

Table 90–2. Mediastinal Masses of Vascular Origin

	Systemic Venous System	Pulmonary Arterial System	Pulmonary Venous System	Systemic Arterial System
Anterior mediastinum				Aortic stenosis Aortic aneurysm (ascending aorta)
Middle mediastinum	Aneurysm of superior vena cava Partial anomalous pulmonary venous return to superior vena cava Azygos vein enlargement	Pulmonary valve stenosis Idiopathic dilatation of pulmonary trunk Congenital absence of pulmonary valve Pulmonary embolism (acute and chronic) Pulmonary arterial hypertension states Anomalous left pulmonary artery	Pulmonary venous varix Pulmonary venous confluence	Aortic stenosis Right aortic arch Aortic aneurysm (transverse aorta) Aneurysm or fistula of coronary artery
Projecting into anterior mediastinum	Aneurysm of the innominate veins Persistent left superior vena cava Hemiazygos vein enlargement	Aneurysm of ductus	Partial anomalous pulmonary venous return to innominate vein Total anomalous pulmonary venous return (supracardiac)	Tortuous innominate artery Cervical aortic arch Coarctation of aorta Aortic aneurysm (transverse aorta)
Paravertebral sulcus				Aortic aneurysm (descending aorta)

Adapted from Kelley, M.J., et al.: Mediastinal masses of vascular origin: a review. J. Thorac. Cardiovasc. Surg. 76:559, 1978.

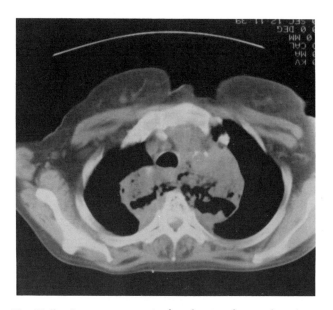

Fig. 90–5. Spontaneous contained perforation of an esophageal carcinoma simulating a primary mediastinal tumor. CT examination reveals pockets of air within the mass.

readily obtainable, because most reports include lesions in both children and adults. In a collected series of 2196 patients, however, which was probably made up mostly of adult patients, the lesions mentioned—in the order of decreasing frequency—were neurogenic tumors, thymic tumors, lymphomas, germ cell tumors, enterogenous cysts, and pericardial cysts (Table 90–4). In my experience as well as that of many of my colleagues, however, thymomas are now the most common mediastinal tumor in adult patients. Mullen and Richardson (1986) found that thymomas constituted 47% of all mediastinal tumors in the anterior compartment in adults.

SIGNS AND SYMPTOMS OF MEDIASTINAL LESIONS

In children, approximately two thirds of the tumors and cysts are symptomatic, whereas in adults, approximately only one third produce symptoms. The signs and symptoms that occur depend on the benignancy or malignancy of the lesion, its size, its location, the presence or absence of infection, the elaboration of specific endocrine or other biochemical products, and the presence of associated disease states.

In infants and children, respiratory symptoms, such as cough, stridor, and dyspnea, are prominent, because even a small mass may, because of its location, compress the airway. Also, because of the relatively small size of the thorax, any mass may readily encroach upon the volume of the lungs. In addition, septic complications with resultant pneumonitis and fever occur frequently.

Table 90–3. Incidence of Mediastinal Tumors and Cysts in Children

	Gross (1953)	Ellis and DuShane (1956)	Heimburger and Battersby (1965)	Jaubert de Beaujeu et al. (1968)	Haller et al. (1969)	Grosfeld et al. (1971)	Whittaker and Lynn (1973)	Pokorny and Sherman (1974)	Bower and Kiesewetter (1977)	Total
Neurogenic tumors	16	19	9	22	18	35	37	35	41	232
Enterogenous cysts	18	10	10	15	10		12	14	17	106
Germ cell tumors	5	16	5	9	8	5	21	4	5	78
Lymphomas			6		8	13	9	27	12	75
Angiomas and lymphangiomas	6	9	5	1	4	1	6	7	5	44
Stem cell tumors		4		1	10	2			5	22
Thymic tumors and cysts	3			3		4	2	3	1	16
Pleuropericardial cysts				1	1				2	4
Miscellaneous	1		1	2	3	2	11			20
Total	49	58	36	54	62	62	98	90	88	597

In children, lethargy, fever, and chest pain often occur with malignant lesions.

Infection of benign cysts causes symptoms in adults as well as in children. At present, such inflammatory complications are noted infrequently. Symptoms and signs from compression of vital structures by benign lesions are also uncommon in the adult because most normal, mobile, mediastinal structures can conform to distortion from pressure. When malignant disease is present, however, not only does distortion occur, but fixation is noted as well. Obstruction and compression of vital structures are then common. Superior vena caval obstruction, dysphagia, cough, and dyspnea may be observed. Direct invasion of adjacent structures, such as the chest wall, pleura, and adjacent nerves, is common with malignant tumors. Specific findings of chest pain, pleural effusion, hoarseness, Horner's syndrome, upper extremity pain, back pain, paraplegia, and diaphragmatic paralysis may occur. In addition, constitutional evidence of malignant disease is sometimes evident.

Certain systemic disease states may be present with both malignant and benign mediastinal tumors. These, as well as other unique findings related to each type of tumor and cyst, will be discussed separately. The diagnosis, treatment, and prognosis will also be considered under the respective, separate headings.

ADDITIONAL INVESTIGATION OF MEDIASTINAL MASSES

When a primary mediastinal mass is recognized on standard roentgenograms of the chest in either an asymptomatic or symptomatic child or adult, the diagnostic possibilities can be narrowed down to a reasonable number by considering the patient's age, the location of the mass, and the associated symptoms and signs present. Standard tomography yields little additional useful information. The use of computed tomography, however, may be rewarding when this exam gives additional details that may not be readily discerned on standard films. Computed tomography is a sensitive method of distinguishing between fatty, vascular, cystic, and soft tissue masses. The differentiation of a cystic structure and a solid one, however, is not always 100%. Mendelson and

Table 90–4. Mediastinal Tumors and Cysts*

	Herlitzka and Gale (1958)	Morrison (1958)	Le Roux (1962)	Boyd and Midell (1968)	Wychulis et al. (1971)	Fontenelle et al. (1971)	Rubush et al. (1973)	Ovrum and Birkeland (1979)	Davis et al. (1987)	Total
Neurogenic tumors	35	101	30	11	212	7	36	19	57	508
Thymoma and thymic cysts	14	47	17	20	225	18	51	10	67	469
Lymphomas	12	33		20	107	14	14	9	62	271
Germ cell tumors	26	36	21	22	99	3	14	5	42	268
Enterogenous cysts	26	29	14	15	83	2	8		50	227
Pericardial cysts	17	13	20	6	72	3	10	7	36	184
Miscellaneous	29	30	3	2	118	17	24	6	40	269
Total	159	289	105	96	916	64	157	56	354	2196

*Excluding substernal thyroid, mediastinal granuloma, and "primary carcinoma of mediastinum."

associates (1983) reported examples of bronchogenic cysts with high Hounsfield numbers. CT also is useful in further evaluating all paravertebral masses that on standard spine films appear to have eroded or enlarged the intervertebral foramen. Intrinsically, the CT scan cannot differentiate between a benign and a malignant tumor, but may on occasion demonstrate invasion into adjacent structures or may reveal pleural or parenchymal metastases. Sones and associates (1982) reported that CT examination provided important additional information compared to standard roentgenograms in their series of patients with mediastinal lesions, and Miller and associates (1984) noted its enhanced value with the use of an intravenous bolus of contrast material during the examination. Despite these data, although computed tomography is valuable, it should not be done routinely for all mediastinal masses when enough information for a diagnostic or therapeutic decision is available without it.

Magnetic resonance imaging may supply additional useful information in separating mediastinal tumors from vessels and bronchi, especially when the use of contrast material is contraindicated. The high signal intensity of fat and other soft tissues contrasts markedly with the low signal intensity of flowing blood and surrounding lung. Furthermore, the availability of sagittal and coronal body section views with MRI may increase the value of this examination, as Dooms and Higgins (1986) noted. It also may be superior to CT in evaluating intraspinal extension or intrathecal spread of paravertebral masses.

Additional contrast studies, i.e., barium swallow and digital and conventional angiograms, may be done in special situations, such as the identification of the artery of Adamkiewicz in some patients with intraspinal canal extension of a paravertebral neurogenic tumor.

DeMeester (personal communication, 1987) suggested ^{67}Ga scans to help differentiate benign from malignant anterior mediastinal masses, uptake being infrequent in the former and common in the latter. Whether this is appropriate or necessary in most instances is undetermined, because in many patients this differentiation can be based reasonably accurately on data obtained by standard evaluation of the patient.

Numerous biochemical markers and hormone levels are elevated in association with specific mediastinal tumors. Alpha fetoprotein levels and beta human chorionic gonadotropic levels are markedly elevated with certain malignant germ cell tumors. Epinephrine and norepinephrine levels may be elevated with either benign or malignant autonomic nerve cell tumors. Other specific markers or elevated hormone levels will be discussed with the various causative tumors. These biochemical studies should be obtained when appropriate, but certainly not routinely.

NEUROGENIC TUMORS

These are reportedly the most common mediastinal masses in both children and adults; 15 to 30% of mediastinal masses are neurogenic tumors. They are discovered slightly more often in women than in men. In children, approximately half of these tumors are malignant, whereas in adults, the incidence of malignant disease is less than 10% and probably only in the range of 1 to 2%. Gale and colleagues (1974) recorded that only 1 of 23 adults with nerve sheath tumor had a malignant variety. Likewise, Davidson and associates (1978) reported only one malignant neurogenic lesion in 38 patients over the age of 21 with such tumors, and Reed and colleagues (1978) noted only 1 malignant tumor in 67 nerve sheath tumors.

Neurogenic tumors arise from cells derived from the neural crest, the important structure in the development of the peripheral nervous system. Ganglion cells of the spinal ganglia and of the autonomic nervous system, the paraganglionic cells of the sympathetic and parasympathetic systems, and the Schwann cells and satellite cells arise from this mass of embryonic tissue. Supporting fibrous connective tissue of mesodermal origin also is involved in some of these tumors.

Because of the varying degrees of maturation, as well as the diversity of cellular types formed, many classifications of neurogenic tumors have been proposed. It seems appropriate, however, to classify these tumors as shown in Table 90–5. Almost all of these are found in the paravertebral sulci along the sympathetic chain or in association with a spinal or intercostal nerve. The right and left paravertebral sulci are involved with equal frequency, and the tumor may occur at any level. Most of these tumors, however, are found in the upper half or third of the chest. A few neurogenic tumors arise in association with either the vagus or phrenic nerves in the visceral compartment. Oosterwijk and Swierenga (1968) reported the involvement of one of these four nerves in 7 of their 111 patients. Rarely, a tumor of the paraganglionic system may be found at the aortic root, in the pericardium, or even in the heart itself. The Askin (1979) tumor may involve the posterior chest wall or even the lung and diaphragm.

In adults, most neurogenic tumors are asymptomatic and are discovered on routine roentgenographic examination of the chest, but cough, dyspnea, chest wall pain, or a Horner's syndrome may be present. In a few patients—approximately 3 to 6%—findings of spinal cord compression are present. Chest pain, cough, dyspnea, and dysphagia are common in infants and children with either benign or malignant lesions. Infants with malignant lesions frequently present with a Horner's syndrome and at times with paraplegia. Constitutional signs and symptoms such as fever and malaise frequently accompany the malignant lesions.

The characteristic roentgenographic feature in an adult is a smoothly rounded, homogenous density abutting the vertebral column (Fig. 90–6). Lobulation is present, at times, and calcifications occasionally appear within the mass. Adjacent bony changes—rib or vertebral body erosion, enlargement of an intervertebral foramen (Fig. 90–7), and splaying of the ribs with widening of the intercostal spaces—occur. These findings usually do not indicate malignant disease but are caused by local pres-

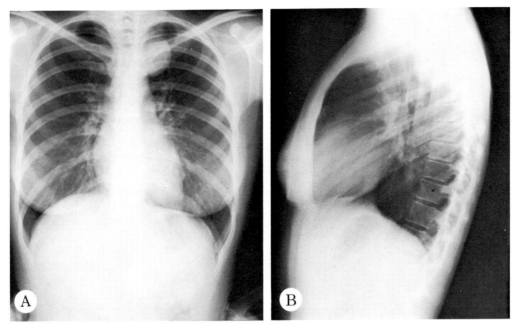

Fig. 90–6. *A* and *B*, PA and lateral roentgenograms of the chest showing a neurilemoma in the left paravertebral sulcus.

Table 90–5. Neurogenic Tumors of the Thorax

Origin	Benign	Malignant
Nerve Sheath	Neurilemoma Neurofibroma	Malignant schwannoma—neurogenic sarcoma
Autonomic Ganglia	Ganglioneuroma	Ganglioneuroblastoma Neuroblastoma

Paraganglionic System
    Sympathetic
    Parasympathetic
	Pheochromocytoma
	Nonchromaffin paraganglioma—chemodectoma
		Malignant pheochromocytoma
		Malignant paraganglioma

Peripheral Neuroectodermal Tumor		Malignant small cell tumor—Askin tumor

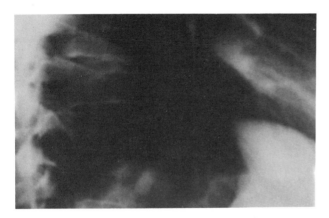

Fig. 90–7. Enlarged, eroded intervertebral foramen from extension of a neurofibroma into the spinal canal. (Reproduced with permission of Shields, T.W., and Reynolds, M.: Neurogenic tumors of the thorax. Surg. Clin. North Am. 68:645, 1988.)

sure changes resulting from growth of the mass. All patients with a paravertebral mass, symptomatic or not, should have roentgenograms of the thoracic spine. When erosion of a vertebral pedicle or enlargement of an intervertebral foramen is identified, computed tomography is then indicated to determine whether there is intraspinal canal extension of the tumor. At present, CT exam is usually done in all without initial spinal roentgenograms (Fig. 90–8). Akwari and associates (1978) reported that 40% of the patients with intraspinal canal extension, which occurs in approximately 10% of all these neurogenic tumors, may be asymptomatic when the lesion is first discovered. As noted, the growth into the canal is best determined by computed tomography or by magnetic resonance imaging, which also may enable one to determine the length of the involvement, but at present contrast myelography is usually done to delineate this feature.

In children, the roentgenographic features resemble those in the adult (Fig. 90–9). Because many of the tumors are malignant and undergo rapid growth, however, the outlines of the tumors may be less distinct than in

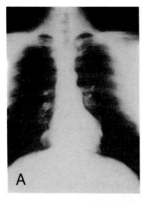
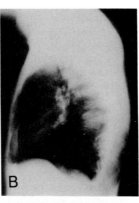

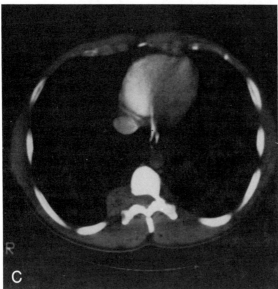

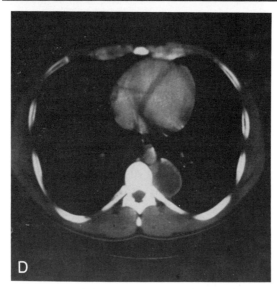

Fig. 90–8. Young adult man with asymptomatic bilateral neurofibromas in association with von Recklinghausen's disease. *A*, PA roentgenogram, smaller lesion on the right and the larger left-sided lesion behind the heart shadow. *B*, Lateral roentgenogram readily showing larger left-sided lesion. *C*, CT exam revealing intraspinal canal extension of lesion on the right. *D*, CT showing no such involvement on the left. (Reproduced with permission of Shields, T.W., and Reynolds, M.: Neurogenic tumors of the thorax. Surg. Clin. North Am. 68:645, 1988.)

adults. Areas of calcification, the result of loss of blood supply and subsequent necrosis, are common within these lesions. Also, these masses are proportionately larger than in the adult, and may distort the trachea and barium-filled esophagus. Occasionally, the mass occupies an entire hemithorax. Intraspinal canal extension also occurs in children, as it does in adults. The impression, however, is that it occurs less frequently in the malignant lesions in the child than in the benign tumors in the adult.

Tumors of Nerve-Sheath Origin

Two benign tumors, the neurilemoma and the neurofibroma, and one malignant tumor, the neurogenic sarcoma—malignant schwannoma—constitute this category of neurogenic tumors.

Both benign tumors occur most often in the third, fourth, and fifth decades of life; together they make up 70% of the intrathoracic neurogenic tumors in adults. Much confusion is apparent in the literature about which of the two is more common. This confusion has occurred because the histologic differentiation between the two has been variously interpreted. At present, most pathologists believe the neurilemoma to be predominant.

Grossly, the neurilemoma is well encapsulated, firm, and grayish tan; it has a whorled pattern on cut section. Areas of degeneration may be prominent. On histologic examination, two types of cellular patterns appear. Antoni type A is a dense, avascular, spindle-cell pattern with distinct palisading (Fig. 90–10). Antoni type B has myxomatous changes associated with multiple cystic areas. Vascular thickening and hyalinized coats of the blood vessels freqently are present. Areas of hemorrhage and calcification also are present. Razzuk and colleagues (1973) described the electron microscopic features of these two cell types. The Antoni type A cells have numerous thin cytoplasmic processes emanating from a cell body with a narrow rim of cytoplasm. The Antoni type B cells lack these processes and have abundant cytoplasm with a complex system of organelles.

The neurofibroma is less common. Grossly, it is bosselated and appears to be well encapsulated, but a true connective-tissue capsule is absent on microscopic examination. Histologically, a tangled network shows schwannian sheath proliferation, with many neurites. The cells are not palisaded. Electron microscopy shows that the tumor is made up of elongated cells with a few thick cytoplasmic processes interspersed with occasional myelinated and unmyelinated axons in an extensive collagenous stroma.

The neurofibromas are often seen in association with generalized neurofibromatosis—von Recklinghausen's disease—and in this situation, the risk of malignant degeneration of the neurofibromas is thought to be as high as 10%, whereas neurilemomas rarely become malignant.

Neurogenic sarcomas or malignant schwannomas tend to occur at both extremes of the age group—the first and second and the sixth and seventh decades—of the patients who have benign nerve-sheath tumors. These ma-

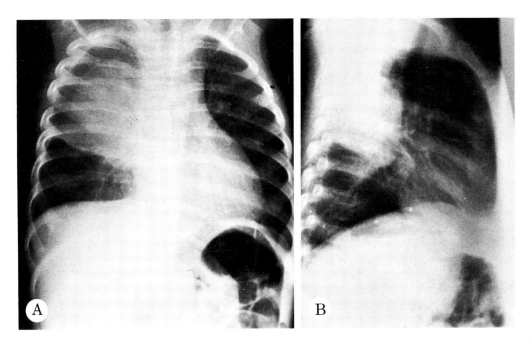

Fig. 90–9. *A* and *B*, PA and lateral roentgenograms of an infant with a large neuroblastoma on the right.

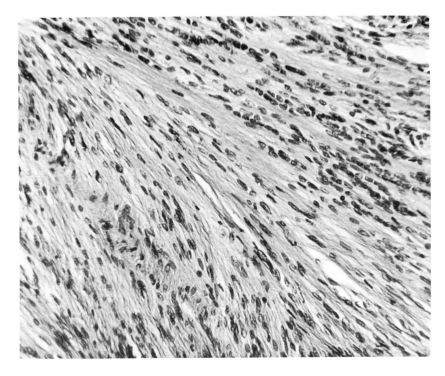

Fig. 90–10. Photomicrograph of a typical neurilemoma.

lignant lesions constitute less than 10% of thoracic neurogenic tumors in adults. Adjacent structures are usually infiltrated and distant metastases occur. Hypercellularity with nuclear pleomorphism and frequent mitotic figures are seen on microscopic examination.

The nerve-sheath tumors are treated by surgical removal. This procedure is accomplished through the appropriate standard posterolateral thoracotomy. The pleura overlying the mass is incised and the tumor freed by both blunt and sharp dissection. Some benign lesions can simply be enucleated, whereas freeing others requires division of one or more nerve trunks, sympathetic or intercostal. Occasionally, intercostal vessels must also be sacrificed. When an intraspinal extension has been identified preoperatively, which it should be, whether it is asymptomatic or not, a one-stage combined approach as LeBrigand (1973) and Akwari (1978), Irger (1980), and Grillo (1983) and their colleagues suggested should be carried out for simultaneous removal of both the thoracic and intraspinal canal extension of the tumor. The various authors have described different incisions and different sequences for removing either portion of the tumor first. I prefer a modified incision similar to that Grillo and associates (1983) described (Fig. 90–11), but prefer to have the neurosurgeon perform the hemilaminectomy with mobilization of the intraspinal canal extension before the intrathoracic portion of the tumor is mobilized.

In patients with a malignant nerve-sheath tumor, surgical resection and postoperative irradiation are indicated.

The morbidity after resection of either a benign or a malignant lesion is related to the injury or necessary resection of associated nerve trunks. Spinal cord complications, fortunately, are rare, but may occur if there is hemorrhage into a residual intraspinal portion of an "hourglass" tumor that was left behind.

Postoperative mortality is infrequent, and the rate should be less than 1 to 2%. The risk of operation is increased if the tumor is large or malignant.

The prognosis is excellent for benign nerve-sheath tumor, and local recurrence is rare. The prognosis with malignant tumors, however, is poor, and death usually occurs within a year following operation.

Tumors of the Autonomic Nervous System

The three specific histologic types of tumors of the autonomic nervous system recognized are ganglioneuroma, ganglioneuroblastoma, and neuroblastoma.

The ganglioneuroma is benign and usually asymptomatic. It is the most common benign neurogenic tumor in children and is also found in the older child and adolescent. The lesion is encapsulated and usually attached to either a sympathetic or intercostal nerve trunk. These tumors infrequently extend intraspinally, although Davidson and associates (1978) described this cell type in seven of their eight patients who had intraspinal canal extension. Microscopic examination reveals mature ganglion cells, singly and in nests, in a stroma composed of Schwann cells and neuromatous and fibrous tissue (Fig. 90–12). Areas of degeneration are evident within the tumor. Calcification may, or may not, be present in these areas.

The ganglioneuroblastoma—partially differentiated ganglioneuroma—occurs in a younger-aged group and is malignant. Symptoms are usually present. A capsule is sometimes recognizable, and attachment to a nerve trunk is common. Histologically an admixture of ganglion cells of varying degrees of maturity, predominantly immature, appears in a stroma like the mature ganglioneuromas. Areas of calcification are usually present.

The neuroblastoma—sympathicoblastoma—is a highly malignant tumor that occurs in young children and infants; most of these tumors are found in children younger than 3 years of age. They comprise over 50% of the neurogenic tumors in the mediastinum of children, and these intrathoracic lesions account for approximately 20% of all neuroblastomas in children. Grossly, the mass may be smooth but often is irregular in outline and involves adjacent structures. Intraspinal extension is unusual, but does occur. Distant metastases to bone and other sites occur frequently.

Grossly, the tumor is reddish to violescent and is vascular. On histologic examination, the tumor is cellular and composed of small, round to oval cells with little cytoplasm and dark, hyperchromatic nuclei. Characteristically, a circular grouping or pseudorosette formation of cells appears around a fine fibrillar network (Fig. 90–13). Areas of degeneration and calcification are common.

The neuroblastomas, as well as the other two autonomic nerve tumors, stain immunohistochemically for neuron-specific enolase—NSE—which Marangos and Schmechel (1980) originally thought was a specific marker for neural elements and their tumors, but as noted in the discussion of small cell tumors of the lung (Chapter 76), this marker is also present in lesions of other cell types as well. In addition to NSE, synapto-

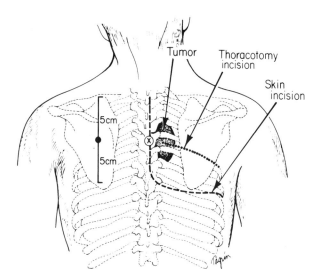

Fig. 90–11. One-stage, single incision for removal of an "hour-glass" neurogenic tumor. (Reproduced with permission of Grillo, H.C., et al.: Combined approach to "dumbbell" intrathoracic and intraspinal neurogenic tumors. Ann. Thorac. Surg. 36:402, 1983.)

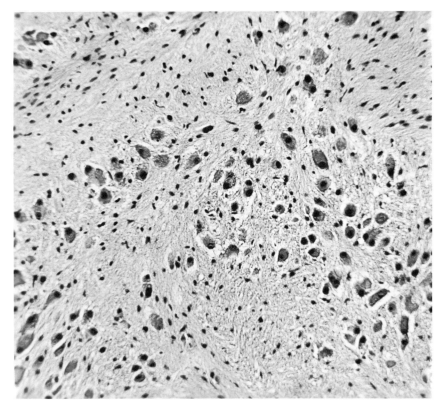

Fig. 90–12. Photomicrograph of a ganglioneuroma.

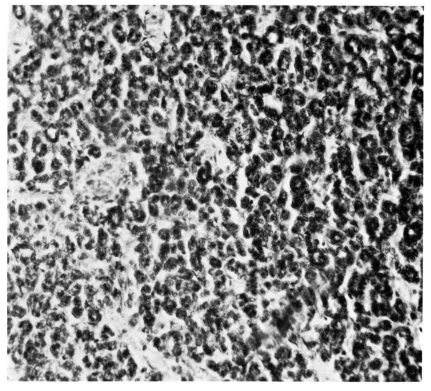

Fig. 90–13. Photomicrograph of a neuroblastoma. Suggestion of pseudorosette formation is seen.

physin can be identified in all these tumors. The presence of this protein or one similar to it is demonstrated by immunofluorescence microscopy on cryostat sections of freshly frozen tissues using a monoclonal antibody to this protein—SY 38; Gould and associates (1987) considered this the "umbrella" marker for neuroendocrine lesions.

Symptoms are most always present in patients with neuroblastomas. Cough, dyspnea, chest pain, Horner's syndrome, paraplegia, fever, and lassitude are common. In some infants, spontaneous abnormal eye movements—"dancing eyes," acute cerebellar ataxia with opsoclonus and chaotic nystagmus—which is thought to be caused by antibody production or other immune response, may be observed. Occasionally, removal of the tumor is followed by a disappearance of the abnormal eye movements.

Children with any one of these autonomic neurogenic tumors may present with diarrhea and abdominal distention or sweating and flushing of the skin, or both. These findings are related to biochemical activity of the tumor with the production of catecholamines—epinephrine and norepinephrine. Even when these symptom complexes are absent, the lesions may produce these substances, and elevated levels of their degradation product, vanillylmandelic acid—VMA—may be identified in the urine. Homovanillic acid—HVA—may also be excreted in the urine. Hamilton and Koop (1965) found elevated levels of VMA in four of seven children with ganglioneuromas and in 85% of those children with neuroblastomas. Seeger and colleagues (1982) reported that catecholamines can be detected in 95% of the neuroblastomas and in fewer of the other two autonomic nerve cell tumors. These levels fall to normal with successful removal of the tumor and may become elevated again with recurrence.

The treatment for these tumors consists of surgical excision by a posterolateral thoracotomy approach. Ganglioneuromas are removed readily. Some ganglioneuroblastomas can be excised completely, but some of these and almost all neuroblastomas can be resected only partially. As much of the tumor as possible, however, must be resected. Patients with either malignant lesion should receive postoperative radiation therapy. The usual amount recommended is 20 to 30 Gy to the tumor bed, but skeletal deformities and spinal cord injury may occur with this dose, particularly in children under 2 years of age, as Zajtchuk and associates (1980) noted. Chemotherapy with vincristine and cyclophosphamide, as well as other agents, such as doxorubicin and cisplatin, is used in most patients. Prednisone is often added to the chemotherapy combination.

The prognosis for patients with ganglioneuromas is excellent. For patients with either ganglioneuroblastomas or neuroblastomas the outlook is guarded, although long-term survivors, those with early-stage disease (Table 90–6), have been recorded with the combined use of surgical resection, radiation therapy, and chemotherapy. Adam and Hochholzer (1981) reported an 88% 5-year actuarial survival rate in 72 patients with various

Table 90–6. Stage Designation of Neuroblastomas

Stage I	Localized disease, tumor confined to the organ or structure of origin.
Stage II	Regional disease, tumor extending in continuity beyond organ or structure of origin but not crossing the midline.
Stage III	Regional disease, tumor extending in continuity beyond the midline.
Stage IV	Disseminated disease, involving skeleton, organs, soft tissues, or distant lymph node groups.
Stage IV-S	Patients who would otherwise be stage I or II but who have remote disease confined to one or more of the following sites: liver, skin, or bone marrow.

Reproduced with permission of Evans, A.E., D'Angilo, G.J., and Randolph, J.: A proposed staging for children with neuroblastoma. Cancer 27:374, 1971.

stages of ganglioneuroblastoma treated by a combination of these methods. Carlsen and associates (1986a) reported an overall survival rate of 22% for all stages of neuroblastoma, but one of 80% for stage I disease. Coldman (1980) and Thomas (1984) and their associates documented, and Carlsen and colleagues (1986a, b) confirmed, that patients with neuroblastoma arising in the thorax have a better prognosis than those in whom the tumor originates in the abdomen. This is attributed to earlier diagnosis of thoracic lesions, which tend to produce local symptoms, unlike the more silent abdominal lesions. Filler and colleagues (1972) noted that even when the thoracically located tumor has spread to produce clinical signs that ordinarily indicate poor prognosis, such tumors in infants frequently could be treated successfully. Catalano and his associates (1978) reported a 63% survival rate in 41 patients with neuroblastomas in the thorax. Patients under the age of 1 had a 90% survival rate and those under the age of 2 an 87% rate. The survival rate was only 34% in those between the ages of 2 and 12. Infants with acute cerebellar ataxia with opsoclonus and chaotic nystagmus are usually under the age of 1, have either stage I or II disease, and as a result experience over a 90% survival rate. The older patients with stage IV—disseminated—disease have the poorest prognosis of all.

Gross and his associates (1959), as well as others, have recorded spontaneous regression of neuroblastomas, with or without treatment. The maturation of neuroblastomas into benign ganglioneuromas was first reported by Cushing and Wolbach in 1927. The explanation is not readily apparent, but this event occurs in 1 to 2% of all children with neuroblastomas. Of course, in such patients the prognosis becomes excellent.

Tumors of the Paraganglionic System

Both chemically active and inactive benign and malignant tumors of the paraganglionic system occur. The inactive lesion is classified as a nonchromaffin paraganglioma—chemodectoma—and the chemically active one as a pheochromocytoma.

The nonchromaffin paragangliomas are rare. The benign lesions are asymptomatic and are found in both the visceral compartment and the paravertebral sulci. The tumor is soft and has an extensive vascular supply. Microscopically, small nests of ovoid cells with uniform or variable-sized nuclei separated by an arrangement of reticulin appear. No mitotic figures are present. The malignant lesions are similar, and malignancy cannot be established histologically. Most paragangliomas are benign—10% are malignant. Olson and Salyer (1978), however, in a review of the literature on aortic body paragangliomas, found a high incidence of aggressive tumor growth in the mediastinum, with serious morbidity or death in just less than half of the patients with an aortic body tumor.

The treatment consists of surgical excision, if this can be accomplished with ease. If the lesion's vascularity makes operative removal too hazardous, biopsy only is indicated, as Ashley and Evans (1966) suggested. The malignant lesions probably should receive postoperative irradiation.

Mediastinal pheochromocytoma is rare. The patient may or may not present with the typical clinical findings of an active pheochromocytoma. If symptoms are present, there may be varying combinations and manifestations of hypertension, hypermetabolism, and diabetes. The hypertension may be paroxysmal or persistent. Any of these conditions plus a paravertebral mass on roentgenographic examination of the chest should alert the physician to the possibility of a pheochromocytoma.

Physiologically, these tumors produce norepinephrine or epinephrine, or both. Vanillylmandelic acid—VMA— is the chief urinary excretion product of these aforementioned substances. Normally, the 24-hour excretion of VMA is between 2 and 9 mg. Higher levels suggest a pheochromocytoma. The urinary and blood levels of the catecholamines can be determined for further confirmation of the tumor. Levels above the normal epinephrine equivalent values for 24-hour urinary catecholamines—50 μg of epinephrine and 150 μg of norepinephrine—establish the diagnosis in more than 90% of the patients with a chemically active tumor.

In the thorax, pheochromocytomas generally are found in the paravertebral sulci along the course of the sympathetic chains. According to Symington and Goodall (1953), the pheochromocytoma is in this mediastinal location in 1% of all patients. Grossly, the pleura overlying the mass is markedly vascular. Maier and Humphreys (1958) emphasized that marked bleeding may occur with incision of the pleura, even when the incision is made at a distance from the mass. The tumor, when exposed, is a soft, glandular growth, often reddish brown. Microscopically, the tissue is composed of groups of epithelial cells separated by capillaries. When fixed with a solution of potassium bichromate, the cytoplasm of these cells is filled with brown granules. These cells contain synaptophysin, the 'umbrella' marker of neuroendocrine differentiation, and react immunocytochemically to the monoclonal antibody SY 38.

The surgical removal of the tumor has the same dangers as removal of such a tumor located elsewhere in the body. Appropriate drugs should be available for control of the possible severe fluctuations of the blood pressure.

Occasionally, the tumor may be hidden in the visceral compartment within the arterial wall or closely applied to the aortopulmonary window. The lesions in the latter two areas are difficult to locate by routine means. Shapiro and associates (1984) reported the value of the use of ^{131}I-metaiodobenzylguanidine—[131]I-MIGB—scintigraphy supplemented with dynamic scanning—rapid sequence—computed tomography in the localization of such lesions. Once they are identified, surgical excision is indicated. When the tumor is within the heart muscle, cardiopulmonary bypass may be necessary for its removal.

The prognosis after removal of these lesions, when they are benign, is good. For malignant pheochromocytoma, the prognosis is poor.

Malignant Small Cell Tumor of the Thoracopulmonary Region

Askin and associates (1979) described a malignant small cell tumor of the thoracopulmonary region in childhood that may present as a paravertebral mass, although it is more common in the posterior chest wall or even in the lung. Many believe that this is a peripheral neuroectodermal tumor—PNET—possibly arising from an intercostal nerve. This position is supported by the identification of neurosecretory granules and cell processes indicative of neuronal differentiation on electron microscopy and more importantly the immunohistochemical demonstration of neuron-specific enolase in these tumors, as Linnoila and colleagues (1986) reported. Whether synaptophysin is present has not been reported.

The Askin tumor—PNET—is seen in older children and young adolescents and is discovered either as a chest wall mass or as a roentgenographic chest mass in a child with thoracic symptoms. It is three times more common in girls than in boys. Wide en bloc excision is the standard therapy, followed by irradiation and chemotherapy when the resection is incomplete. The lesion tends to recur locally, although distant metastases may be observed. Long-term survival is infrequent. Survival is often less than 1 year—Askin and colleagues (1979) noted a median survival of 8 months.

THYMOMAS

Tumors of the thymus are common, perhaps the most common lesion arising in the mediastinum of adults. Rarely are they discovered in children. The inclusion of thymic hyperplasia as a thymic tumor in children is inappropriate. This only tends to confuse the issue of the incidence of true mediastinal tumors in this age group. Thymomas are the most common masses found in the anterior mediastinum. On occasion, a thymoma is discovered in the visceral compartment, especially in the anterior cardiophrenic angle.

Thymomas are discussed in detail in Chapter 91, but several important features should be emphasized here.

First, most thymomas are benign. Second, the benignancy or malignancy of the tumor is most readily determined by the lesion's gross features, that is, presence or absence of invasion into adjacent structures or the presence of distant metastases. Third, many of these tumors are associated with specific disease states: myasthenia gravis, erythrocytic agenesis, acquired agammaglobulinemia, and Cushing's syndrome.

In clinical practice these tumors are appropriately divided into those that initially appear clinically benign—no symptoms or signs of local invasion—and those that are frankly malignant—with chest pain, dyspnea, pleural effusion, superior vena caval syndrome, and so forth or with obvious distant metastases. Of the clinically benign lesions, 20 to 30% are invasive into surrounding structures at operation. The noninvasive—benign—thymoma can be considered stage I, and the asymptomatic, locally invasive lesion stage II. The clinically malignant lesions with local, clinically symptomatic intrathoracic disease can be classified as stage III, and those with distant metastases as stage IV. Stage II patients respond well and stage III patients respond poorly to surgical excision and irradiation. Stage IV disease has generally been considered unusual, but Cohen (1984) and co-workers found distant metastases—to liver, bone, and brain—in approximately one quarter of the patients in their series with invasive thymoma.

Rosai and Higa (1972, 1976) described and Wick and associates (1982) from Mayo Clinic reported carcinoid tumors of the thymus. These tumors are aggressive, and 75% of affected patients die of distant metastases. Long-term survival is infrequent. These tumors, in their clinical behavior, production of amine precursors, decarboxylase-type hormones, metastatic spread, response to therapy, and prognosis are more like small cell tumors of the lung than like carcinoid tumors elsewhere in the body.

GERM CELL TUMORS

Both benign and malignant teratomas, including various malignant mediastinal extragonadal germ-cell tumors—seminoma, embryonal cell carcinoma, choriocarcinomas, and endodermal sinus tumor, the so-called yolk sac tumor—have been classified generically as germ cell tumors. As a group, these germ cell tumors are the fourth most common lesion in the mediastinum of the adult—8 to 15%—and the third in the child—12 to 24%. These are almost always found in the anterior compartment, but a few are located elsewhere within the mediastinum. These tumors may be discovered at any age, but are more common in the second, third, or fourth decade of life. The incidence is approximately the same in men as in women.

Ovrum and Birkeland (1979) and Parker and associates (1983) suggested that the germ cell tumors be classified as benign teratoma—teratodermoids; seminomas; and malignant teratomas—choriocarcinoma, embryonal carcinoma, teratocarcinoma, and endodermal sinus tumor. In the adult, 80 to 85% of the germ cell tumors are

benign, but Lack and colleagues (1985) reported that only 57% of these lesions in patients 16 years of age or younger were benign.

Benign Teratomas—Teratodermoids

Willis (1953) defined teratomas as true tumors composed of multiple tissues foreign to the part in which they are found. The tumors display varying degrees of progressive and uncoordinated growth.

These tumors have been separated into three categories: epidermoid cysts, dermoid cysts, and teratomas. An epidermoid cyst is lined by simple squamous cell epithelium. A dermoid cyst has a squamous epithelial lining containing elements of skin appendages that form hair and sebaceous material (Fig. 90–14). A teratoma is solid or cystic and contains readily recognized cellular elements of two or three germinal layers. On extensive histological investigation of any of these three lesions, however, elements from more than one germinal layer are found. Thus, all three are best classified as teratomas or, as some suggest, teratodermoids. The gross features then can be used to subgroup them into cystic or solid tumors.

Teratomas are thought to originate from totipotential embryonic cells that escaped the influence of the primary

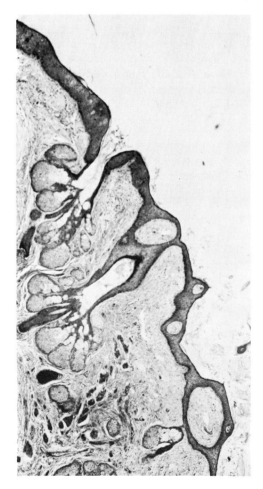

Fig. 90–14. Photomicrograph of the inner wall of a dermoid cyst.

organizers. This event probably occurs near the primitive streak, and therefore, median and paramedian parts are affected. In the mediastinum, teratomas are thought to originate from cells near the third branchial cleft and pouch.

Almost all benign teratomas are found in the anterior mediastinum; in Lewis and associates' (1983) series of 86 patients, this was the site in 97%. A few have been found in the visceral and the paravertebral regions. Morrison (1958) suggested that paravertebral lesions arise from notochordal remnants.

About two thirds of the benign teratomas occurring in adults are asymptomatic. Although many of these lesions are symptomatic in infants and children, Whittaker and Lynn (1973) noted that most are not. Pain in the thorax is the most common complaint. Dyspnea and cough, which may be productive, are the next most common symptoms. In the Mayo series reported by Lewis and associates (1983), these symptoms were present in 61%, 31%, and 28% respectively. Rarely, if a benign cystic teratoma becomes infected, rupture into an adjacent structure may occur. When communication exists with the tracheobronchial tree, hair—trichoptysis—and greasy material are coughed up. With rupture of the cyst into the pleural space, empyema develops. Marsten and his colleagues (1966) and others have reported communication with the pericardium and subsequent tamponade. Erosion into a major vascular structure also has been reported.

Physical findings usually are absent, unless the tumor is malignant. At times, as Le Roux (1962) noted in 5 of 21 patients, when a benign tumor is large, the ribs and costal cartilage overlying the mass may bulge anteriorly. Lewis and associates (1983) found this or a neck mass in 5 of their 86 patients—6%. Roentgenographic examination reveals that the benign teratoma is located in the anterior mediastinum, although on the posteroanterior view, the mass usually projects asymmetrically into either the right or left hemithorax. The outline is smooth and well defined. Le Roux (1960) reported that a calcified rim is present in one third of the lesions, and Lewis and colleagues (1983) found calcification in 26% of their patients (Fig. 90–15). Calcifications within the mass that can be interpreted as rudimentary teeth occasionally appear.

Computed tomography may demonstrate the extent of the lesion better than standard roentgenograms. It also may reveal areas of differing densities consistent with fat, muscle, or other tissue types as well as cystic areas within the mass (Fig. 90–16). Computed tomography, however, is not diagnostic and is not essential in the evaluation of patients suspected of having a benign teratoma.

Benign teratomas are treated by surgical resection. The mass may be approached through either a left or right standard posterolateral thoracotomy, depending upon into which hemithorax the lesion bulges. Most lesions, however, are smaller and less frequently associated with complications than in the past and can readily be approached through a median sternotomy. Excision

is sometimes difficult because of dense adhesions to adjacent intrathoracic structures—pericardium, lung, great vessels, thymus, chest wall, hilar structures, and diaphragm. Complete excision should be attempted and usually can be accomplished, but tissue may need to be left behind to avoid injury to a vital structure.

The prognosis with excision is excellent, even when complete excision is impossible. Postoperative irradiation or other adjuvant measures are not indicated in any of these patients.

Mediastinal Seminomas

The origin of these tumors as well as that of the other malignant extragonadal germ cell tumors of the mediastinum is debated. The two more common views are that they are derived from somatic cells arising from the branchial cleft region in relation to the thymic anlage or that they arise from an extragonadal or extraembryonic yolk sac germ cell whose migration along the urogenital ridge to the gonad has been arrested near the developing thymus. Regardless of these extragonadal mediastinal seminomas' origin, their anatomic relationship to the thymus is striking, and many classified them as a subgroup of thymic tumors.

Bush (1981), Hurt (1982), and Aygum (1984) and their associates reviewed this tumor. The mediastinal seminomas are the most common of the malignant germ cell tumors. In a small series of malignant mediastinal tumors, Adkins and colleagues (1984) found that 13% were seminomas. The tumor is found almost exclusively in young men. It is located in the anterior compartment and is associated with symptoms in 80% of the affected persons. The symptoms are those produced by a malignant anterior mediastinal mass. Roentgenograms of the chest usually reveal a large anterior mediastinal mass (Fig. 90–17). Imaging techniques of the chest add little to the preoperative investigation but computed tomography of the testes may be indicated when the testes are normal to palpation to rule out an occult testicular primary. Alpha-fetoprotein—AFP—and beta-human chorionic gonadotropin—β-HCG—levels should be obtained in all young adult men with suspected malignant anterior mediastinal masses, but these levels are negative in almost all patients with pure seminomatous tumors. Seven percent have an elevated β-HCG level, but AFP has not been reported.

The diagnosis of the seminomatous tumor is established by biopsy of the mass, preferably at the time of surgical excision. All or as much of the tumor as possible should removed as the initial therapeutic maneuver; this is best done through a median sternotomy approach. Postoperatively, irradiation is given at a dose level of 45 to 50 Gy. Chemotherapy is used additionally in those patients with high risk of failure—those patients who present with advanced disease as evidenced by fever, superior vena cava obstruction, or supraclavicular lymph node involvement or those over 35 years of age. Chemotherapy is also indicated in those patients with disseminated disease; the skeletal system and lungs being the most common sites of metastasis. The chemotherapeutic

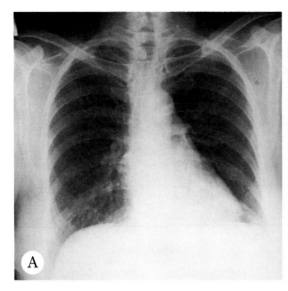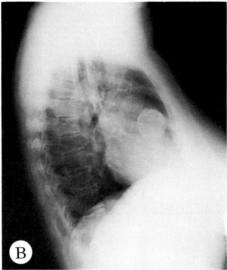

Fig. 90–15. *A* and *B*, PA and lateral roentgenograms of the chest showing a dermoid cyst of the anterior mediastinum. A rim of calcium is present in the wall of the cyst.

regimen used most often consists of varying combinations of vinblastine, bleomycin, and cisplatin.

The prognosis of most patients with pure primary mediastinal seminoma is good; 5-year survival is 50 to 80%. Bush and colleagues (1981) reported an actuarial survival of 69% at 10 years. When death results from the disease, it is usually the result of distant metastases.

Nonseminomatous Malignant Germ Cell Tumors

These tumors as a group are less common than the pure seminomas. They are found almost exclusively in the anterior compartment. Most are seen in young men, but some of these tumors may occur in children as well. The varieties are pure and mixed embryonal carcinomas, teratocarcinomas, choriocarcinomas, and the rare endodermal sinus—yolk sac—tumors. Elevated levels of either β-HCG or AFP, or both, are seen in most of these patients. These studies, as well as abdominal computed tomography, should be obtained in all these patients. Careful examination and computed tomography of the testes is also indicated. Klinefelter's syndrome may be associated with these tumors.

Embryonal Carcinomas

These tumors occur in both children and adults. Clinically and roentgenographically they resemble seminomas. Histologically they resemble pure or mixed embryonal cell carcinoma of the testes.

Endodermal Sinus—Yolk Sac—Tumors

These tumors, unlike the choriocarcinomas, are found in infants and children as well as in adults. They occur only infrequently in the mediastinum and are more commonly seen in the gonads and in sacrococcygeal teratomas. Teilum (1959, 1976) initially described these lesions. Histologically they are variegated, with papillary and tuboalveolar patterns of cystic spaces lined by co-

lumnar and cuboidal epithelium. Glomeruloid structures known as Schiller-Duval bodies and intracytoplasmic eosinophilic hyaline bodies are characteristic findings. Alpha-fetoprotein production is found in endodermal sinus tumors regardless of their location. As Grigor and associates (1977) noted, alpha-fetoprotein production in gonadal or extragonadal germ cell tumors is almost always associated with either embryonal or yolk sac components.

Primary Choriocarcinoma

These tumors occur in the anterior compartment in young adult men. The patient usually presents with cough, chest pain, and gynecomastia. Gynecomastia is present in over half the patients and is believed to result from β-HCG production, which occurs in approximately 60% of these tumors. The hormone presumably is produced by the trophoblastic element of the tumor. As Walden and his associates (1977) pointed out, the measurement of this tumor marker is essential in the management of these patients.

Teratocarcinoma

These are mixed cell lesions. Histologically they resemble malignant teratoma. Germ cell elements may be present. Their presentation and behavior is essentially that of the embryonal and endodermal sinus tumors.

Management of Nonseminomatous Germ Cell Tumors

Almost all of these malignant nonseminomatous germ cell tumors are nonresectable at the time of presentation. Until the 1980s, multimodality therapy, including partial excision, chemotherapy, and irradiation, failed to control these tumors. With the development of more effective chemotherapeutic regimens, better results are being obtained, but as Fevern (1980) and Garnick (1983) and their associates noted, response to even the most aggressive

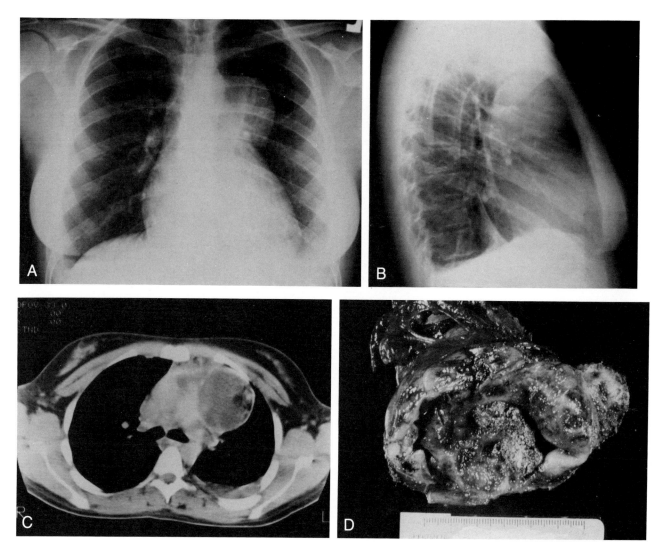

Fig. 90–16. Benign germ cell tumor in an asymptomatic young adult woman. *A* and *B*, PA and lateral roentgenograms of chest show lesion projecting into left hemithorax. *C*, CT scan of chest reveals growth to the right as well as posterior displacement of tracheal bifurcation and the great vessels. *D*, Gross specimen of resected lesion, which was densely adherent to surrounding structures.

approach is less in extragonadal mediastinal primaries than in extragonadal retroperitoneal primaries and even less than in those of testicular origin. Nonetheless, it appears that patients with extragonadal, nonseminomatous germ cell tumors associated with elevated levels of either β-HCG or AFP or both should undergo an intensive course of chemotherapy with multiple drugs, including cisplatin, bleomycin, and vinblastine or etoposide—VP 16-213. Those who respond completely or partially, with disappearance of or fall in the levels of tumor marker and shrinkage of the local tumor, should undergo surgical resection. Chemotherapy with doxorubicin or other drugs may be given postoperatively. The role of adjuvant irradiation is unsettled; Parker (1983) and Kay (1987) and their associates' early results are encouraging. In those patients in whom the levels of the tumor markers remain high, however, surgical intervention is of no benefit and should not be carried out. Irradiation and additional chemotherapy are also of little

avail. Nonresponding patients usually die within 6 months. (See Chapter 98.)

TUMORS OF LYMPH NODES

Neoplastic involvement of mediastinal lymph nodes occurs frequently, and if secondary involvement by metastatic tumor is included, represents the most common mediastinal mass. The actual incidence of primary lymphomas of the mediastinum is, however, difficult to determine, although in Davis and associates' (1987) series from Duke University, lymphomas were the second most common solid masses encountered in the mediastinum. Therefore, the possibility of these lesions must be considered in both children and adults with mediastinal masses. Mullen and Richardson (1986) reported that lymphomas are responsible for 45% of the anterior mediastinal masses seen in children and thus are the most common tumor in this location in this age group. In

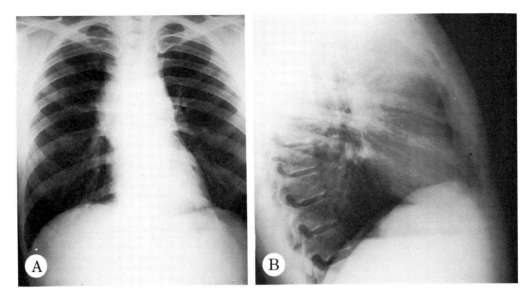

Fig. 90–17. *A* and *B*, PA and lateral laminograms of the chest of a young adult male with a large seminomatous tumor of the anterior mediastinum. (Shields, T.W., Fox, R.T., and Lees, W.M.: Thymic tumors. Arch. Surg. 96:617, 1966.)

adults they reported it to be the second leading cause of anterior mediastinal masses seen in clinical practice.

Most often, the lymph nodes of the anterior compartment are involved (Fig. 90–18), but extension to or primary origin from lymph nodes in the visceral compartment is common. Occasionally, primary involvement of posterior intercostal lymph nodes appears in the paravertebral sulci or as a mass posterior to the esophagus, distending this structure anteriorly and to either the right or left from the midline.

On roentgenographic examination, the mass is usually bilateral and irregular. Distortion and compression of adjacent structures are readily demonstrated by appropriate roentgenographic studies. Arteriography and lymphangiography are sometimes indicated. Computed tomography helps delineate the extent of the mass (Fig. 90–19), but it has little diagnostic specificity.

The age groups involved, as well as the sex ratio, vary with the underlying histopathology of the lesion. Numerous classifications have been proposed, but it is best to classify the malignant lesions as either Hodgkin's disease or non-Hodgkin's lymphoma. Staging of mediastinal lymphoma, as van Heerden and colleagues suggested, is shown in Table 90–7.

Although 20 to 30% of the patients are asymptomatic, 60 to 70% have symptoms of the local malignant disease and 30 to 35% have such systemic manifestations as fever, weight loss, fatigue, and pruritus. Signs of involvement

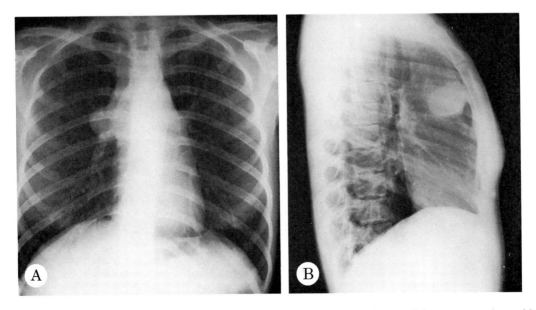

Fig. 90–18. *A* and *B*, PA and lateral chest roentgenograms of a young female with Hodgkin's disease of the anterior mediastinal lymph nodes.

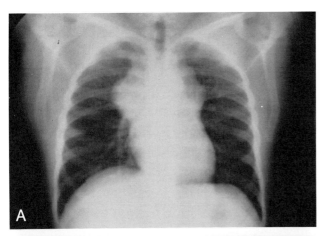

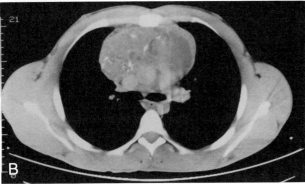

Fig. 90–19. *A*, Roentgenogram of the chest of a symptomatic young adult with a superior vena caval syndrome revealing large, irregular, anterior mediastinal mass. *B*, CT reveals large tumor mass obliterating the vena cava and encroaching upon the great vessels and distorting the tracheal bifurcation. Biopsy revealed a non-Hodgkin's lymphoma.

of adjacent structures are present frequently, and palpable lymph nodes in the neck are noted in 10 to 15% of the patients.

Diagnosis is established by biopsy of cervical nodes or of the mass itself via an anterior mediastinotomy. At times, even a definitive resection of the mediastinal mass may be carried out.

Mediastinal Hodgkin's Disease

The average age of the patient is 30 years, and the sex ratio is about equal. Systemic symptoms—fever, night sweats—are common, although local signs and symptoms are unusual at the time of discovery of the disease. The

Table 90–7. Clinical Staging of Mediastinal Lymphoma

Stage I*	Limited to mediastinum
Stage II*	1. Limited to two contiguous anatomic lymphatic regions (including lymph nodes and thymus)
	2. In more than two anatomic regions above the diaphragm, including lymph nodes, thymus, pleura, lung, and pericardium
Stage III*	Involvement below diaphragm or distant involvement

*Subgroup A with and subgroup B without systemic symptoms.
van Heerden, J.A., et al.: Mediastinal malignant lymphoma. Chest 57:518, 1970.

nodular sclerosing variant is common, and needle biopsy of the mass is rarely diagnostic. Mediastinotomy is usually the diagnostic procedure of choice. Therapy consists of irradiation and combined chemotherapy if relapse occurs. Bergh and associates (1978) wrote that patients with Hodgkin's disease confined to the thymus represent a special clinical situation. In such patients they recommended radical excision with postoperative irradiation as the therapy of choice. Generally, the prognosis for patients with Hodgkin's disease limited to the mediastinum is excellent, as Vaeth and associates (1976) reported. Advanced clinical disease or older age at time of diagnosis generally suggests a poorer prognosis.

Mediastinal Non-Hodgkin's Lymphoma

Non-Hodgkin's lymphoma infrequently originates in the mediastinum; Levitt and co-workers (1982) reported mediastinal origin in only 5.6% of 215 patients with these diseases. The lymphoma is usually of the diffuse histiocytic subtype. Most patients are young adults, although persons in the first five decades of life may develop these tumors. Unlike patients with Hodgkin's disease, over 75% are symptomatic, with dyspnea from tracheal compression and chest pain being common complaints. Superior vena caval obstruction also is common at presentation. Chemotherapy with or without radiation therapy is the treatment of choice. Despite the older literature, resection does not have a place in managing these patients. The prognosis appears to be less favorable than that for patients with Hodgkin's disease, possibly because of the advanced stage of the disease at presentation. Patients under the age of 15 appear to do the poorest of all.

MISCELLANEOUS TUMORS

Vascular Tumors

Various vascular tumors, both benign and malignant, occur in the mediastinum. Although many mediastinal tumors in infants and children are vascular, only one third of 38 mediastinal vascular tumors reviewed by Attar and Cowley (1964) were found in persons younger than 20 years. The other two thirds occurred in older persons, mostly in the fourth and fifth decades of life. The incidence in men and women is approximately equal.

Most vascular tumors occur in the anterior mediastinum and adjacent visceral compartment. The remaining fourth are present in the posterior aspect of the visceral compartment and the paravertebral sulci. Generally, the tumor is solid and discrete, although diffuse infiltrative lesions have been reported. Calcification—phlebolith—occasionally occurs. Bony erosion or enlargement of an intervertebral foramen also may occur.

Approximately 30% of these tumors produce no symptoms. Large masses and malignant lesions are more likely to be symptomatic. Concurrent vascular tumors may be present in the neck or elsewhere.

Various histologic types are seen. Most of these tumors are benign. The benign lesions have been classified as hemangioendotheliomas, capillary hemangiomas, and cavernous hemangiomas; the malignant lesions are designated angiosarcomas or hemangioendotheliosarcomas. Although the malignant lesions occur in all age groups, they are most common in the fourth decade of life.

At thoracotomy, the vascular tumors are often soft, encapsulated, dark purplish masses and may or may not pulsate. Both benign and malignant tumors may infiltrate adjacent structures. Enucleation, when possible, is carried out, but sometimes only partial resection can be accomplished because of infiltration of vital structures even by benign tumors. Blood loss may be extensive. Postoperative irradiation appears to have little value. When the tumor is benign, even if it is not removed in its entirety, the prognosis is favorable. If malignant, the prognosis is poor.

Parathyroid Adenomas

A normal parathyroid gland, usually one of the lower two from either third branchial pouch, may be found within the thymic capsule, in the lower part of the neck, or in the anterior mediastinum in 20% of the population. In a series of 400 patients with parathyroid adenomas, Nathaniels and his colleagues (1970) found that 84 tumors were located in the mediastinum; four fifths of these tumors were in the anterior compartment, and the remaining fifth were in the visceral compartment. These adenomas were associated with the clinical and laboratory findings of hyperparathyroidism. Rarely, the adenoma is discernible by roentgenographic examination of the chest. The barium-filled esophagus is occasionally indented.

High resolution computed tomography is the procedure of choice to localize parathyroid tissue in the neck and upper mediastinum. Both nonenhanced and contrast-enhanced scans should be done. Technetium-thallium subtracting imaging, as Gimlette and Taylor (1985) noted, and ultrasound scanning may also help identify abnormally located parathyroid tissue; Stark and associates (1985) reported that the combination of these noninvasive studies is 91% sensitive in detecting parathyroid lesions. These adenomas are usually found during a cervical exploration. Their blood supply is from the neck, and almost all of them can be removed by way of this approach. If removal by this route is unsuccessful, however, mediastinal exploration is carried out 3 to 4 weeks later through a median sternotomy. Only 5% of the patients require this procedure. The thymus, along with the adjacent tissues, is removed during the exploration.

Carcinoma of a parathyroid gland in the mediastinum has been reported infrequently. It may arise in a displaced gland or may arise in a supernumerary gland, as Kastan and associates (1987) reported. Most patients present with hyperparathyroidism. Excision should be attempted initially through the neck; if this fails, sternotomy should be done.

Ectopic Thyroid

True aberrant thyroid tissue is infrequently found in the anterior mediastinum. The actual incidence of its occurrence is unknown. Usually the patient is asymptomatic and the mass is discovered only on routine roentgenographic study of the chest. The ectopic thyroid tissue is not continuous with the normal gland in the neck. The blood supply is direct from one of the great vessels within the mediastinum. The mass is removed readily, with ligation of its vascular pedicle, through either a median sternotomy or posterolateral thoracotomy approach. Theoretically, the mediastinal thyroid could represent all of the thyroid tissue that the patient has, but scanning of the neck after administration of ^{131}I may reveal a normal cervical gland.

Benign Lymph Node Lesions

Sarcoidosis

Sarcoidosis frequently involves the lymph nodes in the mediastinum, but it is rarely difficult to differentiate this condition from a primary mediastinal tumor. Granulomatous or hamartomatous involvement of mediastinal lymph nodes may, however, appear as a primary mediastinal tumor.

Mediastinal Granulomas

These lesions arise from granulomatous infection of a lymph node or nodes. Histoplasmosis, tuberculosis, and sarcoidosis cause some instances, but the cause usually remains obscure. Mediastinal granulomas occur in any age group and in either sex.

These granulomas are found in the visceral compartment. The paratracheal area, more often on the right than the left, the subcarinal space, and the paraesophageal region are the sites of predilection. Roentgenographic examination reveals these tumors to be solid, discrete lesions of uniform density (Fig. 90–20). Slightly less than half contain variable amounts of calcium. Of those containing calcium, more than two thirds are heavily calcified (Fig. 90–21) and the remainder show stippled calcification.

More than half of the patients have no symptoms; the

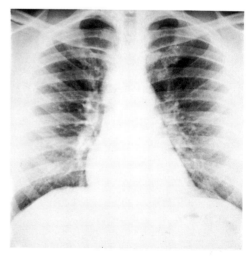

Fig. 90–20. PA roentgenogram of the chest of a young adult male with mediastinal granuloma in the right paratracheal region.

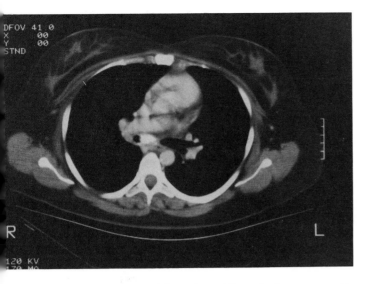

Fig. 90–21. CT exam of chest of a middle-aged white woman with mediastinal granuloma most evident in the subcarinal region. Massive hemoptysis caused by erosion of a bronchial artery into the right main stem bronchus necessitated sleeve resection of the involved area.

others experience coughing, hemoptysis, and recurrent episodes of fever, lithoptysis, and dysphagia. The superior vena cava may be obstructed and a bronchoesophageal fistula may develop (see Chapter 67).

Surgical therapy is indicated to establish the diagnosis in the uncalcified lesions and is chosen as definitive treatment of symptomatic granulomas. Ferguson and Burford (1965) do not recommend prophylactic removal of the asymptomatic heavily calcified granulomas, although half of these eventually produce symptoms. Sakulsky and his associates (1967), however, recommended that all granulomas, symptomatic or not, be removed.

Occasionally, the granuloma can be enucleated, but more frequently, dense adhesions to adjacent structures preclude its total removal. In this circumstance, the capsule is incised and the contents are evacuated. As much of the capsule is removed as can be accomplished easily, and the remaining portion is curetted down to a clean fibrous base. No serious complications attending this technique have been noted.

When the vena cava is obstructed, vascular reconstruction is not recommended, but a bronchoesophageal fistula requires excision of the fistulous tract and closure of both the tracheal and esophageal openings.

The prognosis, once the granuloma is removed, is good, and almost all patients become asymptomatic.

Mediastinal Lymphoid Hamartoma

Mediastinal lymph node hyperplasia, which is also known as Castleman's disease (1956), is a rare benign process that appears as a mediastinal mass. It is found most often in the visceral compartment, although about one fourth occur in either paravertebral sulci.

Usually the patient has no symptoms. Occasionally, as Sethi and Kepes (1971) reported, chronic anemia or dysproteinemia may be associated with this lesion. The lesion may be found in any age group, but more often it occurs in the adolescent or young adult. Its incidence is the same in women as in men.

On roentgenographic examination of the chest, a lymphoid hamartoma appears to be well circumscribed, although its surface frequently is lobulated. Contrast-enhanced CT demonstrates vascular lesions within the mass. Aortograms confirm the marked vascularity of the mass, and a systemic blood supply may be demonstrated (Fig. 90–22).

Grossly, the lesion appears to be encapsulated and composed of conglomerate masses of lympoid tissue. Dense adhesions to adjacent structures often are present. On cut section, the mass is homogeneously grayish red. Microscopically, lymphoid tissue is interspersed with a vascular and fibrous tumor. Zones of mature lymphocytes are arranged concentrically about central zones of larger, eosinophilic cells in a whorled pattern. Areas of hyalinization may be present. The stroma is characterized by its rich vascularity, with capillary proliferation and endothelial thickening of the larger vessels.

Operative removal is indicated, primarily because of the diagnostic difficulties presented. Total removal should be attempted, but vital structures should not be sacrificed. The rich blood supply of the lesion frequently makes the operative removal difficult.

The prognosis for these patients is excellent. Recurrence has not been noted, even though some of the reported surgical excisions were incomplete.

Lipomas

Fatty tumors occur anywhere within the mediastinum but are more commonly located anteriorly. Most are benign and many become large. Even a large lipoma, because of its pliability, rarely causes symptoms.

Roentgenographically, a fatty tumor is less dense than other masses. Examination of the patient in different positions often reveals different contours of the mass because of the effect of gravity on the soft, pliable fatty tissue. With the patient in an upright position, an hourglass or teardrop configuration is occasionally noted. As a rule, the lipoma is easily enucleated. The prognosis is excellent.

Liposarcomas are encountered only rarely. Schweitzer and Aguam (1977) summarized the data of 50 such tumors in the mediastinum. Symptoms are related as a rule to the size and location of the tumor, but as Razzuk and associates (1971) noted, many of these lesions are asymptomatic until the condition is terminal. The tumor may be either well differentiated or poorly differentiated. The latter metastasize to distant sites in 40% of the patients, but the well differentiated tumors rarely do. Surgical excision combined with postoperative radiation therapy appears to be the treatment of choice.

OTHER MESENCHYMAL TUMORS

Fibromas, both benign and malignant, occur in the mediastinum. Pleural effusion may develop with either type. Myxomas, xanthomas, leiomyomas, leiomyosarcomas, rhabdomyosarcomas, and even extraosseous pri-

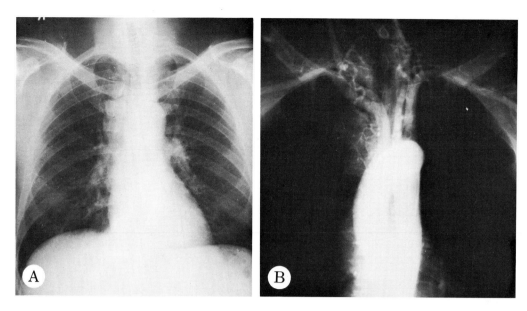

Fig. 90–22. *A*, PA roentgenogram of the chest of a middle-aged adult male with a large right paratracheal mass that proved to be a mediastinal lymphoid hamartoma. *B*, Aortogram reveals the major blood supply to the mass arising from the right internal mammary artery. (Haid, S., and Shields, T.W.: Mediastinal lymphoid hamartoma. Arch. Surg. *101*:442, 1970.)

mary osteogenic sarcoma, as Ikeda and his colleagues (1974) reported, have occurred in the mediastinum.

MEDIASTINAL CYSTS

Various cysts arise within the mediastinum. The largest number of these are located in the visceral compartment, but neither the anterior compartment nor the paravertebral areas are spared.

Roentgenographic examination of the chest usually reveals a well circumscribed, rounded density in one of the mediastinal compartments. On occasion, depending on thickness and rigidity of the capsule, the cyst may assume an ovoid or a teardrop configuration when the patient is examined in the erect position. At times the capsule is calcified. An air-fluid level may be present if a communication exists between the cyst and either the respiratory or gastrointestinal tract. Distortion of the trachea and of the barium-filled esophagus also may appear. If the cyst is attached to the esophagus or within its walls, it may move upward on deglutition.

Enterogenous Cysts

These cysts result from sequestration of cells from the region of the laryngotracheal groove during the development of the tracheobronchial tree from the primitive foregut. Histologically, these legions can be classified as bronchogenic, esophageal, or gastric cysts, depending on the cellular structure of the lining and the cellular contents within the cyst wall (Fig. 90–23). There is a variable combination of cellular elements: ciliated columnar, cuboidal, and flattened epithelium; mucous glands; smooth muscle; fibrous tissue; elastic tissue; and cartilage. Typical intestinal or gastric mucosa occasionally can be identified. The term "enteric duplication" is used when the cyst is highly differentiated. Such cysts may

be contiguous to or even within the wall of the esophagus.

The enterogenous cysts are almost always unilocular and occur in the visceral compartment. They constitute approximately 11% of mediastinal lesions in adults and 24% in children. Sulzer and associates (1970), in reviewing 40 of these cysts, found that all except 5 were associated with the trachea or esophagus. Two thirds of

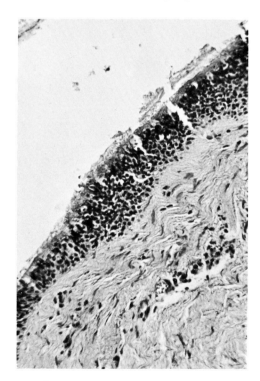

Fig. 90–23. Photomicrograph of the inner lining of an enterogenous cyst of the mediastinum.

these were located in the upper half of the mediastinum and were associated most often with the trachea or the tracheal bifurcation (Fig. 90–24); the remainder were in the lower portion of the mediastinum and were associated with the esophagus.

Almost all of these cysts are asymptomatic in adults, whereas in young children and infants most are symptomatic. In young children and infants the symptoms result from tracheobronchial obstruction. Frequently, severe respiratory distress is noted, and marked dyspnea and cyanosis are often present. Hyperinflation, atelectasis, or infection of either lung occurs. As Eraklis and his colleagues (1969) pointed out, the cyst can be identified only infrequently on routine roentgenographic study of the chest in the symptomatic infant. Computed tomography of the chest may prove to be helpful in identifying these lesions preoperatively, but as Mendelson and colleagues (1983) noted, this may not always reveal its cystic nature.

Early and prompt recognition of the cyst is imperative in the symptomatic infant. If untreated, all these infants die, as Opsahl and Berman (1962) pointed out and Eraklis and his associates (1969) emphasized.

The prognosis with removal of these cysts in infants and children, as well as in adults, is excellent.

Neurenteric Cysts

A second cystic anomaly of the gastrointestinal tract is found in the posterior portion of the visceral compartment extending into either paravertebral region. This is the neurenteric cyst, which contains not only entodermal derivatives but also ectodermal—neurogenic—elements. It most commonly is discovered in infants.

Associated defects of the vertebral column and abnormalities of the spinal canal and its coverings are also found in these patients. Feller and Sternberg (1929) called this combination the split notochord syndrome. The defect is believed to occur during the blastocyst stage of early embryologic development. It is thought that varying degrees of adhesions between the entodermal cells of the yolk sac and the ectodermal cells of the future neural plate occur. As a result, the notochord cannot develop in its normal midline position, and the cells from which it develops are displaced to either side or split, so that two notochordal centers result. Consequently, abnormalities of the vertebral column, spinal canal, and alimentary tract occur in conjunction with each other.

Characteristically, a neurenteric cyst is connected by a stalk to the meninges and spinal cord. The spinal deformities include congenital scoliosis, hemivertebrae, and spina bifida as well as other defects. The cyst also may connect with the gastrointestinal tract and thus represent a portion of a thoracoabdominal duplication of the alimentary tract. Either connecting stalk may be patent.

Roentgenographic examination reveals a posteriorly located mass associated with spinal deformities; tomograms and CT may be necessary to demonstrate the bony abnormalities. At times, depending on the patency of the stalk to the alimentary tract, air may be found in the cyst. Myelography and MRI are indicated to define the deformities of the spinal canal and the possible patency of the stalk connecting the cyst to the spinal canal.

Neurenteric cysts frequently compress adjacent structures and thus cause symptoms, particularly in infants, who generally present with respiratory complaints. In older children, pain or melena are most often the presenting complaints. Gastric mucosa often is present in the cellular lining. As a result, peptic ulceration with pain or bleeding is common.

Surgical excision of the cyst is indicated. The prognosis is good if other associated anomalies are compatible with life.

Mesothelial Cysts

Mesothelial cysts have been referred to variously as pericardial coelomic, pleuropericardial, spring-water, cardiophrenic angle, and simple cysts.

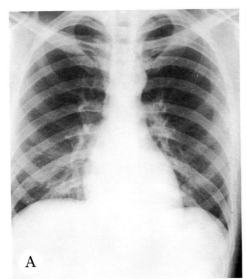
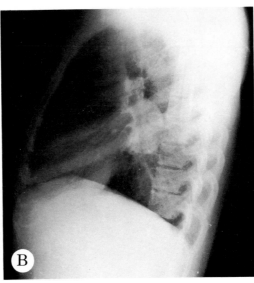

Fig. 90–24. *A and B,* PA and lateral roentgenograms of the chest showing a large bronchogenic cyst located at the tracheal bifurcation.

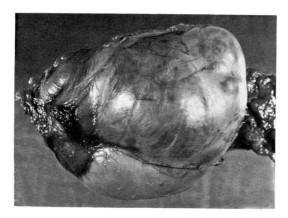

Fig. 90–25. Photograph of a mesothelial—pleuropericardial—cyst of the mediastinum.

Most are found in association with the pericardium, usually in the region of the anterior cardiophrenic angle. A few occur in the hilar area and in the anterior compartment. Lambert (1940) wrote that these cysts result from a failure of fusion of one of the mesenchymal lacunae that normally fuse to form the pericardial sac. Rarely, the cyst may be a true diverticulum of the pericardium, with either a wide or narrow opening. Although the pathogenesis of such a diverticulum may be similar to that described, Lillie and his associates (1950) suggested that it might be an embryologic ventral diverticulum, with persistence of its diverticular connection. In a communication to Drash and Hyer (1950), Kindred advanced a third possible explanation for some of these mesothelial cysts: that some arise from the pleura rather than from the pericardium. This concept was postulated as the result of irregularities or infoldings of the advancing "edge" of the pleural sac during the embryologic expansion of its margins.

Grossly, mesothelial cysts have fibrous walls of varying thickness, are usually unilocular, and contain a clear, watery fluid (Fig. 90–25). Microscopic examination of the wall reveals a single layer of mesothelial cells resting on a loose stroma of connective tissue.

Roentgenographic study usually reveals the cyst to be in a typical location, that is, the anterior cardiophrenic angle, more often the right than the left (Fig. 90–26). On the lateral view, as Ochsner and Ochsner (1966) noted, a teardrop configuration is common, because the cyst tends to conform to the medial aspect of the pulmonary fissure.

The mesothelial cyst is benign, and most authorities now believe that removal is not indicated if precise diagnosis can be reasonably established by the typical position and configuration of the cyst. Needle aspiration of clear, watery fluid from the lesion confirms the diagnosis. If, however, the diagnosis is in doubt or if symptoms are present, resection is indicated.

Teratomatous Cysts

Cystic teratomas, both epidermoids and dermoids, were discussed in the previous section on germ cell tumors.

Cystic Hygromas

As previously mentioned, most cystic hygromas of the mediastinum are extensions of cervical cystic hygromas—lymphangiomas, but occasionally they are isolated mediastinal lesions in either the child or the adult.

The cysts are usually multiloculated, although an isolated mediastinal hygroma may be unilocular (Fig. 90–27). The latter type often is designated simply as a lymphogenous cyst. Both varieties contain a clear yellow or dark-brown fluid.

The cyst usually is found in the anterior compartment, although it frequently extends into the visceral compartment. Removal is usually indicated for diagnostic purposes.

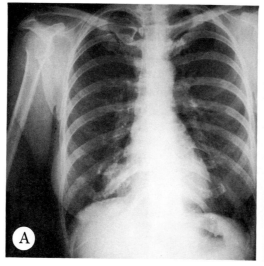
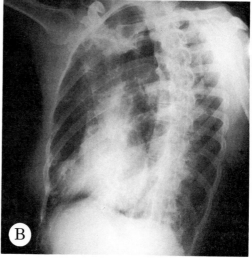

Fig. 90–26. *A* and *B*, PA and oblique roentgenograms of the chest revealing the presence of a pleuropericardial cyst in the right anterior cardiophrenic angle.

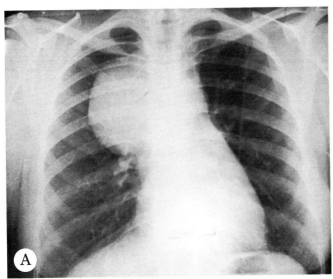
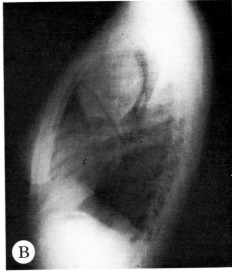

Fig. 90–27. *A* and *B*, PA and lateral chest roentgenograms of a young female with a large isolated, unilocular hygroma of the anterior mediastinum.

Thymic Cysts

Various cystic lesions of the thymus occur. True thymic cysts are thin-walled and unilocular and contain islands of normal thymic tissue within their walls. The lining may be made up of a single layer of low cuboidal cells. These cysts are asymptomatic anterior mediastinal masses and are removed by simple enucleation. Cystic thymomas arise from degeneration within a thymoma. Often, a residual mass is readily identified bulging from the wall of the cyst into the cavity. Such cysts should be considered thymomas and treated as such (Chapter 91).

Thoracic Duct Cysts

These rare mediastinal cysts may arise at any level on the thoracic duct, which lies in the posterior portion of the visceral compartment. Such a cyst may, or may not, communicate with the lumen of the duct. Roentgenographically, the cyst frequently distorts the trachea and the barium-filled esophagus. Theoretically, it could be opacified with contrast material placed into the lymphatic system, but this has not been reported.

Excision of the cyst is indicated, and ligation of the thoracic duct, if required, can be done with impunity.

Miscellaneous Cysts

Simple unilocular cysts may occur anywhere in the mediastinum. Even after removal and histologic examination, these cysts defy specific classification.

REFERENCES

Adam, A., and Hochholzer, L.: Ganglioneuroblastoma of the posterior mediastinum: a clinicopathologic review of 80 cases. Cancer 47:373, 1981.

Adkins, R.B., Jr., Maples, M.D., and Hainsworth, J.D.: Primary malignant mediastinal tumors. Ann. Thorac. Surg. 38:648, 1984.

Akwari, O.E., et al.: Dumbbell neurogenic tumors of the mediastinum. Mayo Clin. Proc. 53:353, 1978.

Ashley, D.J., and Evans, C.J.: Intrathoracic carotid-body tumour (chemodectoma). Thorax 21:184, 1966.

Askin, F.B., et al.: Malignant small cell tumor of the thoracopulmonary region in childhood. Cancer 43:2438, 1979.

Attar, S., and Cowley, R.A.: Hemangioma of the mediastinum. Am. Surg. 30:141, 1964.

Aygum, C., et al.: Primary mediastinal seminoma. Urology 23:109, 1984.

Bergh, N.P., et al.: Tumors of the thymus and thymic region. II. Clinicopathological studies on Hodgkin's disease of the thymus. Ann. Thorac. Surg. 25:99, 1978.

Bush, S.E., Martinez, A., and Bagshaw, M.A.: Primary mediastinal seminoma. Cancer 48:1877, 1981.

Carlsen, N.L., et al.: Prognostic factors in neuroblastomas treated in Denmark from 1943 to 1980: a statistical estimate of prognosis based on 253 cases. Cancer 58:2726, 1986a.

Carlsen, N.L.T., et al.: The prognostic value of different staging systems in neuroblastoma and the completeness of tumor excision. Arch. Dis. Child. 61:832, 1986b.

Castleman, B., Iverson, L., and Menendez, V.P.: Localized mediastinal lymphoid hyperplasia resembling thymoma. Cancer 9:822, 1956.

Catalano, P.W., et al.: Reasonable surgery for thoracic neuroblastoma in infants and children. J. Thorac. Cardiovasc. Surg. 76:459, 1978.

Catinella, F.P., Boyd, A.D., and Spencer, F.C.: Intrathoracic extramedullary hematopoiesis simulating anterior mediastinal tumor. J. Thorac. Cardiovasc. Surg. 89:580, 1985.

Cohen, D.J., et al.: Management of patients with malignant thymoma. J. Thorac. Cardiovasc. Surg. 87:301, 1984.

Coldman, A.J., et al.: Neuroblastoma: influence of age at diagnosis, stage, tumor site, and sex on prognosis. Cancer 46:1896, 1980.

Cushing, H., and Wolbach, S.B.: The transformation of a malignant paravertebral sympathicoblastoma into a benign ganglioneuroma. Am. J. Pathol. 3:203, 1927.

Davidson, K.G., Walbaum, P.R., and McCormack, R.J.M.: Intrathoracic neural tumours. Thorax 33:359, 1978.

Davis, R.D., Jr., et al.: Primary cysts and neoplasms of the mediastinum: recent changes in clinical presentation, methods of diagnosis, management, and results. Ann. Thorac. Surg. 44:229, 1987.

Dooms, G.C., et al.: The potential of magnetic resonance imaging for the evaluation of thoracic arterial diseases. J. Thorac. Cardiovasc. Surg. 92:1088. 1986.

Drash, E.C., and Hyer, H.J.: Mesothelial mediastinal cysts. J. Thorac. Surg. 19:755, 1950.

Eraklis, A.J., Griscom, N.T., and McGovern, J.B.: Bronchogenic cysts of the mediastinum in infancy. N. Engl. J. Med. 281:1150, 1969.

Feller, A., and Sternberg, H.: Zur Kenntnis der Fehlbildungen der Wirbelsaule; die Wirbelkorperspalte und ihre formale Genese. Virchows Arch. Pathol. Anat. *272*:613, 1929.

Ferguson, T.B., and Burford, T.H.: Mediastinal granuloma. Ann. Thorac. Surg. *1*:125, 1965.

Fevern, L.G., Samson, M.K., and Stephens, R.L.: Vinblastine (VLB), bleomycin (BLEO), Cis-Diaminedichoroplatinum (DDP) in disseminated extragonadal germ cell tumors, a Southwest Oncology Group study. Cancer *45*:2543, 1980.

Filler, R.M., et al.: Favorable outlook for children with mediastinal neuroblastoma. J. Pediatr. Surg. *7*:136, 1972.

Gale, A.W., et al.: Neurogenic tumors of the mediastinum. Ann. Thorac. Surg. *17*:434, 1974.

Garnick, M.B., Canellos, G.P., and Richie, J.P.: Treatment and surgical staging of testicular and primary extragonadal germ cell cancer. J.A.M.A. *250*:1733, 1983.

Gimlette, T.M.D., and Taylor, W.H.: Localization of enlarged parathyroid glands by thallium—201 and technetium—99m subtraction imaging. Clin. Nucl. Med. *10*:235, 1985.

Gould, V.E., et al.: Synaptophysin expression in neuroendocrine neoplasms as determined by immunocytochemistry. Am. J. Pathol. *126*:243, 1987.

Grigor, K.M., et al.: Serum alpha-fetoprotein levels in 153 male patients with germ cell tumors. Cancer *33*:252, 1977.

Grillo, H.C., et al.: Combined approach to "dumbbell" intrathoracic and intraspinal neurogenic tumors. Ann. Thorac. Surg. *36*:402, 1983.

Gross, R.E., Farber, S., and Martin, L.W.: Neuroblastoma sympatheticum: a study and report of 217 cases. Pediatrics *23*:1192, 1959.

Hamilton, J.P., and Koop, C.E.: Ganglioneuromas in children. Surg. Gynecol. Obstet. *121*:803, 1965.

Hurt, R.D., et al.: Primary anterior mediastinal seminoma. Cancer *49*:1650, 1982.

Ikeda, T., et al.: Primary osteogenic sarcoma of the mediastinum. Thorax *29*:582, 1974.

Irger, I.M., et al.: Surgical tactics in hour-glass tumor of intervertebral mediastinal localization. Vopr. Neirokhir. (Moscow) *5*:3, 1980.

Johnston, R.H., Jr., et al.: Pancreatic pseudocyst of the mediastinum. Ann. Thorac. Surg. *41*:210, 1986.

Kastan, D.J., et al.: Carcinoma in a mediastinal fifth parathyroid gland. J.A.M.A. *257*:1218, 1987.

Kay, P.H., Wells, F.C., Goldstraw, P.: A multidisciplinary approach to primary nonseminomatous germ cell tumors of the mediastinum. Ann. Thorac. Surg. *44*:578, 1987.

Kelley, M.J., Mannes, E.J., and Ravin, C.E.: Mediastinal masses of vascular origin: a review. J. Thorac. Cardiovasc. Surg. *76*:559, 1978.

Lack, E.E., Weinstein, H.J., and Welch, K.J.: Mediastinal germ cell tumors in children: a clinical and pathological study of 21 cases. J. Thorac. Cardiovasc. Surg. *89*:826, 1985.

Lambert, A.V.S.: Etiology of thin-walled thoracic cysts. J. Thorac. Surg. *10*:1, 1940.

Le Brigand, H.: Nouveau Traite de Technique Chirurgicale, Vol. 3. Paris, Masson, 1973, pp. 658.

Le Roux, B.T.: Mediastinal teratomata. Thorax *15*:333, 1960.

Le Roux, B.T.: Cysts and tumors of the mediastinum. Surg. Gynecol. Obstet. *115*:695, 1962.

Levitt, L.V., Aisenberg, A.C., and Harris, N.L.: Primary non-Hodgkins lymphoma of the mediastinum. Cancer *50*:2486, 1982.

Levowitz, B.S., et al.: Thoracic vertebral chordoma presenting as a posterior mediastinal tumor. Ann. Thorac. Surg. *2*:75, 1966.

Lewis, B.D., et al.: Benign teratomas of the mediastinum. J. Thorac. Cardiovasc. Surg. *86*:727, 1983.

Lillie, W.I., McDonald, J.R.,, and Clagett, O.T.: Pericardial celomic cysts and pericardial diverticula. J. Thorac. Surg. *20*:494, 1950.

Linnoila, R.I., et al.: Evidence for neural origin and PAS-positive variants of the malignant small cell tumor of thoracopulmonary region ("Askin tumor"). Am. J. Surg. Pathol. *10*:124, 1986.

Maier, H.C., and Humphreys, G.H., II: Intrathoracic pheochromocytoma. J. Thorac. Surg. *36*:625, 1958.

Marangos, P.J., and Schmechel, D.: The neurobiology of the brain enolase. *In* Essays in Neurochemistry and Neuropharmacology,

Vol. 4. Edited by M.B.H. Youdin, et al. New York, John Wiley & Sons, Inc., 1980, p. 211.

Marsten, J.L., Cooper, A.G., and Ankeney, J.L.: Acute cardiac tamponade due to perforation of a benign mediastinal teratoma into the pericardial sac. J. Thorac. Cardiovasc. Surg. *51*:700, 1966.

Mendelson, D.S., et al.: Bronchogenic cysts with high CT numbers. Am. J. Radiol. *140*:463, 1983.

Miller, G.A., et al.: CT differentiation of thoracic aortic aneurysm from pulmonary masses adjacent to the mediastinum. J. Comput. Assist. Tomogr. *8*:437, 1984.

Mills, N.L., and Grosfeld, J.L.: One-stage operation for cervicomediastinal cystic hygroma in infancy. J. Thorac. Cardiovasc. Surg. *65*:608, 1973.

Morrison, I.M.: Tumours and cysts of the mediastinum. Thorax *13*:294, 1958.

Mullen, B., and Richardson, J.D.: Primary anterior mediastinal tumors in children and adults. Ann. Thorac. Surg. *42*:338, 1986.

Nathaniels, E.K., Nathaniels, A.M., and Wang, C.: Mediastinal parathyroid tumors. Ann. Surg. *171*:165, 1970.

Ochsner, J.L. and Ochsner, S.F.: Congenitial cysts of the mediastinum. Ann. Surg. *163*:909, 1966.

Olson, J.L., and Salyer, W.R.: Mediastinal paragangliomas (aortic body tumor): a report of four cases and a review of the literature. Cancer *41*:2405, 1978.

Oosterwijk, W.M., and Swierenga, J.: Neurogenic tumours with an intrathoracic localization. Thorax *23*:374, 1968.

Opsahl, T., and Berman, E.J.: Bronchogenic mediastinal cysts in infants. Pediatrics *30*:372, 1962.

Ovrum, E., and Birkeland, S.: Mediastinal tumors and cysts: a review of 191 cases. Scand. J. Thorac. Cardiovasc. Surg. *13*:161, 1979.

Parker, D., Holford, C.P., and Bergent, R.H.: Effective treatment for malignant mediastinal teratoma. Thorax *38*:897, 1983.

Razzuk, M.A., et al.: Liposarcoma of the mediastinum: case report and review of literature. J. Thorac. Cardiovasc. Surg. *61*:819, 1971.

Razzuk, M.A., et al.: Electron microscopical observations on mediastinal neurolemoma, neurofibroma, and ganglioneuroma. Ann. Thorac. Surg. *15*:73, 1973.

Reed, J.C., Hallet, K.K., Feigin, D.S.: Neural tumors of the thorax: subject review from the AFIP. Radiology *126*:9, 1978.

Rosai, J., and Higa, E.: Mediastinal endocrine neoplasm, of probable thymic origin, related to carcinoid tumor: clinicopathologic study of 8 cases. Cancer *29*:1061, 1972.

Rosai, J., et al.: Carcinoid tumors and oat cell carcinomas of the thymus. *In* Pathology Annual. Edited by S.C. Sommers. New York, Appleton-Century-Crofts, 1976, p. 201.

Rosai, J., Higa, E., and Davie, J.: Mediastinal endocrine neoplasm in patients with multiple endocrine adenomatosis. Cancer *29*:1075, 1972.

Sakulsky, S.B., et al.: Mediastinal granuloma. J. Thorac. Cardiovasc. Surg. *54*:279, 1967.

Schweitzer, D.L., and Aguam, A.S.: Primary liposarcoma of the mediastinum: report of a case and review of the literature. J. Thorac. Cardiovasc. Surg. *74*:83, 1977.

Seeger, R.C., Siegel, S.E., and Sidell, N.: Neuroblastoma: clinical perspectives, monoclonal antibodies, and retinoic acid. Ann. Intern. Med. *97*:873, 1982.

Sethi, G., and Kepes, J.J.: Intrathoracic angiomatous lymphoid hamartomas. A report of three cases, one of iron refractory anemia and retarded growth. J. Thorac. Cardiovasc. Surg. *61*:657, 1971.

Shapiro, B., et al.: The location of middle mediastinal pheochromocytomas. J. Thorac. Cardiovasc. Surg. *87*:814, 1984.

Sones, P.J., Jr., et al.: Effectiveness of CT in evaluating intrathoracic masses. Am. J. Radiol. *139*:469, 1982.

Stark, D.D., Gooding, G.A., and Clark, D.H.: Noninvasive parathyroid imaging. Semin. Ultrasound Comput. Tomogr. Mag. Res. *6*:310, 1985.

Sulzer, J., et al.: Forty cases of bronchogenetical cysts of the mediastinum. Ann. Chir. Thorac. Cardiovasc. *9*:261, 1970.

Symington, T., and Goodall, A.L.: Studies in phaeochromocytoma. Glasgow Med. J. *34*:75, 1953.

Teilum, G.: Endodermal sinus tumors of the ovary and testis: comparative morphogenesis of the so-called mesonephroma ovarii

(Schiller) and extraembryonic (yolk sac-allantoic) structures of rat's placenta. Cancer *12*:1092, 1959.

Teilum, G.: Special Tumors of the Ovary and Testis and Related Extragonadal Lesions: Comparative Pathology and Histological Identification, 2nd Ed. Philadelphia, J.B. Lippincott Co., 1976.

Thomas, P.R.M., et al.: An analysis of neuroblastoma at a single institution. Cancer *53*:2079, 1984.

Vaeth, J.M., Moskowitz, S.A., and Green, J.P.: Mediastinal Hodgkin's disease. AJR *126*:123, 1976.

van Heerden, J.A., et al.: Mediastinal malignant lymphoma. Chest *57*:518, 1970.

Walden, P.A.M., et al.: Primary mediastinal trophoblastic teratomas. Thorax *32*:752, 1977.

Whittaker, L.D., and Lynn, H.B.: Mediastinal tumors and cysts in the pediatric patient. Surg. Clin. North Am. *53*:893, 1973.

Wick, M.R., et al.: Primary mediastinal carcinoid tumors. Am. J. Surg. Pathol. *6*:195, 1982.

Willis, R.A.: The Spread of Tumours in the Human Body. London, Butterworth and Co., Ltd., 1953.

YaDeau, R.E., Clagett, O.T., and Divertie, M.B.: Intrathoracic meningocele. J. Thorac. Cardiovasc. Surg. *49*:202, 1965.

Zajtchuk, R., et al.: Intrathoracic ganglioneuroblastoma. J. Thorac. Cardiovasc. Surg. *80*:605, 1980.

CHAPTER 91

SURGERY OF THE THYMUS GLAND

Victor F. Trastek and W. Spencer Payne

The thymus presents a challenge to the surgeon not only as a structure that may be the origin of benign and malignant neoplasms but also also as an organ that is involved in fundamental aspects of cellular immunity and neuromuscular conduction.

The intensive study of the relationship of the thymus to systemic disease and the assessment of thymic surgery as a clinical therapeutic procedure began when Blalock and associates (1939) successfully resected the thymus containing a thymic cyst from a young woman with myasthenia gravis. This patient experienced gradual but complete remission of her neuromuscular disorder.

SURGICAL ANATOMY

Having arisen predominantly from the third branchial cleft, the thymus is situated primarily in the thorax (Fig. 91–1). It is located predominantly in the anterior mediastinum and overlies the pericardium and great vessels at the base of the heart. In accordance with its bilateral origin from branchial pouches, the thymus is a bilobed structure, but the two lobes are rarely symmetrical. The two thymic lobes are fused for a variable distance in the midline. The gland has a roughly H-shaped configuration, resulting from this fusion, the extension of the upper poles of each lobe into the neck and their attachment to the thyroid gland by the thyrothymic ligament, and the attachment of the lower poles down over the pericardium.

The upper portion of the thymus typically lies on the anterior surface of the left innominate vein as this vessel runs obliquely across the superior mediastinum to join the right innominate vein and form the superior vena cava. An enlarged thymus gland may lie adjacent to either the superior vena cava on the right or the pulmonary artery on the left. One or both lobes occasionally lie behind the left innominate vein instead of in front of it, making removal difficult. Other less rare anomalies include partial or complete failure of descent of one or both thymic lobes and aberrant nodules of thymic tissue high in the neck, at the root of a lung, or within pulmonary

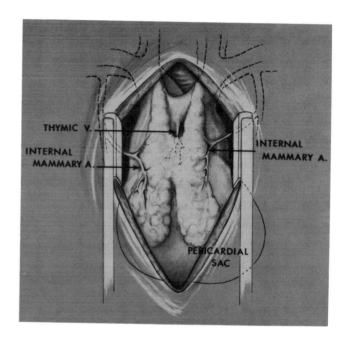

Fig. 91–1. Surgical anatomy of the thymus gland. The thymus lies in the anterior mediastinum overlying the pericardium and great vessels. Arterial supply is predominantly lateral from internal mammary vessels, whereas venous drainage is central into innominate vein.

parenchyma. On rare occasions, parathyroid tissue has been encountered in the thorax embedded in thymic tissue (see Chapter 90).

The arterial blood supply of the thymus is typically through small branches from the inferior thyroid arteries, lateral branches from the internal mammary arteries, and pericardiophrenic branches. Venous drainage is, in part, through small veins accompanying these arteries, but mainly is central, through a venous trunk on the posterior aspect of the gland that drains directly into the left innominate by a single short midline vessel.

Both sympathetic and parasympathetic nerve fibers enter the thymus, but they are believed to innervate only the blood vessels.

The thymus, unlike a lymph node, has no afferent

lymphatic channels, and it is believed that the lymphocytes of the parenchyma do not drain by way of an efferent lymph channel. Indeed, it is believed that lymphatic vessels drain only the capsule and fibrous septa, terminating in mediastinal, pulmonary hilar, and internal mammary nodes.

NORMAL HISTOLOGY

The histologic appearance of the thymus varies greatly with age, and the changes are paralleled by changes in the gross appearance of the gland. At birth, the thymus weighs 10 to 12 g, and normally it enlarges until puberty—to 20 to 50 g; thereafter, it begins to shrink—to 5 to 25 g. In youth the thymus has many lobules, septated by a fibrous capsule and composed of a thick cortex of densely packed lymphocytes, with a more central medulla containing a high proportion of epithelial cells. Unique to the thymus are specialized microscopic structures called "Hassall's corpuscles," which consist of clumps of enlarged epithelial cells arranged in a flattened concentric manner and giving a laminar onion-ring appearance. Less conspicuous, but also in the medulla in relationship to Hassall's corpuscles, are the large so-called myoid cells with striated cytoplasm, suggestive of skeletal muscle. Although many of the other formed blood elements are seen in small numbers in the thymus, true lymphoid follicles with germinal centers are rare. Usually, by the age of 20 years adipose tissue has begun to replace an involuting parenchyma. With further aging, the lobules become smaller and are separated by more fatty tissue, but the basic architecture of cortex and medulla persists throughout life, although the cortex diminishes more rapidly than do medullary elements.

THYMIC FUNCTION

The thymus is essential for the development of cellular immunity. The origin of thymic lymphocytes is most likely extrathymic, in the yolk sac in the embryo and the bone marrow in the adult. These T lymphocytes enter the thymus, proliferate, and gain their cellular immunocompetency. Humoral immunity, mediated through the elaboration of immunoglobins by B lymphocytes, originates in humans by some mammalian equivalent of the avian bursa of Fabricius. Although the origin of these cells is thymic-independent, an interaction between T cells and B cells aids in the production of immunoglobulins.

The proper function of the immune system depends on the normal development of cellular and humoral modalities. The thymic-dependent system consists principally of the thymus and a circulating pool of small T lymphocytes. These lymphocytes act as recognition agents capable of discerning self-antigens from nonself-antigens and producing cell-mediated immune reactions such as are seen in delayed hypersensitivity and allograft reactions. The bursa-dependent system consists of the bursa—or its mammalian equivalent, probably Peyer's patches of small bowel—lymphoid follicles, and plasma cells. This system is responsible for the production of immunoglobulins—IgA, IgG, and IgM—and specific antibodies. Both systems direct the differentiation of lymphoid precursor or stem cells into immunologically competent cells capable of reacting to antigens. Any disturbance in the development of either system can be expected to lead to one of the various immunologic deficiency syndromes. Interestingly, some of these syndromes have been associated with various neoplasms of the thymus as well as with congenital thymic hypoplasias and agenesis. Much of our understanding concerning these conditions is derived from studies, such as that of Good and Gabrielsen (1964), of thymus-related immune deficiency syndromes of infancy. Knowledge gained from experiments in animals is now beginning to lead to therapeutic applications. Indeed, the thymus has been implicated not only in certain immunologic deficiency states but also in certain hematologic, endocrine, autoimmune, collagen, and neuromuscular defects, as well as neoplasia. The mechanisms, nature, and extent of thymic involvement in these conditions remain obscure.

Of particular interest to surgeons are the immunologic consequences of thymectomy, because extirpation is the only commonly used thymic operation. Although thymectomy in certain species, particularly neonatal thymectomy, is often associated with significant alterations in immunity, this relationship has not been observed in either adult or pediatric patients. Although lymphocyte count and tests of immunologic capacity may be diminished by thymectomy in man, as Adner and associates (1966) reported, no particular clinical problems have developed to correlate with these laboratory observations. With the exception of the management of thymic neoplasms and the empiric management of myasthenia gravis, no clear indications for thymectomy exist in clinical practice at present.

MYASTHENIA GRAVIS

Clinical Aspects

Skeletal muscle weakness caused by a defect in neuromuscular conduction is the basic cause for the signs and symptoms of myasthenia gravis (Table 91–1). Any striated muscle group may be affected. Usually, weakness involves more than one group of muscles and is accentuated by repetitive activity and may be absent when the patient has rested. Muscles innervated by cranial nerves are often the first to be affected in the course of the disease. Thus, ptosis of eyelids, diplopia, lack of facial expression with a change in the smile—the myasthenic snarl—dysarthria with nasal tones caused by palatal paresis, diminished timbre of voice, and dysphonia frequently are observed early in the course of the disease. Often patients can bite into food, but as they continue with mastication, the masseters weaken until the patients can no longer chew or close their jaws. Dysphagia may be associated with nasal regurgitation of liquids. Neck and back muscles are often involved, which may result in a need for manual support of the head or

Table 91–1. Modified Clinical Classification of Patients with Myasthenia Gravis

GROUP I

Ocular Myasthenia.

   Involvement of ocular muscles only, with ptosis and diplopia. Very mild. No mortality.

GROUP II

Mild Generalized

   Slow onset, frequently ocular, gradually spreading to skeletal and bulbar muscles. Respiratory system not involved. Response to drug therapy good. Low mortality rate.

Moderate Generalized

   Gradual onset with frequent ocular presentations, progressing to more severe generalized involvement of the skeletal and bulbar muscles. Dysarthria, dysphagia, and difficult mastication more prevalent than in mild generalized myasthenia gravis. Respiratory muscles not involved. Response to drug therapy less satisfactory: patients' activities restricted, but mortality rate low.

Severe Generalized

   Acute fulminating. Rapid onset of severe bulbar and skeletal muscle weakness with early involvement of respiratory muscles. Progress normally complete within 6 months. Percentage of thymomas highest in this group. Response to drug therapy less satisfactory and patients' activities restricted, but mortality rate low.

   Late severe. Severe myasthenia gravis develops at least 2 years after most of group I or group II symptoms. Progression of myasthenia gravis may be either gradual or sudden. Second highest percentage of thymomas. Response to drug therapy poor, and prognosis poor.

Reproduced with permission from Olanow, C.W., and Wechsler, A.S.: The surgical management of myasthenia gravis. *In* Textbook of Surgery: The Biological Basis of Modern Surgical Practice, 13th ed. Edited by D.C. Sabiston, Jr. Philadelphia, W.B. Saunders Co., 1986, p. 2110.

may lead to back pain with activity. Pelvic weakness may result in a "waddling" gait. Weakness of the extremities is common. It may be subtle, with frequent dropping of objects or stumbling, or it may be severe, precluding combing the hair or climbing steps. Perhaps the most serious and alarming involvement is weakness of respiratory muscles. With paresis of intercostal muscles and diaphragm, alveolar ventilation diminishes; cough is ineffective. Respiratory involvement may result in carbon dioxide retention, arterial desaturation, retained tracheobronchial secretions, pulmonary infections, and death.

Although no classic clinical course can be defined, myasthenia gravis is often characterized by frequent, unpredictable, spontaneous exacerbations and remissions. It is frequently aggravated by upper respiratory infections and the premenstrual periods, but it may be ameliorated temporarily by pregnancy or operation. Occasionally, however, pregnancy may aggravate symptoms, especially in the postpartum period. Thyroid dysfunctions can be associated with myasthenia gravis and tend to aggravate symptoms.

Patients with myasthenia gravis are acutely sensitive to quinine and curare, both of which have been used in provocative diagnostic tests. The use of quinine was abandoned because its effect cannot be reversed. Currently, the use of drugs that stimulate neuromuscular

junctions are the preferred diagnostic testing agents. Neostigmine—Prostigmin, edrophonium chloride—Tensilon, and pyridostigmine bromide—Mestinon—are commonly used. The strengthening response to these agents is supportive evidence for myasthenia gravis. Electromyography provides excellent objective confirmation of the clinical diagnosis if the weakness involves skeletal weakness amenable to stimulation of the nerves. The development of diagnostic assays, as Lennon (1982) reported to measure levels of anticholinesterase receptor binding, modulating antibodies, and anti-striated muscle antibodies has added a new modality to help diagnose myasthenia gravis. The elevation of anticholinesterase receptor binding and modulating antibodies occurs in over 90% of patients with proven myasthenia gravis. The anti-striated muscle antibodies are elevated in 30% of patients with myasthenia gravis but in 95% of patients with this disease and an associated thymoma.

Initial medical treatment is usually begun with anticholinesterase medication such as pyridostigmine bromide—Mestinon. If the patient can be stabilized and the medication is well tolerated, this regimen is continued. The role of steroids or immunosuppressive agents for treatment of this disease is controversial and is currently recommended primarily for poorly controlled patients who cannot undergo thymectomy or who have had one previously. An exception is the use of steroids on an every-other-day basis for the treatment of patients with only ocular myasthenia.

Myasthenic crisis is an episode of rapidly progressive exacerbation of the disease, with threatening respiratory symptoms and increased requirement for medication. Such episodes, which are caused solely by exacerbation of myasthenia gravis, should be differentiated from similar clinical episodes of weakness caused by overtreatment, referred to as "cholinergic crisis." Indeed, it is often difficult to distinguish clinically between a myasthenic and a cholinergic crisis. Fortunately, with currently available facilities and techniques for respiratory care, such patients can be carried through episodes of profound weakness without having to depend on medication to restore function. Thus, medication can be withdrawn until the patient's sensitivity to it returns.

In general, patients displaying only well localized, ocular myasthenia generally have a good prognosis for survival. Similarly, those with nondisabling bulbar or peripheral muscle group involvement who respond to anticholinesterase medication have a good prognosis, but those with acute fulminating or late severe symptoms with bulbar or respiratory involvement have a poor prognosis.

Approximately 90% of patients with myasthenia gravis have adult-onset disease, often before the age of 35 years. The disease affects women about twice as often as it affects men. In only about 10% of cases does the onset occur between age 1 year and puberty—so-called juvenile myasthenia. Only 10% of adult patients with the disease have thymic neoplasms (Fig. 91–2), and in our experience, none have been noted at the time of diagnosis of juvenile myasthenia. A rare syndrome, transient

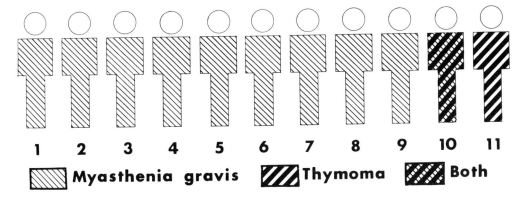

Fig. 91–2. Relationship of myasthenia gravis to thymoma. Approximately 10% of patients with myasthenia gravis have an associated thymoma, whereas nearly half of the patients with thymoma have myasthenia gravis.

noenatal myasthenia, occurs in infants born of myasthenic mothers. The newborn infant has all the usual symptoms of myasthenia gravis and responds well to medication, but the disease disappears spontaneously and permanently within a few weeks after birth. Transient neonatal myasthenia should be clearly differentiated from congenital myasthenia. Whereas the former is a temporary condition, the latter refers to the onset of persistent disease in the first year of life.

Pathophysiology of Myasthenia Gravis

Clinically and physiologically, myasthenia gravis should be differentiated from the myasthenic syndrome. The latter, commonly known as the Eaton-Lambert syndrome, is a rare defect of neuromuscular transmission, often associated with bronchial carcinoma. It occurs predominately in men over 40 years of age and is characterized by weakness and easy fatigability of proximal muscles of the extremities with minimal or no bulbar involvement and decreased or absent deep tendon reflexes.

Neither condition depends on abnormalities of peripheral nerves or the muscles themselves, but Elmqvist and Lambert (1968) described a characteristic pattern of response of muscle to nerve stimulation for both diseases which, in clinical electromyography, has been the key to the differentiation of these conditions.

Several steps are involved in the transmission of an impulse from a motor nerve to a muscle fiber. The propagation of an action potential down a motor nerve fiber triggering the release of acetylcholine from the synaptic vesicles causes depolarization of the muscle end-plate membrane, which activates muscle contraction.

At the resting neuromuscular junction, minute "packages" of acetylcholine are continually being liberated from the motor nerve terminal. The small packages are normally sufficient to elicit miniature end-plate potentials but not enough to trigger a response of muscle fiber. With nerve stimulation, many acetylcholine packages are released; these depolarize the muscle membrane and trigger muscle contraction (Fig. 91–3).

According to Drachman (1978), only a small fraction of the 30 to 40 million receptors per neuromuscular junc-

tion are activated normally in response to a nerve impulse. This receptor excess provides a large safety margin that ensures that neuromuscular transmission can occur, and repetitively if necessary. Any reduction in receptor numbers reduces the probability of interaction.

It now appears that myasthenia gravis is an autoimmune disease in which highly specific humoral antibodies for acetylcholine receptor protein can be assayed in blood and demonstrated on postsynaptic end-plates. Drachman and associates (1980) showed that these antibodies may work through three possible mechanisms: (1) by accelerating the degradation of anticholinesterase receptors through a cross-linking phenomenon, (2) direct blocking of the receptor sites, and (3) actual degradation of the receptor sites, possibly along with the activation of complement. Thus, the reduction in available numbers of receptors probably decreased the physiologic safety margin to which Drachman alludes and interferes with the likelihood of interaction at neuromuscular junctions,

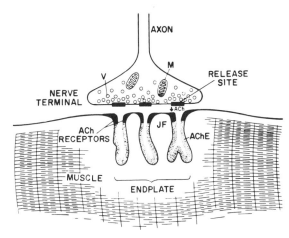

Fig. 91–3. Neuromuscular junction. Vesicles (V) release their acetylcholine (ACh) contents at specialized release sites. After crossing the narrow synaptic space (path indicated by arrow), ACh reaches the ACh receptors, which are most densely situated at the peaks of the junctional folds (JF). Acetylcholinesterase (AChE) in the clefts rapidly hydrolyzes the ACh. M denotes mitochondria. (From Drachman, D.B.: Myasthenia gravis. Part 1. N. Engl. J. Med. 298:136, 1978. By permission of the journal.)

leading to weakness and fatigue. As Lennon (1978) and Williams and Lennon (1986) showed, the thymus is evidently implicated in the production not only of these end-plate antibodies but also of striated muscle antibodies through some aberration in its normal function.

Surgical Aspects

Since Blalock's (1939) original observations, many studies of thymectomy for myasthenia gravis have been reported. Most notable among the early reports were those of Clagett and associates (1949), and Eaton and Clagett (1950, 1955) of the Mayo Clinic; Keynes (1955) of London; and Viets and Schwab (1960) from the Massachusetts General Hospital.

At present, the consensus is that thymectomy is clearly valuable for treating myasthenia gravis, but it is offered largely as an empiric procedure without a clear understanding of its mechanism of action and without a clear means of selecting patients who respond favorably.

At the Mayo Clinic, we now offer thymectomy to men and women, particularly the young and those whose symptoms are of short duration and who have experienced significant disability and poor control with anticholinesterase medication. The condition of such patients must be otherwise satisfactory to tolerate the operation without undue risk. We do not think that patients with ocular symptoms alone or those whose condition is stable and well controlled with medication are candidates for operation, because their prognosis is generally good. At the other extreme, we do not believe that patients in myasthenic crisis are candidates for emergency operations, and we delay thymectomy until better medical control is regained.

Generally, patients accepted for operation are on an optimal medical program that is continued to the morning of surgery, when all medication is discontinued. If the patient cannot be stabilized with medication, then preoperative plasmapheresis will be carried out. The *team approach* to the care of the patient is stressed, with anesthesia, neurology, and the surgical team actively involved pre-, intra-, and postoperatively. Premedication is minimal, usually consisting of atropine and a mild sedative. Myasthenic patients pose no particular anesthetic problem, although muscle relaxants are avoided, and deep anesthesia is maintained by an inhalation agent and short-acting narcotics. Ventilation and the airway are controlled during the operative procedure by an endotracheal tube.

The options for exposure range from a transverse cervical incision, as Kirschner (1969) and Cooper (1988) and their co-workers advocated, to a full median sternotomy plus a cervical incision to allow radical thymectomy, as Jaretzki and associates (1977, 1988) recommended. We prefer performing total thymectomy by a partial sternal-splitting incision (Fig. 91–4). Usually, the upper end of the incision of the skin can be kept well below the sternal notch and is carried to the level of the third interspace. The cut in the manubrium must be complete and is extended to the level of the third intercostal space. Through this relatively short skin incision, with the ster-

num retracted, adequate visualization of the entire intrathoracic portion of the thymus and its cervical extensions can be obtained. If a thymoma is suspected or found incidentally, a full median sternotomy is performed.

By blunt and sharp dissection, the thymus gland is freed from the pericardium and adjacent mediastinal pleura (Fig. 91–4C). The freed lower poles are reflected cephalad and the rather constant arterial supply entering laterally from the internal mammary arteries is easily divided. The thin cervical extensions of each lobe are easily removed with the body of the gland by gentle traction and blunt dissection dividing the thyrothymic ligament. The venous drainage into the left innominate is now easily identified and secured. The phrenic nerves are identified and carefully preserved. After total thymectomy, suction drainage through a catheter placed in the anterior mediastinum and brought to the outside through a cervical stab wound is usually necessary. If pleural spaces are entered, however, drainage through an intercostal tube may be required. The sternal incision is then approximated with wire and the soft tissue and skin are closed, resulting in a relatively comfortable, cosmetically acceptable incision (Fig. 91–4D).

After surgery, the patients are awakened and evaluated closely by the anesthesiologist. Extubation is performed in the recovery room if the respiratory effort and blood gases are satisfactory. Currently, we can extubate nearly all patients after the operation. The patient is then observed closely in the intensive care unit by the surgical, neurology, and respiratory teams. Inspiratory-expiratory pressures and vital capacity are measured every 6 hours to determine the respiratory situation. Aggressive respiratory care is maintained and ambulation begun the day after surgery. Anticholinesterase agents are restarted only if weakness occurs. Initially undertreating with these agents minimizes problems attending oral and tracheal secretions and decreases the possibility of cholinergic crisis. If the patient develops respiratory problems despite this approach, plasmapheresis is instituted. Gracey and associates (1984b) described the successful use of plasmapheresis in treating ventilator-dependent patients with myasthenia gravis. Once patients are out of respiratory danger, they are transferred from intensive care to the general patient floor and their drains are removed at the earliest possible time. Alimentation is started at the first convenient moment.

With the advent of a *team approach* combined with aggressive pre- and postoperative care as outlined, operative mortality has been nearly eliminated. Gracey and associates (1984a) reviewed 53 patients after thymectomy for myasthenia gravis; there were no operative deaths. This type of surgical result has been reported by several others.

Results of Thymectomy for Myasthenia Gravis

Determination of the long-term result of thymectomy for patients with myasthenia gravis is difficult. The natural history of the disease is so variable and its significant determinants so ill defined that it has been difficult to describe results accurately and objectively. Nonetheless,

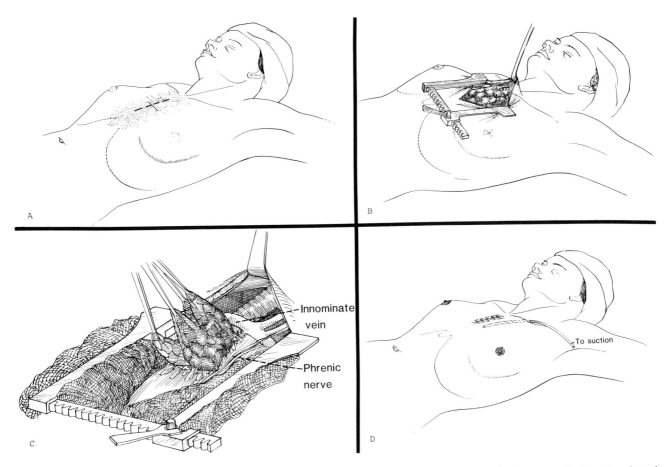

Fig. 91–4. Surgical exposure for thymectomy for myasthenia gravis. *A*, A short midline skin incision is made, keeping well below sternal notch, and carried to third interspace. *B*, Manubrium and sternum are split to third interspace and mediastinum is exposed by spreading sternum and retracting incision cephalad. *C*, After ligation and division of its blood supply, entire thymus is freed from adjacent pericardium and mediastinal pleura by blunt and sharp dissection. Care is taken to remove all thymic tissue, including cervical extensions, while carefully preserving phrenic nerves. *D*, A stable, relatively comfortable, cosmetically acceptable incision results after closure of the wound. Drainage is by small, suction catheter exiting cephalad if pleural cavities have not been violated. A chest tube will be needed if the pleura is entered.

it is apparent, as Howard (personal communication, 1970) summarized, that the adult patients undergoing thymectomy have a higher incidence of complete remissions from this disease, a tendency toward more persistent remissions, and a longevity sigificantly better than that of patients with myasthenia who have not undergone thymectomy.

Among 149 Mayo Clinic patients with juvenile myasthenia gravis—reported by Rodriguez and associates (1983)—whose conditions were followed for a median of 17 years, 50% of the 85 patients who underwent thymectomy obtained complete remission, whereas only 34% of the 64 in the nonoperated group were so improved. Survival was slightly higher after thymectomy, with over 80% alive at 20 years post-thymectomy. Six of the ten deaths in the thymectomy group were secondary to myasthenia gravis, whereas ten of eleven deaths in the nonthymectomy group were from this disease. Although the differences between the results obtained were not statistically significant, it was apparent that more severely ill patients were selected for operation. We thus continue to offer thymectomy to selected patients with juvenile myasthenia gravis.

In a computer-assisted matched retrospective study of 160 adult Mayo Clinic patients, half treated medically and half treated surgically, Buckingham and his associates (1976) found that 33% of patients who underwent thymectomy experienced complete remission, compared with only 8% of those who were treated medically. Significantly fewer late deaths occurred among patients who had thymectomy—11 patients—than among those treated medically—34 patients—during the 21-year average follow-up of this study. These results seemed to apply irrespective of patient age, sex, or duration of disease.

A prospective study of thymectomy in 47 consecutive patients was begun in 1977 and reported by Olanow and associates (1982). All patients were stabilized and underwent thymectomy. Pre- and postoperative acetylcholine receptor antibody titers were obtained. At a mean follow-up of 25.5 months, 83% of patients were free of generalized weakness and 61% were receiving no medications. Thirty patients were asymptomatic. There was no correlation between a reduction in preoperative level of anticholinesterase receptor antibody or in the reduction of the titer of the antibody with clinical improvement.

Whereas the foregoing data pertain to myasthenia gravis without thymoma, the prognosis for patients with thymoma is another aspect of this complex problem. The prognosis for patients with myasthenia gravis with noninvasive thymoma is worse than for those with myasthenia gravis alone. The response rate for those patients who have invasive thymoma and myasthenia gravis is worst of all.

THYMIC NEOPLASMS AND CYSTS

Clinical Aspects

Of 1064 primary mediastinal cysts and neoplasms resected at the Mayo Clinic and reviewed by Wychulis and associates (1971), 231 were of thymic origin. Indeed, thymic cysts and neoplasms were not only the most frequently encountered of the anterior mediastinal tumors but also the commonest tumor resected from the mediastinum. Approximately 10% of thymic tumors are simple benign cysts. Of the neoplasms, about one third are considered invasive.

We have found thymomas in patients as young as age 16 years and as old as 90 years, but most patients are adults—average age of 50 years at the time of diagnosis. Men and women are affected equally.

Symptoms

Nearly 50% of the patients with thymic neoplasms present with myasthenia gravis (Fig. 91–2), and most are adults. In the absence of this complication, most patients with thymoma are asymptomatic. Symptoms, when present, most often include chest pain, dyspnea, cough, weight loss, and fatigue. Chest pain, when present, is an ominous sign, as 70% of these patients have invasive thymomas. Similarly, the presence of dyspnea, superior vena caval obstruction, and pericardial or pleural effusions may suggest invasive disease.

Roentgenographic Appearance

Roentgenographic examination of the thorax has been the most reliable means of detection of thymic tumors (Fig. 91–5A), but little in the appearance of these tumors distinguishes them from other anterior mediastinal tumefactions. Certainly, the presence of an anterior mediastinal tumor in association with myasthenia gravis indicates thymoma. Although standard posteroanterior views of the chest frequently evidence abnormalities in the presence of thymic tumors, lateral views should be obtained, because a thymoma, if small, may be concealed by the silhouette of the heart and great vessels. Indeed, roentgenographic examination of patients with nonsurgically treated myasthenia gravis may help detect thymic tumors that develop after myasthenia gravis has been present for years. Computed tomography with and without contrast medium, helps delineate the extent of a thymic neoplasm. Although usually unable to show if the suspected thymic neoplasm is invasive, it helps in evaluating for metastatic disease and ruling out other significant pathology, such as vascular abnormalities (Fig. 91–5B and C). Magnetic resonance imaging is useful in evaluating mediastinal masses (Fig. 91–5D); whether it will supersede CT is yet to be seen.

Demonstrable calcification within thymic neoplasms is uncommon—10%. Curvilinear and peripheral calcification indicates benignancy. Scattered amorphous calcification within a tumor has been seen in benign and malignant thymomas. Other than their location in the anterior mediastinum, at any point from the neck to the diaphragm, these tumors have few distinguishing characteristics. Some are clearly in the anterior mediastinum but project predominantly into one side of the thorax; others are so large they defy recognition of even anterior mediastinal origin. Rarely, ectopic thymomas have been found in the periphery of a lung or its hilus.

Associated Clinical Syndromes

Thymoma is rare, so its coincidence with other conditions is noteworthy and eventually may lead to further understanding of thymic function in health and disease. In Rosenow and Hurley's (1984) review, 40% of patients with thymoma had a parathymic syndrome, and a third of these had two or more parathymic syndromes (Table 91–2).

Myasthenia Gravis

Approximately half of the patients with thymic tumors have associated myasthenia gravis. These patients tend to be, on average, 10 to 15 years older than patients with myasthenia without tumor and somewhat younger than patients who have thymoma without this complication. Other than these age differences, the clinical features of myasthenia are the same whether or not thymoma is present. Thymoma with myasthenia has not been encountered in juveniles, but a benign mixed cell thymoma developed in adult life in 1 of our 149 patients whose onset of myasthenia occurred before age 16 years.

Although the association of myasthenia with thymoma is usually simultaneous, thymomas have been recognized years after the onset of myasthenia; conversely, myasthenia has developed years after the removal of a thymic neoplasm.

Pure Red Cell Aplasia

The association of thymoma with severe anemia is caused by suppression of erythrogenesis in the marrow is well established. Whereas red cell precursors are greatly reduced or absent, myelopoiesis and megakaryocytopoiesis usually are normal or increased, but Burrows and Carroll (1971) reported pancytopenia. The mechanism of this erythrocyte aplasia is not clear, but Jepson and Vas's (1974) evidence suggests that it is mediated immunologically. In approximately 30% of patients, thymectomy alone has resulted in complete restitution of the abnormalities of the marrow and blood. Of 56 patients with red cell aplasia reviewed by Hirst and Robertson (1967), 7 also had myasthenia gravis and 2 had hypogammaglobulinemia.

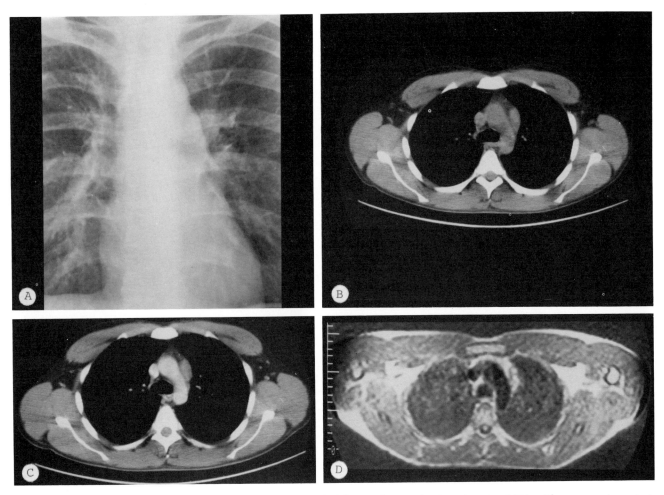

Fig. 91–5. Radiographic manifestations of thymoma. *A*, Projection of solid tumor from mediastinum into the right hemithorax on posteroanterior roentgenogram. *B*, Computed tomography (CT) without contrast medium indicates lesion lies in anterior mediastinum. *C*, Contrast medium injection through the vein shows the tumor is not directly related to the vascular tree, essentially ruling out aneurysm. Relations to other structures, such as pericardium and lung, are delineated. *D*, Magnetic resonance imaging of same tumor provides similar information as CT scan but can be done without contrast medium.

Immunoglobulin Deficiency

The association of thymoma, particularly spindle cell type, and acquired hypogammaglobulinemia, first reported by Good (1954), has been described in about 10% of the patients with such an immunoglobulin deficiency. Plasma cells are diminished or absent in marrow and nodes, and the patient shows little response to most antigens. The syndrome is particularly intriguing because presumably the thymus-dependent immunologic system does not produce humoral antibodies. Thymectomy usually fails to alter the immunoglobulin deficiency.

Endocrinopathies

The relationship of various endocrinopathies with thymoma, including Cushing's syndrome and MEN I and II, has been made more credible by the recognition of the secretory ultrastructure of the epithelial cells. The existence of Kulchitsky cells in the thymus, along with carcinoid tumors of this gland, supports the endocrine influence of some thymomas, as Rosai and colleagues (1976) and Wick and associates (1980) noted.

Pathologic Features

Various nonthymic neoplasms and tumefactions occur in the anterior mediastinum, some of which may be difficult to distinguish clinically from those of thymic origin. Teratomas, seminomas, lymphomas, metastatic malignant neoplasms, substernal goiters, and aneurysms of major arteries can occur in this region of the mediastinum.

Various cysts of the mediastinum also have been diagnosed. Some are of lymphatic origin, whereas others are thought to have developed from Hassall's corpuscles or the branchial clefts. Simple cysts of the thymus should be differentiated clearly from the more commonly encountered cystic thymomas. The latter probably develop from hemorrhage or necrosis in what was previously a solid tumor. In Graeber and associates' (1984) review of 46 patients with cystic lesions of the thymus over a 17-year period, 3 had benign cystic thymoma, 2 had invasive thymoma, 1 had seminoma of the thymus, and 1 had a lymphoblastoma.

Rosai and associates (1976) compiled an excellent sum-

Table 91–2. Conditions Associated with Thymic Neoplasm

Neuromuscular disorder (myasthenia gravis)
Hematologic and protein disorders
  Pure red cell aplasia
  Acquired hypogammaglobulinemia
  Pancytopenia
  Autoimmune hemolytic anemia
  Pernicious anemia*
  Lymphatic leukemia
  Atypical lymphocytosis*
  Multiple myeloma*
  Polycythemia*
  Megakaryocytopenia*
  Hyperglobulinemia purpura*
Endocrine disorders
  Cushing's syndrome (thymic carcinoid)
  Hashimoto's thyroiditis*
  Thyrotoxicosis
  Addison's disease*
  Multiple endocrine neoplasia
Cutaneous disorders
  Mucocutaneous candidiasis
  Pemphigus vulgaris
  Pemphigus erythematosus
  Pemphigus foliaceous
  Lichen planus
  Alopecia areata
Connective tissue diseases
  Systemic lupus erythematosus
  Dermatomyositis and polymyositis*
  Sjögren's syndrome*
  Scleroderma*
Miscellaneous
  Myocarditis (giant cell)
  Nephrotic syndrome
  Myasthenic syndrome*
  Peripheral neuropathy*
  Small bowel disorders*
  Clubbing and hypertrophic osteoarthropathy
  Extrathymic neoplasm

*These diseases have been reported in association with disorders of the thymus, but because of their small numbers and other reasons, the relation may be only coincidental. Reproduced with permission from Rosenow, E.C., III, and Hurley, B.T.: Disorders of the thymus: a review. Arch. Intern. Med. *144:*763, 1984.

Table 91–3. Classification of Thymic Neoplasms

Composed of thymic epithelial cells
  Thymoma (cytologically benign)
    Extent
      Encapsulated
      Invasive
      Metastasizing
    Histology
      Predominantly lymphocytic
      Mixed lymphoepithelial
      Predominantly epithelial
      Spindle cell
  Thymic carcinoma (cytologically malignant)
Composed of other elements
  Thymic carcinoids and neuroendocrine tumors
  Germ cell tumors
  Hodgkin's and non-Hodgkin's lymphomas
  Thymolipoma and thymoliposarcoma

Reproduced with permission of the American Cancer Society from Lewis, J.E., et al: Thymoma: a clinicopathologic review. Cancer *60:*2727, 1987.

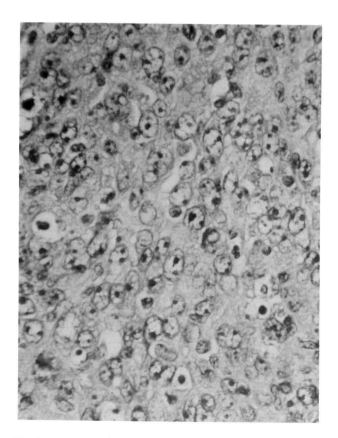

Fig. 91–6. Histopathologic features of thymic carcinoma (cytologically malignant) stained with hematoxylin and eosin. (× 640). Tumor cells of this squamous cell carcinoma of the thymus are large with indistinct borders; nuclei are vesicular with prominent nucleoli and numerous mitotic figures.

mary of the pathology of thymic tumors. Of the many classifications of thymic tumors, the one we use is the one that Bernatz and colleagues (1961) suggested and Lewis and associates (1987) modified (Table 91–3). Neoplasms of the thymus can be divided into those of epithelial cell origin and those whose origin is composed of other elements of the thymus, such as thymic carcinoid, endocrine tumor, germ cell tumor, non-Hodgkin's or Hodgkin's lymphoma, and thymoliposarcoma. Those neoplasms from epithelial cell origin can be further differentiated into cytologically benign thymomas and thymic carcinomas—cytologically malignant tumors resembling carcinoma in other sites (Fig. 91–6). Thymic carcinoma is rare; Wick and associates (1982) noted only 20 patients in a 75-year period at the Mayo Clinic. Most of these cases were of squamous cell carcinomas. Extrathoracic metastases were the rule rather than the exception.

The classification for thymoma is purely descriptive, based on predominant cell type (Fig. 91–7), presence or absence of invasion, or metastases. Indeed, the gross invasive character of a thymoma at operation, or evidence of metastasis, although at times inexact, is probably the single, most important factor to predict future survival. Invasive thymomas can spread by direct extension and less commonly by implantation on mesothelial surfaces. Metastasis outside the thorax, as Lewis and associates (1987) reported, was rare but did occur in extrathoracic lymph nodes, liver, bone, and nervous system. To avoid confusion with thymic carcinomas as defined above, it would appear prudent to discard the term "malignant thymoma." More complicated classifications, in our opinion, have been of little practical assistance. Even histopathologic criteria fail to differentiate the invasive from the encapsulated thymoma. Furthermore, no foolproof pathologic criteria permit clear distinctions between thymoma with and thymoma without myasthenia gravis or other associated conditions (Fig. 91–8).

Surgical Considerations

Surgical resection is the mainstay of treatment for patients with thymoma and should be recommended in all patients who have a mediastinal mass suspected of being thymoma and who can tolerate the proposed procedure. Preoperatively, it is important to rule out vascular abnormalities, metastatic disease to the mediastinum, and lymphoma. This may require a CT scan with contrast medium, MRI, or a needle biopsy. Occasionally, an invasive procedure such as mediastinoscopy or a limited anterior thoracotomy is needed to obtain tissue.

In the absence of myasthenia gravis, the surgical resection of a thymic tumor or cyst entails approximately the same preparation as exploratory thoracotomy for an indeterminate mediastinal tumor. The proper operative approach depends largely on the size and location of the tumor as determined by roentgenographic examination and the presence or absence of associated conditions. A median sternotomy incision is preferred for all tumors situated near the midline. For large tumors that occur chiefly in one pleural space, standard posterolateral thoracotomy is preferable, particularly if the condition suggests a need for lung resection as well. Once the exposure is accomplished and exploration for metastatic disease is completed, the tumor should be resected along with the entire thymus. At any point where adherence or invasion to a surrounding structure is suspected, resection with the thymoma should, if possible, be performed. If the tumor cannot be removed entirely, a debulking proce-

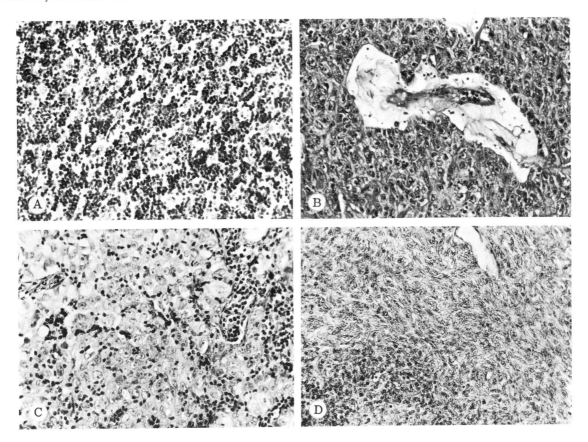

Fig. 91–7. Histopathologic features of thymomas (cytologically benign) stained with hematoxylin and eosin. Four predominant cell types: *A,* Lymphocytic, × 235. *B,* Epithelial, × 155. *C,* Mixed epithelial-lymphocytic, × 235. *D,* Spindle cell, × 235. Histopathologic features fail to show the distinguishing characteristics of benign and malignant neoplasms. The gross invasive character of the tumor at operation is thought to be the best index of malignancy.

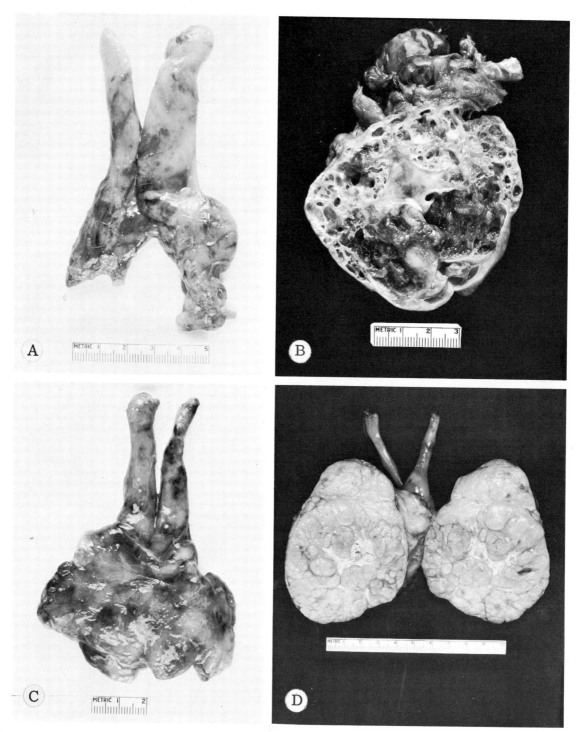

Fig. 91–8. Gross appearance of thymic tissue surgically resected. *A*, Somewhat hyperplastic but not neoplastic thymus removed for myasthenia gravis. *B*, Benign solid thymoma of moderate size from patient with associated myasthenia gravis. *C*, Large benign cystic thymoma from a patient without associated diseases. *D*, Benign thymoma from patient with myasthenia gravis. Note the wide variation in gross appearance of thymomas and that the entire thymus, including cervical extensions, is removed when myasthenia is present.

Table 91–4. Postsurgical Staging for Thymoma

Stage I	Completely encapsulated, no capsular invasion
Stage II	Invasion into surrounding fatty tissue, mediastinal pleura, or capsule
Stage III	Invasion into neighboring structure (pericardium, great vessels, lung, etc.)
Stage IVA	Pleural, pericardial metastasis
Stage IVB	Lymphogenous or hematogenous metastasis

Modified from Masaoka, A., et al.: Follow-up study of thymomas with special reference to their clinical stages. Cancer *48*:2485, 1981.

dure should probably be carried out. Frozen sections during the operative period help assure tumor-free margins. The surgeon should carefully document any gross adherence or invasion present during the resection. Protection of the phrenic nerves is important, but if curative resection requires removal of one phrenic nerve and the patient can tolerate this from a respiratory standpoint, it should be performed.

Postoperative care of the patient is like that for any thoracotomy patient, with attention to respiratory care, removal of tubes when air and fluid drainage have ceased, and early ambulation.

The operative mortality for resection of thymoma remains low. In Lewis and associates' (1987) report from the Mayo Clinic covering 1941 to 1981, 274 patients of 283 reviewed underwent surgical treatment for thymoma, of which 227 had total resection. In this group there were seven deaths, for an operative mortality of 3.1%. Complications occurred in 89 of the patients, with most occurring in patients with myasthenia or prior cardiovascular disease. Although myasthenia gravis has in the past negatively influenced operative survival, with improved pre- and postoperative care this is no longer true.

Survival for patients with thymic carcinoma is poor. Of 20 patients reviewed by Wick and associates (1982) at the Mayo Clinic, 13 underwent resective surgery and there were two operative deaths. The average survival of postoperative patients was 20.3 months. One patient was disease-free 43 months after diagnosis.

Survival of patients with thymoma continues to depend on the stage of invasion or evidence of metastatic disease as determined by the surgeon at the time of surgical intervention (Table 91–4). Lewis and associates (1987) found that invasion or metastasis greatly reduced survival (Fig. 91–9A). Adherence without evidence of invasion led to a slightly worse but not significantly different survival from that of patients with truly encapsulated tumors. Overall survival for all patients in the study, including those not treated surgically or resectable for cure, was 67% at 5 years, 53% at 10 years, and 35% at 20 years (Fig. 91–9B). Cell type *alone* was not believed to be as predictive a factor of survival as invasion (Fig. 91–9C). Although epithelial cell tumors had a poor prognosis, they were also the ones that were most often invasive, whereas spindle cell tumors had the best prognosis and were seldom invasive. Interestingly, 12% of patients with encapsulated tumors did develop local recurrent disease. The mean time of recurrence was 6 years from the date of diagnosis. An unexpected finding was the association of autoimmune-related disorders with tumor recurrence, which has not been previously described. Although patients with associated myasthenia gravis had a worse survival at 5 and 10 years, this was not significant, and the presence of this disease does not indicate poor prognosis (Fig. 91–9D). This has also been shown in Wilkins and Castleman's (1979) Massachusetts General Hospital series.

Nonresectable Invasive Thymoma

Radiation therapy may play a role in the treatment of patients with invasive tumors, both totally and partially resected. Although it remains controversial, several groups, including Shamji and associates (1984) from Toronto, have recommended it.

The role of chemotherapy, adjuvantly or for nonre-

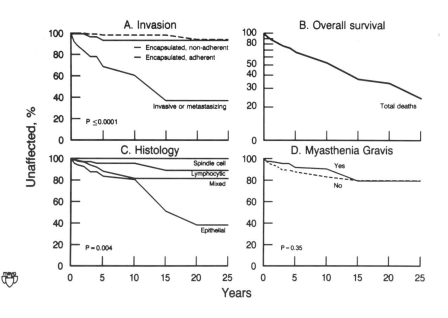

Fig. 91–9. Survival of patients with thymoma. *A*, Survival according to extent of invasion. *B*, Overall survival for all patients. *C*, Survival of thymoma patients according to histologic cell type. *D*, Survival of thymoma patients according to presence or absence of myasthenia gravis. (From Lewis, J.E., et al.: Thymoma: a clinicopathologic review. Cancer [in press]. By permission of the American Cancer Society.)

sectable tumor, is even less clear. Remissions of such neoplasms with the use of multidrug radiation therapy have been reported sporadically. Loehrer and associates (1985) described two patients who developed periods of remission lasting 7 to 8 months. Both developed recurrence.

REFERENCES

Adner, M.M., et al.: Immunologic studies of thymectomized and nonthymectomized patients with myasthenia gravis. Ann. N.Y. Acad. Sci. *135*:536, 1966.

Bernatz, P.E., Harrison, E.G., and Clagett, O.T.: Thymoma: a clinicopathologic study. J. Thorac. Cardiovasc. Surg. *42*:424, 1961.

Blalock, A., et al.: Myasthenia gravis and tumors of the thymic region: report of a case in which the tumor was removed. Ann. Surg. *110*:544, 1939.

Buckingham, J.M., et al.: The value of thymectomy in myasthenia gravis: a computer-assisted matched study. Ann. Surg. *184*:453, 1976.

Burrows, S., and Carroll, R.: Thymoma associated with pancytopenia. Arch. Pathol. *92*:465, 1971.

Clagett, O.T., Eaton, L.M., and Glover, R.P.: Thymectomy for myasthenia gravis: surgical technique. Surgery *26*:852, 1949.

Cooper, J.D., et al.: An improved technique to facilitate transcervical thymectomy for myasthenia gravis. Ann. Thorac. Surg. *45*:242, 1988.

Drachman, D.B.: Myasthenia gravis (parts 1 and 2). N. Engl. J. Med. *298*:136, 186, 1978.

Drachman, D.B., et al.: Mechanisms of acetylcholine receptor loss in myasthenia gravis. J. Neurol. Neurosurg. Psychiatry *43*:601, 1980.

Eaton, L.M., and Clagett, O.T.: Thymectomy in the treatment of myasthenia gravis: results in seventy-two cases compared with one hundred and forty-two control cases. J.A.M.A. *142*:963, 1950.

Eaton, L.M., and Clagett, O.T.: Present status of thymectomy in treatment of myasthenia gravis. Am. J. Med. *19*:703, 1955.

Elmqvist, D., and Lambert, E.H.: Detailed analysis of neuromuscular transmission in a patient with the myasthenic syndrome sometimes associated with bronchogenic carcinoma. Mayo Clin. Proc. *43*:689, 1968.

Good, R.A.: Agammaglobulinemia—a provocative experiment of nature. Bull. Univ. Minn. Hosp. Minn. Med. Found. *26*:1, 1954.

Good, R.A., and Gabrielsen, A.E. (eds.): The Thymus in Immunobiology: Structure, Function, and Role in Disease. New York, Harper & Row, Hoeber Medical Division, 1964.

Gracey, D.R., et al.: Postoperative respiratory care after transsternal thymectomy in myasthenia gravis: a 3-year experience in 53 patients. Chest *86*:67, 1984a.

Gracey, D.R., Howard, F.M., Jr., and Divertie, M.B.: Plasmapheresis in the treatment of ventilator-dependent myasthenia gravis patients: report of four cases. Chest *85*:739, 1984b.

Graeber, G.M., et al.: Cystic lesion of the thymus: an occasionally malignant cervical and/or anterior mediastinal mass. J. Thorac. Cardiovasc. Surg. *87*:295, 1984.

Hirst, E., and Robertson, T.I.: The syndrome of thymoma and erythroblastopenic anemia: a review of 56 cases including 3 case reports. Medicine (Baltimore) *46*:255, 1967.

Jaretzki, A., III, et al.: A rational approach to total thymectomy in the treatment of myasthenia gravis. Ann. Thorac. Surg. *24*:120, 1977.

Jaretzki, A., III, et al.: "Maximal" thymectomy for myasthenia gravis. J. Thorac. Cardiovasc. Surg. *95*:747, 1988.

Jepson, J.H., and Vas, M.: Decreased *in vivo* and *in vitro* erythropoiesis induced by plasma of ten patients with thymoma, lymphosarcoma, or idiopathic erythroblastopenia. Cancer Res. *34*:1325, 1974.

Keynes, G.: Investigations into thymic disease and tumour formation. Br. J. Surg. *42*:449, 1955.

Kirschner, P.A., Osserman, K.E., and Kark, A.E.: Studies in myasthenia gravis: transcervical total thymectomy. J.A.M.A. *209*:906, 1969.

Lennon, V.A.: The immunopathology of myasthenia gravis. Hum. Pathol. *9*:541, 1978.

Lennon, V.A.: Myasthenia gravis: diagnosis by assay of serum antibodies. Mayo Clin. Proc. *57*:723, 1982.

Lewis, J.E., et al.: Thymoma: a clinicopathologic review. Cancer *60*:2727, 1987.

Loehrer, P.J., et al.: Remission of invasive thymoma due to chemotherapy: two patients treated with cyclophosphamide, doxorubicin, and vincristine. Chest *87*:377, 1985.

Olanow, C.W., Wechsler, A.S., and Roses, A.D.: A prospective study of thymectomy and serum acetylcholine receptor antibodies in myasthenia gravis. Ann. Surg. *196*:113, 1982.

Rodriguez, M., et al.: Myasthenia gravis in children: long-term follow-up. Ann. Neurol. *13*:504, 1983.

Rosai, J., et al.: Carcinoid tumors and oat cell carcinomas of the thymus. Pathol. Annu. *11*:201, 1976.

Rosenow, E.C., III, and Hurley, B.T.: Disorders of the thymus: a review. Arch. Intern. Med. *144*:763, 1984.

Shamji, F., et al.: Results of surgical treatment for thymoma. J. Thorac. Cardiovasc. Surg. *87*:43, 1984.

Viets, H.R., and Schwab, R.S.: Thymectomy for Myasthenia Gravis: A Record of Experiences at the Massachusetts General Hospital. Springfield, IL, Charles C Thomas, Publisher, 1960.

Wick, M.R., et al.: Carcinoid tumor of the thymus: a clinicopathologic report of seven cases with a review of the literature. Mayo Clin. Proc. *55*:246, 1980.

Wick, M.R., et al.: Primary thymic carcinomas. Am. J. Surg. Pathol. *6*:613, 1982.

Wilkins, E.W., Jr., and Castleman, B.: Thymoma: a continuing survey at the Massachusetts General Hospital. Ann. Thorac. Surg. *28*:252, 1979.

Williams, C.L., and Lennon, V.A.: Thymic B lymphocyte clones from patients with myasthenia gravis secrete monoclonal striational autoantibodies reacting with myosin, α actinin, or actin. J. Exp. Med. *164*:1043, 1986.

Wychulis, A.R., et al.: Surgical treatment of mediastinal tumors: a 40 year experience. J. Thorac. Cardiovasc. Surg. *62*:379, 1971.

READING REFERENCES

Burnet, F.M.: The Clonal Selection Theory of Acquired Immunity. Nashville, Vanderbilt University Press, 1959.

Lambert, E.H., et al.: Myasthenic syndrome occasionally associated with bronchial neoplasm: neurophysiologic studies. *In* Myasthenia Gravis: The Second International Symposium Proceedings. Edited by H.R. Viets. Springfield, IL, Charles C Thomas, Publisher, 1961, p. 362.

Osserman, K.E.: Myasthenia Gravis. New York, Grune & Stratton, 1958.

Rosai, J., and Levine, G.D.: Tumors of the thymus. *In* Atlas of Tumor Pathology. Series 2, Fascicle 13. Washington, D.C., Armed Forces Institute of Pathology, 1976.

Radiation Therapy

CHAPTER 92

BASIC PRINCIPLES OF RADIATION THERAPY IN CANCER OF THE LUNG AND ESOPHAGUS

Carlos A. Perez

PHYSICAL ASPECTS OF IONIZING RADIATION

Ionizing radiations are special types of electromagnetic or particle energy that produce physical and biochemical events when they interact with atoms of irradiated materials. The different types of ionizing rays differ in the size and charge of the particles involved, or, in the case of x-rays and gamma rays, in their wavelength, frequency, and velocity of propagation in air or tissues.

Ionizing Particles

The several types of ionizing rays are: alpha and beta particles, gamma rays, neutrons, and negative pi-mesons (Fig. 92–1).

Alpha Particles. Equivalent to a nucleus of helium—two protons and two neutrons, these particles have a large mass and a positive charge, and can be stopped by a few sheets of paper or a few centimeters of air.

Beta Particles. These smaller, negatively charged particles—electrons—are more penetrating than alpha rays, but can be stopped by a few millimeters of material of water density or aluminum. In soft tissues, they have a maximum range of about 4 mm per 1 MeV peak.

Gamma Rays. These electromagnetic quanta of energy with the same diffusion characteristics as light are physically and biologically similar to x-rays, except that they originate from a radionuclide. X-rays are artificially produced by bombarding in a vacuum a high atomic number target with electrons. Neither gamma rays nor x-rays are deflected by electronic or magnetic fields.

Neutrons. These particles have a mass similar to that of protons but lack electric charge. They are produced by accelerating a charged particle, such as a deuteron, to high energies and bombarding suitable target material, such as beryllium. Neutrons can also be emitted as by-products of heavy radioactive atomic fission in nuclear reactors. Californium-252 is a neutron source that Atkins (1968) introduced as an aid in interstitial or intracavitary therapy.

Negative Pi-Mesons. These negatively charged particles have a mass 273 times larger than that of electrons.

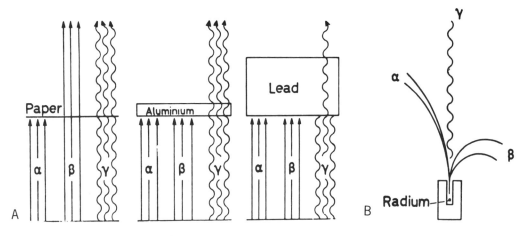

Fig. 92–1. *A*, Schematic representation of the penetrating power of alpha, beta, and gamma radiations. *B*, Deflection in a magnetic field. (Young, M.E.J.: Radiological Physics, 2nd ed. London, H.K. Lewis and Co., Ltd., 1967.)

They are produced by a complex particle acceleration process at high energies—700 to 800 MeV; their use in radiation therapy was suggested by Bond (1971).

Several natural—radium—or artificially produced radioisotopes—cesium-137—^{137}Cs, iodine-125—^{125}I, chromium-51—^{51}Cr, iridium-192—^{192}Ir, cobalt-60—^{60}Co—are used for interstitial or intracavitary procedures. Others, such as ^{131}I and phosphorous-32—^{32}P, are mostly beta emitters and are administered internally or used for intracavitary therapy.

ABSORPTION OF IONIZING RADIATIONS AND HALF-VALUE LAYER

When a photon or electron collides with an electron of another atom in the absorber, the incident ray or photon is either deflected or destroyed, thereby transferring energy to atoms in the absorber. Depending on the energy of the incident photon, the interaction with the electron in the absorbing material produces an event leading either to ionization of atoms or to excitation. The three basic mechanisms of ionization depend on the energy of the incident particles and produce diverse reactions in the nuclei or electrons of the atoms involved in this process: photo-electric effect, Compton scattering effect, and pair production.

The *absorption coefficient* of an absorber is the sum of the various absorption sub-coefficients of the various interactions mentioned previously.

Half-value layer is defined as that thickness of material that decreases by one half the intensity of a beam of ionizing radiation.

RADIOACTIVE DECAY AND PHYSICAL HALF-LIFE

A radioisotope is a disintegrating element that has the same atomic number as the stable element but a different atomic weight or mass, that is, an excess of neutrons in the nucleus. It has the same chemical properties as its stable counterpart, but in disintegrating, it gives off energy that is emitted as ionizing radiation.

The loss of radioactivity, which is characteristic for each radioactive element, is called disintegration or decay. The physical half-life of a radioisotope is the period of time required for half of its radioactivity to disappear.

MEASUREMENT OF IONIZING RADIATIONS

Exposure or given dose is that amount of ionizing radiation delivered to a particular object or a region of a patient, without reference to the nature of the absorbing material.

Absorbed dose is the amount of radiation absorbed by a particular object or a region of a patient, without reference to the nature of the radiation.

Units of Radiation

A roentgen is a unit of radiation exposure. It is defined as that amount of x-radiation or gamma-radiation nec-essary for associated corpuscular emission per 0.001293 g of air to produce in air ions that carry one electrostatic unit or quantity of electricity of either sign.

Rad is the unit of absorbed dose equal to the amount of ionizing radiation that delivers 100 ergs per gram of absorber.

The Gray is equivalent to 100 rads. 1 cGy = 1 rad.

Another unit of radiation is the curie, which is equal to 3.7 × 10^{10} disintegrations per second. The curie, which is used to describe the activity of any radioactive isotope, is approximately the equivalent of the number of disintegrations per second undergone by 1 g of radium, as Johns and Cunningham (1969) noted. A practical unit frequently used is the millicurie—1/1000 of a curie, abbreviated mCi.

Dosimetry in Radiation Therapy

The dose of radiation administered to a patient can be expressed in several ways: the surface dose, maximum or given dose, back-scatter dose, central axis percent depth dose, tumor air ratio, tumor dose, and integral dose (Fig. 92–2).

Surface Dose. As the amount of radiation delivered to the superfical layers of the skin, the surface dose is used only to measure radiation emitted by orthovoltage equipment, which produces the maximum effect at the skin level. It is equal to the sum of the air dose plus the backscatter dose—SD equals AD plus BSD.

Maximum or Given Dose. Because the higher energy of the incident photons and the secondary electrons produced in the absorber—tissues, the point of maximum ionization—electronic equilibrium—usually occurs several millimeters below the skin surface, depending on the effective energy of the beam. This dose is expressed in rads as the maximum dose or, in some institutions, as the given dose. The point of maximum ionization for ^{137}Cs is about 2 mm below the skin, for ^{60}Co, 5 mm, for 4 MeV x-rays, 8 mm, and for 22 MeV x-rays, 4 cm, according to Johns and Cunningham (1969) and Young (1967).

Backscatter Dose. This dose is produced by secondary electrons originating in the absorber and ejected to the surface.

Central Axis Percent Depth Dose. This term expresses the radiation distribution in an absorber as a percentage

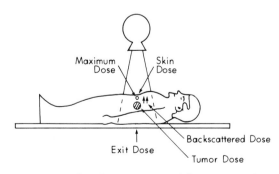

Fig. 92–2. Examples of various types of doses commonly used in radiation therapy. See text for detailed explanation. (Perez, C.A.: Principles of radiation therapy. *In* Clinical Oncology. Edited by J. Horton and G.J. Hill. Philadelphia, W.B. Saunders Co., 1977, p. 129.)

of the surface or maximum ionization dose measured along the central beam at various distances—cm—below the surface. The best compendium of these tables is published in Supplement No. 11 of the British Journal of Radiology (1972).

Tumor Air Ratio. Johns and Cunningham (1969) defined the tumor ratio as the ratio of the absorbed dose to the dose that would be measured at the same point in free air. It is particularly useful in the dose calculations for isocentric techniques as well as in rotational therapy.

Tumor Dose. Sundbom and Asard (1965) defined this dose as the minimal amount of radiation given at a point within or around the tumor.

Integral Dose. The integral dose is the total absorbed energy delivered over the entire volume of the patient during radiation exposure.

Isodose Curves. These two-dimensional representations of the distribution of radiation (Fig. 92–3) can be obtained by direct measurements, by irradiating water phantoms, or by complex mathematical calculations.

EQUIPMENT USED IN CLINICAL RADIATION THERAPY

External beam therapy units are designed to deliver gamma rays—⁶⁰Co teletherapy, x-rays, or electrons. Electron beams have special physical characteristics—for instance, the depth of penetration can be controlled by energy used—and are employed in the treatment of relatively localized lesions.

For a review of the physical aspects of ionizing radiation, the reader is referred to more comprehensive textbooks on this subject—and for the sake of brevity only, a succinct description of the different types of equipment will be given. More detailed information can be found in physics textbooks, such as those by Johns and Cunningham (1969), Tubiana and Lalanne (1967), and Young (1967).

Orthovoltage X-Ray Unit

This machine consists of a glass vacuum tube with a filament—cathode—which, when heated, emits accelerated electrons. These electrons in turn hit a fixed tung-

sten target—anode, resulting in the production of x-rays—usually 200 to 400 kVp. Superficial units in the range of 80 to 100 kVp have aluminum or thin copper filters and are used for superficial lesions, such as skin cancer.

The main disadvantages of this type of equipment are the relative lack of penetration and maximum ionization occurring at the skin level, so that erythema and either dry or moist desquamation appear rapidly even with moderate doses of radiation.

Cobalt-60 Teletherapy Units

The basic machine consists of a shielded head in which the radioactive source is housed, a collimating device, an on-off system, and an electric circuit. These machines produce more penetrating radiation than conventional x-ray machines; the skin is therefore less affected and higher doses can be delivered to deeper tissues than with conventional x-rays.

Linear Accelerators

Linear accelerators are high energy electron accelerators that can be used to produce either electron or x-ray beams. The usual energies for electrons are 4, 6, 8, 10, 12, 18, and 20 MeV. The main feature of the electrons is that in tissues they have a definite range that depends on their energy (Fig. 92–4). Linear accelerators have a high output—200 to 1000 rads per minute at the center of rotation, depending on the type of unit. The beam provides excellent skin-sparing effect and depth of penetration; the dose is more homogeneous than with the ⁶⁰Co unit because of the small focal spot, which generates little penumbra at the edge of the beam.

Betatrons

The betatron accelerates electrons, which may hit a target and produce x-rays; the only difference from a conventional x-ray machine is that this action is done in a circular tube. Betatrons generate high energy, relatively homogenous x-ray beams with sharp edges and no penumbra. As the point of maximum ionization—electronic equilibrium—usually 4 cm below the skin, these machines are excellent for irradiating deep-seated le-

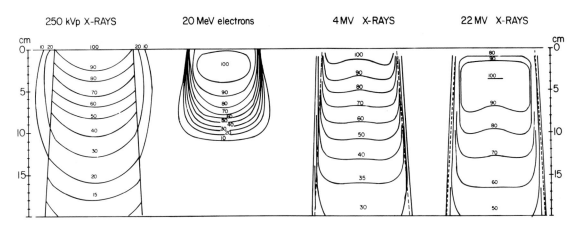

Fig. 92–3. Schematic comparison of external beams of radiation.

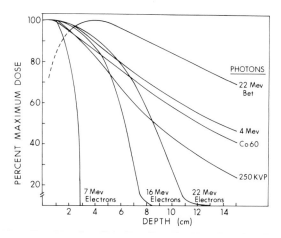

Fig. 92–4. Examples of depth dose curves for a variety of photon and electron beams. Notice the higher doses delivered by 22-MeV betatron photons and the sharp decrease in dose delivered by electron beams. (Perez, C.A.: Principles of radiation therapy. *In* Clinical Oncology. Edited by J. Horton and G.J. Hill. Philadelphia, W.B. Saunders Co., 1977, p. 131.)

sions. The betatron can also be used as a source of electrons. The main disadvantage of this machine is a low output, the small size of the portals, and the lack of rotational capability.

Radioactive Sources and Internally Administered Isotopes

Sometimes it is appropriate to treat a tumor with a source of radiation directly implanted into the tumor—interstitial therapy with [125]I. Likewise, intracavitary administration of radioisotopes is sometimes used to treat malignant pleural effusions—for instance, [32]P.

BIOLOGIC EFFECTS OF IONIZING RADIATIONS AND BIOLOGIC BASIS OF RADIATION THERAPY

When a radioactive particle interacts with an atom, energy is transferred to the electrons in the absorbing material. To eject an electron from an atom, a process called ionization, requires a minimum of 34 electron volts per ion pair in air. If less energy is available, an excitation may occur, in which case the electron is displaced from its orbit without being ejected from the atom. The free electron is either eventually captured by another atom or recaptured by the same or another positive ion. Many of these ionizations occur primarily in the water molecules of the absorber, and this effect is called "indirect." In contrast, the interaction of the incident particle with the atoms or molecules of the absorbing material, without intervention of water molecules, is called "direct." Much of the released energy is absorbed by the water in the tissues and cells, which in turn generates several ions in solution and forms several free radicals—H^+, OH^-, and H_2O_2, for example. These free radicals subsequently combine with other atoms and molecules to produce biochemical effects in the cells (Fig. 92–5).

Kaplan (1963) suggested and Hall (1976) summarized

that the critical target in cell death is the nucleus, probably deoxyribonucleic acid—DNA, and ribonucleic acid—RNA. Ionizing radiation affects these two nucleic acids in at least three different ways: double helix strand breaks, single strand breaks, and base damage, mainly to the pyrimidine bases—cytosine, thymine, and uracil.

These physical and biochemical phenomena take place in fractions of a second at the time of the radiation exposure. Various nuclear and cytoplasmic molecular changes then follow, leading to loss of reproductive ability, metabolic changes, somatic transformation, acceleration of the aging process of the cell, and mutations, among others.

Chromosomes may be disturbed by ionizing radiation, as Evans (1962), Blood and Jijo (1964), and Little (1968) noted, but the damage is not detected in interphase and only appears as the cells go through cell division. Kaplan (1963) reported that the frequency of mutations produced by the single or double strand breaks on the DNA molecule depends not only on the the number of initial breaks but also on the adequacy of the repair mechanisms—reunion or restitution.

Carcinogenesis

Ionizing radiation can induce carcinoma of the skin, leukemia, thyroid cancer, osteosarcoma of bone, fibrosarcomas of soft tissues, and other disorders. The instances of leukemia that have reportedly been caused by prior exposure to radiation include acute leukemias of all types and chronic granulocytic leukemias. Cade (1957) reported malignant tumors of the bone in watchdial painters who ingested radium salts. Bone and soft tissue sarcomas have been observed by Phillips and Sheline (1963) in children who received high doses of radiation for retinoblastoma and also has been reported by Fendel and Feine (1970) in those who received lower doses for adenolymphoid tissue of the nasopharynx. The adult thyroid gland may tolerate as much as 4000 rads without significant changes, but in children who received doses of between 200 and 800 rads to the neck for thymic enlargement, the development many years later of thyroid carcinoma, usually of the papillary type, has been increasingly reported, as Hempelmann and associates (1967) noted.

Cell Kill by Ionizing Radiation

When a cell is hit by an ionizing particle, different kinds of damage may take place. Lethal damage occurs when the cell loses its ability for unlimited proliferation. After the exposure, the cell and its progeny die, although Doggett and his associates (1967) and Tolmach (1961) noted that as many as five to six cell divisions may occur. Potentially lethal damage consists of slightly less severe impairment of the proliferative ability of the cell from which it might recover, but any modification in its environment will interfere with repair and cause the cell to die. Stewart and Fajardo (1972) reported that in humans this happens, for instance, when certain drugs such as hydroxyurea are administered.

Sublethal damage occurs, as Elkind and colleagues

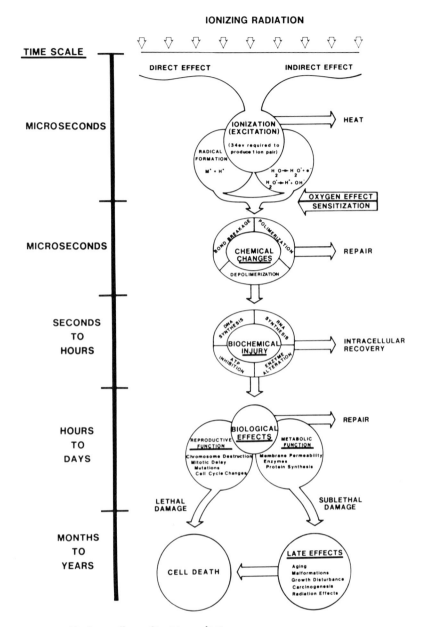

Fig. 92–5. Schematic representation of biologic effects of ionizing radiation.

(1967) noted, when the injury induced by the ionizing radiation can be repaired by the cell. Following exposure to ionizing radiation, the cells exhibit changes in their growth rate, including prolongation of the generation time and mitotic delay. Elkind and Whitmore (1967) discussed these changes, which result from the various types of damage just described.

Cell Survival Curves

A cell survial curve such as that Hewitt and Wilson (1959) described represents the probability of cell kill by various doses of radiation. In biologic terms, cell kill is the loss of unlimited proliferative capacity. It is the inability of the cell to proliferate in an unlimited clonogenic manner that is important in radiation therapy. As Puck and Marcus (1956) pointed out, however, a cell may

appear to be morphologically intact following exposure to radiation, and it may even undergo several more divisions before lysis.

Mathematically speaking, cell survival can be expressed as a complex exponential function in which the fraction of cells killed is independent of the number of cells irradiated. The exponential shape of the cell survival curve indicates that cell kill is a probable event. If this curve is a decreasing straight line, a single hit must affect a single target to kill the cell. Most cell survival curves, however, have an "initial shoulder," suggesting that more than one target must be inactivated by an ionizing event or that one target must be hit several times before the cell is lethally affected. The shoulder seen in the initial portion of the survival curve expresses repair of sublethal damage, but it also reflects the progression of some cells through the cell cycle and some repopulation from the surviving cells. In survival curves with a shoulder, the projection of the straight exponential portion of the curve to dose 0 represents the extrapolation number (Fig. 92–6).

Factors Affecting the Biologic Effects of Ionizing Radiations

Cell Sensitivity to Radiation

Bergonie and Tribondeau (1906) stated that "cells are more sensitive to radiation the greater their mitotic activity." It is not necessary, however, for the cells to be in mitosis at the time of radiation. In addition to the oxygen tension, Sinclair (1968), Terasima and Tolmach (1963), and other investigators have demonstrated in cell cultures and experimental animals that the sensitivity of cells to ionizing radiation and to most chemotherapeutic agents varies according to the phase of the cell cycle in which the cell's exposure to the physical or chemical event occurs.

In clinical practice, a distinction must be made between cell sensitivity to radiation on the one hand and tumor response and curability on the other. Some tumors, such as seminomas, dysgerminomas, lymphomas, and small cell undifferentiated carcinoma, are sensitive to radiation and may disappear after low or moderate doses, but the patient may not necessarily be cured and eventually dies of disseminated disease. Epidermoid carcinoma requires higher doses—6500 to 7500 rads—for tumor control. On the other hand, for a long time it was thought that adenocarcinomas of the breast and prostate were resistant to radiation, yet I and my associates (1980), among others, achieved local control in approximately 70% of patients; many are being cured even though the tumor may take a long time to regress completely.

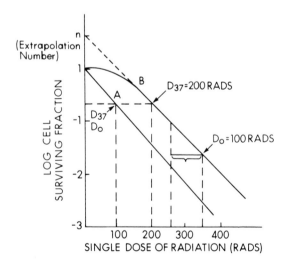

Fig. 92–6. Example of theoretical cell survival curves. Single-hit curve (**A**) is represented by the equation $SF = 1 - e^{D/D_o}$. Multiple-hit survival curve (**B**) with an initial shoulder is represented by the equation $SF = 1 - (1 - e^{D/D_o})^n$. See text for explanation of D_o, D_{37}, and extrapolation number. (Perez, C.A.: Principles of radiation therapy. *In* Clinical Oncology. Edited by J. Horton and G.J. Hill. Philadelphia, W.B. Saunders Co., 1977, p. 131.)

Oxygen Enhancement Effect—Reoxygenation

With sparsely ionizing radiation, such as x-rays or gamma rays, a given biologic effect produced by a given dose is 2 to 3 times greater in the presence of oxygen than if it is absent. Thus augmentation is called the oxygen enhancement ratio—OER. The oxygen must be present during the radiation exposure. This oxygen enhancement effect is absent in high linear energy transfer—LET—radiations, such as alpha particles, and as Alper and Moore (1967) and others noted, is not as marked with fast neutrons and pi-mesons. Although increasing concentrations of oxygen result in more sensitization to radiation, Gray (1961) reported that no significant gain is observed when the oxygen pressure is over 30 mm Hg. The exact mechanism of the oxygen effect has not been fully elucidated, although it is generally agreed that oxygen at the level of the free radicals breaks chemical bonds and initiates a chain of events that results in final biologic damage. In specimens of bronchial carcinoma, Thomlinson (1967) reported no evidence of necrosis pathologically in any tumor with a radius of less than 160 μm; tumors with radii of over 200 μm always had necrotic centers. Suit and Shalek (1963) suggested that the hypoxic cell subpopulations determine the response and probability of control of a tumor to radiation (Fig. 92–7). Fractionated radiation causes a decrease in the size of the tumor and the initial number of cells, as well as new blood vessel proliferation and reoxygenation. Kallman (1972) noted that these changes result in a transfer of hypoxic tumor cells to a more oxygenated compartment, and this transfer in turn eventually leads to complete sterilization of the tumor without significant injury to the surrounding normal tissues. The lack of oxygen enhancement effect in the biologic events induced by high LET particles, as noted by Bond (1971) and Brennan (1969), has caused renewed interest in the clinical applications of these radiations. Kolstad (1971) and Van den Brenk (1968) summarized several clinical trials with hyperbaric oxygen and radiation in tumors of the head and neck, cervix, and urinary bladder.

Linear Energy Transfer

This term represents the energy transferred by an ionizing particle per unit length of pathway. Because most ionizing particles are not monoenergetic, the LET that results from a beam of energy is an average of all the particles or photons in the beam. In addition, at the molecular level, the energy per unit length of track varies. So the LET of an ionizing particle depends in a complex way on the energy and charge of the particle: the greater the charge and the smaller the velocity, the higher the linear energy transfer.

Because of these varying amounts of energy released in an absorber, equal doses of various types of radiation do not produce the same biologic effects on the absorber—or patient. The term relative biologic effect—RBE—was established to compare the biologic effectiveness of a given ionizing radiation with a certain stand-

TUMOR SIZES FOR 90% CHANCE OF CURE (Hewitt's data)

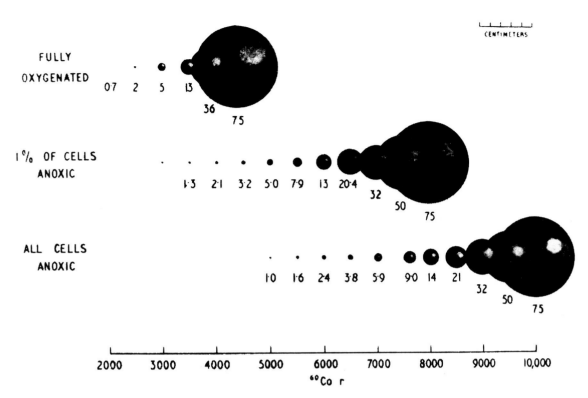

Fig. 92–7. Schematic representation of the effect of hypoxic cells on curability of tumors. A tumor with hypoxic cells, regardless of the proportion, needs a dose of radiation 2 to 3 times greater to achieve the same control rate. Tumor sizes for a 90% chance of cure are illustrated. (Fowler, J., Morgan, R.L., and Wood, C.A.: Pre-therapeutic experiments with the fast neutron beam from the Medical Research Council cyclotron. I. The biological and physical advantages and problems of neutron therapy. Br. J. Radiol. 36:77, 1963.)

ard, which is 250-kV x-rays. For instance, Hall (1961) has recorded that ^{60}Co has a relative biologic effect of about 0.95, and neutrons have an RBE of between 2.0 and 2.5, depending on their energy.

Repair of Radiation Damage—Dose Fractionation

Radiation therapy is given in daily fractions—four or five per week—on the presumption, noted by Cohen (1966) and also by Withers (1970), that, in general, normal cells have a greater and faster capacity to repair sublethal damage than do tumor cells. Because of the cell repair of sublethal damage and cell repopulation between fractions, Ellis (1969) suggested that a patient's chances of survival are greater when the doses of radiation are fractionated, except in the case of high LET particles (Fig. 92–8). This time-dose relationship depends on: individual sensitivity of the cells and their repair ability, size of the radiation fractions, total dose given, time between fractions and of overall treatment, initial hypoxic subpopulation and reoxygenation that takes place throughout the fractionated therapy, and the type of ionizing radiation used.

In analyzing the treatment of a patient, the specifications should include not only the volume of tissue treated and the total dose given, but also the number of fractions and the overall period of time in which they are administered.

Radiosensitizers and Radioprotective Agents

Berry (1965) and Doggett and colleagues (1967) noted that numerous drugs, including the halogenated pyrimidines, dactinomycin, alkylating agents, and others augment the effects of radiation on normal and some tumor tissues. The therapeutic aim of radiosensitizers may be additive or synergistic, depending on the degree of enhancement of effects.

Hypoxic sensitizers have been introduced into clinical trials. These drugs, which potentiate the effects of irradiation on hypoxic cells, must be present at the time of irradiation. Phillips and associates (1978) reported that the main toxicity is peripheral neuropathy.

Simpson and colleagues (1987) reported on a Radiation Therapy Oncology Group—RTOG—trial with misonidazole in locally advanced non-oat cell carcinoma of the lung and various radiation therapy schedules. No significant improvement in tumor control or survival was noted when compared with irradiation alone. Compounds such as SR-2508, with less lipophilicity, allowing larger doses to be administered with the same peripheral

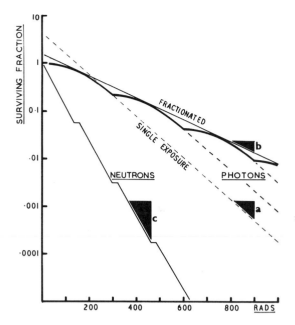

Fig. 92–8. Examples of cell survival curves showing repair with fractionated doses using photons and absence of repair with neutrons (Perez, C.A.: Principles of radiation therapy. *In* Clinical Oncology. Edited by J. Horton and G.J. Hill. Philadelphia, W.B. Saunders Co., 1977, p. 131.)

neuropathy, as Wasserman and associates (1984) reported, will be tested in forthcoming clinical trials.

EFFECTS OF RADIATION ON NORMAL TISSUES

Esophagus

The effects of radiation in the esophagus are caused by damage to the germinal cell layers of the epithelium and the muscular layers and by vascular changes in the underlying tissues. During the first 2 weeks, mucositis and progressive vascular injection may be observed. After 4000 rads, a brisk mucositis and fibrinous exudate appear. These changes are frequently reversible, although with doses over 6000 rads some atrophy of the irradiated mucosa, telangiectasis, fibrosis of the underlying tissues, and esophageal strictures may occur.

Lung

With limited segments of lung receiving irradiation, pneumonitis may develop; the patient may be asymptomatic or complain only of cough or minimal chest discomfort. Rubin and Cassarett (1968) reported that when more than 75% of the pulmonary tissue has been irradiated, with doses over 2000 rads, the patient may develop severe respiratory distress, temperature peaks, and shortness of breath, and he may even die of acute respiratory insufficiency and cor pulmonale. Sputum cultures are negative unless bacterial infection is superimposed—which is common and may be life-threatening. Roentgenograms of the chest show diffuse pulmonary infiltrates that may coalesce and, as Cooper and col-

leagues (1961) noted, may be associated with pleural or interlobar effusions. The underlying pathologic damage consists of alveolar degeneration and hyaline membrane formation, followed by fibrosis of the alveolar wall and interlobar septa, as well as capillary thrombosis and fibrinoid degeneration of the small arterioles. Many of these acute changes are reversible after 3 to 4 weeks with moderate doses of radiation therapy. After larger doses, however, large chronic changes become permanent and can be seen as early as 3 months after radiation treatment. Substantial functional impairment ensues. If the fibrotic process is localized to less than half of one lung, it is generally asymptomatic and can be detected only on roentgenograms of the chest. Decreased pulmonary function frequently occurs following irradiation, particularly if large volumes of the lung are treated with doses over 2000 rads. In the initial phases of radiation therapy, pulmonary capacity may improve because of decreased bronchial obstruction and atelectasis. As Brady and associates (1965) and Deeley (1973) pointed out, however, a progressive decreased ventilatory and diffusing capacity results from alveolar cell degeneration and interstitial fibrosis.

Heart

The probability of radiation-induced heart injury depends on the volume irradiated, the size of the dose, and the number of fractionated doses given. Transient, subacute, or chronic pericarditis may appear with doses over 5000 rads. Stewart and Fajardo (1972) pointed out that this condition may be accompanied by endocardial and myocardial damage. Some of these patients develop endocardial or myocardial fibrosis, and myocardial infarctions have been reported in some young patients.

Most of the patients reported by Stewart and Fajardo (1972) received doses of over 4000 rads to almost the entire volume of the heart. Adequate distribution of doses and selective shielding of the heart substantially decrease these complications. Irradiation of the heart may increase the likelihood of cardiac toxicity from anthracycline antibiotics such as doxorubicin.

Bone Marrow

The acute effects of radiation on the bone marrow, mostly caused by direct cell killing, are related to the volume irradiated and the dose and fractions given. Usually a reduction in the number of lymphocytes occurs—a reflection of the extreme sensitivity of circulating lymphocytes to interphase death. The lymphocyte count remains low for weeks or months; gradually repopulation occurs. The granulocytes decrease 1 to 2 weeks after segmental irradiation, with recovery taking weeks or up to 18 months. Moderate thrombocytopenia is common; if the platelets decrease to less than 20,000, hemorrhages with ecchymosis, hematemesis, and melena, which complicate the fluid and electrolyte imbalance, may occur. The circulating red cells are extremely radioresistant, but chronic irradiation may cause protracted anemia.

Knospe (1966) and Rubin (1973) and their colleagues noted that when the bone marrow is irradiated with doses over 4000 rads, more permanent chronic changes occur. Vascular degeneration, as pointed out by Rubin and Cassarett (1968), and fibrosis, as Lejar and associates (1966) noted, occur, preventing repopulation. These changes are more severe in patients who have previously received bone-marrow-depressing chemotherapeutic agents or in patients who have been treated with these drugs after radiation therapy. Special care should be exercised for patients receiving combination therapy or retreatment after radiation therapy or chemotherapy, and frequent leukocyte and platelet counts are necessary, particularly if the bone marrow is infiltrated with malignant cells.

Spinal Cord

Acute radiation effects in the spinal cord are usually of minimal clinical significance and are caused mostly by transient edema. A transient form of radiation effect on the spinal cord is known as Lhermitte's syndrome; it occurs a few weeks after exposure and is characterized by some electric shock-like sensations that radiate along the spinal cord into the extremities. In most instances the syndrome is reversible and does not correlate with subsequent permanent radiation myelopathy. A more severe type of brain stem or spinal cord injury appears after 6 months or as late as several years after radiation. Radiation myelopathy causes motor and sensory changes referable to the segment injured. If the entire width of the cord is irradiated, complete paraplegia and anesthesia occur as a result of a total transection of the spinal cord. If only half of the cord is irradiated, the neurologic picture is that of Brown-Séquard's syndrome. These permanent changes are secondary to severe capillary degeneration, fibrinoid necrosis of the small arterioles, necrosis of neurons and other oligodendrocytes, accompanied by marked demyelination of the white matter.

Small segments of brain stem or spinal cord may tolerate doses of radiation around 4500 rads, given in weekly increments of 900 rads. With doses of 5000 to 6000 rads per 5 to 6 weeks the probability of radiation myelitis is 10 to 15%. A strong probability exists that higher doses will induce radiation myelopathy more frequently. Also, the greater the length of segment of the spinal cord being irradiated, the more likely the possibility of developing permanent myelopathy.

Table 92–1 presents the accepted tolerated doses for intrathoracic structures in the absence of chemotherapy.

Table 92–1. Radiation Tolerance of Intrathoracic Organs

Intrathoracic Structure	Maximum Tolerated Dose
Ipsilateral normal lung	2000 rads unless required to treat tumor and lymph nodes
Contralateral normal lung	None unless absolutely unavoidable, in which case, 2000 rads TD
Entire heart	4500 rads TD/5 weeks. Less than 50% of heart may receive 5000 rads in 6 weeks
Spinal cord	4000 rads TD/5 weeks (2500 rads TD/1–2 weeks with split course therapy regimen)
Esophagus	5500 rads TD/5 weeks

ADJUVANT CHEMOTHERAPY

Chemotherapy significantly enhances the effect of irradiation. Phillips and Margolis (1972) reported a 50% incidence of radiation penumonitis in patients treated with radiation alone in doses of about 2650 rads in 20 fractions. When dactinomycin was added, the incidence of pneumonitis was 50% with doses of 2050 rads in 20 fractions. Patients receiving bleomycin may develop interstitial pulmonary fibrosis, which can accentuate the similar effects of irradiation.

Johnson and associates (1976) reported instances of severe esophageal fibrosis with stenosis, following the administration of 3000 rads in 2 weeks combined with intensive triple agent chemotherapy—doxorubicin, vincristine, and cyclophosphamide—given the same day every 3 to 4 weeks. Also, the well known cardiotoxicity of doxorubicin coupled with the effects of radiation on the heart, makes this combination more toxic. When these two agents are combined, Chan and colleagues (1976) recommend that no more than a 4500-rad total dose be given to the entire heart, or that a maximum of 450 mg/m² total dose of doxorubicin be administered. Also, the two agents should not be administered simultaneously.

The effects of combined irradiation and chemotherapy on the spinal cord have not been properly evaluated, but it is reasonable to believe that an additive or potentiating effect is present.

REFERENCES

Alper, T., and Moore, J.L.: The interdependence of oxygen enhancement ratios for 250 kvp x-rays and fast neutrons. Br. J. Radiol. *40*:843, 1967.

Atkins, H.L.: The medical use of ²⁵²Cf, californium-252. Proceedings of a symposium sponsored by N.Y. Metropolitan Section of American Nuclear Society. New York, Brookhaven National Laboratory, 1968.

Bergonie, J., and Tribondeau, L.: De quesques resultats de la radiotherapie et essai de fization d'une technique rationelle. C.R. Acad. Sci. *143*:983, 1906.

Berry, R.J.: Modification of radiation effects. Radiol. Clin. North Am. *3*:249, 1965.

Blood, A.D., and Jijo, J.H.: In vivo effects of diagnostic x-irradiation on human chromosomes. N. Engl. J. Med. *270*:1341, 1964.

Bond, V.P.: Negative pions: their possible use in radiotherapy. Am. J. Roentgenol. *111*:9, 1971.

Brady, L.W., Germon, P.A., and Cander, L.: The effects of radiation therapy on pulmonary function in carcinoma of the lung. Radiology *85*:130, 1965.

Brennan, J.T.: Fast neutrons for radiation therapy. Radiol. Clin. North Am. *7*:365, 1969.

Cade, S.: Radiation induced cancer in man. Br. J. Radiol. *30*:393, 1957.

Chan, Y.M., et al.: Co-incident adriamycin (A) and x-ray therapy (XRT) in bronchogenic carcinoma (BC): response and cardiotoxicity (CT). Proc. A.A.C.R. and A.S.C.O. *17*:276, 1976.

Cohen, L.: Radiation response and recovery: radiobiological principles and their relation to clinical practice. *In* Biologic Basis of Radiation Therapy. Edited by E.E. Schwartz, Philadelphia, J.B. Lippincott Co., 1966, p. 208.

Cooper, G., Jr., et al.: Some consequences of pulmonary irradiation. Am. J. Roentgenol. *85*:865, 1961.

Deeley, T.J.: The Chest. *In* Monographs on Oncology, London, Butterworths & Co., Ltd., 1973, p. 84.

Doggett, R., et al.: Combined therapy using chemotherapeutic agents and radiotherapy. *In* Modern Trends in Radiotherapy, Vol. 1. Edited by C. Wood and T.J. Deeley. New York, Appleton-Century-Crofts, 1967, p. 107.

Elkind, M.M., and Whitmore, G.F.: The Radiobiology of Cultured Mammalian Cells. New York, Gordon and Breach Publishers, 1967, p. 7.

Elkind, M.M., et al.: Sub-lethal and lethal radiation damage. Nature 214:1088, 1967.

Ellis, F.: Dose-time and fractionation: a clinical hypothesis. Clin. Radiol. 20:1, 1969.

Evans, H.J.: Chromosome aberrations induced by ionizing radiation. Int. Rev. Cytol. 13:221, 1962.

Fendel, H., and Feine, U.: Late sequelae of therapeutic irradiation for benign condition in childhood. Ann. Radiol. 13:291, 1970.

Gray, L.H.: Radiobiologic basis of oxygen as modifying factor in radiation therapy. Am. J. Roentgenol. 85:803, 1961.

Hall, E.J.: The relative biological efficiency of x-rays generated at 220 kvp and gamma radiation from a cobalt 60 therapy unit. Br. J. Radiol. 34:313, 1961.

Hall, E.J.: Radiobiology for the Radiologist, 2nd ed. New York, Harper & Row, 1976.

Hempelmann, L.H., et al.: Neoplasms in persons treated with x-rays in infancy for thymic enlargement. J. Natl. Cancer Inst. 38:317, 1967.

Hewitt, H.B., and Wilson, C.W.: Survival curve for mammalian leukemia cells irradiation in vivo. Br. J. Cancer 13:69, 1959.

Johns, H.E., and Cunningham, J.R.: The Physics of Radiology, 3rd ed. Springfield, IL, Charles C Thomas, 1969.

Johnson, R.E., Brereton, H.D., and Kent, C.H.: Small cell carcinoma of the lung: attempt to remedy causes of past therapeutic failure. Lancet 2:289, 1976.

Kallman, R.F.: The phenomenon of reoxygenation and its implications for fractionated radiotherapy. Radiology 105:135, 1972.

Kaplan, H.S.: Biochemical basis of reproductive death in irradiated cells. Am. J. Roentgenol. 90:907, 1963.

Knospe, W.H., Blom, J., and Crosby, W.H.: Regeneration of locally irradiated bone marrow. I. Dose-dependent long-term changes in the rat, with particular emphasis upon vascular and stromal reaction. Blood 28:308, 1966.

Kolstad, P.: Oxygen tension and radiocurability. In Modern Radiotherapy—Gynecological Cancer. Edited by T. Deeley. New York, Appleton-Century-Crofts, 1971, p. 155.

Lejar, T.J., et al.: Effects of focal irradiation on human bone marrow. Am. J. Roentgenol. 96:183, 1966.

Little, J.B.: Cellular effects of ionizing radiation. N. Engl. J. Med. 278:308, 1968.

Perez, C.A., et al.: A prospective randomized study of various irradiation doses and fractionation schedules in the treatment of inoperable non-oat cell carcinoma of the lung. Preliminary report by the Radiation Therapy Oncology Group. Cancer 45:2744, 1980.

Phillips, T., and Margolis, L.: Radiation pathology and the clinical response of lung and esophagus. In Frontiers of Radiation Therapy and Oncology, Vol. 6. Edited by J.M. Vaeth. Baltimore, University Park Press, 1972, p. 254.

Phillips, T.L., and Sheline, G.E.: Bone sarcomas following radiation therapy. Radiology 81:992, 1963.

Phillips, T.L., et al.: The hypoxic cell sensitizer program in the United States. Br. J. Cancer 37:(Suppl. III):276, 1978.

Puck, T.T., and Marcus, P.I.: Action of x-rays on mammalian cells. J. Exp. Med. 103:653, 1956.

Rubin, P., and Cassarett, G.: Clinical Radiation Pathology. Philadelphia, W.B. Saunders Co., 1968.

Rubin, P., et al.: Bone marrow regeneration and extension after extended field irradiation in Hodgkin's disease. Cancer 32:699, 1973.

Simpson, J.R., et al.: Large fraction irradiation with or without misonidazole in advanced non-oat cell carcinoma of the lung: a phase III randomized trial of the RTOG. Int. J. Radiat. Oncol. Biol. Phys. 13:861, 1987

Sinclair, W.K.: Cyclic x-ray responses in mammalian cells in vitro. Radiat. Res. 33:620–643, 1968.

Stewart, J.R., and Fajardo, L.F.: Radiation-induced heart disease. In Frontiers of Radiation Therapy and Oncology, Vol. 6. Edited by J.M. Vaeth. Baltimore, University Park Press, 1972, p. 274.

Suit, H.D., and Shalek, R.J.: Response of anoxic C3H mouse mammary carcinoma isotransplants (1–25 MM3) to x-irradiation. J. Natl. Cancer Inst. 31:479, 1963.

Sundbom, L., and Asard, P.E.: Tumor dose concept. Acta Radiol. 3:135, 1965.

Tables of depth dose for use in radiotherapy. Br. J. Radiol. (Suppl. 11), 1972.

Terasima, T., and Tolmach, L.J.: Variations in several responses of hela cells to x-irradiation during division cycle. Biophys. J. 3:11, 1963.

Thomlinson, R.H.: Oxygen therapy-biological considerations. In Modern Trends in Radiotherapy, Vol. 1. Edited by C. Wood and T.J. Deeley. New York, Appleton-Century-Crofts, 1967.

Tolmach, L.J.: Growth patterns in x-irradiated hela cells. Ann. N.Y. Acad. Sci. 95:743, 1961.

Tubiana, M., and Lalanne, C.M.: Treatment by supervoltage machines—telecurie apparatus. In Modern Trends in Radiotherapy, Vol. 1. Edited by C. Wood and T.J. Deeley. Appleton-Century-Crofts, 1967.

Van den Brenk, H.A.S.: Hyperbaric oxygen in radiation therapy. Am. J. Roentgenol. 102:8, 1968.

Wasserman, T.H., Nelson, J.S., and VonGerichten, D.: Neuropathy of nitroimidazole radiosensitizers: Clinical and pathologic description. Int. J. Radiat. Oncol. Biol. Phys. 10:1725, 1984.

Withers, H.R.: Capacity for repair in cells of normal and malignant tissues. In Time and Dose Relationships in Radiation Biology as Applied to Radiotherapy. Upton, New York, Brookhaven National Laboratory Associated Universities, 1970, p. 54.

Young, M.E.J.: Radiological Physics, 2nd ed. Springfield, IL, Charles C Thomas, 1967.

READING REFERENCES

Abramson, N., and Cavanaugh, P.J.: Short-course radiation therapy in carcinoma of the lung. Radiology 96:627, 1970.

Abramson, N., and Cavanaugh, P.J.: Short-course radiation therapy in carcinoma of the lung: a second look. Radiology 108:685, 1973.

Andrews, J.R., and Hollister, H.: Fast neutron beam radiotherapy. Am. J. Roentgenol. 99:954, 1967.

Bennett, D.E., Million, R.R., and Ackerman, L.V.: Bilateral radiation pneumonitis, a complication of the radiotherapy of bronchogenic carcinoma. Cancer 5:1001, 1969.

Berkjis, C.C.: Pathology of Irradiation. Baltimore, Williams & Wilkins, 1971.

Boge, J.R., Edland, R.W., and Matthes, D.C.: Tissue compensators for megavoltage radiotherapy fabricated from hollowed styrofoam filled with wax. Radiology 111:193, 1974.

Clarkson, J.R.: A note on depth doses in fields of irregular shape. Br. J. Radiol. 14:265, 1941.

Cox, J.D., et al.: Dose-time relationships and the local control of small cell carcinoma of the lung. Radiology 128:205, 1978.

Cundiff, J.H., et al.: A method for the calculation of dose in the radiation treatment of Hodgkin's disease. Am. J. Roentgenol. Radium Ther. Nucl. Med. 117:30, 1973.

Eichhorn, H.J., Lessel, A., and Matschke, S.: Comparison between neutron therapy and 60Co gamma ray therapy of bronchial, gastric and oesophagus carcinomata. Eur. J. Cancer 10:361, 1974.

Ellis, F., and Lescrenier, C.: Combined compensator for contours and heterogeneity. Radiology 106:191, 1973.

Fedoruk, S.D., and John, H.E.: Transmission dose measurement for Cobalt 60 radiation with special reference to rotation therapy. Br. J. Radiol. 30:190, 1957.

Fleming, J.S., and Orchard, P.G.: Isocentric radiotherapy treatment planning where the treatment axis is not horizontal. Br. J. Radiol. 47:34, 1974.

Fletcher, G.H.: Clinical dose-response curves of human malignant epithelial tumors. Br. J. Radiol. 46:1, 1973.

Fowler, J.F.: Difference in survival curve shapes for formal multi-target and multi-hit models. Phys. Med. Biol. 9:177, 1964.

Guthrie, R.T., Ptacek, J.J., and Hass, A.C.: Comparative analysis of two regimens of split course radiation in carcinoma of the lung. Am. J. Roentgenol. Radium Ther. Nucl. Med. 117:605, 1973.

Herring, D.F., and Compton, D.M.J.: The degree of precision required in the radiation dose delivered in cancer radiotherapy. Enviro-Med Report, EMI-216, 1970.

Holmes, W.F.: External beam treatment planning with the programmed console. Radiology *94*:391, 1970.

Holsti, L., and Vuorinen, P.: Radiation reaction in the lung after continuous and split-course megavoltage radiotherapy of bronchial carcinoma. Br. J. Radiol. *40*:280, 1967.

International Commission on Radiation Units and Measurements Report 24: Determination of Absorbed Dose in a Patient Irradiated by Beams of X or Gamma Rays in Radiotherapy Procedures. ICRU, Washington, D.C., 1976.

Laughlin, J.S.: Realistic treatment planning. Cancer *22*:716, 1968.

Lee, R.E.: Radiotherapy of bronchogenic carcinoma. Semin. Oncol. *1*:245, 1974.

Levitt, S.H., Bogardus, C.R., and Ladd, G.: Split-dose radiation therapy in the treatment of advanced lung cancer. Radiology *88*:1159, 1967.

Nohl, H.C.: An investigation into the lymphatic and vascular spread of carcinoma of the bronchus. Thorax *11*:172, 1956.

Phillips, R.A., and Tolmach, L.J.: Repair of potentially lethal damage in x-irradiated hela cells. Radiat. Res. *29*:413, 1966.

Powers, W.E., and Tolmach, L.J.: A multicomponent x-ray survival curve for mouse lymphosarcoma cells irradiated in vivo. Nature *197*:710, 1963.

Reinhold, H.S.: Radiations and the microcirculation. *In* Frontiers of Radiation Therapy and Oncology, Vol. 6. Edited by J.M. Vaeth. Baltimore, University Park Press, 1972, p. 44.

Sambrook, D.K.: Split course radiation therapy in malignant tumors. Am. J. Roentgenol. *91*:37, 1964.

Seaman, W.B., and Ackerman, L.V.: The effect of radiation on the esophagus: a clinical and histological study of the effects produced by the betatron. Radiology *68*:534, 1957.

CHAPTER 93

RADIATION THERAPY IN CARCINOMA OF THE LUNG

James D. Cox

Carcinoma of the lung encompasses a group of diseases which, in one manifestation or another, require the aggressive efforts of the thoracic surgeon, the radiation oncologist, and the medical oncologist. Nearly 50% of patients present with disseminated disease; a few patients with small cell carcinoma of the lung present with localized disease and require both systemic therapy and at least local-regional radiation therapy. Approximately one third of all patients with squamous cell carcinoma, adenocarcinoma, or large cell carcinoma of the lung have unresectable disease. Radiation therapy is the only potentially curative treatment in these patients.

Radiation therapy, like surgical resection, is a local-regional treatment. The success of treatment depends upon its proper application to patients whose disease is confined to a primary tumor and regional lymph node metastasis. Radiation therapy can also be used to palliate discrete, symptomatic metastases, more often in the brain or bones, in addition to symptoms arising from the intrathoracic tumor.

Surgery, radiation therapy, and chemotherapy all have important roles in the management of lung cancer. The endpoints used to evaluate the effectiveness of these treatments, however, have differed historically. In surgical management of lung cancer, the focus has been upon the curability of the patient, and the endpoint has usually been survival, less frequently relapse-free survival, at 3 or 5 years. The most common endpoints used in evaluating chemotherapy of lung cancer have been complete and partial response rates and median survival. These are, for practical purposes, palliative endpoints. Two-year survival or relapse-free survival has widely been used to assess the results of treatment of patients with small cell carcinoma of the lung with chemotherapy alone or chemotherapy combined with radiation therapy.

Radiotherapeutic effectiveness has been assessed using both sets of endpoints. The palliative contribution has been reported in terms of response rates and median survival. The lack of sensitive indicators of recurrence after radiation therapy, however, and the recognition that the treatment can cause changes in the irradiated volume that obscure response, raise questions as to the value of "response" as a useful endpoint. Median survival has no necessary relationship to long-term survival. Pretreatment prognostic variables probably outweigh treatment factors in the early survival experience of patients with inoperable non-small cell carcinoma of the lung, and the effectiveness of the treatment can only be determined by survival beyond the median survival—i.e., beyond 9 to 12 months. Definitive—i.e., potentially curative—radiation therapy for squamous cell carcinoma, adenocarcinoma, and large cell carcinoma—non-small cell carcinoma—of the lung has also been reported by Komaki and associates (1985) in terms of long-term—3 or 5 years—survival.

INDICATIONS FOR RADIATION THERAPY FOR BRONCHIAL CARCINOMA BASED ON FAILURE ANALYSES

Failure pattern analyses by Shields (1983) of patients with resectable carcinoma of the lung suggest that a group of patients with squamous cell carcinoma, adenocarcinoma, and large cell carcinoma of the lung could benefit from irradiation of the mediastinum and hila. Patients with T1N0M0 and T2N0M0 fail infrequently in the thorax after complete resection. The presence of regional lymph node metastasis increases considerably the risk of local failure, and it also portends a higher rate of distant metastasis, especially to the brain.

My (1983) failure pattern analyses of patients with inoperable or unresectable carcinoma of the lung showed that the intrathoracic tumor is a major determinant of survival, especially in patients with squamous cell carcinoma who have not had aggressive radiation therapy to the thoracic tumor. These studies also showed that small cell carcinoma disseminated so frequently that systemic treatment was essential in its management. Until the cell types were clearly delineated, it was widely held that all patients with carcinoma of the lung died with disseminated disease. The failure patterns of squamous cell carcinoma, adenocarcinoma, and large cell carcinoma taken together, however, differ considerably from that of small cell carcinoma. Complications of the intrathoracic tumor are the most common cause of death from squamous cell carcinoma of the lung. At the other extreme, small cell carcinoma has such a high propensity for extrathoracic spread that subclinical metastasis must be assumed even with apparently localized tumors. Adenocarcinoma and large cell carcinoma, which constitute nearly 45% of all carcinomas of the lung, are intermediate between squamous and small cell carcinoma; their propensity for extrathoracic spread is higher than squamous carcinoma's, but not as high as small cell carcinoma's; they cause death more frequently from the intrathoracic tumor than small cell carcinoma does, but less frequently than squamous carcinoma.

Thus, squamous cell carcinoma of the lung would seem the most readily managed by definitive radiation therapy when found to be unresectable. I and my associates (1986a), however, suggested that adenocarcinoma/large cell carcinoma—they can be grouped as one because their clinical behaviors are indistinguishable—was actually more radiocurable than squamous cell carcinoma.

EVALUATION BEFORE RADIATION THERAPY

The evaluation of patients with carcinoma of the lung apparently confined to the thorax differs little whether the patient is to be treated with surgical resection or with definitive radiation therapy. The intent of the pretreatment evaluation is to determine the extent of the local and regional manifestations of the intrathoracic tumor, and to investigate the most likely sites of distant metastasis. With rare exceptions, it is inappropriate to undertake a long course of radiation therapy to high total doses, with the attendant risk of morbidity, if distant metastasis is recognized.

A complete blood count, biochemical survey, and posteroanterior and lateral chest roentgenograms are performed routinely. The intrathoracic tumor can be assessed well by high resolution computed tomography with intravenous contrast. Multiple parenchymal lesions, pericardial involvement with effusion, and pleural effusion are signs of intrathoracic dissemination and are contraindications to aggressive local-regional therapy. The liver, adrenal glands, and kidneys, all common sites of distant metastasis at autopsy, can be assessed by high resolution, contrast-enhanced computed tomography of the upper abdomen. Norlund and associates (1985) reported that in patients with small cell carcinoma, adenocarcinoma, and large cell carcinoma, computed tomography of the upper abdomen changes the stage and therefore the treatment plan in 20 to 30% of all patients.

The diagnosis of adenocarcinoma, large cell carcinoma, or small cell carcinoma justifies contrast-enhanced computed tomography of the head to look for occult cerebral metastasis. In patients with no neurologic symptoms, the frequency of occult cerebral metastasis recorded by Jacobs (1977) and Tarver (1984) and their associates ranged from 10 to 20%. The finding of cerebral metastasis, of course, profoundly affects the prognosis as well as the plan of therapy.

SURGICAL ADJUVANT RADIATION THERAPY

Patients who have undergone complete resection and have been found, on histopathologic examination, to have involvement of regional lymph nodes—N1 or N2—are the only ones who have a sufficiently high risk of intrathoracic recurrence to justify the addition of radiation therapy. This explains, at least in part, the failure of studies of preoperative irradiation to demonstrate any benefit; the patients who might have benefited were diluted by those who would not have been expected to benefit. The excellent review by Van Houtte and Henry (1985) summarized trials of both preoperative and postoperative radiation therapy. They concluded that preoperative irradiation has no benefit in patients with clearly operable tumors. Its role might be investigated further for patients with marginally resectable tumors, but no prospective studies to date were specifically targeted to this small group of patients. The same authors reviewed the experiences with postoperative irradiation in patients with hilar or mediastinal lymph node involvement or both. Three- and five-year survival rates in these studies ranged from 16 to 33% in patients with squamous cell carcinoma treated with surgical resection alone versus survival rates of 21 to 52% for surgery plus radiation therapy. The data were even more striking for adenocarcinoma with hilar or mediastinal lymph node involvement: 0 to 8% 5-year survival with surgery alone versus 12 to 62% survival with surgery and postoperative irradiation.

Two prospective randomized trials of postoperative radiation therapy have been conducted. An EORTC trial reported by Israel and associates (1979) suggested a survival benefit of the same order of magnitude as the retrospective studies, i.e., 20 to 25%, but the results were preliminary and not statistically significant. The Lung Cancer Study Group, reported by Holmes and associates (1985), conducted a trial of postoperative radiation therapy versus surgery alone for patients with stage III squamous cell carcinoma of the lung; this study thus mixed patients with and without lymph node involvement and did not study patients with adenocarcinoma/large cell carcinoma, in which the survival benefit may be more pronounced than in patients with squamous cell carcinoma. They found a striking reduction in the frequency of local recurrence within the thorax but no survival benefit.

Therefore, the composite results of surgical adjuvant radiation therapy show no advantage from preoperative irradiation. Patients with regional nodal metastases seem to benefit from postoperative irradiation, but this may not translate into improved survival for those with squamous carcinoma.

DEFINITIVE RADIATION THERAPY FOR SQUAMOUS CELL CARCINOMA, ADENOCARCINOMA, AND LARGE CELL CARCINOMA OF THE LUNG

Radiation therapy is the mainstay of treatment for patients with inoperable squamous cell carcinoma, adenocarcinoma, and large cell carcinoma of the lung. Once the determination has been made that such patients are inoperable or have unresectable tumors, and a thorough evaluation has shown no evidence of distant metastasis, technically sophisticated, high-dose radiation therapy offers the best opportunity for long-term, disease-free survival.

Admittedly, effective treatment of the local regional tumor does not prevent patients from dying of disseminated disease. With the evolution of more effective systemic chemotherapy regimens, it will be important to combine aggressive local-regional radiation therapy with systemic chemotherapy. The experiences to date with small cell carcinoma of the lung limited to the thorax suggest that the importance of effective local-regional radiation therapy will continue or increase with more effective chemotherapeutic regimens.

Determination of the Treatment Volume

Definitive irradiation for lung cancer is predicated upon irradiation of the primary tumor with generous margins, the inclusion of enlarged regional lymph nodes, and the systematic irradiation of anatomic regions that are common sites of lymphatic extension. The entire width of the mediastinum is irradiated in all patients. For upper lobe tumors, the volume extends from the sternal notch superiorly to a point at least 5 cm below the carina, and the lower level of the mediastinal field is extended to the diaphragm for tumors that arise in the lower lobes. A study of protocol compliance versus outcome by Perez and associates (1982), from the Radiation Therapy Oncology Group—RTOG, suggested the need to include both the ipsilateral and contralateral hila.

There has not been a systematic study of supraclavicular irradiation, but data from biopsy studies suggest that possibly one quarter of patients with upper lobe tumor have spread to the scalene or supraclavicular nodes, whereas this risk is less than 10% for tumors arising in the lower lobes. Systematic irradiation of the ipsilateral supraclavicular nodes is considered standard for upper lobe or middle lobe tumors. There may be some justification for irradiating both supraclavicular areas if adenopathy in the superior mediastinum has been demonstrated by computed tomography or bronchoscopy.

Treatment Planning

The process of planning definitive treatment for carcinoma of the lung, following complete assessment of the diagnostic studies, especially the CT scan of the thorax, starts with simulation. The treatment planning simulator is a diagnostic x-ray unit, usually with fluoroscopy, in which the head of the unit can be set to mimic or "simulate" the location of the head of the treatment machine; i.e., the focal spot for diagnostic roentgenograms is set exactly at the same point as the source or target that emits high energy photons. The image intensifier can be moved independently to assess the margins of the field to determine that they adequately encompass the entire volume that is to be treated.

A film of diagnostic quality that shows the intrathoracic anatomy sharply is obtained; the photons from the actual treatment machine are so penetrating that anatomic distinctions between bone and soft tissues are obscured. Correlation of the anatomy displayed on the simulation film with that apparent from the computed tomograms of the chest serves as the basis for defining the exact margins of the volume to be treated. Using the simulation film, an individualized block of a low melting-point alloy of lead is constructed by pouring the molten material into a styrofoam mold. This block is fixed to a plastic tray, which is inserted in the head of the treatment machine so that it is interposed between the source of photons and the patient. When the photons are produced, the field is thus shaped by having photons absorbed in the lead-like material but permitted to pass through where the material is absent. In this manner, normal structures can be protected and only the desired anatomic volume is exposed.

This treatment planning process has become standard in modern departments. There is no reason, any longer, to consider unshaped, square, or rectangular fields the norm. Such careful blocking must be undertaken if the high doses thought necessary to control common epithelial tumors, including those arising in the lung, are to be achieved.

Dose-Time Relationships

The interplay of the individual dose of irradiation—fraction size, the frequency of delivery of the individual dose or fraction, the total dose to the tumor and to normal tissues, and the overall time of treatment, are encompassed by the terms, "dose-time relationships" or "fractionation." In the 1960s and 1970s it was assumed that outcome in the radiation therapy of carcinomas of the lung was not greatly influenced by differing fractionation schemes. Low total doses were used with the rationale that adequate palliation could be achieved without recourse to high doses that might injure normal structures, especially the lung parenchyma. Because the total doses were low, changing the fractionation to a smaller number of large fractions led to the same poor result. Deeley (1967) reported a prospective clinical trial that compared 30 Gy with 40 Gy, both given in 20 fractions in 4 weeks: 12- and 18-month survival data convinced him that the lower dose was at least as effective. A subsequent comparison by Deeley (1974) of 40 Gy in 20 fractions in 4 weeks with 32 Gy in eight fractions—two fractions per week—in 4 weeks confirmed his expectation that both regimens were equal. Thus, a school of thought prevailed that irradiation to low total doses, with or without large-size fractions, was sufficient to relieve distressing symptoms and would cause few deleterious effects on the normal lung.

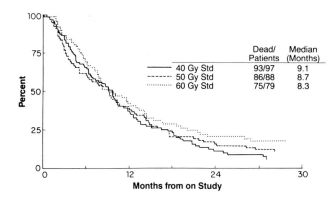

Fig. 93–1. Survival by total dose following radiation therapy for squamous cell carcinoma, adenocarcinoma and large cell carcinoma of the lung: Standard—common—fractionation—2.0 Gy per fraction, 5 fractions per week. From RTOG Protocol 73–01.

The RTOG conducted a landmark study; a multi-center, prospective, centrally randomized trial compared the effectiveness of 40 Gy, 50 Gy, and 60 Gy, delivered as 2.0 Gy per fraction, five fractions per week, for 4, 5, or 6 weeks, respectively. Early analyses of this trial by Perez and associates (1980) revealed a dose-response relationship for tumor control with lower failure rates resulting from higher total doses. Long-term follow-up of the patients in this study, although showing no difference in median survival, showed a highly significant direct relationship between 2- and 3-year survival and total dose (Fig. 93–1). Consequently, a total dose of at least 60 Gy in 30 fractions in 6 weeks is now the standard for definitive treatment. Higher total doses might be used, and certainly should be explored in prospective studies, because the RTOG did not investigate a dose higher than 60 Gy.

A large body of data from the radiation therapy of common epithelial tumors of many sites suggests that fractions larger than 2.0 Gy and treatments less frequent than 5 days per week are disadvantageous. I observed (1985b) that large-dose fractionation could take many forms, including hypofractionation—fewer than five treatments per week, rapid fractionation—large doses 5 days a week for only 3 or 4 weeks, and a split-course radiation therapy—interruption of 1 week or more during the course of radiation therapy—with fractions of 2.0 Gy or less, or larger fractions attempting to compensate for the split, thus combining the split with rapid fractionation.

Studies of hypoxic cell sensitizers which, theoretically, would produce the most effective result from combination with a few large fractions of radiation therapy, have provided important information on the results of hypofractionation. Saunders and associates (1984) randomly assigned 62 patients to receive 35 Gy in six fractions in 3 weeks with and without the nitrofuran, misonidazole. Their careful assessment based on a high autopsy rate showed the fractionation regimen to be ineffective; the overwhelming cause of death was progression of the local-regional tumor. Fewer than 5% of patients had control

of the tumor within the irradiated volume. Also, misonidazole proved to be of no benefit.

A detailed review of the other fractionation schemes is beyond the scope of this chapter, but large-dose fractionation and split-course radiation therapy have been disadvantageous, both in tumor control and in late effects on normal tissues. The disadvantage in tumor control can best be explained by an acceleration of repopulation once the radiation therapy has been started, a more rapid proliferation that cannot be overcome when treatments are insufficiently frequent or are interrupted. The deleterious effect on normal tissues results from the large fractions, which damage preferentially the late-responding normal tissues; the adverse effects on the normal tissues do not appear for several months to several years.

RESULTS OF RADIATION THERAPY FOR INOPERABLE NON-SMALL CELL CARCINOMA OF THE LUNG

Palliation

Slawson and Scott (1979) suggested that symptomatic relief by radiation therapy for local-regional manifestations of squamous cell, adenocarcinoma, and large cell carcinomas of the lung can be predicted fairly accurately. Superior vena caval obstruction can be relieved in more than three quarters of patients. Hemoptysis can be eliminated with similar consistency. Pain in the chest, shoulder, and arm can usually be decreased or eliminated: the more vague and nonspecific the discomfort, the less predictable the relief. By contrast, bronchial obstruction with established atelectasis, usually complicated by obstructive pneumonitis, can be ameliorated in only one quarter of patients. The longer the atelectasis has been established, the greater the opportunity for infectious complications and the less the possibility of effective relief by local radiation therapy. Paralysis of the vocal cord resulting from involvement of the recurrent laryngeal nerve at the aorticopulmonary window, is rarely relieved despite long-term control of the tumor. Whether this is caused by destruction of the nerve by direct invasion or entrapment of the nerve in the tumor and subsequently fibrosis is not clear.

Prolongation of Survival

Radiation therapy of the intrathoracic tumor prolongs survival, even of patients who will eventually die of lung cancer. In a retrospective series of radiation therapy for inoperable or unresectable carcinoma of the lung, Eisert and associates (1976) showed a prolongation of survival for patients whose intrathoracic tumors were controlled with radiation therapy compared with those whose tumors were not controlled. Various fractionation schemes had been used, including common or standard fractionation and hypofractionation. Perez and associates (1986) corroborated this prolongation of survival in a prospective trial conducted by the Radiation Therapy Oncology Group. In addition, a dose response was demonstrated for 2- and 3-year survival (Fig. 93–1). By contrast, I and my associates (1983) reported that patients with tumors limited to the thorax who received no definitive treatment rarely lived 3 years, and fewer than 5% were alive at 2 years.

The Potential for Cure by Radiation Therapy

The most important role for radiation therapy is its potentially curative use in patients who have few or mild symptoms. Komaki and associates (1985) reported the change in 3-year survival rates among patients with inoperable carcinoma of the lung treated at the Medical College of Wisconsin from 1971 to 1978. Of patients treated with radiation therapy alone between 1971 and 1975, 7% of 197 were alive at 3 years, a figure similar to many reports of the results of megavoltage radiation therapy. Of 213 patients treated between 1975 and 1978, 14%—29 patients—were alive after 3 or more years. Long-term observations of the 3-year survivors (Fig. 93–2) showed that 80%—23 patients—were still alive at 5 years—11% of entire group, and two thirds lived 10 years. No patient in this series died of lung cancer after 54 months.

The important gains between the earlier and later time periods were not the result of the treatment of more favorable patients with less extensive disease. Indeed, the patients with more advanced tumors provided the additional long-term survivors (Table 93–1). Only 1% of patients with stage III tumors lived 3 or more years in the earlier time period, compared with 11% of those treated between 1975 and 1978. Most of the improvement in survival was found in patients with mediastinal lymph node involvement.

No patient with the performance status less than 80 on the Karnofsky scale survived three years, compared with 7% whose performance status was 80 to 89, 25% with a performance status 90 to 99, and 70%—seven of ten patients—who were truly asymptomatic, i.e., had a performance status of 100. The patients studied from

1971 through 1978 did not have the benefit of pretreatment evaluation by computed tomography and other sophisticated imaging procedures. This experience should be considered only a baseline for what can be accomplished with contemporary treatment methods and pretreatment selection.

SPECIAL CONSIDERATIONS

Several special circumstances may be encountered among patients with lung cancer that appropriately might lead to the use of radiation therapy.

Apical Sulcus—Pancoast—Tumors

Tumors in the extreme apex of either lung may cause shoulder or arm pain, sensory and motor dysfunction, especially along the distribution of the ulnar nerve, destruction of ribs or, less frequently, vertebral bodies, and Horner's syndrome. Paulson's (1966, 1968) recommendations have been followed for more than two decades: a brief course of preoperative radiation therapy is followed by thoracotomy, mediastinal exploration, and definitive resection if regional lymph node metastasis was not evident (see Chapter 33). This was a justifiable approach when surgical resection was the only tenable treatment. Several series have now demonstrated the efficacy of definitive radiation therapy for these tumors, which seem to have a lesser propensity for extrathoracic dissemination than other presentations of lung cancer. The disadvantages of hypofractionation or split-course radiation therapy have been noted previously. Those patients who receive preoperative irradiation and then are found to have unresectable tumors are placed at a great disadvantage; subsequent radiation therapy with such a long interruption is of little use, and frequently is applied to an already progressing tumor. In the experience of the Memorial Hospital of New York City, Martini and McCormack (1983) reported that fewer than 20% of patients

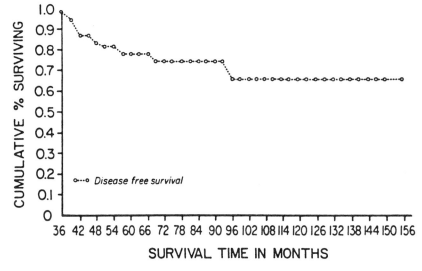

Fig. 93–2. Disease-free survival beyond 3 years after completion of radiotherapy. Reproduced with permission of Komaki, R., et al.: Characteristics of long-term survivors after treatment for inoperable carcinoma of the lung. Am. J. Clin. Oncol. 8:362, 1985.

Table 93–1. Percent of Patients Surviving 36+ Months by Extent of Tumor, Medical College of Wisconsin: 1971–1978

	1971–1975		1975–1978	
	No. of Patients	%	No. of Patients	%
Stage				
I	36	33.3	48	20.8
II	21	4.8	33	18.2
III	140	1.4	132	10.6
Nodal Involvement				
None	72	18.2	81	8.0
Hilar	21	14.3	33	15.2
Mediastinal	86	1.2	82	12.2
Supraclavicular	18	5.6	17	17.6

Modified from Komaki, R., et al: Characteristics of long-term survivors after treatment of inoperable carcinoma of the lung. Am. J. Clin. Oncol. 8:362, 1985.

explored could have complete surgical resection with curative intent. The other 80% of the patients were obligated to have an inferior form of radiation therapy.

Therefore, the most appropriate approach to permit benefit for the entire spectrum of patients with apical sulcus tumors is immediate exploration for those thought to have resectable tumors. If the tumors prove unresectable, the patients can still benefit from the most effective type of radiation therapy.

Superior Vena Caval Obstruction

Obstruction of the superior vena cava almost invariably results from a malignant neoplasm. Lung cancer is, by far, the most frequent neoplasm encountered. Approximately 5% of all patients with carcinoma of the lung present with superior vena caval obstruction. The frequent presentation with dyspnea and swelling of the face, neck, and upper extremities with collateral venous circulation on the upper thorax may be a radiotherapeutic emergency. This presentation, however, is rarely ominous enough to preclude cytologic diagnosis by needle aspirate or even fiber-optic bronchoscopy. The finding of a neoplasm other than lung cancer may change both the therapeutic options and the prognosis. If small cell carcinoma is identified, the treatment programs are different than that for superior vena caval obstruction due to non-small cell lung cancer and are described on pages 1157 and 1158 of this chapter.

The finding of squamous cell carcionoma, adenocarcinoma, or large cell carcinoma of the lung justifies immediate treatment with a few large fractions—3.5 to 4.0 Gy per fraction, followed by common fractionation with 1.8 to 2.0 Gy per fraction. The additional destruction of tumor cells with the initial large fractions is associated with more immediate relief of symptoms than smaller-sized fractions. The number of such large fractions is sufficiently small that the late effects on normal tissues do not become a serious problem. A common approach is the use of three or four large fractions and then a continuation of common fractionation. Over 80% of patients with superior vena caval obstruction experience rapid relief of symptoms. Unfortunately, the remaining

patients probably do not benefit because of thrombosis of the superior vena cava.

Treatment of Metastases

Radiation therapy is frequently useful for the palliation of symptoms from distant metastasis in patients with carcinoma of the lung. Relief of the various symptoms resulting from the intrathoracic tumor has already been reviewed. The most frequent extrathoracic symptoms that can be alleviated by radiation therapy are neurologic dysfunction resulting from metastasis involving the central nervous system—CNS—and pain from metastasis to bones or, less frequently, soft tissues.

CNS Metastasis

Approximately 10% of all patients with cancer of the lung present with cerebral metastasis. Most of these metastases result in neurologic symptoms and signs that suggest the need for further evaluation. Small cell carcinoma, adenocarcinoma, and large cell carcinoma of the lung cause cerebral metastasis so frequently (Table 93–2), that computed tomography or magnetic resonance imaging of the brain is worthwhile even in asymptomatic patients. The yield of occult metastasis is approximately 10%.

Borgelt and associates (1980) suggested that relief of symptoms from brain metastasis by radiation therapy is reasonably consistent and predictable. Seizures and impaired mentation are reversible more frequently than specific motor deficits are.

At least half of all patients who develop brain metastasis from carcinoma of the lung die as a direct result of CNS involvement. The median survival is little more than 3 months. Patients who have cerebral metastasis at the time of initial diagnosis have a somewhat worse prognosis. Patients who develop cerebral metastasis following initial surgical resection or radiation therapy of the intrathoracic tumor have a slightly better prognosis. Indeed, as Komaki and associates (1983) suggested, a few of these patients live for years following aggressive surgical intervention or irradiation for the cerebral metastasis. This is undoubtedly the result of single-organ brain metastasis, i.e., metastasis exclusively to the brain in the

Table 93–2. Frequency of Brain Metastasis at Autopsy by Histopathologic Type of Lung Cancer

Histopathologic Type	Patients with Metastasis/Patients Autopsied	%
Squamous cell	16/123	13
Adenocarcinoma	69/129	54
Large cell	28/54	52
Combined	3/12	25
Non-small cell	116/318	36
Small cell	37/82	45

absence of other extrathoracic dissemination. This phenomenon is more frequent with adenocarcinoma and large cell carcinoma than with squamous cell carcinoma or small cell carcinoma.

Skeletal Metastases

Komaki and associates (1977) reported that at least one third of patients with disseminated lung cancer have symptomatic involvement of the skeletal system, usually manifested as pain. A high probability of pain relief can be expected from palliative irradiation of symptomatic bony metastasis, but complete relief of pain is less frequent than partial relief. Tong and associates (1982) and Blitzer (1985) concur that brief but intensive courses of radiation therapy are indicated for the palliation of pain because it is desirable to reduce as much as possible the amount of time patients spend undergoing treatment when their life expectancy is short. In the uncommon situation where multiple sites of symptomatic metastases are present simultaneously, single-dose, hemibody irradiation can be considered. Treatment of the upper half of the body with 600 or 700 rad in a single fraction or treatment of the lower hemibody with 800 rad in a single fraction, produces remarkable, if short-lived, palliation.

Paraneoplastic Syndromes

Radiation therapy, like surgical resection, can diminish or eliminate paraneoplastic effects. Some paraneoplastic syndromes are more readily reversible than others. Endocrinologic syndromes, including adrenocorticotropic hormone—ACTH—and antidiuretic hormone—ADH—production can be reduced or eliminated by local-regional radiation therapy. Hypercalcemia is more complex and less predictably reversible with radiation therapy. Paraneoplastic neurologic symptoms and signs are infrequently altered by radiation therapy, and hypertrophic pulmonary osteoarthropathy is rarely affected.

Chronic Obstructive Pulmonary Disease and Pulmonary Infection

Chronic obstructive pulmonary disease—COPD—is rarely a contraindication to radiation therapy for inoperable cancer of the lung. Choi and associates (1985) showed by serial pulmonary function studies that judiciously applied radiation therapy rarely causes acute or late pulmonary effects greater than those already caused by the malignant tumor. Effective radiation therapy involves doses higher than those tolerated by the normal lung, so the high dose area must be minimized and confined to a volume that sharply circumscribes the intrathoracic tumor. With careful treatment planning using individualized blocks and multiple sets of fields as described, the primary tumor and regional lymph nodes can be adequately irradiated with few serious effects in the adjacent lung.

Many pulmonary tumors with a significant endobronchial component result in obstruction, distal atelectasis, and subsequent bacterial infection. This is, indeed, an indication for urgent radiation therapy; once atelectasis is well established, reversal is not achieved readily.

Active tuberculosis in a patient with carcinoma of the lung has been considered a contraindication to radiation therapy. With current antituberculous drug therapy, however, treatment for tuberculosis and radiation therapy can both be initiated immediately, if indicated. There is no indication that radiation therapy diminishes the effectiveness of antimicrobial therapy. Anecdotes suggest that radiation therapy has reactivated tuberculosis; this phenomenon, if real, is so rare that it has little practical consequence.

RADIATION EFFECTS ON NORMAL TISSUES OF THE THORAX

A detailed description of radiation effects on normal tissues that might be included during high dose, definitive radiation therapy of lung cancer is discussed in Chapter 92. I and my associates reviewed this subject in 1986.

The most sensitive structure irradiated with the treatment of bronchopulmonary carcinomas is the lung itself. With single doses, 8 to 10 Gy predictably produce radiation pneumonitis. Common fractionation with 1.5 to 1.8 Gy per day permit some repair of radiation effects; pneumonitis occurs in fewer than 5% of patients with total doses of 18 Gy to 20 Gy. As noted, irradiation for lung cancer, which incidentally treats portions of normal lung, usually results in improvement in pulmonary function because of the response of the tumor, followed by some degradation in function resulting from radiation pneumonitis and subsequent scarring. Prior, concurrent, or even subsequent chemotherapy may enhance or recall radiation effects and lower the total dose for radiation-induced inflammation and scarring. Drugs that notably increase radiation effects in the lung include dactino-mycin, bleomycin, carmustine, cyclophosphamide, and methotrexate. To limit the adverse effects of radiation therapy on the lung, the volume irradiated must be limited. Techniques that use multiple field arrangements, "shrinking fields," and individualized blocking are essential.

The most frequent normal tissue to give rise to symptoms during the course of irradiation is the esophagus. The germinal layer of the squamous epithelium lining the esophagus is affected with doses between 15 and 20 Gy. A pseudomembranous inflammation results in symptoms of dysphagia 10 to 14 days after the start of treatment. The symptoms improve even though the treatments continue, but they increase during the fourth week and again during the sixth week because of the cyclic nature of the reaction, resulting from accelerated proliferation of the viable germinal cells. Dietary recommendations and analgesics usually prevent significant weight loss. Late effects of the irradiation on the esophagus—stenosis or complete obstruction—are rare with common fractionation unless one or more of the aforementioned chemotherapeutic agents is combined with the radiation therapy.

Radiation myelopathy is, unquestionably, the most serious potential result of radiation therapy. Experiences with large dose fractionation by Hatlevoll (1983) and Dische (1981) and their associates have resulted in many reported cases of radiation myelopathy. Symptoms consist of weakness of the lower extremities and a Brown-Séquard syndrome beginning 6 to 36 months after completion of radiation therapy. Wollin and Kagan (1976) suggested that this grave, late effect of radiation therapy can be avoided entirely by careful attention to individual fraction size and overall treatment time.

Finally, some portion of the heart must be included within the field of irradiation, with rare exceptions. Stewart and Fajardo (1971) reported that when the entire heart is treated with doses of 40 Gy in 4 to 5 weeks, symptomatic radiation pericarditis is seen in approximately 5% of patients. Because most pulmonary neoplasms arise in the upper lobes, it is usually only necessary to treat the atria and great vessels. When a significant amount of the ventricles must be included within the field of irradiation, the dose must be limited, and treatment plans that sharply confine high doses to a minimal volume must be sought.

RECURRENT CANCER OF THE LUNG

Lung cancer may recur in the thorax following definitive surgery or definitive radiation therapy performed with the intent of complete eradication. In many cases, the recurrence may take the form of diffuse parenchymal metastases or pleural involvement with effusion. Radiation therapy has little, if anything, to offer patients with these manifestations of intrathoracic progression of tumor.

Infrequently, the tumor may progress in the lung or mediastinum adjacent to the site of the primary tumor

or in the regional lymph nodes. This is an indication for local-regional radiation therapy, but the expectations, necessarily, are limited. A tumor that regrows within an operative bed rarely can be controlled. This circumstance is similar to that of macroscopic residual tumor following subtotal resection. The precise reasons for a limited effect of external radiation therapy are not known, but they presumably relate to altered vasculature with broad areas of hypoxia resulting in a tumor less sensitive to the effects of ionizing radiations. Interestingly, Green and Melbye (1982) reported that postirradiation recurrences have a somewhat less grave outlook, and limited success has been achieved with repeat irradiation. Hilaris and Martini (1979) suggested that operative intervention with implants—brachytherapy—may rarely result in benefit. Also Seagren and associates (1985) reported that endobronchial insertion of radioactive sources may be followed by palliation of respiratory symptoms.

RADIATION THERAPY FOR SMALL CELL CARCINOMA

The consistency of overt or subclinical dissemination of small cell carcinoma of the lung was previously noted. Radiation therapy and cytotoxic drugs, administered individually, resulted in frequent responses but little long-term benefit. Combination chemotherapy was demonstrably superior, when measured by rate of response and median survival, and radiation therapy temporarily was thought no longer necessary. Retrospective studies suggested that survival at 2 years or more was superior when radiation therapy of the intrathoracic tumor was integrated with combination chemotherapy. Several prospective, randomized trials were launched to assess the role of thoracic irradiation.

The role of radiation therapy was obscured, not just by selection of endpoints such as response rates and median survival, but by assessment of intrathoracic failure rates that seemed to differ little in studies that compared chemotherapy versus integrated radiation therapy-chemotherapy. I (1985) suggested that it is now more widely recognized that intrathoracic failures are of three types: (1) failure within the irradiated volume is truly a failure of the dose-time relationships used; (2) failure at the margin of the irradiated volume may represent insufficient appreciation of the extent of the original tumor; and (3) failure in the periphery of the pulmonary parenchyma or the pleura which represents failure of the systemic regimen, not the radiation therapy.

Quality control in radiation therapy of small cell carcinoma of the lung profoundly influences the results of treatment. White and colleagues (1982) assessed the importance of compliance with protocol specifications in Southwestern Oncology Group trials; they showed that full compliance with radiation therapy specifications was the single most important prognostic factor. Studies of radiation therapy that have not included assessment of protocol compliance do not contribute meaningfully to the discussion of the proper role of radiation therapy and integrated management of small cell carcinoma.

The optimal means of integrating radiation therapy into the management of small cell carcinoma remains to be defined. Perry and associates (1987) reported studies of the Cancer and Leukemia Group B—CALGB—which suggested that radiation therapy after three or more cycles of chemotherapy was associated with a lesser toxicity and better long-term outcome than when radiation therapy was used with chemotherapy immediately after diagnosis. Bunn and associates (1987) found, in studies at the National Cancer Institute of the United States, that maximal initial therapy with radiation therapy and simultaneous chemotherapy was superior to chemotherapy alone. The alternation of combination chemotherapy and radiation therapy, the latter being used in "split" courses, has been more effective in the studies of Arriagada and associates (1985) from the Institut Gustave-Roussy compared with the studies of Perez and associates from the Southeastern Cancer Study Group—SECSG. Although preliminary, the most encouraging results come from Turrisi and colleagues (1986) who combined two non-cross resistant regimens of chemotherapy with accelerated fractionation—1.5 Gy twice daily to 45 Gy in three weeks. The fact that 50% of their patients are alive and well at 2 years justifies more extensive trials of accelerated fractionation with these chemotherapeutic schedules.

Radiation therapy is thus an important element in integrated management only of patients with small cell carcinoma of the lung clinically confined to the intrathoracic primary tumor and regional lymph nodes. Patients with disseminated disease at presentation respond less favorably to systemic chemotherapy than those with more limited disease, and they have not been shown to benefit from the addition of radiation therapy. Livingston and associates (1984) showed that a subset of these patients, those who have clinical complete responses to combination chemotherapy, fail often enough in the thorax that they constitute an appropriate group for further study of thoracic irradiation with systemic therapy.

CLINICAL RESEARCH IN RADIATION THERAPY OF CANCER OF THE LUNG

Clearly, radiation therapy, as currently used, addresses only part of the multifaceted problem of lung cancer. Efforts are underway to enhance the effectiveness of local radiation therapy in eradication of the intrathoracic tumor. Some of these efforts are based on the hypothesis that a significant fraction of the cells within the tumor are hypoxic and, thus, less sensitive to low linear energy transfer—LET—radiations such as those available from ^{60}Co teletherapy units and linear accelerators. Clinical studies of radiation therapy with high LET radiations in the form of fast neutrons, such as those reported by Laramore and associates (1986), are currently underway with dedicated, hospital-based cyclotrons. Simpson and associates (1987) reported that the first generation of electron-affinic hypoxic cell sensitizers did not

result in increased control of the thoracic tumor, but less toxic drugs that permit higher doses of sensitizers are entering clinical trials.

Alterations of fractionation are worth considering for several reasons. First, fractionation has long been considered the most effective means of overcoming hypoxia, because of reoxygenation of tumor cells between fractions of radiation therapy. Secondly, a dose response with common fractionation has already been demonstrated by the RTOG. Using higher doses with smaller individual fractions delivered more frequently—hyperfractionation—is possible because of the sparing of late effects in normal tissues. The higher doses possible with hyperfractionation may lead to better tumor control. Thirdly, the initial therapeutic insult to a tumor is thought to cause accelerated proliferation even within a tumor that is regressing. Although this may be overcome with hyperfractionation and higher total doses, the accelerated proliferation can be avoided by accelerated fractionation in which most or all of the radiation therapy is accomplished before rapid proliferation commences.

Finally, systemic chemotherapeutic agents, when optimally combined with radiation therapy, not only may enhance tumor control within the irradiated volume, but may reduce or eliminate disease that has disseminated beyond the irradiated volume. Biologic response modifiers, similarly, may enhance effects on the local tumor and simultaneously enhance host defenses to permit eradication of subclinical disease. Although BCG, MER, and levamisole failed to improve the results of radiation therapy, thymosine and interferon offer some promise and are actively under investigation in clinical trials.

CONCLUSIONS

Radiation therapy has an important role in the management of lung cancer. It improves the results in certain subsets of patients who have undergone complete resection when delivered as a postoperative adjuvant. High dose, technically sophisticated radiation therapy is the best hope for cure, at present, of patients with unresectable bronchopulmonary tumors. Radiation therapy is highly effective in relieving most symptoms caused by the primary tumor and has an established role in the palliation of distant metastases. Local-regional irradiation is an integral part of effective management of small cell carcinoma limited to the primary tumor and regional lymph nodes, and it may prove to have a role even in disseminated disease when more effective systemic therapy is at hand. Several clinical trials of high LET radiations, altered fractionation, hypoxic cell sensitizers, systemic chemotherapy and biologic response modifiers, offer the possibility of improving the results of radiation therapy.

REFERENCES

Arriagada, R., et al.: Alternating radiotherapy and chemotherapy with doxorubicin, etoposide, cyclophosphamide, and cisplatin in limited small cell lung cancer. Cancer Treat. Symp. 2:115, 1985.

Blitzer, P.H.: Reanalysis of the RTOG study of the palliation of symptomatic osseous metastasis. Cancer 55:1468, 1985.

Borgelt, B., et al.: The palliation of brain metastases: final result of the first two studies by the Radiation Therapy Oncology Group. Int. J. Radiat. Oncol. Biol. Phys. 6:1, 1980.

Bunn, P.A., Jr., et al: Chemotherapy alone or chemotherapy with chest radiation therapy in limited stage small cell lung cancer. Ann. Intern. Med. 106:655, 1987.

Choi, N.C., Kanarek, D.J., and Kazemi, H.: Physiologic changes in pulmonary function after thoracic radiotherapy for patients with lung cancer and role of regional pulmonary function studies in predicting postradiotherapy pulmonary function before radiotherapy. Cancer Treat. Symp. 2:119, 1985.

Cox, J.D.: Failure analysis of inoperable carcinoma of the lung of all histopathologic types and squamous cell carcinoma of the esophagus. Cancer Treat. Symp. 2:77, 1983.

Cox, J.D.: Importance of endpoints in determining effectiveness of thoracic irradiation for small cell carcinoma of the lung. Cancer Treat. Symp. 2:31, 1985a.

Cox, J.D.: Large dose fractionation (hypofractionation). Cancer 55:2105, 1985b.

Cox, J.D., Komaki, R., and Byhardt, R.: Is immediate chest radiotherapy obligatory for any or all patients with limited stage "non small cell" carcinoma of the lung? Yes. Cancer Treat. Rep. 67:327, 1983.

Cox, J.D., and Yesner, R.A.: Adenocarcinoma of the lung: recent results from the Veterans Administration Lung Group. Am. Rev. Respir. Dis. 120:1025, 1979.

Cox, J.D., et al.: Is adenocarcinoma/large cell carcinoma the most radiocurable type of cancer of the lung? Int. J. Radiat. Oncol. Biol. Phys. 12:1801, 1986.

Cox, J.D., et al.: Complications of radiation therapy and factors in their prevention. World J. Surg. 10:171, 1986.

Deeley, T.J.: The treatment of carcinoma of the bronchus. Br. J. Radiol. 40:801, 1967.

Deeley, T.J.: Radiotherapy for carcinoma of the bronchus. Cancer Treat. Rev. 1:39, 1974.

Dische, S., Martin, W.M.C., and Anderson, P.: Radiation myelopathy in patients treated for carcinoma of bronchus using a six-fraction regime of radiotherapy. Br. J. Radiol. 54:29, 1981.

Eisert, D.R., Cox, J.D., and Komaki, R.: Irradiation for bronchial carcinoma: reasons for failure. I. Analysis as a function of dose time-fractionation. Cancer 37:2665, 1976.

Green, N., and Melbye, R.W.: Lung cancer: retreatment of local recurrence after definitive irradiation. Cancer 49:865, 1982.

Hatlevoll, R., et al.: Myelopathy following radiotherapy of bronchial carcinoma with large single fractions: a retrospective study. Int. J. Radiat. Oncol. Biol. Phys. 9:41, 1983.

Hilaris, B.S., and Martini, N.: Interstitial brachytherapy in cancer of the lung: a 20 year experience: Int. J. Radiat. Oncol. Biol. Phys. 5:1951, 1979.

Holmes, E.C., et al.: A randomized comparison of the effects of adjuvant therapy on resected stages II and III non-small cell carcinoma of the lung. Ann. Surg. 212:335, 1985.

Israel, L., Bonadonna, G., and Sylvester, R.: Controlled study with adjuvant radiotherapy, chemotherapy, immunotherapy, and chemoimmunotherapy in operable squamous carcinoma of the lung. In Lung Cancer: Progress in Therapeutic Research. Edited by F. Muggis and M. Rozencweig. New York, Raven Press, pp. 443–452, 1979.

Jacobs, L., Kinkel, W.R., and Vincent, R.G.: "Silent" brain metastasis from lung carcinoma determined by computerized tomography. Arch. Neurol. 34:690, 1977.

Komaki, R., Cox, J.D., Eisert, D.R.: Irradiation of bronchial carcinoma. II. Pattern of spread and potential for prophylactic irradiation. Int. J. Radiat. Oncol. Biol. Phys. 2:441, 1977.

Komaki, R., et al.: Superior sulcus tumors: results of irradiation of 36 patients. Cancer 48:1563, 1981.

Komaki, R., Cox, J.D., and Stark, R.: Frequency of brain metastasis in adenocarcinoma and large cell carcinoma of the lung: correlation with survival. Int. J. Radiat. Oncol. Biol. Phys. 9:1467, 1983.

Komaki, R., et al.: Characteristics of long-term survivors after treat-

ment of inoperable carcinoma of the lung. Am. J. Clin. Oncol. 8:362, 1985.

Laramore, G.E., et al.: Fast neutron and mixed beam radiotherapy for inoperable non-small cell carcinoma of the lung. Am. J. Clin. Oncol. 9:233, 1986.

Livingston, R.B., et al.: Combined modality treatment of extensive small cell lung cancer: a Southwest Oncology Group study. J. Clin. Oncol. 2:585, 1984.

The Lung Cancer Study Group: Effects of postoperative mediastinal radiation on completely resected stage II and stage III epidermoid cancer of the lung. N. Engl. J. Med. 315:1377, 1986.

Martini, N., and McCormack, P.: Therapy of stage III (nonmetastatic disease). Semin. Oncol. 10:95, 1983.

Norlund, J.D., et al.: Computed tomography in the staging of small cell lung cancer: implications for combined modality therapy. Int. J. Radiat. Oncol. Biol. Phys. 11:1081, 1985.

Paulson, D.L.: The survival rate in superior sulcus tumors treated by presurgical irradiation. JAMA 196:342, 1966.

Paulson, D.L.: Treatment of superior sulcus tumors. In Cancer Therapy by Integrated Radiation and Operation. Edited by B.F. Rush, Jr. and R.H. Greenlaw. Springfield, IL, Charles C Thomas, 1968.

Perez, C.A., et al.: Patterns of tumor recurrence after definitive irradiation for inoperable non-oat cell carcinoma of the lung. Int. J. Radiat. Oncol. Biol. Phys. 6:987, 1980.

Perez, C.A., et al.: Impact of irradiation technique and tumor extent in tumor control and survival of patients with unresectable non-oat cell carcinoma of the lung: report of the Radiation Therapy Oncology Group. Cancer 50:1091, 1982.

Perez, C.A., et al.: Randomized trial of radiotherapy to the thorax in limited small cell carcinoma of the lung treated with multiagent chemotherapy and elective brain irradiation: a preliminary report. J. Clin. Oncol. 2:1200, 1984.

Perez, C.A., et al.: Impact of tumor control on survival in carcinoma of the lung treated with irradiation. Int. J. Radiat. Oncol. Biol. Phys. 12:539, 1986.

Perry, M.C., et al.: Chemotherapy with or without radiation therapy in limited small-cell carcinoma of the lung. N. Engl. J. Med. 316:912, 1987.

Saunders, M.I., et al.: Preliminary tumor control after radiotherapy for carcinoma of the bronchus. Int. J. Radiat. Oncol. Biol. Phys. 10:499, 1984.

Seagren, S.L., Harrell, J.H., and Horn, R.A.: High dose rate intraluminal irradiation in recurrent endobronchial carcinoma. Chest 88:810, 1985.

Shields, T.W.: Treatment failures after surgical resection of thoracic tumors. Cancer Treat. Symp. 2:69, 1983.

Simpson, J.R., et al.: Large fraction irradiation with or without misonidazole in advanced non-oat cell carcinoma of the lung: a phase III randomized trial of the RTOG. Int. J. Radiat. Oncol. Biol. Phys. 13:861, 1987.

Slawson, R.G., and Scott, R.M.: Radiation therapy in bronchogenic carcinoma. Radiology 132:175, 1979.

Stewart, J.R., and Fajardo, L.F.: Radiation induced heart disease. Radiol. Clin. North Am. 9:511, 1971.

Tarver, R.D., Richmond, B.D., and Klatte, E.D.: Cerebral metastases from lung carcinoma: neurological and CT correlation. Radiology 153:689, 1984.

Tong, D., Gillick, L., and Henrickson, F.R.: The palliation of symptomatic osseous metastases: final results of the Radiation Therapy Oncology Group. Cancer 50:893, 1982.

Turrisi, A.T., and Glover, D.J.: The Penn regimen (concurrent twice-daily radiotherapy 2X/D XRT and platinum-etoposide—PE) in limited small cell lung cancer (SCLC). Abstract. Int. J. Radiat. Oncol. Biol. Phys. 12:158, 1986.

Van Houtte, P., and Henry, J.: Preoperative and postoperative radiation therapy in lung cancer. Cancer Treat. Symp. 2:57, 1985.

White, J.E., et al.: The influence of radiation therapy quality control on survival, response, and sites of relapse in oat cell carcinoma of the lung: preliminary report of a Southwest Oncology Group study. Cancer 50:1084, 1982.

Wollin, M., and Kagan, A.R.: Modification of biological dose to normal tissue by daily fractionation. Acta Radiol. 15:481, 1976.

CHAPTER 94

RADIATION THERAPY OF CARCINOMA OF THE ESOPHAGUS

Thomas J. Keane

Guisez (1909) first reported on the use of radiation therapy in the management of carcinoma of the esophagus. This chapter reviews the role of radiation therapy both as a single modality and as a component of the multidisciplinary management of the disease. The primary focus relates to aspects of treatment with curative intent and, unless otherwise indicated, refers to treatment of squamous carcinoma.

TREATMENT WITH CURATIVE INTENT

Radiation therapy shares with surgery a major limitation as a curative modality because it is nonsystemic. It can, at best, only cure those patients whose disease is localized within a volume amenable to a radical dose of radiation before the development of occult distant metastases. In practice, therefore, cure is only possible in those patients whose disease is localized to the primary tumor site, and perhaps a subset of patients with metastases limited to lymph nodes in adjacent tissues. The potential for cure among the latter group has not been reported in the radiation therapy literature because the staging is clinical and the mediastinal nodes are not usually assessed. If, however, the information in the surgical literature is a valid comparison, then the work of Skinner and colleagues (1982) is not encouraging. For all carcinomas in their series, only 2 out of 17 patients survived even when lymph node metastases were confined to one or two nodes.

The proportion of patients in radiation therapy series judged suitable for potentially curative treatment based on clinical staging varies from a high of 63% reported by Pearson (1969) when radiation therapy was virtually the only approach to radical treatment to a much lower proportion of 47 out of 243—19%–reported for curative irradiation alone by Barkley and associates (1981) from the M.D. Anderson Hospital. The degree of selection and the criteria used for such treatment decision-making must be known before any judgement is made about the

value of any radical treatment approach. Many claims for improved treatment represent triumphs of selection rather than triumphs of treatment per se.

FAILURE ANALYSIS FOLLOWING RADIATION THERAPY

In considering possible ways to improve results, it is necessary to review where failures occur following conventional radiation therapy. Table 94–1 shows the results Aisner and co-workers (1983) compiled from several large series. The timing of recurrence is also important, not just clinically but also for the design of randomized clinical studies. Pearson (1969) reported that 73% of local failures occurred in the first year following treatment, 22% in the second year, and no local failures beyond the third year; he also noted that distant metastases occur most often in the first and second year following radiation therapy. Late development of distant metastases beyond 3 years is infrequent.

Clearly, failure to eradicate disease at the primary tumor site is the greatest cause of failure, and any improvement in cure rates must start with improved control of the primary tumor. Of course, not all patients whose primary tumors are controlled survive, because many succumb to distant metastases because they live long enough for such metastases to become apparent.

SURVIVAL FOLLOWING RADICAL RADIATION THERAPY ALONE WITH CURATIVE INTENT

As indicated earlier, the results of treatment depend heavily on the degree of selection for any particular therapy. Particular attention should be paid to the total number of patients receiving radical treatment as a proportion of all patients in any series and also the extent to which surgery and radiation therapy are applied as curative treatments within any center. The best results Pearson

Table 94–1. Sites of Recurrence after Radical Radiation Therapy

| Investigator | No. of Patients | Radiotherapy Dose (rad) | % of Patients with Recurrence | | | | |
			Local	Margin*	Neck	Distant Metastases	Other Sites
Robertson et al.	39	3000–7800	56			36	
Elkon et al.	30	6525	25 +	25	10	25	
			64 +	27	43	66	
			+				
Pierquin et al.	115	4500–8000	82			37	
Pearson†	157	5000	61			23	16
Beatty et al.‡	176	4000–6000	84			47	

*Margin of treatment port
+ Stage I disease
+
+ Stage II and III disease
†Data reported indicate site causing death only
‡Includes 30 patients who had surgery and radiation therapy
Reproduced with permission from Aisner, J., et al.: Patterns of recurrence for carcinoma of the lung and oesophagus. Cancer Treat. Symp. 2:102, 1983.

published (1977) show a 17% 5-year survival rate for a subset of 248 patients representing 40% of all cases treated with curative intent over an 18-year period in Edinburgh. The degree to which this series represents selection can be inferred by the fact that the overall 5-year survival for all patients was between 7 and 9% for the entire period. Newaishey and colleagues (1982) carried out a further analysis of data from Edinburgh for an overlapping time period. When the definition of curative intent was inferred only because of the prescription of a radical dose, the 5-year survival rate among 444 of 848 patients so defined was 9%. This figure is within one standard deviation of the mean 6% 5-year survival rate derived by Earlam and Cunha-Melo (1980) from 49 papers and a total of 8489 patients following radiation therapy of esophageal cancer.

Several prognostic factors appear to be advantageous in terms of survival following radical radiation therapy. Improved survival for women patients has been reported in several series. Newaishey and associates (1982) reported a 5.67% 5-year crude survival for men compared to a figure of 11.6% for women. A comparison of survival patterns suggested that this difference was only apparent after 2 years and only reached statistical significance after 5 years of follow-up. When considered by tumor length, this survival difference was only demonstrated for tumors longer than 5 cm. Most series show an inverse relationship between increasing T stage and survival. Little information indicates whether this trend is associated with decreased local tumor control or the greater propensity for metastases in larger tumors. Tumor location has been considered important in several series, with improved survival for patients with lesions in the cervical and upper third of the thoracic esophagus. Other prognostic factors are disputed and may reflect difficulties with univariate analysis and small numbers of patients. The available evidence suggests that the best survival results with radical radiation therapy are obtained in patients with tumors less than 5 cm long confined to the upper third of the thoracic esophagus.

RADIATION TREATMENT PLANNING

Although a detailed review of the technicalities of treatment planning is beyond the scope of this chapter, it is nevertheless important for surgeons to understand the principles involved to understand the limitations facing the radiation oncologist and to facilitate mutual understanding in the management of this disease.

The aim of radiation treatment is to eradicate tumor while minimizing damage to surrounding normal tissue. This process involves three steps: (1) defining the extent of tumor and adjacent normal structures; (2) defining the target volume to be treated; and (3) accurately delivering a known dose to the target volume while restricting the dose to surrounding normal structures as much as possible.

Defining Tumor Extent

Assuming that staging investigations for disease at distant sites have been completed, the clinical assessment of intrathoracic disease requires endoscopic evaluation of the esophagus and in most cases the respiratory tract. The primary tumor's length and position relative to a recognizable anatomic landmark must be accurately described. Impaired mobility or paresis of the vocal cords, which may indicate spread to mediastinal nodes, should also be noted. I believe that the presence of biopsy-proved disease involving the *mucosa* of the trachea or major bronchi contraindicates curative radiation therapy because a fistula inevitably follows any attempt at radical treatment. Barium studies and computed tomography complement the endoscopic assessment in defining disease extent for treatment planning purposes.

Defining the Target Volume for Radical Treatment

No studies have addressed the question of the optimal target volume that should be irradiated to radical dose levels. Recognizing that the technical difficulties vary according to anatomic location, it is difficult to describe a typical radical dose target volume. The following guidelines, however, appear common to many publications: (1) a 5-cm margin superior and inferior to roentgenologically demonstrated tumor, these margins recognize the propensity for submucosal spread of disease; (2) a minimum 1-cm margin around the lateral margins of the visible tumor, CT-assisted treatment planning can precisely define the target in the horizontal plane. A typical radical dose target volume is shown in Figure 94–1.

Except in tumors of the cervical esophagus, it is generally not possible to encompass a significant proportion of the regional nodes at risk for metastatic spread. Although some regional nodes may be included, the primary goal is to deliver a tumoricidal dose to the visible primary tumor with a margin that allows for possible local extension of disease.

Accurate Dose Delivery and Protection of Critical Normal Tissues

In delivering a radical dose of irradiation to a predetermined volume, the radiation oncologist must pay particular attention to adjacent critical normal tissues. In the case of the esophagus, the critical adjacent normal tissues that may be irradiated are listed in Table 94–2, together with the dose expected to yield a 5% risk for a particular complication within 5 years—TD 5/5. The expected time of onset of each complication is also indicated. Most serious injuries are manifestations of late radiation damage. In the case of the lung, the likelihood of clinical sequelae as a result of exceeding lung tolerance depends on the volume of lung irradiated. Thus, the small volumes of lung that are commonly irradiated beyond tolerance levels are not expected to produce clinical sequelae because the functional reserve of the lung is large. Figure 94–2 shows a typical field arrangement using multiple radiation therapy ports that produces a satisfactory dose distribution to the tumor target volume and the adjacent critical normal tissues.

RADIATION DOSE FOR CURATIVE THERAPY

The optimal radiation dose for curative therapy is that dose that produces the highest cure rate with the lowest rate of normal tissue damage. In practice the latter requirement limits the total dose delivered. In considering dosage information it must be remembered that the biological effect of irradiation varies depending on the daily fraction size and overall treatment time. Typical dose prescriptions vary from 50 to 55 Gy in 20 fractions in 4 weeks to 60 to 70 Gy in 30 to 40 fractions in 6 to 8 weeks—1 Gy = 100 rads. At present there is no compelling evidence for a therapeutic gain for any particular dose fractionation schedule.

PREOPERATIVE RADIATION THERAPY

Many groups have used irradiation preoperatively in efforts to improve resection rates and survival. With two exceptions, all of this experience has been in nonrandomized studies generally using less than curative doses of radiation therapy. Launois and colleagues' (1981) randomized study of 124 patients showed no benefit over surgery alone. This trial, however, is open to criticism on the grounds that the radiation fractionation scheme was unconventional—40 Gy in 8 to 12 days—and also because of low statistical power resulting in a possible type II error—false negative conclusion. The only other randomized study, by Gignoux and colleagues (1982), again using a moderate dose of irradiation but with more patients, failed to demonstrate a survival benefit over surgery alone.

I regard preoperative irradiation as an unproven ap-

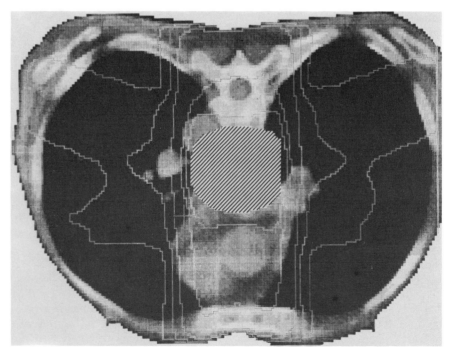

Fig. 94–1. Planning CT scan for typical carcinoma of the mid esophagus. Hatched lines indicate the area receiving radical dose.

Table 94–2. Critical Adjacent Normal Tissues That May Be Irradiated

Critical Normal Tissue	Clinical Manifestation	TD 5/5*	Usual Time of Onset
Spinal Cord	Transverse myelitis Brown-Séquard syndrome	45 Gy	6–36 months
Heart (60% volume)	Asymptomatic Pericardial effusion Constrictive pericarditis	45 Gy	12–60 months
Lung (Single)	Acute pneumonitis	15 Gy (uncorrected for inhomogeneity)	2–6 months
Stomach (Entire organ)	Ulceration Fibrosis, bleeding	45 Gy	6–12 months

*Dose expected to yield a 5% risk of a particular complication within 5 years.
Dose Estimates are approximate
Fractionation of 2 Gy/day 5 days per week

proach in terms of improving survival. Because such management has usually been favored for large or marginally inoperable tumors, large numbers of patients would probably be required to demonstrate statistically a meaningful improvement in survival.

POSTOPERATIVE IRRADIATION ALONE

Postoperative radiation therapy has generally been used when proved or suspected residual disease remains after attempted curative surgery. No randomized studies have been performed, and there is no encouragement in the published literature for any survival benefit. Because a radical dose would be needed for any expected survival benefit, it is difficult with the available evidence to advocate such treatment with its associated potential for morbidity. Radiation therapy using moderate doses to palliate symptoms resulting from residual disease can, of course, be beneficial without major morbidity. In such cases the goal is clearly palliative and a survival benefit is not expected.

COMBINATIONS OF RADIATION THERAPY AND CHEMOTHERAPY

Encouraging reports from several investigators of the treatment of squamous carcinoma at other sites have renewed interest in this approach to the management of squamous carcinoma of the esophagus. Chemotherapy has been applied as an adjuvant to both radiation therapy with curative intent and to preoperative therapy.

CHEMOTHERAPY AS AN ADJUVANT TO CURATIVE RADIATON THERAPY

Radical Radiation Therapy Combined with Chemotherapy

Much of the interest in chemotherapy-radiation therapy combinations centers on concurrent administration

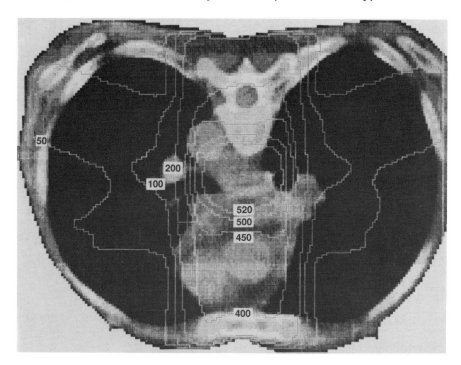

Fig. 94–2. Isodose distribution of a 5-field technique using 25 MV photons. Corrections have been made for lung inhomogeneity. Fields are not equally weighted. Numbers indicate relative percent isodose lines.

of both modalities. In general, the administration of drugs is limited to one or two courses during or close to the time of irradiation. Although the rationale is often not stated, the intent is apparently to improve the radiation effect on the primary tumor rather than influencing systemic disease. The scientific basis for any advantageous drug-radiation therapy interaction remains unclear, but possibilities range from simple additivity of effect to true radiosensitization. Table 94–3 summarizes results from several studies. To date only bleomycin has been studied in a prospective randomized fashion; unfortunately, no evidence of benefit was demonstrated. At present, randomized trials of other combinations listed are in progress under the direction of several cooperative groups.

Preoperative Radiation Therapy Combined with Chemotherapy

The impetus for the many studies of radical radiation therapy and chemotherapy mentioned earlier arose from preoperative studies using similar drug combinations and schedules developed during the late 1970s and reported by Steiger (1981), Franklin (1983), and Leichman (1984) and their associates. All these studies used a modest dose of irradiation—30 Gy in 15 fractions in 3 weeks—combined with 5-fluorouracil infusion and either mitomycin C or cisplatin. Following such protocols, between one half and three quarters of the patients were resected. Approximately one quarter of esophagectomy specimens showed no evidence of residual cancer on pathologic examination. This finding suggested an enhanced antitumor effect for the combination when compared to historical information for radiation therapy alone, which in higher doses—45 Gy—as Marks and associates (1976) reported, showed pathologic evidence of tumor clearance in only 3% of cases. Enthusiam for this finding of high rates of tumor clearance must, however, be tempered with concern about the level of treatment-related mortality, between 18 and 30% in these initial studies. Franklin and associates (1983) reported a 22% 5-year survival rate among patients who were resected, but

when the denominator of all patients entering the study is considered, the 5-year survival rate is only 9%. Leichman and associates (1987) reported no long-term survivors among operated patients in their series using cisplatin and 5-fluorouracil. A benefit for preoperative radiation therapy and chemotherapy has therefore not been established in a prospective randomized study. Only Andersen and associates' (1984) study was randomized; using bleomycin as an adjuvant to preoperative irradiation, they were unable to demonstrate any benefit compared to a control group receiving preoperative radiation therapy alone. Clearly, more prospective studies such as this are necessary.

ADENOCARCINOMA OF THE ESOPHAGUS

Unlike squamous cancer, for which radical radiation therapy is an alternative to surgery, adenocarcinoma is only treated radically when patients are considered unresectable, or inoperable on medical grounds, or when surgery is refused. Adenocarcinomas are less responsive than squamous cancers and the acute morbidity of external beam irradiation to the epigastric area in terms of nausea and vomiting is significant. These considerations and the advanced nature of the cases referred for therapy seriously question any curative role for radiation therapy at present. Palliation may be possible and will be considered later.

Irradiation is occasionally used as an adjuvant to surgery for adenocarcinoma. At present this is most often confined to the use of postoperative treatment in situations where resection margins are positive, residual disease remains, or expectation of recurrence is judged to be high. The place of such treatment remains unproven in terms of demonstrated benefit, and the potential for treatment-related morbidity is high.

PALLIATIVE RADIATION THERAPY

The intent of palliative radiation treatment is to relieve symptoms arising from the local, regional, or systemic

Table 94–3. Drug-Radiation Therapy—RT—Interactions

Study/Reference	No. of Patients	Median Survival in Months	RT Dose
RT + bleomycin vs.	40	6.4	50–60 Gy in 5–6 weeks
RT (randomised)/ Earle et al. (1980)	37	6.2	
RT + DDP + 5 FU + mitomycin C + bleomycin/ Leichman et al. (1987)	20	22	50–Gy in 15 weeks
RT + mitomycin C + 5 FU/ Keane et al. (1985)	35	12	45–50 Gy in 4 weeks or 8 weeks
RT + 5 FU/ Keane (unpublished)	39	17	50–52 Gy in 4 weeks
RT + 5 FU/ Byfield, et al. 1979	6	22	60 Gy in 12 weeks

RT = radiotherapy; DDP = cisplatin; 5-FU = 5-fluorouracil.

spread of disease. This should ideally be achieved with the least amount of treatment-related morbidity in the shortest possible time.

The degree to which irradiation is useful is largely an individual decision by the radiation oncologist in each patient's particular circumstances. In general, squamous carcinomas are more responsive. Esophageal obstruction can be relieved, albeit temporarily, by doses of 20 Gy given in five fractions in 1 week. A decision to treat to radical dose levels may be justifiable when longer-term palliation is required, as is the case in fitter patients with limited evidence of distant metastatic disease. Relief of pain and compressive respiratory symptoms is usually demanded in patients in poor general condition with more advanced disease. Symptom control may be achieved with doses ranging upwards from 8 Gy in a single fraction to higher doses using fractionated treatment. Incurable disease is not in itself an indication for palliative irradiation. The decision to use irradiation should be based on an evaluation of all forms of palliative treatment available. In such circumstances the judicious application of irradiation is undoubtedly of considerable help in achieving symptom control in many patients.

THE FUTURE

Until effective systemic therapies are developed, the major efforts of radiation oncologists will continue to focus on possible ways to improve control rates of the primary tumor without increasing radiation therapy complications. Several strategies aimed at achieving this goal are of interest. The first is the endocavitary application of irradiation to deliver a boost dose to the primary tumor as a supplement to external beam therapy. Although this idea is not new, the possibility now exists for easier and safer application of interstitial radiation sources using specialized endocavitary equipment. These treatment methods are now widely available and suitable for use in many patients. The systematic evaluation of such an approach is in progress in several centers. The second approach is based on new insights into tumor kinetics and the radiobiology of normal tissue injury. These ideas suggest that an alteration of classic daily irradiation fractionation schemes might be beneficial either by accelerating the total time of therapy to counteract tumor repopulation or by using multiple small radiation doses such that total doses of irradiation can be increased without an increase in late damage to normal tissues.

CONCLUSION

Radiation therapy of esophageal cancer remains a difficult challenge for the radiation oncologist. In the absence of effective systemic treatment, improvements in survival are likely to be modest. With the advent of new and, it is hoped, better methods of using radiation therapy, there remains a responsibility for all involved to objectively evaluate such approaches before adopting them as standard treatment.

REFERENCES

Aisner, J., Forastiere, A., and Aroney, R.: Patterns of recurrence for carcinoma of the lung and oesophagus. Cancer Treat. Symp. 2:87, 1983.
Andersen, A.P., et al.: Irradiation chemotherapy and surgery in esophageal cancer: a randomised clinical study. The first Scandanavian trial in esophageal cancer. Radiother. Oncol. 2:179, 1984.
Barkley, H.T., et al.: Radiotherapy in the treatment of carcinoma of the oesophagus. In Gastrointestinal Cancer. Edited by J.R. Stroehlein and M.M. Remsdahl. New York, Raven Press, 1981, p. 171.
Byfield, J., et al.: Infusional 5 Fluorouracil and x-ray therapy for nonresectable esophageal carcinoma. Cancer 22:376, 1979.
Earlam, R., and Cunha-Melo, J.R.: Esophageal squamous cell carcinoma. II. A critical review of radiotherapy. Br. J. Surg. 67:457, 1980.
Earle, J., Gelber, R., and Moertel, C.: A controlled evaluation of combined radiation and bleomycin therapy for squamous cell carcinoma of the esophagus. Int. J. Radiat. Oncol. Biol. Phys. 6:821, 1980.
Franklin, R., Steiger, Z., and Vaishampayan, G.: Combined modality therapy for esophageal squamous carcinoma. Cancer 51:1062, 1983.
Gignoux, M., et al.: A multicentre randomised study comparing preoperative radiotherapy with surgery in cases of resectable oesophageal cancer. Acta. Chir. Belg. 82:373, 1982.
Guisez, J.: Essais de traitement de quelque cas d'epithelioma de l'oesophage par les application locales directes de radium. Bull. Soc. Med. Hop. Paris 27:717, 1909.
Keane, T.J., et al.: Radical radiation therapy with 5 Fluorouracil infusion and mitomycin C for esophageal squamous cell carcinoma. Radiother. Oncol. 4:205, 1985.
Launois, B., et al.: Preoperative radiotherapy for carcinoma of the esophagus. Surg. Gynecol. Obstet. 153:690, 1981.
Leichman, L., Steiger, A., and Seydel, H.G.: Preoperative chemotherapy plus radiation therapy for patients with cancer of the esophagus: a potentially curative approach. J. Clin. Oncol. 2:75, 1984.
Leichman, L., et al.: Nonoperative therapy for squamous cell cancer of the esophagus. J. Clin. Oncol. 5:365, 1987.
Marks, R.D., Schruggs, H.J., and Wallace, K.M.: Preoperative radiation therapy for carcinoma of the esophagus. Cancer 38:84, 1976.
Newaishey, G.A., Read, G.A., and Duncan, W.: Results of radical radiotherapy of squamous carcinoma of the esophagus. Clin. Radiol. 33:347, 1982.
Pearson, J.G.: The value of radiotherapy in the management of esophageal cancer. Am. J. Roentgenol. 105:500, 1969.
Pearson, J.G.: The present status and future potential for radiotherapy in the management of esophageal cancer. Cancer 39:882, 1977.
Rubin, P., and Cassarrett, G.: Clinical Radiation Pathology, Vol. I and II. Philadelphia, W.B. Saunders Co., 1968.
Skinner, D.B., Dowiatshahi, K.D., and DeMeester, T.R.: Potentially curable cancer of the oesophagus. Cancer 50:2571, 1982.
Steiger, Z., Franklin, R., and Wilson, R.F.: Eradication and palliation of squamous cell carcinoma of the esophagus with chemotherapy and surgical therapy. J. Thorac. Cardiovasc. Surg. 82:713, 1981.

READING REFERENCES

Fisher, S.A., and Brady, L.W.: Carcinoma of the esophagus. In Principles and Practice of Radiation Oncology. Edited by C. Perez and L.W. Brady. Philadelphia, J.B. Lippincott Co., 1987, p. 700.
Hanlock, S.L., and Glatstein, E.: Radiation therapy of esophageal cancer. Semin. Oncol. 11:144, 1984.
Moertel, C.G.: The esophagus. In Cancer Medicine, 2nd ed. Edited by J.F. Holland and E. Frei, III. Philadelphia, Lea & Febiger, 1982, p. 1753.

Chemotherapy

CHAPTER 95

PRINCIPLES OF CHEMOTHERAPY

Merrill S. Kies and Steven T. Rosen

Modern chemotherapy depends on the relatively greater sensitivity of tumor cells than normal cells to cell-killing action. Understanding the principles of chemotherapy requires comprehension of the pathophysiology of cancer as well as a working knowledge of the drugs, their mechanisms of action, and their side effects.

CELLULAR AND TUMOR GROWTH

Cancer is a disorder of cell and tissue growth not under normal regulatory controls. Organ dysfunction tends to occur with the accumulation of great tumor bulk, although contrary to what is sometimes presumed, many cancers actually proliferate slowly relative to proliferating normal cells. Because cytotoxic drugs generally depend on cell proliferation for killing effects, this presents a major problem and accounts for the narrow safety margin and considerable inherent toxicity of most commonly used drugs. In fact, cancer cells have no unique features that provide a suitable distinguishing target for drug therapy, and the same parameters describe the biology of tumor and normal tissues.

Cellular Growth Features

The cell cycle time, also known as the *generation time,* is the time required for a cell to move from mitosis to mitosis, to complete a full cell cycle (Fig. 95–1). The cell goes through a growth phase in which DNA is produced—the S phase. After this phase is a gap called G_2. During this phase, the cell is tetraploid, i.e., it contains twice the DNA content, and it continues to synthesize RNA and protein. The cell then undergoes mitosis—M phase—which is followed by a gap called G_1. At this juncture the cell may re-enter the growth—S—phase, accompanied by the necessary RNA and protein synthesis, or may go into a resting phase called G_0.

The cell cycle can be observed through two windows. The first is mitosis, which can be observed morphologically, and the second is S phase, in which the DNA content of the cell doubles. The DNA content can be

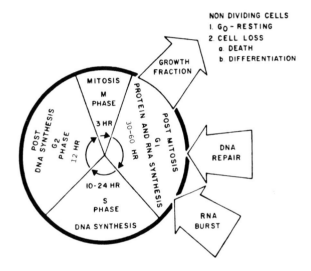

Fig. 95–1. The cell cycle.

measured microfluorometrically. The G_1 phase is the most variable; cells may go either into resting—G_0—phase or into the growth—S—phase. Some average figures for the time in each phase are: M phase—3 hours, G_2—9 to 12 hours, G_1—30 to 60 hours, and S—10 to 24 hours. The time to go through a cell cycle ranges from 50 to 120 hours. In contrast, the cell cycle time of most normal cells is in the range of 24–48 hours.

Tumor Growth

The way the tumor cell mass grows also is germane to tumor kinetics. Several theoretic curves describe growth patterns. Exponential growth, that is, two cells raised to the exponent of two, three, four and so forth, is rapid, but this is not the observed pattern. Similarly, growth of the external surface of a sphere unlimited by other constraints is also rapid, but this is also not the case.

The observed growth pattern is described by the gompertzian growth curve, which shows an initial rapid exponential growth phase and a terminal phase of slowing growth. The implications of this curve are twofold. First, by the time a tumor is evident on physical examination and on chest roentgenograms, slowing of growth has already begun. Whereas in the early part of the curve up to 85% of the cells are in cycle, by the time of diagnosis only 5% of the cells may be cycling. This profoundly affects the effectiveness of chemotherapy, which depends on cell proliferation for cell-killing action. As cells accumulate at the primary site or in a metastasis, all proliferation diminishes, i.e., DNA synthesis slows. Early tumors low on the gompertzian curve tend to have a large growth fraction; late tumors—at diagnosis with most clinical techniques—are generally high in the gompertzian chart and thus have a low fraction of cycling cells.

The doubling time of tumors depends on many factors: the length of the cell cycle, the number of dividing cells, the growth fraction, and cell loss through cell death, metastases, and differentiation. Human tumors in advanced stages demonstrate a range of doubling times, averaging approximately 60 days. With respect to chemotherapy, the percentage of dividing cells probably has more importance. The ideal tumor to treat has a rapid doubling time, a high growth fraction, and a short G_1 phase. The L1210 mouse leukemia model is such a tumor.

The factors that affect tumor growth rates are poorly understood and probably complex. Growth factors, blood supply, nutrients, and changing genetic composition may influence tumor growth. Similarly, mechanisms that slow the entry of the clonogenic fraction into the cell cycle or account for tumor cell death are not well understood. Increasing aneuploidy, thrombosis and hemorrhage, poor oxygenation, and extensive necrosis characterize many fast-growing neoplasms.

A conceptual model of tumor growth is useful in discussing basic chemotherapy strategy (Fig. 95–2). Most chemotherapy drugs interfere in some fashion with DNA synthesis or with the production of precursors for DNA or RNA. Therefore, the strategy of cancer treatment is to shift cells to the cycling pools. A high fraction of cells from sensitive malignancies, such as Burkitt's lymphoma or acute childhood leukemia, are cycling and thus relatively sensitive to drug treatment (Table 95–1). For slower growing solid tumors, such as breast or colon cancer, surgical resection of the primary may leave residual micrometastatic disease, which then theoretically consists of cells more likely to cycle and become susceptible to chemotherapy. Drug treatment, or irradiation, may also be used to reduce tumor bulk and thereby increase the numbers of cells entering into cell cycle.

More than 50% of breast cancer patients are at risk of recurrence, irrespective of the choice of initial therapy, because the disease is frequently systemic at the time of diagnosis. Risk of recurrence is highest in women with demonstrable metastases to axillary nodes, when the primary tumor is found to have low or no estrogen receptor-binding activity, and with larger primary tumor size. This has led to the application of so-called surgical adjuvant therapy with chemotherapy or hormone manipulation in patients at high risk of having disseminated microscopic disease undetectable by routine clinical and roentgenographic techniques. Initial clinical trials comparing treated patients to prospectively randomized control groups receiving standard surgical and radiation therapy alone have shown that the use of systemic cytotoxic therapy given to premenopausal women at high risk of tumor recurrence following surgery increases survival. The hypothesis that micrometastases with higher proliferative indices are sensitive to available cytotoxic drugs is being examined.

CHEMOTHERAPEUTIC AGENTS

Animal and human tumor investigations have shown that most chemotherapeutic agents available today have cell-killing action that follows the principle of first-order kinetics. That is, a fixed percentage of cells are destroyed rather than a fixed number of cells—zero-order kinetics. The percentage cell kill is dose-related, and a larger dose usually kills a larger percentage of cells. A log cell kill denotes reduction of the original number of tumor cells by 10%. A two log kill represents killing 99% of remaining cells. Conceivably, the same dose is required to go from one million cells to one hundred thousand cells as would be required to go from ten cells to one cell. Drug combinations appear to produce higher rates of objective response and longer survival than do single-agent treatments, probably because of the differing mechanisms of action and cytotoxic potentials for multiple drug programs. Indeed, combination chemotherapy is the basis for treatment in cancers curable with chemotherapy, including lymphoma, Hodgkin's disease, and testicular carcinoma.

The host dies of a tumor burden of about 10^{12} cells— 1 kg. The clinical threshold of disease recognition is about 10^9 cells, or 1 g. The aim of chemotherapy is to reduce the tumor burden to 10^4 cells, or fewer, at which time immune factors may be sufficient to control the neoplasm.

Chemotherapy works by interrupting the formation or function of DNA, RNA, and cellular proteins. No unique action takes place on tumor DNA or RNA, and any therapeutic advantage is from quantitative and not qualitative effects relative to normal cells. Tumor cells cycle more

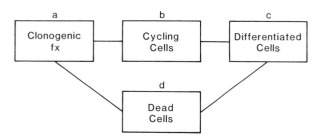

Fig. 95–2. Tumor growth model. Compartment *a* consists of the malignant stem cells, the clonogenic portion. Some are resting in G_0, others are cycling (moving to compartment *b*). Compartment *c* consists of more differentiated or arrested cells, including supportive connective tissue cells and blood vessels. These cells do not reenter the cycling compartment and are thus not important therapeutic targets.

Table 95–1.   Characteristics of Selected Human Cancers Relative to Chemosensitivity

	Malignancy	Histology	Tumor Doubling Time	Growth Fraction
Sensitive	Choriocarcinoma Burkitt's lymphoma Testicular carcinoma	Undifferentiated	30–60 days	50%
Refractory	Non-small cell lung cancer Colon cancer Renal cell cancer	Well differentiated	60–120 days	10%

slowly than their respective normal components, so the timing of chemotherapy is important.

Each chemotherapeutic agent acts at one or more different points of the cell replication cycle. Some agents are phase-specific, such as methotrexate—which acts during the S phase, and vincristine—which acts in the M phase. Cycle-dependent agents act on dividing cells and cycle-independent agents are relatively independent of the stage of cell replication and are most effective in slowly proliferating tumors.

Hydroxyurea and cytarabine–cytosine arabinoside—are cycle-dependent and phase-specific. Methotrexate and 5-fluorouracil are cycle-dependent, phase-specific and less proliferation-dependent. Cyclophosphamide, actinomycin, and carmustine—BCNU—are phase-non-specific and proliferation-dependent. Mechloretha-mine—nitrogen mustard—is cycle-independent, phase-nonspecific, and less proliferation-dependent. Drugs have phase specificity in that their maximal action is in a particular phase of the cell cycle. Vincristine and vinblastine act in the M phase; bleomycin and irradiation act maximally in G_2; doxorubicin—Adriamycin—acts in late S, whereas hydroxyurea and methotrexate act in early S, and actinomycin acts in G_1.

Because the various chemotherapeutic agents have varying times of activity, they are classified by their mechanism of interference with the production of DNA, RNA, or protein (Fig. 95–3). Those agents that act on preformed DNA are often cycle-independent; those that act on forming DNA are cycle-dependent.

The steps in attaining a cytoreductive effect are induction of remission, consolidation, and maintenance. In the first phase, the attempt is made to reduce all evidence of the tumor. If this goal is achieved, a complete remission has been induced. If shrinkage of tumor is greater than 50%, partial remission has been obtained. In general, clinical cure and prolongation of survival only occur if complete remission has been obtained. Consolidation refers to the phase of therapy when full doses are used even though complete remission has been achieved. This phase is an attempt to reduce the cell mass from 10^9 to 10^4 cells. The disease may, of course, still be present in quantities of 1 to 10 g but be below the clinical threshold. Maintenance therapy may or may not be necessary.

Alkylating Agents

The alkylating agents attack preformed DNA. The classic example is mechlorethamine—nitrogen mustard. This compound in solution spontaneously forms an ethylene ammonium ion, and this unstable ion complexes with electron-rich chemical centers, such as the 7 nitrogen of guanine, by a convalent bond. The second, ethyl chloride, portion may attach to a second strand of DNA. Because a double attachment forms, these agents are called bifunctional alkylating agents. Monofunctional alkylating agents are less effective and may be more mutagenic. The classic alkylating agents are busulfan, chlorambucil, melphalan, and thiotepa. Cyclophosphamide must be metabolized by the liver to its active component. Dacarbazine—(3,3-dimethyltriazino)-imidazole-4-carboxamide, DTIC—is a synthetic analog of a purine intermediate, but also acts like an alkylating agent. This agent must also be activated by hepatic microsomal enzymes. Cisplatin is a heavy-metal coordination complex containing a central atom of platinum surrounded by two chloride atoms and two ammonia molecules in the cis position. Its biochemial properties are similar to those of bifunctional alkylating agents; it produces interstrand and intrastrand cross-lengths in DNA, and is apparently cycle-nonspecific.

The nitrosoureas are a class of substituted urea compounds with a nitroso group and an ethyl chloride group attached to one of the urea nitrogens. One portion of the molecule acts like an alkylating agent, whereas the other end—in carmustine the isocyanate group—acts by carbamylation, resulting in inhibition of DNA repair. Carmustine—BCNU—and lomustine—CCNU—are currently available. Streptozotocin is a naturally occurring methyl nitrosourea. Unlike other nitrosoureas it directly inhibits DNA synthesis. It also inhibits pyrimidine nucleotides and enzymes involved in gluconeogenesis. This drug has been useful in treating functioning carcinoid tumors. Mitomycin C is an antitumor antibiotic derived from *Streptomyces caespitosus;* when activated, it is believed to act as a bifunctional or trifunctional agent.

The alkylating agents are usually cross-resistant; when one alkylating agent fails to elicit a response, others are similarly expected to fail.

Even though alkylating agents affect cells in all parts of the cell cycle, the cells appear to be most sensitive in the G_1 and M phase. Resistance to alkylating agents is

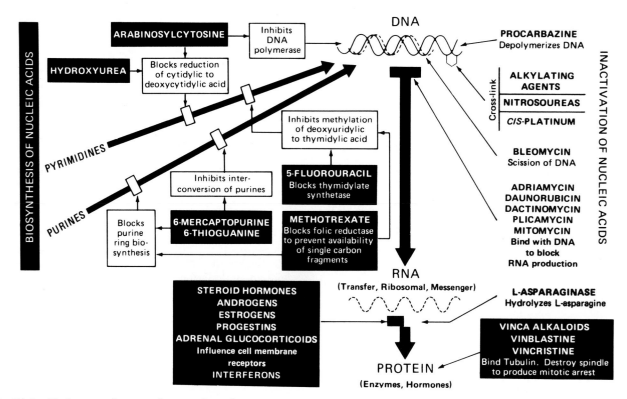

Fig. 95–3. Mechanisms of activity of various chemotherapeutic agents.

explained by an increased capacity of cells to repair sublethal damage to DNA. Chemicals that inhibit DNA repair, such as chloroquine, also delay onset of resistance to tumor systems.

Antitumor Antibiotics

Another group of drugs are cycle-independent but are not alkylating agents. These drugs are believed to act by various mechanisms; bleomycin is one such agent. It is an antibiotic derived from *Streptomyces verticullus*. Its mechanism of action is believed to be direct damage to DNA with fragmentation and strand scission. This drug is somewhat phase-specific in that it works best in the G_2 or M phase.

The anthracycline antibiotics—daunomycin hydrochloride and doxorubicin hydrochloride—have a four-membered ring structure attached to a glucosamine structure. The ring structure intercalates between base pairs and inhibits DNA and RNA production. These drugs have no effect on single-stranded DNA. Damage to DNA may also be mediated by free radical formation. In addition, anthracyclines may react directly with cell membranes to alter function.

Dactinomycin is an antitumor antibiotic also derived from Streptomyces or synthesized chemically. It acts by binding to DNA at guanine moieties. It inhibits DNA-dependent RNA synthesis. It is believed to act in the G_1 phase of the cell cycle.

Plicamycin is used today more often as an agent to lower serum calcium than as an antitumor agent. This effect is believed to be a direct action on osteoclasts. It is thought to complex with DNA in the presence of magnesium to inhibit DNA-directed synthesis of RNA. When used to lower serum calcium, the dose is smaller than the antitumor dose—25 μg/kg.

Procarbazine is a methylhydrazine derivative. It undergoes auto-oxidation and produces free radicals that may depolymerize DNA. This drug is not cross-resistant with other alkylating agents, and readily enters the central nervous system. This drug has multiple drug-drug interactions and must be used carefully.

Antimetabolites

These compounds are chemically similar to naturally occurring metabolites, but differ enough to interfere with normal metabolic pathways. Antimetabolites used in cancer chemotherapy interfere with important enzymatic reactions in the synthesis of nucleic acids, purines, pyrimidines, and their precursors. They also may be incorporated into nucleic acids in place of the corresponding normal nucleotides, which alter important cellular function. Folic acid, pyrimidine, and purine analogs act primarily during the DNA synthesizing phase of the cell cycle—S phase. Some act exclusively in the S phase—for example cytarabine—and others—methotrexate, mercaptopurine—act both in S phase and prior to S phase and thus are self-limiting because they prevent entry of cells into the DNA synthesizing phase. The fluorinated pyrimidines appear to be exceptions; although they act preferentially in cycling cells, they are not phase-specific.

Hydroxyurea inhibits the enzyme ribonucleotide di-phosphate reductase. This enzyme reduces ribonucleotides to their deoxy analogs—cytidine to deoxycytidine, uridine to deoxyuridine. This step is thought to be rate-limiting in the biosynthesis of DNA. This drug does not effect RNA synthesis. Its onset of action is rapid, and it can lower white counts dramatically in acute myeloid leukemia, often within 24 hours.

Methotrexate is the 4-amino-N^{10} methyl analog of folic acid. When converted to the active form, reduced folates participate in the formation of DNA through the conversion of deoxyuridine monophosphate to deoxythymidine monophosphate. This activity is called thymidylate synthetase activity and is inhibited by methotrexate, which competes for the enzyme—dihydrofolate reductase—necessary to convert folate to tetrahydrofolic acid—FH_4—which is then converted to various coenzymes required for one-carbon transfer reactions involved in the synthesis of thymidylate, purines, methionine, and glycine.

Methotrexate undergoes transformation to polyglutamate forms, analogs to polyglutamates of physiologic folates. The polyglutamates bind with equal or greater avidity to dihydrofolate reductase than the parent drug does and after removal of the free drug persist intracellularly longer than the parent compound. Polyglutamate formation may constitute an important determinant of the duration of drug action in both normal and malignant cells. Methotrexate has been used in large doses with leucovorin—5-formyl tetrahydrofolate—rescue in an attempt to accentuate the therapeutic advantage of this agent. The rationale behind this approach is that low dose methotrexate preferentially spares tumor cells, which cannot transport the drug across cell membranes as well as normal cells can. If the drug concentration is raised, a greater dose enters neoplastic cells. Leucovorin, like methotrexate, is preferentially transported into normal cells, thus rescuing them. Any reduced folate may serve as a rescuing agent. Methyl tetrahydrofolate has been used. Other rescuing agents, such as thymidine, carboxypeptidase G_1, and L-asparaginase, have a different mechanism of rescue.

Although the rescuing agent saves the bone marrow, it does not rescue the kidney. Renal toxicity is the main toxicity of high dose methotrexate. One proposed mechanism has been precipitation of the drug or its less soluble metabolite—7-OH methotrexate—in the kidney. To prevent this complication, the patient must be well hydrated, and other drugs that compete for either tubular excretion or protein binding must be avoided. Methotrexate enters third spaces and is slowly released from them. The length of rescue must be extended in patients with ascites or pleural effusions.

Mercaptopurine and 6-thioguanine are analogs that interfere with purine synthesis. 6-Mercaptopurine is a thioanalog of hypoxanthine. Although this agent is not incorporated into DNA, it exerts a strong negative feedback on the rate-limiting step in purine synthesis. The net effect is decreased DNA production. 6-Thioguanine is 2-amino-6-mercaptopurine. It is incorporated into DNA and acts as a false transmitter and thus inhibits nucleic acid synthesis. 6-Mercaptopurine is metabolized by xanthine oxidase, whereas 6-thioguanine is only minimally metabolized by this enzyme. Patients on allopurinol and 6-mercaptopurine must have a dose reduction by 66 to 75% because of the decrease in drug metabolism.

Three antipyrimidine antimetabolites are clinically available: 5-fluorouracil, 5-azacytidine, and cytarabine.

5-Fluorouracil is an analog of thymidine. It must be activated to 5-fluorouracil deoxyuridine 5′ monophosphate—5DUMP—to interfere with the conversion of uridylate to thymidylate. The active form binds to thymidylate synthetase and inhibits the formation of thymidine and DNA. Other metabolites such as 5-FUMP interfere with the production of RNA.

Cytarabine is an analog of the pyrimidine deoxycytidine. It must be converted to the active form ara-C triphosphate. The drug is incorporated into DNA and causes chain termination. It also interferes with DNA polymerase activity. This drug is activated by cytidine kinase and inactivated by cytidine deaminase. It is believed that a low ratio of kinase to deaminase accounts for resistance to this drug. By using the drug in areas of the body with low deaminase activity—the central nervous system—or by using it with tetrahydrouridine—an inhibitor of cytidine deaminase—higher drug levels are obtained.

5-Azacytidine is also an analog of the pyrimidine nucleoside cytidine. This drug is activated by a different kinase than that which activates cytarabine. It is deactivated by the same enzyme. Cross-resistance with cytarabine is absent. Like cytarabine it must be metabolized into its active triphosphate form.

Other Chemotherapeutic Agents

L-Asparaginase

This enzyme is found in guinea pig serum, yeast, and some bacteria. It is both cytotoxic and immunosuppressive. L-asparaginase catalyzes the extracellular breakdown of the amino acid L-asparagine and therefore depletes the body's storage pool. This results in inhibition of protein synthesis. The drug's activity depends on the requirement of some tumor cells for exogenous asparagine to maintain growth.

Vinca Alkaloids

The vinca alkaloids are cycle-dependent inhibitors of mitotic spindle formation. The drugs available in this category are vincristine, vinblastine, and vindesine. Even though their mechanisms of action are believed to be similar, they are not cross-resistant. Like colchicine, these drugs block mitosis with a metaphase arrest. The mechanism of action is thought to be crystallization of the microtubular spindle proteins. Vincristine is less marrow-toxic than vinblastine. It is, however, more neurotoxic.

Podophyllotoxins

The two podophyllotoxins currently in use are etoposides—VP-16—and teniposide—VM-26. These semisynthetic compounds derived from the mayapple plant suppress DNA, RNA, and protein synthesis. These agents have been reported to arrest cells in the late S or G_2 phase, though the mechanism is unclear. Neither VP-16 nor VM-26 bind to microtubular proteins. Bone marrow suppression is their limiting toxicity.

Hormones and Antihormones

Some human tumors arise from tissues normally sensitive to hormones that have cell-surface hormonal receptors. The administration of natural or synthetic hormonal substances can induce lysis or modify the proliferation of sensitive tumor cells. Hormone therapy has had a major impact on the treatment of breast, prostate, and endometrial tumors.

The broad category of antihormone agents contains some of the newer innovations in hormonal anticancer treatment. This group includes the antiestrogenic compounds and the antiadrenal agents. The antiestrogen tamoxifen has shown significant activity in the treatment of breast cancer with minimally associated toxicity. Mitotane—o,p'-DDD—is an antiadrenal compound with direct toxic effects and proven efficacy against adrenocortical carcinoma.

Biologic Response Modifiers

Attempts to enhance the immune response directed against malignancies are fertile ground for investigation. Over the last several years it has become clear that alpha interferons have impressive therapeutic activity in the treatment of hairy cell leukemia, cutaneous T cell lymphomas, and chronic myelocytic leukemia, and also some effectiveness in the treatment of renal cell carcinoma. Interferon alpha-2b, recombinant, has recently been approved for commercial use in the United States. These observations provide the foundation for extensive further investigation of interleukins, other lymphokines, and biologic materials.

Dosage and Routes of Administration

The dosage, routines of administration, and toxic manifestations of the various agents are listed in Table 95–2.

TOXICITY OF SPECIFIC ORGAN SYSTEMS

Bone Marrow Suppression

The most common life-threatening immediate side effect of most drugs is bone marrow suppression, which of course may be associated with infection or bleeding, consequences of leucopenia and thrombopenia, respectively. The extent and timing of myelosuppression is a function of drug schedule and dose, and can reliably be predicted for most patients.

Alopecia

Hair loss is often a major psychologic problem. Vincristine and doxorubicin usually cause total alopecia. Cyclophosphamide causes thinning and alopecia. Hair loss with 5-fluorouracil is milder than with other drugs.

Various stratagems have been invented to prevent alopecia. Immersing the head in ice has been used to prevent this problem. One should realize, however, that the reason that hair is not lost is because the drug has not reached the hair follicle; this area may be fertile soil for metastatic disease.

Cardiac Toxicity

The anthracycline antibiotics cause a cardiomyopathy that most often becomes clinically manifest when they are used in doses of greater than 550 mg/m². This toxicity occurs earlier when mediastinal radiation or cyclophosphamide has been used. The dose not to be exceeded in these patients is 450 mg/m². Several invasive tests—endomyocardial biopsy—and noninvasive tests—systolic time intervals, gated pool scans—have been used to predict toxicity, but they indicate damage only after it has occurred, and none can reliably predict which individuals can tolerate a greater dose. The gated pool scan has allowed greater dosage in one study. This finding is particularly important, because if those patients who would not go into irreversible failure could be identified, larger doses could be used. Wider use of this technique may confirm the initial success as a predictor. Some preliminary evidence suggests that smaller intermittent doses or sustained intravenous infusions are less cardiotoxic.

All patients on anthracyclines have T-wave changes and premature atrial or ventricular beats. This problem is not usually serious and should not lead to discontinuance of therapy.

The cardiomyopathy seen in patients who go into failure is a congestive cardiomyopathy with a decrease in normal myocardial fibers, cellular degeneration, and interstitial edema. Electron microscopy shows Z-band abnormalities.

Cutaneous Toxicity

Particular care must be taken when injecting chemotherapeutic agents, because several agents cause cutaneous necrosis. If this happens, the wound may require skin grafting. Mechlorethamine—nitrogen mustard—is one such agent. Vincristine, vinblastine, actinomycin, doxorubicin, daunomycin, and mitomycin C also cause skin necrosis. Local pain along the vein in the absence of extravasation may occur with carmustine, dacarbazine, doxorubicin, mechlorethamine, and vinblastine. This phenomenon is not merely a subintimal injection that any injection may cause; there may be associated phlebitis, vasospasm, and thrombosis.

Bleomycin has striking skin toxicity; morbilliform rash, urticaria, erythematous swelling, and blistering may occur. The enzyme that degrades this drug is absent in skin and lung, and toxicity predictably occurs in these organs. In addition, after long-term use, a scleroderma-like syndrome may occur in the fingers, causing pitting and pain in the fingertips.

Hyperpigmentation of the skin has been observed with the alkylating agents, busulfan and cyclophosphamide. In addition, many agents cause brown lines in the nail beds. Doxorubicin in particular causes this change. Dac-

Table 95–2. Specific Agents Used in Cancer Chemotherapy

Agents	Principal Route of Administration	Usual Dose	Acute Toxic Signs	Major Toxic Manifestations
Polyfunctional Alkylating Agents				
Mechlorethamine (HN$_2$, Mustargen®)	IV	16 mg/M^2 single or divided doses	N & V	Therapeutic doses moderately depress peripheral blood cell count; excessive doses cause severe bone marrow depression with leukopenia, thrombocytopenia, and bleeding. Maximum toxicity may occur two or three weeks after last dose. Dosage, therefore, must be carefully controlled. Alopecia and hemorrhage cystitis occur occasionally with cyclophosphamide.
Chlorambucil (Leukeran®)	Oral	4–10 mg daily	None	
Melphalan (L-PAM, Alkeran®)	Oral	6–10 mg daily 2–4 mg daily maintenance	None	
Cyclophosphamide (Cytoxan®)	IV Oral	1.0–1.5 g/M^2 50–200 mg daily	N & V	
Thiotepa	IV	16–32 mg/M^2 or 8 mg/M^2 daily × 4–5	None	
Busulfan (Myleran®)	Oral	2–6 mg daily	None	
Antimetabolites				
Methotrexate (Methotrexate®)	Oral IV IM IT	2.5–5.0 mg daily 25–50 mg 1–2 × weekly 200 mg–10 gm with leucovorin rescue 15 mg every 2–5 days	None	Oral and digestive tract ulcerations; bone marrow depression with leukopenia; thrombocytopenia and bleeding. Toxicity enhanced by impaired kidney function.
6-Mercaptopurine (6MP, Purinethol®)	Oral	100 mg/M^2 daily (less if allopurinol is given concurrently)	None	Therapeutic doses usually well tolerated; excessive doses cause bone marrow depression.
6-Thioguanine (6TG, Thioguanine®)	Oral	80 mg/M^2 daily	None	Therapeutic doses usually well tolerated; excessive doses cause bone marrow depression.
5-Fluorouracil (5FU, fluorouracil)	IV	500 mg/M^2 daily × 3 smaller dose 1–2 × weekly for maintenance	None	Stomatitis, GI injury, bone marrow depression, alopecia.
Cytarabine (Ara-C, Cytosar®)	IV	200 mg/M^2 daily × 5 by continuous infusion	N & V	Bone marrow depression, megaloblastosis, leukopenia, thrombocytopenia.
5-Fluorodeoxyuridine (FUDR, floxuridine)	IV IA	16–24 mg/M^2 daily by continuous infusion		Stomatitis, GI injury, bone marrow depression, alopecia.
Antibiotics				
Doxorubicin (Adriamycin®)	IV	50–75 mg/M^2 in single or divided doses every 3 weeks, continuous infusion less cardiotoxic		Stomatitis, GI injury, alopecia, bone marrow depression. Cardiac toxicity at cumulative doses over 500 mg/M^2.
Bleomycin (Blenoxane®)	IV SC	10 U/M^2 daily × 5–7 Maintenance: 1.0–2.0 U daily	N & V, chills, fever	Mucocutaneous ulcerations, alopecia, penumonitis and pulmonary fibrosis at cumulative doses over 400 U.
Dactinomycin (Cosmegen®)	IV	2.5 mg/M^2 in single or divided doses	N & V	Stomatitis, GI injury, alopecia, bone marrow depression.
Daunorubicin (Cerubidine®)	IV	90–180 mg/M^2 in single or divided doses every 3 weeks. Total dose not to exceed 600 mg/M^2	N & V, fever	Bone marrow depression with leukopenia and thrombocytopenia, alopecia, stomatitis, cardiac toxicity at cumulative doses over 600 mg/M^2.
Plicamycin (Mithramycin, Mithracin®)	IV	1 mg/M^2 every other day × 3–4	N & V	Bone marrow depression, particularly thrombocytopenic bleeding, hypocalcemia, hepatic toxicity at large doses.
Mitomycin C (Mutamycin®)	IV	20 mg/M^2 in single dose every 6–8 weeks	N & V	Bone marrow depression, GI injury, hypercalcemia.

Table 95–2. Specific Agents Used in Cancer Chemotherapy *Continued*

Agents	Principal Route of Administration	Usual Dose	Acute Toxic Signs	Major Toxic Manifestations
Steroid and Hormonally Active Compounds				
Androgen				
Testosterone propionate	IM	50–100 mg 3 × weekly	None	Fluid retention, masculinization.
Fluoxymesterone (Halotestin®)	Oral	10–40 mg daily		
Dromostanolone (Drolban®)	IM	100 mg 3 × weekly		
Testolactone (Teslac®)		250 mg 4 × daily		
Methyltestosterone	Oral	50–200 mg daily		
Estrogen				
Diethylstilbestrol	Oral	Breast: 5 mg 3 × daily	Occas.	Fluid retention, feminization.
		Prostate: 1 mg daily	N & V	Uterine bleeding.
Ethinyl estradiol (Estinyl®)	Oral	Breast: 1.0 mg 3 × daily		
		Prostate: 0.1 mg 3 × daily		
Antiestrogen				
Tamoxifen (Nolvadex®)	Oral	10 mg 2 × daily	N & V	Hot flashes.
Leuprolide (Lupron®)	SC	1 mg daily		Hot flashes.
Progestin				
Hydroxyprogesterone caproate (Prodrox®)	IM	1 mg 2 × weekly		
Megestrol Acetate (Megace®)	Oral	40 mg 4 × daily		
Medroxyprogesterone acetate (Provera®)	Oral	100–200 mg daily	None	
	IM	200–600 mg 2 × weekly		
Adrenal Cortical Compounds				
Cortisone acetate	Oral	20–100 mg daily	None	Fluid retention, hypertension, diabetes, increased susceptibility to infection.
Prednisone (Meticorten®)	Oral	15–100 mg daily		
Dexamethasone (Decadron®)	Oral	0.5–4.0 mg daily		
Methylprednisolone sodium succinate (Solu-Medrol®)	IM IV	10–125 mg daily		
Hydrocortisone sodium succinate (Solu-Cortef®)	IV	100–500 mg daily		
Antiadrenal				
Aminoglutethamide	Oral	250–500 mg 4 × daily		Adrenal insufficiency.
Miscellaneous Drugs				
Asparaginase (Elspar®)	IV	8,000 IU/M² 3–7 × weekly for 28 days	N & V, fever, hypersensitivity reactions	Anorexia, weight loss. Somnolence, lethargy, confusion. Hypoproteinemia (including albumin and fibrinogen). Hypolipidemia, abnormal lever function tests, fatty metamorphosis of the liver. Pancreatitis (rare). Azotemia. Granulocytopenia, lymphopenia, and thrombocytopenia (usually mild and transient).
Carmustine (BiCNU®)	IV	200 mg/M²		
Lomustine (CCNU, CeeNU®)	Oral	130 mg/M²	N & V	Bone marrow depression with leukopenia and thrombocytopenia.
Streptozotocin (Zanosar®)	IV	500 mg daily × 5 every 6 weeks	N & V	Hypoglycemia.
Mitotane (o,p′-DDD, Lysodren®)	Oral	2–10 gm daily in divided doses	N & V	Skin eruptions, diarrhea, mental depression, muscle tremors, adrenal insufficiency.
Dacarbazine (DTIC-Dome®)	IV	80–160 mg/M² daily × 10	N & V	Bone marrow depression.
Hydroxyurea (Hydrea®)	Oral	800–1600 mg/M² daily	None	Bone marrow depression.
Etoposide (VP-16) (VR. 16, VePesid®)		50–100 mg/M² daily × 5 every 3 weeks	N & V	Alopecia.
Cisplatin (Cis-Platinum (II) diammine-dichloride)	IV	120 mg/M² every 3 weeks or 20 mg/M² daily × 5 every 3 weeks	N & V	Bone marrow depression, renal tubular damage, deafness.
Procarbazine (lbenzmethyzin) (Matulane®)	Oral	80–160 mg/M² daily	N & V	Bone marrow depression with leukopenia and thrombocytopenia, mental depression.
Vinblastine (Velban®)	IV	4–8 mg/M² weekly	N & V	Alopecia, areflexia, bone marrow depression.
Vincristine (Oncovin®)	IV	1.4 mg/M² weekly	None	Areflexia, muscular weakness, peripheral neuritis, paralytic ileus, mild bone marrow depression.

Key: N & V = nausea and vomiting; IV = intravenous; IM = intramuscular; IT = intrathecal; IA = intra-arterial; SC = subcutaneous
Reproduced with permission from CA-A Cancer Journal for Clinicians, 1987. Krakoff, I.H.: Cancer chemotherapeutic agents. CA 37:93, 1987.

tinomycin and methotrexate have been associated with an erythematous rash. 5-Fluorouracil has been associated with a dry scaling dermatitis.

A facial flush has been seen following plicamycin injection. Initially a pink flush of the neck and head appears, followed by plethora and facial edema. If this reaction occurs, the drug should be discontinued.

Radiation recall dermatitis may be seen with administration of actinomycin, doxorubicin, and perhaps bleomycin.

Fever

Febrile reactions unassociated with infection have been noted with many agents. Bleomycin febrile reactions are common and easily abolished by pretreatment with steroids 1 to 2 hours before injection. Dacarbazine has a peculiar flu-like syndrome with fever myalgias and malaise associated with its administration. This reaction usually occurs 7 days after treatment and may last 1 to 3 weeks. Recurrence with successive courses has been seen. Fever, flush and hypertension—tyramine reactions—seen with procarbazine, are caused by the monoamine oxidase inhibiting properties of this drug. Foods, such as ripe cheese, Chianti wines, beer, and yogurt, and other drugs, such as the tricyclic antidepressants, have elicited this reaction. A disulfiram-like reaction to procarbazine consisting of nausea, vomiting, and flushing has been described following alcohol ingestion when patients have taken this drug. Potentiation of central nervous system depressants, such as barbiturates, phenothiazines, and narcotics, has been observed.

L-Asparaginase catalyzes the hydrolysis of asparagine to aspartic acid, depriving cells of this essential amino acid and interfering with protein synthesis. Preparations come from two sources: *Escherichia coli* and *Erwinia carotovora*. If one elicits an allergic reaction, the other may be used. After treatment, DNA and RNA synthesis decreases. As with other enzyme preparations such as urokinase, vigorous shaking of the preparation may result in loss of some enzyme potency.

Fever with methotrexate occurs in two particular situations. In young patients and children who receive intrathecal methotrexate, an aseptic meningitis-meningismus syndrome with fever is common. Also, fever is a component of methotrexate lung. This condition will be discussed further in the section on pulmonary toxicity. Mechlorethamine is the only alkylating agent to cause fever, which is not common.

Gastrointestinal Toxicity

Nausea and vomiting are common symptoms of chemotherapy. Only melphalan and chlorambucil are rarely associated with nausea and vomiting.

The symptoms are often a reflex to chemotherapy and many patients develop the same symptoms with a placebo, or even before the chemotherapy is given. This anticipatory nausea may be alleviated by use of minor tranquilizers, or perhaps the cannabinoids.

Some agents, such as cytarabine and 5-azacytidine, produce less nausea when they are infused slowly. Agents such as dacarbazine and procarbazine cause less nausea and vomiting when they have been administered for 24 to 48 hours.

Several agents, such as hexamethylmelamine and cisplatin, produce such severe symptoms that some patients refuse therapy. Antiemetics such as the phenothiazines, butyrophenones, metaclopramide, tetrahydrocannabinol—THC—and its derivative nabilone effectively ameliorate toxicity. To maximize efficacy, these agents should be given prophylactically.

Hepatic Toxicity

Many chemotherapeutic agents cause a rise in hepatic enzymes after administration. This reaction, however, is usually not a major problem. Cytarabine, hydroxyurea, and the nitrosoureas are prime examples. Methotrexate, if given by small daily doses, can lead to hepatic fibrosis and cirrhosis. The mean time of drug exposure is about 3 years for fibrosis and 4 years to cirrhosis.

6-Mercaptopurine and plicamycin, however, cause much more damage. 6-Mercaptopurine and its congener azathioprine cause pronouced bile stasis in the liver. Focal necrosis may be seen. This picture resembles that seen after chlorpromazine therapy. The jaundice usually clears rapidly after the drug is discontinued.

Plicamycin is the most hepatotoxic chemotherapeutic agent used today. Dramatic elevations of hepatic enzymes are seen in 100% of patients. The levels of elevation of SGOT, SGPT, and LDH may be in the thousands. A moderate elevation of alkaline phosphatase is seen, and bilirubin elevation does not occur. This acute liver necrosis has a 24-hour onset, a peak at 2 days, and a return to normal over the next 4 to 21 days. Histologically, acute hepatic necrosis is accompanied by vacuolization and fatty metamorphosis. Clotting factors II, V, VII, and X are depressed, leading to a prolonged prothrombin time. In addition, because platelets are depressed, a significant risk of bleeding is present.

L-Asparaginase also leads to mild elevation of hepatic enzymes. This elevation is usually not significant. Although fibrinogen factors II, V, VII, and X decrease, a bleeding diathesis does not usually occur. In fact, paradoxically, a predisposition for thrombosis may develop because of a decreased production of factors necessary for fibrinolysis. The concurrent use of doxorubicin—an agent whose dose must be modified when decreased hepatic function occurs—and streptozotocin has led to excessive hepatic toxicity because of the subclinical damage streptozotocin causes.

Nervous System Toxicity

Vincristine and vinblastine regularly exhibit neurotoxicity. Early changes include loss of the ankle jerk and depression of other deep tendon reflexes. Areflexia occurs in about half the patients receiving weekly injections. This condition is not always a precursor of weakness or paralysis. If the drug is continued in the same dosage, a distal paresthesia occurs. This sensation is usually a precursor of muscle weakness. The paresthesia and weakness are usually distal, rarely extending more proximally than the wrist or ankles. Cranial nerves III, VI, and VII may be involved, and a peculiar type of jaw pain often occurs. Cerebellar ataxia occurs with 5-fluorouracil. This condition is thought to result from a metabolite, fluorocitrate, and may also be seen with hexamethylmelamine. Other central nervous system toxicity symptoms with this drug include paresthesia, sleep disturbance, hallucinations, and seizures. A Parkinson-like syndrome may also be seen. Tinnitus occurs with cisplatin, and eighth nerve toxicity may also be seen with mechlorethamine. Cisplatin may also cause a peripheral neuropathy.

Procarbazine may cause central nervous system depression or stupor in approximately 10% of the patients. A peripheral neuropathy may also occur. L-Asparaginase may cause lethargy, confusion, and occasionally acute psychosis.

Intrathecal methotrexate has been associated with arachnoiditis, neuropathies, and encephalitis. The exact mechanism is not clear. Preservative contaminants and slow drug metabolism have been postulated.

Pulmonary Toxicity

Pulmonary toxicity is being reported for greater numbers of drugs as time passes. The first alkylating agent implicated was busulfan, but all the alkylating agents are suspect. Reports of pulmonary fibrosis have been reported with cyclophosphamide, melphalan, and the nitrosoureas. The presenting symptoms are dyspnea, cough, and fever. The chest roentgenogram demonstrates bilateral infiltrates. The biopsy shows interstitial fibrosis, occasionally vasculitis, and rarely areas of calcification. This type of pulmonary toxicity is irreversible, usually progressive, and often fatal. The mean time to death is 4 to 5 months. Steroids are usually not beneficial.

Reversible pulmonary toxicity occurs with methotrexate, procarbazine, and cytarabine. These drugs are similar in the clinical syndrome. Peripheral eosinophilia and fever are associated with all of these drugs. Use of methotrexate may result in dyspnea, a nonproductive cough, and cyanosis. The roentgenogram shows a confluent interstitial pattern—rarely with small nodular densities. These changes resolve with and often without corticosteroids. Biopsy often shows eosinophilic infiltrate. The alveoli are filled with large mononuclear cells, and arterioles soon cuff with polymorphonuclear cells. Procarbazine was noted in one report to cause fever, cough, and dyspnea. The roentgenogram of the chest may show effusion and interstitial and bilateral basilar infiltrates. This syndrome abates when the drug is stopped and can be reproduced when restarted. Cytarabine has been reported to cause capillary leakage with the subsequent development of noncardiac pulmonary edema.

Bleomycin causes serious pulmonary toxicity. The toxicity is dose-related. Fibrinous intra-alveolar infiltrate, hyaline membrane formation, and interstitial alveolar fibrosis occur, as well as hypertrophy of the type II alveolar pneumocyte and a loss of type I pneumocytes. The pathophysiologic result is a decrease in lung volume. This restrictive defect can be measured by any lung volume

test. The forced vital capacity and the carbon monoxide diffusing capacity are usually decreased. Functional abnormalities occur earlier than roentgenologic evidence. Basilar rales are often the earliest physical sign. Also, changes on gallium scanning are often an early indicator of change. These serious pulmonary changes occur in 3 to 5% of patients with a cumulative dose below 450 mg. The increase is as high as 20% when this dose is exceeded. Notably, patients exposed to both bleomycin and irradiation are particularly susceptible to lung injury.

This toxicity is separate from the anaphylactoid acute reaction with bronchospasm and pulmonary edema. This acute reaction, which often occurs in non-Hodgkin's lymphoma, responds to corticosteroids, whereas the fibrosis does not.

Renal Toxicity

Cyclophosphamide is the only alkylating agent that results in urinary tract toxicity; hemorrhagic cystitis occurs in about 10% of patients treated. The only other drug that produces cystitis is mitotane. Cyclophosphamide causes telangiectasia of the bladder and leads to serious bleeding that may necessitate urinary diversion. Instances of squamous and undifferentiated carcinoma of bladder have been reported in patients on long-term therapy. Continued use in patients with hemorrhagic cystitis may lead to bladder fibrosis. Certain patients seem to be particularly prone to cystitis, in particular women and those patients with prior radiation therapy. In addition, urinary cytologic studies can be bizarre in patients on cyclophosphamide. This aspect does not correlate with the development of neoplasm. Methotrexate in high doses is particularly toxic to the kidney if careful hydration and avoidance of drugs that release it from protein binding or that compete for tubular excretion are not considered. In low doses, methotrexate is not metabolized in the body. In high doses, however, 7-OH methotrexate is formed. This metabolite is less soluble and may precipitate in the renal tubules.

Mitomycin C is toxic to the glomerulus, not the renal tubule. This syndrome occurs in less than 5% of the patients treated. Creatinine level may rise, with no correlation to total dose administered. Pathologically, the lesion is a glomerular sclerosis.

Cisplatin is toxic to the renal tubule. Renal toxicity may be prevented by adequate hydration and diuresis. Hydration with half normal saline and diuresis of 100 ml per hour during therapy and continuing for four hours after the completion of therapy is usually adequate. Changes in glomerular function as well as electrolyte disturbances such as hyponatremia, hypocalcemia, and hypomagnesemia are common. Streptozotocin and other nitrosoureas are also toxic to the renal tubule. The earliest sign is often proteinuria, which is usually followed by a decrease in glomerular filtration, hypophosphatemia, and elevated blood urea nitrogen levels. Renal acidosis and glucosuria may also be seen.

Among the drugs that may be reduced in patients with renal failure are bleomycin, hydroxyurea, 6-mercaptopurine, thioguanine, and dacarbazine. Use of methotrexate and cisplatin should be avoided.

Effect on Serum Electrolytes

A syndrome similar to that of the inappropriate secretion of ADH has been reported with vincristine and high doses of cyclophosphamide. Plicamycin may produce hypocalcemia. A syndrome of seizures and hypocalcemia has been seen following cisplatin therapy.

Hyperkalemia, hyperphosphatemia, and hypocalcemia in association with hyperuricemia may be seen when chemotherapy is given to patients with rapidly proliferating neoplasma, such as Burkitt's lymphoma.

Miscellaneous Side Effects

Sterility is a regularly expected side effect of chemotherapy in both men and women. It is kinetically predictable because germ cells are a rapidly renewing population of cells. Cyclophosphamide regularly produces sterility, as does the MOPP regimen for Hodgkin's disease.

Immunosuppression is also common after chemotherapy, and herpes zoster is seen frequently during therapy. Necrosis of the femoral head has been seen occasionally, especially in the treatment of Hodgkin's disease. A disturbing effect of chemotherapy has been the development of second malignancies. This problem is potentiated when high dose radiation therapy and chemotherapy are used together. Patients with lymphoma and Hodgkin's disease are at highest risk—approaching 10%—at 10 years following treatment.

STRATEGIES IN CHEMOTHERAPY

Several principles guide the selection of drugs to be used in the treatment of individual patients. Single agents that have demonstrated activity are typically combined at optimal doses—usually as high as tolerable—and given in combination with other active agents with relatively nonoverlapping toxicity spectra. Guidelines governing the specific drug regimens sometimes follow cytokinetic principles. An example of this is the usual practice of infusing cytarabine over a period of 5–7 days in the treatment of acute leukemia. Cytarabine is rapidly deaminated in the serum to inactive forms, with a half-life of less than 30 minutes, and for this drug to be effective, continuous infusion or repeating parenteral injections must be given over a period of days. This not only sustains a blood level necessary for cell-killing, but also exposes increasing numbers of acute leukemic cells, which may take days to enter cell cycle, to this agent. For most solid tumors, drugs are scheduled to permit maximal drug dose at frequent repeating intervals. Much work has supported the concept that dose intensity is a major factor in developing effective treatment for chemosensitive tumors.

Many factors influence the effectiveness of chemotherapy, including the general medical condition of the patient, the proliferative characteristics of the tumor, and the distribution of tumor involvement within the body.

A large tumor burden at diagnosis is perhaps the most important limiting feature. Most of the common solid tumors—breast, lung, and gastrointestinal malignancies—are detected when the primary tumor exceeds 10^{10} cancer cells and are high on the gompertzian growth curve.

Tumor cell heterogeneity has been better appreciated in the 1970's and 1980's as it is now clear that a single malignant tumor is often composed of cells heterogeneous for nearly every characteristic studied. Cell size, shape, histologic subtype, cell surface antigens, responsiveness to drugs, and proliferative tendencies vary enormously. Although most malignant tumors appear to originate from a single cell or clone, the descendent cell population apparently diversifies, because of the emergence and selection of new clones from within the original one. Molecular biologic work demonstrates changing genomic constitution over time, which seems to correlate with changes in morphology and in the natural history of the malignancy.

Salmon and associates (1978) described an innovative technique, use of a human tumor stem cell assay, to grow tumor cell clones in soft agar and expose them to various drugs for chemosensitivity testing. Interestingly, only a few cancer cells from a biopsy specimen, typically less than .01% actually grow to develop colonies, even when therapeutic agents are absent. This low plating efficiency probably reflects some limitations of the culture technique, but it also likely is the result of the relatively small number of clonogenic tumor stem cells that exist within any one tumor mass. Thus, human tumors appear to be composed of multiple cell populations with differing potential for proliferation and the production of growth factors and other tumor products.

So-called pleiotropic drug resistance in human cancers and seems to be linked to the expression of a membrane glycoprotein known as the P glycoprotein, which is located on the surface of cancer cells. The physiologic function of this substance is unknown, but its increased surface concentration seems to be associated with decreased accumulation of multiple chemotherapy drugs within these resistant cell populations.

The clonogenic assay has shown promise not only for the identification of active chemotherapy drugs, but also as a means to develop new drugs as studies on drug action can be performed in human cells in vitro under more controlled circumstances than would obtain in in vivo phase II projects. This approach also fosters study of the biology of cancer.

During the last 10 years, combination chemotherapy has proved effective in producing responses in a wide variety of diseases. It has led to cures for some disseminated malignancies (Table 95–1) and effective palliation for a larger number of common cancers. Hodgkin's disease, diffuse large cell lymphoma, testicular carcinoma, and gestational choriocarcinoma are among the adult malignancies that are curable. These malignancies share certain features that earmark cancers most amenable to effective drug therapy. Generally, rapidly growing, poorly differentiated, and relatively uncommon processes have a higher therapeutic index of drug therapy than slower growing, less sensitive, more indolent diseases such as colon cancer have.

New approaches are emerging to counteract problems with low growth fraction and drug resistance. Drug infusions with various agents are now being tested to minimize toxicity and sustain high tissue levels. This approach is designed to expose an increased number of cancer cells entering DNA synthesis to a higher concentration of drug. High dose programs, such as high dose methotrexate with folinic acid rescue or intensive drug and radiation therapy treatments with autologous bone marrow support represent another strategy to deliver highly intensive therapy and, at the same time, protect the patient from what would otherwise be lethal myelosuppressive toxicity. Administration of drugs directly into peritoneal or pleural cavities has demonstrated promise in the treatment of special problems with predominantly involvement of these body cavities. As indicated, experimentation with biologic response modifiers, for example the interferons in the treatment of some leukemias and renal cell carcinoma, may ultimately prove an effective additional modality with or without classical cytotoxic chemotherapy. Hyperthermia, monoclonal antibodies, and other biologic modifiers, such as tumor necrosis factor, are also currently being carefully investigated.

REFERENCE

Salmon, S.E., et al.: Quantitation of differential sensitivity of human tumor stem cells to anticancer drugs. N. Engl. J. Med. 298:1321, 1978.

READING REFERENCES

Chabner, B.A.: Karnofsky Memorial lecture: the oncologic end game. J. Clin. Oncol. 4(5):625, 1986.
Damon, L.E., and Cadman, E.C.: Clinical science review: advances in rational combination chemotherapy. Cancer Invest. 4(5):4211, 1986.
Dexter, D.L., and Leith, J.T.: Review article: tumor heterogeneity and drug resistance. J. Clin. Oncol. 4(2):244, 1986.
Frei, E., III: Position paper: curative cancer chemotherapy. Cancer Res. 45:6523, 1985.
Krakoff, I.H.: Cancer Chemotherapeutic Agents. CA. 37:93, 1987.

CHAPTER 96

CHEMOTHERAPY OF NON-SMALL CELL LUNG CANCER

Martin H. Cohen

The prognosis for most newly diagnosed non-small cell lung cancer patients is dismal. The American Cancer Society's (1988) statistics indicate that fewer than 13% of these individuals survive 5 years. Even when the cancer is resectable, Belcher and Rehahn (1979) found that the 5-year survival is only 25 to 30%. A likely explanation for these poor survival results is that cancer cells have already disseminated, regionally or systemically, by the time diagnosis is established. Direct evidence supporting an early dissemination hypothesis comes from autopsy data collected by Matthews and co-workers (1973) on patients who died within 30 days of a "curative" lung cancer resection. Further support for this hypothesis comes from several sources of data, including: (1) the Ludwig Cancer Study Group's (1987) study of failure patterns of patients with resected stage I and stage II non-small cell lung cancer, (2) Stanley and colleagues' (1981) study of failure patterns after "curative" radiation therapy, and (3) Line and Deeley's (1971) study of disease location at autopsy. Most of the patients in each of these reports had disseminated disease. These data support the concept of early tumor cell dissemination because median survival of lung cancer patients is sufficiently short that, as Geddes (1979) explained, metastases occurring after the time of diagnosis would not have time, before death, to grow large enough to be detectable clinically or at autopsy. If disseminated disease is the major treatment problem in non-small cell lung cancer, systemic treatment—chemotherapy—is needed to control total tumor burden.

Developing effective chemotherapy for non-small cell lung cancer is proving to be difficult. Because lung cancer is common worldwide, numerous studies of single chemotherapy drugs and drug combinations have been done. Thus far no single "best" regimen has emerged. The following discussion will indicate possible causes for poor chemotherapy results and strategies for overcoming these difficulties.

PATHOPHYSIOLOGY

Successful chemotherapy requires that sufficient concentrations of drugs reach neoplastic cells for a sufficient time to exert a lethal injury. The first requirement, therefore, is to ensure that chemotherapy drugs reach all viable, replicating malignant cells within a tumor mass. This may prove to be impossible because of the heterogeneous distribution of blood vessels within a tumor mass. When a tumor is sectioned, an area of central necrosis is almost always visible. In addition, although most of the rim of the tumor appears viable, patchy areas of necrosis may be visible in this region as well. Tomlinson and Gray (1955) reported that microscopic examination of tumor tissue also reveals a heterogeneous distribution of capillaries within the tumor mass. Overall, the number of capillaries per unit area of cancer tissue is less than that seen in the same size area of normal tissue. Because cancer cells are often at a greater distance from a capillary than normal cells are, it is not surprising that focal areas of necrosis are seen throughout malignant tumors. An oxygen gradient must obviously exist from the cells immediately surrounding the capillary to the more peripheral necrotic cells. This gradient was demonstrated in experimental neoplasms by Vaupel and associates (1981) and in human beings by Gatenby and associates (1985) and Mueller-Kleiser and associates (1981). Within tumors, similar gradients would be expected for nutrients, blood-borne growth factors, and chemotherapy drugs. Opposite gradients would exist for carbon dioxide tension and tumor waste products. A good model system for studying the microenvironmental effects of these gradients is the multicellular spheroid, a three-dimensional tumor mass derived from rodent or human cancer cells and grown in vitro. Sutherland (1986) demonstrated that these spheroids show similar oxygen, carbon dioxide, pH, cell proliferation, and drug distribution gradients to those described in human cancers in vivo. They also demonstrated that chemotherapy drugs are either metabolized differently or are metabolically altered in different tumor regions. Thus, Sutherland (1986) showed that doxorubicin is distributed mainly over the nuclei of cells in the oxygenated portion of the tumor but is distributed over the entire cell in hypoxic tumor regions.

There is at present no way to increase tumor vascularity. It is hoped that as chemotherapy is given and as tumor size decreases, residual cancer cells become more closely approximated to tumor capillaries. This must result if tumor blood vessels are not destroyed by chemotherapy. No data on the effect of chemotherapy on tumor vasculature exist, although with chemotherapy vascular toxicity may occur in normal tissues. Examples of such toxicity, summarized by Doll and colleagues (1986), are pulmonary and hepatic veno-occlusive disease, Raynaud's phenomenon, thrombotic microangiopathic syndromes, and acute arterial ischemic episodes—myocardial infarction and cerebrovascular accidents.

In addition to decreased vascular supply there may be impaired microcirculatory blood flow to tumors. A primary determinant of microcirculatory blood flow is red blood cell deformability, the ability of a red blood cell with a 7.5 μm diameter to change its shape sufficiently to traverse capillaries with diameters as small as 3 μm. Failure of red blood cells to deform might cause stasis of microcirculatory blood flow and contribute to the hypoxia, hypercarbia, and acidosis noted in tumor tissue. I (1979, 1981) demonstrated that red blood cell deformability is decreased in experimental cancer and in human patients. I and my colleagues (1984a) further demonstrated that red cell deformability can be improved with various drugs and with appropriate scheduling of chemotherapy, and I and my associates (1984b) reported an 85% response rate in squamous cell lung cancer with this treatment.

The foregoing discussion is concerned with advanced, unresectable cancers. In the surgical adjuvant situation, as Frei (1977) discussed, chemotherapy might be expected to be more efficacious, because smaller tumors have a relative increase in vasculature and more favorable cell kinetics, presumably because of increased oxygen and nutrient supply and more efficient toxic waste removal. As will be discussed later, several single-agent and combination chemotherapy surgical adjuvant studies have already been reported, and two show promising results.

ADJUVANT CHEMOTHERAPY

In developing potential surgical adjuvant treatments, the usual procedure is to first test the regimen in patients with advanced, unresectable disease. To avoid false negative results in these trials it has become standard practice to enroll only patients who have the best chance to benefit from treatment. Host factors that predict increased survival, lessened toxicity from treatment, and increased probability of tumor shrinkage have been identified. Stanley (1980) demonstrated that the most important prognostic factor for survival was performance status. Patients who were fully ambulatory, with or without some disease-related symptoms—Eastern Coopera-

tive Oncology Group performance status 0 to 1, Karnofsky performance status 100 to 80—had significantly prolonged survival and significantly less treatment toxicity than patients whose symptoms confined them to bed during daytime hours. Other important prognostic factors are disease stage, weight loss, and prior therapy. Aisner and Hansen (1981) reported that patients with disease confined to the chest were more likely to respond to treatment than patients with disseminated disease. DeWys and associates (1980) showed that patients who had lost more than 10% of their usual body weight before treatment survived a significantly shorter time than patients with less weight loss. Patients who previously received chemotherapy also have lower response rates and a poorer prognosis than previously untreated patients. Possible explanations for this observation are the induction of pleiotropic drug resistance in residual surviving cells, as Goldie and Coldman (1984) described, or Abrams and colleagues' (1981, 1985) observation that host bone marrow reserve is decreased by prior cytotoxic therapy. Because chemotherapy dose, as Frei and Canellos (1980) reported, and dose-intensity, as Hryniuk and Bush (1984) reported, are important factors in successful chemotherapy, anything that decreases host chemotherapy tolerance might decrease response rates.

Other, possibly less important, prognostic factors include sex and age. In their reviews, Lanzotti and colleagues (1977) and Rossing and Rossing (1982) found that women had a better prognosis than men and patients less than 70 years old had a better prognosis than those over age 70.

EVALUATION OF DRUG REGIMENS

Since the late 1970s, most medical oncologists have recognized the importance of including only good-prognosis patients into trials seeking to discover new "active" treatment regimens.

When evaluating new drug regimens in non-small cell lung cancer patients, how do we determine whether or not we have a useful treatment? The major criterion for selecting active drugs or drug combinations is the response rate, defined by Selawry (1973) and by Eagan and colleagues (1979). Patients are considered to have responded to therapy when the product of the perpendicular diameters of a bidimensionally measurable lesion decreases at least 50% from the pretreatment value or when an evaluable, nonmeasurable lesion is judged by at least two observers to have definitely decreased in size. Survival is a less useful measure of treatment activity because median survival is unaltered unless treatment response rates are greater than 50%, because randomized studies comparing a chemotherapy group with an untreated, control population are inappropriate when a new regimen is first tested for activity, and because comparison of survival of responders and nonresponders to a particular treatment produces, as Anderson and coworkers (1983) discussed, a biased statistical analysis.

RESPONSE RATES

I and Perevodchikova (1978) and Bakowski and Crouch (1983) reviewed response rates for single-agent chemotherapy in non-small cell lung cancer. The studies cited in these reviews include heterogeneous patient populations, but most used standard response criteria. Nine drugs gave response rates between 10 and 20%, including doxorubicin, cisplatin, cyclophosphamide, etoposide—VP-16-213, ifosfamide, methotrexate, mitomycin C, vinblastine, and vindesine. These drugs were subsequently used in various 2- to 5-drug combinations. Drug regimens developed during the early and mid 1970s generally included cyclophosphamide and doxorubicin with or without bleomycin, methotrexate, procarbazine, vincristine, or a nitrosourea—lomustine or methyl-lomustine. Initial single-institution reports of these combinations, such as cyclophosphamide, doxorubicin, methotrexate, and procarbazine—CAMP—or methotrexate, doxorubicin, cyclophosphamide and lomustine—MACC—reported response rates around 40%, suggesting that the various drugs in the combination were at least additive in their activity. Subsequently, as Einhorn and colleagues (1986) reviewed, when these identical regimens were tested in cooperative groups, the response rates fell to 12 to 17%. This decrease in response rate from the original, single-institution trial to a subsequent multicenter trial is a well recognized and often reproduced occurrence. Factors accounting for these discordant results possibly include differences in patient prognostic characteristics from study to study and differences in quantitating the amount of tumor shrinkage that occurred in an indicator lesion to determine if the criteria for response had been met. This factor might be especially important for evaluable lesions, because criteria for definite tumor shrinkage may vary from institution to institution.

Beginning in the late 1970s, cisplatin-containing regimens started to be evaluated. The first was a combination of cyclophosphamide, doxorubicin, and cisplatin—CAP—developed by Eagan and colleagues (1977). The initial response rate to CAP, as Einhorn and colleagues (1986) summarized, was 42%; it was 10% when the regimen was tested in a cooperative group trial.

Treatment toxicity associated with the above regimens could be classified as mild to moderate. Life-threatening toxicity was relatively uncommon and treatment-related mortality was rare. Organ-specific toxicity such as pulmonary, hepatic, neurologic, renal, gastrointestinal—except for nausea and vomiting—occurred infrequently, and when present, was usually mild.

Survival was probably not altered by chemotherapy, although no well designed studies were performed to evaluate this question. Such a study requires an untreated control group that is well matched to the treatment group in prognostic factors and that received supportive care identical to that received by the treatment group. Because many investigators felt that a no-treatment option is unethical, various compromises were made. One such compromise involved treating the control group with low or standard dose single-agent chemotherapy. Thus, Lad and colleagues (1981) randomized patients to CAMP chemotherapy or to low dose lomustine followed by CAMP at progression. Despite differences in response rates—CAMP 30%, lomustine 0%—there was no significant difference in survival. Einhorn and associates (1982) randomized patients between cyclophosphamide, doxorubicin, and methotrexate in combination and the same agents administered sequentially. Again, response rates favored the combination—22% versus 9%—but survival was not statistically different. Similarly, Hoffman and colleagues (1983) found no statistically significant survival difference between the CAMP plus leucovorin versus the component drugs of CAMP administered sequentially.

In the 1980s, the use of high dose cisplatin and mitomycin C-based chemotherapy has been widespread. Other popular drugs, added to one or both of the aforementioned agents, have been vindesine, vinblastine, and etoposide. As Takasugi and Miller (1984), Sculier and Klastersky (1984), Bonomi (1986), and Klastersky (1986) documented, response rates, in single-institution studies, have approached 50 to 60%. As was the case in the 1970s, however, when these regimens were studied in cooperative groups, response rates decreased considerably. The Eastern Cooperative Oncology Group, in a study authored by Ruckdeschel and colleagues (1986), reported a randomized trial comparing CAMP to mitomycin C, vinblastine, and cisplatin; to etoposide and cisplatin; and to vindesine and cisplatin. Response rates varied from 17% to 31%. As expected from these modest response rates, none of the regimens significantly prolonged survival.

Although it is uncertain that the combination chemotherapy regimens of the 1980s are significantly more active than those of the 1970s, they are clearly much more toxic. The use of high dose cisplatin has significantly increased the renal and neurotoxicity of previously used treatments. Further, the hydration required for high dose cisplatin administration has caused congestive heart failure, increased peripheral edema, and exacerbated symptoms in patients with superior vena caval obstruction. Mitomycin C has produced pulmonary toxicity and vascular toxicity in the form of microangiopathic hemolysis. Current regimens also tend to be more myelosuppressive than regimens of the 1970s, so patients require more careful follow-up to prevent complications associated with granulocytopenia or thrombocytopenia, or both. In the aforementioned Eastern Cooperative Oncology group study reported by Ruckdeschel and associates (1986), no treatment-related deaths occurred among 115 CAMP-treated patients. By contrast, 20 deaths occurred among 371 patients treated with one of the 3 cisplatin-containing regimens: 7 on the mitomycin C, vinblastine, and cisplatin arm; 8 on the vindesine and cisplatin arm, and 5 on the VP-16 and cisplastin arm.

Whether any of the current cisplatin-containing regimens prolong survival is also unclear. Einhorn and coworkers (1986) conducted a prospective study in which 124 unresectable non-small cell lung cancer patients were randomized to vindesine alone, to vindesine and cisplatin, or to vindesine, cisplatin, and mitomycin C. Neither of the combination regimens had a significantly better response rate or survival than vindesine alone. These results contrast with those of Elliott and colleagues (1984), who randomized 105 unresectable patients to vindesine alone or with cisplatin. Patients in these two treatment groups had comparable performance status, disease stage, age, sex, and tumor histology. The partial response rate with vindesine and cisplatin treatment was 33%, versus 7% for vindesine alone. Patients receiving combination chemotherapy had a significantly longer median survival than did individuals receiving vindesine alone— 11 months versus 4 months, p = .008. The explanation for the difference between Elliott's and Einhorn's results is uncertain. Drug doses, schedules of drug administration, duration of treatment, and patient prognostic factors were similar in the two studies, although 70% of patients in the Elliott study had squamous cell cancer, compared with 46% with that diagnosis in the Einhorn study.

Finkelstein and co-workers (1986) reviewed long-term results of seven combination chemotherapy regimens tested by the Eastern Cooperative Oncology Group between December, 1979 and June, 1983. Six were cisplatin-containing regimens and the seventh was CAMP. The 893 non-small cell lung cancer patients entered into these studies were ambulatory—ECOG performance status of 2 or less—and had not received prior chemotherapy. One third of the patients had prior radiation therapy. The median survival of all patients was 23.5 weeks. Nineteen percent of patients survived 1 year, nine percent survived 18 months, and four percent survived 2 years. The maximum survival was 3.9 years. There was no correlation between response rate to chemotherapy and survival. The mitomycin C, vinblastine, and cisplatin arm had the highest response rate— 26% and 31% in two separate trials—but had significantly fewer 1-year survivors—12%—than any other regimen. By contrast, the etoposide-cisplatin combination had a response rate of 20%, but 25% of treated patients survived 1 year. Of all patients surviving for one year or more after the start of chemotherapy, only 44% had an objective response to treatment.

RISK-BENEFIT RELATIONSHIP OF CHEMOTHERAPY

Simes (1985) initiated a discussion of risk-benefit relationships for participants in non-small cell lung cancer chemotherapy trials. His database is a 10-year experience—1973 to 1983—of the Eastern Cooperative Oncology Group, including 2714 patients with unresectable disease. Over this time period the response rate to treatment increased modestly, adjusted for performance status and disease stage, from 11% in 1973 to 1976 to 19% in 1980 to 1983. For patients with disease clinically confined to the chest, median survival and percentage of patients surviving 6 months or more increased from 5.2 to 6.6 months and from 45 to 54%, respectively,

during the above time periods. For patients with metastatic disease, median survival increased from 3.6 to 4.9 months and 6-month survival from 30% to 37%. For both groups of patients, 12-month survival was virtually unchanged over the 10-year study period. The cost of these survival increases was a considerable increase in treatment-related toxicity. Severe or worse toxicity occurred in 29% of treated patients in 1973 to 1976 and in 47% of treated patients in 1980 to 1983. Based on these data, Simes (1985) enunciated benefits and risks associated with non-small cell lung cancer chemotherapy. Benefits include possible relief of symptoms, tumor shrinkage, prolongation of survival, psychological benefit from a close physician-patient relationship, and the knowledge that information gained from each individual's treatment might, in the future, benefit others. The risks of undergoing treatment include treatment toxicity that might be severe enough to cause death, the cost and inconvenience of treatment, and the fact that more time might have to be spent in a hospital, either to receive treatment or for treatment-related complications. A final issue, only touched upon in Simes' discussion, was the effect of chemotherapy on quality of survival. Only since the early 1980s have quality-of-life considerations been introduced into clinical trials. Burke and colleagues' (1986) preliminary report evaluated the effects of chemotherapy on pain, cough, hemoptysis, dyspnea, and anorexia using visual analog scales and also evaluated performance status and anxiety levels. Most patients who responded to treatment experienced improvement in symptoms and maintenance of their performance status.

ADJUVANT TREATMENT

The fact that chemotherapy has been modestly active in advanced-disease patients suggested that more benefit might be achieved when the same treatment was used in the adjuvant setting—after resection of all clinically detectable cancer. The rationale for this expectation was discussed earlier. Legha and co-workers (1977) reviewed 15 early adjuvant studies, including single-agent trials with cyclophosphamide, mechlorethamine, and vinblastine; combination chemotherapy studies with cyclophosphamide and methotrexate with or without 5-fluorouracil and vinblastine; and a Japanese trial of chromomycin A_3 plus mitomycin C. These studies either showed no benefit of adjuvant therapy or else suffered from sufficient flaws in randomization, stratification by prognostic variables, or inadequacies of chemotherapy doses to make the study unevaluable. More recent adjuvant trials were reviewed by Holmes (1986), Stanley and Grenchen (1986), and Suemasu (1986). Of all these trials, the two eliciting the most interest, currently, are from the University of Chicago and the Lung Cancer Study Group. In the first, Ferguson and co-workers (1986) retrospectively reviewed 34 consecutive patients with T1N1M0 or T2N1M0 lesions presenting between June, 1974 and December, 1984 who received surgery— 11 patients; surgery plus radiation therapy–7 patients; or surgery, radiation therapy, and CAMP chemotherapy—

16 patients. Treatment assignment was nonrandomized. Prior to 1976, patients received surgery only and after that were offered both chemotherapy and radiation therapy with the option of refusing one or both of these treatments. Median survival for patients treated only with surgery was 13 months, for those receiving surgery and radiation therapy it was 19.2 months, and for all 3 treatments it was 45.5 months. Survival differences between patients receiving surgery only or surgery, radiation therapy, and chemotherapy were significantly different—p < .005. There was no significant survival difference for patients receiving surgery and radiation therapy when compared to patients receiving surgery, radiation therapy, and chemotherapy. In addition to this being a retrospective, nonrandomized study, there were also probable differences in extent or location of disease among the 3 groups, because 73% of surgery-only patients required a pneumonectomy, as compared to 29% of patients in the surgery, radiation therapy arm and 37% in the arm that included chemotherapy.

The Lung Cancer Study Group trial, reported by Holmes and Gail (1986), randomized resected, pathologic stage II and III adenocarcinoma and large cell anaplastic carcinoma patients to cyclophosphamide, doxorubicin, cisplatin—CAP—chemotherapy or to intrapleural BCG plus levamisole. The two patient groups were reasonably balanced for regional node involvement, disease stage, patient age, performance status, and pretreatment weight loss. Twenty-six percent of chemotherapy patients had T1 lesions as opposed to ten percent of immunotherapy-treated patients. The principal finding of this study was that chemotherapy-treated patients had significantly longer disease-free survival than immunotherapy-treated patients had. Survival of the latter group was felt to be identical to that expected for comparable patients treated with surgery alone. At the time the report was published, overall survival was not significantly different between the two groups.

In assessing this study, it must be remembered that disease-free survival is a softer endpoint than overall survival is. Most studies do not have rigorously defined restaging intervals or prescribed tests that must be done at each restaging. Further, and possibly most important, there is little incentive to prove that recurrent disease is present, because few therapeutic options are available at that point of illness. Diagnostic tests may be delayed, therefore, in persons presenting with vague symptoms such as increased cough or weight loss until some other problem requires that restaging be done.

Most authors of adjuvant studies imply in their discussions that additional adjuvant studies should be designed and carried out. The rationale for this suggestion is that better chemotherapy regimens than those used in the aforementioned studies may be available. As indicated previously, this assumption may or may not be true. In any case, if the newer cisplatin or mitomycin C combinations, or both are used, investigators will have to manage substantial treatment-related morbidity and will have to accept the fact that there will be some treatment-related deaths.

SUMMARY

Numerous chemotherapy trials have been conducted in patients with non-small cell lung cancer. Most treatment regimens have been derived empirically. Although newer regimens may be associated with a higher overall response rate than was observed in earlier trials, the complete response rate is still only about 5 to 10% and responses usually last only a few months. Furthermore, better patient selection may account for some percentage of the higher response rates. There is little evidence that chemotherapy prolongs the survival of patients with unresectable disease. Despite the fact that lung cancer response rates are not as high as are achieved in other cancers in which adjuvant chemotherapy seems effective, e.g., breast cancer, as Tormey and colleagues (1982) reported, or osteosarcoma, as Eilber and co-workers (1987) and Holland (1987) reported, the published results of lung cancer adjuvant chemotherapy trials are encouraging. Unfortunately, future trials will probably have to use more toxic treatment regimens. For patients with unresectable disease, current response rates and survival durations will probably not improve significantly until more active chemotherapy drugs are discovered or until a better understanding of the growth biology of these neoplasms leads to new treatment strategies.

REFERENCES

Abrams, R.A., et al.: Amplification of circulating granulocyte-monocyte stem cell numbers following chemotherapy in patients with extensive small cell carcinoma of the lung. Cancer Res. *41*:35, 1981.

Abrams, R.A., et al.: The hematopoietic toxicity of regional radiation therapy. Correlations for combined modality therapy with systemic chemotherapy. Cancer *55*:1429, 1985.

Aisner, J., and Hansen, H.H.: Commentary: current status of chemotherapy for non-small cell lung cancer. Cancer Treat. Rep. *65*:979, 1981.

American Cancer Society: cancer statistics 1988. CA *38*:5, 1988.

Anderson, J.R., Caine, K.C., and Gelber, R.D.: Analysis of survival by tumor response. J. Clin. Oncol. *1*:710, 1983.

Bakowski, M.T., and Crouch, J.C.: Chemotherapy of non-small cell lung cancer: a reappraisal and a look to the future. Cancer Treat. Rev. *10*:159, 1983.

Belcher, J.R., and Rehahn, M.: Late deaths after resection for bronchial carcinoma. Br. J. Dis. Chest *73*:18, 1979.

Bonomi, P.: Brief overview of combination chemotherapy in non-small cell lung cancer. Semin. Oncol. *13*(Suppl. 3):89, 1986.

Burke, M.T., et al.: The palliative influence of response to chemotherapy in patients with stage III non-small cell lung cancer. Proc. Am. Soc. Clin. Oncol. *5*:185, 1986.

Cohen, M.H.: Impairment of red blood cell deformability by tumor growth. J. Natl. Cancer Inst. *63*:525, 1979.

Cohen, M.H.: Influence of tumor burden on red blood cell deformability in small cell lung cancer patients. Ann. Clin. Res. *13*:387, 1981.

Cohen, M.H., and Perevodchikova, N.I.: Single agent chemotherapy of lung cancer. *In* Progress in Cancer Research and Therapy, Vol. 11. Lung Cancer: Progress in Therapeutic Research. Edited by F. Muggia and M. Rozencweig. New York, Raven Press, 1978, p. 343.

Cohen, M.H., et al.: Hormones plus chemotherapy in advanced L1210 leukemia: survival benefit correlated with increased red blood cell deformability. Proc. Am. Assoc. Cancer Res. *25*:318, 1984a.

Cohen, M.H., et al.: An active chemotherapy regimen for squamous cell lung cancer. Cancer Treat. Rep. *68*:475, 1984b.

DeWys, W.D., et al.: Prognostic effect of weight loss prior to chemotherapy in cancer patients. Am. J. Med. *69*:491, 1980.

Doll, D.C., Ringenberg, Q.S., and Yarbro, J.W.: Vascular toxicity associated with antineoplastic agents. J. Clin. Oncol. 4:1405, 1986.

Eagan, R.T., et al.: Platinum based chemotherapy versus dianhydrogalactitol in non-small cell lung cancer. Cancer Treat. Rep. 61:1339, 1977.

Eagan, R.T., Fleming, T.R., and Schoonover, V.: Evaluation of response criteria in advanced lung cancer. Cancer 44:1125, 1979.

Eilber, F., et al.: Adjuvant chemotherapy for osteosarcoma: a randomized prospective trial. J. Clin. Oncol. 5:21, 1987.

Einhorn, L.H., et al.: Random prospective study of cyclophosphamide, doxorubicin, and methotrexate (CAM) combination chemotherapy versus single agent sequential chemotherapy in non-small cell lung cancer. Cancer Treat. Rep. 66:2005, 1982.

Einhorn, L.H., et al.: Random prospective study of vindesine versus vindesine plus high-dose cisplatin versus vindesine plus cisplatin plus mitomycin C in advanced non-small cell lung cancer. J. Clin. Oncol. 4:1037, 1986.

Elliott, J.A., et al.: Vindesine and cisplatin combination chemotherapy compared with vindesine as a single agent in the management of non-small cell lung cancer: a randomized study. Eur. J. Cancer Clin. Oncol. 20:1025, 1984.

Ferguson, M.K., et al.: The role of adjuvant therapy after resection of T1N1M0 and T2N1M0 non-small cell lung cancer. J. Thorac. Cardiovasc. Surg. 91:344, 1986.

Finkelstein, D.M., Ettinger, D.S., and Ruckdeschel, J.C.: Long-term survivors in metastatic non-small cell lung cancer: an Eastern Cooperative Oncology Group study. J. Clin. Oncol. 4:702, 1986.

Frei, E., III: Rationale for combined therapy. Cancer 40:569, 1977.

Frei, E., III, and Canellos, G.P.: Dose: a critical factor in cancer chemotherapy. Am. J. Med. 69:585, 1980.

Gatenby, R.A., et al.: Oxygen tension in human tumors: in vivo mapping using CT-guided probes. Radiology 156:211, 1985.

Geddes, D.M.: The natural history of lung cancer: a review based on rates of tumor growth. Br. J. Dis. Chest 73:1, 1979.

Goldie, J.H., and Coldman, A.J.: The genetic origin of drug resistance in neoplasms: implications for systemic therapy. Cancer Res. 44:3643, 1984.

Hoffman, P., et al.: Metastatic non small cell bronchogenic carcinoma: a randomized trial of sequential versus combination chemotherapy. Eur. J. Cancer Clin. Oncol. 19:33, 1983.

Holland, J.F.: Adjuvant chemotherapy of osteosarcoma: no runs, no hits, two men left on base. J. Clin. Oncol. 5:4, 1987.

Holmes, E.C.: Surgical adjuvant therapy of non-small cell lung cancer. Chest 89:343S, 1986.

Holmes, E.C., and Gail, M.: Surgical adjuvant therapy for stage II and stage II adenocarcinoma and large-cell undifferentiated carcinoma. J. Clin. Oncol. 4:710, 1986.

Hryniuk, W., and Bush, H.: The importance of dose intensity in the chemotherapy of metastatic breast cancer. J. Clin. Oncol. 2:1281, 1984.

Klastersky, J.: Therapy with cisplatin and etoposide in non-small cell lung cancer. Semin. Oncol. 13(Suppl. 3):104, 1986.

Lad, T.E., et al.: Immediate versus postponed combination chemotherapy (CAMP) for unresectable non-small cell lung cancer: a randomized trial. Cancer Treat. Rep. 65:973, 1981.

Lanzotti, V.J., et al.: Survival with inoperable lung cancer: an integration of prognostic variables based on simple clinical criteria. Cancer 39:303, 1977.

Legha, S.A., Muggia, F.M., and Carter, S.K.: Adjuvant chemotherapy in lung cancer: review and prospects. Cancer 39:1415, 1977.

Line, D.H., and Deeley, T.J.: The necropsy findings in carcinoma of the bronchus. Br. J. Dis. Chest 65:238, 1971.

Ludwig Cancer Study Group: Patterns of failure in patients with resected stage I and II non-small cell carcinoma of the lung. Ann. Surg. 205:67, 1987.

Matthews, M.J., et al.: Frequency of residual and metastatic tumor in patients undergoing curative surgical resection for lung cancer. Cancer Chemother. Rep. 4:63, 1973.

Mueller-Klieser, W., et al.: Intracapillary oxyhemoglobin saturation in malignant tumors in humans. Int. J. Radiat. Oncol. Biol. Phys. 7:1397, 1981.

Rossing, T.H., and Rossing, R.G.: Survival in lung cancer: an analysis of the effects of age, sex, resectability, and histopathologic type. Am. Rev. Respir. Dis. 126:771, 1982.

Ruckdeschel, J.C., et al.: A randomized trial of the four most active regimens for metastatic non-small cell lung cancer. J. Clin. Oncol. 4:14, 1986.

Sculier, J.P., and Klastersky, J.: Progress in chemotherapy in non-small cell lung cancer. Eur. J. Cancer Clin. Oncol. 20:1329, 1984.

Selawry, O.S.: Initial therapeutic trial of new drugs in lung cancer. Cancer Chemother. Rep. 4:215, 1973.

Simes, R.J.: Risk-benefit relationships in cancer clinical trials: The ECOG experience in non-small cell lung cancer. J. Clin. Oncol. 3:462, 1985.

Stanley, K.E.: Prognostic factors for survival in patients with inoperable lung cancer. J. Natl. Cancer Inst. 65:25, 1980.

Stanley, K.E., and Grenchen, S.: Experience of the Ludwig Cancer Study Group. Chest 89:343S, 1986.

Stanley, K.E., et al.: Patterns of failure in patients with inoperable carcinoma of the lung. Cancer 47:2725, 1981.

Suemasu, K.: Adjuvant therapy for resectable lung cancer in Japan. Chest 89:344S, 1986.

Sutherland, R.M.: Importance of critical metabolites and cellular interactions in the biology of microregions of tumors. Cancer 58:1668, 1986.

Takasugi, B.J., and Miller, T.P.: Chemotherapy of advanced non-small cell lung cancer. Invest. New Drugs 2:339, 1984.

Tomlinson, R.H., and Gray, L.H.: The histological structure of some human lung cancers and the possible implications for radiotherapy. Br. J. Cancer 9:539, 1955.

Tormey, D.C., et al.: Comparison of induction chemotherapies for metastatic breast cancer: an Eastern Cooperative Oncology Group trial. Cancer 50:1235, 1982.

Vaupel, P.W., Frinak, S., and Bicher, H.I.: Heterogeneous oxygen partial pressure and pH distribution in C3H mouse mammary adenocarcinoma. Cancer Res. 41:2008, 1981.

CHAPTER 97

SMALL CELL LUNG CANCER

Joseph Aisner

Lung cancer is the most common cause of cancer death in the United States. Katlic and Carter (1979) reported that small cell lung cancer—SCLC—accounts for nearly 20 to 25% of all cases of lung cancer and therefore represents a large number of afflicted individuals. This disease has received considerable attention from numerous investigators, including Cohen (1974), Cohen and Matthews (1974), and Muggia (1974), Broder (1977), and Hansen (1985) and their associates, in clinical and laboratory research because of its unique biologic properties, clinical presentation, and response to treatment. Small cell lung cancer has a rapid doubling time and a high labeling index, which are reflected clinically in the relatively short symptomatic presentation—1 to 2 months—and the rapid, fulminant disease process. Small cell lung cancer has been recognized as a distinct clinical-pathologic entity only since the 1960s, and the World Health Organization (1982) and I and Matthews (1985), among others, described various subtypes, including oat cell, fusiform, polygonal, and intermediate cell types. Attempts, such as that of Matthews (1979), to correlate histologic subclassification with outcome have not been successful because of the advanced stage at presentation and the variability of histologic subtype within the same specimen. Yesner and colleagues (1985) attempted to subclassify small cell lung cancer according to small cell, small cell–large cell, and mixed forms. This new subclassification is predicated in part on an observation of Radice and co-workers (1982) that the small cell–large cell form may not have a similar prognosis to the small cell form. In addition, this classification resembles the several forms seen in SCLC cell cultures. I and my associates (1988) noted, however, that the prognostic implications of this new classification system have not been confirmed.

Ihde and colleagues (1981a) observed that regardless of histologic subtype, most patients with SCLC present with regionally advanced or widely disseminated disease. Moreover, Fox and Scadding (1979) reported that in SCLC confined to the chest, regional treatments have not made an important impact on outcome.

A DISSEMINATED DISEASE

Livingston (1980) and Ihde and associates (1981a) noted that at initial presentation, nearly two thirds of patients have disease outside the thorax involving one or more organs. Among those patients without extrathoracic metastases, most have mediastinal involvement and virtually all patients die of metastatic disease. Even among the few patients in the 1960s and early 1970s who were prospectively selected as potentially resectable, Matthews and co-workers (1973) reported that most of such patients died soon after resection, and autopsies showed evidence of disseminated disease. Thus, Mountain's (1978) review of the available thoracic surgery studies suggested that SCLC was a contraindication to initial surgery with curative intent. This led to the use of radiation therapy as the major treatment modality. Irradiation to control regional disease in those patients whose disease was confined to the thorax did produce dramatic tumor shrinkage and slight prolongation of survival, but again, most of these patients died soon afterward of metastatic disease. Fox and Scadding (1979) reported that virtually none of the patients selected for chest irradiation survived 3 years. Small cell lung cancer is therefore considered a disseminated disease regardless of our ability to document all sites of overt or micrometastases. I and my colleagues (1983) noted that the recognition of this concept led to the introduction of chemotherapy for treatment of small cell lung cancer and a shift in the treatment outcomes.

STAGING

With the almost total exclusion of surgery as an initial treatment modality in SCLC, Ihde and Hansen (1981) and Mountain and associates (1974) also recognized and suggested that the TNM system would most likely not be applicable. Most patients present with advanced T and N stages, so the TNM system does not provide sufficient prognostic discrimination. Similarly, the numerical staging was not particularly useful because most patients fell into stage III—stages IIIa and IIIb—and IV by current standards of the new international staging system for lung cancer (see Chapter 76). Therefore, another staging system was developed according to the applicability of chest irradiation, namely the limited/extensive staging system. This staging system, first developed by the Veterans Administration Lung Group and reported by Hyde and colleagues (1965), provides both prognostic discrimination and defines therapeutic options. Limited disease is now usually defined as disease confined to the chest with or without involvement of the mediastinum or with or without involvement of the ipsilateral supraclavicular nodes, namely that disease that could be encompassed by a single irradiation port. Extensive disease is any disease beyond the confines of limited disease. Prospective studies by Maurer and Pajak (1981) and Livingston and associates (1982), however, showed some minor exceptions to the limited/extensive system. For example, Livingston's group (1982) reported that patients whose only evidence of extensive disease is an ipsilateral pleural effusion—regardless of whether it is cytologically positive—have a prognosis similar to that of patients with limited disease. Similarly, Maurer and Pajak (1981) suggested that a single, isolated lesion on bone scan does not carry an adverse prognosis, but these authors failed to show that the positive bone scan was caused by involvement with disease.

Staging techniques, procedures, and categories have been under constant revision. The needs of staging vary with the evolution of treatment. For example, as surgery may find new utility in the treatment of SCLC as a means of local control, modifications of the TNM system may become important. Similarly, if chemotherapy becomes sufficiently successful to control both limited and extensive disease, the staging evaluation might be significantly curtailed. In addition, the staging evaluation can and should be used to develop prognostic information. Currently, patients with limited disease do significantly better in terms of response and survival than those with extensive disease. The latter have essentially no long-term survival. Newer staging approaches may, however, define newer prognostic information. At the University of Maryland Cancer Center, Whitley and colleagues (1984) have been evaluating the role of computed tomography—CT—in the staging of SCLC and have shown that CT scans define the areas of disease not routinely shown with conventional roentgenography and can identify new prognostic signs. These include bronchial narrowing and pericardial thickening (Figs. 97–1 and 97–2). In those patients whose bronchial narrowing was seen on the CT scan, the failure to clear this bronchial narrowing imparted a significantly poorer prognosis and a higher propensity for local treatment failure. This may be the subgroup that benefits most from local chest irradiation. Furthermore, CT scanning can define disease in the abdomen and may be important in radiation port planning. Thus, CT scanning is a useful approach in the staging of patients with SCLC.

An evaluation for the pretreatment staging of patients with SCLC should be designed currently to focus and define areas of overt disease and metastases. Small cell lung cancer can involve virtually any organ or system, but most metastases occur in a relatively common pattern (Table 97–1). Staging should be focused on defining all areas of involvement to anticipate problems. A complete staging evaluation provides parameters for an assessment of treatment outcome and prognosis. At a minimum, the evaluation should include a history and physical examination, serum chemistries—electrolytes, liver profiles—chest roentgenograms, bone marrow aspirates and biopsies, bronchoscopy, isotopic scanning of bone and CT scans of the brain and liver. Because chest irradiation is frequently planned from a CT scan of the chest, and because a CT scan of the chest carried through the liver allows a complete evaluation of any liver disease and an examination of the adrenal glands, computed tomography of the chest and upper abdomen is preferred over an isotopic scan of the liver.

For scanning the brain, Pendergrass and colleagues (1975) showed that a CT scan is considerably more sensitive and accurate than an isotopic scan. Furthermore, Shalen and co-workers (1981) reported that the use of a rapid, high-dose intravenous contrast infusion followed by one immediate CT scan and another after 1.5 hours affords even greater accuracy. Although Wittes and associates (1977) noted that the yield of routine brain scanning in neurologically asymptomatic individuals is relatively low, approximately 4% of the patients have asymptomatic central nervous system—CNS—disease. The brain is a frequent site of metastatic disease, and symptoms may not always resolve with treatment. Thus, Baglan and Marks (1981) believe that irradiation of brain metastases while they are quiescent is most likely to produce a result with the least neurologic impairment.

Small cell lung cancer is also a unique tumor in that it can produce a series of peptide hormones, enzymes, or markers (Table 97–2). Sorenson and colleagues (1985) reviewed this subject. Greco and co-workers (1981), among others, noted that these peptides can be associated with various clinical syndromes such as Cushing's syndrome, syndrome of inappropriate antidiuretic hormone secretion—ADH—with hyponatremia, hypoglycemia, and others. Because the tumor grows rapidly, many of the usual features of these paraneoplastic syndromes may be lacking. For example, with excess adrenocorticotropic hormone—ACTH—the usual facies of Cushing's syndrome are generally absent, and hypertension and hypokalemia are the features that might alert the clinician to the presence of this syndrome. Other clinical paraneoplastic syndromes, such as Eaton-Lambert syndrome, orthostatic hypotension syndromes, and others, can occur in association with SCLC and were reviewed by Doyle and associates (1988). In general, these do not confer any adverse prognosis beyond that of the affected performance status. Some of the markers, such as neuron-specific enolase—NSE—are associated with extensive disease when they are elevated in the plasma. In most circumstances, however, these are no more sensitive than the clinical evaluation.

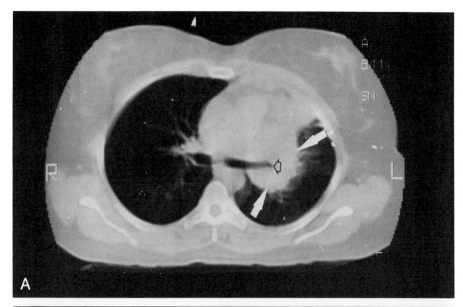

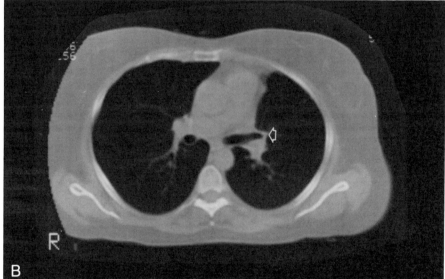

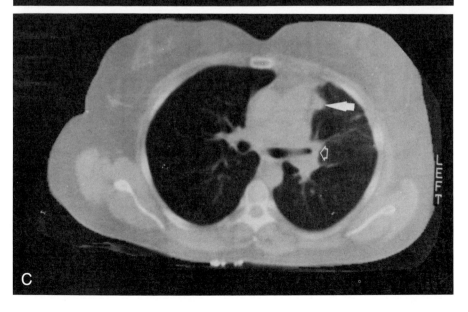

Fig. 97–1. *A,* Initial chest CT scan showing central tumor and mediastinal involvement (solid arrow) and bronchial narrowing (open arrow). *B,* Regression of tumor with persistence of bronchial narrowing (open arrow). Patient judged to be in complete response by all other criteria, including bronchoscopy. *C,* Repeat CT scan showing recurrent disease. Regrowth (solid and open arrow) of tumor (recurrence) is in the area of prior bronchial narrowing (open arrow).

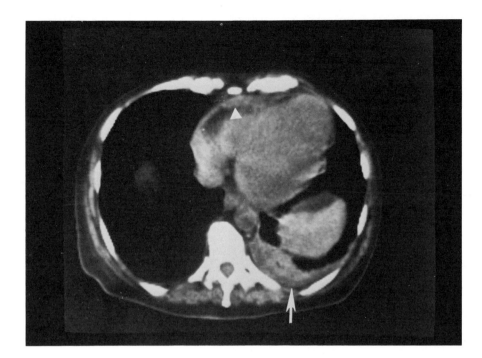

Fig. 97–2. CT scan showing pleural effusion (arrow) and pericardial thickening (wedge). Neither were seen on conventional roentgenograms.

TREATMENT

General

Without treatment, SCLC is rapidly fatal; the median duration of survival is less than 12 weeks. Several factors are know to affect the treatment outcome in SCLC. Stanley (1980), Ihde and Hansen (1981), Maurer and Pajak (1981), and Ihde and associates (1981) reported that these include comorbid disease—e.g., heart and lung diseases in this population, many of whom are heavy smokers; pretreatment performance status; the presence of weight loss; and the extent of disease. The most adverse prognostic factors tend to group together. For example, poor performance status is associated with extensive disease and weight loss. Stanley (1980) and others have shown, however, that these prognostic factors are independent of each other and of treatment in their ability to predict outcome. Other prognostic factors are also often described; but their effect on treatment outcome is variable and not always repeatable. These include age, sex, pretreatment serum sodium levels, and other chemical markers.

Mountain (1978) noted that in previously reported se-

ries surgical resection did not alter either the median or long-term survival; this observation led to discontinuation of initial surgery for cure. Lichter and Ihde (1988) reported that chest irradiation produced a shift in the median survival to about 8 months for patients with limited disease but had no appreciable effect on survival for those with extensive disease. The recognition of the systemic nature of SCLC led to the use of chemotherapy and to a shift in the median survival for all patients and cure for a small percentage. Thus, chemotherapy is now considered the cornerstone of treatment for SCLC, and all other therapies are now considered adjunctive.

Based on the early results from many single institutional studies, the International Association for the Study of Lung Cancer—IASLC—published some guidelines for anticipated results from aggressive treatment, as I

Table 97–1. Small Cell Lung Cancer: Areas of Involvement at Presentation

Organ	Frequency (%)
Lung	95
Lymph nodes	95
Liver	25
Bone	33
Bone marrow	25
Brain	12
Adrenals	15
Others	25

Table 97–2. Hormones and Markers Associated with Small Cell Lung Cancer

Adrenocorticotropic hormone
Antidiuretic hormone
β-endorphin
β-Human chorionic hormone
Calcitonin
Carcinoembryonic antigen
Creatinine kinase BB
Dopa-decarboxylase
Gastrin-releasing peptide—bombesin
Histaminase
Insulin
Neurophysins
Neuron-specific enolase
Neurophysins
Parathormone
Somatostatin
Vasopressin

and my colleagues (1983) reported. First, multiagent chemotherapy should be the initial form of treatment. A delay in the initiation of chemotherapy can allow the micrometastases to grow, become overt, and shift both the stage and the prognosis. Other adjunctive therapies, such as radiation therapy or possibly even surgery, are added subsequently. Second, treatment must be aggressive. Both radiation therapy and chemotherapy have a dose-response effect in this disease. When the treatment is aggressive, patients with limited disease can have a median survival in excess of 15 months, and nearly 20% have long-term, disease-free survival. Patients with extensive disease can have a median survival in excess of 9 months.

Surgery

Although initial surgery with curative intent—as opposed to surgery for diagnosis—has been abandoned for most patients, surgery is beneficial in some circumstances, and there are newer experimental applications of surgery for SCLC. Higgins and associates (1975), in a prospective evaluation of peripheral coin lesions by the Armed Forces and the Veterans Administration Surgical Oncology Group—VASOG, reported that only a small fraction of the proved lung cancers were SCLC. These lesions were removed surgically and no additional therapy was administered. Nevertheless, nearly 40% of these patients were alive 5 years later. Similar results were observed in a prospective trial by the National Cancer Institute of Canada reported by Sagman and colleagues (1988). These data suggest that at least the rare presentation of a T1N0M0 tumor may be amenable to surgical resection. Given the results of such surgery and the outcome of chemotherapy in limited disease, the approach to such isolated pulmonary nodules should probably be resection followed by chemotherapy.

Another approach in the use of surgery has been to add surgical resection after an initial response to chemotherapy. Several studies have shown the technical feasibility of such an approach, and these initial anecdotal studies, reported by Meyer (1982) and Shepherd (1983) and their associates, have suggested that such patients may have a superior survival. These studies were, however, performed on a highly selected group: those with the best performance status, the least comorbid disease, and an excellent response to initial treatment. Based on these preliminary data, several studies, such as the one conducted by Ettinger and colleagues (1985), have been started to evaluate prospectively the role of surgery after chemotherapy in randomized trials. Most of these studies have accrued patients slowly. Prager and co-workers (1984), in an early prospective assessment of the applicability of such a surgical approach, suggested that only a small fraction of patients would be eligible for surgery. Thus, surgery will probably have a limited role in the treatment of SCLC and is currently considered an experimental treatment for SCLC.*

Regardless of the findings of prospective evaluations of surgical series, surgical intervention in SCLC can prove to be useful. Initial surgery has allowed sample acquisition for in-vitro cell growth. Gazdar and Minna (1986) reported that cell cultures derived from short- and long-term cultures have provided considerable information about the biology of this disease. Similarly, surgery after an initial chemotherapy response can provide tissue for study of post-treatment SCLC biology. Because SCLC develops significant drug resistance after initial treatment, such cell cultures may shed considerable light on the mechanisms of drug resistance. In addition, preliminary reports of the findings at postchemotherapy thoracotomies suggest that the areas of prior disease show considerable fibrosis, and Valdivieso and associates (1982), as well as others, reported that nests of non-small cell lung cancer can be seen. This lends further support to Gazdar and colleagues' (1981) hypothesis that all lung cancers are related, and are variable expressions of a similar progenitor cell.

*Editor's note. I agree that surgical resection has a minor role in the management of small cell lung cancer. It may, however, be beneficial not only in peripheral T1 lesions but also in those few patients in whom the extent of the disease after extensive staging can be classified as stage I or II or even some classified as non-N2, IIIa. The editor and associates (1982) in the Veterans Administration Surgical Oncology Group reported that resection of T1N0M0 lesions, both peripheral as well as central, even in the absence of adequate adjuvant chemotherapy, resulted in a 5-year survival rate of 59.5%. With adequate postoperative chemotherapy, Meyer (1986, 1987) reported in a small number of patients with selected stage I and II disease survival rates of 83% and 50%, respectively. Ohta and colleagues reported a 50.8% 5-year survival rate in stage I patients after initial resection followed by adequate chemotherapy. In a series of 112 patients, Karrer and colleagues (1988) reported actuarial survival rates at 36 months after resection followed by intensive chemotherapy of 65% for patients with N0 disease, 52% for those with N1 disease, and 29% for those with N2 disease. The survival curves for stages I, II, and IIIa are seen in Fig. 97–3 and T3N0–1 and AnyTN2 in Fig. 97–4.

Shepherd and associates (1988) reported the results of thoracotomy and resection in 34 patients after preoperative chemotherapy for limited small cell lung cancer. Projected survival rates at 5 years were 71% for stage I and 38% for stage II. Although no survival figure was reported for patients with stage IIIaN2 disease, these authors noted that this subgroup did poorly despite surgical resection—no survival advantage—as was the experience of Myers (1982), Prager (1984), and Ohta (1986) and their associates. In these reports, no patient with resected N2 disease survived 2 years. In many of these reports of resection of N2 disease, however, local recurrence was rarely observed even though no survival benefit was noted.

These aforementioned results of surgical resection either before—which the editor prefers—or after initial adequate chemotherapy in limited, early-stage small cell lung cancer support Davis and colleagues' (1985) observation in a review of a large number of patients with small cell lung cancer that once stage was accounted for, the only factor related to survival beyond 2 years was whether surgical resection had been one of the modalities of treatment. Therefore, until a controlled trial reveals different results, surgical resection of stage I, II, and very selected non-N2 IIIa disease followed or preceded by adjuvant chemotherapy can be recommended as the editor (1988) has previously noted. Whether intensive preoperative chemotherapy can convert originally nonresectable disease to potentially resectable disease remains to be determined. At present, identifiable N2 disease preoperatively—and probably even that identified before chemotherapy—apparently precludes a favorable outcome even with subsequent resection.

Radiation Therapy

Small cell lung cancer is highly sensitive to irradiation. This sensitivity was recognized early and initially led to the use of radiation therapy for all patients with SCLC. Only the subgroup with disease confined within a single radiotherapy port, however, i.e., limited disease, had survival benefit from irradiation. Irradiation can and does produce significant palliation, such as to an area of involved bone, and is the treatment of choice for metastases in the central nervous system—CNS—including prophylactic cranial irradiation—PCI. The focus of radiotherapy is thus its potential for improving local control. For practical purposes, this translates to the use of chest and cranial irradiation.

Considerable experience in the use of chest irradiation for SCLC now allows for some generalizations. First, Cox and associates (1978), Choi and Carey (1976) and Cox (1983) demonstrated a clear dose-response relationship for local control. Cox and associates (1978) and others have clearly demonstrated that 6000 centiGray—cGy—is superior to 4500 cGy, which in turn is superior to 3000 cGy. Second, Cox and co-workers (1978) demonstrated that continuous-course treatment is apparently superior to so-called split-course therapy. Third, the volume of irradiation is important. Failure to irradiate the primary tumor volume can lead to an increased rate of local failure. Cox (1983) further emphasized that there is no doubt that intrathoracic—in-field—recurrences are significantly reduced with the use of chest irradiation. There are, as I and my associates (1983) pointed out, more extrathoracic recurrences, because the areas of micrometastases are not contained within the irradiated field. The dismal outcome of treatment is therefore attributable to the systemic rather than the local disease, and treatment failure is a failure of systemic treatments, not of local control.

One of the difficulties associated with the administration of high-dose chest irradiation is the toxicity to in-field organs, including lungs, esophagus, heart, and spinal cord. Abeloff and Ettinger (1988) reported that radiation pneumonitis, esophagitis, pericarditis, and spinal cord injuries were frequent with the use of high-dose radiation in opposing anterior-posterior, posterior-anterior ports. In the past, these toxicities were dose-limiting, and were particularly dangerous when the radiation treatment was combined with chemotherapy. With modern, three-dimensional, computer-assisted—CT—port planning, these toxicities can be significantly decreased, allowing full dose irradiation to all areas of involvement.

Whereas radiation therapy has only a palliative role in the management of most extrathoracic metastases, it is the treatment of choice for CNS metastases. Nugent and associates (1979) reported that CNS metastases occur in 10 to 15% of patients at presentation and in 30 to 35% during the clinical course of the disease. They also noted that in autopsy series, up to 85% of the patients have CNS involvement. Thus, cranial irradiation can be important. Once CNS metastases occur, they can produce significant and frequently irreversible signs and symptoms.

Bunn and Rosen (1985) reviewed the several studies that have looked at the role of prophylactic cranial irradiation in SCLC, often with conflicting results; some studies suggested that PCI reduces intracranial metastases, whereas others could not demonstrate a significant decrease in the incidence of CNS involvement. None demonstrated a change in survival. At the University of Maryland Cancer Center—UMCC—a randomized trial of PCI was designed. A review of our experience, reported by Aroney and co-workers (1983), showed a significant delay in the onset of CNS metastases and that only the patients who achieved a complete response to treatment derived any benefit from the PCI. Prophylactic cranial irradiation virtually eliminated initial treatment failure in the CNS. Rosen and associates (1983) observed a similar experience at the National Cancer Institute—Navy Oncology Branch. Neither experience showed a significant impact upon survival. A significant impact upon survival is, however, not reasonably expected because (1) CNS metastases occur in about 30% of patients; (2) only about 20% of limited-disease patients achieve long-term survival; and (3) only a large trial could thus detect a significant difference of 5 to 10%. Catane and associates (1981b) reported a poorly understood syndrome of late mental deterioration in association with PCI. It is unclear from the reports whether this is a function of dose fraction, concomitant chemotherapy, or other factors. Most of the reports seem to involve either a nitrosourea, methotrexate, high dose fractions, or concomitant chemotherapy and CNS irradiation. At the UMCC, 3000 cGy over 10 fractions is given predominantly between chemotherapy courses, and our group has not observed any obvious cases of late mental deterioration. Therefore, it is still reasonable to administer PCI to those patients who achieve complete response.

Chemotherapy

Small cell lung cancer has been repeatedly shown to be highly sensitive to chemotherapeutic agents. As I and Abrams (1986), and Broder (1977), Bork (1986), and Smith (1985) and their associates noted, many agents have considerable antineoplastic activity when used as initial therapy or in minimally treated disease (Table 97–3). The activity of these agents is, however, considerably less when they are used in heavily pretreated disease. For example, Bunn (1984) reported that etoposide is one of the most active single agents, with response rates, depending on dose and schedule, that can vary up to 65% for patients with minimally treated disease. When used for patients with heavily pretreated disease, however, Issell and colleagues (1985) reported that the response rate is below 10%. This is manifested clinically as multispecific drug resistance after initial chemotherapy. As I (1988) noted, this emerging drug resistance has led to a dilemma in the approach to the identification of new active agents for SCLC. In the 1980s Cohen and colleagues (1985) reported that few agents with activity in this disease have been identified, perhaps

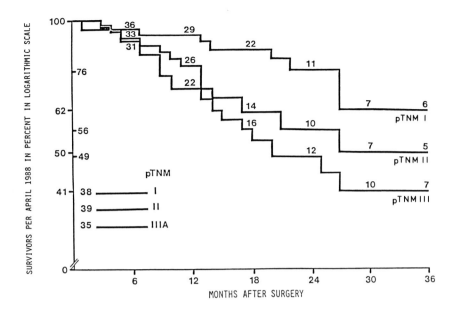

Fig. 97–3. Life-table survival curves for patients with small cell lung cancer pTNM stages I, II, and IIIa managed by initial resection followed by intensive chemotherapy and prophylactic cranial irradiation. (Reproduced with permission of Karrer, K., et al.: The importance of surgery and multimodality treatment for small cell bronchial cancer [SCLC]. Presented at the 14th Annual Meeting of the Western Thoracic Surgical Association, Waikoloa, Hawaii, June 24, 1988.)

because of this multispecific resistance. For example, cisplatin was tested predominantly in previously heavily treated patients and has not been shown to produce a high response rate as a single agent. It therefore would have been rejected as inactive agent if a 20% threshold for activity is used. Nevertheless, I and Abrams (1986) found that it is a highly active agent in combinations. Also, Smith and associates (1985) noted that carboplatinum, a cisplatin analog tested in previously untreated patients, is a highly active single agent. Thus, potentially active agents may be missed with a 20% activity threshold for response in previously treated patients, and as I (1988) pointed out, other strategies for new drug testing should be sought.

Regardless of the single agent activity, the individual

drugs rarely produce complete responses, and the duration of the partial responses tend to be short. Therefore, combination chemotherapy, found to augment response rate and duration of response and survival in the treatment of many human tumors, has been applied to SCLC. In general, the combination of chemotherapeutic agents is based on the use of active agents that have differing mechanisms of action and nonoverlapping toxicities. Many such combination chemotherapy regimens have been tested (Table 97–4), thus leading to considerable improvements in the total response frequency, a high percentage of complete responses, and the demonstration of potential curability. An overview of some of the more successful combination chemotherapy trials allows for some generalizations.

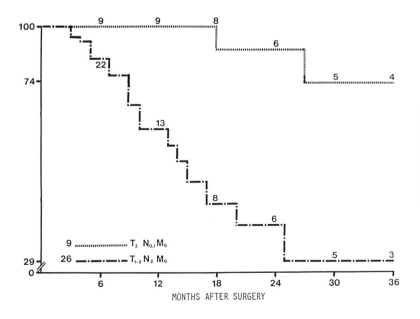

Fig. 97–4. Life-table survival curves for resected small cell lung cancer, stage IIIa: Classification T3N0–1M0 and classification T1–3N2M0. (Reproduced with permission of Karrer, K., et al.: The importance of surgery and multimodality treatment for small cell bronchial cancer [SCLC]. Presented at the 14th Annual Meeting of the Western Thoracic Surgical Association, Waikoloa, Hawaii, June 24, 1988.)

Table 97–3. Activity of Single Agents in Small Cell Lung Cancer

Agent (Abbreviation)	% Activity*
Cyclophosphamide (Cy)	40
Doxorubicin (Ad)	30
Etoposide (Et)	45
Methotrexate (Me)	30
Lomustine (Lo)	15
Carmustine (Bc)	25
Vincristine (On)	35
Vinblastine (Vb)	25
Vindesine (Vd)	25
Cisplatin (Pl)	15
Carboplatin (Cp)	50
Teniposide (Vm)	65
Mechlorethamine (Nm)	35
Procarbazine (Pr)	25†
Hexamethylmelamine (He)	30†

*Compiled approximate response rates do not consider dose or schedule.

†Phase II studies did not verify response rate.

Table 97–4. Combination Chemotherapy Regimens in Small Cell Lung Cancer*

CyAd	CyLo	AdVbPr
CyAdEt	CyLoMeOn	BcOnMePr
CyAdOn	CyLoAdPr	LoOnMePr
CyAdOnEt	CyLoOnPr	EtAdMe
CyAdMeLoOn	CyEt	HeAd
CyAdMeLo	CyEtPt	HeEtMe
CyAdEtPt	CyMeEt	MeAdCyLo
CyAdEtOnPt	CyOnPt	EtPt
CyAdOnMe	CyAdOnHe	AdEt

*See Table 97–3 for abbreviations; abbreviations for these selected chemotherapy regimens are different than the usual acronyms. These regimens were reported as either initial or alternating regimens by Abeloff (1979), Aisner (1982), Hansen (1978), Klastersky (1985), Lowenbraun (1979), and Natale (1985) and their associates and Aisner (1988).

First, three agents are superior to two, and four drugs may be superior to three. Second, the combinations should be given in maximum tolerable doses. Currently, as I and my colleagues (1982) reported, this translates into a regular and predictable toxicity; about 25% of patients experience severe and up to 5% experience lethal toxicity. Virtually every trial with sufficient numbers of cases that tested the concept of dose intensity in this disease has suggested a dose-response curve. In some instances, the authors interpreted a lack of dose effect, but all the long-term survivors received the high-dose regimen. In other instances, the higher dose regimen appeared to be superior, but there were insufficient numbers for statistical significance. Klasa and associates' (1988) overview of randomized trials also supported the concept of a steep dose-response curve for SCLC. Third, combination chemotherapy should probably be continued for about 6 months. The optimal duration of chemotherapy is, however, unknown. Long-term maintenance therapy does not appear to offer any advantage, so more than 12 months of treatment is probably exces-

sive. Finally, the agents chosen for use in combinations can have considerable impact on the results of the treatment. The use of inactive single agents cannot be shown to have an important effect. Similarly, the most active agents, because of the emergence of multispecific drug resistance, should probably be used as initial treatment. For example, multiple studies have now clearly demonstrated the importance of etoposide as part of the initial treatment regimen. Whenever possible, drugs such as etoposide and cisplatin, which, as Schabel and colleagues (1979) noted, have synergistic interactions, would be most desirable in combinations. Therefore, etoposide plus cisplatin may be an important component of combination chemotherapies.

Several theories have evolved regarding methods for optimizing the application of chemotherapy combinations. Norton and Simon (1977) suggested that these include the use of progressively more intensive dosing and Goldie and associates (1982) suggested the addition of multiple agents using an alternation of non-cross-resistant combinations where toxicity would prohibit the use of all the agents together. The former concept has not been adequately tested, whereas the latter, alternating chemotherapies, has received considerable attention. As I (1983) reported, many trials have tested alternating non-cross-resistant combinations with apparently conflicting results. Most studies failed to show a beneficial result for the use of alternating chemotherapies. For example, the trial at the UMCC, reported by me and my associates (1982), alternated CyAdEt with LoOnMePr (see Table 97–3 for abbreviations) and compared this to their use in sequence. The results were clearly within the anticipated standards, but there was no demonstrable difference in favor of the alternating regimen.

Other trials of alternating regimens have been inconsistently interpreted as positive. For example, I and Abrams (1986) and Evan and co-workers (1985a) reported that EtCp is an effective salvage regimen behind CyAdOn, and I and Abrams (1986) noted that some studies alternating between CyAdOn—first—and EtCp have suggested a beneficial result compared to CyAdOn alone. Woods and Levi (1984) reported that when the sequence is reversed, i.e., EtCp is given first, there is no salvage activity for the CyAdOn. This would suggest that there may be alternative explanations for such improvements. One explanation might be that the inclusion of etoposide as part of initial treatment is critical, so that less optimal regimens allow for improvement with crossover treatments, whereas more active regimens might not be improved with such a maneuver. Regardless of the rationale, I (1983) observed that the overall effect of the various alternating regimens has not been strikingly better than that of aggressive single regimens.

Synergistic drug interactions are also important. As Schabel (1979) and Burchenal (1980) and their colleagues suggested, cisplatin is highly synergistic with etoposide, both in animal and human tumors. Thus, this combination has been found to be a potential salvage to some regimens and Evans and associates (1985b) and Woods and Levi (1984) reported that it appears to be a highly active first-line regimen as well. Considering the relative toxicities, Cp plus Et together with chest irradiation and prophylactic cranial irradiation may be a reasonable approach in the nonstudy setting. Based on the previously mentioned observations, however, the use of Cp plus Et would also be a reasonable basis for even more aggressive therapy. At the UMCC, my group added cisplatin to our aggressive three-drug combination of AdCeEt. The resulting four-drug combination proved to be considerably more toxic, and the initial evaluation did not show a higher complete response rate. This led me and my associates (1985) to discontinue the four-drug study. Subsequent follow-up now suggests that the four-drug combination may have produced a marked prolongation of survival, and further confirmatory studies are needed.

Combined Modalities

With the success of combination chemotherapy, I (1982) and Cohen (1983) questioned the role of chest irradiation. It was reasoned that if the disease existed as a systemic process with metastases, regardless of the ability to demonstrate all foci of disease, then local control might not be the most important component in the treatment of SCLC. Lichter and Ihde (1988) summarized several trials that have addressed this question. The early trials failed to show an advantage for the combination of chemotherapy and chest irradiation. In general, the dose of one or the other or both were attenuated to accommodate the other therapy. Furthermore, several studies, as Livingston and associates (1979) noted, suggested an enhanced toxicity from the interactions of the two treatment modalities. Catane and colleagues (1981) reported one study of aggressive combined concurrent modalities that had an exceptionally high rate of pulmonary and esophageal toxicities. This study, however, also suggested that combined concurrent modalities may produce a higher rate of disease control; several of the patients who died of toxicities had no evidence of disease at necropsy. Perry (1987) and Bunn (1987) and their co-workers reported subsequent, prospectively randomized studies of the role of adjuvant chest irradiation that show a defined benefit for the use of the two modalities in combination.

The randomized studies of chest irradiation, using adequate doses, can be divided into two groups: (1) those in which the chest irradiation was given between courses of chemotherapy, the so-called sandwich technique, wherein a rest period is allowed to prevent overlap of any toxicities, and (2) those studies in which the two modalities are given concurrently or in rapid succession such that the treatment effects overlap. In all of these studies, the local—in-field—recurrences are significantly reduced in the combined modality arm compared to the chemotherapy alone arm.

Those studies in which the chest irradiation was administered by a sandwich technique, however, showed no survival advantage to the combined modality arm. In those studies in which the treatment modalities were concurrent or given in rapid succession showed a small but consistent and significant advantage in survival for the combined modality treatment. With the advent of modern computerized treatment portal planning, it should now be possible to administer maximal doses of both modalities. One such study by the Cancer and Leukemia Group B—CALGB—is currently in progress, and I and associates (1987) reported preliminary data that show the feasibility of such an approach.

Despite the significant advantage of the use of combined modalities, most patients still have disease recurrence and die with widespread metastases. Therefore, systemic treatment failure is still the major hurdle to overcome in the treatment strategy. The randomized radiation therapy studies suggest that once systemic treatment becomes more effective, the issue of local control will be more important. Mauch and colleagues (1978) observed this in other diseases, such as Hodgkin's disease, in which chest irradiation is an important part of curative treatment for those with bulky mediastinal disease. Similarly, surgery may become an important treatment for a subgroup of patients once systemic treatment becomes more effective.

Biologic Response Modifiers

The ability to grow SCLC in long-term cell culture, as Gazdar and Minna (1986) and Simms and associates (1980) reported, has permitted the study of the biology of this disease in vitro. As a result, our understanding of the basic biology in the growth and development of this tumor has expanded tremendously. Minna (1984) noted that many of these basic biologic developments have direct implications for the treatment of SCLC. For example, studies by Doyle and colleagues (1985) showed that SCLC cells in culture do not express class I—HLA—histocompatibility antigens, whereas non-SCLC cell lines do express such antigens. Incubation of the SCLC cell lines with the interferons changes the phenotypic expression, and the HLA antigens and β-microglobulin are then expressed. Marley and co-workers (1988) showed that oncogene expression can also be down-regulated with the addition of tumor necrosis factor—TNF—to the interferon in incubation of the cell lines. This may help to explain why the histology sometimes "shifts" after treatment. This ability to alter the expression of recognition antigens may also have important treatment implications, especially after an initial response to chemotherapy. On the basis of such laboratory experiments, the CALGB has initiated a study of gamma-interferon after three courses of aggressive chemotherapy with PtAdCyEt in extensive disease. This approach allows for an initial response from chemotherapy and allows for the testing of a new treatment approach.

Another example of therapeutic concepts derived from the basic science observations comes from the identification of such autocrine growth factors as bombesin in SCLC. Autocrine factors are produced by the SCLC cells themselves and stimulate the growth of the cells in culture. Several such factors have now been described for SCLC, including bombesin—gastrin releasing peptide, insulin-like growth factor, and others. Bombesin has been well described by Cuttita and associates (1985) as an important growth factor. Depletion of bombesin from growth media results in scanty growth, whereas enrichment with bombesin causes luxuriant growth. Interestingly, Aguayo and colleagues (1987) reported finding bombesin in the bronchial lavage of heavy smokers. Cuttita and associates (1985) developed a monoclonal antibody against bombesin that retards the growth of SCLC in cell culture. Even more interestingly, this antibombesin antibody completely inhibits the usually rapid and fulminant growth of SCLC inoculated into nude athymic mice. This observation has already led to a clinical trial of this antibody in advanced disease, and many investigators are awaiting its arrival for treatment as an adjuvant to chemotherapy. A conceptual approach on the integration of the various treatment approaches is illustrated in Fig. 97–5.

Antibodies against specific growth factors or tumor-specific antigens also provide the possibility of linking toxins or high-activity radionuclides to the antibody and delivering high-intensity treatment specifically to the tumors. This entire approach, i.e., the so-called biologic response modifiers, offers a new approach to this disease and the possibility of improving the cure rate in this tumor.

SUMMARY

Small cell lung cancer is a unique form of lung cancer for which significant progress has been made in treatment. Combination chemotherapy is the cornerstone of treatment and should be aggressive. Many active combinations can produce improvements in median and overall survival. Synergistic drug combinations offer the possibility of yet further improvements. Concurrent chest irradiation, given in maximal doses, adds both to local control and survival. Prophylactic cranial irradiation is useful for those patients who achieve complete response. It prolongs the time to CNS relapse and virtually

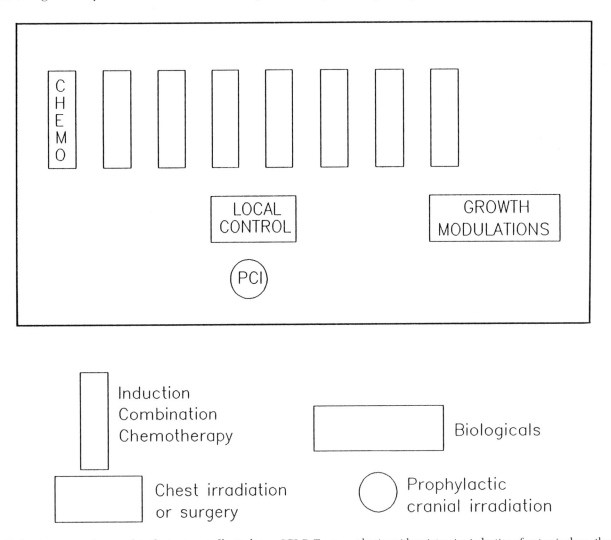

Fig. 97–5. A conceptual approach to the treatment of limited-stage SCLC. Treatment begins with an intensive induction of systemic chemotherapy. This provides for some control of the micrometastases. After three courses, local control modalities including chest irradiation (or surgery) and prophylactic cranial irradiation are added. At least some of the radiation dose is delivered to the original tumor volume. Additional courses of chemotherapy are administered after local control procedures are performed. After maximal tumor reduction, therapy directed at modulating growth of the tumor (e.g., antigrowth factors) is administered.

eliminates initial treatment failure in the CNS. Despite aggressive multimodality treatment, however, most patients have systemic disease recurrence, suggesting that the currently available systemic therapies are not adequate. Should the systemic therapy improve, control of the local intrathoracic disease by either surgery or radiotherapy will become more important. Recent advances in our understanding of the biology of this disease have led to a new category of treatment—biologic response modifiers. These offer the possibility of augmenting the cure rate but need further study. SCLC is a potentially curable disease that has led to considerable clinical and laboratory study. Further systematic study is likely to improve the cure rate from this dreaded disease.

REFERENCES

Abeloff, M.D., and Ettinger, D.S.: Diagnosis and management of medical and surgical problems in the patient with lung cancer. In Lung Cancer: A Comprehensive Treatise. Edited by J.D. Bitran, et al. Orlando, FL, Grune & Stratton, 1988, pp. 411–438.

Abeloff, M.D., et al.: Intensive induction therapy for small cell carcinoma of the lung. Cancer Treat. Rep. 63:519, 1979.

Aguayo, S.M., et al.: Bombesin-like immunoreactivity in bronchoalveolar lavage from smokers and interstitial lung disease. Clin. Res. 35:530A, 1987.

Aisner, J.: Is combined modality treatment of small cell carcinoma of the lung necessary? In Controversies in Oncology. Edited by P.H. Wiernik. New York, John B. Wiley & Sons, 1982, pp. 155–173.

Aisner, J.: Alternating chemotherapy for the treatment of small cell carcinoma of the lung. In Proc. 13th International Congress of Chemotherapy. Vienna, Verlag Egermann, 1983, pp. 221–230.

Aisner, J.: Chemotherapy for small cell carcinoma. In Lung Cancer: A Comprehensive Treatise. Edited by J.D. Bitran, et al. Orlando, FL, Grune & Stratton, 1988a, pp. 307–327.

Aisner, J.: Identification of new drugs in small cell lung cancer: phase II agents first? Cancer Treat. Rep. 71:1131, 1988b.

Aisner, J., and Abrams, J.: Small cell lung cancer: the significance of platinol. Syracuse, NY, Bristol-Meyers Oncology Division, 1986.

Aisner, J., Forastiere, A., and Aroney, R.: Patterns of recurrence for cancer of the lung and esophagus. Cancer Treat. Symp. 2:87, 1983.

Aisner, J., et al.: Combination chemotherapy for small cell carcinoma of the lung: continuous vs. alternating non-cross resistant combinations. Cancer Treat. Rep. 66:221, 1982.

Aisner, J., et al.: Role of chemotherapy in small cell lung cancer: a consensus report of the IASLC workshop. Cancer Treat. Rep. 67:37, 1983.

Aisner, J., et al.: Platinum (P), doxorubicin (A), cyclophosphamide (C) and etoposide (E), PACE, for small cell lung cancer (SCLC). Proc. Am. Soc. Clin. Oncol. 4:181, 1985.

Aisner, J., et al.: Aggressive combination chemotherapy, chest and brain irradiation and warfarin for the treatment of limited disease small cell lung cancer (SCLC). Proc. Am. Soc. Clin. Oncol. 6:179, 1987.

Aisner, S.C., et al.: The clinical significance of variant morphology (small cell/large cell) small cell carcinoma of the lung (SCCL). Proc. Am. Soc. Clin. Oncol. 7:195, 1988.

Aisner, S.C., and Matthews, M.J.: The pathology of lung cancer. In Contemporary Issues in Clinical Oncology: Lung Cancer. Edited by J. Aisner. New York, Churchill Livingstone, 1985, pp. 1–23.

Aroney, R.S., et al.: Alternating non-cross resistant combination chemotherapy for small cell anaplastic carcinoma of the lung. Cancer 49:2449, 1982.

Aroney, R.S., et al.: The value of prophylactic cranial irradiation given at complete remission in small cell lung carcinoma. Cancer Treat. Rep. 67:675, 1983.

Baglan, R.J., and Marks, J.E.: Comparisons of symptomatic and prophylactic irradiation of brain metastases from oat cell carcinoma of the lung. Cancer 47:41, 1981.

Bork, E., et al.: Teniposide (VM-26), an overlooked highly active agent in small cell lung cancer: results of a phase II trial in untreated patients. J. Clin. Oncol. 4:524, 1986.

Broder, L.E., Cohen, M.H., and Selawry, O.S.: Treatment of bronchogenic carcinoma. II. Small cell. Cancer Treat. Rev. 4:219, 1977.

Bunn, P.A., Jr.: The role of chemotherapy in small cell lung cancer. In Etoposide (VP-16) Current Status and New Developments. Edited by B.F. Issell, F.M. Muggia, and S.K. Carter. Orlando, FL, Academic Press, 1984, pp. 141–161.

Bunn, P.A., Jr., and Rosen, S.T.: Central nervous system manifestations of small cell lung cancer. In Contemporary Issues in Oncology: Lung Cancer. Edited by J. Aisner. New York, Churchill Livingstone, 1985, pp. 287–305.

Bunn, P.A., Jr., et al.: Chemotherapy alone or chemotherapy with chest radiation therapy in limited stage small cell lung cancer: a prospective randomized trial. Ann. Intern. Med. 106:655, 1987.

Burchenal, J.H., et al.: Rationale of combination chemotherapy. In Cisplatin: Current Status and New Developments. Edited by S.T. Crooke and S.K. Carter. New York, Academic Press, 1980, pp. 113–123.

Catane, R., Lichter, A., and Lee, Y.J.: Small cell lung cancer: analysis of treatment factors contributing to prolonged survival. Cancer 48:1936, 1981a.

Catane, R., et al.: Follow-up neurological evaluation in patients with small cell lung carcinoma treated with prophylactic cranial irradiation and chemotherapy. Intl. J. Radiat. Oncol. 7:105, 1981b.

Choi, C.H., and Carey, R.W.: Small cell anaplastic carcinoma of the lung: reappraisal of current management. Cancer 37:2651, 1976.

Cohen, E.A., et al.: Phase II studies in small cell lung cancer (SCLC): an analysis of 97 trials. Proc. Am. Soc. Clin. Oncol. 4:190, 1985.

Cohen, M.H.: Signs and symptoms of bronchogenic carcinoma. Semin. Oncol. 1:183, 1974.

Cohen, M.H.: Is thoracic radiation necessary for patients with limited-stage small cell lung cancer? No! Cancer Treat. Rep. 67:217, 1983.

Cohen, M.H., and Matthews, M.J.: Small cell bronchogenic carcinoma: a distinct clinicopathologic entity. Semin. Oncol. 5:234, 1978.

Cohen, M.H., et al.: Intensive chemotherapy of small cell bronchogenic carcinoma. Cancer Treat. Rep. 61:349, 1977.

Cohen, M.H., et al.: Cyclic alternating combination chemotherapy for small cell bronchogenic carcinoma. Cancer Treat. Rep. 63:163, 1979.

Cox, J.D.: Failure analysis of inoperable carcinoma of the lung of all histopathologic types and squamous cell carcinoma of the esophagus. Cancer Treat. Symposia 2:77, 1983.

Cox, J.D., Byhardt, R.W., and Wilson, J.F.: Dose-time relationship and the local control of small cell carcinoma of the lung. Radiology 128:205, 1978.

Cuttita, F., et al.: Bombesin-like peptides can function as autocrine growth factors in human small cell lung cancer. Nature 316:823, 1985.

Dara, P., et al.: Doxorubicin, hexamethylmelamine therapy of small cell carcinoma of the lung. Cancer 48:1944, 1981.

Davis, S., et al.: Long-term survival in small cell carcinoma of the lung: a population experience. J. Clin. Oncol. 3:80, 1985.

Doyle, L.A., et al.: Markedly decreased expression of class I histocompatibility antigens, protein and mRNA in human small cell lung cancer. J. Exp. Med. 161:1135, 1985.

Doyle, A., and Aisner, J.: Clinical presentation of lung cancer. In Thoracic Oncology. Edited by J.A. Roth, J.C. Ruckdeschel, and T.H. Weisenburger. Philadelphia, W.B. Saunders Co. (in press).

Ettinger, D.S., et al.: Prospective evaluation of the role of surgery in limited disease small cell lung cancer: an ECOG pilot study. Proc. Am. Soc. Clin. Oncol. 4:180, 1985.

Evans, W.K., et al.: Etoposide (VP-16) and cisplatin: an effective treatment for relapse in small cell lung cancer. J. Clin. Oncol. 3:65, 1985a.

Evans, W.K., et al.: VP-16 and cisplatin as firstline therapy for small cell lung cancer. J. Clin. Oncol. 3:1471, 1985b.

Feld, R., et al.: Canadian Multicentre randomized trial comparing sequential (S) and alternating (A) administration of two non-cross resistant chemotherapy combinations in patients with limited small cell carcinoma of the lung (SCLC). Proc. Am. Soc. Clin. Oncol. 3:214, 1984.

Fox, W., and Scadding, J.G.: Medical Research Council trial of surgery and radiotherapy for primary treatment of small-celled or oat-celled carcinoma of the bronchus: ten year follow-up. Lancet 2:63, 1979.

Gazdar, A., and Minna, J.D.: Cell lines as an investigational tool for the study of biology of small cell lung cancer. Europe J. Cancer Clin. Oncol. 22:909, 1986.

Gazdar, A., et al.: Small cell carcinoma of the lung: cellular origin and relationship to other pulmonary tumors. In Small Cell Lung Cancer. Edited by F.A. Greco, R.K. Oldham, and P.A. Bunn, Jr. Orlando, FL, Grune & Stratton, 1981, pp. 145–175.

Goldie, J.H., Coldman, A.J., and Gudanskas, G.A.: Rationale for the use of alternating non-cross resistant chemotherapy. Cancer Treat. Rep. 66:439, 1982.

Greco, F.A., et al.: Hormone production and paraneoplastic syndromes. In Small Cell Lung Cancer. Edited by F.A. Greco, R.K. Oldham, and P.A. Bunn, Jr.: Orlando, FL, Grune & Stratton, 1981, pp. 177–223.

Hansen, H.H., Rorth, M., and Aisner, J.: Management of small-cell carcinoma of the lung. In Contemporary Issues in Clinical Oncology: Lung Cancer. Edited by J. Aisner. New York, Churchill Livingstone, 1985, pp. 269–285.

Hansen, H.H., et al.: Chemotherapy of advanced small cell anaplastic carcinoma: superiority of a four-drug regimen to a three-drug regimen. Ann. Intern. Med. 89:177, 1978.

Higgins, G.A., Shields, T.W., and Keehan, R.J.: The solitary pulmonary nodule: ten-year follow-up of the Veterans Administration–Armed Forces Cooperative Study. Arch. Surg. 110:570, 1975.

Hyde, L., et al.: Cell type and natural history of lung cancer. JAMA 193:52, 1965.

Ihde, D.C., and Hansen, H.H.: Staging procedures and prognostic factors in small cell carcinoma of the lung. In Small Cell Lung Cancer. Edited by F.A. Greco, R.K. Oldham, and P.A. Bunn, Jr. Orlando, FL, Grune & Stratton, 1981, pp. 261–283.

Ihde, D.C., et al.: Prognostic implications of stage of disease and sites of metastases in patients with small cell carcinoma of the lung treated with intensive chemotherapy. Am. Rev. Respir. Dis. 123:500, 1981.

Issell, B.F., et al.: Multicenter phase II trial of etoposide in refractory small cell lung cancer. Cancer Treat. Rep. 69:127, 1985.

Karrer, K., et al.: The importance of surgery and multimodality treatment for small cell bronchial carcinoma (SCLC). Presented at 14th annual meeting of the Western Thoracic Surgical Association, Waikoloa, Hawaii, June 24, 1988.

Katalic, M., and Carter, D.: Prognostic implications of histology, size and location of primary tumors. Prog. Cancer Res. Ther. 11:143, 1979.

Klasa, R., Murray, N., and Coldman, A.: Dose intensity (DI) meta-analysis of chemotherapy in small cell carcinoma of the lung (SCCL). Proc. Am. Soc. Clin. Oncol. 7:202, 1988.

Klastersky, J., et al.: Combination chemotherapy with adriamycin, etoposide, and cyclophosphamide for small cell carcinoma of the lung: a study by the EORTC Lung Cancer Working Party (Belgium). Cancer 56:71, 1985.

Lichter, A.S., and Ihde, D.C.: The role of radiation therapy in the treatment of small cell lung cancer. In Lung Cancer: A Comprehensive Treatise. Jacob D. Bitran, editor. Orlando, FL, Grune & Stratton, 1988, pp. 329–353.

Livingston, R.B.: Small cell carcinoma of the lung. Blood 56:575, 1980.

Livingston, R.B., et al.: Unexpected toxicity of combined modality therapy for small cell carcinoma of the lung. Intl. J. Radiat. Oncol. Biol. Phys. 5:1637, 1979.

Livingston, R.B., et al.: Isolated pleural effusions in small cell lung carcinoma: favorable prognosis. Chest 81:208, 1982.

Lowenbraun, S., et al.: The superiority of combination chemotherapy over single-agent chemotherapy in small lung carcinoma. Cancer 44:406, 1979.

Matthews, M.J.: Effects of therapy on the morphology and behavior of small cell carcinoma of the lung: a clinicopathologic study. Prog. Cancer Res. Ther. 11:155, 1979.

Matthews, M.J., et al.: Frequency of residual and metastatic tumor in patients undergoing curative resection of lung cancer. Cancer Chemother. Rep. (Part 3) 4:63, 1973.

Marley, G.O., et al.: Synergy of tumor necrosis factor (TNF) and interferon (INF) in down regulation of c-myc in small cell lung cancer (SCLC) cells. Proc. Am. Soc. Clin. Oncol. 7:50, 1988.

Mauch, P., Goodman, R., and Hellman, S.: The significance of mediastinal involvement in early stage Hodgkin's disease. Cancer 42:1039, 1978.

Maurer, L.H., and Pajak, T.J.: Prognostic factors in small cell carcinoma of the lung: a Cancer and Leukemia Group B study. Cancer Treat. Rep. 65:767, 1981.

Meyer, J.A.: Five-year survival in treated stage I and II small cell carcinoma of the lung. Ann. Thorac. Surg. 42:668, 1986.

Meyer, J.A.: Indications for surgical treatment in small cell carcinoma of the lung. Surg. Clin. N. Am. 67:1103, 1987.

Meyer, J.A., et al.: Phase II trial of extended indications for resection in small cell carcinoma of the lung. J. Thorac. Cardiovasc. Surg. 84:641, 1982.

Minna, J.D.: Recent advances of potential clinical importance in the biology of lung cancer. Proc. Am. Assoc. Cancer Res. 15:393, 1984.

Mountain, C.F.: Clinical biology of small cell bronchogenic carcinoma: relationship to surgical therapy. Semin. Oncol. 5:272, 1978.

Mountain, C.F., Carr, D.T., and Anderson, W.A.D.: A system for the clinical staging of lung cancer. Am. J. Roentgenol. 120:130, 1974.

Muggia, F.M., Krezoski, S.K., and Hansen, H.H.: Cell kinetic studies in patients with small cell carcinoma of the lung. Cancer 34:1683, 1974.

Natale, R.B., et al.: Combination cyclophosphamide, adriamycin, and vincristine rapidly alternating with combination cisplatin and VP-16 in treatment of small cell lung cancer. Am. J. Med. 79:303, 1985.

Norton, L., and Simon, R.: Tumor size, sensitivity to therapy, and design of treatment schedules. Cancer Treat. Rep. 61:1307, 1977.

Nugent, J.L., et al.: CNS metastases in small cell bronchogenic carcinoma: increasing frequency and changing pattern with lengthening survival. Cancer 44:1885, 1979.

Ohta, M., et al.: The role of surgical resection in the management of small cell carcinoma of the lung. Jpn. J. Clin. Oncol. 16:289, 1986.

Pendergrass, H.P., et al.: Relative efficacy of radionuclide imaging and computed tomography of the brain. Radiology 116:26, 1975.

Perry, M.C., et al.: Chemotherapy with or without radiation therapy in limited small cell carcinoma of the lung. N. Engl. J. Med. 316:912, 1987.

Prager, R.L., et al.: The feasibility of "adjuvant surgery" in limited small cell carcinoma: a prospective evaluation. Ann. Thorac. Surg. 38:622, 1984.

Radice, P., et al.: The clinical behavior of "mixed" small/large cell bronchogenic carcinoma, compared to "pure" small cell subtypes. Cancer 50:2894, 1982.

Rosen, S.T., et al.: Role of prophylactic cranial irradiation in prevention of central nervous system metastases in small cell lung cancer: potential benefit restricted to patients in complete response. Am. J. Med. 74:615, 1983.

Sagman, U., et al.: Long-term survival of patients (pts) with small cell cancer (sclc): the Toronto experience. Proc. Am. Soc. Clin. Oncol. 7:203, 1988.

Schabel, F.M., Jr., et al.: Cisdichlorodiammineplatinum (II): combination chemotherapy and cross-resistance studies with tumors of mice. Cancer Treat. Rep. 63:1459, 1979.

Shalen, P.R., et al.: Protocol for delayed contrast enhancement in computed tomography of cerebral neoplasia. Radiology 139:397, 1981.

Shepherd, F.A., et al.: Reduction in local recurrence and improved survival in surgically treated patients with small cell lung cancer. J. Cardiovasc. Surg. 86:498, 1983.

Shepherd, F.A., et al.: A prospective study of adjuvant surgery after chemotherapy for limited small cell lung cancer: a University of Toronto Lung Oncology Group study. J. Thorac. Cardiovasc. Surg. (in press).

Shields, T.W.: Role of surgical resection in small cell carcinoma of the lung. J. Jap. Assoc. Thorac. Surg. 36:665, 1988.

Shields, T.W., et al.: Surgical resection in the management of small cell carcinoma of the lung. J. Thorac. Cardiovasc. Surg. 84:481, 1982.

Simms, E., et al.: Growth of human small cell carcinoma of the lung in serum-free growth factor supplemented medium. Cancer Res. 40:4356, 1980.

Smith, I.E., et al.: Carboplatin: a very active new cisplatin analog in the treatment of small cell lung cancer. Cancer Treat. Rep. 69:43, 1985.

Sorenson, G.D., et al.: Biomarkers in small cell carcinoma of the lung. In Contemporary Issues in Oncology: Lung Cancer. Edited by J. Aisner. New York, Churchill Livingstone, 1985, pp. 203–239.

Stanley, K.: Prognostic factors for survival in patients with inoperable lung cancers. J. Natl. Cancer Inst. 65:25, 1980.

Valdivieso, M., et al.: Increasing importance of adjuvant surgery in the therapy of patients with small cell lung cancer. Proc. Am. Soc. Clin. Oncol. 1:148, 1982.

Whitley, N.O., et al.: Computed tomography of the chest in small cell lung cancer: new potential prognostic signs. Am. J. Roentgenol. 142:885, 1984.

Wittes, R.E., and Yeh, S.D.J.: Indications for liver and brain scans: screening tests for patients with oat cell carcinoma of the lung. JAMA 238:506, 1977.

Woods, R.L., and Levi, J.A.: Chemotherapy for small cell lung cancer (SCLC): a randomized study of maintenance therapy with cyclophosphamide, adriamycin, and vincristine (CAV) after remission induction therapy with cisplatinum (CIS-DDP), VP-16-213 and radiotherapy. Proc. Am. Soc. Clin. Oncol. 3:214, 1984.

World Health Organization: The World Health Organization histological typing of lung tumors, 2nd ed. Am. J. Clin. Pathol. 77:123, 1982.

Yesner, R., et al.: Classification of lung-cancer histology. N. Engl. J. Med. 312:652, 1985.

CHAPTER 98

CHEMOTHERAPY OF MEDIASTINAL GERM CELL TUMORS AND MALIGNANT THYMOMAS

John D. Hainsworth and F. Anthony Greco

Although primary malignancies of the mediastinum are rare, several types deserve specific attention because effective nonsurgical treatments are available. Mediastinal germ cell tumors usually occur in young men and have rarely been amenable to surgical therapy. Within this group of tumors, treatments differ for seminomas and nonseminomas. Seminomas are usually curable either with irradiation or chemotherapy. Intensive cisplatin-based chemotherapy, often combined with postchemotherapy surgical resection of residual disease, has resulted in the cure of many patients with nonseminomatous germ cell tumors. We (F.A.G. and J.D.H.) and associates (1986) recognized that some poorly differentiated carcinomas arising in the mediastinum respond dramatically to similar cisplatin-based chemotherapy. Finally, some malignant thymomas that are either metastatic or locally unresectable have shown prolonged responses to appropriate chemotherapy. This chapter discusses the current therapy of these uncommon but highly treatable neoplasms.

MALIGNANT MEDIASTINAL GERM CELL TUMORS

Primary germ cell tumors arising in the mediastinum are now generally accepted as a distinct clinical entity, and probably arise from primitive rests of totipotential cells that become detached from the blastula or morula during embryogenesis. Little evidence supports the once widely held theory that these tumors are actually metastatic testicular germ tumors with a regressed or undetectable testicular primary. Malignant germ cell tumors of the mediastinum are rare, and constitute 1 to 5% of all germ cell neoplasms, and only 3 to 10% of tumors originating in the mediastinum. Most of these tumors occur in men between the ages of 20 to 35 years; only rarely have these tumors been reported to occur in women.

Mediastinal germ cell tumors and germ cell tumors arising in the testes are histologically identical, and the same range of histologic subtypes has been identified. For purposes of determining optimal treatment, germ cell tumors can be divided into two categories: pure seminoma, and tumors containing nonseminomatous elements—embryonal carcinoma, choriocarcinoma, teratocarcinoma, or yolk sac tumor. Approximately one third of mediastinal germinal tumors are pure seminomas, whereas the remainder contain nonseminomatous elements.

The diagnosis of mediastinal germ cell tumor should be considered in all young men who have a mediastinal mass. In addition to routine physical examination and laboratory studies, initial evaluation should include computed tomography of the chest and abdomen, and determination of the serum levels of human chorionic gonadotropin and alpha-fetoprotein. Any symptoms suggestive of distant metastases should be evaluated with appropriate diagnostic studies. If metastases are obvious, histologic diagnosis should be made using the least invasive approach, because surgical therapy does not play a role in the initial treatment of these patients, and rapid institution of definitive systemic therapy is essential. In patients with tumors that seem localized to the mediastinum, thoracotomy with attempted tumor resection or debulking is sometimes appropriate. Exceptions to this approach include: tumors with obvious involvement of vital mediastinal structures or intrathoracic spread outside the anterior mediastinum, and patients with high serum levels of human chorionic gonadotropin or alpha-fetoprotein. In the second group of patients, the clinical presentation coupled with the elevated marker levels is diagnostic of a nonseminomatous germ cell neoplasm, and initial treatment with combination chemotherapy should proceed immediately.

The treatment and prognosis of mediastinal seminoma and nonseminoma differ; therefore, the treatment of these tumors is considered separately.

Seminoma

Seminomas usually grow slowly and can become large before causing symptoms; tumors 20 to 30 cm in diameter can exist with minimal symptomatology. In some series, 20 to 30% of seminomas were detected by routine chest roentgenogram while still asymptomatic. The remainder of these tumors usually produce symptoms related to compression or impingement on vital mediastinal structures. Although symptoms related to distant metastases are rare at the time of diagnosis, only 30 to 40% of patients have tumors localized to the anterior mediastinum at diagnosis. The lungs and other intrathoracic structures are the most common metastatic sites, and these metastatic lesions can best be detected by computed tomography of the chest. The skeletal system is the most frequently recognized extrathoracic metastatic site.

Because of the rarity of these neoplasms, most reports on therapy have been limited to case reports or small series of patients. It is therefore sometimes difficult to make definitive conclusions concerning the relative efficacy of therapies when more than one modality exists. Curative therapy in seminoma has been reported with several different modalities, including surgical resection, radiation therapy, surgical resection plus radiation therapy, and chemotherapy. The choice of therapy must be made only after careful staging, and with full knowledge of the capabilities of each treatment modality.

Surgical excision of mediastinal seminomas confined to the anterior mediastinum has been attempted since the early 1950s, with multiple reports of long-term survivors. With the increased ability to detect intrathoracic metastases, and the availability of other excellent treatment modalities, primary surgical excision should be restricted to a small subgroup of patients in whom complete surgical excision seems possible. Probably only asymptomatic tumors diagnosed by routine chest roentgenogram are consistently amenable to this approach. Recurrences following "complete" surgical resection have been reported; therefore, resection should never be used as the only therapeutic modality in these patients.

Radiation therapy is highly effective in the treatment of testicular seminomas; 75 to 80% of these patients are cured when irradiation alone is used. Although mediastinal seminomas seem equally sensitive, overall cure rates with irradiation are inferior to those achieved in the treatment of testicular seminoma. Table 98–1 summarizes the results of radiation therapy in reported series containing 5 or more patients. Approximately one third of these patients had partial surgical excision of the mediastinal tumor before radiation therapy. As is evident from Table 98–1, treatment results using these local therapeutic modalities are reasonably good; overall, 49 of 82 patients—60%—in these nine series had long-term, disease-free survival. The lower cure rate when compared to radiation therapy results in testicular seminoma is explained by the more advanced nature of most mediastinal seminomas. At the time of diagnosis, primary lesions in the mediastinum are usually much larger, and more importantly, the incidence of metastases is significantly higher. Most radiation therapy failures result from the appearance of distant metastases, rather than failure to achieve local tumor control.

Radiation therapeutic cures have been reported using various techniques, and curative dosages have ranged from 2000 to 7000 rads. Bush and associates (1981) observed no local relapses when doses over 4500 rads were administered, and therefore recommend 4500 to 5000 rads over 6 weeks delivered by external beam megavoltage irradiation. The irradiated field should cover the mediastinum and both supraclavicular areas.

Surgical debulking before definitive irradiation in the treatment of mediastinal seminomas is controversial. A definite benefit of initial surgery is apparent only when complete surgical excision can be performed. Complete surgical excision followed by radiation therapy is curative in nearly 100% of patients. In contrast, the benefit of partial resection—"debulking"—has not been demonstrated. With currently available radiation therapy techniques, local control has not been a major problem; most treatment failures result from distant metastases.

Systemic combination chemotherapy is another highly

Table 98–1. Mediastinal Seminoma: Results of Treatment with Radiation Therapy

Author (year)	No. of Patients	No. of Patients with Surgical Resection Prior to Radiotherapy (complete or partial)	Radiotherapy Dose (rads)	Number of Disease-Free Survivors (%)
El-Domeiri et al. (1968)	8	2	3000–5000	3 (38%)
Schantz et al. (1972)	12	7	2400–6000	12 (100%)
Martini et al. (1974)	8	1	N.A.	2 (25%)
Cox (1975)	6	0	2000–4000	6 (100%)
Medini et al. (1979)	5	3	3500–4500	3 (60%)
Raghavan et al. (1980)	6	1	3500–4500	3 (50%)
Bush et al. (1981)	13	1	2500–6000	7* (54%)
Hurt et al. (1982)	16	6	3000–4000	9 (56%)
Jain et al. (1984)	8	2	1850–4600	4 (50%)

*2 patients with recurrence are long-term survivors after salvage treatment with further radiotherapy and chemotherapy.

effective treatment for mediastinal seminomas. Einhorn and Donohue (1977) first reported curative therapy in 60 to 70% of metastatic nonseminomatous testicular neoplasms using an intensive cisplatin-based chemotherapy regimen. Subsequent continued improvements in therapy have allowed cures of 80 to 85% of these patients. These same regimens have proven curative in most patients with advanced testicular seminoma, and are also highly effective in the treatment of mediastinal seminoma. Table 98–2 summarizes the limited experience using optimal cisplatin-based combination chemotherapy in the treatment of mediastinal seminoma. Many reported cases have attained complete response and long-term survival, even after radiation therapy failure. Figure 98–1 outlines a standard combination chemotherapy regimen containing bleomycin, etoposide, and cisplatin—BEP—which has proven highly effective in the treatment of both advanced seminoma and nonseminomatous germ cell tumors. Curative chemotherapy for germ cell tumors is brief, 3 to 4 months, but all effective regimens are intensive, and optimal treatment results are obtained only if drugs are given in full prescribed doses and according to schedule. This treatment should always be administered by an experienced medical oncologist.

Only one nonrandomized study, reported by Jain and associates (1984), compares treatment results using irradiation versus combination chemotherapy in patients with mediastinal seminoma. Five of nine patients—56%—treated initially with irradition remain disease-free, as compared to ten of eleven patients—91%—treated with combination chemotherapy. Because the results with radiation therapy are consistent with those achieved in other reported series, the conclusion is made that initial chemotherapy is the treatment of choice for patients with mediastinal seminoma. Although this statement may be true, a categorical statement is difficult to make based on this nonrandomized comparison containing small numbers of patients.

Most patients with mediastinal seminoma can be cured with appropriate therapy, and all patients should be approached with curative intent. Careful pretreatment staging is essential to detect distant metastases, and also to assess the extent of involvement of mediastinal structures. Optimal treatment is well defined in some patient subsets. All patients with small tumors—usually asymptomatic—that appear resectable on the basis of computed tomography of the chest should undergo thoracotomy or median sternotomy with attempted complete resection. Complete tumor excision should be followed by postoperative irradiation—3500 to 4500 rads; close to 100% of these patients are cured with this treatment. The optimal treatment modality is also clear in patients with distant metastases at the time of diagnosis; these patients should undergo initial combination chemotherapy with an intensive cisplatin-based regimen. The BEP regimen outlined in Figure 98–1 is currently widely used; other similar regimens have given comparable results.

Optimal therapy for patients with locally advanced mediastinal seminomas who have no evidence of distant metastases is unclear. Radical debulking procedures for these patients are probably not beneficial. Approximately 60% of these patients can be cured with radiation therapy, most treatment failures result from relapses at distant sites. Some patients whose disease recurs after radiation therapy can be salvaged with combination chemotherapy, but some evidence exists that chemotherapy results are inferior in this group of patients, because of both increased tumor resistance and excessive myelosuppression. The number of patients treated initially with chemotherapy remains small, but the cure rate with this modality is probably high. Although additional evidence is needed before definitive statements can be made, we believe that initial cisplatin-based chemotherapy in this group of patients will prove superior to irradiation.

Table 98–2. Mediastinal Seminoma: Results of Treatment with Cisplatin-Based Combination Chemotherapy

Author (year)	No. of Patients	No. Previously Treated with Radiation Therapy	Treatment Regimen (No. of patients)	Number of Complete Responders (%)	Number of Relapses after Complete Remission
Feun et al. (1980)	2	2	PVB*	0	—
Van Hoesel and Pirado (1980)	1	1	DDP/VLB	1 (100%)	0
Einhorn and Williams (1980)	3	2	PVB + A	2 (66%)	0
Hainsworth et al. (1982)	4	3	PVB	3 (75%)	0
Daugaard et al. (1983b)	1	1	PVB	1 (100%)	0
Clamon (1983)	2	0	PVB	2 (100%)	0
Jain et al. (1984)	11	0	VAB-6 (8) PVB (1) DDP/CTX (2)	10 (91%)	0
Logothetis et al. (1985)	4	N.A.	DDP/CTX (3) CISCA₂ (1)	4 (100%)	0

Key: DDP = cisplatin; VLB = vinblastine; A = doxorubicin; CTX = cyclophosphamide; PVB = Einhorn regimen (cisplatin 20 mg/m² IV × 5 days; vinblastine 0.15 mg/kg days 1, 2; bleomycin 30 units weekly; cycle repeated q 3 weeks × 3 to 4); VAB-6 = multidrug regimen developed at Sloan-Kettering; CISCA₂ = multidrug regimen developed at M.D. Anderson.

*Used lower dosages and longer intervals between dosages than are currently considered optimal.

Cisplatin 20 mg/m² daily × 5 days } Doses repeated
Etoposide 100 mg/m² daily × 5 days } q 3 weeks × 4
Bleomycin 30 units weekly × 12 doses }

Fig. 98–1. Bleomycin/Etoposide/Cisplatin (BEP) Regimen for Treatment of Advanced Germinal Tumors.

Nonseminomatous Mediastinal Germ Cell Tumors

Mediastinal germinal tumors with nonseminomatous elements generally grow more rapidly than pure seminomas. Of these patients, 85 to 95% have at least one site of metastatic disease at diagnosis, and presenting symptoms are frequently caused by distant metastases. The remainder of these patients have symptoms caused by compression or invasion of mediastinal structures, or both. Constitutional symptoms including weight loss, fever, and generalized weakness are more common in these patients than in those with pure seminoma. Common sites of metastases include lung, pleura, lymph nodes—supraclavicular, retroperitoneal—and liver. Neoplasms with elements of choriocarcinoma have a marked hemorrhagic tendency; these patients may present with uncontrolled hemorrhage at a metastatic site, e.g., massive hemoptysis, intracranial hemorrhage, or may have excessive bleeding after a biopsy.

Approximately 90% of patients with nonseminomatous elements have elevated serum levels of human chorionic gonadotropin—HCG—or alpha-fetoprotein—AFP—or both. All patients with elevated levels of AFP have nonseminomatous elements; these patients should be treated as nonseminomatous germinal tumors even if the biopsy shows "pure seminoma." Pretreatment measurement of serum levels of these markers is imperative, not only to aid in the correct diagnosis, but also to assess response to therapy.

Unlike that of mediastinal seminomas, local therapy of nonseminomatous neoplasms is almost always ineffective. In a review of the literature, Cox (1975) found no survivors among 85 patients with mediastinal teratocarcinoma. The failure of local treatment modalities in mediastinal germ cell tumors with nonseminomatous components is explained by the propensity for early metastasis to distant sites, and the relative resistance of these tumors to radiation therapy.

Intensive cisplatin-based regimens developed for the treatment of metastatic nonseminomatous testicular cancer have improved the prognosis of patients with mediastinal nonseminomatous tumors. Table 98–3 summarizes the treatment results of cisplatin-based combination chemotherapy. The overall long-term survival rate in optimally treated patients, i.e., those receiving cisplatin-containing regimens currently considered optimal for the treatment of metastatic testicular malignancies, is 37%. Although these results represent a marked improvement, the long-term survival rate is still lower than in metastatic testicular germinal neoplasms. This difference is probably related to the large bulk of most mediastinal nonseminomatous neoplasms at the time of diagnosis; testicular germinal neoplasms with far-advanced, bulky metastases have comparable long-term survival rates—approximately 40 to 50%. The BEP regimen (Fig. 98–1) is the most widely used chemotherapeutic regimen for these neoplasms; further modifications of this regimen are currently being evaluated in an attempt to further improve the cure rate.

Surgical resection has no role in the initial therapy of these neoplasms, because close to 100% of these neoplasms are either metastatic or locally unresectable. Nonetheless, surgical resection following cisplastin-based combination chemotherapy often plays an integral part in the management of these patients. Surgical resection should be attempted if chemotherapy produces normalization of serum HCG and AFP but only partial roentgenographic resolution of the mediastinal tumor. In this setting, 60 to 80% of patients have either necrotic tumor or benign teratoma in the resected specimen, with no evidence of residual malignancy. The importance of completely resecting residual benign—mature or immature—teratomata in these patients has been recognized; unresected teratomata can cause further problems either by slow local growth, or by subsequent malignant degeneration.

If persistent viable carcinoma is resected following initial chemotherapy, patients should receive further chemotherapy with a salvage regimen, because long-term survival is unusual even following "complete" tumor resection. Patients with persistent elevations in tumor markers following initial chemotherapy should proceed directly to salvage regimens; these patients all have residual viable carcinoma, and surgical intervention almost never results in successful tumor control. Salvage chemotherapy regimens using etoposide, ifosfamide, and cisplatin have resulted in long-term disease-free survival in 20 to 30% of patients who are not cured with initial chemotherapy.

The treatment approach outlined previously applies to all histologic subtypes of nonseminomatous germinal tumors. Although data are limited, some evidence suggests that results are inferior in certain histologic subtypes, including pure choriocarcinoma and pure yolk sac tumor. Kuzur and associates (1982) reported long-term survival in only one of ten patients with pure yolk sac tumor of the mediastinum following treatment with cisplatin-based combination chemotherapy. Logothetis and associates (1985), however, documented long-term survival in three of five patients with pure yolk sac tumor following similar cisplatin-based chemotherapy. Because of the rarity of this tumor, however, definitive conclusions are difficult to make. At present, all patients with mediastinal nonseminomatous germinal neoplasms should receive initial therapy with intensive cisplatin-based regimens, regardless of histology. Further improvements in therapy are necessary; these improvements will probably parallel the development of increasingly effective treatment for patients with far-advanced, poor-prognosis testicular germinal neoplasms.

POORLY DIFFERENTIATED CARCINOMA OF THE MEDIASTINUM

The patient with poorly differentiated—or anaplastic—carcinoma poses difficult problems for both the

Table 98–3. Nonseminomatous Mediastinal Germinal Neoplasms: Results of Treatment with Cisplatin-Based Combination Chemotherapy

Author (year)	No. of Patients	Treatment Regimen (No. of Patients)	Complete Responders (%)	No. of Long-term (> 24 months) Disease-Free Survivors (%)
Feun et al. (1980)	10	PVB*	0	0
Van Hoesel and Pirado (1980)	1	PVB	1 (100%)	1 (100%)
Funes et al. (1981)	13	PVB	6 (46%)	5 (38%)
Vogelzang et al. (1982)	7	PVB (6) VAB-6 (1)	3 (43%)	3 (43%)
Hainsworth et al. (1982)	12	PVB + A	7 (58%)	7 (58%)
Daugaard et al. (1983b)	5	PVB	1 (20%)	1 (20%)
Newlands et al. (1983)	2	POMB/ACE	2 (100%)	2 (100%)
Garnick et al. (1983)	8	PVB	3 (38%)	1 (13%)
Logothetis et al. (1985)	11	CISCA₂ (6) CISCA/VB₄ (5)	N.A.	4 (36%)
Israel et al. (1985)	29 (includes patients with retroperitoneal tumors)	VAB-3 (12) VAB-5 (6) VAB-6 (11)	12 (41%)	5 (17%)†

*Used lower dosages and longer intervals between cisplatin doses than are currently considered optimal.

†When patients treated with optimal regimen (VAB-6) are considered, 4/11 (36%) are long-term survivors.

Key: PVB = Einhorn regimen (see Key, Table 98–2); A = doxorubicin; VAB-3, VAB-5, VAB-6 = multidrug regimens developed at Sloan-Kettering; $CISCA_2$, $CISCA/VB_4$ = multidrug regimens developed at M.D. Anderson; POMB/ACE = cisplatin, vincristine, methotrexate, bleomycin, doxorubicin, cyclophosphamide, etoposide.

clinician and the pathologist. The true nature of these neoplasms is usually unclear, because definitive histopathologic features are absent. The patient with a mediastinal mass in whom the biopsy indicates poorly differentiated carcinoma is often suspected of having metastatic lung cancer with an undetected primary lesion, and palliative radiation therapy is considered. A complete discussion of poorly differentiated carcinoma is beyond the scope of this chapter, but this brief section is included because some patients with poorly differentiated carcinoma in the mediastinum have highly responsive, potentially curable neoplasms and should receive careful attention.

Our interest in poorly differentiated carcinoma in the mediastinum began when Richardson and associates (1981) observed several complete responses to cisplatin-based combination chemotherapy. Most of the initial patients reported were young men with rapidly growing neoplasms and elevated levels of either HCG or AFP. We therefore suspected that these patients actually had mediastinal germinal neoplasms that were unrecognized histologically. Fox and associates (1979) made similar observations independently.

Since that time, we have greatly expanded our experience in treating patients with poorly differentiated carcinoma of unknown primary site. We have now treated a total of 153 patients with this diagnosis; 22 of these patients—14%—had disease located predominantly in the mediastinum. Nineteen patients were men,

three were women; the median age was 46 years. Only 2 of these 22 patients had elevated serum levels of HCG or AFP. Twenty patients received intensive cisplatin-based chemotherapy using regimens proved effective in the treatment of germ cell neoplasms. Seven of twenty patients—35%—had complete response to therapy, and four patients remained disease-free after a follow-up period of 64 to 125 months. We have carefully reviewed the light microscopic histopathology in these patients, and none has been diagnosed subsequently as having an initially unrecognized germinal tumor. In addition, review of the histopathology did not reveal unsuspected malignant lymphoma in any of these patients.

Patients with poorly differentiated carcinoma presenting as mediastinal masses probably have neoplasms of diverse histogenesis. Some patients in this category do indeed have lung cancer, and would not be expected to respond well to chemotherapy. Nevertheless, because a subset of these patients responds dramatically to cisplatin-based chemotherapy, this therapy should be considered for all patients in this group. Responding patients may have histologically atypical mediastinal germ cell neoplasms, but this remains speculative. Better characterization of these neoplasms, both clinically and histologically, may in the future help to identify the chemotherapy-responsive subset.

MALIGNANT THYMOMA

Thymomas are rare, slowly growing tumors that usually occur in adults between 40 and 60 years of age. The histologic appearance of these tumors varies and is characterized by a mixture of lymphocytic and epithelial cells. Classification is based on the predominant cell type; 25 to 35% of thymomas are predominantly lymphocytic, 40 to 45% are predominantly epithelial, and the remainder have mixed populations of these two elements. Although thymomas often grow slowly, and many are encapsulated at the time of surgical excision, all thymomas are potentially invasive, and therefore should be considered malignant. Local invasion of mediastinal structures is the most common mode of spread in thymomas. The most common metastatic sites are pleura and pericardium, probably resulting from shedding of tumor cells from the primary lesion. Blood-borne metastases are unusual, but have been reported in various sites.

Most thymomas are curable with surgical excision alone. At the time of diagnosis 65% are encapsulated, and the recurrence rate following careful excision of these tumors is less than 2%. Many patients with locally invasive thymomas are also cured with surgical resection, but the recurrence rate can be as high as 20 to 25% if no further therapy is administered. Therefore, patients with thymomas should always be evaluated for potentially curative surgery. In this neoplasm, aggressive attempts at resection of locally invasive tumor are warranted, because such procedures cure some patients.

Radiation therapy has been effective in locally unresectable or locally recurrent thymomas following initial excision. Radiation therapy is also routinely recommended for patients who undergo complete excision of locally invasive thymoma, although randomized trials proving the superiority of combined modality therapy are not available. Doses of 3500 to 4500 rads given over 3 to 6 weeks are recommended. Local tumor control is achieved in most patients following radiation therapy.

Data concerning chemotherapy of malignant thymomas are limited, because most patients with this disease are adequately treated with surgical excision and radiation therapy. Trials of chemotherapy have been limited to patients with metastases, or with recurring tumors following local therapy. Most reports of successful chemotherapy of malignant thymomas are limited to single case reports or small series of patients; some cooperative group data became available in the 1980s.

Several reports in the early 1970s documented objective responses of thymomas following treatment with high dose corticosteroids. Most responses were partial, and tumor regrew rapidly after steroids were discontinued. Current evidence indicates that the epithelial cells are the malignant component of malignant thymoma, and the admixed lymphocytes are a reactive, polyclonal population. The objective responses to corticosteroids have been attributed to the lympholytic effect on the benign population of lymphocytes, rather than an antitumor effect on the malignant epithelial population. The fact that all reported steroid responses were in thymomas with lymphoid or mixed histologies supports this hypothesis.

Malignant thymomas have responded to various chemotherapeutic regimens, and the optimal regimen is currently unknown. Interest has focused on cisplatin-containing regimens, because cisplatin when used as a single agent has produced dramatic responses in some patients with metastatic thymoma. Table 98–4 summarizes the results of cisplatin therapy of malignant thymoma. Response rates to cisplatin-based regimens are difficult to determine because few cases have been reported. The response rates of the only two prospective series differed; Fornasiero and colleagues (1984) reported 10 of 11 responses—91% and Loehrer and colleagues (1988) had only 13 of 20 responses—65%. The chemotherapy regimens used were similar; better definition of the response rate awaits further prospective series. At present, it appears that objective tumor regressions are frequent, although few patients—probably 10 to 30%

Table 98–4. Malignant Thymoma: Summary of Treatment Results with Cisplatin-Containing Chemotherapy

Author (year)	No. of Patients	Treatment Regimen	Responses	Duration of Response (months)
SINGLE-AGENT CISPLATIN				
Talley et al. (1973)	1	cisplatin 20–40 mg/m²	PR	13
Needles et al. (1981)	1	cisplatin 120 mg/m²	CR	10+
Shetty and Arora (1981)	1	cisplatin 100 mg/m²	PR	4
Cocconi et al. (1982)	1	cisplatin 100 mg/m²	CR	23+
Giaccone et al. (1985)	1	cisplatin 120 mg/m²	PR	1
CISPLATIN-CONTAINING COMBINATION REGIMENS				
Chahinian et al. (1981)	5	BAP/prednisone	PR 2/5	4, 12
Campbell et al. (1981)	1	CAP	CR	12
Fornasiero et al. (1984)	11	CAVP	CR 4/11	12.5 (median survival)
			PR 6/11	(3 CRs free of disease 11, 30, and 30 months)
Klippstein et al. (1984)	2	AP	CR 2/2	4+, 20
Giaccone et al. (1985)	5	EP	PR 1/5	27+
Loehrer et al. (1988)	22	CAP	CR 3/20	12 (range 4–43+)
			PR 10/20	

Key: P = cisplatin; B = bleomycin; A = doxorubicin; V = vincristine; C = cyclophosphamide; E = etoposide; PR = partial response; CR = complete response.

have complete remissions. Some of the complete remissions have been prolonged (Table 98–4), but follow-up is not sufficient to determine whether chemotherapy is potentially curative in any patient with metastatic thymoma.

Other combination chemotherapy regimens that do not contain cisplatin have also reportedly been effective in small numbers of patients. Evans and associates (1980) reported partial responses in four of five patients following treatment with cyclophosphamide, vincristine, procarbazine, and prednisone—COPP. All of these patients had locally invasive tumors, and following initial chemotherapy-induced regression, these patients underwent definitive local therapy with surgical excision, radiation therapy or both. Two patients experienced long-term disease-free survival following this therapy. All patients had tumors with mixed histologies, and tumor regression may have resulted from the lympholytic capabilities of the prednisone in this regimen. It is also unclear whether the initial chemotherapy contributed to the long-term survival in the two patients who subsequently had surgical excision.

Daugaard and associates (1983a) reported responses in five of nine patients to a combination of cyclophosphamide, vincristine, lomustine, and prednisone. Four patients had complete remission, and one patient remained free of disease 62 months after initiation of therapy.

SUMMARY

Optimal chemotherapy of locally recurrent or metastatic thymoma has not been defined. Some of these neoplasms are highly responsive; complete and partial responses have been reported using several different chemotherapeutic regimens. Based on limited data, the following recommendations can be made: combination chemotherapy regimens are more effective than single agents, and cisplatin should be included in the combination regimen, because this is the only drug that has produced prolonged remissions when used as a single agent. At present, it is unknown whether patients who achieve complete response with chemotherapy have a potential for cure, because long-term follow-up of the few complete responses has not been provided. The use of chemotherapy in malignant thymomas should at present be restricted to patients with metastatic disease and patients in whom primary local treatment with surgical excision or irradiation or both has failed. Although the concept of chemotherapeutic "debulking" of large, marginally resectable mediastinal thymomas is appealing, the efficacy of this approach has not yet been adequately evaluated.

REFERENCES

Bush, S.E., Martinez, A., and Bagshaw, M.A.: Primary mediastinal seminoma. Cancer 48:1877, 1981.
Campbell, M.G., Pollard, R., and Al-Sarraf, M.: A complete response in metastatic malignant thymoma to cis-platinum, doxorubicin, and cyclophosphamide: a case report. Cancer 48:1315, 1981.
Chahinian, A.P., et al.: Treatment of invasive or metastatic thymoma: report of eleven cases. Cancer 47:1752, 1981.
Clamon, G.H.: Management of primary mediastinal seminoma. Chest 83:263, 1983.
Cocconi, G., Boni, C., and Cuomo, A.: Long-lasting response to cis-platinum in recurrent malignant thymoma. Cancer 49:1985, 1982.
Cox, J.D.: Primary malignant germinal tumors of the mediastinum. Cancer 36:1162, 1975.
Daugaard, G., Hansen, H.H., and Rorth, M.: Combination chemotherapy for malignant thymoma. Ann. Intern. Med. 99:189, 1983a.
Daugaard, G., Rorth, M., and Hansen, H.H.: Therapy of extragonadal germ-cell tumors. Eur. J. Clin. Oncol. 19:895, 1983b.
Einhorn, L.H., and Donohue, J.D.: Cis-diamminedichloroplatinum, vinblastine, and bleomycin combination chemotherapy in disseminated testicular cancer. Ann. Intern. Med. 87:293, 1977.
Einhorn, L.H., and Williams, S.D.: Chemotherapy of disseminated seminoma. Cancer Clin. Trials 3:307, 1980.
El-Domeiri, A.A., et al.: Primary seminoma of the anterior mediastinum. Ann. Thorac. Surg. 6:513, 1968.
Evans, W.K., et al.: Combination chemotherapy in invasive thymoma: role of COPP. Cancer 46:1523, 1980.
Feun, L.G., Samson, M.K., and Stephens, R.L.: Vinblastine (VLB), bleomycin (BLEO), cisdiamminedichloroplatinum (DDP) in disseminated extragonadal germ cell tumors: a Southwest Oncology Group study. Cancer 45:2543, 1980.
Fornasiero, A., et al.: Chemotherapy of invasive or metastatic thymoma: report of 11 cases. Cancer Treat. Rep. 68:1205, 1984.
Fox, R.M., Woods, R.L., and Tattersall, M.H.N.: Undifferentiated carcinoma in young men: the atypical teratoma syndrome. Lancet 1:1316, 1979.
Funes, H.C., et al.: Mediastinal germ cell tumors treated with cisplatin, bleomycin, and vinblastine (PVB) (abstract). Proc. Am. Assoc. Cancer Res. 22:474, 1981.
Garnick, M.B., Canellos, G.P., and Richie, J.P.: Treatment and surgical staging of testicular and primary extragonadal germ cell cancer. J.A.M.A. 250:1733, 1983.
Giaccone, G., et al.: Cisplatin-containing chemotherapy in the treatment of invasive thymoma: report of five cases. Cancer Treat. Rep. 69:695, 1985.
Greco, F.A., Vaughn, W.K., and Hainsworth, J.D.: Advanced poorly differentiated carcinoma of unknown primary site: recognition of a treatable syndrome. Ann. Intern. Med. 104:547, 1986.
Hainsworth, J.D., et al.: Advanced extragonadal germ-cell tumors. Successful treatment with combination chemotherapy. Ann. Intern. Med. 97:7, 1982.
Hurt, R.D., et al.: Primary anterior mediastinal seminoma. Cancer 49:1658, 1982.
Israel, A., et al.: The results of chemotherapy for extragonadal germ-cell tumors in the cisplatin era: the Memorial Sloan-Kettering Cancer Center experience (1975 to 1982). J. Clin. Oncol. 3:1073, 1985.
Jain, K.K., et al.: The treatment of extragonadal seminoma. J. Clin. Oncol. 2:820, 1984.
Klippstein, T.H., et al.: High-dose adriamycin (ADM) and cis-platinum (DDP) in advanced soft tissue sarcomas and invasive thymomas. Cancer Chemother. Pharmacol. 13:78, 1984.
Kuzur, M.E., et al.: Endodermal sinus tumor of the mediastinum. Cancer 50:766, 1982.
Loehrer, P.J., et al.: Cisplatin plus adriamycin plus cyclophosphamide in limited and extensive thymoma: preliminary results of an intergroup trial (abstract). Proc. Am. Soc. Clin. Oncol. 7:199, 1988.
Logothetis, C.J., et al.: Chemotherapy of extragonadal germ cell tumors. J. Clin. Oncol. 3:316, 1985.
Martini, N., et al.: Primary mediastinal germ cell tumors. Cancer 33:763, 1974.
Medini, E., et al.: The management of extratesticular seminoma without gonadal involvement. Cancer 44:2032, 1979.
Needles, B., Kemeny, N., and Urmacher, C.: Malignant thymoma: renal metastases responding to cis-platinum. Cancer 48:223, 1981.
Newlands, E.S., et al.: Further advances in the management of malignant teratomas of the testis and other sites. Lancet 1:948, 1983.
Raghavan, D., and Barrett, A.: Mediastinal seminomas. Cancer 46:1187, 1980.

Richardson, R.L., et al.: The unrecognized extragonadal germ cell cancer syndrome. Ann. Intern. Med. 94:181, 1981.

Schantz, A., Sewall, W., and Castleman, B.: Mediastinal germinoma: a study of 21 cases with an excellent prognosis. Cancer 30:1189, 1972.

Shetty, M.R., and Arora, R.K.: Invasive thymoma treated with cisplatin. Cancer Treat. Rep. 65:531, 1981.

Talley, R.W., et al.: Clinical evaluation of toxic effects of cisdiamminedichloroplatinum (NSC-119875)—phase I clinical study. Cancer Chemother. Rep. 57:465, 1973.

Van Hoesel, O.G.C.M., and Piredo, H.M.: Complete remission of mediastinal germ-cell tumors with cis-dichlorodiammine platinum (II) combination chemotherapy. Cancer Treat. Rep. 64:319, 1980.

Vogelzang, N.J., et al.: Mediastinal nonseminomatous germ cell tumors: the role of combined modality therapy. Ann. Thorac. Surg. 33:333, 1982.

Immunotherapy

CHAPTER 99

IMMUNOLOGY OF HUMAN BRONCHIAL CANCER

James A. Radosevich, Roy E. Ritts, and Steven T. Rosen

Since the 1930s, researchers have documented alterations of the immune system in cancer patients. These studies have raised questions concerning the underlying mechanisms of these findings. Since the 1960s, investigators have focused on those alterations of immune function that show potential for enabling the clinician to alter the course of the disease. In addition, the understanding of these altered immunologic functions may provide enhanced diagnostic, prognostic, or therapeutic approaches to cancer.

Many studies have been directed at the unique immunologic aspects of tumor cell lines, transplantable tumors, and virus-induced tumors in experimental animal models. Despite this effort, no direct proof of unique tumor-specific antigens in human cancer exists. Nonetheless, putative tumor associated antigens which are defined by mouse hybridoma monoclonal antibodies—MoAB—have been reported and the data have been summarized by one of us (J.A.R.) and associates (1987). These antigens were thought to be tumor specific, but all have been found to be expressed by other neoplasms, by normal tissue in the adult, or during fetal development. Data by Hellstrom and associates (1970) and by Hoover and co-workers (1981) suggest that the tumor is foreign to the host. Both clinical and experimental findings have promoted the concept that neoplasms can escape detection by or somehow confound the immune system. The loss of a completely functional immune system, and the high incidence of Kaposi's sarcoma among patients with acquired immunodeficiency syndrome—AIDS, as Friendman-Kien and colleagues (1982) reported, supports the concept that the immune system is fundamental in the regulation of neoplastic growth. Thomas (1959) and Burnet (1970) have refined the unifying Ehrlichian doctrine of immunologic defense against invading foreign entities into the immunosurveillance theory. The militaristic analogy of a defensive immune system that fights with a variety of weapons against an invading force of foreign components is often used to depict the concept of immunosurveillance. Within this analogy, neoplastic growth is not a foreign component but rather an alteration of "self"; this alteration may or may not be recognized immunologically as "foreign" and therefore may escape destruction.

THE IMMUNE STATUS OF PATIENTS WITH BRONCHIAL CARCINOMA

Renaud's (1926) observation that patients with cancer had impaired tuberculin response went unsupported until Southam and associates (1957) showed that cancer patients had a cell-mediated immune defect. They demonstrated that these patients showed a delayed rejection of cultured human cell homografts. Levin and colleagues (1964) and Hughes and MacKay (1965) used dinitrofluorobenzene, a de novo antigen, to demonstrate deficiencies in the immune response of cancer patients. Lamb and co-workers (1962) and Solowey and Rappaport (1965) used recall microbial antigens to demonstrate the anergy in patients with solid tumors.

Krant and associates (1968) made the first systematic, prospective study of immune competence in patients with lung cancer. Their data prompted numerous other studies that used their approach for diagnosis and prognosis and their criteria for resectability. They found that patients with bronchial carcinoma who had delayed sensitivity to dinitrochlorobenzene—DNCB—had a better short-term prognosis. This was only true if the diagnosis had not been made more than 6 to 8 months before the positive response to DNCB. A similar correlation could not be derived from tuberculin reactivity data, but the same general pattern of decreased reactivity with disease progression and somewhat better prognosis with an intact response was observed. A progressive leukopenia also was observed in patients with bronchial carcinoma. Although the degree of lymphopenia was correlated with survival time, a cause-and-effect relationship was not ascribed to this event, or to the apparent parallel of loss of delayed-type hypersensitivity—DTH—to DNCB. Elevated IgA levels were also reported, but these findings were not statistically significant.

Comparable findings, particularly with respect to microbial antigens and DNCB reactivities, have been reported by Israel (1967), Takita and Brugarolas (1973), one of us (R.E.R.) and Carr (1974), Wanebo and colleagues (1976), and Holmes and Golub (1976). In a series of studies that controlled for the stage of disease and for potentially immunosuppressive therapy, a general depression of immune function was confirmed. These results supported the notion that these in-vitro tests had clinical utility in predicting the prognosis of lung cancer patients. It is evident from the reported data that anergic and markedly hypoergic patients have shortened disease-free intervals following surgery, poor responses to any modality of treatment, and short survival time when compared with patients who demonstrate a normal response in these tests. Unfortunately, it is also evident from these studies that the reported findings for any particular test is highly variable between institutions. In addition, a test that has been shown to be of clinical significance at one institution may not be at another, and vice versa. These reports, nonetheless, are important for several reasons. They reflect our limited knowledge of the immune system and all of the delicate relationships that it must maintain in normal individuals. These studies also fuel the hopes of eventually being able to manipulate the immune system, by correcting or augmenting the immune system component these tests show is abnormal. They are also important historically, because they demonstrate how the current understanding of basic immunology of that era has been applied to the treatment of cancer of the lung.

An enthusiastic attempt to use DNCB sensitivity as a test of immune function in lung cancer patients has had mixed results. DNCB is a potent hapten when conjugated with a carrier skin protein and can sensitize patients to produce a delayed-type contact skin reactivity upon receiving a challenge dose. The method of sensitization in these studies is unusually uniform, that is, 2000 μg of DNCB in acetone is applied over a 2 cm² area for 48 hours with an occlusive dressing. Rechallenge follows in 2 weeks or more, with graded doses of 5 to 200 μg, which are then scored for induration after 48 hours. No one is naturally or spontaneously reactive to DNCB without prior exposure. A mild to moderate inflammation may result from the sensitizing dose. It is rare that normal individuals cannot be sensitized. Less than 2% of several hundred volunteers tested failed to show evidence of delayed-type reactivity after 2 weeks, the time when the challenge dose is customarily applied. These individuals, however, did subsequently show delayed-type sensitivity after 3 to 4 weeks post challenge. An important aspect of using potent sensitizing contact haptens is that each challenge dose is, in itself, a significant sensitizing dose. It is therefore inappropriate to use the test for clinical applications beyond the first challenge, even in small amounts.

In a series of lung cancer patients, Wanebo and associates (1976) found that 71% of stage I, 89% of stage II, 76% of operable stage III, and 67% inoperable stage III patients reacted to DNCB. Wells and colleagues (1973a, 1973b) studied 25 lung cancer patients and found that only 52% were reactive to DNCB. Seventy percent of the patients capable of responding had resectable disease. Holmes (1976) found that no stage III patients were reactive, and only approximately 2% of the DNCB-positive patients had unresectable disease. Brugarolas and associates (1973) similarly stated that responsiveness to DNCB, in effect, rules out the presence of metastatic disease. One of us (R.E.R.) (1977) and Wanebo (1976) and associates presented data that are contrary to these findings. They show that a significant number of inoperable, untreated, unresectable stage III patients, most with proved metastases to the liver or brain, respond to the first DNCB challenge. Similarly, one of us (R.E.R.) and colleagues (1974, 1977) were unable to discriminate between stages of disease by the use of multiple microbial antigen skin tests, as had been reported by Takita and Brugarolas (1973) and Brugarolas and associates (1973). Additionally, these studies found no prognostic significance in the results of these skin tests, as reported at the 1st Working Party on Lung Cancer by Hersh and co-workers (1976).

It is difficult to explain the conflicting data found by the various groups that used skin reactivity as a simple test of immune function. It is equally difficult to dismiss the positive findings by some of the groups that used this method, because of its potential to be a clinically significant test. Although reading skin contact reactivity to DNCB is difficult for the inexperienced, the skill is easily learned and can be confirmed by biopsy if absolutely necessary. Perhaps differences in the patient populations studied in the quoted references account for the discordance in the data. Therefore, once a procedure is validated and its utility is established in a specific institution, the use of DNCB or recall antigen testing may have important diagnostic and prognostic value for patients seen at that institution. Until multisite studies can provide data to resolve these conflicts, however, any DTH skin tests can only be considered useful if they are used to confirm a clinical judgment of poor condition and poor prognosis.

As one of us (R.E.R.) (1974) noted previously, Wanebo and associates (1976) corroborated the uniformly poor skin test responsiveness to DNCB of patients with small cell lung cancer. This poor response appears to occur irrespective of the stage of disease. It is important to note that early diagnosis of small cell carcinoma is difficult, and therefore these results may reflect the enhanced tumor burden seen in these patients. Both Krant (1968) and Wanebo (1976) and their colleagues found that patients with squamous cell carcinoma lung cancer are more responsive to DNCB than patients with adenocarcinoma are. Wells (1973a) has reported the exact opposite of these findings.

The skin test data from nearly all studies demonstrate that in the presence of metastatic disease immune responsiveness is minimal. Nonetheless, one of us (R.E.R.) and associates (1977) noted that although even occult—stage X—or in-situ disease may be accompanied by a subnormal immune response, 10 to 15% of patients with advanced, metastatic disease may have normal responses. Individual variability in immune function, as seen in skin tests and in-vitro assays, makes immune assessment that uses a single assay at one point in time completely unreliable. Sequential examination of non-specific immune competence using both in-vivo and in-vitro methods may eventually be established to have clinical relevance. It is important to keep in mind that normal values vary with time and result in a consequently wide range of normal values. This variability is further amplified for in-vitro assays because these tests depend on many uncontrollable biologic reagents—fetal calf serum, human serum, plant lectins, etc. Thus, these tests are much less precise and sensitive than most of the clinical laboratory tests used in everyday practice.

In his study, Holmes (1976) interpreted a normal microbial recall DTH and a depressed DNCB as an indication that patients with lung cancer have a defect in the afferent limb of the immune system. The data from Takita and Brugarolas (1973), Brugarolas and Takita (1973), and Concannon (1977), Oldham (1976), Wanebo (1976), and one of us (R.E.R.) (1977) and associates, however, show that both recall and de novo DTH responses are impaired despite a normal inflammatory response. Therefore, it appears unlikely that patients have a defect solely in the afferent or recognition arm of the immune mechanism. Indeed, Hollinshead and colleagues (1974) and Herberman (1974, 1977) reported that lung cancer patients have recognition of presumed tumor-associated antigens even when showing evidence of immunodeficiency.

Several in-vitro assays allow the assessment of both nonspecific and putative lung cancer–associated specific immunity. One assay is the ability of a lymphocyte to undergo blastogenic transformation in response to any number of plant lectins. Phytohemagglutinin—PHA—and concanavalin A—Con A—have been used to stimulate and subsequently assess cell-mediated function. Similarly, allogenic cells have been used. Tests that assay for lymphokine production have also been employed. One example is migration inhibition factor—MIF, a lymphokine that is liberated by specifically sensitized lymphocytes. Several cytolytic tests, leukocyte adherence inhibition, and blastogenesis have been referred to collectively as in-vitro correlates of skin DTH. Holt and coworkers (1976) noted, however, that a battery of such tests do not give parallel or concordant results. This discordance is in part explained by the heterogeneity in the cell populations that respond to the neoplasm. This finding may elucidate the resulting immune response to neoplastic growth. Disparate test results may indicate not only the specific immune perturbations but also the range of these perturbations. Future studies may indicate whether these aberrations in cell function are merely a secondary paraneoplastic event or whether there is a subtle primary derangement that occurs in immune homeostasis. A change of this nature could facilitate the unregulated growth of a normally suppressed cell. The latter notion, if correct, would profoundly alter our concept of neoplasia and would have significant impact on the approach to therapy.

The studies of lymphocyte blastogenesis have been critical to our understanding of immune response in neoplastic induction. Nearly all investigators, such as Ducos (1970), Mekori (1974), Wanebo (1976), and Oldham (1976), and their associates as well as Nelson (1969), one of us (R.E.R.) (1974), and Holmes and Golub (1976), found a depressed PHA and Con A response in patients with lung cancer. Further, it seems reasonably certain that the depression from normal values is proportional to the extent of tumor burden. Statistically significant differences between stages I and II or II and III, however, are not always evident. Furthermore, poor survival, as Wanebo and colleagues (1976) noted, and response to chemotherapy, as Al-Sarraf and associates (1972) reported, have been correlated with marked depression in PHA-induced blastogenesis. These observations have also been reported for squamous cell carcinoma of the head and neck, as Wanebo (1975) and Ryan (1979) and their colleagues reported. This relationship is not seen so definitely in other solid tissue neoplasms, as data suggested by Prichard (1978) and Moertel (1979) and associates. Again, it is important to caution that these assays are currently not sophisticated enough to be used as a single source of information on which to base a diagnosis or prognosis for a particular patient. Patients with far-advanced disease infrequently have a normal response, and occasional patients with minimal disease are markedly immunosuppressed. Serial determinations of multiple immunologic tests in a single patient may give some guidance, particularly if the repeat determinations show marked changes. Caution in interpretation is advised when a sudden depression occurs. Although this change may signal dissemination of the tumor and poor prognosis, it also may be the result of chemotherapy or irradiation. The consensus of investigators seems to be that blastogenesis is a useful nonspecific assessment of the patient's cellular immune status. Studies by one of us (R.E.R.) reported by Moertel and associates (1978, 1979) have indicated that in patients with gastrointestinal malignancies, clinical staging or even a routine laboratory test such as SGOT have a more significant Spearman correlation coefficient with the duration of survival than nonspecific immunologic functions have. Of course, the routine tests are easier to obtain and are more reproducible than nonspecific immune function tests.

Depressed lymphocyte blastogenesis might result from an impressive number of possibilities. An intrinsic cellular defect does exist, but Silk (1967) has reported that serum from cancer patients depresses blastogenesis of lymphocytes from healthy donors. In such sera, one of us (R.E.R.) (1974) noted that inhibitors range from very-low-molecular-weight—less than 3000 daltons—substances to rather large molecules such as alpha-2-macroglobulin, described by Cooperband (1972) and Glasgow (1974) and their co-workers. In addition, fetal proteins identified by Gupta and Good (1977), and blocking antigen–antibody complexes reported by Sjogren and associates (1971) have been described. These components apparently are present occasionally in normal individuals over 60 years of age and in more than half of the tested cancer patients. Jerrells and colleagues (1978) found in lung cancer patients T-suppressor cells that could depress PHA blastogenesis, so an intrinsic functional T-lymphocyte defect may not be the sole indicator in cancer patients. Changes within the subpopulation of cell regulators and humoral inhibitors are important as well. Possibly, some of these humoral suppressors of cell immunity are secreted or induced by the tumor itself. As the tumor burden changes in response to treatments, the complex interaction between these factors is probably influenced. These changes are most likely the cause of the variability seen in a patient's blastogenic potential.

Nearly all immunologic investigations, such as those by Wanebo (1976), Oldham (1976), and Concannon (1977) and their associates as well as by Holmes (1976), Holmes and Golub (1976), and one of us (R.E.R.) and colleagues (1977), of lung cancer patients have found a reduction in the percentage of circulating T cells. No significant alteration in the non-thymic-regulated cells—B cells—has been reported. One of us (R.E.R.) (1977) did show an increase in B cells for 30% of the untreated early stage lung cancer patients. Researchers do not completely agree on the significance of the T- and B-cell reports. Although decreased numbers of T cells may be observed in advanced disease, these differences from normal are often not statistically significant. The correlation between T-cell levels and disease status is poor. West and co-workers (1976) suggested that T-cell rosetting by sheep erythrocytes performed at 29°C—the so-called high-affinity rosette—rather than the customary 9°C may be a more discriminating assay of T-cell numbers in cancer patients. Another procedure, the T-cell rosette inhibition assay, has been reported by Gross and colleagues (1975) to be highly significant. In this study, they compared 29 lung cancer patients to healthy individuals and those with benign lung disease.

Tests of tumor-specific immunity in humans are currently under intense investigation. Because the definitive isolation and identification of a human lung cancer antigen has not been accomplished, existing tests, as Herberman (1974) and Hollinshead and associates (1974) as well as Granlund and one of us (R.E.R.) (1976) noted, must rely on crude extracts and detailed "proof" of their specificity. Bell and Seetharam (1976) and McIntire and colleagues (1979) have identified pure materials that hold promise, but considerable clinical evaluation of these antigens is required.

Hollinshead and associates (1974) reported separating extracts of lung cancer and used these in skin tests. Although these materials are said to elicit reactivity in patients with lung cancer, no available data suggest that they are comparable to those presumed antigens isolated from the lymphocytes of leukemia and lymphoma patients. Herberman (1974) and co-workers (1973) reported that these antigens cause or increase DTH skin reactivity during remission and are negative or decreased upon relapse.

Alth (1973), Boddie (1974, 1975), and Oldham (1976) and their associates showed that an occasional extract of bronchial carcinoma shows activity in leukocyte migration inhibition assays. Similarly, Powell and associates (1975) reported leukocyte adherence inhibition—LAI—tests that have shown specificity. The preliminary data from these studies suggest that these specific immunologic tests may be helpful in the diagnosis of early lung cancer. Likewise, they may have utility in monitoring for recurrence following resection in stage I and II disease, as Shani and colleagues (1978) reported for colorectal carcinoma. Debate continues about the mechanism of the two major methods of performing LAI tests with tumor extracts. The original hemocytometer method of Halliday and Miller (1972) is thought to detect CMI by tumor "antigen" liberation of a lymphokine. The test-tube modification by Grosser and Thomson (1975) is said to measure a cytophilic antibody. Consequently, each approach may have a special utility for clinical application. In addition to their intrinsic value, the LAI techniques also provide a precise approach for measuring blocking factors. The blocking factors are thought to reflect the presence or absence of tumor, as Grosser and Thomson (1976) reported.

It was previously thought that by performing a battery of nonspecific tests of immunologic competence, a series of clinically pertinent profiles that would have diagnostic or prognostic significance might emerge. To date, such clinical correlations have not been found. Moertel and associates (1979) reported that assays of immunologic competence do not yield results that are more compelling as predictors than stage of disease or performance status are.

MONOCLONAL ANTIBODIES

Many monoclonal antibodies have been produced against human pulmonary neoplasms and have been reviewed by two of us (J.A.R., S.T.R.) and associates (1987). Only relatively few of the monoclonal antibodies that are directed at pulmonary neoplasms have been extensively characterized. Current studies are using monoclonal antibodies that have been conjugated with radioisotopes, chemotherapeutic agents, or toxins as imaging and treatment agents. Monoclonal antibodies are valuable in defining specific subtypes of pulmonary neoplasms based on their immunophenotypes. Perhaps the use of these reagents will eventually lead to a panel of antibodies that will more consistently classify this heterogeneous group of neoplasms. It is hoped that the immunophenotype, along with other biologic assessment assays, will provide a more accurate definition of the biologic potential of these tumors. Patients will then be able to be more uniformly selected for clinical trials that use immunotherapy as a form of treatment. It is hoped that this will eventually resolve some of the conflicting data presented earlier and ultimately provide an approach to determining which immunotherapies are effective for lung cancer.

REFERENCES

Al-Sarraf, M., Sardesai, S., and Vaitkeviscius, V.K.: Clinical immunologic responsiveness in malignant disease. II. In vitro lymphocyte response to phytohemagglutinin and the effect of cytotoxic drugs. Oncology 26:357, 1972.

Alth, G., et al.: Aspects of the immunologic treatment of lung cancer. Cancer Chemother. Rep. 4:271, 1973.

Bell, C.E., Jr., and Seetharam, S.: A plasma membrane antigen highly associated with oat-cell carcinoma of the lung and undetectable in normal adult tissue. Int. J. Cancer 18:605, 1976.

Boddie, A.W., Jr., Holmes, E.C., and Roth, J.A.: Inhibition of human leukocyte migration in agarose by KCl extracts of lung cancer. Surg. Forum 25:109, 1974.

Boddie, A.W., Jr., et al.: Inhibition of human leukocyte migration in agarose by KCl extracts of carcinoma of the lung. Int. J. Cancer 15:823, 1975.

Brugarolas, A., and Takita, H.: Immunologic status in lung cancer. Chest 64:427, 1973.

Brugarolas, A., Takita, H., and Vincent, R.: Skin test in bronchogenic carcinoma. II. Its value in the differential diagnosis. J. Surg. Oncol. 5:319, 1973.

Burnet, F.M.: Immunological Surveillance. Sydney, Australia, Pergamon Press, 1970.

Concannon, J.P., et al.: Immunoprofile studies for patients with bronchogenic carcinoma. I. Correlation of pre-therapy studies with stage of disease. Int. J. Radiat. Oncol. Biol. Phys. 2:477, 1974.

Cooperband, S.R., et al.: The effect of immunoregulatory A globulin (IRA) upon lymphocytes in vitro. J. Immunol. 109:154, 1972.

Ducos, J., et al.: Lymphocyte response to P.H.A. in patients with lung cancer. Lancet 1:1111, 1970.

Friedman-Kien, A.E., et al.: Disseminated Kaposi's sarcoma in homosexual men. Ann. Intern. Med. 96:693, 1982.

Glasgow, A.H., et al.: Association of anergy with an immunosuppressive peptide fraction in the serum of patients with cancer. New Engl. J. Med. 291:1263, 1974.

Granlund, D.J., and Ritts, R.E., Jr.: Soluble proteins of human bronchogenic carcinomas. Mayo Clin. Proc. 51:19, 1976.

Gross, R.L., et al.: Abnormal spontaneous rosette formation and rosette inhibition in lung cancer. New Engl. J. Med. 292:439, 1975.

Grosser, N., and Thomson, D.M.P.: Cell-mediated anti-tumor immunity in breast cancer patients evaluated by antigen-induced leukocyte adherence inhibition in test tubes. Cancer Res. 35:2571, 1975.

Grosser, N., and Thomson, D.M.P.: Tube leukocyte (monocyte) adherence inhibition assay for the detection of anti-tumour immunity. III. "Blockade" of monocyte reactivity by excess free antigen and immune complexes in advanced cancer patients. Int. J. Cancer 18:58, 1976.

Gupta, S., and Good, R.A.: Fetoprotein and human lymphocyte subpopulations. J. Immunol. 118:405, 1977.

Halliday, W.J., and Miller, S.: Leukocyte adherence inhibition: A simple test for cell-mediated tumour immunity and serum blocking factors. Int. J. Cancer 9:477, 1972.

Hellstrom, I., et al.: Studies on cellular immunity to human neuroblastoma cells. Int. J. Cancer 6:172, 1970.

Herberman, R.B.: Delayed hypersensitivity response toward autochthonous tumor extracts. Recent Results Cancer Res. 47:140, 1974.

Herberman, R.B.: Immunogenicity of tumor antigens. Biochem. Biophys. Acta Rev. Cancer 473:93, 1977.

Herberman, R.B., et al.: Delayed cutaneous hypersensitivity reactions to extracts of human tumors. Natl. Cancer Inst. Monogr. 37:189, 1973.

Hersh, E.M., et al.: Immunocompetence and prognosis in lung cancer. Proc. Am. Assoc. Cancer Res. and Am. Soc. Clin. Oncol. 17:58, 1976 (Abstract).

Hollinshead, A.C., Steward, T.H.M., and Herberman, R.B.: Delayed hypersensitivity reactions to soluble membrane antigens of human malignant lung cells. J. Natl. Cancer Inst. 52:327, 1974.

Holmes, E.C.: Collective review: immunology and lung cancer. Am. Thorac. Surg. 21:250, 1976.

Holmes, E.C., and Golub, S.H.: Immunologic defects in lung cancer patients. J. Thorac. Cardiovasc. Surg. 71:161, 1976.

Holt, P.G., et al.: Dissociation of correlates of cellular immunity in man: functional heterogeneity within the antigen-reactive cell population? Int. Arch. Allergy Appl. Immunol. 51:560, 1976.

Hoover, H.C., Jr., et al.: Therapy of spontaneous metastases with an autologous tumor vaccine in a guinea pig model. J. Surg. Res. 30:409, 1981.

Hughes, L.E., and MacKay, W.D.: Suppression of the tuberculin response in malignant disease. Br. Med. J. 2:1346, 1965.

Israel, L., et al.: Etude de l'hypersensitilite retardee a la tuberculine chez 130 cancereux adultes. Effets du B.C.G. Pathol. Biol. 15:597, 1967.

Israel, L.: Nonspecific immunostimulation in bronchogenic cancer. Scand. J. Respir. Dis. (Suppl.) 89:95, 1974.

Jerrells, T.R., et al.: Role of suppressor cells in depression of in vitro lymphoproliferative responses of lung cancer and breast cancer patients. J. Natl. Cancer Inst. 61(4):1001, 1978.

Krant, M.J., et al.: Immunologic alterations in bronchogenic cancer: sequential study. Cancer 21:623, 1968.

Lamb, D., et al.: A comparative study of the incidence of anergy in patients with carcinoma, leukemia, Hodgkin's disease, and other lymphomas. J. Immunol. 89:555, 1962.

Levin, A.G., et al.: Delayed hypersensitivity response to DNFB in sick and healthy persons. Ann. N.Y. Acad. Sci. 120:400, 1964.

McIntire, K.R., et al.: Identification of antigens associated with lung cancer suitable for diagnosis and monitoring. In Lung Cancer: Progress in Therapeutic Research. Edited by F. Muggia and M. Rozencweig. New York, Raven Press, 1979, p. 183.

Mekori, T., Shulamith, S., and Robinson, E.: Suppression of the mitogenic response to phytohemagglutinin in malignant neoplasia: correlation with clinical stage and therapy. J. Natl. Cancer Inst. 52:9, 1974.

Moertel, C.G., et al.: A controlled evaluation of combined immunotherapy (MER-BCG) and chemotherapy for advanced colorectal cancer. In Immunotherapy of Cancer: Present Status of Trials in Man. Edited by W.D. Terry and D. Windhorst. New York, Raven Press, 1978, p. 573.

Moertel, C.G., et al.: Non-specific immune determinants in the patient with unresectable gastrointestinal carcinoma. Cancer 43:1483, 1979.

Nelson, H.S.: Delayed hypersensitivity in cancer patients: cutaneous and in vitro lymphocyte response to specific antigens. J. Natl. Cancer Inst. 42:765, 1969.

Oldham, R.K., et al.: Immunological monitoring and immunotherapy in carcinoma of the lung. Int. J. Cancer 18:739, 1976.

Powell, A.E., et al.: Specific responsiveness of leukocytes to soluble extracts of human tumors. Int. J. Cancer 16:905, 1975.

Pritchard, D.J., et al.: A prospective study of immune responsiveness in human melanoma. Cancer 41:2165, 1978.

Radosevich, J.A., et al.: Monoclonal antibody assays for lung cancer. In In Vitro Diagnosis of Human Tumors Using Monoclonal Antibodies. Edited by H.Z. Kupchik, New York, Marcel Dekker, 1987.

Renaud, M.M.: La cuti-reaction a la tuberculine chez les cancereux. Soc. Med. Hosp. Paris 50:1441, 1926.

Ritts, R.E., Jr.: Immunologic factors. Chapter IX. In Bronchial Carcinoma. Edited by T.W. Shields. Springfield, IL, Charles C Thomas, 1974, pp. 82–92 and 129–133.

Ritts, R.E., Jr., and Carr, D.T.: In vivo and in vitro assessment of cellular immune competency in untreated advanced bronchogenic carcinoma. In Neoplasm Immunity: Theory and Application. Edited by R.G. Crispen. Proceedings of a Chicago Symposium, 1974, p. 105.

Ritts, R.E., Jr., et al.: Is the lung cancer patient immunologically competent? An assessment of cellular immunity by extent of tumor burden and histological cell type. In Perspective in Lung Cancer. Edited by T.E. Williams, Jr., H.E. Wilson, and D.S. Yohn. Basel (Switzerland), S. Karger, 1977, p. 47.

Ritts, R.E., Jr., LeDuc, P.V., and Eagan, R.T.: Unpublished data, 1979.

Ryan, R.J., Neel, H.B., III, and Ritts, R.E., Jr.: Unpublished data, 1979.

Shani, A., et al.: A prospective evaluation of the leukocyte adherence inhibition test in colorectal cancer and its correlation with carcinoembryonic antigen levels. Int. J. Cancer 22:113, 1978.

Silk, M.: Effect of plasma from patients with carcinoma on in vitro lymphocyte transformation. Cancer 20:2088, 1967.

Sjogren, H.P., et al.: Suggestive evidence that the "blocking antibodies" of tumor bearing individuals may be antigen-antibody complexes. Proc. Natl. Acad. Sci. 68:1372, 1971.

Solowey, A.C., and Rappaport, A.E.: Immunological responses in cancer patients. Surg. Gynecol. Obstet. *121*:756, 1965.

Southam, C.M., Moore, A.E., and Rhoads, C.P.: Homotransplantation of human cell lines. Science *125*:158, 1957.

Takita, H., and Brugarolas, A.: Skin test in bronchogenic carcinoma: I. Correlation of the immunologic status and the extent of the disease. J. Surg. Oncol. 5:315, 1973.

Thomas, L.: Discussion. *In* Cellular and Humoral Aspects of the Hypersensitive States. Edited by H.S. Lawrence. New York, Hoeber-Harper Book Co., 1959, p. 530.

Wanebo, H.J., et al.: T-cell deficiency in patients with squamous cell cancer of the head and neck. Am. J. Surg. *130*:445, 1975.

Wanebo, H.J., et al.: Immune reactivity in primary carcinoma of the lung and its relations to prognosis. J. Thorac. Cardiovasc. Surg. 72:339, 1976.

Wells, S.A., Burdick, J.F., and Joseph, W.F.: Delayed cutaneous hypersensitivity reactions to tumor cell antigens and to non-specific antigens. J. Thorac. Cardiovasc. Surg. *66*:557, 1973a.

Wells, S.A., Jr., et al.: Demonstration of tumor-associated delayed cutaneous hypersensitivity reactions in patients with lung cancer and in patients with carcinoma of the cervix. Natl. Cancer Inst. Monogr. 37:197, 1973b.

West, W.H., et al.: Modification of the rosette assay between lymphocytes and sheep erythrocytes to study patients with cancer, systemic lupus erythematosus, and other diseases. J. Clin. Immunol. Immunopathol. 5:60, 1976.

CHAPTER 100

IMMUNOTHERAPY OF BRONCHIAL CARCINOMA

Bryan H.R. Stack

Immunotherapy, also called biological response modification, is any method of increasing immunity against tumor cells. Figure 100–1 summarizes the forms of immunotherapy that have been used since the 1960s. Initial investigations concentrated on patients with advanced cancer. It became clear, however, that this form of treatment has only a weak anticancer activity compared with surgery, irradiation, or chemotherapy. It thus came to be used as an adjuvant where one or more of these other treatments had substantially reduced the population of tumor cells. The few positive results of immunotherapy described were after curative resection of bronchial carcinoma.

NONSPECIFIC IMMUNOTHERAPY

This term has been used for methods designed to produce a generalized increase in cell-mediated immunity in the hope of including in this increased activity cells that specifically destroy tumor cells. The two forms of nonspecific immunotherapeutic agents are bacterial antigens and immunorestorant drugs.

BCG Immunotherapy

The most commonly used bacterial antigen has been BCG. This attenuated *Mycobacterium bovis* is widely used in active immunization against tuberculosis. In the United Kingdom, the BCG used in immunotherapy contains approximately 10 times the number of viable organisms per milliliter as that used in tuberculosis prophylaxis.

Baldwin and Pimm (1978) reviewed the use of BCG in immunotherapy and drew attention to the wide variation in properties of the eight different strains in common use at that time. These included the weight of organisms, the number of viable and nonviable organisms per milliliter, and whether the suspension was fresh, freeze-dried, or frozen. This variation has undoubtedly accounted for the wide discrepancy of results from the use of BCG in bronchial carcinoma. Another factor has been difference in the biological activity of batches of the same preparation, as Bennett and associates (1983) described.

Routes of Administration of BCG

Various routes have been used for the administration of BCG (Table 100–1). In some early studies, BCG was injected into the skin of patients with locally advanced inoperable tumors. In some of these, early results were promising, but no difference in survival was found after longer follow-up periods. Later studies concentrated on patients who had undergone resection of the tumor. Whereas intradermal and subcutaneous BCG produced variable results, there was considerable interest in McKneally and colleagues' (1976) report of postoperative intrapleural BCG. In a study of 66 patients there was a marked difference between treatment and control groups in survival and freedom from tumor recurrence during the first few years of follow-up. This difference was sustained through less marked in a report by Maver and colleagues (1982) from the same group (Table 100–2). Subsequent larger studies have failed to confirm this result.

Another local form of immunotherapy has been the injection of BCG directly into tumor tissue by way of a needle passed through chest wall or by way of a bronchoscope. This method, pioneered by Holmes' group (1977), produced an increase in natural killer cell activity among tumor-infiltrating lymphocytes. In a similar

Table 100–1. Routes of Administration of BCG

Into skin	Intradermal percutaneous subdermal by scarification	trunk deltoid thighs
Intrapleural	postoperative into malignant effusions	
Into tumor	percutaneous through bronchoscope	
Oral		
Aerosol		

1217

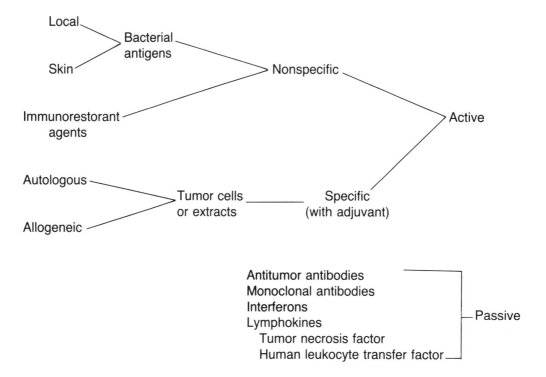

Fig. 100–1. Methods of immunotherapy used in lung cancer. (Adapted from Bronchial Carcinoma. Edited by M. Bates. Berlin, Springer Verlag, 1984, p. 214.)

study, Matthay and colleagues (1986) failed to demonstrate any clinical benefit.

Some workers have combined BCG administration with chemotherapy and radiation therapy. In general, these studies have failed to show any added benefit from the use of BCG.

Toxicity

BCG causes an acute febrile illness lasting 48 hours. This effect is greater in tuberculin-positive patients. Ulceration of the skin has been common, especially where BCG has been injected into the skin of the thighs rather than the deltoid regions. Disseminated BCG infection has been surprisingly rare in bronchial carcinoma patients so treated, although Rosenberg and colleagues

(1974) described this in a patient receiving intralesional BCG for malignant melanoma.

Other mycobacterial preparations that have been tried without lasting clinical effect in bronchial carcinoma have included methanol extraction residue of BCG and oil-droplet attached cell wall skeleton of BCG.

Corynebacterium Parvum

This anaerobic organism, which stimulates cell-mediated immunity in rats, has also been used as an adjuvant to conventional therapy of bronchial carcinoma. The results of subcutaneous and intravenous *C. parvum* added to irradiation and chemotherapy have varied, and in some studies this agent has appeared detrimental. In two important investigations, *C. parvum* has been used

Table 100–2. Results of Local Nonspecific Immunotherapy in Patients Who Have Undergone Resection of Bronchial Carcinoma

	Immunotherapy	Results
Holmes (1981)	Intratumor BCG Tice	Disease free survival over median follow-up of 14 months, BCG group = 55%, control group = 37%
Mountain and Gail (1981)	Intrapleural BCG Tice	No effect on survival in trial involving 425 stage I patients
Maver et al. (1982)	Intrapleural BCG Tice	6 year survival of 30 stage I BCG cases = 60%, controls = 25%, p = 0.048
Ludwig Lung Cancer Study Group (1985)	Intrapleural and intravenous *C. parvum*	Decreased survival in *C. parvum* group in trial involving 405 patients, p = 0.02
Matthay et al. (1986)	Intratumor BCG Tice	No effect on survival in trial involving 85 patients
Ludwig Lung Cancer Study Group (1986)	Intrapleural BCG Tice	No effect on survival, decreased disease free interval in trial involving 407 stage I and II patients

as an adjuvant to surgery. In one randomized prospective trial, Woodruff and Walbaum (1983) gave a single intravenous injection of *C. parvum* 10 days after operation. Thirteen out of twenty-five in the *C. parvum* group, but only five out of twenty-four in the control group, survived 5 years. This difference was not significant. In a trial of postoperative intrapleural and intravenous *C. parvum* involving 405 patients, the Ludwig Lung Cancer Study Group (1985) found that the control group fared better than the *C. parvum* group.

The only established clinical value of *C. parvum* in bronchial carcinoma has been in malignant pleural effusion, as Millar and colleagues (1980) described. It is not clear, however, whether this benefit was achieved by an immunologic rather than a chemical action.

Intravenous *C. parvum* causes an acute febrile reaction, occasionally with hypotension. Severe chest pain and empyema may complicate intrapleural administration.

Immunorestorants

Cell-mediated immunity is depressed for 2 to 4 weeks after surgical operations, during and after irradiation and chemotherapy, and in advanced bronchial carcinoma. The antihelminthic drug levamisole and extracts of animal thymus glands can reverse this depression. In 1980, Amery reported the results of postoperative oral levamisole in a prospective, randomized trial carried out in 211 patients undergoing curative resection and concluded that patients receiving more than 2.1 mg/kg body weight derived clinical benefit. In other studies there was an unacceptably high level of gastrointestinal side effects. In addition, Anthony and colleagues (1979) found an excess of deaths from cardiorespiratory failure in patients treated with this drug. In 2 of these, IgG antibody against myocardial sarcolemma was isolated.

The results of combining immunorestorants with other forms of immunotherapy, radiation therapy, or chemotherapy have varied. This form of treatment has never become part of routine management in any type of bronchial carcinoma.

SPECIFIC IMMUNOTHERAPY

Specific immunotherapy is the injection of tumor-derived material in the hope of stimulating an immunologic response directed specifically against the patient's tumor cells. Stack (1982) and Lachmann (1985) and their colleagues used autologous cells extracted from tumor tissue removed at operation. It was believed that tumor-associated antigens on these cells would be less likely to evoke a transplant rejection response from the host. It later became clear, however, that these tumor-associated antigens were differentiation and not transplantation antigens. Lachmann's group therefore abandoned autologous cells in favor of allogeneic cells. The advantage of the latter method is that, in any major center, a much larger supply of tumor cells is available.

The ability of injected tumor cells to elicit an immunologic response against the patient's tumor has always been enhanced by a nonspecific adjuvant such as BCG to produce a general stimulation of macrophages. Another method used by Takita and associates (1976) is to add neuraminidase to the cell preparation. This cleaves terminal negatively-charged sialic acid residues from membrane glycoproteins. Exposing surface antigens of cells in this way renders them more immunogenic.

Rigorous bacteriologic monitoring of injected material and irradiation of cells before injection reduces the risk of infection and of local growth of implanted cells. Nevertheless, the techniques of cell preparation are crude. Other workers have preferred to use extracts of tumors. For instance, Hollinshead and Stewart (1981) used a preparation extracted from allogeneic cells of the same histologic type with the addition of Freund's complete adjuvant in patients undergoing resection of bronchial carcinoma. This tumor-associated antigen extract also served to assess delayed skin hypersensitivity in patients so treated.

Although some preliminary analyses of specific immunotherapy were promising, this promise has not been fulfilled after longer periods of follow-up (Table 100–3). One exception has been the phase 3 study of tumor-associated antigen by Hollinshead's group (1986). This showed a significant difference in survival of patients 3.5 years after resection of stage 1 tumors. They were also able to demonstrate antibodies to tumor-associated antigen in the sera of patients after the second injection of antigen.

Most tumor cells and extracts have been injected into the skin, but Wiseman and colleagues (1986) introduced autologous tumor cells into the lymphatics of patients with advanced metastatic cancer. In one of the four bronchial carcinoma patients so treated the pulmonary tumor shrank significantly.

PASSIVE IMMUNOTHERAPY

Passive immunotherapy consists of the administration of substances or cells that already have intrinsic immunologic activity against tumor cells. Newman and colleagues (1977) administered tumor-specific immunoglobulin to patients after resection of bronchial carcinoma without significant clinical effect. Since then, most interest has centered on monoclonal antibodies, lymphokines, and interferons.

Monoclonal Antibodies—MoAb

These are antibodies of IgM or IgG class produced by a single clone of cells or a clonally derived cell line. They are formed when spleen cells from mice previously immunized against cells of the tumor under investigation are fused with cells of mouse myeloma to form hybridomas. The immunizing tumor material may be obtained from cell lines, fresh biopsied tumor, or transplants in nude mice. Binding of these MoAb to the cells of individual tumors can be assessed by flow cytometry, immunofluorescence, and labeling of MoAb with radioisotopes.

Table 100–3.   Some Examples of Specific Immunotherapy in Patients Who Have Undergone Resection of Lung Cancer

Authors	Immunotherapy	Clinical Measurements	Treated	Controls	Significance
Perlin et al. (1980)	Irradiated allogeneic tumor cells	Percentage survival at 2 years	72	61	$p = 0.06$
Souter et al. (1981)	Autologous tumor cells with *C. parvum*	Percentage survival at 2 years	56	65	N.S.
Stack et al. (1985)	Irradiated autologous tumor cells and percutaneous BCG	Percentage stage I patients alive and free from tumor recurrence at 5 years	36	32	N.S.
Hollinshead (1986)	Soluble allogeneic lung cancer antigen homogenized with Freund's adjuvant	Cumulative survival at 3.5 years of stage I patients	82	58	$p < 0.05$

Flow Cytometry. This method measures the rate of flow of cells coated with MoAb past a laser beam.

Immunofluorescence. A MoAb is attached to fluorescent dye and the complex is applied to the tumor tissue under investigation. Localization of fluorescence shows the site at which MoAb becomes fixed to surface antigen on tumor cells.

Labeling of MoAb with Radioisotopes. MoAb are labeled with radioisotopes such as ^{131}I or ^{111}In before being injected. This method can be used to localize xenografts of tumor in mice and tumor cells in humans.

MoAb that recognize antigens on the surface of lymphocytes that are active against bronchial carcinoma cells, e.g., natural killer—NK—cells have been developed. They may also bind to antigens specific to histologic types of tumor and to various proteins on the surface of tumor cells.

In a batch of several MoAb produced simultaneously by the same technique, it has been common to identify at least one that is specific for the tumor cell under investigation. Other MoAb produced at the same time, however, also react with cells from tumors of different histologic types of bronchial carcinoma, from tumors of other organs and even from normal tissues.

Diagnostic Applications of MoAb

To Determine the Histologic Type of Malignant Cells in Secretions and Pleural Fluid. For example, Cole and colleagues (1985) developed a MoAb capable of detecting a specific antigen—Leu-7—on the surface of NK cells. This antigen was present in all small cell bronchial carcinoma cell lines tested and 2 of 7 biopsy specimens from small cell carcinoma. It was not found in epidermoid or adenocarcinoma cell lines.

Detection of Tumor Cells in Pleural Effusions, Bronchial Aspirate, and Bone Marrow. Bernal and associates (1985) used MoAb specific for small cell carcinoma to detect cells of this tumor in bone marrow samples extracted for autologous marrow transplant following high dose chemotherapy. Similarly, Postmus' group (1986) detected neuroendocrine-specific differentiation antigen on the surface of cells of the same tumor type.

Detection of Circulating Tumor Antigen. Hirota and colleagues (1985) raised MoAb against tumors of stomach and colon. Sera from 85% of patients with bronchial carcinoma reacted with at least one of the MoAb produced.

Delineation of Tumor Deposits. Mulshine's group (1986) showed that it was possible to demonstrate tumor deposits by injecting radiolabeled MoAb raised against the specific tumor provided that these MoAb were injected in the region of the tumor. Intravenously injected MoAb were merely taken up by the reticuloendothelial system and did not localize accurately in tumor tissue.

Therapeutic Applications of Monoclonal Antibodies

Direct Antitumor Effect. Mabry and colleagues (1985) and Okabe's team (1985) raised MoAb that, when added to cells of small cell bronchial carcinoma labeled with ^{51}Cr, have caused lysis of these cells as shown by release of isotope into culture fluid. Presence of human complement is necessary for this effect.

Localization of Tumor Deposits to Aid Irradiation or Chemotherapy. Injection of MoAb labeled with radioisotopes into the region of tumors allows accurate mapping of their position.

Inhibition of Factors Promoting Tumor Cell Growth. Mulshine and co-workers (1986) raised MoAb against the binding site of bombesin in the tumor cell. As bombesin is an important tumor cell growth factor, this has led to the destruction of cultured tumor cells and of heterotransplants in nude mice. Its effectiveness in patients with bronchial carcinoma is currently under investigation.

Prognostic Value of Monoclonal Antibodies. Rosen and his colleagues (1984) from the U.S. National Cancer Institute—NCI—described the use of MoAb to detect the presence of glycolipid determinants on the surface of small cell carcinoma cells. A more malignant and undifferentiated variant of small cell carcinoma fails to express several of these determinants. This variant also contains greatly amplified c myc oncogenes.

Lymphokines

Lymphokines are proteins produced by primed lymphocytes on contact with antigen. They modulate the behavior of other lymphocytes and of macrophages. Much of the work on these substances has been carried out by Rosenberg and colleagues (1986) of the NCI. They have used interleukin 2—IL 2—obtained by recombinant DNA technology. IL 2 can also be isolated from animal or human lymphocytes as Ito and associates (1984) described.

In the presence of antigen from a cell or molecule that has been digested by a macrophage, IL 2 stimulates helper T cells and thus indirectly cytotoxic T cells and NK cells. Mulé and colleagues (1985) incubated peripheral blood lymphocytes with IL 2 to produce lymphokine-activated killer—LAK—cells. Injection of these cells with IL 2 into immunosuppressed mice bearing transplanted sarcomas reduced the number of pulmonary metastases. This effect was also achieved using a higher concentration of IL 2.

Use of IL 2 and LAK cells in humans is still at an early stage. Rosenberg's team (1986) combined IL 2 and LAK cells in patients with advanced cancer. Four had adenocarcinoma of the lung, and a response was obtained in one of these.

Krigel and colleagues (1986), using IL 2 plus recombinant β ser 17 interferon, observed "stabilization" of progressive disease in patients with non-small cell bronchial carcinoma.

IL 2 increases capillary permeability and therefore causes retention of fluid in the tissues. This leads to weight gain and sometimes dyspnea because of pulmonary edema. Of the 41 patients Rosenberg and associates (1986) described, 32 experienced considerable toxicity, including fever, nausea and vomiting, and confusion.

Use of IL 2 in bronchial carcinoma is in the process of evaluation by research groups including that of Holmes (personal communication, 1986). This research has largely superseded investigation of methods of active immunotherapy previously described.

Interferons

The interferons are a group of proteins manufactured by cells infected with viruses. These proteins are classified as interferons class α, β, and γ (Table 100–4).

As well as directly inhibiting tumor cells, interferons enhance the action of NK cells and activate macrophages.

Beaupain and colleagues (1986) found that human α_2 and γ interferons inhibit growth of pulmonary tumor cells in culture. Nonetheless, although Mattson and associates (1985) observed a minor response to interferon in 3 of 9 patients with limited small cell carcinoma, most early studies have shown no significant clinical effect of these substances in any form of bronchial carcinoma. For example, Jones and colleagues (1983) gave human lymphoblastoid interferon—α—by continuous intravenous infusion for 5 days to 10 patients with limited small cell carcinoma; this produced no clinical response.

Table 100–4. Classes of Interferons

Class	Source	Number of Different Interferons
α	leucocytes	15
β	fibroblasts	1
γ	immune	1

Interferons have been administered by intramuscular injection and by intravenous or subcutaneous infusion. The wide range of toxic effects have included leucopenia and hypocalcemia as well as nonspecific fever, weakness, anorexia, and depression.

At present there is no indication that interferons will be valuable in the treatment of bronchial carcinoma.

Tumor Necrosis Factor

In 1975, Carswell and colleagues described a protein found in the serum of mice treated with BCG or C. parvum and later exposed to bacterial endotoxin. This factor caused hemorrhagic necrosis in certain transplanted tumors in mice. Subsequent studies showed that it delayed growth of cultured mouse cells and then destroyed them. Its ability to inhibit clone formation by cultured tumor cells has been enhanced by interferon, and it seems to be produced by macrophages.

In one phase I study of this substance, Chapman and associates (1986) administered escalating subcutaneous intravenous doses of tumor necrosis factor to 14 patients with advanced cancer, none of whom had bronchial carcinoma. No therapeutic response was observed in the six patients who completed treatment, and considerable toxicity resulted.

CONCLUSION

Research into immunotherapy of bronchial carcinoma is at a watershed. Most researchers who took part in the investigation of different methods of active immunotherapy since the 1960s have now reported their long-term follow-up results. In general, these have been negative, sometimes when earlier analyses had suggested a therapeutic effect. In some instances, immunotherapy even seems to have been detrimental.

The promising new lines of investigation are the uses of monoclonal antibodies and lymphokines. These have reached the stage of administration to patients, and the results will be published during the next few years. It seems likely that their role will be as an additional measure to improve the results of surgery, irradiation, and chemotherapy rather than as a single unsupported form of treatment.

REFERENCES

Amery, W.K.P.C.: Adjuvant levamisole in the treatment of patients with resectable lung cancer. Ann. Clin. Res. 12(Suppl. 27):1, 1980.

Anthony, H.M., et al.: Levamisole and surgery in bronchial carcinoma patients: increase in deaths from cardiorespiratory failure. Thorax 34:4, 1979.

Baldwin, R.W., and Pimm, M.V.: BCG in immunotherapy. Adv. Cancer Res. 28:91, 1978.

Beaupain, R., Billard, C., and Falcoff, E.: Effects of human recombinant interferons -α_2, -β, and -γ on growth and survival of human cancer nodules maintained in continuous organotypic culture. Eur. J. Cancer Clin. Oncol. 22:141, 1986.

Bennett, J.A., et al.: Differences in biological activity among batches of lyophilized Tice BCG and their association with clinical course in stage 1 lung cancer. Cancer Res. 43:4183, 1983.

Bernal, S.D., et al.: Selective cytotoxicity of the SM 1 monoclonal antibody towards small cell carcinoma of the lung. Cancer Res. 45:1026, 1985.

Carswell, E.A., et al.: An endotoxin-induced serum factor that causes necrosis of tumors. Proc. Natl. Acad. Sci. USA 72:3666, 1975.

Chapman, P.B., et al.: Phase I study of recombinant tumor necrosis factor. Proc. ASCO 5:231, 1986.

Cole, S.P.C., et al.: Differential expression of the Leu-7 antigen on human lung tumor cells. Cancer Res. 45:4285, 1985.

Hirota, M., et al.: Detection of tumor-associated antigens in the sera of lung cancer patients by three monoclonal antibodies. Cancer Res. 45:6453, 1985.

Hollinshead, A.C.: Immunotherapy: a report of an adjuvant phase III lung cancer immunotherapy trial. Adv. Oncol. 2:16, 1986.

Hollinshead, A.C., and Stewart, T.H.M.: Specific and nonspecific immunotherapy as an adjuvant to curative surgery for cancer of the lung. Yale J. Biol. Med. 54:367, 1981.

Holmes, E.C.: The immunotherapy of lung cancer. In Lung Cancer, Vol. 1. Edited by R.B. Livingston. The Hague, Martinus Nijhoff, 1981, p. 60.

Holmes, E.C., et al.: New method of immunotherapy for lung cancer. Lancet 2:586, 1977.

Ito, M., et al.: Beneficial effects of interleukin-2 on natural killer activity in lung cancer patients. Anticancer Res. 4:375, 1984.

Jones, D.H., et al.: Human lymphoblastoid interferon in the treatment of small cell lung cancer. Br. J. Cancer 47:361, 1983.

Krigel, R., et al.: A phase I study of recombinant interleukin-2 plus recombinant beta ser 17 interferon. Proc. ASCO 5:225, 1986.

Lachmann, P.J., et al.: A preliminary trial of a novel form of active immunotherapy in squamous cell carcinoma of the lung. Br. J. Cancer 51:415, 1985.

Ludwig Lung Cancer Study Group: Adverse effect of intrapleural Corynebacterium parvum as adjuvant therapy in resected stage I and II non-small cell carcinoma of the lung. J. Thorac. Cardiovasc. Surg. 89:842, 1985.

Ludwig Lung Cancer Study Group: Immunostimulation with intrapleural BCG as adjuvant therapy in resected non-small cell lung cancer. Cancer 58:2411, 1986.

Mabry, M., et al.: Use of SM-1 monoclonal antibody and human complement in selective killing of small cell carcinoma of the lung. J. Clin. Invest. 75:1690, 1985.

Matthay, R.A., et al.: Intratumoral Bacillus Calmette-Guérin immunotherapy prior to surgery for carcinoma of the lung: results of a prospective randomized trial. Cancer Res. 46:5963, 1986.

Mattson, K., et al.: Human leukocyte interferon as part of a combined treatment for previously untreated small cell lung cancer. J. Biol. Response Mod. 4:8, 1985.

Maver, C., et al.: Intrapleural BCG immunotherapy of lung cancer patients. In Adjuvant Therapies of Cancer. Edited by G. Mathé, G. Bonnadonna, and S. Salmon. Berlin, Springer-Verlag, 1982, p.227

McKneally, M.F., Maver, C., and Kausel, H.W.: Regional immunotherapy of lung cancer with intrapleural BCG. Lancet 1:377, 1976.

Millar, J.W., Hunter, A.M., and Horne, N.W.: Intrapleural immunotherapy with Corynebacterium parvum in recurrent malignant pleural effusions. Thorax 35:856, 1980.

Mountain, C.F., and Gail, M.H.: Surgical adjuvant intrapleural BCG treatment for stage I non-small cell lung cancer. J. Thorac. Cardiovasc. Surg. 82:649, 1981.

Mulé, J.J., Shu, S., and Rosenberg, S.A.: The anti-tumor efficacy of lymphokine-activated killer cells and recombinant interleukin 2 in vivo. J. Immunol. 135:646, 1985.

Mulshine, J.: Monoclonal antibodies. Chest 89(Suppl. 4):355S, 1986.

Newman, C.E., et al.: Antibody-drug synergism: an assessment of specific passive immunotherapy in bronchial carcinoma. Lancet 2:163, 1977.

Okabe, T., et al.: Elimination of small cell lung cancer cells in vitro from human bone marrow by a monoclonal antibody. Cancer Res. 45:1930, 1985.

Perlin, E., et al.: Carcinoma of the lung: immunotherapy with intradermal BCG and allogeneic tumor cells. Int. J. Radiat. Oncol. Biol. Phys. 6:1003, 1980.

Postmus, P.E., et al.: Diagnostic application of a monoclonal antibody against small cell lung cancer. Cancer 57:60, 1986.

Rosen, S.T., et al.: Analysis of human small cell lung cancer differentiation antigens using a panel of rat monoclonal antibodies. Cancer Res. 44:2052, 1984.

Rosenberg, E.B., et al.: Systemic infection following BCG therapy. Arch. Intern. Med. 134:769, 1974.

Rosenberg, S.A., et al.: A new approach to the therapy of cancer based on the systemic administration of autologous lymphocyte-activated killer cells and recombinant interleukin-2. Surgery 100:262, 1986.

Souter, R.G., et al.: Failure of specific active immunotherapy in lung cancer. Br. J. Cancer 44:496, 1981.

Stack, B.H.R., et al.: Autologous x-irradiated tumor cells and percutaneous BCG in operable lung cancer. Thorax 37:588, 1982.

Stack, B.H.R., et al.: Long-term results of injection of autologous tumor cells and percutaneous BCG into patients undergoing resection of lung cancer. (abstract) 4th World Conference on Lung Cancer, Toronto, 1985, p. 23.

Takita, H., et al.: Adjuvant immunotherapy in bronchogenic carcinoma. Ann. N.Y. Acad. Sci. 277:345, 1976.

Wiseman, C., et al.: Effect of cyclophosphamide on autologous active specific intralymphatic immunotherapy (ASILI): immunologic and therapeutic results. Proc. ASCO 5:228, 1986.

Woodruff, M., and Walbaum, P.: A phase-II trial of Corynebacterium parvum as adjuvant to surgery in the treatment of operable lung cancer. Cancer Immunol. Immunother. 16:114, 1983.

Index